HARRISON'S Infectious Diseases

Editors

Dennis L. Kasper, MD
William Ellery Channing Professor of Medicine, Professor of Microbiology and Molecular Genetics, Harvard Medical School; Director, Channing Laboratory, Department of Medicine, Brigham and Women's Hospital, Boston

Anthony S. Fauci, MD
Chief, Laboratory of Immunoregulation; Director, National Institute of Allergy and Infectious Diseases, National Institutes of Health, Bethesda

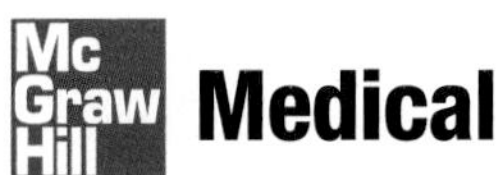

New York Chicago San Francisco Lisbon London Madrid Mexico City
Milan New Delhi San Juan Seoul Singapore Sydney Toronto

The McGraw-Hill Companies

Harrison's Infectious Diseases

Copyright © 2010 by The McGraw-Hill Companies, Inc. All rights reserved. Printed in China. Except as permitted under the United States Copyright Act of 1976, no part of this publication may be reproduced or distributed in any form or by any means, or stored in a data base or retrieval system, without prior written permission of the publisher.

Dr. Fauci's and Dr. Longo's works were performed outside the scope of their employment as U.S. government employees. These works represent their personal and professional views and not necessarily those of the U.S. government.

1 2 3 4 5 6 7 8 9 0 CTP/CTP 14 13 12 11 10

ISBN 978-0-07-170293-5
MHID 0-07-170293-8

This book was set in Bembo by Glyph International. The editors were James F. Shanahan and Kim J. Davis. The production supervisor was Catherine H. Saggese. Project management was provided by Arushi Chawla of Glyph International. The cover design was by Thomas DePierro. Cover, section, and chapter opener illustrations © MedicalRF.com. All rights reserved.

China Translation & Printing Services Ltd. was the printer and binder.

Library of Congress Cataloging-in-Publication Data

Harrison's infectious diseases / editors, Dennis L. Kasper, Anthony S. Fauci.
p. ; cm.
Includes bibliographical references and index.
ISBN-13: 978-0-07-170293-5 (pbk. : alk. paper)
ISBN-10: 0-07-170293-8 (pbk. : alk. paper)
1. Communicable diseases. I. Kasper, Dennis L. II. Fauci, Anthony S., 1940-
III. Harrison, Tinsley Randolph, 1900-1978. IV. Title: Infectious diseases.
[DNLM: 1. Communicable Diseases. WC 100 H323 2010]
RC111.H375 2010
616.9—dc22

2009040803

McGraw-Hill books are available at special quantity discounts to use as premiums and sales promotions, or for use in corporate training programs. To contact a representative please e-mail us at bulksales@mcgraw-hill.com.

CONTENTS

CONTRIBUTORS

Numbers in brackets refer to the chapter(s) written or co-written by the contributor.

ELIAS ABRUTYN, MD†
Professor of Medicine and Public Health, Drexel University College of Medicine, Philadelphia [40, 41]

NEIL M. AMPEL, MD
Professor of Medicine, University of Arizona; Staff Physician, SAVAHCS, Tucson [104]

GORDON L. ARCHER, MD
Professor of Medicine and Microbiology/Immunology; Associate Dean for Research, School of Medicine, Virginia Commonwealth University, Richmond [33]

JOHN C. ATHERTON, MD
Professor of Gastroenterology; Director, Wolfson Digestive Diseases Centre, University of Nottingham, United Kingdom [52]

LINDSEY R. BADEN, MD
Assistant Professor of Medicine, Harvard Medical School, Boston [79]

TAMAR F. BARLAM, MD
Associate Professor of Medicine, Boston University School of Medicine, Boston [14, 48]

MIRIAM J. BARON, MD
Instructor in Medicine, Harvard Medical School, Boston [24]

KENNETH J. BART, MD, MPH, MSHPM
Professor Emeritus, Epidemiology and Biostatistics, San Diego State University, San Diego; Consultant, National Vaccine Program Office, Office of the Secretary, Department of Health and Human Services, Washington [3]

NICHOLAS J. BEECHING, FFTM (RCPS GLAS) DCH, DTM&H
Senior Lecturer in Infectious Diseases, Liverpool School of Tropical Medicine, University of Liverpool; Consultant and Clinical Lead, Tropical and Infectious Disease Unit, Royal Liverpool University Hospital, Liverpool, United Kingdom [58]

JEAN BERGOUNIOUX, MD
Medical Doctor of Pediatrics, Unité de Pathogénie Microbienne Moléculaire, Paris [55]

WILLIAM R. BISHAI, MD, PhD
Professor of Medicine, The Johns Hopkins School of Medicine, Baltimore [38]

MARTIN J. BLASER, MD
Frederick H. King Professor of Internal Medicine; Chair, Department of Medicine; Professor of Microbiology, New York University School of Medicine, New York [52, 56]

GERALD BLOOMFIELD, MD, MPH
Department of Internal Medicine, The Johns Hopkins University School of Medicine, Baltimore [Review and Self-Assessment]

EUGENE BRAUNWALD, MD, MA (Hon), ScD (Hon)
Distinguished Hersey Professor of Medicine, Harvard Medical School; Chairman, TIMI Study Group, Brigham and Women's Hospital, Boston [20]

JOEL G. BREMAN, MD, DTPH
Senior Scientific Advisor, Fogarty International Center, National Institutes of Health, Bethesda [116, 118]

CYNTHIA D. BROWN, MD
Department of Internal Medicine, The Johns Hopkins University School of Medicine, Baltimore [Review and Self-Assessment]

KEVIN E. BROWN, MD
Consultant Medical Virologist, Health Protection Agency, London [85]

JOAN R. BUTTERTON, MD
Assistant Clinical Professor of Medicine, Harvard Medical School; Clinical Associate in Medicine, Massachusetts General Hospital, Boston [25]

STEPHEN B. CALDERWOOD, MD
Morton N. Swartz, MD Academy Professor of Medicine (Microbiology and Molecular Genetics), Harvard Medical School; Chief, Division of Infectious Diseases, Massachusetts General Hospital, Boston [25]

MICHAEL V. CALLAHAN, MD, DTM&H (UK), MSPH
Clinical Associate Physician, Division of Infectious Diseases, Massachusetts General Hospital; Program Manager, Biodefense, Defense Advanced Research Project Agency (DARPA), United States Department of Defense, Washington [9]

GRANT L. CAMPBELL, MD, PhD
Division of Vector-Borne Infectious Diseases, National Center for Infectious Diseases, Centers for Disease Control and Prevention, U.S. Public Health Service, Laporte [60]

JONATHAN R. CARAPETIS, MBBS, PhD
Director, Menzies School of Health Research; Professor, Charles Darwin University, Casuarina, Northern Territory, Australia [37]

ARTURO CASADEVALL, MD, PhD
Professor of Microbiology and Immunology and of Medicine; Chair, Department of Microbiology and Immunology, Albert Einstein College of Medicine, New York [106]

STANLEY W. CHAPMAN, MD
Professor of Medicine and Microbiology; Director, Division of Infectious Diseases; Vice-Chair for Academic Affairs, Department of Medicine, University of Mississippi School of Medicine, Jackson [105, 110]

JEFFREY I. COHEN, MD
Chief, Medical Virology Section, Laboratory of Clinical Infectious Diseases, National Institute of Allergy and Infectious Diseases, National Institutes of Health, Bethesda [82, 94]

†Deceased

RONIT COHEN-PORADOSU, MD
Channing Laboratory, Brigham and Women's Hospital, Boston [65]

MICHAEL J. CORBEL, PhD, DSc(Med), FIBiol
Head, Division of Bacteriology, National Institute for Biological Standards and Control, Potters Bar, United Kingdom [58]

LAWRENCE COREY, MD
Professor of Medicine and Laboratory Medicine; Chair of Medical Virology, University of Washington; Head, Program in Infectious Diseases, Fred Hutchinson Cancer Research Center, Seattle [80]

EMILY DARBY, MD
Senior Fellow, Division of Infectious Diseases, University of Washington, Seattle [61]

CHARLES E. DAVIS, MD
Professor of Pathology and Medicine Emeritus, University of California San Diego School of Medicine; Director Emeritus, Microbiology Laboratory, University of California San Diego Medical Center, San Diego [112]

DAVID W. DENNING, MBBS
Professor of Medicine and Medical Mycology, University of Manchester; Director, Regional Mycology Laboratory, Manchester Education and Research Centre, Wythenshawe Hospital, Manchester, United Kingdom [108]

DAVID T. DENNIS, MD, MPH
Faculty Affiliate, Department of Microbiology, Immunology and Pathology, Colorado State University; Medical Epidemiologist, Division of Influenza, Centers for Disease Control and Prevention, Atlanta [60, 73]

JULES L. DIENSTAG, MD
Carl W. Walter Professor of Medicine and Dean for Medical Education, Harvard Medical School; Physician, Gastrointestinal Unit, Massachusetts General Hospital, Boston [92, 93]

CHARLES A. DINARELLO, MD
Professor of Medicine, University of Colorado Health Science Center, Denver [7]

RAPHAEL DOLIN, MD
Maxwell Finland Professor of Medicine (Microbiology and Molecular Genetics); Dean for Academic and Clinical Programs, Harvard Medical School, Boston [79, 87, 88]

J. STEPHEN DUMLER, MD
Professor, Division of Medical Microbiology, Department of Pathology, The Johns Hopkins University School of Medicine and Immunology, The Johns Hopkins University Bloomberg School of Public Health, Baltimore [75]

JOHN E. EDWARDS, JR., MD
Chief, Division of Infectious Diseases, Harbor/University of California, Los Angeles Medical Center; Professor of Medicine, David Geffen School of Medicine at the University of California, Los Angeles, Torrance [102, 107]

ANTHONY S. FAUCI, MD, DSc (Hon), DM&S (Hon), DHL (Hon), DPS (Hon), DLM (Hon), DMS (Hon)
Chief, Laboratory of Immunoregulation; Director, National Institute of Allergy and Infectious Diseases, National Institutes of Health, Bethesda [6, 89, 90]

GREGORY A. FILICE, MD
Professor of Medicine, University of Minnesota; Chief, Infectious Disease Section, Minneapolis Veterans Affairs Medical Center, Minneapolis [63]

ROBERT FINBERG, MD
Professor and Chair, Department of Medicine, University of Massachusetts Medical School, Worcester [11, 12]

JOYCE FINGEROTH, MD
Associate Professor of Medicine, Harvard Medical School, Boston [12]

DANIEL J. FINK, MD, MPH
Associate Professor of Clinical Pathology, College of Physicians and Surgeons, Columbia University, New York [Appendix]

SUSAN L. GEARHART, MD
Assistant Professor of Colorectal Surgery and Oncology, The Johns Hopkins University School of Medicine, Baltimore [26]

ROBERT H. GELBER, MD
Scientific Director, Leonard Wood Memorial Leprosy Research Center, Cebu, Philippines; Clinical Professor of Medicine and Dermatology, University of California, San Francisco, San Francisco [67]

JEFFREY A. GELFAND, MD
Professor of Medicine, Harvard Medical School; Physician, Department of Medicine, Massachusetts General Hospital, Boston [9, 117]

DALE N. GERDING, MD
Assistant Chief of Staff for Research, Hines VA Hospital, Hines; Professor, Stritch School of Medicine, Loyola University, Maywood [43]

ANNE GERSHON, MD
Professor of Pediatrics, Columbia University College of Physicians and Surgeons, New York [95-97]

ROGER I. GLASS, MD, PhD
Director, Fogarty International Center; Associate Director for International Research, National Institutes of Health, Bethesda [91]

RALPH GONZALES, MD, MSPH
Professor of Medicine, Epidemiology and Biostatistics, University of California, San Francisco, San Francisco [16]

DAVID E. GRIFFITH, MD
Professor of Medicine; William A. and Elizabeth B. Moncrief Distinguished Professor, University of Texas Health Center, Tyler [69]

CHADI A. HAGE, MD
Assistant Professor of Medicine, Indiana University School of Medicine, Roudebush VA Medical Center, Pulmonary-Critical Care and Infectious Diseases, Indianapolis [103]

SCOTT A. HALPERIN, MD
Professor of Pediatrics and of Microbiology and Immunology, Dalhousie University, Halifax, Nova Scotia [50]

GAVIN HART, MD, MPH
Director, STD Services, Royal Adelaide Hospital; Clinical Associate Professor, School of Medicine, Flinders University, Adelaide, Australia [62]

RUDY HARTSKEERL, PhD
Head, FAO/OIE, World Health Organization and National Leptospirosis Reference Centre, KIT Biomedical Research, Royal Tropical Institute, Amsterdam, The Netherlands [72]

BARBARA L. HERWALDT, MD, MPH
Medical Epidemiologist, Division of Parasitic Diseases, Centers for Disease Control and Prevention, Atlanta [119]

MARTIN S. HIRSCH, MD
Professor of Medicine, Harvard Medical School; Professor of Immunology and Infectious Diseases, Harvard School of Public Health; Physician, Massachusetts General Hospital, Boston [83]

ELIZABETH L. HOHMANN, MD
Associate Professor of Medicine and Infectious Diseases, Harvard Medical School, Massachusetts General Hospital, Boston [39]

KING K. HOLMES, MD, PhD
William H. Foege Chair, Department of Global Health; Director, Center for AIDS and STD; Professor of Medicine and Global Health, University of Washington; Head, Infectious Diseases, Harborview Medical Center, Seattle [28]

ALAN C. JACKSON, MD, FRCPC
Professor of Medicine (Neurology) and of Medical Microbiology, University of Manitoba; Section Head of Neurology, Winnipeg Regional Health Authority, Winnipeg, Canada [98]

RICHARD F. JACOBS, MD, FAAP
President, Arkansas Children's Hospital Research Institute; Horace C. Cabe Professor of Pediatrics, University of Arkansas for Medical Sciences, College of Medicine, Little Rock [59]

ERIC C. JOHANNSEN, MD
Assistant Professor, Department of Medicine, Harvard Medical School; Associate Physician, Division of Infectious Diseases, Brigham and Women's Hospital, Boston [98]

JAMES R. JOHNSON, MD
Professor of Medicine, University of Minnesota, Minneapolis [51]

STUART JOHNSON, MD
Associate Professor, Stritch School of Medicine, Loyola University, Maywood; Staff Physician, Hines VA Hospital, Hines [43]

ADOLF W. KARCHMER, MD
Professor of Medicine, Harvard Medical School, Boston [19]

DENNIS L. KASPER, MD, MA (Hon)
William Ellery Channing Professor of Medicine, Professor of Microbiology and Molecular Genetics, Harvard Medical School; Director, Channing Laboratory, Department of Medicine, Brigham and Women's Hospital, Boston [1, 14, 24, 42, 48, 65]

LLOYD H. KASPER, MD
Professor of Medicine and Microbiology/Immunology; Co-Director, Program in Immunotherapeutics, Dartmouth Medical Schoool, Lebanon [121]

ELAINE T. KAYE, MD
Clinical Assistant Professor of Dermatology, Harvard Medical School; Assistant in Medicine, Department of Medicine, Children's Hospital Medical Center, Boston [8, 10]

KENNETH M. KAYE, MD
Associate Professor of Medicine, Harvard Medical School; Associate Physician, Division of Infectious Diseases, Brigham and Women's Hospital, Boston [8, 10]

GERALD T. KEUSCH, MD
Associate Provost and Associate Dean for Global Health, Boston University School of Medicine, Boston [3, 57]

JAY S. KEYSTONE, MD, FRCPC
Professor of Medicine, University of Toronto; Staff Physician, Centre for Travel and Tropical Medicine, Toronto General Hospital, Toronto [4]

ELLIOTT KIEFF, MD, PhD
Harriet Ryan Albee Professor of Medicine and Microbiology and Molecular Genetics, Harvard Medical School; Senior Physician, Brigham and Women's Hospital, Boston [78]

LOUIS V. KIRCHHOFF, MD, MPH
Professor, Departments of Internal Mediciene and Epidemiology, University of Iowa; Staff Physician, Department of Veterans Affairs Medical Center, Iowa City [120]

WALTER J. KOROSHETZ, MD
Deputy Director, National Institute of Neurological Disorders and Stroke, National Institutes of Health, Bethesda [30]

PHYLLIS E. KOZARSKY, MD
Professor of Medicine, Infectious Diseases; Co-Director, Travel and Tropical Medicine, Emory University School of Medicine, Atlanta [4]

ALEXANDER KRATZ, MD, PhD, MPH
Assistant Professor of Clinical Pathology, Columbia University College of Physicians and Surgeons; Associate Director, Core Laboratory, Columbia University Medical Center, New York-Presbyterian Hospital; Director, Allen Pavilion Laboratory, New York [Appendix]

H. CLIFFORD LANE, MD
Clinical Director; Director, Division of Clinical Research; Deputy Director, Clinical Research and Special Projects; Chief, Clinical and Molecular Retrovirology Section, Laboratory of Immunoregulation, National Institute of Allergy and Infectious Diseases, National Institutes of Health, Bethesda [6, 90]

DAN L. LONGO, MD
Scientific Director, National Institute on Aging, National Institutes of Health, Bethesda and Baltimore [89]

FRANKLIN D. LOWY, MD, PhD
Professor of Medicine and Pathology, Columbia University, College of Physicians & Surgeons, New York [35]

SHEILA A. LUKEHART, PhD
Professor of Medicine, University of Washington, Seattle [70, 71]

LAWRENCE C. MADOFF, MD
Associate Professor of Medicine, Harvard Medical School, Boston [1, 23, 32, 42]

ADEL A. F. MAHMOUD, MD, PhD
Professor, Molecular Biology, Princeton University, Princeton [126]

LIONEL A. MANDELL, MD
Professor of Medicine, McMaster University, Hamilton, Ontario [17]

THOMAS MARRIE, MD
Professor, Department of Medicine; Dean, Faculty of Medicine and Dentistry, University of Alberta, Edmonton [75]

ALEXANDER J. McADAM, MD, PhD
Medical Director, Infectious Diseases Diagnostic Division, Children's Hospital, Boston; Assistant Professor, Department of Pathology, Harvard Medical School, Boston [5]

WILLIAM M. McCORMACK, MD
Distinguished Teaching Professor of Medicine; Chief, Infectious Disease Division, SUNY Downstate Medical Center, Brooklyn [76]

BRUCE L. MILLER, MD
AW and Mary Margaret Clausen Distinguished Professor of Neurology, University of California, San Francisco School of Medicine, San Francisco [101]

MARK MILLER, MD
Associate Director for Research, National Institutes of Health, Bethesda [3]

SAMUEL I. MILLER, MD
Professor of Genome Sciences, Medicine, and Microbiology, University of Washington, Seattle [54]

THOMAS A. MOORE, MD
Clinical Professor and Associate Program Director, Department of Medicine, University of Kansas School of Medicine, Wichita [113, 114]

ROBERT S. MUNFORD, MD
Jan and Henri Bromberg Chair in Internal Medicine, University of Texas Southwestern Medical Center, Dallas [15]

JOHN R. MURPHY, PhD
Professor of Medicine and Microbiology; Chief, Section of Molecular Medicine, Boston University School of Medicine, Boston [38]

TIMOTHY F. MURPHY, MD
UB Distinguished Professor, Department of Medicine and Microbiology; Chief, Infectious Diseases, State Univerity of New York, Buffalo [47]

DANIEL M. MUSHER, MD
Chief, Infectious Disease Section, Michael E. DeBakey Veterans Affairs Medical Center; Professor of Medicine and Professor of Molecular Virology and Microbiology, Baylor College of Medicine, Houston [34, 46]

THOMAS B. NUTMAN, MD
Head, Helminth Immunology Section; Head, Clinical Parasitology Unit; Laboratory of Parasitic Diseases, National Institute of Allergy and Infectious Diseases, National Insitutes of Health, Bethesda [124, 125]

RICHARD J. O'BRIEN, MD
Head of Scientific Evaluation, Foundation for Innovative New Diagnostics, Geneva, Switzerland [66]

ANDREW B. ONDERDONK, PhD
Professor of Pathology, Harvard Medical School and Brigham and Women's Hospital, Boston [5]

UMESH D. PARASHAR, MBBS, MPH
Lead, Enteric and Respiratory Viruses Team, Epidemiology Branch, Division of Viral Diseases, National Center for Immunization and Respiratory Diseases, Centers for Disease Control and Prevention, Atlanta [91]

JEFFREY PARSONNET, MD
Associate Professor of Medicine and Microbiology, Dartmouth Medical School, Lebanon [22]

DAVID A. PEGUES, MD
Professor of Medicine, Division of Infectious Diseases, David Geffen School of Medicine at UCLA, Los Angeles [54]

FLORENCIA PEREYRA, MD
Instructor in Medicine, Harvard Medical School; Division of Infectious Disease, Brigham and Women's Hospital, Boston [32]

MICHAEL A. PESCE, PhD
Clinical Professor of Pathology, Columbia University College of Physicians and Surgeons; Director of Specialty Laboratory, New York Presbyterian Hospital, Columbia University Medical Center, New York [Appendix]

CLARENCE J. PETERS, MD
John Sealy Distinguished University Chair in Tropical and Emerging Virology, Director for Biodefense, Center for Biodefense and Emerging Infectious Diseases, University of Texas Medical Branch in Galveston, Galveston [99, 100]

GERALD B. PIER, PhD
Professor of Medicine (Microbiology and Molecular Genetics), Harvard Medical School; Microbiologist, Brigham and Women's Hospital, Boston [2]

RONALD E. POLK, PharmD
Chair, Department of Pharmacy, Professor of Pharmacy and Medicine, School of Pharmacy, Virginia Commonwealth University, Richmond [33]

REUVEN PORAT, MD
Professor of Medicine; Director, Internal Medicine, Tel Aviv Sourasky Medical Center, Sackler Faculty of Medicine, Tel Aviv University, Tel Aviv [7]

DANIEL A. PORTNOY, PhD
Professor of Biochemistry and Molecular Biology, Department of Molecular and Cell Biology, University of California, Berkeley [39]

STANLEY B. PRUSINER, MD
Director, Institute for Neurodegenerative Diseases; Professor, Department of Neurology; Professor, Department of Biochemistry and Biophysics, University of California, San Francisco [101]

SANJAY RAM, MD
Assistant Professor of Medicine, Division of Infectious Diseases and Immunology, University of Massachusetts Medical School, Worcester [45]

REUBEN RAMPHAL, MD
Professor, Division of Infectious Diseases, Department of Medicine, University of Florida College of Medicine, Gainesville [53]

MARIO C. RAVIGLIONE, MD
Director, StopTB Department, World Health Organization, Geneva [66]

SHARON L. REED, MD
Professor of Pathology and Medicine; Director, Microbiology and Virology Laboratories, University of California, San Diego Medical Center, San Diego [112, 115]

RICHARD C. REICHMAN, MD
Professor of Medicine and of Microbiology and Immunology; Director, Infectious Diseases Division, University of Rochester School of Medicine, Rochester [86]

PETER A. RICE, MD
Professor of Medicine, Division of Infectious Diseases and Immunology, University of Massachusetts Medical School, Worcester [45]

KAREN L. ROOS, MD
John and Nancy Nelson Professor of Neurology, Indiana University School of Medicine, Indianapolis [29]

MICHAEL A. RUBIN, MD, PhD
Assistant Professor of Medicine, Division of Epidemiology and Infectious Diseases, Department of Internal Medicine, University of Utah School of Medicine, Salt Lake City [16]

THOMAS A. RUSSO, MD, CM
Professor of Medicine and Microbiology, State University of New York, Buffalo [51, 64]

MIGUEL SABRIA, MD, PhD
Professor of Medicine, Autonomous University of Barcelona; Chief, Infectious Diseases Section, Germans Trias i Pujol Hospital, Barcelona, Spain [49]

MERLE A. SANDE,[†] MD
Professor of Medicine, University of Washington School of Medicine; President, Academic Alliance Foundation, Seattle [16]

PHILIPPE SANSONETTI
Professeur á l'Institut Pasteur, Paris [55]

JOSHUA SCHIFFER, MD
Department of Internal Medicine, The Johns Hopkins University School of Medicine, Baltimore [Review and Self-Assessment]

GORDON E. SCHUTZE, MD
Professor of Pediatrics and Pathology, University of Arkansas for Medical Sciences, College of Medicine; Chief, Pediatric Infectious Diseases, Arkansas Children's Hospital, Little Rock [59]

WILLIAM SILEN, MD
Johnson and Johnson Distinguished Professor of Surgery, Emeritus, Harvard Medical School, Boston [26]

A. GEORGE SMULIAN, MB, BCh
Associate Professor, University of Cincinnati College of Medicine; Chief, Infectious Disease Section, Cincinnati VA Medical Center, Cincinnati [111]

DAVID H. SPACH, MD
Professor of Medicine, Division of Infectious Diseases, University of Washington, Seattle [61]

PETER SPEELMAN, MD, PhD
Professor of Medicine and Infectious Diseases; Head, Division of Infectious Diseases, Tropical Medicine and AIDS; Department of Internal Medicine, Academic Medical Center, University of Amsterdam, The Netherlands [72]

ADAM SPIVAK, MD
Department of Internal Medicine, The Johns Hopkins University School of Medicine, Baltimore [Review and Self-Assessment]

WALTER E. STAMM, MD
Professor of Medicine; Head, Division of Allergy and Infectious Diseases, University of Washington School of Medicine, Seattle [27, 77]

ALLEN C. STEERE, MD
Professor of Medicine, Harvard Medical School, Boston [74]

DENNIS L. STEVENS, MD, PhD
Chief, Infectious Diseases Section, Veteran Affairs Medical Center, Boise; Professor of Medicine, University of Washington School of Medicine, Seattle [21]

STEPHEN E. STRAUS,[†] MD
Senior Investigator, Laboratory of Clinical Investigation, National Institute of Allergy and Infectious Diseases; Director, National Center for Complementary and Alternative Medicine, National Institutes of Health, Bethesda [31]

ALAN M. SUGAR, MD
Professor of Medicine, Boston University School of Medicine; Medical Director, Infectious Diseases Clinical Services, HIV/AIDS Program, and Infection Control, Cape Cod Healthcare, Hyannis [109]

DONNA C. SULLIVAN, PhD
Associate Professor of Medicine and Microbiology, Division of Infectious Diseases, Department of Medicine, University of Mississippi School of Medicine, Jackson [105, 110]

MORTON N. SWARTZ, MD
Professor of Medicine, Harvard Medical School; Chief, Jackson Firm Medical Service and Infectious Disease Unit, Massachusetts General Hospital, Boston [30]

GREGORY TINO, MD
Associate Professor of Medicine, University of Pennsylvania School of Medicine; Chief, Pulmonary Clinical Service Hospital of the University of Pennsylvania, Philadelphia [18]

KENNETH L. TYLER, MD
Reuler-Lewin Family Professor of Neurology and Professor of Medicine and Microbiology, University of Colorado Health Sciences Center; Chief, Neurology Service, Denver Veterans Affairs Medical Center, Denver [29]

EDOUARD VANNIER, PhD
Assistant Professor, Department of Medicine, Division of Infectious Diseases, Tufts-New England Medical Center and Tufts University School of Medicine, Boston [117]

C. FORDHAM von REYN, MD
Professor of Medicine (Infectious Disease) and International Health; Director, DARDAR International Programs, Dartmouth Medical School, Lebanon [68]

MATTHEW K. WALDOR, MD, PhD
Professor of Medicine (Microbiology and Molecular Genetics), Channing Laboratory, Brigham and Women's Hospital, Harvard Medical School, Boston [57]

DAVID H. WALKER, MD
The Carnage and Martha Walls Distinguished University Chair in Tropical Diseases; Professor and Chairman, Department of Pathology; Executive Director, Center for Biodefense and Emerging Infectious Disease, University of Texas Medical Branch, Galveston [75]

RICHARD J. WALLACE, JR., MD
Chairman, Department of Microbiology, University of Texas Health Center at Tyler, Tyler [69]

PETER D. WALZER, MD, MSc
Associate Chief of Staff for Research, Cincinnati VA Medical Center; Professor of Medicine, University of Cincinnati College of Medicine, Cincinnati [111]

FRED WANG, MD
Professor of Medicine, Harvard Medical School, Boston [78, 84]

STEVEN E. WEINBERGER, MD
Senior Vice President for Medical Education Division, American College of Physicians; Senior Lecturer on Medicine, Harvard Medical School; Adjunct Professor of Medicine, University of Pennsylvania School of Medicine, Philadelphia [18]

[†]Deceased.

CHARLES WIENER, MD
Professor of Medicine and Physiology; Vice Chair, Department of Medicine; Director, Osler Medical Training Program, The Johns Hopkins University School of Medicine, Baltimore [Review and Self-Assessment]

ROBERT A. WEINSTEIN, MD
Professor of Medicine, Rush University Medical Center; Chairman, Infectious Diseases, Cook County Hospital; Chief Operating Officer, CORE Center, Chicago [13]

PETER F. WELLER, MD
Professor of Medicine, Harvard Medical School; Co-Chief, Infectious Diseases Division; Chief, Allergy and Inflammation Division; Vice-Chair for Research, Department of Medicine, Beth Israel Deaconess Medical Center, Boston [122-125, 127]

MICHAEL R. WESSELS, MD
Professor of Pediatrics and Medicine (Microbiology and Molecular Genetics), Harvard Medical School; Chief, Division of Infectious Diseases, Children's Hospital, Boston [36]

LEE M. WETZLER, MD
Professor of Medicine, Associate Professor of Microbiology, Boston University School of Medicine, Boston [44]

L. JOSEPH WHEAT, MD
President and Director, MiraVista Diagnostics and MiraBella Technology, Indianapolis [103]

A. CLINTON WHITE, JR., MD
The Paul R. Stalnaker, MD, Distinguished Professor of Internal Medicine; Director, Infectious Disease Division, Department of Internal Medicine, University of Texas Medical Branch, Galveston [127]

NICHOLAS J. WHITE, DSc
Professor of Tropical Medicine, Oxford University, United Kingdom; Mahidol University, Bangkok, Thailand [116, 118]

RICHARD J. WHITLEY, MD
Loeb Scholar in Pediatrics, Professor of Pediatrics, Microbiology, Medicine, and Neurosurgery, University of Alabama, Birmingham [81]

RICHARD WUNDERINK, MD
Professor, Division of Pulmonary and Critical Care, Department of Medicine, Northwestern University Feinberg School of Medicine; Director, Medical Intensive Care Unit, Northwestern Memorial Hospital, Chicago [17]

VICTOR L. YU, MD
Professor of Medicine, University of Pittsburgh, Pittsburgh [49]

PREFACE

Despite enormous advances in diagnosis, treatment, and prevention during the twentieth century, physicians caring for patients with infectious diseases today must cope with extraordinary new challenges, including a never-ending deluge of new information, the rapid evolution of the microorganisms responsible for these diseases, and formidable time and cost constraints. In no other area of medicine is the differential diagnosis so wide, and often the narrowing of the differential to a precise infection caused by a specific organism with established antimicrobial susceptibilities is a matter of great urgency.

To inform crucial decisions about management, today's care providers are typically turning to a variety of sources, including colleagues, print publications, and online services. Our goal in publishing *Harrison's Infectious Diseases* as a stand-alone volume is to provide practitioners with a single convenient source that quickly yields accurate, accessible, up-to-date information to meet immediate clinical needs and that presents this information in the broader context of the epidemiologic, pathophysiologic, and genetic factors that underlie it. The authors of the chapters herein are acknowledged experts in their fields whose points of view represent decades of medical practice and a comprehensive knowledge of the literature. The specific recommendations of these authorities regarding diagnostic options and therapeutic regimens—including drugs of choice, doses, durations, and alternatives—take into account not just the trends and concerns of the moment but also the longer-term factors and forces that have shaped present circumstances and will continue to influence future developments. Among these forces are the changing prevalence, distribution, features, and management alternatives in different regions of the world; accordingly, these topics are addressed from an international perspective.

Prominent among the 127 chapters in this volume, that on HIV infections and AIDS by Anthony S. Fauci and H. Clifford Lane (Chap. 90) is widely considered to be a classic in the field. Its clinically pragmatic focus, along with its comprehensive and analytical approach to the pathogenesis of HIV disease, has led to its use as the sole complete reference on HIV/AIDS in medical schools. A highly practical chapter by Robert A. Weinstein (Chap. 13) addresses health care–associated infections, a topic of enormous significance in terms of patient care in general and antimicrobial resistance in particular. A superb chapter by Richard C. Reichman (Chap. 86) includes critical information and recommendations regarding the recently licensed human papillomavirus vaccine. Thomas A. Russo and James R. Johnson (Chap. 51) take on the complex area of serious infections caused by gram-negative bacilli, including *Escherichia coli*.

With a full-color design, this volume offers abundant illustrations that provide key information in a readily understandable format. Two chapters comprise atlases of images that can be invaluable in clinical assessments: Chap. 10 presents images of rashes associated with fever, while Chap. 118 shows blood smears of the various stages of the parasites causing malaria and babesiosis. Self-assessment questions and answers appear in an appendix at the end of the book.

The Editors thank our authors for their hard work in distilling their experience and the relevant literature into this volume, which we hope you will enjoy using as an authoritative source of current information on infectious diseases.

Dennis L. Kasper, MD

NOTICE

Medicine is an ever-changing science. As new research and clinical experience broaden our knowledge, changes in treatment and drug therapy are required. The authors and the publisher of this work have checked with sources believed to be reliable in their efforts to provide information that is complete and generally in accord with the standards accepted at the time of publication. However, in view of the possibility of human error or changes in medical sciences, neither the authors nor the publisher nor any other party who has been involved in the preparation or publication of this work warrants that the information contained herein is in every respect accurate or complete, and they disclaim all responsibility for any errors or omissions or for the results obtained from use of the information contained in this work. Readers are encouraged to confirm the information contained herein with other sources. For example and in particular, readers are advised to check the product information sheet included in the package of each drug they plan to administer to be certain that the information contained in this work is accurate and that changes have not been made in the recommended dose or in the contraindications for administration. This recommendation is of particular importance in connection with new or infrequently used drugs.

Review and self-assessment questions and answers were selected by Miriam J. Baron, MD, from those prepared by Wiener C, Fauci AS, Braunwald E, Kasper DL, Hauser SL, Longo DL, Jameson JL, Loscalzo J (editors) Bloomfield G, Brown CD, Schiffer J, Spivak A (contributing editors). *Harrison's Principles of Internal Medicine Self-Assessment and Board Review*, 17th ed. New York, McGraw-Hill, 2008, ISBN 978-0-07-149619-3.

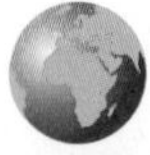
The global icons call greater attention to key epidemiologic and clinical differences in the practice of medicine throughout the world.

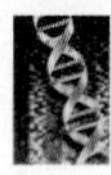
The genetic icons identify a clinical issue with an explicit genetic relationship.

SECTION I

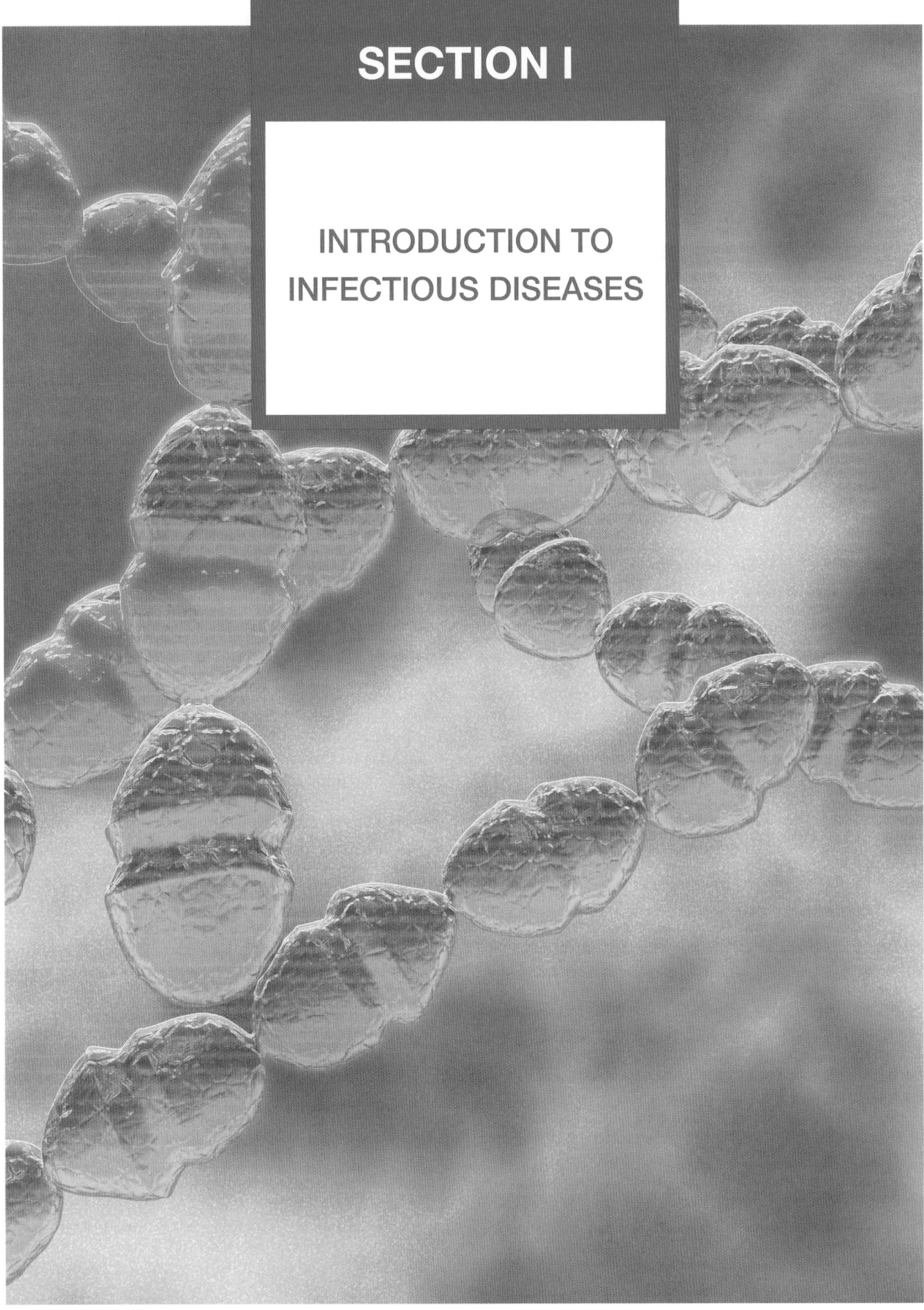

INTRODUCTION TO INFECTIOUS DISEASES

CHAPTER 1

INTRODUCTION TO INFECTIOUS DISEASES: HOST-PATHOGEN INTERACTIONS

Lawrence C. Madoff ■ Dennis L. Kasper

Despite decades of dramatic progress in their treatment and prevention, infectious diseases remain a major cause of death and debility and are responsible for worsening the living conditions of many millions of people around the world. Infections frequently challenge the physician's diagnostic skill and must be considered in the differential diagnoses of syndromes affecting every organ system.

CHANGING EPIDEMIOLOGY OF INFECTIOUS DISEASES

With the advent of antimicrobial agents, some medical leaders believed that infectious diseases would soon be eliminated and become of historic interest only. Indeed, the hundreds of chemotherapeutic agents developed since World War II, most of which are potent and safe, include drugs effective not only against bacteria, but also against viruses, fungi, and parasites. Nevertheless, we now realize that as we developed antimicrobial agents, microbes developed the ability to elude our best weapons and to counterattack with new survival strategies. Antibiotic resistance occurs at an alarming rate among all classes of mammalian pathogens. Pneumococci resistant to penicillin and enterococci resistant to vancomycin have become commonplace. Even *Staphylococcus aureus* strains resistant to vancomycin have appeared. Such pathogens present real clinical problems in managing infections that were easily treatable just a few years ago. Diseases once thought to have been nearly eradicated from the developed world-tuberculosis, cholera, and rheumatic fever, for example-have rebounded with renewed ferocity. Newly discovered and emerging infectious agents appear to have been brought into contact with humans by changes in the environment and by movements of human and animal populations. An example of the propensity for pathogens to escape from their usual niche is the alarming 1999 outbreak in New York of encephalitis due to West Nile virus, which had never previously been isolated in the Americas. In 2003, severe acute respiratory syndrome (SARS) was first recognized. This emerging clinical entity is caused by a novel coronavirus that may have jumped from an animal niche to become a significant human pathogen. By 2006, H5N1 avian influenza, having spread rapidly through poultry farms in Asia and having caused deaths in exposed humans, had reached Europe and Africa, heightening fears of a new influenza pandemic.

Many infectious agents have been discovered only in recent decades (Fig. 1-1). Ebola virus, human metapneumovirus, *Anaplasma phagocytophila* (the agent of human granulocytotropic ehrlichiosis), and retroviruses such as HIV humble us despite our deepening understanding of pathogenesis at the most basic molecular level. Even in developed countries, infectious diseases have made a resurgence. Between 1980 and 1996, mortality from infectious diseases in the United States increased by 64% to levels not seen since the 1940s.

The role of infectious agents in the etiology of diseases once believed to be noninfectious is increasingly recognized. For example, it is now widely accepted that *Helicobacter pylori* is the causative agent of peptic ulcer disease and perhaps of gastric malignancy. Human papillomavirus is likely to be the most important cause of invasive cervical cancer. Human herpesvirus type 8 is believed to be the cause of most cases of Kaposi's sarcoma. Epstein-Barr virus is a cause of certain lymphomas and may play a role in the genesis of Hodgkin's disease. The possibility certainly exists that other diseases of unknown cause, such as rheumatoid arthritis, sarcoidosis, or inflammatory bowel disease, have infectious etiologies. There is even evidence that atherosclerosis may have an infectious component. In contrast, there are data to suggest that decreased exposures to pathogens in childhood may be contributing to an increase in the observed rates of allergic diseases.

Medical advances against infectious diseases have been hindered by changes in patient populations. Immunocompromised hosts now constitute a significant proportion of the seriously infected population. Physicians immunosuppress their patients to prevent the rejection of transplants and to treat neoplastic and inflammatory diseases. Some infections, most notably that caused by HIV, immunocompromise the host in and of themselves. Lesser degrees of immunosuppression are associated with other infections, such as influenza and syphilis. Infectious agents that coexist peacefully with immunocompetent hosts wreak havoc in those who lack a complete immune system. AIDS has brought to prominence once-obscure

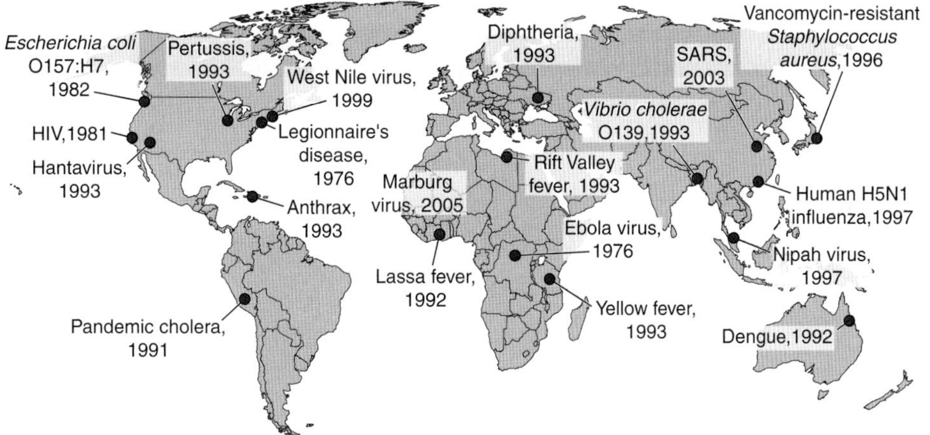

FIGURE 1-1

Map of the world showing examples of geographic locales where infectious diseases were noted to have emerged or resurged. (*Adapted from Addressing Emerging Infectious Disease Threats: A Prevention Strategy for the United States, Department of Health and Human Services, Centers for Disease Control and Prevention, 1994.*)

organisms such as *Pneumocystis*, *Cryptosporidium parvum*, and *Mycobacterium avium*.

HOST FACTORS IN INFECTION

For any infectious process to occur, the pathogen and the host must first encounter each other. Factors such as geography, environment, and behavior thus influence the likelihood of infection. Although the initial encounter between a susceptible host and a virulent organism frequently results in disease, some organisms can be harbored in the host for years before disease becomes clinically evident. For a complete view, individual patients must be considered in the context of the population to which they belong. Infectious diseases do not often occur in isolation; rather, they spread through a group exposed from a point source (e.g., a contaminated water supply) or from one individual to another (e.g., via respiratory droplets). Thus the clinician must be alert to infections prevalent in the community as a whole. A detailed history, including information on travel, behavioral factors, exposures to animals or potentially contaminated environments, and living and occupational conditions, must be elicited. For example, the likelihood of infection by *Plasmodium falciparum* can be significantly affected by altitude, climate, terrain, season, and even time of day. Antibiotic-resistant strains of *P. falciparum* are localized to specific geographic regions, and a seemingly minor alteration in a travel itinerary can dramatically influence the likelihood of acquiring chloroquine-resistant malaria. If such important details in the history are overlooked, inappropriate treatment may result in the death of the patient. Likewise, the chance of acquiring a sexually transmitted disease can be greatly affected by a relatively minor variation in sexual practices, such as the method used for contraception. Knowledge of the relationship between specific risk factors and disease allows the physician to influence a patient's health even before the development of infection by modification of these risk factors and—when a vaccine is available—by immunization.

Many specific host factors influence the likelihood of acquiring an infectious disease. Age, immunization history, prior illnesses, level of nutrition, pregnancy, coexisting illness, and perhaps emotional state all have some impact on the risk of infection after exposure to a potential pathogen. The importance of individual host defense mechanisms, either specific or nonspecific, becomes apparent in their absence, and our understanding of these immune mechanisms is enhanced by studies of clinical syndromes developing in immunodeficient patients (Table 1-1). For example, the higher attack rate of meningococcal disease among people with deficiencies in specific complement proteins of the so-called membrane attack complex (see "Adaptive Immunity" later in the chapter) than in the general population underscores the importance of an intact complement system in the prevention of meningococcal infection.

Medical care itself increases the patient's risk of acquiring an infection in several ways: (1) through contact with pathogens during hospitalization, (2) through breaching of the skin (with intravenous devices or surgical incisions) or mucosal surfaces (with endotracheal tubes or bladder catheters), (3) through introduction of foreign bodies, (4) through alteration of the natural flora with antibiotics, and (5) through treatment with immunosuppressive drugs.

Infection involves complicated interactions of microbe and host and inevitably affects both. In most cases, a pathogenic process consisting of several steps is required for the development of infections. Since the competent host has a complex series of barricades in place to prevent infection, the successful pathogen must use specific strategies at each of these steps. The specific strategies used by bacteria, viruses, and parasites (Chap. 2) have some remarkable conceptual similarities, but the strategic details are unique not only for each class of microorganism, but also for individual species within a class.

TABLE 1-1

INFECTIONS ASSOCIATED WITH SELECTED DEFECTS IN IMMUNITY

HOST DEFECT	DISEASE OR THERAPY ASSOCIATED WITH DEFECT	COMMON ETIOLOGIC AGENT OF INFECTION
Nonspecific Immunity		
Impaired cough	Rib fracture, neuromuscular dysfunction	Bacteria causing pneumonia, aerobic and anaerobic oral flora
Loss of gastric acidity	Achlorhydria, histamine blockade	*Salmonella* spp., enteric pathogens
Loss of cutaneous integrity	Penetrating trauma, athlete's foot	*Staphylococcus* spp., *Streptococcus* spp.
	Burn	*Pseudomonas aeruginosa*
	Intravenous catheter	*Staphylococcus* spp., *Streptococcus* spp., gram-negative rods, coagulase-negative staphylococci
Implantable device	Heart valve	*Streptococcus* spp., coagulase-negative staphylococci, *Staphylococcus aureus*
	Artificial joint	*Staphylococcus* spp., *Streptococcus* spp., gram-negative rods
Loss of normal bacterial flora	Antibiotic use	*Clostridium difficile*, *Candida* spp.
Impaired clearance		
Poor drainage	Urinary tract infection	*Escherichia coli*
Abnormal secretions	Cystic fibrosis	Chronic pulmonary infection with *P. aeruginosa*
Inflammatory Response		
Neutropenia	Hematologic malignancy, cytotoxic chemotherapy, aplastic anemia, HIV infection	Gram-negative enteric bacilli, *Pseudomonas* spp., *Staphylococcus* spp., *Candida* spp.
Chemotaxis	Chédiak-Higashi syndrome, Job's syndrome, protein-calorie malnutrition	*S. aureus*, *Streptococcus pyogenes*, *Haemophilus influenzae*, gram-negative bacilli
	Leukocyte adhesion defects 1 and 2	Bacteria causing skin and systemic infections, gingivitis
Phagocytosis (cellular)	Systemic lupus erythematosus (SLE), chronic myelogenous leukemia, megaloblastic anemia	*Streptococcus pneumoniae*, *H. influenzae*
Splenectomy	—	*H. influenzae*, *S. pneumoniae*, other streptococci, *Capnocytophaga* spp., *Babesia microti*, *Salmonella* spp.
Microbicidal defect	Chronic granulomatous disease	Catalase-positive bacteria and fungi: staphylococci, *E. coli*, *Klebsiella* spp., *P. aeruginosa*, *Aspergillus* spp., *Nocardia* spp.
	Chédiak-Higashi syndrome	*S. aureus*, *S. pyogenes*
	Interferon γ receptor defect, interleukin 12 deficiency, interleukin 12 receptor defect	*Mycobacterium* spp., *Salmonella* spp.
Innate Immunity		
Complement system		
C3	Congenital liver disease, SLE, nephrotic syndrome	*S. aureus*, *S. pneumoniae*, *Pseudomonas* spp., *Proteus* spp.
C5	Congenital	*Neisseria* spp., gram-negative rods
C6, C7, C8	Congenital, SLE	*Neisseria meningitidis*, *N. gonorrhoeae*
Alternative pathway	Sickle cell disease	*S. pneumoniae*, *Salmonella* spp.

(*Continued*)

TABLE 1-1 (*CONTINUED*)

INFECTIONS ASSOCIATED WITH SELECTED DEFECTS IN IMMUNITY

HOST DEFECT	DISEASE OR THERAPY ASSOCIATED WITH DEFECT	COMMON ETIOLOGIC AGENT OF INFECTION
Innate Immunity (*Continued*)		
Toll-like receptor 4	Congenital	Gram-negative bacilli
Interleukin 1 receptor-associated kinase (IRAK) 4	Congenital	*S. pneumoniae*, *S. aureus*, other bacteria
Mannan-binding lectin	Congenital	*N. meningitidis*, other bacteria
Adaptive Immunity		
T lymphocyte deficiency/ dysfunction	Thymic aplasia, thymic hypoplasia, Hodgkin's disease, sarcoidosis, lepromatous leprosy	*Listeria monocytogenes*, *Mycobacterium* spp., *Candida* spp., *Aspergillus* spp., *Cryptococcus neoformans*, herpes simplex virus, varicella-zoster virus
	AIDS	*Pneumocystis*, cytomegalovirus, herpes simplex virus, *Mycobacterium avium-intracellulare*, *C. neoformans*, *Candida* spp.
	Mucocutaneous candidiasis	*Candida* spp.
	Purine nucleoside phosphorylase deficiency	Fungi, viruses
B cell deficiency/dysfunction	Bruton's X-linked agammaglobulinemia	*S. pneumoniae*, other streptococci
	Agammaglobulinemia, chronic lymphocytic leukemia, multiple myeloma, dysglobulinemia	*H. influenzae*, *N. meningitidis*, *S. aureus*, *Klebsiella pneumoniae*, *E. coli*, *Giardia lamblia*, *Pneumocystis*, enteroviruses
	Selective IgM deficiency	*S. pneumoniae*, *H. influenzae*, *E. coli*
	Selective IgA deficiency	*G. lamblia*, hepatitis virus, *S. pneumoniae*, *H. influenzae*
Mixed T and B cell deficiency/ dysfunction	Common variable hypogammaglobulinemia	*Pneumocystis*, cytomegalovirus, *S. pneumoniae*, *H. influenzae*, various other bacteria
	Ataxia-telangiectasia	*S. pneumoniae*, *H. influenzae*, *S. aureus*, rubella virus, *G. lamblia*
	Severe combined immunodeficiency	*S. aureus*, *S. pneumoniae*, *H. influenzae*, *Candida albicans*, *Pneumocystis*, varicella-zoster virus, rubella virus, cytomegalovirus
	Wiskott-Aldrich syndrome	Agents of infections associated with T and B cell abnormalities
	X-linked hyper-IgM syndrome	*Pneumocystis*, cytomegalovirus, *Cryptosporidium parvum*

THE IMMUNE RESPONSE

INNATE IMMUNITY

As they have co-evolved with microbes, higher organisms have developed mechanisms for recognizing and responding to microorganisms. Many of these mechanisms, referred together as *innate immunity*, are evolutionarily ancient, having been conserved from insects to humans. In general, innate immune mechanisms exploit molecular patterns found specifically in pathogenic microorganisms. These "pathogen signatures" are recognized by host molecules that either directly interfere with the pathogen or initiate a response that does so. Innate immunity serves to protect the host without prior exposure to an infectious agent, i.e., before specific or adaptive immunity has had a chance to develop.

Innate immunity also functions as a warning system that activates components of adaptive immunity early in the course of infection.

Toll-like receptors (TLRs) are instructive in illustrating how organisms are detected and send signals to the immune system. There are at least 11 TLRs, each specific to different biologic classes of molecules. For example, even minuscule amounts of lipopolysaccharide (LPS), a molecule found uniquely in gram-negative bacteria, are detected by LPS-binding protein, CD14, and TLR4 (see Fig. 2-3). The interaction of LPS with these components of the innate immune system prompts macrophages, via the transcriptional activator nuclear factor κB (NF-κB), to produce cytokines that lead to inflammation and enzymes that enhance the clearance of microbes. These initial responses serve not only to limit infection but also to initiate specific or adaptive immune responses.

ADAPTIVE IMMUNITY

Once in contact with the host immune system, the microorganism faces the host's tightly integrated cellular and humoral immune responses. Cellular immunity, comprising T lymphocytes, macrophages, and natural killer cells, primarily recognizes and combats pathogens that proliferate intracellularly. Cellular immune mechanisms are important in immunity to all classes of infectious agents, including most viruses and many bacteria (e.g., *Mycoplasma*, *Chlamydophila*, *Listeria*, *Salmonella*, and *Mycobacterium*), parasites (e.g., *Trypanosoma*, *Toxoplasma*, and *Leishmania*), and fungi (e.g., *Histoplasma*, *Cryptococcus*, and *Coccidioides*). Usually, T lymphocytes are activated by macrophages and B lymphocytes, which present foreign antigens along with the host's own major histocompatibility complex antigen to the T-cell receptor. Activated T cells may then act in several ways to fight infection. *Cytotoxic* T cells may directly attack and lyse host cells that express foreign antigens. *Helper* T cells stimulate the proliferation of B cells and the production of immunoglobulins. Antigen-presenting cells and T cells communicate with each other via a variety of signals, acting coordinately to instruct the immune system to respond in a specific fashion. T cells elaborate cytokines (e.g., interferon) that directly inhibit the growth of pathogens or stimulate killing by host macrophages and cytotoxic cells. Cytokines also augment the host's immunity by stimulating the inflammatory response (fever, the production of acute-phase serum components, and the proliferation of leukocytes). Cytokine stimulation does not always result in a favorable response in the host; septic shock (Chap. 15) and toxic shock syndrome (Chaps. 35 and 36) are among the conditions that are mediated by these inflammatory substances.

The immune system has also developed cells that specialize in controlling or downregulating immune responses. For example, T_{reg} cells, a subgroup of CD4+ T cells, prevent autoimmune responses by other T cells and are thought to be important in downregulating immune responses to foreign antigens. There appear to be both naturally occurring and acquired T_{reg} cells.

The reticuloendothelial system comprises monocyte-derived phagocytic cells that are located in the liver (Kupffer cells), lung (alveolar macrophages), spleen (macrophages and dendritic cells), kidney (mesangial cells), brain (microglia), and lymph nodes (macrophages and dendritic cells) and that clear circulating microorganisms. Although these tissue macrophages and polymorphonuclear leukocytes (PMNs) are capable of killing microorganisms without help, they function much more efficiently when pathogens are first *opsonized* (Greek, "to prepare for eating") by components of the complement system such as C3b and/or by antibodies.

Extracellular pathogens, including most encapsulated bacteria (those surrounded by a complex polysaccharide coat), are attacked by the humoral immune system, which includes antibodies, the complement cascade, and phagocytic cells. *Antibodies* are complex glycoproteins (also called *immunoglobulins*) that are produced by mature B lymphocytes, circulate in body fluids, and are secreted on mucosal surfaces. Antibodies specifically recognize and bind to foreign antigens. One of the most impressive features of the immune system is the ability to generate an incredible diversity of antibodies capable of recognizing virtually every foreign antigen yet not reacting with self. In addition to being exquisitely specific for antigens, antibodies come in different structural and functional classes: IgG predominates in the circulation and persists for many years after exposure; IgM is the earliest specific antibody to appear in response to infection; secretory IgA is important in immunity at mucosal surfaces, while monomeric IgA appears in the serum; and IgE is important in allergic and parasitic diseases. Antibodies may directly impede the function of an invading organism, neutralize secreted toxins and enzymes, or facilitate the removal of the antigen (invading organism) by phagocytic cells. Immunoglobulins participate in cell-mediated immunity by promoting the antibody-dependent cellular cytotoxicity functions of certain T lymphocytes. Antibodies also promote the deposition of complement components on the surface of the invader.

The *complement* system consists of a group of serum proteins functioning as a cooperative, self-regulating cascade of enzymes that adhere to—and in some cases disrupt—the surface of invading organisms. Some of these surface-adherent proteins (e.g., C3b) can then act as opsonins for destruction of microbes by phagocytes. The later, "terminal" components (C7, C8, and C9) can directly kill some bacterial invaders (notably, many of the neisseriae) by forming a membrane attack complex and disrupting the integrity of the bacterial membrane, thus causing bacteriolysis. Other complement components, such as C5a, act as chemoattractants for PMNs (see below). Complement activation and deposition occur by either or both of two pathways: the *classic* pathway is activated primarily by immune complexes (i.e., antibody bound to antigen), and the *alternative* pathway is activated by microbial components, frequently in the absence of antibody. PMNs have receptors for both antibody and C3b, and antibody and complement function together to aid in the clearance of infectious agents.

PMNs, short-lived white blood cells that engulf and kill invading microbes, are first attracted to inflammatory sites by chemoattractants such as C5a, which is a product of complement activation at the site of infection. PMNs localize to the site of infection by adhering to cellular adhesion molecules expressed by endothelial cells. Endothelial cells express these receptors, called *selectins* (CD-62, ELAM-1), in response to inflammatory cytokines such as tumor necrosis factor α and interleukin 1. The binding of these selectin molecules to specific receptors on PMNs results in the adherence of the PMNs to the endothelium. Cytokine-mediated upregulation and expression of intercellular adhesion molecule 1 (ICAM 1) on endothelial cells then take place, and this latter receptor binds to β_2 integrins on PMNs, thereby facilitating diapedesis into the extravascular compartment. Once the PMNs are in the extravascular compartment, various molecules (e.g., arachidonic acids) further enhance the inflammatory process.

Approach to the Patient: INFECTIOUS DISEASES

The clinical manifestations of infectious diseases at presentation are myriad, varying from fulminant life-threatening processes to brief and self-limited conditions to indolent chronic maladies. A careful history is essential and must include details on underlying chronic diseases, medications, occupation, and travel. Risk factors for exposure to certain types of pathogens may give important clues to diagnosis. A sexual history may reveal risks for exposure to HIV and other sexually transmitted pathogens. A history of contact with animals may suggest numerous diagnoses, including rabies, Q fever, bartonellosis, *Escherichia coli* O157 infection, or cryptococcosis. Blood transfusions have been linked to diseases ranging from viral hepatitis to malaria to prion disease. A history of exposure to insect vectors (coupled with information about the season and geographic site of exposure) may lead to consideration of such diseases as Rocky Mountain spotted fever, other rickettsial diseases, tularemia, Lyme disease, babesiosis, malaria, trypanosomiasis, and numerous arboviral infections. Ingestion of contaminated liquids or foods may lead to enteric infection with *Salmonella, Listeria, Campylobacter,* amebas, cryptosporidia, or helminths. Since infectious diseases may involve many organ systems, a careful review of systems may elicit important clues as to the disease process.

The physical examination must be thorough, and attention must be paid to seemingly minor details, such as a soft heart murmur that might indicate bacterial endocarditis or a retinal lesion that suggests disseminated candidiasis or cytomegalovirus (CMV) infection. Rashes are extremely important clues to infectious diagnoses and may be the only sign pointing to a specific etiology (Chaps. 8 and 10). Certain rashes are so specific as to be pathognomonic—e.g., the childhood exanthems (measles, rubella, varicella), the target lesion of erythema migrans (Lyme disease), ecthyma gangrenosum (*Pseudomonas aeruginosa*), and eschars (rickettsial diseases). Other rashes, although less specific, may be exceedingly important diagnostic indicators. The prompt recognition of the early scarlatiniform and later petechial rashes of meningococcal infection or of the subtle embolic lesions of disseminated fungal infections in immunosuppressed patients can hasten life-saving therapy. Fever (Chaps. 7, 8, and 9) is a common manifestation of infection and may be its sole apparent indication. Sometimes the pattern of fever or its temporally associated findings may help refine the differential diagnosis. For example, fever occurring every 48–72 h is suggestive of malaria (Chap. 116). The elevation of body temperature in fever (through resetting of the hypothalamic setpoint mediated by cytokines) must be distinguished from elevations in body temperature from other causes, such as drug toxicity (Chap. 9) or heat stroke (Chap. 7).

LABORATORY INVESTIGATIONS

Laboratory studies must be carefully considered and directed toward establishing an etiologic diagnosis in the shortest possible time, at the lowest possible cost, and with the least possible discomfort to the patient. Since mucosal surfaces and the skin are colonized with many harmless or beneficial microorganisms, cultures must be performed in a manner that minimizes the likelihood of contamination with this normal flora while maximizing the yield of pathogens. A sputum sample is far more likely to be valuable when elicited with careful coaching by the clinician than when collected in a container simply left at the bedside with cursory instructions. Gram's stains of specimens should be interpreted carefully and the quality of the specimen assessed. The findings on Gram's staining should correspond to the results of culture; a discrepancy may suggest diagnostic possibilities such as infection due to fastidious or anaerobic bacteria.

The microbiology laboratory must be an ally in the diagnostic endeavor. Astute laboratory personnel will suggest optimal culture and transport conditions or alternative tests to facilitate diagnosis. If informed about specific potential pathogens, an alert laboratory staff will allow sufficient time for these organisms to become evident in culture, even when the organisms are present in small numbers or are slow-growing. The parasitology technician who is attuned to the specific diagnostic considerations relevant to a particular case may be able to detect the rare, otherwise-elusive egg or cyst in a stool specimen. In cases where a diagnosis appears difficult, serum should be stored during the early acute phase of the illness so that a diagnostic rise in titer of antibody to a specific pathogen can be detected later. Bacterial and fungal antigens can sometimes be detected in body fluids, even when cultures are negative or are rendered sterile by antibiotic therapy. Techniques such as the polymerase chain reaction allow the amplification of specific DNA sequences so that minute quantities of foreign nucleic acids can be recognized in host specimens.

℞ Treatment: INFECTIOUS DISEASES

Optimal therapy for infectious diseases requires a broad knowledge of medicine and careful clinical judgment. Life-threatening infections such as bacterial meningitis or sepsis, viral encephalitis, or falciparum malaria must be treated immediately, often before a specific causative organism is identified. Antimicrobial agents must be chosen empirically and must be active against the range of potential infectious agents consistent with the clinical scenario. In contrast, good clinical judgment sometimes dictates withholding of antimicrobial drugs in a self-limited process or until a specific diagnosis is made. The dictum *primum non nocere* should be adhered to, and it should be remembered that all antimicrobial agents carry a risk (and a cost) to the patient. Direct toxicity may be encountered—e.g., ototoxicity due to aminoglycosides, lipodystrophy due to antiretroviral agents, and hepatotoxicity due to antituberculous agents such as isoniazid and rifampin. Allergic reactions are common and can be serious. Since superinfection sometimes follows the eradication of the normal flora and colonization by a resistant organism, one invariant principle is that infectious disease therapy should be directed toward as narrow a spectrum of infectious agents as possible. Treatment specific for the pathogen should result in as little perturbation as possible of the host's microflora. Indeed, future therapeutic agents may act not by killing a microbe, but by interfering with one or more of its virulence factors.

With few exceptions, abscesses require surgical or percutaneous drainage for cure. Foreign bodies, including medical devices, must generally be removed in order to eliminate an infection of the device or of the adjacent tissue. Other infections, such as necrotizing fasciitis, peritonitis due to a perforated organ, gas gangrene, and chronic osteomyelitis, require surgery as the primary means of cure; in these conditions, antibiotics play only an adjunctive role.

The role of immunomodulators in the management of infectious diseases has received increasing attention. Glucocorticoids have been shown to be of benefit in the adjunctive treatment of bacterial meningitis and in therapy for *Pneumocystis* pneumonia in patients with AIDS. The use of these agents in other infectious processes remains less clear and in some cases (in cerebral malaria, for example) is detrimental. Activated protein C (drotrecogin alfa, activated) is the first immunomodulatory agent widely available for the treatment of severe sepsis. Its usefulness demonstrates the interrelatedness of the clotting cascade and systemic immunity. Other agents that modulate the immune response include prostaglandin inhibitors, specific lymphokines, and tumor necrosis factor inhibitors. Specific antibody therapy plays a role in the treatment and prevention of many diseases. Specific immunoglobulins have long been known to prevent the development of symptomatic rabies and tetanus. More recently, CMV immune globulin has been recognized as important not only in preventing the transmission of the virus during organ transplantation, but also in treating CMV pneumonia in bone marrow transplant recipients. There is a strong need for well-designed clinical trials to evaluate each new interventional modality.

PERSPECTIVE

The genetic simplicity of many infectious agents allows them to undergo rapid evolution and to develop selective advantages that result in constant variation in the clinical manifestations of infection. Moreover, changes in the environment and the host can predispose new populations to a particular infection. The dramatic march of West Nile virus from a single focus in New York City in 1999 to locations throughout the North American continent by the summer of 2002 caused widespread alarm, illustrating the fear that new plagues induce in the human psyche. The intentional release of deadly spores of *Bacillus anthracis* via the U.S. Postal Service awakened many from a sense of complacency regarding biologic weapons.

"The terror of the unknown is seldom better displayed than by the response of a population to the appearance of an epidemic, particularly when the epidemic strikes without apparent cause." Edward H. Kass made this statement in 1977 in reference to the newly discovered Legionnaire's disease, but it could apply equally to SARS, H5N1 (avian) influenza, or any other new and mysterious disease. The potential for infectious agents to emerge in novel and unexpected ways requires that physicians and public health officials be knowledgeable, vigilant, and open-minded in their approach to unexplained illness. The emergence of antimicrobial-resistant pathogens (e.g., enterococci that are resistant to all known antimicrobial agents and cause infections that are essentially untreatable) has led some to conclude that we are entering the "postantibiotic era." Others have held to the perception that infectious diseases no longer represent as serious a concern to world health as they once did. The progress that science, medicine, and society as a whole have made in combating these maladies is impressive, and it is ironic that, as we stand on the threshold of an understanding of the most basic biology of the microbe, infectious diseases are posing renewed problems. We are threatened by the appearance of new diseases such as SARS, hepatitis C, and Ebola virus infection and by the reemergence of old foes such as tuberculosis, cholera, plague, and *Streptococcus pyogenes* infection. True students of infectious diseases were perhaps less surprised than anyone else by these developments. Those who know pathogens are aware of their incredible adaptability and diversity. As ingenious and successful as therapeutic approaches may be, our ability to develop methods to counter infectious agents so far has not matched the myriad strategies employed by the sea of microbes that surrounds us. Their sheer numbers and the rate at which they can evolve are daunting. Moreover, environmental changes, rapid global travel, population movements, and medicine itself—through its use of antibiotics and immunosuppressive agents—all increase the impact of infectious diseases. Although new vaccines, new antibiotics, improved global communication, and new modalities for treating and preventing infection will be developed, pathogenic microbes will continue to develop new strategies of their own, presenting us with an unending and dynamic challenge.

FURTHER READINGS

Armstrong G et al: Trends in infectious disease mortality in the United States during the 20th century. JAMA 281:61, 1999

Bartlett JG: Update in infectious diseases. Ann Intern Med 144:49, 2006

Blaser MJ: Introduction to bacteria and bacterial diseases, in *Principles and Practice of Infectious Diseases*, 6th ed, GL Mandell et al (eds). Philadelphia, Elsevier, 2005, p 2319

Henderson DA: Countering the posteradication threat of smallpox and polio. Clin Infect Dis 34:79, 2002

Hoffman J et al: Phylogenetic perspectives in innate immunity. Science 284:1313, 1999

Hung DT et al: Small-molecule inhibitor of *Vibrio cholerae* virulence and intestinal colonization. Science 310:670, 2005

ProMed-Mail: The Program for Monitoring Emerging Diseases. *www.promedmail.org*

Puck JM: Primary immunodeficiency diseases. JAMA 278:1835, 1997

Tyler KL, Nathanson N: Pathogenesis of viral infections, in *Fields Virology*, DM Knipe, PM Howley (eds). Philadelphia, Lippincott Williams & Wilkins, 2001, pp 199-244

Weiss ST: Eat dirt—the hygiene hypothesis and allergic diseases. N Engl J Med 347:930, 2002

CHAPTER 2

MOLECULAR MECHANISMS OF MICROBIAL PATHOGENESIS

Gerald B. Pier

Over the past three decades, molecular studies of the pathogenesis of microorganisms have yielded an explosion of information about the various microbial and host molecules that contribute to the processes of infection and disease. These processes can be classified into several stages: microbial encounter with and entry into the host; microbial growth after entry; avoidance of innate host defenses; tissue invasion and tropism; tissue damage; and transmission to new hosts. *Virulence* is the measure of an organism's capacity to cause disease and is a function of the pathogenic factors elaborated by microbes. These factors promote *colonization* (the simple presence of potentially pathogenic microbes in or on a host), *infection* (attachment and growth of pathogens and avoidance of host defenses), and *disease* (often, but not always, the result of activities of secreted toxins or toxic metabolites). In addition, the host's inflammatory response to infection greatly contributes to disease and its attendant clinical signs and symptoms.

MICROBIAL ENTRY AND ADHERENCE

ENTRY SITES

A microbial pathogen can potentially enter any part of a host organism. In general, the type of disease produced by a particular microbe is often a direct consequence of its route of entry into the body. The most common sites of entry are mucosal surfaces (the respiratory, alimentary, and urogenital tracts) and the skin. Ingestion, inhalation, and sexual contact are typical routes of microbial entry. Other portals of entry include sites of skin injury (cuts, bites, burns, trauma) along with injection via natural (i.e., vector-borne) or artificial (i.e., needlestick) routes. A few pathogens, such as *Schistosoma* spp., can penetrate unbroken skin. The conjunctiva can serve as an entry point for pathogens of the eye.

Microbial entry usually relies on the presence of specific microbial factors needed for persistence and growth in a tissue. Fecal-oral spread via the alimentary tract requires a biology consistent with survival in the varied environments of the gastrointestinal tract (including the low pH of the stomach and the high bile content of the intestine) as well as in contaminated food or water outside the host. Organisms that gain entry via the respiratory tract survive well in small moist droplets produced during sneezing and coughing. Pathogens that enter by venereal routes often survive best on the warm moist environment of the urogenital mucosa and have restricted host ranges (e.g., *Neisseria gonorrhoeae*, *Treponema pallidum*, and HIV).

The biology of microbes entering through the skin is highly varied. Some organisms can survive in a broad range of environments, such as the salivary glands or alimentary tracts of arthropod vectors, the mouths of larger animals, soil, and water. A complex biology allows protozoan parasites such as *Plasmodium*, *Leishmania*, and *Trypanosoma* spp. to undergo morphogenic changes that permit transmission to mammalian hosts during insect feeding for blood meals. Plasmodia are injected as infective sporozoites from the salivary glands during mosquito feeding. *Leishmania* parasites are regurgitated as promastigotes from the alimentary tract of sandflies and are injected by bite into a susceptible host. Trypanosomes are ingested from infected hosts by reduviid bugs, multiply in the insects' gastrointestinal tract, and are released in feces onto the host's skin during subsequent feedings. Most microbes that land directly on intact skin are destined to die, as survival on the skin or in hair follicles requires resistance to fatty acids, low pH, and other antimicrobial factors on skin. Once it is damaged (and particularly if it becomes necrotic), the skin can be a major portal of entry and growth for pathogens and elaboration of their toxic products. Burn wound infections and tetanus are clear examples. After animal bites, pathogens resident in the animal's saliva gain access to the victim's tissues through the damaged skin. Rabies is the paradigm for this pathogenic process; rabies virus grows in striated muscle cells at the site of inoculation.

MICROBIAL ADHERENCE

Once in or on a host, most microbes must anchor themselves to a tissue or tissue factor; the possible exceptions are organisms that directly enter the bloodstream and multiply there. Specific ligands or adhesins for host receptors constitute a major area of study in the field of microbial pathogenesis. Adhesins comprise a wide range of surface structures, not only anchoring the microbe to a tissue and promoting cellular entry where appropriate, but also eliciting host responses critical to the pathogenic process (Table 2-1). Most microbes produce multiple adhesins specific for multiple host receptors. These

TABLE 2-1

EXAMPLES OF MICROBIAL LIGAND-RECEPTOR INTERACTIONS

MICROORGANISM	TYPE OF MICROBIAL LIGAND	HOST RECEPTOR
Viral Pathogens		
Influenza virus	Hemagglutinin	Sialic acid
Measles virus		
Vaccine strain	Hemagglutinin	CD46/moesin
Wild-type strains	Hemagglutinin	Signaling lymphocytic activation molecule (SLAM)
Human herpesvirus type 6	?	CD46
Herpes simplex virus	Glycoprotein C	Heparan sulfate
HIV	Surface glycoprotein	CD4 and chemokine receptors (CCR5 and CXCR4)
Epstein-Barr virus	Envelope protein	CD21 (=CR2)
Adenovirus	Fiber protein	Coxsackie-adenovirus receptor (CAR)
Coxsackievirus	Viral coat proteins	CAR and major histocompatibility class I antigens
Bacterial Pathogens		
Neisseria spp.	Pili	Membrane cofactor protein (CD46)
Pseudomonas aeruginosa	Pili and flagella	Asialo-GM1
	Lipopolysaccharide	Cystic fibrosis transmembrane conductance regulator (CFTR)
Escherichia coli	Pili	Ceramides/mannose and digalactosyl residues
Streptococcus pyogenes	Hyaluronic acid capsule	CD44
Yersinia spp.	Invasin/accessory invasin locus	β_1 Integrins
Bordetella pertussis	Filamentous hemagglutinin	CR3
Legionella pneumophila	Adsorbed C3bi	CR3
Mycobacterium tuberculosis	Adsorbed C3bi	CR3; DC-SIGN[a]
Fungal Pathogens		
Blastomyces dermatitidis	WI-1	Possibly matrix proteins and integrins
Candida albicans	Int1p	Extracellular matrix proteins
Protozoal Pathogens		
Plasmodium vivax	Merozoite form	Duffy Fy antigen
Plasmodium falciparum	Erythrocyte-binding protein 175 (EBA-175)	Glycophorin A
Entamoeba histolytica	Surface lectin	*N*-Acetylglucosamine

[a]A novel dendritic cell–specific C-type lectin.

adhesins are often redundant, are serologically variable, and act additively or synergistically with other microbial factors to promote microbial sticking to host tissues. In addition, some microbes adsorb host proteins onto their surface and utilize the natural host protein receptor for microbial binding and entry into target cells.

Viral Adhesins

(See also Chap. 69) All viral pathogens must bind to host cells, enter them, and replicate within them. Viral coat proteins serve as the ligands for cellular entry, and more than one ligand-receptor interaction may be needed; for example, HIV uses its envelope glycoprotein (gp) 120 to enter host cells by binding to both CD4 and one of two receptors for chemokines (designated CCR5 and CXCR4). Similarly, the measles virus H glycoprotein binds to both CD46 and the membrane-organizing protein moesin on host cells. The gB and gC proteins on herpes simplex virus bind to heparan sulfate; this adherence is not essential for entry, but rather serves to concentrate virions close to the cell surface. This step is followed by attachment to mammalian cells mediated by the viral gD protein. Herpes simplex virus can use a number of eukaryotic cell surface receptors for entry, including the herpesvirus entry mediator (related to the tumor necrosis factor receptor); members of the immunoglobulin superfamily; two proteins called nectin-1 and nectin-2; and modified heparan sulfate.

Bacterial Adhesins

Among the microbial adhesins studied in greatest detail are bacterial pili and flagella (Fig. 2-1). *Pili* or *fimbriae* are commonly used by gram-negative and gram-positive bacteria for attachment to host cells and tissues. In electron micrographs, these hairlike projections (up to several hundred per cell) may be confined to one end of the organism (polar pili) or distributed more evenly over the surface. An individual cell may have pili with a variety of functions. Most pili are made up of a major pilin protein subunit (molecular weight, 17,000-30,000) that polymerizes to form the pilus. Many strains of *Escherichia coli* isolated from urinary tract infections express mannose-binding type 1 pili, whose binding to the integral membrane glycoproteins called *uroplakins* that coat the cells in the bladder epithelium is inhibited by D-mannose. Other strains produce the Pap (pyelonephritis-associated) or P pilus adhesin that mediates binding to digalactose (gal-gal) residues on globosides of the human P blood groups. Both of these types of pili have proteins located at the tips of the main pilus unit that are critical to the binding specificity of the whole pilus unit. It is interesting that, although immunization with the mannose-binding tip protein (FimH) of type 1 pili prevents experimental *E. coli* bladder infections in mice and monkeys, a trial of this vaccine in humans was not successful. *E. coli* cells causing diarrheal disease express pilus-like receptors for enterocytes on the small bowel, along with other receptors termed *colonization factors*.

The type IV pilus, a common type of pilus found in *Neisseria* spp., *Moraxella* spp., *Vibrio cholerae*, *Legionella pneumophila*, *Salmonella enterica* serovar *typhi*, enteropathogenic *E. coli*, and *Pseudomonas aeruginosa*, mediates adherence of these organisms to target surfaces. These pili tend to have a relatively conserved amino-terminal region and a more variable carboxyl-terminal region. For some species (e.g., *N. gonorrhoeae*, *N. meningitidis*, and enteropathogenic *E. coli*), the pili are critical for attachment to mucosal epithelial cells. For others, such as *P. aeruginosa*, the pili only partially mediate the cells' adherence to host tissues. Whereas interference with this stage of colonization would appear to be an effective antibacterial strategy, attempts to develop pilus-based vaccines for human diseases have not been highly successful to date.

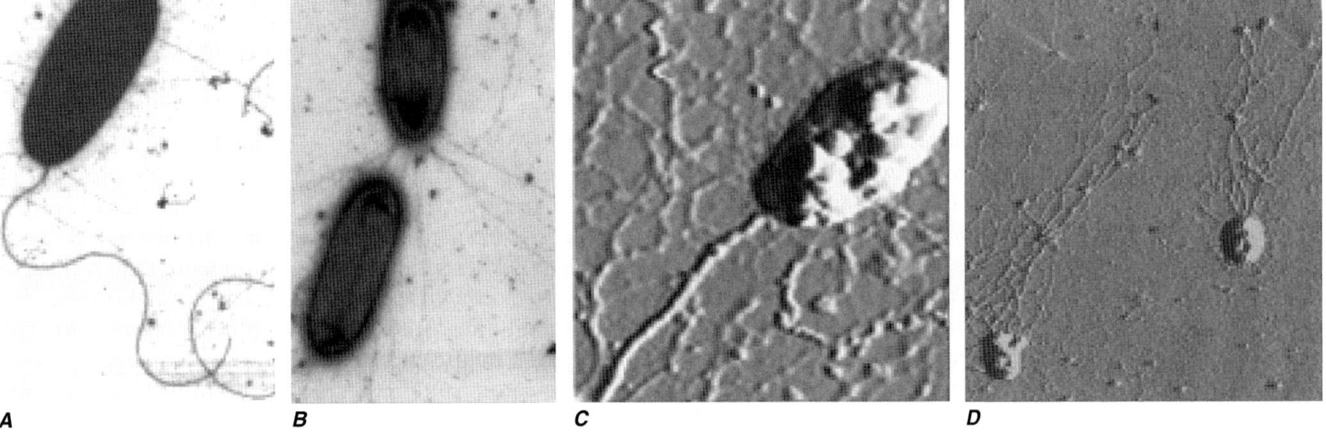

FIGURE 2-1

Bacterial surface structures. *A* and *B*. Traditional electron micrographic images of fixed cells of *Pseudomonas aeruginosa*. Flagella (***A***) and pili (***B***) projecting out from the bacterial poles can be seen. ***C* and *D*.** Atomic force microscopic image of live *P. aeruginosa* freshly planted onto a smooth mica surface. This technology reveals the fine, three-dimensional detail of the bacterial surface structures. (*Images courtesy of Dr. Martin Lee and Dr. Milan Bajmoczi, Harvard Medical School; with permission.*)

Flagella are long appendages attached at either one or both ends of the bacterial cell (polar flagella) or distributed over the entire cell surface (peritrichous flagella). Flagella, like pili, are composed of a polymerized or aggregated basic protein. In flagella, the protein subunits form a tight helical structure and vary serologically with the species. Spirochetes such as *T. pallidum* and *Borrelia burgdorferi* have axial filaments similar to flagella running down the long axis of the center of the cell, and they "swim" by rotation around these filaments. Some bacteria can glide over a surface in the absence of obvious motility structures.

Other bacterial structures involved in adherence to host tissues include specific staphylococcal and streptococcal proteins that bind to human extracellular matrix proteins such as fibrin, fibronectin, fibrinogen, laminin, and collagen. Fibronectin appears to be a commonly used receptor for various pathogens; a particular amino acid sequence in fibronectin (Arg-Gly-Asp, or RGD) is critical for bacterial binding. Binding of the highly conserved *Staphylococcus aureus* surface protein clumping factor A (ClfA) to fibrinogen has been implicated in many aspects of pathogenesis. The conserved outer-core portion of the lipopolysaccharide (LPS) of *P. aeruginosa* mediates binding to the cystic fibrosis transmembrane conductance regulator (CFTR) on airway epithelial cells-an event that appears to be critical for normal host resistance to infection. A number of bacterial pathogens, including coagulase-negative staphylococci, *S. aureus*, and uropathogenic *E. coli* as well as *Yersinia pestis, Y. pseudotuberculosis*, and *Y. enterocolitica*, express a surface polysaccharide composed of poly-*N*-acetylglucosamine. One function of this polysaccharide is to promote binding to materials used in catheters and other types of implanted devices; poly-*N*-acetylglucosamine may be a critical factor in the establishment of device-related infections by pathogens such as staphylococci and *E. coli*. High-powered imaging techniques (e.g., atomic force microscopy) have revealed that bacterial cells have a nonhomogeneous surface that is probably attributable to different concentrations of cell surface molecules, including microbial adhesins, at specific places on the cell surface (Fig 2-1D).

Fungal Adhesins

Several fungal adhesins have been described that mediate colonization of epithelial surfaces, particularly adherence to structures like fibronectin, laminin, and collagen. The product of the *Candida albicans INT1* gene, Int1p, bears similarity to mammalian integrins that bind to extracellular matrix proteins. Transformation of normally nonadherent *Saccharomyces cerevisiae* with this gene allows these yeast cells to adhere to human epithelial cells. The agglutinin-like sequence (ALS) adhesins are large cell-surface glycoproteins mediating adherence of pathogenic *Candida* to host tissues. These adhesins are expressed under certain environmental conditions (often associated with stress) and are crucial for pathogenesis of fungal infections.

For several fungal pathogens that initiate infections after inhalation, the inoculum is ingested by alveolar macrophages, in which the fungal cells transform to pathogenic phenotypes.

Eukaryotic Pathogen Adhesins

Eukaryotic parasites use complicated surface glycoproteins as adhesins, some of which are lectins (proteins that bind to specific carbohydrates on host cells). For example, *Plasmodium vivax* binds (via Duffy-binding protein) to the Duffy blood group carbohydrate antigen Fy on erythrocytes. *Entamoeba histolytica* expresses two proteins that bind to the disaccharide galactose/*N*-acetylgalactosamine. Reports indicate that children with mucosal IgA antibody to one of these lectins are resistant to reinfection with virulent *E. histolytica*. A major surface glycoprotein (gp63) of *Leishmania* promastigotes is needed for these parasites to enter human macrophages—the principal target cell of infection. This glycoprotein promotes complement binding but inhibits complement lytic activity, allowing the parasite to use complement receptors for entry into macrophages; gp63 also binds to fibronectin receptors on macrophages. In addition, the pathogen can express a carbohydrate that mediates binding to host cells. Evidence suggests that, as part of hepatic granuloma formation, *Schistosoma mansoni* expresses a carbohydrate epitope related to the Lewis X blood group antigen that promotes adherence of helminthic eggs to vascular endothelial cells under inflammatory conditions.

HOST RECEPTORS

Host receptors are found both on target cells (e.g., epithelial cells lining mucosal surfaces) and within the mucous layer covering these cells. Microbial pathogens bind to a wide range of host receptors to establish infection (Table 2-1). Selective loss of host receptors for a pathogen may confer natural resistance to an otherwise susceptible population. For example, 70% of individuals in West Africa lack Fy antigens and are resistant to *P. vivax* infection. *S. enterica* serovar *typhi*, the etiologic agent of typhoid fever, uses CFTR to enter the gastrointestinal submucosa after being ingested. As homozygous mutations in *CFTR* are the cause of the life-shortening disease cystic fibrosis, heterozygote carriers (e.g., 4–5% of individuals of European ancestry) may have had a selective advantage due to decreased susceptibility to typhoid fever.

Numerous virus–target cell interactions have been described, and it is now clear that different viruses can use similar host-cell receptors for entry. The list of certain and likely host receptors for viral pathogens is long. Among the host membrane components that can serve as receptors for viruses are sialic acids, gangliosides, glycosaminoglycans, integrins and other members of the immunoglobulin superfamily, histocompatibility antigens, and regulators and receptors for complement components. A notable example of the effect of host receptors on the pathogenesis of infection comes from comparative binding studies of avian influenza A virus subtype H5N1 and influenza A virus strains expressing hemagglutinin subtype H1. The H1-subtype strains, which tend to be highly pathogenic and transmissible from human to human, bind to a receptor composed of two sugar molecules:

sialic acid linked α-2-6 to galactose. This receptor is highly expressed in the airway epithelium. When virus is shed from this surface, its transmission via coughing and aerosol droplets is readily facilitated. In contrast, H5N1 avian influenza virus binds to sialic acid linked α-2-3 to galactose, and this receptor is highly expressed in pneumocytes in the alveoli. Alveolar infection is thought to underlie not only the high mortality rate associated with avian influenza but also the low human-to-human transmissibility rate of this strain, which is not readily transported to the airways (from which it could be expelled by coughing).

MICROBIAL GROWTH AFTER ENTRY

Once established on a mucosal or skin site, pathogenic microbes must replicate before causing full-blown infection and disease. Within cells, viral particles release their nucleic acids, which may be directly translated into viral proteins (positive-strand RNA viruses), transcribed from a negative strand of RNA into a complementary mRNA (negative-strand RNA viruses), or transcribed into a complementary strand of DNA (retroviruses); for DNA viruses, mRNA may be transcribed directly from viral DNA, either in the cell nucleus or in the cytoplasm. To grow, bacteria must acquire specific nutrients or synthesize them from precursors in host tissues. Many infectious processes are usually confined to specific epithelial surfaces—e.g., H1-subtype influenza to the respiratory mucosa, gonorrhea to the urogenital epithelium, and shigellosis to the gastrointestinal epithelium. Although there are multiple reasons for this specificity, one important consideration is the ability of these pathogens to obtain from these specific environments the nutrients needed for growth and survival.

Temperature restrictions also play a role in limiting certain pathogens to specific tissues. Rhinoviruses, a cause of the common cold, grow best at 33°C and replicate in cooler nasal tissues, but not as well in the lung. Leprosy lesions due to *Mycobacterium leprae* are found in and on relatively cool body sites. Fungal pathogens that infect the skin, hair follicles, and nails (dermatophyte infections) remain confined to the cooler, exterior, keratinous layer of the epithelium.

Many bacterial, fungal, and protozoal species grow in multicellular masses referred to as *biofilms*. These masses are biochemically and morphologically quite distinct from the free-living individual cells referred to as *planktonic cells*. Growth in biofilms leads to altered microbial metabolism, production of extracellular virulence factors, and decreased susceptibility to biocides, antimicrobial agents, and host defense molecules and cells. *P. aeruginosa* growing on the bronchial mucosa during chronic infection, staphylococci and other pathogens growing on implanted medical devices, and dental pathogens growing on tooth surfaces to form plaques represent several examples of microbial biofilm growth associated with human disease. Many other pathogens can form biofilms during in vitro growth, and it is increasingly accepted that this mode of growth contributes to microbial virulence and induction of disease.

AVOIDANCE OF INNATE HOST DEFENSES

Because microbes have probably interacted with mucosal/epithelial surfaces since the emergence of multicellular organisms, it is not surprising that multicellular hosts have a variety of innate surface defense mechanisms that can sense when pathogens are present and contribute to their elimination. The skin is acidic and is bathed with fatty acids toxic to many microbes. Skin pathogens such as staphylococci must tolerate these adverse conditions. Mucosal surfaces are covered by a barrier composed of a thick mucous layer that entraps microbes and facilitates their transport out of the body by such processes as mucociliary clearance, coughing, and urination. Mucous secretions, saliva, and tears contain antibacterial factors such as lysozyme and antimicrobial peptides as well as antiviral factors such as interferons. Gastric acidity is inimical to the survival of many ingested pathogens, and most mucosal surfaces—particularly the nasopharynx, the vaginal tract, and the gastrointestinal tract—contain a resident flora of commensal microbes that interfere with the ability of pathogens to colonize and infect a host.

Pathogens that survive these factors must still contend with host endocytic, phagocytic, and inflammatory responses as well as with host genetic factors that determine the degree to which a pathogen can survive and grow. The growth of viral pathogens entering skin or mucosal epithelial cells can be limited by a variety of host genetic factors, including production of interferons, modulation of receptors for viral entry, and age- and hormone-related susceptibility factors; by nutritional status; and even by personal habits such as smoking and exercise.

ENCOUNTERS WITH EPITHELIAL CELLS

Over the past decade, many bacterial pathogens have been shown to enter epithelial cells (Fig. 2-2); the bacteria often use specialized surface structures that bind to receptors, with consequent internalization. However, the exact role and the importance of this process in infection and disease are not well defined for most of these pathogens. Bacterial entry into host epithelial cells is seen as a means for dissemination to adjacent or deeper tissues or as a route to sanctuary to avoid ingestion and killing by professional phagocytes. Epithelial cell entry appears, for instance, to be a critical aspect of dysentery induction by *Shigella*.

Curiously, the less virulent strains of many bacterial pathogens are more adept at entering epithelial cells than are more virulent strains; examples include pathogens that lack the surface polysaccharide capsule needed to cause serious disease. Thus, for *Haemophilus influenzae*, *Streptococcus pneumoniae*, *Streptococcus agalactiae* (group B *Streptococcus*). and *Streptococcus pyogenes*, isogenic mutants or variants lacking capsules enter epithelial cells better than the wild-type, encapsulated parental forms that cause disseminated disease. These observations have led to the proposal that epithelial cell entry may be primarily a

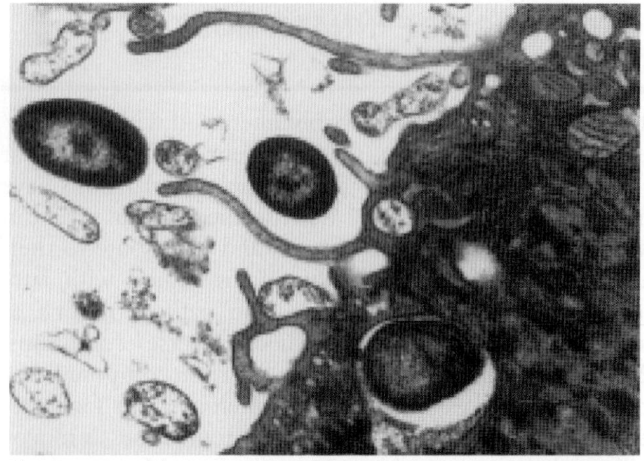

A

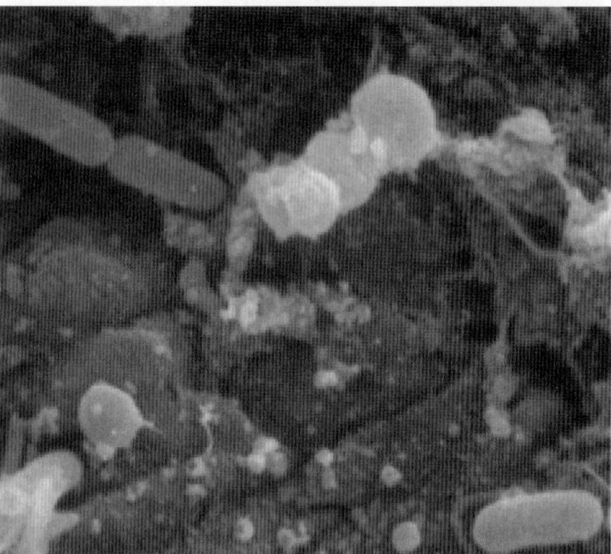

B

FIGURE 2-2

Entry of bacteria into epithelial cells. *A.* Internalization of *P. aeruginosa* by cultured human airway epithelial cells expressing wild-type cystic fibrosis transmembrane conductance regulator (CFTR), the cell receptor for bacterial ingestion. ***B.*** Entry of *P. aeruginosa* into murine tracheal epithelial cells after infection by the intranasal route.

manifestation of host defense, resulting in bacterial clearance by both shedding of epithelial cells containing internalized bacteria and initiation of a protective and nonpathogenic inflammatory response. However, a possible consequence of this process could be the opening of a hole in the epithelium, potentially allowing uningested organisms to enter the submucosa. This scenario has been documented in murine *S. enterica* serovar *typhimurium* infections and in experimental bladder infections with uropathogenic *E. coli*. In the latter system, bacterial pilus–mediated attachment to uroplakins induces exfoliation of the cells with attached bacteria. Subsequently, infection is produced by residual bacterial cells that invade the superficial bladder epithelium, where they can grow intracellularly into biofilm-like masses encased in an extracellular polysaccharide-rich matrix and surrounded by uroplakin. This mode of growth produces structures that have been referred to as *bacterial pods*. At low bacterial inocula, epithelial cell ingestion and subclinical inflammation are probably efficient means to eliminate pathogens; in contrast, at higher inocula, a proportion of surviving bacterial cells enter host tissue through the damaged mucosal surface and multiply, producing disease. Alternatively, failure of the appropriate epithelial cell response to a pathogen may allow the organism to survive on a mucosal surface where, if it avoids other host defenses, it can grow and cause a local infection. Along these lines, as noted above, *P. aeruginosa* is taken into epithelial cells by CFTR, a protein missing or nonfunctional in most severe cases of cystic fibrosis. The major clinical consequence is chronic airway-surface infection with *P. aeruginosa* in 80–90% of patients with cystic fibrosis. The failure of airway epithelial cells to ingest and promote the removal of *P. aeruginosa* via a properly regulated inflammatory response has been proposed as a key component of the hypersusceptibility of these patients to chronic airway infection with this organism.

ENCOUNTERS WITH PHAGOCYTES

Phagocytosis and Inflammation

Phagocytosis of microbes is a major innate host defense that limits the growth and spread of pathogens. Phagocytes appear rapidly at sites of infection in conjunction with the initiation of inflammation. Ingestion of microbes by both tissue-fixed macrophages and migrating phagocytes probably accounts for the limited ability of most microbial agents to cause disease. A family of related molecules called *collectins*, *soluble defense collagens*, or *pattern-recognition molecules* are found in blood (mannose-binding lectins), in lung (surfactant proteins A and D), and most likely in other tissues as well and bind to carbohydrates on microbial surfaces to promote phagocyte clearance. Bacterial pathogens seem to be ingested principally by polymorphonuclear neutrophils (PMNs), whereas eosinophils are frequently found at sites of infection with protozoan or multicellular parasites. Successful pathogens, by definition, must avoid being cleared by professional phagocytes. One of several antiphagocytic strategies employed by bacteria and by the fungal pathogen *Cryptococcus neoformans* is to elaborate large-molecular-weight surface polysaccharide antigens, often in the form of a capsule that coats the cell surface. Most pathogenic bacteria produce such antiphagocytic capsules. On occasion, proteins or polypeptides form capsule-like coatings on organisms such as *Bacillus anthracis*.

Because activation of local phagocytes in tissues is a key step in initiating inflammation and migration of additional phagocytes into infected sites, much attention has been paid to microbial factors that initiate inflammation. Encounters with phagocytes are governed largely by the structure of the microbial constituents that elicit inflammation, and detailed knowledge of these structures for bacterial pathogens has contributed greatly to our understanding of molecular mechanisms of microbial pathogenesis (Fig. 2-3). One of the best-studied systems involves the interaction of LPS from

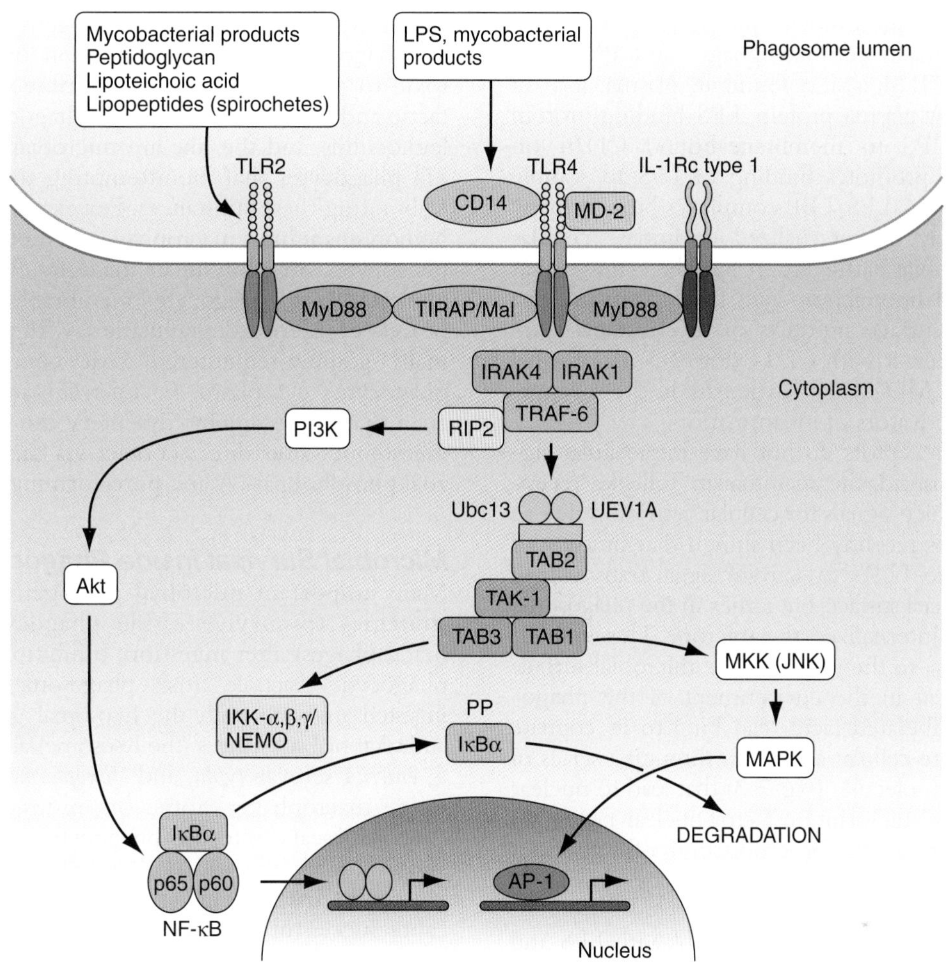

FIGURE 2-3

Cellular signaling pathways for production of inflammatory cytokines in response to microbial products. Various microbial cell-surface constituents interact with CD14, which in turn interacts in a currently unknown fashion with Toll-like receptors (TLRs). Some microbial factors do not need CD14 to interact with TLRs. Associating with TLR4 (and to some extent with TLR2) is MD-2, a cofactor that facilitates the response to lipopolysaccharide (LPS). Both CD14 and TLRs contain extracellular leucine-rich domains that become localized to the lumen of the phagosome upon uptake of bacterial cells; there, the TLRs can bind to microbial products. The TLRs are oligomerized, usually forming homodimers, and then bind to the general adaptor protein MyD88 via the C-terminal Toll/IL-1R (TIR) domains, which also bind to TIRAP (TIR domain-containing adaptor protein), a molecule that participates in the transduction of signals from TLR4. The MyD88/TIRAP complex activates signal-transducing molecules such as IRAK1 and IRAK4 (IL-1Rc-associated kinases 1 and 4); TRAF-6 (tumor necrosis factor receptor–associated factor 6); TAK-1 (transforming growth factor β-activating kinase 1); and TAB1, TAB2, and TAB3 (TAK1-binding proteins 1, 2, and 3). This signaling complex associates with the ubiquitin-conjugating enzyme Ubc13 and the Ubc-like protein UEV1A to catalyze the formation of a polyubiquitin chain on TRAF6. Polyubiquitination of TRAF6 activates TAK1, which, along with TAB2 (a protein that binds to lysine residue 63 in polyubiquitin chains via a conserved zinc-finger domain), phosphorylates the inducible kinase complex IKK-α, -β, and -γ. IKK-γ is also called NEMO [nuclear factor κB (NF-κB) essential modulator]. This large complex then phosphorylates the inhibitory component of NF-κB, IκBα, resulting in release of IκBα from NF-κB. Phosphorylated (PP) IκB is then degraded, and the two components of NF-κB, p50 and p65, translocate to the nucleus, where they bind to regulatory transcriptional sites on target genes, many of which encode inflammatory proteins. In addition to inducing NF-κB nuclear translocation, TAK1 also activates MAP kinase transducers such as the c-Jun N-terminal kinase (JNK) pathway, which can lead to nuclear translocation of the transcription factor AP1. Via the RIP2 protein, TRAF6 bound to IRAK can activate phosphatidylinositol-3 kinase (PI3K) and the regulatory protein Akt to dissociate NF–κB from IκBα, an event followed by translocation of the active NF-κB to the nucleus. *(Figure modified from an original produced by Dr. Terry Means and Dr. Douglas Golenbock.)*

gram-negative bacteria and the glycosylphosphatidylinositol (GPI)-anchored membrane protein CD14 found on the surface of professional phagocytes, including migrating and tissue-fixed macrophages and PMNs. A soluble form of CD14 is also found in plasma and on mucosal surfaces. A plasma protein, LPS-binding protein (LBP), transfers LPS to membrane-bound CD14 on myeloid cells and promotes binding of LPS to soluble CD14. Soluble CD14/LPS/LBP complexes bind to many cell types and may be internalized to initiate cellular responses to microbial pathogens. It has been shown that peptidoglycan and lipoteichoic acid from gram-positive bacteria and cell-surface products of mycobacteria and spirochetes can interact with CD14 (Fig. 2-3). Additional molecules, such as MD-2, also participate in the recognition of bacterial activators of inflammation.

GPI-anchored receptors do not have intracellular signaling domains. Instead, the mammalian Toll-like receptors (TLRs) transduce signals for cellular activation due to LPS binding. It has recently been shown that binding of microbial factors to TLRs to activate signal transduction occurs not on the cell surface, but rather in the phagosome of cells that have internalized the microbe. This interaction is probably due to the release of the microbial surface factor from the cell in the environment of the phagosome, where the liberated factor can bind to its cognate TLRs. TLRs initiate cellular activation through a series of signal-transducing molecules (Fig. 2-3) that lead to nuclear translocation of the transcription factor nuclear factor κB (NF-κB), a master-switch for production of important inflammatory cytokines such as tumor necrosis factor α (TNF-α) and interleukin (IL) 1.

Inflammation can be initiated not only with LPS and peptidoglycan, but also with viral particles and other microbial products such as polysaccharides, enzymes, and toxins. Bacterial flagella activate inflammation by binding of a conserved sequence to TLR5. Some pathogens, including *Campylobacter jejuni*, *Helicobacter pylori*, and *Bartonella bacilliformis*, make flagella that lack this sequence and thus do not bind to TLR5. The result is a lack of efficient host response to infection. Bacteria also produce a high proportion of DNA molecules with unmethylated CpG residues that activate inflammation through TLR9. TLR3 recognizes double-strand RNA, a pattern-recognition molecule produced by many viruses during their replicative cycle. TLR1 and TLR6 associate with TLR2 to promote recognition of acylated microbial proteins and peptides.

The myeloid differentiation factor 88 (MyD88) molecule is a generalized adaptor protein that binds to the cytoplasmic domains of all known TLRs and also to receptors that are part of the IL-1 receptor (IL-1Rc) family. Numerous studies have shown that MyD88-mediated transduction of signals from TLRs and IL-1Rc is critical for innate resistance to infection. Mice lacking MyD88 are more susceptible than normal mice to infection with group B *Streptococcus*, *Listeria monocytogenes*, and *Mycobacterium tuberculosis*. However, it is now appreciated that some of the TLRs (e.g., TLR3 and TLR4) can activate signal transduction via an MyD88-independent pathway.

Additional Interactions of Microbial Pathogens and Phagocytes

Other ways that microbial pathogens avoid destruction by phagocytes include production of factors that are toxic to phagocytes or that interfere with the chemotactic and ingestion function of phagocytes. Hemolysins, leukocidins, and the like are microbial proteins that can kill phagocytes that are attempting to ingest organisms elaborating these substances. For example, staphylococcal hemolysins inhibit macrophage chemotaxis and kill these phagocytes. Streptolysin O made by *S. pyogenes* binds to cholesterol in phagocyte membranes and initiates a process of internal degranulation, with the release of normally granule-sequestered toxic components into the phagocyte's cytoplasm. *E. histolytica*, an intestinal protozoan that causes amebic dysentery, can disrupt phagocyte membranes after direct contact via the release of protozoal phospholipase A and pore-forming peptides.

Microbial Survival inside Phagocytes

Many important microbial pathogens use a variety of strategies to survive inside phagocytes (particularly macrophages) after ingestion. Inhibition of fusion of the phagocytic vacuole (the phagosome) containing the ingested microbe with the lysosomal granules containing antimicrobial substances (the lysosome) allows *M. tuberculosis*, *S. enterica* serovar *typhi*, and *Toxoplasma gondii* to survive inside macrophages. Some organisms, such as *L. monocytogenes*, escape into the phagocyte's cytoplasm to grow and eventually spread to other cells. Resistance to killing within the macrophage and subsequent growth are critical to successful infection by herpes-type viruses, measles virus, poxviruses, *Salmonella*, *Yersinia*, *Legionella*, *Mycobacterium*, *Trypanosoma*, *Nocardia*, *Histoplasma*, *Toxoplasma*, and *Rickettsia*. *Salmonella* spp. use a master regulatory system, in which the *PhoP/PhoQ* genes control other genes, to enter and survive within cells; intracellular survival entails structural changes in the cell envelope LPS.

TISSUE INVASION AND TISSUE TROPISM

TISSUE INVASION

Most viral pathogens cause disease by growth at skin or mucosal entry sites, but some pathogens spread from the initial site to deeper tissues. Virus can spread via the nerves (rabies virus) or plasma (picornaviruses) or within migratory blood cells (poliovirus, Epstein-Barr virus, and many others). Specific viral genes determine where and how individual viral strains can spread.

Bacteria may invade deeper layers of mucosal tissue via intracellular uptake by epithelial cells, traversal of epithelial cell junctions, or penetration through denuded epithelial surfaces. Among virulent *Shigella* strains and invasive *E. coli*, outer-membrane proteins are critical to epithelial cell invasion and bacterial multiplication. *Neisseria* and *Haemophilus* spp. penetrate mucosal cells by poorly understood mechanisms before dissemination into the bloodstream. Staphylococci and streptococci elaborate a variety of extracellular enzymes, such as hyaluronidase, lipases, nucleases, and hemolysins, that are probably important in breaking down cellular and matrix structures and allowing the bacteria access to deeper tissues and blood. Organisms that colonize the gastrointestinal tract can often translocate through the mucosa into the blood and, under circumstances in which host defenses are inadequate, cause bacteremia. *Y. enterocolitica* can invade the mucosa through the activity of the invasin protein. Some bacteria (e.g., *Brucella*) can be carried from a mucosal site to a distant site by phagocytic cells (e.g., PMNs) that ingest but fail to kill the bacteria.

Fungal pathogens almost always take advantage of host immunocompromise to spread hematogenously to deeper tissues. The AIDS epidemic has resoundingly illustrated this principle: The immunodeficiency of many HIV-infected patients permits the development of life-threatening fungal infections of the lung, blood, and brain. Other than the capsule of *C. neoformans*, specific fungal antigens involved in tissue invasion are not well characterized. Both fungal and protozoal pathogens undergo morphologic changes to spread within a host. Yeast-cell forms of *C. albicans* transform into hyphal forms when invading deeper tissues. Malarial parasites grow in liver cells as merozoites and are released into the blood to invade erythrocytes and become trophozoites. *E. histolytica* is found as both a cyst and a trophozoite in the intestinal lumen, through which this pathogen enters the host, but only the trophozoite form can spread systemically to cause amebic liver abscesses. Other protozoal pathogens, such as *T. gondii*, *Giardia lamblia*, and *Cryptosporidium*, also undergo extensive morphologic changes after initial infection to spread to other tissues.

TISSUE TROPISM

The propensity of certain microbes to cause disease by infecting specific tissues has been known since the early days of bacteriology, yet the molecular basis for this propensity is understood somewhat better for viral pathogens than for other agents of infectious disease. Specific receptor-ligand interactions clearly underlie the ability of certain viruses to enter cells within tissues and disrupt normal tissue function, but the mere presence of a receptor for a virus on a target tissue is not sufficient for tissue tropism. Factors in the cell, route of viral entry, viral capacity to penetrate into cells, viral genetic elements that regulate gene expression, and pathways of viral spread in a tissue all affect tissue tropism. Some viral genes are best transcribed in specific target cells, such as hepatitis B genes in liver cells and Epstein-Barr virus genes in B lymphocytes. The route of inoculation of poliovirus determines its neurotropism, although the molecular basis for this circumstance is not understood.

The lesser understanding of the tissue tropism of bacterial and parasitic infections is exemplified by *Neisseria* spp. There is no well-accepted explanation of why *N. gonorrhoeae* colonizes and infects the human genital tract, whereas the closely related species *N. meningitidis* principally colonizes the human oropharynx. *N. meningitidis* expresses a capsular polysaccharide, whereas *N. gonorrhoeae* does not; however, there is no indication that this property plays a role in the different tissue tropisms displayed by these two bacterial species. *N. gonorrhoeae* can use cytidine monophosphate *N*-acetylneuraminic acid from host tissues to add *N*-acetylneuraminic acid (sialic acid) to its lipooligosaccharide (LOS) O side chain, and this alteration appears to make the organism resistant to host defenses. Lactate, present at high levels on genital mucosal surfaces, stimulates sialylation of gonococcal LOS. Bacteria with sialic acid sugars in their capsules, such as *N. meningitidis*, *E. coli* K1, and group B streptococci, have a propensity to cause meningitis, but this generalization has many exceptions. For example, all recognized serotypes of group B streptococci contain sialic acid in their capsules, but only one serotype (III) is responsible for most cases of group B streptococcal meningitis. Moreover, both *H. influenzae* and *S. pneumoniae* can readily cause meningitis, but these organisms do not have sialic acid in their capsules.

TISSUE DAMAGE AND DISEASE

Disease is a complex phenomenon resulting from tissue invasion and destruction, toxin elaboration, and host response. Viruses cause much of their damage by exerting a cytopathic effect on host cells and inhibiting host defenses. The growth of bacterial, fungal, and protozoal parasites in tissue, which may or may not be accompanied by toxin elaboration, can also compromise tissue function and lead to disease. For some bacterial and possibly some fungal pathogens, toxin production is one of the best-characterized molecular mechanisms of pathogenesis, whereas host factors such as IL-1, TNF-α, kinins, inflammatory proteins, products of complement activation, and mediators derived from arachidonic acid metabolites (leukotrienes) and cellular degranulation (histamines) readily contribute to the severity of disease.

VIRAL DISEASE

See Chap. 78.

BACTERIAL TOXINS

Among the first infectious diseases to be understood were those due to toxin-elaborating bacteria. Diphtheria, botulism, and tetanus toxins are responsible for the diseases associated with local infections due to *Corynebacterium diphtheriae*, *Clostridium botulinum*, and *Clostridium tetani*, respectively. Enterotoxins produced by *E. coli*, *Salmonella*, *Shigella*, *Staphylococcus*, and *V. cholerae* contribute to diarrheal disease caused by these organisms. Staphylococci, streptococci, *P. aeruginosa*, and *Bordetella* elaborate various toxins that cause or contribute to disease, including toxic shock syndrome toxin 1 (TSST-1); erythrogenic toxin; exotoxins A, S, T, and U; and pertussis toxin. A number of these toxins (e.g., cholera toxin, diphtheria toxin, pertussis toxin, *E. coli* heat-labile toxin, and *P. aeruginosa* exotoxins A, S, and T) have adenosine diphosphate (ADP)-ribosyltransferase activity—i.e., the toxins enzymatically catalyze the transfer of the ADP-ribosyl portion of nicotinamide adenine diphosphate to target proteins and inactivate them. The staphylococcal enterotoxins, TSST-1, and the streptococcal pyogenic exotoxins behave as superantigens, stimulating certain T cells to proliferate without processing of the protein toxin by antigen-presenting cells. Part of this process involves stimulation of the antigen-presenting cells to produce IL-1 and TNF-α, which have been implicated in many of the clinical features of diseases like toxic shock syndrome and scarlet fever. A number of gram-negative pathogens (*Salmonella*, *Yersinia*, and *P. aeruginosa*) can inject toxins directly into host target cells by means of a complex set of proteins referred to as the type III secretion system. Loss or inactivation of this virulence system usually greatly reduces the capacity of a bacterial pathogen to cause disease.

ENDOTOXIN

The lipid A portion of gram-negative LPS has potent biologic activities that cause many of the clinical manifestations of gram-negative bacterial sepsis, including fever, muscle proteolysis, uncontrolled intravascular coagulation, and shock. The effects of lipid A appear to be mediated by the production of potent cytokines due to LPS binding to CD14 and signal transduction via TLRs, particularly TLR4. Cytokines exhibit potent hypothermic activity through effects on the hypothalamus; they also increase vascular permeability, alter the activity of endothelial cells, and induce endothelial-cell procoagulant activity. Numerous therapeutic strategies aimed at neutralizing the effects of endotoxin are under investigation, but so far the results have been disappointing. One drug, activated protein C (drotrecogin alfa, activated), was found to reduce mortality by ~20% during severe sepsis—a condition that can be induced by endotoxin during gram-negative bacterial sepsis.

INVASION

Many diseases are caused primarily by pathogens growing in tissue sites that are normally sterile. Pneumococcal pneumonia is mostly attributable to the growth of *S. pneumoniae* in the lung and the attendant host inflammatory response, although specific factors that enhance this process (e.g., pneumolysin) may be responsible for some of the pathogenic potential of the pneumococcus. Disease that follows bacteremia and invasion of the meninges by meningitis-producing bacteria such as *N. meningitidis*, *H. influenzae*, *E. coli* K1, and group B streptococci appears to be due solely to the ability of these organisms to gain access to these tissues, multiply in them, and provoke cytokine production, leading to tissue-damaging host inflammation.

Specific molecular mechanisms accounting for tissue invasion by fungal and protozoal pathogens are less well described. Except for studies pointing to factors like capsule and melanin production by *C. neoformans* and (possibly) levels of cell wall glucans in some pathogenic fungi, the molecular basis for fungal invasiveness is not well defined. Melanism has been shown to protect the fungal cell against death caused by phagocyte factors such as nitric oxide, superoxide, and hypochlorite. Morphogenic variation and production of proteases (e.g., the *Candida* aspartyl proteinase) have been implicated in fungal invasion of host tissues.

If pathogens are effectively to invade host tissues (particularly the blood), they must avoid the major host defenses represented by complement and phagocytic cells. Bacteria most often avoid these defenses through their cell surface polysaccharides—either capsular polysaccharides or long O-side-chain antigens characteristic of the smooth LPS of gram-negative bacteria. These molecules can prevent the activation and/or deposition of complement opsonins or limit the access of phagocytic cells with receptors for complement opsonins to these molecules when they are deposited on the bacterial surface below the capsular layer. Another potential mechanism of microbial virulence is the ability of some organisms to present the capsule as an apparent self antigen through molecular mimicry. For example, the polysialic acid capsule of group B *N. meningitidis* is chemically identical to an oligosaccharide found on human brain cells.

Immunochemical studies of capsular polysaccharides have led to an appreciation of the tremendous chemical diversity that can result from the linking of a few monosaccharides. For example, three hexoses can link up in more than 300 different and potentially serologically distinct ways, whereas three amino acids have only six possible peptide combinations. Capsular polysaccharides, which have been used as effective vaccines against meningococcal meningitis as well as against pneumococcal and *H. influenzae* infections, may prove to be of value as vaccines against any organisms that express a nontoxic, immunogenic capsular polysaccharide. In addition, most encapsulated pathogens become virtually avirulent when capsule production is interrupted by genetic manipulation; this observation emphasizes the importance of this structure in pathogenesis.

HOST RESPONSE

The inflammatory response of the host is critical for interruption and resolution of the infectious process, but also is often responsible for the signs and symptoms of disease. Infection promotes a complex series of host responses involving the complement, kinin, and coagulation pathways. The production of cytokines such as IL-1, TNF-α, and other factors regulated in part by the NF-κ*B* transcription factor leads to fever, muscle proteolysis, and other effects, as noted above. An inability to kill or contain the microbe usually results in further damage due to the progression of inflammation and infection. In many chronic infections, degranulation of host inflammatory cells can lead to release of host proteases, elastases, histamines, and other toxic substances that can degrade host tissues. Chronic inflammation in any tissue can lead to the destruction of that tissue and to clinical disease associated with loss of organ function; an example is sterility from pelvic inflammatory disease caused by chronic infection with *N. gonorrhoeae*.

The nature of the host response elicited by the pathogen often determines the pathology of a particular infection. Local inflammation produces local tissue damage, whereas systemic inflammation, such as that seen during sepsis, can result in the signs and symptoms of septic shock. The severity of septic shock is associated with the degree of production of host effectors. Disease due to intracellular parasitism results from the formation of granulomas, wherein the host attempts to wall off the parasite inside a fibrotic lesion surrounded by fused epithelial cells that make up so-called multinucleated giant cells. A number of pathogens, particularly anaerobic bacteria, staphylococci, and streptococci, provoke the formation of an abscess, probably because of the presence of zwitterionic surface polysaccharides such as the capsular polysaccharide of *Bacteroides fragilis*. The outcome of an infection depends on the balance between an effective host response that eliminates a pathogen and an excessive inflammatory response that is associated with an inability to eliminate a pathogen and with the resultant tissue damage that leads to disease.

TRANSMISSION TO NEW HOSTS

As part of the pathogenic process, most microbes are shed from the host, often in a form infectious for susceptible individuals. However, the rate of transmissibility may not necessarily be high, even if the disease is severe in the infected individual, as transmissibility and virulence are not linked traits. Most pathogens exit via the same route by which they entered: respiratory pathogens by aerosols from sneezing or coughing or through salivary spread, gastrointestinal pathogens by fecal-oral spread, sexually transmitted diseases by venereal spread, and vector-borne organisms by either direct contact with the vector through a blood meal or indirect contact with organisms shed into environmental sources such as water. Microbial factors that specifically promote transmission are not well characterized. Respiratory shedding is facilitated by overproduction of mucous secretions, with consequently enhanced sneezing and coughing. Diarrheal toxins such as cholera toxin, *E. coli* heat-labile toxins, and *Shigella* toxins probably facilitate fecal-oral spread of microbial cells in the high volumes of diarrheal fluid produced during infection. The ability to produce phenotypic variants that resist hostile environmental factors (e.g., the highly resistant cysts of *E. histolytica* shed in feces) represents another mechanism of pathogenesis relevant to transmission. Blood parasites such as *Plasmodium* spp. change phenotype after ingestion by a mosquito-a prerequisite for the continued transmission of this pathogen. Venereally transmitted pathogens may undergo phenotypic variation due to the production of specific factors to facilitate transmission, but shedding of these pathogens into the environment does not result in the formation of infectious foci.

In summary, the molecular mechanisms used by pathogens to colonize, invade, infect, and disrupt the host are numerous and diverse. Each phase of the infectious process involves a variety of microbial and host factors interacting in a manner that can result in disease. Recognition of the coordinated genetic regulation of virulence factor elaboration when organisms move from their natural environment into the mammalian host emphasizes the complex nature of the host-parasite interaction. Fortunately, the need for diverse factors in successful infection and disease implies that a variety of therapeutic strategies may be developed to interrupt this process and thereby prevent and treat microbial infections.

FURTHER READINGS

CAMILLI A, BASSLER BL: Bacterial small-molecule signaling pathways. Science 311:1113, 2006

FINLAY BB, MCFADDEN G: Anti-immunology: Evasion of the host immune system by bacterial and viral pathogens. Cell 124:767, 2006

HAN J, ULEVITCH RJ: Limiting inflammatory responses during activation of innate immunity. Nat Immunol 6:1198, 2005

KAWAI T, AKIRA S: Innate immune recognition of viral infection. Nat Immunol 7:131, 2006

KNIREL YA et al: Structural features and structural variability of the lipopolysaccharide of *Yersinia pestis,* the cause of plague. J Endotoxin Res 12:3, 2006

MENDES-GIANNINI MJ et al: Interaction of pathogenic fungi with host cells: Molecular and cellular approaches. FEMS Immunol Med Microbiol 45:383, 2005

PIZARRO-CERDA J, COSSART P: Bacterial adhesion and entry into host cells. Cell 124:715, 2006

SPEAR PG et al: Different receptors binding to distinct interfaces on herpes simplex virus gD can trigger events leading to cell fusion and viral entry. Virology 344:17, 2006

TAKAHASHI K et al: The mannose-binding lectin: A prototypic pattern recognition molecule. Curr Opin Immunol 18:16, 2006

CHAPTER 3

IMMUNIZATION PRINCIPLES AND VACCINE USE

Gerald T. Keusch ■ Kenneth J. Bart ■ Mark Miller

Vaccines play a special role in the health and security of nations. The World Health Organization (WHO) cites immunization and the provision of clean water as the two public health interventions that have had the greatest impact on the world's health, and the World Bank notes that vaccines are among the most cost-effective health interventions available. Over the past century, the integration of immunization into routine health care services in many countries has provided caregivers with some degree of control over disease-related morbidity and mortality, especially among infants and children.

Despite these extraordinary successes, vaccines and their constituents (e.g., the mercury compound thimerosal, formerly used as a preservative) have come under attack in some countries as causes of neurodevelopmental disorders such as autism and attention-deficit hyperactivity disorder, diabetes, and a variety of allergic and autoimmune diseases. Although millions of lives are saved by vaccines each year and countless cases of postinfection disability are averted, some segments of the public are increasingly unwilling to accept any risk whatsoever of vaccine-associated complications (severe or otherwise), and resistance to vaccination is growing.

No medical procedure is absolutely risk-free, and the risk to the individual must always be balanced with benefits to the individual and to the population at large. This dichotomy poses two essential challenges for the medical and public health communities with respect to vaccines: (1) to create more effective and ever-safer vaccines, and (2) to educate patients and the general public more fully about the benefits as well as the risks of vaccine use. Because immunity to infectious diseases is acquired only by infection itself or by immunization, sustained vaccination programs for each birth cohort will continue to be necessary to control vaccine-preventable infectious diseases until and unless their etiologic agents can be eradicated from every region of the world.

An unwavering scientific and public health commitment to immunization is essential in countering public distrust and political pressure to legislate well-intentioned but ill-informed vaccine safety laws in response to the concerns of organized antivaccine advocacy groups. Ironically, it is the public health success of vaccines that has created a significant part of the problem: because the major fatal and disabling diseases of childhood are only rarely seen today in the United States, parents and young practitioners most likely will never have seen tetanus, diphtheria, *Haemophilus influenzae* disease, polio, or measles. Under these circumstances, the risks of immunization can easily (if erroneously) be perceived to outweigh the benefits, and this perception can be fueled by inaccurate information, poor science, and zealous advocacy. Caregivers must be prepared to educate parents about the importance of childhood immunization and to address their concerns effectively.

The medical community must also appreciate public concern about the sheer number of vaccines now licensed and the attendant fear that the more vaccines are administered, the more likely it is that complications and adverse immunologic consequences will occur. More than 50 biologic products are presently licensed in the United States, and dozens of antigens (many of them components of vaccine-combination products) are recommended for routine immunization of infants, children, adolescents, and adults (Figs. 3-1 and 3-2). Moreover, new vaccines are continually becoming available—e.g., human papillomavirus (HPV) vaccine for use in adolescent girls to prevent cervical cancer (Chap. 86) and a herpes zoster vaccine to prevent zoster (Chap. 81). Still other vaccines

Recommended Immunization Schedule for Persons Aged 0–6 Years
UNITED STATES • 2007

A

Vaccine ▼ Age ▶	Birth	1 month	2 months	4 months	6 months	12 months	15 months	18 months	19–23 months	2–3 years	4–6 years
Hepatitis B[1]	HepB	HepB		*see footnote 1*			HepB			HepB Series	
Rotavirus[2]			Rota	Rota	Rota						
Diphtheria, Tetanus, Pertussis[3]			DTaP	DTaP	DTaP		DTaP				DTaP
Haemophilus influenzae type b[4]			Hib	Hib	*Hib*[4]	Hib			Hib		
Pneumococcal[5]			PCV	PCV	PCV	PCV				PCV PPV	
Inactivated Poliovirus			IPV	IPV			IPV				IPV
Influenza[6]								Influenza (Yearly)			
Measles, Mumps, Rubella[7]						MMR					MMR
Varicella[8]						Varicella					Varicella
Hepatitis A[9]							HepA (2 doses)			HepA Series	
Meningococcal[10]										MPSV4	

Range of recommended ages | Catch-up immunization | Certain high-risk groups

FIGURE 3-1

These schedules indicate the recommended ages for routine administration of currently licensed childhood vaccines, as of December 1, 2006, for children aged 0–6 and 7–18 years. For updates see *http://www.cdc.gov/mmwr/preview/mmwrhtml/mm5751a5.htm?s_cid=mm5751a5_*. Any dose not administered at the recommended age should be administered at any subsequent visit, when indicated and feasible. Additional vaccines may be licensed and recommended during the year. Licensed combination vaccines may be used whenever any components of the combination are indicated and other components of the vaccine are not contraindicated and if approved by the Food and Drug Administration for that dose of the series. Providers should consult the respective Advisory Committee on Immunization Practices statement for detailed recommendations. Clinically significant adverse events that follow immunization should be reported to the Vaccine Adverse Event Reporting System (VAERS). Guidance about how to obtain and complete a VAERS form is available at *http://www.vaers.hhs.gov* or by telephone, 800-822-7967.

A. Recommended immunization schedule for persons aged 0–6 years—United States, 2006–2007. **1. Hepatitis B vaccine (HepB).** *(Minimum age: birth)* **At birth:** Administer monovalent HepB to all newborns before hospital discharge. If mother is hepatitis surface antigen (HBsAg)–positive, administer HepB and 0.5 mL of hepatitis B immune globulin (HBIG) within 12 hours of birth. If mother's HBsAg status is unknown, administer HepB within 12 hours of birth. Determine the HBsAg status as soon as possible and if HBsAg-positive, administer HBIG (no later than age 1 week). If mother is HBsAg-negative, the birth dose can only be delayed with physician's order and mother's negative HBsAg laboratory report documented in the infant's medical record. **After the birth dose:** The HepB series should be completed with either monovalent HepB or a combination vaccine containing HepB. The second dose should be administered at age 1–2 months. The final dose should be administered at age ≥24 weeks. Infants born to HBsAg-positive mothers should be tested for HBsAg and antibody to HBsAg after completion of ≥3 doses of a licensed HepB series, at age 9–18 months (generally at the next well-child visit). **4-month dose:** It is permissible to administer 4 doses of HepB when combination vaccines are administered after the birth dose. If monovalent HepB is used for doses after the birth dose, a dose at age 4 months is not needed. **2. Rotavirus vaccine (Rota).** *(Minimum age: 6 weeks)* Administer the first dose at age 6–12 weeks. Do not start the series later than age 12 weeks. Administer the final dose in the series by age 32 weeks. Do not administer a dose later than age 32 weeks. Data on safety and efficacy outside of these age ranges are insufficient. **3. Diphtheria and tetanus toxoids and acellular pertussis vaccine (DTaP).** *(Minimum age: 6 weeks)* The fourth dose of DTaP may be administered as early as age 12 months, provided 6 months have elapsed since the third dose. Administer the final dose in the series at age 4–6 years. **4. *Haemophilus influenzae* type b conjugate vaccine (Hib).** *(Minimum age: 6 weeks)* If PRP-OMP (PedvaxHIB or ComVax [Merck]) is administered at ages 2 and 4 months, a dose at age 6 months is not required. TriHiBit (DTaP/Hib) combination products should not be used for primary immunization but can be used as boosters after any Hib vaccine in children aged ≥12 months. **5. Pneumococcal vaccine.** *(Minimum age: 6 weeks for pneumococcal conjugate vaccine*

(Continued)

Recommended Immunization Schedule for Persons Aged 7–18 Years
UNITED STATES • 2007

Vaccine ▼ / Age ▶	7–10 years	11–12 YEARS	13–14 years	15 years	16–18 years
Tetanus, Diphtheria, Pertussis [1]	see footnote 1	Tdap		Tdap	
Human Papillomavirus [2]	see footnote 2	HPV (3 doses)		HPV Series	
Meningococcal [3]	MPSV4	MCV4		MCV4 [3] MCV4	
Pneumococcal [4]		PPV			
Influenza [5]		Influenza (Yearly)			
Hepatitis A [6]		HepA Series			
Hepatitis B [7]		HepB Series			
Inactivated Poliovirus [8]		IPV Series			
Measles, Mumps, Rubella [9]		MMR Series			
Varicella [10]		Varicella Series			

B

Range of recommended ages — Catch-up immunization — Certain high-risk groups

FIGURE 3-1 (*CONTINUED*)

[PCV]; 2 years for pneumococcal polysaccharide vaccine [PPV]). Administer PCV at ages 24–59 months in certain high-risk groups. Administer PPV to children aged ≥2 years in certain high-risk groups. See MMWR 2000;49(No. RR-9):1–35. **6. Influenza vaccine.** *(Minimum age: 6 months for trivalent inactivated influenza vaccine [TIV]; 5 years for live, attenuated influenza vaccine [LAIV]).* All children aged 6–59 months and close contacts of all children aged 0–59 months are recommended to receive influenza vaccine. Influenza vaccine is recommended annually for children aged ≥59 months with certain risk factors, health care workers, and other persons (including household members) in close contact with persons in groups at high risk. See MMWR 2006;55(No. RR-10):1–41. For healthy persons aged 5–49 years, LAIV may be used as an alternative to TIV. Children receiving TIV should receive 0.25 mL if aged 6–35 months or 0.5 mL if aged ≥3 years. Children aged <9 years who are receiving influenza vaccine for the first time should receive 2 doses (separated by ≥4 weeks for TIV and ≥6 weeks for LAIV). **7. Measles, mumps, and rubella vaccine (MMR).** *(Minimum age: 12 months)* Administer the second dose of MMR at age 4–6 years. MMR may be administered before age 4–6 years, provided ≥4 weeks have elapsed since the first dose and both doses are administered at age ≥12 months. **8. Varicella vaccine.** *(Minimum age: 12 months)* Administer the second dose of varicella vaccine at age 4–6 years. Varicella vaccine may be administered before age 4–6 years, provided that ≥3 months have elapsed since the first dose and both doses are administered at age ≥12 months. If second dose was administered ≥28 days after the first dose, the second dose does not need to be repeated. **9. Hepatitis A vaccine (HepA).** *(Minimum age: 12 months)* HepA is recommended for all children aged 1 year (i.e., aged 12–23 months). The 2 doses in the series should be administered at least 6 months apart. Children not fully vaccinated by age 2 years can be vaccinated at subsequent visits. HepA is recommended for certain other groups of children, including in areas where vaccination programs target older children. See MMWR 2006;55(No. RR-7):1–23. **10. Meningococcal polysaccharide vaccine (MPSV4).** *(Minimum age: 2 years)* Administer MPSV4 to children aged 2–10 years with terminal complement deficiencies or anatomic or functional asplenia and certain other high-risk groups. See MMWR 2005;54(No. RR-7):1–21.

B. Recommended immunization schedule for persons aged 7–18 years—United States, 2006–2007. **1. Tetanus and diphtheria toxoids and acellular pertussis vaccine (Tdap).** *(Minimum age: 10 years for BOOSTRIX and 11 years for ADACEL)* Administer at age 11–12 years for those who have completed the recommended childhood DTP/DTaP vaccination series and have not received a tetanus and diphtheria toxoids vaccine (Td) booster dose. Adolescents aged 13–18 years who missed the 11–12 year Td/Tdap booster dose should also receive a single dose of Tdap if they have completed the recommended childhood DTP/DTaP vaccination series. **2. Human papillomavirus vaccine (HPV).** *(Minimum age: 9 years)* Administer the first dose of the HPV vaccine series to females at age 11–12 years. Administer the second dose 2 months after the first dose and the third dose 6 months after the first dose. Administer the HPV vaccine series to females at age 13–18 years if not previously vaccinated. **3. Meningococcal vaccine.** *(Minimum age: 11 years for meningococcalconjugate vaccine [MCV4]; 2 years for meningococcal polysaccharide vaccine [MPSV4]).* Administer MCV4 at age 11–12 years and to previously unvaccinated adolescents at high school entry (at approximately age 15 years). Administer MCV4 to previously

(Continued)

FIGURE 3-1 (*CONTINUED*)
unvaccinated college freshmen living in dormitories; MPSV4 is an acceptable alternative. Vaccination against invasive meningococcal disease is recommended for children and adolescents aged ≥2 years with terminal complement deficiencies or anatomic or functional asplenia and certain other high-risk groups. See MMWR 2005;54(No. RR-7):1–21. Use MPSV4 for children aged 2–10 years and MCV4 or MPSV4 for older children. **4. Pneumococcal polysaccharide vaccine (PPV).** *(Minimum age: 2 years)* Administer for certain high-risk groups. See MMWR 1997;46(No. RR-8):1–24, and MMWR 2000;49(No. RR-9):1–35. **5. Influenza vaccine.** *(Minimum age: 6 months for trivalent inactivated influenza vaccine [TIV]; 5 years for live, attenuated influenza vaccine [LAIV]).* Influenza vaccine is recommended annually for persons with certain risk factors, health care workers, and other persons (including household members) in close contact with persons in groups at high risk. See MMWR 2006;55 (No. RR–10):1–41. For healthy persons aged 5–49 years, LAIV may be used as an alternative to TIV. Children aged <9 years who are receiving influenza vaccine for the first time should receive 2 doses (separated by ≥4 weeks for TIV and ≥6 weeks for LAIV). **6. Hepatitis A vaccine (HepA).** *(Minimum age: 12 months)* The 2 doses in the series should be administered at least 6 months apart. HepA is recommended for certain other groups of children, including in areas where vaccination programs target older children. See MMWR 2006;55 (No. RR-7):1–23. **7. Hepatitis B vaccine (HepB).** *(Minimum age: birth)* Administer the 3-dose series to those who were not previously vaccinated. A 2-dose series of Recombivax HB is licensed for children aged 11–15 years. **8. Inactivated poliovirus vaccine (IPV).** *(Minimum age: 6 weeks)* For children who received an all-IPV or all-oral poliovirus (OPV) series, a fourth dose is not necessary if the third dose was administered at age ≥4 years. If both OPV and IPV were administered as part of a series, a total of 4 doses should be administered, regardless of the child's current age. **9. Measles, mumps, and rubella vaccine (MMR).** *(Minimum age: 12 months)* If not previously vaccinated, administer 2 doses of MMR during any visit, with ≥4 weeks between the doses. **10. Varicella vaccine.** *(Minimum age: 12 months)* Administer 2 doses of varicella vaccine to persons without evidence of immunity. Administer 2 doses of varicella vaccine to persons aged <13 years at least 3 months apart. Do not repeat the second dose if administered ≥28 days after the first dose. Administer 2 doses of varicella vaccine to persons aged ≥13 years at least 4 weeks apart.

are used in special situations, including responses to outbreaks (e.g., polio), prophylaxis in travelers (e.g., yellow fever), and fulfillment of regional requirements (e.g., Japanese B encephalitis). Of course, for many serious infectious agents, such as eukaryotic pathogens (protozoa and helminths) and HIV, effective and safe vaccines remain only a hope for the future. Current concern about the potential for a human pandemic of H5N1 avian influenza, against which a vaccine product is lacking, underscores the lag time between emerging public health needs and vaccine development programs.

The U.S. government's document *Healthy People 2010 Objectives for the Nation* includes a set of immunization indicators. The goals are for 80% of children to receive diphtheria–tetanus–acellular pertussis (DTaP), poliovirus, measles-mumps-rubella (MMR), *H. influenzae* type b (Hib), and hepatitis B vaccines and for 90% of adults to receive influenza and pneumococcal vaccines by 2010. Unfortunately, even these modest goals may not be attained in the United States.

IMPACT OF IMMUNIZATION

The epidemiologically appropriate use of vaccine resulted in the global eradication of smallpox, permitting the cessation of routine smallpox vaccination. Unfortunately, recent concerns about the potential use of smallpox virus for bioterrorism have led to renewed consideration of the need for routine smallpox immunization and for a new, effective, and much safer smallpox vaccine. Immunization has eliminated naturally transmitted polio-myelitis from the Western Hemisphere, Europe, and the western Pacific. However, polio has recrudesced in some countries in Africa, the Middle East, and parts of Asia because of interruption (for a variety of reasons) of immunization programs. Measles, which affected nearly 100% of children in the prevaccination era, has been effectively eliminated from most of the Western Hemisphere by widespread immunization; a global campaign to reduce measles mortality rates elsewhere is underway. The virtual elimination of rubella and congenital rubella syndrome, neonatal tetanus, and diphtheria in the United States is entirely due to vaccination. The introduction of Hib conjugate vaccines for immunization of infants has all but eliminated invasive Hib infections (including meningitis and pneumonia) among children <5 years of age. This vaccine both elicits durable immunity by the time maternal-derived antibodies dissipate and reduces nasopharyngeal carriage of Hib, thus diminishing the risk of transmission. The introduction of polyvalent pneumococcal polysaccharide conjugate vaccine is beginning to have a significant impact on serious invasive pneumococcal diseases, including otitis media. Vaccine has reduced the incidence of varicella by 70–87% in high-coverage areas. In short, vaccines work.

DEFINITIONS

The terms *vaccination* and *immunization* are often used interchangeably, although technically the former denotes the administration of a vaccine, whereas the latter refers to the induction or provision of immunity by any means, active or passive. Thus vaccination does not guarantee immunization, and immunization may not involve vaccine.

Recommended Adult Immunization Schedule
United States, October 2006–September 2007
Recommended adult immunization schedule, by vaccine and age group

Vaccine ▼ / Age group (yrs) ▶	19–49 years	50–64 years	≥65 years
Tetanus, diphtheria, pertussis (Td/Tdap)[1]*	1-dose Td booster every 10 yrs; Substitute 1 dose of Tdap for Td	1-dose Td booster every 10 yrs; Substitute 1 dose of Tdap for Td	1-dose Td booster every 10 yrs
Human papillomavirus (HPV)[2]*	3 doses (females)		
Measles, mumps, rubella (MMR)[3]*	1 or 2 doses	1 dose	1 dose
Varicella[4]*	2 doses (0, 4–8 wks)	2 doses (0, 4–8 wks)	
Influenza[5]*	1 dose annually	1 dose annually	1 dose annually
Pneumococcal (polysaccharide)[6,7]	1–2 doses	1–2 doses	1 dose
Hepatitis A[8]*	2 doses (0, 6–12 mos, or 0, 6–18 mos)	2 doses (0, 6–12 mos, or 0, 6–18 mos)	2 doses (0, 6–12 mos, or 0, 6–18 mos)
Hepatitis B[9]*	3 doses (0, 1–2, 4–6 mos)	3 doses (0, 1–2, 4–6 mos)	3 doses (0, 1–2, 4–6 mos)
Meningococcal[10]	1 or more doses	1 or more doses	1 or more doses

For all persons in this category who meet the age requirements and who lack evidence of immunity (e.g., lack documentation of vaccination or have no evidence of prior infection)

Recommended if some other risk factor is present (e.g., on the basis of medical, occupational, lifestyle, or other indications)

FIGURE 3-2

Recommended adult immunization schedule, by vaccine and age group—United States, 2006–2007. This schedule indicates the recommended age groups for routine administration of currently licensed vaccines for persons aged ≥19 years, as of October 1, 2006. For updates see *http://www.cdc.gov/mmwr/preview/mmwrhtml/mm5753a6.htm*. Licensed combination vaccines may be used whenever any components of the combination are indicated and when the vaccine's other components are not contraindicated. For detailed recommendations on all vaccines, including those used primarily for travelers or that are issued during the year, consult the manufacturers' package inserts and the complete statements from the Advisory Committee on Immunization Practices (*http://www.cdc.gov/nip/publications/acip-list.htm*). Report all clinically significant postvaccination reactions to the Vaccine Adverse Event Reporting System (VAERS). *Reporting forms and instructions on filing a VAERs report are available at *http://vaers.hhs.gov* or by telephone, 800-822-7967. Information on how to file a Vaccine Injury Compensation Program claim is available at *http://www.hrsa.gov/vaccinecompensation* or by telephone, 800-338-2382. To file a claim for vaccine injury, contact the U.S. Court of Federal Claims, 717 Madison Place, N.W., Washington, DC, 20005; telephone, 202-357-6400. Additional information about the vaccines in this schedule and contraindications for vaccination is also available at *http://www.cdc.gov/nip* or from the CDC-INFO Contact Center at 800-CDC-INFO (800-232-4636) in English and Spanish, 24 hours a day, 7 days a week. **1. Tetanus, diphtheria, and acellular pertussis (Td/Tdap) vaccination.** Adults with uncertain histories of a complete primary vaccination series with diphtheria and tetanus toxoid-containing vaccines should begin or complete a primary vaccination series. A primary series for adults is 3 doses; administer the first 2 doses at least 4 weeks apart and the third dose 6–12 months after the second. Administer a booster dose to adults who have completed a primary series and if the last vaccination was received ≥10 years previously. Tdap or tetanus and diphtheria (Td) vaccine may be used; Tdap should replace a single dose of Td for adults aged <65 years who have not previously received a dose of Tdap (either in the primary series, as a booster, or for wound management). Only one of two Tdap products (Adacel [sanofi pasteur]) is licensed for use in adults. If the person is pregnant and received the last Td vaccination ≥10 years previously, administer Td during the second or third trimester; if the person received the last Td vaccination in <10 years, administer Tdap during the immediate postpartum period. A one-time administration of 1 dose of Tdap with an interval as short as 2 years from a previous Td vaccination is recommended for postpartum women, close contacts of infants aged <12 months, and all health care workers with direct patient contact. In certain situations, Td can be deferred during pregnancy and Tdap substituted in the immediate postpartum period, or Tdap can be given instead of Td to a pregnant woman after an informed discussion with the woman (see *www.cdc.gov/nip/publications/acip-list.htm*). Consult the ACIP statement for recommendations for administering Td asprophylaxis in wound management (*www.cdc.gov/mmwr/preview/mmwrhtml/00041645.htm*).

(*Continued*)

FIGURE 3-2 (*CONTINUED*)

2. Human papillomavirus (HPV) vaccination. HPV vaccination is recommended for all women aged ≤26 years who have not completed the vaccine series. Ideally, vaccine should be administered before potential exposure to HPV through sexual activity; however, women who are sexually active should still be vaccinated. Sexually active women who have not been infected with any of the HPV vaccine types receive the full benefit of the vaccination. Vaccination is less beneficial for women who have already been infected with one or more of the four HPV vaccine types. A complete series consists of 3 doses. The second dose should be administered 2 months after the first dose; the third dose should be administered 6 months after the first dose. Vaccination is not recommended during pregnancy. If a woman is found to be pregnant after initiating the vaccination series, the remainder of the 3-dose regimen should be delayed until after completion of the pregnancy. **3. Measles, mumps, rubella (MMR) vaccination.** *Measles component:* adults born before 1957 can be considered immune to measles. Adults born during or after 1957 should receive ≥1 dose of MMR unless they have a medical contraindication, documentation of ≥1 dose, history of measles based on health care provider diagnosis, or laboratory evidence of immunity. A second dose of MMR is recommended for adults who (1) have been recently exposed to measles or in an outbreak setting; (2) have been previously vaccinated with killed measles vaccine; (3) have been vaccinated with an unknown type of measles vaccine during 1963–1967; (4) are students in postsecondary educational institutions; (5) work in a healthcare facility; or (6) plan to travel internationally. Withhold MMR or other measles-containing vaccines from HIV-infected persons with severe immunosuppression. *Mumps component:* adults born before 1957 can generally be considered immune to mumps. Adults born during or after 1957 should receive 1 dose of MMR unless they have a medical contraindication, history of mumps based on health care provider diagnosis, or laboratory evidence of immunity. A second dose of MMR is recommended for adults who (1) are in an age group that is affected during a mumps outbreak; (2) are students in postsecondary educational institutions; (3) work in a health care facility; or (4) plan to travel internationally. For unvaccinated health care workers born before 1957 who do not have other evidence of mumps immunity, consider giving 1 dose on a routine basis and strongly consider giving a second dose during an outbreak. *Rubella component:* administer 1 dose of MMR vaccine to women whose rubella vaccination history is unreliable or who lack laboratory evidence of immunity. For women of childbearing age, regardless of birth year, routinely determine rubella immunity and counsel women regarding congenital rubella syndrome. Do not vaccinate women who are pregnant or who might become pregnant within 4 weeks of receiving vaccine. Women who do not have evidence of immunity should receive MMR vaccine upon completion or termination of pregnancy and before discharge from the health care facility. **4. Varicella vaccination.** All adults without evidence of immunity to varicella should receive 2 doses of varicella vaccine. Special consideration should be given to those who (1) have close contact with persons at high risk for severe disease (e.g., health care workers and family contacts of immunocompromised persons) or (2) are at high risk for exposure or transmission (e.g., teachers of young children; child care employees; residents and staff members of institutional settings, including correctional institutions; college students; military personnel; adolescents and adults living in households with children; nonpregnant women of childbearing age; and international travelers). Evidence of immunity to varicella in adults includes any of the following: (1) documentation of 2 doses of varicella vaccine at least 4 weeks apart; (2) U.S. born before 1980 (although for health care workers and pregnant women, birth before 1980 should not be considered evidence of immunity); (3) history of varicella based on diagnosis or verification of varicella by a health care provider (for a patient reporting a history of or presenting with an atypical case, a mild case, or both, health care providers should seek either an epidemiologic link with a typical varicella case or evidence of laboratory confirmation, if it was performed at the time of acute disease); (4) history of herpes zoster based on health care provider diagnosis; or (5) laboratory evidence of immunity or laboratory confirmation of disease. Do not vaccinate women who are pregnant or might become pregnant within 4 weeks of receiving the vaccine. Assess pregnant women for evidence of varicella immunity. Women who do not have evidence of immunity should receive dose 1 of varicella vaccine upon completion or termination of pregnancy and before discharge from the health care facility. Dose 2 should be administered 4–8 weeks after dose 1. **5. Influenza vaccination.** *Medical indications:* chronic disorders of the cardiovascular or pulmonary systems, including asthma; chronic metabolic diseases, including diabetes mellitus, renal dysfunction, hemoglobinopathies, or immunosuppression (including immunosuppression caused by medications or HIV); any condition that compromises respiratory function or the handling of respiratory secretions or that can increase the risk of aspiration (e.g., cognitive dysfunction, spinal cord injury, or seizure disorder or other neuromuscular disorder); and pregnancy during the influenza season. No data exist on the risk for severe or complicated influenza disease among persons with asplenia; however, influenza is a risk factor for secondary bacterial infections that can cause severe disease among persons with asplenia. *Occupational indications:* health care workers and employees of long-term–care and assisted living facilities. *Other indications:* residents of nursing homes and other long-term–care and assisted living facilities; persons likely to transmit influenza to persons at high risk (e.g., in-home household contacts and caregivers of children aged 0–59 months, or persons of all ages with high-risk conditions); and anyone who would like to be vaccinated. Healthy, nonpregnant persons aged 5–49 years without high-risk medical conditions who are not contacts of severely immunocompromised persons in special care units can receive either intranasally administered influenza vaccine (FluMist) or inactivated vaccine. Other persons should receive the inactivated vaccine. **6. Pneumococcal polysaccharide vaccination.** *Medical indications:* chronic disorders of the pulmonary system (excluding asthma); cardiovascular

(*Continued*)

FIGURE 3-2 (*CONTINUED*)

diseases; diabetes mellitus; chronic liver diseases, including liver disease as a result of alcohol abuse (e.g., cirrhosis); chronic renal failure or nephrotic syndrome; functional or anatomic asplenia (e.g., sickle cell disease or splenectomy [if elective splenectomy is planned, vaccinate at least 2 weeks before surgery]); immunosuppressive conditions (e.g., congenital immunodeficiency, HIV infection (vaccinate as close to diagnosis as possible when CD4 cell counts are highest), leukemia, lymphoma, multiple myeloma, Hodgkin's disease, generalized malignancy, or organ or bone marrow transplantation); chemotherapy with alkylating agents, antimetabolites, or high-dose, long-term corticosteroids; and cochlear implants. *Other indications:* Alaska Natives and certain American Indian populations and residents of nursing homes or other long-term-care facilities. **7. Revaccination with pneumococcal polysaccharide vaccine.** One-time revaccination after 5 years for persons with chronic renal failure or nephrotic syndrome; functional or anatomic asplenia (e.g., sickle cell disease or splenectomy); immunosuppressive conditions (e.g., congenital immunodeficiency, HIV infection, leukemia, lymphoma, multiple myeloma, Hodgkin's disease, generalized malignancy, or organ or bone marrow transplantation); or chemotherapy with alkylating agents, antimetabolites, or high-dose, long-term corticosteroids. For persons aged ≥65 years, one-time revaccination if they were vaccinated ≥5 years previously and were aged <65 years at the time of primary vaccination. **8. Hepatitis A vaccination.** *Medical indications:* persons with chronic liver disease and persons who receive clotting factor concentrates. *Behavioral indications:* men who have sex with men and persons who use illegal drugs. *Occupational indications:* persons working with hepatitis A virus (HAV)-infected primates or with HAV in a research laboratory setting. *Other indications:* persons traveling to or working in countries that have high or intermediate endemicity of hepatitis A (a list of countries is available at *www.cdc.gov/travel/diseases.htm*) and any person who would like to obtain immunity. Current vaccines should be administered in a 2-dose schedule at either 0 and 6–12 months, or 0 and 6–18 months. If the combined hepatitis A and hepatitis B vaccine is used, administer 3 doses at 0, 1, and 6 months. **9. Hepatitis B vaccination.** *Medical indications:* persons with end-stage renal disease, including patients receiving hemodialysis; persons seeking evaluation or treatment for a sexually transmitted disease (STD); persons with HIV infection; persons with chronic liver disease; and persons who receive clotting factor concentrates. *Occupational indications:* health care workers and public safety workers who are exposed to blood or other potentially infectious body fluids. *Behavioral indications:* sexually active persons who are not in a long-term, mutually monogamous relationship (i.e., persons with >1 sex partner during the previous 6 months); current or recent injection-drug users; and men who have sex with men. *Other indications:* household contacts and sex partners of persons with chronic hepatitis B virus (HBV) infection; clients and staff members of institutions for persons with developmental disabilities; all clients of STD clinics; international travelers to countries with high or intermediate prevalence of chronic HBV infection (a list of countries is available at *www.cdc.gov/travel/ diseases.htm*); and any adult seeking protection from HBV infection. Settings where hepatitis B vaccination is recommended for all adults: STD treatment facilities; HIV testing and treatment facilities; facilities providing drug-abuse treatment and prevention services; health care settings providing services for injection drug users or men who have sex with men; correctional facilities; end-stage renal disease programs and facilities for chronic hemodialysis patients; and institutions and nonresidential daycare facilities for persons with developmental disabilities. *Special formulation indications:* for adult patients receiving hemodialysis and other immunocompromised adults, 1 dose of 40 μg/mL (Recombivax HB) or 2 doses of 20 μg/mL (Engerix-B). **10. Meningococcal vaccination.** *Medical indications:* adults with anatomic or functional asplenia, or terminal complement component deficiencies. *Other indications:* first-year college students living in dormitories; microbiologists who are routinely exposed to isolates of *Neisseria meningitidis*; military recruits; and persons who travel to or live in countries in which meningococcal disease is hyperendemic or epidemic (e.g., the "meningitis belt" of sub-Saharan Africa during the dry season [December–June]), particularly if their contact with local populations will be prolonged. Vaccination is required by the government of Saudi Arabia for all travelers to Mecca during the annual Hajj. Meningococcal conjugate vaccine is preferred for adults with any of the preceding indications who are aged ≤55 years, although meningococcal polysaccharide vaccine (MPSV4) is an acceptable alternative. Revaccination after 5 years might be indicated for adults previously vaccinated with MPSV4 who remain at high risk for infection (e.g., persons residing in areas in which disease is epidemic).

PRINCIPLES OF IMMUNIZATION

The immune system, composed of a variety of cell types and soluble factors, is geared toward the recognition of and response to "foreign" substances termed *antigens*. Vaccines convey antigens from living or killed microorganisms (or protein or carbohydrate molecules derived from these antigens) to elicit immune responses that are generally protective but can occasionally backfire and cause harm to the recipient. Specific immune responses, which interrupt the infectious process, generally take the form of immunoglobulin proteins called *antibodies* and/or activated immune cells that recognize particular antigens from an infectious agent. Immunity is medically induced by active or passive immunization. *Active immunization*—i.e., the administration of a vaccine—induces immunity that is usually long-lasting and is sometimes life-long. In contrast, *passive immunization*—i.e., the administration of exogenously produced immune substances or of protective products made in animals—elicits temporary immunity that dissipates with the turnover of the administered protective substances. Used together, the two methods can produce a complementary effect; this is the case, for example, with the coadministration of hepatitis B vaccine and hepatitis B immune globulin. Caution is required, however: the combination of active and passive immunization can also interfere with the development of immunity—e.g., when measles vaccine is administered within 6 weeks of measles immunoglobulin.

When multiple species or serotypes of an organism exist and share common, cross-reactive antigens, vaccination may induce broad immunity to all or most of the related forms or may result in serotype-specific immunity against the immunizing strain alone. One of the virtues of whole-organism vaccines is their potential to contain all the protective antigens of the organism. This advantage is balanced by the possibility of adverse responses to reactive but nonprotective antigens present in the mix. Because the immune response is genetically controlled, all individuals cannot be expected to respond identically to the same vaccine. Additional vaccine constituents affect immunogenicity, efficacy, and safety and may render one formulation superior to another formulation of the same antigens (see "Adjuvants" later in the chapter).

Approaches to Active Immunization

The two standard approaches to active immunization are (1) the use of live, generally attenuated infectious agents (e.g., measles virus); and (2) the use of inactivated agents (e.g., influenza virus), their constituents (e.g., *Bordetella pertussis*), or their products, which are now commonly obtainable through genetic engineering (e.g., hepatitis B vaccine). For many diseases (e.g., poliomyelitis), both live and inactivated vaccines have been employed, each offering advantages and disadvantages.

Live attenuated vaccines consisting of selected or genetically altered organisms that are avirulent or dramatically attenuated, yet remain immunogenic, typically generate long-lasting immunity. These vaccines are designed to cause a subclinical or mild illness and an immune response that mimics natural infection. They offer the advantage of microbial replication in vivo, which simulates natural infection; they may confer life-long protection with one dose; they can present all potential antigens, including those made only in vivo, thus overcoming immunogenetic restrictions in some hosts; and they can reach the local sites most relevant to the induction of protective immunity.

Nonliving vaccines typically require multiple doses and periodic boosters for the maintenance of immunity. The exceptions to this rule are the pure polysaccharide vaccines, whose effects cannot be boosted by additional exposures because polysaccharides do not elicit immunologic memory. Nonliving vaccines administered parenterally fail to induce mucosal immunity because they lack a delivery system that can effectively transport them to local mucosal antigen-processing cells. Nonetheless, nonliving parenteral vaccines can be extremely efficacious. For example, hepatitis A vaccine appears to be effective in nearly 100% of recipients. Currently available nonliving vaccines consist of inactivated whole organisms (e.g., plague vaccine), detoxified protein exotoxins (e.g., tetanus toxoid), recombinant protein antigens (e.g., hepatitis B vaccine), or carbohydrate antigens—either soluble purified capsular material (e.g., serotype-specific *Streptococcus pneumoniae* polysaccharides) or polysaccharide conjugated to a protein carrier to induce a memory response (e.g., Hib polysaccharide conjugated to a suitable protein moiety).

Despite their many advantages, live vaccines are not always preferable. For example, after several decades of extensive use, live oral polio vaccine (OPV) is no longer recommended in the United States because of the rare but real risk of vaccine-associated polio due to reversion to virulence. However, the WHO continues to recommend OPV for use in the developing world because of lower costs and logistical advantages.

Approaches to Passive Immunization

Passive immunization is generally used to provide temporary immunity in a person exposed to an infectious disease who has not been actively immunized; this situation can arise when active immunization is unavailable (e.g., for respiratory syncytial virus) or when active immunization simply has not been implemented before exposure (e.g., for rabies). Passive immunization is used in the treatment of certain illnesses associated with toxins (e.g., diphtheria), as well as for some snake and spider bites, and as a specific or nonspecific immunosuppressant [Rho(D) immune globulin and antilymphocyte globulin, respectively]. Three types of preparations can be used in passive immunization: (1) standard human immune serum globulin for IM or IV administration; (2) special immune serum globulins with a known content of antibody to specific agents (e.g., hepatitis B virus or varicella-zoster immune globulin); and (3) specific animal antisera and antitoxins.

Postexposure Immunization

For certain infections, active or passive immunization soon after exposure can prevent or attenuate disease expression. Recommended postexposure immunization regimens are shown in Table 3-1. For example, giving either measles immune globulin within 6 days of exposure or measles vaccine within the first few days after exposure may prevent symptomatic infection. Nonimmune pregnant women exposed to rubella can minimize clinical illness by postexposure passive immunization; however, this measure may fail to prevent viremia and infection of the fetus and thus may be followed by the congenital rubella syndrome. Proper immunization for tetanus plays an important role in dirty-wound management. The need for active immunization—with or without passive immunization—depends on the wound's condition and the patient's immunization history. Tetanus is rare among persons with documented receipt of a primary series of tetanus toxoid doses. Tetanus immune globulin is helpful in patients with clinical tetanus, but survivors must be actively immunized since the disease does not stimulate protective levels of antitoxin antibody. Administration of rabies immune globulin plus rabies vaccine in the immediate postexposure period is highly effective in preventing disease. Similarly, for persons who have not been actively immunized, administration of hepatitis A immune globulin within 2 weeks of exposure to hepatitis A virus is likely to prevent clinical illness. Evidence also supports the

TABLE 3-1

RECOMMENDED POSTEXPOSURE IMMUNIZATION WITH IMMUNOGLOBULIN PREPARATIONS IN THE UNITED STATES

DISEASE	INDICATED	COMMENTS
Measles	Yes	Standard human immune globulin is recommended for exposed infants and adults with normal immunocompetence (but with a contraindication to measles vaccine) and for immunocompromised patients exposed to measles (regardless of immunization status). Patients should be actively immunized 3–6 months after immunoglobulin administration. Recommended dose: 0.25–0.50 mL/kg (40–80 mg of IgG/kg) IM; 80 mg of IgG/kg for immunocompromised contact; maximum, 15 mL.
Rubella	No	Efficacy is unreliable; therefore, standard human immune globulin is recommended for administration only to antibody-negative pregnant women in the first trimester who have a documented rubella exposure and will not consider terminating the pregnancy. Recommended dose is 0.55 mL/kg (90 mg of IgG/kg) IM.
Tetanus	Yes	Human tetanus immune globulin (TIG) has replaced equine tetanus antitoxin because of the risk of serum sickness with equine serum. Recommended dose for postexposure prophylaxis is 250–500 units of TIG (10–20 mg of IgG/kg) IM. Recommended dose for treatment of tetanus is 3000–6000 units of TIG IM.
Rabies	Yes	Human rabies immune globulin (RIG) is preferred over equine rabies antiserum because of the risk of serum sickness with equine serum. RIG or antiserum is recommended for nonimmunized individuals with animal bites in whom rabies cannot be ruled out and with other exposures to known rabid animals. Recommended dose of RIG is 20 IU/kg (22 mg of IgG/kg). Recommended dose of antiserum is 40 IU/kg. Rabies vaccine is given as well at 0, 3, 7, 14, and 28 days.
Hepatitis A	Yes	Standard immune serum globulin is given in a single dose of 0.02–0.04 mL/kg or (for continuous exposure) in a dose up to 0.06 mL/kg every 5 months. Postexposure treatment with hepatitis A immune globulin has not been studied.
Varicella	Yes	VariZIG, a new Canadian purified human immune globulin containing high-titer IgG antibody to varicella-zoster virus, is intended for patients without evidence of immunity to varicella who are exposed to infection and who are at high risk for severe disease and complications. It is not currently licensed in the United States but instead has investigational new drug status. VariZIG may be obtained under expanded-access provisions for patients who meet the enrollment criteria and choose to participate. Maximal benefit requires administration within 96 h of exposure. The recommended dose is 125 units/10 kg of body weight, up to a maximum of 625 units.

efficacy of human hepatitis B immune globulin in preventing disease after exposure. Although no high-titer preparation is available for postexposure protection against non-A, non-B hepatitis, standard human immune serum globulin is efficacious. VariZIG, a highly purified preparation of human antibody to varicella-zoster virus (VZV), is licensed in Canada for the prevention of varicella in nonimmune pregnant women who are exposed to infected individuals. At the time of this writing, this product is available in the United States from the Centers for Disease Control and Prevention (CDC) under an investigational new drug (IND) protocol or under an expanded-access program through the U.S. Food and Drug Administration.

THE IMMUNE RESPONSE

Although many constituents of infectious microorganisms and their products (e.g., exotoxins) are or can be rendered immunogenic, only some stimulate protective immune responses that can prevent infection and/or clinical illness or (as in the case of rotavirus) can attenuate illness, providing protection against severe disease but not against infection or mild illness. The immune system is complex, and many factors—including antigen composition and presentation, as well as host characteristics—are critical for stimulation of the desired immune responses.

The Primary Response

The primary response to a vaccine antigen includes an apparent latent period of several days before immune responses can be detected. Although the immune system is rapidly activated, it takes 7–10 days for activated B lymphocytes to produce enough antibody to be detected in the circulation. The primarily IgM antibodies seen initially are rapidly produced but have only a low affinity for the antigen. After the first week, high-affinity IgG antibodies begin to be produced in quantity; this switch from IgM to IgG production requires the participation of CD4+ T-helper lymphocytes—the "middle men" of the immune response. Because precursors for T cells mature within the thymus gland, antigens that stimulate T cells are referred to as *T* or *thymus-dependent* antigens. Circulating antigen-specific T lymphocytes that implement cell-mediated immune responses are identified in the peripheral bloodstream only after several days but begin to increase in number immediately after antigenic stimulation.

Activation of these responses typically requires co-recognition of the antigen by specific molecular species of human leukocyte antigen (HLA), the major histocompatibility complex, which is present on the surface of lymphocytes and macrophages. Some individuals cannot respond to one or more antigens, even when repeatedly exposed, because they do not have the genes for the particular HLA type involved in antigen recognition, processing, and presentation for an immune response. This situation is known as *primary vaccine failure*.

The Secondary Response

Stronger and faster humoral or cell-mediated responses are elicited by a second exposure to the same antigen and are detectable within days of the "booster" dose. The secondary response depends on immunologic memory induced by the primary exposure and is characterized by a marked proliferation of IgG antibody–producing B lymphocytes and/or effector T cells. Pure polysaccharide antigens, such as the first-generation pneumococcal vaccine, evoke immune responses that are independent of T cells and are not enhanced by repeated administration. However, conjugation of the same polysaccharide to a suitable protein converts the carbohydrate antigen into one that is T cell–dependent and able to induce immunologic memory and secondary responses to reexposure. Although levels of vaccine-induced antibodies may decline over time, revaccination or infection generally elicits a rapid (anamnestic) protective secondary response consisting of IgG antibodies, with little or no detectable IgM. Thus a lack of measurable antibody in an immunized individual does not necessarily indicate secondary vaccine failure. Similarly, the mere presence of detectable antibodies after immunization does not ensure clinical protection: the level of circulating antibody may need to exceed a threshold value in order to mediate protection (e.g., 0.01 IU/mL for tetanus antitoxin).

Mucosal Immunity

Some pathogens are confined to and replicate only at mucosal surfaces (e.g., *Vibrio cholerae*), whereas others first encounter the host at a mucosal surface before they invade systemically (e.g., influenza virus). A distinctive immunoglobulin, *secretory IgA*, is produced at mucosal surfaces and is adapted to resist degradation and to function at these sites. Vaccines may be specifically designed to induce secretory IgA and thereby to block the essential initial steps in disease pathogenesis that occur on mucosal surfaces. Given its complexity, mucosal immunology has become a separate branch of the field of immunology.

Measurement of the Immune Response

Immune responses to vaccines are often gauged by the concentration of specific antibody in serum. Although seroconversion (i.e., transition from antibody-negative to antibody-positive status) serves as a dependable indicator of an immune response, it does not necessarily correlate with protection unless serum antibody is the critical mechanism in vivo and the levels achieved are sufficient (e.g., against measles). In some instances, serum antibody correlates with clinical protection but does not directly mediate it (e.g., vibriocidal serum antibodies in cholera).

Herd Immunity

Successful vaccination protects immunized individuals from infection, thereby decreasing the percentage of susceptible persons within a population and reducing the possibility of infection transmission to others. At a definable prevalence of immunity, an infectious organism can no longer circulate freely among the remaining susceptibles. This indirect protection of unvaccinated (nonimmune) persons is called the *herd immunity effect*; through this effect, vaccination programs may confer societal benefits that exceed individual costs. The level of vaccine coverage needed to elicit herd immunity depends on the patterns of interaction among individuals within the population and the biology of the specific infectious agent. For example, measles virus and VZV have high transmission rates and require a higher level of vaccine coverage for herd immunity than do organisms with lower transmission rates, such as *S. pneumoniae*. Wherever herd immunity for poliomyelitis and measles has been induced with vaccines, transmission of infection has ceased; however, herd immunity may wane if immunization programs are interrupted (as was the case for diphtheria in the former Soviet Union) or if a sufficient percentage of individuals refuse to be immunized because of a fear of vaccine-related adverse events (as occurred for pertussis in the United Kingdom and Japan). In either setting, the loss of herd immunity has led to renewed circulation of the organism and subsequent large outbreaks with serious consequences.

PRINCIPLES OF VACCINE USE

Route of Administration

Microbes differ in their routes of infection, patterns of transmission, and predispositions for certain age groups. The route of vaccine administration (oral, intranasal, intradermal, transdermal, subcutaneous, or intramuscular) takes these factors into account in order to maximize protection and minimize adverse events. Vaccine development is more a pragmatic undertaking than an exact science, guided only in part by immunologic principles and shaped largely by the results of clinical trials. Although vaccines can theoretically be given by any route, each vaccine has unique characteristics adapted to a particular route and, in practice, must be given by the licensed route, for which optimal immunogenicity and safety have been documented. For example, vaccines containing adjuvants are designed for injection into the muscle mass. Mucosal administration of vaccines designed for parenteral administration may not induce good systemic responses because such vaccines do not induce mucosal secretory IgA. Administration of hepatitis B vaccine into the gluteal rather than the deltoid muscle may fail to induce an adequate immune response, whereas SC rather than IM administration of DTaP vaccine increases the risk of adverse reactions. Injectable biologicals should be administered at sites where the likelihood of local, neural, vascular, or tissue injury is minimized.

Age

Because age influences the response to vaccines, schedules for immunization are based on age-dependent responses determined empirically in clinical trials. The presence of high levels of maternal antibody and/or the immaturity of the immune system in the early months of life impairs the initial immune response to some vaccines (e.g., measles and pneumococcal polysaccharide vaccines), but not to others (e.g., hepatitis B vaccine). In the elderly, vaccine responses may be diminished because of the natural waning of the immune system, and larger amounts of an antigen may be required to produce the desired response (e.g., in vaccination against influenza). In contrast, in some age groups, the use of substandard amounts of antigen is sufficient for immunity induction and reduces the risk of adverse effects (e.g., a reduced dose of diphtheria toxoid for persons ≥7 years of age). Age-related adverse events are discussed in a later section.

Target Populations and Timing of Administration

Disease attack rates differ across the human life span, and the timing of immunization must consider these variations along with the age-specific response to vaccines, the durability of the immune response, and the logistics for optimal identification and vaccination of the groups at risk. Aside from immunologic parameters, many factors are involved, including demographic features; thus vaccination programs are really as much community as individual endeavors. Schedules for immunization are ultimately derived from careful consideration of the many relevant variables and may ultimately depend on the best opportunities to reach the target groups (e.g., infancy, school entry, puberty, college enrollment, military induction, entry into the workplace). Health care workers administering vaccines or caring for patients with vaccine-preventable diseases have a special responsibility to be adequately immunized themselves and to take all necessary precautions to minimize the risk of spreading infection (e.g., hand washing between immunizations or other interactions with patients). Catch-up immunization schedules for infants and children through the age of 18 years have been approved by the CDC (Fig. 3-3).

For common and highly communicable childhood diseases such as measles, the target population is the universe of susceptible individuals, and the time to immunize is as early in life as is feasible and effective. In the industrialized world, immunization with live-virus vaccine at 12–15 months of age has become the norm because the vaccine protects >95% of children immunized at this age and there is little measles morbidity or mortality among infants <1 year of age. In contrast, under crowded conditions in the developing world, measles remains a significant cause of death among young infants. For optimal benefit in this situation, it is necessary to immunize early enough to narrow the window of vulnerability between the rapid decline of maternal antibody 4–6 months after birth and the development of vaccine-induced active immunity; this choice must be made despite the less efficient immune response in children <1 year old.

Invasive infections due to Hib (meningitis, pneumonia, and epiglottitis) occur primarily in young children, with rates rising sharply after the disappearance of maternally derived antibody. First-generation Hib polysaccharide vaccines often failed when administered during infancy because very young children cannot respond to pure polysaccharides. This problem has been overcome by conjugating the capsular polysaccharide with a protein to create a T cell–dependent antigen, to which infants effectively respond.

In contrast, rubella is primarily a threat to the fetus rather than to infants and young children. The ideal strategy would be to immunize all women of reproductive age before they became pregnant. Because it is difficult to ensure this type of coverage, rubella is included in a combination vaccine with measles and mumps (MMR) that is administered during infancy and boosted at the age of 4–6 years. It is recommended that pregnant women be screened for rubella antibodies and that seronegative women be given rubella vaccine after delivery. Similar considerations apply to the use of the vaccine against HPV that was recently approved in the United States and is intended primarily to prevent cervical cancer in women. Accordingly, it is recommended that the vaccine be given at the age of 11–12 years (or as early as 9 years), so that all are immunized before becoming sexually active.

Some vaccines, such as the influenza and polyvalent pneumococcal polysaccharide products, were originally formulated to prevent pneumonia hospitalizations and deaths among the elderly. These products have been consistently underused, in large part because physicians and otherwise-healthy older individuals ignore the recommendations, but also because vaccines continue to be thought of as interventions for infants and children. There is considerable debate about alternative strategies to reduce the burden of these diseases in the elderly by indirectly protecting them through childhood vaccination, which would reduce transmission. The development of new vaccines and the exploitation of new routes of administration may facilitate this approach; examples include the development of pneumococcal conjugate vaccines and the administration of influenza vaccine by the intranasal route, respectively. The pneumococcal conjugate vaccine has made it possible to immunize young infants at risk of pneumococcal pneumonia, meningitis, and otitis media, but whether immunity will persist or will need boosting in adulthood remains to be determined. What is clear is that the number of recommended vaccines and the strategies for their deployment are undergoing constant revision.

Catch-up Immunization Schedule
for Persons Aged 4 Months–18 Years Who Start Late or Who Are More Than One Month Behind

The table below provides catch-up schedules and minimum intervals between doses for children whose vaccinations have been delayed. A vaccine series does not need to be restarted, regardless of the time that has elapsed between doses. Use the section appropriate for the child's age.

Vaccine	Minimum Age for Dose 1	Minimum Interval Between Doses: Dose 1 to Dose 2	Dose 2 to Dose 3	Dose 3 to Dose 4	Dose 4 to Dose 5
CATCH-UP SCHEDULE FOR PERSONS AGED 4 MONTHS–6 YEARS					
Hepatitis B[1]	Birth	4 weeks	8 weeks (and 16 weeks after first dose)		
Rotavirus[2]	6 wks	4 weeks	4 weeks		
Diphtheria, Tetanus, Pertussis[3]	6 wks	4 weeks	4 weeks	6 months	6 months[3]
Haemophilus influenzae type b[4]	6 wks	**4 weeks** if first dose administered at age < 12 months **8 weeks (as final dose)** if first dose administered at age 12-14 months **No further doses needed** if first dose administered at age ≥ 15 months	**4 weeks**[4] if current age < 12 months **8 weeks (as final dose)**[4] if current age ≥ 12 months and second dose administered at age < 15 months **No further doses needed** if previous dose administered at age ≥ 15 months	**8 weeks (as final dose)** This dose only necessary for children aged 12 months–5 years who received 3 doses before age 12 months	
Pneumococcal[5]	6 wks	**4 weeks** if first dose administered at age < 12 months and current age < 24 months **8 weeks (as final dose)** if first dose administered at age ≥ 12 months or current age 24–59 months **No further doses needed** for healthy children if first dose administered at age ≥ 24 months	**4 weeks** if current age < 12 months **8 weeks (as final dose)** if current age ≥ 12 months **No further doses needed** for healthy children if previous dose administered at age ≥ 24 months	**8 weeks (as final dose)** This dose only necessary for children aged 12 months–5 years who received 3 doses before age 12 months	
Inactivated Poliovirus[6]	6 wks	4 weeks	4 weeks	4 weeks[6]	
Measles, Mumps, Rubella[7]	12 mos	4 weeks			
Varicella[8]	12 mos	3 months			
Hepatitis A[9]	12 mos	6 months			
CATCH-UP SCHEDULE FOR PERSONS AGED 7–18 YEARS					
Tetanus, Diphtheria/ Tetanus, Diphtheria, Pertussis[10]	7 yrs[10]	4 weeks	**8 weeks** if first dose administered at age < 12 months **6 months** if first dose administered at age ≥ 12 months	**6 months** if first dose administered at age < 12 months	
Human Papillomavirus[11]	9 yrs	4 weeks	12 weeks		
Hepatitis A[9]	12 mos	6 months			
Hepatitis B[1]	Birth	4 weeks	8 weeks (and 16 weeks after first dose)		
Inactivated Poliovirus[6]	6 wks	4 weeks	4 weeks	4 weeks[6]	
Measles, Mumps, Rubella[7]	12 mos	4 weeks			
Varicella[8]	12 mos	**4 weeks** if first dose administered at age ≥ 13 years **3 months** if first dose administered at age < 13 years			

FIGURE 3-3

Catch-up immunization schedule for persons aged 4 months-18 years who start late or who are more than 1 month behind. 1. Hepatitis B vaccine (HepB). *(Minimum age: birth)* Administer the 3-dose series to those who were not previously vaccinated. A 2-dose series of Recombivax HB is licensed for children aged 11–15 years. **2. Rotavirus vaccine (Rota).** *(Minimum age: 6 weeks)* Do not start the series later than age 12 weeks. Administer the final dose in the series by age 32 weeks. Do not administer a dose later than age 32 weeks. Data on safety and efficacy outside of these age ranges are insufficient. **3. Diphtheria and tetanus toxoids and acellular pertussis vaccine (DTaP).** *(Minimum age: 6 weeks)* The fifth dose is not necessary if the fourth dose was administered at age ≥4 years. DTaP is not indicated for persons aged ≥7 years. **4. *Haemophilus influenzae* type b conjugate vaccine (Hib).** *(Minimum age: 6 weeks)* Vaccine is not generally recommended for children aged ≥5 years. If current age <12 months and the first 2 doses were PRP-OMP (PedvaxHIB or ComVax [Merck]), the third (and final) dose should be administered at age 12–15 months and at least 8 weeks after the second dose. If first dose was administered at age 7–11 months, administer 2 doses separated by 4 weeks plus a booster at age 12–15 months. **5. Pneumococcal conjugate vaccine (PCV).** *(Minimum age: 6 weeks)* Vaccine is not generally recommended for children aged ≥5 years. **6. Inactivated poliovirus vaccine (IPV).** *(Minimum age: 6 weeks)* For children who received an all-IPV or all-oral poliovirus (OPV) series, a fourth dose is not necessary if third dose was administered at age ≥4 years. If both OPV and IPV were administered as part of a series, a total of 4 doses should be administered, regardless of the child's current age. **7. Measles, mumps, and rubella vaccine (MMR).** *(Minimum age: 12 months)* The second dose of MMR is recommended routinely at age 4–6 years but may be administered earlier if desired. If not previously vaccinated, administer 2 doses of MMR during any visit with ≥4 weeks between the doses. **8. Varicella vaccine.** *(Minimum age: 12 months)* The second dose of varicella vaccine is recommended routinely at age 4–6 years but may be administered earlier if desired. Do not repeat the second dose in persons aged <13 years if

(Continued)

FIGURE 3-3 (*CONTINUED*)

administered ≥28 days after the first dose. **9. Hepatitis A vaccine (HepA).** *(Minimum age: 12 months)* HepA is recommended for certain groups of children, including in areas where vaccination programs target older children. See MMWR 2006;55(No. RR-7):1–23. **10. Tetanus and diphtheria toxoids vaccine (Td) and tetanus and diphtheria toxoids and acellular pertussis vaccine (Tdap).** *(Minimum ages: 7 years for Td, 10 years for BOOSTRIX, and 11 years for ADACEL)* Tdap should be substituted for a single dose of Td in the primary catch-up series or as a booster if age appropriate; use Td for other doses. A 5-year interval from the last Td dose is encouraged when Tdap is used as a booster dose. A booster (fourth) dose is needed if any of the previous doses were administered at age <12 months. Refer to ACIP recommendations for further information. See MMWR 2006;55(No. RR-3). **11. Human papillomavirus vaccine (HPV).** *(Minimum age: 9 years)* Administer the HPV vaccine series to females at age 13–18 years if not previously vaccinated.

Adjuvants

The immune response to some antigens is enhanced by the addition of adjuvants—nonspecific boosters of immune responses. Adjuvants include aluminum salts or, in the case of polysaccharides such as the polyribose phosphate oligosaccharide of Hib, a carrier protein to which the polysaccharide is conjugated. Adjuvants are essential to the efficacy of a number of inactivated vaccines, including diphtheria and tetanus toxoids, acellular pertussis vaccine, and hepatitis B vaccine; they also appear to be required for enhancement of the response to killed H5N1 avian influenza vaccines. The mechanism by which adjuvants enhance immunogenicity is not well defined, but appears to relate to the ability of the adjuvant to activate antigen-presenting cells, frequently through stimulation of Toll-like receptors. Other reported mechanisms for adjuvant effects include rendering of soluble antigens into a particulate form, the mobilization of phagocytes to the site of antigen deposition, and the slowing down of antigen release in order to prolong stimulation of the immune response. Identification of new adjuvants that are safe, more effective, and inexpensive is a high priority for vaccine researchers and manufacturers.

USE OF VACCINES

RECOMMENDATIONS FOR USE

Two or more vaccines should not be mixed in the same syringe in an effort to diminish the number of needle sticks unless such a practice is specifically endorsed by licensure. Disposable needles and syringes must be safely discarded to prevent inadvertent needle stick injury. Although the importance of using a new syringe and needle for each vaccine recipient is obvious, reuse of contaminated equipment is a common reality in resource-poor settings. One-time-use, "auto-destruct" needles and syringes have been designed to prevent this practice, but their use adds to the cost of vaccine delivery.

Wherever effective primary health care systems ensure access to medical services for the majority and the population is educated about the need for and efficacy of vaccines, coverage rates for basic immunizations are usually high, regardless of the route of vaccine administration or the number of doses necessary. However, without systematic attention to the completion of multiple-dose vaccine schedules, coverage rates for second, third, and booster doses may drop off, and the efficacy of immunization may be significantly diminished.

RISK ASSESSMENT

Vaccines are considered safe when the risk of use is judged to be acceptable in relation to the benefits. For vaccines given to healthy individuals for diseases that are no longer common, acceptable risks are set at very low levels—indeed, far lower than for most medical products. However, "safety" does not and cannot ever mean "zero risk." The determination of safety is thus based on a scientific assessment of the data and a considered judgment of all the issues involved, including benefits and risks. Communities and individuals may differ, both among themselves and from health care professionals, in how they perceive the risks, benefits, and acceptability of vaccines and in how they judge the amount of uncertainty that is tolerable. Some parent advocacy groups, such as those that oppose mandatory vaccination, feel that no amount of risk is acceptable, especially for childhood vaccines.

SOURCES OF IMMUNIZATION RECOMMENDATIONS

Harmonized recommendations for vaccine use in the United States are developed by several professional groups. Schedules for immunization of children and adolescents and of adults are shown in Figs. 3-1 and 3-2, respectively. Vaccines recommended for special use are shown in Table 3-2.

As noted above, the number of licensed vaccines and the strategies for their best use change constantly as new products, new indications, and new information become available. The Advisory Committee on Immunization Practices (ACIP) regularly amends immunization recommendations to reflect the evolution of vaccines and vaccination policy in the United States. Changes for 2006 include the following points:

- To implement standing orders to administer hepatitis B vaccine—soon after birth and before hospital discharge—to all infants except those with documented hepatitis B–negative mothers;
- To target adults at high risk for hepatitis B vaccination;
- To use a new tetanus toxoid/reduced-dose diphtheria toxoid plus acellular pertussis combination vaccine (Tdap) formulated for adolescents and adults in place of Td;

TABLE 3-2

SPECIAL VACCINES FOR INFANTS, CHILDREN, AND ADULTS

VACCINE	VACCINE TYPE	ROUTE OF ADMINISTRATION	INDICATIONS	EFFICACY	ADVERSE EVENTS
Anthrax	Inactivated avirulent bacteria	SC (6 doses primary plus annual booster)	For high risk of exposure (e.g., persons in contact with or involved in manufacture of animal hides, furs, bone meal, wool, goat hair) and military risk of biowarfare exposure	90% antibody response; efficacy uncertain	No serious adverse effects known
Tuberculosis (BCG)	Live bacteria (attenuated *Mycobacterium bovis*)	ID	Not generally recommended in United States because of low risk of TB and interference with PPD test Consider for PPD-negative children in prolonged contact with ineffectively treated adult TB patients or those with drug-resistant TB and for health care workers in high-risk settings. Not for immunosuppressed individuals	Variable for adult pulmonary TB; best used to prevent childhood TB, meningitis, and miliary disease	Regional adenitis, disseminated BCG infection in immunocompromised hosts
Cholera	Killed whole bacteria	Oral	Travelers to endemic areas; however, not recommended for use by U.S. citizens because of extremely low risk. Not available in the United States.	60–85%, short duration	Frequent fever and local reactions, pain, swelling
Plague	Inactivated bacteria	IM	Laboratory workers; foresters in endemic areas; ?travelers	90% antibody response; efficacy uncertain	10% local reactions; rare sterile abscess and hypersensitivity
Rabies	Inactivated virus grown in cell culture (human diploid cell or purified chick embryo cell) or grown in cell culture and adsorbed to aluminum phosphate	IM or ID	Preexposure immunization for travelers to high-risk countries, laboratory workers, and veterinarians or postexposure immunization after a bite from a proven or suspected rabies-infected animal	Virtually 100% for pre- or postexposure immunization	25% local reactions; 6% of patients receiving booster doses may develop immune complex reactions with arthropathy, arthritis, angioedema

(*Continued*)

TABLE 3-2 (*CONTINUED*)

SPECIAL VACCINES FOR INFANTS, CHILDREN, AND ADULTS

VACCINE	VACCINE TYPE	ROUTE OF ADMINISTRATION	INDICATIONS	EFFICACY	ADVERSE EVENTS
Yellow fever	Live attenuated virus	SC	Travelers to endemic areas; laboratory workers	High	Rare associated neurologic complications (encephalitis, encephalopathy) or viscerotropic disease (fever; hypotension; respiratory, renal, or hepatic failure; lymphocytopenia; thrombocytopenia; and high risk of death)
Japanese B encephalitis	Inactivated virus	SC	Travelers to endemic areas	80–90%	Anaphylaxis/severe delayed allergic reactions common; recipients should be observed for 10 days
Typhoid	Purified Vi polysaccharide (not for children <2 years of age)	IM	Travelers (≥2 years old) to high-risk areas (southern Asia and other developing areas) except febrile patients	50–80%	Local reactions, mild
	Oral live attenuated Ty21a strain	Oral	Travelers (≥6 years old) to high-risk areas as above, except within 24 h of antibiotic ingestion or in febrile patients	50–80%	Nil

Note: SC, subcutaneous; BCG, bacille Calmette-Guérin; ID, intradermal; PPD, purified protein derivative; TB, tuberculosis.
Source: Recommendations of the Advisory Committee on Immunization Practices of the Centers for Disease Control and Prevention, American Academy of Pediatrics, American College of Physicians.

- To provide meningococcal conjugate vaccine (MCV4) to all children at 11–12 years of age, to unvaccinated adolescents at age 15, and to all college freshmen living in dormitories;
- To administer hepatitis A vaccine to all children at 1 year of age;
- To administer three doses of the newly licensed rotavirus vaccine at 2, 4, and 6 months of age, with the first dose given by 12 weeks of age and the last by 32 weeks of age;
- To immunize children 6 months to 5 years of age with influenza vaccine and to expand routine use of the vaccine for their household contacts and out-of-home caregivers;
- To administer Tdap to protect health care personnel from pertussis and to reduce their potential to transmit nosocomial infections, assigning the highest priority to those who have direct contact with infants <1 year old; and
- To administer HPV vaccine routinely to girls at 11–12 years of age.

VACCINES FOR ROUTINE USE

Infants and Children

It is current practice for all children in the United States to receive DTaP, poliovirus, MMR, Hib, hepatitis B, and varicella vaccines and to receive pneumococcal conjugate, hepatitis A, and rotavirus vaccines in the absence of specific contraindications (Fig. 3-1; *www.cdc.gov/vaccines/vpd-vac/vaccines-list.htm*). Annual influenza seasonal vaccine is recommended for all children 6 months to 5 years old and to other children who have certain risk factors or who reside with persons with certain chronic disorders. In several European countries, meningococcal C conjugate vaccine is routinely recommended for children.

Teenagers

It is now recommended that all adolescents routinely receive quadrivalent meningococcal conjugate vaccine for serogroups A, C, Y, and W135 and the new-formulation Tdap vaccine. Girls should be given HPV vaccine, ideally at the age of 11–12 years, but certainly before becoming sexually active (Fig. 3-1; *www.cdc.gov/vaccines/recs/schedules/teen-schedule.htm*).

Adults, Including College Students

(Fig. 3-2) Immunization recommendations for adults (≥18 years old) fall into four categories: (1) routine vaccines for all adults; (2) vaccines for high-risk exposure groups (health care and other institutional workers, prisoners, students, military personnel, travelers to endemic areas, injection drug users, and men who have sex with men); (3) vaccines for persons at high risk for severe outcomes of infection (pregnant women; the elderly; persons with chronic medical conditions, including diabetes, alcoholism, immunodeficiency, and renal, hepatic, respiratory, or cardiac disease); and (4) vaccines for household contacts of persons in group 3.

Because a substantial proportion of adults in the United States no longer have protective levels of antibodies to tetanus or diphtheria, all adults should receive routine booster doses of Td every 10 years. For those under age 65 years, one-time substitution of Tdap suitable for adults (Adacel, Sanofi-Pasteur) in place of the usual Td booster is recommended. Pregnant women who received their last Td booster >10 years previously may receive Td during the second or third trimester; those boosted <10 years previously (and as recently as 2 years before) should receive Tdap after delivery. Adults who have contact with infants <12 months of age should receive a single dose of Tdap—ideally at least 2 weeks before contact begins—if the most recent Td booster was ≥2 years earlier. If not previously immunized, adults require a primary immunizing course of Td. Young adults without laboratory evidence or a reliable history of past vaccination or disease should be immunized against measles, mumps, rubella, and varicella. A second dose of MMR vaccine is recommended for groups with a higher risk of exposure and for health care workers with certain other indications. Unless they have documented proof of immunity, rubella vaccine should be given to all nonpregnant women of childbearing age. Rubella-susceptible pregnant women should be vaccinated as early as possible in the postpartum period. Live-virus vaccines, such as MMR and varicella vaccines, are contraindicated in pregnant women and immunosuppressed individuals. Routine immunization against polio (with inactivated vaccine) is not recommended for adults unless they are at particular risk of exposure because of travel to the remaining endemic areas. College students, particularly freshmen living in dormitory settings, are at increased risk of meningococcal meningitis, as are military recruits; individuals in both of these groups should be offered the meningococcal polysaccharide or conjugate vaccine for serogroups A, C, Y, and W-135.

Current recommendations also include influenza vaccine for routine annual administration to individuals with chronic illness at any age, to persons living in the same household as chronically ill individuals, and to all adults >50 years of age. Polyvalent pneumococcal polysaccharide vaccine is similarly recommended for adults ≥65 years of age and for all chronically ill persons. Hepatitis B vaccine should be given to adults at high risk from clinical, occupational, behavioral, or travel exposures, including patients undergoing hemodialysis, routine recipients of clotting factors, health care workers exposed to potentially infected blood or blood products, individuals living and working in institutions for the mentally handicapped, travelers to highly endemic countries, persons at excess risk for sexually transmitted diseases, injection drug users, and household contacts of known carriers of hepatitis B surface antigen. Hepatitis A vaccine is recommended for these same groups and for persons with clotting disorders or chronic liver disease. There are a number of other special-use vaccines whose administration is related to travel and occupational exposures (e.g., Japanese B encephalitis, typhoid fever, yellow fever, and rabies); specific recommendations for the use of these vaccines in the United States can be found at *www.cdc.gov/nip/recs/adult-schedule.htm*.

Simultaneous Administration of Multiple Vaccines

There are no contraindications to the simultaneous administration of multiple individual vaccines, although the use of licensed combination vaccines can significantly reduce the required number of injections during the first 2 years of life. Combination DTaP/Hib vaccine should not be used for primary immunization of infants because it results in a blunted, suboptimal response to Hib; the combination may be used for booster immunizations.

Simultaneous administration of the most widely used live and inactivated vaccines has not resulted in impaired antibody responses or in elevated rates of adverse reactions. In fact, this approach increases the likelihood that a child will ultimately be fully immunized. The simultaneous administration of vaccines is useful in any age group when the potential exists for exposure to multiple infectious diseases during travel to endemic countries. Live-virus vaccines may be given together on the same day; if this approach is not feasible, an interval of at least 30 days should be allowed to avoid interference in the response to one or another of the administered vaccine strains.

Because high doses of immune globulin can inhibit the efficacy of measles and rubella vaccines, an interval of at least 3 months is recommended between the administration of immune globulin and that of MMR vaccine or its components. However, postpartum vaccination of rubella-susceptible women should not be delayed because of the administration of anti-Rho(D) immune globulin or any other blood product during the last trimester or at delivery. Should the administration of an immune globulin preparation become necessary after vaccination, it should be postponed, if at all possible, for at least 14 days to allow time for vaccine-virus replication and development of immunity. In general, there is little interaction of immune globulin with inactivated vaccines, and postexposure passive prophylaxis can be given together with hepatitis B vaccine or tetanus toxoid, resulting in both immediate and long-lasting protection.

Adverse Events

Vaccines are generally very safe. Serious adverse events proven to be due to currently licensed vaccines are rare. Concerns about vaccine safety have at times become inflated in conjunction with complacency about the consequences of infections no longer routinely transmitted in the United States. As a result, some parents have refused to have their infants and children immunized.

An *adverse reaction* or *vaccine side effect* is an untoward vaccine effect that is extraneous to the vaccine's primary purpose (to produce immunity). An adverse event can be either a true vaccine reaction or an event whose occurrence is temporally related to a vaccine dose but is entirely unrelated to the vaccine itself. As vaccines are routinely administered through childhood, coincidental events are inevitable. Because our understanding of the underlying biologic mechanisms that cause adverse events remains limited, a few highly publicized claims—unsubstantiated by validated data or analysis—can easily heighten the suspicion that some or all vaccines routinely cause unacceptable adverse events. Antivaccine advocacy groups actively encourage the avoidance of immunization because they believe that vaccines cause certain disorders (e.g., autism). This situation presents a challenge to physicians and public health officials who must educate parents and practitioners about vaccine benefits and risks.

It is true that modern vaccines, although remarkably safe and effective, are associated with adverse events in some recipients and that these events range from frequent and mild to rare and serious or even life-threatening. The decision to recommend a vaccine involves an assessment of the risks of disease and its complications for those who remain unimmunized and the benefit-to-risk ratio of vaccination itself. Because these factors may change over time, the balance between societal benefits and individual risks must be continually evaluated. Valid and invalid contraindications to childhood immunization and appropriate precautions in the use of specific vaccines are reported by the CDC (Table 3-3); updated information can be found at *www.cdc.gov/vaccines/recs/vac-admin/downloads/contraindications_guide.pdf*. A putative link between measles immunization and autism has been the subject of intense international controversy. The Institute of Medicine of the U.S. National Academies of Science has issued four recent reports whose findings (1) fail to support hypotheses that vaccines are associated with multiple sclerosis, neurodevelopmental disorders (e.g., autism), or immune dysfunction; (2) provide no evidence for a temporal association of these conditions with vaccination; and (3) elucidate no biologically plausible basis for the purported relationships.

An illuminating example is the case of Rotashield, a rhesus reassortant rotavirus vaccine, which was introduced for routine use in the United States in the late 1990s. Within 9 months of its introduction, cases of intussusception were reported by the CDC to be temporally associated with the administration of the initial vaccine dose. This report led first to the cessation of the vaccine's use and subsequently to its withdrawal from the market and the discontinuation of its production. The withdrawal of the vaccine in the United States made its use impossible in developing countries, where the risk of any increase in intussusception would have been dramatically outweighed by the benefit of decreased rotavirus mortality rates. It is now apparent that the susceptibility to intussusception is age related, with virtually no events in children <90 days of age. Almost a decade later, a new rotavirus vaccine has been licensed in the United States and recommended for routine use beginning at ≤2 months of age. In the interim, some 4–5 million infants have died of rotavirus diarrhea in the developing world; most of these deaths could have been prevented by the original rhesus rotavirus vaccine.

TABLE 3-3

VALID AND INVALID CONTRAINDICATIONS TO VACCINATION

VACCINE	VALID CONTRAINDICATION[a]	INVALID CONTRAINDICATION
All vaccines in general	Serious allergic reactions (e.g., anaphylaxis) to a previous vaccine dose or a vaccine component *Precaution:* Moderate or severe concurrent illness with or without fever	Mild acute illness with or without fever Mild to moderate local reactions; low-grade or moderate fever after a previous dose Lack of previous physical examination in a well-appearing person Current antimicrobial therapy (except certain live bacterial vaccines) Convalescent phase of illness Premature birth (except hepatitis B in some circumstances) Recent exposure to infectious diseases History of penicillin allergy, other nonvaccine allergies; relatives with allergies; receiving desensitization treatment
DTaP[b]	Severe allergic reaction to a previous dose or a vaccine component Encephalopathy (e.g., coma, decreased level of consciousness, prolonged seizures) within 7 days of a previous dose of DTP or DTaP Progressive neurologic disorder, including infantile spasms, uncontrolled epilepsy, progressive encephalopathy: defer DTaP until neurologic status is clarified and stabilized *Precaution:* Fever of ≥40.5°C at ≤48 h after a previous dose of DTP or DTaP Collapse or shock-like state (i.e., hypotonic hyporesponsive episode ≤48 h after a previous dose of DTP or DTaP) Seizure ≤3 days after a previous dose of DTP or DTaP Persistent, inconsolable crying lasting ≥3 h/≤48 h after a previous dose of DTP or DTaP Moderate or severe acute illness with or without fever	Temperature of <40.5°C; fussiness; mild drowsiness after a prior dose of DTP or DTaP Family history of seizures, sudden infant death syndrome, or adverse event after DTP or DTaP Stable neurologic conditions (e.g., cerebral palsy, well-controlled convulsions, developmental delay)
DT, Td	Severe allergic reaction after a previous dose or to a vaccine component *Precaution:* Guillain-Barré syndrome ≤6 weeks after a previous dose of tetanus toxoid–containing vaccine Moderate or severe acute illness with or without fever	
IPV	Severe allergic reaction to a previous dose or a vaccine component *Precautions:* Pregnancy; moderate or severe acute illness with or without fever	
MMR	Severe allergic reaction to a previous dose or a vaccine component Pregnancy Known severe immunodeficiency (e.g., hematologic and solid tumors, congenital immunodeficiency, long-term immuno-suppressive therapy, or severely symptomatic HIV infection) *Precautions:* Recent (≤11 months) receipt of antibody-containing blood products (specific interval depends on product); history of thrombocytopenia and thrombocytopenic purpura; moderate or severe acute illness with or without fever	Positive tuberculin skin test; simultaneous TB skin testing Breast-feeding Pregnancy of recipient's mother or other close or household contact; recipient is childbearing-age female or immunodeficient family member or household contact; asymptomatic or mildly symptomatic HIV infection; allergy to eggs

(*Continued*)

TABLE 3-3 (*CONTINUED*)

VALID AND INVALID CONTRAINDICATIONS TO VACCINATION

VACCINE	VALID CONTRAINDICATION[a]	INVALID CONTRAINDICATION
Hib	Severe allergic reaction to a previous dose or a vaccine component Age <6 weeks *Precaution:* Moderate or severe acute illness with or without fever	
Hepatitis B	Severe allergic reaction to a previous dose or a vaccine component *Precautions:* Infant weighing <2000 g; moderate or severe acute illness with or without fever	Pregnancy; autoimmune disease (e.g., systemic lupus erythematosus or rheumatoid arthritis)
Hepatitis A	Severe allergic reaction to a previous dose or a vaccine component *Precaution:* Pregnancy; moderate or severe acute illness with or without fever	
Varicella	Severe allergic reaction to a previous dose or a vaccine component Substantial suppression of cellular immunity Pregnancy *Precaution:* Recent (≤11 months) receipt of antibody-containing blood products (specific interval depends on product)	Pregnancy of recipient's mother or another close or household contact Immunodeficient family member or household contact; asymptomatic or mildly symptomatic HIV infection
Pneumococcal conjugate vaccines	Severe allergic reaction to a previous dose or a vaccine component *Precaution:* Moderate or severe acute illness with or without fever	
Influenza	Severe allergic reaction to a previous dose or a vaccine component, including egg protein *Precaution:* Moderate or severe acute illness with or without fever	Nonsevere (e.g., contact) allergy to latex or thimerosal; concurrent administration of warfarin or aminophylline
Pneumococcal polysaccharide vaccines	Severe allergic reaction to a previous dose or a vaccine component *Precaution:* Moderate or severe acute illness with or without fever	

[a]Events or conditions listed as precautions should be reviewed carefully. Benefits and risks of administering a specific vaccine to a person under these circumstances should be considered. If the risk from the vaccine is believed to outweigh the benefit, the vaccine should not be administered. If the benefit of vaccination is believed to outweigh the risk, the vaccine should be administered.
[b]Whether and when to administer DTaP to children with proven or suspected underlying neurologic disorders should be decided on a case-by-case basis.
Note: DTP, diphtheria and tetanus toxoids and whole-cell pertussis vaccine; DTaP, diphtheria and tetanus toxoids and acellular pertussis vaccine; DT, diphtheria and tetanus toxoids; Td, tetanus and reduced-dose diphtheria toxoids, adsorbed; IPV, inactivated polio vaccine; MMR, measles, mumps, and rubella vaccine; Hib, Haemophilus influenzae type b vaccine.
Source: General Recommendations on Immunization. MMWR 51(RR02):1, 2002.

Vaccine components, including protective antigens, animal proteins introduced during vaccine production, and antibiotics or other preservatives or stabilizers, can certainly cause allergic reactions in some recipients. These reactions may be local or systemic, including urticaria and serious anaphylaxis. The most common extraneous allergen is egg protein derived from the growth of measles, mumps, influenza, and yellow fever viruses in embryonated eggs. Gelatin, used as a heat stabilizer, has been implicated in rare but severe allergic reactions. Local or systemic reactions (probably due to antigen-antibody complexes) can result from the too-frequent administration of vaccines such as Td or rabies vaccine. Because live-virus vaccines can interfere with tuberculin test responses, necessary tuberculin testing should be done either on the day of immunization or at least 6 weeks later.

USE OF VACCINES IN SPECIAL CIRCUMSTANCES

Breast Feeding

Neither killed nor live vaccines affect the safety of breast feeding for either mother or infant. Breast-fed infants can be immunized on a normal schedule. Even premature infants can be immunized at their appropriate chronologic age. Seroconversion in response to hepatitis vaccine at birth may be impaired in some premature infants with birth weights of <2000 g. By a chronologic age of 1 month, however, premature infants—regardless of initial birth weight or gestational age—are as likely to respond adequately to vaccines as older and larger infants.

Occupational Exposure

Immunization recommendations for most occupational groups remain to be developed. Specific practices for the immunization of U.S. health care workers against hepatitis B are mandated by the Occupational Safety and Health Administration. Persons employed in caring for patients with chronic diseases can transmit influenza and should be vaccinated annually, independent of age. Rubella is transmitted to and from health care workers in medical facilities, particularly in pediatric practice. Health care workers who might transmit rubella to pregnant patients should be documented to be immune to rubella; susceptible individuals should be promptly immunized. Persons providing health care are also at greater risk from measles and varicella than the general public, and those who are likely to come into contact with measles- and varicella-infected patients should be documented to be immune or be immunized.

HIV Infection and Other Medical Conditions

Limited studies in HIV-infected individuals have found no increase in the risk of adverse events from the use of live or inactivated vaccines. It is not surprising that immune responses may not be as vigorous in immunocompromised individuals as in those with a normal immune system; therefore, persons known to be infected with HIV should be immunized with recommended vaccines in the same manner as individuals with a normal immune system and as early in the course of their disease as possible, before immune function becomes significantly impaired. If MMR immunization is indicated, HIV-infected patients may receive the standard attenuated vaccine; if polio vaccination is required, these patients and their household contacts should receive inactivated polio vaccine.

Albeit prudent, it is not necessary to test for HIV before making decisions about the immunization of asymptomatic individuals from known HIV risk groups. Live attenuated vaccines are contraindicated in other immunocompromised patients, including those with congenital immunodeficiency syndromes, those who have undergone splenectomy, and those who are receiving immunosuppressive therapy. Passive immunization with immunoglobulin preparations or antitoxins can be considered in individual cases, either as postexposure prophylaxis or as part of the treatment of established infection.

Travel

(See also Chap. 4) The International Sanitary Regulations allow countries to impose requirements for yellow fever and killed cholera vaccines as a condition for admission, even though the latter vaccine is not an effective public health tool. Travelers should know whether these vaccines are required for entry into the countries on their itinerary to avoid being turned back or immunized on the spot, with the inherent danger of unsafe injections in poor developing countries. Infants, children, and adults should have all routine immunizations updated before traveling, especially to developing countries, with particular attention to polio, measles, and DTaP or Tdap, depending on age. Immunity to hepatitis A and hepatitis B is advisable for travelers. Special-use vaccines (Table 3-2), including rabies, typhoid, Japanese B encephalitis, and plague vaccines, should be considered for those individuals who expect to go beyond the usual tourist routes or to spend extended periods in rural areas in disease-endemic regions. Most U.S. cities have travel clinics that maintain up-to-date epidemiologic information and can provide the appropriate vaccines. The CDC maintains a useful website for travelers (*www.cdc.gov/travel*).

CURRENT CONTROVERSIES

Even though vaccines are very safe and serious adverse events proven to be due to licensed vaccines are rare, the recent rise in the reporting of autism spectrum disorders has led some parents of affected children to claim that thimerosal—used as a preservative—is the cause of the problem. No study has yet implicated thimerosal or the vaccines in which it has been used as a likely cause of these disorders; however, fully 50% of cases before the Vaccine Injury Compensation Program concern autism allegedly due to mercury. In 1999, thimerosal was removed from single-dose formulations of recommended childhood vaccines in the United States; the exception is influenza vaccine, for which thimerosal-free preparations have been in short supply. There is no evidence that the frequency of autism diagnoses has changed since the discontinuation of thimerosal use, but further observation is necessary. It is important to resolve these controversies, particularly because it may be difficult to ensure product sterility in developing countries—where multidose vials of vaccine are most cost-effective—without the use of preservative.

Disparities in vaccine coverage among the majority and minority communities in the United States persist. Reasons for underimmunization include limited access to health care, lack of insurance, assignment of a low priority to preventive measures, and insufficient knowledge about vaccines and the importance of being vaccinated. The persistence of wild poliovirus in immunocompromised individuals and the reversion of live poliovirus vaccine to virulence in several communities have catalyzed debate about whether it really is possible to eradicate poliovirus from the world (thus allowing the cessation of immunization) or whether the best that can be hoped for is the worldwide elimination of clinical disease, with continued routine immunization to keep the risk low.

The addition of new, individually injectable vaccines to the childhood immunization schedule has heightened parental concerns about multiple injections at a single clinic visit. The continued development and testing of vaccine combinations aim to mitigate these concerns. Even when multiple injections are required, providers must make every effort to administer all indicated vaccines at each visit.

DELIVERY OF VACCINES

Over the past 25 years, considerable progress has been made to ensure that every child in the United States is fully immunized by the time of school entry. All 50 states now require immunization for school entry, and most have laws addressing attendance at preschools and day-care centers. Despite the dramatic impact of immunization and of other improvements in health care on the incidence of vaccine-preventable illness in the United States, many children still are not fully immunized, both in poor communities with inadequate health services and in affluent communities where parental concern about potential adverse events may exceed concern about now-uncommon diseases. The failure to vaccinate preschool children was largely responsible for the resurgence of measles in the United States in 1989–1991, with >55,000 cases and >130 measles-related deaths. Outbreaks of pertussis, mumps, and congenital rubella syndrome have occurred wherever immunization rates among preschool children are low. Although indigenous transmission of polio, measles, and rubella has been eliminated in the United States, the risk of imported infection and spread to vaccine-naïve susceptible persons persists.

ACCESS TO IMMUNIZATION

Four major barriers to infant and childhood immunization have been identified within the health care system: (1) low public awareness and lack of public demand for immunization, (2) inadequate access to immunization services, (3) missed opportunities to administer vaccines, and (4) inadequate resources for public health and preventive programs. National outreach and educational campaigns promote parental awareness of the value of vaccination and encourage health care providers to use every opportunity to vaccinate the children in their care.

HANDLING OF VACCINES

Vaccines must be handled and stored with care. Attention to the entire "cold chain"—from storage, shelf life, reconstitution, and shelf life after reconstitution and opening—is essential to ensuring that clients receive potent vaccines. Vaccines should be kept at 2°–8°C and, with the exception of varicella vaccine and live attenuated influenza vaccine, should not be frozen. The latter two vaccines should be kept frozen at −15°C. Measles vaccine must be protected from light, which inactivates the virus.

STANDARDS FOR IMMUNIZATION PRACTICE

National standards of immunization for childhood, adolescent, and adult practice have been established to define common policies and practices for public health clinics and physicians' private offices (Table 3-4). These standards represent the most desirable immunization practices and highlight the need to distinguish between valid contraindications and conditions that are often considered to be but are not in fact contraindications (www.cdc.gov/vaccines/recs/vac-admin/downloads/contraindications_guide.pdf).

Among the valid contraindications applicable to all vaccines are a history of anaphylaxis or other serious allergic reactions to a vaccine or vaccine component and the presence of a moderate or severe illness, with or without fever. Infants who develop encephalopathy within 72 h of a dose of DTP or DTaP should not receive further doses; those who experience a "precaution" event should not normally receive further doses. Because of theoretical risks to the fetus, pregnant women should not receive MMR or varicella vaccine. Diarrhea, minor respiratory illness (with or without fever), mild to moderate local reactions to a previous dose of vaccine, the concurrent or recent use of antimicrobial agents, mild to moderate malnutrition, and the convalescent phase of an acute illness are not valid contraindications to routine immunization. Failure to vaccinate children because of these conditions is increasingly viewed as a missed opportunity for immunization.

CONTROL OF VACCINE-PREVENTABLE DISEASE

A continuing task of public health practice is to maintain individual and herd immunity, and the job is not over once a population is fully vaccinated. Rather, it is imperative to immunize each subsequent generation as long as the threat

TABLE 3-4

STANDARDS FOR IMMUNIZATION PRACTICE

Child and Adolescent Immunization Practice

1. Immunization services are readily available.
2. Vaccinations are coordinated with other health care services and provided in a "medical home" when possible.
3. Barriers to vaccination are identified and minimized.
4. Patient's costs are minimized.
5. Health care professionals review the vaccination and health status of patients at every encounter to determine which vaccines are indicated.
6. Health care professionals assess for and follow only medically accepted contraindications.
7. Parents/guardians and patients are educated about the benefits and risks of vaccination in a culturally appropriate manner and in easy-to-understand language.
8. Health care professionals follow appropriate procedures for vaccine storage and handling.
9. Up-to-date written vaccination protocols are accessible at all locations where vaccines are administered.
10. Persons who administer vaccines and staff who manage or support vaccine administration are knowledgeable and receive ongoing education.
11. Health care professionals simultaneously administer as many indicated vaccine doses as possible.
12. Vaccination records for patients are accurate, complete, and easily accessible.
13. Health care professionals report adverse events after vaccination promptly and accurately to the VAERS and are aware of the VICP.
14. All personnel who have contact with patients are appropriately vaccinated.
15. Systems are used to remind parents/guardians, patients, and health care professionals when vaccinations are due and to recall patients whose vaccinations are overdue.
16. Office- or clinic-based patient record reviews and vaccination coverage assessments are performed annually.
17. Health care professionals practice community-based approaches.

Adult Immunization Practice

1. Adult immunization services are readily available.
2. Barriers to receiving vaccines are identified and minimized.
3. Patient's out-of-pocket costs are minimized.
4. Health care professionals routinely review the vaccination status of patients.
5. Health care professionals assess for valid contraindications.
6. Patients are educated about risks and benefits of vaccination in easy-to-understand language.
7. Written vaccination protocols are available at all locations where vaccinations are administered.
8. Persons who administer vaccines are properly trained.
9. Health care professionals recommend simultaneous administration of all indicated vaccine doses.
10. Vaccination records for patients are accurate and easily accessible.
11. All personnel who have contact with patients are appropriately vaccinated.
12. Systems are developed and used to remind patients and health care professionals when vaccinations are due and to recall patients whose vaccinations are overdue.
13. Standing orders for vaccinations are employed.
14. Regular assessments of vaccination coverage levels are conducted in the provider's practice.
15. Patient-oriented and community-based approaches are used to reach target populations.

Note: VAERS, Vaccine Adverse Events Reporting System; VICP, Vaccine Injury Compensation Program.
Source: Centers for Disease Control and Prevention, in *Epidemiology and Prevention of Vaccine-Preventable Diseases*, 2006, Appendix H. These standards can be found at *www.cdc.gov/nip/publications*.

of the reintroduction of the disease from anywhere in the world persists. Ongoing surveillance and prompt reporting of disease to local or state health departments are essential to this goal, ensuring a continuing awareness of the possibility of vaccine-preventable illness. Nearly all vaccine-preventable diseases are notifiable, and individual case data are routinely forwarded to the CDC. These data are used to detect outbreaks or other unusual events that require investigation and to evaluate prevention and control policies, practices, and strategies.

INTERNATIONAL CONSIDERATIONS

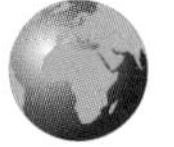

Since the establishment of the Expanded Programme on Immunization (EPI) by the WHO in 1981 and the involvement of UNICEF in the program's implementation, levels of coverage for the recommended basic children's vaccines (bacille Calmette-Guérin, poliomyelitis, DTP/DTaP, and measles) have risen from 5% to ~80% worldwide, although coverage does not necessarily translate into protective immunity. Each year, at least 2.7 million deaths from measles, neonatal tetanus, and pertussis and 200,000 cases of paralysis due to polio are prevented by immunization. Despite the successes of this program, many vaccine-preventable diseases remain prevalent in the developing world. Measles, for example, continues to kill an estimated 500,000 children each year, and diphtheria, whooping cough, polio, and neonatal tetanus still occur at unacceptably high rates. An estimated 20–35% of all deaths of children are due to vaccine-preventable diseases.

In addition to the antigens included in the EPI for routine use in the developing world, others (hepatitis B, Hib, Japanese B encephalitis, yellow fever, meningococcal, mumps, and rubella) are used regionally, depending on disease epidemiology and resources. The rationale for inclusion of hepatitis B vaccine in Africa and Asia is to prevent the subsequent development of hepatocellular carcinoma, which is strongly linked with the persistence of hepatitis B virus from early childhood. The delivery of vaccines in mass campaigns on national immunization days, superseding even civil wars and insurgencies, has resulted in the cessation of transmission of poliomyelitis in the Western Hemisphere, the western Pacific, and Europe and in the virtual elimination of clinical measles from the Western Hemisphere. Periodic vaccination campaigns complement routine infant and childhood vaccination services under the rubric "catch up, follow up, and keep up." Despite these successes, concerns remain about the adequacy of long-term strategies to ensure continuity, the impact of vaccine campaigns on the provision of routine services, and unsafe injection practices.

Because infectious diseases know no geographic or political boundaries, uncontrolled disease anywhere in the world poses a threat to the United States, even without bioterrorism. Vaccines offer the opportunity to effectively control and even eliminate some diseases through individual and herd protection. Vaccines also represent the best societal hope for stopping the pandemic of HIV infection throughout the world and for efficiently controlling malaria and tuberculosis. Issues of cost, liability, risk, and profitability limit the interest of the pharmaceutical industry in the development of vaccines for infectious diseases of the poor.

SOURCES OF INFORMATION ON IMMUNIZATION

- Official vaccine package circulars and Vaccine Administration Statements from the CDC
- Report of the Committee on Infectious Diseases of the American Academy of Pediatrics ("Red Book")
- Recommendations of the Advisory Committee on Immunization Practices, CDC
- Guide for Adult Immunization, American College of Physicians
- Health Information for International Travel (published yearly) and Advisory Memoranda on Travel (published periodically), CDC
- Control of Communicable Diseases in Man, American Public Health Association
- Technical Bulletin of the College of Obstetrics and Gynecology
- National Network for Immunization Information, Infectious Diseases Society of America/Pediatric Infectious Diseases Society/American Academy of Pediatrics/American Nurses Association

FURTHER READINGS

Bonhoeffer J, Heininger U: Immunization: Perception and evidence. Curr Opin Infect Dis 20:237, 2007

Brown NJ et al: Vaccination, seizures and "vaccine damage." Curr Opin Neurol 20:181, 2007

Bruce Aylward R et al: Risk management in a polio-free world. Risk Anal 26:1441, 2006

Fiore AE et al: Prevention and control of influenza: Recommendations of the Advisory Committee on Immunization Practices (ACIP), 2008. MMWR Recomm Rep 57:1, 2008

Goldie S: A public health approach to cervical cancer control: Considerations of screening and vaccination strategies. Int J Gynaecol Obstet 94(Suppl 1):S95, 2006

Jacobson RM et al: Why is evidence-based medicine so harsh on vaccines? An exploration of the method and its natural biases. Vaccine 25:3165, 2007

Kaufmann SH: The contribution of immunology to the rational design of novel antibacterial vaccines. Nat Rev Microbiol 5:491, 2007

Kimmel SR et al: Addressing immunization barriers, benefits, and risks. J Fam Pract 56:S61, 2007

Reeler AV: Anthropological perspectives on injections: A review. Bull World Health Organ 78:135, 2000

Thompson KM, Tebbens RJ: Eradication versus control for poliomyelitis: An economic analysis. Lancet 369:1363, 2007

van der Zeijst BA et al: On the design of national vaccination programmes. Vaccine 25:3143, 2007

CHAPTER 4

HEALTH ADVICE FOR INTERNATIONAL TRAVEL

Jay S. Keystone ■ Phyllis E. Kozarsky

According to the World Tourism Organization, the number of international tourist arrivals in 2004 reached an all-time record of 763 million. This number represents an increase over the 2003 figure of almost 11%—the highest and the only double-digit percentage increase since 1980, when these statistics were first collected. Not only are more people traveling; travelers are seeking more exotic and remote destinations. Studies show that 50–75% of short-term travelers to the tropics or subtropics report some health impairment. Most of these health problems are minor: only 5% require medical attention, and <1% require hospitalization. Although infectious agents contribute substantially to morbidity among travelers, these pathogens account for only ~1% of deaths in this population. Cardiovascular disease and injuries are the most frequent causes of death among travelers from the United States, accounting for 49% and 22% of deaths, respectively. Age-specific rates of death due to cardiovascular disease are similar among travelers and nontravelers. In contrast, rates of death due to injury (the majority from motor vehicle, drowning, or aircraft accidents) are several times higher among travelers. Figure 4-1 summarizes the monthly incidence of health problems during travel in developing countries.

GENERAL ADVICE

Health maintenance recommendations are based not only on the traveler's destination but also on assessment of risk, which is determined by health status, specific itinerary, and lifestyle during travel. Detailed information regarding country-specific risks and recommendations may be obtained from the Centers for Disease Control and Prevention (CDC) publication *Health Information for International Travel* (available at *www.cdc.gov/travel/yb/*).

Fitness for travel is an issue of growing concern in view of the increased numbers of elderly and chronically ill individuals journeying to exotic destinations (see "Travel and Special Hosts" later in the chapter). Since most commercial aircrafts are pressurized to 2500 m (8000 ft) above sea level (corresponding to a PaO_2 of ~55 mmHg), individuals with serious cardiopulmonary problems or anemia should be evaluated before travel. In addition, those who have recently had surgery, a myocardial infarction, a cerebrovascular accident, or a deep-vein thrombosis may be at high risk for adverse events during flight. A summary of current recommendations regarding fitness to fly has been published by the Aerospace Medical Association Air Transport Medicine Committee (*www. asma. org/publications/*). A pretravel health assessment may be advisable for individuals considering particularly adventurous recreational activities, such as mountain climbing and scuba diving.

IMMUNIZATIONS FOR TRAVEL

Immunizations for travel fall into three broad categories: *routine* (childhood/adult boosters that are necessary regardless of travel), *required* (immunizations that are mandated by international regulations for entry into certain areas or for border crossings), and *recommended* (immunizations that are desirable because of travel-related risks). Vaccines commonly given to travelers are listed in Table 4-1.

Routine Immunizations

Diphtheria, Tetanus, and Polio

Diphtheria (Chap. 38) continues to be a problem worldwide. Large outbreaks have occurred over the past decade in the independent states formerly encompassed by the Soviet Union. Serologic surveys show that tetanus (Chap. 40) antitoxin is lacking in many North Americans, especially in women over the age of 50. The risk of polio (Chap. 94) to the international traveler is extremely low, and wild-type poliovirus has been eradicated from the Western Hemisphere and Europe. However, studies in the United States suggest that 12% of adult travelers are unprotected against at least one poliovirus serogroup. Foreign travel offers an ideal opportunity to have these immunizations updated. With the recent increase in pertussis in adults, the diphtheria-tetanus-acellular pertussis (Tdap) combination may replace the Td vaccine as a 10-year booster once an adult polio immunization has been administered.

Measles

Measles (rubeola) continues to be a major cause of morbidity and mortality in the developing world (Chap. 95). Several outbreaks of measles in the United States have been linked to imported cases. The group at highest risk consists of persons born after 1956 and vaccinated before 1980, in many of whom primary vaccination failed.

Influenza

Influenza—possibly the most common vaccine-preventable infection in travelers—occurs year-round in the tropics

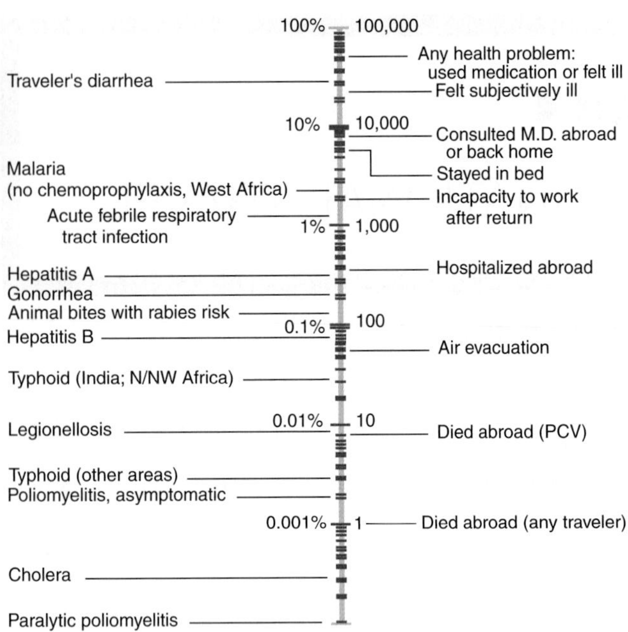

FIGURE 4-1

Incidence rate, per month, of health problems during a stay in developing countries. PCV, Peace Corps volunteer. (*From Steffen R, Lobel HO: Epidemiologic basis for the practice of travel medicine. J Wilderness Med 5:56, 1994. Reprinted with permission from Chapman and Hall, New York.*)

and during the summer months in the Southern Hemisphere (coinciding with the winter months in the Northern Hemisphere). One prospective study showed that influenza developed in 1% of travelers to Southeast Asia per month of stay. Vaccination should be considered for all travelers to these regions, particularly those who are elderly or chronically ill. Travel-related influenza continues to occur during summer months in Alaska and the Northwest Territories of Canada among cruise-ship passengers and staff (Chap. 88).

Pneumococcal Infection

Regardless of travel, pneumococcal vaccine should be administered routinely to the elderly and to persons at high risk of serious infection, including those with chronic heart, lung, or renal disease and those who have been splenectomized or have sickle cell disease (Chap. 34).

Required Immunizations

Yellow Fever

Documentation of vaccination against yellow fever (Chap. 99) may be required as a condition of entry into or passage through countries of Sub-Saharan Africa and equatorial South America, where the disease is endemic or epidemic, or for entry into countries at risk of having the infection introduced. This vaccine is given only

TABLE 4-1

VACCINES COMMONLY USED FOR TRAVEL

VACCINE	PRIMARY SERIES	BOOSTER INTERVAL
Cholera, live oral (CVD 103 - HgR)	1 dose	6 months
Hepatitis A (Havrix), 1440 enzyme immunoassay U/mL	2 doses, 6–12 months apart, IM	None required
Hepatitis A (VAQTA, AVAXIM, EPAXAL)	2 doses, 6–12 months apart, IM	None required
Hepatitis A/B combined (Twinrix)	3 doses at 0, 1, and 6–12 months *or* 0, 7, and 21 days plus booster at 1 year, IM	None required *except* 12 months (once only, for accelerated schedule)
Hepatitis B (Engerix B): accelerated schedule	3 doses at 0, 1, and 2 months *or* 0, 7, and 21 days plus booster at 1 year, IM	12 months, once only
Hepatitis B (Engerix B or Recombivax): standard schedule	3 doses at 0, 1, and 6 months, IM	None required
Immune globulin (hepatitis A prevention)	1 dose IM	Intervals of 3–5 months, depending on initial dose
Japanese encephalitis (JEV, Biken)	3 doses, 1 week apart, SC	12–18 months (first booster), then 4 years
Meningococcus, quadrivalent [Menomune (polysaccharide), Menactra (conjugate)]	1 dose SC	>3 years (optimum booster schedule not yet determined)
Rabies (HDCV), rabies vaccine absorbed (RVA), or purified chick embryo cell vaccine (PCEC)	3 doses at 0, 7, and 21 or 28 days, IM	None required except with exposure
Typhoid Ty21a, oral live attenuated (Vivotif)	1 capsule every other day × 4 doses	5 years
Typhoid Vi capsular polysaccharide, injectable (Typhim Vi)	1 dose IM	2 years
Yellow fever	1 dose SC	10 years

by state-authorized yellow fever centers, and its administration must be documented on an official International Certificate of Vaccination. A registry of U.S. clinics that provide the vaccine is available from the CDC (*www. cdc.gov/travel/*). Recent data suggest that fewer than 50% of travelers entering areas endemic for yellow fever are immunized. Severe adverse events associated with this vaccine have recently increased in incidence. First-time vaccine recipients may present with a syndrome characterized as either neurotropic (1 case per 150,000–250,000 doses) or viscerotropic (1 case per 200,000–300,000 doses; among persons >60 years of age, 1 case per 40,000–50,000). Advanced age and thymic disease seem to increase the risk for these adverse events (*www.cdc.gov/nip/publications/VIS/vis-yf.pdf*).

Meningococcal Meningitis

Protection against meningitis (using one of the quadrivalent vaccines) is required for entry into Saudi Arabia during the Hajj (Chap. 44).

Recommended Immunizations

Hepatitis A and B

Hepatitis A (Chap. 92) is one of the most frequent vaccine-preventable infections of travelers. The risk is six times greater for travelers who stray from the usual tourist routes. The mortality rate for hepatitis A increases with age, reaching almost 3% among individuals over age 50. Of the four hepatitis A vaccines currently available in North America (two in the United States), all are interchangeable and have an efficacy rate of >95%.

Long-stay overseas workers appear to be at considerable risk for hepatitis B infection (Chap. 92). The recommendation that all travelers be immunized against hepatitis B before departure is supported by two recent studies showing that 17% of the assessed travelers who received health care abroad had some type of injection; according to the World Health Organization, nonsterile equipment is used for up to 75% of all injections given in the developing world. A combined hepatitis A and B vaccine is now available in the United States and has been approved for administration on a 3-week accelerated schedule. It seems prudent to consider immunization of all travelers against hepatitis A and B.

Typhoid Fever

The attack rate for typhoid fever (Chap. 54) is 1 case per 30,000 per month of travel to the developing world. However, the attack rates in India, Senegal, and North Africa are tenfold higher and are especially high among travelers to relatively remote destinations and among VFRs (immigrants returning to their homelands to visit friends or relatives). Between 1994 and 1999 in the United States, 77% of imported cases involved the latter group. Both of the available vaccines—one oral (live) and the other injectable (polysaccharide)—have efficacy rates of ~70%. In some countries, a combined hepatitis A/typhoid vaccine is available.

Meningococcal Meningitis

Although the risk of meningococcal disease among travelers has not been quantified, it is likely to be higher among travelers who live with poor indigenous populations in overcrowded conditions (Chap. 44). Either the older polysaccharide vaccine or the newer quadrivalent conjugate vaccine is recommended for persons traveling to Sub-Saharan Africa during the dry season or to areas of the world where there are epidemics. The vaccine, which protects against serogroups A, C, Y, and W-135, has an efficacy rate of >90%.

Japanese Encephalitis

The risk of Japanese encephalitis (Chap. 99), an infection transmitted by mosquitoes in rural Asia and Southeast Asia, is ~1 case per 5000 travelers per month of stay in an endemic area. Most symptomatic infections among U.S. residents have involved military personnel or their families. The vaccine efficacy rate is >90%; serious allergic reactions occur only rarely. The vaccine is recommended for persons staying >1 month in rural endemic areas or for shorter periods if their activities (e.g., camping, bicycling, hiking) in these areas will increase exposure risk. A Vero cell vaccine may be licensed in the United States within the next 2 years.

Cholera

The risk of cholera (Chap. 57) is extremely low, with ~1 case per 500,000 journeys to endemic areas. Cholera vaccine, no longer available in the United States, was rarely recommended but was considered for aid and health care workers in refugee camps or in disaster-stricken/war-torn areas. A more effective oral cholera vaccine is available in other countries.

Rabies

Domestic animals, primarily dogs, are the major transmitters of rabies in developing countries (Chap. 98). Several studies have shown that the risk of rabies posed by a dog bite in an endemic area translates into 1–3.6 cases per 1000 travelers per month of stay. Countries where canine rabies is highly endemic include Mexico, the Philippines, Sri Lanka, India, Thailand, and Vietnam. The three vaccines available in the United States provide >90% protection. Rabies vaccine is recommended for long-stay travelers, particularly children, and persons who may be occupationally exposed to rabies in endemic areas. Even after receipt of a preexposure rabies vaccine series, two postexposure doses are required. Travelers who have had the preexposure series will not require rabies immune globulin (which is often unavailable in developing countries) if they are exposed to the disease.

PREVENTION OF MALARIA AND OTHER INSECT-BORNE DISEASES

It is estimated that more than 30,000 American and European travelers develop malaria each year (Chap. 116). The risk to travelers is highest in Oceania and Sub-Saharan Africa (estimated at 1:5 and 1:50 per month of stay, respectively, among persons not using chemoprophylaxis); intermediate in malarious areas on the Indian subcontinent and in Southeast Asia (1:250–1:1000 per month); and low in South and Central America (1:2500–1:10,000 per month). Of the more than 1000 cases of malaria reported annually in the United States, 90% of those due to *Plasmodium falciparum* occur in travelers returning or immigrating from Africa and Oceania. VFRs are at the highest risk of acquiring malaria. With the worldwide increase in chloroquine- and multidrug-resistant falciparum malaria, decisions about chemoprophylaxis have become more difficult. In addition, the spread of malaria due to primaquine- and chloroquine-resistant strains of *Plasmodium vivax* has added to the complexity of treatment. The case-fatality rate of falciparum malaria in the United States is 4%; however, in only one-third of patients who die is the diagnosis of malaria considered before death.

Several studies indicate that fewer than 50% of travelers adhere to basic recommendations for malaria prevention. Keys to the prevention of malaria include both personal protection measures against mosquito bites (especially between dusk and dawn) and malaria chemoprophylaxis. The former measures include the use of DEET-containing insect repellents, permethrin-impregnated bed-nets and clothing, screened sleeping accommodations, and protective clothing. A new insect repellent containing picaridin as an active ingredient appears to be quite efficacious and is available in the United States only in low-concentration formulations that require frequent reapplications. Thus, in regions where infections such as malaria are transmitted, DEET products (25–50%) are recommended, even for children and infants >2 months of age. Personal protection measures also help prevent other insect-transmitted illnesses, such as dengue fever (Chap. 99). Over the past decade, the incidence of dengue has increased, particularly in the Caribbean region, Latin America, and Southeast Asia. Dengue virus is transmitted by an urban-dwelling mosquito that bites primarily at dawn and dusk.

Table 4-2 lists the currently recommended drugs of choice for prophylaxis of malaria, by destination.

PREVENTION OF GASTROINTESTINAL ILLNESS

Diarrhea, the leading cause of illness in travelers (Chap. 25), is usually a short-lived, self-limited condition; however, 40% of affected individuals need to alter their scheduled activities, and another 20% are confined to bed. The most important determinant of risk is the destination. Incidence rates per 2-week stay have been reported to be as low as 8% in industrialized countries and as high as 55% in parts of Africa, Central and South America, and Southeast Asia. Infants and young adults are at particularly high risk. A recent review suggested that there is little correlation between dietary indiscretions and the occurrence of travelers' diarrhea. Earlier studies of U.S. students in Mexico showed that eating meals in restaurants and cafeterias or consuming food from street vendors was associated with increased risk.

Etiology

(See also Table 25-3) The most frequently identified pathogens causing travelers' diarrhea are toxigenic *Escherichia coli* and enteroaggregative *E. coli* (Chap. 51), although in some parts of the world (notably northern Africa and Southeast Asia) *Campylobacter* infections (Chap. 56) appear to predominate. Other common causative organisms include *Salmonella* (Chap. 54), *Shigella* (Chap. 55), rotavirus (Chap. 91), and norovirus (Chap. 91). The latter virus has caused numerous outbreaks on cruise ships. Except for giardiasis (Chap. 122), parasitic infections are uncommon causes of travelers' diarrhea. A growing problem for travelers is the development of antibiotic resistance among many bacterial pathogens. Examples include strains of *Campylobacter* resistant to quinolones and strains of *E. coli, Shigella,* and *Salmonella* resistant to trimethoprim-sulfamethoxazole.

Precautions

Although the mainstay of prevention of travelers' diarrhea involves food and water precautions, the literature has repeatedly documented dietary indiscretions by 98% of travelers within the first 72 h after arrival at

TABLE 4-2

MALARIA CHEMOSUPPRESSIVE REGIMENS ACCORDING TO GEOGRAPHIC AREA[a]

GEOGRAPHIC AREA	DRUG OF CHOICE	ALTERNATIVES
Central America (north of Panama), Haiti, Dominican Republic, Iraq, Egypt, Turkey, northern Argentina, and Paraguay	Chloroquine	Mefloquine Doxycycline Atovaquone/proguanil
South America including Panama (except northern Argentina and Paraguay); Asia (including Southeast Asia); Africa; and Oceania	Mefloquine Doxycycline Atovaquone-proguanil (Malarone)	Primaquine
Thai-Myanmar and Thai-Cambodian borders	Doxycycline Atovaquone-proguanil (Malarone)	

[a]See CDC's *Health Information for International Travel 2005–2006*.
Note: See also Chap. 116.

their destination. The maxim "Boil it, cook it, peel it, or forget it!" is easy to remember, but apparently difficult to follow. General food and water precautions include eating foods piping hot; avoiding foods that are raw, poorly cooked, or sold by street vendors; and drinking only boiled or commercially bottled beverages, particularly those that are carbonated. Heating kills diarrhea-causing organisms, whereas freezing does not; therefore, ice cubes made from unpurified water should be avoided.

Self-Treatment

(See also Table 25-5) As travelers' diarrhea often occurs despite rigorous food and water precautions, travelers should carry medications for self-treatment. An antibiotic is useful in reducing the frequency of bowel movements and duration of illness in moderate to severe diarrhea. The standard regimen is a 3-day course of a quinolone taken twice daily (or, in the case of some newer formulations, once daily). However, studies have shown that a single double dose of a quinolone may be equally effective. For diarrhea acquired in areas such as Thailand, where >90% of *Campylobacter* infections are quinolone resistant, azithromycin may be a better alternative. Rifaximin, a poorly absorbed rifampin derivative, is highly effective against noninvasive bacterial pathogens such as toxigenic and enteroaggregative *E. coli*.

The current approach to self-treatment of travelers' diarrhea is for the traveler to carry three once-daily doses of an antibiotic and to use as many doses as necessary to resolve the illness. If neither high fever nor blood in the stool accompanies the diarrhea, loperamide may be taken in combination with the antibiotic.

Prophylaxis

Prophylaxis of travelers' diarrhea with bismuth subsalicylate is widely used but is only ~60% effective. For certain individuals (e.g., athletes, persons with a repeated history of travelers' diarrhea, and persons with chronic diseases), a single daily dose of a quinolone or azithromycin or a once-daily rifaximin regimen during travel of <1 month's duration is 75–90% efficacious in preventing travelers' diarrhea.

Illness after Return

Although extremely common, acute travelers' diarrhea is usually self-limited or amenable to antibiotic therapy. Persistent bowel problems after the traveler returns home have a less well-defined etiology and may require medical attention from a specialist. Infectious agents (e.g., *Giardia lamblia*, *Cyclospora cayetanensis*, *Entamoeba histolytica*) appear to be responsible for only a small proportion of cases with persistent bowel symptoms. By far the most frequent causes of persistent diarrhea after travel are postinfectious sequelae such as lactose intolerance or irritable bowel syndrome. A recent meta-analysis showed that postinfectious irritable bowel syndrome may occur in as many as 4–13% of cases. When no infectious etiology can be identified, a trial of metronidazole therapy for presumed giardiasis, a strict lactose-free diet for 1 week, or a several-week trial of high-dose hydrophilic mucilloid (plus lactulose for persons with constipation) relieves the symptoms of many patients.

PREVENTION OF OTHER TRAVEL-RELATED PROBLEMS

Travelers are at high risk for *sexually transmitted diseases* (Chap. 28). Surveys have shown that large numbers engage in casual sex, and there is a reluctance to use condoms consistently. An increasing number of travelers are being diagnosed with *schistosomiasis* (Chap. 126). Travelers should be cautioned to avoid bathing, swimming, or wading in freshwater lakes, streams, or rivers in parts of tropical South America, the Caribbean, Africa, and Southeast Asia. Prevention of *travel-associated injury* depends mostly on common-sense precautions. Riding on motorcycles (especially without helmets) and in overcrowded public vehicles is not recommended; individuals should not travel in developing countries by road after dark, particularly in rural areas. In addition to its association with motor vehicle accidents, excessive alcohol use has been a significant factor in drownings, assaults, and injuries. Travelers are cautioned to avoid walking barefoot because of the risk of hookworm and *Strongyloides* infections (Chap. 124) and snakebites.

THE TRAVELER'S MEDICAL KIT

A traveler's medical kit is strongly advisable. The contents may vary widely, depending on the itinerary, duration of stay, style of travel, and local medical facilities. Although many medications are available abroad (often over the counter), directions for their use may be nonexistent or in a foreign language, or a product may be outdated or counterfeit. For example, a recent multicountry study in Southeast Asia showed that a mean of 53% (range, 21–92%) of antimalarial products were counterfeit or contained inadequate amounts of active drug. In the medical kit, the short-term traveler should consider carrying an analgesic; an antidiarrheal agent and an antibiotic for self-treatment of travelers' diarrhea; antihistamines; a laxative; oral rehydration salts; a sunscreen with a skin-protection factor of at least 30; a DEET-containing insect repellent for the skin; an insecticide for clothing (permethrin); and, if necessary, an antimalarial drug. To these medications, the long-stay traveler might add a broad-spectrum general-purpose antibiotic (levofloxacin or azithromycin), an antibacterial eye and skin ointment, and a topical antifungal cream. Regardless of the duration of travel, a first-aid kit containing such items as scissors, tweezers, and bandages should be considered. A practical approach to self-treatment of infections in the long-stay traveler who carries a once-daily dose of antibiotics is to use 3 tablets "below the waist" (bowel and bladder infections) and 6 tablets "above the waist" (skin and respiratory infections).

TRAVEL AND SPECIAL HOSTS

PREGNANCY AND TRAVEL

A woman's medical history and itinerary, the quality of medical care at her destinations, and her degree of flexibility determine whether travel is wise during pregnancy. According to the American College of Obstetrics and Gynecology, the safest part of pregnancy in which to travel is between 18 and 24 weeks, when there is the least danger of spontaneous abortion or premature labor. Some obstetricians prefer that women stay within a few hundred miles of home after the 28th week of pregnancy in case problems arise. In general, however, healthy women may be advised that it is acceptable to travel.

Relative contraindications to international travel during pregnancy include a history of miscarriage, premature labor, incompetent cervix, or toxemia. General medical problems such as diabetes, heart failure, severe anemia, or a history of thromboembolic disease should also prompt the pregnant woman to postpone her travels. Finally, regions in which the pregnant woman and her fetus may be at excessive risk (e.g., those at high altitudes and those where live-virus vaccines are required or where multidrug-resistant malaria is endemic) are not ideal destinations during any trimester.

Malaria

Malaria during pregnancy carries a significant risk of morbidity and death. Levels of parasitemia are highest and failure to clear the parasites after treatment is most frequent among primigravidae. Severe disease, with complications such as cerebral malaria, massive hemolysis, and renal failure, is especially likely in pregnancy. Fetal sequelae include spontaneous abortion, stillbirth, preterm delivery, and congenital infection.

Travelers' Diarrhea

Pregnant travelers must be extremely cautious regarding their food and beverage intake. Dehydration due to travelers' diarrhea can lead to inadequate placental blood flow. Infections such as toxoplasmosis, hepatitis E, and listeriosis can also have serious sequelae in pregnancy.

The mainstay of therapy for travelers' diarrhea is rehydration. Loperamide may be used if necessary. For self-treatment, azithromycin may be the best option. Although quinolones are increasingly being used safely during pregnancy and rifaximin is poorly absorbed from the gastrointestinal tract, they are not approved for this indication.

Because of the major problems encountered when infants are given local foods and beverages, women are strongly encouraged to breast-feed when traveling with a neonate. A nursing mother with travelers' diarrhea should not stop breast-feeding, but should increase her fluid intake.

Air Travel and High-Altitude Destinations

Commercial air travel is not a risk to the healthy pregnant woman or to the fetus. The higher radiation levels reported at altitudes of >10,500 m (>35,000 ft) should pose no problem to the healthy pregnant traveler. Since each airline has a policy regarding pregnancy and flying, it is best to check with the specific carrier when booking reservations. Domestic air travel is usually permitted until the 36th week, whereas international air travel is generally curtailed after the 32nd week.

There are no known risks for pregnant women who travel to high-altitude destinations and stay for short periods. However, there are likewise no data on the safety of pregnant women at altitudes of >4500 m (15,000 ft).

THE HIV-INFECTED TRAVELER

(See also Chap. 90) The HIV-infected traveler is at special risk of serious infections due to a number of pathogens that may be more prevalent at travel destinations than at home. However, the degree of risk depends primarily on the state of the immune system at the time of travel. For persons whose CD4+ T cell counts are normal or >500/μL, no data suggest a greater risk during travel than for persons without HIV infection. Individuals with AIDS (CD4+ T cell counts of <200/μL) and others who are symptomatic need special counseling and should visit a travel medicine practitioner before departure, especially when traveling to the developing world.

Several countries now routinely deny entry to HIV-positive individuals, even though these restrictions do not appear to decrease rates of transmission of the virus. In general, HIV testing is required of those individuals who wish to stay abroad >3 months or who intend to work or study abroad. Some countries will accept an HIV serologic test done within 6 months of departure, whereas others will not accept a blood test done at any time in the traveler's home country. Border officials often have the authority to make inquiries of individuals entering a country and to check the medications they are carrying. If a drug such as zidovudine is identified, the person may be barred from entering the country. Information on testing requirements for specific countries is available from consular offices but is subject to frequent change.

Immunizations

All of the HIV-infected traveler's routine immunizations should be up to date (Chap. 3). The response to immunization may be impaired at CD4+ T cell counts of <200/μL (and in some cases at even higher counts). Thus HIV-infected persons should be vaccinated as early as possible to ensure adequate immune responses to all vaccines. In patients receiving highly active antiretroviral therapy, at least 3 months must elapse before regenerated CD4+ T cells can be considered fully functional; therefore, in these patients, vaccinations should be delayed. However, when the risk of illness is high or the sequelae of illness are serious, immunization is recommended. In certain circumstances, it may be prudent to check the adequacy of the serum antibody response before departure.

Because of the increased risk of infections due to *Streptococcus pneumoniae* and other bacterial pathogens that cause pneumonia after influenza, pneumococcal polysaccharide and influenza vaccines should be administered. The estimated rates of response to influenza vaccine are

>80% among persons with asymptomatic HIV infection and <50% among those with AIDS.

In general, live attenuated vaccines are contraindicated for persons with immune dysfunction. Because measles (rubeola) can be a severe and lethal infection in HIV-positive patients, these patients should receive the measles vaccine (or the combination measles-mumps-rubella vaccine) unless the CD4+ T cell count is <200/μL. Between 18% and 58% of symptomatic HIV-infected vaccinees develop adequate antibody titers, and 50–100% of asymptomatic HIV-infected persons seroconvert.

It is recommended that the live yellow fever vaccine not be given to HIV-infected travelers. Although the potential adverse effects of a live vaccine in an HIV-infected individual are always a consideration, there appear to have been no reported cases of illness in those who have inadvertently received this vaccine. Nonetheless, if the CD4+ T cell count is <200/μL, an alternative itinerary that poses no risk of exposure to yellow fever is recommended. If the traveler is passing through or traveling to an area where the vaccine is required but the disease risk is low, a physician's waiver should be issued.

A transient increase in viremia (lasting days to weeks) has been demonstrated in HIV-infected individuals after immunization against influenza, pneumococcal infection, and tetanus (Chap. 90). However, at this point, there is no evidence that this transient increase is detrimental.

Gastrointestinal Illness

Decreased levels of gastric acid, abnormal gastrointestinal mucosal immunity, other complications of HIV infection, and medications taken by HIV-infected patients make travelers' diarrhea especially problematic in these individuals. Travelers' diarrhea is likely to occur more frequently, be more severe, be accompanied by bacteremia, and be more difficult to treat. Although uncommon, *Cryptosporidium, Isospora belli, and Microsporidium* infections are associated with increased morbidity and mortality in AIDS patients.

The HIV-infected traveler must be careful to consume only appropriately prepared foods and beverages and may benefit from antibiotic prophylaxis for travelers' diarrhea. Sulfonamides (as used to prevent pneumocystosis) are ineffective because of widespread resistance.

Other Travel-Related Infections

Data are lacking on the severity of many vector-borne diseases in HIV-infected individuals. Malaria is especially severe in asplenic persons and in those with AIDS. The HIV load doubles during malaria, with subsidence in ~8–9 weeks; the significance of this increase in viral load is unknown.

Visceral leishmaniasis (Chap. 119) has been reported in numerous HIV-infected travelers. Diagnosis may be difficult, given that splenomegaly and hyperglobulinemia are often lacking and serologic results are frequently negative. Sandfly bites may be prevented by evening use of insect repellents.

Certain respiratory illnesses, such as histoplasmosis and coccidioidomycosis, cause greater morbidity and mortality among patients with AIDS. Although tuberculosis is common among HIV-infected persons (especially in developing countries), its acquisition by the short-term HIV-infected traveler has not been reported as a major problem.

Medications

Adverse events due to medications and drug interactions are common and raise complex issues for HIV-infected persons. Rates of cutaneous reaction (e.g., increased cutaneous sensitivity to sulfonamides) are unusually high among patients with AIDS. Since zidovudine is metabolized by hepatic glucuronidation, inhibitors of this process may elevate serum levels of the drug. Concomitant administration of the antimalarial drug mefloquine and the antiretroviral agent ritonavir may result in decreased plasma levels of ritonavir. In contrast, no significant influence of concomitant mefloquine administration on plasma levels of indinavir or nelfinavir was detected in two HIV-infected travelers. There is a strong theoretical concern that the antimalarial drugs lumefantrine (combined with artemisinin in Coartem and Riamet) and halofantrine may interact with HIV protease inhibitors and nonnucleoside reverse transcriptase inhibitors since the latter are known to be potent inhibitors of cytochrome P450.

CHRONIC ILLNESS, DISABILITY, AND TRAVEL

Chronic health problems need not prevent travel, but special measures can make the journey safer and more comfortable.

Heart Disease

Cardiovascular events are the main cause of deaths among travelers and of in-flight emergencies on commercial aircraft. Extra supplies of all medications should be kept in carry-on luggage, along with a copy of a recent electrocardiogram and the name and telephone number of the traveler's physician at home. Pacemakers are not affected by airport security devices, although electronic telephone checks of pacemaker function cannot be transmitted by international satellites. Travelers with electronic defibrillators should carry a note to that effect and ask for hand screening. A traveler may benefit from supplemental oxygen; since oxygen delivery systems are not standard, supplementary oxygen should be ordered by the traveler's physician well before flight time. Travelers may benefit from aisle seating and should walk, perform stretching and flexing exercises, consider wearing support hose, and remain hydrated during the flight to prevent venous thrombosis and pulmonary embolism.

Chronic Lung Disease

Chronic obstructive pulmonary disease is one of the most common diagnoses in patients who require emergency-department evaluation for symptoms occurring during airline flights. The best predictor of the development of in-flight problems is the sea-level PaO_2. A PaO_2 of at least 72 mmHg corresponds to an in-flight arterial PaO_2 of ~55 mmHg when the cabin is pressurized to 2500 m (8000 ft). If the traveler's baseline PaO_2 is <72 mmHg, the provision of supplemental oxygen should be considered. Contraindications to flight include active bronchospasm, lower respiratory infection, lower-limb deep-vein phlebitis, pulmonary hypertension, and recent thoracic surgery (within the preceding 3 weeks) or pneumothorax. Decreased outdoor activity at the destination should be considered if air pollution is excessive.

Diabetes Mellitus

Alterations in glucose control and changes in insulin requirements are common problems among patients with diabetes who travel. Changes in time zone, in the amount and timing of food intake, and in physical activity demand vigilant assessment of metabolic control. The traveler with diabetes should pack medication (including a bottle of regular insulin for emergencies), insulin syringes and needles, equipment and supplies for glucose monitoring, and snacks in carry-on luggage. Insulin is stable for ~3 months at room temperature but should be kept as cool as possible. The name and telephone number of the home physician and a card and bracelet listing the patient's medical problems and the type and dose of insulin used should accompany the traveler. In traveling eastward (e.g., from the United States to Europe), the morning insulin dose on arrival may need to be decreased. The blood glucose can then be checked during the day to determine whether additional insulin is required. For flights westward, with lengthening of the day, an additional dose of regular insulin may be required.

Other Special Groups

Other groups for whom special travel measures are encouraged include patients undergoing dialysis, those with transplants, and those with other disabilities. Up to 13% of travelers have some disability, but few advocacy groups and tour companies dedicate themselves to this growing population. Medication interactions are a source of serious concern for these travelers, and appropriate medical information should be carried, along with the home physician's name and telephone number. Some travelers taking glucocorticoids carry stress doses in case they become ill. Immunization of these immunocompromised travelers may result in less than adequate protection. Thus the traveler and the physician must carefully consider which destinations are appropriate.

PROBLEMS AFTER RETURN

The most common medical problems encountered by travelers after their return home are diarrhea, fever, respiratory illnesses, and skin diseases (Fig. 4-2). Frequently ignored problems are fatigue and emotional stress, especially in long-stay travelers. The approach to diagnosis requires some knowledge of geographic medicine, in particular, the epidemiology and clinical presentation of infectious disorders. A geographic history should focus on the traveler's exact itinerary, including dates of arrival and departure; exposure history (food indiscretions, drinking-water sources, freshwater contact, sexual activity, animal contact, insect bites); location and style of travel (urban vs rural, first-class hotel accommodation vs camping); immunization history; and use of antimalarial chemosuppression.

DIARRHEA

See "Prevention of Gastrointestinal Illness" earlier in the chapter.

FEVER

Fever in a traveler who has returned from a malarious area should be considered a medical emergency because death from *P. falciparum* malaria can follow an illness of only several days' duration. Although "fever from the tropics" does not always have a tropical cause, malaria should be the first diagnosis considered. The risk of *P. falciparum* malaria is highest among travelers returning from Africa or Oceania and among those who become symptomatic within the first 2 months after return. Other important causes of fever after travel include viral hepatitis (hepatitis A and E), typhoid fever, bacterial enteritis, arboviral infections (e.g., dengue fever), rickettsial infections (including tick and scrub typhus and Q fever), and—in rare instances—leptospirosis, acute HIV infection, and amebic liver abscess. A cooperative study by GeoSentinel (an emerging infectious disease surveillance group established by the CDC and the International Society of Travel Medicine) showed that, among 3907 febrile returned travelers, malaria was acquired most often from Africa, dengue from Southeast Asia and the Caribbean, typhoid fever from southern Asia, and rickettsial infections (tick typhus) from southern Africa (Table 4-3). In at least 25% of cases, no etiology can be found, and the illness resolves spontaneously. Clinicians should keep in mind that no present-day antimalarial agent guarantees protection from malaria and that some immunizations (notably, that against typhoid fever) are only partially protective.

When no specific diagnosis is forthcoming, the following investigations, where applicable, are suggested: complete blood count, liver function tests, thick/thin blood films for malaria (repeated twice if necessary), urinalysis, urine and blood cultures (repeated once), chest x-ray, and collection of an acute-phase serum sample to be held for subsequent examination along with a paired convalescent-phase serum sample.

SKIN DISEASES

Pyodermas, sunburn, insect bites, skin ulcers, and cutaneous larva migrans are the most common skin conditions affecting travelers after their return home. In those with persistent skin ulcers, a diagnosis of cutaneous

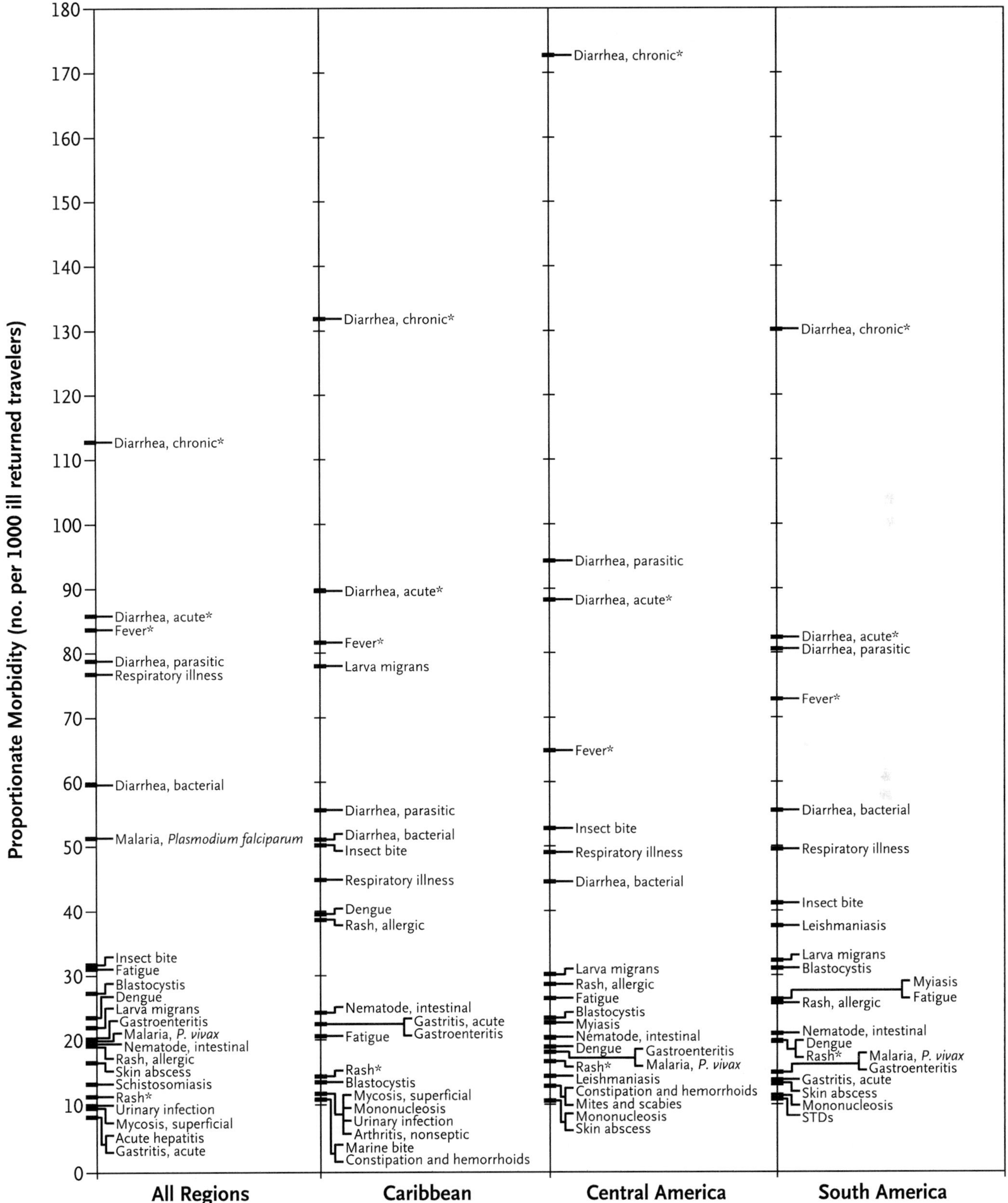

FIGURE 4-2

Proportionate morbidity among ill travelers returning from the developing world, according to region of travel. The proportions (not incidence rates) are shown for each of the top 22 specific diagnoses among all ill returned travelers within each region.

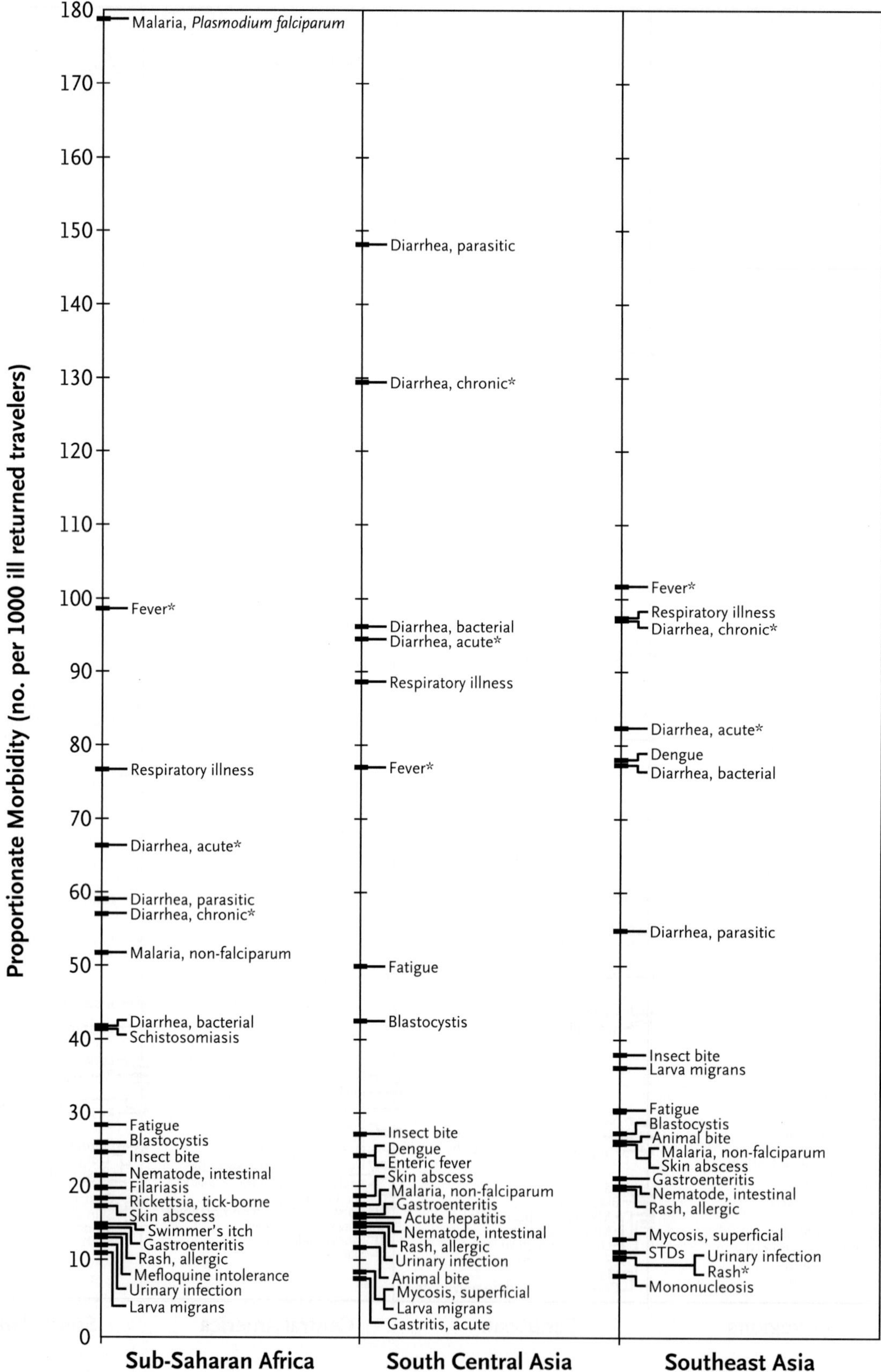

FIGURE 4-2 (*CONTINUED*)
STDs, sexually transmitted diseases. Asterisks indicate syndromic diagnoses for which specific etiologies could not be assigned. (*Reprinted with permission from Freedman et al. © 2006 Massachusetts Medical Society.*)

TABLE 4-3

ETIOLOGY AND GEOGRAPHIC DISTRIBUTION (PERCENT) OF SYSTEMIC FEBRILE ILLNESS IN RETURNED TRAVELERS (*N* = 3907)

ETIOLOGY	CARIB	CAM	SAM	SSA	SCA	SEA
Malaria	<1	13	13	**62**	14	13
Dengue	**23**	12	14	<1	14	**32**
Mononucleosis	7	7	8	1	2	3
Rickettsia	0	0	0	**6**	1	2
Salmonella	2	3	2	<1	**14**	3

Note: Carib, Caribbean; CAm, Central America; SAm, South America; SSA, Sub-Saharan Africa; SCA, South Central Asia; SEA, Southeast Asia. Bold type is for emphasis only.
Source: Revised from Table 2 in Freedman et al, 2006. Used with permission from the Massachusetts Medical Society.

leishmaniasis, mycobacterial infection, or fungal infection should be considered. Careful, complete inspection of the skin is important in detecting the rickettsial eschar in a febrile patient or the central breathing hole in a "boil" due to myiasis.

EMERGING INFECTIOUS DISEASES

In recent years, travel and commerce have fostered the worldwide spread of HIV infection, led to the reemergence of cholera as a global health threat, and created considerable fear about the possible spread of severe acute respiratory syndrome (SARS) and avian influenza (H5N1). For travelers, there are more realistic concerns. One of the largest outbreaks of dengue fever ever documented is now raging in Latin America; schistosomiasis is being described in previously unaffected lakes in Africa; and antibiotic-resistant strains of sexually transmitted and enteric pathogens are emerging at an alarming rate in the developing world. In addition, concerns have been raised about the potential for bioterrorism involving not only standard strains of unusual agents but mutant strains as well. Time will tell whether travelers (as well as persons at home) will routinely be vaccinated against diseases such as anthrax and smallpox. As Nobel laureate Dr. Joshua Lederberg pointed out, "The microbe that felled one child in a distant continent yesterday can reach yours today and seed a global pandemic tomorrow." The vigilant clinician understands that the importance of a thorough travel history cannot be overemphasized.

FURTHER READINGS

Chen LH, Keystone JS: New strategies for the prevention of malaria in travelers. Infect Dis Clin North Am 19:185, 2005

DuPont AW, DuPont HL: Travelers' diarrhea: Modern concepts and new developments. Curr Treat Options Gastroenterol 9:13, 2006

Freedman DO et al (GeoSentinel Surveillance Network): Spectrum of disease and relation to place of exposure among ill returned travelers. N Engl J Med 354:119, 2006

Keystone JS et al: *Travel Medicine*. Philadelphia, Mosby, 2004

Meltzer E et al: Eosinophilia among returning travelers: A practical approach. Am J Trop Med Hyg 78:702, 2008

Okhuysen PC: Current concepts in travelers' diarrhea: Epidemiology, antimicrobial resistance and treatment. Curr Opin Infect Dis 18: 522, 2005

Ryan ET et al: Illness after international travel. N Engl J Med 347: 505, 2002

Shlim DR: Update in traveler's diarrhea. Infect Dis Clin North Am 19:137, 2005

Sohail MR, Fischer PR: Health risks to air travelers. Infect Dis Clin North Am 19:67, 2005

Wilson ME, Chen LH: Dermatologic infectious diseases in international travelers. Curr Infect Dis Rep 6:54, 2004

Websites of Interest: Chronic renal failure: *www.kidney.org*. Diabetes: *www.diabetesmonitor.com/other-14.htm*. Dialysis: *www. dialysisfinder.com*. Disability: *www.access-able.com*. HIV: *www.aegis.com*.

CHAPTER 5

LABORATORY DIAGNOSIS OF INFECTIOUS DISEASES

Alexander J. McAdam ■ Andrew B. Onderdonk

The laboratory diagnosis of infection requires the demonstration—either direct or indirect—of viral, bacterial, fungal, or parasitic agents in tissues, fluids, or excreta of the host. Clinical microbiology laboratories are responsible for processing these specimens and also for determining the antibiotic susceptibility of bacterial and fungal pathogens. Traditionally, detection of pathogenic agents has relied largely on either the microscopic visualization of pathogens in clinical material or the growth of microorganisms in the laboratory. Identification is generally based on phenotypic characteristics, such as fermentation profiles for bacteria, cytopathic effects in tissue culture for viral agents, and microscopic morphology for fungi and parasites. These techniques are reliable but are often time-consuming. Increasingly, the use of nucleic acid probes is becoming a standard method for detection, quantitation, and/or identification in the clinical microbiology laboratory, gradually replacing phenotypic characterization and microscopic visualization methods.

DETECTION METHODS

Reappraisal of the methods employed in the clinical microbiology laboratory has led to the development of strategies for detection of pathogenic agents through nonvisual biologic signal detection systems. Much of this methodology is based on the use of either electronic detection systems involving relatively inexpensive but sophisticated computers or nucleic acid probes directed at specific DNA or RNA targets. This chapter discusses both the methods that are currently available and those that are being developed.

BIOLOGIC SIGNALS

A *biologic signal* is a material that can be reproducibly differentiated from other substances present in the same physical environment. Key issues in the use of a biologic (or electronic) signal are distinguishing it from background noise and translating it into meaningful information. Examples of biologic signals applicable to clinical microbiology include structural components of bacteria, fungi, and viruses; specific antigens; metabolic end products; unique DNA or RNA base sequences; enzymes; toxins or other proteins; and surface polysaccharides.

DETECTION SYSTEMS

A detector is used to sense a signal and to discriminate between the signal and background noise. Detection systems range from the trained eyes of a technologist assessing morphologic variations to sensitive electronic instruments, such as gas-liquid chromatographs coupled to computer systems for signal analysis. The sensitivity with which signals can be detected varies widely. It is essential to use a detection system that discerns small amounts of signal even when biologic background noise is present—i.e., that is both sensitive and specific. Common detection systems include immunofluorescence, chemiluminescence for DNA/RNA probes, flame ionization detection of short- or long-chain fatty acids, and detection of substrate utilization or end-product formation as color changes, of enzyme activity as a change in light absorbance, of turbidity changes as a measure of growth, of cytopathic effects in cell lines, and of particle agglutination as a measure of antigen presence.

AMPLIFICATION

Amplification enhances the sensitivity with which weak signals can be detected. The most common microbiologic amplification technique is growth of a single bacterium into a discrete colony on an agar plate or into a suspension containing many identical organisms. The advantage of growth as an amplification method is that it requires only an appropriate growth medium; the disadvantage is the amount of time required for amplification. More rapid specific amplification of biologic signals can be achieved with techniques such as polymerase chain reaction (PCR) or ligase chain reaction (LCR, for DNA/RNA), enzyme immunoassays (EIAs, for antigens and antibodies), electronic amplification (for gas-liquid chromatography assays), antibody capture methods (for concentration and/or separation), and selective filtration or centrifugation. Although a variety of methods are available for the amplification and detection of biologic signals in research, thorough testing is required before these methods are validated as diagnostic assays.

DIRECT DETECTION

MICROSCOPY

The field of microbiology has been defined largely by the development and use of the microscope. The examination of specimens by microscopic methods rapidly provides useful diagnostic information. Staining techniques permit organisms to be seen more clearly.

The simplest method for microscopic evaluation is the wet mount, which is used, for example, to examine cerebrospinal fluid (CSF) for the presence of *Cryptococcus neoformans*, with India ink as a background against which to visualize large-capsuled yeast cells. Wet mounts with dark-field illumination are also used to detect spirochetes from genital lesions and to reveal *Borrelia* or *Leptospira* in blood. Skin scrapings and hair samples can be examined with use of either 10% KOH wet-mount preparations or the calcofluor white method and ultraviolet illumination to detect fungal elements as fluorescing structures. Staining of wet mounts—e.g., with lactophenol cotton blue stain for fungal elements—is often used for morphologic identification. These techniques enhance signal detection and decrease the background, making it easier to identify specific fungal structures.

STAINING

Gram's Stain

Without staining, bacteria are difficult to see at the magnifications (400× to 1000×) used for their detection. Although simple one-step stains can be used, differential stains are more common. Gram's stain differentiates between organisms with thick peptidoglycan cell walls (gram-positive) and those with thin peptidoglycan cell walls and outer membranes that can be dissolved with alcohol or acetone (gram-negative). Cellular morphology and Gram's stain characteristics can often be used to categorize stained organisms into groups such as streptococci, staphylococci, and clostridia (Fig. 5-1).

Gram's stain is particularly useful for examining sputum for polymorphonuclear leukocytes (PMNs) and bacteria. Sputum specimens from immunocompetent patients with ≥25 PMNs and <10 epithelial cells per low-power field often provide clinically useful information. However, the presence in "sputum" samples of >10 epithelial cells per low-power field and of multiple bacterial types suggests contamination with oral microflora. Despite the difficulty of discriminating between normal microflora and pathogens, Gram's stain may prove useful for specimens from areas with a large resident microflora if a useful biologic marker (signal) is available. Gram's staining of vaginal swab specimens can be used to detect epithelial cells covered with gram-positive bacteria in the absence of lactobacilli and the presence of gram-negative rods—a scenario regarded as a sign of bacterial vaginosis. Similarly, examination of stained stool specimens for leukocytes is useful as a screening procedure before testing for *Clostridium difficile* toxin or other enteric pathogens.

The examination of CSF and joint, pleural, or peritoneal fluid with Gram's stain is useful for determining whether bacteria and/or PMNs are present. The sensitivity is such that $>10^4$ bacteria per milliliter should be detected. Centrifugation is often performed before staining to concentrate specimens thought to contain low numbers of organisms. The pellet is examined after staining. This simple method is particularly useful for examination of CSF for bacteria and white blood cells or of sputum for acid-fast bacilli (AFB).

Gram-Negative Organisms

	GRx only	Oxidase +	Oxidase –	Fastidious	Anaerobic	Curved
Rod		*Pseudomonas* *Aeromonas* *Pasteurella* Others	Enterobacteriaceae Others	*Haemophilus* *Legionella* *Bordetella* *Brucella* *Francisella* Others	*Bacteroides* *Prevotella* *Fusobacterium* Others	*Vibrio* *Campylobacter*
Coccus	*Neisseria* *Branhamella*				*Veillonella* *Acidaminococcus* *Megasphaera*	

Gram-Positive Organisms

	Branching	Spores	Acid-Fast	Catalase +	Catalase –
Rod	*Nocardia* *Actinomyces* *Bifidobacterium*	*Clostridium* *Bacillus*	*Mycobacterium*	*Corynebacterium* *Listeria* Others	*Lactobacillus* Others
Coccus				*Staphylococcus* *Micrococcus* Others	*Streptococcus*

FIGURE 5-1
Interpretation of Gram's stain.

Acid-Fast Stain

The acid-fast stain identifies organisms that retain carbol fuchsin dye after acid/organic solvent disruption (e.g., *Mycobacterium* spp.). Modifications of this procedure allow the differentiation of *Actinomyces* from *Nocardia* or other weakly (or partially) acid-fast organisms. The acid-fast stain is applied to sputum, other fluids, and tissue samples when AFB (e.g., *Mycobacterium* spp.) are suspected. The identification of the pink/red AFB against the blue background of the counterstain requires a trained eye, since few AFB may be detected in an entire smear, even when the specimen has been concentrated by centrifugation. An alternative method is the auramine-rhodamine combination fluorescent dye technique.

Fluorochrome Stains

Fluorochrome stains, such as acridine orange, are used to identify white blood cells, yeasts, and bacteria in body fluids. Other specialized stains, such as Dappe's stain, may be used for the detection of mycoplasmas in cell cultures. Capsular, flagellar, and spore stains are used for identification or demonstration of characteristic structures.

Immunofluorescent Stains

The *direct* immunofluorescent antibody technique uses antibody coupled to a fluorescing compound, such as fluorescein, and directed at a specific antigenic target to visualize organisms or subcellular structures. When samples are examined under appropriate conditions, the fluorescing compound absorbs ultraviolet light and reemits light at a higher wavelength visible to the human eye. In the *indirect* immunofluorescent antibody technique, an unlabeled (target) antibody binds a specific antigen. The specimen is then stained with fluorescein-labeled polyclonal antibody directed at the target antibody. Because each unlabeled target antibody attached to the appropriate antigen has multiple sites for attachment of the second antibody, the visual signal can be intensified (i.e., amplified). This form of staining is called *indirect* because a two-antibody system is used to generate the signal for detection of the antigen. Both direct and indirect methods detect viral antigens (e.g., cytomegalovirus, herpes simplex virus, and respiratory viruses) within cultured cells or clinical specimens as well as many difficult-to-grow bacterial agents (e.g., *Legionella pneumophila*) directly in clinical specimens.

MACROSCOPIC ANTIGEN DETECTION

Latex agglutination assays and EIAs are rapid and inexpensive methods for identifying organisms, extracellular toxins, and viral agents by means of protein and polysaccharide antigens. Such assays may be performed directly on clinical samples or after growth of organisms on agar plates or in viral cell cultures. The biologic signal in each case is the antigen to be detected. Monoclonal or polyclonal antibodies coupled to a reporter (such as latex particles or an enzyme) are used for detection of antibody-antigen binding reactions.

Techniques such as direct agglutination of bacterial cells with specific antibody are simple but relatively insensitive, whereas latex agglutination and EIAs are more sensitive. Some cell-associated antigens, such as capsular polysaccharides and lipopolysaccharides, can be detected by agglutination of a suspension of bacterial cells when antibody is added; this method is useful for typing of the somatic antigens of *Shigella* and *Salmonella*. In systems such as EIAs, which employ antibodies coupled to an enzyme, an antigen-antibody reaction results in the conversion of a colorless substrate to a colored product. Because the coupling of an enzyme to the antibody can amplify a weak biologic signal, the sensitivity of such assays is often high. In each instance, the basis for antigen detection is antigen-antibody binding, with the detection system changed to accommodate the biologic signal. Most such assays provide information as to whether antigen is present but do not quantify the antigen. EIAs are also useful for detecting bacterial toxins—e.g., *C. difficile* toxins A and B in stool.

Rapid and simple tests for antigens of group A *Streptococcus*, influenza virus, and respiratory syncytial virus can be used in the clinic setting, without a specialized diagnostic laboratory. Such tests are usually reasonably specific but may have only modest sensitivity.

DETECTION OF PATHOGENIC AGENTS BY CULTURE

SPECIMEN COLLECTION AND TRANSPORT

To culture bacterial, mycotic, or viral pathogens, an appropriate sample must be placed into the proper medium for growth (amplification). The success of efforts to identify a specific pathogen often depends on the collection and transport process coupled to a laboratory-processing algorithm suitable for the specific sample/agent. In some instances, it is better for specimens to be plated at the time of collection rather than first being transported to the laboratory (e.g., urethral swabs being cultured for *Neisseria gonorrhoeae* or sputum specimens for pneumococci). In general, the more rapidly a specimen is plated onto appropriate media, the better the chance for isolating bacterial pathogens. Deep tissue or fluid (pus) samples are more likely to give useful culture results than are superficial swab specimens. Table 5-1 lists procedures for collection and transport of common specimens. Because there are many pathogen-specific paradigms for these procedures, it is important to seek advice from the microbiology laboratory when in doubt about a particular situation.

ISOLATION OF BACTERIAL PATHOGENS

Isolation of suspect pathogens from clinical material relies on the use of artificial media that support bacterial growth in vitro. Such media are composed of agar, which is not metabolized by bacteria; nutrients to support the growth of the species of interest; and sometimes substances to inhibit the growth of other bacteria. Broth is employed for growth (amplification) of organisms from specimens with few bacteria, such as peritoneal dialysis fluid, CSF, or samples in which anaerobes or other fastidious organisms may be present. The

TABLE 5-1

INSTRUCTIONS FOR COLLECTION AND TRANSPORT OF SPECIMENS FOR CULTURE

TYPE OF CULTURE (SYNONYMS)	SPECIMEN	MINIMUM VOLUME	CONTAINER	OTHER CONSIDERATIONS
Blood				
Blood, routine (blood culture for aerobes, anaerobes, and yeasts)	Whole blood	10 mL in each of 2 bottles for adults and children; 5 mL, if possible, in aerobic bottles for infants; less for neonates	See below.[a]	See below.[b]
Blood for fungi/ *Mycobacterium* spp.	Whole blood	10 mL in each of 2 bottles, as for routine blood cultures, or in Isolator tube requested from laboratory	Same as for routine blood culture	Specify "hold for extended incubation," since fungal agents may require ≥4 weeks to grow.
Blood, Isolator (lysis centrifugation)	Whole blood	10 mL	Isolator tubes	Use mainly for isolation of fungi, *Mycobacterium,* or other fastidious aerobes and for elimination of antibiotics from cultured blood in which organisms are concentrated by centrifugation.
Respiratory Tract				
Nose	Swab from nares	1 swab	Sterile culturette or similar transport system containing holding medium	Swabs made of calcium alginate may be used.
Throat	Swab of posterior pharynx, ulcerations, or areas of suspected purulence	1 swab	Sterile culturette or similar swab specimen collection system containing holding medium	See below.[c]
Sputum	Fresh sputum (not saliva)	2 mL	Commercially available sputum collection system or similar sterile container with screw cap	*Cause for rejection:* Care must be taken to ensure that the specimen is sputum and not saliva. Examination of Gram's stain, with number of epithelial cells and PMNs noted, can be an important part of the evaluation process. Induced sputum specimens should not be rejected.
Bronchial aspirates	Transtracheal aspirate, bronchoscopy specimen, or bronchial aspirate	1 mL of aspirate or brush in transport medium	Sterile aspirate or bronchoscopy tube, bronchoscopy brush in a separate sterile container	Special precautions may be required, depending on diagnostic considerations (e.g., *Pneumocystis*).

(*Continued*)

TABLE 5-1 (*CONTINUED*)

INSTRUCTIONS FOR COLLECTION AND TRANSPORT OF SPECIMENS FOR CULTURE

TYPE OF CULTURE (SYNONYMS)	SPECIMEN	MINIMUM VOLUME	CONTAINER	OTHER CONSIDERATIONS
Stool				
Stool for routine culture; stool for *Salmonella, Shigella,* and *Campylobacter*	Rectal swab or (preferably) fresh, randomly collected stool	1 g of stool or 2 rectal swabs	Plastic-coated cardboard cup or plastic cup with tight-fitting lid. Other leak-proof containers are also acceptable.	If *Vibrio* spp. are suspected, the laboratory must be notified, and appropriate collection/ transport methods should be used.
Stool for *Yersinia, E. coli* O157	Fresh, randomly collected stool	1 g	Plastic-coated cardboard cup or plastic cup with tight-fitting lid	*Limitations:* Procedure requires enrichment techniques.
Stool for *Aeromonas* and *Plesiomonas*	Fresh, randomly collected stool	1 g	Plastic-coated cardboard cup or plastic cup with tight-fitting lid	*Limitations:* Stool should not be cultured for these organisms unless also cultured for other enteric pathogens.
Urogenital Tract				
Urine	Clean-voided urine specimen or urine collected by catheter	0.5 mL	Sterile, leak-proof container with screw cap or special urine transfer tube	See below.[d]
Urogenital secretions	Vaginal or urethral secretions, cervical swabs, uterine fluid, prostatic fluid, etc.	1 swab or 0.5 mL of fluid	Vaginal and rectal swabs transported in Amies transport medium or similar holding medium for group B *Streptococcus*; direct inoculation preferred for *Neisseria gonorrhoeae*	Vaginal swab samples for "routine culture" should be discouraged whenever possible unless a particular pathogen is suspected. For detection of multiple organisms (e.g., group B *Streptococcus, Trichomonas, Chlamydia,* or *Candida* spp.), 1 swab per test should be obtained.
Body Fluids, Aspirates, and Tissues				
Cerebrospinal fluid (lumbar puncture)	Spinal fluid	1 mL for routine cultures; ≥5 mL for *Mycobacterium*	Sterile tube with tight-fitting cap	Do not refrigerate; transfer to laboratory as soon as possible.
Body fluids	Aseptically aspirated body fluids	1 mL for routine cultures	Sterile tube with tight-fitting cap. Specimen may be left in syringe used for collection if the syringe is capped before transport.	For some body fluids (e.g., peritoneal lavage samples), increased volumes are helpful for isolation of small numbers of bacteria.
Biopsy and aspirated materials	Tissue removed at surgery, bone, anticoagulated bone marrow, biopsy samples, or other specimens from normally sterile areas	1 mL of fluid or a 1-g piece of tissue	Sterile "culturette"-type swab or similar transport system containing holding medium. Sterile bottle or jar should be used for tissue specimens.	Accurate identification of specimen and source is critical. Enough tissue should be collected for both microbiologic and histopathologic evaluations.

Wounds	Purulent material or abscess contents obtained from wound or abscess without contamination by normal microflora	2 swabs or 0.5 mL of aspirated pus	Culturette swab or similar transport system or sterile tube with tight-fitting screw cap. For simultaneous anaerobic cultures, send specimen in anaerobic transport device or closed syringe.	*Collection:* Abscess contents or other fluids should be collected in a syringe (rather than with a swab) when possible to provide an adequate sample volume and an anaerobic environment.
Special Recommendations				
Fungi	Specimen types listed above may be used. When urine or sputum is cultured for fungi, a first-morning specimen is usually preferred.	1 mL or as specified above for individual listing of specimens. Large volumes may be useful for urinary fungi.	Sterile, leak-proof container with tight-fitting cap	*Collection:* Specimen should be transported to microbiology laboratory within 1 h of collection. Contamination with normal flora from skin, rectum, vaginal tract, or other body surfaces should be avoided.
Mycobacterium (acid-fast bacilli)	Sputum, tissue, urine, body fluids	10 mL of fluid or small piece of tissue. Swabs should not be used.	Sterile container with tight-fitting cap	Detection of *Mycobacterium* spp. is improved by use of concentration techniques. Smears and cultures of pleural, peritoneal, and pericardial fluids often have low yields. Multiple cultures from the same patient are encouraged. Culturing in liquid media shortens the time to detection.
Legionella	Pleural fluid, lung biopsy, bronchoalveolar lavage fluid, bronchial/transbronchial biopsy. Rapid transport to laboratory is critical.	1 mL of fluid; any size tissue sample, although a 0.5-g sample should be obtained when possible.	—	—
Anaerobic organisms	Aspirated specimens from abscesses or body fluids	1 mL of aspirated fluid, 1 g of tissue, or 2 swabs	An appropriate anaerobic transport device is required.[e]	Specimens cultured for obligate anaerobes should be cultured for facultative bacteria as well. Fluid or tissue is preferred to swabs.

(*Continued*)

TABLE 5-1 (*CONTINUED*)

INSTRUCTIONS FOR COLLECTION AND TRANSPORT OF SPECIMENS FOR CULTURE

TYPE OF CULTURE (SYNONYMS)	SPECIMEN	MINIMUM VOLUME	CONTAINER	OTHER CONSIDERATIONS
Special Recommendations (*Continued*)				
Viruses[f]	Respiratory secretions, wash aspirates from respiratory tract, nasal swabs, blood samples (including buffy coats), vaginal and rectal swabs, swab specimens from suspicious skin lesions, stool samples (in some cases)	1 mL of fluid, 1 swab, or 1 g of stool in each appropriate transport medium	Fluid or stool samples in sterile containers or swab samples in viral culturette devices (kept on ice but not frozen) are generally suitable. Plasma samples and buffy coats in sterile collection tubes should be kept at 4–8°C. If specimens are to be shipped or kept for a long time, freezing at −80°C is usually adequate.	Most samples for culture are transported in holding medium containing antibiotics to prevent bacterial overgrowth and viral inactivation. Many specimens should be kept cool but not frozen, provided they are transported promptly to the laboratory. Procedures and transport media vary with the agent to be cultured and the duration of transport.

Note: It is absolutely essential that the microbiology laboratory be informed of the site of origin of the sample to be cultured and of the infections that are suspected. This information determines the selection of culture media and the length of culture time.

[a]For samples from adults, two bottles (smaller for pediatric samples) should be used: one with dextrose phosphate, tryptic soy, or another appropriate broth and the other with thioglycollate or another broth containing reducing agents appropriate for isolation of obligate anaerobes. For children, from whom only limited volumes of blood can be obtained, only an aerobic culture should be done unless there is specific concern about anaerobic sepsis (e.g., with abdominal infections). For special situations (e.g., suspected fungal infection, culture-negative endocarditis, or mycobacteremia), different blood collection systems may be used (Isolator systems; see table).

[b]*Collection*: An appropriate disinfecting technique should be used on both the bottle septum and the patient. Do not allow air bubbles to get into anaerobic broth bottles. *Special considerations*: There is no more important clinical microbiology test than the detection of blood-borne pathogens. The rapid identification of bacterial and fungal agents is a major determinant of patients' survival. Bacteria may be present in blood either continuously (as in endocarditis, overwhelming sepsis, and the early stages of salmonellosis and brucellosis) or intermittently (as in most other bacterial infections, in which bacteria are shed into the blood on a sporadic basis). Most blood culture systems employ two separate bottles containing broth medium: one that is vented in the laboratory for the growth of facultative and aerobic organisms and a second that is maintained under anaerobic conditions. In cases of suspected continuous bacteremia/fungemia, two or three samples should be drawn before the start of therapy, with additional sets obtained if fastidious organisms are thought to be involved. For intermittent bacteremia, two or three samples should be obtained at least 1 h apart during the first 24 h.

[c]Normal microflora includes alpha-hemolytic streptococci, saprophytic *Neisseria* spp., diphtheroids, and *Staphylococcus* spp. Aerobic culture of the throat ("routine") includes screening for and identification of beta-hemolytic *Streptococcus* spp. and other potentially pathogenic organisms. Although considered components of the normal microflora, organisms such as *Staphylococcus aureus*, *Haemophilus influenzae*, and *Streptococcus pneumoniae* will be identified by most laboratories, if requested. When *Neisseria gonorrhoeae* or *Corynebacterium diphtheriae* is suspected, a special culture request is recommended.

[d](1) Clean-voided specimens, midvoid specimens, and Foley or indwelling catheter specimens that yield ≥50,000 organisms/mL and from which no more than three species are isolated should have organisms identified. Neither indwelling catheter tips nor urine from the bag of a catheterized patient should be cultured. (2) Straight-catheterized, bladder-tap, and similar urine specimens should undergo a complete workup (identification and susceptibility testing) for all potentially pathogenic organisms, regardless of colony count. (3) Certain clinical problems (e.g., acute dysuria in women) may warrant identification and susceptibility testing of isolates present at concentrations of <50,000 organisms/mL.

[e]Aspirated specimens in capped syringes or other transport devices designed to limit oxygen exposure are suitable for the cultivation of obligate anaerobes. A variety of commercially available transport devices may be used. Contamination of specimens with normal microflora from the skin, rectum, vaginal vault, or another body site should be avoided. Collection containers for aerobic culture (such as dry swabs) and inappropriate specimens (such as refrigerated samples; expectorated sputum; stool; gastric aspirates; and vaginal, throat, nose, and rectal swabs) should be rejected as unsuitable.

[f]Laboratories generally use diverse methods to detect viral agents, and the specific requirements for each specimen should be checked before a sample is sent.

general use of liquid medium for all specimens is not worthwhile.

Two basic strategies are used to isolate pathogenic bacteria. The first is to employ enriched media that support the growth of any bacteria that may be present in a sample such as blood or CSF, which contain no bacteria under normal conditions. Broths that allow the growth of small numbers of organisms may be subcultured to solid media when growth is detected. The second strategy is to use selective media to isolate (amplify) specific bacterial species from stool, genital tract secretions, or sputum—sites that contain many bacteria under normal conditions. Antimicrobial agents or other inhibitory substances are incorporated into the agar medium to inhibit growth of all but the bacteria of interest. After incubation, organisms that grow on such media are further characterized to determine whether they are pathogens. Selection for organisms that may be pathogens from the normal microflora shortens the time required for diagnosis (Fig. 5-2).

ISOLATION OF VIRAL AGENTS

(See also Chap. 78) Pathogenic viral agents often are sought by culture when the presence of serum antibody is not a criterion for active infection or when an increase in serum antibody may not be detected during infection. The biologic signal—virus—is amplified to a detectable level. Although a number of techniques are available, an essential element is a monolayer of cultured mammalian cells sensitive to infection with the suspected virus. These cells serve as the amplification system by allowing the proliferation of viral particles. Virus may be detected by direct observation of the cultured cells for cytopathic effects or by immunofluorescent detection of viral antigens after incubation. Conventional viral culture is useful for detection of rapidly propagated agents, such as herpes simplex virus. Viruses that grow more slowly (e.g., cytomegalovirus and varicella-zoster virus) can be detected quickly by shell-vial culture, in which the specimen is centrifuged on a monolayer of cells that is then incubated for 1–2 days and

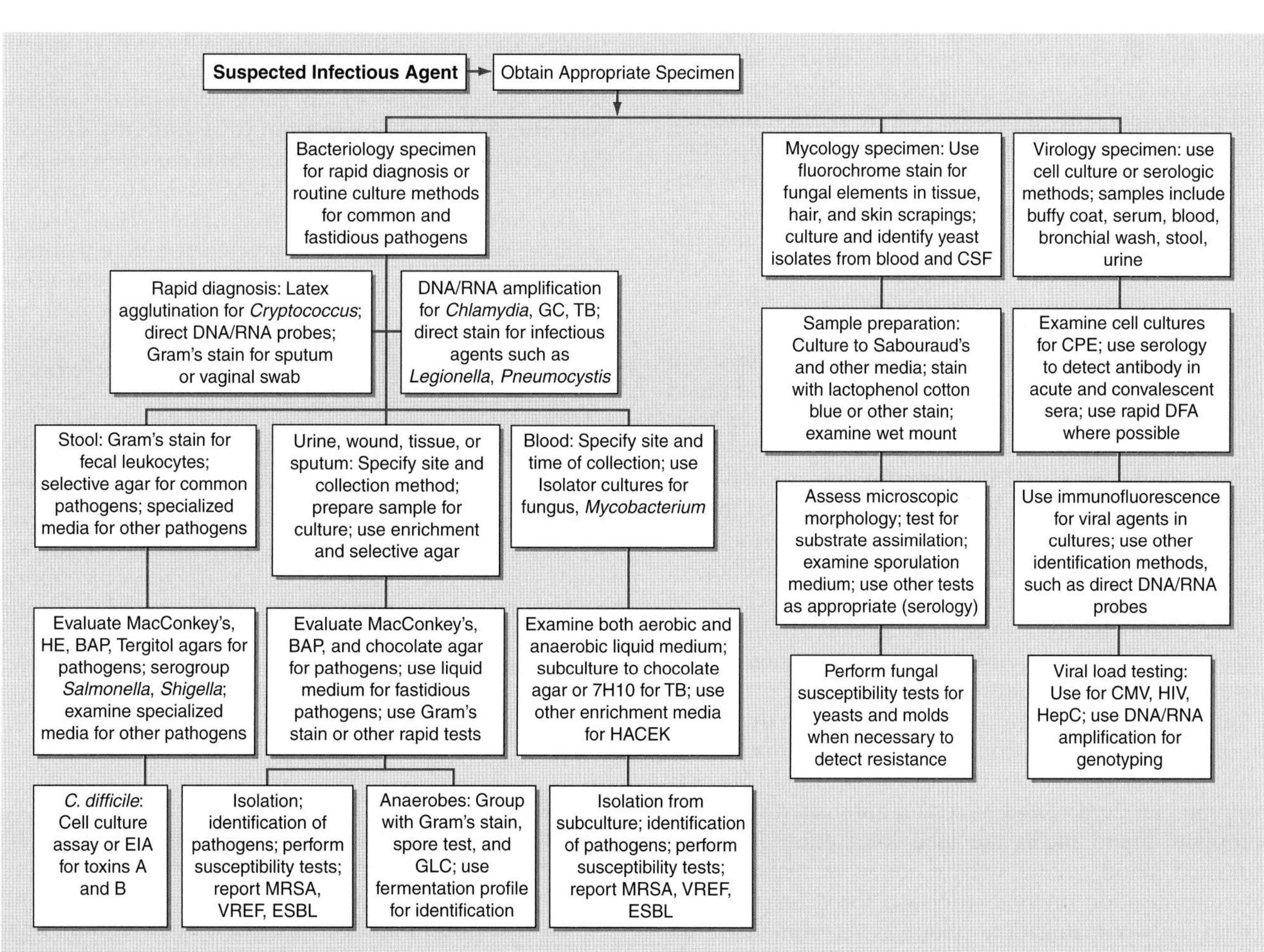

FIGURE 5-2

Common specimen-processing algorithms used in clinical microbiology laboratories. BAP, blood agar plate; CMV, cytomegalovirus; CPE, cytopathic effects; CSF, cerebrospinal fluid; DFA, direct immunofluorescence assay; EIA, enzyme immunoassays; ESBL, extended spectrum beta-lactamase; GC, gonorrhea culture; GLC, gas-liquid chromatography; HACEK, *Haemophilus* spp., *Actinobacillus actinomycetemcomitans*, *Cardiobacterium hominis*, *Eikenella corrodens*, and *Kingella* spp.; HE, Hektoen enteric; HepC, hepatitis C; HIV, human immunodeficiency virus; MRSA, methicillin-resistant *Staphylococcus aureus*; TB, tuberculosis; VREF, vancomycin-resistant *Enterococcus faecium*.

finally stained for viral antigens with fluorochrome-conjugated antibodies.

AUTOMATION OF MICROBIAL DETECTION IN BLOOD

The detection of microbial pathogens in blood is difficult because the number of organisms present in the sample is often low and the organisms' integrity and ability to replicate may be damaged by humoral defense mechanisms or antimicrobial agents. Over the years, systems that rely on the detection of gas (usually CO_2) produced by bacteria and yeasts in blood culture medium have allowed the automation of the detection procedure. The most common systems involve either (1) the measurement of gas pressure in the headspace to indicate bacterial gas production or consumption or (2) the use of reflectance optics, with a light-emitting diode and photodiode employed to detect a color change in a CO_2-sensitive indicator built into the bottom of the culture bottle. These systems measure CO_2 concentration as indicative of microbial growth. Such methods are no more sensitive than the human eye in detecting a positive culture; however, because the bottles in an automated system are monitored more frequently, a positive culture is often detected more rapidly than by manual techniques, and important information, including the result of Gram's stain and preliminary susceptibility assays, can be obtained sooner. One advantage of automated blood culture systems is that the bottles are scanned continuously in a noninvasive monitoring procedure, and thus the likelihood of laboratory contamination is decreased.

Several factors affect the yield of blood culture from bacteremic patients. Increasing the volume of blood tested increases the chance of a positive culture. An increase from 10 to 20 mL of blood increases the proportion of positive cultures by ~30%; however, this effect is less pronounced in patients with bacterial endocarditis. Obtaining multiple cultures (up to three per 24-h period) also increases the chance of detecting a bacterial pathogen. Prolonged culture and blind subculture for detection of most fastidious bacteria (e.g., *Haemophilus, Actinobacillus, Cardiobacterium, Eikenella*, and *Kingella* spp.) are not needed with automated blood culture systems.

Automated systems have also been applied to the detection of microbial growth from specimens other than blood, such as peritoneal and other normally sterile fluids. *Mycobacterium* spp. can be detected in certain automated systems if appropriate liquid media are used for culture. Although automated blood culture systems are more sensitive than lysis-centrifugation methods (Isolator) for yeasts and most bacteria, lysis-centrifugation culture is recommended for filamentous fungi, *Histoplasma capsulatum*, and some fastidious bacteria (*Legionella* and *Bartonella*).

DETECTION OF PATHOGENIC AGENTS BY SEROLOGIC METHODS

Measurement of serum antibody provides an indirect marker for past or current infection with a specific viral agent or other pathogens, including *Brucella, Legionella, Rickettsia*, and *Helicobacter pylori*. The biologic signal is usually either IgM or IgG antibody directed at surface-expressed antigen. The detection systems include those used for bacterial antigens (agglutination reactions, immunofluorescence, and EIA) and unique systems such as hemolysis inhibition and complement fixation. Serologic methods generally fall into two categories: those that determine protective antibody levels and those that measure changing antibody titers during infection. Determination of an antibody response as a measure of current immunity is important in the case of viral agents for which there are vaccines, such as rubella virus or varicella-zoster virus; assays for this purpose normally use one or two dilutions of serum for a qualitative determination of protective antibody levels. Quantitative serologic assays to detect increases in antibody titers most often employ paired serum samples obtained at the onset of illness and 10–14 days later (i.e., acute- and convalescent-phase samples). Since the incubation period before symptoms are noted may be long enough for an antibody response to occur, the demonstration of acute-phase antibody alone is often insufficient to establish the diagnosis of active infection as opposed to past exposure. In such circumstances, IgM may be useful as a measure of an early, acute-phase antibody response. A fourfold increase in total antibody titer or in EIA activity between the acute- and convalescent-phase samples is also regarded as evidence for active infection.

For certain viral agents, such as Epstein-Barr virus, the antibodies produced may be directed at different antigens during different phases of the infection. For this reason, most laboratories test for antibody directed at both viral capsid antigens and antigens associated with recently infected host cells to determine the stage of infection.

IDENTIFICATION METHODS

Once bacteria are isolated, characteristics that are readily detectable after growth on agar media (colony size, color, hemolytic reactions, odor, microscopic appearance) may suggest a species, but definitive identification requires additional tests. Identification methods include classic biochemical phenotyping, which is still the most common approach, and more sophisticated methods, such as gas chromatography and nucleic acid tests.

CLASSIC PHENOTYPING

Classic phenotypic identification of bacteria entails tests for protein or carbohydrate antigens, the production of specific enzymes, the ability to metabolize specific substrates and carbon sources (such as carbohydrates), or the production of certain metabolites. Rapid versions of some of these tests are available, and many common organisms can be identified on the first day of growth. Other organisms, particularly gram-negative bacteria, require more extensive testing, either manual or automated.

Automated systems allow rapid phenotypic identification of bacterial pathogens. Most such systems are based on biotyping techniques, in which isolates are grown on multiple substrates and the reaction pattern is compared with known patterns for various bacterial species. This procedure is relatively fast, and commercially available systems include miniaturized fermentation, coding to simplify recording of results, and probability calculations for the most likely pathogens. If the biotyping approach is automated and the reading process is coupled to computer-based data analysis, rapidly growing organisms (such as Enterobacteriaceae) can be identified within hours of detection on agar plates.

Several systems use preformed enzymes for even speedier identification (within 2–3 h). Such systems do not rely on bacterial growth per se to determine whether a substrate has been used. They employ a heavy inoculum in which specific bacterial enzymes are present in amounts sufficient to convert substrate to product rapidly. In addition, some systems use fluorogenic substrate/end-product detection methods to increase sensitivity (through signal amplification).

GAS-LIQUID CHROMATOGRAPHY

Gas-liquid chromatography is often used to detect metabolic end products of bacterial fermentations. One common application is identification of short-chain fatty acids produced by obligate anaerobes during glucose fermentation. Because the types and relative concentrations of volatile acids differ among the various genera and species that make up this group of organisms, such information serves as a metabolic "fingerprint" for a particular isolate.

Gas-liquid chromatography can be coupled to a sophisticated signal-analysis software system for identification and quantitation of long-chain fatty acids (LCFAs) in the outer membranes and cell walls of bacteria and fungi. For any given species, the types and relative concentrations of LCFAs are distinctive enough to allow differentiation even from closely related species. An organism may be identified definitively within a few hours after detection of growth on appropriate media. LCFA analysis is one of the most advanced procedures currently available for phenotypic characterization.

NUCLEIC ACID TESTS

Techniques for the detection and quantitation of specific DNA and RNA base sequences in clinical specimens have become powerful tools for the diagnosis of bacterial, viral, parasitic, and fungal infections. Nucleic acid tests are used for four purposes. First, they are used to detect, and sometimes to quantify, specific pathogens in clinical specimens. Second, such tests are used for identification of organisms (usually bacteria) that are difficult to identify by conventional methods. Third, nucleic acid tests are used to determine whether two or more isolates of the same pathogen are closely related (belonging to the same "clone" or "strain"). Last, nucleic acid tests are used to predict the sensitivity of organisms (typically viruses) to chemotherapeutic agents. Current technology encompasses a wide array of methods for amplification and signal detection, some of which have been approved by the U.S. Food and Drug Administration (FDA) for clinical diagnosis.

Use of nucleic acid tests generally involves lysis of intact cells or viruses and denaturation of the DNA or RNA to render it single-stranded. Probe(s) or primer(s) complementary to the pathogen-specific target sequence may be hybridized to the target sequence in a solution or on a solid support, depending on the system employed. In situ hybridization of a probe to a target is also possible and allows the use of probes with agents present in tissue specimens. Once the probe(s) or primer(s) have been hybridized to the target (biologic signal), a variety of strategies may be employed to detect, amplify, and/or quantify the target-probe complex (Fig. 5-3).

PROBES FOR DIRECT DETECTION OF PATHOGENS IN CLINICAL SPECIMENS

Nucleic acid probes are used for direct detection of pathogens in clinical specimens without amplification of the target strand of DNA or RNA. Such tests detect a relatively short sequence of bases specific for a particular pathogen on single-stranded DNA or RNA by hybridization of a complementary sequence of bases (probe) coupled to a "reporter" system that serves as the signal for detection. Nucleic acid probes are available commercially for direct detection of various bacterial and parasitic pathogens, including *Chlamydia trachomatis, N. gonorrhoeae,* and group A *Streptococcus.* A combined assay to detect and differentiate agents of vaginitis/vaginosis (*Gardnerella vaginalis, Trichomonas vaginalis,* and *Candida* spp.) has also been approved. An assortment of probes are available for confirming the identity of cultured pathogens, including some dimorphic molds, *Mycobacterium* spp., and other bacteria (e.g., *Campylobacter* spp., *Streptococcus* spp., and *Staphylococcus aureus*). Probes for the direct detection of bacterial pathogens are often aimed at highly conserved 16S ribosomal RNA sequences, of which there are many more copies than there are of any single genomic DNA sequence in a bacterial cell. The sensitivity and specificity of probe assays for direct detection are comparable to those of more traditional assays, including EIA and culture.

In an alternative probe assay, called *hybrid capture,* an RNA probe anneals to a DNA target, and the resulting DNA/RNA hybrid is captured on a solid support by antibody specific for DNA/RNA hybrids (concentration/amplification) and detected by chemiluminescent-labeled antibody specific for DNA/RNA hybrids. Hybrid capture assays are available for *C. trachomatis, N. gonorrhoeae,* cytomegalovirus, and human papillomavirus.

Many laboratories have developed their own probes for pathogens; however, unless a method-validation protocol for diagnostic testing has been performed, federal law in the United States restricts the use of such probes to research.

NUCLEIC ACID AMPLIFICATION TEST STRATEGIES

In theory, a single target nucleic acid sequence can be amplified to detectable levels. There are several strategies for nucleic acid amplification tests (NAATs), including PCR, LCR, strand displacement amplification, and self-sustaining sequence replication. In each case, exponential amplification of a pathogen-specific DNA or RNA sequence depends on primers that anneal to the target

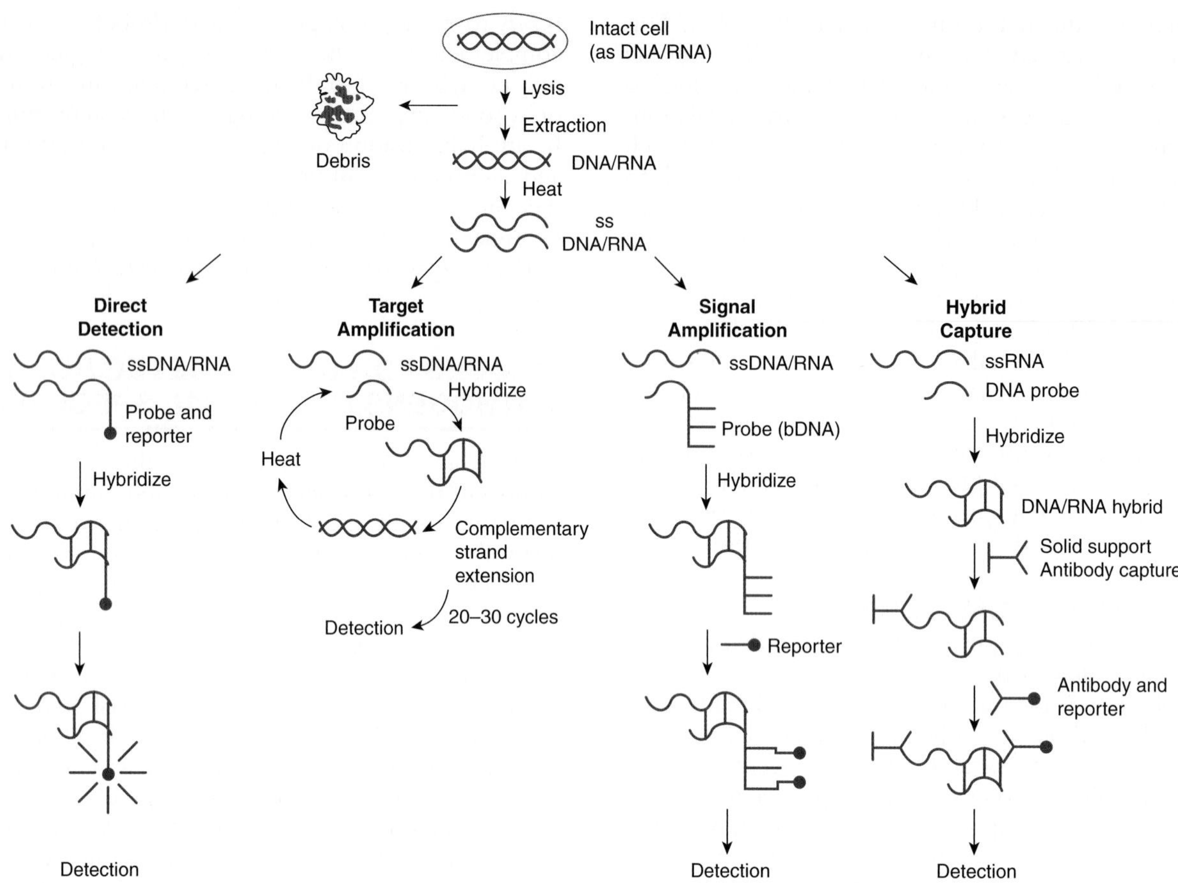

FIGURE 5-3

Strategies for amplification and/or detection of a target-probe complex. DNA or RNA extracted from microorganisms is heated to create single-stranded (ss) DNA/RNA containing appropriate target sequences. These target sequences may be hybridized directly (direct detection) with probes attached to reporter molecules; they may be amplified by repetitive cycles of complementary strand extension (polymerase chain reaction) before attachment of a reporter probe; or the original target-probe signal may be amplified via hybridization with an additional probe containing multiple copies of a secondary reporter target sequence (branched-chain DNA, or bDNA). DNA/RNA hybrids can also be "captured" on a solid support (hybrid capture), with antibody directed at the DNA/RNA hybrids used to concentrate them and a second antibody coupled to a reporter molecule attached to the captured hybrid.

sequence. The amplified nucleic acid can be detected after the reaction is complete or (in *real-time* detection) as amplification proceeds. PCR, the first and still most common NAAT, requires repeated heating of the DNA to separate the two complementary strands of the double helix, hybridization of a primer sequence to the appropriate target sequence, target amplification using the PCR for complementary strand extension, and signal detection via a labeled probe. Methods for the monitoring of PCR after each amplification cycle—via either incorporation of fluorescent dyes into the DNA during primer extension or use of fluorescent probes capable of fluorescence resonance energy transfer—have now decreased the period required to detect a specific target. The sensitivity of NAATs is far greater than that of traditional assay methods such as culture. However, the care with which the assays are performed is important, because cross-contamination of clinical material with DNA or RNA from other sources (even at low levels) can cause false-positive results. An alternative NAAT employs transcription-mediated amplification, in which an RNA target sequence is converted to DNA, which is then exponentially transcribed into RNA target. The advantage of this method is that only a single heating/annealing step is required for amplification. At present, amplification assays for *Mycobacterium tuberculosis, N. gonorrhoeae, C. trachomatis, Mycoplasma hominis*, group B *Streptococcus*, and methicillin-resistant *S. aureus* are on the market. Again, many laboratories have used commercially available *taq* polymerase, probe sequences, and analyte-specific reagents (ASRs) to develop "in-house" assays for diagnostic use. Issues related to quality control, interpretation of results, sample processing, and regulatory requirements have slowed the commercial development of many diagnostic assay kits.

Identification of otherwise difficult-to-identify bacteria involves an initial amplification of a highly conserved region of 16S rDNA by PCR. Automated sequencing of several hundred bases is then performed, and the sequence information is compared with large databases containing sequence information for thousands of different organisms. Although 16S sequencing is not as rapid as other methods and is still relatively expensive for routine use in the clinical microbiology laboratory, it is becoming the definitive method for identification of unusual or difficult-to-cultivate organisms.

QUANTITATIVE NUCLEIC ACID TEST STRATEGIES

With the advent of newer therapeutic regimens for HIV-associated disease, cytomegalovirus infection, and hepatitis B and C virus infections, the response to therapy has been monitored by determining both genotype and "viral load" at various times after treatment initiation. Quantitative NAATs are available for HIV (PCR), cytomegalovirus (PCR), hepatitis B (PCR), and hepatitis C (PCR and transcription-mediated amplification, or TMA). Many laboratories have validated and perform quantitative assays for these and other pathogens (e.g., Epstein-Barr virus), using ASRs for NAATs.

Branched-chain DNA (bDNA) testing is an alternative to NAATs for quantitative nucleic acid testing. In such testing, bDNA attaches to a site different from the target-binding sequence of the original probe. Chemiluminescent-labeled oligonucleotides can then bind to multiple repeating sequences on the bDNA. The amplified bDNA signal is detected by chemiluminescence. bDNA assays for viral load of HIV, hepatitis B virus, and hepatitis C virus have been approved by the FDA. The advantage of bDNA over PCR is that only a single heating/annealing step is required to hybridize the target-binding probe to the target sequence for amplification.

APPLICATION OF NUCLEIC ACID TESTS

In addition to the applications already discussed, nucleic acid tests are used to detect and identify difficult-to-grow or noncultivable bacterial pathogens, such as *Mycobacterium*, *Legionella*, *Ehrlichia*, *Rickettsia*, *Babesia*, *Borrelia*, and *Tropheryma whippelii*. In addition, methods for rapid detection of agents of public health concern, such as *Bacillus anthracis*, smallpox virus, and *Yersinia pestis*, have been developed.

Nucleic acid tests are also used to determine how close the relationship is among different isolates of the same species of pathogen. The demonstration that bacteria of a single clone have infected multiple patients in the context of a possible means of transmission (e.g., a health care provider) offers confirmatory evidence for an outbreak. Pulse-field gel electrophoresis remains the usual gold standard for bacterial strain analysis. This method involves the use of restriction enzymes that recognize rare sequences of nucleotides to digest the bacterial DNA, resulting in large DNA fragments. These fragments are separated by gel electrophoresis with variable polarity of the electrophoretic current and then are visualized. Similar band patterns (i.e., differences in ″ 3 bands) suggest that different bacterial isolates are closely related, or clonal. Simpler methods of strain typing include sequencing of single or multiple genes and PCR-based amplification of repetitive DNA sequences in the bacterial chromosome.

Future applications of nucleic acid testing will likely include the replacement of culture for identification of many pathogens with solid-state DNA/RNA chip technology, in which thousands of unique nucleic acid sequences can be detected on a single silicon chip.

SUSCEPTIBILITY TESTING OF BACTERIA

A principal responsibility of the clinical microbiology laboratory is to determine which antimicrobial agents inhibit a specific bacterial isolate. Such testing is used to screen for infection control problems, such as methicillin-resistant *S. aureus* or vancomycin-resistant *Enterococcus faecium*. Two approaches are useful. The first is a qualitative assessment of susceptibility, with responses categorized as susceptible, resistant, or intermediate. This approach can involve either the placement of paper disks containing antibiotics on an agar surface inoculated with the bacterial strain to be tested (Kirby-Bauer or disk/agar diffusion method), with measurement of the zones of growth inhibition after incubation, or the use of broth cultures containing a set concentration of antibiotic (breakpoint method). These methods have been carefully calibrated against quantitative methods and clinical experience with each antibiotic, and zones of inhibition and breakpoints have been calculated on a species-by-species basis.

The second approach is to inoculate the test strain of bacteria into a series of broth cultures (or agar plates) with increasing concentrations of antibiotic. The lowest concentration of antibiotic that inhibits visual microbial growth in this test system is known as the *minimum inhibitory concentration* (MIC). If tubes in which no growth is seen are subcultured, the minimum concentration of antibiotic required to kill 99.9% of the starting inoculum can also be determined (*minimum bactericidal concentration*, or MBC). The MIC value can be given a categorical interpretation of susceptible, resistant, or intermediate and so is more widely used than the MBC. Quantitative susceptibility testing by the microbroth dilution technique, a miniaturized version of the broth dilution technique using microwell plates, lends itself to automation and is commonly used in larger clinical laboratories.

A novel version of the disk/agar diffusion method employs a quantitative diffusion gradient, or Epsilometer (E-test), and uses an absorbent strip with a known gradient of antibiotic concentrations along its length. When the strip is placed on the surface of an agar plate seeded with a bacterial strain to be tested, antibiotic diffuses into the medium, and bacterial growth is inhibited. The MIC is estimated as the lowest concentration that inhibits visible growth.

For some organisms, such as obligate anaerobes, routine susceptibility testing generally is not performed because of the difficulty of growing the organisms and the predictable sensitivity of most isolates to specific antibiotics.

SUSCEPTIBILITY TESTING OF FUNGAL AGENTS

With the advent of many new agents for treating yeasts and systemic fungal agents, the need for testing of individual isolates for susceptibility to specific antifungal agents has increased. In the past, few laboratories participated in such testing because of a lack of standard methods like those available for testing bacterial agents. However, several systems have now been approved for antifungal susceptibility testing. These methods, which determine the minimal fungicidal concentration (MFC), are similar to the broth microdilution methods used to determine the MIC for bacteria. The E-test method is approved for testing the susceptibility of yeasts to fluconazole, itraconazole, and flucytosine, and disk diffusion can be used to test the susceptibility of *Candida* spp. to fluconazole and voriconazole. Methods for determining the MFC against fungal agents such as *Aspergillus* spp. are technically difficult, and most clinical laboratories refer requests for such testing to reference laboratories.

ANTIVIRAL TESTING

See Chap. 78.

FURTHER READINGS

AIRES DE SOUSA M, DE LENCASTRE H: Bridges from hospitals to the laboratory: Genetic portraits of methicillin-resistant *Staphylococcus aureus* clones. FEMS Immunol Med Microbiol 40:101, 2004

BARON EJ et al: Prolonged incubation and extensive subculturing do not increase recovery of clinically significant microorganisms from standard automated blood cultures. Clin Infect Dis 41: 1677, 2005

CALIENDO AM et al: Distinguishing cytomegalovirus (CMV) infection and disease with CMV nucleic acid assays. J Clin Microbiol 40:1581, 2002

COCKERHILL FR et al: Optimal testing parameters for blood cultures. Clin Infect Dis 38:1724, 2004

DOMIATI-SAAD R, SCHEUERMANN RH: Nucleic acid testing for viral burden and viral genotyping. Clin Chim Acta 363:197, 2005

MAGIORAKOS AP, HADLEY S: Impact of real-time fungal susceptibility on clinical practices. Curr Opin Infect Dis 17:511, 2004

PANCHOLI P et al: Rapid detection of cytomegalovirus infection in transplant patients. Expert Rev Mol Diagn 4:231, 2004

PFALLER MA et al: Clinical evaluation of a frozen commercially prepared microdilution panel for antifungal susceptibility testing of seven antifungal agents, including the new triazoles posaconazole, ravuconazole and voriconazole. J Clin Microbiol 40:1694, 2002

SERVOSS JC, FRIEDMAN LS: Serologic and molecular diagnosis of hepatitis B virus. Clin Liver Dis 8:267, 2004

YEGHIAZARIAN T et al: Quantitation of human immunodeficiency virus type 1 RNA levels in plasma by using small-volume-format branched-DNA assays. J Clin Microbiol 36:2096, 1998

CHAPTER 6

MICROBIAL BIOTERRORISM

H. Clifford Lane ■ Anthony S. Fauci

Descriptions of the use of microbial pathogens as potential weapons of war or terrorism date from ancient times. Among the most frequently cited of such episodes are the poisoning of water supplies in the sixth century B.C. with the fungus *Claviceps purpurea* (rye ergot) by the Assyrians, the hurling of the dead bodies of plague victims over the walls of the city of Kaffa by the Tartar army in 1346, and the efforts by the British to spread smallpox via contaminated blankets to the native American population loyal to the French in 1767. Although the use of chemical weapons in wartime took place in the not-too-distant past, the tragic events of September 11, 2001, followed closely by the anthrax attacks through the U.S. Postal System, dramatically changed the mindset of the American public regarding both our vulnerability to microbial bioterrorist attacks and the seriousness and intent of the Federal government to protect its citizens against future attacks. Modern science has revealed methods of deliberately spreading or enhancing disease in ways not appreciated by our ancestors. The combination of basic research, good medical practice, and constant vigilance will be needed to defend against such attacks.

Although the potential impact of a bioterrorist attack could be enormous, leading to thousands of deaths and extensive morbidity, acts of bioterrorism would be expected to produce their greatest impact through the fear and terror they generate. In contrast to biowarfare, where the primary goal is destruction of the enemy through mass casualties, an important goal of bioterrorism is to destroy the morale of a society through fear and uncertainty. Although the actual biologic impact of a single act may be small, the degree of disruption created by the realization that such an attack is possible may be enormous. This was readily apparent with the impact on the U.S. Postal System and the functional interruption of the activities of the legislative branch of government after the anthrax attacks noted above. Thus the key to the defense against these attacks is a highly functioning system of public health surveillance and education so that attacks can be quickly recognized and effectively contained. This is complemented by the availability of appropriate countermeasures in the form of diagnostics, therapeutics, and vaccines, both in response to and in anticipation of bioterrorist attacks.

The Working Group for Civilian Biodefense has put together a list of key features that characterize the elements of biologic agents that make them particularly effective as weapons (Table 6-1). Included among these are the ease of spread and transmission of the agent as well as the presence of an adequate database to allow newcomers to the field to quickly apply the good science of others to bad intentions of their own. Agents of bioterrorism may be used in their naturally occurring forms, or they can be deliberately modified to provide maximal impact. Among the approaches to maximizing the deleterious effects of biologic agents are the genetic modification of microbes for the purposes of antimicrobial resistance or evasion by the immune system, creation of fine-particle aerosols, chemical treatment to stabilize and prolong infectivity, and alteration of host range through changes in surface proteins. Certain of these approaches fall under the category of *weaponization*, which is a term generally used to describe the processing of microbes or toxins in a manner that would ensure a devastating effect of a release. For example, weaponization of anthrax by the Soviets comprised the production of vast amounts of spores in a form that maintained aerosolization for prolonged periods of time; the spores were of appropriate size to reach the lower respiratory tract easily and could be delivered in a massive release, such as via widely dispersed bomblets.

The U.S. Centers for Disease Control and Prevention (CDC) classifies potential biologic threats into three categories: A, B, and C (Table 6-2). Category A agents are the highest-priority pathogens. They pose the greatest risk to national security because they (1) can be easily disseminated or transmitted from person to person, (2) result in high mortality rates and have the potential for major public health impact, (3) might cause public panic and social disruption, and (4) require special action for public health preparedness. Category B agents are the second highest-priority pathogens and include those that are moderately easy to disseminate, result in moderate morbidity rates and low mortality rates, and require specifically enhanced diagnostic capacity. Category C agents are the third highest priority. These include certain emerging pathogens, to which the general population lacks immunity, that could be engineered for mass dissemination in the future because of availability, ease of production, ease of dissemination, potential for high morbidity and mortality, and major public health impact. A potential pandemic strain of influenza, such as avian influenza, is one such example. It should be pointed out, however, that these designations are empirical, and, depending on evolving circumstances such as intelligence-based threat assessments, the priority rating of any given microbe or toxin could change. The CDC classification system also largely reflects the severity of illness produced by a given agent, rather than its accessibility to potential terrorists.

TABLE 6-1

KEY FEATURES OF BIOLOGIC AGENTS USED AS BIOWEAPONS

1. High morbidity and mortality
2. Potential for person-to-person spread
3. Low infective dose and highly infectious by aerosol
4. Lack of rapid diagnostic capability
5. Lack of universally available effective vaccine
6. Potential to cause anxiety
7. Availability of pathogen and feasibility of production
8. Environmental stability
9. Database of prior research and development
10. Potential to be "weaponized"

Source: From L Borio et al: JAMA 287:2391, 2002; with permission.

TABLE 6-2

CDC CATEGORY A, B, AND C AGENTS

Category A

Anthrax (*Bacillus anthracis*)
Botulism (*Clostridium botulinum* toxin)
Plague (*Yersinia pestis*)
Smallpox (*Variola major*)
Tularemia (*Francisella tularensis*)
Viral hemorrhagic fevers
  Arenaviruses: Lassa, New World (Machupo, Junin, Guanarito, and Sabia)
  Bunyaviridae: Crimean Congo, Rift Valley
  Filoviridae: Ebola, Marburg

Category B

Brucellosis (*Brucella* spp.)
Epsilon toxin of *Clostridium perfringens*
Food safety threats (e.g., *Salmonella* spp., *Escherichia coli* 0157:H7, *Shigella*)
Glanders (*Burkholderia mallei*)
Melioidosis (*B. pseudomallei*)
Psittacosis (*Chlamydophila psittaci*)
Q fever (*Coxiella burnetii*)
Ricin toxin from *Ricinus communis* (castor beans)
Staphylococcal enterotoxin B
Typhus fever (*Rickettsia prowazekii*)
Viral encephalitis [alphaviruses (e.g., Venezuelan, eastern, and western equine encephalitis)]
Water safety threats (e.g., *Vibrio cholerae, Cryptosporidium parvum*)

Category C

Emerging infectious diseases threats such as Nipah, hantavirus, SARS coronavirus, and pandemic influenza.

Source: Centers for Disease Control and Prevention and the National Institute of Allergy and Infectious Diseases.

CATEGORY A AGENTS

ANTHRAX

Bacillus Anthracis as a Bioweapon

Anthrax may be the prototypic disease of bioterrorism. Although rarely, if ever, spread from person to person, the illness embodies the other major features of a disease introduced through terrorism, as outlined in Table 6-1. U.S. and British government scientists studied anthrax as a potential biologic weapon beginning approximately at the time of World War II (WWII). Offensive bioweapons activity including bioweapons research on microbes and toxins in the United States ceased in 1969 as a result of two executive orders by President Richard M. Nixon. The 1972 Biological and Toxin Weapons Convention Treaty outlawed research of this type worldwide. Clearly, the Soviet Union was in direct violation of this treaty until at least the Union dissolved in the late 1980s. It is well documented that during this post-treaty period, the Soviets produced and stored tons of anthrax spores for potential use as a bioweapon. At present there is suspicion that research on anthrax as an agent of bioterrorism is ongoing by several nations and extremist groups. One example of this is the release of anthrax spores by the Aum Shrinrikyo cult in Tokyo in 1993. Fortunately, there were no casualties associated with this episode because of the inadvertent use of a nonpathogenic strain of anthrax by the terrorists.

The potential impact of anthrax spores as a bioweapon was clearly demonstrated in 1979 after the accidental release of spores into the atmosphere from a Soviet Union bioweapons facility in Sverdlosk, Russia. Although actual figures are not known, at least 77 cases of anthrax were diagnosed with certainty, of which 66 were fatal. These victims were exposed in an area within 4 km downwind of the facility, and deaths due to anthrax were also noted in livestock up to 50 km further downwind. Based on recorded wind patterns, the interval between the time of exposure and development of clinical illness ranged from 2–43 days. The majority of cases were within the first 2 weeks. Death typically occurred within 1–4 days after the onset of symptoms. It is likely that the widespread use of postexposure penicillin prophylaxis limited the total number of cases. The extended period of time between exposure and disease in some individuals supports the data from nonhuman primate studies suggesting the anthrax spores can lie dormant in the respiratory tract for at least 4–6 weeks without evoking an immune response. This extended period of microbiologic latency after exposure poses a significant challenge for management of victims in the postexposure period.

In September 2001, the American public was exposed to anthrax spores as a bioweapon delivered through the U.S. Postal System. The CDC identified 22 confirmed or suspected cases of anthrax as a consequence of this attack. These included 11 patients with inhalational anthrax, of whom 5 died, and 11 patients with cutaneous anthrax (7 confirmed), all of whom survived (Fig. 6-1). Cases occurred in individuals who opened contaminated letters as well as in postal workers involved in the processing of mail. A minimum of five letters mailed from Trenton, NJ, served as the vehicles for these attacks. One of these letters was reported to contain 2 g of material, equivalent to 100 billion to 1 trillion weapon-grade spores. Since studies performed in the 1950s using monkeys exposed

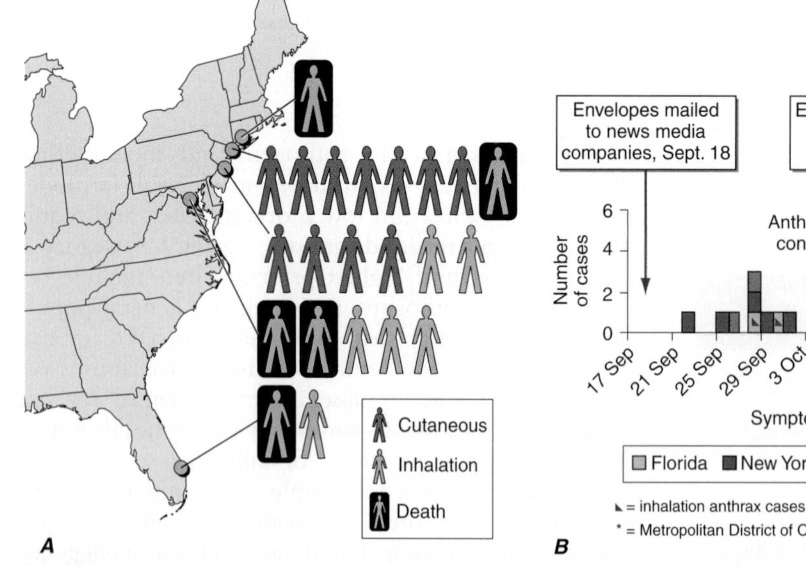

FIGURE 6-1

Confirmed anthrax cases associated with bioterrorism: United States, 2001. ***A.*** Geographic location, clinical manifestation, and outcome of the 11 cases of confirmed inhalational and 11 cases of confirmed cutaneous anthrax. ***B.*** Epidemic curve for 18 confirmed cases of inhalational and cutaneous anthrax and additional 4 cases of suspected cutaneous anthrax. (*From DB Jernigan et al: Investigation of bioterrorism-related anthrax, US 2001: Epidemiologic findings. Emerg Infect Dis 8:1019, 2002; with permission.*)

to aerosolized anthrax suggested that ~10,000 spores were required to produce lethal disease in 50% of animals exposed to this dose (the LD_{50}), the contents of one letter had the theoretical potential, under optimal conditions, of causing illness or death in up to 50 million individuals when one considers an LD_{50} of 10,000 spores. The strain used in this attack was the Ames strain. Although it was noted to have an inducible beta-lactamase and to constitutively express a cephalosporinase, it was susceptible to all antibiotics standard for *B. anthracis*.

Microbiology and Clinical Features

Anthrax is caused by *B. anthracis*, a gram-positive, nonmotile, spore-forming rod that is found in soil and predominantly causes disease in herbivores such as cattle, goats, and sheep. Anthrax spores can remain viable for decades. The remarkable stability of these spores makes them an ideal bioweapon, and their destruction in decontamination activities can be a challenge. Naturally occurring human infection is generally the result of contact with anthrax-infected animals or animal products such as goat hair. Although an LD_{50} of 10,000 spores is a generally accepted number, it has also been suggested that as few as one to three spores may be adequate to cause disease in some settings. Advanced technology is likely to be necessary to generate spores of the optimal size (1–5 μm) to travel to the alveolar spaces as a bioweapon.

The three major clinical forms of anthrax are gastrointestinal, cutaneous, and inhalational. *Gastrointestinal anthrax* typically results from the ingestion of contaminated meat; the condition is rarely seen and is unlikely to be the result of a bioterrorism event. The lesion of *cutaneous anthrax* typically begins as a papule after the introduction of spores through an opening in the skin. This papule then evolves to a painless vesicle followed by the development of a coal-black, necrotic eschar (Fig. 6-2). It is the Greek word for coal (*anthrax*) that gives the organism and the disease its name. Cutaneous anthrax was ~20% fatal before the availability of antibiotics. *Inhalational anthrax* is the form most likely to be responsible for death in the setting of a bioterrorist attack. It occurs after the inhalation of spores that become deposited in the alveolar spaces. These spores are phagocytosed by macrophages and transported to the mediastinal and peribronchial lymph nodes where they germinate, leading to active bacterial growth and elaboration of the bacterial products edema toxin and lethal toxin. Subsequent hematogenous spread of bacteria is accompanied by cardiovascular collapse and death. The earliest symptoms are typically a viral-like prodrome with fever, malaise, and abdominal and/or chest symptoms that progress over the course of a few days to a moribund state. A characteristic finding is mediastinal widening and pleural effusions on chest x-ray (Fig. 6-3). Although initially thought to be 100% fatal, the experiences at Sverdlosk in 1979 and in the United States in 2001 (see below) indicate that, with prompt initiation of antibiotic therapy, survival is possible. The characteristics of the 11 cases of inhalational anthrax diagnosed in the United States in 2001 after exposure to contaminated letters postmarked September 18 or October 9, 2001, followed the classic pattern established for this illness, with patients presenting with a rapidly progressive course characterized by fever, fatigue or malaise, nausea or vomiting, cough, and shortness of breath. At presentation, the total white blood cell counts were ~10,000 cells/μL; transaminases tended to be elevated, and all 11 had abnormal findings on chest x-ray and CT. Radiologic findings included infiltrates, mediastinal widening, and hemorrhagic pleural effusions. For cases in which the dates of exposure were known, symptoms appeared within 4–6 days. Death occurred within 7 days of diagnosis in the 5 fatal cases (overall mortality rate 55%). Rapid diagnosis and prompt initiation of antibiotic therapy were key to survival.

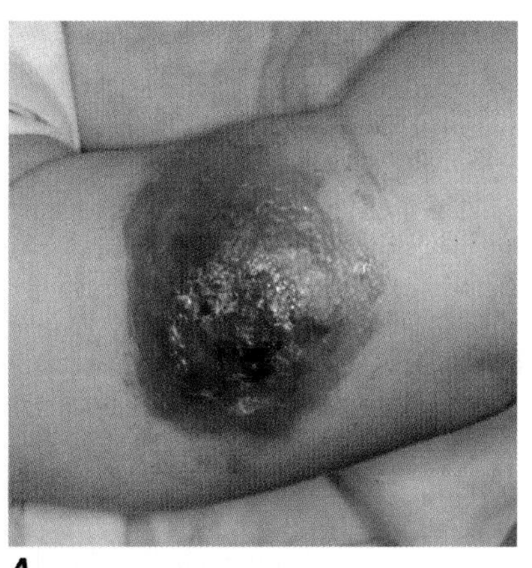
A

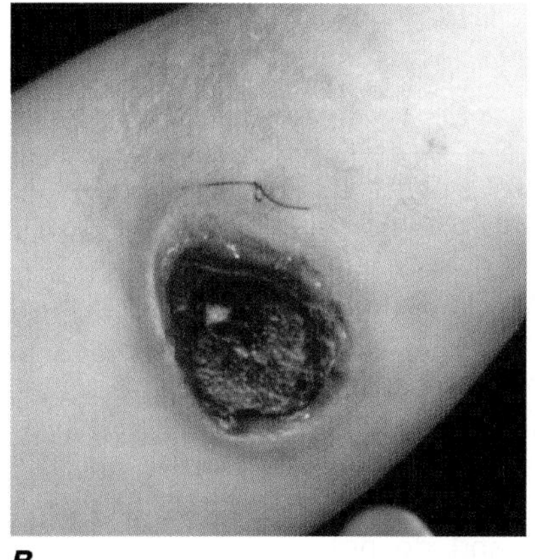
B

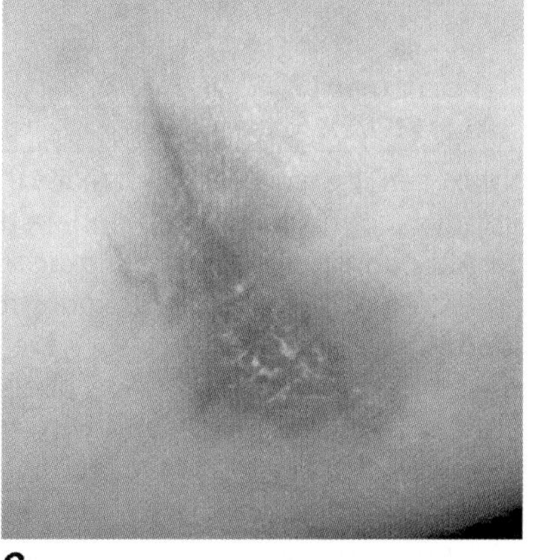
C

FIGURE 6-2

Clinical manifestations of a pediatric case of cutaneous anthrax associated with the bioterrorism attack of 2001. The lesion progresses from vesicular on day 5 (***A***) to necrotic with the classic black eschar on day 12 (***B***) to a healed scar 2 months later (***C***). (*Photographs provided by Dr. Mary Wu Chang and (A) reprinted with permission of the New England Journal of Medicine.*)

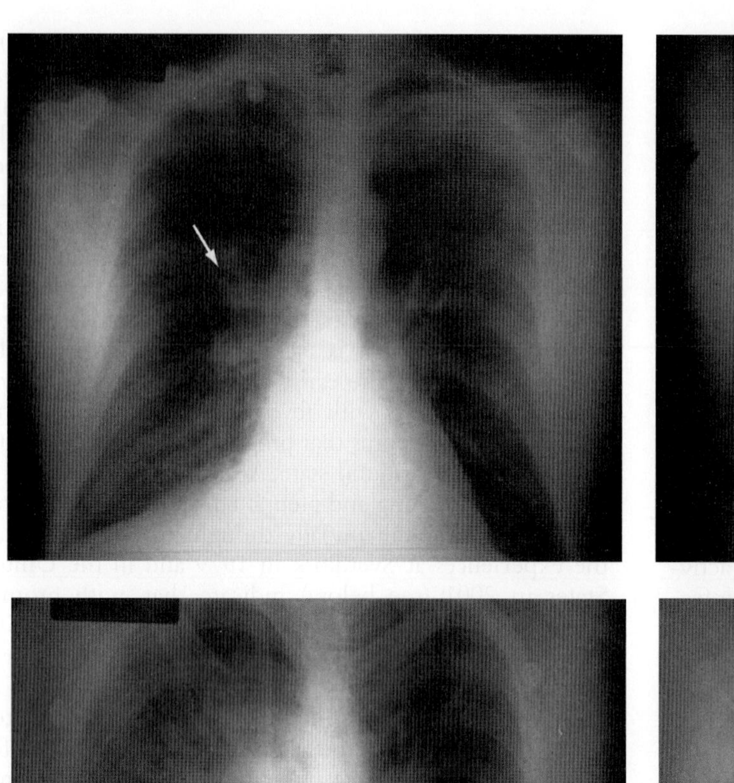
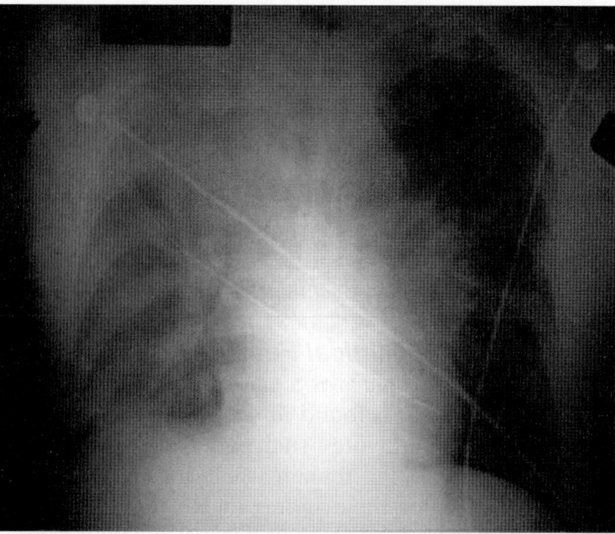
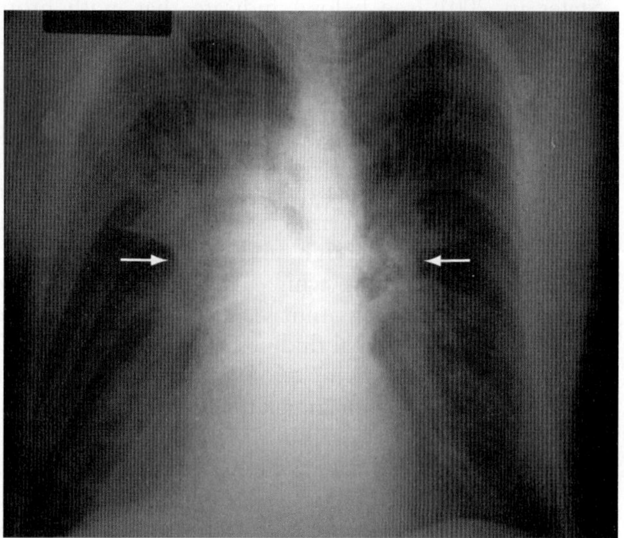
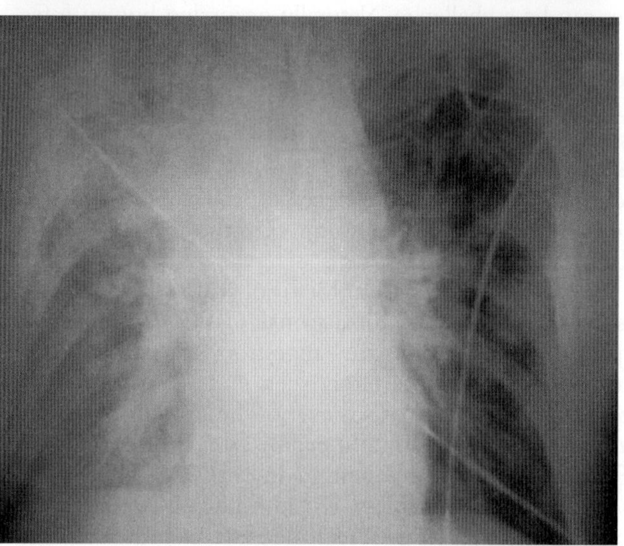

FIGURE 6-3

Progression of chest x-ray findings in a patient with inhalational anthrax. Findings evolved from subtle hilar prominence and right perihilar infiltrate to a progressively widened mediastinum, marked perihilar infiltrates, peribronchial cuffing, and air bronchograms. (*From L Borio et al: Death due to bioterrorism-related inhalational anthrax. JAMA 286:2554, 2001; with permission.*)

℞ Treatment: ANTHRAX

Anthrax can be successfully treated if the disease is promptly recognized and appropriate therapy is initiated early. Although penicillin, ciprofloxacin, and doxycycline are the currently licensed antibiotics for this indication, clindamycin and rifampin also have in vitro activity against the organism and have been used as part of treatment regimens. Until sensitivity results are known, suspected cases are best managed with a combination of broadly active agents (Table 6-3). Patients with inhalational anthrax are not contagious and do not require special isolation procedures.

Vaccination and Prevention

The first successful vaccine for anthrax was developed for animals by Louis Pasteur in 1881. At present, the single vaccine licensed for human use is a product produced from the cell-free culture supernatant of an attenuated, nonencapsulated strain of *B. anthracis* (Stern's strain), referred to as *anthrax vaccine adsorbed* (AVA). Clinical trials for safety in humans and efficacy in animals are currently underway to evaluate the role of recombinant protective antigen (one of the major components, along with lethal factor and edema factor, of *B. anthracis* toxins) as an alternative to AVA. In a postexposure setting in nonhuman primates, a 2-week course of AVA plus ciprofloxacin was found to be superior to ciprofloxacin alone in preventing the development of clinical disease and death. Although the current recommendation for postexposure prophylaxis is 60 days of antibiotics, it would seem prudent to include immunization with anthrax vaccine if available. Given the potential for *B. anthracis* to be engineered to express penicillin resistance, the empirical regimen of choice in this setting is either ciprofloxacin or doxycycline.

TABLE 6-3

CLINICAL SYNDROMES, PREVENTION, AND TREATMENT STRATEGIES FOR DISEASES CAUSES BY CATEGORY A AGENTS

AGENT	CLINICAL SYNDROME	INCUBATION PERIOD	DIAGNOSIS	TREATMENT	PROPHYLAXIS
Bacillus anthracis (anthrax)	Cutaneous lesion: Papule to eschar Inhalational disease: Fever, malaise, chest and abdominal discomfort Pleural effusion, widened mediastinum on chest x-ray	1–12 days 1–60 days	Culture, Gram's stain, PCR, Wright's stain of peripheral smear	Postexposure: Ciprofloxacin, 500 mg, PO bid × 60 d *or* Doxycycline, 100 mg PO bid × 60 d also (Amoxicillin, 500 mg PO q8h, likely to be effective if strain penicillin sensitive) *Active disease:* Ciprofloxacin, 400 mg IV q12h *or* Doxycycline, 100 mg IV q12 *plus* Clindamycin, 900 mg IV q8h and/or rifampin, 300 mg IV q12h; switch to PO when stable × 60 d total *Antitoxin strategies:* Neutralizing monoclonal and polyclonal antibodies are under study	Anthrax vaccine adsorbed Recombinant protective antigen vaccines are under study
Yersinia pestis (pneumonic plague)	Fever, cough, dyspnea, hemoptysis Infiltrates and consolidation on chest x-ray	1–6 days	Culture, Gram's stain, direct fluorescent antibody, PCR	Gentamicin, 2.0 mg/kg IV loading then 1.7 mg/kg q8h IV *or* Streptomycin, 1.0 g q12h IM *or* IV Alternatives include doxycycline, 100 mg bid PO or IV; chloramphenicol 500 mg qid PO or IV	Doxycycline, 100 mg PO bid (ciprofloxacin may also be active) Formalin-fixed vaccine (FDA licensed; not available)
Variola major (smallpox)	Fever, malaise, headache, backache, emesis Maculopapular to vesicular to pustular skin lesions	7–17 days	Culture, PCR, electron microscopy	Supportive measures; consideration for cidofovir, antivaccinia immunoglobulin	Vaccinia immunization

(*Continued*)

TABLE 6-3 (*CONTINUED*)

CLINICAL SYNDROMES, PREVENTION, AND TREATMENT STRATEGIES FOR DISEASES CAUSES BY CATEGORY A AGENTS

AGENT	CLINICAL SYNDROME	INCUBATION PERIOD	DIAGNOSIS	TREATMENT	PROPHYLAXIS
Francisella tularensis (tularemia)	Fever, chills, malaise, myalgia, chest discomfort, dyspnea, headache, skin rash, pharyngitis, conjunctivitis Hilar adenopathy on chest x-ray	1–14 days	Gram's stain, culture, immunohistochemistry, PCR	Streptomycin, 1 g IM bid *or* Gentamicin, 5 mg/kg per day div q8h IV for 14 days *or* Doxycycline, 100 mg IV bid *or* Chloramphenicol, 15 mg/kg IV qid *or* Ciprofloxacin, 400 mg IV bid	Doxycycline, 100 mg PO bid × 14 days *or* Ciprofloxacin, 500 mg PO bid × 14 days
Viral hemorrhagic fevers	Fever, myalgia, rash, encephalitis, prostration	2–21 days	RT-PCR, serologic testing for antigen or antibody Viral isolation by CDC or U.S. Army Medical Institute of Infectious Diseases	Supportive measures Ribavirin 30 mg/kg up to 2 g × 1, followed by 16 mg/kg IV up to 1 g q6h for 4 days, followed by 8 mg/kg IV up to 0.5 g q8h × 6 days	No known chemoprophylaxis Consideration for ribavirin in high-risk situations Vaccine exists for yellow fever
Botulinum toxin (*Clostridium botulinum*)	Dry mouth, blurred vision, ptosis, weakness, dysarthria, dysphagia, dizziness, respiratory failure, progressive paralysis, dilated pupils	12–72 h	Mouse bioassay, toxin immunoassay	Supportive measures including ventilation 5000–9000 IU equine antitoxin	Administration of antitoxin

Note: CDC, U.S. Centers for Disease Control and Prevention; FDA, U.S. Food and Drug Administration; PCR, polymerase chain reaction; RT-PCR, reverse transcriptase PCR.

PLAGUE

See also Chap. 60.

Yersinia Pestis as a Bioweapon

Although it lacks the environmental stability of anthrax, the highly contagious nature and high mortality of plague make it a close to ideal agent of bioterrorism, particularly if delivered in a weaponized form. Occupying a unique place in history, plague has been alleged to have been used as a biologic weapon for centuries. The catapulting of plague-infected corpses into besieged fortresses is a practice that was first noted in 1346 during the assault of the city of Kaffa by the Tartars. Although unlikely to have resulted in disease transmission, some believe that this event may have played a role in the start of the Black Death pandemic of the fourteenth and fifteenth centuries in Europe. Given that plague was already moving across Asia toward Europe at this time, it is unclear whether such an allegation is accurate. During WWII, the infamous Unit 731 of the Japanese army was reported to have repeatedly dropped plague-infested fleas over parts of China, including Manchuria. These drops were associated with subsequent outbreaks of plague in the targeted areas. After WWII, the United States and the Soviet Union conducted programs of research on how to create aerosolized *Y. pestis* that could be used as a bioweapon to cause primary pneumonic plague. As mentioned above, plague was thought to be an excellent bioweapon due to the fact that, in addition to causing infection in those inhaling the aerosol, significant numbers of secondary cases of primary pneumonic plague would likely occur due to the contagious nature of the disease and person-to-person transmission via respiratory aerosol. Secondary reports of research conducted during that time suggest that organisms remain viable for up to 1 h and can be dispersed for distances up to 10 km. Although the offensive bioweapons program in the United States was terminated before production of sufficient quantities of plague organisms for use as a weapon, it is believed that Soviet scientists did manufacture quantities sufficient for such a purpose. It has also been reported that more than 10 Soviet Institutes and >1000 scientists were working with plague as a biologic weapon. Of concern is the fact that, in 1995, a microbiologist in Ohio was arrested for having obtained *Y. pestis* in the mail from the American Type Culture Collection, using a credit card and a false letterhead. In the wake of this incident, the U.S. Congress passed a law in 1997 requiring that anyone intending to send or receive any of 42 different agents that could potentially be used as bioweapons first register with the CDC.

Microbiology and Clinical Features

Plague is caused by *Y. pestis*, a nonmotile, gram-negative bacillus that exhibits bipolar, or "safety pin," staining with Wright's, Giemsa's, or Wayson's stains. It has had a major impact on the course of history, thus adding to the element of fear evoked by its mention. The earliest reported plague epidemic was in 224 B.C. in China. The most infamous pandemic began in Europe in the fourteenth century, during which time one-third to one-half of the entire population of Europe was killed. During a plague outbreak in India in 1994, even though the number of confirmed cases was relatively small, it is estimated that 500,000 individuals fled their homes in fear of this disease.

The clinical syndromes of plague generally reflect the mode of infection. *Bubonic plague* is the consequence of an insect bite; primary *pneumonic plague* arises through the inhalation of bacteria. Most of the plague seen in the world today is bubonic plague and is the result of a bite by a plague-infected flea. In part as a consequence of past pandemics, plague infection of rodents exists widely in nature, including in the southwestern United States, and each year thousands of cases of plague occur worldwide through contact with infected animals or fleas. After inoculation of regurgitated bacteria into the skin by a flea bite, organisms travel through the lymphatics to regional lymph nodes, where they are phagocytized but not destroyed. Inside the cell, they multiply rapidly, leading to inflammation, painful lymphadenopathy with necrosis, fever, bacteremia, septicemia, and death. The characteristic enlarged, inflamed lymph nodes, or *buboes*, give this form of plague its name. In some instances, patients may develop bacteremia without lymphadenopathy after infection, a condition referred to as *primary septicemic plague*. Extensive ecchymoses may develop due to disseminated intravascular coagulation, and gangrene of the digits and/or nose may develop in patients with advanced septicemic plague. It is thought that this appearance of some patients gave rise to the term *Black Death* in reference to the plague epidemic of the fourteenth and fifteenth centuries. Some patients may develop pneumonia (secondary pneumonic plague) as a complication of bubonic or septicemic plague. These patients may then transmit the agent to others via the respiratory route, causing cases of primary pneumonic plague. Primary pneumonic plague is the manifestation most likely to occur as the result of a bioterrorist attack, with an aerosol of bacteria spread over a wide area or a particular environment that is densely populated. In this setting, patients would be expected to develop fever, cough with hemoptysis, dyspnea, and gastrointestinal symptoms 1–6 days after exposure. Clinical features of pneumonia would be accompanied by pulmonary infiltrates and consolidation on chest x-ray. In the absence of antibiotics, the mortality of this disease is on the order of 85%, and death usually occurs within 2–6 days.

℞ Treatment: PLAGUE

Streptomycin, tetracycline, and doxycycline are licensed by the U.S. Food and Drug Administration (FDA) for the treatment of plague. Multiple additional antibiotics licensed for other infections are commonly used and are likely effective. Among these are aminoglycosides such as gentamicin, cephalosporins, trimethoprim/sulfamethoxazole, chloramphenicol, and ciprofloxacin (Table 6-3). A multidrug-resistant strain of *Y. pestis* was identified in 1995 from a patient with bubonic plague in Madagascar. Although this organism was resistant to streptomycin, ampicillin, chloramphenicol, sulfonamides, and tetracycline, it retained its susceptibility to other aminoglycosides and cephalosporins. Given the subsequent identification of a similar organism in 1997 coupled with the fact that this resistance is plasmid-mediated, it seems likely that genetically modifying *Y. pestis* to a multidrug-resistant form is possible. Unlike patients with inhalational anthrax (see above), patients with pulmonary plague should be cared for under conditions of strict respiratory isolation comparable to that used for multidrug-resistant tuberculosis.

Vaccination and Prevention

A formalin-fixed, whole-organism vaccine was licensed by the FDA for the prevention of plague. That vaccine is no longer being manufactured, but its potential value as a current countermeasure against bioterrorism would likely have been modest at best, as it was ineffective against animal models of primary pneumonic plague. Efforts are underway to develop a second generation of vaccines that will protect against aerosol challenge. Among the candidates being tested are recombinant forms of the F1 and V antigens of *Y. pestis*. It is likely that doxycycline or ciprofloxacin would provide coverage in a chemoprophylaxis setting. Unlike the case with anthrax, in which one has to be concerned about the persistence of ungerminated spores in the respiratory tract, the duration of prophylaxis against plague need only extend to 7 days after exposure.

SMALLPOX

Variola Virus as a Bioweapon

Given that most of the world's population was vaccinated against smallpox, variola virus would not have been considered a good candidate as a bioweapon 30 years ago. However, with the cessation of immunization programs in the United States in 1972 and throughout the world in 1980 due to the successful global eradication of smallpox, close to 50% of the U.S. population is fully susceptible to smallpox today. Given its infectious nature and the 10–30% mortality in unimmunized individuals, the deliberate spread of this virus could have a devastating effect on our society and unleash a previously conquered deadly disease. It is estimated that an initial infection of 50–100 persons in a first-generation of cases could expand by a factor of 10–20 with each succeeding generation in the absence of any effective containment measures. Although the likely implementation of an effective public health response makes this scenario unlikely, it does illustrate the potential damage and disruption that can result from a smallpox outbreak.

In 1980, the World Health Organization (WHO) recommended that all immunization programs be terminated; that representative samples of variola virus be transferred to two locations: one at the CDC in Atlanta, GA, in the United States and the other at the Institute of Virus Preparations in the Soviet Union; and that all other stocks of smallpox be destroyed. Several years later, it was recommended that these two authorized collections be destroyed. However, these latter recommendations were placed on hold in the wake of increased concerns of the use of *variola virus* as a biologic weapon and thus the need to maintain an active program of defensive research. Many of these concerns were based on allegations made by former Soviet officials that extensive programs had been in place in that country for the production and weaponization of large quantities of smallpox virus. The dismantling of these programs with the fall of the Soviet Union and the subsequent weakening of security measures led to fears that stocks of *V. major* may have made their way to other countries or terrorist organizations. In addition, accounts that efforts had been taken to produce recombinant strains of *Variola* that would be more virulent and more contagious than the wild-type virus have led to an increase in the need to be vigilant for the reemergence of this often fatal-infectious disease.

Microbiology and Clinical Features

Smallpox is caused by one of two variants of variola virus, *V. major* and *V. minor*. Variola is a double-strand DNA virus and member of the Orthopoxvirus genus of the Poxviridae family. Infections with *V. minor* are generally less severe than those of *V. major*, with milder constitutional symptoms and lower mortality rates; thus *V. major* is the only one considered to be a viable bioweapon. Infection with *V. major* typically occurs after contact with an infected person from the time that a maculopapular rash appears on the skin and oropharynx, through the resolution and scabbing of the pustular lesions. Infection occurs principally during close contact, through the inhalation of saliva droplets containing virus from the oropharyngeal exanthem. Aerosolized material from contaminated clothing or linen can also spread infection. Several days after exposure, a primary viremia is believed to occur that results in dissemination of virus to lymphoid tissues. A secondary viremia occurs ~4 days later that leads to localization of infection in the dermis. Approximately 12–14 days after the initial exposure, the patient develops high fever, malaise, vomiting, headache, backache, and a maculopapular rash that begins on the face and extremities and spreads to the trunk (centripetal), with lesions in the same developmental stage in any given location. This is in contrast to the rash of varicella (chickenpox) that begins on the trunk and face and spreads to the extremities (centrifugal), with lesions at all stages of development. The lesions are initially maculopapular and evolve to vesicles that eventually become pustules and then scabs. The oral mucosa also develops maculopapular lesions that evolve to ulcers. The lesions appear over a period of 1–2 days and evolve at the same rate. Although virus can be isolated from the scabs on the skin, the conventional thinking is that once the scabs have formed, the patient is no longer contagious. Smallpox is associated with a 10–30% mortality, with patients typically dying of severe systemic illness during the second week of symptoms. Historically, ~5–10% of naturally occurring smallpox cases take either of two highly virulent atypical forms, classified as *hemorrhagic* and *malignant*. These are difficult to recognize because of their atypical presentations. The hemorrhagic form is uniformly fatal and begins with the relatively abrupt onset of a severely prostrating illness characterized by high fevers and severe headache and back and abdominal pain. This form of the illness resembles a severe systemic inflammatory syndrome, in which patients have a high viremia, but die without developing the characteristic rash. Cutaneous erythema develops accompanied by petechiae and hemorrhages into the skin and mucous membranes. Death usually occurs within 5–6 days. The malignant, or "flat," form of smallpox is frequently fatal and has an onset similar to the hemorrhagic form, but with confluent skin lesions developing more slowly and never progressing to the pustular stage.

℞ Treatment: SMALLPOX

Given the infectious nature of smallpox and the extreme vulnerability of contemporary society, patients who are suspected cases should be handled with strict isolation procedures. Although laboratory confirmation of a suspected case by culture and electron microscopy is essential, it is equally important that appropriate precautions be employed when obtaining samples for culture and laboratory testing. All health care and laboratory workers caring for patients should have been recently immunized with vaccinia, and all samples should be transported in doubly sealed containers. Patients should be cared for in negative-pressure rooms with strict isolation precautions.

There is no licensed specific therapy for smallpox, and historic treatments have focused solely on supportive care. Although several antiviral agents, including cidofovir, that are licensed for other diseases have in vitro activity against *V. major*, they have never been tested in the setting of human disease. For this reason, it is difficult to predict whether or not they would be effective in cases of smallpox and, if effective, whether or not they would be of value in patients with advanced disease. Research programs studying the efficacy of new antiviral compounds against *V. major* are currently underway.

Vaccination and Prevention

In 1796 Edward Jenner demonstrated that deliberate infection with cowpox virus could prevent illness on subsequent exposure to smallpox. Today, smallpox is a preventable disease after immunization with vaccinia. The current dilemma facing our society regarding assessment of the risk and/or benefit of smallpox vaccination is that the degree of risk that someone will deliberately and effectively release smallpox into our society is unknown. As a prudent first step in preparedness for a smallpox attack, virtually all members of the U.S. armed services have received primary or booster immunizations with vaccinia. In addition, tens of thousands of civilian health care workers who comprise smallpox-response teams at the state and local public health level have been vaccinated.

Initial fears regarding the immunization of a segment of the American population with vaccinia when there are more individuals receiving immunosuppressive drugs and other immunocompromised patients than ever before have largely been dispelled as data are generated from the current military and civilian immunization campaigns. Adverse event rates for the first 450,000 immunizations are similar to and, in certain categories of adverse events, even lower than those from historic data, in which most severe sequelae of vaccination occurred in young infants (Table 6-4). In addition, 11 patients

TABLE 6-4

COMPLICATIONS FROM 438,134 ADMINISTRATIONS OF VACCINIA DURING THE U.S. DEPARTMENT OF DEFENSE (DoD) SMALLPOX IMMUNIZATION CAMPAIGN INITIATED IN DECEMBER 2002

COMPLICATION	NUMBER OF CASES	DoD RATE PER MILLION VACCINEES (95% CONFIDENCE INTERVAL)	HISTORIC RATE PER MILLION VACCINEES
Mild or temporary:			
Generalized vaccinia, mild	35	67 (52, 85)	45 to 212[a]
Inadvertent inoculation, self	62	119 (98, 142)	606[a]
Vaccinia transfer to contact	28	53 (40, 69)	8 to 27[a]
Moderate or serious:			
Encephalitis	1	2.2 (0.6, 7.2)	2.6 to 8.7[a]
Acute myopericarditis	69	131 (110, 155)	100[b]
Eczema vaccinatum	0	0 (0, 3.7)	2 to 35[a]
Progressive vaccinia	0	0 (0, 3.7)	1 to 7[a]
Death[c]	1	1.9 (0.2, 5.6)	1 to 2[a]

[a]Based on adolescent and adult smallpox vaccinations from 1968 studies, both primary and revaccinations.
[b]Based on case series in Finnish military recruits given the Finnish strain of smallpox vaccine.
[c]Potentially attributable to vaccination; after lupus-like illness.
Source: From JD Grabenstein and W Winkenwerder: *http://www.smallpox.mil/event/SPSafetySum.asp*

with early-stage HIV infection have been inadvertently immunized without problem. One significant concern during the recent immunization campaign, however, has been the description of a syndrome of myopericarditis, which was not appreciated during prior immunization campaigns with vaccinia.

TULAREMIA

See also Chap. 59.

Francisella tularensis as a Bioweapon

Tularemia has been studied as an agent of bioterrorism since the mid-twentieth century. It has been speculated by some that the outbreak of tularemia among German and Soviet soldiers during fighting on the Eastern Front during WWII was the consequence of a deliberate release. Unit 731 of the Japanese Army studied the use of tularemia as a bioweapon during WWII. Large preparations were made for mass productive of *F. tularensis* by the United States, but no stockpiling of any agent took place. Stocks of *F. tularensis* were reportedly generated by the Soviet Union in the mid-1950s. It has also been suggested that the Soviet program extended into the era of molecular biology and that some strains were engineered to be resistant to common antibiotics. *F. tularensis* is an extremely infectious organism, and human infections have occurred from merely examining an uncovered petri dish streaked with colonies. Given these facts, it is reasonable to conclude that this organism might be utilized as a bioweapon through either an aerosol or contamination of food or drinking water.

Microbiology and Clinical Features

Although similar in many ways to anthrax and plague, tularemia, also referred to as rabbit fever or deer fly fever, is neither as lethal nor as fulminant as either of these other two category A bacterial infections. It is, however, extremely infectious, and as few as 10 organisms can lead to establishment of infection. Despite this fact, it is not spread from person to person. Tularemia is caused by *F. tularensis*, a small, nonmotile, gram-negative coccobacillus. Although it is not a spore-forming organism, it is a hardy bacterium that can survive for weeks in the environment. Infection typically comes from insect bites or contact with organisms in the environment. Large waterborne outbreaks have been recorded. It is most likely that the outbreak among German and Russian soldiers and Russian civilians noted above during WWII represented a large waterborne tularemia outbreak in a *Tularensis*-enzootic area devastated by warfare.

Humans can become infected through a variety of environmental sources. Infection is most common in rural areas where a variety of small mammals may serve as reservoirs. Human infections in the summer are often the result of insect bites from ticks, flies, or mosquitoes that have bitten infected animals. In colder months infections are most likely the result of direct contact with infected mammals and are most common in hunters. In these settings infection typically presents as a systemic illness with an area of inflammation and necrosis at the site of tissue entry. Drinking of contaminated water may lead to an oropharyngeal form of tularemia characterized by pharyngitis with cervical and/or retropharyngeal lymphadenopathy (Chap. 59). The most likely mode of dissemination of tularemia as a biologic weapon would be as an aerosol, as has occurred in a number of natural outbreaks in rural areas, including Martha's Vineyard in the United States. Approximately 1–14 days after exposure by this route, one would expect to see inflammation of the airways with pharyngitis, pleuritis, and bronchopneumonia. Typical symptoms would include the abrupt onset of fever, fatigue, chills, headache, and malaise (Table 6-3). Some patients might experience conjunctivitis with ulceration, pharyngitis, and/or cutaneous exanthems. A pulse-temperature dissociation might be present. Approximately 50% of patients would show a pulmonary infiltrate on chest x-ray. Hilar adenopathy might also be present, and a small percentage of patients could have adenopathy without infiltrates. The highly variable presentation makes acute recognition of aerosol-disseminated tularemia very difficult. The diagnosis would likely be made by immunohistochemistry or culture of infected tissues or blood. Untreated, mortality rates range from 5–15% for cutaneous routes of infection and 30–60% for infection by inhalation. Since the advent of antibiotic therapy, these rates have dropped to <2%.

℞ Treatment: TULAREMIA

Both streptomycin and doxycycline are licensed for treatment of tularemia. Other agents likely to be effective include gentamicin, chloramphenicol, and ciprofloxacin (Table 6-3). Given the potential for genetic modification of this organism to yield antibiotic-resistant strains, broad-spectrum coverage should be the rule until sensitivities have been determined. As mentioned above, special isolation procedures are not required.

Vaccination and Prevention

There are no vaccines currently licensed for the prevention of tularemia. Although a live, attenuated strain of the organism has been used in the past with some reported success, there are inadequate data to support its widespread use at this time. Development of a vaccine for this agent is an important part of the current biodefense research agenda. In the absence of an effective vaccine, postexposure chemoprophylaxis with either doxycycline or ciprofloxacin appears to be a reasonable approach (Table 6-3).

VIRAL HEMORRHAGIC FEVERS

See also Chaps. 99 and 100.

Hemorrhagic Fever Viruses as Bioweapons

Several of the hemorrhagic fever viruses have been reported to have been weaponized by the Soviet Union and the United States. Nonhuman primate studies indicate that infection can be established with very few virions and that infectious aerosol preparations can be produced. Under the guise of wanting to aid victims of an Ebola outbreak, members of the Aum Shrinrikyo cult in Japan were reported to have traveled to central Africa in 1992 in an attempt to obtain Ebola virus for use in a bioterrorist attack. Thus, although there has been no evidence that these agents have ever been used in a biologic attack, there is clear interest in their potential for this purpose.

Microbiology and Clinical Features

The viral hemorrhagic fevers are a group of illnesses caused by any one of a number of similar viruses (Table 6-2). These viruses are all enveloped, single-strand RNA viruses that are thought to depend upon a rodent or insect host reservoir for long-term survival. They tend to be geographically restricted according to the migration patterns of their hosts. Great apes are not a natural reservoir for Ebola virus, but large numbers of these animals in Sub-Saharan Africa have died from Ebola infection over the past decade. Humans can become infected with hemorrhagic fever viruses if they come into contact with an infected host or other infected animals. Person-to-person transmission, largely through direct contact with virus-containing body fluids, has been documented for Ebola, Marburg, and Lassa virus and rarely for the New World arenaviruses. Although there is no clear evidence of respiratory spread among humans, these viruses have been shown in animal models to be highly infectious by the aerosol route. This, coupled with mortality rates as high as 90%, makes them excellent candidate agents of bioterrorism.

The clinical features of the viral hemorrhagic fevers vary depending upon the particular agent (Table 6-3). Initial signs and symptoms typically include fever, myalgia, prostration, and disseminated intravascular coagulation with thrombocytopenia and capillary hemorrhage. These findings are consistent with a cytokine-mediated systemic inflammatory syndrome. A variety of different maculopapular or erythematous rashes may be seen. Leukopenia, temperature-pulse dissociation, renal failure, and seizures may also be part of the clinical presentation. Outbreaks of most of these diseases are sporadic and unpredictable. As a consequence, most studies of pathogenesis have been performed using laboratory animals. The diagnosis should be suspected in anyone with temperature >38.3°C for <3 weeks who also exhibits at least 2 of the following: hemorrhagic or purpuric rash, epistaxis, hematemesis, hemoptysis, or hematochezia in the absence of any other identifiable cause. In this setting, samples of blood should be sent after consultation to the CDC or the U.S. Army Medical Research Institute of Infectious Diseases for serologic testing for antigen and antibody as well as reverse transcriptase polymerase chain reaction (RT-PCR) testing for hemorrhagic fever viruses. All samples should be handled with double-bagging. Given how little is known regarding the human-to-human transmission of these viruses, appropriate isolation measures would include full-barrier precautions with negative-pressure rooms and use of N95 masks or powered air-purifying respirators (PAPRs). Unprotected skin contact with cadavers has been implicated in the transmission of certain hemorrhagic fever viruses such as Ebola, so it is recommended that autopsies be performed using the strictest measures for protection and that burial or cremation be performed promptly without embalming.

℞ Treatment: VIRAL HEMORRHAGIC FEVERS

There are no approved and effective antiviral therapies for this class of viruses (Table 6-3). Although there are anecdotal reports of the efficacy of ribavirin, interferon-α, or hyperimmune immunoglobulin, definitive data are lacking. The best data for ribavirin are in arenavirus (Lassa and New World) infections. In some in vitro systems, specific immunoglobulin has been reported to enhance infectivity, and thus these potential treatments must be approached with caution.

Vaccination and Prevention

A live attenuated virus vaccine is available in limited quantities for prevention of yellow fever. There are no other licensed and effective vaccines for these agents. Studies are currently underway examining the potential role of DNA, recombinant viruses, and attenuated viruses as vaccines for several of these infections. Among the most promising at present are vaccines for Argentine, Ebola, Rift Valley, and Kyasanur Forest viruses.

BOTULISM TOXIN (*CLOSTRIDIUM BOTULINUM*)

See also Chap. 41.

Botulinum Toxin as a Bioweapon

In a bioterrorist attack, botulinum toxin would likely be dispersed as an aerosol or as contamination of a food supply. Although contamination of a water supply is possible, it is likely that any toxin would be rapidly inactivated by the chlorine used to purify drinking water. Similarly, toxin can be inactivated by heating any food to >85°C for >5 min. Without external facilitation, the environmental decay rate is estimated at 1% per minute, and thus the time interval between weapon release and ingestion or inhalation needs to be rather short. The Japanese biologic warfare group, Unit 731, is reported to have conducted experiments on botulism poisoning in prisoners in the 1930s. The United States and the Soviet Union both acknowledged producing botulinum toxin, and there is some evidence that the

Soviet Union attempted to create recombinant bacteria containing the gene for botulinum toxin. In records submitted to the United Nations, Iraq admitted to having produced 19,000 L of concentrated toxin—enough toxin to kill the entire population of the world three times over. By many accounts, botulinum toxin was the primary focus of the pre-1991 Iraqi bioweapons program. In addition to these examples of state-supported research into the use of botulinum toxin as a bioweapon, the Aum Shrinrikyo cult unsuccessfully attempted on a least three occasions to disperse botulism toxin into the civilian population of Tokyo.

Microbiology and Clinical Features

Unique among the category A agents for not being a live microorganism, botulinum toxin is one of the most potent toxins ever described and is thought by some to be the most poisonous substance in existence. It is estimated that 1 g of botulinum toxin would be sufficient to kill 1 million individuals if adequately dispersed. Botulinum toxin is produced by the gram-positive, spore-forming anaerobe *C. botulinum* (Chap. 42). Its natural habitat is soil. There are seven antigenically distinct forms of botulinum toxin, designated A–G. The majority of naturally occurring human cases are of types A, B, and E. Antitoxin directed toward one of these will have little to no activity against the others. The toxin is a 150-kDa zinc-containing protease that prevents the intracellular fusion of acetylcholine vesicles with the motor neuron membrane, thus preventing the release of acetylcholine. In the absence of acetylcholine-dependent triggering of muscle fibers, a flaccid paralysis develops. Although botulism does not spread from person to person, the ease of production of the toxin coupled with its high morbidity and 60–100% mortality make it a close to ideal bioweapon.

Botulism can result from the presence of *C. botulinum* infection in a wound or the intestine, the ingestion of contaminated food, or the inhalation of aerosolized toxin. The latter two forms are the most likely modes of transmission for bioterrorism. Once toxin is absorbed into the bloodstream it binds to the neuronal cell membrane, enters the cell, and cleaves one of the proteins required for the intracellular binding of the synaptic vesicle to the cell membrane, thus preventing release of the neurotransmitter to the membrane of the adjacent muscle cell. Patients initially develop multiple cranial nerve palsies that are followed by a descending flaccid paralysis. The extent of the neuromuscular compromise is dependent upon the level of toxemia. The majority of patients experience diplopia, dysphagia, dysarthria, dry mouth, ptosis, dilated pupils, fatigue, and extremity weakness. There are minimal true central nervous system effects, and patients rarely show significant alterations in mental status. Severe cases can involve complete muscular collapse, loss of the gag reflex, and respiratory failure, requiring weeks or months of ventilator support. Recovery requires the regeneration of new motor neuron synapses with the muscle cell, a process that can take weeks to months. In the absence of secondary infections, which may be common during the protracted recovery phase of this illness, patients remain afebrile. The diagnosis is suspected on clinical grounds and confirmed by a mouse bioassay or toxin immunoassay.

℞ Treatment: BOTULISM

Treatment for botulism is mainly supportive and may require intubation, mechanical ventilation, and parenteral nutrition (Table 6-3). If diagnosed early enough, administration of equine antitoxin may reduce the extent of nerve injury and decrease the severity of disease. At present, antitoxins are available on a limited basis as a licensed bivalent product with activity against toxin types A and B and as an experimental product with activity against toxin type E. In the event of attack with another toxin type, an investigational antitoxin with activity against all seven toxin types is also available through the U.S. Army. A single dose of antitoxin is usually adequate to neutralize any circulating toxin. Given that these preparations are all derived from horse serum, one needs to be vigilant for hypersensitivity reactions, including serum sickness and anaphylaxis after their administration. Once the damage to the nerve axon has been done, however, there is little possible in the way of specific therapy. At this point, vigilance for secondary complications such as infections during the protracted recovery phase is of the utmost importance. Due to their ability to worsen neuromuscular blockade, aminoglycosides and clindamycin should be avoided in the treatment of these infections.

Vaccination and Prevention

A botulinum toxoid preparation has been used as a vaccine for laboratory workers at high risk of exposure and in certain military situations; however, it is not currently available in quantities that could be used for the general population. At present, early recognition of the clinical syndrome and use of appropriate equine antitoxin is the mainstay of prevention of full-blown disease in exposed individuals. The development of human monoclonal antibodies as a replacement for equine antitoxin antibodies is an area of active research interest.

CATEGORY B AND C AGENTS

The category B agents include those that are easy or moderately easy to disseminate and result in moderate morbidity and low mortality rates. A listing of the current category B agents is provided in Table 6-2. As can be seen, it includes a wide array of microorganisms and products of microorganisms. Several of these agents have been used in bioterrorist attacks, although never with the impact of the agents described above. Among the more notorious of these was the contamination of salad bars in Oregon in 1984 with *Salmonella typhimurium* by the religious cult Rajneeshee. In this outbreak, which many consider to be the first bioterrorist attack against U.S. citizens, >750 individuals were poisoned and 40 were hospitalized in an effort to influence a local election. The intentional nature of this outbreak went unrecognized for more than a decade.

Category C agents are the third highest-priority agents in the biodefense agenda. These agents include emerging pathogens to which little or no immunity exists in the general population, such as the severe acute respiratory syndrome (SARS) coronavirus or pandemic-potential strains of influenza that could be obtained from nature and deliberately disseminated. These agents are characterized as being relatively easy to produce and disseminate and as having high morbidity and mortality rates as well as a significant public health impact. There is no running list of category C agents at the present time.

PREVENTION AND PREPAREDNESS

As noted above, a large and diverse array of agents has the potential to be used in a bioterrorist attack. In contrast to the military situation with biowarfare, where the primary objective is to inflict mass casualties on a healthy and prepared militia, the objectives of bioterrorism are to harm civilians, as well as to create fear and disruption among the civilian population. Although the military needs only to prepare their troops to deal with the limited number of agents that pose a legitimate threat of biowarfare, the public health system needs to prepare the entire civilian population to deal with the multitude of agents and settings that could be utilized in a bioterrorism attack. This includes anticipating issues specific to the very young and the very old, the pregnant patient, and the immunocompromised individual. The challenges in this regard are enormous and immediate. Although military preparedness emphasizes vaccines toward a limited number of agents, civilian preparedness needs to rely upon rapid diagnosis and treatment of a wide array of conditions.

The medical profession must maintain a high index of suspicion that unusual clinical presentations or the clustering of cases of a rare disease may not be a chance occurrence but rather the first sign of a bioterrorist event. This is particularly true when such diseases occur in traditionally healthy populations, when surprisingly large numbers of rare conditions occur, and when diseases commonly seen in rural settings appear in urban populations. Given the importance of rapid diagnosis and early treatment for many of these conditions, it is essential that the medical care team report any suspected cases of bioterrorism immediately to local and state health authorities and/or to the CDC (888-246-2675). Recent enhancements have been made to the public health surveillance network to facilitate the rapid sharing of information among public health agencies.

At present, a series of efforts are taking place to ensure the biomedical security of the civilian population of the United States. The Public Health Service is moving toward a larger, more highly trained, fully deployable force. A Strategic National Stockpile (SNS) has been created by the CDC to provide rapid access to quantities of pharmaceuticals, antidotes, vaccines, and other medical supplies that may be of value in the event of biologic or chemical terrorism. The SNS has two basic components. The first of these consists of "push packages" that can be deployed anywhere in the United States within 12 h. These push packages are a preassembled set of supplies, pharmaceuticals, and medical equipment ready for immediate delivery to the field. They provide treatment for a variety of conditions given the fact that an actual threat may not have been precisely identified at the time of stockpile deployment. The contents of the push packages are constantly updated to ensure that they reflect current needs as determined by national security threat assessments; they include antibiotics for treatment of anthrax, plague, and tularemia as well as a cache of vaccine to deal with a smallpox threat. The second component of the SNS comprises inventories managed by specific vendors and consists of the provision of additional pharmaceuticals, supplies, and/or products tailored to the specific attack.

The number of FDA-approved and -licensed drugs and vaccines for category A and B agents is currently limited and not reflective of the pharmacy of today. In an effort to speed the licensure of additional drugs and vaccines for these diseases, the FDA has proposed a new rule for the licensure of such countermeasures against agents of bioterrorism when adequate and well-controlled clinical efficacy studies cannot be ethically conducted in humans. Thus, for indications in which field trials of prophylaxis or therapy for naturally occurring disease are not feasible, the FDA is proposing to rely on evidence solely from laboratory animal studies. For this rule to apply, it must be shown that (1) there are reasonably well-understood pathophysiologic mechanisms for the condition and its treatment; (2) the effect of the intervention is independently substantiated in at least two animal species, including species expected to react with a response predictive for humans; (3) the animal study endpoint is clearly related to the desired benefit in humans; and (4) the data in animals allow selection of an effective dose in humans.

Finally, an initiative referred to as Project BioShield has been established to facilitate biodefense research within the federal government, create a stable source of funding for the purchase of countermeasures against agents of bioterrorism, and create a category of "emergency use authorization" to allow the FDA to approve the use of unlicensed treatments during times of extraordinary unmet needs, as might be present in the context of a bioterrorist attack.

Although the prospect of a deliberate attack on civilians with disease-producing agents may seem to be an act of incomprehensible evil, history shows us that it is something that has been done in the past and will likely be done again in the future. It is the responsibility of health care providers to be aware of this possibility, to be able to recognize early signs of a potential bioterrorist attack and alert the public health system, and to respond quickly to provide care to the individual patient. Among the websites with current information on microbial bioterrorism are *www.bt.cdc.gov*, *www.niaid.nih.gov*, *www. jhsph.edu/preparedness*, and *www.cns.miis.edu/research/cbw/index.htm*.

FURTHER READINGS

Alibek K, Handelman S: *Biohazard: The Chilling True Story of the Largest Covert Biological Weapons in the World, Told from the Inside by the Man Who Ran It*. New York, Random House, 1999

Beigel JH et al: Avian influenza A (H5N1) infection in humans. N Engl J Med 353:1375, 2005

Croddy E (with C Perey-Armendariz and J Hart): *Chemical and Biological Warfare: A Comprehensive Survey for the Concerned Citizen*. New York, Copernicus Books, 2001

Doolan DL et al: The US Capitol bioterrorism anthrax exposures: Clinical, epidemiological, and immunological characteristics. J Infect Dis 195:174, 2007

Henderson DA et al (eds): *Bioterrorism: Guidelines for Medical and Public Health Management*. Chicago, JAMA and Archives Journals, AMA Press, 2002

Jernigan JA et al: Bioterrorism-related inhalational anthrax: The first 10 cases reported in the United States. Emerg Infect Dis 7:933, 2001

Wilkening DA: Sverdlovsk revisited: Modeling human inhalation anthrax. Proc Natl Acad Sci USA 103:20, 2006

SECTION II

FEVER AND APPROACH TO THE FEBRILE PATIENT

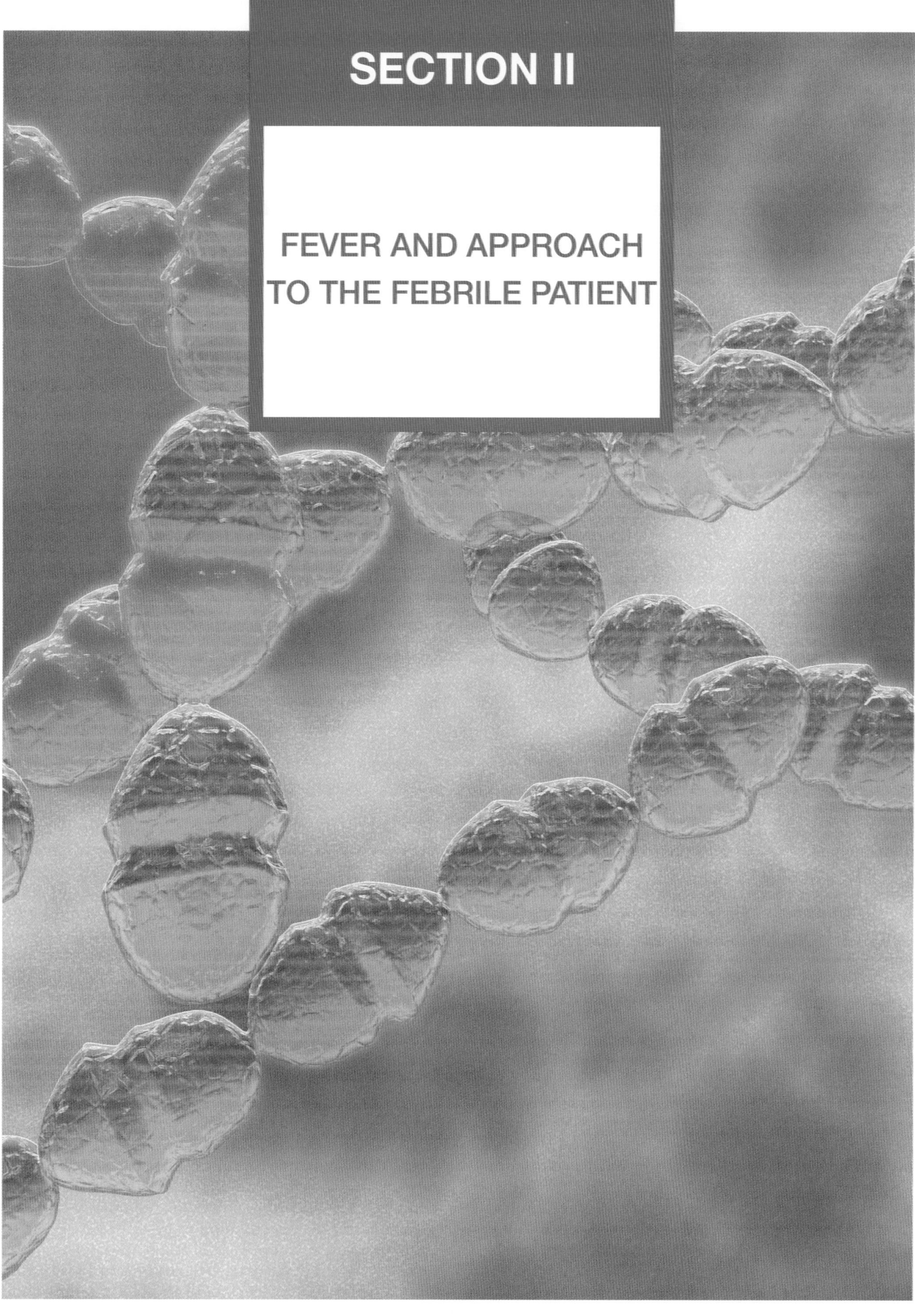

CHAPTER 7

FEVER AND HYPERTHERMIA

Charles A. Dinarello ■ Reuven Porat

Body temperature is controlled by the hypothalamus. Neurons in both the preoptic anterior hypothalamus and the posterior hypothalamus receive two kinds of signals: one from peripheral nerves that transmit information from warmth/cold receptors in the skin and the other from the temperature of the blood bathing the region. These two types of signals are integrated by the thermoregulatory center of the hypothalamus to maintain normal temperature. In a neutral temperature environment, the metabolic rate of humans produces more heat than is necessary to maintain the core body temperature at 37°C.

A normal body temperature is ordinarily maintained, despite environmental variations, because the hypothalamic thermoregulatory center balances the excess heat production derived from metabolic activity in muscle and the liver with heat dissipation from the skin and lungs. According to studies of healthy individuals 18–40 years of age, the mean oral temperature is 36.8° ± 0.4°C (98.2° ± 0.7°F), with low levels at 6 A.M. and higher levels at 4–6 P.M. The maximum normal oral temperature is 37.2°C (98.9°F) at 6 A.M. and 37.7°C (99.9°F) at 4 P.M.; these values define the 99th percentile for healthy individuals. In light of these studies, *an A.M. temperature of >37.2°C (>98.9°F) or a P.M. temperature of >37.7°C (>99.9°F) would define a fever.* The normal daily temperature variation is typically 0.5°C (0.9°F). However, in some individuals recovering from a febrile illness, this daily variation can be as great as 1.0°C. During a febrile illness, the diurnal variation is usually maintained, but at higher, febrile levels. The daily temperature variation appears to be fixed in early childhood; in contrast, elderly individuals can exhibit a reduced ability to develop fever, with only a modest fever even in severe infections.

Rectal temperatures are generally 0.4°C (0.7°F) higher than oral readings. The lower oral readings are probably attributable to mouth breathing, which is a factor in patients with respiratory infections and rapid breathing. Lower-esophageal temperatures closely reflect core temperature. Tympanic membrane (TM) thermometers measure radiant heat from the tympanic membrane and nearby ear canal and display that absolute value (unadjusted mode) or a value automatically calculated from the absolute reading on the basis of nomograms relating the radiant temperature measured to actual core temperatures obtained in clinical studies (adjusted mode). These measurements, although convenient, may be more variable than directly determined oral or rectal values. Studies in adults show that readings are lower with unadjusted-mode than with adjusted-mode TM thermometers and that unadjusted-mode TM values are 0.8°C (1.6°F) lower than rectal temperatures.

In women who menstruate, the A.M. temperature is generally lower in the 2 weeks before ovulation; it then rises by ~0.6°C (1°F) with ovulation and remains at that level until menses occur. Body temperature can be elevated in the postprandial state. Pregnancy and endocrinologic dysfunction also affect body temperature.

FEVER VERSUS HYPERTHERMIA

FEVER

Fever is an elevation of body temperature that exceeds the normal daily variation and occurs *in conjunction with an increase in the hypothalamic set point* (e.g., from 37°C to 39°C). This shift of the set point from "normothermic" to febrile levels very much resembles the resetting of the home thermostat to a higher level in order to raise the ambient temperature in a room. Once the hypothalamic set point is raised, neurons in the vasomotor center are activated and vasoconstriction commences. The individual first notices vasoconstriction in the hands and feet. Shunting of blood away from the periphery to the internal organs essentially decreases heat loss from the skin, and the person feels cold. For most fevers, body temperature increases by 1°–2°C. Shivering, which increases heat production from the muscles, may begin at this time; however, shivering is not required if heat conservation mechanisms raise blood temperature sufficiently. Nonshivering heat production from the liver also contributes to increasing core temperature. In humans, behavioral adjustments (e.g., putting on more clothing or bedding) help raise body temperature by decreasing heat loss.

The processes of heat conservation (vasoconstriction) and heat production (shivering and increased nonshivering thermogenesis) continue until the temperature of the blood bathing the hypothalamic neurons matches the new thermostat setting. Once that point is reached, the hypothalamus maintains the temperature at the febrile level by the same mechanisms of heat balance that function in the afebrile state. When the hypothalamic set point is again reset downward (in response to either a reduction in the concentration of pyrogens or the use of antipyretics), the processes of heat loss through vasodilation and sweating are initiated. Loss of heat by sweating and vasodilation continues until the blood temperature at the hypothalamic level matches the lower setting. Behavioral changes (e.g., removal of clothing) facilitate heat loss.

A fever of >41.5°C (>106.7°F) is called *hyperpyrexia*. This extraordinarily high fever can develop in patients with severe infections, but most commonly occurs in patients with central nervous system (CNS) hemorrhages. In the preantibiotic era, fever due to a variety of infectious diseases rarely exceeded 106°F, and there has been speculation that this natural "thermal ceiling" is mediated by neuropeptides functioning as central antipyretics.

In rare cases, the hypothalamic set point is elevated as a result of local trauma, hemorrhage, tumor, or intrinsic hypothalamic malfunction. The term *hypothalamic fever* is sometimes used to describe elevated temperature caused by abnormal hypothalamic function. However, most patients with hypothalamic damage have *sub*normal, not *supra*normal, body temperatures.

HYPERTHERMIA

Although most patients with elevated body temperature have fever, there are circumstances in which elevated temperature represents not fever but hyperthermia (Table 7-1). Hyperthermia is characterized by an uncontrolled increase in body temperature that exceeds the body's ability to lose heat. The setting of the hypothalamic thermoregulatory center is unchanged. In contrast to fever in infections, hyperthermia does not involve pyrogenic molecules (see "Pyrogens" later in the chapter). Exogenous heat exposure and endogenous heat production are two mechanisms by which hyperthermia can result in dangerously high internal temperatures. Excessive heat production can easily cause hyperthermia despite physiologic and behavioral control of body temperature. For example, work or exercise in hot environments can produce heat faster than peripheral mechanisms can lose it.

Heat stroke in association with a warm environment may be categorized as exertional or nonexertional. *Exertional heat stroke* typically occurs in individuals exercising at elevated ambient temperatures and/or humidities. In a dry environment and at maximal efficiency, sweating can dissipate ~600 kcal/h, requiring the production of >1 L of sweat. Even in healthy individuals, dehydration or the use of common medications (e.g., over-the-counter antihistamines with anticholinergic side effects) may precipitate exertional heat stroke. *Nonexertional heat stroke* typically occurs in either very young or elderly individuals, particularly during heat waves. According to the Centers for Disease Control and Prevention, there were 7000 deaths attributed to heat injury in the United States from 1979 to 1997. The elderly, the bedridden, persons taking anticholinergic or antiparkinsonian drugs or diuretics, and individuals confined to poorly ventilated and non–air-conditioned environments are most susceptible.

Drug-induced hyperthermia has become increasingly common as a result of the increased use of prescription psychotropic drugs and illicit drugs. Drug-induced hyperthermia may be caused by monoamine oxidase inhibitors (MAOIs), tricyclic antidepressants, and amphetamines and by the illicit use of phencyclidine (PCP), lysergic acid diethylamide (LSD), methylenedioxymethamphetamine (MDMA, "ecstasy"), or cocaine.

Malignant hyperthermia occurs in individuals with an inherited abnormality of skeletal-muscle sarcoplasmic reticulum that causes a rapid increase in intracellular calcium levels in response to halothane and other inhalational anesthetics or to succinylcholine. Elevated temperature, increased muscle metabolism, muscle rigidity, rhabdomyolysis, acidosis, and cardiovascular instability develop within minutes. This rare condition is often fatal. The *neuroleptic malignant syndrome* occurs in the setting of neuroleptic agent use (antipsychotic phenothiazines, haloperidol, prochlorperazine, metoclopramide) or the withdrawal of dopaminergic drugs and is characterized by "lead-pipe" muscle rigidity, extrapyramidal side effects, autonomic dysregulation, and hyperthermia. This disorder appears to be caused by the inhibition of central dopamine receptors in the hypothalamus, which results in increased heat generation and decreased heat dissipation. The *serotonin syndrome*, seen with selective serotonin uptake inhibitors (SSRIs), MAOIs, and other serotonergic medications, has many overlapping features, including

TABLE 7-1

CAUSES OF HYPERTHERMIA SYNDROMES

Heat Stroke
Exertional: Exercise in higher-than-normal heat and/or humidity Nonexertional: Anticholinergics, including antihistamines; antiparkinsonian drugs; diuretics; phenothiazines
Drug-Induced Hyperthermia
Amphetamines, cocaine, phencyclidine (PCP), methylenedioxymethamphetamine (MDMA; "ecstasy"), lysergic acid diethylamide (LSD), salicylates, lithium, anticholinergics, sympathomimetics
Neuroleptic Malignant Syndrome
Phenothiazines; butyrophenones, including haloperidol and bromperidol; fluoxetine; loxapine; tricyclic dibenzodiazepines; metoclopramide; domperidone; thiothixene; molindone; withdrawal of dopaminergic agents
Serotonin Syndrome
Selective serotonin reuptake inhibitors (SSRIs), monoamine oxidase inhibitors (MAOIs), tricyclic antidepressants
Malignant Hyperthermia
Inhalational anesthetics, succinylcholine
Endocrinopathy
Thyrotoxicosis, pheochromocytoma
Central Nervous System Damage
Cerebral hemorrhage, status epilepticus, hypothalamic injury

Source: After FJ Curley, RS Irwin, JM Rippe et al (eds): *Intensive Care Medicine*, 3d ed. Boston, Little, Brown, 1996.

hyperthermia, but may be distinguished by the presence of diarrhea, tremor, and myoclonus rather than the lead-pipe rigidity of the neuroleptic malignant syndrome. Thyrotoxicosis and pheochromocytoma can also cause increased thermogenesis.

It is important to distinguish between fever and hyperthermia since hyperthermia can be rapidly fatal and characteristically does not respond to antipyretics. In an emergency situation, however, making this distinction can be difficult. For example, in systemic sepsis, fever (hyperpyrexia) can be rapid in onset, and temperatures can exceed 40.5°C. Hyperthermia is often diagnosed on the basis of the events immediately preceding the elevation of core temperature—e.g., heat exposure or treatment with drugs that interfere with thermoregulation. In patients with heat stroke syndromes and in those taking drugs that block sweating, the skin is hot but dry, whereas in fever, the skin can be cold as a consequence of vasoconstriction. Antipyretics do not reduce the elevated temperature in hyperthermia, whereas in fever—and even in hyperpyrexia—adequate doses of either aspirin or acetaminophen usually result in some decrease in body temperature.

PATHOGENESIS OF FEVER

PYROGENS

The term *pyrogen* is used to describe any substance that causes fever. *Exogenous* pyrogens are derived from outside the patient; most are microbial products, microbial toxins, or whole microorganisms. The classic example of an exogenous pyrogen is the lipopolysaccharide (endotoxin) produced by all gram-negative bacteria. Pyrogenic products of gram-positive organisms include the enterotoxins of *Staphylococcus aureus* and the group A and B streptococcal toxins, also called *superantigens*. One staphylococcal toxin of clinical importance is that associated with isolates of *S. aureus* from patients with toxic shock syndrome. These products of staphylococci and streptococci cause fever in experimental animals when injected intravenously at concentrations of 1–10 μg/kg. Endotoxin is a highly pyrogenic molecule in humans: when injected intravenously into volunteers, a dose of 2–3 ng/kg produces fever, leukocytosis, acute-phase proteins, and generalized symptoms of malaise.

PYROGENIC CYTOKINES

Cytokines are small proteins (molecular mass, 10,000–20,000 Da) that regulate immune, inflammatory, and hematopoietic processes. For example, the elevated leukocytosis seen in several infections with an absolute neutrophilia is the result of the cytokines interleukin (IL) 1 and IL-6. Some cytokines also cause fever; formerly referred to as *endogenous pyrogens*, they are now called *pyrogenic cytokines*. The pyrogenic cytokines include IL-1, IL-6, tumor necrosis factor (TNF), ciliary neurotropic factor (CNTF), and interferon α. (IL-18, a member of the IL-1 family, does not appear to be a pyrogenic cytokine.) Other pyrogenic cytokines probably exist. Each cytokine is encoded by a separate gene, and each pyrogenic cytokine has been shown to cause fever in laboratory animals and in humans. When injected into humans, IL-1 and TNF produce fever at low doses (10–100 ng/kg); in contrast, for IL-6, a dose of 1–10 μg/kg is required for fever production.

A wide spectrum of bacterial and fungal products induce the synthesis and release of pyrogenic cytokines, as do viruses. However, fever can be a manifestation of disease in the absence of microbial infection. For example, inflammatory processes, trauma, tissue necrosis, or antigen-antibody complexes can induce the production of IL-1, TNF, and/or IL-6, which—individually or in combination—trigger the hypothalamus to raise the set point to febrile levels.

ELEVATION OF THE HYPOTHALAMIC SET POINT BY CYTOKINES

During fever, levels of prostaglandin E_2 (PGE_2) are elevated in hypothalamic tissue and the third cerebral ventricle. The concentrations of PGE_2 are highest near the circumventricular vascular organs (organum vasculosum of lamina terminalis)—networks of enlarged capillaries surrounding the hypothalamic regulatory centers. Destruction of these organs reduces the ability of pyrogens to produce fever. Most studies in animals have failed to show, however, that pyrogenic cytokines pass from the circulation into the brain itself. Thus it appears that both exogenous and endogenous pyrogens interact with the endothelium of these capillaries and that this interaction is the first step in initiating fever—i.e., in raising the set point to febrile levels.

The key events in the production of fever are illustrated in Fig. 7-1. As has been mentioned, several cell types can produce pyrogenic cytokines. Pyrogenic cytokines such

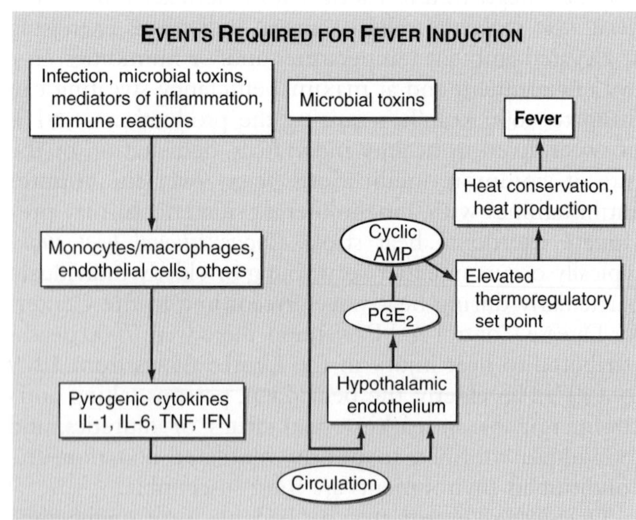

FIGURE 7-1

Chronology of events required for the induction of fever. AMP, adenosine 5′-monophosphate; IFN, interferon; IL, interleukin; PGE_2, prostaglandin E_2; TNF, tumor necrosis factor.

as IL-1, IL-6, and TNF are released from the cells and enter the systemic circulation. Although the systemic effects of these circulating cytokines lead to fever by inducing the synthesis of PGE_2, they also induce PGE_2 in peripheral tissues. The increase in PGE_2 in the periphery accounts for the nonspecific myalgias and arthralgias that often accompany fever. It is thought that some systemic PGE_2 escapes destruction by the lung and gains access to the hypothalamus via the internal carotid. However, it is the elevation of PGE_2 in the brain that starts the process of raising the hypothalamic set point for core temperature.

There are four receptors for PGE_2, and each signals the cell in different ways. Of the four receptors, the third (EP-3) is essential for fever: when the gene for this receptor is deleted in mice, no fever follows the injection of IL-1 or endotoxin. Deletion of the other PGE_2 receptor genes leaves the fever mechanism intact. Although PGE_2 is essential for fever, it is not a neurotransmitter. Rather, the release of PGE_2 from the brain side of the hypothalamic endothelium triggers the PGE_2 receptor on glial cells, and this stimulation results in the rapid release of cyclic adenosine 5′-monophosphate (cyclic AMP), which is a neurotransmitter. As shown in Fig. 7-1, the release of cyclic AMP from the glial cells activates neuronal endings from the thermoregulatory center that extend into the area. The elevation of cyclic AMP is thought to account for changes in the hypothalamic set point either directly or indirectly (by inducing the release of neurotransmitters). Distinct receptors for microbial products are located on the hypothalamic endothelium. These receptors are called *Toll-like receptors* and are similar in many ways to IL-1 receptors. The direct activation of Toll-like receptors also results in PGE_2 production and fever.

PRODUCTION OF CYTOKINES IN THE CNS

Several viral diseases produce active infection in the brain. Glial and possibly neuronal cells synthesize IL-1, TNF, and IL-6. CNTF is also synthesized by neural as well as neuronal cells. What role in the production of fever is played by these cytokines produced in the brain itself? In experimental animals, the concentrations of cytokine required to cause fever are several orders of magnitude lower with direct injection into the brain than with IV injection. Therefore, CNS production of these cytokines apparently can raise the hypothalamic set point, bypassing the circumventricular organs involved in fever caused by circulating cytokines. CNS cytokines may account for the hyperpyrexia of CNS hemorrhage, trauma, or infection.

Approach to the Patient: FEVER OR HYPERTHERMIA

PHYSICAL EXAMINATION Attention must be paid to the chronology of events and to other signs and symptoms preceding the fever. The temperature may be taken orally or rectally, but the site used should be consistent. Axillary temperatures are notoriously unreliable. Electronic devices for measuring tympanic membrane temperatures are reliable and preferred over oral temperature measurements in patients with pulmonary disease such as acute infection or asthma.

LABORATORY TESTS The workup should include a complete blood count; a differential count should be performed manually or with an instrument sensitive to the identification of eosinophils, juvenile or band forms, toxic granulations, and Döhle's bodies, the last three of which are suggestive of bacterial infection. Neutropenia may be present with some viral infections.

Measurement of circulating cytokines in patients with fever is of little use since levels of pyrogenic cytokines in the circulation often are below the detection limit of the assay or do not coincide with the fever. Although some studies have shown correlations between circulating IL-6 levels and peak febrile elevations, the most valuable measurements in patients with fever are C-reactive protein level and erythrocyte sedimentation rate. These markers of pathologic processes are particularly helpful in identifying disease in patients with small elevations in body temperature.

FEVER IN RECIPIENTS OF ANTICYTOKINE THERAPY As of this writing, more than 750,000 patients in the United States are receiving chronic anticytokine therapy for Crohn's disease, rheumatoid arthritis, or psoriasis. Does such therapy mask infection by preventing fever? With the increasing use of anticytokines to reduce the activity of IL-1, IL-6, IL-12, and TNF, the effect of these agents on the febrile response must be considered.

The blocking of cytokine activity has the distinct clinical drawback of lowering the level of host defenses against both routine bacterial and opportunistic infections. The opportunistic infections reported in patients given neutralizing antibodies to TNF-α (infliximab or adalimumab) are similar to those reported in the HIV-1–infected population (e.g., new infection with or reactivation of *Mycobacterium tuberculosis*, with dissemination). A soluble receptor for TNF, etanercept, is also associated with opportunistic infections, but less so than the neutralizing antibodies.

In nearly all reported cases of infection associated with anticytokine therapy, fever is among the presenting signs. However, the extent to which the febrile response is reduced in these patients remains unknown. Fever in a patient who develops an infection during anticytokine treatment is likely to be due to the direct action of microbial products on the hypothalamic thermoregulatory center, with induction of PGE_2. For example, blocking the activity of IL-1 or TNF during experimental endotoxin-induced fever in volunteers does not affect the febrile response.

℞ Treatment: FEVER AND HYPERTHERMIA

THE DECISION TO TREAT FEVER Most fevers are associated with self-limited infections, such as common viral diseases. The use of antipyretics is not contraindicated in these infections: there is no significant clinical evidence that antipyretics delay the resolution of viral or bacterial infections, nor is there evidence that fever facilitates recovery from infection or acts as an adjuvant to the immune system. In fact, peripheral PGE_2 production is a potent immunosuppressant. In short, treatment of fever and its symptoms does no harm and does not slow the resolution of common viral and bacterial infections.

However, in bacterial infections, withholding antipyretic therapy can be helpful in evaluating the effectiveness of a particular antibiotic therapy, particularly in the absence of cultural identification of the infecting organism. The routine use of antipyretics can mask an inadequately treated bacterial infection. Withholding antipyretics in some cases may facilitate the diagnosis of an unusual febrile disease. For example, the usual times of peak and trough temperatures may be reversed in typhoid fever and disseminated tuberculosis. Temperature-pulse dissociation (relative bradycardia) occurs in typhoid fever, brucellosis, leptospirosis, some drug-induced fevers, and factitious fever. In newborns, the elderly, patients with chronic renal failure, and patients taking glucocorticoids, fever may not be present despite infection, or core temperature may be hypothermic. Hypothermia is often observed in patients with septic shock.

Some infections have characteristic patterns in which febrile episodes are separated by intervals of normal temperature. For example, *Plasmodium vivax* causes fever every third day, whereas fever occurs every fourth day with *P. malariae*. Other relapsing fevers are related to *Borrelia* infections, with days of fever followed by a several-day afebrile period and then a relapse of days of fever. In the Pel-Ebstein pattern, fever lasting 3–10 days is followed by afebrile periods of 3–10 days; this pattern can be classic for Hodgkin's disease and other lymphomas. In cyclic neutropenia, fevers occur every 21 days and accompany the neutropenia. There is no periodicity of fever in patients with familial Mediterranean fever.

Recurrent fever is documented at some point in most autoimmune diseases and all autoinflammatory diseases. The autoinflammatory diseases include adult and juvenile Still's disease, familial Mediterranean fever, hyper-IgD syndrome, familial cold-induced autoinflammatory syndrome, neonatal-onset multisystem autoinflammatory disease, Blau's syndrome, Schnitzler's syndrome, Muckle-Wells syndrome, and TNF receptor–associated periodic syndrome. Besides recurrent fevers, neutrophilia and serosal inflammation characterize these diseases. The fevers associated with these illnesses are dramatically reduced by blocking of IL-1β activity. Anticytokines therefore reduce fever in autoimmune and autoinflammatory diseases. Although fevers in autoinflammatory diseases are mediated by IL-1β, patients also respond to antipyretics.

MECHANISMS OF ANTIPYRETIC AGENTS The reduction of fever by lowering of the elevated hypothalamic set point is a direct function of reducing the level of PGE_2 in the thermoregulatory center. The synthesis of PGE_2 depends on the constitutively expressed enzyme cyclooxygenase. The substrate for cyclooxygenase is arachidonic acid released from the cell membrane, and this release is the rate-limiting step in the synthesis of PGE_2. Therefore, inhibitors of cyclooxygenase are potent antipyretics. The antipyretic potency of various drugs is directly correlated with the inhibition of brain cyclooxygenase. Acetaminophen is a poor cyclooxygenase inhibitor in peripheral tissue and lacks noteworthy anti-inflammatory activity; in the brain, however, acetaminophen is oxidized by the p450 cytochrome system, and the oxidized form inhibits cyclooxygenase activity. Moreover, in the brain, the inhibition of another enzyme, COX-3, by acetaminophen may account for the antipyretic effect of this agent. However, COX-3 is not found outside the CNS.

Oral aspirin and acetaminophen are equally effective in reducing fever in humans. Nonsteroidal anti-inflammatory drugs (NSAIDs) such as ibuprofen and specific inhibitors of COX-2 are also excellent antipyretics. Chronic, high-dose therapy with antipyretics such as aspirin or any NSAID does not reduce normal core body temperature. Thus PGE_2 appears to play no role in normal thermoregulation.

As effective antipyretics, glucocorticoids act at two levels. First, similar to the cyclooxygenase inhibitors, glucocorticoids reduce PGE_2 synthesis by inhibiting the activity of phospholipase A_2, which is needed to release arachidonic acid from the cell membrane. Second, glucocorticoids block the transcription of the mRNA for the pyrogenic cytokines. Limited experimental evidence indicates that ibuprofen and COX-2 inhibitors reduce IL-1–induced IL-6 production and may contribute to the antipyretic activity of NSAIDs.

REGIMENS FOR THE TREATMENT OF FEVER The objectives in treating fever are first to reduce the elevated hypothalamic set point and second to facilitate heat loss. Reducing fever with antipyretics also reduces systemic symptoms of headache, myalgias, and arthralgias.

Oral aspirin and NSAIDs effectively reduce fever but can adversely affect platelets and the gastrointestinal tract. Therefore, acetaminophen is preferred to all of these agents as an antipyretic. In children, acetaminophen must be used because aspirin increases the risk of Reye's syndrome. If the patient cannot take oral antipyretics, parenteral preparations of NSAIDs and rectal suppository preparations of various antipyretics can be used.

Treatment of fever in some patients is highly recommended. Fever increases the demand for oxygen (i.e., for every increase of 1°C over 37°C, there is a 13% increase in oxygen consumption) and can aggravate preexisting cardiac, cerebrovascular, or pulmonary insufficiency. Elevated temperature can induce mental changes in patients with organic brain disease. Children with a history of febrile or nonfebrile seizure should be aggressively treated to reduce fever, although it is unclear what triggers the febrile seizure, and there is no correlation between absolute temperature elevation and onset of a febrile seizure in susceptible children.

In hyperpyrexia, the use of cooling blankets facilitates the reduction of temperature; however, cooling blankets should not be used without oral antipyretics. In hyperpyretic patients with CNS disease or trauma, reducing core temperature mitigates the ill effects of high temperature on the brain.

TREATING HYPERTHERMIA A high core temperature in a patient with an appropriate history (e.g., environmental heat exposure or treatment with anticholinergic or neuroleptic drugs, tricyclic antidepressants, succinylcholine, or halothane) along with appropriate clinical findings (dry skin, hallucinations, delirium, pupil dilation, muscle rigidity, and/or elevated levels of creatine phosphokinase) suggests hyperthermia. Attempts to lower the already normal hypothalamic set point are of little use. Physical cooling with sponging, fans, cooling blankets, and even ice baths should be initiated immediately in conjunction with the administration of IV fluids and appropriate pharmacologic agents (see below). If insufficient cooling is achieved by external means, internal cooling can be achieved by gastric or peritoneal lavage with iced saline. In extreme circumstances, hemodialysis or even cardiopulmonary bypass with cooling of blood may be performed.

Malignant hyperthermia should be treated immediately with cessation of anesthesia and IV administration of dantrolene sodium. The recommended dose of dantrolene is 1–2.5 mg/kg given intravenously every 6 h for at least 24–48 h—until oral dantrolene can be administered, if needed. Procainamide should also be administered to patients with malignant hyperthermia because of the likelihood of ventricular fibrillation in this syndrome. Dantrolene at similar doses is indicated in the neuroleptic malignant syndrome and in drug-induced hyperthermia and may even be useful in the hyperthermia of the serotonin syndrome and thyrotoxicosis. The neuroleptic malignant syndrome may also be treated with bromocriptine, levodopa, amantadine, or nifedipine or by induction of muscle paralysis with curare and pancuronium. Tricyclic antidepressant overdose may be treated with physostigmine.

ACKNOWLEDGMENT

The substantial contributions of Jeffrey A. Gelfand to this chapter in previous editions of Harrison's Principles of Internal Medicine are gratefully acknowledged.

FURTHER READINGS

De Koning HD et al: Beneficial response to anakinra and thalidomide in Schnitzler's syndrome. Ann Rheum Dis 65:542, 2006

Dinarello CA: Infection, fever, and exogenous and endogenous pyrogens: Some concepts have changed. J Endotoxin Res 10:202, 2004

Hawkins PN et al: Spectrum of clinical features in Muckle-Wells syndrome and response to anakinra. Arthritis Rheum 50:607, 2004

Hoffman HM et al: Prevention of cold-associated acute inflammation in familial cold autoinflammatory syndrome by interleukin-1 receptor antagonist. Lancet 364:1779, 2004

Keane J et al: Tuberculosis associated with infliximab, a tumor necrosis factor-α-neutralizing agent. N Engl J Med 345:1098, 2001

Laupland KB: Fever in the critically ill medical patient. Crit Care Med 37(7 Suppl):S273, 2009

Pascual V et al: Role of interleukin-1 (IL-1) in the pathogenesis of systemic onset juvenile idiopathic arthritis and clinical response to IL-1 blockade. J Exp Med 201:1479, 2005

Simon A, van der Meer JW: Pathogenesis of familial periodic fever syndromes or hereditary autoinflammatory syndromes. Am J Physiol Regul Integr Comp Physiol 292:R86, 2007

——— et al: Beneficial response to interleukin-1 receptor antagonist in TRAPS. Am J Med 117:208, 2004

Wallis RS et al: Differential effects of TNF blockers on TB immunity. Ann Rheum Dis 64(Suppl3):132, 2005

——— et al: Granulomatous infectious diseases associated with tumor necrosis factor antagonists. Clin Infect Dis 38:1261, 2004

CHAPTER 8

FEVER AND RASH

Elaine T. Kaye ■ Kenneth M. Kaye

The acutely ill patient with fever and rash often presents a diagnostic challenge for physicians. The distinctive appearance of an eruption in concert with a clinical syndrome may facilitate a prompt diagnosis and the institution of life-saving therapy or critical infection-control interventions. Representative images of many of the rashes discussed in this chapter are included in Chap. 10.

Approach to the Patient: FEVER AND RASH

A thorough history of patients with fever and rash includes the following relevant information: immune status, medications taken within the previous month, specific travel history, immunization status, exposure to domestic pets and other animals, history of animal (including arthropod) bites, existence of cardiac abnormalities, presence of prosthetic material, recent exposure to ill individuals, and exposure to sexually transmitted diseases. The history should also include the site of onset of the rash and its direction and rate of spread.

A thorough physical examination entails close attention to the rash, with an assessment and precise definition of its salient features. First, it is critical to determine the *type* of lesions that make up the eruption. *Macules* are flat lesions defined by an area of changed color (i.e., a blanchable erythema). *Papules* are raised, solid lesions <5 mm in diameter; *plaques* are lesions >5 mm in diameter with a flat, plateau-like surface; and *nodules* are lesions >5 mm in diameter with a more rounded configuration. *Wheals* (urticaria, hives) are papules or plaques that are pale pink and may appear annular (ringlike) as they enlarge; classic (nonvasculitic) wheals are transient, lasting only 24–48 h in any defined area. *Vesicles* (<5 mm) and *bullae* (>5 mm) are circumscribed, elevated lesions containing fluid. *Pustules* are raised lesions containing purulent exudate; vesicular processes such as varicella or herpes simplex may evolve to pustules. *Nonpalpable purpura* is a flat lesion that is due to bleeding into the skin; if <3 mm in diameter, the purpuric lesions are termed *petechiae*; if >3 mm, they are termed *ecchymoses*. *Palpable purpura* is a raised lesion that is due to inflammation of the vessel wall (vasculitis) with subsequent hemorrhage. An *ulcer* is a defect in the skin extending at least into the upper layer of the dermis, and an *eschar* (tâche noire) is a necrotic lesion covered with a black crust.

Other pertinent features of rashes include their *configuration* (i.e., annular or target), the *arrangement* of their lesions, and their *distribution* (i.e., central or peripheral). For further discussion, see Chap. 14.

CLASSIFICATION OF RASH

This chapter reviews rashes that reflect systemic disease, but it does not include localized skin eruptions (i.e., cellulitis, impetigo) that may also be associated with fever (Chap. 21). Rashes are classified herein on the basis of the morphology and distribution of lesions. For practical purposes, this classification system is based on the most typical disease presentations. However, morphology may vary as rashes evolve, and the presentation of diseases with rashes is subject to many variations. For instance, the classic petechial rash of Rocky Mountain spotted fever (RMSF; Chap. 75) may initially consist of blanchable erythematous macules distributed peripherally; at times, the rash associated with RMSF may not be predominantly acral, or a rash may not develop at all.

Diseases with fever and rash may be classified by type of eruption: centrally distributed maculopapular, peripheral, confluent desquamative erythematous, vesiculobullous, urticarial, nodular, purpuric, ulcerated, or eschar (Table 8-1). For a more detailed discussion of each disease associated with a rash, the reader is referred to the chapter dealing with that specific disease. (Reference chapters are cited in the text and listed in Table 8-1.)

CENTRALLY DISTRIBUTED MACULOPAPULAR ERUPTIONS

Centrally distributed rashes, in which lesions are primarily truncal, are the most common type of eruption. The rash of *rubeola* (measles) starts at the hairline 2–3 days into the illness and moves down the body, sparing the palms and soles (Chap. 95). It begins as discrete erythematous lesions, which become confluent as the rash spreads. Koplik's spots (1- to 2-mm white or bluish lesions with an erythematous halo on the buccal mucosa) are pathognomonic for measles and are generally seen during the first 2 days of symptoms. They should not be confused with Fordyce's spots (ectopic sebaceous glands), which have no erythematous halos and are found in the mouth of healthy individuals. Koplik's spots may briefly overlap with the measles exanthem.

Rubella (German measles) also spreads from the hairline downward; unlike that of measles, however, the rash of rubella tends to clear from originally affected areas as it migrates, and it may be pruritic (Chap. 96). Forchheimer's spots (palatal petechiae) may develop but are nonspecific since they also develop in mononucleosis (Chap. 82) and scarlet fever (Chap. 36). Postauricular and suboccipital adenopathy and arthritis are common among adults with German measles. Exposure of pregnant women to ill individuals should be avoided, as rubella causes severe congenital abnormalities. Numerous strains of enteroviruses (Chap. 94), primarily echoviruses and coxsackieviruses, cause nonspecific syndromes of fever and eruptions that may mimic rubella or measles. Patients with infectious mononucleosis caused by Epstein-Barr virus (Chap. 82) or with primary infection caused by HIV (Chap. 90) may exhibit pharyngitis, lymphadenopathy, and a nonspecific maculopapular exanthem.

The rash of *erythema infectiosum* (fifth disease), which is caused by human parvovirus B19, primarily affects children 3–12 years old; it develops after fever has resolved as a bright, blanchable erythema on the cheeks ("slapped cheeks") with perioral pallor (Chap. 85). A more diffuse rash (often pruritic) appears the next day on the trunk and extremities and then rapidly develops into a lacy reticular eruption that may wax and wane (especially with temperature change) over 3 weeks. Adults with fifth disease often have arthritis, and fetal hydrops can develop in association with this condition in pregnant women.

Exanthem subitum (roseola) is caused by human herpesvirus 6 and is most common among children <3 years of age (Chap. 83). As in erythema infectiosum, the rash usually appears after fever has subsided. It consists of 2- to 3-mm rose-pink macules and papules that rarely coalesce,

TABLE 8-1

DISEASES ASSOCIATED WITH FEVER AND RASH

DISEASE	ETIOLOGY	DESCRIPTION	GROUP AFFECTED/ EPIDEMIOLOGIC FACTORS	CLINICAL SYNDROME	CHAPTER
Centrally Distributed Maculopapular Eruptions					
Acute meningococcemia[a]	—	—	—	—	44
Rubeola (measles, first disease)	Paramyxovirus	Discrete lesions that become confluent as rash spreads from hairline downward, sparing palms and soles; lasts ≥3 days; Koplik's spots	Nonimmune individuals	Cough, conjunctivitis, coryza, severe prostration	95
Rubella (German measles, third disease)	Togavirus	Spreads from hairline downward, clearing as it spreads; Forchheimer's spots	Nonimmune individuals	Adenopathy, arthritis	96
Erythema infectiosum (fifth disease)	Human parvovirus B19	Bright-red "slapped-cheek" appearance followed by lacy reticular rash that waxes and wanes over 3 weeks; rarely, papular-purpuric "gloves-and-socks" syndrome on hands and feet	Most common in children aged 3–12 years; occurs in winter and spring	Mild fever; arthritis in adults; rash after resolution of fever	85
Exanthem subitum (roseola, sixth disease)	Human herpesvirus 6	Diffuse maculopapular eruption (sparing face); resolves within 2 days	Usually affects children <3 years old	Rash after resolution of fever; similar to Boston exanthem (echovirus 16)	83
Primary HIV infection	HIV	Nonspecific diffuse macules and papules; may be urticarial; oral or genital ulcers in some cases	Individuals recently infected with HIV	Pharyngitis, adenopathy, arthralgias	90
Infectious mononucleosis	Epstein-Barr virus	Diffuse maculopapular eruption (10–15% of cases; 90% if ampicillin is given); urticaria in some cases; periorbital edema (50%); palatal petechiae (25%)	Adolescents, young adults	Hepatosplenomegaly, pharyngitis, cervical lymphadenopathy, atypical lymphocytosis, heterophile antibody	82
Other viral exanthems	Echoviruses 2, 4, 9, 11, 16, 19, and 25; coxsackieviruses A9, B1, and B5; etc.	Skin findings mimicking rubella or measles	Affect children more commonly than adults	Nonspecific viral syndromes	94
Exanthematous drug-induced eruption	Drugs (antibiotics, anticonvulsants, diuretics, etc.)	Intensely pruritic, bright-red macules and papules, symmetric on trunk and extremities; may become confluent	Occurs 2–3 d after exposure in previously sensitized individuals; otherwise, after 2–3 weeks (but can occur anytime, even shortly after drug is discontinued)	Variable findings: fever and eosinophilia	...
Epidemic typhus	*Rickettsia prowazekii*	Maculopapular eruption appearing in axillae, spreading to trunk and later to extremities; usually spares face, palms, soles; evolves from blanchable macules to confluent eruption with petechiae; rash evanescent in recrudescent typhus (Brill-Zinsser's disease)	Exposure to body lice; occurrence of recrudescent typhus as relapse after 30–50 years	Headache, myalgias; 10–40% mortality if untreated; milder clinical presentation in recrudescent form	75

(*Continued*)

TABLE 8-1 (*CONTINUED*)

DISEASES ASSOCIATED WITH FEVER AND RASH

DISEASE	ETIOLOGY	DESCRIPTION	GROUP AFFECTED/ EPIDEMIOLOGIC FACTORS	CLINICAL SYNDROME	CHAPTER
Centrally Distributed Maculopapular Eruptions (*Continued*)					
Endemic (murine) typhus	*Rickettsia typhi*	Maculopapular eruption, usually sparing palms, soles	Exposure to rat or cat fleas	Headache, myalgias	75
Scrub typhus	*Orientia tsutsugamushi*	Diffuse macular rash starting on trunk; eschar at site of mite bite	Endemic in South Pacific, Australia, Asia; transmitted by mites	Headache, myalgias, regional adenopathy; mortality up to 30% if untreated	75
Rickettsial spotted fevers	*Rickettsia conorii* (boutonneuse fever), *Rickettsia australis* (North Queensland tick typhus), *Rickettsia sibirica* (Siberian tick typhus), and others	Eschar common at bite site; maculopapular (rarely, vesicular and petechial) eruption on proximal extremities, spreading to trunk and face	Exposure to ticks; *R. conorii* in Mediterranean region, India, Africa; *R. australis* in Australia; *R. sibirica* in Siberia, Mongolia	Headache, myalgias, regional adenopathy	75
Human monocytotropic ehrlichiosis[b]	*Ehrlichia chaffeensis*	Maculopapular eruption (40% of cases), involves trunk and extremities; may be petechial	Tick-borne; most common in U.S. Southeast, southern Midwest, and mid-Atlantic regions	Headache, myalgias, leukopenia	75
Leptospirosis	*Leptospira interrogans*	Maculopapular eruption; conjunctivitis; scleral hemorrhage in some cases	Exposure to water contaminated with animal urine	Myalgias; aseptic meningitis; *fulminant form*: icterohemorrhagic fever (Weil's disease)	72
Lyme disease	*Borrelia burgdorferi*	Papule expanding to erythematous annular lesion with central clearing (erythema chronicum migrans or ECM; average diameter, 15 cm), sometimes with concentric rings, sometimes with indurated or vesicular center; multiple secondary ECM lesions in some cases	Bite of tick vector	Headache, myalgias, chills, photophobia occurring acutely; CNS disease, myocardial disease, arthritis weeks to months later in some cases	74
Typhoid fever	*Salmonella typhi*	Transient, blanchable erythematous macules and papules, 2–4 mm, usually on trunk (rose spots)	Ingestion of contaminated food or water (rare in United States)	Variable abdominal pain and diarrhea; headache, myalgias, hepatosplenomegaly	54
Dengue fever[c]	Dengue virus (4 serotypes; flaviviruses)	Rash in 50% of cases; initially diffuse flushing; midway through illness, onset of maculopapular rash, which begins on trunk and spreads centrifugally to extremities and face; pruritus, hyperesthesia in some cases; after defervescence, petechiae on extremities in some cases	Occurs in tropics and subtropics; transmitted by mosquito	Headache, musculoskeletal pain ("breakbone fever"); leukopenia; occasionally biphasic ("saddleback") fever	99
Rat-bite fever (sodoku)	*Spirillum minus*	Eschar at bite site; then blotchy violaceous or red-brown rash involving trunk and extremities	Rat bite; primarily found in Asia; rare in United States	Regional adenopathy, recurrent fevers if untreated	...
Relapsing fever	*Borrelia* species	Central rash at end of febrile episode; petechiae in some cases	Exposure to ticks or body lice	Recurrent fever, headache, myalgias, hepatosplenomegaly	73

(*Continued*)

TABLE 8-1 (*CONTINUED*)

DISEASES ASSOCIATED WITH FEVER AND RASH

DISEASE	ETIOLOGY	DESCRIPTION	GROUP AFFECTED/ EPIDEMIOLOGIC FACTORS	CLINICAL SYNDROME	CHAPTER
Centrally Distributed Maculopapular Eruptions (*Continued*)					
Erythema marginatum (rheumatic fever)	Group A *Streptococcus*	Erythematous annular papules and plaques occurring as polycyclic lesions in waves over trunk, proximal extremities; evolving and resolving within hours	Patients with rheumatic fever	Pharyngitis preceding polyarthritis, carditis, subcutaneous nodules, chorea	37
Systemic lupus erythematosus	Autoimmune disease	Macular and papular erythema, often in sun-exposed areas; discoid lupus lesions (local atrophy, scale, pigmentary changes); periungual telangiectasis; malar rash; vasculitis sometimes causing urticaria, palpable purpura; oral erosions in some cases	Most common in young to middle-aged women; flares precipitated by sun exposure	Arthritis; cardiac, pulmonary, renal, hematologic, and vasculitic disease	...
Still's disease	Autoimmune disease	Transient 2- to 5-mm erythematous papules appearing at height of fever on trunk, proximal extremities; lesions evanescent	Children and young adults	High spiking fever, polyarthritis, splenomegaly; erythrocyte sedimentation rate, >100 mm/h	...
Arcanobacterial pharyngitis	*Arcanobacterium (Corynebacterium) haemolyticum*	Diffuse, erythematous, maculopapular eruption involving trunk and proximal extremities; may desquamate	Children and young adults	Exudative pharyngitis, lymphadenopathy	38
Peripheral Eruptions					
Chronic meningococcemia, disseminated gonococcal infection[a], human parvovirus B19 infection[g]	—	—	—	—	44, 45, 85
Rocky Mountain spotted fever	*Rickettsia rickettsii*	Rash beginning on wrists and ankles and spreading centripetally; appears on palms and soles later in disease; lesion evolution from blanchable macules to petechiae	Tick vector; widespread but more common in southeastern and southwest-central United States	Headache, myalgias, abdominal pain; mortality up to 40% if untreated	75
Secondary syphilis	*Treponema pallidum*	Coincident primary chancre in 10% of cases; copper-colored, scaly papular eruption, diffuse but prominent on palms and soles; rash never vesicular in adults; condyloma latum, mucous patches, and alopecia in some cases	Sexually transmitted	Fever, constitutional symptoms	70

(*Continued*)

TABLE 8-1 (*CONTINUED*)

DISEASES ASSOCIATED WITH FEVER AND RASH

DISEASE	ETIOLOGY	DESCRIPTION	GROUP AFFECTED/ EPIDEMIOLOGIC FACTORS	CLINICAL SYNDROME	CHAPTER
Peripheral Eruptions (*Continued*)					
Atypical measles	Paramyxovirus	Maculopapular eruption beginning on distal extremities and spreading centripetally; may evolve into vesicles or petechiae; edema of extremities; Koplik's spots absent	Individuals contracting measles who received killed measles vaccine in 1963–1967 in United States without subsequent live vaccine	Headache, nodular pneumonia	95
Hand-foot-and-mouth disease	Coxsackievirus A16 most common cause	Tender vesicles, erosions in mouth; 0.25-cm papules on hands and feet with rim of erythema evolving into tender vesicles	Summer and fall; primarily children <10 years old; multiple family members	Transient fever	94
Erythema multiforme	Drugs, infection, idiopathic causes	Target lesions (central erythema surrounded by area of clearing and another rim of erythema) up to 2 cm; symmetric on knees, elbows, palms, soles; may become diffuse; may involve mucosal surfaces; life-threatening in maximal form (Stevens-Johnson's syndrome)	Drug intake (i.e., sulfa, phenytoin, penicillin); herpes simplex virus or *Mycoplasma pneumoniae* infection	Varies with predisposing factor	—[d]
Rat-bite fever (Haverhill fever)	*Streptobacillus moniliformis*	Maculopapular eruption over palms, soles, and extremities; tends to be more severe at joints; eruption sometimes becoming generalized; may be purpuric; may desquamate	Rat bite, ingestion of contaminated food	Myalgias; arthritis (50%); fever recurrence in some cases	...
Bacterial endocarditis	*Streptococcus*, *Staphylococcus*, etc.	*Subacute course*: Osler's nodes (tender pink nodules on finger or toe pads); petechiae on skin and mucosa; splinter hemorrhages. *Acute course* (*Staphylococcus aureus*): Janeway lesions (painless erythematous or hemorrhagic macules, usually on palms and soles)	Abnormal heart valve, intravenous drug use	New heart murmur	19
Confluent Desquamative Erythemas					
Scarlet fever (second disease)	Group A *Streptococcus* (pyrogenic exotoxins A, B, C)	Diffuse blanchable erythema beginning on face and spreading to trunk and extremities; circumoral pallor; "sandpaper" texture to skin; accentuation of linear erythema in skin folds (Pastia's lines); enanthem of white evolving into red "strawberry" tongue; desquamation in second week	Most common in children aged 2–10 years; usually follows group A streptococcal pharyngitis	Fever, pharyngitis, headache	36

(*Continued*)

TABLE 8-1 (*CONTINUED*)

DISEASES ASSOCIATED WITH FEVER AND RASH

DISEASE	ETIOLOGY	DESCRIPTION	GROUP AFFECTED/ EPIDEMIOLOGIC FACTORS	CLINICAL SYNDROME	CHAPTER
Confluent Desquamative Erythemas (*Continued*)					
Kawasaki's disease	Idiopathic causes	Rash similar to scarlet fever (scarlatiniform) or erythema multiforme; fissuring of lips, strawberry tongue; conjunctivitis; edema of hands, feet; desquamation later in disease	Children <8 years	Cervical adenopathy, pharyngitis, coronary artery vasculitis	...
Streptococcal toxic shock syndrome	Group A *Streptococcus* (associated with pyrogenic exotoxin A and/or B or certain M types)	When present, rash often scarlatiniform	May occur in setting of severe group A streptococcal infections, such as necrotizing fasciitis, bacteremia, pneumonia	Multiorgan failure, hypotension; 30% mortality rate	36
Staphylococcal toxic shock syndrome	*S. aureus* (toxic shock syndrome toxin 1, enterotoxin B or C)	Diffuse erythema involving palms; pronounced erythema of mucosal surfaces; conjunctivitis; desquamation 7–10 days into illness	Colonization with toxin-producing *S. aureus*	Fever >39°C (102°F), hypotension, multiorgan dysfunction	35
Staphylococcal scalded-skin syndrome	*S. aureus*, phage group II	Diffuse tender erythema, often with bullae and desquamation; Nikolsky's sign	Colonization with toxin-producing *S. aureus*; occurs in children <10 years old (termed "Ritter's disease" in neonates) or adults with renal dysfunction	Irritability; nasal or conjunctival secretions	35
Exfoliative erythroderma syndrome	Underlying psoriasis, eczema, drug eruption, mycosis fungoides	Diffuse erythema (often scaling) interspersed with lesions of underlying condition	Usually occurs in adults over age 50; more common in men	Fever, chills (i.e., difficulty with thermoregulation); lymphadenopathy	...
Stevens-Johnson's syndrome (SJS), toxic epidermal necrolysis (TEN)	Drugs, other causes (infection, neoplasm, graft-vs-host disease)	Diffuse erythema or target-like lesions progressing to bullae, with sloughing and necrosis of entire epidermis; Nikolsky's sign. *TEN:* maximal form of SJS. *SJS:* maximal form of erythema multiforme	Uncommon in children; more common in patients with HIV infection or graft-vs-host disease	Dehydration, sepsis sometimes resulting from lack of normal skin integrity; 25% mortality	...
Vesiculobullous Eruptions					
Hand-foot-and-mouth syndrome[e]; staphylococcal scalded-skin syndrome; toxic epidermal necrolysis[f]	—	—	—	—	—[d]

(*Continued*)

CHAPTER 8

Fever and Rash

TABLE 8-1 (*CONTINUED*)

DISEASES ASSOCIATED WITH FEVER AND RASH

DISEASE	ETIOLOGY	DESCRIPTION	GROUP AFFECTED/ EPIDEMIOLOGIC FACTORS	CLINICAL SYNDROME	CHAPTER
Vesiculobullous Eruptions (*Continued*)					
Varicella (chickenpox)	Varicella-zoster virus	Macules (2–3 mm) evolving into papules, then vesicles (sometimes umbilicated), on an erythematous base ("dewdrops on a rose petal"); pustules then forming and crusting; lesions appearing in crops; may involve scalp, mouth; intensely pruritic	Usually affects children; 10% of adults susceptible; most common in late winter and spring	Malaise; generally mild disease in healthy children; more severe disease with complications in adults and immunocompromised children	81
Pseudomonas "hot-tub" folliculitis	*Pseudomonas aeruginosa*	Pruritic, erythematous follicular, papular, vesicular, or pustular lesions that may involve axillae, buttocks, abdomen, and especially areas occluded by bathing suits; can manifest as tender isolated nodules on palmar or plantar surfaces (the latter designated "*Pseudomonas* hot-foot syndrome")	Bathers in hot tubs or swimming pools; occurs in outbreaks	Earache, sore eyes and/or throat; generally self-limited	53
Variola (smallpox)	Variola major virus	Red macules on tongue, palate evolving to papules and vesicles; skin macules evolving to papules, then vesicles, then pustules over 1 week, with subsequent lesion crusting; lesions initially appearing on face and spreading centrifugally from trunk to extremities; differs from varicella in that (1) skin lesions in any given area are at same stage of development and (2) there is a prominent distribution of lesions on face and extremities (including palms, soles) as opposed to prominent rash on trunk	Nonimmune individuals exposed to smallpox	Prodrome of fever, headache, backache, myalgias; vomiting in 50% of cases	6
Primary herpes simplex virus (HSV) infection	HSV	Erythema rapidly followed by hallmark *grouped vesicles* that may evolve into pustules; painful lesions that may ulcerate, especially on mucosal surfaces; lesions at site of inoculation: commonly gingivostomatitis for HSV-1 and genital lesions for HSV-2; recurrent disease milder (e.g., herpes labialis does not involve oral mucosa)	Primary infection most common in children and young adults for HSV-1 and in sexually active young adults for HSV-2; no fever in recurrent infection	Regional lymphadenopathy	80

(*Continued*)

TABLE 8-1 (*CONTINUED*)

DISEASES ASSOCIATED WITH FEVER AND RASH

DISEASE	ETIOLOGY	DESCRIPTION	GROUP AFFECTED/ EPIDEMIOLOGIC FACTORS	CLINICAL SYNDROME	CHAPTER
Vesiculobullous Eruptions (*Continued*)					
Disseminated herpesvirus infection	Varicella-zoster virus or HSV	Generalized vesicles that can evolve to pustules and ulcerations; individual lesions similar for varicella-zoster and HSV. *Zoster cutaneous dissemination*: >25 lesions extending outside involved dermatome. *HSV*: extensive, progressive mucocutaneous lesions in some cases; HSV lesions sometimes disseminate in eczematous skin (eczema herpeticum); HSV visceral dissemination may occur with only limited skin lesions	Immunosuppressed individuals, eczema	Visceral organ involvement (especially liver) in some cases	29, 80, 81
Rickettsialpox	*Rickettsia akari*	Eschar found at site of mite bite; generalized rash involving face, trunk, extremities; may involve palms and soles; <100 papules and plaques (2–10 mm); tops of lesions develop vesicles that may evolve into pustules	Seen in urban settings; transmitted by mouse mites	Headache, myalgias, regional adenopathy; mild disease	75
Disseminated *Vibrio vulnificus* infection	*V. vulnificus*	Erythematous lesions evolving into hemorrhagic bullae and then into necrotic ulcers	Patients with cirrhosis, diabetes, renal failure; exposure by ingestion of contaminated saltwater seafood	Hypotension; 50% mortality	57
Ecthyma gangrenosum	*P. aeruginosa*, other gram-negative rods, fungi	Indurated plaque evolving into hemorrhagic bulla or pustule that sloughs, resulting in eschar formation; erythematous halo; most common in axillary, groin, perianal regions	Usually affects neutropenic patients; occurs in up to 28% of individuals with *Pseudomonas* bacteremia	Clinical signs of sepsis	53
Urticarial Eruptions					
Urticarial vasculitis	Serum sickness, often due to infection (including hepatitis B viral, enteroviral, parasitic), drugs (including penicillins, sulfonamides, salicylates, barbiturates); connective tissue disease; idiopathic causes	Erythematous, circumscribed areas of edema; occasionally indurated; pruritic or burning; lesions sometimes purpuric; individual lesions lasting up to 5 days	In serum sickness, occurs 8–14 days after antigen exposure in nonsensitized individuals; may occur within 36 h in sensitized individuals	Malaise, lymphadenopathy, myalgias, arthralgias	—[d]

(Continued)

TABLE 8-1 (CONTINUED)

DISEASES ASSOCIATED WITH FEVER AND RASH

DISEASE	ETIOLOGY	DESCRIPTION	GROUP AFFECTED/ EPIDEMIOLOGIC FACTORS	CLINICAL SYNDROME	CHAPTER
Nodular Eruptions					
Disseminated infection	Fungi (e.g., candidiasis, histoplasmosis, cryptococcosis, sporotrichosis, coccidioidomycosis); mycobacteria	Subcutaneous nodules (up to 3 cm); fluctuance, draining common with mycobacteria; necrotic nodules (extremities, periorbital or nasal regions) common with *Aspergillus*, *Mucor*	Immunocompromised hosts (i.e., bone marrow transplant recipients, patients undergoing chemotherapy, HIV-infected patients, alcoholics)	Features vary with organism	—[d]
Erythema nodosum (septal panniculitis)	Infections (e.g., streptococcal, fungal, mycobacterial, yersinial); drugs (e.g., sulfas, penicillins, oral contraceptives); sarcoidosis; idiopathic causes	Large, violaceous, nonulcerative, subcutaneous nodules; exquisitely tender; usually on lower legs but also on upper extremities	More common in females 15–30 years old	Arthralgias (50%); features vary with associated condition	—[d]
Sweet's syndrome (acute febrile neutrophilic dermatosis)	Yersinial infection; lymphoproliferative disorders; idiopathic causes	Tender red or blue edematous nodules giving impression of vesiculation; usually on face, neck, upper extremities; when on lower extremities, may mimic erythema nodosum	More common in women and in persons 30–60 years old; 20% of cases associated with malignancy (men and women equally affected in this group)	Headache, arthralgias, leukocytosis	...
Bacillary angiomatosis	*Bartonella henselae* or *Bartonella quintana*	Many forms, including erythematous, smooth vascular nodules; friable, exophytic lesions; erythematous plaques (may be dry, scaly); subcutaneous nodules (may be erythematous)	Usually in HIV infection	Peliosis of liver and spleen in some cases; lesions may involve multiple organs; bacteremia	61
Purpuric Eruptions					
Rocky Mountain spotted fever, rat-bite fever, endocarditis[e]; epidemic typhus[g]; dengue fever[c]; human parvovirus B19 infection[g]	—	—	—	—	—[d]
Acute meningococcemia	*Neisseria meningitidis*	Initially pink maculopapular lesions evolving into petechiae; petechiae rapidly becoming numerous, sometimes enlarging and becoming vesicular; trunk, extremities most commonly involved; may appear on face, hands, feet; may include purpura fulminans reflecting disseminated intravascular coagulation (see below)	Most common in children, individuals with asplenia or terminal complement component deficiency (C5-C8)	Hypotension, meningitis (sometimes preceded by upper respiratory infection)	44

(Continued)

TABLE 8-1 (*CONTINUED*)

DISEASES ASSOCIATED WITH FEVER AND RASH

DISEASE	ETIOLOGY	DESCRIPTION	GROUP AFFECTED/ EPIDEMIOLOGIC FACTORS	CLINICAL SYNDROME	CHAPTER
Purpuric Eruptions (*Continued*)					
Purpura fulminans	Severe disseminated intravascular coagulation	Large ecchymoses with sharply irregular shapes evolving into hemorrhagic bullae and then into black necrotic lesions	Individuals with sepsis (e.g., involving *N. meningitidis*), malignancy, or massive trauma; asplenic patients at high risk for sepsis	Hypotension	15, 44
Chronic meningococcemia	*N. meningitidis*	Variety of recurrent eruptions, including pink maculopapular; nodular (usually on lower extremities); petechial (sometimes developing vesicular centers); purpuric areas with pale blue-gray centers	Individuals with complement deficiencies	Fevers, sometimes intermittent; arthritis, myalgias, headache	44
Disseminated gonococcal infection	*Neisseria gonorrhoeae*	Papules (1–5 mm) evolving over 1–2 days into hemorrhagic pustules with gray necrotic centers; hemorrhagic bullae occurring rarely; lesions (usually fewer than 40) distributed peripherally near joints (more commonly on upper extremities)	Sexually active individuals (more often females), some with complement deficiency	Low-grade fever, tenosynovitis, arthritis	45
Enteroviral petechial rash	Usually echovirus 9 or coxsackievirus A9	Disseminated petechial lesions (may also be maculopapular, vesicular, or urticarial)	Often occurs in outbreaks	Pharyngitis, headache; aseptic meningitis with echovirus 9	94
Viral hemorrhagic fever	Arboviruses and arenaviruses	Petechial rash	Residence in or travel to endemic areas or other virus exposure	Triad of fever, shock, hemorrhage from mucosa or gastrointestinal tract	99, 100
Thrombotic thrombocytopenic purpura/ hemolytic-uremic syndrome	Idiopathic, *Escherichia coli* O157:H7 (Shiga's toxin), drugs	Petechiae	Individuals with *E. coli* O157:H7 gastroenteritis (especially children), cancer chemotherapy, HIV infection, autoimmune diseases; pregnant/ postpartum women	Fever (not always present), hemolytic anemia, thrombocytopenia, renal dysfunction, neurologic dysfunction; coagulation studies normal	51, 55
Cutaneous small-vessel vasculitis (leukocytoclastic vasculitis)	Infections (including group A *Streptococcus*, viral hepatitis), drugs, chemicals, food allergens, idiopathic causes	Palpable purpuric lesions appearing in crops on legs or other dependent areas; may become vesicular or ulcerative; usually resolve over 3–4 weeks	Occurs in a wide spectrum of diseases, including connective tissue disease, cryoglobulinemia, malignancy, Henoch-Schönlein's purpura (HSP); more common in children	Fever, malaise, arthralgias, myalgias; systemic vasculitis in some cases; renal, joint, and gastrointestinal involvement commonly seen in HSP	...

(*Continued*)

TABLE 8-1 (*CONTINUED*)

DISEASES ASSOCIATED WITH FEVER AND RASH

DISEASE	ETIOLOGY	DESCRIPTION	GROUP AFFECTED/ EPIDEMIOLOGIC FACTORS	CLINICAL SYNDROME	CHAPTER
Eruptions with Ulcers and/or Eschars					
Scrub typhus, rickettsial spotted fevers, rat-bite fever[g]; rickettsialpox, ecthyma gangrenosum[h]	—	—	—	—	—[d]
Tularemia	*Francisella tularensis*	Ulceroglandular form: erythematous, tender papule evolves into necrotic, tender ulcer with raised borders; in 35% of cases, eruptions (maculopapular, vesiculopapular, acneiform, urticarial, erythema nodosum, or erythema multiforme) may occur	Exposure to ticks, biting flies, infected animals	Fever, headache, lymphadenopathy	59
Anthrax	*Bacillus anthracis*	Pruritic papule enlarging and evolving into a 1- by 3-cm painless ulcer surrounded by vesicles and then developing a central eschar with edema; residual scar	Exposure to infected animals or animal products or other exposure to anthrax spores	Lymphadenopathy, headache	6

[a]See "Purpuric eruptions."
[b]In human granulocytotropic ehrlichiosis, or anaplasmosis (caused by *Anaplasma phagocytophila*; most common in the upper midwestern and northeastern regions of the United States), rash is rare.
[c]See "Viral hemorrhagic fever" under "Purpuric eruptions" for dengue hemorrhagic fever/dengue shock syndrome.
[d]See etiology-specific chapters.
[e]See "Peripheral eruptions."
[f]See "Confluent desquamative erythemas."
[g]See "Centrally distributed maculopapular eruptions."
[h]See "Vesiculobullous eruptions."

occur initially on the trunk and sometimes on the extremities (sparing the face), and fade within 2 days.

Although drug reactions have many manifestations, including urticaria, exanthematous *drug-induced eruptions* are most common and are often difficult to distinguish from viral exanthems. Eruptions elicited by drugs are usually more intensely erythematous and pruritic than viral exanthems, but this distinction is not reliable. A history of new medications and an absence of prostration may help to distinguish a drug-related rash from an eruption of another etiology. Rashes may persist for up to 2 weeks after administration of the offending agent is discontinued. Certain populations are more prone than others to drug rashes. Of HIV-infected patients, 50–60% develop a rash in response to sulfa drugs; 90% of patients with mononucleosis due to Epstein-Barr virus develop a rash when given ampicillin.

Rickettsial illnesses (Chap. 75) should be considered in the evaluation of individuals with centrally distributed maculopapular eruptions. The usual setting for *epidemic typhus* is a site of war or natural disaster in which people are exposed to body lice. A diagnosis of recrudescent typhus should be considered in European immigrants to the United States. However, an indigenous form of typhus, presumably transmitted by flying squirrels, has been reported in the southeastern United States. *Endemic typhus* or *leptospirosis* (the latter caused by a spirochete; Chap. 72) may be seen in urban environments where rodents proliferate. Outside the United States, other rickettsial diseases cause a spotted-fever syndrome and should be considered in residents of or travelers to endemic areas. Similarly, *typhoid fever*, a nonrickettsial disease caused by *Salmonella typhi* (Chap. 54), is usually acquired during travel outside the United States. Dengue fever, caused by a mosquito-transmitted flavivirus, occurs in tropical and subtropical regions of the world (Chap. 99).

Some centrally distributed maculopapular eruptions have distinctive features. Erythema chronicum migrans (ECM), the rash of Lyme disease (Chap. 74), typically manifests as singular or multiple annular plaques. Untreated ECM lesions usually fade within a month but may persist for more than a year. *Erythema marginatum*, the rash of acute rheumatic fever (Chap. 37), has a distinctive pattern of enlarging and shifting transient annular lesions.

Collagen vascular diseases may cause fever and rash. Patients with *systemic lupus erythematosus* typically develop a sharply defined, erythematous eruption in a butterfly distribution on the cheeks (malar rash) as well as many other skin manifestations. *Still's disease* manifests as an evanescent salmon-colored rash on the trunk and proximal extremities that coincides with fever spikes.

PERIPHERAL ERUPTIONS

These rashes are alike in that they are most prominent peripherally or begin in peripheral (acral) areas before spreading centripetally. Early diagnosis and therapy are critical in RMSF (Chap. 75) because of its grave prognosis if untreated. Lesions evolve from macular to petechial, start on the wrists and ankles, spread centripetally, and appear on the palms and soles only later in the disease. The rash of *secondary syphilis* (Chap. 70), which may be generalized but is prominent on the palms and soles, should be considered in the differential diagnosis of pityriasis rosea, especially in sexually active patients. *Atypical measles* (Chap. 95) is seen in individuals contracting measles who received the killed measles vaccine between 1963 and 1967 in the United States and who were not subsequently protected with the live vaccine. *Hand-foot-and-mouth disease* (Chap. 94), most commonly caused by coxsackievirus A16, is distinguished by tender vesicles distributed peripherally and in the mouth; outbreaks commonly occur within families. The classic target lesions of *erythema multiforme* (EM) appear symmetrically on the elbows, knees, palms, soles, and face. In severe cases, these lesions spread diffusely and involve mucosal surfaces. Stevens-Johnson's syndrome is considered a maximal form of erythema multiforme and is life-threatening. Lesions may develop on the hands and feet in *endocarditis* (Chap. 19).

CONFLUENT DESQUAMATIVE ERYTHEMAS

These eruptions consist of diffuse erythema frequently followed by desquamation. The eruptions caused by group A *Streptococcus* or *Staphylococcus aureus* are toxin mediated. *Scarlet fever* (Chap. 36) usually follows pharyngitis; patients have a facial flush, a "strawberry" tongue, and accentuated petechiae in body folds (Pastia's lines). *Kawasaki's disease* presents in the pediatric population as fissuring of the lips, a strawberry tongue, conjunctivitis, adenopathy, and sometimes cardiac abnormalities. *Streptococcal toxic shock syndrome* (Chap. 36) manifests with hypo-tension, multiorgan failure, and often a severe group A streptococcal infection (e.g., necrotizing fasciitis). *Staphylococcal toxic shock syndrome* (Chap. 35) also presents with hypotension and multiorgan failure, but usually only *S. aureus* colonization—not a severe *S. aureus* infection—is documented. *Staphylococcal scalded-skin syndrome* (Chap. 35) is seen primarily in children and in immunocompromised adults. Generalized erythema is often evident during the prodrome of fever and malaise; profound tenderness of the skin is distinctive. In the exfoliative stage, the skin can be induced to form bullae with light lateral pressure (Nikolsky's sign). In a mild form, a scarlatiniform eruption mimics scarlet fever, but the patient does not exhibit a strawberry tongue or circumoral pallor. In contrast to the staphylococcal scalded-skin syndrome, in which the cleavage plane is superficial in the epidermis, *toxic epidermal necrolysis*, a maximal variant of Stevens-Johnson's syndrome, involves sloughing of the entire epidermis, resulting in severe disease. *Exfoliative erythroderma syndrome* is a serious reaction associated with systemic toxicity that is often due to eczema, psoriasis, mycosis fungoides, or a severe drug reaction.

VESICULOBULLOUS ERUPTIONS

Varicella (Chap. 81) is highly contagious, often occurring in winter or spring. At any point in time, within a given region of the body, varicella lesions are in different stages of development. In immunocompromised hosts, varicella vesicles may lack the characteristic erythematous base or may appear hemorrhagic. Lesions of *Pseudomonas* "hot-tub" folliculitis (Chap. 53) are also pruritic and may appear similar to those of varicella. However, hot-tub folliculitis generally occurs in outbreaks after bathing in hot tubs or swimming pools, and lesions occur in regions occluded by bathing suits. Lesions of *variola* (smallpox; Chap. 6) also appear similar to those of varicella but are all at the same stage of development in a given region of the body. Variola lesions are most prominent on the face and extremities, whereas varicella lesions are most prominent on the trunk. Herpes simplex virus infection (Chap. 80) is characterized by hallmark grouped vesicles on an erythematous base. Primary herpes infection is accompanied by fever and toxicity, whereas recurrent disease is milder. *Rickettsialpox* (Chap. 75) is often documented in urban settings and is characterized by vesicles. It can be distinguished from varicella by an eschar at the site of the mouse-mite bite and the papule/plaque base of each vesicle. Disseminated *Vibrio vulnificus* infection (Chap. 57) or *ecthyma gangrenosum* due to *Pseudomonas aeruginosa* (Chap. 53) should be considered in immunosuppressed individuals with sepsis and hemorrhagic bullae.

URTICARIAL ERUPTIONS

Individuals with classic urticaria ("hives") usually have a hypersensitivity reaction without associated fever. In the presence of fever, urticarial eruptions are usually due to *urticarial vasculitis*. Unlike individual lesions of classic urticaria, which last up to 48 h, these lesions may last up to 5 days. Etiologies include serum sickness (often induced by drugs such as penicillins, sulfas, salicylates, or barbiturates), connective-tissue disease (e.g., systemic lupus erythematosus or Sjögren's syndrome), and infection (e.g., with hepatitis B virus, enteroviruses, or parasites). Malignancy may be associated with fever and chronic urticaria.

NODULAR ERUPTIONS

In immunocompromised hosts, nodular lesions often represent disseminated infection. Patients with disseminated *candidiasis* (often due to *Candida tropicalis*) may have a triad of fever, myalgias, and eruptive nodules (Chap. 107). Disseminated *cryptococcosis* lesions (Chap. 106) may resemble molluscum contagiosum (Chap. 84). Necrosis of nodules should raise the suspicion of *aspergillosis* (Chap. 108) or *mucormycosis* (Chap. 109). *Erythema nodosum* presents with exquisitely tender nodules on the lower extremities. *Sweet's syndrome* should be considered in individuals with multiple nodules and plaques, often so edematous that they give the appearance of vesicles or bullae. Sweet's syndrome may affect either healthy individuals or persons with lymphoproliferative disease.

PURPURIC ERUPTIONS

Acute meningococcemia (Chap. 44) classically presents in children as a petechial eruption, but initial lesions may appear as blanchable macules or urticaria. RMSF should be considered in the differential diagnosis of acute meningococcemia. *Echovirus 9 infection* (Chap. 94) may mimic acute meningococcemia; patients should be treated as if they have bacterial sepsis since prompt differentiation of these conditions may be impossible. Large ecchymotic areas of *purpura fulminans* (Chaps. 44 and 15) reflect severe underlying disseminated intravascular coagulation, which may be due to infectious or noninfectious causes. The lesions of *chronic meningococcemia* (Chap. 44) may have a variety of morphologies, including petechial. Purpuric nodules may develop on the legs and resemble erythema nodosum but lack its exquisite tenderness. Lesions of *disseminated gonococcemia* (Chap. 45) are distinctive, sparse, countable hemorrhagic pustules, usually located near joints. The lesions of chronic meningococcemia and those of gonococcemia may be indistinguishable in terms of appearance and distribution. *Viral hemorrhagic fever* (Chaps. 99 and 100) should be considered in patients with an appropriate travel history and a petechial rash. *Thrombotic thrombocytopenic purpura* and *hemolytic-uremic syndrome* (Chaps. 51 and 55) are closely related and are noninfectious causes of fever and petechiae. *Cutaneous small-vessel vasculitis* (*leukocytoclastic vasculitis*) typically manifests as palpable purpura and has a wide variety of causes.

ERUPTIONS WITH ULCERS OR ESCHARS

The presence of an ulcer or eschar in the setting of a more widespread eruption can provide an important diagnostic clue. For example, the presence of an eschar may suggest the diagnosis of scrub typhus or rickettsialpox (Chap. 75) in the appropriate setting. In other illnesses (e.g., anthrax; Chap. 6), an ulcer or eschar may be the only skin manifestation.

FURTHER READINGS

CHERRY JD: Contemporary infectious exanthems. Clin Infect Dis 16:199, 1993

———: Cutaneous manifestations of systemic infections, in *Textbook of Pediatric Infectious Diseases*, vol. 1, 4th ed, RD Feigin, JD Cherry (eds). Philadelphia, Saunders, 1998, pp 713–737

EICHENFIELD LF et al (eds): *Textbook of Neonatal Dermatology*. Philadelphia, Saunders, 2001

FREEDBERG IM et al (eds): *Fitzpatrick's Dermatology in General Medicine*, 6th ed. New York, McGraw-Hill, 2003

LEVIN S, GOODMAN LJ: An approach to acute fever and rash (AFR) in the adult. Curr Clin Top Infect Dis 15:19, 1995

PALLER AS, MANCINI AJ (eds): *Hurwitz Clinical Pediatric Dermatology*, 3d ed. Philadelphia, Elsevier Saunders, 2006

SCHLOSSBERG D: Fever and rash. Infect Dis Clin North Am 10:101, 1996

WEBER DJ et al: The acutely ill patient with fever and rash, in *Principles and Practice of Infectious Diseases*, vol 1, 6th ed, GL Mandell et al (eds). Philadelphia, Elsevier Churchill Livingstone, 2005, pp 729–746

WENNER HA: Virus diseases associated with cutaneous eruptions. Prog Med Virol 16:269, 1973

WOLFF K, JOHNSON RAJ: *Fitzpatrick's Color Atlas and Synopsis of Clinical Dermatology*, 5th ed. New York, McGraw-Hill, 2005

CHAPTER 9

FEVER OF UNKNOWN ORIGIN

Jeffrey A. Gelfand ■ Michael V. Callahan

DEFINITION AND CLASSIFICATION

Fever of unknown origin (FUO) was defined by Petersdorf and Beeson in 1961 as (1) temperatures of >38.3°C (>101°F) on several occasions; (2) a duration of fever of >3 weeks; and (3) failure to reach a diagnosis despite 1 week of inpatient investigation. Although this classification has stood for more than 30 years, Durack and Street have proposed a new system for classification of FUO:

(1) classic FUO; (2) nosocomial FUO; (3) neutropenic FUO; and (4) FUO associated with HIV infection.

Classic FUO corresponds closely to the earlier definition of FUO, differing only with regard to the prior requirement for 1 week's study in the hospital. The newer definition is broader, stipulating three outpatient visits or 3 days in the hospital without elucidation of a cause or 1 week of "intelligent and invasive" ambulatory investigation. In *nosocomial FUO*, a temperature of ≥38.3°C (≥101°F) develops on several occasions in a hospitalized patient who is receiving acute care and in whom infection was not manifest or incubating on admission. Three days of investigation, including at least 2 days' incubation of cultures, is the minimum requirement for this diagnosis. *Neutropenic FUO* is defined as a temperature of ≥38.3°C (≥101°F) on several occasions in a patient whose neutrophil count is <500/μL or is expected to fall to that level in 1–2 days. The diagnosis of neutropenic FUO is invoked if a specific cause is not identified after 3 days of investigation, including at least 2 days' incubation of cultures. *HIV-associated FUO* is defined by a temperature of ≥38.3°C (≥101°F) on several occasions over a period of >4 weeks for outpatients or >3 days for hospitalized patients with HIV infection. This diagnosis is invoked if appropriate investigation over 3 days, including 2 days' incubation of cultures, reveals no source.

Adoption of these categories of FUO in the literature has allowed a more rational compilation of data regarding these disparate groups. In the remainder of this chapter, the discussion will focus on classic FUO in the adult unless otherwise specified.

CAUSES OF CLASSIC FUO

Table 9-1 summarizes the findings of several large studies of FUO carried out since the advent of the antibiotic era, including a prospective study of 167 adult patients with FUO encompassing all eight university hospitals in the Netherlands and using a standardized protocol in which the first author reviewed every patient. Coincident with the widespread use of antibiotics, increasingly useful diagnostic technologies—both noninvasive and invasive—have been developed. Newer studies reflect not only changing patterns of disease, but also the impact of diagnostic techniques that make it possible to eliminate many patients with specific illness from the FUO category. The ubiquitous use of potent broad-spectrum antibiotics may have decreased the number of infections causing FUO. The wide availability of ultrasonography, CT, MRI, radionuclide scanning, and positron emission tomography (PET) scanning has enhanced the detection of localized infections and of occult neoplasms and lymphomas in patients previously thought to have FUO. Likewise, the widespread availability of highly specific and sensitive immunologic testing has reduced the number of undetected cases of systemic lupus erythematosus and other autoimmune diseases.

Infections, especially extrapulmonary tuberculosis, remain the leading diagnosable cause of FUO. Prolonged mononucleosis syndromes caused by Epstein-Barr virus, cytomegalovirus (CMV), or HIV are conditions whose consideration as a cause of FUO is sometimes confounded by delayed antibody responses. Intraabdominal abscesses (sometimes poorly localized) and renal, retroperitoneal, and paraspinal abscesses continue to be difficult to diagnose. Renal malacoplakia, with submucosal plaques or nodules involving the urinary tract, may cause FUO and is often fatal if untreated. It is associated with intracellular bacterial infection, is seen most often in patients with defects of intracellular bacterial killing, and is treated with fluoroquinolones or trimethoprim-sulfamethoxazole. Occasionally, other organs may be involved. Osteomyelitis, especially where prosthetic devices have been implanted, and infective endocarditis must be considered. Although true culture-negative infective endocarditis is rare, one may be misled by slow-growing organisms of the HACEK group (*Haemophilus aphrophilus*, *Actinobacillus actinomycetemcomitans*, *Cardiobacterium hominis*, *Eikenella corrodens*, and *Kingella kingae*; Chap. 48), *Bartonella* spp. (previously *Rochalimaea*), *Legionella* spp., *Coxiella burnetii*, *Chlamydophila psittaci*, and fungi. Prostatitis, dental abscesses, sinusitis, and cholangitis continue to be sources of occult fever.

TABLE 9-1

CLASSIC FUO IN ADULTS

AUTHORS (YEAR OF PUBLICATION)	YEARS OF STUDY	NO. OF CASES	INFECTIONS (%)	NEOPLASMS (%)	NONINFECTIOUS INFLAMMATORY DISEASES (%)	MISCELLANEOUS CAUSES (%)	UNDIAGNOSED CAUSES (%)
Petersdorf and Beeson (1961)	1952–1957	100	36	19	19[a]	19[a]	7
Larson and Featherstone (1982)	1970–1980	105	30	31	16[a]	11[a]	12
Knockaert and Vanneste (1992)	1980–1989	199	22.5	7	23[a]	21.5[a]	25.5
de Kleijn et al. (1997, Part I)	1992–1994	167	26	12.5	24	8	30

[a]Authors' raw data retabulated to conform to altered diagnostic categories.

Source: Modified from de Kleijn et al., 1997 (Part I).

Fungal disease, most notably histoplasmosis involving the reticuloendothelial system, may cause FUO. FUO with headache should prompt examination of spinal fluid for *Cryptococcus neoformans*. Malaria (which may result from transfusion, the failure to take a prescribed prophylactic agent, or infection with a drug-resistant strain) continues to be a cause, particularly of asynchronous FUO. A related protozoan infection, babesiosis, may cause FUO and is increasing in geographic distribution and in incidence, especially among the elderly and immunosuppressed.

In most earlier series, neoplasms were the next most common cause of FUO after infections (Table 9-1). In more recent series, a decrease in the percentage of FUO cases due to malignancy was attributed to improvement in diagnostic technologies—in particular, high-resolution tomography, MRI, PET scanning, and tumor antigen assays. This observation does not diminish the importance of considering neoplasia in the initial diagnostic evaluation of a patient with fever. A number of patients in these series had temporal arteritis, adult Still's disease, drug-related fever, and factitious fever. In recent series, ~25–30% of cases of FUO have remained undiagnosed. The general term *noninfectious inflammatory diseases* applies to systemic rheumatologic or vasculitic diseases such as polymyalgia rheumatica, lupus, and adult Still's disease, as well as to granulomatous diseases such as sarcoidosis and Crohn's and granulomatous hepatitis.

In the elderly, multisystem disease is the most frequent cause of FUO, with giant-cell arteritis being the leading etiologic entity in this category. In patients >50 years of age, this disease accounts for 15–20% of FUO cases. Tuberculosis is the most common infection causing FUO in the elderly, and colon cancer is an important cause of FUO with malignancy in this age group.

Many diseases have been grouped in the various studies as "miscellaneous." On this list are drug fever, pulmonary embolism, factitious fever, the hereditary periodic fever syndromes (familial Mediterranean fever, hyper-IgD syndrome, tumor necrosis factor receptor–associated periodic syndrome, familial cold urticaria, and the Muckle-Wells syndrome), and Fabry's disease.

A drug-related etiology must be considered in any case of prolonged fever. Any febrile pattern may be elicited by a drug. Virtually all classes of drugs cause fever, but antimicrobial agents (especially β-lactam antibiotics), cardiovascular drugs (e.g., quinidine), antineoplastic drugs, and drugs acting on the central nervous system (e.g., phenytoin) are particularly common causes.

It is axiomatic that, as the duration of fever increases, the likelihood of an infectious cause decreases, even for the more indolent infectious etiologies (e.g., brucellosis, paracoccidioidomycosis, and malaria due to *Plasmodium malariae*). In a series of 347 patients referred to the National Institutes of Health from 1961 to 1977, only 6% had an infection (Table 9-2). A significant proportion (9%) had factitious fevers—i.e., fevers due either to false elevations of temperature or to self-induced disease. A substantial number of these factitious cases were in young women in the health professions. It is worth noting that 8% of the patients with prolonged fevers (some of whom had completely normal liver function studies) had granulomatous hepatitis, and 6% had adult Still's disease. After prolonged investigation, 19% of cases still had no specific diagnosis. A total of 27% of patients had no actual fever during inpatient observation or had an exaggerated circadian temperature rhythm without chills, elevated pulse, or other abnormalities.

TABLE 9-2

CAUSES OF FUO LASTING >6 MONTHS

CAUSE	CASES, %
None identified	19
Miscellaneous causes	13
Factitious causes	9
Granulomatous hepatitis	8
Neoplasm	7
Still's disease	6
Infection	6
Collagen vascular disease	4
Familial Mediterranean fever	3
No fever[a]	27

[a]No actual fever observed during 2–3 weeks of inpatient observation. Includes patients with exaggerated circadian rhythm.

Source: From a study of 347 patients referred to the National Institutes of Health from 1961 to 1977 with a presumptive diagnosis of FUO of >6 months' duration (R Aduan et al. Prolonged fever of unknown origin. Clin Res 26:558A, 1978).

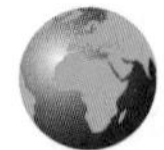

More than 200 conditions may be considered in the differential diagnosis of classic FUO in adults; the most common of these are listed in Table 9-3. This list applies strictly to the United States. Geographic considerations are paramount. For example, in Japan, human T-cell lymphotropic virus type I is a consideration; in China, infection plays a greater role and tuberculosis is prominent; and in Spain, visceral leishmaniasis may be a more common cause of FUO. The frequency of global travel underscores the need for a detailed travel history, and the continuing emergence of new infectious diseases makes this listing potentially incomplete. The possibility of international and domestic terrorist activity involving the intentional release of infectious agents, many of which cause illnesses presenting with prolonged fever, underscores the need for obtaining an insightful environmental, occupational, and professional history, with early notification of public health authorities in cases of suspicious etiology (Chap. 6).

SPECIALIZED DIAGNOSTIC STUDIES

Classic FUO

A stepwise flow chart depicting the diagnostic workup and therapeutic management of FUO is provided in Fig. 9-1. In this flow chart, reference is made to "potentially diagnostic clues," as outlined by de Kleijn and colleagues; these clues may be key findings in the history (e.g., travel), localizing signs, or key symptoms.

TABLE 9-3

CAUSES OF FUO IN ADULTS IN THE UNITED STATES

Infections

- Localized pyogenic infections
  - Appendicitis
  - Cat-scratch disease
  - Cholangitis
  - Cholecystitis
  - Dental abscess
  - Diverticulitis/abscess
  - Lesser sac abscess
  - Liver abscess
  - Mesenteric lymphadenitis
  - Osteomyelitis
  - Pancreatic abscess
  - Pelvic inflammatory disease
  - Perinephric/intrarenal abscess
  - Prostatic abscess
  - Renal malacoplakia
  - Sinusitis
  - Subphrenic abscess
  - Suppurative thrombophlebitis
  - Tuboovarian abscess
- Intravascular infections
  - Bacterial aortitis
  - Bacterial endocarditis
  - Vascular catheter infection
- Systemic bacterial infections
  - Bartonellosis
  - Brucellosis
  - Campylobacter infection
  - Cat-scratch disease/bacillary angiomatosis (*Bartonella henselae*)
  - Gonococcemia
  - Legionnaires' disease
  - Leptospirosis
  - Listeriosis
  - Lyme disease
  - Melioidosis
  - Meningococcemia
  - Rat-bite fever
  - Relapsing fever
  - Salmonellosis
  - Syphilis
  - Tularemia
  - Typhoid fever
  - Vibriosis
  - Yersinia infection
- Mycobacterial infections
  - *M. avium/M. intracellulare* infections
  - Other atypical mycobacterial infections
  - Tuberculosis
- Other bacterial infections
  - Actinomycosis
  - Bacillary angiomatosis
  - Nocardiosis
  - Whipple's disease
- Rickettsial infections
  - Anaplasmosis
  - Ehrlichiosis
  - Murine typhus
  - Q fever
  - Rickettsialpox
  - Rocky Mountain spotted fever
- Mycoplasmal infections
- Chlamydial infections
  - Lymphogranuloma venereum
  - Psittacosis
  - TWAR (*Chlamydophila pneumoniae*) infection
- Viral infections
  - Colorado tick fever
  - Coxsackievirus group B infection
  - Cytomegalovirus infection
  - Dengue
  - Epstein-Barr virus infection
  - Hepatitis A, B, C, D, and E
  - Human herpesvirus 6 infection
  - Human immunodeficiency virus infection
  - Lymphocytic choriomeningitis
  - Parvovirus B19 infection
- Fungal infections
  - Aspergillosis
  - Blastomycosis
  - Candidiasis
  - Coccidioidomycosis
  - Cryptococcosis
  - Histoplasmosis
  - Mucormycosis
  - Paracoccidioidomycosis
  - Pneumocystis infection
  - Sporotrichosis
- Parasitic infections
  - Amebiasis
  - Babesiosis
  - Chagas' disease
  - Leishmaniasis
  - Malaria
  - Strongyloidiasis
  - Toxocariasis
  - Toxoplasmosis
  - Trichinosis
- Presumed infections, agent undetermined
  - Kawasaki's disease (mucocutaneous lymph node syndrome)
  - Kikuchi's necrotizing lymphadenitis

Neoplasms

- Malignant
  - Colon cancer
  - Gall bladder carcinoma
  - Hepatoma
  - Hodgkin's lymphoma
  - Immunoblastic T-cell lymphoma
  - Leukemia
  - Lymphomatoid granulomatosis
  - Malignant histiocytosis
  - Non-Hodgkin's lymphoma
  - Pancreatic cancer
  - Renal cell carcinoma
  - Sarcoma
- Benign
  - Atrial myxoma
  - Castleman's disease
  - Renal angiomyolipoma

Habitual Hyperthermia

(Exaggerated circadian rhythm)

Collagen Vascular/Hypersensitivity Diseases

- Adult Still's disease
- Behçet's disease
- Erythema multiforme
- Erythema nodosum
- Giant-cell arteritis/polymyalgia rheumatica
- Hypersensitivity pneumonitis
- Hypersensitivity vasculitis
- Mixed connective-tissue disease
- Polyarteritis nodosa
- Relapsing polychondritis
- Rheumatic fever
- Rheumatoid arthritis
- Schnitzler's syndrome
- Systemic lupus erythematosus
- Takayasu's aortitis
- Weber-Christian disease
- Wegener's granulomatosis

Granulomatous Diseases

- Crohn's disease
- Granulomatous hepatitis
- Midline granuloma
- Sarcoidosis

Miscellaneous Conditions

- Aortic dissection
- Drug fever
- Gout
- Hematomas
- Hemoglobinopathies
- Laennec's cirrhosis
- PFPA syndrome: periodic fever, adenitis, pharyngitis, aphthae
- Postmyocardial infarction syndrome
- Recurrent pulmonary emboli
- Subacute thyroiditis (de Quervain's)
- Tissue infarction/necrosis

Inherited and Metabolic Diseases

- Adrenal insufficiency
- Cyclic neutropenia
- Deafness, urticaria, and amyloidosis
- Fabry's disease
- Familial cold urticaria
- Familial Mediterranean fever
- Hyperimmunoglobulinemia D and periodic fever
- Muckle-Wells syndrome
- Tumor necrosis factor receptor–associated periodic syndrome
- Type V hypertriglyceridemia

Thermoregulatory Disorders

- Central
  - Brain tumor
  - Cerebrovascular accident
  - Encephalitis
  - Hypothalamic dysfunction
- Peripheral
  - Hyperthyroidism
  - Pheochromocytoma

Factitious Fevers

"Afebrile" FUO (<38.3°C)

Source: Modified from RK Root, RG Petersdorf, in JD Wilson et al (eds): *Harrison's Principles of Internal Medicine*, 12th ed. New York, McGraw-Hill, 1991.

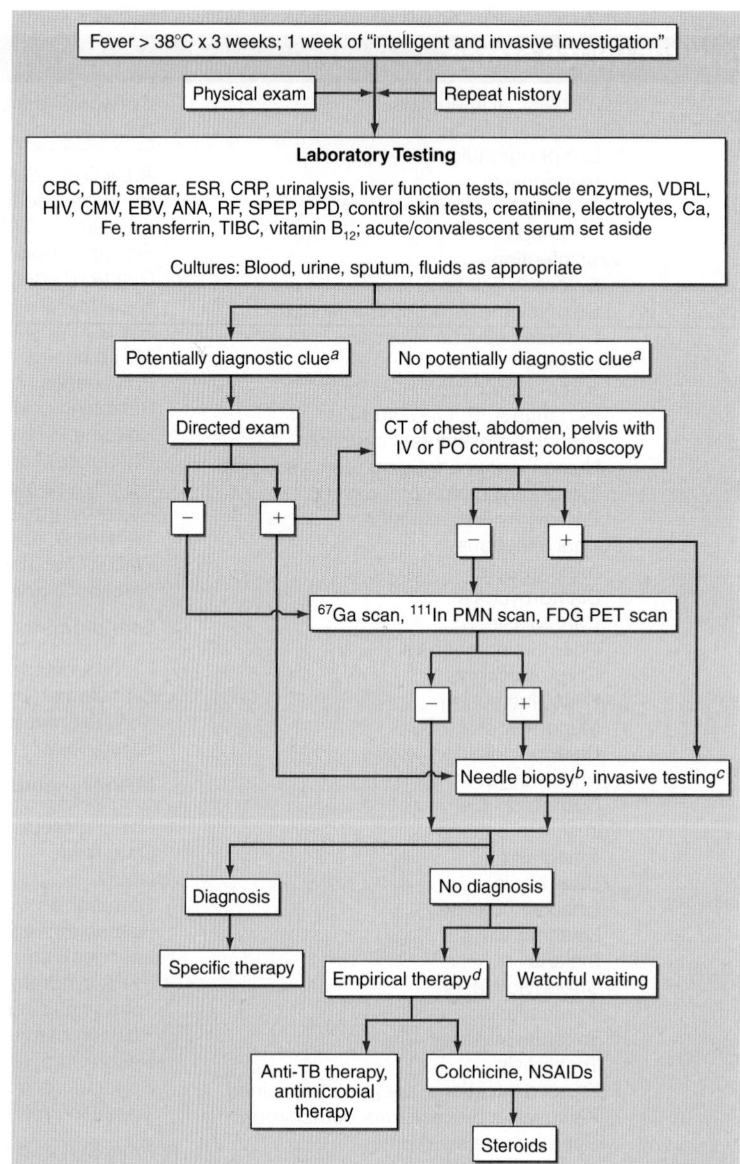

FIGURE 9-1

Approach to the patient with classic FUO. [a]"Potentially diagnostic clues," as outlined by de Kleijn and colleagues (1997, Part II), may be key findings in the history, localizing signs, or key symptoms. [b]Needle biopsy of liver as well as any other tissue indicated by "potentially diagnostic clues." [c]Invasive testing could involve laparoscopy. [d]Empirical therapy is a last resort, given the good prognosis of most patients with FUO persisting without a diagnosis. ANA, antinuclear antibody; CBC, complete blood count; CMV, cytomegalovirus; CRP, C-reactive protein; CT, computed tomography; Diff, differential; EBV, Epstein-Barr virus; ESR, erythrocyte sedimentation rate; FDG, fluorodeoxyglucose F18; NSAIDs, nonsteroidal anti-inflammatory drugs; PET, positron emission tomography; PMN, polymorphonuclear leukocyte; PPD, purified protein derivative; RF, rheumatoid factor; SPEP, serum protein electrophoresis; TB, tuberculosis; TIBC, total iron-binding capacity; VDRL, Venereal Disease Research Laboratory test.

Certain specific diagnostic maneuvers become critical in dealing with prolonged fevers. If factitious fever is suspected, electronic thermometers should be used, temperature-taking should be supervised, and simultaneous urine and body temperatures should be measured. Thick blood smears should be examined for *Plasmodium*; thin blood smears, prepared with proper technique and quality stains and subjected to expert microscopy, should be used to speciate *Plasmodium* and to identify *Babesia*, *Trypanosoma*, *Leishmania*, *Rickettsia*, and *Borrelia*. Any tissue removed during prior relevant surgery should be reexamined; slides should be requested, and, if need be, paraffin blocks of fixed pathologic material should be reexamined and additional special studies performed. Relevant x-rays should be reexamined; reviewing of prior radiologic reports may be insufficient. Serum should be set aside in the laboratory as soon as possible and retained for future examination for rising antibody titers.

Febrile agglutinins is a vague term that in most laboratories refers to serologic studies for salmonellosis, brucellosis, and rickettsial diseases. These studies are seldom useful, having low sensitivity and variable specificity. Multiple blood samples (no fewer than three and rarely more than six, including samples for anaerobic culture) should be cultured in the laboratory for at least 2 weeks to ensure that any HACEK group organisms that may be present have ample time to grow (Chap. 48). Lysis-centrifugation blood culture techniques should be employed in cases where prior antimicrobial therapy or fungal or atypical mycobacterial infection is suspected. Blood culture media should be supplemented with L-cysteine or pyridoxal to assist in the isolation of nutritionally variant streptococci. It should be noted that sequential cultures positive for multiple organisms may reflect self-injection of contaminated substances. Urine cultures, including cultures for mycobacteria, fungi, and CMV, are indicated. In the setting of recurrent fevers with lymphocytic meningitis (Mollaret's meningitis), cerebrospinal fluid can be tested for herpesvirus, with use of the polymerase chain reaction (PCR) to amplify and detect viral nucleic acid (Chap. 80). A recent report described a highly multiplexed oligonucleotide microarray using PCR amplification and containing probes for all recognized vertebrate virus species and for 135 bacterial, 73 fungal, and 63 parasitic genera and species. The eventual clinical validation of such microarrays will further diminish rates of undiagnosed FUO of infectious etiology.

In any FUO workup, the erythrocyte sedimentation rate (ESR) should be determined. Striking elevation of the ESR and anemia of chronic disease are frequently seen in association with giant-cell arteritis or polymyalgia rheumatica—common causes of FUO in patients >50 years of age. Still's disease is suggested by elevations of ESR, leukocytosis, and anemia and is often accompanied by arthralgias, polyserositis (pleuritis, pericarditis), lymphadenopathy, splenomegaly, and rash. The C-reactive protein level may be a useful cross-reference for the ESR and is a more sensitive and specific indicator of an "acute-phase" inflammatory metabolic response. Antinuclear antibody, antineutrophil cytoplasmic antibody, rheumatoid factor, and serum cryoglobulins should be measured to rule out other collagen vascular diseases and vasculitis. Elevated levels of angiotensin-converting enzyme in serum may point to sarcoidosis. With rare exceptions, the intermediate-strength purified protein derivative (PPD) skin test should be used to screen for tuberculosis in patients with classic FUO. Concurrent control tests, such as the mumps skin test antigen (Aventis-Pasteur, Swiftwater, PA), should be employed. It should be kept in mind that both the PPD skin test and control tests may yield negative results in miliary tuberculosis, sarcoidosis, Hodgkin's disease, malnutrition, or AIDS.

Noninvasive procedures should include an upper gastrointestinal contrast study with small-bowel follow-through and colonoscopy to examine the terminal ileum and cecum. Colonoscopy is especially strongly indicated in the elderly. Chest x-rays should be repeated if new symptoms arise. Sputum should be induced with an ultrasonic nebulizer for cultures and cytology. If there are pulmonary signs or symptoms, bronchoscopy with bronchoalveolar lavage for cultures and cytology should be considered. High-resolution spiral CT of the chest and abdomen should be performed with both IV and oral contrast. If a spinal or paraspinal lesion is suspected, however, MRI is preferred. MRI may be superior to CT in demonstrating intraabdominal abscesses and aortic dissection, but the relative utility of MRI and CT in the diagnosis of FUO is unknown. At present, abdominal CT with contrast should be used unless MRI is specifically indicated. Arteriography may be useful for patients in whom systemic necrotizing vasculitis is suspected. Saccular aneurysms may be seen, most commonly in renal or hepatic vessels, and may permit diagnosis of arteritis when biopsy is difficult. Ultrasonography of the abdomen is useful for investigation of the hepatobiliary tract, kidneys, spleen, and pelvis. Echocardiography may be helpful in an evaluation for bacterial endocarditis, pericarditis, nonbacterial thrombotic endocarditis, and atrial myxomas. Transesophageal echocardiography is especially sensitive for these lesions.

Radionuclide scanning procedures using technetium (Tc) 99m sulfur colloid, gallium (Ga) 67 citrate, or indium (In) 111–labeled leukocytes may be useful in identifying and/or localizing inflammatory processes. In one study, Ga scintigraphy yielded useful diagnostic information in almost one-third of cases, and it was suggested that this procedure might actually be used before other imaging techniques if no specific organ is suspected of being abnormal. It is likely that PET scanning, which provides quicker results (hours vs days), will prove even more sensitive and specific than ^{67}Ga scanning in FUO. ^{99m}Tc bone scan should be undertaken to look for osteomyelitis or bony metastases; ^{67}Ga scan may be used to identify sarcoidosis or *Pneumocystis* infection (Chap. 111) in the lungs or Crohn's disease in the abdomen. ^{111}In-labeled white blood cell (WBC) scan may be used to locate abscesses. With these scans, false-positive and false- negative findings are common. Fluorodeoxyglucose F18 (FDG) PET scanning appears to be superior to other forms of nuclear imaging. The FDG used in PET scans accumulates in tumors and at sites of inflammation and has even been shown to accumulate reliably at sites of vasculitis. Where available, FDG PET scanning should therefore be chosen over ^{67}Ga scanning in the diagnosis of FUO.

Biopsy of the liver and bone marrow should be considered in the workup of FUO if the studies mentioned above are unrevealing and if fever is prolonged. Granulomatous hepatitis has been diagnosed by liver biopsy, even when liver enzymes are normal and no other diagnostic clues point to liver disease. All biopsy specimens should be cultured for bacteria, mycobacteria, and fungi. Likewise, in the absence of clues pointing to the bone marrow, bone marrow biopsy (not simple aspiration) for histology and culture has yielded diagnoses late in the workup. When possible, a section of the tissue block should be retained for further sections or stains. PCR technology makes it possible in some cases to identify and speciate mycobacterial DNA in paraffin-embedded, fixed tissues at some research centers. Thus, in some cases, a retrospective diagnosis can be made on the basis of studies of long-fixed pathologic tissues. In a patient over age 50 (or occasionally in a younger patient) with the appropriate symptoms and laboratory findings, "blind biopsy" of one or both temporal arteries may yield a diagnosis of arteritis. Tenderness or decreased pulsation, if noted, should guide the selection of a site for biopsy. Lymph node biopsy may be helpful if nodes are enlarged, but inguinal nodes are often palpable and are seldom diagnostically useful.

Exploratory laparotomy has been performed when all other diagnostic procedures fail but has largely been replaced by imaging and guided-biopsy techniques. Laparoscopic biopsy may provide more adequate guided sampling of lymph nodes or liver, with less invasive morbidity.

Nosocomial FUO

(See also Chap. 13) The primary considerations in diagnosing nosocomial FUO are the underlying susceptibility of the patient coupled with the potential complications of hospitalization. The original surgical or procedural field is the place to begin a directed physical and laboratory examination for abscesses, hematomas, or infected foreign bodies. More than 50% of patients with nosocomial FUO are infected. Intravascular lines, septic phlebitis, and prostheses are all suspect. In this setting, the best approach is to focus on sites where occult infections may be sequestered, such as the sinuses of intubated patients or a prostatic abscess in a man with a urinary catheter. *Clostridium difficile* colitis may be associated with fever and leukocytosis before the onset of diarrhea. In ~25% of patients with nosocomial FUO, the fever has a noninfectious cause. Among these causes are acalculous cholecystitis, deep-vein thrombophlebitis, and pulmonary embolism. Drug fever, transfusion reactions, alcohol/drug withdrawal, adrenal insufficiency, thyroiditis, pancreatitis, gout, and pseudogout are among the many possible causes to consider. As in classic FUO, repeated meticulous physical examinations, coupled with focused diagnostic techniques, are imperative. Multiple blood, wound, and fluid cultures are mandatory. The pace of diagnostic tests is accelerated, and the threshold for procedures—CT scans, ultrasonography, ^{111}In WBC scans, noninvasive venous studies—is low. Even so, 20% of cases of nosocomial FUO may go undiagnosed.

Like diagnostic measures, therapeutic maneuvers must be swift and decisive, as many patients are already critically ill. IV lines must be changed (and cultured), drugs stopped for 72 h, and empirical therapy started if bacteremia is a threat. In many hospital settings, empirical antibiotic coverage for nosocomial FUO now includes vancomycin for coverage of methicillin-resistant *Staphylococcus aureus*, as well as broad-spectrum gram-negative coverage with piperacillin/tazobactam, ticarcillin/clavulanate, imipenem, or meropenem. Practice guidelines covering many of these issues have been published jointly by the Infectious Diseases Society of America (IDSA) and the Society for Critical Care Medicine and can be accessed on the IDSA website (*www.journals.uchicago. edu/IDSA/guidelines*).

Neutropenic FUO

(See also Chap. 11) Neutropenic patients are susceptible to focal bacterial and fungal infections, to bacteremic infections, to infections involving catheters (including septic thrombophlebitis), and to perianal infections. *Candida* and *Aspergillus* infections are common. Infections due to herpes simplex virus or CMV are sometimes causes of FUO in this group. Although the duration of illness may be short in these patients, the consequences of untreated infection may be catastrophic; 50–60% of febrile neutropenic patients are infected, and 20% are bacteremic. The IDSA has published extensive practice guidelines covering these critically ill neutropenic patients; these guidelines appear on the website cited in the previous section. In these patients, severe mucositis, quinolone prophylaxis, colonization with methicillin-resistant *S. aureus*, obvious catheter-related infection, or hypotension dictates the use of vancomycin plus ceftazidime, cefepime, or a carbapenem with or without an aminoglycoside to provide empirical coverage for bacterial sepsis.

HIV-Associated FUO

HIV infection alone may be a cause of fever. Infection due to *Mycobacterium avium* or *Mycobacterium intracellulare*, tuberculosis, toxoplasmosis, CMV infection, *Pneumocystis* infection, salmonellosis, cryptococcosis, histoplasmosis, non-Hodgkin's lymphoma, and (of particular importance) drug fever are all possible causes of FUO. Mycobacterial infection can be diagnosed by blood cultures and by liver, bone marrow, and lymph node biopsies. Chest CT should be performed to identify enlarged mediastinal nodes. Serologic studies may reveal cryptococcal antigen, and ^{67}Ga scan may help identify *Pneumocystis* pulmonary infection. FUO has an infectious etiology in >80% of HIV-infected patients, but drug fever and lymphoma remain important considerations. Treatment of HIV-associated FUO depends on many factors and is discussed in Chap. 90.

℞ Treatment: FEVER OF UNKNOWN ORIGIN

The focus here is on classic FUO. Other modifiers of FUO—neutropenia, HIV infection, a nosocomial setting—all vastly affect the risk equation and dictate therapy based on the probability of various causes of fever and on the calculated risks and benefits of a guided empirical approach. The age and physical state of the patient are factors as well: the frail elderly patient may merit a trial of empirical therapy earlier than the robust young adult.

The emphasis in patients with classic FUO is on continued observation and examination, with the avoidance of "shotgun" empirical therapy. Antibiotic therapy (even that for tuberculosis) may irrevocably alter the ability to culture fastidious bacteria or mycobacteria and delineate ultimate cause. However, vital-sign instability or neutropenia is an indication for empirical therapy with a fluoroquinolone plus piperacillin or the regimen mentioned above (see "Nosocomial FUO"), for example. Cirrhosis, asplenia, intercurrent immunosuppressive drug use, or recent exotic travel may all tip the balance toward earlier empirical anti-infective therapy. If the PPD skin test is positive or if granulomatous hepatitis or other granulomatous disease is present with anergy (and sarcoid seems unlikely), then a therapeutic trial with isoniazid and rifampin (and possibly a third drug) should be undertaken, with treatment usually continued for up to 6 weeks. A failure of the fever to respond over this period suggests an alternative diagnosis.

The response of rheumatic fever and Still's disease to aspirin and nonsteroidal anti-inflammatory drugs (NSAIDs) may be dramatic. The effects of glucocorticoids on temporal arteritis, polymyalgia rheumatica, and granulomatous hepatitis are equally dramatic. Colchicine is highly effective in preventing attacks of familial Mediterranean fever but is of little use once an attack is well underway. The ability of glucocorticoids and NSAIDs to mask fever while permitting the spread of infection dictates that their use be avoided unless infection has been largely ruled out and unless inflammatory disease is both probable and debilitating or threatening.

When no underlying source of FUO is identified after prolonged observation (>6 months), the prognosis is generally good, however vexing the fever may be to the patient. Under such circumstances, debilitating symptoms are treated with NSAIDs, and glucocorticoids are the last resort. The initiation of empirical therapy does not mark the end of the diagnostic workup; rather, it commits the physician to continued thoughtful reexamination and evaluation. Patience, compassion, equanimity, and intellectual flexibility are indispensable attributes for the clinician in dealing successfully with FUO.

ACKNOWLEDGMENT

Sheldon M. Wolff, MD, now deceased, was an author of a previous version of this chapter in Harrison's Principles of Internal Medicine. It is to his memory that the chapter is dedicated. The substantial contributions of Charles A. Dinarello, MD, to this chapter in previous editions are gratefully acknowledged.

FURTHER READINGS

BLEEKER-ROVERS CP et al: A prospective multicenter study on fever of unknown origin: The yield of a structured diagnostic protocol. Medicine 86:26, 2007

CUNHA BA: Fever of unknown origin: Clinical overview of classic and current concepts. Infect Dis Clin North Am 21:867, 2007

CUNHA BA: Fever of unknown origin: Focused diagnostic approach based on clinical clues from the history, physical examination, and laboratory tests. Infect Dis Clin North Am 21:1137, 2007

DE KLEIJN EM et al: Fever of unknown origin (FUO): I. A prospective multicenter study of 167 patients with FUO, using fixed epidemiologic entry criteria. Medicine 76:392, 1997

——— et al: Fever of unknown origin (FUO): II. Diagnostic procedures in a prospective multicenter study of 167 patients. Medicine 76:401, 1997

GOTO M et al: A retrospective review of 226 hospitalized patients with fever. Intern Med 46:17, 2007

HIRSCHMANN JV: Fever of unknown origin in adults. Clin Infect Dis 24:291, 1997

HOT A et al: Fever of unknown origin in HIV/AIDS patients. Infect Dis Clin North Am 21:1013, 2007

HUGHES WT et al: 2002 guidelines for the use of antimicrobial agents in neutropenic patients with cancer. Clin Infect Dis 34:730, 2002

KNOCKAERT DC et al: Fever of unknown origin in adults: 40 years on. J Intern Med 253:263, 2003

MOURAD O et al: A comprehensive evidence-based approach to fever of unknown origin. Arch Intern Med 163:545, 2003

O'GRADY NP et al: Practice guidelines for evaluating new fever in critically ill adult patients. Clin Infect Dis 26:1042, 1998

TOLIA J, SMITH LG: Fever of unknown origin: Historical and physical clues to making the diagnosis. Infect Dis Clin North Am 21:917, 2007

ZENONE T: Fever of unknown origin in adults: Evaluation of 144 cases in a non-university hospital. Scand J Infect Dis 38:632, 2006

CHAPTER 10

ATLAS OF RASHES ASSOCIATED WITH FEVER

Kenneth M. Kaye ■ Elaine T. Kaye

Given the extremely broad differential diagnosis, the presentation of a patient with fever and rash often poses a thorny diagnostic challenge for even the most astute and experienced clinician. Rapid narrowing of the differential by prompt recognition of a rash's key features can result in appropriate and sometimes life-saving therapy. This atlas presents high-quality images of a variety of rashes that have an infectious etiology and are commonly associated with fever.

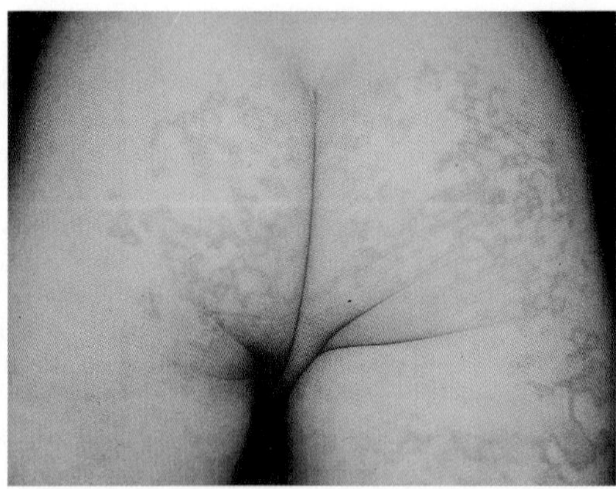

FIGURE 10-1
Lacy reticular rash of **erythema infectiosum** (fifth disease).

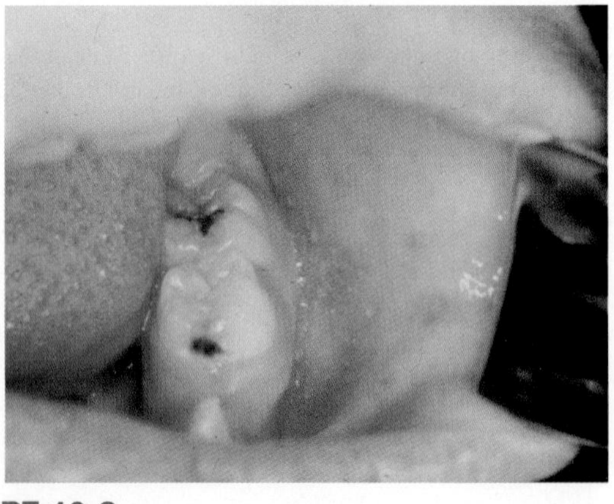

FIGURE 10-2
Koplik's spots, which manifest as white or bluish lesions with an erythematous halo on the buccal mucosa, usually occur in the first 2 days of measles symptoms and may briefly overlap the measles exanthem. The presence of the erythematous halo differentiates Koplik's spots from Fordyce's spots (ectopic sebaceous glands), which occur in the mouths of healthy individuals. (*Source: CDC. Photo selected by Kenneth M. Kaye, MD.*)

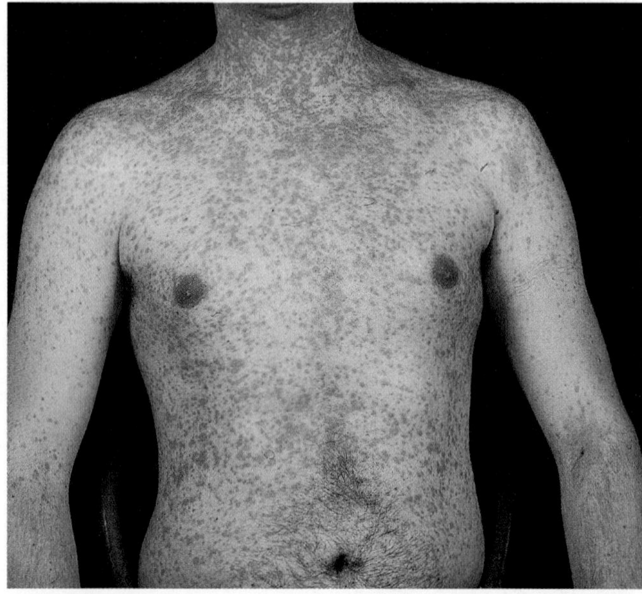

FIGURE 10-3
In **measles,** discrete erythematous lesions become confluent on the face and neck over 2–3 days as the rash spreads downward to the trunk and arms, where lesions remain discrete. (*Reprinted from K Wolff, RA Johnson: Color Atlas & Synopsis of Clinical Dermatology, 5th ed. New York, McGraw-Hill, 2005, p 788.*)

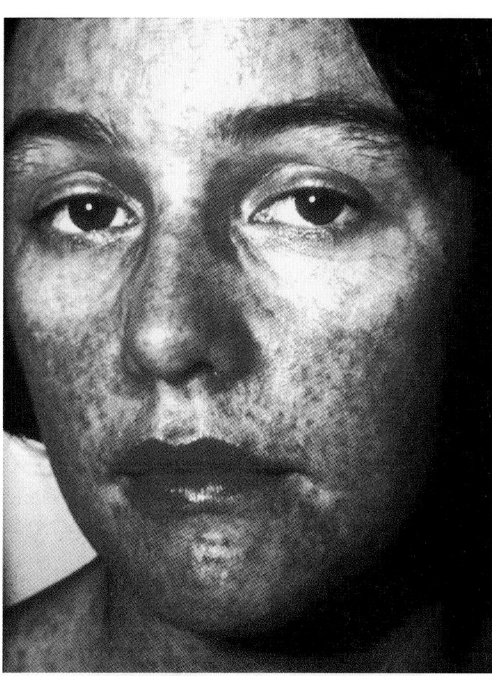

FIGURE 10-4
In **rubella,** an erythematous exanthem spreads from the hairline downward and clears as it spreads. (*Photo courtesy of Stephen E. Gellis, MD; with permission.*)

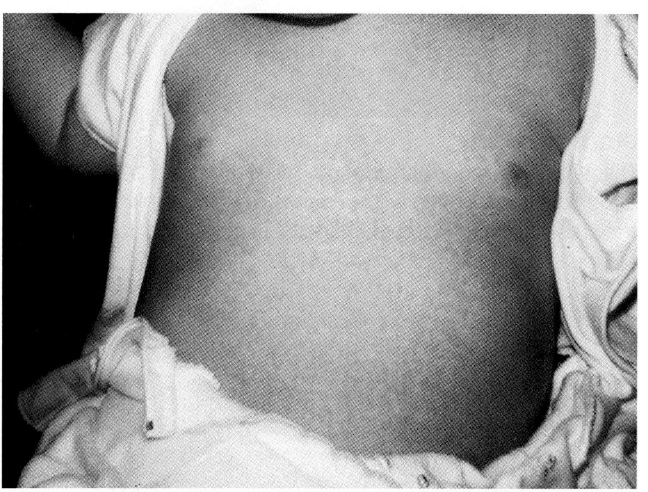

FIGURE 10-5
Exanthem subitum occurs most commonly in young children. A diffuse maculopapular exanthem follows resolution of fever. (*Photo courtesy of Stephen E. Gellis, MD; with permission.*)

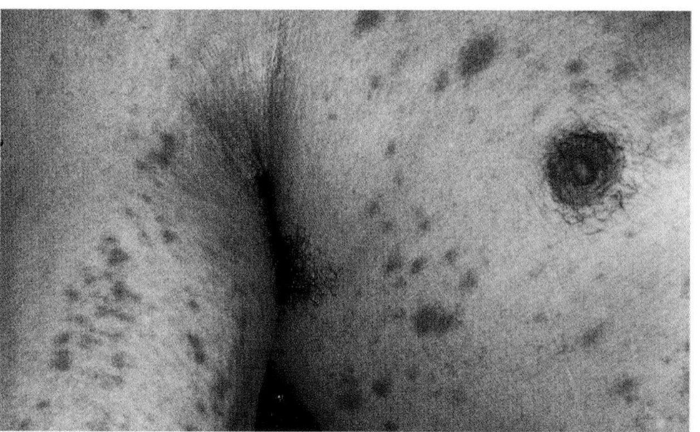

FIGURE 10-6
Erythematous macules and papules are apparent on the trunk and arm of this patient with **primary HIV infection.** (*Reprinted from K Wolff, RA Johnson: Color Atlas & Synopsis of Clinical Dermatology, 5th ed. New York, McGraw-Hill, 2005.*)

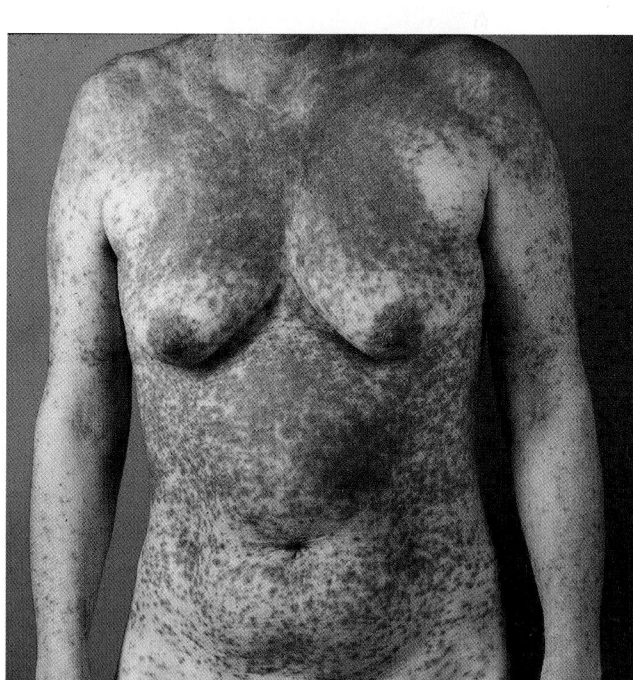

FIGURE 10-7
This **exanthematous drug-induced eruption** consists of brightly erythematous macules and papules, some which are confluent, distributed symmetrically on the trunk and extremities. Ampicillin caused this rash. (*Reprinted from K Wolff, RA Johnson: Color Atlas & Synopsis of Clinical Dermatology, 5th ed. New York, McGraw-Hill, 2005.*)

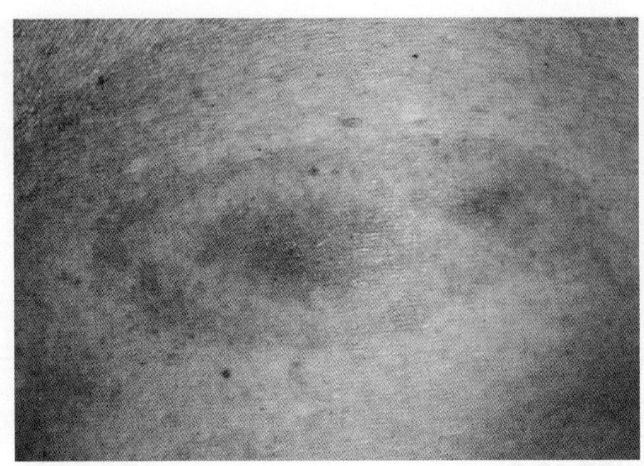

FIGURE 10-8
Erythema chronicum migrans is the early cutaneous manifestation of Lyme disease and is characterized by erythematous annular patches, often with a central erythematous papule at the tick bite site. (*Courtesy of Yale Resident's Slide Collection; with permission.*)

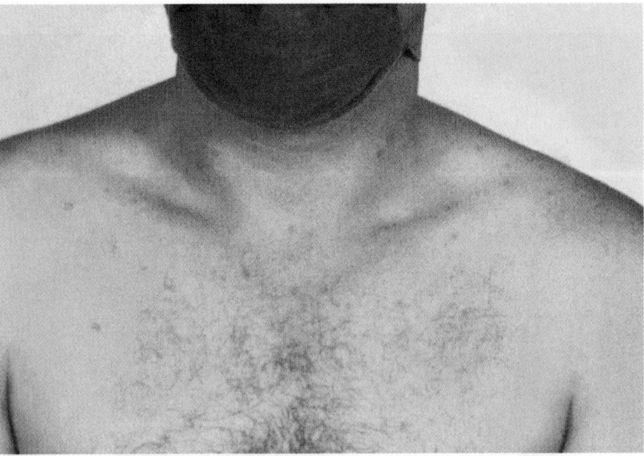

FIGURE 10-9
Rose spots are evident as erythematous macules on the trunk of this patient with **typhoid fever.**

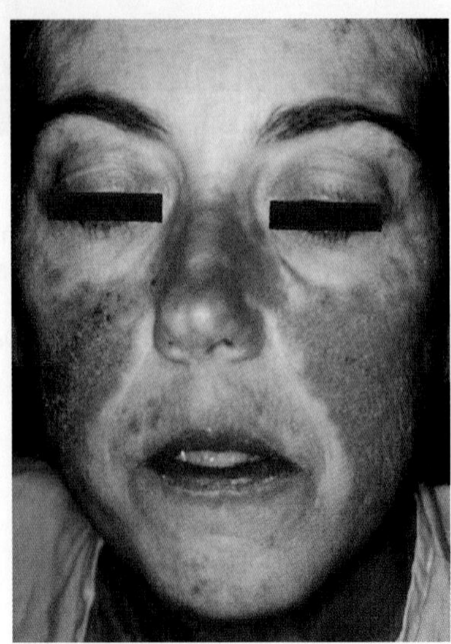

FIGURE 10-10
Systemic lupus erythematosus showing prominent, scaly, malar erythema. Involvement of other sun-exposed sites is also common.

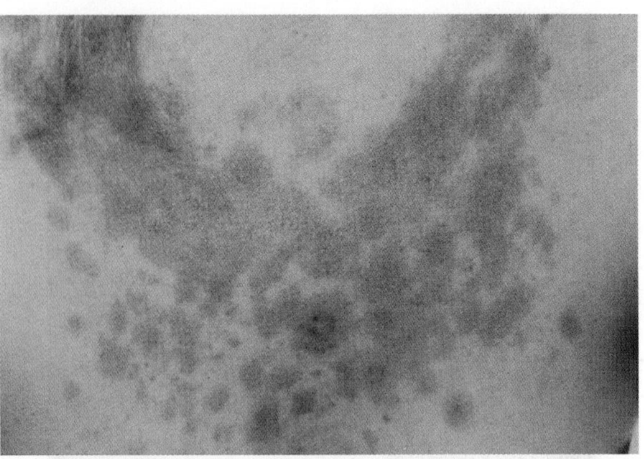

FIGURE 10-11
Acute lupus erythematosus on the upper chest, with brightly erythematous and slightly edematous coalescence papules and plaques. (*Courtesy of Robert Swerlick, MD; with permission.*)

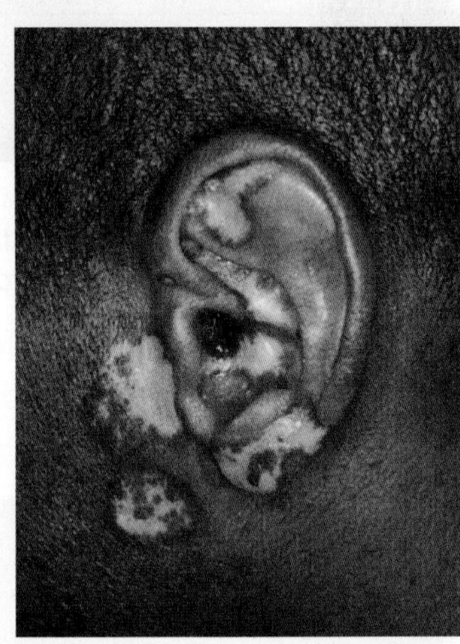

FIGURE 10-12
Discoid lupus erythematosus. Violaceous, hyperpigmented, atrophic plaques, often with evidence of follicular plugging (which may result in scarring), are characteristic of this cutaneous form of lupus. (*Courtesy of Marilynne McKay, MD; with permission.*)

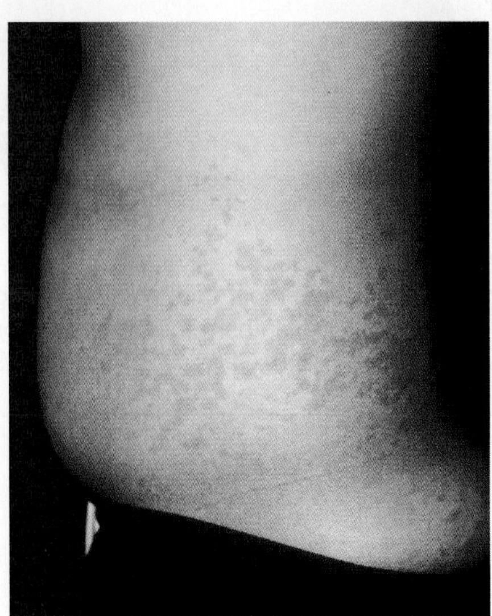

FIGURE 10-13
The rash of **Still's disease** typically exhibits evanescent, erythematous papules that appear at the height of fever on the trunk and proximal extremities. (*Courtesy of Stephen E. Gellis, MD; with permission.*)

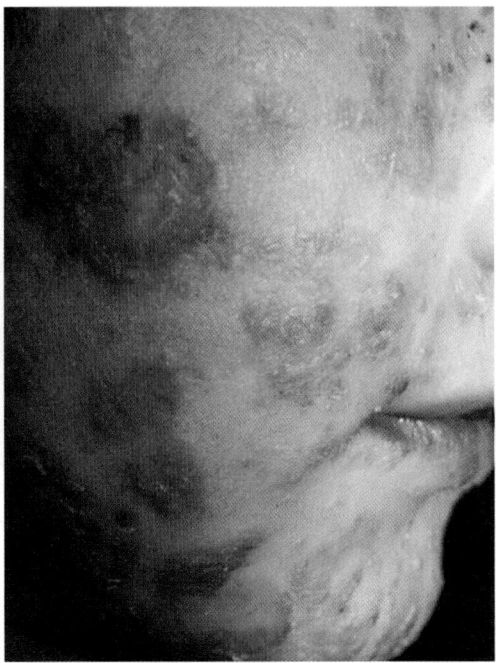

FIGURE 10-14
Impetigo contagiosa is a superficial streptococcal or *Staphylococcus aureus* infection consisting of honey-colored crusts and erythematous weeping erosions. Occasionally, bullous lesions may be seen. (*Courtesy of Mary Spraker, MD; with permission.*)

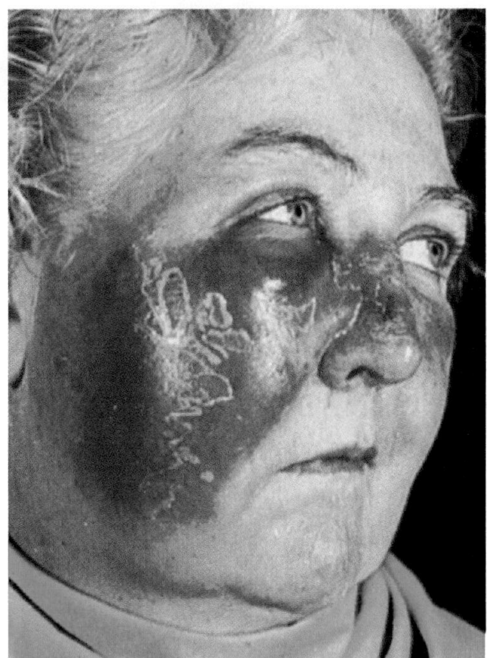

FIGURE 10-15
Erysipelas is a streptococcal infection of the superficial dermis and consists of well-demarcated, erythematous, edematous, warm plaques.

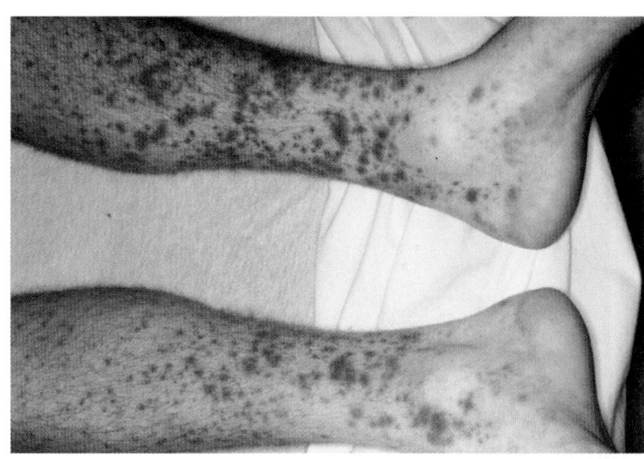

A

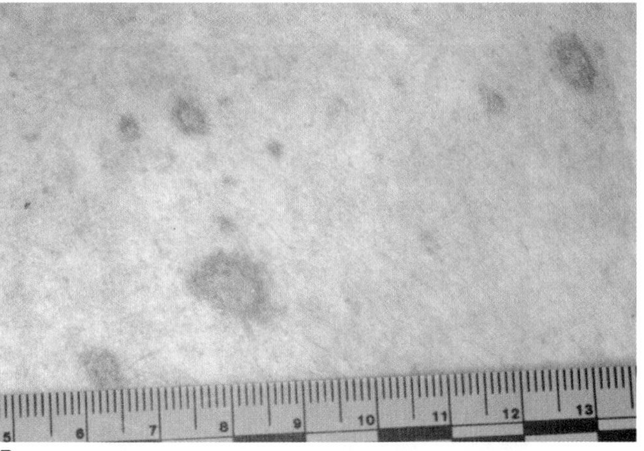

B

FIGURE 10-16
A. Petechial lesions of **Rocky Mountain spotted fever** on the lower legs and soles of a young, otherwise-healthy patient. ***B.*** Close-up of lesions from the same patient. (*Photos courtesy of Lindsey Baden, MD; with permission.*)

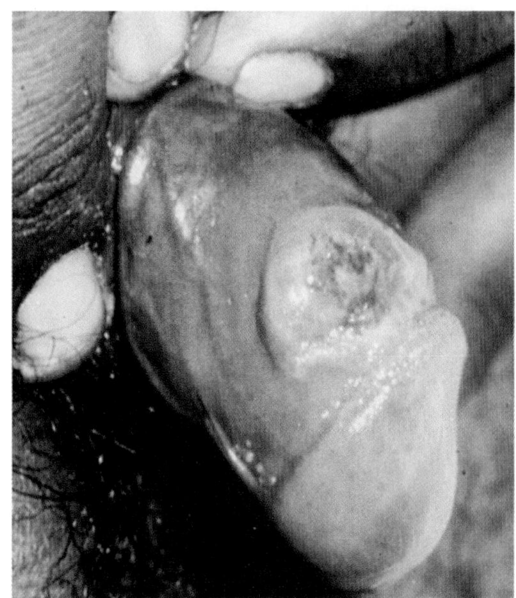

FIGURE 10-17
Primary syphilis with a firm, nontender chancre.

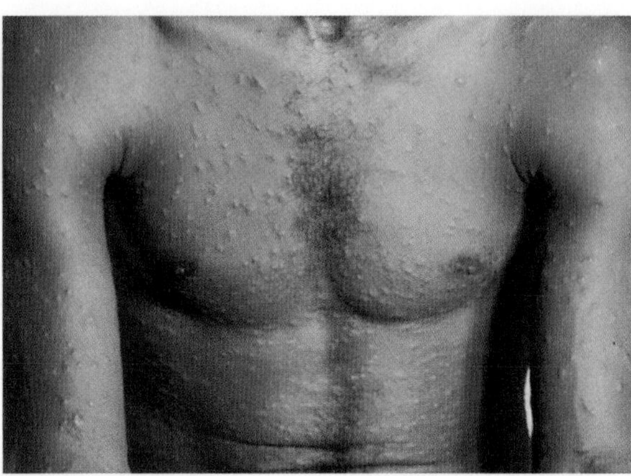

FIGURE 10-18
Secondary syphilis demonstrating the papulosquamous truncal eruption.

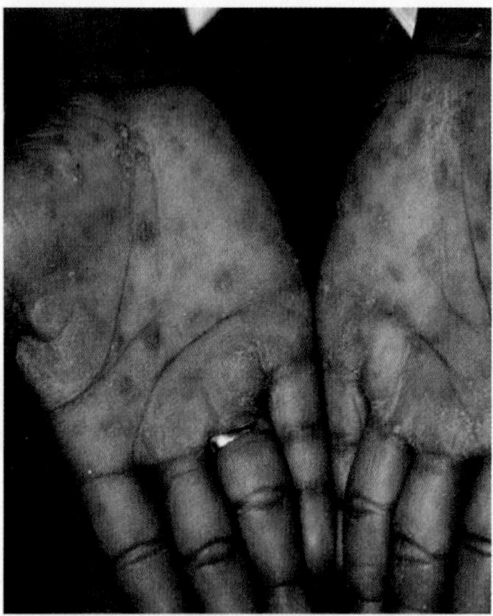

FIGURE 10-19
Secondary syphilis commonly affects the palms and soles with scaling, firm, red-brown papules.

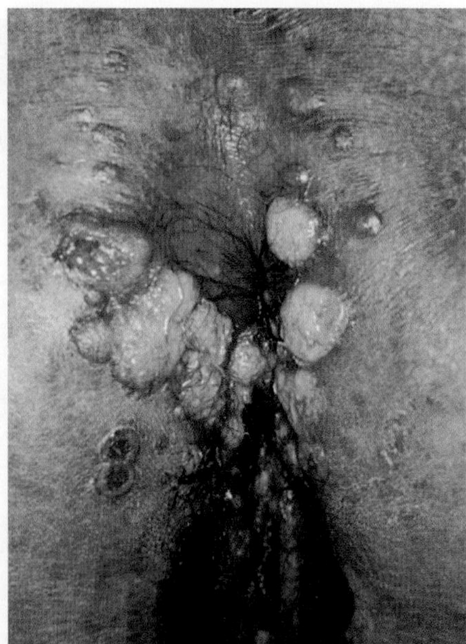

FIGURE 10-20
Condylomata lata are moist, somewhat verrucous intertriginous plaques seen in secondary syphilis.

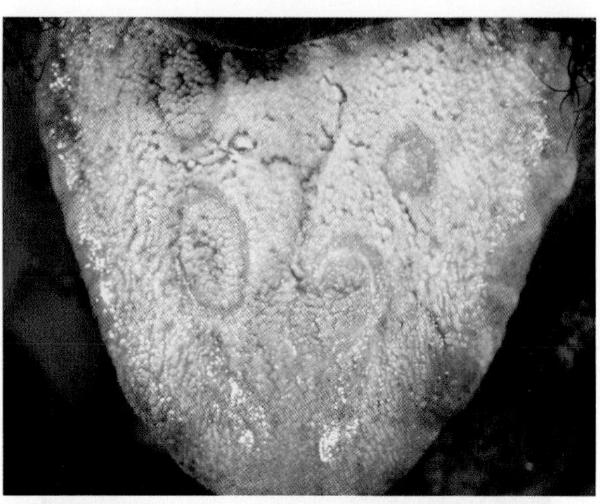

FIGURE 10-21
Mucous patches on the tongue of a patient with **secondary syphilis.** *(Courtesy of Ron Roddy; with permission.)*

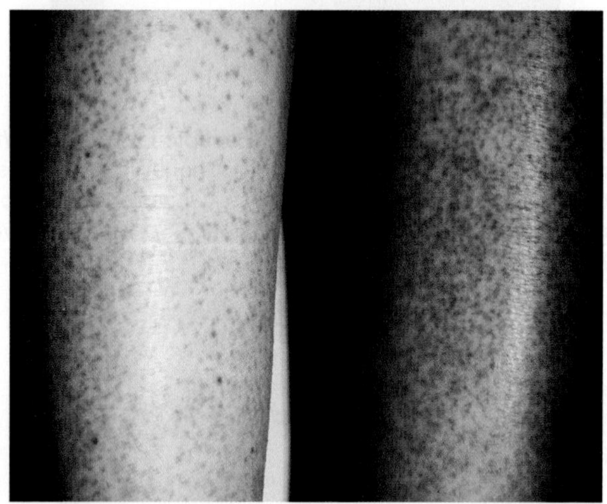

FIGURE 10-22
Petechial lesions in a patient with **atypical measles.** *(Photo courtesy of Stephen E. Gellis, MD; with permission.)*

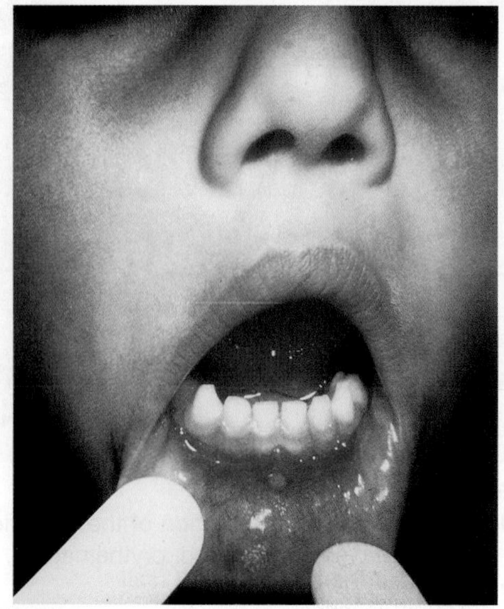

FIGURE 10-23
Tender vesicles and erosions in the mouth of a patient with **hand-foot-and-mouth disease.** *(Courtesy of Stephen E. Gellis, MD; with permission.)*

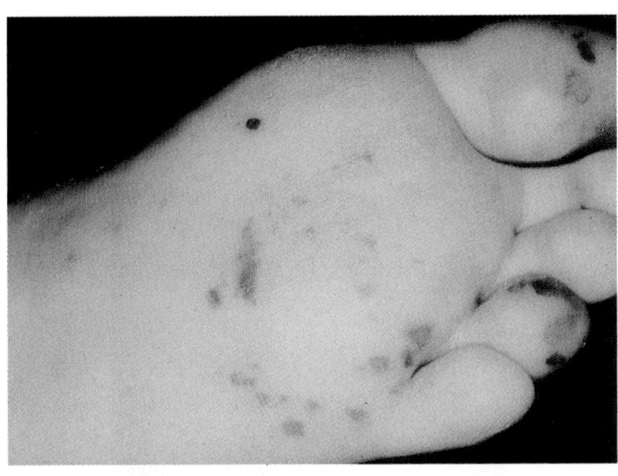

FIGURE 10-24
Septic emboli with hemorrhage and infarction due to acute *Staphylococcus aureus* **endocarditis.** (*Courtesy of Lindsey Baden, MD; with permission.*)

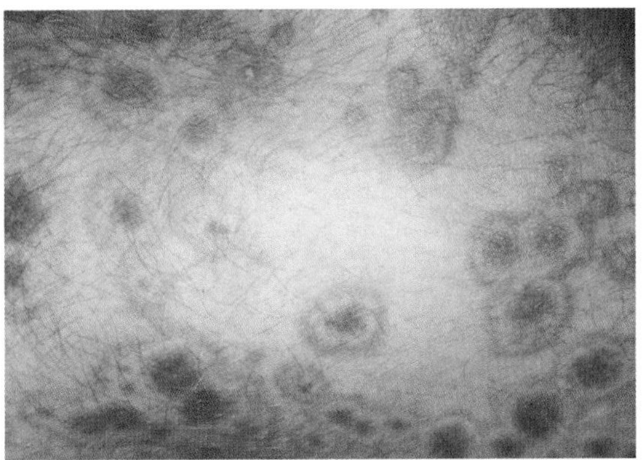

FIGURE 10-25
Erythema multiforme is characterized by multiple erythematous plaques with a target or iris morphology and usually represents a hypersensitivity reaction to drugs or infections (especially herpes simplex virus). (*Courtesy of the Yale Resident's Slide Collection; with permission.*)

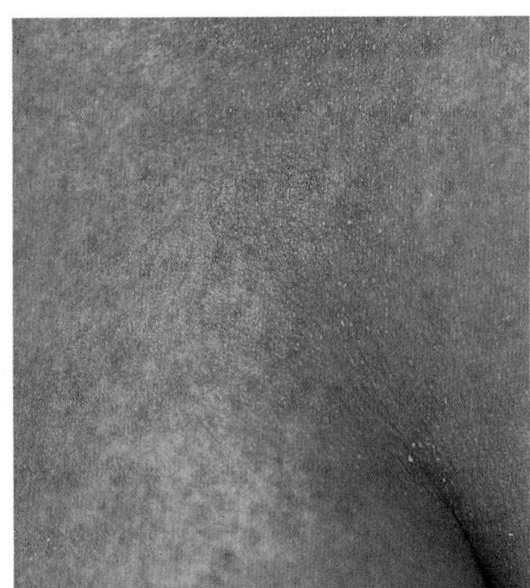

FIGURE 10-26
Scarlet fever exanthem. Finely punctuated erythema has become confluent (scarlatiniform); accentuation of linear erythema in body folds (Pastia's lines) is seen here. (*Reprinted from K Wolff, RA Johnson: Color Atlas & Synopsis of Clinical Dermatology, 5th ed. New York, McGraw-Hill, 2005.*)

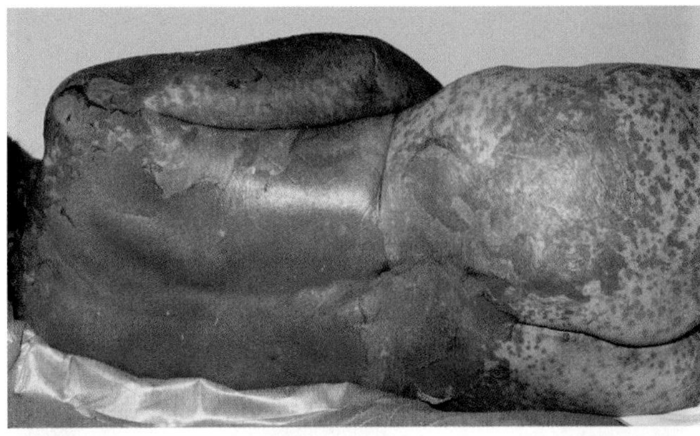

FIGURE 10-27
Erythema progressing to bullae with resulting sloughing of the entire thickness of the epidermis occurs in **toxic epidermal necrolysis.** This reaction was due to a sulfonamide. (*Reprinted from K Wolff, RA Johnson: Color Atlas & Synopsis of Clinical Dermatology, 5th ed. New York, McGraw-Hill, 2005.*)

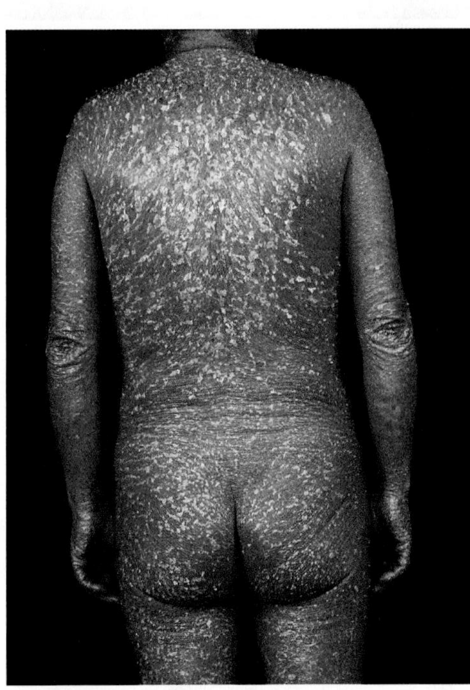

FIGURE 10-28
Diffuse erythema and scaling are present in this patient with psoriasis and the **exfoliative erythroderma syndrome.** (*Reprinted from K Wolff, RA Johnson: Color Atlas & Synopsis of Clinical Dermatology, 5th ed. New York, McGraw-Hill, 2005.*)

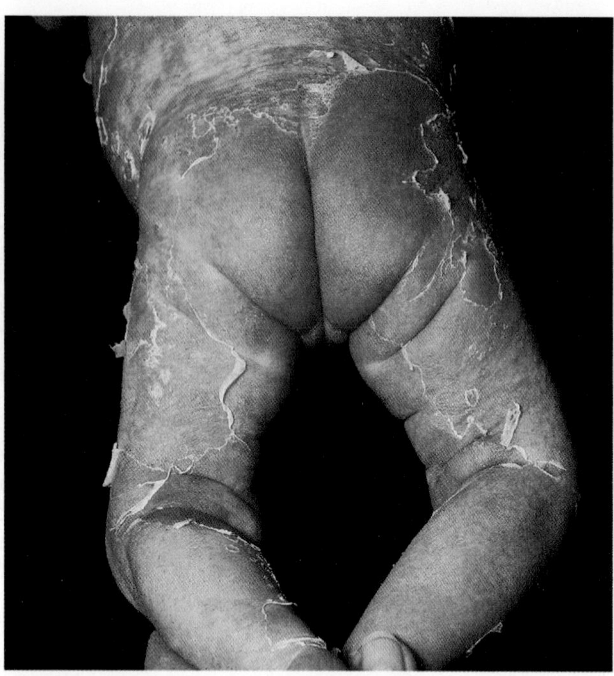

FIGURE 10-29
This infant with **staphylococcal scalded skin syndrome** demonstrates generalized desquamation. (*Reprinted from K Wolff, RA Johnson: Color Atlas & Synopsis of Clinical Dermatology, 5th ed. New York, McGraw-Hill, 2005.*)

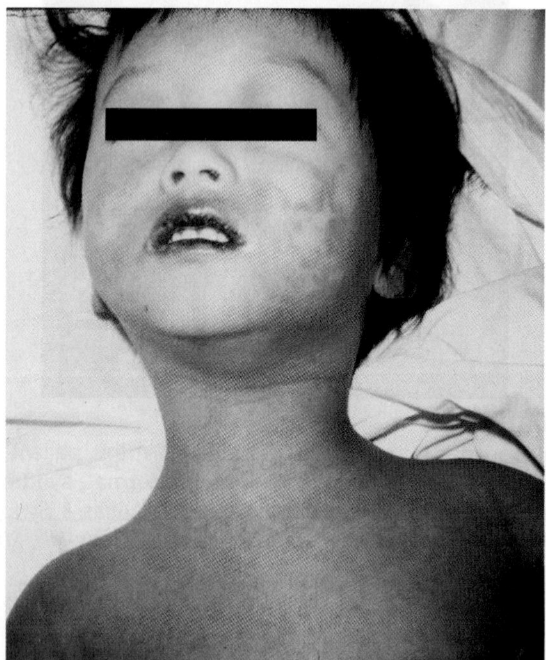

FIGURE 10-30
Fissuring of the lips and an erythematous exanthem are evident in this patient with **Kawasaki's disease.** (*Courtesy of Stephen E. Gellis, MD; with permission.*)

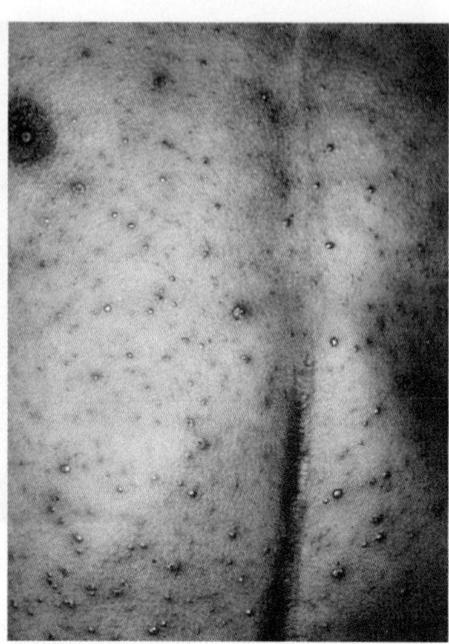

FIGURE 10-31
Numerous **varicella** lesions at various stages of evolution: vesicles on an erythematous base, umbilical vesicles, and crusts. (*Courtesy of R. Hartman; with permission.*)

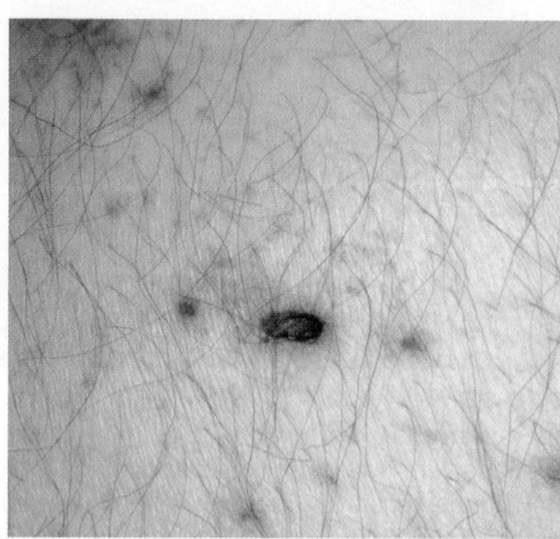

FIGURE 10-32
Close-up of lesions of **disseminated zoster.** Note lesions at different stages of evolution, including pustules and crusting. (*Photo courtesy of Lindsey Baden, MD; with permission.*)

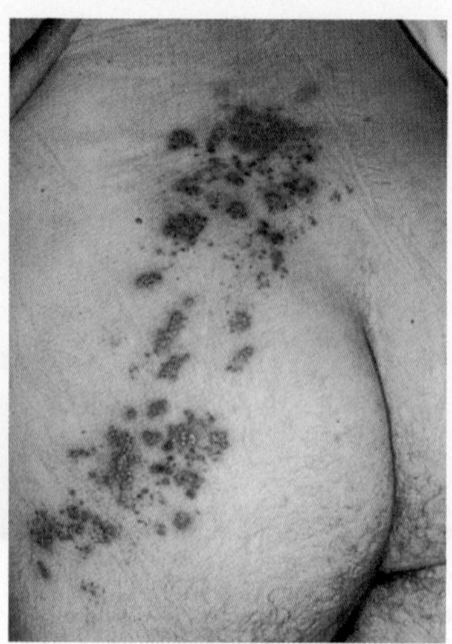

FIGURE 10-33
Herpes zoster is seen in this HIV-infected patient as hemorrhagic vesicles and pustules on an erythematous base grouped in a dermatomal distribution.

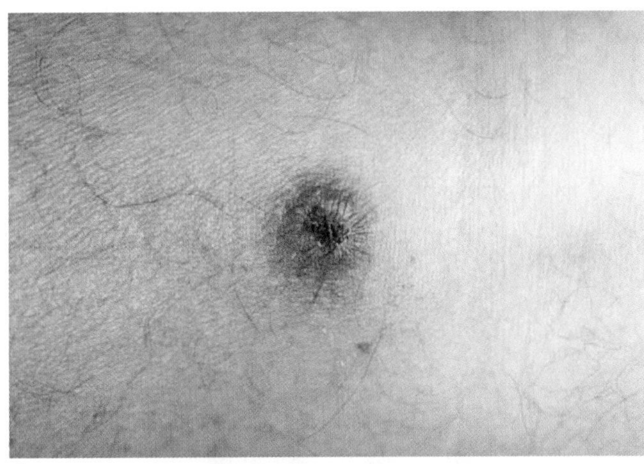

A

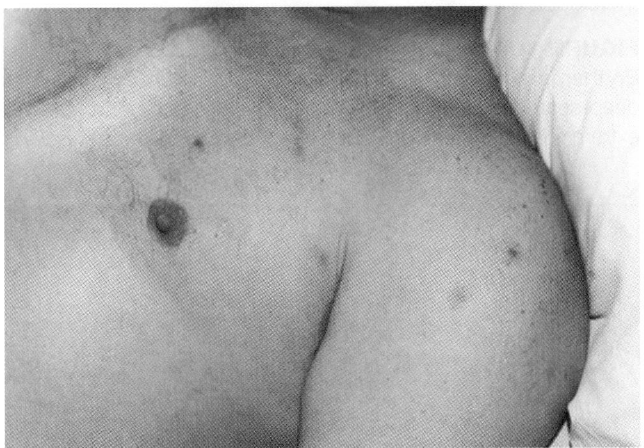

B

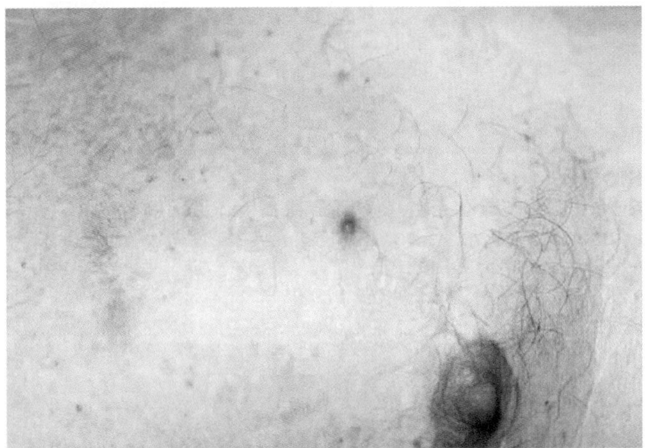

C

FIGURE 10-34
A. Eschar at the site of the mite bite in a patient with **rickettsialpox. *B.*** Papulovesicular lesions on the trunk of the same patient. ***C.*** Close-up of lesions from the same patient. (*Reprinted from A Krusell et al: Emerg Infect Dis 8:727, 2002. Photos obtained by Kenneth M. Kaye, MD.*)

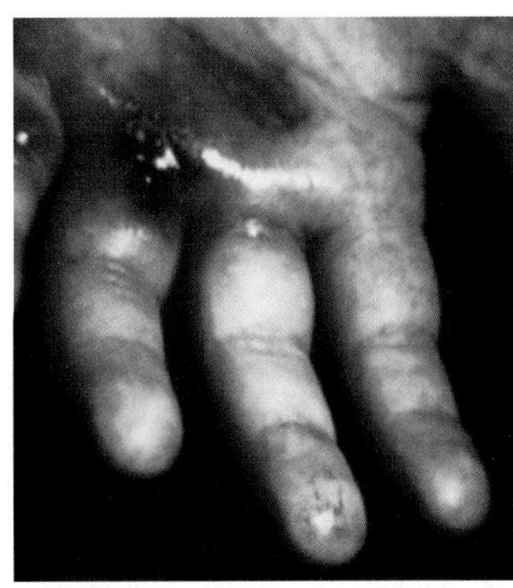

FIGURE 10-35
Ecthyma gangrenosum in a neutropenic patient with *Pseudomonas aeruginosa* bacteremia.

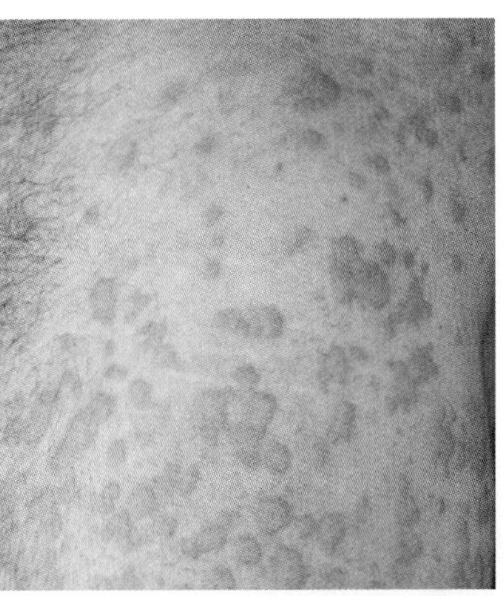

FIGURE 10-36
Urticaria showing characteristic discrete and confluent, edematous, erythematous papules and plaques.

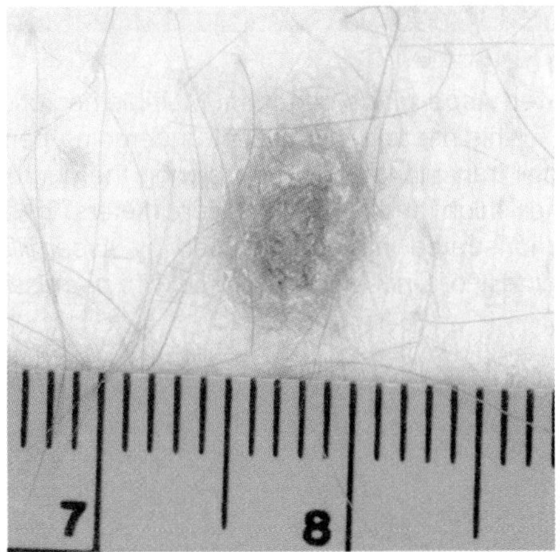

FIGURE 10-37
Disseminated cryptococcal infection. A liver transplant recipient developed six cutaneous lesions similar to the one shown. Biopsy and serum antigen testing demonstrated *Cryptococcus.* Important features of the lesion include a benign-appearing fleshy papule with central umbilication resembling molluscum contagiosum. (*Photo courtesy of Lindsey Baden, MD; with permission.*)

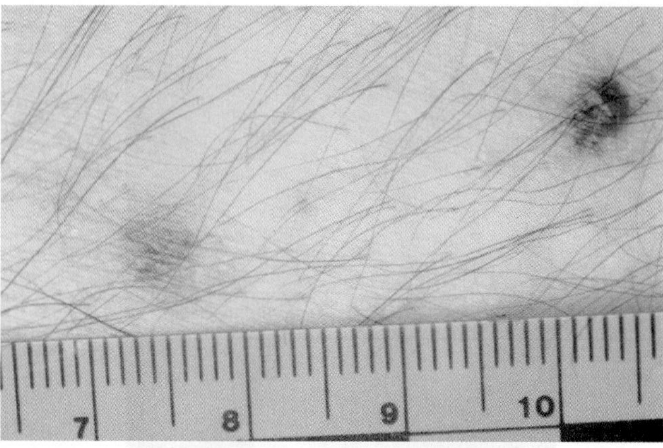

FIGURE 10-38
Disseminated candidiasis. Tender, erythematous, nodular lesions developed in a neutropenic patient with leukemia who was undergoing induction chemotherapy. (*Photo courtesy of Lindsey Baden, MD; with permission.*)

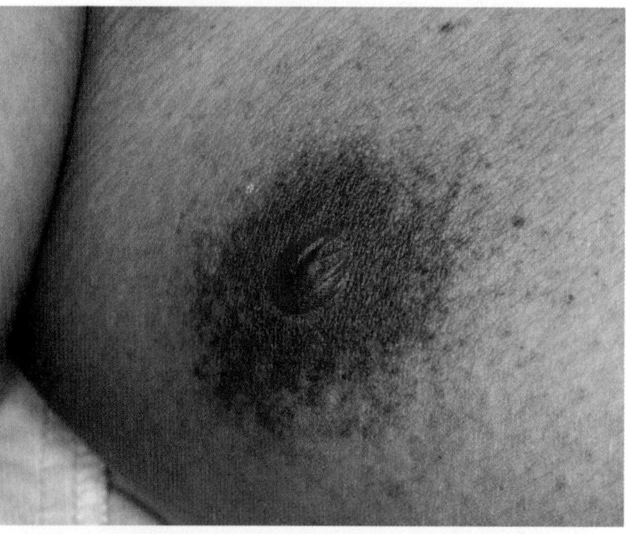

FIGURE 10-39
Disseminated *Aspergillus* infection. Multiple necrotic lesions developed in this neutropenic patient undergoing hematopoietic stem-cell transplantation. The lesion in the photograph is on the inner thigh and is several centimeters in diameter. Biopsy demonstrated infarction caused by *Aspergillus fumigatus*. (*Courtesy of Lindsey Baden, MD; with permission.*)

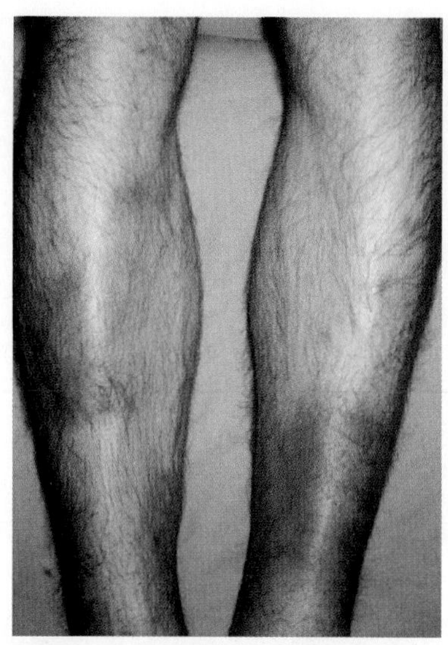

FIGURE 10-40
Erythema nodosum is a panniculitis characterized by tender deep-seated nodules and plaques usually located on the lower extremities. (*Courtesy of Robert Swerlick, MD; with permission.*)

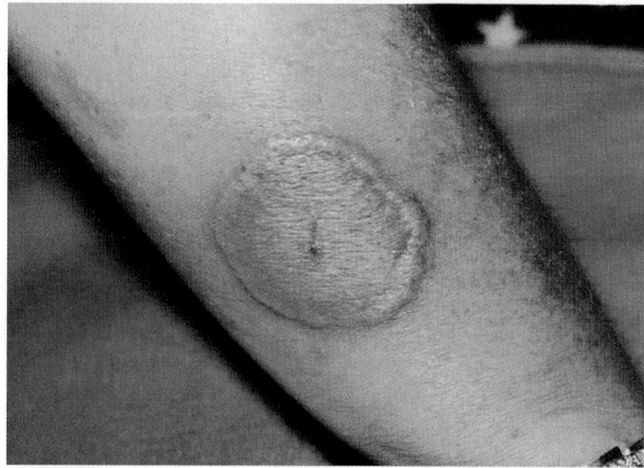

FIGURE 10-41
Sweet's syndrome: an erythematous indurated plaque with a pseudo-vesicular border. (*Courtesy of Robert Swerlick, MD; with permission.*)

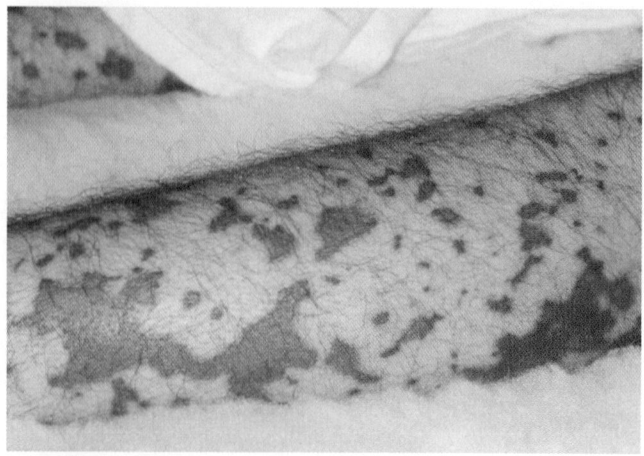

FIGURE 10-42
Fulminant meningococcemia with extensive angular purpuric patches. (*Courtesy of Stephen E. Gellis, MD; with permission.*)

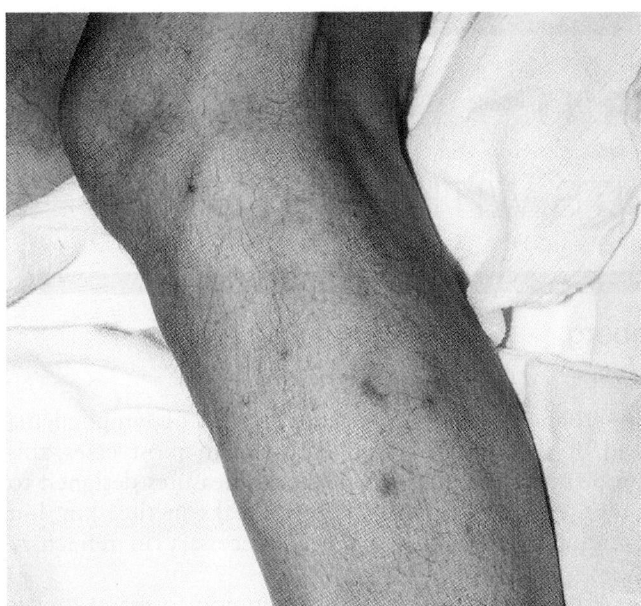

FIGURE 10-43
Erythematous papular lesions are seen on the leg of this patient with **chronic meningococcemia.** (*Courtesy of Kenneth M. Kaye, MD, and Elaine T. Kaye, MD; with permission.*)

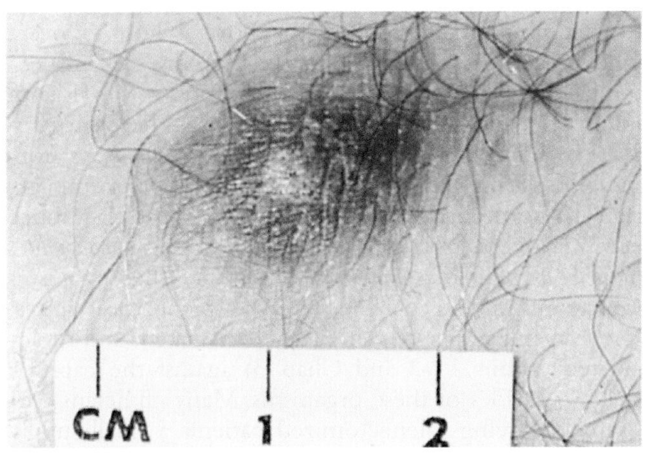

FIGURE 10-44
Disseminated gonococcemia in the skin is seen as hemorrhagic papules and pustules with purpuric centers in a centrifugal distribution. (*Courtesy of Daniel M. Musher, MD; with permission.*)

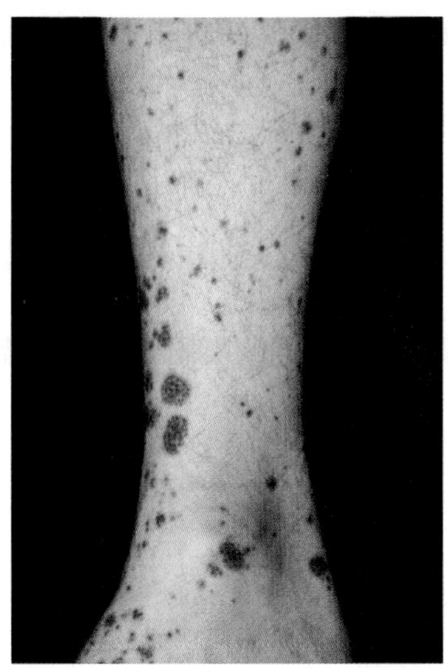

FIGURE 10-45
Palpable purpuric papules on the lower legs are seen in this patient with **cutaneous small-vessel vasculitis.** (*Courtesy of Robert Swerlick, MD; with permission.*)

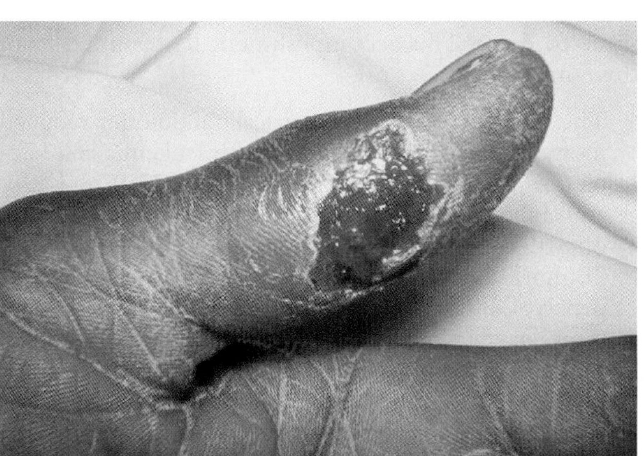

FIGURE 10-46
The thumb of a patient with a necrotic ulcer of **tularemia.** (*From the Centers for Disease Control and Prevention.*)

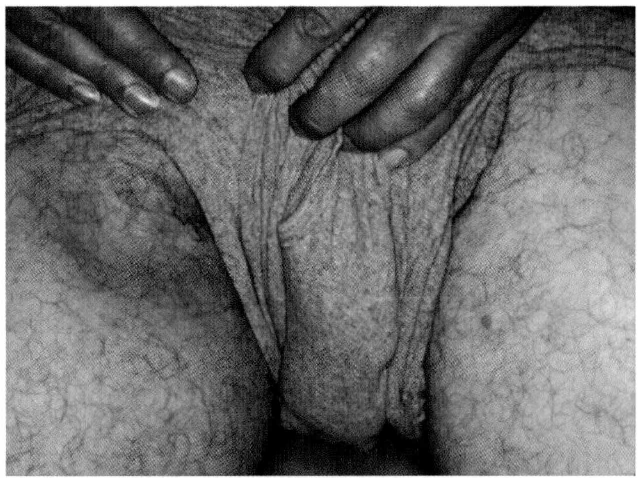

FIGURE 10-47
This 50-year-old man developed high fever and massive inguinal lymphadenopathy after a small ulcer healed on his foot. **Tularemia** was diagnosed. (*Courtesy of Lindsey Baden, MD; with permission.*)

CHAPTER 11

INFECTIONS IN PATIENTS WITH CANCER

Robert Finberg

Infections are a common cause of death and an even more common cause of morbidity in patients with a wide variety of neoplasms. Autopsy studies show that most deaths from acute leukemia and half of deaths from lymphoma are caused directly by infection. With more intensive chemotherapy, patients with solid tumors have also become more likely to die of infection. Fortunately, an evolving approach to prevention and treatment of infectious complications of cancer has decreased rates of infection-associated mortality and will probably continue to do so. This accomplishment has resulted from three major steps:

1. The concept of "early empirical" antibiotics reduced mortality rates among patients with leukemia and bacteremia from 84% in 1965 to 44% in 1972. With better availability (and early use) of broad-spectrum antibiotics, this figure has recently dropped to 20–36%.
2. "Empirical" antifungal therapy has lowered the incidence of disseminated fungal infection; in trial settings, mortality rates now range from 7–21%. An antifungal agent is administered—on the basis of likely fungal infection—to neutropenic patients who, after 4–7 days of antibiotic therapy, remain febrile but have no positive cultures.
3. Use of antibiotics for afebrile neutropenic patients as broad-spectrum prophylaxis against infections promises to decrease both mortality and morbidity even further.

A physical predisposition to infection in patients with cancer (Table 11-1) can be a result of the neoplasm's production of a break in the skin. For example, a squamous cell carcinoma may cause local invasion of the epidermis, which allows bacteria to gain access to the subcutaneous tissue and permits the development of cellulitis. The artificial closing of a normally patent orifice can also predispose to infection: Obstruction of a ureter by a tumor can cause urinary tract infection, and obstruction of the bile duct can cause cholangitis. Part of the host's normal defense against infection depends on the continuous emptying of a viscus; without emptying, a few bacteria present as a result of bacteremia or local transit can multiply and cause disease.

A similar problem can affect patients whose lymph node integrity has been disrupted by radical surgery, particularly patients who have had radical node dissections. A common clinical problem after radical mastectomy is the development of cellulitis (usually caused by streptococci or staphylococci) because of lymphedema and/or inadequate lymph drainage. In most cases, this problem can be addressed by local measures designed to prevent fluid accumulation and breaks in the skin, but antibiotic prophylaxis has been necessary in refractory cases.

A life-threatening problem common to many cancer patients is the loss of the reticuloendothelial capacity to clear microorganisms after splenectomy. Splenectomy may be performed as part of the management of hairy cell leukemia, chronic lymphocytic leukemia (CLL), and chronic myelocytic leukemia (CML) and in Hodgkin's disease. Even after curative therapy for the underlying disease, the lack of a spleen predisposes such patients to rapidly fatal infections. The loss of the spleen through trauma similarly predisposes the normal host to overwhelming infection for life after splenectomy. The splenectomized patient should be counseled about the risks of infection with certain organisms, such as the protozoan *Babesia* (Chap. 117) and *Capnocytophaga canimorsus* (formerly dysgonic fermenter 2, or DF-2), a bacterium carried in the mouths of animals (Chaps. 5 and 48). Since encapsulated bacteria (*Streptococcus pneumoniae*, *Haemophilus influenzae*, and *Neisseria meningitidis*) are the organisms most commonly associated with postsplenectomy sepsis, splenectomized persons should be vaccinated (and revaccinated; Table 11-2 and Chap. 3) against the capsular polysaccharides of these organisms. Many clinicians recommend giving splenectomized patients a small supply of antibiotics effective against *S. pneumoniae*, *N. meningitidis*, and *H. influenzae* to avert rapid, overwhelming sepsis in the event that they cannot present for medical attention immediately after the onset of fever or other symptoms of bacterial infection. A few amoxicillin/clavulanic acid tablets are a reasonable choice for this purpose.

The level of suspicion of infections with certain organisms should depend on the type of cancer diagnosed (Table 11-3). Diagnosis of multiple myeloma or CLL should alert the clinician to the possibility of hypogammaglobulinemia. Although immuno-globulin replacement therapy can be effective, in most cases prophylactic antibiotics are a cheaper, more convenient method of eliminating bacterial infections in CLL patients with hypogammaglobulinemia. Patients with acute lymphocytic leukemia (ALL), patients with non-Hodgkin's lymphoma, and all cancer patients treated with high-dose glucocorticoids (or glucocorticoid-containing chemotherapy

TABLE 11-1

DISRUPTION OF NORMAL BARRIERS THAT MAY PREDISPOSE TO INFECTIONS IN PATIENTS WITH CANCER

TYPE OF DEFENSE	SPECIFIC LESION	CELLS INVOLVED	ORGANISM	CANCER ASSOCIATION	DISEASE
Physical barrier	Breaks in skin	Skin epithelial cells	Staphylococci, streptococci	Head and neck, squamous cell carcinoma	Cellulitis, extensive skin infection
Emptying of fluid collections	Occlusion of orifices: ureters, bile duct, colon	Luminal epithelial cells	Gram-negative bacilli	Renal, ovarian, biliary tree, metastatic diseases of many cancers	Rapid, overwhelming bacteremia; urinary tract infection
Lymphatic function	Node dissection	Lymph nodes	Staphylococci, streptococci	Breast cancer surgery	Cellulitis
Splenic clearance of microorganisms	Splenectomy	Splenic reticuloendothelial cells	*Streptococcus pneumoniae*, *Haemophilus influenzae*, *Neisseria meningitidis*, *Babesia*, *Capnocytophaga canimorsus*	Hodgkin's disease, leukemia, idiopathic thrombocytopenic purpura	Rapid, overwhelming sepsis
Phagocytosis	Lack of granulocytes	Granulocytes (neutrophils)	Staphylococci, streptococci, enteric organisms, fungi	Hairy cell, acute myelocytic, and acute lymphocytic leukemias	Bacteremia
Humoral immunity	Lack of antibody	B cells	*S. pneumoniae*, *H. influenzae*, *N. meningitidis*	Chronic lymphocytic leukemia, multiple myeloma	Infections with encapsulated organisms, sinusitis, pneumonia
Cellular immunity	Lack of T cells	T cells and macrophages	*Mycobacterium tuberculosis*, *Listeria*, herpesviruses, fungi, other intracellular parasites	Hodgkin's disease, leukemia, T-cell lymphoma	Infections with intracellular bacteria, fungi, parasites

regimens) should receive antibiotic prophylaxis for *Pneumocystis* infection (Table 11-3) for the duration of their chemotherapy. In addition to exhibiting susceptibility to certain infectious organisms, patients with cancer are likely to manifest their infections in characteristic ways.

SYSTEM-SPECIFIC SYNDROMES

SKIN-SPECIFIC SYNDROMES

Skin lesions are common in cancer patients, and the appearance of these lesions may permit the diagnosis of systemic bacterial or fungal infection. Although cellulitis caused by skin organisms such as *Streptococcus* or *Staphylococcus* is common, neutropenic patients—i.e., those with <500 functional polymorphonuclear leukocytes (PMNs)/μL—and patients with impaired blood or lymphatic drainage may develop infections with unusual organisms. Innocent-looking macules or papules may be the first sign of bacterial or fungal sepsis in immunocompromised patients (Fig. 11-1). In the neutropenic host, a macule progresses rapidly to ecthyma gangrenosum, a usually painless, round, necrotic lesion consisting of a central black or gray-black eschar with surrounding erythema. Ecthyma gangrenosum, which is located in nonpressure areas (as distinguished from necrotic lesions associated with lack of circulation), is often associated with *Pseudomonas aeruginosa* bacteremia (Chap. 53), but may be caused by other bacteria.

Candidemia (Chap. 107) is also associated with a variety of skin conditions and commonly presents as a maculopapular rash. Punch biopsy of the skin may be the best method for diagnosis.

Cellulitis, an acute spreading inflammation of the skin, is most often caused by infection with group A *Streptococcus* or *Staphylococcus aureus*, virulent organisms normally found on the skin (Chap. 21). Although cellulitis tends to be circumscribed in normal hosts, it may spread rapidly in neutropenic patients. A tiny break in the skin may lead to spreading cellulitis, which is characterized by pain and erythema; in the affected patients, signs of infection (e.g., purulence) are often lacking. What might be a furuncle in a normal host may require amputation because of uncontrolled infection in a patient presenting

TABLE 11-2

VACCINATION OF CANCER PATIENTS RECEIVING CHEMOTHERAPY

	USE IN INDICATED PATIENTS		
VACCINE	**INTENSIVE CHEMOTHERAPY**	**HODGKIN'S DISEASE**	**HEMATOPOIETIC STEM-CELL TRANSPLANTATION**
Diphtheria-tetanus[a]	Primary series and boosters as necessary	No special recommendation	12, 14, and 24 months after transplantation
Poliomyelitis[b]	Complete primary series and boosters	No special recommendation	12, 14, and 24 months after transplantation
Haemophilus influenzae type b conjugate	Primary series and booster for children	Immunization before treatment and booster 3 months afterward	12, 14, and 24 months after transplantation
Hepatitis A	Not routinely recommended	Not routinely recommended	Not routinely recommended
Hepatitis B	Complete series	No special recommendation	12, 14, and 24 months after transplantation
23-Valent pneumococcal polysaccharide[c]	Every 5 years	Immunization before treatment and booster 3 months afterward	12 and 24 months after transplantation
4-Valent meningococcal conjugate[d]	Should be administered to splenectomized patients and patients living in endemic areas, including college students in dormitories	Should be administered to splenectomized patients and patients living in endemic areas, including college students in dormitories	Should be administered to splenectomized patients and patients living in endemic areas, including college students in dormitories
Influenza	Seasonal immunization	Seasonal immunization	Seasonal immunization
Measles/mumps/rubella	Contraindicated	Contraindicated during chemotherapy	After 24 months in patients without graft-versus-host disease
Varicella-zoster virus	Contraindicated[e]	Contraindicated	Contraindicated

[a]The Td (tetanus-diphtheria) combination is currently recommended for adults. Pertussis vaccines have not been recommended for people >6 years of age in the past. However, recent data indicate that the Tdap (tetanus–diphtheria–acellular pertussis) product is both safe and efficacious in adults.
[b]Live-virus vaccine is contraindicated; inactivated vaccine should be used.
[c]The seven-serotype pneumococcal conjugate vaccine is currently recommended only for children. It is anticipated that future vaccines will include more serotypes and will be recommended for adults.
[d]Currently licensed for people 11–55 years of age.
[e]Contact the manufacturer for more information on use in children with acute lymphocytic leukemia.

TABLE 11-3

INFECTIONS ASSOCIATED WITH SPECIFIC TYPES OF CANCER

CANCER	**UNDERLYING IMMUNE ABNORMALITY**	**ORGANISMS CAUSING INFECTION**
Multiple myeloma	Hypogammaglobulinemia	*Streptococcus pneumoniae*, *Haemophilus influenzae*, *Neisseria meningitidis*
Chronic lymphocytic leukemia	Hypogammaglobulinemia	*S. pneumoniae*, *H. influenzae*, *N. meningitidis*
Acute myelocytic or lymphocytic leukemia	Granulocytopenia, skin and mucous-membrane lesions	Extracellular gram-positive and gram-negative bacteria, fungi
Hodgkin's disease	Abnormal T-cell function	Intracellular pathogens (*Mycobacterium tuberculosis*, *Listeria*, *Salmonella*, *Cryptococcus*, *Mycobacterium avium*)
Non-Hodgkin's lymphoma and acute lymphocytic leukemia	Glucocorticoid chemotherapy, T- and B-cell dysfunction	*Pneumocystis*
Colon and rectal tumors	Local abnormalities[a]	*Streptococcus bovis* (bacteremia)
Hairy cell leukemia	Abnormal T-cell function	Intracellular pathogens (*M. tuberculosis*, *Listeria*, *Cryptococcus*, *M. avium*)

[a]The reason for this association is not well defined.

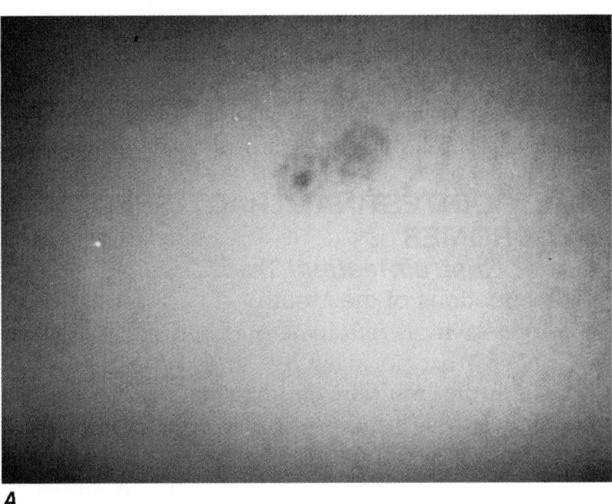

A

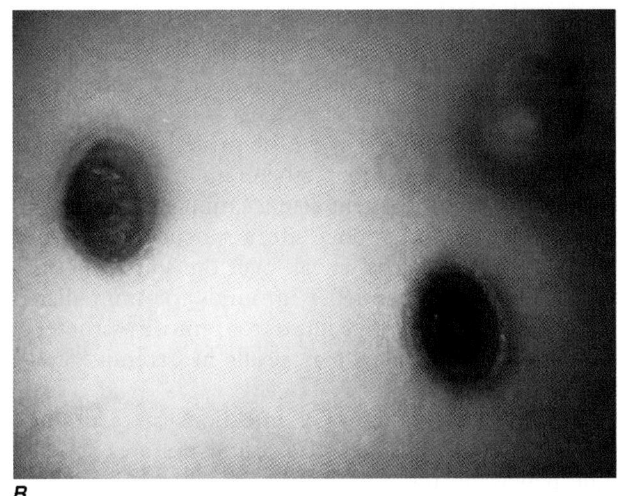

B

FIGURE 11-1

A.* Papules related to *Escherichia coli bacteremia in a neutropenic patient with acute lymphocytic leukemia. ***B.*** The same lesion the following day.

with leukemia. A dramatic response to an infection that might be trivial in a normal host can mark the first sign of leukemia. Fortunately, granulocytopenic patients are likely to be infected with certain types of organisms (Table 11-4); thus the selection of an antibiotic regimen is somewhat easier than it might otherwise be (see "Antibacterial Therapy" later in the chapter). It is essential to recognize cellulitis early and to treat it aggressively. Patients who are neutropenic or have previously received antibiotics for other reasons may develop cellulitis with unusual organisms (e.g., *Escherichia coli*, *Pseudomonas*, or fungi). Early treatment, even of innocent-looking lesions, is essential to prevent necrosis and loss of tissue. Debridement to prevent spread may sometimes be necessary early in the course of disease, but it can often be performed after chemotherapy, when the PMN count increases.

TABLE 11-4

ORGANISMS LIKELY TO CAUSE INFECTIONS IN GRANULOCYTOPENIC PATIENTS

Gram-positive cocci	Non-*aeruginosa*
Staphylococcus epidermidis	*Pseudomonas* spp.[a]
Staphylococcus aureus	*Enterobacter* spp.
Viridans *Streptococcus*	*Serratia* spp.
Enterococcus faecalis	*Acinetobacter* spp.[a]
Streptococcus pneumoniae	*Citrobacter* spp.
Gram-negative bacilli	Gram-positive bacilli
Escherichia coli	Diphtheroids
Klebsiella spp.	JK bacillus[a]
Pseudomonas aeruginosa	Fungi
	Candida spp.
	Aspergillus spp.

[a]Often associated with intravenous catheters.

Sweet's syndrome, or *febrile neutrophilic dermatosis*, was originally described in women with elevated white blood cell (WBC) counts. The disease is characterized by the presence of leukocytes in the lower dermis, with edema of the papillary body. Ironically, this disease now is usually seen in neutropenic patients with cancer, most often in association with acute leukemia, but also in association with a variety of other malignancies. Sweet's syndrome usually presents as red or bluish-red papules or nodules that may coalesce and form sharply bordered plaques. The edema may suggest vesicles, but on palpation the lesions are solid, and vesicles probably never arise in this disease. The lesions are most common on the face, neck, and arms. On the legs, they may be confused with erythema nodosum. The development of lesions is often accompanied by high fevers and an elevated erythrocyte sedimentation rate. Both the lesions and the temperature elevation respond dramatically to glucocorticoid administration. Treatment begins with high doses of glucocorticoids (60 mg/d of prednisone) followed by tapered doses over the next 2–3 weeks.

Data indicate that *erythema multiforme* with mucous membrane involvement is often associated with herpes simplex virus (HSV) infection and is distinct from Stevens-Johnson syndrome, which is associated with drugs and tends to have a more widespread distribution. Since cancer patients are both immunosuppressed (and therefore susceptible to herpes infections) and heavily treated with drugs (and therefore subject to Stevens-Johnson syndrome), both of these conditions are common in this population.

Cytokines, which are used as adjuvants or primary treatments for cancer, can themselves cause characteristic rashes, further complicating the differential diagnosis. This phenomenon is a particular problem in bone marrow transplant recipients (Chap. 12), who, in addition to having the usual chemotherapy-, antibiotic-, and cytokine-induced rashes, are plagued by graft-versus-host disease.

CATHETER-RELATED INFECTIONS

Because IV catheters are commonly used in cancer chemotherapy and are prone to infection (Chap. 13), they pose a major problem in the care of patients with cancer. Some catheter-associated infections can be treated with antibiotics, whereas in others, the catheter must be removed (Table 11-5). If the patient has a "tunneled" catheter (which consists of an entrance site, a subcutaneous tunnel, and an exit site), a red streak over the subcutaneous part of the line (the tunnel) is grounds for immediate removal of the catheter. Failure to remove catheters under these circumstances may result in extensive cellulitis and tissue necrosis.

More common than tunnel infections are exit-site infections, often with erythema around the area where the line penetrates the skin. Most authorities (Chap. 35) recommend treatment (usually with vancomycin) for an exit-site infection caused by a coagulase-negative *Staphylococcus*. Treatment of coagulase-positive staphylococcal infection is associated with a poorer outcome, and it is advisable to remove the catheter if possible. Similarly, many clinicians remove catheters associated with infections due to *P. aeruginosa* and *Candida* species, since such infections are difficult to treat and bloodstream infections with these organisms are likely to be deadly. Catheter infections caused by *Burkholderia cepacia*, *Stenotrophomonas* spp., *Agrobacterium* spp., and *Acinetobacter baumannii* as well as *Pseudomonas* spp. other than *aeruginosa* are likely to be very difficult to eradicate with antibiotics alone. Similarly, isolation of *Bacillus*, *Corynebacterium*, and *Mycobacterium* spp. should prompt removal of the catheter.

GASTROINTESTINAL TRACT–SPECIFIC SYNDROMES

Upper Gastrointestinal Tract Disease

Infections of the Mouth

The oral cavity is rich in aerobic and anaerobic bacteria (Chap. 65) that normally live in a commensal relationship with the host. The antimetabolic effects of chemotherapy cause a breakdown of host defenses, leading to ulceration of the mouth and the potential for invasion by resident bacteria. Mouth ulcerations afflict most patients receiving chemotherapy and have been associated with viridans streptococcal bacteremia. The use of keratinocyte growth factor (palifermin) in a daily dose of 60 μg/kg for 3 days before chemotherapy and total-body irradiation is of proven value in preventing mucosal ulceration after stem-cell transplantation. Fluconazole is clearly effective in the treatment of both local infections (thrush) and systemic infections (esophagitis) due to *Candida albicans*. Newer azoles (such as voriconazole) are similarly effective.

TABLE 11-5

APPROACH TO CATHETER INFECTIONS IN IMMUNOCOMPROMISED PATIENTS

CLINICAL PRESENTATION	CATHETER REMOVAL	ANTIBIOTICS	COMMENTS
Evidence of Infection, Negative Blood Cultures			
Exit-site erythema	Not necessary if infection responds to treatment	Usually begin treatment for gram-positive cocci.	Coagulase-negative staphylococci are most common.
Tunnel-site erythema	Required	Treat for gram-positive cocci pending culture results.	Failure to remove the catheter may lead to complications.
Blood Culture–Positive Infections			
Coagulase-negative staphylococci	Line removal optimal but may be unnecessary if patient is clinically stable and responds to antibiotics	Usually start with vancomycin. (Linezolid, quinupristin/dalfopristin, and daptomycin are all appropriate.)	If there are no contraindications to line removal, this course of action is optimal. If the line is removed, antibiotics may not be necessary.
Other gram-positive cocci (e.g., *Staphylococcus aureus*, *Enterococcus*); gram-positive rods (*Bacillus*, *Corynebacterium* spp.)	Recommended	Treat with antibiotics to which the organism is sensitive, with duration based on the clinical setting.	The incidence of metastatic infections after *S. aureus* infection and the difficulty of treating enterococcal infection make line removal the recommended course of action. In addition, gram-positive rods do not respond readily to antibiotics alone.
Gram-negative bacteria	Recommended	Use an agent to which the organism is shown to be sensitive.	Organisms like *Stenotrophomonas*, *Pseudomonas*, and *Burkholderia* are notoriously hard to treat.
Fungi	Recommended	—	Fungal infections of catheters are extremely difficult to treat.

Noma (*cancrum oris*), commonly seen in malnourished children, is a penetrating disease of the soft and hard tissues of the mouth and adjacent sites, with resulting necrosis and gangrene. It has a counterpart in immunocompromised patients and is thought to be due to invasion of the tissues by *Bacteroides*, *Fusobacterium*, and other normal inhabitants of the mouth. Noma is associated with debility, poor oral hygiene, and immunosuppression.

Viruses, particularly HSV, are a prominent cause of morbidity in immunocompromised patients, in whom they are associated with severe mucositis. The use of acyclovir, either prophylactically or therapeutically, is of value.

Esophageal Infections

The differential diagnosis of esophagitis (usually presenting as substernal chest pain upon swallowing) includes herpes simplex and candidiasis, both of which are readily treatable.

Lower Gastrointestinal Tract Disease

Hepatic candidiasis (Chap. 107) results from seeding of the liver (usually from a gastrointestinal source) in neutropenic patients. It is most common in patients being treated for acute leukemia and usually presents symptomatically around the time the neutropenia resolves. The characteristic picture is that of persistent fever unresponsive to antibiotics; abdominal pain and tenderness or nausea; and elevated serum levels of alkaline phosphatase in a patient with hematologic malignancy who has recently recovered from neutropenia. The diagnosis of this disease (which may present in an indolent manner and persist for several months) is based on the finding of yeasts or pseudohyphae in granulomatous lesions. Hepatic ultrasound or CT may reveal bull's-eye lesions. In some cases, MRI reveals small lesions not visible by other imaging modalities. The pathology (a granulomatous response) and the timing (with resolution of neutropenia and an elevation in granulocyte count) suggest that the host response to *Candida* is an important component of the manifestations of disease. In many cases, although organisms are visible, cultures of biopsied material may be negative. The designation *hepatosplenic candidiasis* or *hepatic candidiasis* is a misnomer because the disease often involves the kidneys and other tissues; the term *chronic disseminated candidiasis* may be more appropriate. Because of the risk of bleeding with liver biopsy, diagnosis is often based on imaging studies (MRI, CT). Amphotericin B is traditionally used for therapy (often for several months, until all manifestations of disease have disappeared), but fluconazole may be useful for outpatient therapy. The use of other antifungal agents and combination therapy is less well studied.

Typhlitis

Typhlitis (also referred to as necrotizing colitis, neutropenic colitis, necrotizing enteropathy, ileocecal syndrome, and cecitis) is a clinical syndrome of fever and right-lower-quadrant tenderness in an immunosuppressed host. This syndrome is classically seen in neutropenic patients after chemotherapy with cytotoxic drugs. It may be more common among children than among adults and appears to be much more common among patients with acute myelocytic leukemia (AML) or ALL than among those with other types of cancer; a similar syndrome has been reported in patients infected with HIV type 1. Physical examination reveals right-lower-quadrant tenderness, with or without rebound tenderness. Associated diarrhea (often bloody) is common, and the diagnosis can be confirmed by the finding of a thickened cecal wall on CT, MRI, or ultrasonography. Plain films may reveal a right-lower-quadrant mass, but CT with contrast or MRI is a much more sensitive means of making the diagnosis. Although surgery is sometimes attempted to avoid perforation from ischemia, most cases resolve with medical therapy alone. The disease is sometimes associated with positive blood cultures (which usually yield aerobic gram-negative bacilli), and therapy is recommended for a broad spectrum of bacteria (particularly gram-negative bacilli, which are likely to be found in the bowel flora). Surgery is indicated in the case of perforation.

Clostridium Difficile–*Induced Diarrhea*

Patients with cancer are predisposed to the development of *C. difficile* diarrhea (Chap. 43) as a consequence of chemotherapy alone. Thus they may have positive toxin tests before receiving antibiotics. Obviously, such patients are also subject to *C. difficile*– induced diarrhea as a result of antibiotic pressure. *C. difficile* should always be considered as a possible cause of diarrhea in cancer patients who have received antibiotics.

CENTRAL NERVOUS SYSTEM–SPECIFIC SYNDROMES

Meningitis

The presentation of meningitis in patients with lymphoma or CLL, patients receiving chemotherapy (particularly with glucocorticoids) for solid tumors, and patients who have received bone marrow transplants suggests a diagnosis of cryptococcal or listerial infection. As noted previously, splenectomized patients are susceptible to rapid, overwhelming infection with encapsulated bacteria (including *S. pneumoniae*, *H. influenzae*, and *N. meningitidis*). Similarly, patients who are antibody-deficient (such as patients with CLL, those who have received intensive chemotherapy, or those who have undergone bone marrow transplantation) are likely to have infections caused by these bacteria. Other cancer patients, however, because of their defective cellular immunity, are likely to be infected with other pathogens (Table 11-3).

Encephalitis

The spectrum of disease resulting from viral encephalitis is expanded in immunocompromised patients. A predisposition to infections with intracellular organisms similar to those encountered in patients with AIDS (Chap. 90) is seen in cancer patients receiving (1) high-dose cytotoxic chemotherapy, (2) chemotherapy affecting T-cell function (e.g., fludarabine), or (3) antibodies that eliminate

TABLE 11-6

DIFFERENTIAL DIAGNOSIS OF CENTRAL NERVOUS SYSTEM INFECTIONS IN PATIENTS WITH CANCER

	UNDERLYING PREDISPOSITION	
FINDINGS ON CT OR MRI	**PROLONGED NEUTROPENIA**	**DEFECTS IN CELLULAR IMMUNITY[a]**
Mass lesions	*Aspergillus* brain abscess *Nocardia* brain abscess *Cryptococcus* brain abscess	Toxoplasmosis EBV-LPD
Diffuse encephalitis	PML (J-C virus)	Infection with VZV, CMV, HSV, HHV-6, J-C virus (PML), *Listeria*

[a]High-dose glucocorticoid therapy, cytotoxic chemotherapy.

Note: CMV, cytomegalovirus; EBV-LPD, Epstein-Barr virus lymphoproliferative disease; HHV-6, human herpesvirus type 6; HSV, herpes simplex virus; PML, progressive multifocal leukoencephalopathy; VZV, varicella-zoster virus.

TABLE 11-7

DIFFERENTIAL DIAGNOSIS OF CHEST INFILTRATES IN IMMUNOCOMPROMISED PATIENTS

	CAUSE OF PNEUMONIA	
INFILTRATE	**INFECTIOUS**	**NONINFECTIOUS**
Localized	Bacteria, *Legionella*, mycobacteria	Local hemorrhage or embolism, tumor
Nodular	Fungi (e.g., *Aspergillus* or *Mucor*), *Nocardia*	Recurrent tumor
Diffuse	Viruses (especially CMV), *Chlamydophila*, *Pneumocystis*, *Toxoplasma gondii*, mycobacteria	Congestive heart failure, radiation pneumonitis, drug-induced lung injury, diffuse alveolar hemorrhage (described after BMT)

Note: BMT, bone marrow transplantation; CMV, cytomegalovirus.

T cells (e.g., anti-CD3) or cytokine activity. Infection with varicella-zoster virus (VZV) has been associated with encephalitis that may be caused by VZV-related vasculitis. Chronic viral infections may also be associated with dementia and encephalitic presentations, and a diagnosis of progressive multifocal leukoencephalopathy should be considered when a patient who has received chemotherapy presents with dementia (Table 11-6). Other abnormalities of the central nervous system (CNS) that may be confused with infection include normal-pressure hydrocephalus and vasculitis resulting from CNS irradiation. It may be possible to differentiate these conditions by MRI.

Brain Masses

Mass lesions of the brain most often present as headache with or without fever or neurologic abnormalities. Infections associated with mass lesions may be caused by bacteria (particularly *Nocardia*), fungi (particularly *Cryptococcus* or *Aspergillus*), or parasites (*Toxoplasma*). Epstein-Barr virus (EBV)–associated lymphoproliferative disease may also present as single or multiple mass lesions of the brain. A biopsy may be required for a definitive diagnosis.

PULMONARY INFECTIONS

Pneumonia (Chap. 17) in immunocompromised patients may be difficult to diagnose because conventional methods of diagnosis depend on the presence of neutrophils. Bacterial pneumonia in neutropenic patients may present without purulent sputum—or, in fact, without any sputum at all—and may not produce physical findings suggestive of chest consolidation (rales or egophony).

In granulocytopenic patients with persistent or recurrent fever, the chest x-ray pattern may help to localize an infection and thus to determine which investigative tests and procedures should be undertaken and which therapeutic options should be considered (Table 11-7). The difficulties encountered in the management of pulmonary infiltrates relate in part to the difficulties of performing diagnostic procedures on the patients involved. When platelet counts can be increased to adequate levels by transfusion, microscopic and microbiologic evaluation of the fluid obtained by endoscopic bronchial lavage is often diagnostic. Lavage fluid should be cultured for *Mycoplasma*, *Chlamydophila*, *Legionella*, *Nocardia*, more common bacterial pathogens, and fungi. In addition, the possibility of *Pneumocystis* pneumonia should be considered, especially in patients with ALL or lymphoma who have not received prophylactic trimethoprim-sulfamethoxazole (TMP-SMX). The characteristics of the infiltrate may be helpful in decisions about further diagnostic and therapeutic maneuvers. Nodular infiltrates suggest fungal pneumonia (e.g., that caused by *Aspergillus* or *Mucor*). Such lesions may best be approached by visualized biopsy procedures.

Aspergillus spp. (Chap. 108) can colonize the skin and respiratory tract or cause fatal systemic illness. Although *Aspergillus* may cause aspergillomas in a previously existing cavity or may produce allergic bronchopulmonary aspergillosis, the major problem posed by this genus in neutropenic patients is invasive disease due to *A. fumigatus* or *A. flavus*. The organisms enter the host after colonization of the respiratory tract, with subsequent invasion of the blood vessels. The disease is likely to present as a thrombotic or embolic event because of the organisms' ability to invade blood vessels. The risk of infection with *Aspergillus* is correlated directly with the duration of neutropenia. In prolonged neutropenia, positive surveillance cultures for colonization of the nasopharynx with *Aspergillus* may predict the development of disease.

Patients with *Aspergillus* infection often present with pleuritic chest pain and fever, which are sometimes accompanied by cough. Hemoptysis may be an ominous sign. Chest x-rays may reveal new focal infiltrates or nodules. Chest CT may reveal a characteristic halo consisting of a mass-like infiltrate surrounded by an area of low attenuation. The presence of a "crescent sign" on a chest x-ray or a chest CT scan, in which the mass progresses to central cavitation, is characteristic of invasive *Aspergillus* infection but may develop as the lesions are resolving.

In addition to causing pulmonary disease, *Aspergillus* may invade through the nose or palate, with deep sinus penetration. The appearance of a discolored area in the nasal passages or on the hard palate should prompt a search for invasive *Aspergillus*. This situation is likely to require surgical debridement. Catheter infections with *Aspergillus* usually require both removal of the catheter and antifungal therapy.

Diffuse interstitial infiltrates suggest viral, parasitic, or *Pneumocystis* pneumonia. If the patient has a diffuse interstitial pattern on chest x-ray, it may be reasonable to institute empirical treatment with TMP-SMX (for *Pneumocystis*) and a quinolone (for *Chlamydophila*, *Mycoplasma*, and *Legionella*) or an erythromycin derivative (e.g., azithromycin) while considering invasive diagnostic procedures. Noninvasive procedures, such as staining of sputum smears for *Pneumocystis*, serum cryptococcal antigen tests, and urine testing for *Legionella* antigen, may be helpful. In transplant recipients who are seropositive for cytomegalovirus (CMV), a determination of CMV load in the serum should be considered. Viral load studies (which allow physicians to quantitate viruses) have superseded simple measurement of serum IgG, which merely documents prior exposure to virus. Infections with viruses that cause only upper respiratory symptoms in immunocompetent hosts, such as respiratory syncytial virus (RSV), influenza viruses, and parainfluenza viruses, may be associated with fatal pneumonitis in immunocompromised hosts. An attempt at early diagnosis by nasopharyngeal aspiration should be considered so that appropriate treatment can be instituted.

Bleomycin is the most common cause of chemotherapy-induced lung disease. Other causes include alkylating agents (such as cyclophosphamide, chlorambucil, and melphalan), nitrosoureas [carmustine (BCNU), lomustine (CCNU), and methyl-CCNU], busulfan, procarbazine, methotrexate, and hydroxyurea. Both infectious and noninfectious (drug- and/or radiation-induced) pneumonitis can cause fever and abnormalities on chest x-ray; thus the differential diagnosis of an infiltrate in a patient receiving chemotherapy encompasses a broad range of conditions (Table 11-7). Since the treatment of radiation pneumonitis (which may respond dramatically to glucocorticoids) or drug-induced pneumonitis is different from that of infectious pneumonia, a biopsy may be important in the diagnosis. Unfortunately, no definitive diagnosis can be made in ~30% of cases, even after bronchoscopy.

Open-lung biopsy is the "gold standard" of diagnostic techniques. Biopsy via a visualized thoracostomy can replace an open procedure in many cases. When a biopsy cannot be performed, empirical treatment can be undertaken with a quinolone or erythromycin (or an erythromycin derivative such as azithromycin) and TMP-SMX (in the case of diffuse infiltrates) or with amphotericin B or other antifungal agents (in the case of nodular infiltrates). The risks should be weighed carefully in these cases. If inappropriate drugs are administered, empirical treatment may prove toxic or ineffective; either of these outcomes may be riskier than biopsy.

CARDIOVASCULAR INFECTIONS

Patients with Hodgkin's disease are prone to persistent infections by *Salmonella*, sometimes (and particularly often in elderly patients) affecting a vascular site. The use of IV catheters deliberately lodged in the right atrium is associated with a high incidence of bacterial endocarditis, presumably related to valve damage followed by bacteremia. Nonbacterial thrombotic endocarditis has been described in association with a variety of malignancies (most often solid tumors) and may follow bone marrow transplantation as well. The presentation of an embolic event with a new cardiac murmur suggests this diagnosis. Blood cultures are negative in this disease of unknown pathogenesis.

ENDOCRINE SYNDROMES

Infections of the endocrine system have been described in immunocompromised patients. *Candida* infection of the thyroid may be difficult to diagnose during the neutropenic period. It can be defined by indium-labeled WBC scans or gallium scans after neutrophil counts increase. CMV infection can cause adrenalitis with or without resulting adrenal insufficiency. The presentation of a sudden endocrine anomaly in an immunocompromised patient may be a sign of infection in the involved end organ.

MUSCULOSKELETAL INFECTIONS

Infection that is a consequence of vascular compromise, resulting in gangrene, can occur when a tumor restricts the blood supply to muscles, bones, or joints. The process of diagnosis and treatment of such infection is similar to that in normal hosts, with the following caveats:

1. *In terms of diagnosis,* a lack of physical findings resulting from a lack of granulocytes in the granulocytopenic patient should make the clinician more aggressive in obtaining tissue rather than relying on physical signs.
2. *In terms of therapy,* aggressive debridement of infected tissues may be required, but it is usually difficult to operate on patients who have recently received chemotherapy, both because of a lack of platelets (which results in bleeding complications) and because of a lack of WBCs (which may lead to secondary infection). A blood culture positive for *Clostridium perfringens*—an organism commonly associated with gas gangrene—can have a number of meanings (Chap. 42). Bloodstream infections with intestinal organisms such as *Streptococcus bovis* and *C. perfringens* may arise spontaneously from lower gastrointestinal lesions (tumor or polyps); alternatively, these lesions may be harbingers of invasive disease. The clinical setting must be considered in order to define the appropriate treatment for each case.

RENAL AND URETERAL INFECTIONS

Infections of the urinary tract are common among patients whose ureteral excretion is compromised (Table 11-1). *Candida*, which has a predilection for the kidney, can invade either from the bloodstream or in a retrograde manner (via the ureters or bladder) in immunocompromised patients. The presence of "fungus balls" or persistent candiduria suggests invasive disease. Persistent funguria (with *Aspergillus* as well as *Candida*) should prompt a search for a nidus of infection in the kidney.

Certain viruses are typically seen only in immunosuppressed patients. BK virus (polyomavirus hominis 1) has been documented in the urine of bone marrow transplant recipients and, like adenovirus, may be associated with hemorrhagic cystitis. BK-induced cystitis usually remits with decreasing immunosuppression. Anecdotal reports have described the treatment of infections due to adenovirus and BK virus with cidofovir.

ABNORMALITIES THAT PREDISPOSE TO INFECTION

(Table 11-1)

THE LYMPHOID SYSTEM

It is beyond the scope of this chapter to detail how all the immunologic abnormalities that result from cancer or from chemotherapy for cancer lead to infections. Disorders of the immune system are discussed in other sections of this book. As has been noted, patients with antibody deficiency are predisposed to overwhelming infection with encapsulated bacteria (including *S. pneumoniae*, *H. influenzae*, and *N. meningitidis*). Infections that result from the lack of a functional cellular immune system are described in Chap. 90. It is worth mentioning, however, that patients undergoing intensive chemotherapy for any form of cancer will have not only defects due to granulocytopenia but also lymphocyte dysfunction, which may be profound. Thus these patients—especially those receiving glucocorticoid-containing regimens or drugs that inhibit T-cell activation or cytokine induction—should be given prophylaxis for *Pneumocystis* pneumonia.

THE HEMATOPOIETIC SYSTEM

Initial studies in the 1960s revealed a dramatic increase in the incidence of infections (fatal and nonfatal) among cancer patients with a granulocyte count of <500/μL. More recent studies have cited a figure of 48.3 infections per 100 neutropenic patients (<1000 granulocytes/μL) with hematologic malignancies and solid tumors, or 46.3 infections per 1000 days at risk.

Neutropenic patients are unusually susceptible to infection with a wide variety of bacteria; thus antibiotic therapy should be initiated promptly to cover likely pathogens if infection is suspected. Indeed, early initiation of antibacterial agents is mandatory to prevent deaths. These patients are susceptible to gram-positive and gram-negative organisms found commonly on the skin and in the bowel (Table 11-4). Because treatment with narrow-spectrum agents leads to infection with organisms not covered by the antibiotics used, the initial regimen should target pathogens likely to be initial causes of bacterial infection in neutropenic hosts (Fig. 11-2).

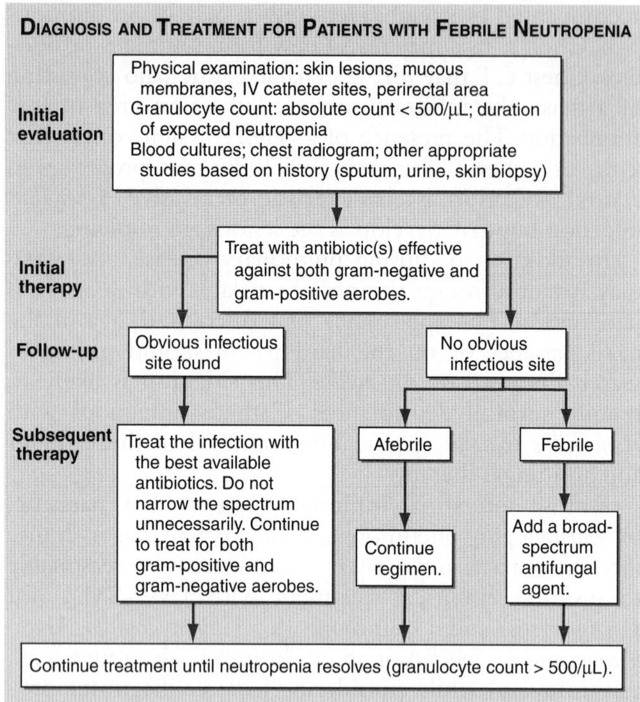

FIGURE 11-2
Algorithm for the diagnosis and treatment of febrile neutropenic patients.

℞ Treatment: INFECTIONS IN CANCER PATIENTS

ANTIBACTERIAL THERAPY Hundreds of antibacterial regimens have been tested for use in patients with cancer. The major risk of infection is related to the degree of neutropenia seen as a consequence of either the disease or the therapy. Many of the relevant studies involved small populations in which the outcomes were generally good, and most lacked the statistical power to detect differences among the regimens studied. Each febrile neutropenic patient should be approached as a unique problem, with particular attention given to previous infections and recent antibiotic exposures. Several general guidelines are useful in the initial treatment of neutropenic patients with fever (Fig. 11-2):

1. In the initial regimen, it is necessary to use antibiotics active against both gram-negative and gram-positive bacteria (Table 11-4).
2. An aminoglycoside or an antibiotic without good activity against gram-positive organisms (e.g., ciprofloxacin or aztreonam) alone is not adequate in this setting.
3. The agents used should reflect both the epidemiology and the antibiotic resistance pattern of the hospital.

4. If the pattern of resistance justifies its use, a single third-generation cephalosporin constitutes an appropriate initial regimen in many hospitals.
5. Most standard regimens are designed for patients who have not previously received prophylactic antibiotics. The development of fever in a patient who has received antibiotics affects the choice of subsequent therapy, which should target resistant organisms and organisms known to cause infections in patients being treated with the antibiotics already administered.
6. Randomized trials have indicated the safety of oral antibiotic regimens in the treatment of "low-risk" patients with fever and neutropenia. Outpatients who are expected to remain neutropenic for <10 days and who have no concurrent medical problems (such as hypotension, pulmonary compromise, or abdominal pain) can be classified as low risk and treated with a broad-spectrum oral regimen.
7. Several large-scale studies indicate that prophylaxis with a fluoroquinolone (ciprofloxacin or levofloxacin) decreases morbidity and mortality rates among afebrile patients who are anticipated to have neutropenia of long duration.

The initial antibacterial regimen should be refined on the basis of culture results (Fig. 11-2). Blood cultures are the most relevant on which to base therapy; surface cultures of skin and mucous membranes may be misleading. In the case of gram-positive bacteremia or another gram-positive infection, it is important that the antibiotic be optimal for the organism isolated. Although it is not desirable to leave the patient unprotected, the addition of more and more antibacterial agents to the regimen is not appropriate unless there is a clinical or microbiologic reason to do so. Planned progressive therapy (the serial, empirical addition of one drug after another without culture data) is not efficacious in most settings and may have unfortunate consequences. Simply adding another antibiotic for fear that a gram-negative infection is present is a dubious practice. The synergy exhibited by β-lactams and aminoglycosides against certain gram-negative organisms (especially *P. aeruginosa*) provides the rationale for using two antibiotics in this setting, but recent analyses suggest that efficacy is not enhanced by the addition of aminoglycosides, whereas toxicity may be increased. Mere "double coverage," with the addition of a quinolone or another antibiotic that is not likely to exhibit synergy, has not been shown to be of benefit and may cause additional toxicities and side effects. Cephalosporins can cause bone marrow suppression, and vancomycin is associated with neutropenia in some healthy individuals (Chap. 33). Furthermore, the addition of multiple cephalosporins may induce β-lactamase production by some organisms; cephalosporins and double β-lactam combinations should probably be avoided altogether in *Enterobacter* infections.

ANTIFUNGAL THERAPY Fungal infections in cancer patients are most often associated with neutropenia. Neutropenic patients are predisposed to the development of invasive fungal infections, most commonly those due to *Candida* and *Aspergillus* species and occasionally those caused by *Fusarium*, *Trichosporon*, and *Bipolaris*. Cryptococcal infection, which is common among patients taking immunosuppressive agents, is uncommon among neutropenic patients receiving chemotherapy for AML. Invasive candidal disease is usually caused by *C. albicans* or *C. tropicalis* but can be caused by *C. krusei*, *C. parapsilosis*, and *C. glabrata*.

For decades it has been common clinical practice to add amphotericin B to antibacterial regimens if a neutropenic patient remains febrile despite 4–7 days of treatment with antibacterial agents. The rationale for the empirical addition of amphotericin B is that it is difficult to culture fungi before they cause disseminated disease and that mortality rates from disseminated fungal infections in granulocytopenic patients are high. Before the introduction of newer azoles into clinical practice, amphotericin B was the mainstay of antifungal therapy. The insolubility of amphotericin B has resulted in the marketing of several lipid formulations that are less toxic than the amphotericin B deoxycholate complex. However, because of the high cost of the lipid preparations, their use at many centers is reserved for patients who fail to respond to standard amphotericin B. Since the side effects of the formulations differ, unnecessary switching from one to another is not recommended.

Although fluconazole is efficacious in the treatment of infections due to many *Candida* spp., its use against serious fungal infections in immunocompromised patients is limited by its narrow spectrum: it has no activity against *Aspergillus* or against several non-*albicans Candida* spp. The release of newer broad-spectrum azoles (such as voriconazole and posaconazole) has provided another option for the treatment of *Aspergillus* infection (including CNS infection, in which amphotericin B has usually failed). In fact, experience indicates that these drugs may well supplant amphotericin B as the mainstay of treatment because of their lesser toxicity and better penetration into cerebrospinal fluid and other sites. Clinicians should be aware that the spectrum of each azole is somewhat different and that no drug can be assumed to be efficacious against all fungi. For example, although voriconazole is active against *Pseudallescheria boydii*, amphotericin B is not; however, voriconazole has no activity against *Mucor*. Recent studies suggest a role for posaconazole as a prophylactic agent in patients with prolonged neutropenia. For a full discussion of antifungal therapy, see Chap. 102.

Echinocandins (such as caspofungin) are useful in the treatment of infections caused by azole-resistant *Candida*. Studies in progress are assessing the use of these agents in combinations to determine whether treatment with multiple antifungal agents leads to better outcomes.

ANTIVIRAL THERAPY The availability of a variety of agents active against herpes-group viruses, including some new agents with a broader spectrum of activity, has heightened focus on the treatment of viral infections, which pose a major problem in cancer patients. Viral diseases caused by the herpes group are prominent. Serious (and sometimes fatal) infections due to HSV and CMV are well documented, and VZV infections may be fatal to patients receiving chemotherapy. The roles of human herpesvirus (HHV) 6, HHV-7, and HHV-8 (Kaposi's sarcoma herpesvirus) in cancer patients are being defined (Chap. 83). Although clinical experience is most extensive with acyclovir, which can be used therapeutically or prophylactically, a number of derivative drugs offer advantages over this agent (Table 11-8).

In addition to the herpes group, several respiratory viruses (especially RSV) may cause serious disease in cancer patients. Although vaccination with influenza vaccine is recommended (see below), it may be ineffective in this patient population. The availability of antiviral drugs with activity against influenza viruses gives the clinician additional options for the treatment of these patients (Table 11-9).

OTHER THERAPEUTIC MODALITIES Another way to address the problems of the febrile neutropenic patient is to replenish the neutrophil population. Although granulocyte transfusions are efficacious in the treatment of refractory gram-negative bacteremia, they do not have a documented role in prophylaxis. Because of the expense, the risk of leukoagglutinin reactions (which has probably been decreased by improved cell-separation procedures), and the risk of transmission of CMV from unscreened donors (which has been reduced by the use of filters), granulocyte transfusion is reserved for patients unresponsive to antibiotics. This modality is efficacious for documented gram-negative bacteremia refractory to antibiotics, particularly in situations where granulocyte numbers will be depressed for only a short period. The demonstrated usefulness of granulocyte colony-stimulating factor (G-CSF) in mobilizing neutrophils and advances in preservation techniques may make this option more useful than in the past.

A variety of cytokines, including G-CSF and granulocyte-macrophage colony-stimulating factor, enhance granulocyte recovery after chemotherapy and consequently shorten the period of maximal vulnerability to fatal infections. The role of these cytokines in routine practice is still a matter of some debate. Most authorities recommend their use only when neutropenia is both severe and prolonged. The cytokines themselves may have adverse effects, including fever, hypoxemia, and pleural effusions or serositis in other areas. Since there is little evidence that their routine administration lessens the risk of death and since they are still expensive, the use of these cytokines has not become the standard of

TABLE 11-8

ANTIVIRAL AGENTS ACTIVE AGAINST HERPESVIRUSES

AGENT	DESCRIPTION	SPECTRUM	TOXICITY	OTHER ISSUES
Acyclovir	Inhibits HSV polymerase	HSV, VZV (± CMV, EBV)	Rarely has side effects; crystalluria can occur at high doses	Long history of safety; original antiviral agent
Famciclovir	Prodrug of penciclovir (a guanosine analogue)	HSV, VZV (± CMV)	Associated with cancer in rats	Longer effective half-life than acyclovir
Valacyclovir	Prodrug of acyclovir; better absorption	HSV, VZV (± CMV)	Associated with thrombotic microangiopathy in one study of immunocompromised patients	Better oral absorption and longer effective half-life than acyclovir; can be given as a single daily dose for prophylaxis
Ganciclovir	More potent polymerase inhibitor; more toxic than acyclovir	HSV, VZV, CMV, HHV-6	Bone marrow suppression	Neutropenia may respond to G-CSF or GM-CSF
Valganciclovir	Prodrug of ganciclovir; better absorption	HSV, VZV, CMV, HHV-6	Bone marrow suppression	—
Cidofovir	Nucleotide analogue of cytosine	HSV, VZV, CMV; good in vitro activity against adenovirus and others	Nephrotoxic marrow suppression	Given IV once a week
Foscarnet	Phosphonoformic acid; inhibits viral DNA polymerase	HSV, VZV, CMV, HHV-6	Nephrotoxic; electrolyte abnormalities common	IV only

Note: ±, agent has some activity but not enough for the treatment of infections; CMV, cytomegalovirus; EBV, Epstein-Barr virus; G-CSF, granulocyte colony-stimulating factor; GM-CSF, granulocyte-macrophage colony-stimulating factor; HHV, human herpesvirus; HSV, herpes simplex virus; VZV, varicella-zoster virus.

TABLE 11-9

OTHER ANTIVIRAL AGENTS USEFUL IN THE TREATMENT OF INFECTIONS IN CANCER PATIENTS

AGENT	DESCRIPTION	SPECTRUM	TOXICITY	OTHER ISSUES
Amantadine, rimantadine	Interfere with uncoating	Influenza A only	5–10% fewer CNS effects with rimantadine	May be given prophylactically
Zanamivir	Neuraminidase inhibitor	Influenza A and B	Usually well tolerated	Inhalation only
Oseltamivir	Neuraminidase inhibitor	Influenza A and B	Usually well tolerated	PO dosing
Pleconaril	Blocks enterovirus binding and uncoating	90% of enteroviruses, 80% of rhinoviruses	Generally well tolerated	Decreases duration of meningitis; available for compassionate use only
Interferons	Cytokines with broad spectrum of activity	Used locally for warts, systemically for hepatitis	Fever, myalgias, bone marrow suppression	Not shown to be helpful in CMV infection; use limited by toxicity
Ribavirin	Purine analogue (precise mechanism of action unknown)	Broad theoretical spectrum; documented use, against RSV Lassa fever virus, and hepatitis viruses (with interferon)	IV form causes anemia	Given by aerosol for RSV infection (efficacy in doubt); approved for use in children with heart/lung disease

Note: CMV, cytomegalovirus; CNS, central nervous system; RSV, respiratory syncytial virus.

care in all centers. The role of other cytokines (such as macrophage colony-stimulating factor for monocytes or interferon-γ) in preventing or treating infections in granulocytopenic patients is under investigation.

Once neutropenia has resolved, patients are not at increased risk of infection. However, depending on what drugs they receive, patients who continue on chemotherapeutic protocols remain at high risk for certain diseases. Any patient receiving more than a maintenance dose of glucocorticoids (including many treatment regimens for diffuse lymphoma) should also receive prophylactic TMP-SMX because of the risk of *Pneumocystis* infection; those with ALL should receive such prophylaxis for the duration of chemotherapy.

PREVENTION OF INFECTION IN CANCER PATIENTS

EFFECT OF THE ENVIRONMENT

Outbreaks of fatal *Aspergillus* infection have been associated with construction projects and materials in several hospitals. The association between spore counts and risk of infection suggests the need for a high-efficiency air-handling system in hospitals that care for large numbers of neutropenic patients. The use of laminar-flow rooms and prophylactic antibiotics has decreased the number of infectious episodes in severely neutropenic patients. However, because of the expense of such a program and the failure to show that it dramatically affects mortality rates, most centers do not routinely use laminar flow to care for neutropenic patients. Some centers use "reverse isolation," in which health care providers and visitors to a patient who is neutropenic wear gowns and gloves. Since most of the infections these patients develop are due to organisms that colonize the patients' own skin and bowel, the validity of such schemes is dubious, and limited clinical data do not support their use. Hand washing by all staff caring for neutropenic patients should be required to prevent the spread of resistant organisms.

The presence of large numbers of bacteria (particularly *P. aeruginosa*) in certain foods, especially fresh vegetables, has led some authorities to recommend a special "low-bacteria" diet. A diet consisting of cooked and canned food is satisfactory to most neutropenic patients and does not involve elaborate disinfection or sterilization protocols. However, there are no studies to support even this type of dietary restriction. Counseling of patients to avoid leftovers, deli foods, and unpasteurized dairy products is recommended.

PHYSICAL MEASURES

Although few studies address this issue, patients with cancer are predisposed to infections resulting from anatomic compromise (e.g., lymphedema resulting from node dissections after radical mastectomy). Surgeons who specialize in cancer surgery can provide specific guidelines for the care of such patients, and patients benefit from commonsense advice about how to prevent infections in vulnerable areas.

IMMUNOGLOBULIN REPLACEMENT

Many patients with multiple myeloma or CLL have immunoglobulin deficiencies as a result of their disease, and all allogeneic bone marrow transplant recipients are hypogammaglobinemic for a period after transplantation. However, current recommendations reserve intravenous immunoglobulin (IVIg) replacement therapy for those patients with severe (<400 mg/dL), prolonged hypogammaglobulinemia. Antibiotic prophylaxis has been shown to be cheaper and efficacious in preventing infections in most CLL patients with hypogammaglobulinemia. Routine use of IVIg replacement is not recommended.

SEXUAL PRACTICES

The use of condoms is recommended for severely immunocompromised patients. Any sexual practice that results in oral exposure to feces is not recommended. Neutropenic patients should be advised to avoid any practice that results in trauma, as even microscopic cuts may result in bacterial invasion and fatal sepsis.

ANTIBIOTIC PROPHYLAXIS

Several studies indicate that the use of oral fluoroquinolones prevents infection and decreases mortality rates among severely neutropenic patients. Fluconazole prevents *Candida* infections when given prophylactically to patients receiving bone marrow transplants. The use of broader-spectrum antifungal agents (e.g., posaconazole) appears to be more efficacious. Prophylaxis for *Pneumocystis* is mandatory for patients with ALL and for all cancer patients receiving glucocorticoid-containing chemotherapy regimens.

VACCINATION OF CANCER PATIENTS

In general, patients undergoing chemotherapy respond less well to vaccines than do normal hosts. Their greater need for vaccines thus leads to a dilemma in their management. Purified proteins and inactivated vaccines are almost never contraindicated and should be given to patients even during chemotherapy. For example, all adults should receive diphtheria-tetanus toxoid boosters at the indicated times as well as seasonal influenza vaccine. However, if possible, vaccination should not be undertaken concurrent with cytotoxic chemotherapy. If patients are expected to be receiving chemotherapy for several months and vaccination is indicated (for example, influenza vaccination in the fall), the vaccine should be given midcycle—as far apart in time as possible from the antimetabolic agents that will prevent an immune response. The meningococcal and pneumococcal polysaccharide vaccines should be given to patients before splenectomy, if possible. The *H. influenzae* type b conjugate vaccine should be administered to all splenectomized patients.

In general, live virus (or live bacterial) vaccines should not be given to patients during intensive chemotherapy because of the risk of disseminated infection. Recommendations on vaccination are summarized in Table 11-2.

FURTHER READINGS

BOHLIUS J et al: Granulopoiesis-stimulating factors to prevent adverse effects in the treatment of malignant lymphoma. Cochrane Database Syst Rev 3:CD003189, 2004

GAFTER-GVILI A et al: Antibiotic prophylaxis for bacterial infections in afebrile neutropenic patients following chemotherapy. Cochrane Database Syst Rev 4:CD004386, 2005

HALL K et al: Diagnosis and management of long-term central venous catheter infections. J Vasc Interv Radiol 15:327, 2004

PAUL M et al: Empirical antibiotic monotherapy for febrile neutropenia: Systematic review and meta-analysis of randomized controlled trials. J Antimicrob Chemother 57:176, 2006

SUNG L et al: Meta-analysis: Effect of prophylactic hematopoietic colony-stimulating factors on mortality and outcomes of infection. Ann Intern Med 147:400, 2007

ULLMANN AJ et al: Posaconazole or fluconazole for prophylaxis in severe graft-versus-host disease. N Engl J Med 356:335, 2007

CHAPTER 12

INFECTIONS IN TRANSPLANT RECIPIENTS

Robert Finberg ■ Joyce Fingeroth

The evaluation of infections in transplant recipients involves consideration of both the donor and the recipient of the transplanted organ. Infections after transplantation are complicated by the use of drugs that are necessary to enhance the likelihood of survival of the transplanted organ, but that also cause the host to be immunocompromised. Thus what might have been a latent or asymptomatic infection in an immunocompetent donor or in the recipient before therapy can become a life-threatening problem when the recipient becomes immunosuppressed.

PRETRANSPLANTATION EVALUATION

A variety of organisms have been transmitted by organ transplantation (Table 12-1). Careful attention to the sterility of the medium used to process the organ combined with meticulous microbiologic evaluation reduces rates of transmission of bacteria that may be present or grow in the organ culture medium. From 2% to >20% of donor kidneys are estimated to be contaminated with bacteria—in most cases, with the organisms that colonize the skin or grow in the tissue culture medium used

TABLE 12-1

ORGANISMS TRANSMITTED BY ORGAN TRANSPLANTATION AND THEIR PRIMARY SITES OF REACTIVATION DISEASE[a]

	BLOOD	LUNGS	HEART	BRAIN	LIVER/SPLEEN	SKIN
Viruses						
Cytomegalovirus[b]	+	+	±	±	+	±
Epstein-Barr virus[c]	+	+	±	±	+	±
Herpes simplex virus		+		±	+	+
Human herpesvirus type 6	+	+		+		+
Kaposi's sarcoma–associated herpesvirus	+	±			±	+
Hepatitis B and C viruses					+	
Rabies virus[d]				+		
West Nile virus	+			+		
Fungi						
Candida albicans	+	+			+	+
Histoplasma capsulatum	+	+			+	+
Cryptococcus neoformans	+	+		+	±	+
Parasites						
Toxoplasma gondii[e]		+	+	+		
Strongyloides stercoralis[f,g]		+				
Trypanosoma cruzi[g]			+			
Plasmodium falciparum[g]	+					
Prion Diseases						
Creutzfeldt-Jakob disease (CJD)[h]				+		
Variant CJD/bovine spongiform encephalopathy[i]				+		

[a]+, well documented; ±, probably occurs.
[b]Cytomegalovirus reactivation is prone to occur in the transplanted organ. The same may be true for Kaposi's sarcoma–associated herpesvirus.
[c]Epstein-Barr virus reactivation usually presents as an extranodal proliferation of transformed B cells and can be present either as a diffuse disease or as a mass lesion in a single organ.
[d]Rabies virus has been transmitted through corneal transplants.
[e]*T. gondii* usually causes disease in the brain. In hematopoietic stem-cell transplant recipients, acute pulmonary disease may also occur. Heart transplant recipients develop disease in the allograft.
[f]*Strongyloides* "hyperinfection" may present with pulmonary disease—often associated with gram-negative bacterial pneumonia.
[g]Although transmission with organs has been described, it is unusual.
[h]CJD (sporadic and familial) has been transmitted with corneal transplants. Whether it can be transmitted with blood is not known.
[i]Variant CJD can be transmitted with transfused non-leukodepleted blood, posing a theoretical risk to transplant recipients.

to bathe the donor kidney while it awaits implantation. The reported rate of bacterial contamination of transplanted stem cells (bone marrow, peripheral blood, cord blood) is as high as 17% but is most commonly ~1%. The use of enrichment columns and monoclonal-antibody depletion procedures results in a higher incidence of contamination. In one series of patients receiving contaminated products, 14% had fever or bacteremia, but none died. Results of cultures performed at the time of cryopreservation and at the time of thawing were helpful in guiding therapy for the recipient.

In many transplantation centers, transmission of infections that may be latent or clinically inapparent in the donor organ has resulted in the development of specific donor-screening protocols. In addition to ordering serologic studies focused on viruses such as herpes-group viruses [herpes simplex virus types 1 and 2 (HSV-1, HSV-2), varicella-zoster virus (VZV), cytomegalovirus (CMV), human herpesvirus (HHV) type 6, Epstein-Barr virus (EBV), and Kaposi's sarcoma–associated herpesvirus (KSHV)] as well as hepatitis B and C viruses, human immunodeficiency virus (HIV), human T-cell lymphotropic virus type I, and West Nile virus, donors should be screened for parasites such as *Toxoplasma gondii and Trypanosoma cruzi* (the latter particularly in Latin America). Clinicians caring for prospective organ donors should also consider assessing stool for parasites, should examine chest radiographs for evidence of granulomatous disease, and should perform purified protein derivative (PPD) skin testing or obtain blood for immune cell–based assays that detect active or latent *Mycobacterium tuberculosis* infection. An investigation of the donor's dietary habits (e.g., consumption of raw meat or fish or of unpasteurized dairy products), occupations or avocations (e.g., gardening or spelunking), and travel history (e.g., travel to areas with endemic fungi) is also mandatory. It is expected that the recipient will have been likewise assessed. Because of immune dysfunction resulting from chemotherapy or underlying chronic disease, however, direct testing of the recipient may prove less reliable. This chapter considers aspects of infection unique to various transplantation settings.

INFECTIONS IN HEMATOPOIETIC STEM-CELL TRANSPLANT (HSCT) RECIPIENTS

Transplantation of hematopoietic stem cells from bone marrow or from peripheral or cord blood for cancer, immunodeficiency, or autoimmune disease results in a transient state of complete immunologic incompetence. Immediately after transplantation, both phagocytes and adaptive immune cells (T and B cells) are absent, and the host is extremely susceptible to infection. The reconstitution that follows transplantation has been likened to maturation of the immune system in neonates. The analogy does not entirely predict infections seen in HSCT recipients, however, because the new cells mature in an old host who has several latent infections already. Nevertheless, most infections occur in a predictable time frame after transplantation (Table 12-2).

BACTERIAL INFECTIONS

In the first month after hematopoietic stem-cell transplantation, infectious complications are similar to those in granulocytopenic patients receiving chemotherapy for acute leukemia (Chap. 11). Because of the anticipated 1- to 3-week duration of neutropenia and the high rate of bacterial infection in this population, many centers give prophylactic antibiotics to patients upon initiation of myeloablative therapy. Quinolones decrease the incidence of gram-negative bacteremia among these patients. Bacterial infections are common in the first few days after hematopoietic stem-cell transplantation. The organisms involved are predominantly those found on the skin or in IV catheters (*Staphylococcus aureus*, coagulase-negative staphylococci) and aerobic bacteria that colonize the bowel (*Escherichia coli*, *Klebsiella*, *Pseudomonas*). Beyond the first few days of neutropenia, infections with filamentous bacteria such as *Nocardia* become more common. Episodes of bacteremia due to encapsulated organisms mark the late posttransplantation period (>6 months after hematopoietic stem-cell reconstitution).

Chemotherapy and use of broad-spectrum antibiotics place HSCT patients at risk for diarrhea and colitis caused by *Clostridium difficile* overgrowth and toxin production.

FUNGAL INFECTIONS

Beyond the first week after transplantation, fungal infections become increasingly common, particularly among patients who have received broad-spectrum antibiotics. As in most granulocytopenic patients, *Candida* infections are most commonly seen in this setting. With increased use of prophylactic fluconazole, infections with resistant fungi—in particular, *Aspergillus* and other molds (*Fusarium*, *Scedosporium*, *Penicillium*)—have become more common, prompting some centers to replace fluconazole with agents such as caspofungin, voriconazole, and posaconazole. The role of antifungal prophylaxis with these different agents, in contrast to empirical treatment for suspected or documented infection, remains controversial (Chap. 11). In patients with graft-versus-host disease (GVHD) who require prolonged or indefinite courses of glucocorticoids and other immunosuppressive agents [e.g., cyclosporine, FK506 (tacrolimus), mycophenolate, rapamycin (sirolimus), antithymocyte globulin, or anti-CD52 antibody (alemtuzumab, an antilymphocyte and antimonocyte monoclonal antibody)], there is a high risk of fungal infection

TABLE 12-2

COMMON SOURCES OF INFECTIONS AFTER HEMATOPOIETIC STEM CELL TRANSPLANTATION

	PERIOD AFTER TRANSPLANTATION		
INFECTION SITE	**EARLY (<1 MONTH)**	**MIDDLE (1–4 MONTHS)**	**LATE (>6 MONTHS)**
Disseminated	Aerobic gram-negative, gram-positive bacteria	*Nocardia* *Candida, Aspergillus*	Encapsulated bacteria (*Streptococcus pneumoniae, Haemophilus influenzae, Neisseria meningitidis*)
Skin and mucous membranes	HSV	HHV-6	VZV
Lungs	Aerobic gram-negative, gram-positive bacteria *Candida, Aspergillus* HSV	CMV, seasonal respiratory viruses *Pneumocystis* *Toxoplasma*	*Pneumocystis*
Gastrointestinal tract		CMV	
Kidney		BK virus, adenovirus	BK virus
Brain	HHV-6	HHV-6 *Toxoplasma*	*Toxoplasma* JC virus
Bone marrow	HHV-6		

Note: CMV, cytomegalovirus; HHV-6, human herpesvirus type 6; HSV, herpes simplex virus; VZV, varicella-zoster virus.

(usually with *Candida* or *Aspergillus*), even after engraftment and resolution of neutropenia. These patients are also at high risk for reactivation of latent fungal infection (histoplasmosis, coccidioidomycosis, blastomycosis) in areas where endemic fungi reside and if they have been involved in activities such as gardening or caving. Prolonged use of central venous catheters for parenteral nutrition (lipids) increases the risk of fungemia with *Malassezia*. Some centers administer prophylactic antifungal agents to these patients. Because of the high and prolonged risk of *Pneumocystis jiroveci* pneumonia (especially among patients being treated for hematologic malignancies), most patients receive maintenance prophylaxis with trimethoprim-sulfamethoxazole (TMP-SMX) starting 1 month after engraftment and continuing for at least 1 year.

PARASITIC INFECTIONS

The regimen just described for the fungal pathogen *Pneumocystis* may also protect patients seropositive for the parasite *T. gondii*, which may cause pneumonia or, more commonly, central nervous system (CNS) lesions. The advantages of maintaining HSCT recipients on daily TMP-SMX for 1 year after transplantation include some protection against *Listeria monocytogenes* and nocardial disease as well as late infections with *Streptococcus pneumoniae* and *Haemophilus influenzae*, which are a consequence of the inability of the immature immune system to respond to polysaccharide antigens.

VIRAL INFECTIONS

HSCT recipients are susceptible to infection with a variety of viruses, including primary and reactivation syndromes caused by most HHVs (Table 12-3) and acute infections caused by viruses that circulate in the community.

TABLE 12-3

COMMON HERPESVIRUS SYNDROMES IN TRANSPLANT RECIPIENTS

VIRUS	REACTIVATION DISEASE
Herpes simplex virus type 1	Oral lesions Esophageal lesions Pneumonia (only in hematopoietic stem-cell transplant recipients) Hepatitis
Herpes simplex virus type 2	Anogenital lesions Hepatitis
Varicella-zoster virus	Zoster (potentially disseminated)
Cytomegalovirus	Associated graft rejection Fever Bone marrow failure Pneumonitis Gastrointestinal disease Other
Epstein-Barr virus	B-cell lymphoproliferative disease/lymphoma Oral hairy leukoplakia (rare)
Human herpesvirus type 6	Fever Delayed monocyte/platelet engraftment Encephalitis (controversial)
Human herpesvirus type 7	Undefined
Kaposi's sarcoma–associated virus	Kaposi's sarcoma Primary effusion lymphoma (rare) Multicentric Castleman's disease (rare) Marrow aplasia

Herpes Simplex Virus

Within the first 2 weeks after transplantation, most patients who are seropositive for HSV-1 excrete the virus from the oropharynx. The ability to isolate HSV declines with time. Administration of prophylactic acyclovir (or valacyclovir) to seropositive HSCT recipients has been shown to reduce mucositis and prevent HSV pneumonia (a rare condition reported almost exclusively in allogeneic HSCT recipients). Both esophagitis (usually due to HSV-1) and anogenital disease (commonly induced by HSV-2) may be prevented with acyclovir prophylaxis. For further discussion, see Chap. 80.

Varicella-Zoster Virus

Reactivation of herpes zoster may occur within the first month, but more commonly occurs several months after transplantation. Reactivation rates are ~40% for allogeneic recipients and 25% for autologous recipients. Localized zoster can spread rapidly in an immunosuppressed patient. Fortunately, disseminated disease can usually be controlled with high doses of acyclovir. Because of frequent dissemination among patients with skin lesions, acyclovir is given prophylactically in some centers to prevent severe disease. Low doses of acyclovir (400 mg orally, three times daily) appear to be effective in preventing reactivation of VZV. However, acyclovir can also suppress the development of VZV-specific immunity. Thus its administration for only 6 months after transplantation does not prevent zoster from occurring when treatment is stopped. Some data suggest that administration of low doses of acyclovir for an entire year after transplantation is effective and may eliminate most cases of posttransplantation zoster. For further discussion, see Chap. 81.

Cytomegalovirus

The onset of CMV disease (interstitial pneumonia, bone marrow suppression, graft failure, hepatitis/colitis) usually begins 30–90 days after transplantation, when the granulocyte count is adequate but immunologic reconstitution has not occurred. CMV disease rarely develops earlier than 14 days after transplantation and may become evident as late as 4 months after the procedure. It is of greatest concern in the second month after transplantation, particularly in allogeneic HSCT recipients. In cases in which the donor marrow is depleted of T cells (to prevent GVHD or eliminate a T-cell tumor), the disease may be manifested earlier. The use of alemtuzumab to prevent GVHD in nonmyeloablative transplantation has been associated with an increase in CMV disease. Patients who receive ganciclovir for prophylaxis, preemptive treatment, or treatment (see below) may develop recurrent CMV infection even later than 4 months after transplantation, as treatment appears to delay the development of the normal immune response to CMV infection. Although CMV disease may present as isolated fever, granulocytopenia, thrombocytopenia, or gastrointestinal disease, the foremost cause of death from CMV infection in the setting of hematopoietic stem-cell transplantation is pneumonia.

With the standard use of CMV-negative or filtered blood products, primary CMV infection should be a risk in allogeneic transplantation only when the donor is CMV-seropositive and the recipient is CMV-seronegative. Reactivation disease or superinfection with another strain from the donor is also common in CMV-positive recipients, and most seropositive patients who undergo hematopoietic stem-cell transplantation excrete CMV, with or without clinical findings. Serious CMV disease is much more common among allogeneic than autologous recipients and is often associated with GVHD. In addition to pneumonia and marrow suppression (and, less often, graft failure), manifestations of CMV disease in HSCT recipients include fever with or without arthralgias, myalgias, hepatitis, and esophagitis. CMV ulcerations occur in both the lower and the upper gastrointestinal tract, and it may be difficult to distinguish diarrhea due to GVHD from that due to CMV infection. The finding of CMV in the liver of a patient with GVHD does not necessarily mean that CMV is responsible for hepatic enzyme abnormalities. It is interesting that the ocular and neurologic manifestations of CMV infections are uncommon in these patients.

Management of CMV disease in HSCT recipients includes strategies directed at prophylaxis and preemptive therapy (suppression of silent replication) and at treatment of disease. Prophylaxis results in a lower incidence of disease at the cost of treating many patients who otherwise would not require therapy. Because of the high fatality rate associated with CMV pneumonia in these patients and the difficulty of early diagnosis of CMV infection, prophylactic IV ganciclovir (or oral valganciclovir) has been used in some centers and has been shown to abort CMV disease during the period of maximal vulnerability (from engraftment to day 120 after transplantation). Ganciclovir also prevents HSV reactivation and reduces the risk of VZV reactivation; thus acyclovir prophylaxis should be discontinued when ganciclovir is administered. The foremost problem with the administration of ganciclovir relates to adverse effects, which include dose-related bone marrow suppression (thrombocytopenia, leukopenia, anemia, and pancytopenia). Because the frequency of CMV pneumonia is lower among autologous HSCT recipients (2–7%) than among allogeneic HSCT recipients (10–40%), prophylaxis in the former group will not become the rule until a less toxic oral antiviral agent becomes available. Promising new drugs that are now being assessed in clinical trials include maribavir, a benzimidazole ribonucleoside that inhibits a viral protein kinase activity (UL97).

Like prophylaxis, preemptive treatment, which targets patients with polymerase chain reaction (PCR) evidence of CMV, entails the unnecessary treatment of many individuals (on the basis of a laboratory test that is not highly predictive of disease) with drugs that have adverse effects. Currently, because of the neutropenia associated with ganciclovir in HSCT recipients, a preemptive approach—that is, treatment of those patients in whose blood CMV is detected by an antigen or nucleic acid amplification test—is used at most centers. This approach is almost as effective as prophylaxis and causes less toxicity. Quantitative viral load assays, which are not dependent on circulating polymorphonuclear leukocytes, have supplanted antigen-based assays and are used by most centers. A positive test (or increasing viral load) prompts the initiation of preemptive therapy. When prophylaxis or preemptive therapy is stopped, late disease may occur, although by then the patient is often equipped with improved graft function and is better able to combat disease.

Treatment of CMV pneumonia in HSCT recipients (unlike that in other clinical settings) involves both IV immune globulin (IVIg) and ganciclovir. In patients who cannot tolerate ganciclovir, foscarnet is a useful alternative, although it may produce nephrotoxicity and electrolyte imbalance. When neither ganciclovir nor foscarnet is clinically tolerated, cidofovir can be used; however, its efficacy is less well established, and its side effects include nephrotoxicity. Case reports have suggested that the immunosuppressive agent leflunomide may be active in this setting, but controlled studies are lacking. Maribavir is under investigation for treatment as well as prophylaxis. Transfusion of CMV-specific T cells from the donor decreased viral load in a small series of patients; this result suggests that immunotherapy may play a role in the treatment of this disease in the future.

For further discussion, see Chap. 83.

Human Herpesviruses 6 and 7

HHV-6, the cause of roseola in children, is a ubiquitous herpesvirus that reactivates (as determined by quantitative plasma PCR) in ~50% of HSCT recipients 2–4 weeks after transplantation. Reactivation is more common among patients requiring glucocorticoids for GVHD and among those receiving second transplants. Reactivation of HHV-6 (primarily type B) appears to be associated with delayed monocyte and platelet engraftment. Although encephalitis developing after transplantation has been associated with HHV-6 in cerebrospinal fluid (CSF), the causality of the association is not well defined. In several cases, plasma viremia was detected long before the onset of encephalitis; nevertheless, patients with encephalitis did tend to have very high viral loads in plasma at the time of CNS illness. HHV-6 DNA is sometimes found in lung samples after transplantation. However, its role in pneumonitis is also unclear. Although HHV-6 has been shown to be susceptible to foscarnet (and possibly to ganciclovir) in vitro, the efficacy of antiviral treatment has not been well studied. Little is known about the related herpesvirus HHV-7 or its role in posttransplantation infection. For further discussion, see Chap. 83.

Epstein-Barr Virus

Primary EBV infection can be fatal to HSCT recipients; EBV reactivation can cause EBV–B-cell lymphoproliferative disease (EBV-LPD), which may also be fatal to patients taking immunosuppressive drugs. Latent EBV infection of B cells leads to several interesting phenomena in HSCT recipients. The marrow ablation that occurs as part of the HSCT procedure may sometimes eliminate latent EBV from the host. Infection can then be reacquired immediately after transplantation by transfer of infected donor B cells. Rarely, transplantation from a seronegative donor may result in cure. The recipient is then at risk for a second primary infection.

EBV-LPD can develop in the recipient's B cells (if any survive marrow ablation) but is more likely to be a consequence of outgrowth of infected donor cells. Both lytic and latent EBV replication are more likely during immunosuppression (e.g., they are associated with GVHD and the use of antibodies to T cells). Although less likely in autologous transplantation, reactivation can occur in T-cell–depleted autologous recipients (e.g., patients being given antibodies to T cells for the treatment of a T-cell lymphoma with marrow depletion). EBV-LPD, which can become apparent as early as 1–3 months after engraftment, can cause high fevers and cervical adenopathy resembling the symptoms of infectious mononucleosis but more commonly presents as an extranodal mass. The incidence of EBV-LPD among allogeneic HSCT recipients is 0.6–1%, which contrasts with figures of ~5% for renal transplant recipients and up to 20% for cardiac transplant patients. In all cases, EBV-LPD is more likely to occur with high-dose, prolonged immunosuppression, especially that caused by the use of antibodies to T cells, glucocorticoids, and calcineurin inhibitors (e.g., cyclosporine, FK506).

PCR can be used to monitor EBV production after hematopoietic stem-cell transplantation. High or increasing viral loads predict an enhanced likelihood of developing EBV-LPD and should prompt rapid reduction of immunosuppression and search for a focus of disease. If reduction of immunosuppression does not have the desired effect, administration of a monoclonal antibody to CD20 (rituximab or others) for the treatment of B-cell lymphomas that express this surface protein has elicited dramatic responses and currently constitutes first-line therapy for CD20-positive EBV-LPD. However, long-term suppression of new antibody responses accompanies therapy, and recurrences are not infrequent. Additional B-cell–directed antibodies, including anti-CD22, are under study. The role of antivirals is uncertain because no available agents have been documented to have activity against the different forms of latent EBV infection. Preventing lytic replication in these patients would theoretically produce a statistical decrease in the frequency of latent disease by decreasing the number of virions available to cause additional infection. In case reports and small animal studies, ganciclovir and/or high-dose zidovudine together with other agents has been used to eradicate EBV-LPD and CNS lymphomas, another EBV-associated complication of transplantation. Both interferon and retinoic acid have been employed in the treatment of EBV-LPD, as has IVIg, but no large prospective studies have assessed the efficacy of any of these agents. Several additional drugs are undergoing preclinical evaluation. Standard chemotherapeutic regimens have been used as a last resort, even though patients' tolerance and long-term results have been disappointing. EBV-specific T cells generated from the donor have been used experimentally to prevent and to treat EBV-LPD in allogeneic recipients, and efforts are underway to increase the activity and specificity of ex vivo–generated T cells.

For further discussion, see Chap. 82.

Human Herpesvirus 8

The EBV-related gammaherpesvirus KSHV, which is causally associated with Kaposi's sarcoma, with primary effusion lymphoma, and with multicentric Castleman's disease, has rarely resulted in disease in HSCT recipients, although some cases of virus-associated marrow aplasia have been reported in the peritransplantation period. The relatively low seroprevalence of KSHV in the population and the limited duration of profound T-cell suppression after hematopoietic stem-cell transplantation provide a probable explanation for the currently low incidence of KSHV disease. For further discussion, see Chap. 83.

Other (Nonherpes) Viruses

The diagnosis of pneumonia in HSCT recipients poses some special problems. Because patients have undergone treatment with multiple chemotherapeutic agents and sometimes irradiation, their differential diagnosis should include—in addition to bacterial and fungal pneumonia—CMV pneumonitis, pneumonia of other viral etiologies, parasitic pneumonia, diffuse alveolar hemorrhage, and chemical- or radiation-associated pneumonitis. Since fungi and viruses [e.g., influenza A and B viruses, respiratory syncytial virus (RSV), parainfluenza virus (types 1, 2, and 3), metapneumoviruses, and adenoviruses] are also causes of pneumonia in this setting, it is important to diagnose CMV specifically (see "Cytomegalovirus" earlier in the chapter). *M. tuberculosis* has been an uncommon cause of pneumonia among HSCT recipients in Western countries (accounting for <0.1–0.2% of cases) but is common in Hong Kong (5.5%) and in countries where the prevalence of tuberculosis is high. The recipient's exposure history is clearly critical in an assessment of posttransplantation infections.

Both RSV and parainfluenza viruses, particularly type 3, can cause severe or even fatal pneumonia in HSCT recipients. Infections with both of these agents sometimes occur as disastrous nosocomial epidemics. Preemptive treatment of upper airway infection and therapy for established lower tract invasion with aerosolized ribavirin and/or the anti-RSV monoclonal antibody palivizumab have been reported to lessen the severity of RSV disease in some studies. (RespiGam, a polyclonal anti-RSV preparation, is no longer available.) However, no large prospective studies establishing the efficacy of these agents in HSCT recipients have been performed. Aerosolized ribavirin is difficult to administer. Antibody in particular may prove more active in immunocompromised hosts, but relevant evaluation is lacking.

Influenza also occurs in HSCT recipients and generally mirrors the presence of infection in the community. Progression to pneumonia is more common when infection occurs early after transplantation and when the recipient is lymphopenic. Several drugs are available for the treatment of influenza. Amantadine and rimantadine have limited effects, primarily reducing symptoms and shortening the duration of illness caused by sensitive strains of influenza A virus. The neuraminidase inhibitors oseltamivir (oral) and zanamivir (aerosolized) are active against both influenza A virus and influenza B virus and are a reasonable treatment option. Parenteral forms of neuraminidase inhibitors are undergoing clinical trials. An important preventive measure is immunization of household members, hospital staff members, and other frequent contacts.

Human metapneumovirus, a paramyxovirus, can sometimes cause severe pneumonia and respiratory failure in HSCT recipients; however, mild or even asymptomatic infection may be more common. At present, the overall contribution of human metapneumovirus to the burden of lower respiratory tract disease in HSCT recipients is unknown.

Adenovirus can be isolated from HSCT recipients at rates varying from 5–18%. Although hemorrhagic cystitis, pneumonia, gastroenteritis, and fatal disseminated infection have been reported, adenovirus infection, which (like CMV infection) usually occurs in the first or second month after transplantation, is often asymptomatic. A role for cidofovir therapy has been suggested, but the efficacy of this agent is unproven.

Infections with parvovirus B19 (presenting as anemia or occasionally as pancytopenia) and enteroviruses (sometimes fatal) can occur. Parvovirus infection may possibly respond to IVIg (Chap. 85). Intranasal pleconaril, a capsid-binding agent, is being studied for the treatment of enterovirus infection.

Rhinoviruses and coronaviruses are frequent co-pathogens in HSCT recipients; however, whether they independently contribute to significant pulmonary infection is not known. Rotaviruses are a common cause of gastroenteritis in these patients. The polyomavirus BK virus is found at high titers in the urine of patients who are profoundly immunosuppressed. BK viruria may be associated with hemorrhagic cystitis in these patients. Compared with the incidence among patients with impaired T-cell function due to HIV infection, progressive multifocal leukoencephalopathy caused by the related JC virus is rare among HSCT recipients (Chap. 29). When transmitted by mosquitoes or by blood transfusion, West Nile virus can cause encephalitis and death after hematopoietic stem-cell transplantation.

INFECTIONS IN SOLID ORGAN TRANSPLANT (SOT) RECIPIENTS

Morbidity and mortality among SOT recipients are reduced by the use of effective antibiotics. The organisms that cause acute infections in recipients of SOT are different from those that infect HSCT recipients because SOT recipients do not go through a period of neutropenia. As the transplantation procedure involves major surgery, however, SOT recipients are subject to infections at anastomotic sites and to wound infections. Compared with HSCT recipients, SOT patients are immunosuppressed for longer periods (often permanently). Thus they are susceptible to many of the same organisms as patients with chronically impaired T-cell immunity (Chap. 11, especially Table 11-1).

During the early period (<1 month after transplantation), infections are most commonly caused by extracellular bacteria (staphylococci, streptococci, enterococci, *E. coli*, other gram-negative organisms), which often originate in surgical wound or anastomotic sites. The type of transplant largely determines the spectrum of infection.

In subsequent weeks, the consequences of the administration of agents that suppress cell-mediated immunity become apparent, and acquisition or reactivation of viruses and parasites (from the recipient or from the transplanted organ) can occur. CMV infection is often a problem, particularly in the first 6 months after transplantation, and may present as severe systemic disease or as infection of the transplanted organ. HHV-6 reactivation (assessed by plasma PCR) occurs within the first 2–4 weeks after transplantation and may be associated with fever, leukopenia, and possibly encephalitis. Data suggest that replication of HHV-6 and HHV-7 may exacerbate CMV-induced disease. CMV is associated not only with generalized immunosuppression, but also with organ-specific, rejection-related syndromes: glomerulopathy in kidney transplant recipients, bronchiolitis obliterans in lung transplant recipients, vasculopathy in heart transplant recipients, and the vanishing bile duct syndrome in liver transplant recipients. A complex interplay between increased CMV replication and enhanced graft rejection is well established: Increasing immunosuppression leads to increased CMV replication, which is associated with graft rejection. For this reason, considerable attention has been focused on the diagnosis, prophylaxis, and treatment of CMV infection in SOT recipients. Early transmission of West Nile virus to transplant recipients from an organ donor has been reported; however, the risk of West Nile acquisition has been reduced by implementation of screening procedures.

Beyond 6 months after transplantation, infections characteristic of patients with defects in cell-mediated immunity—e.g., infections with *Listeria*, *Nocardia*, *Rhodococcus*, various fungi, and other intracellular pathogens—may be a problem. International patients and global travelers may experience reactivation of dormant infections with trypanosomes, *Leishmania*, *Plasmodium*, *Strongyloides*, and other parasites. Elimination of these late infections will not be possible until the patient develops specific tolerance to the transplanted organ in the absence of drugs that lead to generalized immunosuppression. Meanwhile, vigilance, prophylaxis/preemptive therapy (when indicated), and rapid diagnosis and treatment of infections can be lifesaving in SOT recipients, who, unlike most HSCT recipients, continue to be immunosuppressed.

SOT recipients are susceptible to EBV-LPD from as early as 2 months to many years after transplantation. The prevalence of this complication is increased by potent and prolonged use of T-cell–suppressive drugs. Decreasing the degree of immunosuppression may in some cases reverse the condition. Among SOT patients, those with heart and lung transplants—who receive the most intensive immunosuppressive regimens—are most likely to develop EBV-LPD, particularly in the lungs. Although the disease usually originates in recipient B cells, several cases of donor origin, particularly in the transplanted organ, have been noted. High organ-specific content of B lymphoid tissues (e.g., bronchial-associated lymphoid tissue in the lung), anatomic factors (e.g., lack of access of host T cells to the transplanted organ because of disturbed lymphatics), and differences in major histocompatibility loci between the host T cells and the organ (e.g., lack of cell migration or lack of effective T-cell/macrophage cooperation) may result in defective elimination of EBV-infected B cells. SOT recipients are also highly susceptible to the development of Kaposi's sarcoma and less frequently to the B-cell proliferative disorders associated with KSHV, such as primary effusion lymphoma and multicentric Castleman's disease. Kaposi's sarcoma is much more common (in fact, 550–1000 times more common than in the general population), can develop very rapidly after transplantation, and can also occur in the allograft. However, because the seroprevalence of KSHV is very low in Western countries, Kaposi's sarcoma is not often observed.

KIDNEY TRANSPLANTATION

(See Table 12-4)

Early Infections

Bacteria often cause infections that develop in the period immediately after kidney transplantation. There is a role for perioperative antibiotic prophylaxis, and many centers give cephalosporins to decrease the risk of postoperative complications. Urinary tract infections developing soon after transplantation are usually related to anatomic alterations resulting from surgery. Such early infections may require prolonged treatment (e.g., 6 weeks of antibiotic administration for pyelonephritis). Urinary tract infections that occur >6 months after transplantation may be treated for shorter periods because they do not seem to be associated with the high rate of pyelonephritis or relapse seen with infections that occur in the first 3 months.

Prophylaxis with TMP-SMX [1 double-strength tablet (800 mg of sulfamethoxazole, 160 mg of trimethoprim) per day] for the first 4–6 months after transplantation decreases the incidence of early and middle-period infections (see below, Table 12-4, and Table 12-5).

Middle-Period Infections

Because of continuing immunosuppression, kidney transplant recipients are predisposed to lung infections characteristic of those in patients with T-cell deficiency (i.e., infections with intracellular bacteria, mycobacteria, nocardiae, fungi, viruses, and parasites). The high mortality rates associated with *Legionella pneumophila* infection (Chap. 49) led to the closing of renal transplant units in hospitals with endemic legionellosis.

About 50% of all renal transplant recipients presenting with fever 1–4 months after transplantation have evidence of CMV disease; CMV itself accounts for the fever in more than two-thirds of cases and thus is the predominant pathogen during this period. CMV infection (Chap. 83) may also present as arthralgias, myalgias, or organ-specific symptoms. During this period, this infection may represent primary disease (in the case of a seronegative recipient of a kidney from a seropositive donor) or may represent reactivation disease or superinfection. Patients may have atypical lymphocytosis. Unlike immunocompetent patients, however, they often do not have lymphadenopathy or splenomegaly. Therefore, clinical suspicion and laboratory confirmation are necessary for diagnosis. The clinical syndrome may be accompanied by bone marrow suppression (particularly leukopenia). CMV also causes glomerulopathy

TABLE 12-4

COMMON INFECTIONS AFTER KIDNEY TRANSPLANTATION

	PERIOD AFTER TRANSPLANTATION		
INFECTION SITE	**EARLY (<1 MONTH)**	**MIDDLE (1–4 MONTHS)**	**LATE (>6 MONTHS)**
Urinary tract	Bacteria (*Escherichia coli*, *Klebsiella*, Enterobacteriaceae, *Pseudomonas*, *Enterococcus*) associated with bacteremia and pyelonephritis; *Candida*	CMV (fever, bone marrow suppression, hepatitis); BK virus (nephropathy, graft failure, vasculopathy)	Bacteria (late urinary tract infections usually not associated with bacteremia); BK virus (nephropathy, graft failure, generalized vasculopathy)
Lungs	Bacteria (*Legionella* in endemic settings)	CMV disease; *Pneumocystis; Legionella*	*Nocardia*; invasive fungi
Central nervous system		*Listeria* (meningitis); *Toxoplasma gondii*	CMV disease; *Listeria* (meningitis); *Cryptococcus* (meningitis); *Nocardia*

Note: CMV, cytomegalovirus.

TABLE 12-5

PROPHYLAXIS OF INFECTIONS IN TRANSPLANT RECIPIENTS

RISK FACTOR	ORGANISM	PROPHYLACTIC ANTIBIOTICS	EXAMINATION(S)[a]
Travel to or residence in area with known risk of fungal infection	*Coccidioides, Histoplasma, Blastomyces*	Consider imidazoles	Chest radiography, antigen testing, serology
Latent viruses	HSV, VZV, EBV, CMV	Acyclovir after hematopoietic stem-cell transplantation to prevent HSV and VZV; ganciclovir to prevent CMV in some settings	Serologic test for HSV, VZV, CMV, HHV-6, EBV, KSHV
Latent fungi and parasites	*Pneumocystis jiroveci, Toxoplasma gondii*	Trimethoprim-sulfamethoxazole (dapsone or atovaquone)	Serology for *Toxoplasma*
History of exposure to tuberculosis or latent tuberculosis	*Mycobacterium tuberculosis*	Isoniazid if recent conversion for positive chest imaging and/or no previous treatment	Chest imaging; PPD and/or cell-based assay

[a]Serologic examination, PPD testing, and interferon assays may be less reliable after transplantation.

Note: CMV, cytomegalovirus; EBV, Epstein-Barr virus; HHV-6, human herpesvirus type 6; HSV, herpes simplex virus; KSHV, Kaposi's sarcoma–associated herpesvirus; PPD, purified protein derivative; VZV, varicella-zoster virus.

and is associated with an increased incidence of other opportunistic infections. Because of the frequency and severity of disease, a considerable effort has been made to prevent and treat CMV infection in renal transplant recipients. An immune globulin preparation enriched with antibodies to CMV was used by many centers in the past in an effort to protect the group at highest risk for severe infection (seronegative recipients of seropositive kidneys). However, with the development of highly effective oral antiviral agents, CMV immune globulin is no longer used. Ganciclovir (valganciclovir) is beneficial when prophylaxis is indicated and for the treatment of serious CMV disease. One study showed a significant (50%) reduction in CMV disease and rejection at 6 months among patients who received prophylactic valacyclovir (an acyclovir congener) for the first 90 days after renal transplantation. Acyclovir (valacyclovir) is less efficacious, but is also less toxic than ganciclovir (valganciclovir). The availability of valganciclovir and valacyclovir has allowed most centers to move to oral prophylaxis for transplant recipients. Additional oral prophylactic agents, such as maribavir, are in clinical study.

Infection with the other herpes-group viruses may become evident within 6 months after transplantation or later. Early after transplantation, HSV may cause either oral or anogenital lesions that are usually responsive to acyclovir. Large ulcerating lesions in the anogenital area may lead to bladder and rectal dysfunction as well as predisposing to bacterial infection. VZV may cause fatal disseminated infection in nonimmune kidney transplant recipients, but in immune patients, reactivation zoster usually does not disseminate outside the dermatome; thus disseminated VZV infection is a less fearsome complication in kidney transplantation than in hematopoietic stem-cell transplantation. HHV-6 reactivation may take place and (although usually asymptomatic) may be associated with fever, rash, marrow suppression, or encephalitis.

EBV disease is more serious; it may present as an extranodal proliferation of B cells that invade the CNS, nasopharynx, liver, small bowel, heart, and other organs, including the transplanted kidney. The disease is diagnosed by the finding of a mass of proliferating EBV-positive B cells. The incidence of EBV-LPD is higher among patients who acquire EBV infection from the donor and among patients given high doses of cyclosporine, FK506, glucocorticoids, and anti–T-cell antibodies. Disease may regress once immunocompetence is restored. KSHV infection can be transmitted with the donor kidney, although it more often represents latent infection of the recipient. Kaposi's sarcoma often appears within 1 year after transplantation, although the range of onset is wide (1 month to ~20 years). Avoidance of immunosuppressive agents that inhibit calcineurin has been associated with less outgrowth of EBV and less CMV replication. The use of rapamycin (sirolimus) has led to regression of Kaposi's sarcoma.

The papovaviruses BK virus and JC virus (polyomavirus hominis types 1 and 2) have been cultured from the urine of kidney transplant recipients (as they have from that of HSCT recipients) in the setting of profound immunosuppression. High levels of BK virus replication detected by PCR in urine and blood are predictive of pathology, particularly in the setting of renal transplantation. Excretion of BK virus and BK viremia are associated with the development of ureteral strictures, polyomavirus-associated nephropathy (1–10% of renal transplant recipients), and (less commonly) generalized vasculopathy. Timely reduction of immunosuppression is critical and can reduce rates of graft loss related to polyomavirus-associated nephropathy from 90% to 10–30%. A possible role for treatment with cidofovir (given by the IV route and by bladder instillation), leflunomide, quinolones, and (most recently) lactoferrin has been reported, but the efficacy of these agents has not been substantiated through adequate clinical study. JC virus is associated with rare cases of progressive multifocal leukoencephalopathy. Adenoviruses may persist with continued immunosuppression in these patients, but disseminated disease like that which occurs in HSCT recipients is much less common.

Kidney transplant recipients are also subject to infections with other intracellular organisms. These patients may develop pulmonary infections with *Nocardia*, *Aspergillus*, and *Mucor* as well as infections with other pathogens in which the T-cell/macrophage axis plays an important role. In patients without IV catheters, *L. monocytogenes* is a common cause of bacteremia ≥1 month after renal transplantation and should be seriously considered in renal transplant recipients presenting with fever and headache. Kidney transplant recipients may develop *Salmonella* bacteremia, which can lead to endovascular infections and require prolonged therapy. Pulmonary infections with *Pneumocystis* are common unless the patient is maintained on TMP-SMX prophylaxis. *Nocardia* infection (Chap. 63) may present in the skin, bones, and lungs or in the CNS, where it usually takes the form of single or multiple brain abscesses. Nocardiosis generally occurs ≥1 month after transplantation and may follow immunosuppressive treatment for an episode of rejection. Pulmonary findings are nonspecific: localized disease with or without cavities is most common, but the disease may disseminate. The diagnosis is made by culture of the organism from sputum or from the involved nodule. As with *Pneumocystis*, prophylaxis with TMP-SMX is often efficacious in the prevention of disease. The occurrence of *Nocardia* infections >2 years after transplantation suggests that a long-term prophylactic regimen may be justified.

Toxoplasmosis can occur in seropositive patients but is less common than in other transplant settings, usually developing in the first few months after kidney transplantation. Again, TMP-SMX is helpful in prevention. In endemic areas, histoplasmosis, coccidioidomycosis, and blastomycosis may cause pulmonary infiltrates or disseminated disease.

Late Infections

Late infections (>6 months after kidney transplantation) may involve the CNS and include CMV retinitis as well as other CNS manifestations of CMV disease. Patients (particularly those whose immunosuppression has been increased) are at risk for subacute meningitis due to *Cryptococcus neoformans*. Cryptococcal disease may present in an insidious manner (sometimes as a skin infection before the development of clear CNS findings). *Listeria* meningitis may have an acute presentation and requires prompt therapy to avoid a fatal outcome.

Patients who continue to take glucocorticoids are predisposed to ongoing infection. "Transplant elbow" is a recurrent bacterial infection in and around the elbow that is thought to result from a combination of poor tensile strength of the skin of steroid-treated patients and steroid-induced proximal myopathy that requires patients to push themselves up with their elbows to get out of chairs. Bouts of cellulitis (usually caused by *S. aureus*) recur until patients are provided with elbow protection.

Kidney transplant recipients are susceptible to invasive fungal infections, including those due to *Aspergillus* and *Rhizopus*, which may present as superficial lesions before dissemination. Mycobacterial infection (particularly that with *Mycobacterium marinum*) can be diagnosed by skin examination. Infection with *Prototheca wickerhamii* (an achlorophyllic alga) has been diagnosed by skin biopsy. Warts caused by human papillomaviruses (HPVs) are a late consequence of persistent immunosuppression; imiquimod or other forms of local therapy are usually satisfactory.

Although BK virus replication and virus-associated disease can be detected far earlier, the median time to clinical diagnosis of polyomavirus-associated nephropathy is ~300 days, qualifying it as a late-onset disease. With establishment of better screening procedures (e.g., blood PCR), it is likely that this disease will be detected earlier (see "Middle-Period Infections" earlier in the chapter).

HEART TRANSPLANTATION

Early Infections

Sternal wound infection and mediastinitis are early complications of heart transplantation. An indolent course is common, with fever or a mildly elevated white blood cell count preceding the development of site tenderness or drainage. Clinical suspicion based on evidence of sternal instability and failure to heal may lead to the diagnosis. Common microbial residents of the skin (e.g., *S. aureus*, including methicillin-resistant strains, and *Staphylococcus epidermidis*) as well as gram-negative organisms (e.g., *Pseudomonas aeruginosa*) and fungi (e.g., *Candida*) are often involved. In rare cases, mediastinitis in heart transplant recipients can also be due to *Mycoplasma hominis* (Chap. 76). Since this organism requires an anaerobic environment for growth and may be difficult to see on conventional medium, the laboratory should be alerted that *M. hominis* infection is suspected. *M. hominis* mediastinitis has been cured with a combination of surgical debridement (sometimes requiring muscle-flap placement) and the administration of clindamycin and tetracycline. Organisms associated with mediastinitis may be cultured from accompanying pericardial fluid.

Middle-Period Infections

T. gondii (Chap. 121) residing in the heart of a seropositive donor may be transmitted to a seronegative recipient. Thus serologic screening for *T. gondii* infection is important before and in the months after cardiac transplantation. Rarely, active disease can be introduced at the time of transplantation. The overall incidence of toxoplasmosis is so high in the setting of heart transplantation that some prophylaxis is always warranted. Although alternatives are available, the most frequently used agent is TMP-SMX, which prevents infection with *Pneumocystis* as well as with *Nocardia* and several other bacterial pathogens. CMV also has been transmitted by heart transplantation. CNS infections can be caused by *Toxoplasma*, *Nocardia*, and *Aspergillus*. *L. monocytogenes* meningitis should be considered in heart transplant recipients with fever and headache.

CMV infection is associated with poor outcomes after heart transplantation. The virus is usually cultivable 1–2 months after transplantation, causes early signs and laboratory abnormalities (usually fever and atypical lymphocytosis or leukopenia and thrombocytopenia) at 2–3 months, and can produce severe disease (e.g., pneumonia) at 3–4 months. Seropositive recipients usually develop cultivable virus faster than patients whose primary CMV infection is a consequence of transplantation. Between 40 and 70% of patients develop symptomatic CMV disease in the form of (1) CMV pneumonia, the most likely form to be fatal; (2) CMV esophagitis and gastritis, sometimes accompanied by abdominal pain with or without ulcerations and bleeding; and (3) the CMV syndrome, consisting of CMV in the blood along with fever, leukopenia, thrombocytopenia, and hepatic enzyme abnormalities. Ganciclovir is efficacious in the treatment of CMV infection; prophylaxis with ganciclovir or possibly with other antiviral agents, as described for renal transplantation, may reduce the overall incidence of CMV-related disease. When prophylaxis is stopped, late-onset disease may occur. In fact, because of the expanded use of prophylaxis, this scenario is increasingly common, particularly in patients with ongoing GVHD.

Late Infections

EBV infection usually presents as a lymphoma-like proliferation of B cells late after heart transplantation, particularly in patients maintained on intense immunosuppressive therapy. A subset of heart and heart-lung transplant recipients may develop early fulminant EBV-LPD (within 2 months). Treatment includes the reduction of immunosuppression (if possible), the use of glucocorticoid and calcineurin inhibitor–sparing regimens, and the consideration of therapy with anti–B-cell antibodies (rituximab and possibly others). Immunomodulatory and antiviral agents continue to be studied, and aggressive chemotherapy is a last resort, as discussed earlier for HSCT recipients. KSHV-associated disease, including Kaposi's sarcoma and primary effusion lymphoma, has been reported in heart transplant recipients. Treatment with rapamycin (sirolimus) may prevent both rejection and outgrowth of KSHV-infected cells. Prophylaxis for *Pneumocystis* infection is required for these patients (see "Lung Transplantation, Late Infections" later in the chapter).

LUNG TRANSPLANTATION

Early Infections

It is not surprising that lung transplant recipients are predisposed to the development of pneumonia. The combination of ischemia and the resulting mucosal damage, together with accompanying denervation and lack of lymphatic drainage, probably contributes to the high rate of pneumonia (66% in one series). The prophylactic use of high doses of broad-spectrum antibiotics for the first 3–4 days after surgery may decrease the incidence of pneumonia. Gram-negative pathogens (Enterobacteriaceae and *Pseudomonas* species) are troublesome in the first 2 weeks after surgery (the period of maximal vulnerability). Pneumonia can also be caused by *Candida* (possibly as a result of colonization of the donor lung), *Aspergillus*, and *Cryptococcus*.

Mediastinitis may occur at an even higher rate among lung transplant recipients than among heart transplant recipients and most commonly develops within 2 weeks of surgery. In the absence of prophylaxis, pneumonitis due to CMV (which may be transmitted as a consequence of transplantation) usually presents between 2 weeks and 3 months after surgery, with primary disease occurring later than reactivation disease.

Middle-Period Infections

The incidence of CMV infection, either reactivated or primary, is 75–100% if either the donor or the recipient is seropositive for CMV. CMV-induced disease appears to be most severe in recipients of lung and heart-lung transplants. Whether this severity relates to the mismatch in lung antigen-presenting and host immune cells or is attributable to other (nonimmunologic) factors is not known. More than half of lung transplant recipients with symptomatic CMV disease have pneumonia. Difficulty in distinguishing the radiographic picture of CMV infection from other infections and organ rejection further complicates therapy. CMV can also cause bronchiolitis obliterans in lung transplants. The development of pneumonitis related to HSV has led to the prophylactic use of acyclovir. Such prophylaxis may also decrease rates of CMV disease, but ganciclovir is more active against CMV and is also active against HSV. The prophylaxis of CMV infection with IV ganciclovir—or increasingly with valganciclovir, the oral alternative—is recommended for lung transplant recipients. Antiviral alternatives are discussed in the earlier section on hematopoietic stem-cell transplantation. Although the overall incidence of serious disease is decreased during prophylaxis, late disease may occur when prophylaxis is stopped—a pattern observed increasingly in recent years. With recovery from peritransplantation complications and, in many cases, a decrease in immunosuppression, the recipient is often better equipped to combat late infection.

Late Infections

The incidence of *Pneumocystis* infection (which may present with a paucity of findings) is high among lung and heart-lung transplant recipients. Some form of prophylaxis for *Pneumocystis* pneumonia is indicated in all organ transplant situations (Table 12-5). Prophylaxis with TMP-SMX for 12 months after transplantation may be sufficient to prevent *Pneumocystis* disease in patients whose degree of immunosuppression is not increased.

As in other transplant recipients, infection with EBV may cause either a mononucleosis-like syndrome or EBV-LPD. The tendency of the B-cell blasts to present in the lung appears to be greater after lung transplantation than after the transplantation of other organs. Reduction of immunosuppression and switching of regimens, as discussed in earlier sections, causes remission in some cases, but airway compression can be fatal, and more rapid intervention may therefore become necessary. The approach to EBV-LPD is similar to that described in other sections.

LIVER TRANSPLANTATION

Early Infections

As in other transplantation settings, early bacterial infections are a major problem after liver transplantation. Many centers administer systemic broad-spectrum antibiotics for the first 24 h or sometimes longer after surgery, even in the absence of documented infection. However, despite prophylaxis, infectious complications are common and are correlated with the duration of the surgical procedure and the type of biliary drainage. An operation lasting >12 h is associated with an increased likelihood of infection. Patients who have a choledochojejunostomy with drainage of the biliary duct to a Roux-en-Y jejunal bowel loop have more fungal infections than those whose bile is drained via a choledochocholedochostomy with anastomosis of the donor common bile duct to the recipient common bile duct.

Peritonitis and intraabdominal abscesses are common complications of liver transplantation. Bacterial peritonitis or localized abscesses may result from biliary leaks. Early leaks are even more common (incidence, ~17%) with live-donor liver transplants (LDLTs). Peritonitis in liver transplant recipients is often polymicrobial, commonly involving enterococci, aerobic gram-negative bacteria, staphylococci, anaerobes, *Candida*, or other invasive fungi. Only one-third of patients with intraabdominal abscesses have bacteremia. Abscesses within the first month after surgery may occur not only in and around the liver, but also in the spleen, pericolic area, and pelvis. Treatment includes antibiotic administration and drainage as necessary.

Liver transplant patients have a high incidence of fungal infections, and the occurrence of fungal (often candidal) infection is correlated with preoperative use of glucocorticoids, long duration of treatment with antibacterial agents, and posttransplantation use of immunosuppressive agents.

Middle-Period Infections

The development of postsurgical biliary stricture predisposes patients to cholangitis. The incidence of strictures is increased in LDLT (~17% of liver transplant recipients); therefore, cholangitis is also more common among these patients. Transplant recipients who develop cholangitis may have high spiking fevers and rigors but often lack the characteristic signs and symptoms of classic cholangitis, including abdominal pain and jaundice. Although these findings may suggest graft rejection, rejection is typically accompanied by marked elevation of liver function enzymes. In contrast, in cholangitis in transplant recipients, results of liver function tests (with the possible exception of alkaline phosphatase levels) are often within the normal range. Definitive diagnosis of cholangitis in liver transplant recipients requires documentation of bacteremia or demonstration of aggregated neutrophils in bile duct biopsy specimens. Unfortunately, invasive studies of the biliary tract (either T-tube cholangiography or endoscopic retrograde cholangiopancreatography) may themselves lead to cholangitis. For this reason, many clinicians recommend an empirical trial of therapy with antibiotics covering gram-negative organisms and anaerobes before these procedures are undertaken, as well as antibiotic coverage if they are eventually performed.

Reactivation of viral hepatitis is a common complication of liver transplantation (Chap. 92). Recurrent hepatitis B and C infections, for which transplantation may be performed, are problematic. To prevent hepatitis B virus reinfection, prophylaxis with an optimal antiviral agent or combination of agents (lamivudine, adefovir, entecavir) and hepatitis B immune globulin is currently recommended, although the optimal dose, route, and duration of therapy remain controversial. Success in preventing reinfection with hepatitis B virus has increased in recent years; in contrast, reinfection of the graft with hepatitis C virus occurs in all patients, with a variable time frame. Studies of aggressive pretransplantation treatment of selected recipients with antiviral agents and prophylactic/preemptive regimens are ongoing. However, early initiation of treatment for histologically documented disease with a combination of ribavirin and pegylated interferon has produced sustained responses at rates in the range of 25–40%.

As in other transplantation settings, reactivation disease with herpes-group viruses is common (Table 12-3). Herpesviruses can be transmitted in donor organs. Although CMV hepatitis occurs in ~4% of liver transplant recipients, it is usually not so severe as to require retransplantation. Without prophylaxis, CMV disease develops in the majority of seronegative recipients of organs from CMV-positive donors, but fatality rates are lower among liver transplant recipients than among lung or heart-lung transplant recipients. Disease due to CMV can also be associated with the vanishing bile duct syndrome after liver transplantation. Patients respond to treatment with ganciclovir; prophylaxis with oral forms of ganciclovir or high-dose acyclovir may decrease the frequency of disease. A role for HHV-6 reactivation in posttransplantation fever and leukopenia has been proposed, although the more severe sequelae described in hematopoietic stem-cell transplantation are unusual. HHV-6 and HHV-7 appear to exacerbate CMV disease in this setting. EBV-LPD after liver transplantation shows a propensity for involvement of the liver, and such disease may be of donor origin. See previous sections for discussion of EBV infections in solid organ transplantation.

PANCREAS TRANSPLANTATION

Transplantation of the pancreas can be complicated by early bacterial and yeast infections. Most pancreatic transplants are drained into the bowel, whereas the remaining transplants (~20%) are drained into the bladder. A cuff of duodenum is used in the anastomosis between the pancreatic graft and either the gut or the bladder. Bowel drainage poses a risk of early abdominal and allograft infections with enteric bacteria and yeasts. These infections often result in loss of the graft. Bladder drainage causes a high rate of urinary tract infection and sterile cystitis; however, infection can usually be cured with appropriate antimicrobial agents. In both procedures, prophylactic antimicrobial agents are commonly used at the time of surgery. An alternative method—the transplantation of islet cells only—may eliminate the problems characteristically posed by wound and urinary tract sepsis in pancreatic transplant recipients.

Issues related to the development of CMV infection, EBV-LPD, and infections with opportunistic pathogens in patients receiving a pancreatic transplant are similar to those in other SOT recipients.

MISCELLANEOUS INFECTIONS IN SOLID ORGAN TRANSPLANTATION

Indwelling IV Catheter Infections

The prolonged use of indwelling IV catheters for administration of medications, blood products, and nutrition is common in diverse transplantation settings and poses a risk of local and bloodstream infections. Significant insertion-site infection is most commonly caused by *S. aureus*. Bloodstream infection most frequently develops within a week of catheter placement or in patients who become neutropenic. Coagulase-negative staphylococci are the most common isolates from the blood.

For further discussion of differential diagnosis and therapeutic options, see Chap. 11.

Tuberculosis

The incidence of tuberculosis occurring within the first 12 months after solid organ transplantation is greater than that observed after hematopoietic stem-cell transplantation (0.23–0.79%) and ranges broadly worldwide (1.2–15%), reflecting the prevalences of tuberculosis in local populations. Lesions suggesting prior tuberculosis on chest x-ray, older age, diabetes, chronic liver disease, GVHD, and intense immunosuppression are predictive of tuberculosis reactivation and development of disseminated disease in a host with latent disease. Tuberculosis has rarely been transmitted from the donor organ. In contrast to the low mortality rate among HSCT recipients, mortality rates among SOT patients are reported to be as high as 30%. Vigilance is indicated, as the presentation of disease is often extrapulmonary (gastrointestinal, genitourinary, central nervous, endocrine, musculoskeletal, laryngeal) and atypical, sometimes manifesting as a fever of unknown origin. A careful history and a direct evaluation of both the recipient and the donor before transplantation are optimal. Skin testing of the recipient with PPD may be unreliable because of chronic disease and/or immunosuppression, but newer cell-based assays that measure interferon and/or cytokine production may prove more sensitive in the future. Isoniazid toxicity has not been a significant problem except in the setting of liver transplantation. Therefore, appropriate prophylaxis should proceed. An assessment of the need to treat latent disease should include careful consideration of the possibility of a false-negative test result. Pending final confirmation of suspected tuberculosis, aggressive multidrug treatment in accordance with the guidelines of the Centers for Disease Control and Prevention (CDC), the Infectious Diseases Society of America, and the American Thoracic Society is indicated because of the high mortality rates among these patients. Altered drug metabolism (e.g., upon co-administration of rifampin and certain immunosuppressive agents) can be managed with careful monitoring of drug levels and appropriate dose adjustment. Close follow-up of hepatic enzymes is warranted, particularly during treatment with isoniazid, pyrazinamide, and/or rifampin. Drug-resistant tuberculosis is especially problematic in these individuals (Chap. 66).

Virus-Associated Malignancies

In addition to malignancy associated with gammaherpesvirus infection (EBV, KSHV) and simple warts (HPV), other tumors that are virus-associated or suspected of being virus-associated are more likely to develop in transplant recipients, particularly those who require long-term immunosuppression, than in the general population. The interval to tumor development is usually >1 year. Transplant recipients develop nonmelanoma skin or lip cancers that, in contrast to de novo skin cancers, have a high ratio of squamous cells to basal cells. HPV may play a major role in these lesions. Cervical and vulvar carcinomas, quite clearly associated with HPV, develop with increased frequency in female transplant recipients. Among renal transplant recipients, rates of melanoma are modestly increased, and rates of cancers of the kidney and bladder are increased.

VACCINATION OF TRANSPLANT RECIPIENTS

In addition to receiving antibiotic prophylaxis, transplant recipients should be vaccinated against likely pathogens (Table 12-6). In the case of HSCT recipients, optimal responses cannot be achieved until after immune reconstitution, despite previous immunization of both donor and recipient. Recipients of allogeneic HSCTs must be reimmunized if they are to be protected against pathogens. The situation is less clear-cut in the case of autologous transplantation. T and B cells in the peripheral blood may reconstitute the immune response if they are transferred in adequate numbers. However, cancer patients (particularly those with Hodgkin's disease, in whom vaccination has been extensively studied) who are undergoing chemotherapy do not respond normally to immunization, and titers of antibodies to infectious agents fall more rapidly than in healthy individuals. Therefore, even immunosuppressed patients who have not had HSCTs may need booster vaccine injections. If memory cells are specifically eliminated as part of a stem-cell "cleanup" procedure, it will be necessary to reimmunize the recipient with a new primary series. Optimal times for immunizations of different transplant populations are being evaluated. Yearly immunization of household and other contacts (including health care personnel) against influenza benefits the patient by preventing local spread.

In the absence of compelling data regarding optimal timing, it is reasonable to administer the pneumococcal and *H. influenzae* type b conjugate vaccines to both autologous and allogeneic HSCT recipients beginning 12 months after transplantation. A series that includes both the 7-valent pneumococcal conjugate vaccine and the

TABLE 12-6

VACCINATION FOR HEMATOPOIETIC STEM-CELL TRANSPLANT (HSCT) OR SOLID ORGAN TRANSPLANT (SOT) RECIPIENTS

	TYPE OF TRANSPLANTATION	
VACCINE	**HSCT**	**SOT[a]**
Streptococcus pneumoniae, *Haemophilus influenzae*,	Immunize after transplantation (optimal timing not established)	Immunize before transplantation and every 5 years for Pneumovax (others not established)
Neisseria meningitidis	Use Prevnar Preimmunize donor (graft)[b] See CDC recommendations	See CDC recommendations
Seasonal influenza	Vaccinate in the fall Vaccinate close contacts	Vaccinate in the fall Vaccinate close contacts
Poliomyelitis	Administer inactivated vaccine	Administer inactivated vaccine
Measles/mumps/rubella	Immunize 24 months after transplantation if patient does not have graft-versus-host disease	Immunize before transplantation with attenuated vaccine
Tetanus, diphtheria	Reimmunize after transplantation with primary series See CDC recommendations	Immunize before transplantation; give boosters at 10 years or as required; primary series not required
Hepatitis B and A	Reimmunize after transplantation See CDC recommendations	Immunize before transplantation as appropriate
Human papillomavirus	Recommendations pending	Recommendations pending

[a]Immunizations should be given before transplantation whenever possible.
[b]Studies indicate that it is possible to "immunize the graft" before transplantation.

23-valent Pneumovax is now recommended (following CDC guidelines). The pneumococcal and *H. influenzae* type b vaccines are particularly important for patients who have undergone splenectomy. In addition, diphtheria, tetanus, acellular pertussis, and inactivated polio vaccines can all be given at these same intervals (12 months and, as required, 24 months after transplantation). *Neisseria meningitidis* polysaccharide (a new conjugate vaccine) is now available and will probably be recommended in the future. Some authorities recommend a new primary series for tetanus/ diphtheria/pertussis and inactivated polio vaccine beginning 12 months after transplantation. Because of the risk of spread, household contacts of HSCT recipients (or of patients immunosuppressed as a result of chemotherapy) should receive only inactivated polio vaccine. Live-virus measles/mumps/rubella vaccine can be given to autologous HSCT recipients 24 months after transplantation and to most allogeneic HSCT recipients at the same point if they are not receiving maintenance therapy with immunosuppressive drugs and do not have ongoing GVHD. The risk of spread from a household contact is lower for MMR vaccine than for polio vaccine. Neither patients nor their household contacts should be vaccinated with vaccinia unless they have been exposed to the smallpox virus. Among patients who have active GVHD and/or are taking high maintenance doses of glucocorticoids, it may be prudent to avoid all live-virus vaccines. Vaccination to prevent hepatitis B and hepatitis A also seems advisable.

In the case of SOT recipients, administration of all the usual vaccines and of the indicated booster doses should be completed before immunosuppression, if possible, to maximize responses. For patients taking immunosuppressive agents, the administration of pneumococcal vaccine should be repeated every 5 years. No data are available for the meningococcal vaccine, but it is probably reasonable to administer it along with the pneumococcal vaccine. *H. influenzae* conjugate vaccine is safe and should be efficacious in this population; therefore, its administration before transplantation is recommended. Booster doses of this vaccine are not recommended for adults. SOT recipients who continue to receive immunosuppressive drugs should not receive live-virus vaccines. A person in this group who is exposed to measles should be given immune globulin. Similarly, an immunocompromised patient who is seronegative for varicella and who comes into contact with a person who has chickenpox should be given varicella-zoster immune globulin as soon as possible (and certainly within 96 h) or, if this is not possible, should be started immediately on a 10- to 14-day course of acyclovir therapy. Upon the discontinuation of treatment, clinical disease may still occur in a small number of patients; thus vigilance is indicated. Rapid re-treatment should limit the symptoms of disease. Household contacts of transplant recipients can receive live attenuated VZV vaccine, but vaccinees should avoid direct contact with the patient if a rash develops. Virus-like particle (VLP) vaccines (not live attenuated) have recently been licensed for the prevention of infection with several HPV serotypes most commonly implicated in cervical and anal carcinomas and in anogenital and laryngeal warts. For example, the tetravalent vaccine contains HPV serotypes 6, 11, 16, and 18. At present, no information is available about the safety, immunogenicity, or efficacy of this vaccine in transplant recipients.

Immunocompromised patients who travel may benefit from some but not all vaccines (Chaps. 3 and 4). In general, these patients should receive any killed or inactivated vaccine preparation appropriate to the area they are visiting; this recommendation includes the vaccines for Japanese encephalitis, hepatitis A and B, poliomyelitis, meningococcal infection, and typhoid. The live typhoid vaccines are not recommended for use in most immunocompromised patients, but inactivated or purified polysaccharide typhoid vaccine can be used. Live yellow fever vaccine should not be administered. On the other hand, primary immunization or boosting with the purified-protein hepatitis B vaccine is indicated if patients are likely to be exposed. Patients who will reside for >6 months in areas where hepatitis B is common (Africa, Southeast Asia, the Middle East, Eastern Europe, parts of South America, and the Caribbean) should receive hepatitis B vaccine. Inactivated hepatitis A vaccine should also be used in the appropriate setting (Chap. 3). A combined vaccine is now available that provides dual protection against hepatitis A and hepatitis B. If hepatitis A vaccine is not administered, travelers should consider receiving passive protection with immune globulin (the dose depending on the duration of travel in the high-risk area).

FURTHER READINGS

BOUZA E et al: Fever of unknown origin in solid organ transplant recipients. Infect Dis Clin North Am 21:1033, 2007

CENTERS FOR DISEASE CONTROL AND PREVENTION: Chagas disease after organ transplantation—Los Angeles, California, 2006. MMWR Morb Mortal Wkly Rep 55:798, 2006

CORNELY OA et al: Posaconazole vs. fluconazole or itraconazole prophylaxis in patients with neutropenia. N Engl J Med 356:348, 2007

DYKEWICZ CA: Cytomegalovirus infection after liver transplantation: Summary of the guidelines for preventing opportunistic infections among hematopoietic stem cell transplant recipients. Clin Infect Dis 33:139, 2001

HIRSCH HH, SUTHANTHIRAN M: The natural history, risk factors and outcomes of polyomavirus BK–associated nephropathy after renal transplantation. Nat Clin Pract Nephrol 2:240, 2006

KOTTON CN et al: Prevention of infection in adult travelers after solid organ transplantation. Am J Transplant 5:8, 2004

MUNOZ P et al: *Mycobacterium tuberculosis* infection in recipients of solid organ transplants. Clin Infect Dis 40:581, 2005

ZERR DM et al: Clinical outcomes of human herpesvirus 6 reactivation after hematopoietic stem cell transplantation. Clin Infect Dis 40:932, 2005

CHAPTER 13

HEALTH CARE–ASSOCIATED INFECTIONS

Robert A. Weinstein

The costs of hospital-acquired (nosocomial) and other health care–associated infections are great. It is estimated that these infections affect >2 million patients, cost $4.5 billion, and contribute to 88,000 deaths in U.S. hospitals annually. Efforts to lower infection risks have been challenged by the growing numbers of immunocompromised patients; antibiotic-resistant bacteria, fungal, and viral superinfections; and invasive devices and procedures. Nevertheless, evidence-based guidelines for prevention and control are available (Table 13-1); according to some estimates, consistent application of these guidelines may reduce the risk of health care–associated infection by more than one-third, and the growing viewpoint of consumer advocates is that almost all such infections are preventable. This chapter reviews health care–acquired and device-related infections and the basic surveillance, prevention, control, and treatment activities that have been developed to deal with these problems.

ORGANIZATION, RESPONSIBILITIES, AND INCREASING SCRUTINY OF INFECTION-CONTROL PROGRAMS

The standards of the Joint Commission require all accredited hospitals to have an active program for surveillance, prevention, and control of nosocomial infections. Education of physicians in infection control and health care epidemiology is required in infectious disease fellowship programs and is available by online courses. Diagnosis-related reimbursement has led hospital administrators to place increased emphasis on infection control.

TABLE 13-1

SOURCES OF INFECTION-CONTROL GUIDANCE AND OVERSIGHT

ORGANIZATION	ROLE	MAJOR CONSTITUENTS	WEBSITE
JCAHO	Regulatory	Hospitals, long-term care facilities, laboratories	http://www.jointcommission.org
CAP	Regulatory	Laboratories	http://www.cap.org
OSHA	Regulatory	Workers	http://www.osha.gov
CMS (formerly HCFA)	Regulatory	Medicare/Medicaid providers	http://www.cms.hhs.gov
CDC			
DHQP	Advisory	Health care facilities and personnel	http://www.cdc.gov/ncidod/hip/default.htm
HICPAC	Advisory	Health care facilities and personnel	http://www.cdc.gov/ncidod/hip/HICPAC/hicpac.htm
NIOSH	Advisory	Workers	http://www.cdc.gov/niosh/homepage.htm
AHRQ	Advisory	Broad (e.g., health care personnel)	http://www.ahrq.org
NQF	Advisory	Broad (e.g., health care personnel)	http://www.qualityforum.org
IOM	Advisory	Broad (e.g., health care personnel)	http://www.iom.edu
IDSA	Professional society	Infectious disease physicians/ researchers	http://www.idsociety.org
SHEA	Professional society	Hospital epidemiologists	http://www.shea-online.org
APIC	Professional society	Infection-control practitioners	http://www.apic.org
MedQIC	Quality improvement	Broad (e.g., health care personnel)	http://www.medqic.org
IHI	Quality improvement	Broad (e.g., health care personnel)	http://www.ihi.org

Note: JCAHO, Joint Commission; CAP, College of American Pathologists; OSHA, Occupational Safety & Health Administration; CMS, Centers for Medicare & Medicaid Services; HCFA, Health Care Financing Administration; CDC, Centers for Disease Control and Prevention; DHQP, Division of Healthcare Quality Promotion; HICPAC, Healthcare Infection Control Practices Advisory Committee; NIOSH, National Institute for Occupational Safety and Health; AHRQ, Agency for Healthcare Research and Quality; NQF, National Quality Forum; IOM, Institute of Medicine; IDSA, Infectious Diseases Society of America; SHEA, Society for Healthcare Epidemiology of America, Inc.; APIC, Association for Professionals in Infection Control and Epidemiology, Inc.; MedQIC, Medicare Quality Improvement Community; IHI, Institute for Healthcare Improvement.

Federal concerns over "patient safety" have led to legislation that would limit reimbursement for hospital costs resulting from at least two (yet-to-be-determined) nosocomial infections. The patient safety movement has prompted major national efforts to improve, measure, and publicly report on processes of patient care (e.g., timely administration and appropriateness of perioperative antibiotic prophylaxis) and patient outcomes (e.g., surgical wound infection rates).

SURVEILLANCE

Traditionally, infection-control practitioners have surveyed inpatients for infections acquired in hospitals (defined as those neither present nor incubating at the time of admission). Surveillance involves review of microbiology laboratory results, "shoe-leather" epidemiology on nursing wards, and application of standardized definitions of infection. Some infection-control programs use computerized hospital databases for algorithm-driven electronic surveillance (e.g., of vascular catheter and surgical wound infections). Commercial health care information systems that facilitate these functions are considered "value-added" products.

Most hospitals aim surveillance at infections associated with a high level of morbidity or expense. Quality-improvement activities in infection control have led to increased surveillance of personnel compliance with infection-control policies (e.g., adherence to influenza vaccination recommendations). The growing number of states that require public reporting of processes for prevention of health care–associated infection and/or patient outcomes has added new complexity to what hospitals measure and how they measure it.

Results of surveillance are expressed as rates. In general, 5–10% of patients develop nosocomial infections—a rate that, as patient advocates emphasize, has remained unchanged for 20–30 years. However, such broad statistics have little value unless qualified by duration of risk, site of infection, patient population, and exposure to risk factors. Meaningful denominators for infection rates include the number of patients exposed to a specific risk (e.g., patients using mechanical ventilators) or the number of intervention days (e.g., 1000 patient-days on a ventilator).

Temporal trends in rates should be reviewed, and rates should be compared with regional and national benchmarks. However, even comparison rates generated by the National Healthcare Safety Network (NHSN) have not been validated independently and represent a nonrandom sample of hospitals. [NHSN is the successor to the National Nosocomial Infections Surveillance System, a program of the Centers for Disease Control and Prevention (CDC) that collected data from more than 350 hospitals that use standardized definitions of nosocomial infections.] Interhospital comparisons may be misleading because of the wide range in risk factors and severity of underlying illnesses. Although systems for making adjustments for these factors either are rudimentary or have not been well validated, process measures (e.g., adherence to hand hygiene) do not usually require risk adjustment, and outcome measures (e.g., cardiac surgery wound infection rates) can identify hospitals with higher infection rates (e.g., in the top quartile) for further evaluation. Moreover, temporal analysis of an individual hospital's process and infection outcome rates helps to determine whether control measures are succeeding and where increased efforts should be focused.

EPIDEMIOLOGIC BASIS AND GENERAL MEASURES FOR PREVENTION AND CONTROL

Nosocomial infections follow basic epidemiologic patterns that can help to direct prevention and control measures. Nosocomial pathogens have reservoirs, are transmitted by predictable routes, and require susceptible hosts. Reservoirs and sources exist in the inanimate environment (e.g., tap water contaminated with *Legionella*) and in the animate environment (e.g., infected or colonized health care workers, patients, and hospital visitors). The mode of transmission usually is either cross-infection (e.g., indirect spread of pathogens from one patient to another on the inadequately cleaned hands of hospital personnel) or autoinoculation (e.g., aspiration of oropharyngeal flora into the lung along an endotracheal tube). Occasionally, pathogens (e.g., group A streptococci and many respiratory viruses) are spread from person to person via infectious droplets released by coughing or sneezing. Much less common—but often devastating in terms of epidemic risk—is true airborne spread of droplet nuclei (as in nosocomial chickenpox) or common-source spread by contaminated materials (e.g., contaminated IV fluids). Factors that increase host susceptibility include underlying conditions and the many medical–surgical interventions and procedures that bypass or compromise normal host defenses.

Through their programs, hospitals' infection-control committees must determine general and specific control measures. Given the prominence of cross-infection, hand hygiene is the single most important preventive measure in hospitals. Health care workers' rates of adherence to hand-hygiene recommendations are abysmally low (<50%). Reasons cited include inconvenience, time pressures, and skin damage from frequent washing. Sinkless alcohol rubs are quick and highly effective and actually improve hand condition since they contain emollients and allow the retention of natural protective oils that would be removed with repeated rinsing. Use of alcohol hand rubs between patient contacts is now recommended for all health care workers except when the hands are visibly soiled, in which case washing with soap and water is still required.

NOSOCOMIAL AND DEVICE-RELATED INFECTIONS

The fact that 25–50% or more of nosocomial infections are due to the combined effect of the patient's own flora and invasive devices highlights the importance of improvements in the use and design of such devices. Intensive education and "bundling" of evidence-based interventions (Table 13-2) can reduce infection rates through

TABLE 13-2

EXAMPLES OF "BUNDLED INTERVENTIONS" TO PREVENT COMMON HEALTH CARE–ASSOCIATED INFECTIONS AND OTHER ADVERSE EVENTS

Prevention of Central Venous Catheter Infections
Educate personnel about catheter insertion and care.
Use chlorhexidine to prepare the insertion site.
Use maximum barrier precautions during catheter insertion.
Ask daily: Is the catheter needed?
Prevention of Ventilator-Associated Pneumonia and Complications
Elevate head of bed to 30–45 degrees.
Give "sedation vacation" and assess readiness to extubate daily.
Use peptic ulcer disease prophylaxis.
Use deep-vein thrombosis prophylaxis (unless contraindicated).
Prevention of Surgical-Site Infections
Administer prophylactic antibiotics within 1 h before surgery; discontinue within 24 h.
Limit any hair removal to the time of surgery; use clippers or do not remove hair at all.
Maintain normal perioperative glucose levels (cardiac surgery patients).[a]
Maintain perioperative normothermia (colorectal surgery patients).[a]
Prevention of Urinary Tract Infections
Place bladder catheters only when absolutely needed (e.g., to relieve obstruction), not solely for the provider's convenience.
Use aseptic technique for catheter insertion and urinary tract instrumentation.
Minimize manipulation or opening of drainage systems.
Remove bladder catheters as soon as is feasible.

[a]These components of care are supported by clinical trials and experimental evidence in the specified populations; they may prove valuable for other surgical patients as well.

Source: Adapted from information presented at the following websites: *www.cdc.gov/ncidod/dhqp/gl_intravascular.html*; *www.cdc.gov/ncidod/dhqp/gl_hcpneumonia.html*; *www.cdc.gov/ncidod/dhqp/gl_surgicalsite.html*; *www.cdc.gov/ncidod/dhqp/gl_catheter_assoc. html*; *www.ihi. org*; *www. medqic.org/scip*.

improved asepsis in handling and earlier removal of invasive devices, but the maintenance of such gains requires ongoing efforts. It is especially noteworthy that turnover or shortages of trained personnel jeopardize safe and effective patient care and have been associated with increased infection rates.

Urinary Tract Infections

Urinary tract infections (UTIs) account for as many as 40–45% of nosocomial infections; up to 3% of bacteriuric patients develop bacteremia. Although UTIs contribute only 10–15% to prolongation of hospital stay and to extra costs, these infections are important reservoirs and sources for spread of antibiotic-resistant bacteria in hospitals. Almost all nosocomial UTIs are associated with preceding instrumentation or indwelling bladder catheters, which create a 3–10% risk of infection each day. UTIs generally are caused by pathogens that spread up the periurethral space from the patient's perineum or gastrointestinal tract—the most common pathogenesis in women—or via intraluminal contamination of urinary catheters, usually due to cross-infection by caregivers who are irrigating catheters or emptying drainage bags. Pathogens come occasionally from inadequately disinfected urologic equipment and rarely from contaminated supplies.

Hospitals should closely monitor essential performance measures for preventing nosocomial UTIs (Table 13-2). Sealed catheter–drainage tube junctions can help to prevent breaks in the system. Approaches to the prevention of UTIs also have included use of topical meatal antimicrobials, drainage bag disinfectants, and anti-infective catheters. None of the latter three measures is considered routine. In fact, a recent meta-analysis suggests that silver alloy–coated anti-infective catheters do not reduce the incidence of bacteriuria from that occurring with silicone catheters.

Administration of systemic antimicrobial agents for other purposes decreases the risk of UTI during the first 4 days of catheterization, after which resistant bacteria or yeasts emerge as pathogens. Selective decontamination of the gut is also associated with a reduced risk. Again, however, neither approach is routine.

Irrigation of catheters, with or without antimicrobial agents, may actually increase the risk of infection. A condom catheter for men without bladder obstruction may be more acceptable than an indwelling catheter, but the infection risks with the two types are similar unless the condom catheter is carefully maintained. The role of suprapubic catheters in preventing infection is not well defined.

Treatment of UTIs is based on the results of quantitative urine cultures (Chap. 27). The most common pathogens are *Escherichia coli*, nosocomial gram-negative bacilli, enterococci, and *Candida*. Several caveats apply in the treatment of institutionally acquired infection. First, in patients with chronic indwelling bladder catheters, especially those in long-term care facilities, "catheter flora"—microorganisms living on encrustations within the catheter lumen—may differ from actual urinary tract pathogens. Therefore, for suspected infection in the setting of chronic catheterization (especially in women), it is useful to replace the bladder catheter and to obtain a freshly voided urine specimen. Second, as in all nosocomial infections, at the time treatment is initiated on the basis of a positive culture, it is useful to repeat the culture to verify the persistence of infection. Third, the frequency with which UTIs occur may lead to the erroneous assumption that this site alone is the source of infection in a febrile hospitalized patient. Fourth, recovery of *Staphylococcus aureus* from urine cultures may result from hematogenous seeding and may indicate an occult systemic infection. Finally, although *Candida* is now the most common pathogen in nosocomial UTIs in patients on intensive care units (ICUs), treatment of candiduria is often unsuccessful and is recommended only when there is upper-pole invasion, obstruction, neutropenia, or immunosuppression.

Pneumonia

Pneumonia accounts for 15–20% of nosocomial infections but has been responsible for 24% of extra hospital days and 39% of extra costs—i.e., 6 days and the associated costs per episode. Almost all cases of bacterial nosocomial pneumonia are caused by aspiration of endogenous or hospital-acquired oropharyngeal (and occasionally gastric) flora. Nosocomial pneumonias are associated with more deaths than are infections at any other body site. However, attributable mortality for ventilator-associated pneumonia—the most common and lethal form of nosocomial pneumonia—is in the 6–14% range; this figure suggests that the risk of dying from nosocomial pneumonia is affected greatly by other factors, including comorbidities, inadequate antibiotic treatment, and the involvement of specific pathogens (particularly *Pseudomonas aeruginosa* and *Acinetobacter*). Surveillance and accurate diagnosis of pneumonia are often problematic in hospitals because many patients, especially those in the ICU, have abnormal chest roentgenographs, fever, and leukocytosis potentially attributable to multiple causes. Viral pneumonias, which are particularly important in pediatric and immunocompromised patients, are discussed in the virology section and in Chap. 17.

Risk factors for nosocomial pneumonia, particularly ventilator-associated pneumonia, include those events that increase colonization by potential pathogens (e.g., prior antimicrobial therapy, contaminated ventilator circuits or equipment, or decreased gastric acidity), those that facilitate aspiration of oropharyngeal contents into the lower respiratory tract (e.g., intubation, decreased levels of consciousness, or presence of a nasogastric tube), and those that reduce host defense mechanisms in the lung and permit overgrowth of aspirated pathogens (e.g., chronic obstructive pulmonary disease, old age, or upper abdominal surgery).

Control measures for pneumonia (Table 13-2) are aimed at the remediation of risk factors in general patient care (e.g., minimizing aspiration-prone supine positioning) and at meticulous aseptic care of respirator equipment (e.g., disinfecting or sterilizing all inline reusable components such as nebulizers, replacing tubing circuits at intervals of >48 h—rather than more frequently—to lessen the number of breaks in the system, and teaching aseptic technique for suctioning). The benefits of selective decontamination of the oropharynx and gut with nonabsorbable antimicrobial agents and/or use of short-course postintubation systemic antibiotics have been controversial. Among the logical preventive measures that require further investigation are the use of endotracheal tubes that provide channels for subglottic drainage of secretions and the use of noninvasive mechanical ventilation whenever feasible. It is noteworthy that reducing the rate of ventilator-associated pneumonia most often has not reduced overall ICU mortality; this fact suggests that this infection is a marker for patients with an otherwise-heightened risk of death.

The most likely pathogens for nosocomial pneumonia and treatment options are discussed in Chap. 17. Several considerations regarding diagnosis and treatment are worth emphasizing. Clinical criteria for diagnosis (e.g., fever, leukocytosis, development of purulent secretions, new or changing radiographic infiltrates, changes in oxygen requirement or ventilator settings) have high sensitivity but relatively low specificity. These criteria are most useful for selecting patients for bronchoscopic or nonbronchoscopic procedures that yield lower respiratory tract samples protected from upper-tract contamination; quantitative cultures of such specimens have diagnostic sensitivities in the range of 80%. Early-onset nosocomial pneumonia, which manifests within the first 4 days of hospitalization, is most often caused by community-acquired pathogens, such as *Streptococcus pneumoniae* and *Haemophilus* species. Late-onset pneumonias most commonly are due to *S. aureus*, *P. aeruginosa*, *Enterobacter* species, *Klebsiella pneumoniae*, or *Acinetobacter*—a pathogen of increasing concern in many ICUs. When invasive techniques are used to diagnose ventilator-associated pneumonia, the proportion of isolates accounted for by gram-negative bacilli decreases from 50–70% to 35–45%. Infection is polymicrobial in as many as 20–40% of cases. The role of anaerobic bacteria in ventilator-associated pneumonia is not well defined. A recent study suggested that 8 days is an appropriate duration of therapy for nosocomial pneumonia, with a longer duration (15 days in this study) when the pathogen is *Acinetobacter* or *P. aeruginosa*. Finally, in febrile patients (particularly those who have endotracheal and/or nasogastric tubes), more occult sources of respiratory tract infection, especially bacterial sinusitis and otitis media, should be considered.

Surgical Wound Infections

Wound infections account for up to 20–30% of nosocomial infections but contribute up to 57% of extra hospital days and 42% of extra costs. The average wound infection has an incubation period of 5–7 days (longer than many postoperative stays), and many procedures are now performed on an outpatient basis. Thus the incidence of wound infections has become difficult to assess. These infections usually are caused by the patient's endogenous or hospital-acquired skin and mucosal flora and occasionally are due to airborne spread of skin squames that may be shed into the wound from members of the operating-room team. True airborne spread of infection through droplet nuclei is rare in operating rooms unless there is a "disseminator" (e.g., of group A streptococci or staphylococci) among the staff. In general, the most common risks for postoperative wound infection are related to the surgeon's technical skill, the patient's underlying diseases (e.g., diabetes mellitus, obesity) or advanced age, and inappropriate timing of antibiotic prophylaxis. Additional risk factors include the presence of drains, prolonged preoperative hospital stays, shaving of the operative site by razor the day before surgery, a long duration of surgery, and infection at remote sites (e.g., untreated UTI).

The substantial literature related to risk factors for surgical-site infections and the recognized morbidity and cost of these infections have led to national prevention efforts—the Surgical Infection Prevention (SIP) Project, the Institute for Healthcare Improvement (IHI) 100,000 Lives Campaign, and the Surgical Care Improvement Project (SCIP)—and to recommendations for "bundling" of evidence-based preventive measures (Table 13-2). Additional measures include attention to technical surgical issues and operating-room asepsis (e.g., avoiding open or prophylactic drains) and preoperative therapy for active infection. Reporting of surveillance results to surgeons has been associated with reductions in infection rates. The use of preoperative intranasal mupirocin to eliminate that reservoir for *S. aureus*, preoperative antiseptic bathing, and supplemental intra- and postoperative oxygen remain controversial because of conflicting study results.

The increasingly extensive review of infection rates by regulatory agencies and third-party payers emphasizes the importance of stratifying rates by patient-related risk factors and of developing meaningful systems for wound surveillance after the patient's discharge from the hospital or clinic (when >50% of infections first become apparent) or for use of surrogate markers of wound infection (e.g., prolonged postoperative antibiotic courses).

The epidemic of mad cow disease, centered in the United Kingdom, and associated human cases of variant Creutzfeldt-Jakob disease (Chap. 101) caused by disinfection-resistant prion agents have led to revised recommendations for decontaminating surgical instruments, especially those used for operations on the central nervous system or in patients with dementing illness of unknown etiology.

The process of diagnosing and treating wound infections begins with a careful assessment of the surgical site in the febrile postoperative patient. Clinical findings range from obvious cellulitis or abscess formation to subtler clues, such as a sternal "click" after open heart surgery. Diagnosis of deeper organ-space infections or subphrenic abscesses requires a high index of suspicion and the use of CT or MRI. Diagnosis of infections of prosthetic devices, such as orthopedic implants, may be particularly difficult and often requires the use of interventional radiographic techniques to obtain periprosthetic specimens for culture. The most common pathogens in postoperative wound infections are *S. aureus*, coagulase-negative staphylococci, and enteric and anaerobic bacteria. In rapidly progressing postoperative infections, which manifest within 24–48 h of a surgical procedure, the level of suspicion regarding group A streptococcal or clostridial infection (Chaps. 36 and 42) should be high. Treatment of postoperative wound infections requires drainage or surgical excision of infected or necrotic material and antibiotic therapy aimed at the most likely or laboratory-confirmed pathogens.

Infections Related to Vascular Access and Monitoring

Intravascular devices are common causes of local site infection and cause up to 50% of nosocomial bacteremias; central vascular catheters (CVCs) account for 80–90% of these infections. National estimates indicate that as many as 200,000 bloodstream infections associated with CVCs occur each year in the United States, with an attributable mortality of 12–25% and an estimated cost of $25,000 per episode; one-third to one-half of these episodes occur in ICUs. With increasing care of seriously ill patients in the community, vascular catheter–associated bloodstream infections acquired in outpatient settings may become as frequent as those acquired in hospitals. This possibility emphasizes the need to broaden surveillance activities.

Catheter-related bloodstream infections derive largely from the cutaneous microflora of the insertion site, with pathogens migrating extraluminally to the catheter tip, usually during the first week after insertion. In addition, contamination of hubs of CVCs or of the ports of "needleless" systems may lead to intraluminal infection over longer periods, particularly with surgically implanted or cuffed catheters. Intrinsic contamination of infusate, although rare, is the most common cause of epidemic device-related bloodstream infection; extrinsic contamination may cause up to half of endemic bacteremias related to arterial infusions used for hemodynamic monitoring. The most common pathogens isolated from vascular device–associated bacteremias include coagulase-negative staphylococci, *S. aureus* (with up to 50% or more of isolates in the United States resistant to methicillin), enterococci, nosocomial gram-negative bacilli, and *Candida*. Many pathogens, especially staphylococci, produce extracellular polysaccharide biofilms that facilitate attachment to catheters and provide sanctuary from antimicrobial agents. "Quorum-sensing" proteins help bacterial cells communicate during biofilm development.

Infections related to vascular catheters and monitoring devices may be the most preventable of nosocomial infections. Evidence-based bundles of control measures (Table 13-2) have been strikingly effective, eliminating all infections in one ICU study. Hospitals should periodically monitor adherence to these performance indicators. Use of antimicrobial- or antiseptic-impregnated CVCs does not appear necessary if the prevention bundle is fully implemented. Additional control measures for infections associated with vascular access include using a chlorhexidine-impregnated patch at the skin-catheter junction; avoiding the femoral site for catheterization because of higher risk of infection (most likely related to the density of the skin flora); moving peripheral catheters to a new site at specified intervals (e.g., every 72–96 h), which may be facilitated by use of an IV therapy team; and applying disposable transducers for pressure monitoring and aseptic technique for accessing transducers or other vascular ports. Improvements in composition of semitransparent access-site dressings and potential nursing benefits (ease of bathing and site inspection, protection of site from secretions) favor the use of such coverings. Unresolved issues include the best frequency for rotation of CVC sites (given that guidewire-assisted catheter changes at the same site do not lessen and may even increase infection risk); the appropriate role of mupirocin ointment, a topical antibiotic with excellent antistaphylococcal activity, in site care; the relative degrees of risk posed by peripherally inserted central catheters (PICC) lines; and the risk-benefit of prophylactic use of heparin (to avoid catheter thrombi, which may be associated with increased risk of infection) or of vancomycin or alcohol (as catheter flushes or "locks"—i.e., concentrated anti-infective solutions instilled into the catheter lumen) for high-risk patients.

Vascular device–related infection is suspected on the basis of the appearance of the catheter site or the presence of fever or bacteremia without another source in patients with vascular catheters. The diagnosis is confirmed by the recovery of the same species of microorganism from peripheral-blood cultures (preferably two cultures drawn from peripheral veins by separate venipunctures) and from semiquantitative or quantitative cultures of the vascular catheter tip. Less commonly used diagnostic measures include differential time to positivity (>2 h) for blood drawn through the vascular access device compared with a sample from a peripheral vein or differences in quantitative cultures (a 5- to 10-fold or greater "step-up") for blood samples drawn simultaneously from a peripheral vein and from a CVC. When infusion-related sepsis is considered (e.g., because of the abrupt onset of fever or shock temporally related to infusion therapy), a sample of the infusate or blood product should be retained for culture.

Therapy for vascular access–related infection is directed at the pathogen recovered from the blood and/or infected site. Important considerations in treatment are the need for an echocardiogram (to evaluate the patient for bacterial endocarditis), the duration of therapy, and the need to remove potentially infected catheters. In one report, approximately one-fourth of patients with intravascular catheter–associated *S. aureus* bacteremia who were studied by transesophageal echocardiography had evidence of endocarditis; this test may be useful in determining the appropriate duration of treatment.

Detailed consensus guidelines for the management of intravascular catheter–related infections have been published and recommend catheter removal in most cases of bacteremia or fungemia due to nontunneled CVCs. When attempting to salvage a potentially infected catheter, some clinicians use the "antibiotic lock" technique, which may facilitate penetration of infected biofilms, in addition to systemic antimicrobial therapy. In one study of hemodialysis catheters, only about one-third of salvage attempts were successful, although delayed removal did not appear to increase the risk of complications.

Often, a potentially infected CVC may be exchanged over a guidewire. If cultures of the removed catheter tip are positive, the replacement catheter will be moved to a new site; if the tip cultures are negative, the replacement catheter may remain in the original site but may be at increased risk of subsequent infection due to this manipulation.

The authors of the consensus guidelines advise that the decision to remove a tunneled catheter or implanted device suspected of being the source of bacteremia or fungemia should be based on the severity of the patient's illness, the strength of the evidence that the device is infected, an assessment of the specific pathogens, and the presence of local or systemic complications. For patients with track-site infection, successful therapy without catheter removal is unusual. For patients with suppurative venous thrombophlebitis, excision of the affected vein is usually required.

ISOLATION TECHNIQUES

Written policies for the isolation of infectious patients are a standard component of infection-control programs. In 1996, the CDC revised its isolation guidelines to make them simpler; to recognize the importance of all body fluids, secretions, and excretions in the transmission of nosocomial pathogens; and to focus precautions on the major routes of infection transmission. These policies are currently being updated by the CDC to include integrated guidelines for control of multidrug-resistant organisms.

Standard precautions are designed for the care of all patients in hospitals and aim to reduce the risk of transmission of microorganisms from both recognized and unrecognized sources. These precautions include gloving as well as hand cleansing for potential contact with (1) blood; (2) all other body fluids, secretions, and excretions, whether or not they contain visible blood; (3) nonintact skin; and (4) mucous membranes. Depending on exposure risks, standard precautions also include use of masks, eye protection, and gowns.

Precautions for the care of patients with potentially contagious clinical syndromes (e.g., acute diarrhea) or with suspected or diagnosed colonization or infection with transmissible pathogens are based on probable routes of transmission: *airborne*, *droplet*, and *contact*. Sets of precautions may be combined for diseases that have more than one route of transmission (e.g., varicella).

Because some prevalent antibiotic-resistant pathogens, particularly vancomycin-resistant enterococci (VRE), may be present on *intact* skin of patients in hospitals, some experts recommend gloving for all contact with patients who are acutely ill and/or from high-risk units, such as ICUs. Wearing gloves does not replace the need for hand hygiene because hands occasionally become contaminated during wearing or removal of gloves. Some studies have suggested that use of gowns and gloves compared with routine care of patients (i.e., using neither of these barriers) decreases the risk of nosocomial infection; however, the benefit of gowning by personnel beyond that conferred by gloving and hand hygiene is controversial. Nevertheless, requiring increased precaution levels can improve the compliance of health care workers with isolation recommendations by 30%.

EPIDEMIC AND EMERGING PROBLEMS

Outbreaks and emerging pathogens are always big news but probably account for <5% of nosocomial infections. Concern about emerging pathogens often prompts authorities to require hospitals to develop contingency and response plans. The investigation and control of nosocomial epidemics require that infection-control personnel develop a case definition, confirm that an outbreak really exists (since many apparent epidemics are actually pseudo-outbreaks due to surveillance or laboratory artifacts), review aseptic practices and disinfectant use, determine the extent of the outbreak, perform an epidemiologic investigation to determine modes of transmission, work closely with microbiology personnel to culture for common sources or personnel carriers as appropriate and to type epidemiologically important isolates, and heighten surveillance to judge the effect of control measures. Control measures generally include reinforcing routine aseptic practices and hand hygiene during a search for compliance problems that may have fostered the outbreak, ensuring appropriate isolation of cases (and instituting cohort isolation and nursing if needed), and implementing further controls on the basis of the investigation's findings. Examples of some emerging and potential epidemic problems follow.

Viral Respiratory Infections: SARS and Influenza

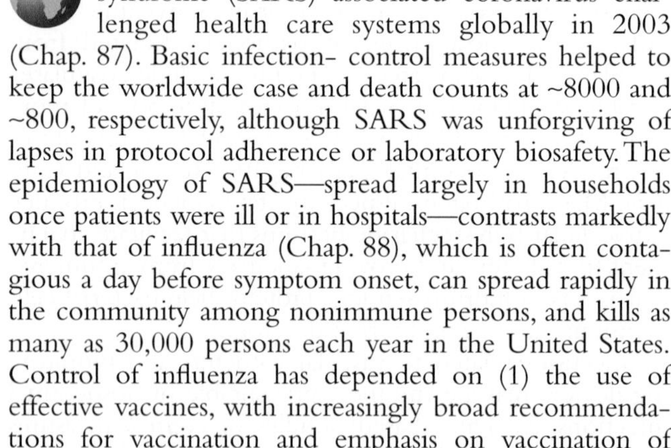

Infections caused by the severe acute respiratory syndrome (SARS)–associated coronavirus challenged health care systems globally in 2003 (Chap. 87). Basic infection- control measures helped to keep the worldwide case and death counts at ~8000 and ~800, respectively, although SARS was unforgiving of lapses in protocol adherence or laboratory biosafety. The epidemiology of SARS—spread largely in households once patients were ill or in hospitals—contrasts markedly with that of influenza (Chap. 88), which is often contagious a day before symptom onset, can spread rapidly in the community among nonimmune persons, and kills as many as 30,000 persons each year in the United States. Control of influenza has depended on (1) the use of effective vaccines, with increasingly broad recommendations for vaccination and emphasis on vaccination of health care workers; (2) the use of antiviral medications for early treatment and for prophylaxis as part of outbreak control, especially in high- risk settings like nursing homes or hospitals; and (3) infection control (surveillance and droplet precautions) for symptomatic patients.

Concerns about avian (H5N1) and pandemic influenza have led to recommendations for "respiratory hygiene and cough etiquette" and "source containment" (e.g., use of face masks and spatial separation) for outpatients with potentially infectious respiratory illnesses; to the concept of "social distancing" (e.g., closing community venues such as shopping malls) in the event of a pandemic; and to debate about the level of avian influenza respiratory protection required for health care workers—i.e., whether to use the higher-efficiency N95 respirators recommended for airborne isolation rather than the surgical masks used for droplet precautions.

Nosocomial Diarrhea

A new, more virulent strain of *Clostridium difficile* has emerged in North America, and overall rates of *C. difficile*–associated diarrhea (Chap. 43) have increased in U.S. hospitals during the past few years. The potential role of exposure to newer fluoroquinolone antibiotics in driving these changes is being investigated. *C. difficile* control measures include judicious use of all antibiotics; heightened suspicion for "atypical" presentations (e.g., toxic megacolon or leukemoid reaction without diarrhea); and early diagnosis, treatment, and contact precautions.

Outbreaks of norovirus infection (Chap. 91) in U.S. and European health care facilities appear to be increasing in frequency, with the virus often introduced by ill visitors or health care workers. This pathogen should be suspected when nausea and vomiting are prominent aspects of bacterial culture–negative diarrheal syndromes. Contact precautions may need to be augmented by aggressive environmental cleaning (given the persistence of norovirus on inanimate objects) and active exclusion of ill staff and visitors.

Chickenpox

Infection-control practitioners institute a varicella exposure investigation and control plan whenever health care workers either (1) are exposed to chickenpox (Chap. 81) in the community or through patients with initially unrecognized infections or (2) work during the 24 h before developing chickenpox. The names of exposed workers and patients are obtained; medical histories are reviewed, and (if necessary) serologic tests for immunity are conducted; physicians are notified of susceptible exposed patients; postexposure prophylaxis with varicella-zoster immune globulin (VZIG) is considered for immunocompromised or pregnant contacts (see Table 81-1); varicella vaccine is recommended or preemptive use of acyclovir is considered as an alternative strategy in other susceptible persons; and susceptible exposed employees are furloughed during the at-risk period for disease (8–21 days or—if VZIG has been administered—28 days). Routine varicella vaccination of children and susceptible employees can markedly decrease risk and frequency of exposures.

Tuberculosis

Important measures for the control of tuberculosis (Chap. 66) include prompt recognition, isolation, and treatment of cases; recognition of atypical presentations (e.g., lower-lobe infiltrates without cavitation); use of negative-pressure, 100% exhaust, private isolation rooms with closed doors and 6–12 or more air changes per hour; use of N95 "respirators" (approved by the National Institute for Occupational Safety and Health) by caregivers entering isolation rooms; possible use of high-efficiency particulate air filter units and/or ultraviolet lights for disinfecting air when other engineering controls are not feasible or reliable; and follow-up skin-testing of susceptible personnel who have been exposed to infectious patients before isolation. The use of new serologic tests, rather than skin tests, in the diagnosis of latent tuberculosis for infection control purposes is being studied.

Group A Streptococcal Infections

The potential for an outbreak of group A streptococcal infection (Chap. 36) should be considered when even a single nosocomial case occurs. Most outbreaks involve surgical wounds and are due to the presence of an asymptomatic carrier in the operating room. Investigation can be confounded by carriage at extrapharyngeal sites such as the rectum and vagina. Health care workers in whom carriage has been linked to nosocomial transmission of group A streptococci are removed from the patient-care setting and are not permitted to return until carriage has been eliminated by antimicrobial therapy.

Fungal Infections

Fungal spores are common in the environment, particularly on dusty surfaces. When dusty areas are disturbed during hospital repairs or renovation, the spores become airborne. Inhalation of spores by immunosuppressed (especially neutropenic) patients creates a risk of pulmonary and/or paranasal sinus infection and disseminated aspergillosis (Chap. 108). Routine surveillance among neutropenic patients for infections with filamentous fungi, such as *Aspergillus* and *Fusarium*, helps hospitals to determine whether they are facing unduly extensive environmental risks. As a matter of routine, hospitals should inspect and clean air-handling equipment, review all planned renovations with infection-control personnel and subsequently construct appropriate barriers, remove immunosuppressed patients from renovation sites, and consider the use of high-efficiency particulate air intake filters for rooms housing immunosuppressed patients.

Legionellosis

Nosocomial *Legionella* pneumonia (Chap. 49) is most often due to contamination of potable water and predominantly affects immunosuppressed patients, particularly those receiving glucocorticoid medication. The risk varies greatly within and among geographic regions, depending on the extent of hospital hot-water contamination and on specific hospital practices (e.g., inappropriate use of nonsterile water in respiratory therapy equipment). Laboratory-based surveillance for nosocomial *Legionella* should be performed, and a diagnosis of legionellosis should probably be considered more often than it is. If cases are detected, environmental samples (e.g., tap water) should be cultured. If cultures yield *Legionella* and if typing of clinical and environmental isolates reveals a correlation, eradication measures should be pursued. An alternative approach is to periodically culture tap water in wards housing high-risk patients. If *Legionella* is found, a concerted effort should be made to culture samples from all patients with nosocomial pneumonia for *Legionella*.

Antibiotic-Resistant Bacteria

Control of antibiotic resistance, particularly in outbreaks (Table 13-3), depends on close laboratory surveillance,

TABLE 13-3

CONTROLLING ANTIBIOTIC RESISTANCE: APPROACHES TO CONSIDER

Conduct surveillance for antibiotic resistance.
Perform molecular typing (e.g., pulsed-field gel electrophoresis) when rates increase.
For clonal expansion (e.g., single-strain outbreaks): Stress hand hygiene (alcohol hand rub and universal gloving); monitor adherence and give feedback.
For polyclonal expansion (e.g., multistrain outbreaks): Stress antibiotic prudence (consider antibiotic rotation for ICUs); monitor adherence and give feedback.
For continued problems: Obtain patient-surveillance cultures and isolate or provide cohort nursing for colonized/infected patients.
Control device-related infections.
Enlist administrative support proactively.

Source: Adapted from: RA Weinstein, Emerg Infect Dis 7:188, 2001; see also *www.cdc.gov/ncidod/dhqp/pdf/ar/mdroGuideline2006.pdf.*

with early detection of problems; on aggressive reinforcement of routine asepsis (e.g., hand hygiene); on implementation of barrier precautions for all colonized and/or infected patients; on use of patient-surveillance cultures to more fully ascertain the extent of patient colonization; and on timely initiation of an epidemiologic investigation when rates increase. Colonized personnel who are implicated in nosocomial transmission and patients who pose a threat may be decontaminated. In a few ICUs, selective decontamination of patients has been used successfully as a temporary emergency control measure for outbreaks of infection due to gram-negative bacilli. Other promising ICU control measures include daily bathing of patients with chlorhexidine and enforcement of environmental cleaning; in recent trials, each of these measures reduced cross-transmission of VRE. The value of "search-and-destroy" methods—i.e., the use of active surveillance cultures to detect and isolate the "resistance iceberg" of patients colonized with methicillin-resistant *S. aureus* (MRSA) or VRE—in non-outbreak settings has been controversial but is credited with elimination of nosocomial MRSA in the Netherlands and Denmark.

Currently, several antibiotic resistance problems are of particular health care concern. First, the emergence of community-acquired MRSA has been dramatic in many countries, with as many as 50% of community-acquired "staph infections" in some U.S. cities now caused by strains resistant to β-lactam antibiotics (Chap. 35). The potential incursion of these strains into hospitals and the resulting impact on control of nosocomial MRSA infections are of enormous concern. Second, in the ongoing global reemergence of nosocomial multidrug-resistant gram-negative bacilli, new problems include plasmid-mediated resistance to fluoroquinolones, metallo-β-lactamase-mediated resistance to carbapenems, and panresistant strains of *Acinetobacter*. Many of these multidrug-resistant strains are susceptible only to colistin, which has led to a "rediscovery" and renewed use of this drug. Finally, clinical infections with MRSA strains exhibiting high-level vancomycin resistance due to VRE-derived plasmids have been reported in several patients in the United States, often in the setting of prolonged or repeated treatment with vancomycin and/or VRE colonization. The detection of any of these current problems should trigger an epidemiologic investigation and aggressive infection-control measures.

Because the excessive use of broad-spectrum antibiotics underlies many resistance problems, aggressive antibiotic-control policies must be considered a cornerstone of resistance-control efforts. Recommendations for "antibiotic stewardship" are being promulgated by the Infectious Diseases Society of America. Although the efficacy of antibiotic-control measures in reducing rates of antimicrobial resistance has not been proven in prospective controlled trials, it seems worthwhile to restrict the use of particular agents to narrowly defined indications in order to limit selective pressure on the nosocomial flora.

Bioterrorism and Other "Surge-Event" Preparedness

The horrific attack on the World Trade Center in New York City on September 11, 2001; the subsequent mailings of anthrax spores in the United States; and recently exposed terrorist plans and activities in the United Kingdom and elsewhere have made bioterrorism a prominent source of concern to hospital infection-control programs. The essentials for hospital preparedness (Table 13-4) entail education, internal and external communication, and risk assessment. Up-to-date information on a variety of bioterrorism-associated issues is available from the CDC (*www.bt.cdc.gov*).

EMPLOYEE HEALTH SERVICE ISSUES

An institution's employee health service is a critical component of its infection-control efforts. New employees should be processed through the service, where a contagious-disease history can be taken; evidence of immunity to a variety of diseases, such as hepatitis B, chickenpox, measles, mumps, and rubella, can be sought; immunizations for hepatitis B, measles, mumps, rubella, and varicella can be given as needed, and a reminder about the need for yearly influenza immunization can be imparted; baseline and "booster" purified protein derivative of tuberculin skin-testing or serologic testing for tuberculosis can be performed; and education about personal responsibility for infection control can be initiated. Evaluations of employees should be codified to meet the requirements of accrediting and regulatory agencies.

The employee health service must have protocols for dealing with workers who have been exposed to contagious diseases, such as those percutaneously or mucosally exposed to the blood of patients infected with HIV or hepatitis B or C virus. For example, postexposure HIV

TABLE 13-4

HIGHLIGHTS OF HOSPITAL PREPAREDNESS FOR BIOTERRORISM AND OTHER "SURGE EVENTS"

Emergency Department: Educate (bioterrorism diagnoses, case definitions, and appropriate syndrome-based isolation precautions)
Laboratory: Identify protocols and laboratory safety procedures for agents of bioterrorism
Pharmacy: Develop medication and vaccine par stock, allocation, and delivery plans
Nursing: Assess bed and isolation surge capacity; help develop contingency plans to free bed space (e.g., early discharges)
Hospital Police: Plan for responsibilities as first responders and providers of risk assessment
Engineering/Buildings and Grounds: Evaluate air-handling systems and ensure familiarity with shutoffs and controls; educate about environmental decontamination
Outpatient Areas: Develop plans for delivery of prophylactic medications and/or vaccines
Public Health: Open lines of communication, education, and surveillance
The Community: Plan for infection-control practitioners to serve as liaisons for emergency departments, laboratories, and community providers
Administration: Perform resource assessment (e.g., medical supplies, transportation capabilities, potable water, sanitation facilities, provider backup, bed-space backup); oversee development of an incident command system
"Morale Officer": Keep staff functioning

prophylaxis with a combination of two or three antiretroviral agents is recommended; free consultation is available from the CDC PEPLine (888-HIV-4911). Protocols are also needed for dealing with caregivers who have common contagious diseases (such as chickenpox, group A streptococcal infections, respiratory infections, and infectious diarrhea) and for those who have less common but high-visibility public health problems (such as chronic hepatitis B or C or HIV infection) for which exposure-control guidelines have been published by the CDC and by the Society for Healthcare Epidemiology of America.

FURTHER READINGS

Bratzler DW, Hunt DR: The Surgical Infection Prevention and Surgical Care Improvement Projects: National initiatives to improve outcomes for patients having surgery. Clin Infect Dis 43:322, 2006

Centers for Disease Control and Prevention: Guidelines for preventing opportunistic infections among hematopoietic stem cell transplant recipients: Recommendations of CDC, the Infectious Diseases Society of America, and the American Society of Blood and Marrow Transplantation. MMWR 49(RR-10):1, 2000

———: Guideline for hand hygiene in health-care settings: Recommendations of the Healthcare Infection Control Practices Advisory Committee and the HICPAC/SHEA/APIC/IDSA Hand Hygiene Task Force. MMWR 51(RR-16):1, 2002

———: Environmental infection control guidelines. Recommendations of the Healthcare Infection Control Practices Advisory Committee. MMWR 52(RR10):1, 2003

Hota B, Weinstein RA: Basics work: Preventing infections in ICUs in developing countries. Crit Care Med 33:2133, 2005

Kollef M: SMART approaches for reducing nosocomial infections in the ICU. Chest 134:447, 2008

McKibben L et al: Guidance on public reporting of healthcare-associated recommendations of the Healthcare Infection Control Practices Advisory Committee. Infect Control Hosp Epidemiol 26:580, 2005

Mermel LA et al: Guidelines for the management of intravascular catheter–related infections. Clin Infect Dis 32:1249, 2001

Strausbaugh LJ et al: Preventing transmission of multidrug-resistant bacteria in health care settings: A tale of two guidelines. Clin Infect Dis 42:828, 2006

Weinstein RA et al: Infection control report cards—securing patient safety. N Engl J Med 353:225, 2005

———, Bonten MJ: Controlling antibiotic resistant bacteria: What's an intensivist to do? Crit Care Med 33:2446, 2005

CHAPTER 14

APPROACH TO THE ACUTELY ILL INFECTED FEBRILE PATIENT

Tamar F. Barlam ■ Dennis L. Kasper

The physician treating the acutely ill febrile patient must be able to recognize infections that require emergent attention. If such infections are not adequately evaluated and treated at initial presentation, the opportunity to alter an adverse outcome may be lost. In this chapter, the clinical presentations of and approach to patients with relatively common infectious disease emergencies are discussed. These infectious processes and their treatments are discussed in detail in other chapters. Noninfectious causes of fever are not covered in this chapter; information on the approach to fever of unknown origin, including that eventually shown to be of noninfectious etiology, is presented in Chap. 9.

Approach to the Patient: ACUTE FEBRILE ILLNESS

A physician must have a consistent approach to acutely ill patients. Even before the history is elicited and a physical examination performed, an immediate assessment of the patient's general appearance yields valuable information. The perceptive physician's subjective sense that a patient is septic or toxic often proves accurate. Visible agitation or anxiety in a febrile patient can be a harbinger of critical illness.

HISTORY Presenting symptoms are frequently nonspecific. Detailed questions should be asked about the onset and duration of symptoms and about changes in severity or rate of progression over time. Host factors and comorbid conditions may enhance the risk of infection with certain organisms or of a more fulminant course than is usually seen. Lack of splenic function, alcoholism with significant liver disease, intravenous drug use, HIV infection, diabetes, malignancy, and chemotherapy all predispose to specific infections and frequently to increased severity. The patient should be questioned about factors that might help identify a nidus for invasive infection, such as recent upper respiratory tract infections, influenza, or varicella; prior trauma; disruption of cutaneous barriers due to lacerations, burns, surgery, or decubiti; and the presence of foreign bodies, such as nasal packing after rhinoplasty, barrier contraceptives, tampons, arteriovenous fistulas, or prosthetic joints. Travel, contact with pets or other animals, or activities that might result in tick exposure can lead to diagnoses that would not otherwise be considered. Recent dietary intake, medication use, social or occupational contact with ill individuals, vaccination history, recent sexual contacts, and menstrual history may be relevant. A review of systems should focus on any neurologic signs or sensorium alterations, rashes or skin lesions, and focal pain or tenderness and should also include a general review of respiratory, gastrointestinal, or genitourinary symptoms.

PHYSICAL EXAMINATION A complete physical examination should be performed, with special attention to several areas that are sometimes given short shrift in routine examinations. Assessment of the patient's general appearance and vital signs, skin and soft tissue examination, and the neurologic evaluation are of particular importance.

The patient may appear either anxious and agitated or lethargic and apathetic. Fever is usually present, although elderly patients and compromised hosts [e.g., patients who are uremic or cirrhotic and those who are taking glucocorticoids or nonsteroidal anti-inflammatory drugs (NSAIDs)] may be afebrile despite serious underlying infection. Measurement of blood pressure, heart rate, and respiratory rate helps determine the degree of hemodynamic and metabolic compromise. The patient's airway must be evaluated to rule out the risk of obstruction from an invasive oropharyngeal infection.

The etiologic diagnosis may become evident in the context of a thorough skin examination (Chap. 8). Petechial rashes are typically seen with meningococcemia or Rocky Mountain spotted fever (RMSF); erythroderma is associated with toxic shock syndrome (TSS) and drug fever. The soft tissue and muscle examination is critical. Areas of erythema or duskiness, edema, and tenderness may indicate underlying necrotizing fasciitis, myositis, or myonecrosis. The neurologic examination must include a careful assessment of mental status for signs of early encephalopathy. Evidence of nuchal rigidity or focal neurologic findings should be sought.

DIAGNOSTIC WORKUP After a quick clinical assessment, diagnostic material should be obtained rapidly and antibiotic and supportive treatment begun. Blood (for cultures; baseline complete blood count with differential; measurement of serum electrolytes, blood urea nitrogen, serum creatinine, and serum glucose; and liver function tests) can be obtained at the time an intravenous line is placed and before antibiotics are administered. Three sets of blood cultures should be performed for patients with possible acute endocarditis. Asplenic patients should have a blood smear examined to confirm the presence of Howell-Jolly bodies (indicating the absence of splenic function) and a buffy coat examined for bacteria; these patients can have $>10^6$ organisms per milliliter of blood (compared with 10^4/mL in patients with an intact spleen). Blood smears from patients at risk for severe parasitic disease, such as malaria or babesiosis, must be examined for the diagnosis and quantitation of parasitemia. Blood smears may also be diagnostic in ehrlichiosis.

Patients with possible meningitis should have cerebrospinal fluid (CSF) obtained before the initiation of antibiotic therapy. Focal findings, depressed mental status, or papilledema should be evaluated by brain imaging before lumbar puncture, which, in this setting, could initiate herniation. *Antibiotics should be administered before imaging but after blood for cultures has been drawn.* If CSF cultures are negative, blood cultures will provide the diagnosis in 50–70% of cases.

Focal abscesses necessitate immediate CT or MRI as part of an evaluation for surgical intervention. Other diagnostic procedures, such as cultures of wounds or scraping of skin lesions, should not delay the initiation of treatment for more than minutes. Once emergent evaluation, diagnostic procedures, and (if appropriate) surgical consultation (see below) have been completed, other laboratory tests can be conducted. Appropriate radiography, computed axial tomography, MRI, urinalysis, erythrocyte sedimentation rate (ESR) determination, and transthoracic or transesophageal echocardiography may all prove important.

℞ Treatment: THE ACUTELY ILL PATIENT

In the acutely ill patient, empirical antibiotic therapy is critical and should be administered without undue delay. Increased prevalence of antibiotic resistance in community-acquired bacteria must be considered when antibiotics are selected. Table 14-1 lists first-line treatments for infections considered in this chapter. In addition to the rapid initiation of antibiotic therapy, several of these infections require urgent surgical attention. Neurosurgical evaluation for subdural empyema or spinal epidural abscess, otolaryngologic surgery for possible mucormycosis, and cardiothoracic surgery for critically ill patients with acute endocarditis are as important as antibiotic therapy. For infections such as necrotizing fasciitis and clostridial myonecrosis, rapid surgical intervention supersedes other diagnostic or therapeutic maneuvers.

Adjunctive treatments may reduce morbidity and mortality and include dexamethasone for bacterial meningitis; intravenous immunoglobulin (IVIg) for TSS and necrotizing fasciitis caused by group A *Streptococcus*; low-dose hydrocortisone and fludrocortisone for septic shock; and drotrecogin alfa (activated), also known as recombinant human activated protein C, for meningococcemia and severe sepsis. Adjunctive therapies should usually be initiated within the first hours of treatment; however, dexamethasone for bacterial meningitis must be given before or at the time of the first dose of antibiotic.

SPECIFIC PRESENTATIONS

The infections considered below according to common clinical presentation can have rapidly catastrophic outcomes, and their immediate recognition and treatment can be life-saving. Recommended empirical therapeutic regimens are presented in Table 14-1.

SEPSIS WITHOUT AN OBVIOUS FOCUS OF PRIMARY INFECTION

These patients initially have a brief prodrome of nonspecific symptoms and signs that progresses quickly to hemodynamic instability with hypotension, tachycardia, tachypnea, respiratory distress, and altered mental status. Disseminated intravascular coagulation (DIC) with clinical evidence of a hemorrhagic diathesis is a poor prognostic sign.

Septic Shock

(See also Chap. 15) Patients with bacteremia leading to septic shock may have a primary site of infection (e.g., pneumonia, pyelonephritis, or cholangitis) that is not evident initially. Elderly patients with comorbid conditions, hosts compromised by malignancy and neutropenia, and patients who have recently undergone a surgical procedure or hospitalization are at increased risk for an adverse outcome. Gram-negative bacteremia with organisms such as *Pseudomonas aeruginosa* or *Escherichia coli* and gram-positive infection with organisms such as *Staphylococcus aureus* or group A streptococci can present as intractable hypotension and multiorgan failure. Treatment can usually be initiated empirically on the basis of the presentation (Table 15-3). Adjunctive therapy with either drotrecogin alfa (activated) or glucocorticoids should be considered for patients with severe sepsis.

Overwhelming Infection in Asplenic Patients

(See also Chap. 15) Patients without splenic function are at risk for overwhelming bacterial sepsis. Asplenic adult patients succumb to sepsis at 58 times the rate of the general population; 50–70% of cases occur within the first 2 years after splenectomy, with a mortality rate of up to 80%, but the increased risk persists throughout life. In asplenia, encapsulated bacteria cause the majority of infections. Adults, who are more likely to have antibody to these organisms, are at lower risk than children. *Streptococcus pneumoniae* is the most common isolate, causing 50–70% of cases, but the risk of infection with *Haemophilus influenzae* or *Neisseria meningitidis* is also high. Severe clinical manifestations of infections due to *E. coli*, *S. aureus*, group B streptococci, *P. aeruginosa*, *Capnocytophaga*, *Babesia*, and *Plasmodium* have been described.

Babesiosis

(See also Chap. 117) A history of recent travel to endemic areas raises the possibility of infection with *Babesia*. Between 1 and 4 weeks after a tick bite, the patient experiences chills, fatigue, anorexia, myalgia, arthralgia, shortness of breath, nausea, and headache; ecchymosis and/or petechiae are occasionally seen. The tick that most commonly transmits *Babesia*, *Ixodes scapularis*, also transmits *Borrelia burgdorferi* (the agent of Lyme disease) and *Ehrlichia*; co-infection can occur, resulting in more severe disease. Infection with the European species *Babesia divergens* is more frequently fulminant than that due to the U.S. species *Babesia microti*. *B. divergens* causes a febrile syndrome with hemolysis, jaundice, hemoglobinemia, and renal failure and is associated with a mortality rate of >50%. Severe babesiosis is especially common in asplenic hosts but does occur in hosts with normal splenic function, particularly at >60 years of age. Complications include renal failure, acute respiratory failure, and DIC.

Other Sepsis Syndromes

Tularemia (Chap. 59) is seen throughout the United States but occurs primarily in Arkansas, Oklahoma, and Missouri. This disease is associated with wild rabbit, tick, and tabanid fly contact. The uncommon typhoidal form can be associated with gram-negative septic shock and a mortality rate of >30%. In the United States, plague

TABLE 14-1

EMPIRICAL TREATMENT FOR COMMON INFECTIOUS DISEASE EMERGENCIES

CLINICAL SYNDROME	POSSIBLE ETIOLOGIES	TREATMENT	COMMENTS	SEE CHAP.
Sepsis without a Clear Focus				
Septic shock	*Pseudomonas* spp., gram-negative enteric bacilli, *Staphylococcus* spp., *Streptococcus* spp.	Vancomycin (1 g q12h) ***plus*** Gentamicin (5 mg/kg per day) ***plus either*** Piperacillin/tazobactam (3.375 g q4h) ***or*** Cefepime (2 g q12h)	Adjust treatment when culture data become available. Drotrecogin alfa (activated)[a] or low-dose hydrocortisone and fludrocortisone[b] may improve outcome in patients with septic shock.	15, 35, 36, 51, 53
Overwhelming post-splenectomy sepsis	*Streptococcus pneumoniae*, *Haemophilus influenzae*, *Neisseria meningitidis*	Ceftriaxone (2 g q12h) ***plus*** Vancomycin (1 g q12h)	If a β-lactam–sensitive strain is identified, vancomycin can be discontinued.	15
Babesiosis	*Babesia microti* (United States), *B. divergens* (Europe)	***Either:*** Clindamycin (600 mg tid) ***plus*** Quinine (650 mg tid) ***or*** Atovaquone (750 mg q12h) ***plus*** Azithromycin (500-mg loading dose, then 250 mg/d)	Atovaquone and azithromycin are as effective as clindamycin and quinine and are associated with fewer side effects. Treatment with doxycycline (100 mg bid[c]) for potential coinfection with *Borrelia burgdorferi* or *Ehrlichia* spp. may be prudent.	113, 117
Sepsis with Skin Findings				
Meningococcemia	*N. meningitidis*	Penicillin (4 mU q4h) ***or*** Ceftriaxone (2 g q12h)	Consider protein C replacement in fulminant meningococcemia.	44, 75
Rocky Mountain spotted fever (RMSF)	*Rickettsia rickettsii*	Doxycycline (100 mg bid)	If both meningococcemia and RMSF are being considered, use chloramphenicol alone (50–75 mg/kg per day in four divided doses) ***or*** ceftriaxone (2 g q12h) ***plus*** doxycycline (100 mg bid[c]) If RMSF is diagnosed, doxycycline is the proven superior agent.	
Purpura fulminans	*S. pneumoniae*, *H. influenzae*, *N. meningitidis*	Ceftriaxone (2 g q12h) ***plus*** Vancomycin (1 g q12h)	If a β-lactam–sensitive strain is identified, vancomycin can be discontinued.	15, 44
Erythroderma: toxic shock syndrome	Group A *Streptococcus*, *Staphylococcus aureus*	Vancomycin (1 g q12h) ***plus*** Clindamycin (600 mg q8h)	If a penicillin- or oxacillin-sensitive strain is isolated, those agents are superior to vancomycin (penicillin, 2 mU q4h; or oxacillin, 2 g q4h). The site of toxigenic bacteria should be debrided; IV immunoglobulin can be used in severe cases.[d]	35, 36
Sepsis with Soft Tissue Findings				
Necrotizing fasciitis	Group A *Streptococcus*, mixed aerobic/anaerobic flora	Penicillin (2 mU q4h) ***plus*** Clindamycin (600 mg q8h) ***plus*** Gentamicin (5 mg/kg per day)	Urgent surgical evaluation is critical. If community-acquired methicillin-resistant *S. aureus* is a concern, vancomycin (1 g q12h) can be substituted for penicillin while culture data are pending.	21, 36

(*Continued*)

TABLE 14-1 (*CONTINUED*)

EMPIRICAL TREATMENT FOR COMMON INFECTIOUS DISEASE EMERGENCIES

CLINICAL SYNDROME	POSSIBLE ETIOLOGIES	TREATMENT	COMMENTS	SEE CHAP.
Sepsis with Soft Tissue Findings (*Continued*)				
Clostridial myonecrosis	*Clostridium perfringens*	Penicillin (2 mU q4h) ***plus*** Clindamycin (600 mg q8h)	Urgent surgical evaluation is critical.	42
Neurologic Infections				
Bacterial meningitis	*S. pneumoniae*, *N. meningitidis*	Ceftriaxone (2 g q12h) ***plus*** Vancomycin (1 g q12h)	If a β-lactam–sensitive strain is identified, vancomycin can be discontinued. If the patient is >50 years old or has comorbid disease, add ampicillin (2 g q4h) for *Listeria* coverage. Dexamethasone (10 mg q6h × 4 days) improves outcome in adult patients with meningitis (especially pneumococcal) and cloudy CSF, positive CSF Gram's stain, or a CSF leukocyte count >1000/μL.	29
Brain abscess, suppurative intracranial infections	*Streptococcus* spp., *Staphylococcus* spp., anaerobes, gram-negative bacilli	Vancomycin (1 g q12h) ***plus*** Metronidazole (500 mg q8h) ***plus*** Ceftriaxone (2 g q12h)	Urgent surgical evaluation is critical. If a penicillin- or oxacillin-sensitive strain is isolated, those agents are superior to vancomycin (penicillin, 4 mU q4h; or oxacillin, 2 g q4h).	29
Cerebral malaria	*Plasmodium falciparum*	Quinine (650 mg tid) ***plus*** Tetracycline (250 mg tid)	Do not use glucocorticoids.	113, 116
Spinal epidural abscess	*Staphylococcus* spp., gram-negative bacilli	Vancomycin (1 g q12h) ***plus*** Ceftriaxone (2 g q24h)	Surgical evaluation is essential. If a penicillin- or oxacillin-sensitive strain is isolated, those agents are superior to vancomycin (penicillin, 4 mU q4h; or oxacillin, 2 g q4h).	...
Focal Infections				
Acute bacterial endocarditis	*S. aureus*, β-hemolytic streptococci, HACEK group,[e] *Neisseria* spp., *S. pneumoniae*	Ceftriaxone (2 g q12h) ***plus*** Vancomycin (1 g q12h)	Adjust treatment when culture data become available. Surgical evaluation is essential.	19

[a]Drotrecogin alfa (activated) is administered at a dose of 24 μg/kg per hour for 96 h. It has been approved for use in patients with severe sepsis and a high risk of death as defined by an Acute Physiology and Chronic Health Evaluation II (APACHE II) score of ≥25 and/or multiorgan failure.

[b]Hydrocortisone (50-mg IV bolus q6h) with fludrocortisone (50-μg tablet daily for 7 days) may improve outcomes of severe sepsis, particularly in the setting of relative adrenal insufficiency.

[c]Tetracyclines can be antagonistic in action to β-lactam agents. Adjust treatment as soon as the diagnosis is confirmed.

[d]The optimal dose of IV immunoglobulin has not been determined, but the median dose in observational studies is 2 g/kg (total dose administered over 1–5 days).

[e]*Haemophilus aphrophilus, H. paraphrophilus, H. parainfluenzae, Actinobacillus actinomycetemcomitans, Cardiobacterium hominis, Eikenella corrodens,* and *Kingella kingae*.

(Chap. 60) occurs primarily in New Mexico, Arizona, and Colorado after contact with ground squirrels, prairie dogs, or chipmunks. Plague can occur with greater frequency outside the United States, especially in developing countries in Africa and Asia. The septic form is particularly rare and is associated with shock, multiorgan failure, and a 30% mortality rate. These rare infections should be considered in the appropriate epidemiologic setting. The Centers for Disease Control and Prevention lists tularemia and plague, along with anthrax, as important agents that might be used for bioterrorism (Chap. 6).

SEPSIS WITH SKIN MANIFESTATIONS

(See also Chap. 8) Maculopapular rashes may reflect early meningococcal or rickettsial disease but are usually associated with nonemergent infections. Exanthems are usually viral. Primary HIV infection commonly presents with a rash that is typically maculopapular and involves the upper part of the body but can spread to the palms and soles. The patient is usually febrile and can have lymphadenopathy, severe headache, dysphagia, diarrhea, myalgias, and arthralgias. Recognition of this syndrome provides an opportunity to prevent transmission and to institute treatment and monitoring early on.

Petechial rashes caused by viruses are seldom associated with hypotension or a toxic appearance, although severe measles can be an exception. In other settings, petechial rashes require more urgent attention.

Meningococcemia

(See also Chap. 44) Almost three-quarters of patients with bacteremic *N. meningitidis* infection have a rash. Meningococcemia most often affects young children (i.e., those 6 months to 5 years old). In Sub-Saharan Africa, the high prevalence of serogroup A meningococcal disease has been a threat to public health for more than a century. In addition, epidemic outbreaks occur every 8–12 years. In the United States, sporadic cases and outbreaks occur in day-care centers, schools (grade school through college), and army barracks. Household members of index cases are at 400–800 times greater risk of disease than the general population. Patients may exhibit fever, headache, nausea, vomiting, myalgias, changes in mental status, and meningismus. However, the rapidly progressive form of disease is not usually associated with meningitis. The rash is initially pink, blanching, and maculopapular, appearing on the trunk and extremities, but then becomes hemorrhagic, forming petechiae. Petechiae are first seen at the ankles, wrists, axillae, mucosal surfaces, and palpebral and bulbar conjunctiva, with subsequent spread to the lower extremities and trunk. A cluster of petechiae may be seen at pressure points—e.g., where a blood pressure cuff has been inflated. In rapidly progressive meningococcemia (10–20% of cases), the petechial rash quickly becomes purpuric and patients develop DIC, multiorgan failure, and shock. Of these patients, 50–60% die, and survivors often require extensive debridement or amputation of gangrenous extremities. Hypotension with petechiae for <12 h is associated with significant mortality. The mortality rate can exceed 90% among patients without meningitis who have rash, hypotension, and a normal or low white blood cell (WBC) count and ESR. Cyanosis, coma, oliguria, metabolic acidosis, and elevated partial thromboplastin time are also associated with a fatal outcome. Correction of protein C deficiency may improve outcome. Antibiotics given in the office by the primary care provider before hospital evaluation and admission may improve prognosis; this observation suggests that early initiation of treatment may be life-saving.

Rocky Mountain Spotted Fever

(See also Chap. 75) RMSF is a tickborne disease caused by *Rickettsia rickettsii* that occurs throughout North and South America. A history of known tick bite is common; however, if such a history is lacking, a history of travel or outdoor activity (e.g., camping in tick-infested areas) can be ascertained. For the first 3 days, headache, fever, malaise, myalgias, nausea, vomiting, and anorexia are present. By day 3, half of patients have skin findings. Blanching macules develop initially on the wrists and ankles and then spread over the legs and trunk. The lesions become hemorrhagic and are frequently petechial. The rash spreads to palms and soles later in the course. The centripetal spread is a classic feature of RMSF. However, 10–15% of patients with RMSF never develop a rash. The patient can be hypotensive and develop noncardiogenic pulmonary edema, confusion, lethargy, and encephalitis progressing to coma. The CSF contains 10–100 cells/μL, usually with a predominance of mononuclear cells. The CSF glucose level is often normal; the protein concentration may be slightly elevated. Renal and hepatic injury and bleeding secondary to vascular damage are noted. Untreated infection has a mortality rate of 30%.

Although RMSF is the most severe rickettsial disease, other rickettsial diseases cause significant morbidity and mortality worldwide. *Mediterranean spotted fever* caused by *Rickettsia conorii* is found in Africa, southwestern and south-central Asia, and southern Europe. Patients have fever, flulike symptoms, and an inoculation eschar at the site of the tick bite. A maculopapular rash develops within 1–7 days, involving the palms and soles but sparing the face. Elderly patients or those with diabetes, alcoholism, uremia, or congestive heart failure are at risk for severe disease characterized by neurologic involvement, respiratory distress, and gangrene of the digits. Mortality rates associated with this severe form of disease approach 50%. *Epidemic typhus*, caused by *Rickettsia prowazekii*, is transmitted in louse-infested environments and emerges in conditions of extreme poverty, war, and natural disaster. Patients experience a sudden onset of high fevers, severe headache, cough, myalgias, and abdominal pain. A maculopapular rash develops (primarily on the trunk) in more than half of patients and can progress to petechiae and purpura. Serious signs include delirium, coma, seizures, noncardiogenic pulmonary edema, skin necrosis, and peripheral gangrene.

Mortality rates approached 60% in the preantibiotic era and continue to exceed 10–15% in contemporary outbreaks. *Scrub typhus*, caused by *Orientia tsutsugamushi*—a separate genus in the family Rickettsiaceae—is transmitted by larval mites or chiggers and is one of the most common infections in southeastern Asia and the western Pacific. The organism is found in areas of heavy scrub vegetation (e.g., along riverbanks). Patients present with fever and lymphadenopathy, may have an inoculation eschar, and may develop a maculopapular rash. Severe cases progress to pneumonia, meningoencephalitis, DIC, and renal failure. Mortality rates range from 1% to 35%.

If recognized in a timely fashion, rickettsial disease is very responsive to treatment. Doxycycline (100 mg twice daily for 3–14 days) is the treatment of choice for both adults and children. The newer macrolides and chloramphenicol may be suitable alternatives.

Purpura Fulminans

(See also Chaps. 15 and 44) Purpura fulminans is the cutaneous manifestation of DIC and presents as large ecchymotic areas and hemorrhagic bullae. Progression of petechiae to purpura, ecchymoses, and gangrene is associated with congestive heart failure, septic shock, acute renal failure, acidosis, hypoxia, hypotension, and death. Purpura fulminans has been associated primarily with *N. meningitidis* but, in splenectomized patients, may be associated with *S. pneumoniae* and *H. influenzae*. Several small studies have suggested that correction of the protein C deficiency evident in meningococcal purpura fulminans with drotrecogin alfa (activated) may dramatically improve outcome.

Ecthyma Gangrenosum

Septic shock caused by *P. aeruginosa* or *Aeromonas hydrophila* can be associated with ecthyma gangrenosum (see Fig. 53-1): hemorrhagic vesicles surrounded by a rim of erythema with central necrosis and ulceration. These gram-negative bacteremias are most common among patients with neutropenia, extensive burns, and hypogammaglobulinemia.

Other Emergent Infections Associated with Rash

Vibrio vulnificus and other noncholera *Vibrio* bacteremic infections (Chap. 57) can cause focal skin lesions and overwhelming sepsis in hosts with liver disease. After ingestion of contaminated shellfish, there is a sudden onset of malaise, chills, fever, and hypotension. The patient develops bullous or hemorrhagic skin lesions, usually on the lower extremities, and 75% of patients have leg pain. The mortality rate can be as high as 50–60%. *Capnocytophaga canimorsus* can cause septic shock in asplenic patients. Infection with this fastidious gram-negative rod typically presents after a dog bite as fever, chills, myalgia, vomiting, diarrhea, dyspnea, confusion, and headache. Findings can include an exanthem or erythema multiforme, cyanotic mottling or peripheral cyanosis, petechiae, and ecchymosis. About 30% of patients with this fulminant form die of overwhelming sepsis and DIC, and survivors may require amputation because of gangrene.

Erythroderma

TSS (Chaps. 35 and 36) is usually associated with erythroderma. The patient presents with fever, malaise, myalgias, nausea, vomiting, diarrhea, and confusion. There is a sunburn-type rash that may be subtle and patchy but is usually diffuse and is found on the face, trunk, and extremities. Erythroderma, which desquamates after 1–2 weeks, is more common in *Staphylococcus*-associated than in *Streptococcus*-associated TSS. Hypotension develops rapidly—often within hours—after the onset of symptoms. Multiorgan failure is seen. Early renal failure may precede hypotension and distinguishes this syndrome from other septic shock syndromes. Commonly there is no indication of a primary focal infection, although possible cutaneous or mucosal portals of entry for the organism can be ascertained when a careful history is taken. Colonization rather than overt infection of the vagina or a postoperative wound, for example, is typical with staphylococcal TSS, and the mucosal areas appear hyperemic but not infected. The diagnosis of TSS is defined by the clinical criteria of fever, rash, hypotension, and multiorgan involvement. The mortality rate is 5% for menstruation-associated TSS, 10–15% for nonmenstrual TSS, and 30–70% for streptococcal TSS.

Viral Hemorrhagic Fevers

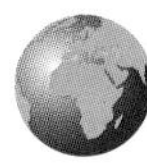

Viral hemorrhagic fevers (Chaps. 99 and 100) are zoonotic illnesses caused by viruses that reside in either animal reservoirs or arthropod vectors. These diseases occur worldwide and are restricted to areas where the host species live. They are caused by four major groups of viruses: Arenaviridae (e.g., Lassa fever in Africa), Bunyaviridae (e.g., Rift Valley fever in Africa or hantavirus hemorrhagic fever with renal syndrome in Asia), Filoviridae (e.g., Ebola and Marburg virus infections in Africa), and Flaviviridae (e.g., yellow fever in Africa and South America and dengue in Asia, Africa, and the Americas). Lassa fever as well as Ebola and Marburg virus infections are also transmitted from person to person. The vectors for most viral fevers are found in rural areas; dengue and yellow fever are important exceptions. After a prodrome of fever, myalgias, and malaise, patients develop evidence of vascular damage, petechiae, and local hemorrhage. Shock, multifocal hemorrhaging, and neurologic signs (e.g., seizures or coma) predict a poor prognosis. Although supportive care to maintain blood pressure and intravascular volume is key, ribavirin may be useful against Arenaviridae and Bunyaviridae. Dengue (Chap. 99) is the most common arboviral disease worldwide. More than a quarter of a million cases of dengue hemorrhagic fever occur each year, with 25,000 deaths. Patients have a triad of symptoms: hemorrhagic manifestations, evidence of plasma leakage, and platelet counts <100,000/μL. Mortality rates are 10–20%. If dengue shock syndrome develops, mortality can reach 40%. Immediate supportive care and volume-replacement therapy are life-saving.

SEPSIS WITH A SOFT TISSUE/MUSCLE PRIMARY FOCUS

See also Chap. 21.

Necrotizing Fasciitis

This infection may arise at a site of minimal trauma or postoperative incision and may also be associated with recent varicella, childbirth, or muscle strain. The most common causes of necrotizing fasciitis are group A streptococci alone (Chap. 36) and a mixed facultative and anaerobic flora (Chap. 21). Diabetes mellitus, peripheral vascular disease, and intravenous drug use are associated risk factors. Use of NSAIDs has been reported to allow progression of skin or soft tissue infections; however, prospective studies have not shown that NSAIDs increase the risk of disease or exacerbate established infection. The patient may have bacteremia and hypotension without other organ-system failure. Physical findings are minimal compared with the severity of pain and the degree of fever. The examination is often unremarkable except for soft tissue edema and erythema. The infected area is red, hot, shiny, swollen, and exquisitely tender. In untreated infection, the overlying skin develops blue-gray patches after 36 h, and cutaneous bullae and necrosis develop after 3–5 days. Necrotizing fasciitis due to a mixed flora, but not that due to group A streptococci, can be associated with gas production. Without treatment, pain decreases because of thrombosis of the small blood vessels and destruction of the peripheral nerves—an ominous sign. The mortality rate is 25–30% overall, >70% in association with TSS, and nearly 100% without surgical intervention. Life-threatening necrotizing fasciitis may also be due to *Clostridium perfringens* (Chap. 42); in this condition, the patient is extremely toxic and the mortality rate is high. Within 48 h, rapid tissue invasion and systemic toxicity associated with hemolysis and death ensue. The distinction between this entity and clostridial myonecrosis is made by muscle biopsy. Necrotizing fasciitis caused by community-acquired methicillin-resistant *S. aureus* (MRSA) was recently described. The MRSA-infected patients required extensive surgical debridement, but there were no deaths.

Clostridial Myonecrosis

(See also Chap. 42) Myonecrosis is often associated with trauma or surgery but can be spontaneous. The incubation period is usually 12–24 h long, and massive necrotizing gangrene develops within hours of onset. Systemic toxicity, shock, and death can occur within 12 h. The patient's pain and toxic appearance are out of proportion to physical findings. On examination, the patient is febrile, apathetic, tachycardic, and tachypneic and may express a feeling of impending doom. Hypotension and renal failure develop later, and hyperalertness is evident preterminally. The skin over the affected area is bronze-brown, mottled, and edematous. Bullous lesions with serosanguineous drainage and a mousy or sweet odor can be present. Crepitus can occur secondary to gas production in muscle tissue. The mortality rate is >65% with spontaneous myonecrosis, which is often associated with *Clostridium septicum* and underlying malignancy. The mortality rates associated with trunk and limb infection are 63% and 12%, respectively, and any delay in surgical treatment increases the risk of death.

NEUROLOGIC INFECTIONS WITH OR WITHOUT SEPTIC SHOCK

Bacterial Meningitis

(See also Chap. 29) Bacterial meningitis is one of the most common infectious disease emergencies involving the central nervous system. Although hosts with cell-mediated immune deficiency (including transplant recipients, diabetic patients, elderly patients, and cancer patients receiving certain chemotherapeutic agents) are at particular risk for *Listeria monocytogenes* meningitis, most cases in adults are due to *S. pneumoniae* (30–50%) and *N. meningitidis* (10–35%). The classic presentation of headache, meningismus, and fever is seen in only one-half to two-thirds of patients. The elderly can present without fever or meningeal signs despite lethargy and confusion. Cerebral dysfunction is evidenced by confusion, delirium, and lethargy that can progress to coma. A fulminant presentation with sepsis and brain edema occurs in some cases; papilledema at presentation is unusual and suggests another diagnosis (e.g., an intracranial lesion). Focal signs, including cranial nerve palsies (IV, VI, VII), can be seen in 10–20% of cases; 50–70% of patients have bacteremia. A poor outcome is associated with coma, hypotension, meningitis due to *S. pneumoniae*, respiratory distress, a CSF glucose level of <0.6 mmol/L (<10 mg/dL), a CSF protein level of >2.5 g/L, a peripheral WBC count of <5000/μL, and a serum sodium level of <135 mmol/L.

Suppurative Intracranial Infections

(See also Chap. 29) In suppurative intracranial infections, rare intracranial lesions present along with sepsis and hemodynamic instability. Rapid recognition of the toxic patient with central neurologic signs is crucial to improvement of the dismal prognosis of these entities. *Subdural empyema* arises from the paranasal sinus in 60–70% of cases. Microaerophilic streptococci and staphylococci are the predominant etiologic organisms. The patient is toxic, with fever, headache, and nuchal rigidity. Of all patients, 75% have focal signs, and 6–20% die. Despite improved survival rates, 15–44% of patients are left with permanent neurologic deficits. *Septic cavernous sinus thrombosis* follows a facial or sphenoid sinus infection; 70% of cases are due to staphylococci, and the remainder is due primarily to aerobic or anaerobic streptococci. A unilateral or retroorbital headache progresses to a toxic appearance and fever within days. Three-quarters of patients have unilateral periorbital edema that becomes bilateral and then progresses to ptosis, proptosis, ophthalmoplegia, and papilledema. The mortality rate is as high as 30%. *Septic thrombosis of the superior sagittal sinus* spreads from the ethmoid or maxillary sinuses and is caused by *S. pneumoniae*, other streptococci, and staphylococci. The fulminant course is characterized by headache, nausea, vomiting, rapid progression to confusion and coma, nuchal rigidity, and brainstem signs. If the sinus is totally thrombosed, the mortality rate exceeds 80%.

Brain Abscess

(See also Chap. 29) Brain abscess often occurs without systemic signs. Almost half of patients are afebrile, and presentations are more consistent with a space-occupying lesion in the brain; 70% of patients have headache, 50% have focal neurologic signs, and 25% have papilledema. Abscesses can present as single or multiple lesions resulting from contiguous foci or hematogenous infection, such as endocarditis. The infection progresses over several days from cerebritis to an abscess with a mature capsule. More than half of infections are polymicrobial, with an etiology consisting of aerobic bacteria (primarily streptococcal species) and anaerobes. Abscesses arising hematogenously are especially apt to rupture into the ventricular space, causing a sudden and severe deterioration in clinical status and high mortality. Otherwise, mortality is low, but morbidity is high (30–55%). Patients presenting with stroke and a parameningeal infectious focus, such as sinusitis or otitis, may have a brain abscess, and physicians must maintain a high level of suspicion. Prognosis worsens in patients with a fulminant course, delayed diagnosis, abscess rupture into the ventricles, multiple abscesses, or abnormal neurologic status at presentation.

Cerebral Malaria

(See also Chap. 116) This entity should be urgently considered if patients who have recently traveled to areas endemic for malaria present with a febrile illness and lethargy or other neurologic signs. Fulminant malaria is caused by *Plasmodium falciparum* and is associated with temperatures of >40°C (>104°F), hypotension, jaundice, adult respiratory distress syndrome, and bleeding. By definition, any patient with a change in mental status or repeated seizure in the setting of fulminant malaria has cerebral malaria. In adults, this nonspecific febrile illness progresses to coma over several days; occasionally, coma occurs within hours and death within 24 h. Nuchal rigidity and photophobia are rare. On physical examination, symmetric encephalopathy is typical, and upper motor neuron dysfunction with decorticate and decerebrate posturing can be seen in advanced disease. Unrecognized infection results in a 20–30% mortality rate.

Spinal Epidural Abscesses

Patients with spinal epidural abscesses often present with back pain and develop neurologic deficits late in their course. At-risk patients include those with diabetes mellitus; intravenous drug use; chronic alcohol abuse; recent spinal trauma, surgery, or epidural anesthesia; and other comorbid conditions, such as HIV infection. The thoracic or lumbar spine is the most common location; cervical spine infections are associated with worse outcomes. Staphylococci are the most common etiologic agents. This diagnosis must immediately be considered in patients with a history of antecedent back pain and new neurologic symptoms. Almost 60% of patients have fever, and almost 90% have back pain. Paresthesia, bowel and bladder dysfunction, radicular pain, and weakness are frequent neurologic complaints, and examination of the patient may reveal abnormal reflexes and motor and sensory deficits. The ESR and leukocyte counts are usually elevated. Rapid recognition and treatment, which may include surgical drainage, can prevent or minimize permanent neurologic sequelae.

OTHER FOCAL SYNDROMES WITH A FULMINANT COURSE

Infection at virtually any primary focus (e.g., osteomyelitis, pneumonia, pyelonephritis, or cholangitis) can result in bacteremia and sepsis. TSS has been associated with focal infections such as septic arthritis, peritonitis, sinusitis, and wound infection. Rapid clinical deterioration and death can be associated with destruction of the primary site of infection, as is seen in endocarditis and in necrotizing infections of the oropharynx (in which edema suddenly compromises the airway).

Rhinocerebral Mucormycosis

(See also Chap. 109) Patients with diabetes or malignancy are at risk for invasive rhinocerebral mucormycosis. Patients present with low-grade fever, dull sinus pain, diplopia, decreased mental status, decreased ocular motion, chemosis, proptosis, dusky or necrotic nasal turbinates, and necrotic hard-palate lesions that respect the midline. Without rapid recognition and intervention, the process continues on an inexorable invasive course, with high mortality.

Acute Bacterial Endocarditis

(See also Chap. 19) This entity presents with a much more aggressive course than subacute endocarditis. Bacteria such as *S. aureus*, *S. pneumoniae*, *L. monocytogenes*, *Haemophilus* spp., and streptococci of groups A, B, and G attack native valves. Mortality rates range from 10% to 40%. The host may have comorbid conditions such as underlying malignancy, diabetes mellitus, intravenous drug use, or alcoholism. The patient presents with fever, fatigue, and malaise <2 weeks after onset of infection. On physical examination, a changing murmur and congestive heart failure may be noted. Hemorrhagic macules on palms or soles (*Janeway's lesions*) sometimes develop. Petechiae, Roth's spots, splinter hemorrhages, and splenomegaly are unusual. Rapid valvular destruction, particularly of the aortic valve, results in pulmonary edema and hypotension. Myocardial abscesses can form, eroding through the septum or into the conduction system and causing life-threatening arrhythmias or high-degree conduction block. Large friable vegetations can result in major arterial emboli, metastatic infection, or tissue infarction. Emboli can lead to stroke, changes in mental status, visual disturbances, aphasia, ataxia, headache, meningismus, brain abscess, cerebritis, spinal cord infarct with paraplegia, arthralgia, osteomyelitis, splenic abscess, septic arthritis, and hematuria. Older patients with *S. aureus* endocarditis are especially likely to present with nonspecific symptoms—a circumstance that delays diagnosis and worsens prognosis. Rapid intervention is crucial for a successful outcome.

Inhalational Anthrax

(See also Chap. 6) Inhalational anthrax, the most severe form of disease caused by *Bacillus anthracis*, had not been reported in the United States for more than 25 years until the recent use of this organism as an agent of bioterrorism (Chap. 6). Patients presented with malaise, fever, cough, nausea, drenching sweats, shortness of breath, and headache. Rhinorrhea was unusual. All patients had abnormal chest roentgenograms at presentation. Pulmonary infiltrates, mediastinal widening, and pleural effusions were the most common findings. Hemorrhagic meningitis was seen in 38% of these patients. Survival was more likely when antibiotics were given during the prodromal period and if multidrug regimens were used. In the absence of urgent intervention with antimicrobial agents and supportive care, inhalational anthrax progresses rapidly to hypotension, cyanosis, and death.

Avian Influenza (H5N1) Infection

(See also Chap. 88) Human cases of avian influenza were first reported in Hong Kong. Recent cases have occurred primarily in Southeast Asia, particularly Vietnam. However, evidence of a rapidly expanding geographic distribution of the virus throughout the world is of grave concern. Avian influenza should be considered in patients with severe respiratory tract illness, particularly if they have been exposed to poultry. To date, human- to-human transmission is rare. Patients present with high fever, an influenza-like illness, and lower respiratory tract symptoms. Watery diarrhea may develop and may precede respiratory symptoms. Dyspnea develops a median of 5 days after the onset of symptoms and can progress to respiratory distress syndrome, multiorgan failure, and death within 9–10 days after the onset of illness. Early antiviral treatment with neuraminidase inhibitors should be initiated along with aggressive supportive measures.

Hantavirus Pulmonary Syndrome

(See also Chap. 99) Hantavirus pulmonary syndrome (HPS) has been documented in the United States (primarily the southwestern states), Canada, and South America. Most cases occur in rural areas and are associated with exposure to rodents. Patients present with a nonspecific viral prodrome of fever, malaise, myalgias, nausea, vomiting, and dizziness that may progress to pulmonary edema and respiratory failure. HPS causes myocardial depression and increased pulmonary vascular permeability; therefore, careful fluid resuscitation and use of pressor agents are crucial. Aggressive cardiopulmonary support during the first few hours of illness can be life-saving.

CONCLUSION

Acutely ill febrile patients with the syndromes discussed in this chapter require close observation, aggressive supportive measures, and—in most cases—admission to intensive care units. The most important task of the physician is to distinguish these patients from other infected febrile patients who will not progress to fulminant disease. The alert physician must recognize the acute infectious disease emergency and then proceed with appropriate urgency.

FURTHER READINGS

Beigel JH et al: Avian influenza A (H5N1) infection in humans. N Engl J Med 353:1374, 2005

Darouiche RO: Spinal epidural abscess. N Engl J Med 355:2012, 2006

Hasham S et al: Necrotising fasciitis. BMJ 330:830, 2005

Idro R et al: Pathogenesis, clinical features, and neurological outcome of cerebral malaria. Lancet Neurol 4:827, 2005

Kyaw MH et al: Evaluation of severe infection and survival after splenectomy. Am J Med 119:276.e1, 2006

Nguyen HB et al: Severe sepsis and septic shock: Review of the literature and emergency department management guidelines. Ann Emerg Med 48:28, 2006

Osborn MK, Steinberg JP: Subdural empyema and other suppurative complications of paranasal sinusitis. Lancet Infect Dis 7:62, 2007

Stephens DS et al: Epidemic meningitis, meningococcemia, and *Neisseria meningitidis*. Lancet 369:2196, 2007

van de Beek D et al: Community-acquired bacterial meningitis in adults. N Engl J Med 354:44, 2006

Wills BA et al: Comparison of three fluid solutions for resuscitation in dengue shock syndrome. N Engl J Med 353:877, 2005

CHAPTER 15

SEVERE SEPSIS AND SEPTIC SHOCK

Robert S. Munford

DEFINITIONS

(See Table 15-1) Animals mount both local and systemic responses to microbes that traverse epithelial barriers and invade underlying tissues. Fever or hypothermia, leukocytosis or leukopenia, tachypnea, and tachycardia are the cardinal signs of the systemic response often called the *systemic inflammatory response syndrome* (SIRS). SIRS may have an infectious or a noninfectious etiology. If infection is suspected or proven, a patient with SIRS is said to have *sepsis*. When sepsis is associated with dysfunction of organs

TABLE 15-1

DEFINITIONS USED TO DESCRIBE THE CONDITION OF SEPTIC PATIENTS	
Bacteremia	Presence of bacteria in blood, as evidenced by positive blood cultures
Septicemia	Presence of microbes or their toxins in blood
Systemic inflammatory response syndrome (SIRS)	Two or more of the following conditions: (1) fever (oral temperature >38°C) or hypothermia (<36°C); (2) tachypnea (>24 breaths/min); (3) tachycardia (heart rate >90 beats/min); (4) leukocytosis (>12,000/μL), leukopenia (<4,000/μL), or >10% bands; may have a noninfectious etiology
Sepsis	SIRS that has a proven or suspected microbial etiology
Severe sepsis (similar to "sepsis syndrome")	Sepsis with one or more signs of organ dysfunction—for example: 1. *Cardiovascular:* Arterial systolic blood pressure ≤90 mmHg or mean arterial pressure ≤70 mmHg that responds to administration of intravenous fluid 2. *Renal:* Urine output <0.5 mL/kg per hour for 1 h despite adequate fluid resuscitation 3. *Respiratory:* Pa_{O_2}/Fi_{O_2} ≤250 or, if the lung is the only dysfunctional organ, ≤200 4. *Hematologic:* Platelet count <80,000/μL or 50% decrease in platelet count from highest value recorded over previous 3 days 5. *Unexplained metabolic acidosis:* A pH ≤7.30 or a base deficit ≥ 5.0 mEq/L and a plasma lactate level >1.5 times upper limit of normal for reporting lab 6. *Adequate fluid resuscitation:* Pulmonary artery wedge pressure ≥12 mmHg or central venous pressure ≥ 8 mmHg
Septic shock	Sepsis with hypotension (arterial blood pressure <90 mmHg systolic, or 40 mmHg less than patient's normal blood pressure) for at least 1 h despite adequate fluid resuscitation; *or* Need for vasopressors to maintain systolic blood pressure ≥90 mmHg *or* mean arterial pressure ≥70 mmHg
Refractory septic shock	Septic shock that lasts for >1 h and does not respond to fluid or pressor administration
Multiple-organ dysfunction syndrome (MODS)	Dysfunction of more than one organ, requiring intervention to maintain homeostasis

Source: Adapted from the American College of Chest Physicians/Society of Critical Care Medicine Consensus Conference Committee and Bernard et al. Published in Crit Care Med, with permission.

distant from the site of infection, the patient has *severe sepsis*. Severe sepsis may be accompanied by hypotension or evidence of hypoperfusion. When hypotension cannot be corrected by infusing fluids, the diagnosis is *septic shock*. These definitions were proposed by consensus conference committees in 1992 and 2001 and are now widely used; there is evidence that the different stages form a continuum. As sepsis progresses to septic shock, the risk of dying increases substantially. Sepsis is usually reversible, whereas patients with septic shock often succumb despite aggressive therapy.

ETIOLOGY

Severe sepsis can be a response to any class of microorganism. Microbial invasion of the bloodstream is not essential for the development of severe sepsis, since local inflammation can also elicit distant organ dysfunction and hypotension. In fact, blood cultures yield bacteria or fungi in only ~20–40% of cases of severe sepsis and 40–70% of cases of septic shock. Individual gram-negative or gram-positive bacteria account for ~70% of these isolates; the remainder are fungi or a mixture of microorganisms (Table 15-2). In patients whose blood cultures are negative, the etiologic agent is often established by culture or microscopic examination of infected material from a local site. In some case series, a majority of patients with a clinical picture of severe sepsis or septic shock have had negative microbiologic data.

EPIDEMIOLOGY

The septic response is a contributing factor in >200,000 deaths per year in the United States. The incidence of severe sepsis and septic shock has increased over the past 20 years, and the annual number of cases is now >700,000 (~3 per 1000 population). Approximately two-thirds of the cases occur in patients with significant underlying illness. Sepsis-related incidence and mortality rates increase with age and preexisting comorbidity. The rising incidence of severe sepsis in the United States is attributable to the aging of the population, the increasing longevity of patients with chronic diseases, and the relatively high frequency with which sepsis develops in patients with AIDS. The widespread use of antimicrobial agents, immunosuppressive drugs, indwelling catheters and mechanical devices, and mechanical ventilation also plays a role.

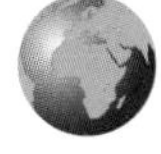

Invasive bacterial infections are prominent causes of death around the world, particularly among young children. In Sub-Saharan Africa, for example, careful screening for positive blood cultures found that community-acquired bacteremia accounted for at least one-fourth of deaths of children >1 year of age. Nontyphoidal *Salmonella* species, *Streptococcus pneumoniae*, *Haemophilus influenzae*, and *Escherichia coli* were the most commonly isolated bacteria. Bacteremic children often had HIV infection or were severely malnourished.

TABLE 15-2

MICROORGANISMS INVOLVED IN EPISODES OF SEVERE SEPSIS AT EIGHT ACADEMIC MEDICAL CENTERS

MICROORGANISMS	EPISODES WITH BLOODSTREAM INFECTION, % (*n* = 436)	EPISODES WITH DOCUMENTED INFECTION BUT NO BLOODSTREAM INFECTION, % (*n* = 430)	TOTAL EPISODES, % (*n* = 866)
Gram-negative bacteria[a]	35	44	40
Gram-positive bacteria[b]	40	24	31
Fungi	7	5	6
Polymicrobial	11	21	16
Classic pathogens[c]	<5	<5	<5

[a]Enterobacteriaceae, pseudomonads, *Haemophilus* spp., other gram-negative bacteria.

[b]*Staphylococcus aureus*, coagulase-negative staphylococci, enterococci, *Streptococcus pneumoniae*, other streptococci, other gram-positive bacteria.

[c]Such as *Neisseria meningitidis*, *S. pneumoniae*, *H. influenzae*, and *Streptococcus pyogenes*.

Source: Adapted from Sands et al.

PATHOPHYSIOLOGY

Most cases of severe sepsis are triggered by bacteria or fungi that do not ordinarily cause systemic disease in immunocompetent hosts (Table 15-2). These microbes probably exploit deficiencies in innate host defenses (e.g., phagocytes, complement, and natural antibodies) to survive within the body. Microbial pathogens, in contrast, are able to circumvent innate defenses by elaborating toxins or other virulence factors. In both cases, the body can fail to kill the invaders despite mounting a vigorous inflammatory reaction that can result in severe sepsis. The septic response may also be induced by microbial exotoxins that act as superantigens (e.g., toxic shock syndrome toxin 1; Chap. 35).

Host Mechanisms for Sensing Microbes

Animals have exquisitely sensitive mechanisms for recognizing and responding to conserved microbial molecules. Recognition of the lipid A moiety of lipopolysaccharide (LPS, also called *endotoxin*; Chap. 2) is the best-studied example. A host protein (LPS-binding protein, or LBP) binds lipid A and transfers the LPS to CD14 on the surfaces of monocytes, macrophages, and neutrophils. LPS then is passed to MD-2, which interacts with Toll-like receptor (TLR) 4 to form a molecular complex that transduces the LPS recognition signal to the interior of the cell. This signal rapidly triggers the production and release of mediators, such as tumor necrosis factor (TNF; see below), that amplify the LPS signal and transmit it to other cells and tissues. Bacterial peptidoglycan and lipoteichoic acids elicit responses in animals that are generally similar to those induced by LPS; whereas these molecules also bind CD14, they interact with different TLRs. Having numerous TLR-based receptor complexes (10 different TLRs have been identified so far in humans) allows animals to recognize many conserved microbial molecules. The ability of some of the TLRs to serve as receptors for host ligands (e.g., hyaluronans, heparan sulfate, saturated fatty acids) raises the possibility that these molecules play a role in producing noninfectious sepsis-like states. Other host pattern-recognition proteins that are important for sensing microbial invasion and initiating host inflammation include the intracellular NOD1 and NOD2 proteins, which recognize discrete fragments of bacterial peptidoglycan; complement (principally the alternative pathway); mannose-binding lectin; and C-reactive protein.

The ability to recognize certain microbial molecules may influence both the potency of the host defense and the pathogenesis of severe sepsis. For example, MD-2–TLR4 best senses LPS that has a hexaacyl lipid A moiety (i.e., one with six fatty acyl chains). Most of the commensal aerobic and facultatively anaerobic gram-negative bacteria that trigger severe sepsis and shock (including *E. coli*, *Klebsiella*, and *Enterobacter*) make this lipid A structure. When they invade human hosts, often through breaks in an epithelial barrier, infection is typically localized to the subepithelial tissue. Bacteremia, if it occurs, is intermittent and low-grade, as these bacteria are efficiently cleared from the bloodstream by TLR4-expressing Kupffer cells and splenic macrophages. These mucosal commensals seem to induce severe sepsis most often by triggering severe local tissue inflammation rather than by circulating within the bloodstream. In contrast, gram-negative bacteria that do not make hexaacyl lipid A (*Yersinia pestis*, *Francisella tularensis*, *Vibrio vulnificus*, *Pseudomonas aeruginosa*, and *Burkholderia pseudomallei*, among others) are poorly recognized by MD-2–TLR4. These bacteria usually enter the body via nonmucosal routes—e.g., as a result of bites, cuts, or inhalation—and initially induce relatively little inflammation. When they do trigger severe sepsis, it is often in the setting of massive bacterial growth throughout the body. Engineering a virulent strain of *Y. pestis* to produce hexaacyl lipid A has rendered it avirulent in mice; this result attests to the importance of TLR4-based bacterial recognition in host defense. For most gram-negative bacteria, the pathogenesis of sepsis thus depends, at least in part, on whether the bacterium's LPS is sensed by the host receptor MD-2–TLR4.

Local and Systemic Host Responses to Invading Microbes

Recognition of microbial molecules by tissue phagocytes triggers the production and/or release of numerous host molecules (cytokines, chemokines, prostanoids, leukotrienes, and others) that increase blood flow to the infected tissue, enhance the permeability of local blood vessels, recruit neutrophils to the site of infection, and elicit pain. These phenomena are familiar elements of local inflammation, the body's frontline innate immune mechanism for eliminating microbial invaders. Systemic responses are activated by neural and/or humoral communication with the hypothalamus and brainstem; these responses enhance local defenses by increasing blood flow to the infected area, augmenting the number of circulating neutrophils, and elevating blood levels of numerous molecules (such as the microbial recognition proteins discussed above) that have anti-infective functions.

Cytokines and Other Mediators

Cytokines can exert endocrine, paracrine, and autocrine effects. TNF-α stimulates leukocytes and vascular endothelial cells to release other cytokines (as well as additional TNF-α), to express cell- surface molecules that enhance neutrophil-endothelial adhesion at sites of infection, and to increase prostaglandin and leukotriene production. Whereas blood levels of TNF-α are not elevated in individuals with localized infections, they increase in most patients with severe sepsis or septic shock. Moreover, IV infusion of TNF-α can elicit the characteristic abnormalities of SIRS. In animals, larger doses of TNF-α induce shock, disseminated intravascular coagulation (DIC), and death.

Although TNF-α is a central mediator, it is only one of many proinflammatory molecules that contribute to innate host defense. Chemokines, most prominently interleukin (IL) 8, attract circulating neutrophils to the infection site. IL-1β exhibits many of the same activities as TNF-α. TNF-α, IL-1β, interferon (IFN) γ, IL-12, and other cytokines probably interact synergistically with one another and with additional mediators. High-mobility group B-1, a transcription factor, can also be released from cells and interact with microbial products to induce host responses late in the course of the septic response.

Coagulation Factors

Intravascular thrombosis, a hallmark of the local inflammatory response, may help wall off invading microbes and prevent infection and inflammation from spreading to other tissues. Intravascular fibrin deposition, thrombosis, and DIC can also be important features of the systemic response. IL-6 and other mediators promote intravascular coagulation initially by inducing blood monocytes and vascular endothelial cells to express tissue factor. When tissue factor is expressed on cell surfaces, it binds to factor VIIa to form an active complex that can convert factors X and IX to their enzymatically active forms. The result is activation of both extrinsic and intrinsic clotting pathways, culminating in the generation of fibrin. Clotting is also favored by impaired function of the protein C–protein S inhibitory pathway and depletion of antithrombin and protein C, whereas fibrinolysis is prevented by increased plasma levels of plasminogen activator inhibitor 1. Thus there may be a striking propensity toward intravascular fibrin deposition, thrombosis, and bleeding; this propensity has been most apparent in patients with intravascular endothelial infections such as meningococcemia (Chap. 44). Contact-system activation occurs during sepsis but contributes more to the development of hypotension than to DIC.

Control Mechanisms

Elaborate control mechanisms operate within both local sites of inflammation and the systemic circulation.

Local Control Mechanisms

Host recognition of invading microbes within subepithelial tissues typically ignites immune responses that rapidly kill the invader and then subside to allow tissue recovery. The anti-inflammatory forces that put out the fire and clean up the battleground include molecules that neutralize or inactivate microbial signals. Among these molecules are LPS; intracellular factors (e.g., suppressor of cytokine signaling 3) that diminish the production of proinflammatory mediators by neutrophils and macrophages; anti-inflammatory cytokines (IL-10, IL-4); and molecules derived from essential polyunsaturated fatty acids (lipoxins, resolvins, and protectins) that promote tissue restoration.

Systemic Control Mechanisms

The signaling apparatus that links microbial recognition to cellular responses in tissues is less active in the blood. For example, whereas LBP plays a role in recognizing the presence of LPS, in plasma it also prevents LPS signaling by transferring LPS molecules into plasma lipoprotein particles, which sequester the lipid A moiety so that it cannot interact with cells. At the high concentrations found in blood, LBP also inhibits monocyte responses to LPS, and the soluble (circulating) form of CD14 strips off LPS that has bound to monocyte surfaces.

Systemic responses to infection also diminish cellular responses to microbial molecules. Circulating levels of anti-inflammatory cytokines (e.g., IL-6 and IL-10) increase even in patients with mild infections. Glucocorticoids inhibit cytokine synthesis by monocytes in vitro; the increase in blood cortisol levels early in the systemic response presumably plays a similarly inhibitory role. Epinephrine inhibits the TNF-α response to endotoxin infusion in humans while augmenting and accelerating the release of IL-10; prostaglandin E_2 has a similar "reprogramming" effect on the responses of circulating monocytes to LPS and other bacterial agonists. Cortisol, epinephrine, IL-10, and C-reactive protein reduce the ability of neutrophils to attach to vascular endothelium, favoring their demargination and thus contributing to leukocytosis while preventing neutrophil-endothelial adhesion in uninflamed organs. The available evidence thus suggests that the body's systemic responses to injury and infection normally prevent inflammation within organs distant from a site of infection.

The acute-phase response increases the blood concentrations of numerous molecules that have anti-inflammatory actions. Blood levels of IL-1 receptor antagonist (IL-1Ra) often greatly exceed those of circulating IL-1β, for example, and this excess may result in inhibition of the binding of IL-1β to its receptors. High levels of soluble TNF receptors neutralize TNF-α that enters the circulation. Other acute-phase proteins are protease inhibitors; these may neutralize proteases released from neutrophils and other inflammatory cells.

Organ Dysfunction and Shock

As the body's responses to infection intensify, the mixture of circulating cytokines and other molecules becomes very complex: elevated blood levels of more than 50 molecules have been found in patients with septic shock. Although high concentrations of both pro- and anti-inflammatory molecules are found, the net mediator balance in the plasma of these extremely sick patients may actually be anti-inflammatory. For example, blood leukocytes from patients with severe sepsis are often hyporesponsive to agonists such as LPS. In patients with severe sepsis, persistence of leukocyte hyporesponsiveness has been associated with an increased risk of dying. Apoptotic death of B cells, follicular dendritic cells, and CD4+ T lymphocytes also may contribute significantly to the immunosuppressive state.

Endothelial Injury

Most investigators have favored widespread vascular endothelial injury as the major mechanism for multiorgan dysfunction. In keeping with this idea, one study found high numbers of vascular endothelial cells in the peripheral blood of septic patients. Leukocyte-derived mediators and platelet-leukocyte-fibrin thrombi may contribute to vascular injury, but the vascular endothelium also seems to play an active role. Stimuli such as TNF-α induce vascular endothelial cells to produce and release cytokines, procoagulant molecules, platelet-activating factor (PAF), nitric oxide, and other mediators. In addition, regulated cell-adhesion molecules promote the adherence of neutrophils to endothelial cells. Although these responses can attract phagocytes to infected sites and activate their antimicrobial arsenals, endothelial cell activation can also promote increased vascular permeability, microvascular thrombosis, DIC, and hypotension.

Tissue oxygenation may decrease as the number of functional capillaries is reduced by luminal obstruction due to swollen endothelial cells, decreased deformability of circulating erythrocytes, leukocyte-platelet-fibrin thrombi, or compression by edema fluid. On the other hand, studies using orthogonal polarization spectral imaging of the microcirculation in the tongue found that sepsis-associated derangements in capillary flow could be reversed by applying acetylcholine to the surface of the tongue or giving nitroprusside intravenously; these observations suggest a neuroendocrine basis for the loss of capillary filling. Oxygen utilization by tissues may also be impaired by a state of "hibernation" in which ATP production is diminished as oxidative phosphorylation decreases because of mitochondrial dysfunction; nitric oxide or its metabolites may be responsible for inducing this response.

Remarkably, poorly functioning "septic" organs usually appear normal at autopsy. There is typically very little necrosis or thrombosis, and apoptosis is largely confined to lymphoid organs and the gastrointestinal tract. Moreover, organ function usually returns to normal if patients recover. These points suggest that organ dysfunction during severe sepsis has a basis that is principally biochemical, not anatomic.

Septic Shock

The hallmark of septic shock is a decrease in peripheral vascular resistance that occurs despite increased levels of vasopressor catecholamines. Before this vasodilatory phase, many patients experience a period during which oxygen delivery to tissues is compromised by myocardial depression, hypovolemia, and other factors. During this "hypodynamic" period, the blood lactate concentration is elevated, and central venous oxygen saturation is low. Fluid administration is usually followed by the hyperdynamic, vasodilatory phase during which cardiac output is normal (or even high) and oxygen consumption is independent of oxygen delivery. The blood lactate level may be normal or increased, and normalization of the central venous oxygen saturation (SvO_2) may reflect either improved oxygen delivery or left-to-right shunting.

Prominent hypotensive molecules include nitric oxide, β-endorphin, bradykinin, PAF, and pro-stacyclin. Agents that inhibit the synthesis or action of each of these mediators can prevent or reverse endotoxic shock in animals. However, in clinical trials, neither a PAF receptor antagonist nor a bradykinin antagonist improved survival rates among patients with septic shock, and a nitric oxide synthetase inhibitor, L-N^G-methylarginine HCl, actually increased the mortality rate.

Severe Sepsis: A Single Pathogenesis?

In some cases, circulating bacteria and their products almost certainly elicit multiorgan dysfunction and hypotension by directly stimulating inflammatory responses within the vasculature. In patients with fulminant meningococcemia, for example, mortality rates have correlated well with blood endotoxin levels and with the occurrence of DIC (Chap. 44). In most patients with nosocomial infections, in contrast, circulating bacteria or bacterial molecules may reflect uncontrolled infection at a local tissue site and have little or no direct impact on distant organs; in these patients, inflammatory mediators or neural signals arising from the local site seem to be the key triggers for severe sepsis and septic shock. In a large series of patients with positive blood cultures, the risk of developing severe sepsis was strongly related to the site of primary infection: bacteremia arising from a pulmonary or abdominal source was eightfold more likely to be associated with severe sepsis than was bacteremic urinary tract infection, even after the investigators controlled for age, the kind of bacteria isolated from the blood, and other factors. A third pathogenesis may be represented by severe sepsis due to superantigen-producing *Staphylococcus aureus* or *Streptococcus pyogenes*, since the T-cell activation induced by these toxins produces a cytokine profile that differs substantially from that elicited by gram-negative bacterial infection.

In summary, the pathogenesis of severe sepsis may differ according to the infecting microbe, the ability of the host's innate defense mechanisms to sense it, the site of the primary infection, the presence or absence of immune defects, and the prior physiologic status of the host. Genetic factors may also be important. For example, studies in different ethnic groups have identified associations between allelic polymorphisms in TLR4, caspase 12L, TNF-α, and IFN-γ genes and the risk of developing severe sepsis. Further studies in this area are needed.

CLINICAL MANIFESTATIONS

The manifestations of the septic response are usually superimposed on the symptoms and signs of the patient's underlying illness and primary infection. The rate at which signs and symptoms develop may differ from patient to patient, and there are striking individual variations in presentation. For example, some patients with sepsis are normo- or hypothermic; the absence of fever is most common in neonates, in elderly patients, and in persons with uremia or alcoholism.

Hyperventilation is often an early sign of the septic response. Disorientation, confusion, and other manifestations of encephalopathy may also develop early on, particularly in the elderly and in individuals with preexisting neurologic impairment. Focal neurologic signs are uncommon, although preexisting focal deficits may become more prominent.

Hypotension and DIC predispose to acrocyanosis and ischemic necrosis of peripheral tissues, most commonly the digits. Cellulitis, pustules, bullae, or hemorrhagic lesions may develop when hematogenous bacteria or fungi seed the skin or underlying soft tissue. Bacterial toxins may also be distributed hematogenously and elicit diffuse cutaneous reactions. On occasion, skin lesions may suggest specific pathogens. When sepsis is accompanied by cutaneous petechiae or purpura, infection with *Neisseria meningitidis* (or, less commonly, *H. influenzae*) should be suspected (Fig. 44-1); in a patient who has been bitten by a tick while in an endemic area, petechial lesions also suggest Rocky Mountain spotted fever (Fig. 75-1). A cutaneous lesion seen almost exclusively in neutropenic patients is ecthyma gangrenosum, usually caused by *P. aeruginosa*. It is a bullous lesion, surrounded by edema that undergoes central hemorrhage and necrosis (Fig. 53-1). Histopathologic examination shows bacteria in and around the wall of a small vessel, with little or no neutrophilic response. Hemorrhagic or bullous lesions in a septic patient who has recently eaten raw oysters suggest *V. vulnificus* bacteremia, whereas such lesions in a patient who has recently suffered a dog bite may indicate bloodstream infection due to *Capnocytophaga canimorsus* or *C. cynodegmi*. Generalized erythroderma in a septic patient suggests the toxic shock syndrome due to *S. aureus* or *S. pyogenes*.

Gastrointestinal manifestations such as nausea, vomiting, diarrhea, and ileus may suggest acute gastroenteritis. Stress ulceration can lead to upper gastrointestinal bleeding. Cholestatic jaundice, with elevated levels of serum bilirubin (mostly conjugated) and alkaline phosphatase, may precede other signs of sepsis. Hepatocellular or canalicular dysfunction appears to underlie most cases, and the results of hepatic function tests return to normal with resolution of the infection. Prolonged or severe hypotension may induce acute hepatic injury or ischemic bowel necrosis.

Many tissues may be unable to extract oxygen normally from the blood, so that anaerobic metabolism occurs despite near-normal mixed venous oxygen saturation. Blood lactate levels rise early because of increased glycolysis as well as impaired clearance of the resulting lactate and pyruvate by the liver and kidneys. The blood glucose concentration often increases, particularly in patients with diabetes, although impaired gluconeogenesis and excessive insulin release on occasion produce hypoglycemia. The cytokine-driven acute-phase response inhibits the synthesis of transthyretin while enhancing the production of C-reactive protein, fibrinogen, and complement components. Protein catabolism is often markedly accelerated. Serum albumin levels decline as a result of decreased hepatic synthesis and the movement of albumin into interstitial spaces, which is promoted by arterial vasodilation.

MAJOR COMPLICATIONS

Cardiopulmonary Complications

Ventilation-perfusion mismatching produces a fall in arterial P_{O_2} early in the course. Increasing alveolar capillary permeability results in an increased pulmonary water content, which decreases pulmonary compliance and interferes with oxygen exchange. Progressive diffuse pulmonary infiltrates and arterial hypoxemia (Pa_{O_2}/FI_{O_2}, compliance and interferes with <200) indicate the development of the acute respiratory distress syndrome (ARDS). ARDS develops in ~50% of patients with severe sepsis or septic shock. Respiratory muscle fatigue can exacerbate hypoxemia and hypercapnia. An elevated pulmonary capillary wedge pressure (>18 mmHg) suggests fluid volume overload or cardiac failure rather than ARDS. Pneumonia caused by viruses or by *Pneumocystis* may be clinically indistinguishable from ARDS.

Sepsis-induced hypotension (see "Septic Shock" earlier in the chapter) usually results initially from a generalized maldistribution of blood flow and blood volume and from hypovolemia that is due, at least in part, to diffuse capillary leakage of intravascular fluid. Other factors that may decrease effective intravascular volume include dehydration from antecedent disease or insensible fluid losses, vomiting or diarrhea, and polyuria. During early septic shock, systemic vascular resistance is usually elevated and cardiac output may be low. After fluid repletion, in contrast, cardiac output typically increases and systemic vascular resistance falls. Indeed, normal or increased cardiac output and decreased systemic vascular resistance distinguish septic shock from cardiogenic, extracardiac obstructive, and hypovolemic shock; other processes that can produce this combination include anaphylaxis, beriberi, cirrhosis, and overdoses of nitroprusside or narcotics.

Depression of myocardial function, manifested as increased end-diastolic and systolic ventricular volumes with a decreased ejection fraction, develops within 24 h in most patients with severe sepsis. Cardiac output is maintained despite the low ejection fraction because ventricular dilatation permits a normal stroke volume. In survivors, myocardial function returns to normal over several days. Although myocardial dysfunction may contribute to hypotension, refractory hypotension is usually due to a low systemic vascular resistance, and death results from refractory shock or the failure of multiple organs rather than from cardiac dysfunction per se.

Renal Complications

Oliguria, azotemia, proteinuria, and nonspecific urinary casts are frequently found. Many patients are inappropriately polyuric; hyperglycemia may exacerbate this tendency. Most renal failure is due to acute tubular necrosis induced by hypotension or capillary injury, although some patients also have glomerulonephritis, renal cortical necrosis, or interstitial nephritis. Drug-induced renal damage may complicate therapy, particularly when hypotensive patients are given aminoglycoside antibiotics.

Coagulopathy

Although thrombocytopenia occurs in 10–30% of patients, the underlying mechanisms are not understood. Platelet counts are usually very low (<50,000/μL) in patients with DIC; these low counts may reflect diffuse endothelial injury or microvascular thrombosis.

Neurologic Complications

When the septic illness lasts for weeks or months, "critical-illness" polyneuropathy may prevent weaning from ventilatory support and produce distal motor weakness. Electrophysiologic studies are diagnostic. Guillain-Barré syndrome, metabolic disturbances, and toxin activity must be ruled out.

LABORATORY FINDINGS

Abnormalities that occur early in the septic response may include leukocytosis with a left shift, thrombocytopenia, hyperbilirubinemia, and proteinuria. Leukopenia may develop. The neutrophils may contain toxic granulations, Döhle's bodies, or cytoplasmic vacuoles. As the septic response becomes more severe, thrombocytopenia worsens (often with prolongation of the thrombin time, decreased fibrinogen, and the presence of D-dimers, suggesting DIC), azotemia and hyperbilirubinemia become more prominent, and levels of aminotransferases rise. Active hemolysis suggests clostridial bacteremia, malaria, a drug reaction, or DIC; in the case of DIC, microangiopathic changes may be seen on a blood smear.

During early sepsis, hyperventilation induces respiratory alkalosis. With respiratory muscle fatigue and the accumulation of lactate, metabolic acidosis (with increased anion gap) typically supervenes. Evaluation of arterial blood gases reveals hypoxemia, which is initially correctable with supplemental oxygen but whose later refractoriness to 100% oxygen inhalation indicates right-to-left shunting. The chest radiograph may be normal or may show evidence of underlying pneumonia, volume overload, or the diffuse infiltrates of ARDS. The electrocardiogram may show only sinus tachycardia or nonspecific ST–T-wave abnormalities.

Most diabetic patients with sepsis develop hyperglycemia. Severe infection may precipitate diabetic ketoacidosis, which may exacerbate hypotension. Hypoglycemia occurs rarely. The serum albumin level, initially within the normal range, declines as sepsis continues. Hypocalcemia is rare.

DIAGNOSIS

There is no specific diagnostic test for the septic response. Diagnostically sensitive findings in a patient with suspected or proven infection include fever or hypothermia, tachypnea, tachycardia, and leukocytosis or leukopenia (Table 15-1); acutely altered mental status, thrombocytopenia, an elevated blood lactate level, or hypotension also should suggest the diagnosis. The septic response can be quite variable, however. In one study, 36% of patients with severe sepsis had a normal temperature, 40% had a normal respiratory rate, 10% had a normal pulse rate, and 33% had normal white blood cell counts. Moreover, the systemic responses of uninfected patients with other conditions may be similar to those characteristic of sepsis. Noninfectious etiologies of SIRS (Table 15-1) include pancreatitis, burns, trauma, adrenal insufficiency, pulmonary embolism, dissecting or ruptured aortic aneurysm, myocardial infarction, occult hemorrhage, cardiac tamponade, post–cardiopulmonary bypass syndrome, anaphylaxis, and drug overdose.

Definitive etiologic diagnosis requires isolation of the microorganism from blood or a local site of infection. At least two blood samples (10 mL each) should be obtained (from different venipuncture sites) for culture. Because gram-negative bacteremia is typically low-grade (<10 organisms/mL of blood), prolonged incubation of cultures may be necessary; *S. aureus* grows more readily and is detectable in blood cultures within 48 h in most instances. In many cases, blood cultures are negative; this result can reflect prior antibiotic administration, the presence of slow-growing or fastidious organisms, or the absence of microbial invasion of the bloodstream. In these cases, Gram's staining and culture of material from the primary site of infection or of infected cutaneous lesions may help establish the microbial etiology. The skin and mucosae should be examined carefully and repeatedly for lesions that might yield diagnostic information. With overwhelming bacteremia (e.g., pneumococcal sepsis in splenectomized individuals, fulminant meningococcemia, or infection with *V. vulnificus, B. pseudomallei*, or *Y. pestis*), microorganisms are sometimes visible on buffy coat smears of peripheral blood.

℞ Treatment: SEVERE SEPSIS AND SEPTIC SHOCK

Patients in whom sepsis is suspected must be managed expeditiously. This task is best accomplished by personnel who are experienced in the care of the critically ill. Successful management requires urgent measures to treat the infection, to provide hemodynamic and respiratory support, and to eliminate the offending microorganism. Most emergency centers now aim to initiate these measures within 1 h of the patient's presentation with severe sepsis or shock. Rapid assessment and diagnosis are therefore essential.

ANTIMICROBIAL AGENTS Antimicrobial chemotherapy should be initiated as soon as samples of blood and other relevant sites have been cultured. A large retrospective review of patients who developed septic shock found that the interval between the onset of hypotension and the administration of appropriate antimicrobial chemotherapy was the major determinant of outcome; a delay of as little as 1 h was associated with lower survival rates.

It is important, pending culture results, to initiate empirical antimicrobial therapy that is effective against both gram-positive and gram-negative bacteria (Table 15-3). Maximal recommended doses of antimicrobial drugs should be given intravenously, with adjustment for impaired renal function when necessary. Available information about patterns of antimicrobial susceptibility among bacterial isolates from the community, the hospital, and the patient should be taken into account. When culture results become available, the regimen can often be simplified, as a single antimicrobial agent is usually adequate for the treatment of a known pathogen. Meta-analyses have concluded that, with one exception, combination antimicrobial therapy is not superior to monotherapy for treating gram-negative bacteremia; the exception is that aminoglycoside monotherapy for *P. aeruginosa* bacteremia is less effective than the combination of an aminoglycoside with an antipseudomonal β-lactam agent. Most patients require antimicrobial therapy for at least 1 week; the duration of treatment is typically influenced by factors such as the site of tissue infection, the adequacy of surgical drainage, the patient's underlying disease, and the antimicrobial susceptibility of the bacterial isolate(s).

REMOVAL OF THE SOURCE OF INFECTION Removal or drainage of a focal source of infection is essential. Sites of occult infection should be sought

TABLE 15-3

INITIAL ANTIMICROBIAL THERAPY FOR SEVERE SEPSIS WITH NO OBVIOUS SOURCE IN ADULTS WITH NORMAL RENAL FUNCTION

CLINICAL CONDITION	ANTIMICROBIAL REGIMENS (INTRAVENOUS THERAPY)
Immunocompetent adult	The many acceptable regimens include (1) ceftriaxone (2 g q24h) ***or*** ticarcillin-clavulanate (3.1 g q4–6h) ***or*** piperacillin-tazobactam (3.375 g q4–6h); (2) imipenem-cilastatin (0.5 g q6h) or meropenem (1 g q8h) ***or*** cefepime (2 g q12h). Gentamicin ***or*** tobramycin (5–7 mg/kg q24h) may be ***added*** to either regimen. If the patient is allergic to β-lactam agents, use ciprofloxacin (400 mg q12h) ***or*** levofloxacin (500–750 mg q12h) ***plus*** clindamycin (600 mg q8h). If the institution ***or*** the community has a high prevalence of MRSA isolates, add vancomycin (15 mg/kg q12h) to each of the above regimens.
Neutropenia[a] (<500 neutrophils/μL)	Regimens include (1) imipenem-cilastatin (0.5 g q6h) ***or*** meropenem (1 g q8h) ***or*** cefepime (2 g q8h); (2) ticarcillin-clavulanate (3.1 g q4h) ***or*** piperacillin-tazobactam (3.375 g q4h) ***plus*** tobramycin (5–7 mg/kg q24h). Vancomycin (15 mg/kg q12h) should be added if the patient has an infected vascular catheter, if staphylococci are suspected, if the patient has received quinolone prophylaxis, if the patient has received intensive chemotherapy that produces mucosal damage, if the institution has a high incidence of MRSA infections, or if there is a high prevalence of MRSA isolates in the community.
Splenectomy	Cefotaxime (2 g q6–8h) ***or*** ceftriaxone (2 g q12h) should be used. If the local prevalence of cephalosporin-resistant pneumococci is high, ***add*** vancomycin. If the patient is allergic to β-lactam drugs, vancomycin (15 mg/kg q12h) ***plus*** ciprofloxacin (400 mg q12h) ***or*** levofloxacin (750 mg q12h) ***or*** aztreonam (2 g q8h) should be used.
IV drug user	Nafcillin or oxacillin (2 g q8h) ***plus*** gentamicin (5–7 mg/kg q24h). If the local prevalence of MRSA is high or if the patient is allergic to β-lactam drugs, vancomycin (15 mg/kg q12h) with gentamicin should be used.
AIDS	Cefepime (2 g q8h), ticarcillin-clavulanate (3.1 g q4h), ***or*** piperacillin-tazobactam (3.375 g q4h) ***plus*** tobramycin (5–7 mg/kg q24h) should be used. If the patient is allergic to β-lactam drugs, ciprofloxacin (400 mg q12h) ***or*** levofloxacin (750 mg q12h) ***plus*** vancomycin (15 mg/kg q12h) ***plus*** tobramycin should be used.

[a]Adapted in part from WT Hughes et al: Clin Infect Dis 25:551, 1997.
Note: MRSA, methicillin-resistant *Staphylococcus aureus*.

carefully. Indwelling IV catheters should be removed and the tip rolled over a blood agar plate for quantitative culture; after antibiotic therapy has been initiated, a new catheter should be inserted at a different site. Foley and drainage catheters should be replaced. The possibility of paranasal sinusitis (often caused by gram-negative bacteria) should be considered if the patient has undergone nasal intubation. In patients with abnormalities on chest radiographs, CT of the chest may identify unsuspected parenchymal, mediastinal, or pleural disease. In the neutropenic patient, cutaneous sites of tenderness and erythema, particularly in the perianal region, must be carefully sought. In patients with sacral or ischial decubitus ulcers, it is important to exclude pelvic or other soft tissue pus collections with CT or MRI. In patients with severe sepsis arising from the urinary tract, sonography or CT should be used to rule out ureteral obstruction, perinephric abscess, and renal abscess.

HEMODYNAMIC, RESPIRATORY, AND METABOLIC SUPPORT The primary goals are to restore adequate oxygen and substrate delivery to the tissues as quickly as possible and to improve tissue oxygen utilization and cellular metabolism. Adequate organ perfusion is thus essential. Initial management of hypotension should include the administration of IV fluids, typically beginning with 1–2 L of normal saline over 1–2 h. To avoid pulmonary edema, the pulmonary capillary wedge pressure should be maintained at 12–16 mmHg or the central venous pressure at 8–12 cm H_2O. The urine output rate should be kept at >0.5 mL/kg per hour by continuing fluid administration; a diuretic such as furosemide may be used if needed. In about one-third of patients, hypotension and organ hypoperfusion respond to fluid resuscitation; a reasonable goal is to maintain a mean arterial blood pressure of >65 mmHg (systolic pressure, >90 mmHg) and a cardiac index of ≥4 L/min per m^2. If these guidelines cannot be met by volume infusion, vasopressor therapy is indicated. Circulatory adequacy is also assessed by clinical parameters (mentation, urine output, skin perfusion) and, when possible, by measurements of oxygen delivery and consumption.

A study of "early goal-directed therapy" (EGDT) found that prompt resuscitation based on maintenance of the SvO_2 at >70% was associated with significantly improved survival of patients who were admitted to an emergency department with severe sepsis. The treatment algorithm included rapid administration of fluids, antibiotics, and vasopressor support; erythrocyte transfusion (to maintain the hematocrit above 30%); and administration of dobutamine if fluids, erythrocytes, and pressors did not result in an SvO_2 of >70%. The extent to which the different components of the EGDT algorithm contribute to the overall effect has not been examined in controlled trials. In particular, neither the use of SvO_2 to manage therapy nor the need for continuous SvO_2 monitoring with a pulmonary artery catheter has been formally confirmed. A multicenter study (sponsored by the National Institutes of Health) of the efficacy of the EGDT approach is in progress.

In patients with septic shock, plasma vasopressin levels increase transiently but then decrease dramatically. Studies have found that vasopressin infusion can reverse septic shock in some patients, reducing or eliminating the need for catecholamine pressors. An adequately powered and randomized trial of vasopressin infusion has not been performed. Vasopressin is a potent vasoconstrictor that may be most useful in patients who have vasodilatory shock and relative resistance to other pressor hormones.

Adrenal insufficiency is very likely when the plasma cortisol level is <15 μg/dL in a patient with severe sepsis. Generally accepted criteria for *partial* adrenal insufficiency have not been devised; major problems have been the inability to raise cortisol levels in extremely stressed individuals above high baseline values in response to cosyntropin (α^{1-24}–ACTH) and the high frequency of hypoalbuminemia, which decreases total but not free (active) plasma cortisol levels. Adrenal insufficiency should be strongly considered in septic patients with refractory hypotension, fulminant meningococcal bacteremia, disseminated tuberculosis, AIDS, or prior use of glucocorticoids, megestrol, etomidate, or ketoconazole. Hydrocortisone (50 mg IV every 6 h) may be given as a trial therapeutic intervention. If clinical improvement occurs over 24–48 h, most experts would continue hydrocortisone therapy, tapering and discontinuing it after 5–7 days. Improved recommendations regarding hydrocortisone therapy may come from the European CORTICUS trial.

Ventilator therapy is indicated for progressive hypoxemia, hypercapnia, neurologic deterioration, or respiratory muscle failure. Sustained tachypnea (respiratory rate, >30 breaths/min) is frequently a harbinger of impending respiratory collapse; mechanical ventilation is often initiated to ensure adequate oxygenation, to divert blood from the muscles of respiration, to prevent aspiration of oropharyngeal contents, and to reduce the cardiac afterload. The results of recent studies favor the use of low tidal volumes (6 mL/kg of ideal body weight, or as low as 4 mL/kg if the plateau pressure exceeds 30 cmH_2O). Patients undergoing mechanical ventilation require careful sedation, with daily interruptions; elevation of the head of the bed helps to prevent nosocomial pneumonia. Stress-ulcer prophylaxis with a histamine H_2-receptor antagonist may decrease the risk of gastrointestinal hemorrhage in ventilated patients.

The use of erythrocyte transfusion continues to be debated. In the study of EGDT, packed erythrocytes were given to raise the hematocrit to 30% if the patient's SvO_2 was <70%. The extent to which this intervention contributed to the improvement reported in patients who received the EGDT regimen is uncertain.

Bicarbonate is sometimes administered for severe metabolic acidosis (arterial pH <7.2), but there is little evidence that it improves either hemodynamics or the response to vasopressor hormones. DIC, if complicated by major bleeding, should be treated with transfusion of fresh-frozen plasma and platelets. Successful treatment of the underlying infection is essential to reverse both acidosis and DIC. Patients who are hypercatabolic and have acute renal failure may benefit greatly from hemodialysis or hemofiltration.

GENERAL SUPPORT In patients with prolonged severe sepsis (i.e., that lasting more than 2 or 3 days), nutritional supplementation may reduce the impact of protein hypercatabolism; the available evidence, which is not strong, favors the enteral delivery route. Prophylactic heparinization to prevent deep venous thrombosis is indicated for patients who do not have active bleeding or coagulopathy. Recovery is also assisted by preventing skin breakdown, nosocomial infections, and stress ulcers.

Investigators in Belgium reported in 2001 that maintaining blood glucose levels in the normal range (80–110 mg/dL) greatly improved survival rates among patients who had just undergone major surgery and had received IV glucose feeding for the previous 24 h. The same group then studied intensive glucose control in critically ill medical patients and found a survival benefit only for patients who remained in the intensive care unit for ≥3 days. Hypoglycemia was much more common in the intensive-insulin group. Until more experience with intensive glucose control is reported, it seems reasonable to maintain glucose levels of <150 mg/dL during the first 3 days of severe sepsis and then to target the normoglycemic range if the patient remains in the intensive care unit for a longer period. Frequent monitoring of blood glucose levels is indicated to avoid hypoglycemia during intensive insulin therapy.

OTHER MEASURES Despite aggressive management, many patients with severe sepsis or septic shock die. Numerous interventions have been tested for their ability to improve survival in patients with severe sepsis. The list includes endotoxin-neutralizing proteins, inhibitors of cyclooxygenase or nitric oxide synthase, anticoagulants, polyclonal immunoglobulins, glucocorticoids, and antagonists to TNF-α, IL-1, PAF, and bradykinin. Unfortunately, none of these agents has improved rates of survival among patients with severe sepsis/septic shock in more than one large, randomized, placebo-controlled clinical trial. This lack of reproducibility has had many contributing factors, including (1) heterogeneity in the patient populations studied and the inciting microbes and (2) the nature of the "standard" therapy also used. A dramatic example of this problem was seen in a trial of tissue factor pathway inhibitor (Fig. 15-1). Whereas the drug appeared to improve survival rates after 722 patients had been studied ($p = .006$), it did not do so in the next 1032 patients, and the overall result was negative. This inconsistency, even within a carefully selected patient population, argues strongly that a sepsis intervention should show significant survival benefit in more than one placebo-controlled clinical trial before it is accepted as part of routine clinical practice.

Recombinant activated protein C (aPC) was the first drug to be approved by the U.S. Food and Drug Administration (FDA) for the treatment of patients with severe sepsis or septic shock. In a single randomized controlled

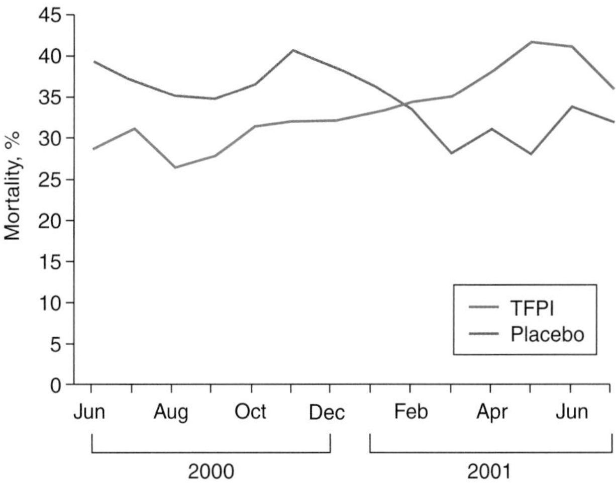

FIGURE 15-1
Mortality rates among patients who received tissue factor pathway inhibitor (TFPI) or placebo, shown as the running average over the course of the clinical trial. The drug seemed highly efficacious at the interim analysis in December 2000, but this trend reversed later in the trial. Demonstrating that therapeutic agents for sepsis have consistent, reproducible efficacy has been extremely difficult, even within well-defined patient populations. (*Reprinted with permission from Abraham et al.*)

trial in which drug or placebo was given within 24 h of the patient's first sepsis-related organ dysfunction, 28-day mortality was significantly lower among recipients of aPC than among patients who received placebo (24.7% vs 30.8%; $p < .005$). In addition, aPC recipients were more likely than placebo recipients to have severe bleeding (3.5% vs 2%). Survival improved only for patients who had an APACHE II score of ≥25 during the 24 h before initiation of aPC infusion. Midtrial changes in the protocol and drug were followed by improvement in the apparent efficacy of aPC. The FDA approved aPC for use in adults (>18 years of age) who meet the APACHE II criterion and have a low risk of hemorrhage-related side effects.

aPC is administered as a constant IV infusion of 24 μg/kg per hour for 96 h. Each patient's clotting parameters must be monitored carefully. aPC should not be given to patients who have platelet counts of <30,000/μL or to patients who have dysfunction of one organ system and have had surgery during the previous 30 days. Treatment with aPC should not be started >24 h after the onset of severe sepsis, nor should it be used in the patient subsets—e.g., patients with pancreatitis or AIDS—that were excluded from the clinical trial.

Although the theoretical rationale for treating septic patients with anticoagulants is strong and studies have found that aPC may have anti-inflammatory and anti-apoptotic properties in vitro, two additional randomized, placebo-controlled trials of aPC were stopped when interim analyses showed lack of efficacy. One trial was in children, and the other was in adults with APACHE II scores of ≤25. aPC has not been tested again in the patient population for which it was approved by the FDA: adults with high APACHE II scores.

Some experts have advocated "bundling" of multiple therapeutic maneuvers into a unified, algorithmic approach to management that would become the standard of care for severe sepsis. The proposed *resuscitation* (6-h) bundle incorporates most of the elements discussed above for acute (EGDT) resuscitation. The *management* (24-h) bundle includes three measures of uncertain or marginal benefit: tight control of blood glucose, administration of low-dose hydrocortisone, and treatment with aPC. Bundling of therapies obscures the efficacy and toxicity of the individual interventions and allows little room for individualizing therapy. The use of bundling in an industry-sponsored marketing program for aPC (the Surviving Sepsis Campaign) has also been criticized.

A careful retrospective analysis found that the apparent efficacy of all sepsis therapeutics studied to date has been greatest among the patients at greatest risk of dying before treatment; conversely, use of many of these drugs has been associated with increased mortality rates among patients who are less ill. The authors proposed that neutralizing one of many different mediators may help patients who are very sick, whereas disrupting the mediator balance may be harmful to those whose adaptive defense mechanisms are still working. This analysis suggests that if more aggressive early resuscitation improves survival rates among sicker patients, it should become more difficult to show additional benefit from other therapies; that is, if early resuscitation improves patients' status, moving them into a "less severe illness" category, the addition of another agent is less likely to be beneficial.

PROGNOSIS

Approximately 20–35% of patients with severe sepsis and 40–60% of patients with septic shock die within 30 days. Others die within the ensuing 6 months. Late deaths often result from poorly controlled infection, immunosuppression, complications of intensive care, failure of multiple organs, or the patient's underlying disease.

Prognostic stratification systems such as APACHE II indicate that factoring in the patient's age, underlying condition, and various physiologic variables can yield estimates of the risk of dying of severe sepsis. Of the individual covariates, the severity of underlying disease most strongly influences the risk of dying. Septic shock is also a strong predictor of short- and long-term mortality. Case-fatality rates are similar for culture-positive and culture-negative severe sepsis.

PREVENTION

Prevention offers the best opportunity to reduce morbidity and mortality. In developed countries, most episodes of severe sepsis and septic shock are complications of nosocomial infections. These cases might be prevented by reducing the number of invasive procedures undertaken, by limiting the use (and duration of use) of indwelling vascular and bladder catheters, by reducing the incidence and duration of profound neutropenia (<500 neutrophils/μL), and by more aggressively treating localized nosocomial infections. Indiscriminate use of antimicrobial agents and glucocorticoids should be avoided, and optimal infection-control measures (Chap. 13) should be used. Several studies point to associations between allelic polymorphisms in specific genes and risk of severe sepsis; if these associations prove to be broadly applicable, such polymorphisms can be used prospectively to identify high-risk patients and to target preventive and/or therapeutic measures to them. Studies indicate that 50–70% of patients who develop nosocomial severe sepsis or septic shock have experienced a less severe stage of the septic response (e.g., SIRS, sepsis) on at least 1 previous day in the hospital. Research is needed to develop adjunctive agents that can damp the septic response before organ dysfunction or hypotension occurs.

FURTHER READINGS

Abraham E et al: Efficacy and safety of tifacogin (recombinant tissue factor pathway inhibitor) in severe sepsis: A randomized controlled trial. JAMA 290:238, 2003

Arafah BM: Hypothalamic pituitary adrenal function during critical illness: Limitations of current assessment methods. J Clin Endocrinol Metab 91:3725, 2006

Berkley JA et al: Bacteremia among children admitted to a rural hospital in Kenya. N Engl J Med 352:39, 2005

Brunkhorst FM et al: Intensive insulin therapy and pentastarch resuscitation in severe sepsis. N Engl J Med 358:125, 2008

Dellinger RP et al: Surviving Sepsis Campaign: International guidelines for management of severe sepsis and septic shock: 2008. Crit Care Med 36:296, 2008

Eichacker P et al: Risk and the efficacy of anti-inflammatory agents: Retrospective and confirmatory studies of sepsis. Am J Respir Crit Care Med 166:1197, 2002

Harbath S et al: Does antibiotic selection impact patient outcome? Clin Infect Dis 44:87, 2007

Hotchkiss RS, Nicholson DW: Apoptosis and caspases regulate death and inflammation in sepsis. Nat Rev Immunol 6:813, 2006

Kumar A et al: Duration of hypotension before initiation of effective antimicrobial therapy is the critical determinant of survival in human septic shock. Crit Care Med 34:1589, 2006

Munford RS: Severe sepsis and septic shock: The role of gram-negative bacteremia. Annu Rev Pathol Mech Dis 1:467, 2006

Otero RM et al: Early goal-directed therapy in severe sepsis and septic shock revisited: Concepts, controversies, and contemporary findings. Chest 130:1579, 2006

Russell JA: Management of sepsis. N Engl J Med 355:1699, 2006

Sands KE et al: Epidemiology of sepsis syndrome in 8 academic medical centers. JAMA 278:234, 1997

Sprung CL et al: Hydrocortisone therapy for patients with septic shock. N Engl J Med 358:111, 2008

Turgeon AF et al: Meta-analysis: Intravenous immunoglobulin in critically ill adult patients with sepsis. Ann Intern Med 146:193, 2007

SECTION III

INFECTIONS IN ORGAN SYSTEMS

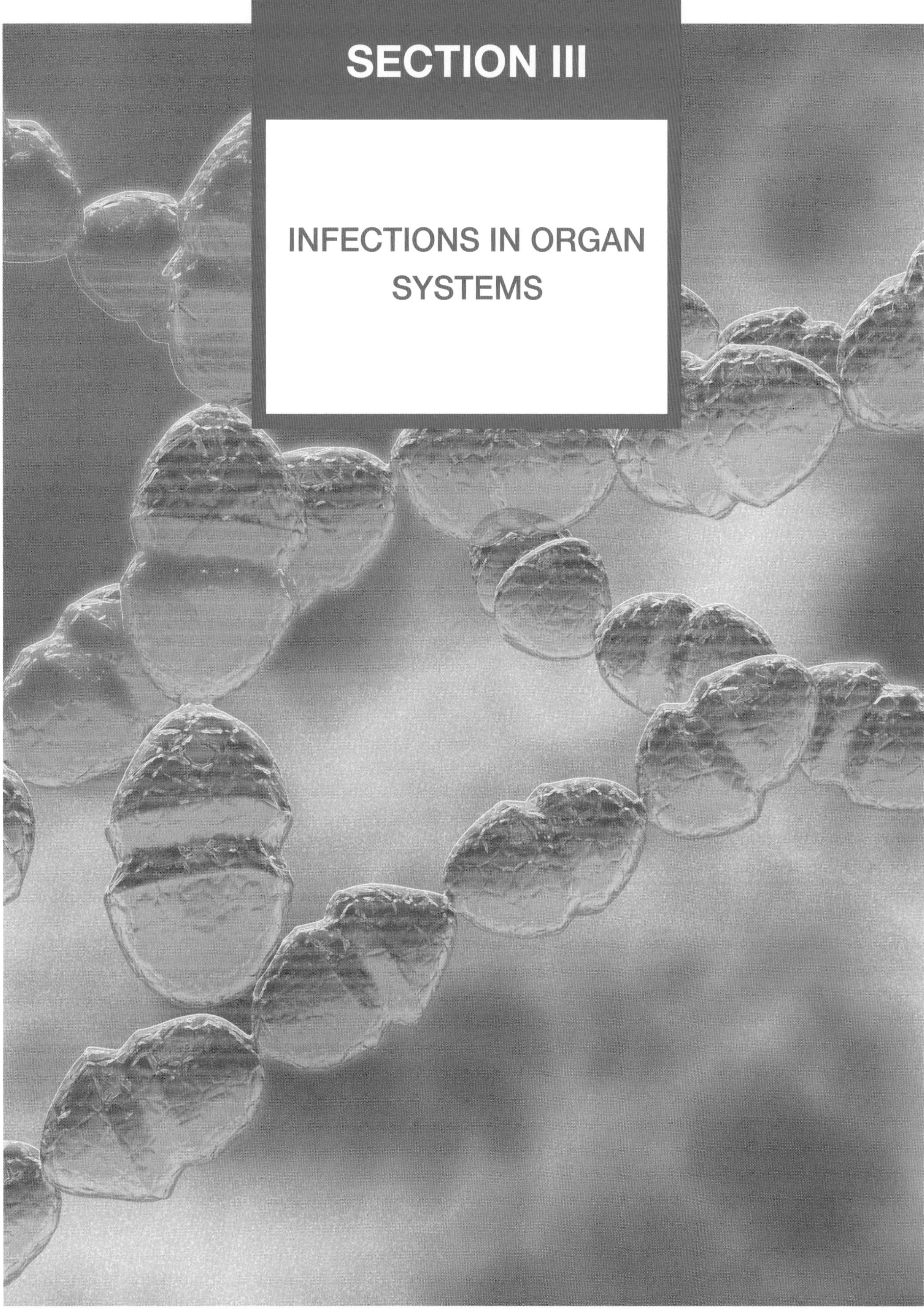

CHAPTER 16

PHARYNGITIS, SINUSITIS, OTITIS, AND OTHER UPPER RESPIRATORY TRACT INFECTIONS

Michael A. Rubin ■ Ralph Gonzales ■ Merle A. Sande†

Infections of the upper respiratory tract (URIs) have a tremendous impact on public health. They are among the most common reasons for visits to primary care providers, and, although the illnesses are typically mild, their high incidence and transmission rates place them among the leading causes of time lost from work or school. Even though the minority (~25%) of cases are caused by bacteria, URIs are the leading diagnoses for which antibiotics are prescribed on an outpatient basis in the United States. The enormous consumption of antibiotics for these illnesses has contributed to the rise in antibiotic resistance among common community-acquired pathogens such as *Streptococcus pneumoniae*—a trend that in itself has had an enormous influence on public health.

Although most URIs are caused by viruses, distinguishing patients with primary viral infection from those with primary bacterial infection is difficult. Signs and symptoms of bacterial and viral URIs are, in fact, indistinguishable. Because routine, rapid testing is neither available nor practical for most syndromes, acute infections are diagnosed largely on clinical grounds. Thus the judicious use of antibiotics in this setting is challenging.

NONSPECIFIC INFECTIONS OF THE UPPER RESPIRATORY TRACT

Nonspecific URIs are a broadly defined group of disorders that collectively constitute the leading cause of ambulatory care visits in the United States. By definition, nonspecific URIs have no prominent localizing features. They are identified by a variety of descriptive names, including *acute infective rhinitis, acute rhinopharyngitis/nasopharyngitis, acute coryza,* and *acute nasal catarrh,* as well as by the inclusive label *common cold.*

Etiology

The large assortment of URI classifications reflects the wide variety of causative infectious agents and the varied manifestations of common pathogens. Nearly all nonspecific URIs are caused by viruses spanning multiple virus families and many antigenic types. For instance, there are at least 100 immunotypes of rhinovirus (Chap. 87), the most common cause of URI (~30–40% of cases); other causes include influenza virus (three immunotypes; Chap. 88) as well as parainfluenza virus (four immunotypes), coronavirus (at least three immunotypes), and adenovirus (47 immunotypes) (Chap. 87). Respiratory syncytial virus (RSV) also accounts for a small percentage of cases each year, as do some viruses not typically associated with URIs (e.g., enteroviruses, rubella virus, and varicella-zoster virus). Even with sophisticated diagnostic and culture techniques, a substantial proportion (25–30%) of cases have no assigned pathogen.

Clinical Manifestations

The signs and symptoms of nonspecific URI are similar to those of other URIs but lack a pronounced localization to one particular anatomic location, such as the sinuses, pharynx, or lower airway. Nonspecific URI is commonly described as an acute, mild, and self-limited catarrhal syndrome, with a median duration of ~1 week. Signs and symptoms are diverse and frequently variable across patients. The principal signs and symptoms of nonspecific URI include rhinorrhea (with or without purulence), nasal congestion, cough, and sore throat. Other manifestations, such as fever, malaise, sneezing, and hoarseness, are more variable, with fever more common among infants and young children. Occasionally, clinical features reflect the underlying viral pathogen; myalgias and fatigue, for example, are sometimes seen with influenza and parainfluenza infections, whereas conjunctivitis may suggest infection with adenovirus or enterovirus. Findings on physical examination are frequently nonspecific and unimpressive. Between 0.5 and 2% of colds are complicated by secondary bacterial infections (e.g., rhinosinusitis, otitis media, and pneumonia), particularly in high-risk populations such as infants, elderly persons, and chronically ill patients. Secondary bacterial infections are usually associated with a prolonged course of illness, increased severity of illness, and localization of signs and symptoms. Purulent secretions from the nares or throat have often been used as an indication of sinusitis or pharyngitis. However, these secretions are also seen in nonspecific URI and, in the absence of other clinical features, are poor predictors of bacterial infection.

†Deceased.

℞ Treatment: UPPER RESPIRATORY INFECTIONS

Antibiotics have no role in the treatment of uncomplicated nonspecific URI. In the absence of clinical evidence of bacterial infection, treatment remains entirely symptom-based, with use of decongestants and nonsteroidal anti-inflammatory drugs. Other therapies directed at specific symptoms are often useful, including dextromethorphan for cough and lozenges with topical anesthetic for sore throat. Clinical trials of zinc, vitamin C, echinacea, and other alternative remedies have revealed no consistent benefit for the treatment of nonspecific URI.

INFECTIONS OF THE SINUS

Sinusitis refers to an inflammatory condition involving the four paired structures surrounding the nasal cavities. Although most cases of sinusitis involve more than one sinus, the maxillary sinus is most commonly involved; next in frequency are the ethmoid, frontal, and sphenoid sinuses. Each sinus is lined with a respiratory epithelium that produces mucus, which is transported out by ciliary action through the sinus ostium and into the nasal cavity. Normally, mucus does not accumulate in the sinuses, which remain sterile despite their adjacency to the bacterium-filled nasal passages. When the sinus ostia are obstructed, however, or when ciliary clearance is impaired or absent, the secretions can be retained, producing the typical signs and symptoms of sinusitis. The retained secretions may become infected with a variety of pathogens, including viruses, bacteria, and fungi. Sinusitis affects a tremendous proportion of the population, accounts for millions of visits to primary care physicians each year, and is the fifth leading diagnosis for which antibiotics are prescribed. It is typically classified by duration of illness (acute vs. chronic); by etiology (infectious vs. noninfectious); and, when infectious, by the offending pathogen type (viral, bacterial, or fungal).

ACUTE SINUSITIS

Acute sinusitis—defined as sinusitis of <4 weeks' duration—constitutes the vast majority of sinusitis cases. Most cases are diagnosed in the ambulatory care setting and occur primarily as a consequence of a preceding viral URI. Differentiating acute bacterial and viral sinusitis on clinical grounds is difficult. Therefore, it is perhaps unsurprising that antibiotics are prescribed frequently (in 85–98% of all cases) for this condition.

Etiology

A number of infectious and noninfectious factors can contribute to acute obstruction of the sinus ostia or impairment of ciliary clearance, with consequent sinusitis. Noninfectious causes include allergic rhinitis (with either mucosal edema or polyp obstruction), barotrauma (e.g., from deep-sea diving or air travel), or chemical irritants. Illnesses such as nasal and sinus tumors (e.g., squamous cell carcinoma) or granulomatous diseases (e.g., Wegener's granulomatosis or rhinoscleroma) can also produce obstruction of the sinus ostia, whereas conditions leading to altered mucus content (e.g., cystic fibrosis) can cause sinusitis through impaired mucus clearance. In the hospital setting, nasotracheal intubation is a major risk factor for nosocomial sinusitis in intensive care units.

Acute infectious sinusitis can be caused by a variety of organisms, including viruses, bacteria, and fungi. Viral rhinosinusitis is far more common than bacterial sinusitis, although relatively few studies have sampled sinus aspirates for the presence of different viruses. In those studies that have done so, the viruses most commonly isolated—both alone and with bacteria—have been rhinovirus, parainfluenza virus, and influenza virus. Bacterial causes of sinusitis have been better described. Among community-acquired cases, *S. pneumoniae* and nontypable *Haemophilus influenzae* are the most common pathogens, accounting for 50–60% of cases. *Moraxella catarrhalis* causes disease in a significant percentage (20%) of children but less often in adults. Other streptococcal species and *Staphylococcus aureus* cause only a small percentage of cases, although there is increasing concern about community strains of methicillin-resistant *S. aureus* (MRSA) as an emerging cause. Anaerobes are occasionally found in association with infections of the roots of premolar teeth that spread into the adjacent maxillary sinuses. The role of *Chlamydophila pneumoniae* and *Mycoplasma pneumoniae* in the pathogenesis of acute sinusitis is still unclear. Nosocomial cases are commonly associated with bacteria found in the hospital environment, including *S. aureus*, *Pseudomonas aeruginosa*, *Serratia marcescens*, *Klebsiella pneumoniae*, and *Enterobacter* species. Often, these infections are polymicrobial and involve organisms that are highly resistant to numerous antibiotics. Fungi are also established causes of sinusitis, although most acute cases are in immunocompromised patients and represent invasive, life-threatening infections. The best-known example is rhinocerebral mucormycosis caused by fungi of the order Mucorales, which includes *Rhizopus*, *Rhizomucor*, *Mucor*, *Absidia*, and *Cunninghamella*. These infections usually occur in diabetic patients with ketoacidosis but also develop in transplant recipients, patients with hematologic malignancies, and patients receiving chronic glucocorticoid or deferoxamine therapy. Other hyaline molds, such as *Aspergillus* and *Fusarium* species, are also occasional causes of this disease.

Clinical Manifestations

Most cases of acute sinusitis present after or in conjunction with a viral URI, and it can be difficult to discriminate the clinical features of one from the other. A large proportion of patients with colds have sinus inflammation, although bacterial sinusitis complicates only 0.2–2% of these viral infections. Common presenting symptoms of sinusitis include nasal drainage and congestion, facial pain or pressure, and headache. Thick, purulent or discolored nasal discharge is often thought to indicate bacterial sinusitis but also occurs early in viral infections such as the common cold and is not specific to bacterial infection. Other nonspecific manifestations include cough, sneezing, and fever. Tooth pain, most often involving the upper molars, is associated with bacterial sinusitis, as is halitosis.

In acute sinusitis, sinus pain or pressure often localizes to the involved sinus (particularly the maxillary sinus) and can be worse when the patient bends over or is supine. Although rare, manifestations of advanced sphenoid or ethmoid sinus infection can be profound, including severe frontal or retroorbital pain radiating to the occiput, thrombosis of the cavernous sinus, and signs of orbital cellulitis. Acute focal sinusitis is uncommon but should be considered in the patient with severe symptoms over the maxillary sinus and fever, regardless of illness duration. Similarly, advanced frontal sinusitis can present with a condition known as *Pott's puffy tumor*, with soft tissue swelling and pitting edema over the frontal bone from a communicating subperiosteal abscess. Life-threatening complications include meningitis, epidural abscess, and cerebral abscess.

Patients with acute fungal sinusitis (such as mucormycosis) often present with symptoms related to pressure effects, particularly when the infection has spread to the orbits and cavernous sinus. Signs such as orbital swelling and cellulitis, proptosis, ptosis, and decreased extraocular movement are common, as is retroorbital or periorbital pain. Nasopharyngeal ulcerations, epistaxis, and headaches are also frequent, and involvement of cranial nerves V and VII has been described in more advanced cases. Bony erosion may be evident on examination. Oftentimes, the patient does not appear seriously ill despite the rapidly progressive nature of these infections.

Patients with acute nosocomial sinusitis are often critically ill and thus do not manifest the typical clinical features of sinus disease. This diagnosis should be suspected, however, when hospitalized patients who have appropriate risk factors (e.g., nasotracheal intubation) develop fever of unknown origin.

Diagnosis

Distinguishing viral from bacterial sinusitis in the ambulatory setting is usually difficult, given the relatively low sensitivity and specificity of the common clinical features. One clinical feature that has been used to help guide diagnostic and therapeutic decision making is illness duration. Because acute bacterial sinusitis is uncommon in patients whose symptoms have lasted <7 days, several authorities now recommend reserving this diagnosis for patients with "persistent" symptoms (i.e., symptoms lasting >7 days in adults or >10–14 days in children) accompanied by purulent nasal discharge (Table 16-1). Even among the patients who meet these criteria, only 40–50% have true bacterial sinusitis. The use of CT or sinus radiography is not recommended for routine cases, particularly early in the course of illness (i.e., at <7 days), given the high prevalence of similar abnormalities among cases of acute viral rhinosinusitis. In the evaluation of persistent, recurrent, or chronic sinusitis, CT of the sinuses is the radiographic study of choice.

The clinical history and/or setting can often identify cases of acute anaerobic bacterial sinusitis, acute fungal sinusitis, or sinusitis from noninfectious causes (e.g., allergic rhinosinusitis). In the case of an immunocompromised patient with acute fungal sinus infection, immediate examination by an otolaryngologist is required. Biopsy specimens from involved areas should be examined by a pathologist for evidence of fungal hyphal elements and tissue invasion. Cases of suspected acute nosocomial sinusitis should be confirmed by sinus CT. Because therapy should target the offending organism, a sinus aspirate should be obtained, if possible, for culture and susceptibility testing.

℞ Treatment: ACUTE SINUSITIS

Most patients with a diagnosis of acute rhinosinusitis based on clinical grounds improve without antibiotic therapy. The preferred initial approach in patients with mild to moderate symptoms of short duration is therapy aimed at facilitating sinus drainage, such as oral and topical decongestants, nasal saline lavage, and—in patients with a history of chronic sinusitis or allergies—nasal glucocorticoids. Adult patients who do not improve after 7 days, children who do not improve after 10–14 days, and patients with more severe symptoms (regardless of duration) should be treated with antibiotics (Table 16-1). Empirical therapy should consist of the narrowest-spectrum agent active against the most common bacterial pathogens, including *S. pneumoniae* and *H. influenzae*—e.g., amoxicillin. No clinical trials support the use of broad-spectrum agents for routine cases of bacterial sinusitis, even in the current era of drug-resistant *S. pneumoniae*. Up to 10% of patients do not respond to initial antimicrobial therapy; sinus aspiration and/or lavage by an otolaryngologist should be considered in these cases. Antibiotic prophylaxis to prevent episodes of recurrent acute bacterial sinusitis is not recommended.

Surgical intervention and IV antibiotic administration are usually reserved for patients with severe disease or those with intracranial complications, such as abscess or orbital involvement. Immunocompromised patients with acute invasive fungal sinusitis usually require extensive surgical debridement and treatment with IV antifungal agents active against fungal hyphal forms, such as amphotericin B. Specific therapy should be individualized according to the fungal species and the individual patient's characteristics.

Treatment of nosocomial sinusitis should begin with broad-spectrum antibiotics to cover common pathogens such as *S. aureus* and gram-negative bacilli. Therapy should then be tailored to the results of culture and susceptibility testing of sinus aspirates.

CHRONIC SINUSITIS

Chronic sinusitis is characterized by symptoms of sinus inflammation lasting >12 weeks. This illness is most commonly associated with either bacteria or fungi, and clinical cure in most cases is very difficult. Many patients have undergone treatment with repeated courses of antibacterial agents and multiple sinus surgeries, increasing their risk of colonization with antibiotic-resistant pathogens

TABLE 16-1

GUIDELINES FOR THE DIAGNOSIS AND TREATMENT OF ACUTE SINUSITIS

AGE GROUP	DIAGNOSTIC CRITERIA	TREATMENT RECOMMENDATIONS[a]
Adults	Moderate symptoms (e.g., nasal purulence/congestion or cough) for >7 d *or* Severe symptoms of any duration, including unilateral/focal facial swelling or tooth pain	*Initial therapy* Amoxicillin, 500 mg PO tid or 875 mg PO bid, *or* TMP-SMX, 1 DS tablet PO bid for 10–14 d *Exposure to antibiotics within 30 d or >30% prevalence of penicillin-resistant S. pneumoniae* Amoxicillin, 1000 mg PO tid, *or* Amoxicillin/clavulanate (extended release), 2000 mg PO bid, *or* Antipneumococcal fluoroquinolone (e.g., levofloxacin, 500 mg PO qd) *Recent treatment failure* Amoxicillin/clavulanate (extended release), 2000 mg PO bid, *or* Amoxicillin, 1500 mg bid, plus clindamycin, 300 mg PO qid, *or* Antipneumococcal fluoroquinolone (e.g., levofloxacin, 500 mg PO qd)
Children	Moderate symptoms (e.g., nasal purulence/congestion or cough) for >10–14 d *or* Severe symptoms of any duration, including fever (>102°F), unilateral/focal facial swelling or pain	*Initial therapy* Amoxicillin, 45–90 mg/kg qd (up to 2 g) PO in divided doses (bid or tid), *or* Cefuroxime axetil, 30 mg/kg qd PO in divided doses (bid), *or* Cefdinir, 14 mg/kg PO qd *Exposure to antibiotics within 30 d, recent treatment failure, or >30% prevalence of penicillin-resistant S. pneumoniae* Amoxicillin, 90 mg/kg qd (up to 2 g) PO in divided doses (bid), plus clavulanate, 6.4 mg/kg qd PO in divided doses (bid) (extra-strength suspension), *or* Cefuroxime axetil, 30 mg/kg qd PO in divided doses (bid), *or* Cefdinir, 14 mg/kg PO qd

[a]Unless otherwise specified, the duration of therapy is generally 10 d, with appropriate follow-up.
Note: DS, double-strength; TMP-SMX, trimethoprim-sulfamethoxazole.
Sources: American Academy of Pediatrics Subcommittee on Management of Sinusitis and Committee on Quality Improvement, 2001; Hickner et al, 2001; Piccirillo, 2004; and Sinus and Allergy Health Partnership, 2004.

and of surgical complications. Patients often suffer significant morbidity, sometimes over many years.

In *chronic bacterial sinusitis*, infection is thought to be due to the impairment of mucociliary clearance from repeated infections rather than to persistent bacterial infection. However, the pathogenesis of this condition is poorly understood. Although certain conditions (e.g., cystic fibrosis) can predispose patients to chronic bacterial sinusitis, most patients with this infection do not have obvious underlying conditions that result in the obstruction of sinus drainage, the impairment of ciliary action, or immune dysfunction. Patients experience constant nasal congestion and sinus pressure, with intermittent periods of greater severity, which may persist for years. CT can be helpful in determining the extent of disease and the response to therapy. The management team should include an otolaryngologist to conduct endoscopic examinations and obtain tissue samples for histologic examination and culture.

Chronic fungal sinusitis is a disease of immunocompetent hosts and is usually noninvasive, although slowly progressive invasive disease is sometimes seen. Noninvasive disease, which is typically associated with hyaline molds such as *Aspergillus* species and dematiaceous molds such as *Curvularia* or *Bipolaris* species, can present as a number of different scenarios. In mild, indolent disease, which usually occurs in the setting of repeated failures of antibacterial therapy, only nonspecific mucosal changes may be seen on sinus CT. Endoscopic surgery is usually curative in these patients, with no need for antifungal therapy. Another form of disease presents with long-standing, often unilateral symptoms and opacification of a single sinus on imaging studies as a result of a mycetoma (fungus ball) within the sinus. Treatment for this condition is also surgical, although systemic antifungal therapy may be warranted in the rare case where bony erosion occurs. A third form of disease, known as *allergic fungal sinusitis*, is seen in patients with a history of nasal polyposis and asthma, who often have had multiple sinus surgeries. Patients with this condition produce a thick, eosinophilic mucus with the consistency of peanut butter that contains sparse fungal hyphae on histologic examination. Patients often present with pansinusitis.

℞ Treatment: CHRONIC SINUSITIS

Treatment of chronic bacterial sinusitis can be challenging and consists primarily of repeated culture-guided courses of antibiotics, sometimes for 3–4 weeks at a time; administration of intranasal glucocorticoids; and mechanical irrigation of the sinus with sterile saline solution. When this management approach fails, sinus surgery may be indicated and sometimes provides significant, albeit short-term, alleviation. Treatment of chronic fungal sinusitis consists of surgical removal of impacted mucus. Recurrence, unfortunately, is common.

INFECTIONS OF THE EAR AND MASTOID

Infections of the ear and associated structures can involve both the middle and external ear, including the skin, cartilage, periosteum, ear canal, and tympanic and mastoid cavities. Both viruses and bacteria are known causes of these infections, some of which result in significant morbidity if not treated appropriately.

INFECTIONS OF THE EXTERNAL EAR STRUCTURES

Infections involving the structures of the external ear are often difficult to differentiate from noninfectious inflammatory conditions with similar clinical manifestations. Clinicians should consider inflammatory disorders as a possible cause of external ear irritation, particularly in the absence of local or regional adenopathy. Aside from the more salient causes of inflammation, such as trauma, insect bite, and overexposure to sunlight or extreme cold, the differential diagnosis should include less common conditions, such as autoimmune disorders (e.g., lupus or relapsing polychondritis) and vasculitides (e.g., Wegener's granulomatosis).

Auricular Cellulitis

Auricular cellulitis is an infection of the skin overlying the external ear and typically follows minor local trauma. It presents with the typical signs and symptoms of a skin/soft tissue infection, with tenderness, erythema, swelling, and warmth of the external ear (particularly the lobule), but without apparent involvement of the ear canal or inner structures. Treatment consists of warm compresses and oral antibiotics such as dicloxacillin that are active against typical skin and soft tissue pathogens (specifically, *S. aureus* and streptococci). IV antibiotics, such as a first-generation cephalosporin (e.g., cefazolin) or a penicillinase-resistant penicillin (e.g., nafcillin), are occasionally needed for more severe cases.

Perichondritis

Perichondritis, an infection of the perichondrium of the auricular cartilage, typically follows local trauma (e.g., ear piercing, burns, or lacerations). Occasionally, when the infection spreads down to the cartilage of the pinna itself, patients may also have chondritis. The infection may closely resemble auricular cellulitis, with erythema, swelling, and extreme tenderness of the pinna, although the lobule is less often involved in perichondritis. The most common pathogens are *P. aeruginosa* and *S. aureus*, although other gram-negative and gram-positive organisms are occasionally involved. Treatment consists of systemic antibiotics active against both *P. aeruginosa* and *S. aureus*. An antipseudomonal penicillin (e.g., piperacillin) or a combination of a penicillinase-resistant penicillin plus an antipseudomonal quinolone (e.g., nafcillin plus ciprofloxacin) is typically used. Incision and drainage may be helpful for culture and for resolution of infection, which often takes weeks. When perichondritis fails to respond to adequate antimicrobial therapy, clinicians should consider a noninfectious inflammatory etiology; for example, relapsing polychondritis is often mistaken for infectious perichondritis.

Otitis Externa

The term *otitis externa* refers to a collection of diseases involving primarily the auditory meatus. Otitis externa usually results from a combination of heat, retained moisture, and desquamation and maceration of the epithelium of the outer ear canal. The disease exists in several forms: localized, diffuse, chronic, and invasive. All forms are predominantly bacterial in origin, with *P. aeruginosa* and *S. aureus* the most common pathogens.

Acute localized otitis externa (*furunculosis*) can develop in the outer third of the ear canal, where skin overlies cartilage and hair follicles are numerous. As in furunculosis elsewhere on the body, *S. aureus* is the usual pathogen, and treatment typically consists of an oral antistaphylococcal penicillin (e.g., dicloxacillin), with incision and drainage in cases of abscess formation.

Acute diffuse otitis externa is also known as *swimmer's ear*, although it can develop in patients who have not recently been swimming. Heat, humidity, and the loss of protective cerumen lead to excessive moisture and elevation of the pH in the ear canal, which in turn lead to skin maceration and irritation. Infection may then occur; the predominant pathogen is *P. aeruginosa*, although other gram-negative and gram-positive organisms have been recovered from patients with this condition. The illness often starts with itching and progresses to severe pain, which is usually triggered by manipulation of the pinna or tragus. The onset of pain is generally accompanied by the development of an erythematous, swollen ear canal, often with scant white, clumpy discharge. Treatment consists of cleansing the canal to remove debris and to enhance the activity of topical therapeutic agents—usually hypertonic saline or mixtures of alcohol and acetic acid. Inflammation can also be decreased by adding glucocorticoids to the treatment regimen or by using Burow's solution (aluminum acetate in water). Antibiotics are most effective when given topically. Otic mixtures provide adequate pathogen coverage; these preparations usually combine neomycin with polymyxin, with or without glucocorticoids.

Chronic otitis externa is caused primarily by repeated local irritation, most commonly arising from persistent drainage from a chronic middle-ear infection. Other causes of repeated irritation, such as insertion of cotton swabs or other foreign objects into the ear canal, can lead to this condition, as can rare chronic infections such as syphilis, tuberculosis, or leprosy. Chronic otitis externa typically presents as erythematous, scaling dermatitis in which the predominant symptom is pruritus rather than pain; this condition must be differentiated from several others that produce a similar clinical picture, such as atopic dermatitis, seborrheic dermatitis, psoriasis, and dermatomycosis. Therapy consists of identifying and treating or removing the offending process, although successful resolution is frequently difficult.

Invasive otitis externa, also known as *malignant* or *necrotizing* otitis externa, is an aggressive and potentially life-threatening disease that occurs predominantly in elderly diabetic patients and other immunocompromised patients. The disease begins in the external canal, progresses slowly over weeks to months, and often is difficult to distinguish from a severe case of chronic otitis externa because of the presence of purulent otorrhea and an erythematous swollen ear and external canal. Severe, deep-seated otalgia is often noted and can help differentiate invasive from chronic otitis externa. The characteristic finding on examination is granulation tissue in the posteroinferior wall of the external canal, near the junction of bone and cartilage. If left unchecked, the infection can migrate to the base of the skull (resulting in skull-base osteomyelitis) and on to the meninges and brain, with a high associated mortality rate. Cranial nerve involvement is occasionally seen, with the facial nerve usually affected first and most often. Thrombosis of the sigmoid sinus can occur if the infection extends to that area. CT, which can reveal osseous erosion of the temporal bone and skull base, can be used to help determine the extent of disease, as can gallium and technetium-99 scintigraphy studies. *P. aeruginosa* is by far the most common pathogen, although *S. aureus*, *Staphylococcus epidermidis*, *Aspergillus*, *Actinomyces*, and some gram-negative bacteria have also been associated with this disease. In all cases, the external ear canal should be cleansed, and a biopsy specimen of the granulation tissue within the canal (or of deeper tissues) should be obtained for culture of the offending organism. IV antibiotic therapy is directed specifically toward the recovered pathogen. For *P. aeruginosa*, the regimen typically includes an antipseudomonal penicillin or cephalosporin (e.g., piperacillin or ceftazidime) with an aminoglycoside. A fluoroquinolone antibiotic is frequently used in place of the aminoglycoside and can even be administered orally, given the excellent bioavailability of this drug class. In addition, antibiotic drops containing an agent active against *Pseudomonas* (e.g., ciprofloxacin) are usually prescribed and are combined with glucocorticoids to reduce inflammation. Cases of invasive *Pseudomonas* otitis externa recognized in the early stages can sometimes be treated with oral and otic fluoroquinolones alone, albeit with close follow-up. Extensive surgical debridement, once an important component of the treatment approach, is now rarely indicated.

INFECTIONS OF MIDDLE-EAR STRUCTURES

Otitis media is an inflammatory condition of the middle ear that results from dysfunction of the eustachian tube in association with a number of illnesses, including URIs and chronic rhinosinusitis. The inflammatory response to these conditions leads to the development of a sterile transudate within the middle-ear and mastoid cavities. Infection may occur if bacteria or viruses from the nasopharynx contaminate this fluid, producing an acute (or sometimes chronic) illness.

Acute Otitis Media

Acute otitis media results when pathogens from the nasopharynx are introduced into the inflammatory fluid collected in the middle ear (e.g., by nose blowing during a URI). The proliferation of these pathogens in this space leads to the development of the typical signs and symptoms of acute middle-ear infection. The diagnosis of acute otitis media requires the demonstration of fluid in the middle ear (with tympanic membrane immobility) and the accompanying signs or symptoms of local or systemic illness (Table 16-2).

Etiology

Acute otitis media typically follows a viral URI. The causative viruses (most commonly RSV, influenza virus, rhinovirus, and enterovirus) can themselves cause subsequent acute otitis media; more often, they predispose the patient to bacterial otitis media. Studies using tympanocentesis have consistently found *S. pneumoniae* to be the most important bacterial cause, isolated in up to 35% of cases. *H. influenzae* (nontypable strains) and *M. catarrhalis* are also common bacterial causes of acute otitis media, and concern is increasing about community strains of MRSA as an emerging etiologic agent. Viruses, such as those mentioned above, have been recovered either alone or with bacteria in 17–40% of cases.

Clinical Manifestations

Fluid in the middle ear is typically demonstrated or confirmed with pneumatic otoscopy. In the absence of fluid, the tympanic membrane moves visibly with the application of positive and negative pressure, but this movement is dampened when fluid is present. With bacterial infection, the tympanic membrane can also be erythematous, bulging, or retracted and occasionally can spontaneously perforate. The signs and symptoms accompanying infection can be local or systemic, including otalgia, otorrhea, diminished hearing, fever, or irritability. Erythema of the tympanic membrane is often evident but is nonspecific, as it is frequently seen in association with inflammation of the upper respiratory mucosa (e.g., during examination of young children). Other signs and symptoms that are occasionally reported include vertigo, nystagmus, and tinnitus.

TABLE 16-2

GUIDELINES FOR THE DIAGNOSIS AND TREATMENT OF ACUTE OTITIS MEDIA

ILLNESS SEVERITY	DIAGNOSTIC CRITERIA	TREATMENT RECOMMENDATIONS
Mild to moderate	Fluid in the middle ear, evidenced by decreased tympanic membrane mobility, air/fluid level behind tympanic membrane, bulging tympanic membrane, purulent otorrhea *and* Acute onset of signs and symptoms of middle-ear inflammation, including fever, otalgia, decreased hearing, tinnitus, vertigo, erythematous tympanic membrane	*Initial therapy*[a] Observation alone (symptom relief only)[b] *or* Amoxicillin, 80–90 mg/kg qd (up to 2 g) PO in divided doses (bid or tid), *or* Cefdinir, 14 mg/kg qd PO in 1 dose or divided doses Cefuroxime, 30 mg/kg qd PO in divided doses (bid), *or* Azithromycin, 10 mg/kg qd PO on day 1 followed by 5 mg/kg qd PO for 4 d *Exposure to antibiotics within 30 d or recent treatment failure*[a,c] Amoxicillin, 90 mg/kg qd (up to 2 g) PO in divided doses (bid), plus clavulanate, 6.4 mg/kg qd PO in divided doses (bid), *or* Ceftriaxone, 50 mg/kg IV/IM qd for 3 d, *or* Clindamycin, 30–40 mg/kg qd PO in divided doses (tid)
Severe	As above, with temperature ≥39.0°C *or* Moderate to severe otalgia	*Initial therapy*[a] Amoxicillin, 90 mg/kg qd (up to 2 g) PO in divided doses (bid), plus clavulanate, 6.4 mg/kg qd PO in divided doses (bid), *or* Ceftriaxone, 50 mg/kg IV/IM qd for 3 d *Exposure to antibiotics within 30 d or recent treatment failure*[a,c] Ceftriaxone, 50 mg/kg IV/IM qd for 3 d, *or* Clindamycin, 30–40 mg/kg qd PO in divided doses (tid), *or* Consider tympanocentesis with culture

[a]Duration (unless otherwise specified): 10 d for patients <6 years old and patients with severe disease; 5–7 d (with consideration of observation only in previously healthy individuals with mild disease) for patients ≥6 years old.

[b]Observation (deferring antibacterial treatment for 48–72 h and limiting management to symptom relief) is an option for mild to moderate disease in children 6 months to 2 years of age with an uncertain diagnosis and for children ≥2 years of age.

[c]Failure to improve and/or clinical worsening after 48–72 h of observation or treatment.

Sources: American Academy of Pediatrics Subcommittee on Management of Acute Otitis Media, 2004; Dowell et al, 1998.

℞ Treatment: ACUTE OTITIS MEDIA

There has been considerable debate on the usefulness of antibiotics for the treatment of acute otitis media. Although most cases resolve clinically 1 week after the onset of illness, antibiotics appear to be of some benefit. A higher proportion of treated than of untreated patients are free of illness 3–5 days after diagnosis. The difficulty of predicting which patients will benefit from antibiotic therapy has led to different approaches. In the Netherlands, for instance, physicians typically manage acute otitis media with initial observation, administering anti-inflammatory agents for aggressive pain management and reserving antibiotics for high-risk patients, patients with complicated disease, or patients who do not improve after 48–72 h. In contrast, many experts in the United States continue to recommend antibiotic therapy for children <6 months old in light of the higher frequency of secondary complications in this young and functionally immunocompromised population. However, observation without antimicrobial therapy is now generally considered a reasonable option in the United States for mild to moderate disease in children 6 months to 2 years of age with an uncertain diagnosis and for children ≥2 years of age (Table 16-2).

Given that most studies of the etiologic agents of acute otitis media consistently document similar pathogen profiles, therapy is generally empirical, except in those few cases where tympanocentesis is warranted—e.g., cases in newborns, cases refractory to therapy, and cases in patients who are severely ill or immunodeficient. Despite resistance to penicillin and amoxicillin in roughly one-quarter of *S. pneumoniae* isolates, one-third of *H. influenzae* isolates, and nearly all *M. catarrhalis* isolates, outcome studies continue to find that amoxicillin is as successful as any other agent, and it remains the drug of first choice in recommendations from multiple sources (Table 16-2). Therapy for uncomplicated acute otitis media is typically administered for 5–7 days to patients ≥6 years old; longer courses (e.g., 10 days) should be reserved for children <6 years old and patients with severe disease, in whom short-course therapy may be inadequate.

A switch in regimen is recommended if there is no clinical improvement by the third day of therapy, given the possibility of infection with a β-lactamase-producing strain of *H. influenzae* or *M. catarrhalis* or with a strain of penicillin-resistant *S. pneumoniae*. Decongestants and antihistamines are frequently used as adjunctive agents to reduce congestion and relieve obstruction of the eustachian tube, but clinical trials have yielded no significant evidence of benefit with either class of agents.

Recurrent Acute Otitis Media

Recurrent acute otitis media (more than three episodes within 6 months or four episodes within 12 months) is generally due to relapse or reinfection, although data indicate that the majority of early recurrences are new infections. In general, the same pathogens responsible for acute otitis media cause recurrent disease; even so, the recommended treatment consists of antibiotics active against β-lactamase-producing organisms. Antibiotic prophylaxis [e.g., with trimethoprim-sulfamethoxazole (TMP-SMX) or amoxicillin] can reduce recurrences in patients with recurrent acute otitis media by an average of one episode per year, but this benefit is small compared with the cost of the drug and the high likelihood of colonization with antibiotic-resistant pathogens. Other approaches, including placement of tympanostomy tubes, adenoidectomy, and tonsillectomy plus adenoidectomy, are of questionable overall value, given the relatively small benefit compared with the potential for complications.

Serous Otitis Media

In serous otitis media (otitis media with effusion), fluid is present in the middle ear for an extended period and in the absence of signs and symptoms of infection. In general, acute effusions are self-limited; most resolve in 2–4 weeks. In some cases, however (in particular after an episode of acute otitis media), effusions can persist for months. These chronic effusions are often associated with a significant hearing loss in the affected ear. In younger children, persistent effusions and decreased hearing can be associated with impairment of language acquisition skills. The great majority of cases of otitis media with effusion resolve spontaneously within 3 months without antibiotic therapy. Antibiotic therapy or myringotomy with insertion of tympanostomy tubes is typically reserved for patients in whom bilateral effusion (1) has persisted for at least 3 months and (2) is associated with significant bilateral hearing loss. With this conservative approach and the application of strict diagnostic criteria for acute otitis media and otitis media with effusion, it is estimated that 6–8 million courses of antibiotics could be avoided each year in the United States.

Chronic Otitis Media

Chronic suppurative otitis media is characterized by persistent or recurrent purulent otorrhea in the setting of tympanic membrane perforation. Usually, there is also some degree of conductive hearing loss. This condition can be categorized as active or inactive. Inactive disease is characterized by a central perforation of the tympanic membrane, which allows drainage of purulent fluid from the middle ear. When the perforation is more peripheral, squamous epithelium from the auditory canal may invade the middle ear through the perforation, forming a mass of keratinaceous debris (*cholesteatoma*) at the site of invasion. This mass can enlarge and has the potential to erode bone and promote further infection, which can lead to meningitis, brain abscess, or paralysis of cranial nerve VII. Treatment of chronic active otitis media is surgical; mastoidectomy, myringoplasty, and tympanoplasty can be performed as outpatient surgical procedures, with an overall success rate of ~80%. Chronic inactive otitis media is more difficult to cure, usually requiring repeated courses of topical antibiotic drops during periods of drainage. Systemic antibiotics may offer better cure rates, but their role in the treatment of this condition remains unclear.

Mastoiditis

Acute mastoiditis was relatively common among children before the introduction of antibiotics. Because the mastoid air cells connect with the middle ear, the process of fluid collection and infection is usually the same in the mastoid as in the middle ear. Early and frequent treatment of acute otitis media is most likely the reason that the incidence of acute mastoiditis has declined to only 1.2–2.0 cases per 100,000 person-years in countries with high prescribing rates for acute otitis media. In countries like the Netherlands, where antibiotics are used sparingly for acute otitis media, the incidence rate of acute mastoiditis is roughly twice that in countries like the United States. However, neighboring Denmark has a rate of acute mastoiditis similar to that in the Netherlands but an antibiotic-prescribing rate for acute otitis media more similar to that in the United States.

In typical acute mastoiditis, purulent exudate collects in the mastoid air cells (Fig. 16-1), producing pressure that may result in erosion of the surrounding bone and the formation of abscess-like cavities that are usually evident on CT. Patients typically present with pain, erythema, and swelling of the mastoid process along with displacement of the pinna, usually in conjunction with the typical signs and symptoms of acute middle-ear infection. Rarely, patients can develop severe complications if the infection tracks under the periosteum of the temporal bone to cause a subperiosteal abscess, erodes through the mastoid tip to cause a deep neck abscess, or extends posteriorly to cause septic thrombosis of the lateral sinus.

Purulent fluid should be cultured whenever possible to help guide antimicrobial therapy. Initial empirical therapy is usually directed against the typical organisms associated with acute otitis media, such as *S. pneumoniae*, *H. influenzae*, and *M. catarrhalis*. Some patients with more severe or prolonged courses of illness should be treated for infection with *S. aureus* and gram-negative bacilli (including *Pseudomonas*). Broad empirical therapy is usually narrowed once culture results become available. Most patients can be treated conservatively with IV antibiotics;

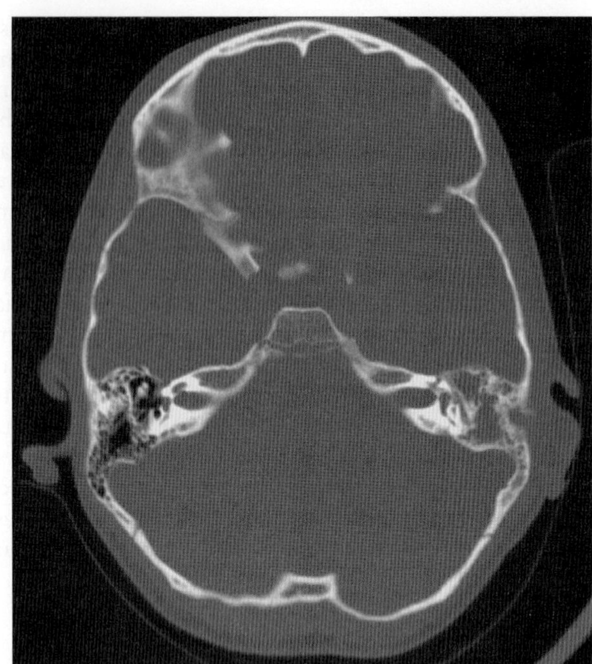

FIGURE 16-1
Acute mastoiditis. Axial CT image shows an acute fluid collection within the mastoid air cells on the left.

surgery (cortical mastoidectomy) can be reserved for complicated cases and those in which conservative treatment has failed.

INFECTIONS OF THE PHARYNX AND ORAL CAVITY

Oropharyngeal infections range from mild, self-limited viral illnesses to serious, life-threatening bacterial infections. The most common presenting symptom is sore throat—one of the most frequent reasons for ambulatory care visits by both adults and children. Although sore throat is a symptom in many noninfectious illnesses as well, the overwhelming majority of patients with a new sore throat have acute pharyngitis of viral or bacterial etiology.

ACUTE PHARYNGITIS

Millions of visits to primary care providers each year are for sore throat; the majority of cases of acute pharyngitis are caused by typical respiratory viruses. The most important source of concern is infection with group A β-hemolytic *Streptococcus* (*S. pyogenes*), which is associated with acute glomerulonephritis and acute rheumatic fever. The risk of rheumatic fever can be reduced by timely penicillin therapy.

Etiology

A wide variety of organisms cause acute pharyngitis. The relative importance of the different pathogens can only be estimated, since a significant proportion of cases (~30%) have no identified cause. Together, respiratory viruses are the most common identifiable cause of acute pharyngitis, with rhinoviruses and coronaviruses accounting for large proportions of cases (~20% and at least 5%, respectively). Influenza virus, parainfluenza virus, and adenovirus also account for a measurable share of cases, the latter as part of the more clinically severe syndrome of pharyngoconjunctival fever. Other important but less common viral causes include herpes simplex virus (HSV) types 1 and 2, coxsackievirus A, cytomegalovirus (CMV), and Epstein-Barr virus (EBV). Acute HIV infection can present as acute pharyngitis and should be considered in high-risk populations.

Acute bacterial pharyngitis is typically caused by *S. pyogenes*, which accounts for ~5–15% of all cases of acute pharyngitis in adults; rates vary with the season and with utilization of the health care system. Group A streptococcal pharyngitis is primarily a disease of children 5–15 years of age; it is uncommon among children <3 years old, as is rheumatic fever. Streptococci of groups C and G account for a minority of cases, although these serogroups are nonrheumatogenic. The remaining bacterial causes of acute pharyngitis are seen infrequently (<1% each) but should be considered in appropriate exposure groups because of the severity of illness if left untreated; these etiologic agents include *Neisseria gonorrhoeae*, *Corynebacterium diphtheriae*, *Corynebacterium ulcerans*, *Yersinia enterocolitica*, and *Treponema pallidum* (in secondary syphilis). Anaerobic bacteria can also cause acute pharyngitis (*Vincent's angina*) and can contribute to more serious polymicrobial infections, such as peritonsillar or retropharyngeal abscess (see below). Atypical organisms such as *M. pneumoniae* and *C. pneumoniae* have been recovered from patients with acute pharyngitis; whether these agents are commensals or causes of acute infection is debatable.

Clinical Manifestations

Although the signs and symptoms accompanying acute pharyngitis are not reliable predictors of the etiologic agent, the clinical presentation occasionally suggests that one etiology is more likely than another. Acute pharyngitis due to respiratory viruses such as rhinovirus or coronavirus is usually not severe and is typically associated with a constellation of coryzal symptoms better characterized as nonspecific URI. Findings on physical examination are uncommon; fever is rare, and tender cervical adenopathy and pharyngeal exudates are not seen. In contrast, acute pharyngitis from influenza virus can be severe and is much more likely to be associated with fever as well as with myalgias, headache, and cough. The presentation of pharyngoconjunctival fever due to adenovirus infection is similar. Since pharyngeal exudate may be present on examination, this condition can be difficult to differentiate from streptococcal pharyngitis. However, adenoviral pharyngitis is distinguished by the presence of conjunctivitis in one-third to one-half of patients. Acute pharyngitis from primary HSV infection can also mimic streptococcal pharyngitis in some cases, with pharyngeal inflammation and exudate, but the presence of vesicles and shallow ulcers on the palate can help differentiate the two diseases. This HSV syndrome is distinct from pharyngitis caused by coxsackievirus (*herpangina*), which is associated with small vesicles that develop on the soft palate and uvula and then rupture to form shallow white ulcers. Acute exudative pharyngitis coupled with fever, fatigue, generalized lymphadenopathy, and (on occasion) splenomegaly is characteristic of infectious mononucleosis due to EBV or CMV. Acute primary infection with HIV is frequently associated with fever and acute pharyngitis as well as with myalgias, arthralgias, malaise, and occasionally a nonpruritic maculopapular rash, which later may be followed by lymphadenopathy and mucosal ulcerations without exudate.

The clinical features of acute pharyngitis caused by streptococci of groups A, C, and G are all similar, ranging from a relatively mild illness without many accompanying symptoms to clinically severe cases with profound pharyngeal pain, fever, chills, and abdominal pain. A hyperemic pharyngeal membrane with tonsillar hypertrophy and exudate is usually seen, along with tender anterior cervical adenopathy. Coryzal manifestations, including cough, are typically absent; when present, they suggest a viral etiology. Strains of *S. pyogenes* that generate erythrogenic toxin can also produce scarlet fever characterized by an erythematous rash and strawberry tongue. The other types of acute bacterial pharyngitis (e.g., gonococcal, diphtherial, and yersinial) often present as exudative pharyngitis with or without other clinical features. Their etiologies are often suggested only by the clinical history.

Diagnosis

The primary goal of diagnostic testing is to separate acute streptococcal pharyngitis from pharyngitis of other etiologies (particularly viral) so that antibiotics can be prescribed more efficiently for patients to whom they may be beneficial. The most appropriate standard for the diagnosis of streptococcal pharyngitis, however, has not been definitively established. Throat swab culture is generally regarded as such. However, this method cannot distinguish between infection and colonization, and it takes 24–48 h to yield results that vary according to technique and culture conditions. Rapid antigen-detection tests offer good specificity (>90%) but lower sensitivity when implemented in routine practice. The sensitivity has also been shown to vary across the clinical spectrum of disease (65–90%). Several clinical prediction systems (Table 16-3) can increase the sensitivity of rapid antigen-detection tests to >90% in controlled settings. Since the sensitivities achieved in routine clinical practice are often lower, several medical and professional societies continue to recommend that all negative rapid antigen-detection tests in children be confirmed by a throat culture to limit transmission and complications of illness caused by group A streptococci. The Centers for Disease Control and Prevention, the Infectious Diseases Society of America, the American College of Physicians, and the American Academy of Family Physicians do not recommend backup culture when adults have negative results in a high-sensitivity, rapid antigen-detection test, however, given the lower prevalence and smaller benefit in this age group.

Cultures and rapid diagnostic tests for other causes of acute pharyngitis, such as influenza virus, adenovirus, HSV, EBV, CMV, and *M. pneumoniae*, are available in some locations and can be used when these infections are suspected. The diagnosis of acute EBV infection depends primarily on the detection of antibodies to the

TABLE 16-3

GUIDELINES FOR THE DIAGNOSIS AND TREATMENT OF ACUTE PHARYNGITIS

AGE GROUP	DIAGNOSTIC CRITERIA	TREATMENT RECOMMENDATIONS[a]
Adults	*Clinical suspicion of streptococcal pharyngitis* (e.g., fever, tonsillar swelling, exudate, enlarged/tender anterior cervical lymph nodes, absence of cough or coryza)[b] *with:* History of rheumatic fever *or* Documented household exposure *or* Positive rapid strep screen	Penicillin V, 500 mg PO tid, *or* Amoxicillin, 500 mg PO bid, *or* Erythromycin, 250 mg PO qid, *or* Benzathine penicillin G, single dose of 1.2 million units IM
Children	*Clinical suspicion of streptococcal pharyngitis* (e.g., tonsillar swelling, exudate, enlarged/tender anterior cervical lymph nodes, absence of coryza) *with:* History of rheumatic fever *or* Documented household exposure *or* Positive rapid strep screen *or* Positive throat culture (for patients with negative rapid strep screen)	Amoxicillin, 45 mg/kg qd PO in divided doses (bid or tid), *or* Penicillin VK, 50 mg/kg qd PO in divided doses (bid), *or* Cephalexin, 50 mg/kg qd PO in divided doses (qid), *or* Benzathine penicillin G, single dose of 25,000 units/kg IM

[a]Unless otherwise specified, the duration of therapy is generally 10 d, with appropriate follow-up.
[b]Some organizations support treating adults who have these symptoms and signs without administering a rapid streptococcal antigen test.
Sources: Cooper et al, 2001; Schwartz et al, 1998.

virus with a heterophile agglutination assay (monospot slide test) or enzyme-linked immunosorbent assay. Testing for HIV RNA or antigen (p24) should be performed when acute primary HIV infection is suspected. If other bacterial causes are suspected (particularly *N. gonorrhoeae*, *C. diphtheriae*, or *Y. enterocolitica*), specific cultures should be requested since these organisms may be missed on routine throat swab culture.

Rx Treatment: PHARYNGITIS

Antibiotic treatment of pharyngitis due to *S. pyogenes* confers numerous benefits, including a decrease in the risk of rheumatic fever. The magnitude of this benefit is fairly small, however, since rheumatic fever is now a rare disease, even among untreated patients. When therapy is started within 48 h of illness onset, however, symptom duration is also decreased. An additional benefit of therapy is the potential to reduce the spread of streptococcal pharyngitis, particularly in areas of overcrowding or close contact. Antibiotic therapy for acute pharyngitis is therefore recommended in cases where *S. pyogenes* is confirmed as the etiologic agent by rapid antigen-detection test or throat swab culture. Otherwise, antibiotics should be given in routine cases only when another bacterial cause has been identified. Effective therapy for streptococcal pharyngitis consists of either a single dose of IM benzathine penicillin or a full 10-day course of oral penicillin (Table 16-3). Erythromycin can be used in place of penicillin, although resistance to erythromycin among *S. pyogenes* strains in some parts of the world (particularly Europe) can prohibit the use of this drug. Newer (and more expensive) antibiotics are also active against streptococci but offer no greater efficacy than the above agents. Testing for cure is unnecessary and may reveal only chronic colonization. There is no evidence to support antibiotic treatment of group C or G streptococcal pharyngitis or of pharyngitis in which *Mycoplasma* or *Chlamydophila* has been recovered. Penicillin prophylaxis (benzathine penicillin G, 1.2 million units IM every 3–4 weeks) is indicated for patients at risk of recurrent rheumatic fever.

Treatment of viral pharyngitis is entirely symptom-based except in infection with influenza virus or HSV. For influenza, a number of therapeutic agents exist, including amantadine, rimantadine, and the two newer agents oseltamivir and zanamivir. All of these agents need to be started within 36–48 h of symptom onset to reduce illness duration meaningfully. Of these agents, only oseltamivir and zanamivir are active against both influenza A and influenza B and therefore can be used when local infection patterns are unknown. Oropharyngeal HSV infection sometimes responds to treatment with antiviral agents such as acyclovir, although these drugs are often reserved for immunosuppressed patients.

Complications

Although rheumatic fever is the best-known complication of acute streptococcal pharyngitis, the risk of its following acute infection remains quite low. Other complications include acute glomerulonephritis and numerous suppurative conditions, such as peritonsillar abscess (*quinsy*), otitis media, mastoiditis, sinusitis, bacteremia, and pneumonia—all of which occur at low rates. Although antibiotic treatment of acute streptococcal pharyngitis can prevent the development of rheumatic fever, there is no evidence that it can prevent acute glomerulonephritis. Some evidence supports antibiotic use to prevent the suppurative complications of streptococcal pharyngitis, particularly peritonsillar abscess, which can also involve oral anaerobes such as *Fusobacterium*. Abscesses are usually accompanied by severe pharyngeal pain, dysphagia, fever, and dehydration; in addition, medial displacement of the tonsil and lateral displacement of the uvula are often evident on examination. Although early use of IV antibiotics (e.g., clindamycin; penicillin G with metronidazole) may obviate the need for surgical drainage in some cases, treatment typically involves needle aspiration or incision and drainage.

ORAL INFECTIONS

Aside from periodontal disease such as gingivitis, infections of the oral cavity most commonly involve HSV or *Candida* species. In addition to causing painful cold sores on the lips, HSV can infect the tongue and buccal mucosa, causing the formation of irritating vesicles. Although topical antiviral agents (e.g., acyclovir and penciclovir) can be used externally for cold sores, oral or IV acyclovir is often needed for primary infections, extensive oral infections, and infections in immunocompromised patients. Oropharyngeal candidiasis (*thrush*) is caused by a variety of *Candida* species, most often *C. albicans*. Thrush occurs predominantly in neonates, immunocompromised patients (especially those with AIDS), and recipients of prolonged antibiotic or glucocorticoid therapy. In addition to sore throat, patients often report a burning tongue, and physical examination reveals friable white or gray plaques on the gingiva, tongue, and oral mucosa. Treatment, which usually consists of an oral antifungal suspension (nystatin or clotrimazole) or oral fluconazole, is frequently successful. In the uncommon cases of fluconazole-refractory thrush that are seen in some patients with AIDS, other therapeutic options include oral formulations of itraconazole, amphotericin B, or voriconazole, as well as the IV echinocandins (caspofungin, micafungin, and anidulafungin).

Vincent's angina, also known as *acute necrotizing ulcerative gingivitis* or *trench mouth*, is a unique and dramatic form of gingivitis characterized by painful, inflamed gingiva with ulcerations of the interdental papillae that bleed easily. Since oral anaerobes are the cause, patients typically have halitosis and frequently present with fever, malaise, and lymphadenopathy. Treatment consists of debridement and oral administration of penicillin plus metronidazole, with clindamycin alone as an alternative.

Ludwig's angina is a rapidly progressive, potentially fulminant cellulitis that involves the sublingual and submandibular spaces and that typically originates from an infected or recently extracted tooth, most commonly the lower second and third molars. Improved dental care has substantially reduced the incidence of this disorder. Infection in these areas leads to dysphagia, odynophagia, and "woody" edema in the sublingual region, forcing the tongue up and back with the potential for airway obstruction. Fever, dysarthria, and drooling may also be noted, and patients may speak in a "hot potato" voice. Intubation or tracheostomy may be necessary to secure the airway, as asphyxiation is the most common cause of death. Patients should be monitored closely and treated promptly with IV antibiotics directed against streptococci and oral anaerobes. Recommended agents include ampicillin/sulbactam and high-dose penicillin plus metronidazole.

Postanginal septicemia (*Lemierre's disease*) is a rare anaerobic oropharyngeal infection caused predominantly by *Fusobacterium necrophorum*. The illness typically starts as a sore throat (most commonly in adolescents and young adults), which may present as exudative tonsillitis or peritonsillar abscess. Infection of the deep pharyngeal tissue allows organisms to drain into the lateral pharyngeal space, which contains the carotid artery and internal jugular vein. Septic thrombophlebitis of the internal jugular vein can result, with associated pain, dysphagia, and neck swelling and stiffness. Sepsis usually occurs 3–10 days after the onset of sore throat and is often coupled with metastatic infection to the lung and other distant sites. Occasionally, the infection can extend along the carotid sheath and into the posterior mediastinum, resulting in mediastinitis, or it can erode into the carotid artery, with the early sign of repeated small bleeds into the mouth. The mortality rate from these invasive infections can be as high as 50%. Treatment consists of IV antibiotics (penicillin G or clindamycin) and surgical drainage of any purulent collections. The concomitant use of anticoagulants to prevent embolization remains controversial but is often advised.

INFECTIONS OF THE LARYNX AND EPIGLOTTIS

LARYNGITIS

Laryngitis is defined as any inflammatory process involving the larynx and can be caused by a variety of infectious and noninfectious processes. The vast majority of laryngitis cases seen in clinical practice in developed countries are acute. Acute laryngitis is a common syndrome caused predominantly by the same viruses responsible for many other URIs. In fact, most cases of acute laryngitis occur in the setting of a viral URI.

Etiology

Nearly all major respiratory viruses have been implicated in acute viral laryngitis, including rhinovirus, influenza virus, parainfluenza virus, adenovirus, coxsackievirus, coronavirus, and RSV. Acute laryngitis can also be associated with acute bacterial respiratory infections, such as those caused by group A *Streptococcus* or *C. diphtheriae* (although diphtheria has been all but eliminated in the United States). Another bacterial pathogen thought to play a role (albeit unclear) in the pathogenesis of acute laryngitis is *M. catarrhalis*, which has been recovered on nasopharyngeal culture from a significant percentage of people with acute laryngitis. Chronic laryngitis of infectious etiology is much less common in developed than in developing countries. Laryngitis due to *Mycobacterium tuberculosis* is often difficult to distinguish from laryngeal cancer, in part because of the frequent absence of signs, symptoms, and radiographic findings typical of pulmonary disease. *Histoplasma* and *Blastomyces* may cause laryngitis, often as a complication of systemic infection. *Candida* species can cause laryngitis as well, often in association with thrush or esophagitis and particularly in immunosuppressed patients. Rare cases of chronic laryngitis are due to *Coccidioides* and *Cryptococcus*.

Clinical Manifestations

Laryngitis is characterized by hoarseness and can also be associated with reduced vocal pitch or aphonia. As acute laryngitis is caused predominantly by respiratory viruses, these symptoms usually occur in association with other symptoms and signs of URI, including rhinorrhea, nasal congestion, cough, and sore throat. Direct laryngoscopy often reveals diffuse laryngeal erythema and edema, along with vascular engorgement of the vocal folds. In addition, chronic disease (e.g., tuberculous laryngitis) often includes mucosal nodules and ulcerations visible on laryngoscopy; these lesions are sometimes mistaken for laryngeal cancer.

℞ Treatment: LARYNGITIS

Acute laryngitis is usually treated with humidification and voice rest alone. Antibiotics are not recommended except when group A *Streptococcus* is cultured, in which case penicillin is the drug of choice. The choice of therapy for chronic laryngitis depends on the pathogen, whose identification usually requires biopsy with culture. Patients with laryngeal tuberculosis are highly contagious because of the large number of organisms that are easily aerosolized. These patients should be managed in the same way as patients with active pulmonary disease.

CROUP

The term *croup* actually denotes a group of diseases collectively referred to as "croup syndrome," all of which are acute and predominantly viral respiratory illnesses characterized by marked swelling of the subglottic region of the larynx. Croup primarily affects children <6 years old. For a detailed discussion of this entity, the reader is referred to a text of pediatric medicine.

EPIGLOTTITIS

Acute epiglottitis (supraglottitis) is an acute, rapidly progressive cellulitis of the epiglottis and adjacent structures that can result in complete—and potentially fatal—airway obstruction in both children and adults. Before the widespread use of *H. influenzae* type b (Hib) vaccine, this entity was much more common among children, with a peak incidence at ~3.5 years of age. In some countries, mass vaccination against Hib has reduced the annual incidence of acute epiglottitis in children by >90%; in contrast, the annual incidence in adults has changed little since the introduction of Hib vaccine. Because of the danger of airway obstruction, acute epiglottitis constitutes a medical emergency, particularly in children, and prompt diagnosis and airway protection are of utmost importance.

Etiology

After the introduction of the Hib vaccine in the mid-1980s, disease incidence among children in the United States declined dramatically. Nevertheless, lack of vaccination or vaccine failure has meant that many pediatric cases seen today are still due to Hib. In adults and (more recently) in children, a variety of other bacterial pathogens have been associated with epiglottitis, the most common being group A *Streptococcus*. Other pathogens seen less frequently include *S. pneumoniae*, *Haemophilus parainfluenzae*, and *S. aureus*. Viruses have not yet been established as causes of acute epiglottitis.

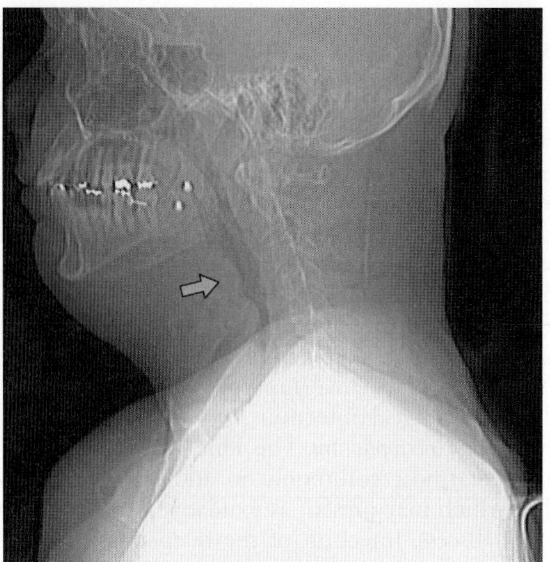

FIGURE 16-2
Acute epiglottitis. In this lateral soft tissue radiograph of the neck, the arrow indicates the enlarged edematous epiglottis (the "thumbprint sign").

Clinical Manifestations and Diagnosis

Epiglottitis typically presents more acutely in young children than in adolescents or adults. On presentation, most children have had symptoms for <24 h, including high fever, severe sore throat, tachycardia, systemic toxicity, and (in many cases) drooling while sitting forward. Symptoms and signs of respiratory obstruction may also be present and may progress rapidly. The somewhat milder illness in adolescents and adults often follows 1–2 days of severe sore throat and is commonly accompanied by dyspnea, drooling, and stridor. Physical examination of patients with acute epiglottitis may reveal moderate or severe respiratory distress, with inspiratory stridor and retractions of the chest wall. These findings *diminish* as the disease progresses and the patient tires. Conversely, oropharyngeal examination reveals infection that is much less severe than would be predicted from the symptoms—a finding that should alert the clinician to a cause of symptoms and obstruction that lies beyond the tonsils. The diagnosis is often made on clinical grounds, although direct fiberoptic laryngoscopy is frequently performed in a controlled environment (e.g., an operating room) in order to visualize and culture the typical edematous "cherry-red" epiglottis and to facilitate placement of an endotracheal tube. Direct visualization in an examination room (e.g., with a tongue blade and indirect laryngoscopy) is not recommended because of the risk of immediate laryngospasm and complete airway obstruction. Lateral neck radiographs and laboratory tests can assist in the diagnosis but may delay the critical securing of the airway and cause the patient to be moved or repositioned more than is necessary, thereby increasing the risk of further airway compromise. Neck radiographs typically reveal an enlarged edematous epiglottis (the "thumbprint sign," Fig. 16-2), usually with a dilated hypopharynx and normal subglottic structures. Laboratory tests characteristically document mild to moderate leukocytosis, with a predominance of neutrophils. Blood cultures are positive in a significant proportion of cases.

℞ Treatment: EPIGLOTTITIS

Security of the airway is always of primary concern in acute epiglottitis, even if the diagnosis is only suspected. Mere observation for signs of impending airway obstruction is not routinely recommended, particularly in children. Many adults have been managed with observation only since the illness is perceived to be milder in this age group, but some data suggest that this approach may be risky and probably should be reserved only for adult patients who have yet to develop dyspnea or stridor. Once the airway has been secured and specimens of blood and epiglottis tissue have been obtained for culture, treatment with IV antibiotics should be given to cover the most likely organisms, particularly *H. influenzae*. Because rates of ampicillin resistance in this organism have risen significantly in recent years, therapy with a β-lactam/β-lactamase inhibitor combination or a second- or third-generation cephalosporin is recommended. Typically, ampicillin/sulbactam, cefuroxime, cefotaxime, or ceftriaxone is given, with clindamycin and TMP-SMX reserved for patients allergic to β-lactams. Antibiotic therapy should be continued for 7–10 days and should be tailored, if necessary, to the organism recovered in culture. If the household contacts of a patient with *H. influenzae* epiglottitis include an unvaccinated child under the age of 4, all members of the household (including the patient) should receive prophylactic rifampin for 4 days to eradicate carriage of *H. influenzae*.

INFECTIONS OF THE DEEP NECK STRUCTURES

Deep neck infections are usually extensions of infection from other primary sites, most often within the pharynx or oral cavity. Many of these infections are life-threatening but are difficult to detect at early stages when they may be more easily managed. Three of the most clinically relevant spaces in the neck are the submandibular (and sublingual) space, the lateral pharyngeal (or parapharyngeal) space, and the retropharyngeal space. These spaces communicate with one another and with other important structures in the head, neck, and thorax, providing pathogens with easy access to areas including the mediastinum, carotid sheath, skull base, and meninges. Once infection reaches these sensitive areas, mortality rates can be as high as 20–50%.

Infection of the submandibular and/or sublingual space typically originates from an infected or recently extracted lower tooth. The result is the severe, life-threatening infection referred to as Ludwig's angina (see "Oral Infections" earlier in the chapter). Infection of the lateral pharyngeal (or parapharyngeal) space is most often a complication of common infections of the oral cavity and upper respiratory tract, including tonsillitis, peritonsillar abscess, pharyngitis, mastoiditis, or periodontal infection. This space, located deep to the lateral wall of the pharynx, contains a number of sensitive structures, including the carotid artery, internal jugular vein, cervical sympathetic chain, and portions of cranial nerves IX through XII; at its distal end, it opens into the posterior mediastinum. Involvement of this space with infection can therefore be rapidly fatal. Examination may reveal some tonsillar displacement, trismus, and neck rigidity, but swelling of the lateral pharyngeal wall can easily be missed. The diagnosis can be confirmed by CT. Treatment consists of airway management, operative drainage of fluid collections, and at least 10 days of IV therapy with an antibiotic active against streptococci and oral anaerobes (e.g., ampicillin/ sulbactam). A particularly severe form of this infection involving the components of the carotid sheath (postanginal septicemia, Lemierre's disease) is described above (see "Oral Infections"). Infection of the retropharyngeal space can also be extremely dangerous, as this space runs posterior to the pharynx from the skull base to the superior mediastinum. Infections in this space are more common among children <5 years old because of the presence of several small retropharyngeal lymph nodes that typically atrophy by the age of 4 years. Infection is usually a consequence of extension from another site of infection, most commonly acute pharyngitis. Other sources include otitis media, tonsillitis, dental infections, Ludwig's angina, and anterior extension of vertebral osteomyelitis. Retropharyngeal space infection can also follow penetrating trauma to the posterior pharynx (e.g., from an endoscopic procedure). Infections are commonly polymicrobial, involving a mixture of aerobes and anaerobes; group A β-hemolytic streptococci and *S. aureus* are the most common pathogens. *M. tuberculosis* was a frequent cause in the past but now is rarely involved in the United States.

Patients with retropharyngeal abscess typically present with sore throat, fever, dysphagia, and neck pain and are often drooling because of difficulty and pain with swallowing. Examination may reveal tender cervical adenopathy, neck swelling, and diffuse erythema and edema of the posterior pharynx as well as a bulge in the posterior pharyngeal wall that may not be obvious on routine inspection. A soft tissue mass is usually demonstrable by lateral neck radiography or CT. Because of the risk of airway obstruction, treatment begins with securing of the airway, which is followed by a combination of surgical drainage and IV antibiotic administration. Initial empirical therapy should cover streptococci, oral anaerobes, and *S. aureus*; ampicillin/sulbactam, clindamycin alone, or clindamycin plus ceftriaxone is usually effective. Complications result primarily from extension to other areas; for example, rupture into the posterior pharynx may lead to aspiration pneumonia and empyema. Extension may also occur to the lateral pharyngeal space and mediastinum, resulting in mediastinitis and pericarditis, or into nearby major blood vessels. All these events are associated with a high mortality rate.

FURTHER READINGS

American Academy of Pediatrics Subcommittee on Management of Acute Otitis Media: Diagnosis and management of acute otitis media. Pediatrics 113:1451, 2004

American Academy of Pediatrics Subcommittee on Management of Sinusitis and Committee on Quality Improvement: Clinical practice guideline: Management of sinusitis. Pediatrics 108:798, 2001

Ahovuo-Saloranta A et al: Antibiotics for acute maxillary sinusitis. Cochrane Database Syst Rev 2:CD000243, 2008

Carfrae MJ, Kesser BW: Malignant otitis externa. Otolaryngol Clin North Am 41:537, 2008

Cooper RJ et al: Principles of appropriate antibiotic use for acute pharyngitis in adults: Background. Ann Intern Med 134:509, 2001

Dowell SF et al: Otitis media—principles of judicious use of antimicrobial agents. Pediatrics 101:165, 1998

Gerber MA et al: Prevention of rheumatic fever and diagnosis and treatment of acute streptococcal pharyngitis: A scientific statement from the American Heart Association Rheumatic Fever, Endocarditis, and Kawasaki Disease Committee of the Council on Cardiovascular Disease in the Young, the Interdisciplinary Council on Functional Genomics and Translational Biology, and the Interdisciplinary Council on Quality of Care and Outcomes Research: Endorsed by the American Academy of Pediatrics. Circulation 119:1541, 2009

Gonzales R et al: Principles of appropriate antibiotic use for treatment of nonspecific upper respiratory tract infections in adults: Background. Ann Intern Med 134:490, 2001

Hickner JM et al: Principles of appropriate antibiotic use for acute rhinosinusitis in adults: Background. Ann Intern Med 134:498, 2001

Ongkasuwan J et al: Pneumococcal mastoiditis in children and the emergence of multidrug-resistant serotype 19A isolates. Pediatrics 122:34, 2008

Paradise JL et al: Tympanostomy tubes and developmental outcomes at 9 to 11 years of age. N Engl J Med 356:248, 2007

Pfoh E et al: Burden and economic cost of group A streptococcal pharyngitis. Pediatrics 121:229, 2008

PICCIRILLO JF: Acute bacterial sinusitis. N Engl J Med 351:902, 2004
RAFEI K et al: Airway infectious disease emergencies. Pediatr Clin North Am 53:215, 2006
SCHWARTZ B et al: Pharyngitis—principles of judicious use of antimicrobial agents. Pediatrics 101:171, 1998
SINUS AND ALLERGY HEALTH PARTNERSHIP: Antimicrobial treatment guidelines for acute bacterial rhinosinusitis. Otolaryngol Head Neck Surg 130:1, 2004
VAN ZUIJLEN DA et al: National differences in incidence of acute mastoiditis: Relationship to prescribing patterns of antibiotics for acute otitis media? Pediatr Infect Dis J 20:140, 2001
WENZEL RP et al: Acute bronchitis. N Engl J Med 355:2125, 2006
YOUNG J et al: Antibiotics for adults with clinically diagnosed acute rhinosinusitis: A meta-analysis of individual patient data. Lancet 371:908, 2008

CHAPTER 17

PNEUMONIA

Lionel A. Mandell ■ Richard Wunderink

DEFINITION

Pneumonia is an infection of the pulmonary parenchyma. Despite being the cause of significant morbidity and mortality, pneumonia is often misdiagnosed, mistreated, and underestimated. In the past, pneumonia was typically classified as community-acquired, hospital-acquired, or ventilator-associated. Over the last decade or two, however, patients presenting to the hospital have often been found to be infected with multidrug-resistant (MDR) pathogens previously associated with hospital-acquired pneumonia. Factors responsible for this phenomenon include the development and widespread use of potent oral antibiotics, earlier transfer of patients out of acute-care hospitals to their homes or various lower-acuity facilities, increased use of outpatient IV antibiotic therapy, general aging of the population, and more extensive immunomodulatory therapies. The potential involvement of these MDR pathogens has led to a revised classification system in which infection is categorized as either community-acquired pneumonia (CAP) or health care–associated pneumonia (HCAP), with subcategories of HCAP including hospital-acquired pneumonia (HAP) and ventilator-associated pneumonia (VAP). The conditions associated with HCAP and the likely pathogens are listed in Table 17-1 (see also Chap. 13).

Although the new classification system has been helpful in designing empirical antibiotic strategies, it is not without disadvantages. For instance, not all MDR pathogens are associated with all risk factors (Table 17-1). Therefore, this system represents a distillation of multiple risk factors, and each patient must be considered individually. For example, the risk of infection with MDR pathogens for a nursing home resident with dementia who can independently dress, ambulate, and eat is quite different from the risk for a patient who is in a chronic vegetative state with a tracheostomy and a percutaneous feeding tube in place. In addition, risk factors for MDR infection do not preclude the development of pneumonia caused by the usual CAP pathogens.

This chapter deals with pneumonia in patients who are not considered to be immunocompromised. Pneumonia in immunocompromised patients is discussed in other chapters, including Chaps. 11, 12, and 90.

PATHOPHYSIOLOGY

Pneumonia results from the proliferation of microbial pathogens at the alveolar level and the host's response to those pathogens. Microorganisms gain access to the lower respiratory tract in several ways. The most common is by aspiration from the oropharynx. Small-volume aspiration occurs frequently during sleep (especially in the elderly) and in patients with decreased levels of consciousness. Many pathogens are inhaled as contaminated droplets. Rarely, pneumonia occurs via hematogenous spread (e.g., from tricuspid endocarditis) or by contiguous extension from an infected pleural or mediastinal space.

Mechanical factors are critically important in host defense. The hairs and turbinates of the nares catch larger inhaled particles before they reach the lower respiratory tract, and the branching architecture of the tracheobronchial tree traps particles on the airway lining, where mucociliary clearance and local antibacterial factors either clear or kill the potential pathogen. The gag reflex and the cough mechanism offer critical protection from aspiration. In addition, the normal flora adhering to mucosal cells of the oropharynx, whose components are remarkably constant, prevents pathogenic bacteria from binding and thereby decreases the risk of pneumonia caused by these more virulent bacteria.

When these barriers are overcome or when the microorganisms are small enough to be inhaled to the alveolar level, resident alveolar macrophages are extremely efficient at clearing and killing pathogens. Macrophages are assisted

TABLE 17-1

CLINICAL CONDITIONS ASSOCIATED WITH AND LIKELY PATHOGENS IN HEALTH CARE-ASSOCIATED PNEUMONIA

	PATHOGEN			
CONDITION	**MRSA**	***PSEUDOMONAS AERUGINOSA***	***ACINETOBACTER* SPP.**	**MDR ENTEROBACTERIACEAE**
Hospitalization for ≥48 h	X	X	X	X
Hospitalization for ≥2 days in prior 3 months	X	X	X	X
Nursing home or extended-care facility residence	X	X	X	X
Antibiotic therapy in preceding 3 months		X		X
Chronic dialysis	X			
Home infusion therapy	X			
Home wound care	X			
Family member with MDR infection	X			X

Note: MDR, multidrug-resistant; MRSA, methicillin-resistant *Staphylococcus aureus*.

by local proteins (e.g., surfactant proteins A and D) that have intrinsic opsonizing properties or antibacterial or antiviral activity. Once engulfed, the pathogens—even if they are not killed by macrophages—are eliminated via either the mucociliary elevator or the lymphatics and no longer represent an infectious challenge. Only when the capacity of the alveolar macrophages to ingest or kill the microorganisms is exceeded does clinical pneumonia become manifest. In that situation, the alveolar macrophages initiate the inflammatory response to bolster lower respiratory tract defenses. The host inflammatory response, rather than the proliferation of microorganisms, triggers the clinical syndrome of pneumonia. The release of inflammatory mediators, such as interleukin (IL) 1 and tumor necrosis factor (TNF), results in fever. Chemokines, such as IL-8 and granulocyte colony-stimulating factor, stimulate the release of neutrophils and their attraction to the lung, producing both peripheral leukocytosis and increased purulent secretions. Inflammatory mediators released by macrophages and the newly recruited neutrophils create an alveolar capillary leak equivalent to that seen in the acute respiratory distress syndrome (ARDS), although in pneumonia this leak is localized (at least initially). Even erythrocytes can cross the alveolar-capillary membrane, with consequent hemoptysis. The capillary leak results in a radiographic infiltrate and rales detectable on auscultation, and hypoxemia results from alveolar filling. Moreover, some bacterial pathogens appear to interfere with the hypoxic vasoconstriction that would normally occur with fluid-filled alveoli, and this interference can result in severe hypoxemia. Increased respiratory drive in the systemic inflammatory response syndrome (SIRS) leads to respiratory alkalosis. Decreased compliance due to capillary leak, hypoxemia, increased respiratory drive, increased secretions, and, occasionally, infection-related bronchospasm all lead to dyspnea. If severe enough, the changes in lung mechanics secondary to reductions in lung volume and compliance and the intrapulmonary shunting of blood may cause the patient's death.

PATHOLOGY

Classic pneumonia evolves through a series of pathologic changes. The initial phase is one of *edema*, with the presence of a proteinaceous exudate—and often of bacteria—in the alveoli. This phase is rarely evident in clinical or autopsy specimens because it is so rapidly followed by a *red hepatization* phase. The presence of erythrocytes in the cellular intraalveolar exudate gives this second stage its name, but neutrophils are also present and are important from the standpoint of host defense. Bacteria are occasionally seen in cultures of alveolar specimens collected during this phase. In the third phase, *gray hepatization*, no new erythrocytes are extravasating, and those already present have been lysed and degraded. The neutrophil is the predominant cell, fibrin deposition is abundant, and bacteria have disappeared. This phase corresponds with successful containment of the infection and improvement in gas exchange. In the final phase, *resolution*, the macrophage is the dominant cell type in the alveolar space, and the debris of neutrophils, bacteria, and fibrin has been cleared, as has the inflammatory response.

This pattern has been described best for pneumococcal pneumonia and may not apply to pneumonias of all etiologies, especially viral or *Pneumocystis* pneumonia. In VAP, respiratory bronchiolitis may precede the development of a radiologically apparent infiltrate. Because of the microaspiration mechanism, a bronchopneumonia pattern is most common in nosocomial pneumonias, whereas a lobar pattern is more common in bacterial CAP. Despite the radiographic appearance, viral and *Pneumocystis* pneumonias represent alveolar rather than interstitial processes.

COMMUNITY-ACQUIRED PNEUMONIA

ETIOLOGY

The extensive list of potential etiologic agents in CAP includes bacteria, fungi, viruses, and protozoa. Newly identified pathogens include hantaviruses, metapneumoviruses,

TABLE 17-2

MICROBIAL CAUSES OF COMMUNITY-ACQUIRED PNEUMONIA, BY SITE OF CARE

	HOSPITALIZED PATIENTS	
OUTPATIENTS	**NON-ICU**	**ICU**
Streptococcus pneumoniae	*S. pneumoniae*	*S. pneumoniae*
Mycoplasma pneumoniae	*M. pneumoniae*	*Staphylococcus aureus*
Haemophilus influenzae	*Chlamydophila pneumoniae*	*Legionella* spp.
C. pneumoniae	*H. influenzae*	Gram-negative bacilli
Respiratory viruses[a]	*Legionella* spp.	*H. influenzae*
	Respiratory viruses[a]	

[a]Influenza A and B viruses, adenoviruses, respiratory syncytial viruses, parainfluenza viruses.

Note: Pathogens are listed in descending order of frequency. ICU, intensive care unit.

the coronavirus responsible for the severe acute respiratory syndrome (SARS), and community-acquired strains of methicillin-resistant *Staphylococcus aureus* (MRSA). Most cases of CAP, however, are caused by relatively few pathogens (Table 17-2). Although *Streptococcus pneumoniae* is most common, other organisms must also be considered in light of the patient's risk factors and severity of illness. In most cases, it is most useful to think of the potential causes as either "typical" bacterial pathogens or "atypical" organisms. The former category includes *S. pneumoniae, Haemophilus influenzae*, and (in selected patients) *S. aureus* and gram-negative bacilli such as *Klebsiella pneumoniae* and *Pseudomonas aeruginosa*. The "atypical" organisms include *Mycoplasma pneumoniae, Chlamydophila pneumoniae*, and *Legionella* spp. as well as respiratory viruses such as influenza viruses, adenoviruses, and respiratory syncytial viruses (RSVs). Data suggest that a virus may be responsible in up to 18% of cases of CAP that require admission to the hospital. The atypical organisms cannot be cultured on standard media, nor can they be seen on Gram's stain. The frequency and importance of atypical pathogens such as *M. pneumoniae* and *C. pneumoniae* in outpatients and *Legionella* in inpatients have significant implications for therapy. These organisms are intrinsically resistant to all β-lactam agents and must be treated with a macrolide, a fluoroquinolone, or a tetracycline. In ~10–15% of CAP cases that are polymicrobial, the etiology often includes a combination of typical and atypical pathogens.

Anaerobes play a significant role only when an episode of aspiration has occurred days to weeks before presentation for pneumonia. The combination of an unprotected airway (e.g., in patients with alcohol or drug overdose or a seizure disorder) and significant gingivitis constitutes the major risk factor. Anaerobic pneumonias are often complicated by abscess formation and significant empyemas or parapneumonic effusions.

S. aureus pneumonia is well known to complicate influenza infection. Recently, however, MRSA strains have been reported as primary causes of CAP. Although this entity is still relatively uncommon, clinicians must be aware of its potentially serious consequences, such as necrotizing pneumonia. Two important developments have led to this problem: the spread of MRSA from the hospital setting to the community and the emergence of genetically distinct strains of MRSA in the community. These novel community-acquired MRSA (CA-MRSA) strains have infected healthy individuals who have had no association with health care.

Unfortunately, despite a careful history and physical examination, as well as routine radiographic studies, it is usually impossible to predict the pathogen in a case of CAP with any degree of certainty; in more than half of cases, a specific etiology is never determined. Nevertheless, it is important to consider epidemiologic and risk factors that might suggest certain pathogens (Table 17-3).

TABLE 17-3

EPIDEMIOLOGIC FACTORS SUGGESTING POSSIBLE CAUSES OF COMMUNITY-ACQUIRED PNEUMONIA

FACTOR	POSSIBLE PATHOGEN(S)
Alcoholism	*Streptococcus pneumoniae*, oral anaerobes, *Klebsiella pneumoniae, Acinetobacter* spp., *Mycobacterium tuberculosis*
COPD and/or smoking	*Haemophilus influenzae, Pseudomonas aeruginosa, Legionella* spp., *S. pneumoniae, Moraxella catarrhalis, Chlamydophila pneumoniae*
Structural lung disease (e.g., bronchiectasis)	*P. aeruginosa, Burkholderia cepacia, Staphylococcus aureus*
Dementia, stroke, decreased level of consciousness	Oral anaerobes, gram-negative enteric bacteria
Lung abscess	CA-MRSA, oral anaerobes, endemic fungi, *M. tuberculosis*, atypical mycobacteria
Travel to Ohio or St. Lawrence river valleys	*Histoplasma capsulatum*
Travel to southwestern United States	Hantavirus, *Coccidioides* spp.
Travel to Southeast Asia	*Burkholderia pseudomallei*, avian influenza virus
Stay in hotel or on cruise ship in previous 2 weeks	*Legionella* spp.
Local influenza activity	Influenza virus, *S. pneumoniae, S. aureus*
Exposure to bats or birds	*H. capsulatum*
Exposure to birds	*Chlamydophila psittaci*
Exposure to rabbits	*Francisella tularensis*
Exposure to sheep, goats, parturient cats	*Coxiella burnetii*

Note: CA-MRSA, community-acquired methicillin-resistant *Staphylococcus aureus*; COPD, chronic obstructive pulmonary disease.

EPIDEMIOLOGY

In the United States, ~80% of the 4 million CAP cases that occur annually are treated on an outpatient basis, and ~20% are treated in the hospital. CAP results in more than 600,000 hospitalizations, 64 million days of restricted activity, and 45,000 deaths annually. The overall yearly cost associated with CAP is estimated at $9–10 billion (U.S.). The incidence rates are highest at the extremes of age. Although the overall annual figure in the United States is 12 cases per 1000 persons, the figure is 12–18 per 1000 among children <4 years of age and 20 per 1000 among persons >60 years of age.

The risk factors for CAP in general and for pneumococcal pneumonia in particular have implications for treatment regimens. Risk factors for CAP include alcoholism, asthma, immunosuppression, institutionalization, and an age of ≥70 years versus 60–69 years. Risk factors for pneumococcal pneumonia include dementia, seizure disorders, heart failure, cerebrovascular disease, alcoholism, tobacco smoking, chronic obstructive pulmonary disease, and HIV infection. CA-MRSA infection is more likely in Native Americans, homeless youths, men who have sex with men, prison inmates, military recruits, children in day-care centers, and athletes such as wrestlers. The Enterobacteriaceae tend to affect patients who have recently been hospitalized and/or received antibiotic therapy or who have comorbidities such as alcoholism, heart failure, or renal failure. *P. aeruginosa* may also infect these patients as well as those with severe structural lung disease. Risk factors for *Legionella* infection include diabetes, hematologic malignancy, cancer, severe renal disease, HIV infection, smoking, male gender, and a recent hotel stay or ship cruise. (Many of these risk factors would now reclassify as HCAP some cases that were previously designated CAP.)

CLINICAL MANIFESTATIONS

CAP can vary from indolent to fulminant in presentation and from mild to fatal in severity. The various signs and symptoms, which depend on the progression and severity of the infection, include both constitutional findings and manifestations limited to the lung and its associated structures. In light of the pathobiology of the disease, many of the findings are to be expected.

The patient is frequently febrile, with a tachycardic response, and may have chills and/or sweats and cough that is either nonproductive or productive of mucoid, purulent, or blood-tinged sputum. In accordance with the severity of infection, the patient may be able to speak in full sentences or may be very short of breath. If the pleura is involved, the patient may experience pleuritic chest pain. Up to 20% of patients may have gastrointestinal symptoms such as nausea, vomiting, and/or diarrhea. Other symptoms may include fatigue, headache, myalgias, and arthralgias.

Findings on physical examination vary with the degree of pulmonary consolidation and the presence or absence of a significant pleural effusion. An increased respiratory rate and use of accessory muscles of respiration are common. Palpation may reveal increased or decreased tactile fremitus, and the percussion note can vary from dull to flat, reflecting underlying consolidated lung and pleural fluid, respectively. Crackles, bronchial breath sounds, and possibly a pleural friction rub may be heard on auscultation. The clinical presentation may not be so obvious in the elderly, who may initially display new-onset or worsening confusion and few other manifestations. Severely ill patients who have septic shock secondary to CAP are hypotensive and may have evidence of organ failure.

DIAGNOSIS

When confronted with possible CAP, the physician must ask two questions: Is this pneumonia, and, if so, what is the etiology? The former question is typically answered by clinical and radiographic methods, whereas the latter requires the aid of laboratory techniques.

Clinical Diagnosis

The differential diagnosis includes both infectious and noninfectious entities such as acute bronchitis, acute exacerbations of chronic bronchitis, heart failure, pulmonary embolism, and radiation pneumonitis. The importance of a careful history cannot be overemphasized. For example, known cardiac disease may suggest worsening pulmonary edema, whereas underlying carcinoma may suggest lung injury secondary to radiation. Epidemiologic clues, such as recent travel to areas with known endemic pathogens, may alert the physician to specific possibilities (Table 17-3).

Unfortunately, the sensitivity and specificity of the findings on physical examination are less than ideal, averaging 58% and 67%, respectively. Therefore, chest radiography is often necessary to help differentiate CAP from other conditions. Radiographic findings serve as a baseline and may include risk factors for increased severity (e.g., cavitation or multilobar involvement). Occasionally, radiographic results suggest an etiologic diagnosis. For example, pneumatoceles suggest infection with *S. aureus*, and an upper-lobe cavitating lesion suggests tuberculosis. CT is rarely necessary but may be of value in a patient with suspected postobstructive pneumonia caused by a tumor or foreign body. For cases managed on an outpatient basis, the clinical and radiologic assessment is usually all that is done before treatment is started since most laboratory test results are not available soon enough to influence initial management. In certain cases, however (e.g., influenza virus infection), the availability of rapid point-of-care diagnostic tests and access to specific drugs for treatment and prevention can be very important.

Etiologic Diagnosis

The etiology of pneumonia usually cannot be determined on the basis of clinical presentation; instead, the physician must rely upon the laboratory for support. Except for the 2% of CAP patients who are admitted to the intensive care unit (ICU), no data exist to show that treatment directed at a specific pathogen is statistically superior to empirical therapy. The benefits of establishing a microbial etiology can therefore be questioned, particularly in light of the cost of diagnostic testing. However, a number of reasons can be advanced for attempting an etiologic diagnosis. Identification of an unexpected pathogen allows narrowing of the initial empirical regimen, which decreases antibiotic selection pressure and may lessen the risk of resistance. Pathogens with important public safety implications, such as *Mycobacterium tuberculosis* and influenza virus, may be found in some cases. Finally, without culture and susceptibility data, trends in resistance cannot be followed accurately, and appropriate empirical therapeutic regimens are harder to devise.

Gram's Stain and Culture of Sputum

The main purpose of the sputum Gram's stain is to ensure that a sample is suitable for culture. However, Gram's staining may also help to identify certain pathogens (e.g., *S. pneumoniae*, *S. aureus*, and gram-negative bacteria) by their characteristic appearance. To be adequate for culture, a sputum sample must have >25 neutrophils and <10 squamous epithelial cells per low-power field. The sensitivity and specificity of the sputum Gram's stain and culture are highly variable; even in cases of proven bacteremic pneumococcal pneumonia, the yield of positive cultures from sputum samples is ≤50%.

Some patients, particularly elderly individuals, may not be able to produce an appropriate expectorated sputum sample. Others may already have started a course of antibiotics, which can interfere with results, at the time a sample is obtained. The inability to produce sputum can be a consequence of dehydration, and the correction of this condition may result in increased sputum production and a more obvious infiltrate on chest radiography. For patients admitted to the ICU and intubated, a deep-suction aspirate or bronchoalveolar lavage sample should be sent to the microbiology laboratory as soon as possible. Since the etiologies in severe CAP are somewhat different from those in milder disease (Table 17-2), the greatest benefit of staining and culturing respiratory secretions is to alert the physician of unsuspected and/or resistant pathogens and to permit appropriate modification of therapy. Other stains and cultures may be useful as well. For suspected tuberculosis or fungal infection, specific stains are available. Cultures of pleural fluid obtained from effusions >1 cm in height on a lateral decubitus chest radiograph may also be helpful.

Blood Cultures

The yield from blood cultures, even those obtained before antibiotic therapy, is disappointingly low. Only ~5–14% of cultures of blood from patients hospitalized with CAP are positive, and the most frequently isolated pathogen is *S. pneumoniae*. Since recommended empirical regimens all provide pneumococcal coverage, a blood culture positive for this pathogen has little, if any, effect on clinical outcome. However, susceptibility data may allow a switch from a broader-spectrum regimen (e.g., a fluoroquinolone or β-lactam plus a macrolide) to penicillin in appropriate cases. Because of the low yield and the lack of significant impact on outcome, blood cultures are no longer considered *de rigueur* for all hospitalized CAP patients. Certain high-risk patients—including those with neutropenia secondary to pneumonia, asplenia, or complement deficiencies; chronic liver disease; or severe CAP—should have blood cultured.

Antigen Tests

Two commercially available tests detect pneumococcal and certain *Legionella* antigens in urine. The test for *Legionella pneumophila* detects only serogroup 1, but this serogroup accounts for most community-acquired cases of Legionnaires' disease. The sensitivity and specificity of the *Legionella* urine antigen test are as high as 90% and 99%, respectively. The pneumococcal urine antigen test is also quite sensitive and specific (80% and >90%, respectively). Although false-positive results can be obtained with samples from colonized children, the test is generally reliable. Both tests can detect antigen even after the initiation of appropriate antibiotic therapy and after weeks of illness. Other antigen tests include a rapid test for influenza virus and direct fluorescent antibody tests for influenza virus and RSV, although the test for RSV is only poorly sensitive.

Polymerase Chain Reaction

Polymerase chain reaction (PCR) tests are available for a number of pathogens, including *L. pneumophila* and mycobacteria. In addition, a multiplex PCR can detect the nucleic acid of *Legionella* spp., *M. pneumoniae*, and *C. pneumoniae*. However, the use of these PCR assays is generally limited to research studies.

Serology

A fourfold rise in specific IgM antibody titer between acute- and convalescent-phase serum samples is generally considered diagnostic of infection with the pathogen in question. In the past, serologic tests were used to help identify atypical pathogens, as well as some typical but relatively unusual organisms, such as *Coxiella burnetii*. Recently, however, they have fallen out of favor because of the time required to obtain a final result for the convalescent-phase sample.

℞ Treatment: COMMUNITY-ACQUIRED PNEUMONIA

SITE OF CARE The decision to hospitalize a patient with CAP must take into consideration diminishing health care resources and rising costs of treatment. The cost of inpatient management exceeds that of outpatient treatment by a factor of 20 and accounts for most CAP-related expenditures. Certain patients clearly can be managed at home, and others clearly require treatment in the hospital, but the choice is sometimes difficult. Tools that objectively assess the risk of adverse outcomes, including severe illness and death, may minimize unnecessary hospital admissions and help to identify patients who will benefit from hospital care. There are currently two sets of criteria: the Pneumonia Severity Index (PSI), a prognostic model used to identify patients at low risk of dying; and the CURB-65 criteria, a severity-of-illness score.

To determine the PSI, points are given for 20 variables, including age, coexisting illness, and abnormal physical and laboratory findings. On the basis of the resulting score, patients are assigned to one of five classes, with the following mortality rates: class 1, 0.1%; class 2, 0.6%; class 3, 2.8%; class 4, 8.2%; and class 5, 29.2%. Clinical trials have demonstrated that routine use of the PSI results in lower admission rates for class 1 and class 2 patients. Patients in classes 4 and 5 should be admitted to the hospital, whereas those in class 3 should ideally be admitted to an observation unit until a further decision can be made.

The CURB-65 criteria include five variables: confusion (C); urea >7 mmol/L (U); respiratory rate ≥30/min (R); blood pressure, systolic ≤90 mmHg or diastolic ≤60 mmHg (B); and age ≥65 years (65). Patients with a score of 0, among whom the 30-day mortality rate is 1.5%, can be treated outside the hospital. With a score of 2, the 30-day mortality rate is 9.2%, and patients should be admitted to the hospital. Among patients with scores of ≥3, mortality rates are 22% overall; these patients may require admission to an ICU.

At present, it is difficult to say which assessment tool is superior. The PSI is less practical in a busy emergency-room setting because of the need to assess 20 variables. Although the CURB-65 criteria are easily remembered, they have not been studied as extensively. Whichever system is used, these objective criteria must always be tempered by careful consideration of factors relevant to individual patients, including the ability to comply reliably with an oral antibiotic regimen and the resources available to the patient outside the hospital.

RESISTANCE Antimicrobial resistance is a significant problem that threatens to diminish our therapeutic armamentarium. Misuse of antibiotics results in increased antibiotic selection pressure that can affect resistance locally or even globally by clonal dissemination. For CAP, the main resistance issues currently involve *S. pneumoniae* and CA-MRSA.

S. Pneumoniae In general, pneumococcal resistance is acquired (1) by direct DNA incorporation and remodeling resulting from contact with closely related oral commensal bacteria, (2) by the process of natural transformation, or (3) by mutation of certain genes.

Pneumococcal strains are classified as sensitive to penicillin if the minimal inhibitory concentration (MIC) is ≤0.06 μg/mL, as intermediate if the MIC is 0.1–1.0 μg/mL, and as resistant if the MIC is ≥2 μg/mL. Strains resistant to drugs from three or more antimicrobial classes with different mechanisms of action are considered MDR isolates. Pneumococcal resistance to β-lactam drugs is due solely to the presence of low-affinity penicillin-binding proteins. The propensity for pneumococcal resistance to penicillin to be associated with reduced susceptibility to other drugs, such as macrolides, tetracyclines, and trimethoprim-sulfamethoxazole (TMP-SMX), is of concern. In the United States, 58.9% of penicillin-resistant pneumococcal isolates from blood cultures are also resistant to macrolides. Penicillin is an appropriate agent for the treatment of pneumococcal infection caused by strains with MICs of ≤1 μg/mL. For infections caused by pneumococcal strains with penicillin MICs of 2–4 μg/mL, the data are conflicting; some studies suggest no increase in treatment failure with penicillin, whereas others suggest increased rates of death or complications. For strains of *S. pneumoniae* with intermediate levels of resistance, higher doses of the drug should be used. Risk factors for drug-resistant pneumococcal infection include recent antimicrobial therapy, an age of <2 years or >65 years, attendance at day-care centers, recent hospitalization, and HIV infection. Fortunately, resistance to penicillin appears to be reaching a plateau.

In contrast, resistance to macrolides is increasing through several mechanisms, including target-site modification and the presence of an efflux pump. Target-site modification is caused by ribosomal methylation in 23S rRNA encoded by the *ermB* gene and results in resistance to macrolides, lincosamides, and streptogramin B–type antibiotics. This *MLSB phenotype* is associated with high-level resistance, with typical MICs of ≥64 μg/mL. The efflux mechanism encoded by the *mef* gene (*M phenotype*) is usually associated with low-level resistance (MICs, 1–32 μg/mL). These two mechanisms account for ~45% and ~65%, respectively, of resistant pneumococcal isolates in the United States. Some pneumococcal isolates with both the *erm* and *mef* genes have been identified, but the exact significance of this finding is unknown. High-level resistance to macrolides is more common in Europe, whereas lower-level resistance seems to predominate in North America. Although clinical failures with macrolides have been reported, many experts think that these drugs still have a role to play in the management of pneumococcal pneumonia in North America.

Pneumococcal resistance to fluoroquinolones (e.g., ciprofloxacin and levofloxacin) has been reported. Changes can occur in one or both target sites (topoisomerases II and IV); changes in these two sites usually result from mutations in the *gyrA* and *parC* genes, respectively. The increasing number of pneumococcal isolates that, although susceptible to fluoroquinolones, already have a mutation in one target site is of concern. Such organisms may be more likely to undergo a second step mutation that will render them fully resistant to fluoroquinolones. In addition, an efflux pump may play a role in pneumococcal resistance to fluoroquinolones.

CA-MRSA CAP due to MRSA may be caused by infection with the classic hospital-acquired strains or with the more recently identified, genotypically and phenotypically distinct community-acquired strains. Most infections with the former strains have been acquired either directly or indirectly by contact with the health care environment and, although classified as HAP in the past, would now be classified as HCAP. In some hospitals, CA-MRSA strains are displacing the classic hospital-acquired strains—a trend suggesting that the newer strains may be more robust.

Methicillin resistance in *S. aureus* is determined by the *mecA* gene, which encodes for resistance to all β-lactam drugs. At least five *staphylococcal chromosomal cassette* mec (SCCmec) types have been described. The typical hospital-acquired strain usually has type II or III, whereas CA-MRSA has a type IV SCC*mec* element. CA-MRSA isolates tend to be less resistant than the older hospital-acquired strains and are often susceptible to TMP-SMX, clindamycin, and tetracycline in addition to vancomycin and linezolid. However, CA-MRSA strains may also carry genes for superantigens, such as enterotoxins B and C and Panton-Valentine leukocidin, a membrane-tropic toxin that can create cytolytic pores in polymorphonuclear neutrophils, monocytes, and macrophages.

Gram-Negative Bacilli A detailed discussion of resistance among gram-negative bacilli is beyond the scope of this chapter (see Chap. 51). Fluoroquinolone resistance among isolates of *Escherichia coli* from the community appears to be increasing. *Enterobacter* spp. are typically resistant to cephalosporins; the drugs of choice for use against these bacteria are usually fluoroquinolones or carbapenems. Similarly, when infections due to bacteria producing extended-spectrum β-lactamases (ESBLs) are documented or suspected, a fluoroquinolone or a carbapenem should be used; these MDR strains are more likely to be involved in HCAP.

INITIAL ANTIBIOTIC MANAGEMENT Since the physician rarely knows the etiology of CAP at the outset of treatment, initial therapy is usually empirical and is designed to cover the most likely pathogens (Table 17-4). In all cases, antibiotic treatment should be initiated as expeditiously as possible.

The CAP treatment guidelines in the United States (summarized in Table 17-4) represent joint statements from the Infectious Diseases Society of America (IDSA) and the American Thoracic Society (ATS); the Canadian guidelines come from the Canadian Infectious Disease Society and the Canadian Thoracic Society. In these guidelines, coverage is always provided for the pneumococcus and the atypical pathogens. In contrast, guidelines from some European countries do not always include atypical coverage based on local epidemiologic data. The U.S.-Canadian approach is supported by retrospective data from almost 13,000 patients >65 years of age. Atypical pathogen coverage provided by a macrolide or a fluoroquinolone has been associated with a significant reduction in mortality rates compared with those for β-lactam coverage alone.

Therapy with a macrolide or a fluoroquinolone within the previous 3 months is associated with an increased likelihood of infection with a macrolide- or fluoroquinolone-resistant strain of *S. pneumoniae*. For this reason, a fluoroquinolone-based regimen should be used for patients recently given a macrolide, and vice versa (Table 17-4). Telithromycin, a ketolide derived from the macrolide class, differs from the macrolides in that it binds to bacteria more avidly and at two sites rather than one. This drug is active against pneumococci resistant to penicillins, macrolides, and fluoroquinolones. Its future role in the outpatient management of CAP will depend on the evaluation of its safety by the U.S. Food and Drug Administration.

TABLE 17-4

EMPIRICAL ANTIBIOTIC TREATMENT OF COMMUNITY-ACQUIRED PNEUMONIA

Outpatients

Previously healthy and no antibiotics in past 3 months

- A macrolide [clarithromycin (500 mg PO bid) or azithromycin (500 mg PO once, then 250 mg od)] ***or***
- Doxycycline (100 mg PO bid)

Comorbidities or antibiotics in past 3 months: select an alternative from a different class

- A respiratory fluoroquinolone [moxifloxacin (400 mg PO od), gemifloxacin (320 mg PO od), levofloxacin (750 mg PO od)] ***or***
- A β-lactam [preferred: high-dose amoxicillin (1 g tid) or amoxicillin/clavulanate (2 g bid); alternatives: ceftriaxone (1–2 g IV od), cefpodoxime (200 mg PO bid), cefuroxime (500 mg PO bid)] *plus* a macrolide[a]

In regions with a high rate of "high-level" pneumococcal macrolide resistance,[b] consider alternatives listed above for patients with comorbidities.

Inpatients, non-ICU

- A respiratory fluoroquinolone [moxifloxacin (400 mg PO or IV od), gemifloxacin (320 mg PO od), levofloxacin (750 mg PO or IV od)]
- A β-lactam[c] [cefotaxime (1–2 g IV q8h), ceftriaxone (1–2 g IV od), ampicillin (1–2 g IV q4–6h), ertapenem (1 g IV od in selected patients)] ***plus*** a macrolide[d] [oral clarithromycin or azithromycin (as listed above for previously healthy patients) or IV azithromycin (1 g once, then 500 mg od)]

Inpatients, ICU

- A β-lactam[e] [cefotaxime (1–2 g IV q8h), ceftriaxone (2 g IV od), ampicillin-sulbactam (2 g IV q8h)] ***plus***
- Azithromycin or a fluoroquinolone (as listed above for inpatients, non-ICU)

Special concerns

If *Pseudomonas* is a consideration

- An antipneumococcal, antipseudomonal β-lactam [piperacillin/tazobactam (4.5 g IV q6h), cefepime (1–2 g IV q12h), imipenem (500 mg IV q6h), meropenem (1 g IV q8h)] *plus* either ciprofloxacin (400 mg IV q12h) or levofloxacin (750 mg IV od)
- The above β-lactams *plus* an aminoglycoside [amikacin (15 mg/kg od) or tobramycin (1.7 mg/kg od) and azithromycin]
- The above β-lactams[f] *plus* an aminoglycoside *plus* an antipneumococcal fluoroquinolone

If CA-MRSA is a consideration

- Add linezolid (600 mg IV q12h) or vancomycin (1 g IV q12h)

Note: CA-MRSA, community-acquired methicillin-resistant *Staphylococcus aureus*; ICU, intensive care unit.

[a]Doxycycline (100 mg PO bid) is an alternative to the macrolide.

[b]Minimal inhibitory concentrations of >16 μg/mL in 25% of isolates.

[c]A respiratory fluoroquinolone should be used for penicillin-allergic patients.

[d]Doxycycline (100 mg IV q12h) is an alternative to the macrolide.

[e]For penicillin-allergic patients, use a respiratory fluoroquinolone and aztreonam (2 g IV q8h).

[f]For penicillin-allergic patients, substitute aztreonam.

Once the etiologic agent(s) and susceptibilities are known, therapy may be altered to target the specific pathogen(s). However, this decision is not always straightforward. If blood cultures yield *S. pneumoniae* sensitive to penicillin after 2 days of treatment with a macrolide plus a β-lactam or a fluoroquinolone, should therapy be switched to penicillin? Penicillin alone would not be effective in the potential 15% of cases with atypical co-infection. No standard approach exists. Some experts would argue that pneumococcal coverage by a switch to penicillin is appropriate, whereas others would opt for continued coverage of both the pneumococcus and atypical pathogens. One compromise would be to continue atypical coverage with either a macrolide or a fluoroquinolone for a few more days and then to complete the treatment course with penicillin alone. In all cases, the individual patient and the various risk factors must be considered.

Management of bacteremic pneumococcal pneumonia is also controversial. Data from nonrandomized studies suggest that combination therapy (e.g., with a macrolide and a β-lactam) is associated with a lower mortality rate than monotherapy, particularly in severely ill patients. The exact reason is unknown, but explanations include possible atypical co-infection or the immunomodulatory effects of the macrolides.

For patients with CAP who are admitted to the ICU, the risk of infection with *P. aeruginosa* or CA-MRSA is increased, and coverage should be considered when a patient has risk factors or a Gram's stain suggestive of these pathogens (Table 17-4). The main risk factors for *P. aeruginosa* infection are structural lung disease (e.g., bronchiectasis) and recent treatment with antibiotics or glucocorticoids. If CA-MRSA infection is suspected, either linezolid or vancomycin should be added to the initial empirical regimen.

Although hospitalized patients have traditionally received initial therapy by the IV route, some drugs—particularly the fluoroquinolones—are very well absorbed and can be given orally from the outset to select patients. For patients initially treated IV, a switch to oral treatment is appropriate as long as the patient can ingest and absorb the drugs, is hemodynamically stable, and is showing clinical improvement.

The duration of treatment for CAP has recently generated considerable interest. Patients have usually been treated for 10–14 days, but recent studies with fluoroquinolones and telithromycin suggest that a 5-day course is sufficient for otherwise uncomplicated CAP. A longer course is required for patients with bacteremia, metastatic infection, or infection with a particularly virulent pathogen, such as *P. aeruginosa* or CA-MRSA. Longer- term therapy should also be considered if initial treatment was ineffective and in most cases of severe CAP. Data from studies with azithromycin, which suggest 3–5 days of treatment for outpatient-managed CAP, cannot be extrapolated to other drugs because of the extremely long half-life of azithromycin.

Patients may be discharged from the hospital once they are clinically stable and have no active medical problems requiring ongoing hospital care. The site of residence after discharge (in a nursing home, at home with family, at home alone) is an important consideration, particularly for elderly patients.

GENERAL CONSIDERATIONS In addition to appropriate antimicrobial therapy, certain general considerations apply in dealing with either CAP or HAP. Adequate hydration, oxygen therapy for hypoxemia, and assisted ventilation when necessary are critical to the success of therapy. Patients with severe CAP who remain hypotensive despite fluid resuscitation may have adrenal insufficiency and may respond to glucocorticoid treatment. Immunomodulatory therapy in the form of drotrecogin alfa (activated) should be considered for CAP patients with persistent septic shock and Acute Physiology and Chronic Health Evaluation (APACHE) II scores of ≥25, particularly if the infection is caused by *S. pneumoniae*.

Failure to Improve Patients who are slow to respond to therapy should be reevaluated at about day 3 (sooner if their condition is worsening rather than simply not improving), and a number of possible scenarios should be considered. (1) Is this a noninfectious condition? (2) If this is an infection, is the correct pathogen being targeted? (3) Is this a superinfection with a new nosocomial pathogen? A number of noninfectious conditions can mimic pneumonia, including pulmonary edema, pulmonary embolism, lung carcinoma, radiation and hypersensitivity pneumonitis, and connective tissue disease involving the lungs. If the patient has CAP and treatment is aimed at the correct pathogen, the lack of response may be explained in a number of ways. The pathogen may be resistant to the drug selected, or a sequestered focus (e.g., a lung abscess or empyema) may be blocking access of the antibiotic(s) to the pathogen. Alternatively, the patient may be getting either the wrong drug or the correct drug at the wrong dose or frequency of administration. It is also possible that CAP is the correct diagnosis but that a different pathogen (e.g., *M. tuberculosis* or a fungus) is the cause. In addition, nosocomial superinfections—both pulmonary and extrapulmonary—are possible explanations for persistence. In all cases of delayed response or deteriorating condition, the patient must be carefully reassessed and appropriate studies initiated. These studies may include such diverse procedures as CT and bronchoscopy.

Complications As in other severe infections, common complications of severe CAP include respiratory failure, shock and multiorgan failure, bleeding diatheses, and exacerbation of comorbid illnesses. Three particularly noteworthy conditions are metastatic infection, lung abscess, and complicated pleural effusion. Metastatic infection (e.g., brain abscess or endocarditis), although unusual, deserves immediate attention by the physician, with a detailed workup and proper treatment. Lung abscess may occur in association with aspiration or with infection caused by a single CAP pathogen, such CA-MRSA,

P. aeruginosa, or (rarely) *S. pneumoniae*. Aspiration pneumonia is typically a mixed polymicrobial infection involving both aerobes and anaerobes. In either scenario, drainage should be established, and antibiotics that cover the known or suspected pathogens should be administered. A significant pleural effusion should be tapped for both diagnostic and therapeutic purposes. If the fluid has a pH of <7, a glucose level of <2.2 mmol/L, and a lactate dehydrogenase concentration of >1000 U/L or if bacteria are seen or cultured, then the fluid should be drained; a chest tube is usually required.

Follow-Up Fever and leukocytosis usually resolve within 2 and 4 days, respectively, in otherwise healthy patients with CAP, but physical findings may persist longer. Chest radiographic abnormalities are slowest to resolve and may require 4–12 weeks to clear, with the speed of clearance depending on the patient's age and underlying lung disease. For a patient whose condition is improving and who (if hospitalized) has been discharged, a follow-up radiograph can be done ~4–6 weeks later. If relapse or recurrence is documented, particularly in the same lung segment, the possibility of an underlying neoplasm must be considered.

PROGNOSIS

The prognosis of CAP depends on the patient's age, comorbidities, and site of treatment (inpatient or outpatient). Young patients without comorbidity do well and usually recover fully after ~2 weeks. Older patients and those with comorbid conditions can take several weeks longer to recover fully. The overall mortality rate for the outpatient group is <1%. For patients requiring hospitalization, the overall mortality rate is estimated at 10%, with ~50% of the deaths directly attributable to pneumonia.

PREVENTION

The main preventive measure is vaccination. The recommendations of the Advisory Committee on Immunization Practices should be followed for influenza and pneumococcal vaccines. In the event of an influenza outbreak, unprotected patients at risk from complications should be vaccinated immediately and given chemoprophylaxis with either oseltamivir or zanamivir for 2 weeks—i.e., until vaccine-induced antibody levels are sufficiently high. Because of an increased risk of pneumococcal infection, even among patients without obstructive lung disease, smokers should be strongly encouraged to stop smoking.

HEALTH CARE–ASSOCIATED PNEUMONIA

VENTILATOR-ASSOCIATED PNEUMONIA

Most research on VAP has focused on illness in the hospital setting (see also Chap. 13). However, the information and principles based on this research can be applied to HCAP not associated with ventilator use as well. The main rationale for the new designation *HCAP* is that the pathogens and treatment strategies for VAP are more similar to those for HAP than to those for pure CAP. The greatest difference between VAP and HCAP/HAP—and the greatest similarity of VAP to CAP—is the return to dependence on expectorated sputum for a microbiologic diagnosis, which is further complicated by the frequent colonization with pathogens among patients in the hospital or other health care–associated settings.

Etiology

Potential etiologic agents of VAP include both MDR and non-MDR bacterial pathogens (**Table 17-5**). The non-MDR group is nearly identical to the pathogens found in severe CAP (Table 17-2); it is not surprising that such pathogens predominate if VAP develops in the first 5–7 days of the hospital stay. However, if patients have other risk factors for HCAP, MDR pathogens are a consideration, even early in the hospital course. The relative frequency of individual MDR pathogens can vary significantly from hospital to hospital and even between different critical care units within the same institution. Many hospitals have problems with *P. aeruginosa* and MRSA, but other MDR pathogens are often institution-specific.

Less commonly, fungal and viral pathogens cause VAP, most frequently affecting severely immunocompromised patients. Rarely, community-associated viruses cause miniepidemics, usually when introduced by ill health care workers.

Epidemiology

Pneumonia is a common complication among patients requiring mechanical ventilation. Prevalence estimates vary between 6 and 52 cases per 100 patients, depending on the population studied. On any given day in the ICU,

TABLE 17-5

MICROBIOLOGIC CAUSES OF VENTILATOR-ASSOCIATED PNEUMONIA

NON-MDR PATHOGENS	MDR PATHOGENS
Streptococcus pneumoniae	*Pseudomonas aeruginosa*
Other *Streptococcus* spp.	MRSA
Haemophilus influenzae	*Acinetobacter* spp.
MSSA	Antibiotic-resistant Enterobacteriaceae
Antibiotic-sensitive Enterobacteriaceae	*Enterobacter* spp.
Escherichia coli	ESBL-positive strains
Klebsiella pneumoniae	*Klebsiella* spp.
Proteus spp.	*Legionella pneumophila*
Enterobacter spp.	*Burkholderia cepacia*
Serratia marcescens	*Aspergillus* spp.

Note: ESBL, extended-spectrum β-lactamase; MDR, multidrug-resistant; MRSA, methicillin-resistant *Staphylococcus aureus*; MSSA, methicillin-sensitive *S. aureus*.

an average of 10% of patients will have pneumonia—VAP in the overwhelming majority of cases. The frequency of diagnosis is not static but changes with the duration of mechanical ventilation, with the highest hazard ratio in the first 5 days and a plateau in additional cases (1% per day) after ~2 weeks. However, the cumulative rate among patients who remain ventilated for as long as 30 days is as high as 70%. These rates often do not reflect the recurrence of VAP in the same patient. Once a ventilated patient is transferred to a chronic care facility or to home, the incidence of pneumonia drops significantly, especially in the absence of other risk factors for pneumonia.

Three factors are critical in the pathogenesis of VAP: colonization of the oropharynx with pathogenic microorganisms, aspiration of these organisms from the oropharynx into the lower respiratory tract, and compromise of the normal host defense mechanisms. Most risk factors and their corresponding prevention strategies pertain to one of these three factors (Table 17-6).

The most obvious risk factor is the endotracheal tube (ET), which bypasses the normal mechanical factors preventing aspiration. Although the presence of an ET may prevent large-volume aspiration, microaspiration is actually enhanced by secretions pooling above the cuff. The ET and the concomitant need for suctioning can damage the tracheal mucosa, thereby facilitating tracheal colonization. In addition, pathogenic bacteria can form a glycocalyx biofilm on the ET surface that protects them from both antibiotics and host defenses. The bacteria can also be dislodged during suctioning and can reinoculate the trachea, or tiny fragments of glycocalyx can embolize to distal airways, carrying bacteria with them.

In a high percentage of critically ill patients, the normal oropharyngeal flora is replaced by pathogenic microorganisms. The most important risk factors are antibiotic selection pressure, cross-infection from other infected/colonized patients or contaminated equipment, and malnutrition.

How the lower respiratory tract defenses become overwhelmed remains poorly understood. Almost all intubated patients experience microaspiration and are at least transiently colonized with pathogenic bacteria. However, only around one-third of colonized patients develop VAP. Severely ill patients with sepsis and trauma appear to enter a state of immunoparalysis several days after admission to the ICU—a time that corresponds to the greatest risk of developing VAP. The mechanism of this immunosuppression is not clear, although several factors have been suggested. Hyperglycemia affects neutrophil function, and recent trials suggest that keeping the blood sugar close to normal with exogenous insulin may have beneficial effects, including a decreased risk of infection. More frequent transfusions, especially of leukocyte-depleted red blood cells, also affect the immune response positively.

TABLE 17-6

PATHOGENIC MECHANISMS AND CORRESPONDING PREVENTION STRATEGIES FOR VENTILATOR-ASSOCIATED PNEUMONIA

PATHOGENIC MECHANISM	PREVENTION STRATEGY
Oropharyngeal colonization with pathogenic bacteria	
Elimination of normal flora	Avoidance of prolonged antibiotic courses
Large-volume oropharyngeal aspiration around time of intubation	Short course of prophylactic antibiotics for comatose patients[a]
Gastroesophageal reflux	Postpyloric enteral feeding[b]; avoidance of high gastric residuals, prokinetic agents
Bacterial overgrowth of stomach	Avoidance of gastrointestinal bleeding due to prophylactic agents that raise gastric pH[b]; selective decontamination of digestive tract with nonabsorbable antibiotics[b]
Cross-infection from other colonized patients	Hand washing, especially with alcohol-based hand rub; intensive infection control education[a]; isolation; proper cleaning of reusable equipment
Large-volume aspiration	Endotracheal intubation; avoidance of sedation; decompression of small-bowel obstruction
Microaspiration around endotracheal tube	
Endotracheal intubation	Noninvasive ventilation[a]
Prolonged duration of ventilation	Daily awakening from sedation,[a] weaning protocols[a]
Abnormal swallowing function	Early percutaneous tracheostomy[a]
Secretions pooled above endotracheal tube	Head of bed elevated[a]; continuous aspiration of subglottic secretions with specialized endotracheal tube[a]; avoidance of reintubation; minimization of sedation and patient transport
Altered lower respiratory host defenses	Tight glycemic control[a]; lowering of hemoglobin transfusion threshold; specialized enteral feeding formula

[a]Strategies demonstrated to be effective in at least one randomized controlled trial.
[b]Strategies with negative randomized trials or conflicting results.

Clinical Manifestations

The clinical manifestations of VAP are generally the same as for all other forms of pneumonia: fever, leukocytosis, increase in respiratory secretions, and pulmonary consolidation on physical examination, along with a new or changing radiographic infiltrate. The frequency of abnormal chest radiographs before the onset of pneumonia in intubated patients and the limitations of portable radiographic technique make interpretation of radiographs more difficult than in patients who are not intubated. Other clinical features may include tachypnea, tachycardia, worsening oxygenation, and increased minute ventilation.

Diagnosis

No single set of criteria is reliably diagnostic of pneumonia in a ventilated patient. The inability to identify such patients compromises efforts to prevent and treat VAP and even calls into question estimates of the impact of VAP on mortality rates.

Application of clinical criteria consistently results in overdiagnosis of VAP, largely because of three common findings in at-risk patients: (1) tracheal colonization with pathogenic bacteria in patients with ETs, (2) multiple alternative causes of radiographic infiltrates in mechanically ventilated patients, and (3) the high frequency of other sources of fever in critically ill patients. The differential diagnosis of VAP includes a number of entities, such as atypical pulmonary edema, pulmonary contusion and/or hemorrhage, hypersensitivity pneumonitis, ARDS, and pulmonary embolism. Clinical findings in ventilated patients with fever and/or leukocytosis may have alternative causes, including antibiotic-associated diarrhea, sinusitis, urinary tract infection, pancreatitis, and drug fever. Conditions mimicking pneumonia are often documented in patients in whom VAP has been ruled out by accurate diagnostic techniques. Most of these alternative diagnoses do not require antibiotic treatment, require antibiotics different from those used to treat VAP, or require some additional intervention, such as surgical drainage or catheter removal, for optimal management.

This diagnostic dilemma has led to debate and controversy. The major question is whether a quantitative-culture approach as a means of eliminating false-positive clinical diagnoses is superior to the clinical approach enhanced by principles learned from quantitative-culture studies. The recent IDSA/ATS guidelines for HCAP suggest that either approach is clinically valid.

Quantitative-Culture Approach

The essence of the quantitative-culture approach is to discriminate between colonization and true infection by determining the bacterial burden. The more distal in the respiratory tree the diagnostic sampling, the more specific the results and therefore the lower the threshold of growth necessary to diagnose pneumonia and exclude colonization. For example, a quantitative endotracheal aspirate yields proximate samples, and the diagnostic threshold is 10^6 cfu/mL. The protected specimen brush method, in contrast, obtains distal samples and has a threshold of 10^3 cfu/mL. Conversely, sensitivity declines as more distal secretions are obtained, especially when they are collected blindly (i.e., by a technique other than bronchoscopy). Additional tests that may increase the diagnostic yield include Gram's stain, differential cell counts, staining for intracellular organisms, and detection of local protein levels elevated in response to infection.

Several studies have compared patient cohorts managed by the various quantitative-culture methods. Although these studies documented issues of relative sensitivity and specificity, outcomes were not significantly different for the various groups of patients. The IDSA/ATS guidelines have suggested that all these methods are appropriate and that the choice depends on availability and local expertise.

The Achilles heel of the quantitative approach is the effect of antibiotic therapy. With sensitive microorganisms, a single antibiotic dose can reduce colony counts below the diagnostic threshold. Recent changes in antibiotic therapy are the most significant. After ≥3 days of consistent antibiotic therapy for another infection before suspicion of pneumonia, the accuracy of diagnostic tests for pneumonia is unaffected. Conversely, colony counts above the diagnostic threshold during antibiotic therapy suggest that the current antibiotics are ineffective. Even the normal host response may be sufficient to reduce quantitative-culture counts below the diagnostic threshold by the time of sampling. In short, expertise in quantitative-culture techniques is critical, with a specimen obtained as soon as pneumonia is suspected and before antibiotic therapy is initiated or changed.

In a study comparing the quantitative with the clinical approach, use of bronchoscopic quantitative cultures resulted in significantly less antibiotic use at 14 days after study entry and lower rates of mortality and severity-adjusted mortality at 28 days. In addition, more alternative sites of infection were found in patients randomized to the quantitative-culture strategy. A critical aspect of this study was that antibiotic treatment was initiated only in patients whose gram-stained respiratory sample was positive or who displayed signs of hemodynamic instability. Fewer than half as many patients were treated for pneumonia in the bronchoscopy group, and only one-third as many microorganisms were cultured.

Clinical Approach

The lack of specificity of a clinical diagnosis of VAP has led to efforts to improve the diagnostic criteria. The Clinical Pulmonary Infection Score (CPIS) was developed by weighting of the various clinical criteria usually used for the diagnosis of VAP (Table 17-7). Use of the CPIS allows the selection of low-risk patients who may need only short-course antibiotic therapy or no treatment at all. Moreover, studies have demonstrated that the absence of bacteria in gram-stained endotracheal aspirates makes pneumonia an unlikely cause of fever or pulmonary infiltrates. These findings, coupled with a heightened awareness of the alternative diagnoses possible in patients with suspected VAP, can prevent inappropriate treatment for this disease. Furthermore, data show that the absence of an MDR pathogen in tracheal aspirate cultures eliminates the need for MDR coverage when empirical antibiotic therapy is narrowed. Since the most likely explanations for the mortality benefit of bronchoscopic quantitative cultures are decreased antibiotic selection pressure (which reduces the risk of subsequent infection with MDR pathogens) and identification

TABLE 17-7

CLINICAL PULMONARY INFECTION SCORE (CPIS)

CRITERION	SCORE
Fever (°C)	
≥38.5 but ≤38.9	1
>39 or <36	2
Leukocytosis	
<4000 or >11,000/μL	1
Bands >50%	1 (additional)
Oxygenation (mmHg)	
Pa_{O_2}/FI_{O_2} <250 and no ARDS	2
Chest radiograph	
Localized infiltrate	2
Patchy or diffuse infiltrate	1
Progression of infiltrate (no ARDS or CHF)	2
Tracheal aspirate	
Moderate or heavy growth	1
Same morphology on Gram's stain	1 (additional)
Maximal score[a]	12

[a]The progression of the infiltrate is not known and tracheal aspirate culture results are often unavailable at the time of the original diagnosis; thus the maximal score is initially 8–10.

Note: ARDS, acute respiratory distress syndrome; CHF, congestive heart failure.

of alternative sources of infection, a clinical diagnostic approach that incorporates such principles may result in similar outcomes.

℞ Treatment: VENTILATOR-ASSOCIATED PNEUMONIA

Many studies have demonstrated higher mortality rates with inappropriate than with appropriate empirical antibiotic therapy. The key to appropriate antibiotic management of VAP is an appreciation of the patterns of resistance of the most likely pathogens in any given patient.

RESISTANCE If it were not for the risk of infection with MDR pathogens (Table 17-1), VAP could be treated with the same antibiotics used for severe CAP. However, antibiotic selection pressure leads to the frequent involvement of MDR pathogens by selecting either for drug-resistant isolates of common pathogens (MRSA and ESBL-positive Enterobacteriaceae) or for intrinsically resistant pathogens (*P. aeruginosa* and *Acinetobacter* spp.). Frequent use of β-lactam drugs, especially cephalosporins, appears to be the major risk factor for infection with MRSA and ESBL-positive strains.

P. aeruginosa has demonstrated the ability to develop resistance to all routinely used antibiotics. Unfortunately, even if initially sensitive, *P. aeruginosa* isolates have also shown a propensity to develop resistance during treatment. Occasionally, derepression of resistance genes may be the cause of the selection of resistant clones within the large bacterial inoculum associated with most pneumonias. *Acinetobacter, Stenotrophomonas maltophilia*, and *Burkholderia cepacia* are intrinsically resistant to many of the empirical antibiotic regimens listed in Table 17-8. VAP caused by these pathogens emerges during treatment of other infections, and resistance is always evident at initial diagnosis.

EMPIRICAL THERAPY Recommended options for empirical therapy are listed in Table 17-8. Treatment should be started once diagnostic specimens have been obtained. The major factor in the selection of agents is the presence of risk factors for MDR pathogens. Choices among the various options listed depend on local patterns of resistance and the patient's prior antibiotic exposure.

The majority of patients *without* risk factors for MDR infection can be treated with a single agent. The major difference from CAP is the markedly lower incidence of atypical pathogens in VAP; the exception is *Legionella*, which can be a nosocomial pathogen, especially when there are deficiencies in the treatment of a hospital's potable water supply.

The standard recommendation for patients *with* risk factors for MDR infection is for three antibiotics: two directed at *P. aeruginosa* and one at MRSA. The choice of a β-lactam agent provides the greatest variability in coverage, yet the use of the broadest-spectrum agent—a carbapenem—still represents inappropriate initial therapy in 10–15% of cases.

TABLE 17-8

EMPIRICAL ANTIBIOTIC TREATMENT OF HEALTH CARE–ASSOCIATED PNEUMONIA

Patients without Risk Factors for MDR Pathogens

Ceftriaxone (2 g IV q24h) ***or***
Moxifloxacin (400 mg IV q24h), ciprofloxacin (400 mg IV q8h), or levofloxacin (750 mg IV q24h) ***or***
Ampicillin/sulbactam (3 g IV q6h) ***or***
Ertapenem (1 g IV q24h)

Patients with Risk Factors for MDR Pathogens

1. A β-lactam:
   Ceftazidime (2 g IV q8h) or cefepime (2 g IV q8–12h) ***or***
   Piperacillin/tazobactam (4.5 g IV q6h), imipenem (500 mg IV q6h or 1 g IV q8h), or meropenem (1 g IV q8h) ***plus***
2. A second agent active against gram-negative bacterial pathogens:
   Gentamicin or tobramycin (7 mg/kg IV q24h) or amikacin (20 mg/kg IV q24h) ***or***
   Ciprofloxacin (400 mg IV q8h) or levofloxacin (750 mg IV q24h) ***plus***
3. An agent active against gram-positive bacterial pathogens:
   Linezolid (600 mg IV q12h) ***or***
   Vancomycin (15 mg/kg, up to 1 g IV, q12h)

Note: MDR, multidrug-resistant.

SPECIFIC TREATMENT Once an etiologic diagnosis is made, broad-spectrum empirical therapy can be modified to address the known pathogen specifically. For patients with MDR risk factors, antibiotic regimens can be reduced to a single agent in more than half of cases and to a two-drug combination in more than one-quarter. Only a minority of cases require a complete course with three drugs. A negative tracheal-aspirate culture or growth below the threshold for quantitative cultures, especially if the sample was obtained before any antibiotic change, strongly suggests that antibiotics should be discontinued. Identification of other confirmed or suspected sites of infection may require ongoing antibiotic therapy, but the spectrum of pathogens (and the corresponding antibiotic choices) may be different from those for VAP. If the CPIS decreases over the first 3 days, antibiotics should be stopped after 8 days. An 8-day course of therapy is just as effective as a 2-week course and is associated with less frequent emergence of antibiotic-resistant strains.

The major controversy regarding specific therapy for VAP concerns the need for ongoing combination treatment of *Pseudomonas* infection. No randomized controlled trials have demonstrated a benefit of combination therapy with a β-lactam and an aminoglycoside, nor have subgroup analyses in other trials found a survival benefit with such a regimen. The unacceptably high rates of clinical failure and death for VAP caused by *P. aeruginosa* despite combination therapy (see "Failure to Improve," below) indicate that better regimens are needed—including, perhaps, aerosolized antibiotics.

VAP caused by MRSA is associated with a 40% clinical failure rate when treated with standard-dose vancomycin. One proposed solution is the use of high-dose individualized treatment, but the risk-to-benefit ratio of this approach is not known. Linezolid appears to be more efficacious than the standard dose of vancomycin, especially in patients with renal insufficiency.

FAILURE TO IMPROVE Treatment failure is not uncommon in VAP, especially in that caused by MDR pathogens. In addition to the 40% failure rate for MRSA infection treated with vancomycin, VAP due to *Pseudomonas* has a 50% failure rate, no matter what the regimen. The causes of clinical failure vary with the pathogen(s) and the antibiotic(s). Inappropriate therapy can usually be minimized by use of the recommended triple-drug regimen (Table 17-8). However, the emergence of β-lactam resistance during therapy is an important problem, especially in infection with *Pseudomonas* and *Enterobacter* spp. Recurrent VAP caused by the same pathogen is possible because the biofilm on ETs allows reintroduction of the microorganism. However, studies of VAP caused by *Pseudomonas* show that approximately half of recurrent cases are caused by a new strain. Inadequate local levels of vancomycin are the likely cause of treatment failure in VAP due to MRSA.

Treatment failure is very difficult to diagnose. Pneumonia due to a new superinfection, the presence of extrapulmonary infection, and drug toxicity must be considered in the differential diagnosis of treatment failure. Serial CPIS appears to track the clinical response accurately, whereas repeat quantitative cultures may clarify the microbiologic response. A persistently elevated or rising CPIS value by day 3 of therapy is likely to indicate failure. The most sensitive component of the CPIS is improvement in oxygenation.

COMPLICATIONS Apart from death, the major complication of VAP is prolongation of mechanical ventilation, with corresponding increases in length of stay in the ICU and in the hospital. In most studies, an additional week of mechanical ventilation because of VAP is common. The additional expense of this complication warrants costly and aggressive efforts at prevention.

In rare cases, some types of necrotizing pneumonia (e.g., that due to *P. aeruginosa*) result in significant pulmonary hemorrhage. More commonly, necrotizing infections result in the long-term complications of bronchiectasis and parenchymal scarring leading to recurrent pneumonias. The long-term complications of pneumonia are underappreciated. Pneumonia results in a catabolic state in a patient already nutritionally at risk. The muscle loss and general debilitation from an episode of VAP often require prolonged rehabilitation and, in the elderly, commonly result in an inability to return to independent function and the need for nursing home placement.

FOLLOW-UP Clinical improvement, if it occurs, is usually evident within 48–72 h of the initiation of antimicrobial treatment. Because findings on chest radiography often worsen initially during treatment, they are less helpful than clinical criteria as an indicator of clinical response in severe pneumonia. Although no hard and fast rules govern the frequency of follow-up chest radiography in seriously ill patients with pneumonia, assessment every few days in a responding patient seems appropriate. Once the patient has improved substantially and has stabilized, follow-up radiographs may not be necessary for a few weeks.

Prognosis

VAP is associated with significant mortality. Crude mortality rates of 50–70% have been reported, but the real issue is attributable mortality. Many patients with VAP have underlying diseases that would result in death even if VAP did not occur. Attributable mortality exceeded 25% in one matched-cohort study. Patients who develop VAP are at least twice as likely to die as those who do not. Some of the variability in reported figures is clearly related to the type of patient and ICU studied. VAP in trauma patients is not associated with attributable mortality, possibly because many of the patients were otherwise healthy before being injured. However, the causative pathogen also plays a major role. Generally, MDR pathogens are associated with significantly greater attributable mortality than non-MDR pathogens. Pneumonia caused by some pathogens (e.g., *S. maltophilia*) is simply a marker for a patient whose immune system is so compromised that death is almost inevitable.

Prevention

(Table 17-6) Because of the significance of the ET as a risk factor for VAP, the most important preventive intervention is to avoid endotracheal intubation or at least to minimize its duration. Successful use of noninvasive ventilation via a nasal or full-face mask avoids many of the problems associated with ETs. Strategies that minimize the duration of ventilation have also been highly effective in preventing VAP.

Unfortunately, a tradeoff in risks is sometimes required. Aggressive attempts to extubate early may result in reintubation(s), which pose a risk of VAP. Heavy continuous sedation increases the risk, but self-extubation because of too little sedation is also a risk. The tradeoff is probably best illustrated by antibiotic therapy. Short-course antibiotic prophylaxis can decrease the risk of VAP in comatose patients requiring intubation, and data suggest that antibiotics decrease VAP rates in general. However, the major benefit appears to be a decrease in the incidence of early-onset VAP, which is usually caused by the less pathogenic non-MDR microorganisms. Conversely, prolonged courses of antibiotics consistently increase the risk of VAP caused by the more lethal MDR pathogens. Despite its virulence and associated mortality, VAP caused by *Pseudomonas* is rare among patients who have not recently received antibiotics.

Minimizing the amount of microaspiration around the ET cuff is also a strategy for avoidance of VAP. Simply elevating the head of the bed (at least 30° above horizontal but preferably 45°) decreases VAP rates. Specially modified ETs that allow removal of the secretions pooled above the cuff may also prevent VAP. The risk-to-benefit ratio of transporting the patient outside the ICU for diagnostic tests or procedures should be carefully considered, since VAP rates are increased among transported patients.

Emphasis on the avoidance of agents that raise gastric pH and on oropharyngeal decontamination has been diminished by the equivocal and conflicting results of more recent clinical trials. The role in the pathogenesis of VAP that is played by the overgrowth of bacterial components of the bowel flora in the stomach has also been downplayed. MRSA and the nonfermenters *P. aeruginosa* and *Acinetobacter* spp. are not normally part of the bowel flora but reside primarily in the nose and on the skin, respectively. Therefore, an emphasis on controlling overgrowth of the bowel flora may be relevant only in certain populations, such as liver transplant recipients and patients who have undergone other major intraabdominal procedures or who have bowel obstruction.

In outbreaks of VAP due to specific pathogens, the possibility of a breakdown in infection control measures (particularly contamination of reusable equipment) should be investigated. Even high rates of pathogens that are already common in a particular ICU may be a result of cross-infection. Education and reminders of the need for consistent infection control practices can minimize this risk.

HOSPITAL-ACQUIRED PNEUMONIA

(See also Chap. 13) Although significantly less well studied than VAP, HAP in nonintubated patients, both inside and outside the ICU, is similar to VAP. The main differences are in the higher frequency of non-MDR pathogens and the better underlying host immunity in nonintubated patients. The lower frequency of MDR pathogens allows monotherapy in a larger proportion of cases of HAP than of VAP.

The only pathogens that may be more common in the non-VAP population are anaerobes. The greater risk of macroaspiration by nonintubated patients and the lower oxygen tensions in the lower respiratory tract of these patients increase the likelihood of a role for anaerobes. As in the management of CAP, specific therapy targeting anaerobes probably is not indicated unless gross aspiration is a concern.

Diagnosis is even more difficult for HAP in the nonintubated patient than for VAP. Lower respiratory tract samples appropriate for culture are considerably more difficult to obtain from nonintubated patients. Many of the underlying diseases that predispose a patient to HAP are also associated with an inability to cough adequately. Since blood cultures are infrequently positive (<15% of cases), the majority of patients with HAP do not have culture data on which antibiotic modifications can be based. Therefore, de-escalation of therapy is less likely in patients with risk factors for MDR pathogens. Despite these difficulties, the better host defenses in non-ICU patients result in lower mortality rates than are documented for VAP. In addition, the risk of antibiotic failure is lower in HAP.

FURTHER READINGS

AARTS MA et al: Empiric antibiotic therapy for suspected ventilator-associated pneumonia: A systematic review and meta-analysis of randomized trials. Crit Care Med 36:108, 2008

AMERICAN THORACIC SOCIETY/INFECTIOUS DISEASES SOCIETY OF AMERICA: Guidelines for the management of adults with hospital-acquired, ventilator-associated, and healthcare-associated pneumonia. Am J Respir Crit Care Med 171:388, 2005

CHASTRE J, FAGON JY: Ventilator-associated pneumonia. Am J Respir Crit Care Med 165:867, 2002

FAGON JY et al: Invasive and noninvasive strategies for management of suspected ventilator-associated pneumonia. A randomized trial. Ann Intern Med 132:621, 2000

FINE MJ et al: A prediction rule to identify low-risk patients with community-acquired pneumonia. N Engl J Med 336:243, 1997

KLOMPAS M: Does this patient have ventilator-associated pneumonia? JAMA 297:1583, 2007

LIM WS et al: Defining community acquired pneumonia severity on presentation to hospital: An international derivation and validation study. Thorax 58:377, 2003

MANDELL LA et al: Infectious Diseases Society of America/American Thoracic Society consensus guidelines on the management of community-acquired pneumonia in adults. Clin Infect Dis 44(Suppl 2): S27, 2007

SINGH N et al: Short-course empiric antibiotic therapy for patients with pulmonary infiltrates in the intensive care unit. A proposed solution for indiscriminate antibiotic prescription. Am J Respir Crit Care Med 162:505, 2000

VANDERKOOI OG et al: Predicting antimicrobial resistance in invasive pneumococcal infections. Clin Infect Dis 40:1288, 2005

CHAPTER 18

BRONCHIECTASIS AND LUNG ABSCESS

Gregory Tino ■ Steven E. Weinberger

BRONCHIECTASIS

DEFINITION

Bronchiectasis is an abnormal and permanent dilatation of bronchi. It may be either focal, involving airways supplying a limited region of pulmonary parenchyma, or diffuse, involving airways in a more widespread distribution. Recent studies have estimated there to be about 110,000 patients with bronchiectasis in the United States. It is a disorder that typically affects older individuals; approximately two-thirds of patients are women.

PATHOLOGY

The bronchial dilatation of bronchiectasis is associated with destructive and inflammatory changes in the walls of medium-sized airways, often at the level of segmental or subsegmental bronchi. Airway inflammation is primarily mediated by neutrophils and results in up-regulation of enzymes such as elastase and matrix metalloproteinases. The normal structural components of the wall, including cartilage, muscle, and elastic tissue, are destroyed and may be replaced by fibrous tissue. The dilated airways frequently contain pools of thick, purulent material, whereas more peripheral airways are often occluded by secretions or obliterated and replaced by fibrous tissue. Additional microscopic features include bronchial and peribronchial inflammation and fibrosis, ulceration of the bronchial wall, squamous metaplasia, and mucous gland hyperplasia. The parenchyma normally supplied by the affected airways is abnormal, containing varying combinations of fibrosis, emphysema, bronchopneumonia, and atelectasis. As a result of the inflammation, vascularity of the bronchial wall increases, with associated enlargement of the bronchial arteries and anastomoses between the bronchial and pulmonary arterial circulations.

Three different patterns of bronchiectasis have been described. In *cylindrical bronchiectasis*, the involved bronchi appear uniformly dilated and end abruptly at the point that smaller airways are obstructed by secretions. In *varicose bronchiectasis*, the affected bronchi have an irregular or beaded pattern of dilatation resembling varicose veins. In *saccular (cystic) bronchiectasis*, the bronchi have a ballooned appearance at the periphery, ending in blind sacs without recognizable bronchial structures distal to the sacs.

ETIOLOGY AND PATHOGENESIS

Bronchiectasis is a consequence of inflammation and destruction of the structural components of the bronchial wall. Infection is the usual cause of the inflammation; microorganisms such as *Pseudomonas aeruginosa* and *Haemophilus influenzae* produce pigments, proteases, and other toxins that injure the respiratory epithelium and impair mucociliary clearance. The host inflammatory response induces epithelial injury, largely as a result of mediators released from neutrophils. As protection against infection is compromised, the dilated airways become more susceptible to colonization and growth of bacteria. Thus a reinforcing cycle can result, with inflammation producing airway damage, impaired clearance of microorganisms, and further infection, which then completes the cycle by inciting more inflammation.

Infectious Causes

Adenovirus and influenza virus are the main viruses that cause bronchiectasis in association with lower respiratory tract involvement. Virulent bacterial infections, especially with potentially necrotizing organisms such as *Staphylococcus aureus*, *Klebsiella*, and anaerobes, remain important causes of bronchiectasis when antibiotic treatment of a pneumonia is not given or is significantly delayed. Infection with *Bordetella pertussis*, particularly in childhood, has also been classically associated with chronic suppurative airways disease. Bronchiectasis has been reported in patients with HIV infection, perhaps at least partly due to recurrent bacterial infection. Tuberculosis, a major cause of bronchiectasis worldwide, can produce airway dilatation by a necrotizing effect on pulmonary parenchyma and airways and indirectly as a consequence of airway obstruction from bronchostenosis or extrinsic compression by lymph nodes. Nontuberculous mycobacteria are frequently cultured from patients with bronchiectasis, often as secondary infections or colonizing organisms. However, it has also been recognized that these organisms, especially those of the *Mycobacterium avium* complex, can serve as primary pathogens associated with the development and/or progression of bronchiectasis.

Impaired host defense mechanisms are often involved in the predisposition to recurrent infections. The major cause of localized impairment of host defenses is endobronchial obstruction. Bacteria and secretions cannot be cleared adequately from the obstructed airway, which develops recurrent or chronic infection. Slowly growing endobronchial neoplasms such as carcinoid tumors may be associated with bronchiectasis. Foreign-body aspiration is another important cause of endobronchial obstruction, particularly in children. Airway obstruction can also result from bronchostenosis, from impacted secretions, or from extrinsic compression by enlarged lymph nodes.

Generalized impairment of pulmonary defense mechanisms occurs with immunoglobulin deficiency, primary ciliary disorders, or cystic fibrosis (CF). Infections and bronchiectasis are therefore often more diffuse. With panhypogammaglobulinemia, the best described of the immunoglobulin disorders associated with recurrent infection and bronchiectasis, patients often also have a history of sinus or skin infections. Selective deficiency of an IgG subclass, especially IgG2, has also been described in a small number of patients with bronchiectasis.

The primary disorders associated with ciliary dysfunction, termed *primary ciliary dyskinesia*, are responsible for 5–10% of cases of bronchiectasis. Primary ciliary dyskinesia is inherited in an autosomal recessive fashion. Numerous defects are encompassed under this category, including structural abnormalities of the dynein arms, radial spokes, and microtubules; mutations in heavy and intermediate chain dynein have been described in a small number of patients. The cilia become dyskinetic; their coordinated, propulsive action is diminished, and bacterial clearance is impaired. The clinical effects include recurrent upper and lower respiratory tract infections, such as sinusitis, otitis media, and bronchiectasis. Because normal sperm motility also depends on proper ciliary function, males are generally infertile. Additionally, since visceral rotation during development depends upon proper ciliary motion, the positioning of normally lateralized organs becomes random. As a result, approximately half of patients with primary ciliary dyskinesia fall into the subgroup of *Kartagener's syndrome*, in which situs inversus accompanies bronchiectasis and sinusitis.

In CF, the tenacious secretions in the bronchi are associated with impaired bacterial clearance, resulting in colonization and recurrent infection with a variety of organisms, particularly mucoid strains of *P. aeruginosa*, but also *S. aureus*, *H. influenzae*, *Escherichia coli*, and *Burkholderia cepacia*.

Noninfectious Causes

Some cases of bronchiectasis are associated with exposure to a toxic substance that incites a severe inflammatory response. Examples include inhalation of a toxic gas such as ammonia or aspiration of acidic gastric contents, though the latter problem is often also complicated by aspiration of bacteria. An immune response in the airway may also trigger inflammation, destructive changes, and bronchial dilatation. This mechanism is presumably important for bronchiectasis with allergic bronchopulmonary aspergillosis (ABPA), which is due at least in part to an immune response to *Aspergillus* organisms that have colonized the airway.

In α_1-antitrypsin deficiency, the usual respiratory complication is the early development of panacinar emphysema, but affected individuals may occasionally have bronchiectasis. In the *yellow nail syndrome*, which is due to hypoplastic lymphatics, the triad of lymphedema, pleural effusion, and yellow discoloration of the nails is accompanied by bronchiectasis in approximately 40% of patients.

CLINICAL MANIFESTATIONS

Patients typically present with persistent or recurrent cough and purulent sputum production. Repeated, purulent respiratory tract infections should raise clinical suspicion for bronchiectasis. Hemoptysis occurs in 50–70% of cases and can be due to bleeding from friable, inflamed airway mucosa. More significant, even massive bleeding is often a consequence of bleeding from hypertrophied bronchial arteries. Systemic symptoms such as fatigue, weight loss, and myalgias can also occur.

When a specific infectious episode initiates bronchiectasis, patients may describe a severe pneumonia followed by chronic cough and sputum production. Alternatively, patients without a dramatic initiating event often describe the insidious onset of symptoms. In some cases, patients are either asymptomatic or have a nonproductive cough, often associated with "dry" bronchiectasis in an upper lobe. Dyspnea or wheezing generally reflects either widespread bronchiectasis or underlying chronic obstructive pulmonary disease. With exacerbations of infection, the amount of sputum increases, and it becomes more purulent and often more bloody; systemic symptoms, including fever, may also be prominent.

Physical examination of the chest overlying an area of bronchiectasis is quite variable. Any combination of crackles, rhonchi, and wheezes may be heard, all of which reflect the damaged airways containing significant secretions. As with other types of chronic intrathoracic infection, clubbing may be present. Patients with severe diffuse disease, particularly those with chronic hypoxemia, may have associated cor pulmonale and right ventricular failure.

RADIOGRAPHIC AND LABORATORY FINDINGS

Though the chest radiograph is important in the evaluation of suspected bronchiectasis, the findings are often nonspecific. At one extreme, the radiograph may be normal with mild disease. Alternatively, patients with saccular bronchiectasis may have prominent cystic spaces, either with or without air-liquid levels, corresponding to the dilated airways. These may be difficult to distinguish from enlarged airspaces due to bullous emphysema or from regions of honeycombing in patients with severe interstitial lung disease. Other findings are due to dilated airways with thickened walls, which result from peribronchial inflammation. These dilated airways are often crowded together in parallel. When seen longitudinally, the airways appear as "tram tracks"; when seen in cross-section, they produce "ring shadows." Because the dilated airways may be filled with secretions, the lumen may appear dense rather than radiolucent, producing an opaque tubular or branched tubular structure.

CT, especially with high-resolution images 1.0–1.5-mm thick, provides an excellent view of dilated airways (Fig. 18-1). Consequently, it is now the standard technique for detecting or confirming the diagnosis of bronchiectasis.

Examination of sputum often reveals an abundance of neutrophils and colonization or infection with a variety of possible organisms. Appropriate staining and

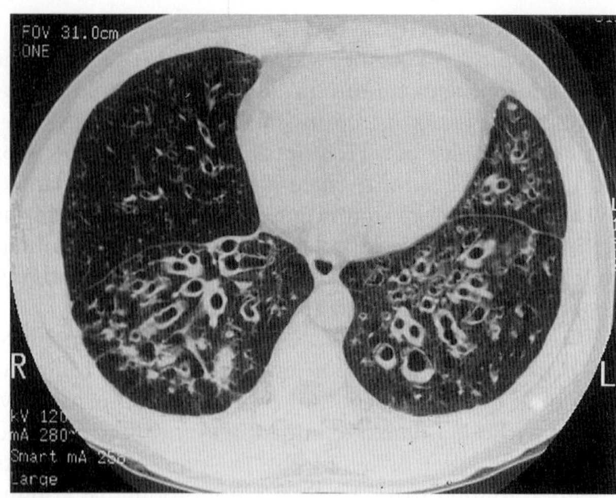

FIGURE 18-1
High-resolution CT scan of bronchiectasis showing dilated airways in both lower lobes and in the lingula. When seen in cross-section, the dilated airways have a ringlike appearance. *(From SE Weinberger: Principles of Pulmonary Medicine, 4th ed. Philadelphia, Saunders, 2004, with permission.)*

culturing of sputum often provide a guide to antibiotic therapy.

When bronchiectasis is focal, fiberoptic bronchoscopy may reveal an underlying endobronchial obstruction. In other cases, upper lobe involvement may be suggestive of either tuberculosis or ABPA. With more widespread disease, measurement of sweat chloride levels for CF, structural or functional assessment of nasal or bronchial cilia or sperm for primary ciliary dyskinesia, and quantitative assessment of immunoglobulins may explain recurrent airway infection.

Pulmonary function tests may demonstrate airflow obstruction as a consequence of diffuse bronchiectasis or associated chronic obstructive lung disease. Bronchial hyperreactivity, e.g., to methacholine challenge, and some reversibility of the airflow obstruction with inhaled bronchodilators are relatively common.

Figure 18-2 illustrates a diagnostic approach based on clinical suspicion and radiographic findings. As the differential diagnosis for focal versus diffuse bronchiectasis is different, the radiographic distribution of disease can serve as a starting point of the diagnostic workup. This algorithm should not imply that all studies be obtained in all patients with bronchiectasis. Rather, the workup should be dictated by a careful assessment of the clinical scenario. In a patient with focal bronchiectasis, for example, documentation of a prior pneumonia in the same location may suffice. Evaluation for immunoglobulin deficiency and CF should be considered for young patients with bronchiectasis and sino-pulmonary disease.

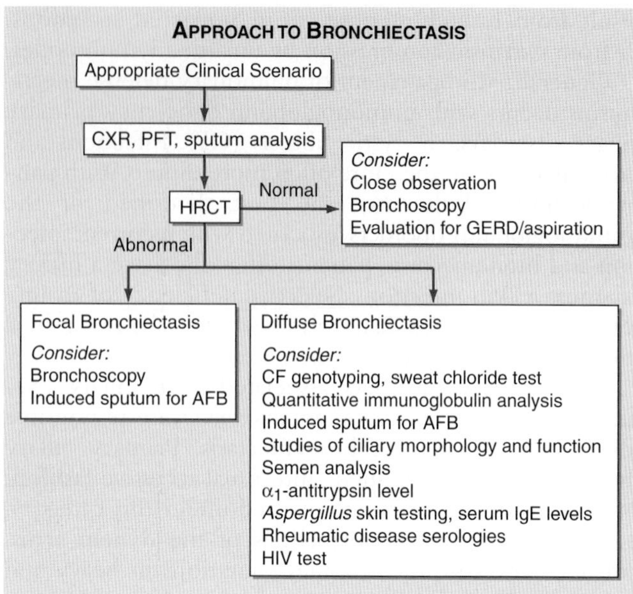

FIGURE 18-2
Diagnostic approach to bronchiectasis. AFB, acid-fast bacilli; CXR, chest X-ray; GERD, gastroesophageal reflux disease; HRCT, high-resolution computed tomography; PFT, pulmonary function testing.

℞ Treatment: BRONCHIECTASIS

Therapy has several major goals: (1) treatment of infection, particularly during acute exacerbations; (2) improved clearance of tracheobronchial secretions; (3) reduction of inflammation; and (4) treatment of an identifiable underlying problem.

Antibiotics are the cornerstone of bronchiectasis management. For patients with infrequent exacerbations characterized by an increase in quantity and purulence of the sputum, antibiotics are used only during acute episodes. Although choice of an antibiotic should be guided by Gram's stain and culture of sputum, empiric coverage (e.g., with amoxicillin, trimethoprim-sulfamethoxazole, or levofloxacin) is often given initially. Infection with *P. aeruginosa* is of particular concern, as it appears to be associated with greater rate of deterioration of lung function and worse quality of life. When *Pseudomonas* is present, oral therapy with a quinolone or parenteral therapy with an aminoglycoside, carbapenem, or third-generation cephalosporin is appropriate based on antibiotic sensitivity patterns. There are no firm guidelines for length of therapy, but a 10–14-day course or longer is typically administered.

A variety of mechanical methods and devices accompanied by appropriate positioning can facilitate drainage in patients with copious secretions. Though commonly employed and probably beneficial, these airway-clearance techniques have been poorly studied, and their efficacy is not proven. Pharmacologic agents are also employed to promote bronchopulmonary hygiene. Mucolytic agents to thin secretions and allow better clearance are controversial. Aerosolized recombinant DNase, which decreases viscosity of sputum by breaking down DNA released from neutrophils, has been shown to improve pulmonary function in CF but may be deleterious and should be avoided in bronchiectasis not associated with CF. Bronchodilators to improve obstruction and aid clearance of secretions are particularly useful in patients with airway hyperreactivity and reversible airflow obstruction.

Although surgical therapy was common in the past, more effective antibiotic and supportive therapy has largely replaced surgery. However, when bronchiectasis is localized and the morbidity is substantial despite adequate medical therapy, surgical resection of the involved region of lung should be considered.

When massive hemoptysis, often originating from the hypertrophied bronchial circulation, does not resolve with conservative therapy, including rest and antibiotics, therapeutic options are either surgical resection or bronchial arterial embolization. Although resection may be successful if disease is localized, embolization is preferable with widespread disease.

LUNG ABSCESS

Lung abscess is defined as pulmonary parenchymal necrosis and cavitation resulting from infection. The development of a lung abscess implies a high microorganism burden as well as inadequate microbial clearance from the airways. Aspiration is the most common cause; factors that portend an increased risk of aspiration include esophageal dysmotility, seizure disorders, and neurologic conditions causing bulbar dysfunction. Other predisposing conditions for lung abscess include periodontal disease and alcoholism.

MICROBIOLOGY

Anaerobic bacteria are the most common causative organisms for lung abscess. Aerobic or facultative bacteria such as *S. aureus, Klebsiella pneumoniae, Nocardia sp.,* and gram-negative organisms, as well as nonbacterial pathogens like fungi and parasites, may also cause abscess formation. In the immunocompromised host, aerobic bacteria and opportunistic pathogens may predominate. Multiple isolates are more commonly seen in all patients when anaerobic and aerobic cultures are done.

CLINICAL MANIFESTATIONS

The symptoms of lung abscess are typical of pulmonary infection in general and may include cough, purulent sputum production, pleuritic chest pain, fever, and hemoptysis. In anaerobic infection, the clinical course may evolve over an extended period of time, and some patients may be asymptomatic. More acute presentations are typical of infection with aerobic bacteria.

Physical examination is often unrevealing. Rales or evidence of consolidation may be present. Fetid breath and poor dentition may be diagnostic clues. Clubbing or hypertrophic pulmonary osteoarthropathy may occur in chronic cases.

The chest radiograph classically reveals one or two thick-walled cavities in dependent areas of the lung, particularly the upper lobes and posterior segments of the lower lobes (Fig. 18-3). An air-fluid level is often present.

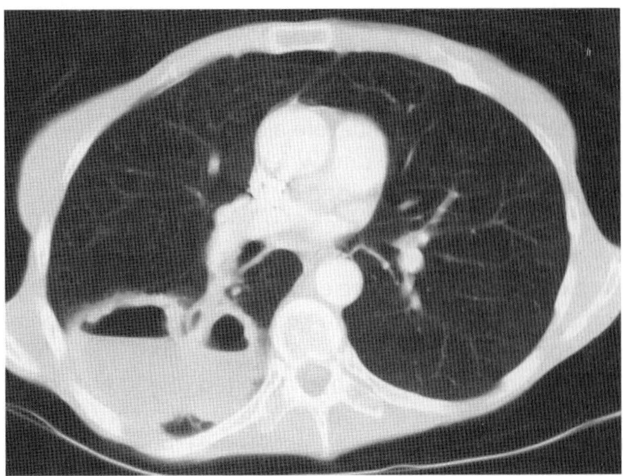

FIGURE 18-3
Cross-sectional CT image from a patient with an anaerobic lung abscess showing two contiguous thick-walled cavitary lesions in the right lower lobe with air-fluid levels. *(From WT Miller Jr: Diagnostic Thoracic Imaging. New York, McGraw-Hill, 2006, with permission.)*

CT of the chest is helpful in defining the size and location of the abscess, as well as to evaluate for additional cavities and the presence of pleural disease. Cavitary lesions in nondependent regions like the right middle lobe or anterior segments of the upper lobes should raise the possibility of other etiologies, including malignancy.

Laboratory studies may reveal leukocytosis, anemia, and an elevated erythrocyte sedimentation rate.

DIAGNOSIS

The diagnosis of lung abscess is based on clinical symptoms, identification of predisposing conditions, and chest radiographic findings. The differential diagnosis includes mycobacterial infection, pulmonary sequestration, malignancy, pulmonary infarction, and an infected bulla.

Identification of a causative organism is an ideal but challenging goal. Anaerobic bacteria are particularly difficult to isolate. Blood, sputum cultures, and, when appropriate, pleural fluid cultures should be obtained from patients with lung abscess. The role of fiberoptic bronchoscopy with bronchoalveolar lavage or protected-specimen brush for diagnosis or drainage of lung abscess is controversial. The relatively low yield, especially with anaerobic lung abscess, should be balanced against the risk of rupture of the abscess cavity with spillage into the airways. Bronchoscopy is perhaps most useful to rule out airway obstruction, mycobacterial infection, or malignancy. Other less commonly utilized methods for microbiologic sampling are transtracheal or transthoracic aspiration.

℞ Treatment: LUNG ABSCESS

For many years, penicillin was the mainstay of empiric antibiotic therapy for lung abscess. Due to the emergence of β-lactamase–producing organisms, clindamycin

(150–300 mg every 6 h) is now standard therapy. Other agents, such as carbapenems and β-lactam/β-lactamase inhibitor combinations, may be useful in selected cases. Metronidazole alone is associated with a high treatment failure rate. When possible, the choice of antibiotics should be guided by microbiologic results.

The duration of treatment for lung abscess is controversial. Four to six weeks of antibiotic therapy is typically employed, though a more extended course is favored by some experts. Treatment failure suggests the possibility of a noninfectious etiology.

Although surgery has had a limited role in treatment in the antibiotic era, indications include refractory hemoptysis, inadequate response to medical therapy, or the need for a tissue diagnosis when there is concern for a noninfectious etiology.

In general, outcomes for patients with classic anaerobic lung abscess are favorable, with a 90–95% cure rate. Higher mortality rates have been reported in immunocompromised patients, those with significant comorbidities, and infection with *P. aeruginosa*, *S. aureus*, and *K. pneumoniae*.

FURTHER READINGS

BARKER AF: Bronchiectasis. N Engl J Med 346:1383, 2002

LIGHT RW: Parapneumonic effusions and empyema. Proc Am Thorac Soc 3:75, 2006

MANSHARAMANI N et al: Lung abscess in adults: Clinical comparison of immunocompromised to non-immunocompromised patients. Respir Med 96:178, 2002

MANSHARAMANI N, KOZIEL H: Chronic lung sepsis: Lung abscess, bronchiectasis, and empyema. Curr Opin Pulm Med 9:181, 2003

NOONE PG et al: Primary ciliary dyskinesia: Diagnostic and phenotypic features. Am J Respir Crit Care Med 169:459, 2004

PASTEUR MC et al: An investigation into causative factors in patients with bronchiectasis. Am J Respir Crit Care Med 162:1277, 2000

ROSEN MJ: Chronic cough due to bronchiectasis. ACCP evidence-based clinical practice guidelines. Chest 129:122S, 2006

SCHEINBERG P, SHORE E: A pilot study of the safety and efficacy of tobramycin solution for inhalation in patients with severe bronchiectasis. Chest 127:1420, 2005

WEYCKER D et al: Prevalence and economic burden of bronchiectasis. Clin Pulm Med 12:205, 2005

WILLS P, GREENSTONE M: Inhaled hyperosmolar agents for bronchiectasis. Cochrane Database Syst Rev 2:CD002996, 2006

CHAPTER 19

INFECTIVE ENDOCARDITIS

Adolf W. Karchmer

The prototypic lesion of infective endocarditis, the *vegetation* (Fig. 19-1), is a mass of platelets, fibrin, microcolonies of microorganisms, and scant inflammatory cells. Infection most commonly involves heart valves (either native or prosthetic), but may also occur on the low-pressure side of the ventricular septum at the site of a defect, on the mural endocardium where it is damaged by aberrant jets of blood or foreign bodies, or on intracardiac devices themselves. The analogous process involving arteriovenous shunts, arterioarterial shunts (patent ductus arteriosus), or a coarctation of the aorta is called *infective endarteritis*.

Endocarditis may be classified according to the temporal evolution of disease, the site of infection, the cause of infection, or a predisposing risk factor, such as injection drug use. Although each classification criterion provides therapeutic and prognostic insight, none is sufficient alone. *Acute endocarditis* is a hectically febrile illness that rapidly damages cardiac structures, hematogenously seeds extracardiac sites, and, if untreated, progresses to death within weeks. *Subacute endocarditis* follows an indolent course; causes structural cardiac damage only slowly, if at all; rarely metastasizes; and is gradually progressive unless complicated by a major embolic event or ruptured mycotic aneurysm.

In developed countries, the incidence of endocarditis ranges from 2.6 to 7.0 cases per 100,000 population per year and remained relatively stable from 1950 to 2000. Although rates of congenital heart diseases remain constant, other predisposing conditions in developed countries have shifted from chronic rheumatic heart disease to illicit IV drug use, degenerative valve disease, intracardiac devices, and health care–associated infection. The incidence of endocarditis is notably increased among the elderly. In reported series, 10–30% of endocarditis cases involve prosthetic valves. The risk of prosthesis infection is greatest during the first 6 months after valve replacement; gradually declines to a low, stable rate thereafter; and is similar for mechanical and bioprosthetic devices.

ETIOLOGY

Although many species of bacteria and fungi cause sporadic episodes of endocarditis, only a few bacterial species cause the majority of cases (Table 19-1). The

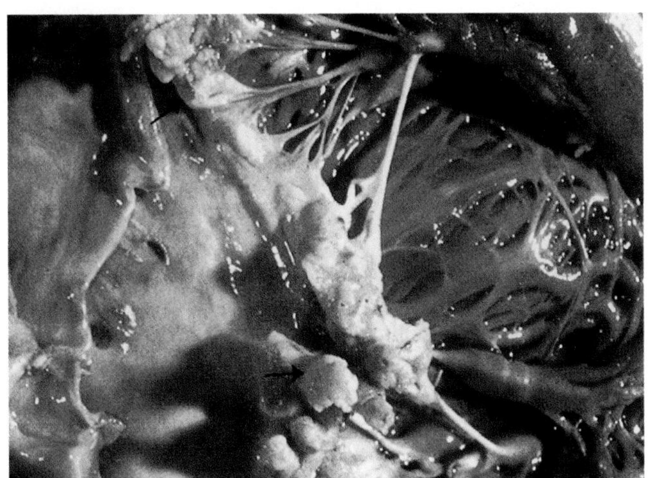

FIGURE 19-1
Vegetations (*arrows*) due to viridans streptococcal endocarditis involving the mitral valve.

pathogens vary somewhat with the clinical types of endocarditis, in part because of different portals of entry. The oral cavity, skin, and upper respiratory tract are the respective primary portals for the viridans streptococci, staphylococci, and HACEK organisms (*Haemophilus*, *Aggregatibacter* (*Actinobacillus*), *Cardiobacterium*, *Eikenella*, and *Kingella*) causing community-acquired native valve endocarditis. *Streptococcus bovis* originates from the gastrointestinal tract, where it is associated with polyps and colonic tumors, and enterococci enter the bloodstream from the genitourinary tract. Health care–associated native valve endocarditis is the consequence of bacteremia arising from intravascular catheter infections, nosocomial wound and urinary tract infections, and chronic invasive procedures such as hemodialysis. Endocarditis complicates 6–25% of episodes of catheter-associated *Staphylococcus aureus* bacteremia; the higher rates are detected by careful transesophageal echocardiography (TEE) screening (see "Echocardiography" later in the chapter).

Prosthetic valve endocarditis arising within 2 months of valve surgery is generally the result of intraoperative contamination of the prosthesis or a bacteremic postoperative complication. The nosocomial nature of these infections is reflected in their primary microbial causes: coagulase-negative staphylococci (CoNS), *S. aureus*, facultative gram-negative bacilli, diphtheroids, and fungi. The portals of entry and organisms causing cases beginning >12 months after surgery are similar to those in community-acquired native valve endocarditis. Epidemiologic evidence

TABLE 19-1

ORGANISMS CAUSING MAJOR CLINICAL FORMS OF ENDOCARDITIS

	PERCENT OF CASES							
	NATIVE VALVE ENDOCARDITIS		PROSTHETIC VALVE ENDOCARDITIS AT INDICATED TIME OF ONSET (MONTHS) AFTER VALVE SURGERY			ENDOCARDITIS IN INJECTION DRUG USERS		
ORGANISM	COMMUNITY-ACQUIRED (*n* = 683)	HEALTH CARE–ASSOCIATED (*n* = 128)	<2 (*n* = 144)	2–12 (*n* = 31)	>12 (*n* = 194)	RIGHT-SIDED (*n* = 346)	LEFT-SIDED (*n* = 204)	TOTAL (*n* = 675)[a]
Streptococci[b]	32	8	1	9	31	5	15	12
Pneumococci	1	—	—	—	—	—	—	—
Enterococci	8	16	8	12	11	2	24	9
Staphylococcus aureus	35	44[c]	22	12	18	77	23	57
Coagulase-negative staphylococci	4	15	33	32	11	—	—	—
Fastidious gram-negative coccobacilli (HACEK group)[d]	3	—	—	—	6	—	—	—
Gram-negative bacilli	3	5	13	3	6	5	13	7
Candida spp.	1	6	8	12	1	—	12	4
Polymicrobial/ miscellaneous	6	1	3	6	5	8	10	7
Diphtheroids	—	—	6	—	3	—	—	0.1
Culture-negative	5	5	5	6	8	3	3	3

[a]The total number of cases is larger than the sum of right- and-left-sided cases because the location of infection was not specified in some cases.
[b]Includes viridans streptococci; *Streptococcus bovis*; other non–group A, groupable streptococci; and *Abiotrophia* spp. (nutritionally variant, pyridoxal-requiring streptococci).
[c]Methicillin resistance is common among these *S. aureus* strains.
[d]Includes *Haemophilus* spp., *Aggregatibacter* (*Actinobacillus*) *actinomycetemcomitans, Cardiobacterium hominis, Eikenella* spp., and *Kingella* spp.
Note: Data are compiled from multiple studies.

suggests that prosthetic valve endocarditis due to CoNS that presents 2–12 months after surgery often represents delayed-onset nosocomial infection. At least 85% of CoNS strains that cause prosthetic valve endocarditis within 12 months of surgery are methicillin-resistant; the rate of methicillin resistance decreases to 25% among CoNS strains causing prosthetic valve endocarditis that presents >1 year after valve surgery.

Transvenous pacemaker lead– and/or implanted defibrillator–associated endocarditis is usually nosocomial. The majority of episodes occur within weeks of implantation or generator change and are caused by *S. aureus* or CoNS.

Endocarditis occurring among injection drug users, especially when infection involves the tricuspid valve, is commonly caused by *S. aureus* strains, many of which are methicillin-resistant. Left-sided valve infections in addicts have a more varied etiology and involve abnormal valves, often ones damaged by prior episodes of endocarditis. A number of these cases are caused by *Pseudomonas aeruginosa* and *Candida* species, and sporadic cases are due to unusual organisms such as *Bacillus*, *Lactobacillus*, and *Corynebacterium* species. Polymicrobial endocarditis is more common among injection drug users than among patients who do not inject drugs. The presence of HIV in the former population does not significantly influence the causes of endocarditis.

From 5 to 15% of patients with endocarditis have negative blood cultures; in one-third to one-half of these cases, cultures are negative because of prior antibiotic exposure. The remainder of these patients are infected by fastidious organisms, such as nutritionally variant organisms (now designated *Granulicatella* and *Abiotrophia* species), HACEK organisms, and *Bartonella* species. Some fastidious organisms that cause endocarditis do so in characteristic epidemiologic settings (e.g., *Coxiella burnetii* in Europe, *Brucella* species in the Middle East). *Tropheryma whipplei* causes an indolent, culture-negative, afebrile form of endocarditis.

PATHOGENESIS

Unless it is injured, the endothelium is resistant to infection by most bacteria and to thrombus formation. Endothelial injury (e.g., at the site of impact of high-velocity blood jets or on the low-pressure side of a cardiac structural lesion) causes aberrant flow and allows either direct infection by virulent organisms or the development of an uninfected platelet-fibrin thrombus—a condition called *nonbacterial thrombotic endocarditis* (NBTE). The thrombus subsequently serves as a site of bacterial attachment during transient bacteremia. The cardiac conditions most commonly resulting in NBTE are mitral regurgitation, aortic stenosis, aortic regurgitation, ventricular septal defects, and complex congenital heart disease. These conditions result from rheumatic heart disease (particularly in the developing world, where rheumatic fever remains prevalent), mitral valve prolapse, degenerative heart disease, and congenital malformations. NBTE also arises as a result of a hypercoagulable state; this phenomenon gives rise to the clinical entity of *marantic endocarditis* (uninfected vegetations seen in patients with malignancy and chronic diseases) and to bland vegetations complicating systemic lupus erythematosus and the antiphospholipid antibody syndrome.

Organisms that cause endocarditis generally enter the bloodstream from mucosal surfaces, the skin, or sites of focal infection. Except for more virulent bacteria (e.g., *S. aureus*) that can adhere directly to intact endothelium or exposed subendothelial tissue, microorganisms in the blood adhere to sites at NBTE. If resistant to the bactericidal activity of serum and the microbicidal peptides released locally by platelets, the organisms proliferate and induce a procoagulant state at the site by eliciting tissue factor from adherent monocytes or, in the case of *S. aureus*, from monocytes and from intact endothelium. Fibrin deposition combines with platelet aggregation, stimulated by tissue factor and independently by proliferating microorganisms, to generate an infected vegetation. The organisms that commonly cause endocarditis have surface adhesin molecules, collectively called microbial surface components recognizing adhesin matrix molecules (MSCRAMMs), that mediate adherence to NBTE sites or injured endothelium. Fibronectin-binding proteins present on many gram-positive bacteria, clumping factor (a fibrinogen- and fibrin-binding surface protein) on *S. aureus*, and glucans or FimA (a member of the family of oral mucosal adhesins) on streptococci facilitate adherence. Fibronectin-binding proteins are required for *S. aureus* invasion of intact endothelium; thus these surface proteins may facilitate infection of previously normal valves. In the absence of host defenses, organisms enmeshed in the growing platelet-fibrin vegetation proliferate to form dense microcolonies. Organisms deep in vegetations are metabolically inactive (nongrowing) and relatively resistant to killing by antimicrobial agents. Proliferating surface organisms are shed into the bloodstream continuously.

The pathophysiologic consequences and clinical manifestations of endocarditis—other than constitutional symptoms, which probably result from cytokine production—arise from damage to intracardiac structures; embolization of vegetation fragments, leading to infection or infarction of remote tissues; hematogenous infection of sites during bacteremia; and tissue injury due to the deposition of circulating immune complexes or immune responses to deposited bacterial antigens.

CLINICAL MANIFESTATIONS

The clinical syndrome of infective endocarditis is highly variable and spans a continuum between acute and subacute presentations. Native valve endocarditis (whether acquired in the community or in association with health care), prosthetic valve endocarditis, and endocarditis due to injection drug use share clinical and laboratory manifestations (Table 19-2). The causative microorganism is primarily responsible for the temporal course of endocarditis. β-Hemolytic streptococci, *S. aureus*, and pneumococci typically result in an acute course, although *S. aureus* occasionally causes subacute disease. Endocarditis caused by *Staphylococcus lugdunensis* (a coagulase-negative species)

TABLE 19-2

CLINICAL AND LABORATORY FEATURES OF INFECTIVE ENDOCARDITIS

FEATURE	FREQUENCY, %
Fever	80–90
Chills and sweats	40–75
Anorexia, weight loss, malaise	25–50
Myalgias, arthralgias	15–30
Back pain	7–15
Heart murmur	80–85
New/worsened regurgitant murmur	10–40
Arterial emboli	20–50
Splenomegaly	15–50
Clubbing	10–20
Neurologic manifestations	20–40
Peripheral manifestations (Osler's nodes, subungual hemorrhages, Janeway's lesions, Roth's spots)	2–15
Petechiae	10–40
Laboratory manifestations	
Anemia	70–90
Leukocytosis	20–30
Microscopic hematuria	30–50
Elevated erythrocyte sedimentation rate	>90
Elevated C-reactive protein level	>90
Rheumatoid factor	50
Circulating immune complexes	65–100
Decreased serum complement	5–40

or by enterococci may present acutely. Subacute endocarditis is typically caused by viridans streptococci, enterococci, CoNS, and the HACEK group. Endocarditis caused by *Bartonella* species and the agent of Q fever, *C. burnetii*, is exceptionally indolent.

The clinical features of endocarditis are nonspecific. However, these symptoms in a febrile patient with valvular abnormalities or a behavior pattern that predisposes to endocarditis (e.g., injection drug use) suggest the diagnosis, as do bacteremia with organisms that frequently cause endocarditis, otherwise-unexplained arterial emboli, and progressive cardiac valvular incompetence. In patients with subacute presentations, fever is typically low-grade and rarely exceeds 39.4°C (103°F); in contrast, temperatures of 39.4°–40°C (103°–104°F) are often noted in acute endocarditis. Fever may be blunted or absent in patients who are elderly or severely debilitated or who have marked cardiac or renal failure.

Cardiac Manifestations

Although heart murmurs are usually indicative of the predisposing cardiac pathology rather than of endocarditis, valvular damage and ruptured chordae may result in new regurgitant murmurs. In acute endocarditis involving a normal valve, murmurs are heard on presentation in only 30–45% of patients but ultimately are detected in 85%. Congestive heart failure develops in 30–40% of patients; it is usually a consequence of valvular dysfunction but occasionally is due to endocarditis-associated myocarditis or an intracardiac fistula. Heart failure due to aortic valve dysfunction progresses more rapidly than does that due to mitral valve dysfunction. Extension of infection beyond valve leaflets into adjacent annular or myocardial tissue results in perivalvular abscesses, which in turn may cause fistulae (from the root of the aorta into cardiac chambers or between cardiac chambers) with new murmurs. Abscesses may burrow from the aortic valve annulus through the epicardium, causing pericarditis. Extension of infection into paravalvular tissue adjacent to either the right or the noncoronary cusp of the aortic valve may interrupt the conduction system in the upper interventricular septum, leading to varying degrees of heart block. Although perivalvular abscesses arising from the mitral valve may potentially interrupt conduction pathways near the atrioventricular node or in the proximal bundle of His, such interruption occurs infrequently. Emboli to a coronary artery may result in myocardial infarction; nevertheless, embolic transmural infarcts are rare.

Noncardiac Manifestations

The classic nonsuppurative peripheral manifestations of subacute endocarditis are related to the duration of infection and, with early diagnosis and treatment, have become infrequent. In contrast, septic embolization mimicking some of these lesions (subungual hemorrhage, Osler's nodes) is common in patients with acute *S. aureus* endocarditis (Fig. 19-2). Musculoskeletal symptoms, including nonspecific inflammatory arthritis and back pain, usually remit promptly with treatment but must be distinguished from focal metastatic infection. Hematogenously seeded focal infection may involve any organ but most often is clinically evident in the skin, spleen, kidneys, skeletal system, and meninges. Arterial emboli are clinically apparent in up to 50% of patients. Vegetations

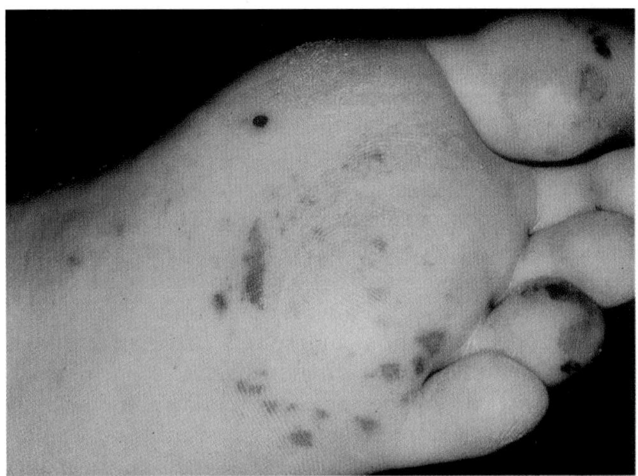

FIGURE 19-2
Septic emboli with hemorrhage and infarction due to acute *Staphylococcus aureus* endocarditis. (*Used with permission of L. Baden.*)

>10 mm in diameter (as measured by echocardiography) and those located on the mitral valve are more likely to embolize than are smaller or nonmitral vegetations. Embolic events—often with infarction—involving the extremities, spleen, kidneys, bowel, or brain are often noted at presentation. With effective antibiotic treatment, the frequency of embolic events decreases from 13 per 1000 patient-days during the initial week to 1.2 per 1000 patient-days after the third week. Emboli occurring late during or after effective therapy do not in themselves constitute evidence of failed antimicrobial treatment. Neurologic symptoms, most often resulting from embolic strokes, occur in up to 40% of patients. Other neurologic complications include aseptic or purulent meningitis, intracranial hemorrhage due to hemorrhagic infarcts or ruptured mycotic aneurysms, seizures, and encephalopathy. (*Mycotic aneurysms* are focal dilations of arteries occurring at points in the artery wall that have been weakened by infection in the vasa vasorum or where septic emboli have lodged.) Microabscesses in brain and meninges occur commonly in *S. aureus* endocarditis; surgically drainable intracerebral abscesses are infrequent.

Immune complex deposition on the glomerular basement membrane causes diffuse hypocomplementemic glomerulonephritis and renal dysfunction, which typically improve with effective antimicrobial therapy. Embolic renal infarcts cause flank pain and hematuria but rarely cause renal dysfunction.

Manifestations of Specific Predisposing Conditions

In almost 50% of patients who have endocarditis associated with injection drug use, infection is limited to the tricuspid valve. These patients present with fever, faint or no murmur, and (in 75% of cases) prominent pulmonary findings related to septic emboli, including cough, pleuritic chest pain, nodular pulmonary infiltrates, and occasionally pyopneumothorax. Infection involving valves on the left side of the heart presents with the typical clinical features of endocarditis.

Health care–associated endocarditis (defined as that which is nosocomial, arises after recent hospitalization, or is a direct consequence of long-term indwelling devices) has typical manifestations if it is not associated with a retained intracardiac device. Endocarditis associated with flow-directed pulmonary artery catheters is often cryptic, with symptoms masked by comorbid critical illness, and is commonly diagnosed at autopsy. Transvenous pacemaker lead– and/or implanted defibrillator–associated endocarditis may be associated with obvious or cryptic generator pocket infection and results in fever, minimal murmur, and pulmonary symptoms due to septic emboli.

Late-onset prosthetic valve endocarditis presents with typical clinical features. Cases arising within 60 days of valve surgery (early onset) lack peripheral vascular manifestations, and typical symptoms may be obscured by comorbidity associated with recent surgery. In both early-onset and more delayed presentations, paravalvular infection is common and often results in partial valve dehiscence, regurgitant murmurs, congestive heart failure, or disruption of the conduction system.

DIAGNOSIS

The Duke Criteria

The diagnosis of infective endocarditis is established with certainty only when vegetations obtained at cardiac surgery, at autopsy, or from an artery (an embolus) are examined histologically and microbiologically. Nevertheless, a highly sensitive and specific diagnostic schema—known as the *Duke criteria*—has been developed on the basis of clinical, laboratory, and echocardiographic findings (Table 19-3). Documentation of two major criteria, of one major and three minor criteria, or of five minor criteria allows a clinical diagnosis of definite endocarditis. The diagnosis of endocarditis is rejected if an alternative diagnosis is established, if symptoms resolve and do not recur with ≤4 days of antibiotic therapy, or if surgery or autopsy after ≤4 days of antimicrobial therapy yields no histologic evidence of endocarditis. Illnesses not classified as definite endocarditis or rejected are considered cases of possible infective endocarditis when either one major and one minor criterion or three minor criteria are identified. Requiring the identification of clinical features of endocarditis for classification as possible infective endocarditis increases the specificity of the schema without significantly reducing its sensitivity.

The roles of bacteremia and echocardiographic findings in the diagnosis of endocarditis are appropriately emphasized in the Duke criteria. The requirement for multiple positive blood cultures over time is consistent with the continuous low-density bacteremia characteristic of endocarditis (≤100 organisms/mL). Among patients with untreated endocarditis who ultimately have a positive blood culture, 95% of all blood cultures are positive; in 98% of these cases, one of the initial two sets of cultures yields the microorganism. The diagnostic criteria attach significance to the species of organism isolated from blood cultures. To fulfill a major criterion, the isolation of an organism that causes both endocarditis and bacteremia in the absence of endocarditis (e.g., *S. aureus*, enterococci) must take place repeatedly (i.e., persistent bacteremia) and in the absence of a primary focus of infection. Organisms that rarely cause endocarditis but commonly contaminate blood cultures (e.g., diphtheroids, CoNS) must be isolated repeatedly if their isolation is to serve as a major criterion.

Blood Cultures

Isolation of the causative microorganism from blood cultures is critical not only for diagnosis, but also for determination of antimicrobial susceptibility and planning of treatment. In the absence of prior antibiotic therapy, three blood culture sets (with two bottles per set), separated from each other by at least 1 h, should be obtained from different venipuncture sites over 24 h. If the cultures remain negative after 48–72 h, two or three additional blood culture sets should be obtained, and the laboratory should be consulted for advice regarding optimal

TABLE 19-3

THE DUKE CRITERIA FOR THE CLINICAL DIAGNOSIS OF INFECTIVE ENDOCARDITIS

Major Criteria

1. Positive blood culture
   - Typical microorganism for infective endocarditis from two separate blood cultures
     - Viridans streptococci, *Streptococcus bovis*, HACEK group, *Staphylococcus aureus, or*
     - Community-acquired enterococci in the absence of a primary focus, *or*
   - Persistently positive blood culture, defined as recovery of a microorganism consistent with infective endocarditis from:
     - Blood cultures drawn >12 h apart; *or*
     - All of three or a majority of four or more separate blood cultures, with first and last drawn at least 1 h apart
   - Single positive blood culture for *Coxiella burnetii* or phase I IgG antibody titer of >1:800
2. Evidence of endocardial involvement
   - Positive echocardiogram[a]
     - Oscillating intracardiac mass on valve or supporting structures or in the path of regurgitant jets or in implanted material, in the absence of an alternative anatomic explanation, *or*
     - Abscess, *or*
     - New partial dehiscence of prosthetic valve, *or*
   - New valvular regurgitation (increase or change in preexisting murmur not sufficient)

Minor Criteria

1. Predisposition: predisposing heart condition or injection drug use
2. Fever ≥38.0°C (≥100.4°F)
3. Vascular phenomena: major arterial emboli, septic pulmonary infarcts, mycotic aneurysm, intracranial hemorrhage, conjunctival hemorrhages, Janeway's lesions
4. Immunologic phenomena: glomerulonephritis, Osler's nodes, Roth's spots, rheumatoid factor
5. Microbiologic evidence: positive blood culture but not meeting major criterion as noted previously[b] or serologic evidence of active infection with organism consistent with infective endocarditis

[a]Transesophageal echocardiography is recommended for assessing possible prosthetic valve endocarditis or complicated endocarditis.
[b]Excluding single positive cultures for coagulase-negative staphylococci and diphtheroids, which are common culture contaminants, and organisms that do not cause endocarditis frequently, such as gram-negative bacilli.
Note: HACEK, *Haemophilus* spp., *Actinobacillus actinomycetemcomitans, Cardiobacterium hominis, Eikenella corrodens, Kingella* species.
Source: Adapted from Li et al., with permission from the University of Chicago Press.

culture techniques. Empirical antimicrobial therapy should not be administered initially to hemodynamically stable patients with subacute endocarditis, especially those who have received antibiotics within the preceding 2 weeks; thus, if necessary, additional blood culture sets can be obtained without the confounding effect of empirical treatment. Patients with acute endocarditis or with deteriorating hemodynamics who may require urgent surgery should be treated empirically immediately after three sets of blood cultures are obtained over several hours.

Non-Blood-Culture Tests

Serologic tests can be used to implicate causally some organisms that are difficult to recover by blood culture: *Brucella, Bartonella, Legionella*, and *C. burnetii*. Pathogens can also be identified in surgically recovered vegetations or emboli by culture, by microscopic examination with special stains (i.e., the periodic acid–Schiff stain for *T. whipplei*), and by use of polymerase chain reaction (PCR) to recover unique microbial DNA or 16S rRNA that, when sequenced, allows identification of organisms.

Echocardiography

Imaging with echocardiography allows anatomic confirmation of infective endocarditis, sizing of vegetations, detection of intracardiac complications, and assessment of cardiac function (Fig. 19-3). Transthoracic echocardiography (TTE) is noninvasive and exceptionally specific; however, it cannot image vegetations <2 mm in diameter, and in 20% of patients it is technically inadequate because of emphysema or body habitus. Thus TTE detects vegetations in only 65% of patients with definite clinical endocarditis; i.e., it has a sensitivity of 65%. Moreover, TTE is not adequate for evaluating prosthetic valves or detecting intracardiac complications. TEE is safe and significantly more sensitive than TTE. It detects vegetations in >90% of patients with definite endocarditis; nevertheless, false-negative studies are noted in 6–18% of endocarditis patients. TEE is the optimal method for the diagnosis of prosthetic endocarditis or the detection of myocardial abscess, valve perforation, or intracardiac fistulae.

Experts favor echocardiographic evaluation of all patients with a clinical diagnosis of endocarditis; however, the test should not be used to screen patients with a low probability of endocarditis (e.g., patients with unexplained fever). An American Heart Association approach to the use of echocardiography for evaluation of patients with suspected endocarditis is illustrated in Fig. 19-4. A negative TEE when endocarditis is likely does not exclude the diagnosis, but rather warrants repetition of the study in 7–10 days.

Other Studies

Many laboratory studies that are not diagnostic—i.e., complete blood count, creatinine determination, liver function tests, chest radiography, and electrocardiography—are nevertheless important in the management of patients with endocarditis. The erythrocyte sedimentation rate, C-reactive protein level, and circulating immune complex titer are commonly increased in endocarditis (Table 19-2).

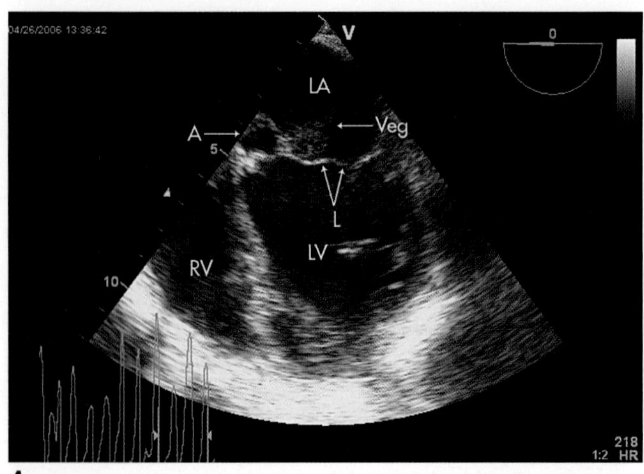

A

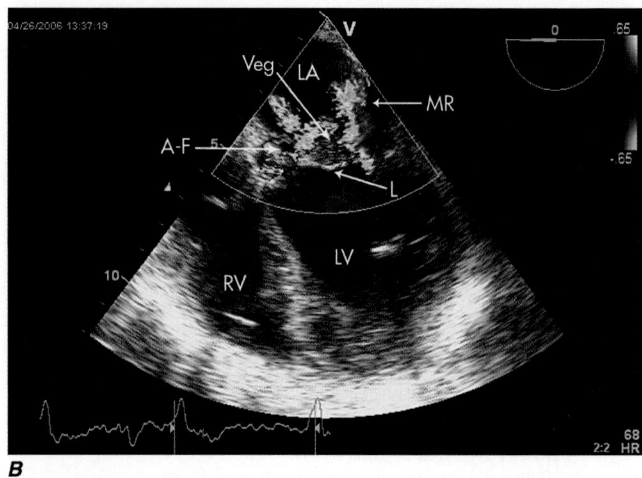

B

FIGURE 19-3

Imaging of a mitral valve infected with *Staphylococcus aureus* by low-esophageal four-chamber-view transesophageal echocardiography (TEE). ***A.*** Two-dimensional echocardiogram showing a large vegetation with an adjacent echolucent abscess cavity. ***B.*** Color-flow Doppler image showing severe mitral regurgitation through both the abscess-fistula and the central valve orifice. A, abscess; A-F, abscess-fistula; L, valve leaflets; LA, left atrium; LV, left ventricle; MR, mitral central valve regurgitation; RV, right ventricle; veg, vegetation. (*With permission of Andrew Burger, MD.*)

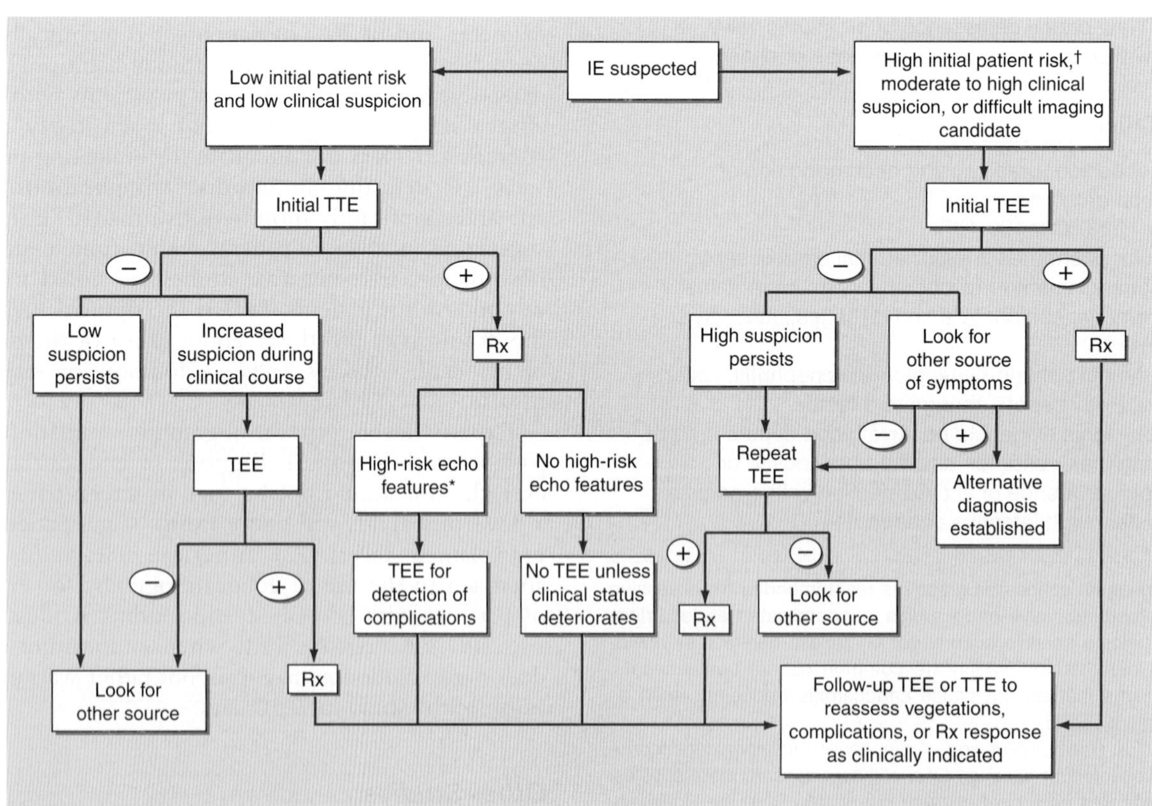

FIGURE 19-4

The diagnostic use of transesophageal and transtracheal echocardiography (TEE and TTE, respectively). †High initial patient risk for endocarditis as listed in Table 19-8 or evidence of intracardiac complications (new regurgitant murmur, new electrocardiographic conduction changes, or congestive heart failure). *High-risk echocardiographic features include large vegetations, valve insufficiency, paravalvular infection, or ventricular dysfunction. Rx indicates initiation of antibiotic therapy. [*Reproduced with permission from Diagnosis and Management of Infective Endocarditis and Its Complications* (*Circulation 1998; 98:2936-2948. © 1998 American Heart Association.*)]

Cardiac catheterization is useful primarily to assess coronary artery patency in older individuals who are to undergo surgery for endocarditis.

℞ Treatment: INFECTIVE ENDOCARDITIS

ANTIMICROBIAL THERAPY It is difficult to eradicate bacteria from the avascular vegetation in infective endocarditis because this site is relatively deficient in host defenses and because the largely nongrowing, metabolically inactive bacteria are less easily killed by antibiotics. To cure endocarditis, all bacteria in the vegetation must be killed; therefore, therapy must be bactericidal and prolonged. Antibiotics are generally given parenterally and must reach high serum concentrations that will, through passive diffusion, lead to effective concentrations in the depths of the vegetation. The choice of effective therapy requires precise knowledge of the susceptibility of the causative microorganisms. The decision to initiate treatment before a cause is defined must balance the need to establish a microbiologic diagnosis against the potential progression of disease or the need for urgent surgery (see "Blood Cultures" earlier in the chapter). The individual vulnerabilities of the patient should be weighed in the selection of therapy—e.g., simultaneous infection at other sites (such as meningitis), allergies, end-organ dysfunction, interactions with concomitant medications, and risks of adverse events.

Although given for several weeks longer, the regimens recommended for the treatment of endocarditis involving prosthetic valves (except for staphylococcal infections) are similar to those used to treat native valve infection (Table 19-4). Recommended doses and durations of therapy should be adhered to unless alterations are required by adverse events.

Organism-Specific Therapies

Streptococci To select the optimal therapy for streptococcal endocarditis, the minimum inhibitory concentration (MIC) of penicillin for the causative isolate must be determined (Table 19-4). The 2-week penicillin/gentamicin or ceftriaxone/gentamicin regimens should not be used to treat complicated native valve infection or prosthetic valve endocarditis. The regimen recommended for relatively penicillin-resistant streptococci is advocated for treatment of endocarditis caused by organisms of group B, C, or G. Endocarditis caused by nutritionally variant organisms (*Granulicatella* or *Abiotrophia* species) and *Gemella morbillorum* is treated with the regimen for moderately penicillin-resistant streptococci, as is prosthetic valve endocarditis caused by these organisms or by streptococci with a penicillin MIC of >0.1 μg/mL (Table 19-4).

Enterococci Enterococci are resistant to oxacillin, nafcillin, and the cephalosporins and are only inhibited—not killed—by penicillin, ampicillin, teicoplanin (not available in the United States), and vancomycin. To kill enterococci requires the synergistic interaction of a cell wall–active antibiotic (penicillin, ampicillin, vancomycin, or teicoplanin) that is effective at achievable serum concentrations and an aminoglycoside (gentamicin or streptomycin) to which the isolate does not exhibit high-level resistance. An isolate's resistance to cell wall–active agents or its ability to replicate in the presence of gentamicin at ≥500 μg/mL or streptomycin at 1000–2000 μg/mL—a phenomenon called *high-level aminoglycoside resistance*—indicates that the ineffective antimicrobial agent cannot participate in the interaction to produce killing. High-level resistance to gentamicin predicts that tobramycin, netilmicin, amikacin, and kanamycin also will be ineffective. In fact, even when enterococci are not highly resistant to gentamicin, it is difficult to predict the ability of these other aminoglycosides to participate in synergistic killing; consequently, they should not in general be used to treat enterococcal endocarditis.

Enterococci causing endocarditis must be tested for high-level resistance to streptomycin and gentamicin, β-lactamase production, and susceptibility to penicillin and ampicillin (MIC ≤16 μg/mL) and to vancomycin (MIC ≤8 μg/mL). If the isolate produces β-lactamase, ampicillin/sulbactam or vancomycin can be used as the cell wall–active component; if the penicillin/ampicillin MIC is >16 μg/mL, vancomycin can be considered; and if the vancomycin MIC is >8 μg/mL, penicillin or ampicillin may be considered. In the absence of high-level resistance, gentamicin or streptomycin should be used as the aminoglycoside (Table 19-4). If there is high-level resistance to both these drugs, no aminoglycoside should be given; instead, an 8- to 12-week course of a single cell wall–active agent is suggested—or, for *E. faecalis*, high doses of ampicillin plus either ceftriaxone or cefotaxime. If this alternative therapy fails or the isolate is resistant to all of the commonly used agents, surgical treatment is advised. The role of newer agents potentially active against multidrug-resistant enterococci [quinupristin/dalfopristin (*E. faecium* only), linezolid, and daptomycin] in the treatment of endocarditis has not been established. Although the dose of gentamicin used to achieve bactericidal synergy in treating enterococcal endocarditis is smaller than that used in standard therapy, nephrotoxicity is not uncommon during treatment for 4–6 weeks. Regimens wherein the aminoglycoside component of treatment has been truncated at 2–3 weeks because of toxicity have been curative. Thus discontinuation of the aminoglycoside is recommended when toxicity develops in patients with enterococcal endocarditis who have responded satisfactorily to therapy.

Staphylococci The regimens used to treat staphylococcal endocarditis (Table 19-4) are based not on coagulase production, but rather on the presence or absence of a prosthetic valve or foreign device, the native valve(s) involved, and the resistance of the isolate to penicillin and methicillin. Penicillinase is produced by 95% of staphylococci; thus all isolates should be considered penicillin-resistant until shown not to produce this enzyme. Similarly, methicillin resistance has become so prevalent

TABLE 19-4

ANTIBIOTIC TREATMENT FOR INFECTIVE ENDOCARDITIS CAUSED BY COMMON ORGANISMS[a]

ORGANISM	DRUG (DOSE, DURATION)	COMMENTS
Streptococci		
Penicillin-susceptible[b] streptococci, *S. bovis*	• Penicillin G (2–3 mU IV q4h for 4 weeks)	—
	• Ceftriaxone (2 g/d IV as a single dose for 4 weeks)	Can use ceftriaxone in patients with nonimmediate penicillin allergy
	• Vancomycin[c] (15 mg/kg IV q12h for 4 weeks)	Use vancomycin in patients with severe or immediate β-lactam allergy
	• Penicillin G (2–3 mU IV q4h) *or* ceftriaxone (2 g IV qd) for 2 weeks *plus* gentamicin[d] (3 mg/kg qd IV or IM, as a single dose[e] or divided into equal doses q8h for 2 weeks)	Avoid 2-week regimen when risk of aminoglycoside toxicity is increased and in prosthetic valve or complicated endocarditis
Relatively penicillin-resistant[f] streptococci	• Penicillin G (4 mU IV q4h) *or* ceftriaxone (2 g IV qd) for 4 weeks *plus* gentamicin[d] (3 mg/kg qd IV or IM, as a single dose[e] or divided into equal doses q8h for 2 weeks)	Penicillin alone at this dose for 6 weeks or with gentamicin during initial 2 weeks preferred for prosthetic valve endocarditis caused by streptococci with penicillin MIC ≤0.1 μg/mL
	• Vancomycin[c] as noted above for 4 weeks	—
Moderately penicillin-resistant[g] streptococci, nutritionally variant organisms, or *Gemella morbillorum*	• Penicillin G (4–5 mU IV q4h) *or* ceftriaxone (2 g IV qd) for 6 weeks *plus* gentamicin[d] (3 mg/kg qd IV or IM as a single dose[e] or divided into equal doses q8h for 6 weeks)	Preferred for prosthetic valve endocarditis caused by streptococci with penicillin MICs of >0.1 μg/mL
	• Vancomycin[c] as noted above for 4 weeks	—
Enterococci[h]		
	• Penicillin G (4–5 mU IV q4h) *plus* gentamicin[d] (1 mg/kg IV q8h), both for 4–6 weeks	Can use streptomycin (7.5 mg/kg q12h) in lieu of gentamicin if there is not high-level resistance to streptomycin
	• Ampicillin (2 g IV q4h) *plus* gentamicin[d] (1 mg/kg IV q8h), both for 4–6 weeks	—
	• Vancomycin[c] (15 mg/kg IVq12h) *plus* gentamicin[d] (1 mg/kg IV q8h), both for 4–6 weeks	Use vancomycin plus gentamicin for penicillin-allergic patients, or desensitize to penicillin
Staphylococci		
Methicillin-susceptible, infecting native valves (no foreign devices)	• Nafcillin or oxacillin (2 g IV q4h for 4–6 weeks) *plus* (optional) gentamicin[d] (1 mg/kg IM or IV q8h for 3–5 days)	Can use penicillin (4 mU q4h) if isolate is penicillin-susceptible (does not produce β-lactamase)
	• Cefazolin (2 g IV q8h for 4–6 weeks) *plus* (optional) gentamicin[d] (1 mg/kg IM or IV q8h for 3–5 days)	Can use cefazolin regimen for patients with nonimmediate penicillin allergy
	• Vancomycin[c] (15 mg/kg IV q12h for 4–6 weeks)	Use vancomycin for patients with immediate (urticarial) or severe penicillin allergy
Methicillin-resistant, infecting native valves (no foreign devices)	• Vancomycin[c] (15 mg/kg IV q12h for 4–6 weeks)	No role for routine use of rifampin
Methicillin-susceptible, infecting prosthetic valves	• Nafcillin or oxacillin (2 g IV q4h for 6–8 weeks) *plus* gentamicin[d] (1 mg/kg IM or IV q8h for 2 weeks) *plus* rifampin[i] (300 mg PO q8h for 6–8 weeks)	Use gentamicin during initial 2 weeks; determine susceptibility to gentamicin before initiating rifampin (see text); if patient is highly allergic to penicillin, use regimen for methicillin-resistant staphylococci; if β-lactam allergy is of the minor, nonimmediate type, can substitute cefazolin for oxacillin/nafcillin

(*Continued*)

TABLE 19-4 (*CONTINUED*)

ANTIBIOTIC TREATMENT FOR INFECTIVE ENDOCARDITIS CAUSED BY COMMON ORGANISMS[a]

ORGANISM	DRUG (DOSE, DURATION)	COMMENTS
Staphylococci (*Continued*)		
Methicillin-resistant, infecting prosthetic valves	• Vancomycin[c] (15 mg/kg IV q12h for 6–8 weeks) *plus* gentamicin[d] (1 mg/kg IM or IV q8h for 2 weeks) *plus* rifampin[i] (300 mg PO q8h for 6–8 weeks)	Use gentamicin during initial 2 weeks; determine gentamicin susceptibility before initiating rifampin (see text)
HACEK Organisms		
	• Ceftriaxone (2 g/d IV as a single dose for 4 weeks)	Can use another third-generation cephalosporin at comparable dosage
	• Ampicillin/sulbactam (3 g IV q6h for 4 weeks)	—

[a]Doses are for adults with normal renal function. Doses of gentamicin, streptomycin, and vancomycin must be adjusted for reduced renal function. Ideal body weight is used to calculate doses of gentamicin and streptomycin per kilogram (men = 50 kg + 2.3 kg per inch over 5 feet; women = 45.5 kg + 2.3 kg per inch over 5 feet).
[b]MIC, ≤0.1 μg/mL.
[c]Desirable peak vancomycin level 1 h after completion of a 1-h infusion is 30–45 μg/mL.
[d]Aminoglycosides should not be administered as single daily doses for enterococcal endocarditis and should be introduced as part of the initial treatment. Target peak and trough serum concentrations of divided-dose gentamicin 1 h after a 20- to 30-min infusion or IM injection are ~3.5 μg/mL and ≤1 μg/mL, respectively; target peak and trough serum concentrations of streptomycin (timing as with gentamicin) are 20–35 μg/mL and <10 μg/mL, respectively.
[e]Netilmicin (4 mg/kg qd, as a single dose) can be used in lieu of gentamicin.
[f]MIC, >0.1 μg/mL and <0.5 μg/mL.
[g]MIC, ≥0.5 μg/mL and <8.0 μg/mL.
[h]Antimicrobial susceptibility must be evaluated; see text.
[i]Rifampin increases warfarin and dicumarol requirements for anticoagulation.

among staphylococci, including *S. aureus*, that therapy should be initiated with a regimen for methicillin-resistant organisms and subsequently revised if the strain proves to be susceptible to methicillin. The addition of gentamicin (if the isolate is susceptible) to a β-lactam antibiotic to enhance therapy for native mitral or aortic valve endocarditis is optional. Its addition hastens eradication of bacteremia but does not improve survival rates. If added, gentamicin should be limited to the initial 3–5 days of therapy to minimize nephrotoxicity. Gentamicin generally is not added to the vancomycin regimen in this setting. The efficacy of linezolid or daptomycin as an alternative to vancomycin for left-sided, methicillin-resistant *S. aureus* (MRSA) endocarditis has not been established.

Methicillin-susceptible *S. aureus* endocarditis that is uncomplicated and limited to the tricuspid or pulmonic valve—a condition occurring almost exclusively in injection drug users—can often be treated with a 2-week course that combines oxacillin or nafcillin (but not vancomycin) with gentamicin. Prolonged fevers (≥5 days) during therapy suggest that these patients should receive standard therapy. Right-sided endocarditis caused by MRSA is treated for 4 weeks with standard doses of vancomycin or daptomycin (6 mg/kg as a single daily dose).

Staphylococcal prosthetic valve endocarditis is treated for 6–8 weeks with a multidrug regimen. Rifampin is an essential component because it kills staphylococci that are adherent to foreign material. Two other agents (selected on the basis of susceptibility testing) are combined with rifampin to prevent in vivo emergence of resistance. Because many staphylococci (particularly MRSA and *S. epidermidis*) are resistant to gentamicin, the utility of gentamicin or an alternative agent should be established before rifampin treatment is begun. If the isolate is resistant to gentamicin, another aminoglycoside or a fluoroquinolone (chosen in light of susceptibility results) or another active agent should be substituted for gentamicin.

Other Organisms In the absence of meningitis, endocarditis caused by *Streptococcus pneumoniae* with a penicillin MIC of ≤1.0 can be treated with IV penicillin (4 million units every 4 h), ceftriaxone (2 g/d as a single dose), or cefotaxime (at a comparable dosage). Infection caused by pneumococcal strains with a penicillin MIC of ≥2.0 should be treated with vancomycin. Until the strain's susceptibility to penicillin is established, therapy should consist of vancomycin plus ceftriaxone, especially if concurrent meningitis is suspected. *P. aeruginosa* endocarditis is treated with an antipseudomonal penicillin (ticarcillin or piperacillin) and high doses of tobramycin (8 mg/kg per day in three divided doses). Endocarditis caused by Enterobacteriaceae is treated with a potent β-lactam antibiotic plus an aminoglycoside.

Corynebacterial endocarditis is treated with penicillin plus an aminoglycoside (if the organism is susceptible to the aminoglycoside) or with vancomycin, which is highly bactericidal for most strains. Therapy for *Candida* endocarditis consists of amphotericin B plus flucytosine and early surgery; long-term (if not indefinite) suppression with an oral azole is advised. Caspofungin treatment of *Candida* endocarditis has been effective in sporadic cases; nevertheless, the role of echinocandins in this setting has not been established.

Empirical Therapy In designing and executing therapy without culture data (i.e., before culture results are known or when cultures are negative), clinical and epidemiologic clues to etiology must be weighed, and both the pathogens associated with the specific endocarditis syndrome and the hazards of suboptimal therapy must be considered. Thus empirical therapy for acute endocarditis in an injection drug user should cover MRSA and gram-negative bacilli. The initiation of treatment with vancomycin plus gentamicin immediately after blood is obtained for cultures covers these as well as many other potential causes. In the treatment of culture-negative episodes, marantic endocarditis must be excluded and fastidious organisms sought serologically. In the absence of confounding prior antibiotic therapy, it is unlikely that *S. aureus*, CoNS, or enterococcal infection will present with negative blood cultures. Thus, in this situation, these organisms are not the determinants of therapy for subacute endocarditis. Pending the availability of diagnostic data, blood culture–negative subacute native valve endocarditis is treated with ceftriaxone plus gentamicin; these two antimicrobial agents plus vancomycin should be used if prosthetic valves are involved.

Outpatient Antimicrobial Therapy Fully compliant patients who have sterile blood cultures, are afebrile during therapy, and have no clinical or echocardiographic findings that suggest an impending complication may complete therapy as outpatients. Careful follow-up and a stable home setting are necessary, as are predictable IV access and use of antimicrobial agents that are stable in solution.

Monitoring Antimicrobial Therapy The serum bactericidal titer—the highest dilution of the patient's serum during therapy that kills 99.9% of the standard inoculum of the infecting organism—is no longer recommended for assessment of standard regimens. However, in the treatment of endocarditis caused by unusual organisms, this measurement, although not standardized and difficult to interpret, may provide a patient-specific assessment of in vivo antibiotic effect. Serum concentrations of aminoglycosides and vancomycin should be monitored.

Antibiotic toxicities, including allergic reactions, occur in 25–40% of patients and commonly arise during the third week of therapy. Blood tests to detect renal, hepatic, and hematologic toxicity should be performed periodically.

In most patients, effective antibiotic therapy results in subjective improvement and resolution of fever within 5–7 days. Blood cultures should be repeated daily until sterile, rechecked if there is recrudescent fever, and performed again 4–6 weeks after therapy to document cure. Blood cultures become sterile within 2 days after the start of appropriate therapy when infection is caused by viridans streptococci, enterococci, or HACEK organisms. In *S. aureus* endocarditis, β-lactam therapy results in sterile cultures in 3–5 days, whereas positive cultures may persist for 7–9 days with vancomycin treatment. When fever persists for 7 days despite appropriate antibiotic therapy, patients should be evaluated for paravalvular abscess and for extracardiac abscesses (spleen, kidney) or complications (embolic events). Recrudescent fever raises the question of these complications, but also of drug reactions or complications of hospitalization. Serologic abnormalities (e.g., in C-reactive protein level, erythrocyte sedimentation rate, rheumatoid factor) resolve slowly and do not reflect response to treatment. Vegetations become smaller with effective therapy, but at 3 months after cure, half are unchanged and 25% are slightly larger.

SURGICAL TREATMENT Intracardiac and central nervous system complications of endocarditis are important causes of morbidity and death associated with this infection. In some cases, effective treatment for these complications requires surgery. Most of the clinical indications for surgical treatment of endocarditis are not absolute (Table 19-5). The risks and benefits as well as the timing of surgical treatment must therefore be individualized (Table 19-6).

Intracardiac Surgical Indications Most surgical interventions are warranted by intracardiac findings, detected most reliably by TEE. Because of the highly invasive nature of prosthetic valve endocarditis, as many as 40% of affected patients merit surgical treatment. In many patients, coincident rather than single intracardiac events necessitate surgery.

Congestive Heart Failure Moderate to severe refractory congestive heart failure caused by new or worsening valve dysfunction is the major indication for cardiac surgical treatment of endocarditis. Of patients with moderate to severe heart failure due to valve dysfunction who are treated medically, 60–90% die within 6 months. In this setting, surgical treatment improves outcome, with mortality rates of 20% in native valve endocarditis and 35–55% in prosthetic valve infection. Surgery can relieve functional stenosis due to large vegetations or restore competence to damaged regurgitant valves.

Perivalvular Infection This complication, which occurs in 10–15% of native valve and 45–60% of prosthetic valve infections, is suggested by persistent unexplained fever during appropriate therapy, new electrocardiographic conduction disturbances, and pericarditis. Extension can occur from any valve but is most common with aortic valve infection. TEE with color Doppler is the test of choice to detect perivalvular abscesses (sensitivity, ≥85%). Although occasional perivalvular infections

TABLE 19-5

INDICATIONS FOR CARDIAC SURGICAL INTERVENTION IN PATIENTS WITH ENDOCARDITIS

Surgery required for optimal outcome
- Moderate to severe congestive heart failure due to valve dysfunction
- Partially dehisced unstable prosthetic valve
- Persistent bacteremia despite optimal antimicrobial therapy
- Lack of effective microbicidal therapy (e.g., fungal or *Brucella* endocarditis)
- *S. aureus* prosthetic valve endocarditis with an intracardiac complication
- Relapse of prosthetic valve endocarditis after optimal antimicrobial therapy

Surgery to be strongly considered for improved outcome[a]
- Perivalvular extension of infection
- Poorly responsive *S. aureus* endocarditis involving the aortic or mitral valve
- Large (>10-mm diameter) hypermobile vegetations with increased risk of embolism
- Persistent unexplained fever (≥10 days) in culture-negative native valve endocarditis
- Poorly responsive or relapsed endocarditis due to highly antibiotic-resistant enterococci or gram-negative bacilli

[a]Surgery must be carefully considered; findings are often combined with other indications to prompt surgery.

are cured medically, surgery is warranted when fever persists, fistulae develop, prostheses are dehisced and unstable, and invasive infection relapses after appropriate treatment. Cardiac rhythm must be monitored since high-grade heart block may require insertion of a pacemaker.

Uncontrolled Infection Continued positive blood cultures or otherwise-unexplained persistent fevers (in patients with either blood culture–positive or –negative endocarditis) despite optimal antibiotic therapy may reflect uncontrolled infection and may warrant surgery. Surgical treatment is also advised for endocarditis caused by organisms against which clinical experience indicates that effective antimicrobial therapy is lacking. This category includes infections caused by yeasts, fungi, *P. aeruginosa*, other highly resistant gram-negative bacilli, *Brucella* species, and probably *C. burnetii*.

S. Aureus *Endocarditis* Mortality rates for *S. aureus* prosthetic valve endocarditis exceed 70% with medical treatment but are reduced to 25% with surgical treatment. In patients with intracardiac complications associated with *S. aureus* prosthetic valve infection, surgical treatment reduces the mortality rate twentyfold. Surgical treatment should be considered for patients with *S. aureus* native aortic or mitral valve infection who have TTE-demonstrable vegetations and remain septic during the initial week of therapy. Isolated tricuspid valve endocarditis, even with persistent fever, rarely requires surgery.

TABLE 19-6

TIMING OF CARDIAC SURGICAL INTERVENTION IN PATIENTS WITH ENDOCARDITIS

	INDICATION FOR SURGICAL INTERVENTION	
TIMING	**STRONG SUPPORTING EVIDENCE**	**CONFLICTING EVIDENCE, BUT MAJORITY OF OPINIONS FAVOR SURGERY**
Emergent (same day)	Acute aortic regurgitation plus preclosure of mitral valve Sinus of Valsalva abscess ruptured into right heart Rupture into pericardial sac	
Urgent (within 1–2 days)	Valve obstruction by vegetation Unstable (dehisced) prosthesis Acute aortic or mitral regurgitation with heart failure (New York Heart Association class III or IV) Septal perforation Perivalvular extension of infection with/without new electrocardiographic conduction system changes Lack of effective antibiotic therapy	Major embolus plus persisting large vegetation (>10 mm in diameter)
Elective (earlier usually preferred)	Progressive paravalvular prosthetic regurgitation Valve dysfunction plus persisting infection after ≥7–10 days of antimicrobial therapy Fungal (mold) endocarditis	Staphylococcal PVE Early PVE (≤2 months after valve surgery) Fungal endocarditis (*Candida* spp.) Antibiotic-resistant organisms

Note: PVE, prosthetic valve endocarditis.
Source: Adapted from L Olaison, G Pettersson: Infect Dis Clin North Am 16:453, 2002.

Prevention of Systemic Emboli Death and persisting morbidity due to emboli are largely limited to patients suffering occlusion of cerebral or coronary arteries. Echocardiographic determination of vegetation size and anatomy, although predictive of patients at high risk of systemic emboli, does not identify those patients in whom the benefits of surgery to prevent emboli clearly exceed the risks of the surgical procedure and an implanted prosthetic valve. Net benefits favoring surgery are most likely when the risk of embolism is high and other surgical benefits can be achieved simultaneously—e.g., repair of a moderately dysfunctional valve or debridement of a paravalvular abscess. Reduced overall risks of surgical intervention (e.g., use of vegetation resection and valve repair to avoid insertion of a prosthesis) make the benefit-to-risk ratio more favorable and this intervention more attractive.

Timing of Cardiac Surgery In general, when indications for surgical treatment of infective endocarditis are identified, surgery should not be delayed simply to permit additional antibiotic therapy, since this course of action increases the risk of death (Table 19-6). Delay is justified only when infection is controlled and congestive heart failure is fully compensated with medical therapy. After 14 days of recommended antibiotic therapy, excised valves are culture-negative in 99% and 50% of patients with streptococcal and *S. aureus* endocarditis, respectively. Recrudescent endocarditis involving a new implanted prosthetic valve follows surgery in 2% of patients with culture-positive native valve endocarditis and in 6–15% of patients with active prosthetic valve endocarditis. These risks are more acceptable than the high mortality rates that result when surgery is inappropriately delayed or not performed.

Among patients who have experienced a neurologic complication of endocarditis, further neurologic deterioration can occur as a consequence of cardiac surgery. The risk of significant neurologic exacerbation is related to the interval between the complication and the surgery. Whenever feasible, cardiac surgery should be delayed for 2–3 weeks after a nonhemorrhagic embolic stroke and for 4 weeks after a hemorrhagic embolic stroke. A ruptured mycotic aneurysm should be clipped and cerebral edema allowed to resolve before cardiac surgery.

Antibiotic Therapy after Cardiac Surgery Bacteria visible in Gram-stained preparations of excised valves do not necessarily indicate a failure of antibiotic therapy. Organisms have been detected on Gram's stain—or their DNA has been detected by PCR—in excised valves from 45% of patients who have successfully completed the recommended therapy for endocarditis. In only 7% of these patients are the organisms, most of which are unusual and antibiotic resistant, cultured from the valve. Despite the detection of organisms or their DNA, relapse of endocarditis after surgery is uncommon. Thus, for uncomplicated native valve infection caused by susceptible organisms in conjunction with negative valve cultures, the duration of preoperative plus postoperative treatment should equal the total duration of recommended therapy, with ~2 weeks of treatment administered after surgery. For endocarditis complicated by paravalvular abscess, partially treated prosthetic valve infection, or cases with culture-positive valves, a full course of therapy should be given postoperatively.

Extracardiac Complications Splenic abscess develops in 3–5% of patients with endocarditis. Effective therapy requires either image-guided percutaneous drainage or splenectomy. Mycotic aneurysms occur in 2–15% of endocarditis patients; half of these cases involve the cerebral arteries and present as headaches, focal neurologic symptoms, or hemorrhage. Cerebral aneurysms should be monitored by angiography. Some will resolve with effective antimicrobial therapy, but those that persist, enlarge, or leak should be treated surgically if possible. Extracerebral aneurysms present as local pain, a mass, local ischemia, or bleeding; these aneurysms are treated by resection.

OUTCOME

Older age, severe comorbid conditions, delayed diagnosis, involvement of prosthetic valves or the aortic valve, an invasive (*S. aureus*) or antibiotic-resistant (*P. aeruginosa*, yeast) pathogen, intracardiac complications, and major neurologic complications adversely impact outcome. Death and poor outcome often are related not to failure of antibiotic therapy, but rather to the interactions of comorbidities and endocarditis-related end-organ complications. Overall survival rates for patients with native valve endocarditis caused by viridans streptococci, HACEK organisms, or enterococci (susceptible to synergistic therapy) are 85–90%. For *S. aureus* native valve endocarditis in patients who do not inject drugs, survival rates are 55–70%, whereas 85–90% of injection drug users survive this infection. Prosthetic valve endocarditis beginning within 2 months of valve replacement results in mortality rates of 40–50%, whereas rates are only 10–20% in later-onset cases.

PREVENTION

Antibiotic prophylaxis has been recommended by the American Heart Association in conjunction with selected procedures considered to entail a risk for bacteremia and endocarditis. The benefits of prophylaxis, however, are not established and in fact may be modest: only 50% of patients presenting with native valve endocarditis know that they have a predisposing valve lesion, most endocarditis cases do not follow a procedure, and 35% of cases are caused by organisms not targeted by prophylaxis. Dental treatments, the procedures most widely accepted as predisposing to endocarditis, are no more frequent during the 3 months preceding endocarditis than in uninfected matched controls. Furthermore, the frequency and magnitude of bacteremia associated with dental procedures and routine daily activities (e.g., tooth brushing and flossing) are similar. Because patients undergo dental procedures infrequently, exposure of endocarditis-vulnerable cardiac structures to bacteremia-causing oral cavity organisms is notably greater from routine daily activities than from dental care. It is estimated that annual exposure of heart valves to bacteremia-causing organisms may be 5.6 million times greater from routine daily activity than from a tooth extraction. The relation of gastrointestinal and genitourinary procedures to subsequent endocarditis is more tenuous than that of dental procedures.

Antibiotic prophylaxis, if 100% effective, likely prevents only a small number of cases of endocarditis; nevertheless, it is possible that rare cases are prevented. Weighing the potential benefits, potential adverse events, and costs associated with antibiotic prophylaxis, the expert committee of the American Heart Association has dramatically restricted the recommendations for antibiotic prophylaxis. Prophylactic antibiotics (Table 19-7) are advised only for those patients at highest risk for severe morbidity or death from endocarditis (Table 19-8). Prophylaxis is recommended only for dental procedures wherein there is manipulation of gingival tissue or the periapical region of the teeth or perforation of the oral mucosa (including surgery on the respiratory tract). Although prophylaxis is not advised for patients undergoing gastrointestinal or genitourinary tract procedures, it is recommended that effective treatment be given to these high-risk patients before or when they undergo procedures on an infected genitourinary tract or on infected skin and related soft tissue. Maintaining good dental hygiene is also advised. (For further details, see *http://www.americanheart.org/presenter.jhtml?identifier=3047083.*)

TABLE 19-7

ANTIBIOTIC REGIMENS FOR PROPHYLAXIS OF ENDOCARDITIS IN ADULTS WITH HIGH-RISK CARDIAC LESIONS[a,b]

A. Standard oral regimen
   1. Amoxicillin 2.0 g PO 1 h before procedure
B. Inability to take oral medication
   1. Ampicillin 2.0 g IV or IM within 1 h before procedure
C. Penicillin allergy
   1. Clarithromycin or azithromycin 500 mg PO 1 h before procedure
   2. Cephalexin[c] 2.0 g PO 1 h before procedure
   3. Clindamycin 600 mg PO 1 h before procedure
D. Penicillin allergy, inability to take oral medication
   1. Cefazolin[c] or ceftriaxone[c] 1.0 g IV or IM 30 min before procedure
   2. Clindamycin 600 mg IV or IM 1 h before procedure

[a]Dosing for children: for amoxicillin, ampicillin, cephalexin, or cefadroxil, use 50 mg/kg PO; cefazolin, 25 mg/kg IV; clindamycin, 20 mg/kg PO, 25 mg/kg IV; clarithromycin, 15 mg/kg PO; and vancomycin, 20 mg/kg IV.

[b]For high-risk lesions, see Table 19-8. Prophylaxis is not advised for other lesions.

[c]Do not use cephalosporins in patients with immediate hypersensitivity (urticaria, angioedema, anaphylaxis) to penicillin.

Source: W Wilson et al: Circulation, published online April 19, 2007.

TABLE 19-8

HIGH-RISK CARDIAC LESIONS FOR WHICH ENDOCARDITIS PROPHYLAXIS IS ADVISED BEFORE DENTAL PROCEDURES

Prosthetic heart valves
Prior endocarditis
Unrepaired cyanotic congenital heart disease, including palliative shunts or conduits
Completely repaired congenital heart defects during the 6 months after repair
Incompletely repaired congenital heart disease with residual defects adjacent to prosthetic material
Valvulopathy developing after cardiac transplantation

Source: W Wilson et al: Circulation, published online April 19, 2007.

FURTHER READINGS

American College of Cardiology/American Heart Association Task Force on Practice Guidelines et al: ACC/AHA 2006 guidelines for the management of patients with valvular heart disease: A report of the American College of Cardiology/American Heart Association Task Force on Practice Guidelines (writing committee to revise the 1998 Guidelines for the Management of Patients with Valvular Heart Disease): Developed in collaboration with the Society of Cardiovascular Anesthesiologists: Endorsed by the Society for Cardiovascular Angiography and Interventions and the Society of Thoracic Surgeons. Circulation 114:e84, 2006

Baddour LM et al: Diagnosis, antimicrobial therapy, and management of complications. A statement for healthcare professionals from the Committee on Rheumatic Fever, Endocarditis, and Kawasaki Disease, Council on Cardiovascular Disease in the Young, and the Councils on Clinical Cardiology, Stroke, and Cardiovascular Surgery and Anesthesia, American Heart Association. Circulation 111:e394, 2005

Durack DT (ed): Infective endocarditis. Infect Dis Clin North Am 16:255, 2002

Fowler VG Jr et al: Endocarditis and intravascular infections, in *Principles and Practice of Infectious Diseases*, 6th ed, GL Mandell et al (eds). Philadelphia, Elsevier Churchill Livingstone, 2005, pp 975–1021

Gavaldà J et al: Brief communication: Treatment of *Enterococcus faecalis* endocarditis with ampicillin plus ceftriaxone. Ann Intern Med 146:574, 2007

Horstkotte D et al: Guidelines on prevention, diagnosis and treatment of infective endocarditis. Executive summary, The Task Force on Infective Endocarditis of the European Society of Cardiology. Eur Heart J 25:267, 2004

Karchmer AW: Infective endocarditis, in *Heart Disease*, 8th ed, E Braunwald et al (eds). Philadelphia, Elsevier Saunders, 2007, in press

———, Longworth DL: Infections of intracardiac devices. Cardiol Clin 21:253, 2003

Li JS et al: Proposed modifications to the Duke criteria for the diagnosis of infective endocarditis. Clin Infect Dis 30:633, 2000

Moreillon P, Que YA: Infective endocarditis. Lancet 363:139, 2004

Morpeth S et al: Non-HACEK gram-negative bacillus endocarditis. Ann Intern Med 147:829, 2007

Morris AJ et al: Bacteriological outcome after valve surgery for active infective endocarditis: Implications for duration of treatment after surgery (abstract). Clin Infect Dis 41:187, 2005

VERHAGEN DW et al: Prognostic value of serial C-reactive protein measurements in left-sided native valve endocarditis. Arch Intern Med 168:302, 2008

VIKRAM HR et al: Impact of valve surgery on 6-month mortality in adults with complicated, left-sided native valve endocarditis: A propensity analysis. JAMA 290:3207, 2003

WILSON W et al: Prevention of infective endocarditis: Guidelines from the American Heart Association. A guideline from the American Heart Association Rheumatic Fever, Endocarditis, and Kawasaki Disease Committee, Council on Cardiovascular Disease in the Young, and the Council on Clinical Cardiology, Council on Cardiovascular Surgery and Anesthesia, and the Quality of Care and Outcomes Research Interdisciplinary Working Group. J Am Dent Assoc 138:739, 2007

CHAPTER 20

PERICARDIAL DISEASE

Eugene Braunwald

NORMAL FUNCTIONS OF THE PERICARDIUM

The normal pericardium is a double-layered sac; the visceral pericardium is a serous membrane that is separated by a small quantity (15–50 mL) of fluid, an ultrafiltrate of plasma, from the fibrous parietal pericardium. The normal pericardium, by exerting a restraining force, prevents sudden dilation of the cardiac chambers, especially of the right atrium and ventricle, during exercise and with hypervolemia. It also restricts the anatomic position of the heart, minimizes friction between the heart and surrounding structures, prevents displacement of the heart and kinking of the great vessels, and probably retards the spread of infections from the lungs and pleural cavities to the heart. Notwithstanding the foregoing, total absence of the pericardium, either congenital or after surgery, does not produce obvious clinical disease. In partial left pericardial defects, the main pulmonary artery and left atrium may bulge through the defect; very rarely, herniation and subsequent strangulation of the left atrium may cause sudden death.

ACUTE PERICARDITIS

Acute pericarditis, by far the most common pathologic process involving the pericardium, may be classified both clinically and etiologically (Table 20-1). Pain, a pericardial friction rub, electrocardiographic changes, and pericardial effusion with cardiac tamponade and paradoxical pulse are cardinal manifestations of many forms of acute pericarditis.

Chest pain is an important but not invariable symptom in various forms of acute pericarditis; it is usually present in the acute infectious types and in many of the forms presumed to be related to hypersensitivity or autoimmunity. Pain is often absent in slowly developing tuberculous, postirradiation, neoplastic, or uremic pericarditis. The pain of acute pericarditis is often severe, retrosternal and left precordial, and referred to the neck, arms, or the left shoulder. Often the pain is pleuritic, consequent to accompanying pleural inflammation, i.e., sharp and aggravated by inspiration, coughing, and changes in body position, but sometimes it is a steady, constricting pain that radiates into either arm or both arms and resembles that of myocardial ischemia; therefore, confusion with acute myocardial infarction (AMI) is common. Characteristically, however, pericardial pain may be relieved by sitting up and leaning forward and is intensified by lying supine. The differentiation of AMI from acute pericarditis becomes perplexing when, with acute pericarditis, serum biomarkers of myocardial damage such as creatine kinase and troponin rise, presumably because of concomitant involvement of the epicardium in the inflammatory process (an epi-myocarditis) with resulting myocyte necrosis. However, these elevations, if they occur, are quite modest, given the extensive electrocardiographic ST-segment elevation in pericarditis. This dissociation is useful in the differentiation between these conditions.

The *pericardial friction rub,* audible in about 85% of patients, may have up to three components per cardiac cycle, is high-pitched, and is described as rasping, scratching, or grating; it can be elicited sometimes only when the diaphragm of the stethoscope is applied firmly to the chest wall at the left lower sternal border. It is heard most frequently at end-expiration with the patient upright and leaning forward. The rub is often inconstant, and the loud to-and-fro leathery sound may disappear within a few hours, possibly to reappear on the following day. A pericardial rub is heard throughout the respiratory cycle, whereas a pleural rub disappears when respiration is suspended.

TABLE 20-1

CLASSIFICATION OF PERICARDITIS

Clinical Classification

I. Acute pericarditis (<6 weeks)
  A. Fibrinous
  B. Effusive (serous or sanguineous)
II. Subacute pericarditis (6 weeks to 6 months)
  A. Effusive-constrictive
  B. Constrictive
III. Chronic pericarditis (>6 months)
  A. Constrictive
  B. Effusive
  C. Adhesive (nonconstrictive)

Etiologic Classification

I. Infectious pericarditis
  A. Viral (coxsackievirus A and B, echovirus, mumps, adenovirus, hepatitis, HIV)
  B. Pyogenic (pneumococcus, *Streptococcus, Staphylococcus, Neisseria, Legionella*)
  C. Tuberculous
  D. Fungal (histoplasmosis, coccidioidomycosis, *Candida,* blastomycosis)
  E. Other infections (syphilitic, protozoal, parasitic)
II. Noninfectious pericarditis
  A. Acute myocardial infarction
  B. Uremia
  C. Neoplasia
    1. Primary tumors (benign or malignant, mesothelioma)
    2. Tumors metastatic to pericardium (lung and breast cancer, lymphoma, leukemia)
  D. Myxedema
  E. Cholesterol
  F. Chylopericardium
  G. Trauma
    1. Penetrating chest wall
    2. Nonpenetrating
  H. Aortic dissection (with leakage into pericardial sac)
  I. Postirradiation
  J. Familial Mediterranean fever
  K. Familial pericarditis
    1. Mulibrey nanism[a]
  L. Acute idiopathic
  M. Whipple's disease
  N. Sarcoidosis
III. Pericarditis presumably related to hypersensitivity or autoimmunity
  A. Rheumatic fever
  B. Collagen vascular disease (SLE, rheumatoid arthritis, ankylosing spondylitis, scleroderma, acute rheumatic fever, Wegener's granulomatosis)
  C. Drug-induced (e.g., procainamide, hydralazine, phenytoin, isoniazid, minoxidil, anticoagulants, methysergide)
  D. Postcardiac injury
    1. Postmyocardial infarction (Dressler's syndrome)
    2. Postpericardiotomy
    3. Posttraumatic

[a]An autosomal recessive syndrome, characterized by growth failure, muscle hypotonia, hepatomegaly, ocular changes, enlarged cerebral ventricles, mental retardation, ventricular hypertrophy, and chronic constrictive pericarditis.

The *electrocardiogram* (ECG) in acute pericarditis without massive effusion usually displays changes secondary to acute subepicardial inflammation (Fig. 20-1). It typically evolves through four stages. In stage 1, there is widespread elevation of the ST segments, often with upward concavity, involving two or three standard limb leads and V_2 to V_6, with reciprocal depressions only in aVR and sometimes V_1, as well as PR-segment depression. Usually there are no significant changes in QRS complexes. In stage 2, after several days, the ST segments return to normal, and only then, or even later, do the T waves become inverted (stage 3). Ultimately, weeks or months after the onset of acute pericarditis, the ECG returns to normal in stage 4. In contrast, in AMI, ST elevations are convex, and reciprocal depression is usually more prominent; QRS changes occur, particularly the development of Q waves, as well as notching and loss of R-wave amplitude; and T-wave inversions are usually seen within hours *before* the ST segments have become isoelectric. Sequential ECGs are useful in distinguishing acute pericarditis from AMI. In the latter, elevated ST segments return to normal within hours.

Early repolarization is a normal variant and may also be associated with widespread ST-segment elevation, most prominent in left precordial leads. However, in this condition, the T waves are usually tall and the ST/T ratio is <0.25; importantly, this ratio is higher in acute pericarditis. Depression of the PR segment (below the TP segment) is also common and reflects atrial involvement.

PERICARDIAL EFFUSION

In acute pericarditis, effusion is usually associated with pain and/or the above-mentioned ECG changes, as well as with an enlargement of the cardiac silhouette. Pericardial effusion is especially important clinically when it develops within a relatively short time, as it may lead to cardiac tamponade (see below). Differentiation from cardiac enlargement may be difficult on physical examination, but heart sounds may be fainter with pericardial effusion. The friction rub may disappear, and the apex impulse may vanish, but sometimes it remains palpable, albeit medial to the left border of cardiac dullness. The base of the left lung may be compressed by pericardial fluid, producing *Ewart's sign*, a patch of dullness and increased fremitus (and egophony) beneath the angle of the left scapula. The chest roentgenogram may show a "water bottle" configuration of the cardiac silhouette (Fig. 20-2) but may also be normal.

Diagnosis

Echocardiography is the most effective imaging technique available since it is sensitive, specific, simple, noninvasive, may be performed at the bedside, and can identify accompanying cardiac tamponade (see below) (Fig. 20-3). The presence of pericardial fluid is recorded by two-dimensional transthoracic echocardiography as a relatively echo-free space between the posterior pericardium and left ventricular epicardium in patients with small effusions, and as a space between the anterior right ventricle and the parietal pericardium just beneath the anterior chest wall in those with larger effusions. In the latter the

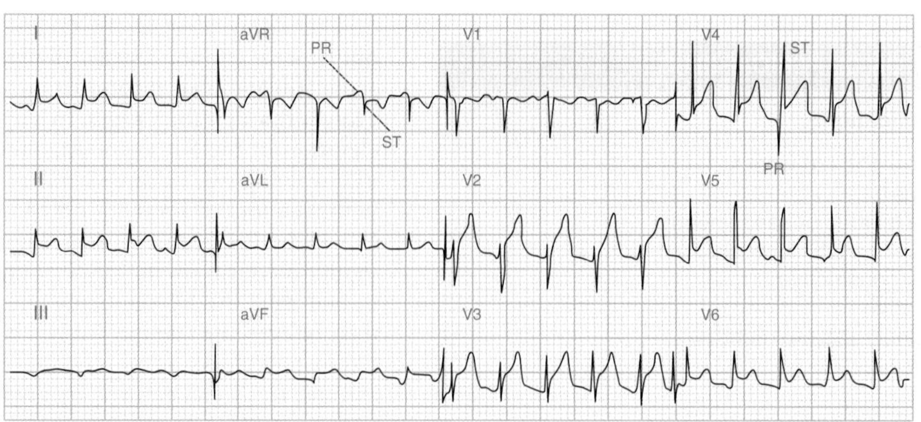

FIGURE 20-1
Acute pericarditis often produces diffuse ST-segment elevations (in this case in leads I, II, aVF, and V_2 to V_6) due to a ventricular current of injury. Note also the characteristic PR-segment deviation (opposite in polarity to the ST segment) due to a concomitant atrial injury current.

heart may swing freely within the pericardial sac. When severe, the extent of this motion alternates and may be associated with electrical alternans. Echocardiography allows localization and estimation of the quantity of pericardial fluid.

The diagnosis of pericardial fluid or thickening may be confirmed by computed tomography (CT) or magnetic resonance imaging (MRI) (Fig. 20-4). These techniques may be superior to echocardiography in detecting loculated pericardial effusions, pericardial thickening, and the presence of pericardial masses.

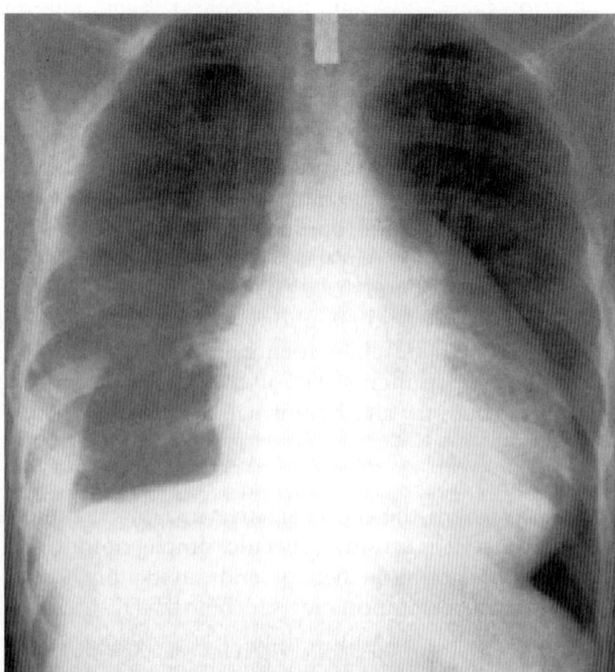

FIGURE 20-2
Chest radiogram from a patient with a pericardial effusion showing typical "water bottle" heart. There is also a right pleural effusion.[*From SS Kabbani, M LeWinter, in MH Crawford et al (eds): Cardiology. London, Mosby, 2001.*]

CARDIAC TAMPONADE

The accumulation of fluid in the pericardial space in a quantity sufficient to cause serious obstruction to the inflow of blood to the ventricles results in cardiac tamponade. This complication may be fatal if it is not recognized and treated promptly. The three most common causes of tamponade are neoplastic disease, idiopathic pericarditis,

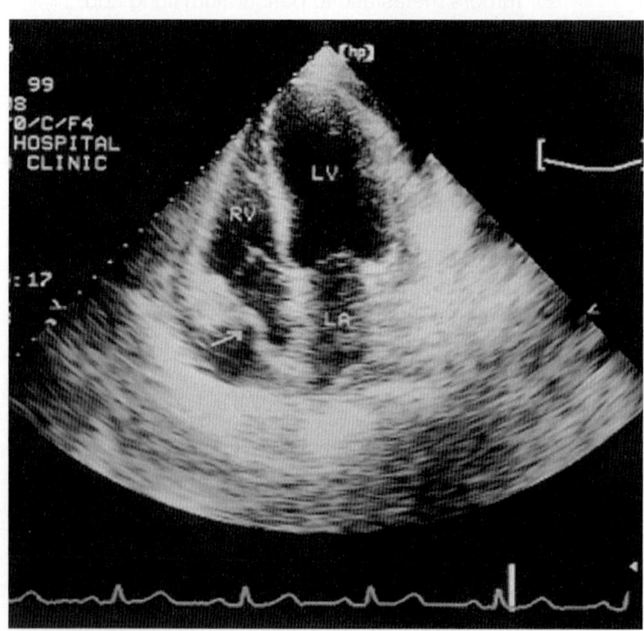

FIGURE 20-3
Apical four-chamber echocardiogram recorded in a patient with a moderate pericardial effusion and evidence of hemodynamic compromise. The frame is recorded in early ventricular systole, immediately after atrial contraction. Note that the right atrial wall is indented inward and its curvature is frankly reversed (*arrow*), implying elevated intrapericardial pressure above right atrial pressure. LA, left atrium; LV, left ventricle; RV, right ventricle. [*From WF Armstrong: Echocardiography, in DP Zipes et al (eds): Braunwald's Heart Disease, 7th ed. Philadelphia, Elsevier, 2005.*]

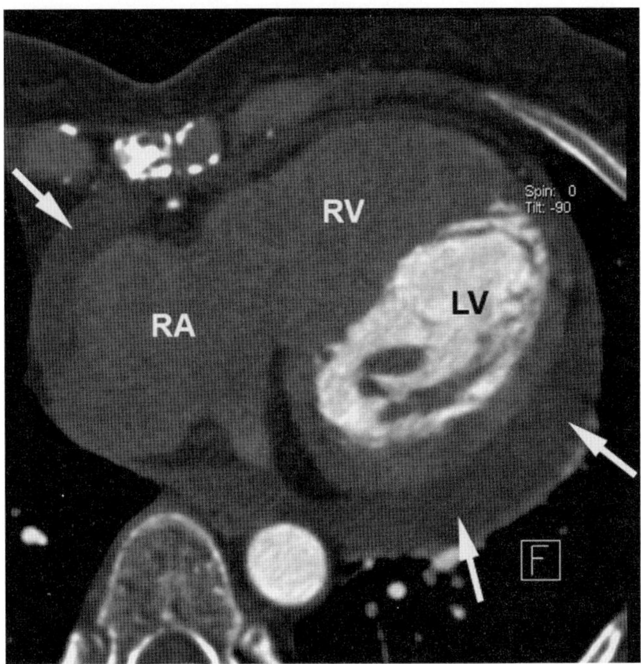

FIGURE 20-4

Chronic pericardial effusion in a 54-year-old female patient with Hodgkin's disease seen in contrast-enhanced 64-slice CT. The arrows point at the pericardial effusion (LV, left ventricle; RV, right ventricle; RA, right atrium). Due to the timing of the scan relative to contrast injection, only the blood in the left ventricle is contrast-enhanced, hence the low attenuation in the right-sided chambers. (*Courtesy of Stephan Achenbach, MD; with permission.*)

and pericardial effusion secondary to renal failure. Tamponade may also result from bleeding into the pericardial space either after cardiac operations and trauma (including cardiac perforation during cardiac catheterization, percutaneous coronary intervention, or insertion of pacemaker wires) or from tuberculosis and hemopericardium. The latter may occur when a patient with any form of acute pericarditis is treated with anticoagulants.

The three principal features of tamponade (*Beck's triad*) are hypotension, soft or absent heart sounds, and jugular venous distention with a prominent x descent but an absent y descent. There are both limitation of ventricular filling and reduction of cardiac output. The quantity of fluid necessary to produce this critical state may be as small as 200 mL when the fluid develops rapidly or >2000 mL in slowly developing effusions when the pericardium has had the opportunity to stretch and adapt to an increasing volume. The volume of fluid required to produce tamponade also varies directly with the thickness of the ventricular myocardium and inversely with the thickness of the parietal pericardium.

Tamponade may also develop more slowly, and under these circumstances the clinical manifestations may resemble those of heart failure, including dyspnea, orthopnea, and hepatic engorgement. A high index of suspicion for cardiac tamponade is required since, in many instances, no obvious cause for pericardial disease is apparent, and it should be considered in any patient with hypotension and elevation of jugular venous pressure. Otherwise unexplained enlargement of the cardiac silhouette (especially in subacute or chronic tamponade), reduction in amplitude of the QRS complexes, and *electrical alternans* of the P, QRS, or T waves each should raise the suspicion of cardiac tamponade.

Table 20-2 lists the features that distinguish acute cardiac tamponade from constrictive pericarditis.

Paradoxical Pulse

This important clue to the presence of cardiac tamponade consists of a greater than normal (10 mmHg) inspiratory decline in systolic arterial pressure. When severe, it may be detected by palpating weakness or disappearance of the arterial pulse during inspiration, but usually sphygmomanometric measurement of systolic pressure during slow respiration is required.

Since both ventricles share a tight incompressible covering, i.e., the pericardial sac, the inspiratory enlargement of the right ventricle in cardiac tamponade compresses and reduces left ventricular volume; leftward bulging of the interventricular septum further reduces the left ventricular cavity as the right ventricle enlarges during inspiration. Thus in cardiac tamponade the normal inspiratory augmentation of right ventricular volume causes an exaggerated reciprocal reduction in left ventricular volume. Also, respiratory distress increases the fluctuations in intrathoracic pressure, which exaggerates the mechanism just described. Right ventricular infarction may resemble cardiac tamponade with hypotension, elevated jugular venous pressure, an absent y descent in the jugular venous pulse, and, occasionally, pulsus paradoxus. The differences between these two conditions are shown in Table 20-2.

Paradoxical pulse occurs not only in cardiac tamponade, but also in approximately one-third of patients with constrictive pericarditis (see below). This physical finding is not pathognomonic of pericardial disease because it may be observed in some cases of hypovolemic shock, acute and chronic obstructive airways disease, and pulmonary embolus.

Low-pressure tamponade refers to mild tamponade in which the intrapericardial pressure is increased from its slightly subatmospheric levels to +5 to +10 mmHg; in some instances, hypovolemia coexists. As a consequence, the central venous pressure is normal or only slightly elevated, whereas arterial pressure is unaffected and there is no paradoxical pulse. The patients are asymptomatic or complain of mild weakness and dyspnea. The diagnosis is aided by echocardiography, and both hemodynamic and clinical manifestations improve after pericardiocentesis.

Diagnosis

Since immediate treatment of cardiac tamponade may be life-saving, prompt measures to establish the diagnosis by echocardiography should be undertaken (Fig. 20-3). When pericardial effusion causes tamponade, Doppler ultrasound shows that tricuspid and pulmonic valve flow velocities increase markedly during inspiration, whereas

TABLE 20-2

FEATURES THAT DISTINGUISH CARDIAC TAMPONADE FROM CONSTRICTIVE PERICARDITIS AND SIMILAR CLINICAL DISORDERS

CHARACTERISTIC	TAMPONADE	CONSTRICTIVE PERICARDITIS	RESTRICTIVE CARDIOMYOPATHY	RVMI
Clinical				
Pulsus paradoxus	Common	Usually absent	Rare	Rare
Jugular veins				
Prominent *y* descent	Absent	Usually present	Rare	Rare
Prominent *x* descent	Present	Usually present	Present	Rare
Kussmaul's sign	Absent	Present	Absent	Present
Third heart sound	Absent	Absent	Rare	May be present
Pericardial knock	Absent	Often present	Absent	Absent
Electrocardiogram				
Low ECG voltage	May be present	May be present	May be present	Absent
Electrical alternans	May be present	Absent	Absent	Absent
Echocardiography				
Thickened pericardium	Absent	Present	Absent	Absent
Pericardial calcification	Absent	Often present	Absent	Absent
Pericardial effusion	Present	Absent	Absent	Absent
RV size	Usually small	Usually normal	Usually normal	Enlarged
Myocardial thickness	Normal	Normal	Usually increased	Normal
Right atrial collapse and RVDC	Present	Absent	Absent	Absent
Increased early filling, ↑mitral flow velocity	Absent	Present	Present	May be present
Exaggerated respiratory variation in flow velocity	Present	Present	Absent	Absent
CT/MRI				
Thickened/calcific pericardium	Absent	Present	Absent	Absent
Cardiac catheterization				
Equalization of diastolic pressures	Usually present	Usually present	Usually absent	Absent or present
Cardiac biopsy helpful?	No	No	Sometimes	No

Note: RV, right ventricle; RVMI, right ventricular myocardial infarction; RVDC, right ventricular diastolic collapse; ECG, electrocardiograph.
Source: From GM Brockington et al: Cardiol Clin 8:645, 1990, with permission.

pulmonic vein, mitral, and aortic flow velocities diminish. Often the right ventricular cavity is reduced in diameter, and there is late diastolic inward motion (collapse) of the right ventricular free wall and of the right atrium. Transesophageal echocardiography may be necessary to diagnose a loculated or hemorrhagic effusion responsible for cardiac tamponade.

℞ Treatment: CARDIAC TAMPONADE

Patients with acute pericarditis should be observed frequently for the development of an effusion; if a large effusion is present, the patient should be hospitalized and watched closely for signs of tamponade. Arterial and venous pressures and heart rate should be monitored or followed carefully and serial echocardiograms obtained.

PERICARDIOCENTESIS If manifestations of tamponade appear, echocardiographically guided pericardiocentesis using an apical, parasternal, or, most commonly, a subxiphoid approach must be carried out at once, as reduction of the elevated intrapericardial pressure may be life-saving. Intravenous saline may be administered as the patient is being readied for the procedure. Intrapericardial pressure should be measured before fluid is withdrawn, and the pericardial cavity should be drained as completely as possible. A small, multiholed catheter advanced over the needle inserted into the pericardial cavity may be left in place to allow draining of the pericardial space if fluid reaccumulates. Surgical drainage through a limited (subxiphoid) thoracotomy may be required in recurrent tamponade, when it is necessary to remove loculated effusions, and/or when it is necessary to obtain tissue for diagnosis.

Pericardial fluid obtained from an effusion often has the physical characteristics of an exudate. Bloody fluid is most commonly due to neoplasm in the United States and tuberculosis in developing nations but may also be found in the effusion of rheumatic fever, post-cardiac injury, and post-myocardial infarction, as well as in the pericarditis associated with renal failure or dialysis. Transudative pericardial effusions may occur in heart failure.

The pericardial fluid should be analyzed for red and white blood cells, and cytologic studies for cancer, microscopic studies, and cultures should be obtained.

The presence of DNA of *Mycobacterium tuberculosis* determined by polymerase chain reaction or an elevated adenosine deaminase activity (>30 U/L) strongly supports the diagnosis of tuberculous pericarditis (Chap. 66).

VIRAL OR IDIOPATHIC FORM OF ACUTE PERICARDITIS

In some cases of this common disorder, coxsackievirus A or B or the virus of influenza, echovirus, mumps, herpes simplex, chickenpox, adenovirus, cytomegalovirus, Epstein-Barr, or HIV has been isolated from pericardial fluid and/or appropriate elevations in viral antibody titers have been noted. In many instances, acute pericarditis occurs in association with illnesses of known viral origin and, presumably, are caused by the same agent. Commonly, there is an antecedent infection of the respiratory tract, but in many patients such an association is not evident, and viral isolation and serologic studies are negative. Pericardial effusion is a common cardiac manifestation of HIV; it is usually secondary to infection (often mycobacterial) or neoplasm, most frequently lymphoma. In full-blown AIDS, pericardial effusion is associated with a shortened survival (Chap. 90).

Most frequently, a viral causation cannot be established; the term *idiopathic acute pericarditis* is then appropriate. Viral or idiopathic acute pericarditis occurs at all ages but is more frequent in young adults, and is often associated with pleural effusions and pneumonitis. The almost simultaneous development of fever and precordial pain, often 10–12 days after a presumed viral illness, constitutes an important feature in the differentiation of acute pericarditis from AMI, in which pain precedes fever. The constitutional symptoms are usually mild to moderate, and a pericardial friction rub is often audible. The disease ordinarily runs its course in a few days to 4 weeks. The ST-segment alterations in the ECG usually disappear after 1 or more weeks, but the abnormal T waves may persist for several years and be a source of confusion in persons without a clear history of pericarditis.

Pleuritis and pneumonitis frequently accompany pericarditis. Accumulation of some pericardial fluid is common, and both tamponade and constrictive pericarditis are possible complications. Recurrent (relapsing) pericarditis occurs in about one-fourth of patients with acute idiopathic pericarditis. In a smaller number, there are multiple recurrences.

℞ Treatment: IDIOPATHIC ACUTE PERICARDITIS

Hyperimmune globulin has been reported to be beneficial in cytomegalovirus, adenovirus, and parvovirus pericarditis, whereas interferon α has been reported to be so in coxsackie B pericarditis. In acute idiopathic pericarditis there is no specific therapy, but bed rest and anti-inflammatory treatment with aspirin (2–4 g/d) may be given. If this is ineffective, one of the nonsteroidal anti-inflammatory drugs (NSAIDs), such as ibuprofen (400–800 mg qid) or colchicine (0.6 mg bid), is often effective. Glucocorticoids (e.g., prednisone, 40–80 mg daily) usually suppress the clinical manifestations of the acute illness and may be useful in patients in whom purulent bacterial pericarditis has been excluded and in patients with pericarditis secondary to connective tissue disorders and renal failure (see below). Anticoagulants should be avoided since their use could cause bleeding into the pericardial cavity and tamponade.

After the patient has been asymptomatic and afebrile for about a week, the dose of the NSAID may be tapered gradually. Colchicine may prevent recurrences, but when recurrences are multiple, frequent, disabling, continue beyond 2 years, and are not controlled by pulses of high doses of glucocorticoids, pericardiectomy may be carried out in an attempt to terminate the illness.

Postcardiac Injury Syndrome

Acute pericarditis may appear under a variety of circumstances that have one common feature: previous injury to the myocardium with blood in the pericardial cavity. The syndrome may develop after a cardiac surgery (postpericardiotomy syndrome); after cardiac trauma, blunt or penetrating; or after perforation of the heart with a catheter. Rarely, it follows AMI.

The clinical picture mimics acute viral or idiopathic pericarditis. The principal symptom is the pain of acute pericarditis, which usually develops 1 to 4 weeks after the cardiac injury (1 to 3 days after AMI) but sometimes appears only after an interval of months. Recurrences are common and may occur up to 2 years or more after the injury. Fever with temperature up to 40°C, pericarditis, pleuritis, and pneumonitis are the outstanding features, and the bout of illness usually subsides in 1 or 2 weeks. The pericarditis may be of the fibrinous variety or it may be a pericardial effusion, which is often serosanguineous, but rarely causes tamponade. Leukocytosis, an increased sedimentation rate, and electrocardiographic changes typical of acute pericarditis may also occur.

The mechanisms responsible for this syndrome have not been identified, but they are probably the result of a hypersensitivity reaction to antigen which originates from injured myocardial tissue and/or pericardium. Circulating myocardial antisarcolemmal and antifibrillar autoantibodies occur frequently, but their precise role has not been defined. Viral infection may also play an etiologic role, since antiviral antibodies are often elevated in patients who develop this syndrome after cardiac surgery.

Often no treatment is necessary aside from aspirin and analgesics. The management of pericardial effusion and tamponade is discussed above. When the illness is followed by a series of disabling recurrences, therapy with an NSAID, colchicine, or a glucocorticoid is usually effective.

DIFFERENTIAL DIAGNOSIS

Since there is no specific test for *acute idiopathic pericarditis*, the diagnosis is one of exclusion. Consequently, all other disorders that may be associated with acute fibrinous pericarditis must be considered. A common diagnostic error is mistaking acute viral or idiopathic pericarditis for AMI and vice versa. When acute fibrinous pericarditis is associated with AMI, it is characterized by fever, pain, and a friction rub in the first 4 days after the development of the infarct. ECG abnormalities (such as the appearance of Q waves, brief ST-segment elevations with reciprocal changes, and earlier T-wave changes in AMI) and the extent of the elevations of myocardial enzymes are helpful in differentiating pericarditis from AMI.

Pericarditis secondary to post-cardiac injury is differentiated from acute idiopathic pericarditis chiefly by timing. If it occurs within a few days or weeks of an AMI, a chest blow, a cardiac perforation, or cardiac operation, it may be justified to conclude that the two are probably related. If the infarct has been silent or the chest blow forgotten, the relationship to the pericarditis may not be recognized.

It is important to distinguish *pericarditis due to collagen vascular disease* from acute idiopathic pericarditis. Most important in the differential diagnosis is the pericarditis due to systemic lupus erythematosus (SLE) or drug-induced (procainamide or hydralazine) lupus. Pain is often present in pericarditis due to collagen vascular disease. Sometimes in SLE the pericarditis appears as an asymptomatic effusion and, rarely, tamponade develops. When pericarditis occurs in the absence of any obvious underlying disorder, the diagnosis of SLE may be suggested by a rise in the titer of antinuclear antibodies. Acute pericarditis is an occasional complication of *rheumatoid arthritis, scleroderma,* and *polyarteritis nodosa,* and other evidence of these diseases is usually obvious. Asymptomatic pericardial effusion is also frequent in these disorders. It is important to question every patient with acute pericarditis about the ingestion of procainamide, hydralazine, isoniazid, cromolyn, and minoxidil, since these drugs can cause this syndrome. The pericarditis of *acute rheumatic fever* is generally associated with evidence of severe pancarditis and with cardiac murmurs (Chap. 37).

Pyogenic (purulent) pericarditis is usually secondary to cardiothoracic operations, by extension of infection from the lungs or pleural cavities, from rupture of the esophagus into the pericardial sac, or rupture of a ring abscess in a patient with infective endocarditis, or can occur if septicemia complicates aseptic pericarditis. It is accompanied by fever, chills, septicemia, and evidence of infection elsewhere and generally has a poor prognosis. The diagnosis is made by examination of the pericardial fluid. Acute pericarditis may also complicate the viral, pyogenic, mycobacterial, and fungal infections that occur with HIV infection.

Pericarditis of renal failure occurs in up to one-third of patients with chronic uremia *(uremic pericarditis)*, is also seen in patients undergoing chronic dialysis with normal levels of blood urea and creatinine, and is termed *dialysis-associated pericarditis*. These two forms of pericarditis may be fibrinous and are generally associated with an effusion that may be sanguineous. A friction rub is common, but pain is usually absent or mild. Treatment with a nonsteroidal anti-inflammatory drug and intensification of dialysis are usually adequate. Occasionally, tamponade occurs and pericardiocentesis is required. When the pericarditis of renal failure is recurrent or persistent, a pericardial window should be created or pericardiectomy may be necessary.

Pericarditis due to *neoplastic diseases* results from extension or invasion of metastatic tumors (most commonly carcinoma of the lung and breast, malignant melanoma, lymphoma, and leukemia) to the pericardium; pain, atrial arrhythmias, and tamponade are complications that occur occasionally. Diagnosis is made by pericardial fluid cytology or pericardial biopsy. *Mediastinal irradiation* for neoplasm may cause acute pericarditis and/or chronic constrictive pericarditis after eradication of the tumor. Unusual causes of acute pericarditis include syphilis, fungal infection (histoplasmosis, blastomycosis, aspergillosis, and candidiasis), and parasitic infestation (amebiasis, toxoplasmosis, echinococcosis, trichinosis).

CHRONIC PERICARDIAL EFFUSIONS

Chronic pericardial effusions are sometimes encountered in patients without an antecedent history of acute pericarditis. They may cause few symptoms per se, and their presence may be detected by finding an enlarged cardiac silhouette on chest roentgenogram. Tuberculosis is a common cause (Chap. 66).

Other Causes

Myxedema may be responsible for chronic pericardial effusion that is sometimes massive but rarely, if ever, causes cardiac tamponade. The cardiac silhouette is markedly enlarged, and an echocardiogram distinguishes cardiomegaly from pericardial effusion. The diagnosis of myxedema can be confirmed by tests for thyroid function. Myxedematous pericardial effusion responds to thyroid hormone replacement.

Neoplasms, SLE, rheumatoid arthritis, mycotic infections, radiation therapy to the chest, pyogenic infections, and chylopericardium may also cause chronic pericardial effusion and should be considered and specifically sought in such patients.

Aspiration and analysis of the pericardial fluid are often helpful in diagnosis. Pericardial fluid should be analyzed as described on p. 227. Grossly sanguineous pericardial fluid results most commonly from a neoplasm, tuberculosis, renal failure, or slow leakage from an aortic aneurysm. Pericardiocentesis may resolve large effusions, but pericardiectomy may be required with recurrence. Intrapericardial instillation of sclerosing agents or antineoplastic agents (e.g., bleomycin) may be used to prevent reaccumulation of fluid.

CHRONIC CONSTRICTIVE PERICARDITIS

This disorder results when the healing of an acute fibrinous or serofibrinous pericarditis or the resorption of a chronic pericardial effusion is followed by obliteration of the pericardial cavity with the formation of granulation tissue. The latter gradually contracts and forms a firm scar, encasing the heart and interfering with filling of the ventricles. In developing nations where the condition is prevalent, a high percentage of cases is of tuberculous origin, but in North America this is now an infrequent cause. Chronic constrictive pericarditis may follow acute or relapsing viral or idiopathic pericarditis, trauma with organized blood clot, cardiac surgery of any type, mediastinal irradiation, purulent infection, histoplasmosis, neoplastic disease (especially breast cancer, lung cancer, and lymphoma), rheumatoid arthritis, SLE, and chronic renal failure with uremia treated by chronic dialysis. In many patients, the cause of the pericardial disease is undetermined, and in them an asymptomatic or forgotten bout of viral pericarditis, acute or idiopathic, may have been the inciting event.

The basic physiologic abnormality in patients with chronic constrictive pericarditis is the inability of the ventricles to fill because of the limitations imposed by the rigid, thickened pericardium or the tense pericardial fluid. In constrictive pericarditis, ventricular filling is unimpeded during early diastole, but it is reduced abruptly when the elastic limit of the pericardium is reached, whereas in cardiac tamponade, ventricular filling is impeded throughout diastole. In both conditions, ventricular end-diastolic and stroke volumes are reduced and the end-diastolic pressures in both ventricles and the mean pressures in the atria, pulmonary veins, and systemic veins are all elevated to similar levels, i.e., within 5 mmHg of one another. Despite these hemodynamic changes, myocardial function may be normal or only slightly impaired in chronic constrictive pericarditis. However, the fibrotic process may extend into the myocardium and cause myocardial scarring, and atrophy, and venous congestion may then be due to the combined effects of the pericardial and myocardial lesions.

In constrictive pericarditis, the right and left atrial pressure pulses display an M-shaped contour, with prominent *x* and *y* descents; the *y* descent, which is absent or diminished in cardiac tamponade, is the most prominent deflection in constrictive pericarditis; it reflects rapid early filling of the ventricles. The *y* descent is interrupted by a rapid rise in atrial pressure during early diastole, when ventricular filling is impeded by the constricting pericardium. These characteristic changes are transmitted to the jugular veins, where they may be recognized by inspection. In constrictive pericarditis, the ventricular pressure pulses in both ventricles exhibit characteristic "square root" signs during diastole. These hemodynamic changes, although characteristic, are not pathognomonic of constrictive pericarditis and may also be observed in cardiomyopathies characterized by restriction of ventricular filling (Table 20-2).

CLINICAL AND LABORATORY FINDINGS

Weakness, fatigue, weight gain, increased abdominal girth, abdominal discomfort, a protuberant abdomen, and edema are common. The patient often appears chronically ill, and in advanced cases there are anasarca, skeletal muscle wasting, and cachexia. Exertional dyspnea is common, and orthopnea may occur, although it is usually not severe. Acute left ventricular failure (acute pulmonary edema) is very uncommon. The cervical veins are distended and may remain so even after intensive diuretic treatment, and venous pressure may fail to decline during inspiration (*Kussmaul's sign*). The latter is frequent in chronic pericarditis but may also occur in tricuspid stenosis, right ventricular infarction, and restrictive cardiomyopathy.

The pulse pressure is normal or reduced. In about one-third of cases, a paradoxical pulse (p. 226) can be detected. Congestive hepatomegaly is pronounced and may impair hepatic function and cause jaundice; ascites is common and is usually more prominent than dependent edema. The apical pulse is reduced and may retract in systole (*Broadbent's sign*). The heart sounds may be distant; an early third heart sound, i.e., a pericardial knock, occurring 0.09–0.12 s after aortic valve closure at the cardiac apex, is often conspicuous; it occurs with the abrupt cessation of ventricular filling. A systolic murmur of tricuspid regurgitation may be present.

The *ECG* frequently displays low voltage of the QRS complexes and diffuse flattening or inversion of the T waves. Atrial fibrillation is present in about one-third of patients. The *chest roentgenogram* shows a normal or slightly enlarged heart; pericardial calcification is most common in tuberculous pericarditis.

Inasmuch as the usual physical signs of cardiac disease (murmurs, cardiac enlargement) may be inconspicuous or absent in chronic constrictive pericarditis, hepatic enlargement and dysfunction associated with jaundice and intractable ascites may lead to a mistaken diagnosis of hepatic cirrhosis. This error can be avoided if the neck veins are inspected carefully in patients with ascites and hepatomegaly. Given a clinical picture resembling hepatic cirrhosis, but with the added feature of distended neck veins, careful search for thickening of the pericardium by CT or MRI should be carried out and may disclose this curable or remediable form of heart disease.

The two-dimensional transthoracic *echocardiogram* typically shows pericardial thickening, dilatation of the inferior vena cava and hepatic veins, and a sharp halt in ventricular filling in early diastole, with normal ventricular systolic function and flattening of the left ventricular posterior wall. Atrial enlargement may be seen, especially in patients with long-standing constrictive physiology. There is a distinctive pattern of transvalvular flow velocity on Doppler flow-velocity echocardiography. During inspiration there is an exaggerated reduction in blood flow velocity in the pulmonary veins and across the mitral valve and a leftward shift of the ventricular septum; the opposite occurs during expiration. Diastolic flow velocity in the vena cavae into the right atrium and across the tricuspid valve increases in an exaggerated manner during inspiration and declines during expiration (Fig. 20-5). However, echocardiography cannot definitively exclude the diagnosis of constrictive pericarditis. MRI and CT scanning (Fig. 20-6) are more accurate than echocardiography in establishing or excluding the presence of a thickened pericardium. Pericardial thickening and even pericardial calcification, however, are not synonymous with constrictive pericarditis since they may occur without seriously impairing ventricular filling.

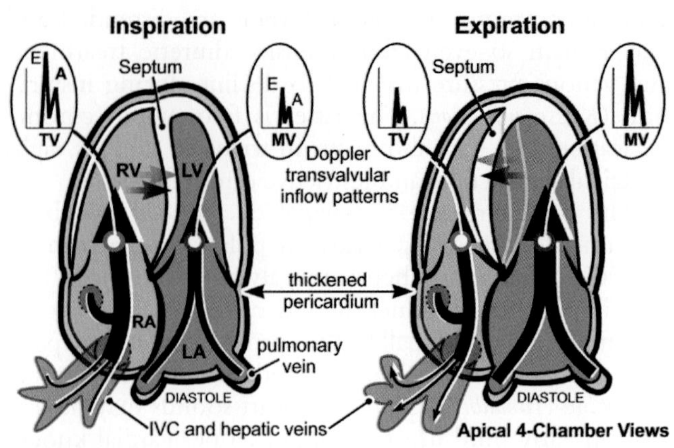

FIGURE 20-5

Constrictive pericarditis Doppler schema of respirophasic changes in mitral and tricuspid inflow. Reciprocal patterns of ventricular filling are assessed on pulsed Doppler examination of mitral (MV) and tricuspid (TV) inflow. (*Courtesy of Bernard E. Bulwer, MD; with permission*.)

DIFFERENTIAL DIAGNOSIS

Like chronic constrictive pericarditis, cor pulmonale may be associated with severe systemic venous hypertension but little pulmonary congestion; the heart is usually not enlarged, and a paradoxical pulse may be present. However, in cor pulmonale, advanced parenchymal pulmonary disease is usually obvious and venous pressure *falls* during inspiration, i.e., Kussmaul's sign is negative. *Tricuspid stenosis* may also simulate chronic constrictive pericarditis; congestive hepatomegaly, splenomegaly, ascites, and venous distention may be equally prominent. However, in tricuspid stenosis, a characteristic murmur as well as the murmur of accompanying mitral stenosis are usually present. In tricuspid stenosis, a paradoxical pulse and a steep, deep *y* descent in the jugular venous pulse do *not* occur, serving to differentiate it from chronic constrictive pericarditis.

Because constrictive pericarditis can be corrected surgically, it is important to distinguish chronic constrictive pericarditis from restrictive cardiomyopathy, which has a similar physiologic abnormality, i.e., restriction of ventricular filling. In many of these patients, the ventricular wall is thickened on echocardiographic examination (Table 20-2). The features favoring the diagnosis of restrictive cardiomyopathy over chronic constrictive pericarditis include a well-defined apex beat, cardiac enlargement, and pronounced orthopnea with attacks of acute left ventricular failure, left ventricular hypertrophy, gallop sounds (in place of a pericardial knock), bundle branch block, and, in some cases, abnormal Q waves on the ECG. The typical echocardiographic features of constrictive pericarditis (see above) are useful in the differential diagnosis in chronic constrictive pericarditis (Fig. 20-5). CT scanning (usually with contrast) and MRI are key in distinguishing between restrictive cardiomyopathy and chronic constrictive pericarditis. In the former, the ventricular walls are hypertrophied, whereas in the latter, the pericardium is thickened and sometimes calcified. When a patient has progressive, disabling, and unresponsive congestive heart failure and displays any of the features of constrictive heart disease, Doppler echocardiography to record respiratory effects on transvalvular flow and an MRI or CT scan should be obtained to detect or exclude constrictive pericarditis, since the latter is usually curable.

℞ Treatment: CONSTRICTIVE PERICARDITIS

Pericardial resection is the only definitive treatment of constrictive pericarditis, but dietary sodium restriction and diuretics are useful during preoperative preparation. Coronary arteriography should be carried out preoperatively in patients older than 50 years to exclude unsuspected coronary disease. The benefits derived

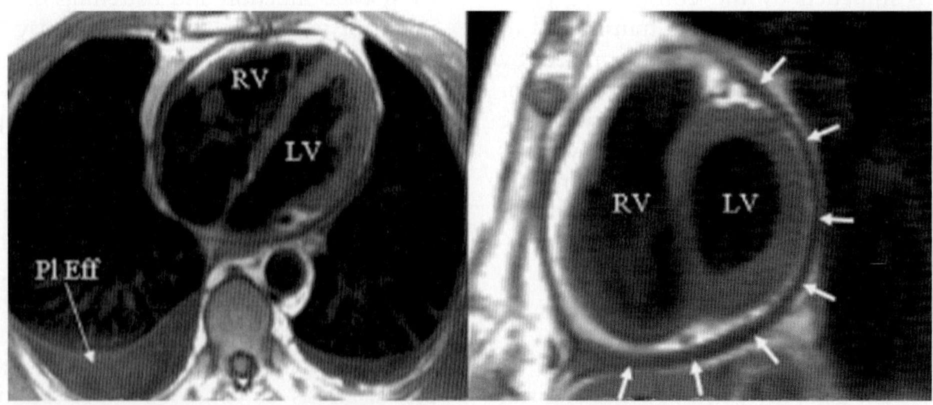

FIGURE 20-6

Cardiovascular magnetic resonance in a patient with constrictive pericarditis. On the right is a basal short-axis view of the ventricles showing a thickened pericardium encasing the heart (*arrows*). On the left is a transaxial view, again showing the thickened pericardium, particularly over the right heart, but also a pleural effusion (Pl Eff). LV, left ventricle; RV, right ventricle. [*From D Pennell: Cardiovascular magnetic resonance, in DP Zipes et al (eds): Braunwald's Heart Disease, 7th ed. Philadelphia, Elsevier, 2005.*]

from cardiac decortication are usually progressive over a period of months. The risk of this operation depends on the extent of penetration of the myocardium by the calcific process, by the severity of myocardial atrophy, by the extent of secondary impairment of hepatic and/or renal function, and by the patient's general condition. Operative mortality is in the range of 5–10%; the patients with the most severe disease are at highest risk. Therefore, surgical treatment should be carried out relatively early in the course.

Subacute Effusive-Constrictive Pericarditis

This form of pericardial disease is characterized by the combination of a tense effusion in the pericardial space and constriction of the heart by thickened pericardium. It shares a number of features both with chronic pericardial effusion producing cardiac compression and with pericardial constriction. It may be caused by tuberculosis (see below), multiple attacks of acute idiopathic pericarditis, radiation, traumatic pericarditis, renal failure, scleroderma, and neoplasms. The heart is generally enlarged, and a paradoxical pulse and a prominent x descent (without a prominent y descent) are present in the atrial and jugular venous pressure pulses. After pericardiocentesis, the physiologic findings may change from those of cardiac tamponade to those of pericardial constriction, with a "square root" sign in the ventricular pressure pulse and a prominent y descent in the atrial and jugular venous pressure pulses. Furthermore, the intrapericardial pressure and the central venous pressure may decline, but not to normal. The diagnosis can be established by pericardiocentesis followed by pericardial biopsy. In many patients, the condition progresses to the chronic constrictive form of the disease. Wide excision of both the visceral and parietal pericardium is usually effective therapy.

Tuberculous Pericardial Disease

This chronic infection is a common cause of chronic pericardial effusion, although less so in the United States than in Africa, Asia, the Middle East, and other parts of the developing world where active tuberculosis is endemic (Chap. 66). The clinical picture is that of a chronic, systemic illness in a patient with pericardial effusion. It is important to consider this diagnosis in a patient with known tuberculosis, with HIV, and with fever, chest pain, weight loss, and enlargement of the cardiac silhouette of undetermined origin. Inasmuch as treatment is quite effective, overlooking a tuberculous pericardial effusion may have serious consequences. If the etiology of chronic pericardial effusion remains obscure, despite detailed analysis of the pericardial fluid (see earlier), a pericardial biopsy, preferably by a limited thoracotomy, should be performed. If definitive evidence is then still lacking but the specimen shows granulomata with caseation, antituberculous chemotherapy (Chap. 66) is indicated.

If the biopsy specimen shows a thickened pericardium, pericardiectomy should be carried out in order to prevent the development of constriction, a serious complication of tuberculosis that occurs in about one-half of patients with tuberculous pericardial effusion despite treatment with chemotherapy and glucocorticoids. Tubercular cardiac constriction should be treated surgically while the patient is receiving antituberculous chemotherapy. In many patients, subacute effusive-constrictive pericarditis develops.

OTHER DISORDERS OF THE PERICARDIUM

Pericardial cysts appear as rounded or lobulated deformities of the cardiac silhouette, most commonly at the right cardiophrenic angle. They do not cause symptoms, and their major clinical significance lies in the possibility of confusion with a tumor, ventricular aneurysm, or massive cardiomegaly. *Tumors* involving the pericardium are most commonly secondary to malignant neoplasms originating in or invading the mediastinum, including carcinoma of the bronchus and breast, lymphoma, and melanoma. The most common *primary* malignant tumor is the mesothelioma. The usual clinical picture of malignant pericardial tumor is an insidiously developing, often bloody, pericardial effusion. Surgical exploration is required to establish a definitive diagnosis and to carry out definitive or, more commonly, palliative treatment.

FURTHER READINGS

AXEL L: Assessment of pericardial disease by magnetic resonance and computed tomography. J Magn Reson Imaging 19:816, 2004

HOIT BD: Management of effusive and constrictive pericardial heart disease. Circulation 105:2939, 2002

LANGE RA, HILLIS LD: Acute pericarditis. N Engl J Med 351:2195, 2004

LEWINTER M, KABBANI S: Pericardial diseases, in *Braunwald's Heart Disease*, 8th ed, D Zipes et al (eds). Philadelphia, Saunders, 2008

MAISCH B et al: Guidelines on the diagnosis and management of pericardial diseases executive summary: the Task Force on the Diagnosis and Management of Pericardial Diseases of the European Society of Cardiology. Eur Heart J 25:587, 2004

MAYOSI BM et al: Tuberculous pericarditis. Circulation 112:3608, 2005

PARIKH SV et al: Purulent pericarditis: Report of 2 cases and review of the literature. Medicine (Baltimore) 88:52, 2009

RAJAGOPALAN N et al: Comparison of new Doppler echocardiographic methods to differentiate constrictive pericardial heart disease and restrictive cardiomyopathy. Am J Cardiol 87:86, 2001

CHAPTER 21

INFECTIONS OF THE SKIN, MUSCLE, AND SOFT TISSUES

Dennis L. Stevens

ANATOMIC RELATIONSHIPS: CLUES TO THE DIAGNOSIS OF SOFT TISSUE INFECTIONS

Protection against infection of the epidermis depends on the mechanical barrier afforded by the stratum corneum, since the epidermis itself is devoid of blood vessels (Fig. 21-1). Disruption of this layer by burns or bites, abrasions, foreign bodies, primary dermatologic disorders (e.g., herpes simplex, varicella, ecthyma gangrenosum), surgery, or vascular or pressure ulcer allows penetration of bacteria to the deeper structures. Similarly, the hair follicle can serve as a portal either for components of the normal flora (e.g., *Staphylococcus*) or for extrinsic bacteria (e.g., *Pseudomonas* in hot-tub folliculitis). Intracellular infection of the squamous epithelium with vesicle formation may arise from cutaneous inoculation, as in infection with herpes simplex virus (HSV) type 1; from the dermal capillary plexus, as in varicella and infections due to other viruses associated with viremia; or from cutaneous nerve roots, as in herpes zoster. Bacteria infecting the epidermis, such as *Streptococcus pyogenes*, may be translocated laterally to deeper structures via lymphatics, an event that results in the rapid superficial spread of erysipelas. Later, engorgement or obstruction of lymphatics causes flaccid edema of the epidermis, another characteristic of erysipelas.

The rich plexus of capillaries beneath the dermal papillae provides nutrition to the stratum germinativum, and physiologic responses of this plexus produce important clinical signs and symptoms. For example, infective vasculitis of the plexus results in petechiae, Osler's nodes, Janeway's lesions, and palpable purpura, which, if present, are important clues to the existence of endocarditis (Chap. 19). In addition, metastatic infection within this plexus can result in cutaneous manifestations of disseminated fungal infection (Chap. 107), gonococcal infection (Chap. 45), *Salmonella* infection (Chap. 54), *Pseudomonas* infection (i.e., ecthyma gangrenosum; Chap. 53), meningococcemia (Chap. 44), and staphylococcal infection (Chap. 35). The plexus also provides bacteria with access to the circulation, thereby facilitating local spread or bacteremia. The postcapillary venules of this plexus are a major site of polymorphonuclear leukocyte sequestration, diapedesis, and chemotaxis to the site of cutaneous infection.

Exaggeration of these physiologic mechanisms by excessive levels of cytokines or bacterial toxins causes leukostasis, venous occlusion, and pitting edema. Edema with purple bullae, ecchymosis, and cutaneous anesthesia suggests loss of vascular integrity and necessitates exploration of the deeper structures for evidence of necrotizing fasciitis or myonecrosis. An early diagnosis requires a high level of suspicion in instances of unexplained fever and of pain and tenderness in the soft tissue, even in the absence of acute cutaneous inflammation.

Table 21-1 indicates the chapters in which the infections described below are discussed in greater detail. Many of these infections are illustrated in the chapters cited or in Chap. 10 (Atlas of Rashes Associated With Fever).

INFECTIONS ASSOCIATED WITH VESICLES

(Table 21-1) Vesicle formation due to infection is caused by viral proliferation within the epidermis. In varicella and variola, viremia precedes the onset of a diffuse centripetal rash that progresses from macules to vesicles, then to pustules, and finally to scabs over the course

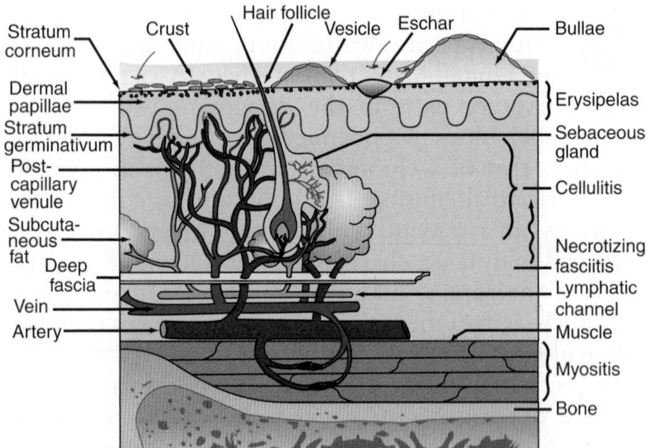

FIGURE 21-1
Structural components of the skin and soft tissue, superficial infections, and infections of the deeper structures. The rich capillary network beneath the dermal papillae plays a key role in the localization of infection and in the development of the acute inflammatory reaction.

TABLE 21-1

SKIN AND SOFT TISSUE INFECTIONS

LESION, CLINICAL SYNDROME	INFECTIOUS AGENT	CHAPTER(S)
Vesicles		
Smallpox	Variola virus	6
Chickenpox	Varicella-zoster virus	81
Shingles (herpes zoster)	Varicella-zoster virus	81
Cold sores, herpetic whitlow, herpes gladiatorum	Herpes simplex virus	80
Hand-foot-and-mouth disease	Coxsackievirus A16	94
Orf	Parapoxvirus	84
Molluscum contagiosum	Pox-like virus	84
Rickettsialpox	*Rickettsia akari*	75
Blistering distal dactylitis	*Staphylococcus aureus* or *Streptococcus pyogenes*	35, 36
Bullae		
Staphylococcal scalded-skin syndrome	*S. aureus*	35
Necrotizing fasciitis	*S. pyogenes*, *Clostridium* spp., mixed aerobes and anaerobes	36, 42, 65
Gas gangrene	*Clostridium* spp.	42
Halophilic vibrio	*Vibrio vulnificus*	57
Crusted lesions		
Bullous impetigo/ecthyma	*S. aureus*	35
Impetigo contagiosa	*S. pyogenes*	36
Ringworm	Superficial dermatophyte fungi	110
Sporotrichosis	*Sporothrix schenckii*	110
Histoplasmosis	*Histoplasma capsulatum*	103
Coccidioidomycosis	*Coccidioides immitis*	104
Blastomycosis	*Blastomyces dermatitidis*	105
Cutaneous leishmaniasis	*Leishmania* spp.	119
Cutaneous tuberculosis	*Mycobacterium tuberculosis*	66
Nocardiosis	*Nocardia asteroides*	63
Folliculitis		
Furunculosis	*S. aureus*	35
Hot-tub folliculitis	*Pseudomonas aeruginosa*	53
Swimmer's itch	*Schistosoma* spp.	126
Acne vulgaris	*Propionibacterium acnes*	...
Papular and nodular lesions		
Fish-tank or swimming-pool granuloma	*Mycobacterium marinum*	68
Creeping eruption (cutaneous larva migrans)	*Ancylostoma braziliense*	123
Dracunculiasis	*Dracunculus medinensis*	125
Cercarial dermatitis	*Schistosoma mansoni*	126
Verruca vulgaris	Human papillomaviruses 1, 2, 4	86
Condylomata acuminata (anogenital warts)	Human papillomaviruses 6, 11, 16, 18	86
Onchocerciasis nodule	*Onchocerca volvulus*	125
Cutaneous myiasis	*Dermatobia hominis*	...
Verruca peruana	*Bartonella bacilliformis*	61
Cat-scratch disease	*Bartonella henselae*	61
Lepromatous leprosy	*Mycobacterium leprae*	67
Secondary syphilis (papulosquamous, nodular, and condylomata lata lesions)	*Treponema pallidum*	70
Tertiary syphilis (nodular gummatous lesions)	*T. pallidum*	70
Ulcers with or without eschars		
Anthrax	*Bacillus anthracis*	6
Ulceroglandular tularemia	*Francisella tularensis*	6, 59
Bubonic plague	*Yersinia pestis*	6, 60
Buruli ulcer	*Mycobacterium ulcerans*	68
Leprosy	*M. leprae*	67
Cutaneous tuberculosis	*M. tuberculosis*	66
Chancroid	*Haemophilus ducreyi*	47
Primary syphilis	*T. pallidum*	70

(Continued)

TABLE 21-1 (CONTINUED)

SKIN AND SOFT TISSUE INFECTIONS

LESION, CLINICAL SYNDROME	INFECTIOUS AGENT	CHAPTER(S)
Erysipelas	*S. pyogenes*	36
Cellulitis	*Staphylococcus* spp., *Streptococcus* spp., various other bacteria	Various
Necrotizing fasciitis		
Streptococcal gangrene	*S. pyogenes*	36
Fournier's gangrene	Mixed aerobic and anaerobic bacteria	65
Staphylococcal necrotizing fasciitis	Methicillin-resistant *S. aureus*	35
Myositis and myonecrosis		
Pyomyositis	*S. aureus*	35
Streptococcal necrotizing myositis	*S. pyogenes*	36
Gas gangrene	*Clostridium* spp.	42
Nonclostridial (crepitant) myositis	Mixed aerobic and anaerobic bacteria	65
Synergistic nonclostridial anaerobic myonecrosis	Mixed aerobic and anaerobic bacteria	65

of 1–2 weeks. Vesicles of varicella have a "dewdrop" appearance and develop in crops randomly about the trunk, extremities, and face over 3–4 days. Herpes zoster occurs in a single dermatome; the appearance of vesicles is preceded by pain for several days. Zoster may occur in persons of any age but is most common among immunosuppressed individuals and elderly patients, whereas most cases of varicella occur in young children. Vesicles due to HSV are found on or around the lips (HSV-1) or genitals (HSV-2) but may appear on the head and neck of young wrestlers (herpes gladiatorum) or on the digits of health care workers (herpetic whitlow). Recurrent herpes labialis (HSV-1) and herpes genitalis commonly follow primary infection. Coxsackievirus A16 characteristically causes vesicles on the hands, feet, and mouth of children. Orf is caused by a DNA virus related to smallpox virus and infects the fingers of individuals who work around goats and sheep. Molluscum contagiosum virus induces flaccid vesicles on the skin of healthy and immunocompromised individuals. Although variola (smallpox) in nature was eradicated as of 1977, recent terrorist events have renewed interest in this devastating infection (Chap. 6). Viremia beginning after an incubation period of 12 days is followed by a diffuse maculopapular rash, with rapid evolution to vesicles, pustules, and then scabs. Secondary cases can occur among close contacts.

Rickettsialpox begins after mite-bite inoculation of *Rickettsia akari* into the skin. A papule with a central vesicle evolves to form a 1- to 2.5-cm painless crusted black eschar with an erythematous halo and proximal adenopathy. Although more common in the northeastern United States and the Ukraine in 1940–1950, rickettsialpox has recently been described in Ohio, Arizona, and Utah. Blistering dactylitis is a painful, vesicular, localized *Staphylococcus aureus* or group A streptococcal infection of the pulps of the distal digits of the hands.

INFECTIONS ASSOCIATED WITH BULLAE

(Table 21-1) Staphylococcal scalded-skin syndrome (SSSS) in neonates is caused by a toxin (exfoliatin) from phage group II *S. aureus*. SSSS must be distinguished from toxic epidermal necrolysis (TEN), which occurs primarily in adults, is drug-induced, and is associated with a higher mortality rate. Punch biopsy with frozen section is useful in making this distinction since the cleavage plane is the stratum corneum in SSSS and the stratum germinativum in TEN (Fig. 21-1). Intravenous γ-globulin is a promising treatment for TEN. Necrotizing fasciitis and gas gangrene also induce bulla formation (see "Necrotizing Fasciitis" later in the chapter). Halophilic vibrio infection can be as aggressive and fulminant as necrotizing fasciitis; a helpful clue in its diagnosis is a history of exposure to waters of the Gulf of Mexico or the Atlantic seaboard or (in a patient with cirrhosis) the ingestion of raw seafood. The etiologic organism (*Vibrio vulnificus*) is highly susceptible to tetracycline.

INFECTIONS ASSOCIATED WITH CRUSTED LESIONS

(Table 21-1) Impetigo contagiosa is caused by *S. pyogenes*, and bullous impetigo is due to *S. aureus*. Both skin lesions may have an early bullous stage but then appear as thick crusts with a golden-brown color. Epidemics of impetigo caused by methicillin-resistant *S. aureus* (MRSA) have been reported. Streptococcal lesions are most common among children 2–5 years of age, and epidemics may occur in settings of poor hygiene, particularly among children of lower socioeconomic status in tropical climates. It is important to recognize impetigo contagiosa because of its relationship to poststreptococcal glomerulonephritis. Rheumatic fever is not a complication of skin infection caused by *S. pyogenes*. Superficial dermatophyte infection (ringworm) can occur on any skin surface, and skin scrapings with KOH staining are diagnostic. Primary infections with dimorphic fungi such as *Blastomyces dermatitidis* and *Sporothrix schenckii* can initially present as crusted skin lesions resembling ringworm. Disseminated infection with *Coccidioides immitis* can also involve the skin, and biopsy and culture should be performed on crusted lesions in patients from endemic areas. Crusted nodular lesions caused by *Mycobacterium chelonei* have been described in HIV-seropositive patients. Treatment with clarithromycin looks promising.

FOLLICULITIS

(Table 21-1) Hair follicles serve as portals for a number of bacteria, although *S. aureus* is the most common cause of localized folliculitis. Sebaceous glands empty into hair follicles and ducts and, if blocked, form sebaceous cysts, which may resemble staphylococcal abscesses or may become secondarily infected. Infection of sweat glands (hidradenitis suppurativa) can also mimic infection of hair follicles, particularly in the axillae. Chronic folliculitis is uncommon except in acne vulgaris, where constituents of the normal flora (e.g., *Propionibacterium acnes*) may play a role.

Diffuse folliculitis occurs in two settings. Hot-tub folliculitis is caused by *Pseudomonas aeruginosa* in waters that are insufficiently chlorinated and maintained at temperatures of 37–40°C. Infection is usually self-limited, although bacteremia and shock have been reported. Swimmer's itch occurs when a skin surface is exposed to water infested with freshwater avian schistosomes. Warm water temperatures and alkaline pH are suitable for mollusks that serve as intermediate hosts between birds and humans. Free-swimming schistosomal cercariae readily penetrate human hair follicles or pores but quickly die and elicit a brisk allergic reaction, causing intense itching and erythema.

PAPULAR AND NODULAR LESIONS

(Table 21-1) Raised lesions of the skin occur in many different forms. *Mycobacterium marinum* infections of the skin may present as cellulitis or as raised erythematous nodules. Erythematous papules are early manifestations of cat-scratch disease (with lesions developing at the primary site of inoculation of *Bartonella henselae*) and bacillary angiomatosis (also caused by *B. henselae*). Raised serpiginous or linear eruptions are characteristic of cutaneous larva migrans, which is caused by burrowing larvae of dog or cat hookworms (*Ancylostoma braziliense*) and which humans acquire through contact with soil that has been contaminated with dog or cat feces. Similar burrowing raised lesions are present in dracunculiasis caused by migration of the adult female nematode *Dracunculus medinensis*. Nodules caused by *Onchocerca volvulus* measure 1–10 cm in diameter and occur mostly in persons bitten by *Simulium* flies in Africa. The nodules contain the adult worm encased in fibrous tissue. Migration of microfilariae into the eyes may result in blindness. Verruca peruana is caused by *Bartonella bacilliformis*, which is transmitted to humans by the sandfly *Phlebotomus*. This condition can take the form of single gigantic lesions (several centimeters in diameter) or multiple small lesions (several millimeters in diameter). Numerous subcutaneous nodules may also be present in cysticercosis caused by larvae of *Taenia solium*. Multiple erythematous papules develop in schistosomiasis; each represents a cercarial invasion site. Skin nodules as well as thickened subcutaneous tissue are prominent features of lepromatous leprosy. Large nodules or gummas are features of tertiary syphilis, whereas flat papulosquamous lesions are characteristic of secondary syphilis. Human papillomavirus may cause singular warts (verruca vulgaris) or multiple warts in the anogenital area (condylomata acuminata). The latter are major problems in HIV-infected individuals.

ULCERS WITH OR WITHOUT ESCHARS

(Table 21-1) Cutaneous anthrax begins as a pruritic papule, which develops within days into an ulcer with surrounding vesicles and edema and then into an enlarging ulcer with a black eschar. Cutaneous anthrax may cause chronic nonhealing ulcers with an overlying dirty-gray membrane, although lesions may also mimic psoriasis, eczema, or impetigo. Ulceroglandular tularemia may have associated ulcerated skin lesions with painful regional adenopathy. Although buboes are the major cutaneous manifestation of plague, ulcers with eschars, papules, or pustules are also present in 25% of cases.

Mycobacterium ulcerans typically causes chronic skin ulcers on the extremities of individuals living in the tropics. *Mycobacterium leprae* may be associated with cutaneous ulcerations in patients with lepromatous leprosy related to Lucio's phenomenon, in which immune-mediated destruction of tissue bearing high concentrations of *M. leprae* bacilli occurs, usually several months after initiation of effective therapy. *Mycobacterium tuberculosis* may also cause ulcerations, papules, or erythematous macular lesions of the skin in both normal and immunocompromised patients.

Decubitus ulcers are due to tissue hypoxia secondary to pressure-induced vascular insufficiency and may become secondarily infected with components of the skin and gastrointestinal flora, including anaerobes. Ulcerative lesions on the anterior shins may be due to pyoderma gangrenosum, which must be distinguished from similar lesions of infectious etiology by histologic evaluation of biopsy sites. Ulcerated lesions on the genitals may be either painful (chancroid) or painless (primary syphilis).

ERYSIPELAS

(Table 21-1) Erysipelas is due to *S. pyogenes* and is characterized by an abrupt onset of fiery-red swelling of the face or extremities. The distinctive features of erysipelas are well-defined indurated margins, particularly along the nasolabial fold; rapid progression; and intense pain. Flaccid bullae may develop during the second or third day of illness, but extension to deeper soft tissues is rare. Treatment with penicillin is effective; swelling may progress despite appropriate treatment, although fever, pain, and the intense red color diminish. Desquamation of the involved skin occurs 5–10 days into the illness. Infants and elderly adults are most commonly afflicted, and the severity of systemic toxicity varies.

CELLULITIS

(Table 21-1) Cellulitis is an acute inflammatory condition of the skin that is characterized by localized pain, erythema, swelling, and heat. Cellulitis may be caused by indigenous flora colonizing the skin and appendages (e.g., *S. aureus* and *S. pyogenes*) or by a wide variety of exogenous bacteria. Because the exogenous bacteria involved in cellulitis occupy unique niches in nature, a thorough history (including epidemiologic data) provides important clues to etiology. When there is drainage, an open wound, or an obvious portal of entry, Gram's stain and culture provide a definitive diagnosis. In the absence of these findings, the bacterial etiology of cellulitis is difficult to establish, and in some cases staphylococcal and streptococcal cellulitis may have similar features. Even with needle aspiration of the leading edge or a punch biopsy of the cellulitis tissue itself, cultures are positive in only 20% of cases. This observation suggests that relatively low numbers of bacteria may cause cellulitis and that the expanding area of erythema within the skin may be a direct effect of extracellular toxins or of the soluble mediators of inflammation elicited by the host.

Bacteria may gain access to the epidermis through cracks in the skin, abrasions, cuts, burns, insect bites, surgical incisions, and intravenous catheters. Cellulitis caused by *S. aureus* spreads from a central localized infection, such as an abscess, folliculitis, or an infected foreign body (e.g., a splinter, a prosthetic device, or an intravenous catheter). MRSA is rapidly replacing methicillin-sensitive *S. aureus* (MSSA) as a cause of cellulitis in both inpatient and outpatient settings. In contrast, cellulitis due to *S. pyogenes* is a more rapidly spreading, diffuse process frequently associated with lymphangitis and fever. Recurrent streptococcal cellulitis of the lower extremities may be caused by organisms of group A, C, or G in association with chronic venous stasis or with saphenous venectomy for coronary artery bypass surgery. Streptococci also cause recurrent cellulitis among patients with chronic lymphedema resulting from elephantiasis, lymph node dissection, or Milroy's disease. Recurrent staphylococcal cutaneous infections are more common among individuals who have eosinophilia and elevated serum levels of IgE (Job's syndrome) and among nasal carriers of staphylococci. Cellulitis caused by *Streptococcus agalactiae* (group B *Streptococcus*) occurs primarily in elderly patients and those with diabetes mellitus or peripheral vascular disease. *Haemophilus influenzae* typically causes periorbital cellulitis in children in association with sinusitis, otitis media, or epiglottitis. It is unclear whether this form of cellulitis will (like meningitis) become less common as a result of the impressive efficacy of the *H. influenzae* type b vaccine.

Many other bacteria also cause cellulitis. Fortunately, these organisms occur in such characteristic settings that a good history provides useful clues to the diagnosis. Cellulitis associated with cat bites and, to a lesser degree, with dog bites is commonly caused by *Pasteurella multocida*, although in the latter case *Staphylococcus intermedius* and *Capnocytophaga canimorsus* (formerly DF-2) must also be considered. Sites of cellulitis and abscesses associated with dog bites and human bites also contain a variety of anaerobic organisms, including *Fusobacterium*, *Bacteroides*, aerobic and anaerobic streptococci, and *Eikenella corrodens*. *Pasteurella* is notoriously resistant to dicloxacillin and nafcillin but is sensitive to all other β-lactam antimicrobial agents, as well as to quinolones, tetracycline, and erythromycin. Ampicillin/clavulanate, ampicillin/sulbactam, and cefoxitin are good choices for the treatment of animal or human bite infections. *Aeromonas hydrophila* causes aggressive cellulitis in tissues surrounding lacerations sustained in freshwater (lakes, rivers, and streams). This organism remains sensitive to aminoglycosides, fluoroquinolones, chloramphenicol, trimethoprim-sulfamethoxazole, and third-generation cephalosporins; it is resistant to ampicillin, however.

P. aeruginosa causes three types of soft tissue infection: ecthyma gangrenosum in neutropenic patients, hot-tub folliculitis, and cellulitis after penetrating injury. Most commonly, *P. aeruginosa* is introduced into the deep tissues when a person steps on a nail. Treatment includes surgical inspection and drainage, particularly if the injury also involves bone or joint capsule. Choices for empirical treatment while antimicrobial susceptibility data are awaited include an aminoglycoside, a third-generation cephalosporin (ceftazidime, cefoperazone, or cefotaxime), a semisynthetic penicillin (ticarcillin, mezlocillin, or piperacillin), or a fluoroquinolone (although drugs of the last class are not indicated for the treatment of children <13 years old).

Gram-negative bacillary cellulitis, including that due to *P. aeruginosa*, is most common among hospitalized, immunocompromised hosts. Cultures and sensitivity tests are critically important in this setting because of multidrug resistance (Chap. 53).

The gram-positive aerobic rod *Erysipelothrix rhusiopathiae* is most often associated with fish and domestic swine and causes cellulitis primarily in bone renderers and fishmongers. *E. rhusiopathiae* remains susceptible to most β-lactam antibiotics (including penicillin), erythromycin, clindamycin, tetracycline, and cephalosporins but is resistant to sulfonamides, chloramphenicol, and vancomycin. Its resistance to vancomycin, which is unusual among gram-positive bacteria, is of potential clinical significance since this agent is sometimes used in empirical therapy for skin infection. Fish food containing the water flea *Daphnia* is sometimes contaminated with *M. marinum*, which can cause cellulitis or granulomas on skin surfaces exposed to the water in aquariums or injured in swimming pools. Rifampin plus ethambutol has been an effective therapeutic combination in some cases, although no comprehensive studies have been undertaken. In addition, some strains of *M. marinum* are susceptible to tetracycline or to trimethoprim-sulfamethoxazole.

NECROTIZING FASCIITIS

(Table 21-1) Necrotizing fasciitis, formerly called streptococcal gangrene, may be associated with group A *Streptococcus* or mixed aerobic-anaerobic bacteria or may occur as part of gas gangrene caused by *Clostridium perfringens*. Strains of MRSA that produce the Panton-Valentine leukocidin have been reported to cause necrotizing fasciitis. Early diagnosis may be difficult when pain or unexplained fever is the only presenting manifestation. Swelling then develops and is followed by brawny edema and tenderness. With progression, dark-red induration of the epidermis appears, along with bullae filled with blue or purple fluid. Later the skin becomes friable and takes on a bluish, maroon, or black color. By this stage, thrombosis of blood vessels in the dermal papillae (Fig. 21-1) is extensive. Extension of infection to the level of the deep fascia causes this tissue to take on a brownish-gray appearance. Rapid spread occurs along fascial planes, through venous channels and lymphatics. Patients in the later stages are toxic and frequently manifest shock and multiorgan failure.

Necrotizing fasciitis caused by mixed aerobic-anaerobic bacteria begins with a breach in the integrity of a mucous membrane barrier, such as the mucosa of the gastrointestinal or genitourinary tract. The portal can be a malignancy, diverticulum, hemorrhoid, anal fissure, or urethral tear. Other predisposing factors include peripheral vascular disease, diabetes mellitus, surgery, and penetrating injury to the abdomen. Leakage into the perineal area results in a syndrome called *Fournier's gangrene*, characterized by massive swelling of the scrotum and penis with extension into the perineum or the abdominal wall and legs.

Necrotizing fasciitis caused by *S. pyogenes* has increased in frequency and severity since 1985. It often begins deep at the site of a nonpenetrating minor trauma, such as a bruise or a muscle strain. Seeding of the site via transient bacteremia is likely, although most patients deny antecedent streptococcal infection. Alternatively, *S. pyogenes* may reach the deep fascia from a site of cutaneous infection or penetrating trauma. Toxicity is severe, and renal impairment may precede the development of shock. In 20–40% of cases, myositis occurs concomitantly, and, as in gas gangrene (see later), serum creatine phosphokinase levels may be markedly elevated. Necrotizing fasciitis due to mixed aerobic-anaerobic bacteria may be associated with gas in deep tissue, but gas usually is not present when the cause is *S. pyogenes* or MRSA. Prompt surgical exploration down to the deep fascia and muscle is essential. Necrotic tissue must be surgically removed, and Gram's staining and culture of excised tissue are useful in establishing whether group A streptococci, mixed aerobic-anaerobic bacteria, MRSA, or *Clostridium* species are present (see "Treatment" later in the chapter).

MYOSITIS/MYONECROSIS

(Table 21-1) Muscle involvement can occur with viral infection (e.g., influenza, dengue, or coxsackievirus B infection) or parasitic invasion (e.g., trichinellosis, cysticercosis, or toxoplasmosis). Although myalgia can occur in most of these infections, severe muscle pain is the hallmark of pleurodynia (coxsackievirus B), trichinellosis, and bacterial infection. Acute rhabdomyolysis predictably occurs with clostridial and streptococcal myositis, but may also be associated with influenza virus, echovirus, coxsackievirus, Epstein-Barr virus, and *Legionella* infections.

Pyomyositis is usually due to *S. aureus*, is common in tropical areas, and generally has no known portal of entry. Infection remains localized, and shock does not develop unless organisms produce toxic shock syndrome toxin 1 or certain enterotoxins and the patient lacks antibodies to the toxin produced by the infecting organisms. In contrast, *S. pyogenes* may induce primary myositis (referred to as *streptococcal necrotizing myositis*) in association with severe systemic toxicity. Myonecrosis occurs concomitantly with necrotizing fasciitis in ~50% of cases. Both are part of the streptococcal toxic shock syndrome.

Gas gangrene usually follows severe penetrating injuries that result in interruption of the blood supply and introduction of soil into wounds. Such cases of traumatic gangrene are usually caused by the clostridial species *C. perfringens*, *C. septicum*, and *C. histolyticum*. Rarely, latent or recurrent gangrene can occur years after penetrating trauma; dormant spores that reside at the site of previous injury are most likely responsible. Spontaneous nontraumatic gangrene among patients with neutropenia, gastrointestinal malignancy, diverticulosis, or recent radiation therapy to the abdomen is caused by several clostridial species, of which *C. septicum* is the most commonly involved. The tolerance of this anaerobe to oxygen probably explains why it can initiate infection spontaneously in normal tissue anywhere in the body.

Synergistic nonclostridial anaerobic myonecrosis, also known as necrotizing cutaneous myositis and synergistic necrotizing cellulitis, is a variant of necrotizing fasciitis caused by mixed aerobic and anaerobic bacteria with the exclusion of clostridial organisms (see "Necrotizing Fasciitis" earlier in the chapter).

DIAGNOSIS

This chapter has emphasized the physical appearance and location of lesions within the soft tissues as important diagnostic clues. The temporal progression of the lesions as well as the patient's travel history, animal exposure or bite history, age, underlying disease status, and lifestyle are also crucial considerations in the formulation of a narrowed differential diagnosis. However, even the astute clinician may find it challenging to diagnose all infections of the soft tissues by history and inspection alone. Soft tissue radiography, computed tomography (Fig. 21-2), and magnetic resonance imaging may be useful in determining the depth of infection and should be performed in patients with rapidly progressing lesions or evidence of systemic inflammatory response syndrome. These tests are particularly valuable for defining a localized abscess or detecting gas in tissue. Unfortunately,

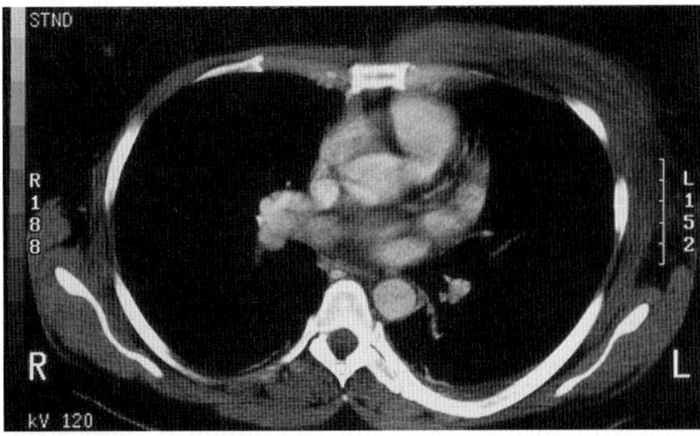

FIGURE 21-2
Computed tomography showing edema and inflammation of the left chest wall in a patient with necrotizing fasciitis and myonecrosis caused by group A *Streptococcus*.

TABLE 21-2

TREATMENT OF COMMON INFECTIONS OF THE SKIN

DIAGNOSIS/CONDITION	PRIMARY TREATMENT	ALTERNATIVE TREATMENT	SEE ALSO CHAP(S).
Animal bite (prophylaxis or early infection)[a]	Amoxicillin/clavulanate, 875/125 mg PO bid	Doxycycline, 100 mg PO bid	32
Animal bite[a] (established infection)	Ampicillin/sulbactam, 1.5–3.0 g IV q6h	Clindamycin, 600–900 mg IV q8h *plus* Ciprofloxacin, 400 mg IV q12h *or* Cefoxitin, 2 g IV q6h	32
Bacillary angiomatosis	Erythromycin, 500 mg PO qid	Doxycycline, 100 mg PO bid	61
Herpes simplex (primary genital)	Acyclovir, 400 mg PO tid for 10 days	Famciclovir, 250 mg PO tid for 5–10 days *or* Valacyclovir, 1000 mg PO bid for 10 days	80
Herpes zoster (immunocompetent host >50 years of age)	Acyclovir, 800 mg PO 5 times daily for 7–10 days	Famciclovir, 500 mg PO tid for 7–10 days *or* Valacyclovir, 1000 mg PO tid for 7 days	81
Cellulitis (staphylococcal or streptococcal[b,c])	Nafcillin or oxacillin, 2 g IV q4–6h	Cefazolin, 1–2 g q8h *or* Ampicillin/sulbactam, 1.5–3.0 g IV q6h *or* Erythromycin, 0.5–1.0 g IV q6h *or* Clindamycin, 600–900 mg IV q8h	35, 36
MRSA skin infection[d]	Vancomycin, 1 g IV q12h	Linezolid, 600 mg IV q12h	35
Necrotizing fasciitis (group A streptococcal[b])	Clindamycin, 600–900 mg IV q6–8h *plus* Penicillin G, 4 million units IV q4h	Clindamycin, 600–900 mg IV q6–8h *plus* Cephalosporin (first- or second-generation)	36
Necrotizing fasciitis (mixed aerobes and anaerobes)	Ampicillin, 2 g IV q4h *plus* Clindamycin, 600–900 mg IV q6–8h *plus* Ciprofloxacin, 400 mg IV q6–8h	Vancomycin, 1 g IV q6h *plus* Metronidazole, 500 mg IV q6h *plus* Ciprofloxacin, 400 mg IV q6–8h	65
Gas gangrene	Clindamycin, 600–900 mg IV q6–8h *plus* Penicillin G, 4 million units IV q4–6h	Clindamycin, 600–900 mg IV q6–8h *plus* Cefoxitin, 2 g IV q6h	42

[a]*Pasteurella multocida*, a species commonly associated with both dog and cat bites, is resistant to cephalexin, dicloxacillin, clindamycin, and erythromycin. *Eikenella corrodens*, a bacterium commonly associated with human bites, is resistant to clindamycin, penicillinase-resistant penicillins, and metronidazole but is sensitive to trimethoprim-sulfamethoxazole and fluoroquinolones.

[b]The frequency of erythromycin resistance in group A *Streptococcus* is currently ~5% in the United States but has reached 70–100% in some other countries. Most, but not all, erythromycin-resistant group A streptococci are susceptible to clindamycin. Approximately 90–95% of *Staphylococcus aureus* strains are sensitive to clindamycin.

[c]Severe hospital-acquired *S. aureus* infections or community-acquired *S. aureus* infections that are not responding to the β-lactam antibiotics recommended in this table may be caused by methicillin-resistant strains, requiring a switch to vancomycin or linezolid.

[d]Some strains of methicillin-resistant *S. aureus* (MRSA) remain sensitive to tetracycline and trimethoprim-sulfamethoxazole. Daptomycin (4 mg/kg IV q24h) or tigecycline (100-mg loading dose followed by 50 mg IV q12h) are alternative treatments for MRSA.

they may reveal only soft tissue swelling and thus are not specific for fulminant infections such as necrotizing fasciitis or myonecrosis caused by group A *Streptococcus* (Fig. 21-2), where gas is not found in lesions.

Aspiration of the leading edge or punch biopsy with frozen section may be helpful if the results are positive, but false-negative results occur in ~80% of cases. There is some evidence that aspiration alone may be superior to injection and aspiration with normal saline. Frozen sections are especially useful in distinguishing SSSS from TEN and are quite valuable in cases of necrotizing fasciitis. Open surgical inspection with debridement as indicated is clearly the best way to determine the extent and severity of infection and to obtain material for Gram's staining and culture. Such an aggressive approach is important and may be lifesaving if undertaken early in the course of fulminant infections where there is evidence of systemic toxicity.

℞ Treatment: INFECTIONS OF THE SKIN, MUSCLE, AND SOFT TISSUES

A full description of the treatment of all the clinical entities described herein is beyond the scope of this chapter. As a guide to the clinician in selecting appropriate treatment, the antimicrobial agents useful in the most common and the most fulminant cutaneous infections are listed in Table 21-2.

Early and aggressive surgical exploration is essential in patients with suspected necrotizing fasciitis, myositis, or gangrene in order to (1) visualize the deep structures, (2) remove necrotic tissue, (3) reduce compartment pressure, and (4) obtain suitable material for Gram's staining and for aerobic and anaerobic cultures. Appropriate empirical antibiotic treatment for mixed aerobic-anaerobic infections could consist of ampicillin/sulbactam, cefoxitin, or the following combination: (1) clindamycin (600–900 mg intravenously every 8 h) or metronidazole (750 mg every 6 h) plus (2) ampicillin or ampicillin/sulbactam (2–3 g intravenously every 6 h) plus (3) gentamicin (1.0–1.5 mg/kg every 8 h). Group A streptococcal and clostridial infection of the fascia and/or muscle carries a mortality rate of 20–50% with penicillin treatment. In experimental models of streptococcal and clostridial necrotizing fasciitis/myositis, clindamycin has exhibited markedly superior efficacy, but no comparative trials have been performed in humans. Hyperbaric oxygen treatment may also be useful in gas gangrene due to clostridial species. Antibiotic treatment should be continued until all signs of systemic toxicity have resolved, all devitalized tissue has been removed, and granulation tissue has developed (Chaps. 36, 42, and 65).

In summary, infections of the skin and soft tissues are diverse in presentation and severity and offer a great challenge to the clinician. This chapter provides an approach to diagnosis and understanding of the pathophysiologic mechanisms involved in these infections. More in-depth information is found in chapters on specific infections.

FURTHER READINGS

ANAYA DA et al: Necrotizing soft-tissue infection: Diagnosis and management. Clin Infect Dis 44:705, 2007

BISNO AI, STEVENS DL: Streptococcal infections in skin and soft tissues. N Engl J Med 334:240, 1996

BREMAN JG, HENDERSON DA: Diagnosis and management of smallpox. N Engl J Med 346:1300, 2002

CARPENTER CF, CHAMBERS HF: Daptomycin: Another novel agent for treating infections due to drug-resistant gram-positive pathogens. Clin Infect Dis 38:994, 2004

ELLIS-GROSSE EJ et al: The efficacy and safety of tigecycline in the treatment of skin and skin-structure infections: Results of 2 double-blind phase 3 comparison studies with vancomycin-aztreonam. Clin Infect Dis 41(Suppl 5):S341, 2005

FRIDKIN SK et al: Methicillin-resistant *Staphylococcus aureus* disease in three communities. N Engl J Med 352:1436, 2005

MILLER LG et al: Necrotizing fasciitis caused by community-associated methicillin-resistant *Staphylococcus aureus* in Los Angeles. N Engl J Med 352:1445, 2005

NORRBY-TEGLUND A, STEVENS DL: Novel therapies in streptococcal toxic shock syndrome: Attenuation of virulence factor expression and modulation of host response. Curr Opin Infect Dis 11:285, 1998

STEVENS DL: Streptococcal toxic shock syndrome associated with necrotizing fasciitis. Annu Rev Med 51:271, 2000

———: Necrotizing soft tissue infections. Curr Treat Opt Infect Dis 2:359, 2000

TALAN DA et al: Bacteriologic analysis of infected dog and cat bites. Emergency Medicine Animal Bite Infection Study Group. N Engl J Med 340:85, 1999

CHAPTER 22

OSTEOMYELITIS

Jeffrey Parsonnet

Osteomyelitis, an infection of bone, is caused most commonly by pyogenic bacteria and mycobacteria. As a useful framework for evaluating a patient and planning treatment, cases are classified on the basis of the causative agent; the route by which organisms gain access to bone; the duration of infection; the anatomic location of infection; and the local and systemic host factors that have a bearing on pathogenesis and outcome.

PATHOGENESIS AND PATHOLOGY

Microorganisms enter bone by hematogenous dissemination, by spread from a contiguous focus of infection, or by a penetrating wound. Trauma, ischemia, and foreign bodies enhance the susceptibility of bone to microbial invasion by exposing sites to which bacteria can bind and by impeding host defenses. Phagocytes attempt to contain the infection and, in the process, release enzymes that lyse bone. Bacteria escape host defenses by adhering tightly to damaged bone, by entering and persisting within osteoblasts, and by coating themselves and underlying surfaces with a protective polysaccharide-rich biofilm. Pus spreads into vascular channels, raising intraosseous pressure and impairing the flow of blood; as the untreated infection becomes chronic, ischemic necrosis of bone results in the separation of large devascularized fragments (*sequestra*). When pus breaks through the cortex, subperiosteal or soft tissue abscesses form, and the elevated periosteum deposits new bone (an *involucrum*) around the sequestrum.

Microorganisms, infiltrates of neutrophils, and congested or thrombosed blood vessels are the principal histologic findings of acute osteomyelitis. The distinguishing feature of chronic osteomyelitis is necrotic bone, which is characterized by the absence of living osteocytes. Mononuclear cells predominate in chronic infections, and granulation and fibrous tissues replace bone that has been resorbed by osteoclasts. In the chronic stage, organisms may be too few to be seen on staining.

HEMATOGENOUS OSTEOMYELITIS

Hematogenous infection accounts for ~20% of cases of osteomyelitis and primarily affects children, in whom the long bones are infected, and older adults and IV drug users, in whom the spine is the most common site of infection.

ACUTE HEMATOGENOUS OSTEOMYELITIS

Infection usually involves a single bone, most commonly the tibia, femur, or humerus in children and vertebral bodies in injection drug users and older adults. Bacteria settle in the well-perfused metaphysis of growing bones, a network of venous sinusoids slows the flow of blood, and fenestrations in capillaries allow organisms to escape into the extravascular space. Because vascular anatomy changes with age, hematogenous infection of long bones is uncommon during adulthood and, when it occurs, usually involves the diaphysis.

On presentation, the child with osteomyelitis usually appears acutely ill, with fever, chills, localized pain and tenderness, and—in many cases—restriction of movement or difficulty bearing weight. Overlying erythema and swelling indicate extension of pus through the cortex. During infancy and after puberty, infection may spread through the epiphysis into the joint space. In children of other ages, extension of infection through the cortex results in involvement of joints if the metaphysis is intracapsular. Thus septic arthritis of the elbow, shoulder, and hip may complicate osteomyelitis of the proximal radius, humerus, and femur, respectively. In children, the source of bacteremia is usually inapparent. A history is often obtained of recent blunt trauma to the area involved; presumably, this event results in a small intraosseous hematoma or vascular obstruction that predisposes to infection. Adults with hematogenous osteomyelitis may present either in the context of an infection elsewhere (e.g., the respiratory or urinary tract, a heart valve, or an intravascular catheter site) or without an obvious source of bacteremia.

Plain radiographs obtained early in the course of infection may show soft tissue swelling, but the first change in bone—a periosteal reaction—is not evident until at least 10 days after the onset of infection. Lytic changes can be detected only after 2–6 weeks, when 50–75% of bone density has been lost. Rarely, a well-circumscribed lytic lesion, or *Brodie's abscess*, is seen in a child who has been in pain for several months but has had no fever.

VERTEBRAL OSTEOMYELITIS

The vertebrae are the most common sites of hematogenous osteomyelitis in adults. Organisms reach the well-perfused vertebral body via spinal arteries and quickly spread from the end plate into the disk space and then to the adjacent vertebral body. Sources of bacteremia include the urinary tract (especially among men over age 50), dental abscesses, soft tissue infections, and contaminated IV lines, but the source of bacteremia is not evident in more than half of patients. Diabetes mellitus requiring insulin injection, a recent invasive medical procedure, hemodialysis, and injection drug use carry an increased risk of spinal infection. Many patients have a history of degenerative joint disease involving the spine, and some report an episode of trauma preceding the onset of infection. Penetrating injuries and surgical procedures involving the spine may cause nonhematogenous vertebral osteomyelitis or infection localized to a disk.

Most patients with vertebral osteomyelitis report neck or back pain; patients may describe atypical pain in the chest, the abdomen, or an extremity that is due to irritation of nerve roots. Symptoms are localized to the lumbar spine more often than to the thoracic spine (>50% vs 35% of cases) or the cervical spine in pyogenic infections, but the thoracic spine is involved most commonly in tuberculous spondylitis (Pott's disease). More than 50% of patients experience a subacute illness in which a vague, dull pain gradually intensifies over 2–3 months. Fever is usually low-grade or absent, but some patients recall having had an episode of fever and chills before or at the onset of pain. An acute presentation with high fever and toxicity is less common and suggests ongoing bacteremia. Percussion over the involved vertebra elicits tenderness, and physical examination may reveal spasm of the paraspinal muscles and limitation of motion.

Laboratory findings at the time of presentation include a normal or modestly elevated white blood cell count, anemia, and, almost invariably, an increased erythrocyte sedimentation rate (ESR) and C-reactive protein (CRP) level. Blood cultures are positive only 20–50% of the time.

By the time the patient seeks medical attention, plain radiographs often show irregular erosions in the end plates of adjacent vertebral bodies and narrowing of the intervening disk space. This radiographic pattern is virtually diagnostic of bacterial infection because tumors and other diseases of the spine rarely cross the disk space. CT or MRI may demonstrate epidural, paraspinal, retropharyngeal, mediastinal, retroperitoneal, or psoas abscesses that originate in the spine.

A spinal epidural abscess may evolve suddenly or over several weeks; the classic clinical presentation is spinal pain progressing to radicular pain and/or weakness. Irreversible paralysis may result from failure to recognize epidural abscess before the development of neurologic deficits. MRI is the best procedure for detection of epidural abscess and should be performed in all cases of vertebral osteomyelitis accompanied by subjective weakness or objective neurologic abnormalities.

MICROBIOLOGY

More than 95% of cases of hematogenous osteomyelitis are caused by a single organism, with *Staphylococcus aureus* accounting for 50% of cases. Other common pathogens in children are group A streptococci and, during the neonatal period, group B streptococci and *Escherichia coli*. In adults, vertebral osteomyelitis is caused by *E. coli* and other enteric bacilli in ~25% of cases. *S. aureus*, *Pseudomonas aeruginosa*, *Serratia*, and *Candida albicans* infections are associated with injection drug use and may involve the sacroiliac, sternoclavicular, or pubic joints as well as the spine. *Salmonella* spp. and *S. aureus* are the major causes of long-bone osteomyelitis complicating sickle cell anemia and other hemoglobinopathies. Tuberculosis and brucellosis affect the spine more often than other bones. Other common sites of tuberculous osteomyelitis include the small bones of the hands and feet, the metaphyses of long bones, the ribs, and the sternum.

Unusual causes of hematogenous osteomyelitis include disseminated histoplasmosis, coccidioidomycosis, and blastomycosis in endemic areas. Immunocompromised persons may rarely develop osteomyelitis due to atypical mycobacteria, *Bartonella henselae*, or opportunistic fungi. Hematogenous osteomyelitis with *Mycobacterium bovis* has been reported after intravesicular instillation of bacille Calmette-Guérin (BCG) for cancer of the bladder. The etiology of chronic relapsing multifocal osteomyelitis, an inflammatory condition of children that is characterized by recurrent episodes of painful lytic lesions in multiple bones, has not been identified.

OSTEOMYELITIS SECONDARY TO A CONTIGUOUS FOCUS OF INFECTION

CLINICAL FEATURES

This broad category of osteomyelitis accounts for ~80% of all cases and occurs most commonly in adults. It includes infections introduced by penetrating injuries, such as bites, puncture wounds, and open fractures; by surgical procedures; and by direct extension of infection from adjacent soft tissues. Generalized vascular insufficiency and the presence of a foreign body are important predisposing factors and also make infection more difficult to cure.

Frequently, the diagnosis of this type of osteomyelitis is not made until the infection has already become chronic. The pain, fever, and inflammatory signs due to bony infection may be attributed to the original injury, to underlying bone or joint disease (such as degenerative arthritis), or to overlying soft tissue infection. Osteomyelitis may become apparent only weeks or months later, when a sinus tract develops, a surgical wound breaks down, or a fracture fails to heal. It may be impossible to distinguish radiographic abnormalities due to osteomyelitis from those due to the precipitating condition.

A special type of contiguous-focus osteomyelitis occurs in the setting of peripheral vascular disease and nearly always involves the small bones of the feet of adults with diabetes. This type of infection is a major cause of morbidity for patients with diabetes and results in many thousands of amputations per year. Diabetic neuropathy exposes the foot to frequent trauma and pressure sores, and the patient may be unaware of infection as it spreads into bone. Poor tissue perfusion impairs normal inflammatory responses and wound healing and creates a milieu that is conducive to anaerobic infections. It is often during the evaluation of a nonhealing ulcer, a swollen toe, or acute cellulitis that a radiograph provides the first evidence of osteomyelitis. If bone is palpable during examination of the base of an ulcer with a blunt surgical probe, osteomyelitis is likely.

MICROBIOLOGY

S. aureus is a pathogen in more than half of cases of contiguous-focus osteomyelitis. However, in contrast to hematogenous osteomyelitis, these infections are often polymicrobial and are more likely to involve gram-negative and anaerobic bacteria. Hence a mixture of staphylococci, streptococci, enteric organisms, and anaerobic bacteria may be isolated from a diabetic foot infection or pelvic osteomyelitis underlying a decubitus ulcer. Aerobic and anaerobic bacteria cause osteomyelitis after surgery or soft tissue infection of the oropharynx, paranasal sinuses, gastrointestinal tract, or female genital tract. A human bite may result in mixed infection of the hand, with anaerobes included among the etiologic agents. *S. aureus* is the principal cause of postoperative infections, coagulase-negative staphylococci are common pathogens after implantation of orthopedic appliances, and these organisms as well as gram-negative enteric bacilli, atypical mycobacteria, and *Mycoplasma* may cause sternal osteomyelitis after cardiac surgery. Infection with *P. aeruginosa* is frequently associated with puncture wounds of the foot, especially when a nail passes through a sneaker, and *Pasteurella multocida* infection commonly follows cat bites.

CHRONIC OSTEOMYELITIS

With prompt treatment, <5% of cases of acute hematogenous osteomyelitis progress to chronic osteomyelitis. Chronic infection is more likely to develop in contiguous-focus than in hematogenous osteomyelitis. The presence of a foreign body makes establishment of chronic infection especially likely.

A protracted clinical course, long periods of quiescence, and recurrent exacerbations are characteristic of chronic osteomyelitis. Sinus tracts between bone and skin may drain purulent material and occasionally pieces of necrotic bone. An increase in drainage, pain, or swelling signals an exacerbation, which is usually accompanied by increases in CRP level and ESR. Fever is unusual except when obstruction of a sinus tract leads to soft tissue infection. Rare late complications include pathologic fractures, squamous cell carcinoma of the sinus tract, and amyloidosis.

DIAGNOSIS

Early diagnosis of acute osteomyelitis is critical because prompt antibiotic therapy may prevent necrosis of bone. The ESR and the CRP level are elevated in most cases of active osteomyelitis, including those in which constitutional symptoms and leukocytosis are lacking. These findings are not specific to osteomyelitis, however, and the ESR is occasionally normal in early infections. Baseline values are often useful in monitoring the efficacy of treatment.

A variety of radiologic tests are available for evaluation of osteomyelitis (Table 22-1). Evaluation usually begins with plain radiographs because of their ready availability, although they typically show no abnormalities during early infection. Three-phase bone scans (^{99}Tc-methylene diphosphonate) offer high sensitivity but are often of low specificity, especially in the presence of underlying bone abnormalities. There is a lack of consensus over the optimal use of other radionuclide studies, and there is considerable variation between institutions in their use. Use of MRI (Fig. 22-1) is expanding because of its high sensitivity and specificity as well as its ability to demonstrate associated soft tissue abnormalities, but this modality is not available at all institutions.

The role of diagnostic imaging in chronic osteomyelitis is to detect active infection and delineate the extent of debridement necessary to remove necrotic bone and abnormal soft tissues. CT is more sensitive than plain films for the detection of sequestra, sinus tracts, and soft tissue abscesses. Both CT and ultrasound are useful for guiding percutaneous aspiration of subperiosteal and soft tissue fluid collections. Sequential technetium and gallium or indium scans may help determine whether infection is active and may distinguish infection from noninflammatory bone changes. MRI provides superior information about the anatomic extent of infection, but does not always distinguish osteomyelitis from healing fractures and tumors. MRI is particularly useful in distinguishing cellulitis from osteomyelitis in the diabetic foot; however, no imaging modality consistently distinguishes infection from neuropathic osteopathy.

Appropriate samples for microbiologic studies should be obtained in all cases of suspected osteomyelitis before the initiation of antimicrobial therapy. Blood cultures are indicated in acute cases and are positive in more than one-third of cases of hematogenous osteomyelitis in children and 25% of cases of vertebral osteomyelitis in adults. The presence of sepsis occasionally requires initiation of empirical therapy after blood samples alone have been

TABLE 22-1

DIAGNOSTIC IMAGING STUDIES FOR OSTEOMYELITIS

TYPE OF STUDY	COMMENTS
Plain radiographs	Insensitive, especially in early osteomyelitis. May show periosteal elevation after 10 days, lytic changes after 2–6 weeks. Useful to look for anatomic abnormalities (e.g., fractures, bony variants, or deformities), foreign bodies, and soft tissue gas.
Three-phase bone scan (^{99m}Tc-MDP)	Characteristic finding in osteomyelitis: increased uptake in all three phases of scan. Highly sensitive (~95%) in acute infection; somewhat less sensitive if blood flow to bone is poor. Specificity moderate if plain films are normal, but poor in presence of neuropathic arthropathy, fractures, tumor, infarction.
Other radionuclide scans	Examples: ^{67}Ga-citrate, ^{111}In-labeled WBCs. ^{111}In-WBCs more specific than gallium but not always available. Often used in conjunction with bone scan because its greater specificity for inflammation than ^{99m}Tc-MDP helps to distinguish infectious from noninfectious processes. Lack of consensus over role; often supplanted by MRI when the latter is available.
Ultrasound	May detect subperiosteal fluid collection or soft tissue abscess adjacent to bone, but largely supplanted by CT and MRI.
CT	Limited role in acute osteomyelitis. In chronic osteomyelitis, excellent for detection of sequestra, cortical destruction, soft tissue abscesses, and sinus tracts. Use limited in the presence of a metallic foreign body.
MRI	As sensitive as ^{99m}Tc-MDP bone scan for acute osteomyelitis (~95%); detects changes in water content of marrow before disruption of cortical bone. High specificity (~87%), with better anatomic detail than nuclear studies. Procedure of choice for vertebral osteomyelitis because of high sensitivity for epidural abscess. Use may be limited by a metallic foreign body.

Note: ^{99m}Tc-MDP, technetium-99m methylene diphosphonate; ^{67}Ga, gallium-67; ^{111}In, indium-111; WBCs, white blood cells.

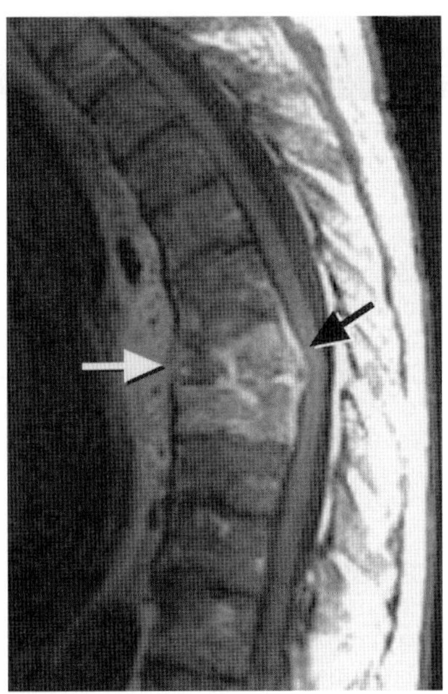

FIGURE 22-1
Osteomyelitis of the thoracic spine demonstrated on a sagittal, fat-suppressed T1-weighted magnetic resonance image after the administration of IV gadolinium. At T8–T9, there is involvement of the adjacent vertebral bodies and intervening disk. Abnormally enhancing inflammatory tissue extends from the disk space anteriorly (*white arrow*) as well as posteriorly into the epidural space, compressing the thecal sac (*black arrow*).

obtained for culture. If blood cultures are negative, samples from needle aspiration of pus in bone or soft tissues or from a bone biopsy should be obtained for culture; in the case of vertebral osteomyelitis, these samples can usually be obtained percutaneously with the guidance of fluoroscopy or CT.

The results of culture of swabs of a sinus tract or the base of an ulcer correlate poorly with those of samples of the infected bone. For this reason, in cases of chronic osteomyelitis and contiguous-focus osteomyelitis, samples for aerobic and anaerobic culture should be obtained by percutaneous needle aspiration through uninfected tissue, percutaneous biopsy, or intraoperative biopsy at the time of surgical debridement. Coagulase-negative staphylococci and other organisms of low virulence should not automatically be disregarded as contaminants, especially in the presence of prosthetic materials. Special culture media may be necessary for the isolation of mycobacteria, fungi, and fastidious pathogens. In some cases, histopathologic examination of biopsy specimens may be the only way to confirm a diagnosis of osteomyelitis.

℞ Treatment: OSTEOMYELITIS

ANTIBIOTIC THERAPY (Table 22-2) Antibiotics should be administered only after appropriate specimens have been obtained for culture. Use of bactericidal agents has been recommended, although controlled data for this recommendation are lacking. Antibiotics should be given at a high dose; thus, for most agents, parenteral administration is required. Empirical therapy is guided by findings on Gram's staining of a specimen from the bone or abscess or is chosen to cover the most likely pathogens; such therapy should usually include high doses of an agent active against *S. aureus* (such as oxacillin, nafcillin, cefazolin, or vancomycin) or—if gram-negative organisms are likely to be involved—a third-generation cephalosporin, an aminoglycoside, or a fluoroquinolone. Empirical therapy should also include an agent active against anaerobes in the setting of a decubitus ulcer or diabetic foot infection.

Specific therapy is ultimately based on in vitro susceptibility testing of the organism(s) isolated from bone or blood. Outpatient parenteral antimicrobial therapy (OPAT) is appropriate for motivated and medically stable patients and represents a significant advance in management. Antibiotics that require infrequent dosing, such as ceftriaxone, ertapenem, daptomycin, and vancomycin, may facilitate home therapy, but these choices often have an overly broad spectrum of activity. Fortunately, many antibiotics can be given automatically by means of a portable infusion pump, which decreases the disruption otherwise caused by frequent administration of a drug. Use of a peripherally inserted central catheter (PICC line) also greatly facilitates outpatient drug administration. OPAT requires close coordination of nursing, pharmacy, and physician care, with clear delineations of responsibility for monitoring of safety and efficacy.

After administration of parenteral therapy for 5–10 days and after resolution of signs of active infection, oral antibiotics have been used with great success in children with hematogenous osteomyelitis. The doses of oral penicillins or cephalosporins required for the treatment of pediatric osteomyelitis are high, and adults may not tolerate such doses as well as children. With the exception of the fluoroquinolones, rifampin, and linezolid, few data support the use of oral antibiotics for adults with osteomyelitis. For treatment of infection due to Enterobacteriaceae, oral administration of a fluoroquinolone has been as successful as IV administration of β-lactam antibiotics. Caution should be exercised in the use of fluoroquinolones as the sole agents for treatment of infection due to *S. aureus* or *P. aeruginosa* because resistance may develop during therapy. Addition of oral rifampin (300 mg bid) to a fluoroquinolone has yielded encouraging results in infections due to *S. aureus*, but potential drug toxicity and drug interactions make this option desirable only for selected patients, such as those for whom parenteral therapy poses unacceptable logistical or financial hardship. Oral administration of metronidazole (500 mg every 8 h) results in high drug levels in serum and can take the place of IV regimens for the treatment of *Bacteroides* infections. The bacteriostatic drug linezolid (600 mg by mouth every 12 h) has been used successfully in uncontrolled studies involving moderate numbers of patients with infection caused by methicillin-resistant *S. aureus* (MRSA) and vancomycin-resistant enterococci, but data are currently insufficient

TABLE 22-2

SELECTION OF ANTIBIOTICS FOR TREATMENT OF ACUTE OSTEOMYELITIS

	SUGGESTED REGIMEN[a]	
ORGANISM	**PRIMARY**	**ALTERNATIVES[b]**
Staphylococcus aureus		
Penicillin-resistant, methicillin-sensitive (MSSA)	Nafcillin or oxacillin, 2 g IV q4h	Cefazolin, 1 g IV q8h; ceftriaxone, 1 g IV q24h; clindamycin, 900 mg IV q8h[c]
Penicillin-sensitive	Penicillin, 3–4 million U IV q4h	Cefazolin, ceftriaxone, clindamycin (as above)
Methicillin-resistant (MRSA)	Vancomycin, 15 mg/kg IV q12h; rifampin, 300 mg PO q12h (see text)	Clindamycin[c] (as above); linezolid, 600 mg IV or PO q12h[d]; daptomycin, 4–6 mg/kg IV q24h[d]
Streptococci (including *S. milleri*, β-hemolytic streptococci)	Penicillin (as above)	Cefazolin, ceftriaxone, clindamycin (as above)
Gram-negative aerobic bacilli		
Escherichia coli, other "sensitive" species	Ampicillin, 2 g IV q4h; cefazolin, 1 g IV q8h	Ceftriaxone, 1 g IV q24h; parenteral or oral fluoroquinolone (e.g., ciprofloxacin, 400 mg IV or 750 mg PO q12h)[e]
Pseudomonas aeruginosa	Extended-spectrum β-lactam agent (e.g., piperacillin, 3–4 g IV q4–6h; or ceftazidime, 2 g IV q12h) *plus* tobramycin, 5–7 mg/kg q24h[f]	May substitute parenteral or oral fluoroquinolone for β-lactam agents (if patient is allergic) or for tobramycin (in relation to nephrotoxicity)
Enterobacter spp., other "resistant" species	Extended-spectrum β-lactam agent IV or fluoroquinolone IV or PO[e] (as above)	
Mixed infections possibly involving anaerobic bacteria	Ampicillin/sulbactam, 1.5–3 g IV q6h; piperacillin/tazobactam, 3.375 g IV q6h	Carbapenem antibiotic or a combination of a fluoroquinolone plus clindamycin (as above) or metronidazole, 500 mg PO tid

[a]Duration of treatment is discussed in the text.
[b]Cephalosporins may be used for the treatment of patients allergic to penicillin whose reaction did not consist of anaphylaxis or urticaria (immediate-type hypersensitivity).
[c]Because of the possibility of inducible resistance, clindamycin must be used with caution for the treatment of strains resistant to erythromycin. Consult clinical microbiology laboratory.
[d]Experience is limited; there are anecdotal reports of efficacy.
[e]Oral fluoroquinolones must not be coadministered with divalent cations (calcium, magnesium, iron, aluminum), which block the drugs' absorption.
[f]Tobramycin levels and renal function must be monitored closely to minimize the risks of nephro- and ototoxicity.

to recommend the routine use of this agent. Data do not support the routine use of the serum minimal bactericidal concentration in guiding therapy.

Osteomyelitis caused by MRSA is a growing problem that poses unique challenges in terms of treatment. Vancomycin has historically been the drug of choice for MRSA osteomyelitis, but only because of a lack of acceptable alternatives. The drug is less effective than β-lactam agents in treating infections caused by methicillin-susceptible *S. aureus* (MSSA), and this low efficacy extends to infections caused by MRSA. Vancomycin should not be used for treatment of osteomyelitis caused by MSSA, and oral rifampin should be coadministered with vancomycin when the latter drug is used for MRSA infection, unless there are compelling contraindications. Linezolid has performed reasonably well in uncontrolled studies of staphylococcal osteomyelitis. However, side effects and hematologic toxicity are common with this agent; thus in the absence of controlled studies, its routine use is discouraged. Daptomycin, a bactericidal drug with favorable pharmacokinetics, has also been used successfully. Unfortunately, because resistance can develop during therapy (with resultant treatment failure), the routine use of this drug is not recommended. Trimethoprim-sulfamethoxazole, clindamycin, and tetracycline derivatives (doxycycline and minocycline) are often used—seemingly to good advantage—as "continuation therapy" for MRSA osteomyelitis after a course of a parenteral agent, but no controlled data are available to support this approach.

ACUTE HEMATOGENOUS OSTEOMYELITIS

Early treatment of acute hematogenous osteomyelitis of childhood with 4–6 weeks of an appropriate antibiotic is usually successful; treatment for <3 weeks has resulted in a tenfold greater rate of failure. Surgical intervention in childhood cases is indicated for intraosseous or subperiosteal abscesses, concomitant septic arthritis, and lack of improvement of the acute signs of infection in 24–48 h. Acute hematogenous osteomyelitis of bones other than the spine in adults often requires surgical debridement.

VERTEBRAL OSTEOMYELITIS A 6- to 8-week course of treatment with an appropriate antibiotic is usually sufficient to cure vertebral osteomyelitis. Failure of the ESR to drop by two-thirds or more of its pretreatment level or of the CRP level to normalize is an indication for reevaluation and (possibly) longer treatment. Surgery is seldom necessary, even in cases of many months' duration, except in instances of spinal instability, new or progressive neurologic deficits, or large soft-tissue abscesses that cannot be drained percutaneously. All but small and asymptomatic epidural abscesses should be surgically drained. Patients should maintain bed rest until back pain has declined to the point at which ambulation is possible. Body casts are no longer used except for comfort.

CONTIGUOUS-FOCUS OSTEOMYELITIS Even when diagnosed early, contiguous-focus osteomyelitis usually requires surgery in addition to 4–6 weeks of appropriate antibiotic therapy because of underlying soft tissue infection or damage to bone from an injury or surgery. A 2-week course of antibiotics after thorough debridement and soft tissue coverage has yielded adequate results in the treatment of superficial osteomyelitis involving only the outer cortex of bone.

CHRONIC OSTEOMYELITIS The risks and benefits of aggressive therapy for chronic osteomyelitis should be weighed before any attempt is made to eradicate the infection. Some patients with extensive disease prefer to live with their infections rather than undergo multiple surgical procedures, take prolonged courses of antimicrobial therapy, and face the risk of loss of an extremity. Such persons often benefit from intermittent courses of oral antibiotics to suppress acute exacerbations.

Once the decision has been made to treat chronic osteomyelitis aggressively, the patient's nutritional and metabolic status should be optimized to expedite healing of soft tissues and bone. Antibiotic administration should be started several days before surgery to reduce inflammation if the etiology of the infection is known; if not, antibiotic therapy should be withheld until debridement. A 4- to 6-week course of appropriate antibiotic therapy is given postoperatively on the basis of the susceptibility pattern of organisms isolated from bone. A subsequent prolonged course of oral antibiotic therapy is often prescribed, especially in the setting of a foreign body, but controlled data for this approach are lacking. There are insufficient data to recommend either the routine use of hyperbaric oxygen or the use of antibiotic-impregnated methacrylate beads or other depots to deliver high levels of antibiotics to the bone. The success of therapy for chronic osteomyelitis still rests largely on the complete surgical removal of necrotic bone and abnormal soft tissues. In the past, the inability to repair large defects in bone and soft tissue limited the extent of debridement. Muscle flaps and skin grafts are now used routinely to cover large soft-tissue defects and to fill dead space, and bone grafts and vascularized bone transfer may restore a seriously compromised bone to a functional state.

In infections of recent fractures requiring internal fixators, such devices are often left in place and the infection is controlled by limited debridement and "suppressive" antibiotic therapy. Definitive surgical/antimicrobial therapy is delayed until bony union of the fracture has been achieved. If there is persistent nonunion of the fracture or loosening of the fixator, the appliance must be removed, the bone debrided, and an external fixator or a new internal fixator applied.

Osteomyelitis of the small bones of the feet in persons with vascular disease usually requires surgical treatment. The effectiveness of the surgery is limited by the blood supply to the site and the body's ability to heal the wound. Revascularization of the extremity is indicated if the vascular disease involves large arteries. In cases of decreased perfusion due to small-vessel disease, foot-sparing surgery may fail, and the best option is often suppressive therapy or amputation. The duration of antibiotic therapy depends on the surgical procedure performed. When the infected bone is removed entirely but residual infection of soft tissues remains, antibiotic therapy should be given for 2 weeks; if amputation eliminates infected bone and soft tissue, standard surgical prophylaxis is given; otherwise, postoperative antibiotics must be given for 4–6 weeks.

ACKNOWLEDGMENT

The substantial contributions of Dr. James H. Maguire to this chapter in previous editions of Harrison's Principles of Internal Medicine are gratefully acknowledged.

FURTHER READINGS

BUTALIA S et al: Does this patient with diabetes have osteomyelitis of the lower extremity? JAMA 299:806, 2008

DAROUICHE RO: Spinal epidural abscess. N Engl J Med 355:2012, 2006

KAIM AH et al: Imaging of chronic posttraumatic osteomyelitis. Eur Radiol 12:1193, 2002

KHATRI G et al: Effect of bone biopsy in guiding antimicrobial therapy for osteomyelitis complicating open wounds. Am J Med Sci 321:367, 2001

LEW DP, WALDVOGEL FA: Osteomyelitis. N Engl J Med 336:999, 1997

LIPSKY BA: Osteomyelitis of the foot in diabetic patients. Clin Infect Dis 25:1318, 1997

MCHENRY MC et al: Vertebral osteomyelitis: Long-term outcome for 253 patients from 7 Cleveland-area hospitals. Clin Infect Dis 34:1342, 2002

RISSING JP: Antimicrobial therapy for chronic osteomyelitis in adults: Role of the quinolones. Clin Infect Dis 25:1327, 1997

TICE AD et al: Outcomes of osteomyelitis among patients treated with outpatient parenteral antimicrobial therapy. Am J Med 114:723, 2003

TSUKAYAMA DT: Pathophysiology of posttraumatic osteomyelitis. Clin Orthop 360:22, 1999

ZARROUK V et al: Imaging does not predict the clinical outcome of bacterial osteomyelitis. Rheumatology 46:292, 2007

CHAPTER 23

INFECTIOUS ARTHRITIS

Lawrence C. Madoff

INTRODUCTION

Although *Staphylococcus aureus*, *Neisseria gonorrhoeae*, and other bacteria are the most common causes of infectious arthritis, various mycobacteria, spirochetes, fungi, and viruses also infect joints (Table 23-1). Since acute bacterial infection can rapidly destroy articular cartilage, all inflamed joints must be evaluated without delay to exclude noninfectious processes and to determine appropriate antimicrobial therapy and drainage procedures. For more detailed information on infectious arthritis due to specific organisms, the reader is referred to the chapters on those organisms.

Acute bacterial infection typically involves a single joint or a few joints. Subacute or chronic monarthritis or oligoarthritis suggests mycobacterial or fungal infection; episodic inflammation is seen in syphilis, Lyme disease, and the reactive arthritis that follows enteric infections and chlamydial urethritis. Acute polyarticular inflammation occurs as an immunologic reaction during the course of endocarditis, rheumatic fever, disseminated neisserial infection, and acute hepatitis B. Bacteria and viruses occasionally infect multiple joints, the former most commonly in persons with rheumatoid arthritis.

Approach to the Patient: INFECTIOUS ARTHRITIS

Aspiration of synovial fluid—an essential element in the evaluation of potentially infected joints—can be performed without difficulty in most cases by the insertion of a large-bore needle into the site of maximal fluctuance or tenderness or by the route of easiest access. Ultrasonography or fluoroscopy may be used to guide aspiration of difficult-to-localize effusions of the hip and, occasionally, the shoulder and other joints. Normal synovial fluid contains <180 cells (predominantly mononuclear cells) per microliter. Synovial cell counts averaging 100,000/μL (range, 25,000–250,000/μL), with >90% neutrophils, are characteristic of acute bacterial infections. Crystal-induced, rheumatoid, and other noninfectious inflammatory arthritides are usually associated with <30,000–50,000 cells/μL; cell counts of 10,000–30,000/μL, with 50–70% neutrophils and the remainder lymphocytes, are common in mycobacterial and fungal infections. Definitive diagnosis of an infectious process relies on identification of the pathogen in stained smears of synovial fluid, isolation of the pathogen from cultures of synovial fluid and blood, or detection of microbial nucleic acids and proteins by polymerase chain reaction (PCR)–based assays and immunologic techniques.

ACUTE BACTERIAL ARTHRITIS

Pathogenesis

Bacteria enter the joint from the bloodstream; from a contiguous site of infection in bone or soft tissue; or by direct inoculation during surgery, injection, animal or human bite, or trauma. In hematogenous infection, bacteria escape from synovial capillaries, which have no limiting basement membrane, and within hours provoke neutrophilic infiltration of the synovium. Neutrophils and bacteria enter the joint space; later, bacteria adhere to articular cartilage. Degradation of cartilage begins within 48 h as a result of increased intraarticular pressure, release of proteases and cytokines from chondrocytes and synovial macrophages, and invasion of the cartilage by bacteria and inflammatory cells. Histologic studies reveal bacteria lining the synovium and cartilage as well as abscesses extending into the synovium, cartilage, and—in severe cases—subchondral bone. Synovial proliferation results in the formation of a pannus over the cartilage, and thrombosis of inflamed synovial vessels develops. Bacterial factors that appear important in the pathogenesis of infective arthritis include various surface-associated adhesins in *S. aureus* that permit adherence to cartilage and endotoxins that promote chondrocyte-mediated breakdown of cartilage.

Microbiology

The hematogenous route of infection is the most common route in all age groups, and nearly every bacterial pathogen is capable of causing septic arthritis. In infants, group B streptococci, gram-negative enteric bacilli, and *S. aureus* are the usual pathogens. Since the advent of the *Haemophilus influenzae* vaccine, *S. aureus*, *Streptococcus pyogenes* (group A *Streptococcus*), and (in some centers) *Kingella kingae* have predominated among children <5 years of age. Among young adults and adolescents, *N. gonorrhoeae* is the most commonly implicated organism. *S. aureus* accounts for most nongonococcal isolates in adults of all ages; gram-negative bacilli, pneumococci, and β-hemolytic streptococci—particularly groups A and B, but also groups C, G, and F—are involved in up to one-third

TABLE 23-1

DIFFERENTIAL DIAGNOSIS OF ARTHRITIS SYNDROMES

ACUTE MONARTICULAR ARTHRITIS	CHRONIC MONARTICULAR ARTHRITIS	POLYARTICULAR ARTHRITIS
Staphylococcus aureus	*Mycobacterium tuberculosis*	*Neisseria meningitidis*
Streptococcus pneumoniae	Nontuberculous mycobacteria	*N. gonorrhoeae*
β-Hemolytic streptococci	*Borrelia burgdorferi*	Nongonococcal bacterial arthritis
Gram-negative bacilli	*Treponema pallidum*	Bacterial endocarditis
Neisseria gonorrhoeae	*Candida* species	*Candida* species
Candida species	*Sporothrix schenckii*	Poncet's disease (tuberculous rheumatism)
Crystal-induced arthritis	*Coccidioides immitis*	Hepatitis B virus
Fracture	*Blastomyces dermatitidis*	Parvovirus B19
Hemarthrosis	*Aspergillus* species	HIV
Foreign body	*Cryptococcus neoformans*	Human T-lymphotropic virus type I
Osteoarthritis	*Nocardia* species	Rubella virus
Ischemic necrosis	*Brucella* species	Arthropod-borne viruses
Monarticular rheumatoid arthritis	Legg-Calvé-Perthes disease	Sickle cell disease flare
	Osteoarthritis	Reactive arthritis
		Serum sickness
		Acute rheumatic fever
		Inflammatory bowel disease
		Systemic lupus erythematosus
		Rheumatoid arthritis/Still's disease
		Other vasculitides
		Sarcoidosis

of cases in older adults, especially those with underlying comorbid illnesses.

Infections after surgical procedures or penetrating injuries are due most often to *S. aureus* and occasionally to other gram-positive bacteria or gram-negative bacilli. Infections with coagulase-negative staphylococci are unusual except after the implantation of prosthetic joints or arthroscopy. Anaerobic organisms, often in association with aerobic or facultative bacteria, are found after human bites and when decubitus ulcers or intraabdominal abscesses spread into adjacent joints. Polymicrobial infections complicate traumatic injuries with extensive contamination. Bites and scratches from cats and other animals may introduce *Pasteurella multocida* into joints, and bites from humans may introduce *Eikenella corrodens* or other components of the oral flora.

Nongonococcal Bacterial Arthritis

Epidemiology

Although hematogenous infections with virulent organisms such as *S. aureus*, *H. influenzae*, and pyogenic streptococci occur in healthy persons, there is an underlying host predisposition in many cases of septic arthritis. Patients with rheumatoid arthritis have the highest incidence of infective arthritis (most often secondary to *S. aureus*) because of chronically inflamed joints, glucocorticoid therapy, and frequent breakdown of rheumatoid nodules, vasculitic ulcers, and skin overlying deformed joints. Diabetes mellitus, glucocorticoid therapy, hemodialysis, and malignancy all carry an increased risk of infection with *S. aureus* and gram-negative bacilli. Tumor necrosis factor (TNF) inhibitors (etanercept and infliximab), increasingly used for the treatment of rheumatoid arthritis, predispose to mycobacterial infections and possibly to other pyogenic bacterial infections and could be associated with septic arthritis in this population. Pneumococcal infections complicate alcoholism, deficiencies of humoral immunity, and hemoglobinopathies. Pneumococci, *Salmonella*, and *H. influenzae* cause septic arthritis in persons infected with HIV. Persons with primary immunoglobulin deficiency are at risk for mycoplasmal arthritis, which results in permanent joint damage if treatment with tetracycline and IV immunoglobulin (IVIg) replacement is not administered promptly. IV drug users acquire staphylococcal and streptococcal infections from their own flora and acquire pseudomonal and other gram-negative infections from drugs and injection paraphernalia.

Clinical Manifestations

Some 90% of patients present with involvement of a single joint—most commonly the knee; less frequently the hip; and still less often the shoulder, wrist, or elbow. Small joints of the hands and feet are more likely to be affected after direct inoculation or a bite. Among IV drug users, infections of the spine, sacroiliac joints, or sternoclavicular joints (Fig. 23-1) are more common than infections of the appendicular skeleton. Polyarticular infection is most common among patients with rheumatoid arthritis and may resemble a flare of the underlying disease.

The usual presentation consists of moderate to severe pain that is uniform around the joint, effusion, muscle spasm, and decreased range of motion. Fever in the range of 38.3°–38.9°C (101°–102°F) and sometimes higher is

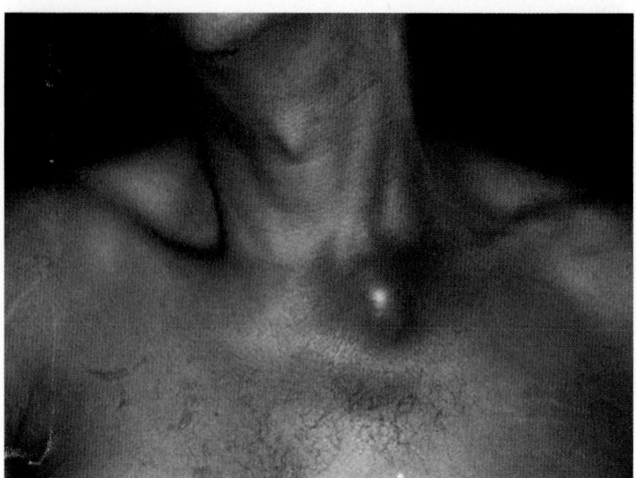

FIGURE 23-1

Acute septic arthritis of the sternoclavicular joint. A man in his 40s with a history of cirrhosis presented with a new onset of fever and lower neck pain. He had no history of IV drug use or previous catheter placement. Jaundice and a painful swollen area over his left sternoclavicular joint were evident on physical exam. Cultures of blood drawn at admission grew group B *Streptococcus*. The patient recovered after treatment with IV penicillin. *(Courtesy of Francisco M. Marty, MD, Brigham & Women's Hospital, Boston; with permission.)*

common but may be lacking, especially in persons with rheumatoid arthritis, renal or hepatic insufficiency, or conditions requiring immunosuppressive therapy. The inflamed, swollen joint is usually evident on examination except in the case of a deeply situated joint, such as the hip, shoulder, or sacroiliac joint. Cellulitis, bursitis, and acute osteomyelitis, which may produce a similar clinical picture, should be distinguished from septic arthritis by their greater range of motion and less-than-circumferential swelling. A focus of extraarticular infection, such as a boil or pneumonia, should be sought. Peripheral-blood leukocytosis with a left shift and elevation of the erythrocyte sedimentation rate (ESR) or C-reactive protein level are common.

Plain radiographs show evidence of soft tissue swelling, joint-space widening, and displacement of tissue planes by the distended capsule. Narrowing of the joint space and bony erosions indicate advanced infection and a poor prognosis. Ultrasound is useful for detecting effusions in the hip, and CT or MRI can demonstrate infections of the sacroiliac joint, the sternoclavicular joint, and the spine very well.

Laboratory Findings

Specimens of peripheral blood and synovial fluid should be obtained before antibiotics are administered. Blood cultures are positive in up to 50–70% of *S. aureus* infections but are less frequently positive in infections due to other organisms. The synovial fluid is turbid, serosanguineous, or frankly purulent. Gram-stained smears confirm the presence of large numbers of neutrophils. Levels of total protein and lactate dehydrogenase in synovial fluid are elevated, and the glucose level is depressed; however, these findings are not specific for infection, and measurement of these levels is not necessary to make the diagnosis. The synovial fluid should be examined for crystals, because gout and pseudogout can resemble septic arthritis clinically, and infection and crystal-induced disease occasionally occur together. Organisms are seen on synovial fluid smears in nearly three-quarters of infections with *S. aureus* and streptococci and in 30–50% of infections due to gram-negative and other bacteria. Cultures of synovial fluid are positive in >90% of cases. Inoculation of synovial fluid into bottles containing liquid media for blood cultures increases the yield of culture, especially if the pathogen is a fastidious organism or the patient is taking an antibiotic. Although not yet widely available, PCR-based assays for bacterial DNA will also be useful for the diagnosis of partially treated or culture-negative bacterial arthritis.

℞ Treatment: NONGONOCOCCAL BACTERIAL ARTHRITIS

Prompt administration of systemic antibiotics and drainage of the involved joint can prevent destruction of cartilage, postinfectious degenerative arthritis, joint instability, or deformity. Once samples of blood and synovial fluid have been obtained for culture, empirical antibiotics should be given that are directed against bacteria visualized on smears or against the pathogens that are likely, given the patient's age and risk factors. Initial therapy should consist of the IV administration of bactericidal agents; direct instillation of antibiotics into the joint is not necessary to achieve adequate levels in synovial fluid and tissue. An IV third-generation cephalosporin such as cefotaxime (1 g every 8 h) or ceftriaxone (1–2 g every 24 h) provides adequate empirical coverage for most community-acquired infections in adults when smears show no organisms. Either oxacillin or nafcillin (2 g every 4 h) is used if there are gram-positive cocci on the smear. If methicillin-resistant *S. aureus* is a possible pathogen (e.g., when it is widespread in the community or in hospitalized patients), IV vancomycin (1 g every 12 h) should be given. In addition, an aminoglycoside or third-generation cephalosporin should be given to IV drug users or other patients in whom *Pseudomonas aeruginosa* may be the responsible agent.

Definitive therapy is based on the identity and antibiotic susceptibility of the bacteria isolated in culture. Infections due to staphylococci are treated with oxacillin, nafcillin, or vancomycin for 4 weeks. Pneumococcal and streptococcal infections due to penicillin-susceptible organisms respond to 2 weeks of therapy with penicillin G (2 million units IV every 4 h); infections caused by *H. influenzae* and by strains of *S. pneumoniae* that are resistant to penicillin are treated with cefotaxime or ceftriaxone for 2 weeks. Most enteric gram-negative infections can be cured in 3–4 weeks by a second- or third-generation cephalosporin given IV or by a fluoroquinolone, such as levofloxacin (500 mg IV or PO every 24 h). *P. aeruginosa* infection should be treated for at least 2 weeks with a combination regimen of an aminoglycoside plus either an extended-spectrum penicillin, such as mezlocillin (3 g IV every 4 h), or an antipseudomonal cephalosporin, such as ceftazidime (1 g IV every 8 h). If tolerated, this regimen is continued for an additional 2 weeks; alternatively, a fluoroquinolone, such as ciprofloxacin (750 mg PO twice daily), is given by itself or with the penicillin or cephalosporin in place of the aminoglycoside.

Timely drainage of pus and necrotic debris from the infected joint is required for a favorable outcome. Needle aspiration of readily accessible joints such as the knee may be adequate if loculations or particulate matter in the joint does not prevent its thorough decompression. Arthroscopic drainage and lavage may be employed initially or within several days if repeated needle aspiration fails to relieve symptoms, decrease the volume of the effusion and the synovial white cell count, and clear bacteria from smears and cultures. In some cases, arthrotomy is necessary to remove loculations and debride infected synovium, cartilage, or bone. Septic arthritis of the hip is best managed with arthrotomy, particularly in young children, in whom infection threatens the viability of the femoral head. Septic joints do not require immobilization except for pain control before symptoms are alleviated by treatment. Weight bearing should be avoided until signs of inflammation have subsided, but frequent passive motion of the joint is indicated to maintain full mobility. Although addition of glucocorticoids to antibiotic treatment improves the outcome of *S. aureus* arthritis in experimental animals, no clinical trials have yet evaluated this approach in humans.

Gonococcal Arthritis

Epidemiology

Although its incidence has declined in recent years, gonococcal arthritis (Chap. 45) has accounted for up to 70% of episodes of infectious arthritis in persons <40 years of age in the United States. Arthritis due to *N. gonorrhoeae* is a consequence of bacteremia arising from gonococcal infection or, more frequently, from asymptomatic gonococcal mucosal colonization of the urethra, cervix, or pharynx. Women are at greatest risk during menses and during pregnancy and overall are two to three times more likely than men to develop disseminated gonococcal infection (DGI) and arthritis. Persons with complement deficiencies, especially of the terminal components, are prone to recurrent episodes of gonococcemia. Strains of gonococci that are most likely to cause DGI include those that produce transparent colonies in culture, have the type IA outer-membrane protein, or are of the AUH-auxotroph type.

Clinical Manifestations and Laboratory Findings

The most common manifestation of DGI is a syndrome of fever, chills, rash, and articular symptoms. Small numbers of papules that progress to hemorrhagic pustules develop on the trunk and the extensor surfaces of the distal extremities. Migratory arthritis and tenosynovitis of the knees, hands, wrists, feet, and ankles are prominent. The cutaneous lesions and articular findings are believed to be the consequence of an immune reaction to circulating gonococci and immune-complex deposition in tissues. Thus cultures of synovial fluid are consistently negative, and blood cultures are positive in <45% of patients. Synovial fluid may be difficult to obtain from inflamed joints and usually contains only 10,000–20,000 leukocytes/μL.

True gonococcal septic arthritis is less common than the DGI syndrome and always follows DGI, which is unrecognized in one-third of patients. A single joint, such as the hip, knee, ankle, or wrist, is usually involved. Synovial fluid, which contains >50,000 leukocytes/μL, can be obtained with ease; the gonococcus is only occasionally evident in gram-stained smears, and cultures of synovial fluid are positive in <40% of cases. Blood cultures are almost always negative.

Because it is difficult to isolate gonococci from synovial fluid and blood, specimens for culture should be obtained from potentially infected mucosal sites. Cultures and gram-stained smears of skin lesions are occasionally positive. All specimens for culture should be plated onto Thayer-Martin agar directly or in special transport media at the bedside and transferred promptly to the microbiology laboratory in an atmosphere of 5% CO_2, as generated in a candle jar. PCR-based assays are extremely sensitive in detecting gonococcal DNA in synovial fluid. A dramatic alleviation of symptoms within 12–24 h after the initiation of appropriate antibiotic therapy supports a clinical diagnosis of the DGI syndrome if cultures are negative.

℞ Treatment: GONOCOCCAL ARTHRITIS

Initial treatment consists of ceftriaxone (1 g IV or IM every 24 h) to cover possible penicillin-resistant organisms. Once local and systemic signs are clearly resolving and if the sensitivity of the isolate permits, the 7-day course of therapy can be completed with an oral agent such as ciprofloxacin (500 mg twice daily) if sensitivity allows. If penicillin-susceptible organisms are isolated, amoxicillin (500 mg three times daily) may be used. Suppurative arthritis usually responds to needle aspiration of involved joints and 7–14 days of antibiotic treatment. Arthroscopic lavage or arthrotomy is rarely required. Patients with DGI should be treated for *Chlamydia trachomatis* infection unless this infection is ruled out by appropriate testing.

It is noteworthy that arthritis symptoms similar to those seen in DGI occur in meningococcemia. A dermatitis-arthritis syndrome, purulent monarthritis, and reactive polyarthritis have been described. All respond to treatment with IV penicillin.

SPIROCHETAL ARTHRITIS

Lyme Disease

Lyme disease (Chap. 74) due to infection with the spirochete *Borrelia burgdorferi* causes arthritis in up to 70% of persons who are not treated. Intermittent arthralgias and myalgias—but not arthritis—occur within days or weeks of inoculation of the spirochete by the *Ixodes* tick. Later, there are three patterns of joint disease: (1) Fifty percent of untreated persons experience intermittent episodes of monarthritis or oligoarthritis involving the knee and/or other large joints. The symptoms wax and wane without treatment over months, and each year 10–20% of patients report loss of joint symptoms. (2) Twenty percent of untreated persons develop a pattern of waxing and waning arthralgias. (3) Ten percent of untreated patients develop chronic inflammatory synovitis resulting in erosive lesions and destruction of the joint. Serologic tests for IgG antibodies to *B. burgdorferi* are positive in >90% of persons with Lyme arthritis, and a PCR-based assay detects *Borrelia* DNA in 85%.

℞ Treatment: LYME ARTHRITIS

Lyme arthritis generally responds well to therapy. A regimen of oral doxycycline (100 mg twice daily for 30 days), oral amoxicillin (500 mg four times daily for 30 days), or parenteral ceftriaxone (2 g/d for 2–4 weeks) is recommended. Patients who do not respond to a total of 2 months of oral therapy or 1 month of parenteral therapy are unlikely to benefit from additional antibiotic therapy and are treated with anti-inflammatory agents or synovectomy. Failure of therapy is associated with host features such as the HLA-DR4 genotype, persistent reactivity to outer-surface protein A (OspA), and the presence of human leukocyte function–associated antigen 1 (hLFA-1), which cross-reacts with OspA.

Syphilitic Arthritis

Articular manifestations occur in different stages of syphilis (Chap. 70). In early congenital syphilis, periarticular swelling and immobilization of the involved limbs (Parrot's pseudoparalysis) complicate osteochondritis of long bones. Clutton's joint, a late manifestation of congenital syphilis that typically develops between the ages of 8 and 15 years, is caused by chronic painless synovitis with effusions of large joints, particularly the knees and elbows. Secondary syphilis may be associated with arthralgias; with symmetric arthritis of the knees and ankles and occasionally of the shoulders and wrists; and with sacroiliitis. The arthritis follows a subacute to chronic course with a mixed mononuclear and neutrophilic synovial-fluid pleocytosis (typical cell counts, 5000–15,000/μL). Immunologic mechanisms may contribute to the arthritis, and symptoms usually improve rapidly with penicillin therapy. In tertiary syphilis, Charcot's joint is a result of sensory loss due to tabes dorsalis. Penicillin is not helpful in this setting.

MYCOBACTERIAL ARTHRITIS

Tuberculous arthritis (Chap. 66) accounts for ~1% of all cases of tuberculosis and for 10% of extrapulmonary cases. The most common presentation is chronic granulomatous monarthritis. An unusual syndrome, Poncet's disease, is a reactive symmetric form of polyarthritis that affects persons with visceral or disseminated tuberculosis. No mycobacteria are found in the joints, and symptoms resolve with antituberculous therapy.

Unlike tuberculous osteomyelitis (Chap. 22), which typically involves the thoracic and lumbar spine (50% of cases), tuberculous arthritis primarily involves the large weight-bearing joints, in particular the hips, knees, and ankles, and only occasionally involves smaller non–weight-bearing joints. Progressive monarticular swelling and pain develop over months or years, and systemic symptoms are seen in only half of all cases. Tuberculous arthritis occurs as part of a disseminated primary infection or through late reactivation, often in persons with HIV infection or other immunocompromised hosts. Coexistent active pulmonary tuberculosis is unusual.

Aspiration of the involved joint yields fluid with an average cell count of 20,000/μL, with ~50% neutrophils. Acid-fast staining of the fluid yields positive results in fewer than one-third of cases, and cultures are positive in 80%. Culture of synovial tissue taken at biopsy is positive in ~90% of cases and shows granulomatous inflammation in most. DNA amplification methods such as PCR can shorten the time to diagnosis to 1 or 2 days. Radiographs reveal peripheral erosions at the points of synovial attachment, periarticular osteopenia, and eventually joint-space narrowing. Therapy for tuberculous arthritis is the same as that for tuberculous pulmonary disease, requiring the administration of multiple agents for 6–9 months. Therapy is more prolonged in immunosuppressed individuals, such as those infected with HIV.

Various atypical mycobacteria (Chap. 68) found in water and soil may cause chronic indolent arthritis. Such disease results from trauma and direct inoculation associated with farming, gardening, or aquatic activities. Smaller joints, such as the digits, wrists, and knees, are usually involved. Involvement of tendon sheaths and bursae is typical. The mycobacterial species involved include *Mycobacterium marinum*, *M. avium-intracellulare*, *M. terrae*, *M. kansasii*, *M. fortuitum*, and *M. chelonae*. In persons who have HIV infection or are receiving immunosuppressive therapy, hematogenous spread to the joints has been reported for *M. kansasii*, *M. avium-intracellulare*, and *M. haemophilum*. Diagnosis usually requires biopsy and culture, and therapy is based on antimicrobial susceptibility patterns.

FUNGAL ARTHRITIS

Fungi are an unusual cause of chronic monarticular arthritis. Granulomatous articular infection with the endemic dimorphic fungi *Coccidioides immitis*, *Blastomyces dermatitidis*, and (less commonly) *Histoplasma capsulatum* (Fig. 23-2) results from hematogenous seeding or direct

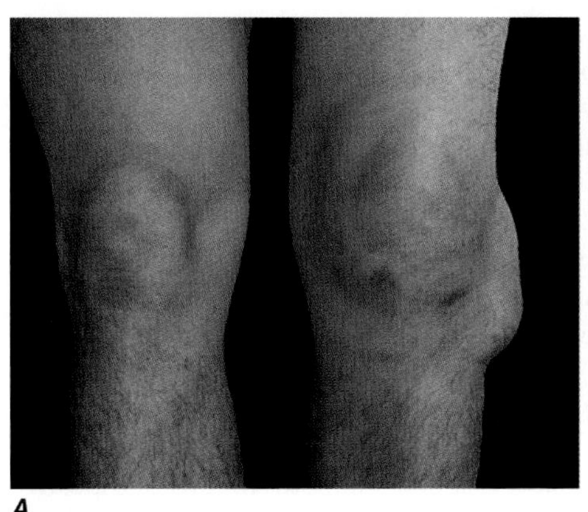
A

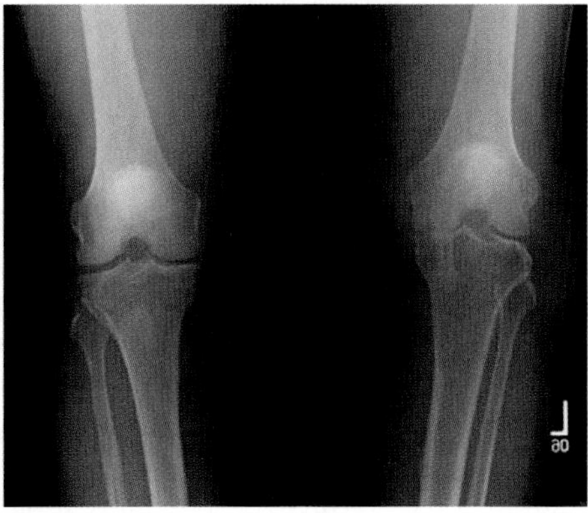
B

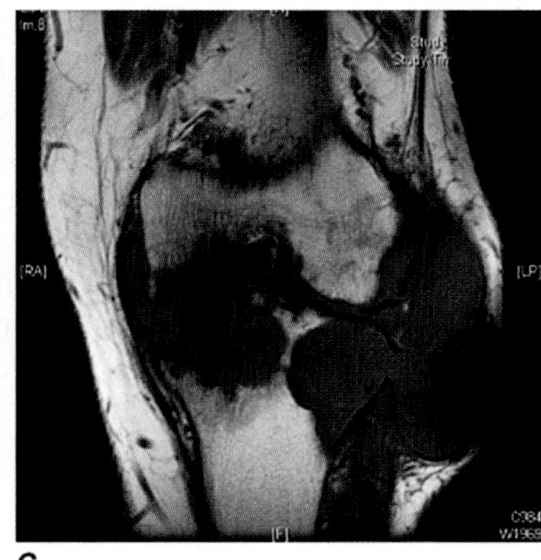
C

FIGURE 23-2

Chronic arthritis caused by *Histoplasma capsulatum* in the left knee. ***A.*** A man in his 60s from El Salvador presented with a history of progressive knee pain and difficulty walking for several years. He had undergone arthroscopy for a meniscal tear 7 years before presentation (without relief) and had received several intraarticular glucocorticoid injections. The patient developed significant deformity of the knee over time, including a large effusion in the lateral aspect. ***B.*** An x-ray of the knee showed multiple abnormalities, including severe medial femorotibial joint-space narrowing, several large subchondral cysts within the tibia and the patellofemoral compartment, a large suprapatellar joint effusion, and a large soft-tissue mass projecting laterally over the knee. ***C.*** MRI further defined these abnormalities and demonstrated the cystic nature of the lateral knee abnormality. Synovial biopsies demonstrated chronic inflammation with giant cells, and cultures grew *H. capsulatum* after 3 weeks of incubation. All clinical cystic lesions and the effusion resolved after 1 year of treatment with itraconazole. The patient underwent a left total knee replacement for definitive treatment. (*Courtesy of Francisco M. Marty, MD, Brigham & Women's Hospital, Boston; with permission.*)

extension from bony lesions in persons with disseminated disease. Joint involvement is an unusual complication of sporotrichosis (infection with *Sporothrix schenckii*) among gardeners and other persons who work with soil or sphagnum moss. Articular sporotrichosis is six times more common among men than among women, and alcoholics and other debilitated hosts are at risk for polyarticular infection.

Candida infection involving a single joint—usually the knee, hip, or shoulder—results from surgical procedures, intraarticular injections, or (among critically ill patients with debilitating illnesses, such as diabetes mellitus or hepatic or renal insufficiency, and patients receiving immunosuppressive therapy) hematogenous spread. *Candida* infections in IV drug users typically involve the spine, sacroiliac joints, or other fibrocartilaginous joints. Unusual cases of arthritis due to *Aspergillus* species, *Cryptococcus neoformans*, *Pseudallescheria boydii*, and the dematiaceous fungi have also resulted from direct inoculation or disseminated hematogenous infection in immunocompromised persons.

The synovial fluid in fungal arthritis usually contains 10,000–40,000 cells/μL, with ~70% neutrophils. Stained specimens and cultures of synovial tissue often confirm the diagnosis of fungal arthritis when studies of synovial fluid give negative results. Treatment consists of drainage and lavage of the joint and systemic administration of an antifungal agent directed at a specific pathogen. The doses and duration of therapy are the same as for disseminated disease (see Section 7). Intraarticular instillation of amphotericin B has been used in addition to IV therapy.

VIRAL ARTHRITIS

Viruses produce arthritis by infecting synovial tissue during systemic infection or by provoking an immunologic reaction that involves joints. As many as 50% of women report persistent arthralgias and 10% report frank arthritis within 3 days of the rash that follows natural infection with rubella virus and within 2–6 weeks after receipt of live-virus vaccine. Episodes of symmetric inflammation of fingers, wrists, and knees uncommonly recur for >1 year, but a syndrome of chronic fatigue, low-grade fever, headaches, and myalgias can persist for months or years. IVIg has been helpful in selected cases. Self-limited monarticular or migratory polyarthritis may develop within 2 weeks of the parotitis of mumps; this sequela is more common among men than among women. Approximately 10% of children and 60% of women develop arthritis after infection with parvovirus B19. In adults, arthropathy sometimes occurs without fever or rash. Pain and stiffness, with less prominent swelling (primarily of the hands but also of the knees, wrists, and ankles), usually resolve within weeks, although a small proportion of patients develop chronic arthropathy.

About 2 weeks before the onset of jaundice, up to 10% of persons with acute hepatitis B develop an immune complex–mediated, serum sickness–like reaction with maculopapular rash, urticaria, fever, and arthralgias. Less common developments include symmetric arthritis involving the hands, wrists, elbows, or ankles and morning stiffness that resembles a flare of rheumatoid arthritis. Symptoms resolve at the time jaundice develops. Many persons with chronic hepatitis C infection report persistent arthralgia or arthritis, both in the presence and in the absence of cryoglobulinemia. Painful arthritis involving larger joints often accompanies the fever and rash of several arthropod-borne viral infections, including those caused by chikungunya, O'nyong-nyong, Ross River, Mayaro, and Barmah Forest viruses. Symmetric arthritis involving the hands and wrists may occur during the convalescent phase of infection with lymphocytic choriomeningitis virus. Patients infected with an enterovirus frequently report arthralgias, and echovirus has been isolated from patients with acute polyarthritis.

Several arthritis syndromes are associated with HIV infection. Reiter's syndrome with painful lower-extremity oligoarthritis often follows an episode of urethritis in HIV-infected persons. HIV-associated Reiter's syndrome appears to be extremely common among persons with the HLA-B27 haplotype, but sacroiliac joint disease is unusual and is seen mostly in the absence of HLA-B27. Up to one-third of HIV-infected persons with psoriasis develop psoriatic arthritis. Painless monarthropathy and persistent symmetric polyarthropathy occasionally complicate HIV infection. Chronic persistent oligoarthritis of the shoulders, wrists, hands, and knees occurs in women infected with human T-cell lymphotropic virus type I. Synovial thickening, destruction of articular cartilage, and leukemic-appearing atypical lymphocytes in synovial fluid are characteristic, but progression to T-cell leukemia is unusual.

PARASITIC ARTHRITIS

Arthritis due to parasitic infection is rare. The guinea worm *Dracunculus medinensis* may cause destructive joint lesions in the lower extremities as migrating gravid female worms invade joints or cause ulcers in adjacent soft tissues that become secondarily infected. Hydatid cysts infect bones in 1–2% of cases of infection with *Echinococcus granulosus*. The expanding destructive cystic lesions may spread to and destroy adjacent joints, particularly the hip and pelvis. In rare cases, chronic synovitis has been associated with the presence of schistosomal eggs in synovial biopsies. Monarticular arthritis in children with lymphatic filariasis appears to respond to therapy with diethylcarbamazine, even in the absence of microfilariae in synovial fluid. Reactive arthritis has been attributed to hookworm, *Strongyloides*, *Cryptosporidium*, and *Giardia* infection in case reports, but confirmation is required.

POSTINFECTIOUS OR REACTIVE ARTHRITIS

Reiter's syndrome, a reactive polyarthritis, develops several weeks after ~1% of cases of nongonococcal urethritis and 2% of enteric infections, particularly those due to *Yersinia enterocolitica*, *Shigella flexneri*, *Campylobacter jejuni*, and *Salmonella* species. Only a minority of these patients have the other findings of classic Reiter's syndrome, including urethritis, conjunctivitis, uveitis, oral ulcers, and rash. Studies have identified microbial DNA or antigen in synovial fluid or blood, but the pathogenesis of this condition is poorly understood.

Reiter's syndrome is most common among young men (except after *Yersinia* infection) and has been linked to the HLA-B27 locus as a potential genetic predisposing factor. Patients report painful, asymmetric oligoarthritis affecting mainly the knees, ankles, and feet. Low-back pain is common, and radiographic evidence of sacroiliitis is found in patients with long-standing disease. Most patients recover within 6 months, but prolonged recurrent disease is more common in cases after chlamydial urethritis. Anti-inflammatory agents help to relieve symptoms, but the role of prolonged antibiotic therapy in eliminating microbial antigen from the synovium is controversial.

Migratory polyarthritis and fever constitute the usual presentation of acute rheumatic fever in adults (Chap. 37). This presentation is distinct from that of poststreptococcal reactive arthritis, which also follows infections with group A *Streptococcus* but is not migratory, lasts beyond the typical 3-week maximum of acute rheumatic fever, and responds poorly to aspirin.

INFECTIONS IN PROSTHETIC JOINTS

Infection complicates 1–4% of total joint replacements. The majority of infections are acquired intraoperatively or immediately postoperatively as a result of wound breakdown or infection; less commonly, these joint infections develop later after joint replacement and are the result of hematogenous spread or direct inoculation. The presentation may be acute, with fever, pain, and local signs of inflammation, especially in infections due to *S. aureus*, pyogenic streptococci, and enteric bacilli. Alternatively, infection may persist for months or years without causing constitutional symptoms when less virulent organisms, such as coagulase-negative staphylococci or diphtheroids, are involved. Such indolent infections are usually acquired during joint implantation and are discovered during evaluation of chronic unexplained pain or after a radiograph shows loosening of the prosthesis; the ESR and C-reactive protein level are usually elevated in such cases.

The diagnosis is best made by needle aspiration of the joint; accidental introduction of organisms during aspiration must be meticulously avoided. Synovial fluid pleocytosis with a predominance of polymorphonuclear leukocytes is highly suggestive of infection, since other inflammatory processes uncommonly affect prosthetic joints. Culture and Gram's stain usually yield the responsible pathogen. Use of special media for unusual pathogens such as fungi, atypical mycobacteria, and *Mycoplasma* may be necessary if routine and anaerobic cultures are negative.

℞ Treatment: PROSTHETIC JOINT INFECTIONS

Treatment includes surgery and high doses of parenteral antibiotics, which are given for 4–6 weeks because bone is usually involved. In most cases, the prosthesis must be replaced to cure the infection. Implantation of a new prosthesis is best delayed for several weeks or months because relapses of infection occur most commonly within this time frame. In some cases, reimplantation is not possible, and the patient must manage without a joint, with a fused joint, or even with amputation. Cure of infection without removal of the prosthesis is occasionally possible in cases that are due to streptococci or pneumococci and that lack radiologic evidence of loosening of the prosthesis. In these cases, antibiotic therapy must be initiated within several days of the onset of infection, and the joint should be drained vigorously either by open arthrotomy or arthroscopically. In selected patients who prefer to avoid the high morbidity associated with joint removal and reimplantation, suppression of the infection with antibiotics may be a reasonable goal. A high cure rate with retention of the prosthesis has been reported when the combination of oral rifampin and ciprofloxacin is given for 3–6 months to persons with staphylococcal prosthetic joint infection of short duration. This approach, which is based on the ability of rifampin to kill organisms adherent to foreign material and in the stationary growth phase, requires confirmation in prospective trials.

Prevention

To avoid the disastrous consequences of infection, candidates for joint replacement should be selected with care. Rates of infection are particularly high among patients with rheumatoid arthritis, persons who have undergone previous surgery on the joint, and persons with medical conditions requiring immunosuppressive therapy. Perioperative antibiotic prophylaxis, usually with cefazolin, and measures to decrease intraoperative contamination, such as laminar flow, have lowered the rates of perioperative infection to <1% in many centers. After implantation, measures should be taken to prevent or rapidly treat extraarticular infections that might give rise to hematogenous spread to the prosthesis. The effectiveness of prophylactic antibiotics for the prevention of hematogenous infection after dental procedures has not been demonstrated; in fact, viridans streptococci and other components of the oral flora are extremely unusual causes of prosthetic joint infection. Accordingly, the American Dental Association and the American Academy of Orthopaedic Surgeons do not recommend antibiotic prophylaxis for most dental patients with total joint replacements. They do, however, recommend prophylaxis for patients who may be at high risk of hematogenous infection, including those with inflammatory arthropathies, immunosuppression, type 1 diabetes mellitus, joint replacement within 2 years, previous prosthetic joint infection, malnourishment, or hemophilia. The recommended regimen is amoxicillin (2 g PO) 1 h before dental procedures associated with a high incidence of bacteremia. Clindamycin (600 mg PO) is suggested for patients allergic to penicillin.

ACKNOWLEDGMENT

The contributions of James H. Maguire and the late Scott J. Thaler to this chapter in earlier editions of Harrison's Principles of Internal Medicine are gratefully acknowledged.

FURTHER READINGS

BARDIN T: Gonococcal arthritis. Best Pract Res Clin Rheumatol 17:201, 2003

DONATTO KC: Orthopedic management of septic arthritis. Rheum Dis Clin North Am 24:275, 1998

FRANSSILA R, HEDMAN K: Infection and musculoskeletal conditions: Viral causes of arthritis. Best Pract Res Clin Rheumatol 20:1139, 2006

HARRINGTON JT: Mycobacterial and fungal arthritis. Curr Opin Rheumatol 10:335, 1998

MARGARETTEN ME et al: Does this adult patient have septic arthritis? JAMA 297:1478, 2007

MATHEWS CJ, COAKLEY G: Septic arthritis: Current diagnostic and therapeutic algorithm. Curr Opin Rheumatol 20:457, 2008

MEDINA RODRIGUEZ F: Rheumatic manifestations of human immunodeficiency virus infection. Rheum Dis Clin North Am 29:145, 2003

MEEHAN AM et al: Outcome of penicillin-susceptible streptococcal prosthetic joint infection treated with debridement and retention of the prosthesis. Clin Infect Dis 36:845, 2003

SHIRTLIFF ME, MADER JT: Acute septic arthritis. Clin Microbiol Rev 15:527, 2002

SIMON F et al: Chikungunya infection: An emerging rheumatism among travelers returned from Indian Ocean islands. Report of 47 cases. Medicine (Baltimore) 86:123, 2007

STENGEL D et al: Systematic review and meta-analysis of antibiotic therapy for bone and joint infections. Lancet Infect Dis 1:175, 2001

TARKOWSKI A: Infection and musculoskeletal conditions: Infectious arthritis. Best Pract Res Clin Rheumatol 20:1029, 2006

ZIMMERLI W et al: Prosthetic-joint infections. N Engl J Med 351:145, 2004

CHAPTER 24

INTRAABDOMINAL INFECTIONS AND ABSCESSES

Miriam J. Baron ■ Dennis L. Kasper

Intraperitoneal infections generally arise because a normal anatomic barrier is disrupted. This disruption may occur when the appendix, a diverticulum, or an ulcer ruptures; when the bowel wall is weakened by ischemia, tumor, or inflammation (e.g., in inflammatory bowel disease); or with adjacent inflammatory processes, such as pancreatitis or pelvic inflammatory disease, in which enzymes (in the former case) or organisms (in the latter) may leak into the peritoneal cavity. Whatever the inciting event, once inflammation develops and organisms usually contained within the bowel or another organ enter the normally sterile peritoneal space, a predictable series of events takes place. Intraabdominal infections occur in two stages: peritonitis and—if the patient survives this stage and goes untreated—abscess formation. The types of microorganisms predominating in each stage of infection are responsible for the pathogenesis of disease.

PERITONITIS

Peritonitis is a life-threatening event that is often accompanied by bacteremia and sepsis syndrome (Chap. 15). The peritoneal cavity is large but is divided into compartments. The upper and lower peritoneal cavities are divided by the transverse mesocolon; the greater omentum extends from the transverse mesocolon and from the lower pole of the stomach to line the lower peritoneal cavity. The pancreas, duodenum, and ascending and descending colon are located in the anterior retroperitoneal space; the kidneys, ureters, and adrenals are found in the posterior retroperitoneal space. The other organs, including liver, stomach, gallbladder, spleen, jejunum, ileum, transverse and sigmoid colon, cecum, and appendix, are within the peritoneal cavity. The cavity is lined with a serous membrane that can serve as a conduit for fluids—a property exploited in peritoneal dialysis (Fig. 24-1). A small amount of serous fluid is normally present in the peritoneal space, with a protein content (consisting mainly of albumin) of <30 g/L and <300 white blood cells (WBCs, generally mononuclear cells) per microliter. In bacterial infections, leukocyte recruitment into the infected peritoneal cavity consists of an early influx of polymorphonuclear leukocytes (PMNs) and a prolonged subsequent phase of mononuclear cell migration. The phenotype of the infiltrating leukocytes during the course of inflammation is regulated primarily by resident-cell chemokine synthesis.

PRIMARY (SPONTANEOUS) BACTERIAL PERITONITIS

Peritonitis is either primary (without an apparent source of contamination) or secondary. The types of organisms found and the clinical presentations of these two processes are different. In adults, primary bacterial peritonitis (PBP) occurs most commonly in conjunction with cirrhosis of the liver (frequently the result of alcoholism). However, the disease has been reported in adults with metastatic malignant disease, postnecrotic cirrhosis, chronic active hepatitis, acute viral hepatitis, congestive heart failure, systemic lupus erythematosus, and lymphedema, as well as in patients with no underlying disease. Although PBP virtually always develops in patients with preexisting ascites, it is, in general, an uncommon event, occurring in ≤10% of cirrhotic patients. The cause of PBP has not been established definitively but is believed to involve hematogenous spread of organisms in a patient in whom a diseased liver and altered portal circulation result in a defect in the usual filtration function. Organisms multiply in ascites, a good medium for growth. The proteins of the complement cascade have been found in peritoneal fluid, with lower levels in cirrhotic patients than in patients with ascites of other etiologies. The opsonic and phagocytic properties of PMNs are diminished in patients with advanced liver disease.

The presentation of PBP differs from that of secondary peritonitis. The most common manifestation is fever, which is reported in up to 80% of patients. Ascites is found but virtually always predates infection. Abdominal pain, an acute onset of symptoms, and peritoneal irritation during physical examination can be helpful diagnostically, but the absence of any of these findings does not exclude this often-subtle diagnosis. Nonlocalizing symptoms (such as malaise, fatigue, or encephalopathy) without another clear etiology should also prompt consideration of PBP in a susceptible patient. It is vital to sample the peritoneal fluid of any cirrhotic patient with ascites and fever. The finding of >250 PMNs/μL is diagnostic for PBP, according to Conn (*http://jac.oxfordjournals.org/cgi/content/full/47/3/369*). This criterion does not apply to secondary peritonitis (see below). The microbiology of PBP is also distinctive. Although enteric gram-negative bacilli such as *Escherichia coli* are most commonly encountered, gram-positive organisms such as streptococci, enterococci, or even pneumococci are sometimes found. In PBP, a single organism is typically isolated;

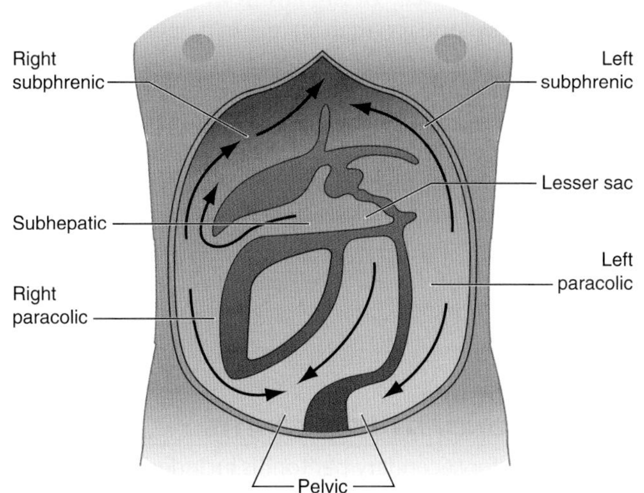

FIGURE 24-1

Diagram of the intraperitoneal spaces, showing the circulation of fluid and potential areas for abscess formation. Some compartments collect fluid or pus more often than others. These compartments include the pelvis (the lowest portion), the subphrenic spaces on the right and left sides, and Morrison's pouch, which is a posterosuperior extension of the subhepatic spaces and is the lowest part of the paravertebral groove when a patient is recumbent. The falciform ligament separating the right and left subphrenic spaces appears to act as a barrier to the spread of infection; consequently, it is unusual to find bilateral subphrenic collections. [*Reprinted with permission from B Lorber (ed): Atlas of Infectious Diseases, vol VII: Intra-abdominal Infections, Hepatitis, and Gastroenteritis. Philadelphia, Current Medicine, 1996, p 1.13.*]

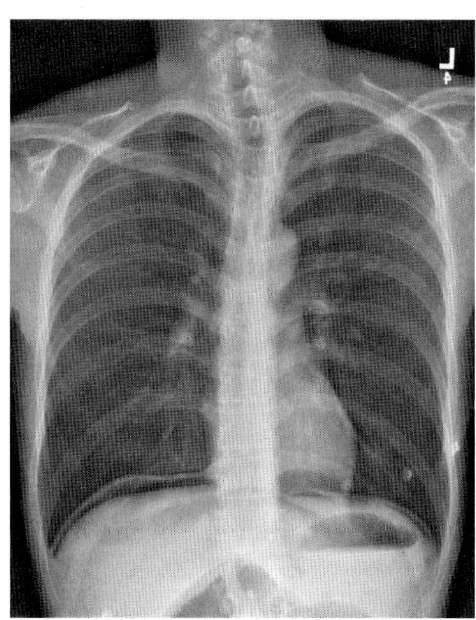

FIGURE 24-2

Pneumoperitoneum. Free air under the diaphragm on an upright chest film suggests the presence of a bowel perforation and associated peritonitis. (*Image courtesy of Dr. John Braver; with permission.*)

anaerobes are found less frequently in PBP than in secondary peritonitis, in which a mixed flora including anaerobes is the rule. In fact, if PBP is suspected and multiple organisms including anaerobes are recovered from the peritoneal fluid, the diagnosis must be reconsidered and a source of secondary peritonitis sought.

The diagnosis of PBP is not easy. It depends on the exclusion of a primary intraabdominal source of infection. Contrast-enhanced CT is useful in identifying an intraabdominal source for infection. It may be difficult to recover organisms from cultures of peritoneal fluid, presumably because the burden of organisms is low. However, the yield can be improved if 10 mL of peritoneal fluid is placed directly into a blood culture bottle. Since bacteremia frequently accompanies PBP, blood should be cultured simultaneously. No specific radiographic studies are helpful in the diagnosis of PBP. A plain film of the abdomen would be expected to show ascites. Chest and abdominal radiography should be performed in patients with abdominal pain to exclude free air, which signals a perforation (Fig. 24-2).

℞ Treatment: PRIMARY BACTERIAL PERITONITIS

Treatment for PBP is directed at the isolate from blood or peritoneal fluid. Gram's staining of peritoneal fluid often gives negative results in PBP. Therefore, until culture results become available, therapy should cover gram-negative aerobic bacilli and gram-positive cocci. Third-generation cephalosporins such as cefotaxime (2 g q8h, administered IV) provide reasonable initial coverage in moderately ill patients. Broad-spectrum antibiotics, such as penicillin/β-lactamase inhibitor combinations (e.g., piperacillin/tazobactam, 3.375 g q6h IV for adults with normal renal function) or ceftriaxone (2 g q24h IV), are also options. Empirical coverage for anaerobes is not necessary. After the infecting organism is identified, therapy should be narrowed to target the specific pathogen. Patients with PBP usually respond within 72 h to appropriate antibiotic therapy. Antimicrobial therapy can be administered for as little as 5 days if rapid improvement occurs and blood cultures are negative, but a course of up to 2 weeks may be required for patients with bacteremia and for those whose improvement is slow. Persistence of WBCs in the ascitic fluid after therapy should prompt a search for additional diagnoses.

Prevention

PBP has a high rate of recurrence. Up to 70% of patients experience a recurrence within 1 year. Antibiotic prophylaxis reduces this rate to <20%. Prophylactic regimens for adults with normal renal function include fluoroquinolones (ciprofloxacin, 750 mg weekly; norfloxacin, 400 mg/d) or trimethoprim-sulfamethoxazole (one double-strength tablet daily). However, long-term administration of broad-spectrum antibiotics in this setting has been shown to increase the risk of severe staphylococcal infections.

SECONDARY PERITONITIS

Secondary peritonitis develops when bacteria contaminate the peritoneum as a result of spillage from an intraabdominal viscus. The organisms found almost always constitute a mixed flora in which facultative gram-negative bacilli and anaerobes predominate, especially when the contaminating source is colonic. Early in the course of infection, when the host response is directed toward containment of the infection, exudate containing fibrin and PMNs is found. Early death in this setting is attributable to gram-negative bacillary sepsis and to potent endotoxins circulating in the bloodstream (Chap. 15). Gram-negative bacilli, particularly *E. coli*, are common bloodstream isolates, but *Bacteroides fragilis* bacteremia also occurs. The severity of abdominal pain and the clinical course depend on the inciting process. The organisms isolated from the peritoneum also vary with the source of the initial process and the normal flora at that site. Secondary peritonitis can result primarily from chemical irritation and/or bacterial contamination. For example, as long as the patient is not achlorhydric, a ruptured gastric ulcer will release low-pH gastric contents that will serve as a chemical irritant. The normal flora of the stomach comprises the same organisms found in the oropharynx (Chap. 65), but in lower numbers. Thus the bacterial burden in a ruptured ulcer is negligible compared with that in a ruptured appendix. The normal flora of the colon below the ligament of Treitz contains ~10^{11} anaerobic organisms/g of feces but only 10^8 aerobes/g; therefore, anaerobic species account for 99.9% of the bacteria. Leakage of colonic contents (pH 7–8) does not cause significant chemical peritonitis, but infection is intense because of the heavy bacterial load.

Depending on the inciting event, local symptoms may occur in secondary peritonitis—for example, epigastric pain from a ruptured gastric ulcer. In appendicitis (Chap. 26), the initial presenting symptoms are often vague, with periumbilical discomfort and nausea followed in a number of hours by pain more localized to the right lower quadrant. Unusual locations of the appendix (including a retrocecal position) can complicate this presentation further. Once infection has spread to the peritoneal cavity, pain increases, particularly with infection involving the parietal peritoneum, which is innervated extensively. Patients usually lie motionless, often with knees drawn up to avoid stretching the nerve fibers of the peritoneal cavity. Coughing and sneezing, which increase pressure within the peritoneal cavity, are associated with sharp pain. There may or may not be pain localized to the infected or diseased organ from which secondary peritonitis has arisen. Patients with secondary peritonitis generally have abnormal findings on abdominal examination, with marked voluntary and involuntary guarding of the anterior abdominal musculature. Later findings include tenderness, especially rebound tenderness. In addition, there may be localized findings in the area of the inciting event. In general, patients are febrile, with marked leukocytosis and a left shift of the WBCs to band forms.

Although recovery of organisms from peritoneal fluid is easier in secondary than in primary peritonitis, a tap of the abdomen is rarely the procedure of choice in secondary peritonitis. An exception is in cases involving trauma, where the possibility of a hemoperitoneum may need to be excluded early. Emergent studies (such as abdominal CT) to find the source of peritoneal contamination should be undertaken if the patient is hemodynamically stable; unstable patients may require surgical intervention without prior imaging.

℞ Treatment: SECONDARY PERITONITIS

Treatment for secondary peritonitis includes early administration of antibiotics aimed particularly at aerobic gram-negative bacilli and anaerobes (see below). Mild to moderate disease can be treated with many drugs covering these organisms, including broad-spectrum penicillin/β-lactamase inhibitor combinations (e.g., ticarcillin/clavulanate, 3.1 g q4–6h IV) or cefoxitin (2 g q4–6h IV). Patients in intensive care units should receive imipenem (500 mg q6h IV), meropenem (1 g q8h IV), or combinations of drugs, such as ampicillin plus metronidazole plus ciprofloxacin. The role of enterococci and *Candida* spp. in mixed infections is controversial. Secondary peritonitis usually requires both surgical intervention to address the inciting process and antibiotics to treat early bacteremia, to decrease the incidence of abscess formation and wound infection, and to prevent distant spread of infection. Although surgery is rarely indicated in PBP in adults, it may be life-saving in secondary peritonitis.

Peritonitis may develop as a complication of abdominal surgeries. These infections may be accompanied by localizing pain and/or nonlocalizing symptoms such as fever, malaise, anorexia, and toxicity. As a nosocomial infection, postoperative peritonitis may be associated with organisms such as staphylococci, components of the gram-negative hospital microflora, and the microbes that cause PBP and secondary peritonitis, as described above.

PERITONITIS IN PATIENTS UNDERGOING CAPD

A third type of peritonitis arises in patients who are undergoing continuous ambulatory peritoneal dialysis (CAPD). Unlike PBP and secondary peritonitis, which are caused by endogenous bacteria, CAPD-associated peritonitis usually involves skin organisms. The pathogenesis of infection is similar to that of intravascular device–related infection, in which skin organisms migrate along the catheter, which both serves as an entry point and exerts the effects of a foreign body. Exit-site or tunnel infection may or may not accompany CAPD-associated peritonitis. Like PBP, CAPD-associated peritonitis is usually caused by a single organism. Peritonitis is, in fact, the most common reason for discontinuation of CAPD. Improvements in equipment design, especially the Y-set connector, have resulted in a decrease from one case of peritonitis per 9 months of CAPD to one case per 15 months.

The clinical presentation of CAPD peritonitis resembles that of secondary peritonitis in that diffuse pain and peritoneal signs are common. The dialysate is usually cloudy and contains >100 WBCs/μL, >50% of which are neutrophils. The most common organisms are *Staphylococcus* spp., which accounted for ~45% of cases in one recent series. Historically, coagulase-negative staphylococcal species were identified most commonly in these infections, but more recently these isolates have been decreasing in frequency. *Staphylococcus aureus* is more often involved among patients who are nasal carriers of the organism than among those who are not, and this organism is the most common pathogen in overt exit-site infections. Gram-negative bacilli and fungi such as *Candida* spp. are also found. Vancomycin-resistant enterococci and vancomycin-intermediate *S. aureus* have been reported to produce peritonitis in CAPD patients. The finding of more than one organism in dialysate culture should prompt evaluation for secondary peritonitis. As with PBP, culture of dialysate fluid in blood culture bottles improves the yield. To facilitate diagnosis, several hundred milliliters of removed dialysis fluid should be concentrated by centrifugation before culture.

℞ Treatment: CAPD PERITONITIS

Empirical therapy for CAPD peritonitis should be directed at *S. aureus*, coagulase-negative *Staphylococcus*, and gram-negative bacilli until the results of cultures are available. Guidelines issued in 2005 suggest that agents should be chosen on the basis of local experience with resistant organisms. In some centers, a first-generation cephalosporin such as cefazolin (for gram-positive bacteria) and a fluoroquinolone or a third-generation cephalosporin such as ceftazidime (for gram-negative bacteria) may be reasonable; in areas with high rates of infection with methicillin-resistant *S. aureus*, vancomycin should be used instead of cefazolin, and gram-negative coverage may need to be broadened. Broad coverage including vancomycin should be particularly considered for toxic patients and for those with exit-site infections. Loading doses are administered intraperitoneally; doses depend on the dialysis method and the patient's renal function. Antibiotics are given either continuously (i.e., with each exchange) or intermittently (i.e., once daily, with the dose allowed to remain in the peritoneal cavity for at least 6 h). If the patient is severely ill, IV antibiotics should be added at doses appropriate for the patient's degree of renal failure. The clinical response to an empirical treatment regimen should be rapid; if the patient has not responded after 48 h of treatment, catheter removal should be considered.

TUBERCULOUS PERITONITIS

See Chap. 66.

INTRAABDOMINAL ABSCESSES

INTRAPERITONEAL ABSCESSES

Abscess formation is common in untreated peritonitis if overt gram-negative sepsis either does not develop or develops but is not fatal. In experimental models of abscess formation, mixed aerobic and anaerobic organisms have been implanted intraperitoneally. Without therapy directed at anaerobes, animals develop intraabdominal abscesses. As in humans, these experimental abscesses may stud the peritoneal cavity, lie within the omentum or mesentery, or even develop on the surface of or within viscera such as the liver.

Pathogenesis and Immunity

There is often disagreement about whether an abscess represents a disease state or a host response. In a sense, it represents both: although an abscess is an infection in which viable infecting organisms and PMNs are contained in a fibrous capsule, it is also a process by which the host confines microbes to a limited space, thereby preventing further spread of infection. In any event, abscesses do cause significant symptoms, and patients with abscesses can be quite ill. Experimental work has helped to define both the host cells and the bacterial virulence factors responsible—most notably, in the case of *B. fragilis*. This organism, although accounting for only 0.5% of the normal colonic flora, is the anaerobe most frequently isolated from intraabdominal infections, is especially prominent in abscesses, and is the most common anaerobic bloodstream isolate. On clinical grounds, therefore, *B. fragilis* appears to be uniquely virulent. Moreover, *B. fragilis* acts alone to cause abscesses in animal models of intraabdominal infection, whereas most other *Bacteroides* species must act synergistically with a facultative organism to induce abscess formation.

Of the several virulence factors identified in *B. fragilis*, one is critical: the capsular polysaccharide complex (CPC) found on the bacterial surface. The CPC comprises at least eight distinct surface polysaccharides. Structural analysis of these polysaccharides has shown an unusual motif of oppositely charged sugars. Polysaccharides having these *zwitterionic* characteristics, such as polysaccharide A (PSA), evoke a host response in the peritoneal cavity that localizes bacteria into abscesses. *B. fragilis* and PSA have been found to adhere to primary mesothelial cells in vitro; this adherence, in turn, stimulates the production of tumor necrosis factor α (TNF-α) and intercellular adhesion molecule 1 (ICAM-1) by peritoneal macrophages. Although abscesses characteristically contain PMNs, the process of abscess induction depends on the stimulation of T lymphocytes by these unique zwitterionic polysaccharides. The stimulated CD4+ T lymphocytes secrete leukoattractant cytokines and chemokines. The alternative pathway of complement and fibrinogen also participate in abscess formation.

Although antibodies to the CPC enhance bloodstream clearance of *B. fragilis*, CD4+ T cells are critical in immunity to abscesses. When administered subcutaneously, *B. fragilis* PSA has immunomodulatory characteristics and stimulates CD4+ T-regulatory cells via an interleukin (IL) 2–dependent mechanism to produce IL-10. IL-10 downregulates the inflammatory response, thereby preventing abscess formation.

Clinical Presentation

Of all intraabdominal abscesses, 74% are intraperitoneal or retroperitoneal and are not visceral. Most intraperitoneal abscesses result from fecal spillage from a colonic source, such as an inflamed appendix. Abscesses can also arise from other processes. They usually form within weeks of the development of peritonitis and may be found in a variety of locations—from omentum to mesentery, pelvis to psoas muscles, and subphrenic space to a visceral organ such as the liver, where they may develop either on the surface of the organ or within it. Periappendiceal and diverticular abscesses occur commonly. Diverticular abscesses are least likely to rupture. Infections of the female genital tract and pancreatitis are also among the more common causative events. When abscesses occur in the female genital tract—either as a primary infection (e.g., tuboovarian abscess) or as an infection extending into the pelvic cavity or peritoneum—*B. fragilis* figures prominently among the organisms isolated. *B. fragilis* is not found in large numbers in the normal vaginal flora. For example, it is encountered less commonly in pelvic inflammatory disease and endometritis without an associated abscess. In pancreatitis with leakage of damaging pancreatic enzymes, inflammation is prominent. Therefore, clinical findings such as fever, leukocytosis, and even abdominal pain do not distinguish pancreatitis itself from complications such as pancreatic pseudocyst, pancreatic abscess, or intraabdominal collections of pus. Especially in cases of necrotizing pancreatitis, in which the incidence of local pancreatic infection may be as high as 30%, needle aspiration under CT guidance is performed to sample fluid for culture. Many centers prescribe preemptive antibiotics for patients with necrotizing pancreatitis. Imipenem is frequently used for this purpose since it reaches high tissue levels in the pancreas (although it is not unique in this regard). If needle aspiration yields infected fluid, most experts agree that surgery is superior to percutaneous drainage.

Diagnosis

Scanning procedures have considerably facilitated the diagnosis of intraabdominal abscesses. Abdominal CT probably has the highest yield, although ultrasonography is particularly useful for the right upper quadrant, kidneys, and pelvis. Both indium-labeled WBCs and gallium tend to localize in abscesses and may be useful in finding a collection. Since gallium is taken up in the bowel, indium-labeled WBCs may have a slightly greater yield for abscesses near the bowel. Neither indium-labeled WBC nor gallium scans serve as a basis for a definitive diagnosis, however; both need to be followed by other, more specific studies, such as CT, if an area of possible abnormality is identified. Abscesses contiguous with or contained within diverticula are particularly difficult to diagnose with scanning procedures. Occasionally, a barium enema may detect a diverticular abscess not diagnosed by other procedures, although barium should not be injected if a perforation is suspected. If one study is negative, a second study sometimes reveals a collection. Although exploratory laparotomy has been less commonly used since the advent of CT, this procedure still must be undertaken on occasion if an abscess is strongly suspected on clinical grounds.

℞ Treatment: INTRAPERITONEAL ABSCESSES

An algorithm for the management of patients with intraabdominal (including intraperitoneal) abscesses is presented in Fig. 24-3. The treatment of intraabdominal infections involves the determination of the initial focus of infection, the administration of broad-spectrum antibiotics targeting the organisms involved, and the performance of a drainage procedure if one or more definitive abscesses have formed. Antimicrobial therapy, in general, is adjunctive to drainage and/or surgical correction of an underlying lesion or process in intraabdominal abscesses. Unlike the intraabdominal abscesses resulting from most causes, for which drainage of some kind is generally required, abscesses associated with diverticulitis usually wall off locally after rupture of a diverticulum, so that surgical intervention is not routinely required.

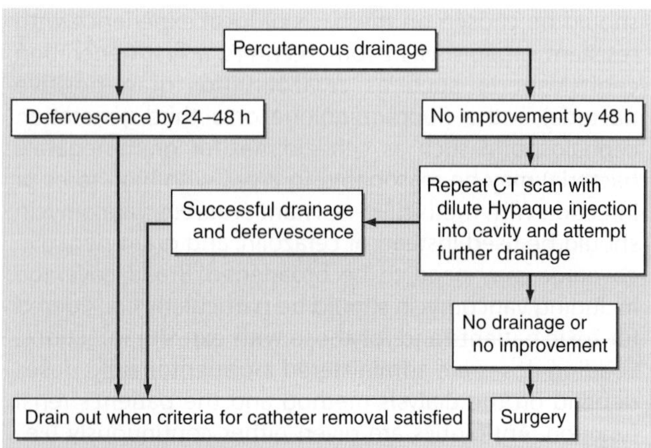

FIGURE 24-3

Algorithm for the management of patients with intraabdominal abscesses using percutaneous drainage. Antimicrobial therapy should be administered concomitantly. [*Reprinted with permission from B Lorber (ed): Atlas of Infectious Diseases, vol VII: Intra-abdominal Infections, Hepatitis, and Gastroenteritis. Philadelphia, Current Medicine, 1996, p 1.30, as adapted from OD Rotstein, RL Simmons, in SL Gorbach et al (eds): Infectious Diseases. Philadelphia, Saunders, 1992, p 668.*]

A number of agents exhibit excellent activity against aerobic gram-negative bacilli. Since mortality in intraabdominal sepsis is linked to gram-negative bacteremia, empirical therapy for intraabdominal infection always needs to include adequate coverage of gram-negative aerobic, facultative, and anaerobic organisms. Even if anaerobes are not cultured from clinical specimens, they still must be covered by the therapeutic regimen. Empirical antibiotic therapy should be the same as that discussed above for secondary peritonitis.

VISCERAL ABSCESSES

Liver Abscesses

The liver is the organ most subject to the development of abscesses. In one study of 540 intraabdominal abscesses, 26% were visceral. Liver abscesses made up 13% of the total number, or 48% of all visceral abscesses. Liver abscesses may be solitary or multiple; they may arise from hematogenous spread of bacteria or from local spread from contiguous sites of infection within the peritoneal cavity. In the past, appendicitis with rupture and subsequent spread of infection was the most common source for a liver abscess. Currently, associated disease of the biliary tract is most common. Pylephlebitis (suppurative thrombosis of the portal vein), usually arising from infection in the pelvis but sometimes from infection elsewhere in the peritoneal cavity, is another common source for bacterial seeding of the liver.

Fever is the most common presenting sign of liver abscess. Some patients, particularly those with associated disease of the biliary tract, have symptoms and signs localized to the right upper quadrant, including pain, guarding, punch tenderness, and even rebound tenderness. Nonspecific symptoms, such as chills, anorexia, weight loss, nausea, and vomiting, may also develop. Only 50% of patients with liver abscesses, however, have hepatomegaly, right-upper-quadrant tenderness, or jaundice; thus half of patients have no symptoms or signs to direct attention to the liver. Fever of unknown origin (FUO) may be the only manifestation of liver abscess, especially in the elderly. Diagnostic studies of the abdomen, especially the right upper quadrant, should be a part of any FUO workup. The single most reliable laboratory finding is an elevated serum concentration of alkaline phosphatase, which is documented in 70% of patients with liver abscesses. Other tests of liver function may yield normal results, but 50% of patients have elevated serum levels of bilirubin, and 48% have elevated concentrations of aspartate aminotransferase. Other laboratory findings include leukocytosis in 77% of patients, anemia (usually normochromic, normocytic) in 50%, and hypoalbuminemia in 33%. Concomitant bacteremia is found in one-third of patients. A liver abscess is sometimes suggested by chest radiography, especially if a new elevation of the right hemidiaphragm is seen; other suggestive findings include a right basilar infiltrate and a right pleural effusion.

Imaging studies are the most reliable methods for diagnosing liver abscesses. These studies include ultrasonography, CT (Fig. 24-4), indium-labeled WBC or gallium scan, and MRI. More than one such study may be required. Organisms recovered from liver abscesses vary with the source. In liver infection arising from the biliary tree, enteric gram-negative aerobic bacilli and enterococci are common isolates. Unless previous surgery has been performed, anaerobes are not generally involved in liver abscesses arising from biliary infections. In contrast, in liver abscesses arising from pelvic and other intraperitoneal sources, a mixed flora including both aerobic and anaerobic species is common; *B. fragilis* is the species most frequently isolated. With hematogenous spread of infection, usually only a single organism is encountered; this species may be *S. aureus* or a streptococcal species such as *S. milleri*. Results of cultures obtained from drain sites are not reliable for defining the etiology of infections. Liver abscesses may also be caused by *Candida* spp.; such abscesses usually follow fungemia in patients receiving chemotherapy for cancer and often present when PMNs return after a period of neutropenia. Amebic liver abscesses are not an uncommon problem (Chap. 115). Amebic serologic testing gives positive results in >95% of cases; thus a negative result helps to exclude this diagnosis.

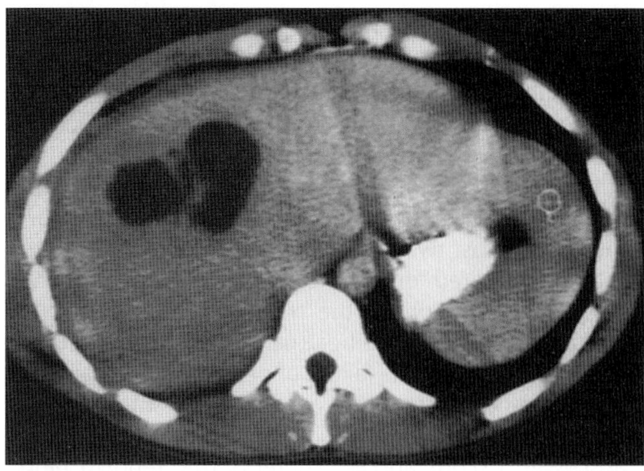

FIGURE 24-4
Multilocular liver abscess on CT scan. Multiple or multilocular abscesses are more common than solitary abscesses. [*Reprinted with permission from B Lorber (ed): Atlas of Infectious Diseases, Vol VII: Intra-abdominal Infections, Hepatitis, and Gastroenteritis. Philadelphia, Current Medicine, 1996, Fig. 1.22.*]

℞ Treatment: LIVER ABSCESSES

(See Fig. 24-3) Although drainage—either percutaneous (with a pigtail catheter kept in place) or surgical—is the mainstay of therapy for intraabdominal abscesses (including liver abscesses), there is growing interest in medical management alone for pyogenic liver abscesses. The drugs used for empirical therapy include the same ones used in intraabdominal sepsis and secondary bacterial peritonitis. Usually, a diagnostic aspirate of abscess contents should be obtained before the initiation of empirical therapy, with antibiotic choices adjusted when the results of Gram's staining and culture become available. Cases treated without definitive drainage generally require longer courses of antibiotic therapy. When percutaneous drainage was compared with open surgical drainage, the average length of hospital stay for the former was almost twice that for the latter, although both the time required for fever to resolve and the mortality rate were the same for the two procedures. Mortality was appreciable despite treatment, averaging 15%. Several factors predict the failure of percutaneous drainage and therefore may favor primary surgical intervention. These factors include the presence of multiple, sizable abscesses; viscous abscess contents that tend to plug the catheter; associated disease (e.g., disease of the biliary tract) requiring surgery; or the lack of a clinical response to percutaneous drainage in 4–7 days.

Treatment of candidal liver abscesses often entails initial administration of amphotericin B or liposomal amphotericin, with subsequent fluconazole therapy (Chap. 107).

In some cases, therapy with fluconazole alone (6 mg/kg daily) may be used—e.g., in clinically stable patients whose infecting isolate is susceptible to this drug.

Splenic Abscesses

Splenic abscesses are much less common than liver abscesses. The incidence of splenic abscesses has ranged from 0.14 to 0.7% in various autopsy series. The clinical setting and the organisms isolated usually differ from those for liver abscesses. The degree of clinical suspicion for splenic abscess needs to be high, as this condition is frequently fatal if left untreated. Even in the most recently published series, diagnosis was made only at autopsy in 37% of cases. Although splenic abscesses may arise occasionally from contiguous spread of infection or from direct trauma to the spleen, hematogenous spread of infection is more common. Bacterial endocarditis is the most common associated infection (Chap. 19). Splenic abscesses can develop in patients who have received extensive immunosuppressive therapy (particularly those with malignancy involving the spleen) and in patients with hemoglobinopathies or other hematologic disorders (especially sickle cell anemia).

Although ~50% of patients with splenic abscesses have abdominal pain, the pain is localized to the left upper quadrant in only half of these cases. Splenomegaly is found in ~50% of cases. Fever and leukocytosis are generally present; the development of fever preceded diagnosis by an average of 20 days in one series. Left-sided chest findings may include abnormalities to auscultation, and chest radiographic findings may include an infiltrate or a left-sided pleural effusion. CT scan of the abdomen has been the most sensitive diagnostic tool. Ultrasonography can yield the diagnosis but is less sensitive. Liver-spleen scan or gallium scan may also be useful. Streptococcal species are the most common bacterial isolates from splenic abscesses, followed by *S. aureus*—presumably reflecting the associated endocarditis. An increase in the prevalence of gram-negative aerobic isolates from splenic abscesses has been reported; these organisms often derive from a urinary tract focus, with associated bacteremia, or from another intraabdominal source. *Salmonella* species are seen fairly commonly, especially in patients with sickle cell hemoglobinopathy. Anaerobic species accounted for only 5% of isolates in the largest collected series, but the reporting of a number of "sterile abscesses" may indicate that optimal techniques for the isolation of anaerobes were not employed.

℞ Treatment: SPLENIC ABSCESSES

Because of the high mortality figures reported for splenic abscesses, splenectomy with adjunctive antibiotics has traditionally been considered standard treatment and remains the best approach for complex, multilocular abscesses or multiple abscesses. However, percutaneous drainage has worked well for single, small (<3-cm) abscesses in some studies and may also be useful for patients with high surgical risk. Patients undergoing splenectomy should be vaccinated against encapsulated organisms (*Streptococcus pneumoniae, Haemophilus influenzae, Neisseria meningitidis*). The most important factor in successful treatment of splenic abscesses is early diagnosis.

Perinephric and Renal Abscesses

Perinephric and renal abscesses are not common: The former accounted for only ~0.02% of hospital admissions and the latter for ~0.2% in Altemeier's series of 540 intraabdominal abscesses. Before antibiotics became available, most renal and perinephric abscesses were hematogenous in origin, usually complicating prolonged bacteremia, with *S. aureus* most commonly recovered. Now, in contrast, >75% of perinephric and renal abscesses arise from a urinary tract infection. Infection ascends from the bladder to the kidney, with pyelonephritis occurring before abscess development. Bacteria may directly invade the renal parenchyma from medulla to cortex. Local vascular channels within the kidney may also facilitate the transport of organisms. Areas of abscess developing within the parenchyma may rupture into the perinephric space. The kidneys and adrenal glands are surrounded by a layer of perirenal fat that, in turn, is surrounded by Gerota's fascia, which extends superiorly to the diaphragm and inferiorly to the pelvic fat. Abscesses extending into the perinephric space may track through Gerota's fascia into the psoas or transversalis muscles, into the anterior peritoneal cavity, superiorly to the subdiaphragmatic space, or inferiorly to the pelvis. Of the risk factors that have been associated with the development of perinephric abscesses, the most important is concomitant nephrolithiasis obstructing urinary flow. Of patients with perinephric abscess, 20–60% have renal stones. Other structural abnormalities of the urinary tract, prior urologic surgery, trauma, and diabetes mellitus have also been identified as risk factors.

The organisms most frequently encountered in perinephric and renal abscesses are *E. coli*, *Proteus* spp., and *Klebsiella* spp. *E. coli*, the aerobic species most commonly found in the colonic flora, seems to have unique virulence properties in the urinary tract, including factors promoting adherence to uroepithelial cells. The urease of *Proteus* spp. splits urea, thereby creating a more alkaline and more hospitable environment for bacterial proliferation. *Proteus* spp. are frequently found in association with large struvite stones caused by the precipitation of magnesium ammonium sulfate in an alkaline environment. These stones serve as a nidus for recurrent urinary tract infection. Although a single bacterial species is usually recovered from a perinephric or renal abscess, multiple species may also be found. If a urine culture is not contaminated with periurethral flora and is found to contain more than one organism, a perinephric abscess or renal abscess should be considered in the differential diagnosis. Urine cultures may also be polymicrobial in cases of bladder diverticulum.

Candida spp. can cause renal abscesses. This fungus may spread to the kidney hematogenously or by ascension from the bladder. The hallmark of the latter route of infection is ureteral obstruction with large fungal balls.

The presentation of perinephric and renal abscesses is quite nonspecific. Flank pain and abdominal pain are common. At least 50% of patients are febrile. Pain may be referred to the groin or leg, particularly with extension of infection. The diagnosis of perinephric abscess, like that of splenic abscess, is frequently delayed, and the mortality rate in some series is appreciable, although lower than in the past. Perinephric or renal abscess should be most seriously considered when a patient presents with symptoms and signs of pyelonephritis and remains febrile after 4 or 5 days of treatment. Moreover, when a urine culture yields a polymicrobial flora, when a patient is known to have renal stones, or when fever and pyuria coexist with a sterile urine culture, these diagnoses should be entertained.

Renal ultrasonography and abdominal CT are the most useful diagnostic modalities. If a renal or perinephric abscess is diagnosed, nephrolithiasis should be excluded, especially when a high urinary pH suggests the presence of a urea-splitting organism.

℞ Treatment: PERINEPHRIC AND RENAL ABSCESSES

Treatment for perinephric and renal abscesses, like that for other intraabdominal abscesses, includes drainage of pus and antibiotic therapy directed at the organism(s) recovered. For perinephric abscesses, percutaneous drainage is usually successful.

Psoas Abscesses

The psoas muscle is another location in which abscesses are encountered. Psoas abscesses may arise from a hematogenous source, by contiguous spread from an intraabdominal or pelvic process, or by contiguous spread from nearby bony structures (e.g., vertebral bodies). Associated osteomyelitis due to spread from bone to muscle or from muscle to bone is common in psoas abscesses. When Pott's disease was common, *Mycobacterium tuberculosis* was a frequent cause of psoas abscess. Currently, either *S. aureus* or a mixture of enteric organisms including aerobic and anaerobic gram-negative bacilli is usually isolated from psoas abscesses in the United States. *S. aureus* is most likely to be isolated when a psoas abscess arises from hematogenous spread or a contiguous focus of osteomyelitis; a mixed enteric flora is the most likely etiology when the abscess has an intraabdominal or pelvic source. Patients with psoas abscesses frequently present with fever, lower abdominal or back pain, or pain referred to the hip or knee. CT is the most useful diagnostic technique.

℞ Treatment: PSOAS ABSCESSES

Treatment includes surgical drainage and the administration of an antibiotic regimen directed at the inciting organism(s).

ACKNOWLEDGMENT
The substantial contributions of Dori F. Zaleznik, MD, to this chapter in previous editions are gratefully acknowledged.

FURTHER READINGS

Brook I: Microbiology and management of abdominal infections. Dig Dis Sci 53:2585, 2008

Campillo B et al: Epidemiology of severe hospital-acquired infections in patients with liver cirrhosis: Effect of long-term administration of norfloxacin. Clin Infect Dis 26:1066, 1998

Chen W et al: Clinical outcome and prognostic factors of patients with pyogenic liver abscess requiring intensive care. Crit Care Med 36:1184, 2008

Gibson FC III et al: Cellular mechanism of intraabdominal abscess formation by *Bacteroides fragilis*. J Immunol 160:5000, 1998

Johanssen EC, Madoff LC: Infections of the liver and biliary system, in *Principles and Practice of Infectious Diseases*, 6th ed, GL Mandell et al (eds). Philadelphia, Elsevier Churchill Livingstone, 2005, pp 951–959

Levison ME, Bush LM: Peritonitis and intraperitoneal abscesses, in *Principles and Practice of Infectious Diseases*, 6th ed, GL Mandell et al (eds). Philadelphia, Elsevier Churchill Livingstone, 2005, pp 927–945

Pappas PG et al: Guidelines for treatment of candidiasis. Clin Infect Dis 38:161, 2004

Piraino B et al: Peritoneal dialysis–related infections recommendations: 2005 update. Perit Dial Int 25:107, 2005

Rahimian J et al: Pyogenic liver abscess: Recent trends in etiology and mortality. Clin Infect Dis 39:1654, 2004

Solomkin JS et al: Guidelines for the selection of anti-infective agents for complicated intra-abdominal infections. Clin Infect Dis 37:997, 2003

Tzianabos AO, Kasper DL: Anaerobic infections: General concepts, in *Principles and Practice of Infectious Diseases*, 6th ed, GL Mandell et al (eds). Philadelphia, Elsevier Churchill Livingstone, 2005, pp 2810–2816

Tzianabos AO et al: T cells activated by zwitterionic molecules prevent abscesses induced by pathogenic bacteria. J Biol Chem 275:6733, 2000

van Ruler O et al: Comparison of on-demand vs planned relaparotomy strategy in patients with severe peritonitis: A randomized trial. JAMA 298:865, 2007

CHAPTER 25

ACUTE INFECTIOUS DIARRHEAL DISEASES AND BACTERIAL FOOD POISONING

Joan R. Butterton ■ Stephen B. Calderwood

Ranging from mild annoyances during vacations to devastating dehydrating illnesses that can kill within hours, acute gastrointestinal illnesses rank second only to acute upper respiratory illnesses as the most common diseases worldwide. In children <5 years old, attack rates range from 2 to 3 illnesses per child per year in developed countries to as high as 10–18 illnesses per child per year in developing countries. In Asia, Africa, and Latin America, acute diarrheal illnesses are not only a leading cause of morbidity in children—with an estimated 1 billion cases per year—but also a major cause of death. These illnesses are responsible for 4–6 million deaths per year, or a sobering total of 12,600 deaths per day. In some areas, >50% of childhood deaths are directly attributable to acute diarrheal illnesses. In addition, by contributing to malnutrition and thereby reducing resistance to other infectious agents, gastrointestinal illnesses may be indirect factors in a far greater burden of disease.

The wide range of clinical manifestations of acute gastrointestinal illnesses is matched by the wide variety of infectious agents involved, including viruses, bacteria, and parasitic pathogens (Table 25-1). This chapter discusses factors that enable gastrointestinal pathogens to cause disease, reviews host defense mechanisms, and delineates an approach to the evaluation and treatment of patients presenting with acute diarrhea. Individual organisms causing acute gastrointestinal illnesses are discussed in detail in subsequent chapters.

PATHOGENIC MECHANISMS

Enteric pathogens have developed a variety of tactics to overcome host defenses. Understanding the virulence factors employed by these organisms is important in the diagnosis and treatment of clinical disease.

Inoculum Size

The number of microorganisms that must be ingested to cause disease varies considerably from species to species. For *Shigella*, enterohemorrhagic *Escherichia coli*, *Giardia lamblia*, or *Entamoeba*, as few as 10–100 bacteria or cysts can produce infection, whereas 10^5–10^8 *Vibrio cholerae* organisms must be ingested orally to cause disease. The infective dose of *Salmonella* varies widely, depending on the species, host, and food vehicle. The ability of organisms to overcome host defenses has important implications for transmission; *Shigella*, enterohemorrhagic *E. coli*, *Entamoeba*, and *Giardia* can spread by person-to-person contact, whereas under some circumstances, *Salmonella* may have to grow in food for several hours before reaching an effective infectious dose.

Adherence

Many organisms must adhere to the gastrointestinal mucosa as an initial step in the pathogenic process; thus organisms that can compete with the normal bowel flora and colonize the mucosa have an important advantage in causing disease. Specific cell-surface proteins involved in attachment of bacteria to intestinal cells are important virulence determinants. *V. cholerae*, for example, adheres to the brush border of small-intestinal enterocytes via specific surface adhesins, including the toxin-coregulated pilus and other accessory colonization factors. Enterotoxigenic *E. coli*, which causes watery diarrhea, produces an adherence protein called *colonization factor antigen* that is necessary for colonization of the upper small intestine by the organism before the production of enterotoxin. Enteropathogenic *E. coli*, an agent of diarrhea in young children, and enterohemorrhagic *E. coli*, which causes hemorrhagic colitis and the hemolytic-uremic syndrome, produce virulence determinants that allow these organisms to attach to and efface the brush border of the intestinal epithelium.

Toxin Production

The production of one or more exotoxins is important in the pathogenesis of numerous enteric organisms. Such toxins include *enterotoxins*, which cause watery diarrhea by acting directly on secretory mechanisms in the intestinal mucosa; *cytotoxins*, which cause destruction of mucosal cells and associated inflammatory diarrhea; and *neurotoxins*, which act directly on the central or peripheral nervous system.

The prototypical enterotoxin is cholera toxin, a heterodimeric protein composed of one A and five B subunits. The A subunit contains the enzymatic activity of the

TABLE 25-1

GASTROINTESTINAL PATHOGENS CAUSING ACUTE DIARRHEA

MECHANISM	LOCATION	ILLNESS	STOOL FINDINGS	EXAMPLES OF PATHOGENS INVOLVED
Noninflammatory (enterotoxin)	Proximal small bowel	Watery diarrhea	No fecal leukocytes; mildor no increase in fecal lactoferrin	*Vibrio cholerae*, enterotoxigenic *Escherichia coli* (LT and/or ST), enteroaggregative *E. coli*, *Clostridium perfringens*, *Bacillus cereus*, *Staphylococcus aureus*, *Aeromonas hydrophila*, *Plesiomonas shigelloides*, rotavirus, norovirus, enteric adenoviruses, *Giardia lamblia*, *Cryptosporidium* spp., *Cyclospora* spp., microsporidia
Inflammatory (invasion or cytotoxin)	Colon or distal small bowel	Dysentery or inflammatory diarrhea	Fecal polymorphonuclear leukocytes; substantial increase in fecal lactoferrin	*Shigella* spp., *Salmonella* spp., *Campylobacter jejuni*, enterohemorrhagic *E. coli*, enteroinvasive *E. coli*, *Yersinia enterocolitica*, *Vibrio parahaemolyticus*, *Clostridium difficile*, ?*A. hydrophila*, ?*P. shigelloides*, *Entamoeba histolytica*
Penetrating	Distal small bowel	Enteric fever	Fecal mononuclear leukocytes	*Salmonella typhi*, *Y. enterocolitica*, ?*Campylobacter fetus*

Note: LT, heat-labile enterotoxin; ST, heat-stable enterotoxin.
Source: After Guerrant and Steiner.

toxin, whereas the B subunit pentamer binds holotoxin to the enterocyte surface receptor, the ganglioside G_{M1}. After the binding of holotoxin, a fragment of the A subunit is translocated across the eukaryotic cell membrane into the cytoplasm, where it catalyzes the ADP-ribosylation of a GTP-binding protein and causes persistent activation of adenylate cyclase. The end result is an increase of cyclic AMP in the intestinal mucosa, which increases Cl^- secretion and decreases Na^+ absorption, leading to loss of fluid and the production of diarrhea.

Enterotoxigenic strains of *E. coli* may produce a protein called *heat-labile enterotoxin* (LT) that is similar to cholera toxin and causes secretory diarrhea by the same mechanism. Alternatively, enterotoxigenic strains of *E. coli* may produce *heat-stable enterotoxin* (ST), one form of which causes diarrhea by activation of guanylate cyclase and elevation of intracellular cyclic GMP. Some enterotoxigenic strains of *E. coli* produce both LT and ST.

Bacterial cytotoxins, in contrast, destroy intestinal mucosal cells and produce the syndrome of dysentery, with bloody stools containing inflammatory cells. Enteric pathogens that produce such cytotoxins include *Shigella dysenteriae* type 1, *Vibrio parahaemolyticus*, and *Clostridium difficile*. *S. dysenteriae* type 1 and Shiga toxin–producing strains of *E. coli* produce potent cytotoxins and have been associated with outbreaks of hemorrhagic colitis and hemolytic-uremic syndrome.

Neurotoxins are usually produced by bacteria outside the host and therefore cause symptoms soon after ingestion. Included are the staphylococcal and *Bacillus cereus* toxins, which act on the central nervous system to produce vomiting.

Invasion

Dysentery may result not only from the production of cytotoxins, but also from bacterial invasion and destruction of intestinal mucosal cells. Infections due to *Shigella* and enteroinvasive *E. coli* are characterized by the organisms' invasion of mucosal epithelial cells, intraepithelial multiplication, and subsequent spread to adjacent cells. *Salmonella* causes inflammatory diarrhea by invasion of the bowel mucosa but generally is not associated with the destruction of enterocytes or the full clinical syndrome of dysentery. *Salmonella typhi* and *Yersinia enterocolitica* can penetrate intact intestinal mucosa, multiply intracellularly in Peyer's patches and intestinal lymph nodes, and then disseminate through the bloodstream to cause enteric fever, a syndrome characterized by fever, headache, relative bradycardia, abdominal pain, splenomegaly, and leukopenia.

HOST DEFENSES

Given the enormous number of microorganisms ingested with every meal, the normal host must combat a constant influx of potential enteric pathogens. Studies of infections in patients with alterations in defense mechanisms have led to a greater understanding of the variety of ways in which the normal host can protect itself against disease.

Normal Flora

The large numbers of bacteria that normally inhabit the intestine act as an important host defense by preventing colonization by potential enteric pathogens. Persons with fewer intestinal bacteria, such as infants who have not yet developed normal enteric colonization or patients receiving antibiotics, are at significantly greater risk of developing infections with enteric pathogens. The composition of the intestinal flora is as important as the number of organisms present. More than 99% of the normal colonic flora is made up of anaerobic bacteria, and the acidic pH and volatile fatty acids produced by these organisms appear to be critical elements in resistance to colonization.

Gastric Acid

The acidic pH of the stomach is an important barrier to enteric pathogens, and an increased frequency of infections due to *Salmonella*, *G. lamblia*, and a variety of helminths has been reported among patients who have undergone gastric surgery or are achlorhydric for some other reason. Neutralization of gastric acid with antacids or H_2 blockers—a common practice in the management of hospitalized patients—similarly increases the risk of enteric colonization. In addition, some microorganisms can survive the extreme acidity of the gastric environment; rotavirus, for example, is highly stable to acidity.

Intestinal Motility

Normal peristalsis is the major mechanism for clearance of bacteria from the proximal small intestine. When intestinal motility is impaired (e.g., by treatment with opiates or other antimotility drugs, anatomic abnormalities, or hypomotility states), the frequency of bacterial overgrowth and infection of the small bowel with enteric pathogens is increased. Some patients whose treatment for *Shigella* infection consists of diphenoxylate hydrochloride with atropine (Lomotil) experience prolonged fever and shedding of organisms, whereas patients treated with opiates for mild *Salmonella* gastroenteritis have a higher frequency of bacteremia than those not treated with opiates.

Immunity

Both cellular immune responses and antibody production play important roles in protection from enteric infections. The wide spectrum of viral, bacterial, parasitic, and fungal gastrointestinal infections in patients with AIDS highlights the significance of cell-mediated immunity in protection from these pathogens. Humoral immunity is also important and consists of systemic IgG and IgM as well as secretory IgA. The mucosal immune system may be the first line of defense against many gastrointestinal pathogens. The binding of bacterial antigens to the luminal surface of M cells in the distal small bowel and the subsequent presentation of antigens to subepithelial lymphoid tissue lead to the proliferation of sensitized lymphocytes. These lymphocytes circulate and populate all of the mucosal tissues of the body as IgA-secreting plasma cells.

Genetic Determinants

The mechanisms underlying genetic variation in host susceptibility remain poorly understood. People with blood group O show increased susceptibility to cholera, shigellosis, and norovirus infection. A polymorphism in the interleukin 8 gene is associated with increased risk of diarrhea from enteroaggregative *E. coli*.

Approach to the Patient: INFECTIOUS DIARRHEA OR BACTERIAL FOOD POISONING

The approach to the patient with possible infectious diarrhea or bacterial food poisoning is shown in Fig. 25-1.

HISTORY The answers to questions with high discriminating value can quickly narrow the range of potential causes of diarrhea and help determine whether treatment is needed. Important elements of the narrative history are detailed in Fig. 25-1.

PHYSICAL EXAMINATION The examination of patients for signs of dehydration provides essential information about the severity of the diarrheal illness and the need for rapid therapy. Mild dehydration is indicated by thirst, dry mouth, decreased axillary sweat, decreased urine output, and slight weight loss. Signs of moderate dehydration include an orthostatic fall in blood pressure, skin tenting, and sunken eyes (or, in infants, a sunken fontanelle). Signs of severe dehydration range from hypotension and tachycardia to confusion and frank shock.

DIAGNOSTIC APPROACH After the severity of illness is assessed, the clinician must distinguish between *inflammatory* and *noninflammatory* disease. Using the history and epidemiologic features of the case as guides, the clinician can then rapidly evaluate the need for further efforts to define a specific etiology and for therapeutic intervention. Examination of a stool sample may supplement the narrative history. Grossly bloody or mucoid stool suggests an inflammatory process. A test for fecal leukocytes (preparation of a thin smear of stool on a glass slide, addition of a drop of methylene blue, and examination of the wet mount) can suggest inflammatory disease in patients with diarrhea, although the predictive value of this test is still debated. A test for fecal lactoferrin, which is a marker of fecal leukocytes, is more sensitive and is available in latex agglutination and enzyme-linked immunosorbent assay formats. Causes of acute infectious diarrhea, categorized as inflammatory and noninflammatory, are listed in Table 25-1.

POST-DIARRHEA COMPLICATIONS Chronic complications may follow the resolution of an acute diarrheal episode. The clinician should inquire about prior diarrheal illness if the conditions listed in Table 25-2 are observed.

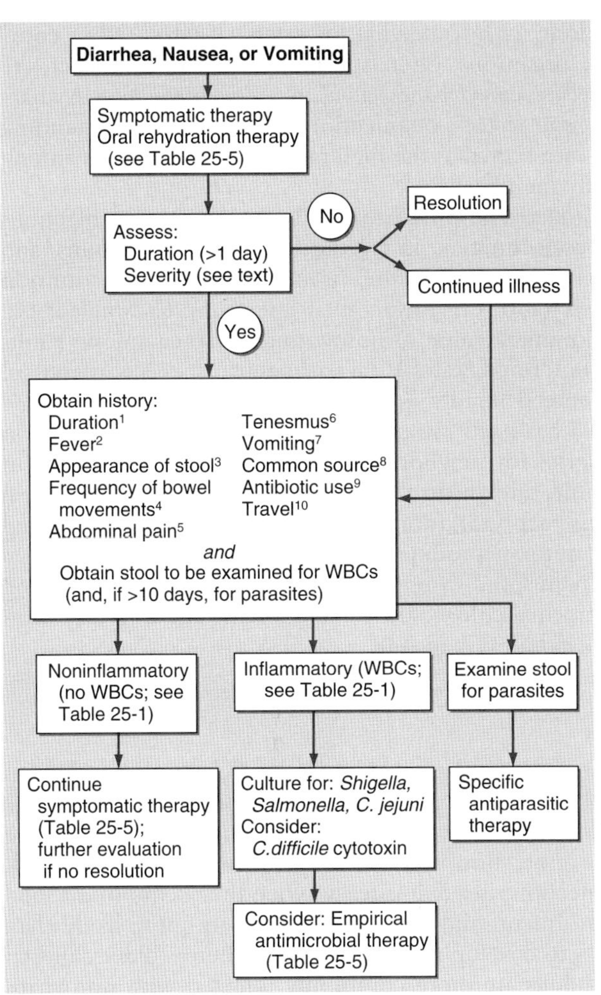

FIGURE 25-1

Clinical algorithm for the approach to patients with community-acquired infectious diarrhea or bacterial food poisoning. Key to superscripts: **1.** Diarrhea lasting >2 weeks is generally defined as chronic; in such cases, many of the causes of acute diarrhea are much less likely, and a new spectrum of causes needs to be considered. **2.** Fever often implies invasive disease, although fever and diarrhea may also result from infection outside the gastrointestinal tract, as in malaria. **3.** Stools that contain blood or mucus indicate ulceration of the large bowel. Bloody stools without fecal leukocytes should alert the laboratory to the possibility of infection with Shiga toxin–producing enterohemorrhagic *Escherichia coli*. Bulky white stools suggest a small-intestinal process that is causing malabsorption. Profuse "rice-water" stools suggest cholera or a similar toxigenic process. **4.** Frequent stools over a given period can provide the first warning of impending dehydration. **5.** Abdominal pain may be most severe in inflammatory processes like those due to *Shigella*, *Campylobacter*, and necrotizing toxins. Painful abdominal muscle cramps, caused by electrolyte loss, can develop in severe cases of cholera. Bloating is common in giardiasis. An appendicitis-like syndrome should prompt a culture for *Yersinia enterocolitica* with cold enrichment. **6.** Tenesmus (painful rectal spasms with a strong urge to defecate but little passage of stool) may be a feature of cases with proctitis, as in shigellosis or amebiasis. **7.** Vomiting implies an acute infection (e.g., a toxin-mediated illness or food poisoning) but can also be prominent in a variety of systemic illnesses (e.g., malaria) and in intestinal obstruction. **8.** Asking patients whether anyone else they know is sick is a more efficient means of identifying a common source than is constructing a list of recently eaten foods. If a common source seems likely, specific foods can be investigated. See text for a discussion of bacterial food poisoning. **9.** Current antibiotic therapy or a recent history of treatment suggests *Clostridium difficile* diarrhea (Chap. 43). Stop antibiotic treatment if possible and consider tests for *C. difficile* toxins. Antibiotic use may increase the risk of other infections, such as salmonellosis. **10.** See text (and Chap. 4) for a discussion of traveler's diarrhea. (*After Guerrant and Steiner; RL Guerrant, DA Bobak: N Engl J Med 325:327, 1991; with permission.*)

TABLE 25-2

POST-DIARRHEA COMPLICATIONS OF ACUTE INFECTIOUS DIARRHEAL ILLNESS

COMPLICATION	COMMENTS
Chronic diarrhea • Lactase deficiency • Small-bowel bacterial overgrowth • Malabsorption syndromes (tropical and celiac sprue)	Occurs in ~1% of travelers with acute diarrhea • Protozoa account for ~1/3 of cases
Initial presentation or exacerbation of inflammatory bowel disease	May be precipitated by traveler's diarrhea
Irritable bowel syndrome	Occurs in ~10% of travelers with traveler's diarrhea
Reiter's syndrome (reactive arthritis)	Particularly likely after infection with invasive organisms (*Shigella*, *Salmonella*, *Campylobacter*)
Hemolytic-uremic syndrome (hemolytic anemia, thrombocytopenia, and renal failure)	Follows infection with Shiga toxin–producing bacteria (*Shigella dysenteriae* type 1 and enterohemorrhagic *Escherichia coli*)

EPIDEMIOLOGY

Travel History

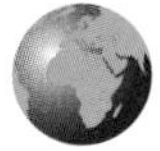

Of the several million people who travel from temperate industrialized countries to tropical regions of Asia, Africa, and Central and South America each year, 20–50% experience a sudden onset of abdominal cramps, anorexia, and watery diarrhea; thus *traveler's diarrhea* is the most common travel-related illness (Chap. 4). The time of onset is usually 3 days to 2 weeks after the traveler's arrival in a tropical area; most cases begin within the first 3–5 days. The illness is generally self-limited, lasting 1–5 days. The high rate of diarrhea among travelers to underdeveloped areas is related to the ingestion of contaminated food or water.

The organisms that cause traveler's diarrhea vary considerably with location (Table 25-3). In all areas, enterotoxigenic and enteroaggregative *E. coli* are the most common isolates from persons with the classic secretory traveler's diarrhea syndrome.

Location

Day-care centers have particularly high attack rates of enteric infections. Rotavirus is most common among children <2 years old, with attack rates of 75–100% among those exposed. *G. lamblia* is more common among older

TABLE 25-3

EPIDEMIOLOGY OF TRAVELER'S DIARRHEA

ETIOLOGIC AGENT	APPROXIMATE PERCENTAGE OF CASES	COMMENTS
Enterotoxigenic *Escherichia coli*	15–50	Single most important agent, particularly in summertime in semitropical areas; percentage of cases ranges from 15% in Asia to 50% in Latin America
Enteroaggregative *E. coli*	20–35	Emerging enteric pathogen of worldwide distribution
Shigella and enteroinvasive *E. coli*	10–25	Major causes of fever and dysentery
Salmonella	5–10	Causes fever and dysentery
Campylobacter jejuni	3–15	More common in winter in semitropical areas; more common in Asia
Aeromonas	5	Important in Thailand
Plesiomonas	5	Related to tropical travel and seafood consumption
Vibrio cholerae	0–10	Most common in India and Asia; also common in Central and South America
Rotavirus and norovirus	10–40	Latin America, Asia, and Africa; norovirus associated with seafood ingestion on cruise ships
Entamoeba histolytica	5	Particularly important in Mexico and Thailand
Giardia lamblia	<2	Zoonotic reservoirs in northern United States; affects hikers and campers who drink from freshwater streams; contaminates water supplies in Russia
Cryptosporidium	2	Affects travelers to Russia, Mexico, and Africa; causes large-scale urban outbreaks in United States
Cyclospora	<1	Affects travelers to Nepal, Haiti, and Peru; contaminates water or food
Unknown	20	Illness improves with antibacterial therapy, implicating bacterial diarrhea

Source: After Dupont.

children, with somewhat lower attack rates. Other common organisms, often spread by fecal-oral contact, are *Shigella*, *Campylobacter jejuni*, and *Cryptosporidium*. A characteristic feature of infection among children attending day-care centers is the high rate of secondary cases among family members.

Similarly, hospitals are sites in which enteric infections are concentrated. In medical intensive-care units and pediatric wards, diarrhea is one of the most common manifestations of nosocomial infections. *C. difficile* is the predominant cause of nosocomial diarrhea among adults in the United States. Viral pathogens, especially rotavirus, can spread rapidly in pediatric wards. Enteropathogenic *E. coli* has been associated with outbreaks of diarrhea in nurseries for newborns. One-third of elderly patients in chronic-care institutions develop a significant diarrheal illness each year; more than half of these cases are caused by cytotoxin-producing *C. difficile*. Antimicrobial therapy can predispose to pseudomembranous colitis by altering the normal colonic flora and allowing the multiplication of *C. difficile* (Chap. 43).

Age

Most of the morbidity and mortality from enteric pathogens involves children <5 years of age. Breast-fed infants are protected from contaminated food and water and derive some protection from maternal antibodies, but their risk of infection rises dramatically when they begin to eat solid foods. Infants and younger children are more likely than adults to develop rotavirus disease, whereas older children and adults are more commonly infected with norovirus. Other organisms with higher attack rates among children than among adults include enterotoxigenic, enteropathogenic, and enterohemorrhagic *E. coli*; *C. jejuni*; and *G. lamblia*. In children, the incidence of *Salmonella* infections is highest among those <1 year of age, whereas the attack rate for *Shigella* infections is greatest among those 6 months to 4 years of age.

Bacterial Food Poisoning

If the history and the stool examination indicate a noninflammatory etiology of diarrhea and there is evidence of a common-source outbreak, questions concerning the ingestion of specific foods and the time of onset of the diarrhea after a meal can provide clues to the bacterial cause of the illness. Potential causes of bacterial food poisoning are shown in Table 25-4.

Bacterial disease caused by an enterotoxin elaborated outside the host, such as that due to *Staphylococcus aureus* or *B. cereus*, has the shortest incubation period (1–6 h) and generally lasts <12 h. Most cases of staphylococcal food poisoning are caused by contamination from infected human carriers. Staphylococci can multiply at a wide range of temperatures; thus, if food is left to cool slowly and remains at room temperature after cooking, the organisms will have the opportunity to form enterotoxin. Outbreaks after picnics where potato salad, mayonnaise, and cream pastries have been served offer classic

TABLE 25-4

BACTERIAL FOOD POISONING

INCUBATION PERIOD, ORGANISM	SYMPTOMS	COMMON FOOD SOURCES
1–6 h		
Staphylococcus aureus	Nausea, vomiting, diarrhea	Ham, poultry, potato or egg salad, mayonnaise, cream pastries
Bacillus cereus	Nausea, vomiting, diarrhea	Fried rice
8–16 h		
Clostridium perfringens	Abdominal cramps, diarrhea (vomiting rare)	Beef, poultry, legumes, gravies
B. cereus	Abdominal cramps, diarrhea (vomiting rare)	Meats, vegetables, dried beans, cereals
>16 h		
Vibrio cholerae	Watery diarrhea	Shellfish
Enterotoxigenic *Escherichia coli*	Watery diarrhea	Salads, cheese, meats, water
Enterohemorrhagic *E. coli*	Bloody diarrhea	Ground beef, roast beef, salami, raw milk, raw vegetables, apple juice
Salmonella spp.	Inflammatory diarrhea	Beef, poultry, eggs, dairy products
Campylobacter jejuni	Inflammatory diarrhea	Poultry, raw milk
Shigella spp.	Dysentery	Potato or egg salad, lettuce, raw vegetables
Vibrio parahaemolyticus	Dysentery	Mollusks, crustaceans

examples of staphylococcal food poisoning. Diarrhea, nausea, vomiting, and abdominal cramping are common, whereas fever is less so.

B. cereus can produce either a syndrome with a short incubation period—the *emetic* form, mediated by a staphylococcal type of enterotoxin—or one with a longer incubation period (8–16 h)—the *diarrheal* form, caused by an enterotoxin resembling *E. coli* LT, in which diarrhea and abdominal cramps are characteristic but vomiting is uncommon. The emetic form of *B. cereus* food poisoning is associated with contaminated fried rice; the organism is common in uncooked rice, and its heat-resistant spores survive boiling. If cooked rice is not refrigerated, the spores can germinate and produce toxin. Frying before serving may not destroy the preformed, heat-stable toxin.

Food poisoning due to *Clostridium perfringens* also has a slightly longer incubation period (8–14 h) and results from the survival of heat-resistant spores in inadequately cooked meat, poultry, or legumes. After ingestion, toxin is produced in the intestinal tract, causing moderately severe abdominal cramps and diarrhea; vomiting is rare, as is fever. The illness is self-limited, rarely lasting >24 h.

Not all food poisoning has a bacterial cause. Nonbacterial agents of short-incubation food poisoning include capsaicin, which is found in hot peppers, and a variety of toxins found in fish and shellfish.

LABORATORY EVALUATION

Many cases of noninflammatory diarrhea are self-limited or can be treated empirically, and in these instances, the clinician may not need to determine a specific etiology. Potentially pathogenic *E. coli* cannot be distinguished from normal fecal flora by routine culture, and tests to detect enterotoxins are not available in most clinical laboratories. In situations in which cholera is a concern, stool should be cultured on thiosulfate–citrate–bile salts–sucrose (TCBS) agar. A latex agglutination test has made the rapid detection of rotavirus in stool practical for many laboratories, whereas reverse-transcriptase polymerase chain reaction and specific antigen enzyme immunoassays have been developed for the identification of norovirus. At least three stool specimens should be examined for *Giardia* cysts or stained for *Cryptosporidium* if the level of clinical suspicion regarding the involvement of these organisms is high.

All patients with fever and evidence of inflammatory disease acquired outside the hospital should have stool cultured for *Salmonella*, *Shigella*, and *Campylobacter*. *Salmonella* and *Shigella* can be selected on MacConkey's agar as non–lactose-fermenting (colorless) colonies or can be grown on *Salmonella-Shigella* agar or in selenite enrichment broth, both of which inhibit most organisms except these pathogens. Evaluation of nosocomial diarrhea should initially focus on *C. difficile*; stool culture for other pathogens in this setting has an extremely low yield and is not cost-effective. Toxins A and B produced by pathogenic strains of *C. difficile* can be detected by rapid enzyme immunoassays and latex agglutination tests (Chap. 43). Isolation of *C. jejuni* requires inoculation of fresh stool onto selective growth medium and incubation at 42°C in a microaerophilic atmosphere. In many laboratories in the United States, *E. coli* O157:H7 is among the most common pathogens isolated from visibly bloody stools. Strains of this enterohemorrhagic serotype can be identified in specialized laboratories by serotyping but also can be identified presumptively in hospital laboratories as lactose-fermenting, indole-positive colonies of sorbitol nonfermenters (white colonies) on sorbitol MacConkey plates. Fresh stools should be examined for amebic cysts and trophozoites.

℞ Treatment: INFECTIOUS DIARRHEA OR BACTERIAL FOOD POISONING

In many cases, a specific diagnosis is not necessary or not available to guide treatment. The clinician can proceed with the information obtained from the history, stool examination, and evaluation of dehydration severity. Empirical regimens for the treatment of traveler's diarrhea are listed in Table 25-5.

The mainstay of treatment is adequate rehydration. The treatment of cholera and other dehydrating diarrheal diseases was revolutionized by the promotion of oral rehydration solutions, the efficacy of which depends on the fact that glucose-facilitated absorption of sodium and water in the small intestine remains intact in the presence of cholera toxin. The use of oral rehydration solutions has reduced mortality due to cholera from >50% (in untreated cases) to <1%. The World Health Organization recommends a solution containing 3.5 g sodium chloride, 2.5 g sodium bicarbonate, 1.5 g potassium chloride, and 20 g glucose (or 40 g sucrose) per liter of water. Oral rehydration solutions containing rice or cereal as the carbohydrate source may be even more effective than glucose-based solutions, and the addition of L-histidine may reduce the frequency and volume of stool output. Patients who are severely dehydrated or in

TABLE 25-5

TREATMENT OF TRAVELER'S DIARRHEA ON THE BASIS OF CLINICAL FEATURES

CLINICAL SYNDROME	SUGGESTED THERAPY
Watery diarrhea (no blood in stool, no fever), 1 or 2 unformed stools per day without distressing enteric symptoms	Oral fluids (Pedialyte, Lytren, or flavored mineral water) and saltine crackers
Watery diarrhea (no blood in stool, no fever), 1 or 2 unformed stools per day with distressing enteric symptoms	Bismuth subsalicylate (for adults): 30 mL or 2 tablets (262 mg/tablet) every 30 min for 8 doses; or loperamide[a]: 4 mg initially followed by 2 mg after passage of each unformed stool, not to exceed 8 tablets (16 mg) per day (prescription dose) or 4 caplets (8 mg) per day (over-the-counter dose); drugs can be taken for 2 days
Watery diarrhea (no blood in stool, no distressing abdominal pain, no fever), >2 unformed stools per day	Antibacterial drug[b] plus (for adults) loperamide[a] (see dose above)
Dysentery (passage of bloody stools) or fever (>37.8°C)	Antibacterial drug[b]
Vomiting, minimal diarrhea	Bismuth subsalicylate (for adults; see dose above)
Diarrhea in infants (<2 y old)	Fluids and electrolytes (Pedialyte, Lytren); continue feeding, especially with breast milk; seek medical attention for moderate dehydration, fever lasting >24 h, bloody stools, or diarrhea lasting more than several days
Diarrhea in pregnant women	Fluids and electrolytes; can consider attapulgite, 3 g initially, with dose repeated after passage of each unformed stool or every 2 h (whichever is earlier), for a total dosage of 9 g/d; seek medical attention for persistent or severe symptoms
Diarrhea despite trimethoprim-sulfamethoxazole prophylaxis	Fluoroquinolone—with loperamide[a] (see dose above) if no fever and no blood in stool, alone in cases of fever/dysentery
Diarrhea despite fluoroquinolone prophylaxis	Bismuth subsalicylate (see dose above) for mild to moderate disease; consult physician for moderate to severe disease or if disease persists

[a]Loperamide should not be used by patients with fever or dysentery; its use may prolong diarrhea in patients with infection due to Shigella or other invasive organisms.

[b]The recommended antibacterial drugs are as follows:

Travel to high-risk country other than Thailand:

Adults: (1) A fluoroquinolone such as ciprofloxacin, 750 mg as a single dose or 500 mg bid for 3 days; levofloxacin, 500 mg as a single dose or 500 mg qd for 3 days; or norfloxacin, 800 mg as a single dose or 400 mg bid for 3 days. (2) Azithromycin, 1000 mg as a single dose or 500 mg qd for 3 days. (3) Rifaximin, 200 mg tid or 400 mg bid for 3 days (not recommended for use in dysentery).

Children: Azithromycin, 10 mg/kg on day 1, 5 mg/kg on days 2 and 3 if diarrhea persists.

Alternative agent: furazolidone, 7.5 mg/kg per day in four divided doses for 5 days.

Travel to Thailand (with risk of fluoroquinolone-resistant *Campylobacter*):

Adults: Azithromycin (at above dose for adults). Alternative agent: a fluoroquinolone (at above doses for adults).

Children: Same as for children traveling to other areas (see above).

All patients should take oral fluids (Pedialyte, Lytren, or flavored mineral water) plus saltine crackers. If diarrhea becomes moderate or severe, if fever persists, or if bloody stools or dehydration develops, the patient should seek medical attention.

Source: After Dupont.

whom vomiting precludes the use of oral therapy should receive IV solutions such as Ringer's lactate.

Although most secretory forms of traveler's diarrhea—usually due to enterotoxigenic and enteroaggregative *E. coli*—can be treated effectively with rehydration, bismuth subsalicylate, or antiperistaltic agents, antimicrobial agents can shorten the duration of illness from 3–4 days to 24–36 h. Changes in diet have not been shown to have an impact on the duration of illness, whereas the efficacy of probiotics continues to be debated.

Antibiotic treatment for children who present with bloody diarrhea raises special concerns. Laboratory studies of enterohemorrhagic *E. coli* strains have demonstrated that a number of antibiotics induce replication of Shiga toxin–producing lambdoid bacteriophages, significantly increasing toxin production by these strains. Clinical studies have supported these laboratory results, and antibiotics are not recommended for the treatment of enterohemorrhagic *E. coli* infections in children.

PROPHYLAXIS

Improvements in hygiene to limit fecal-oral spread of enteric pathogens will be necessary if the prevalence of diarrheal diseases is to be significantly reduced in developing countries. Travelers can reduce their risk of diarrhea by eating only hot, freshly cooked food; by avoiding raw vegetables, salads, and unpeeled fruit; and by drinking only boiled or treated water and avoiding ice. Historically, few travelers to tourist destinations adhere to these dietary restrictions. However, an intensive hygienic effort in Jamaica involving government, hotel, and tourism agencies led to a decrease in the incidence of traveler's diarrhea by 72% from 1996 to 2002.

Bismuth subsalicylate is an inexpensive agent for the prophylaxis of traveler's diarrhea; it is taken at a dosage of 2 tablets (525 mg) four times a day. Treatment appears to be effective and safe for up to 3 weeks. Prophylactic antimicrobial agents, although effective, are not generally recommended for the prevention of traveler's diarrhea, except when travelers are immunosuppressed or have other underlying illnesses that place them at high risk for morbidity from gastrointestinal infection. The risk of side effects and the possibility of developing an infection with a drug-resistant organism or with more harmful, invasive bacteria make it more reasonable to institute an empirical short course of treatment if symptoms develop. The recent availability of effective nonabsorbed antibiotics such as rifaximin may lead to new prophylactic options.

The possibility of exerting a major impact on the worldwide morbidity and mortality associated with diarrheal diseases has led to intense efforts to develop effective vaccines against the common bacterial and viral enteric pathogens. Recent research has yielded promising advances in the development of vaccines against rotavirus, *Shigella*, *V. cholerae*, *S. typhi*, and enterotoxigenic *E. coli*.

FURTHER READINGS

Al-Abri SS et al: Traveller's diarrhoea. Lancet Infect Dis 5:349, 2005

Bartlett JG: Clinical practice. Antibiotic-associated diarrhea. N Engl J Med 346:334, 2002

Centers for Disease Control and Prevention: Preliminary FoodNet data on the incidence of infection with pathogens transmitted commonly through food—10 states, 2008. MMWR Morb Mortal Wkly Rep 58:333, 2009

DuPont HL: Travelers' diarrhea, in *Infections of the Gastrointestinal Tract*, 2d ed, MJ Blaser et al (eds). Philadelphia, Lippincott Williams & Wilkins, 2002, Chap 19

Grimwood K, Buttery JP: Clinical update: Rotavirus gastroenteritis and its prevention. Lancet 370:302, 2007

Guerrant RL, Steiner TS: Principles and syndromes of enteric infection, in *Mandell, Douglas and Bennett's Principles and Practice of Infectious Diseases*, 5th ed, GL Mandell et al (eds). Philadelphia, Churchill Livingstone, 2000, Chap 81

Koo HL, DuPont HL: Current and future developments in travelers' diarrhea therapy. Expert Rev Anti Infect Ther 4:417, 2006

Musher DM, Musher BL: Contagious acute gastrointestinal infections. N Engl J Med 351:2417, 2004

Okhuysen PC: Current concepts in travelers' diarrhea: Epidemiology, antimicrobial resistance and treatment. Curr Opin Infect Dis 18:522, 2005

Sazawal S et al: Efficacy of probiotics in prevention of acute diarrhoea: A meta-analysis of masked, randomised, placebo-controlled trials. Lancet Infect Dis 6:374, 2006

Shah N et al: Global etiology of travelers' diarrhea: Systematic review from 1973 to the present. Am J Trop Med Hyg 80:609, 2009

Tauxe RV et al: Foodborne disease, in *Mandell, Douglas and Bennett's Principles and Practice of Infectious Diseases*, 5th ed, GL Mandell et al (eds). Philadelphia, Churchill Livingstone, 2000, Chap 87

Wong CS et al: The risk of the hemolytic-uremic syndrome after antibiotic treatment of *Escherichia coli* O157:H7 infections. N Engl J Med 342:1930, 2000

CHAPTER 26

ACUTE APPENDICITIS AND PERITONITIS

Susan L. Gearhart ■ William Silen

ACUTE APPENDICITIS

INCIDENCE AND EPIDEMIOLOGY

With more than 250,000 appendectomies performed annually, appendicitis is the most common abdominal surgical emergency in the United States. The peak incidence of acute appendicitis is in the second and third decades of life; it is relatively rare at the extremes of age. However, perforation is more common in infancy and in the elderly, during which periods mortality rates are highest. Males and females are equally affected, except between puberty and age 25, when males predominate in a 3:2 ratio. The incidence of appendicitis has remained stable in the United States over the last 30 years, whereas the incidence of appendicitis is much lower in underdeveloped countries, especially parts of Africa, and in lower socioeconomic groups. The mortality rate in the United States decreased eightfold between 1941 and 1970 but has remained at <1 per 100,000 since then.

PATHOGENESIS

Appendicitis is believed to occur as a result of appendiceal luminal obstruction. Obstruction is most commonly caused by a fecalith, which results from accumulation and inspissation of fecal matter around vegetable fibers. Enlarged lymphoid follicles associated with viral infections (e.g., measles), inspissated barium, worms (e.g., pinworms, *Ascaris*, and *Taenia*), and tumors (e.g., carcinoid or carcinoma) may also obstruct the lumen. Other common pathological findings include appendiceal ulceration. The cause of the ulceration is unknown, although a viral etiology has been postulated. Infection with *Yersinia* organisms may cause the disease, since high complement fixation antibody titers have been found in up to 30% of cases of proven appendicitis. Luminal bacteria multiply and invade the appendiceal wall as venous engorgement and subsequent arterial compromise result from the high intraluminal pressures. Finally, gangrene and perforation occur. If the process evolves slowly, adjacent organs such as the terminal ileum, cecum, and omentum may wall off the appendiceal area so that a localized abscess will develop, whereas rapid progression of vascular impairment may cause perforation with free access to the peritoneal cavity. Subsequent rupture of primary appendiceal abscesses may produce fistulas between the appendix and bladder, small intestine, sigmoid, or cecum. Occasionally, acute appendicitis may be the first manifestation of Crohn's disease.

Although chronic infection of the appendix with tuberculosis, amebiasis, and actinomycosis may occur, a useful clinical aphorism states that *chronic appendiceal inflammation is not usually the cause of prolonged abdominal pain of weeks' or months' duration*. In contrast, recurrent acute appendicitis does occur, often with complete resolution of inflammation and symptoms between attacks. Recurrent acute appendicitis may also occur if a long appendiceal stump is left after initial appendectomy.

CLINICAL MANIFESTATIONS

The sequence of abdominal discomfort and anorexia associated with acute appendicitis is pathognomonic. The pain is described as being located in the periumbilical region initially and then migrating to the right lower quadrant. This classic sequence of symptoms occurs in only 66% of patients. However, in a male patient these symptoms are sufficient to advise surgical exploration. The differential diagnoses for periumbilical and right lower quadrant pain are listed in Table 26-1. The periumbilical abdominal pain is of the visceral type, resulting from distention of the appendiceal lumen. This pain is carried on slow-conducting C fibers and is usually poorly localized in the periumbilical or epigastric region. In general, this visceral pain is mild, often cramping and usually lasting 4–6 h, but it may not be noted by stoic individuals. As inflammation spreads to the parietal peritoneal surfaces, the pain becomes somatic, steady, and more severe and aggravated by motion or cough. Parietal afferent nerves are A delta fibers, which are fast-conducting and unilateral. These fibers localize the pain to the *right lower quadrant*. *Anorexia* is very common; a hungry patient does not have acute appendicitis. *Nausea* and *vomiting* occur in 50–60% of cases, but vomiting is usually self-limited. Change in bowel habit is of little diagnostic value, since any or no alteration may be observed, although the presence of diarrhea caused by an inflamed appendix in juxtaposition to the sigmoid may cause diagnostic difficulties. Urinary frequency and dysuria occur if the appendix lies adjacent to the bladder.

Physical findings vary with time after onset of the illness and according to the location of the appendix, which may be situated deep in the pelvic cul-de-sac; in the right lower quadrant in any relation to the peritoneum, cecum, and small intestine; in the right upper

TABLE 26-1

THE ANATOMIC ORIGIN OF PERIUMBILICAL AND RIGHT LOWER QUADRANT PAIN IN THE DIFFERENTIAL DIAGNOSIS OF APPENDICITIS

Periumbilical	
Appendicitis	
Small-bowel obstruction	
Gastroenteritis	
Mesenteric ischemia	
Right Lower Quadrant	
Gastrointestinal causes	Gynecologic causes
Appendicitis	Ovarian tumor/torsion
Inflammatory bowel disease	Pelvic inflammatory disease
Right-sided diverticulitis	Renal causes
Gastroenteritis	Pyelonephritis
Inguinal hernia	Perinephritic abscess
	Nephrolithiasis

quadrant (especially during pregnancy); or even in the left lower quadrant. *The diagnosis cannot be established unless tenderness can be elicited.* Although tenderness is sometimes absent in the early visceral stage of the disease, it ultimately always develops and is found in any location corresponding to the position of the appendix. Typically, tenderness to palpation will often occur at McBurney's point, anatomically located on a line one-third of the way between the anterior iliac spine and the umbilicus. Abdominal tenderness may be completely absent if a retrocecal or pelvic appendix is present, in which case the sole physical finding may be tenderness in the flank or on rectal or pelvic examination. Referred rebound tenderness is often present and is most likely to be absent early in the illness. Flexion of the right hip and guarded movement by the patient are due to parietal peritoneal involvement. Hyperesthesia of the skin of the right lower quadrant and a positive psoas or obturator sign are often late findings and are rarely of diagnostic value.

The temperature is usually normal or slightly elevated [37.2°–38°C (99°–100.5°F)], but a temperature >38.3°C (101°F) should suggest perforation. Tachycardia is commensurate with the elevation of the temperature. Rigidity and tenderness become more marked as the disease progresses to perforation and localized or diffuse peritonitis. Distention is rare unless severe diffuse peritonitis has developed. A mass may develop if localized perforation has occurred but will not usually be detectable before 3 days after onset. Earlier presence of a mass suggests carcinoma of the cecum or Crohn's disease. Perforation is rare before 24 h after onset of symptoms, but the rate may be as high as 80% after 48 h.

Although moderate leukocytosis of 10,000–18,000 cells/μL is frequent (with a concomitant left shift), the absence of leukocytosis does not rule out acute appendicitis. Leukocytosis of >20,000 cells/μL suggests probable perforation. Anemia and blood in the stool suggest a primary diagnosis of carcinoma of the cecum, especially in elderly individuals. The urine may contain a few white or red blood cells without bacteria if the appendix lies close to the right ureter or bladder. Urinalysis is most useful in excluding genitourinary conditions that may mimic acute appendicitis.

Radiographs are rarely of value except when an opaque fecalith (5% of patients) is observed in the right lower quadrant (especially in children). Consequently, abdominal films are not routinely obtained unless other conditions such as intestinal obstruction or ureteral calculus may be present. The diagnosis may also be established by the ultrasonic demonstration of an enlarged and thick-walled appendix. Ultrasound is most useful to exclude ovarian cysts, ectopic pregnancy, or tuboovarian abscess. Several studies have recently demonstrated the benefit of contrast-enhanced or nonenhanced CT over ultrasound and plain radiographs in the diagnosis of acute appendicitis. The findings on CT will include a thickened appendix with periappendiceal stranding and often the presence of a fecalith (Figs. 26-1 and 26-2). The reported positive predictive value of CT is 95–97% and the overall accuracy is 90–98%. Furthermore, nonvisualization of the appendix on CT is associated with the findings of a normal appendix 98% of the time. Free peritoneal air is uncommon, even in perforated appendicitis.

Although the typical historic sequence and physical findings are present in 50–60% of cases, a wide variety of atypical patterns of disease are encountered, especially at the age extremes and during pregnancy. Infants under 2 years of age have a 70–80% incidence of perforation and generalized peritonitis. This is thought to be the result of a delay in diagnosis. Any infant or child with diarrhea, vomiting, and abdominal pain is highly suspect. Fever is much more common in this age group, and abdominal distention is often the only physical finding. In the elderly, pain and tenderness are often blunted, and thus the diagnosis is also frequently delayed and leads to

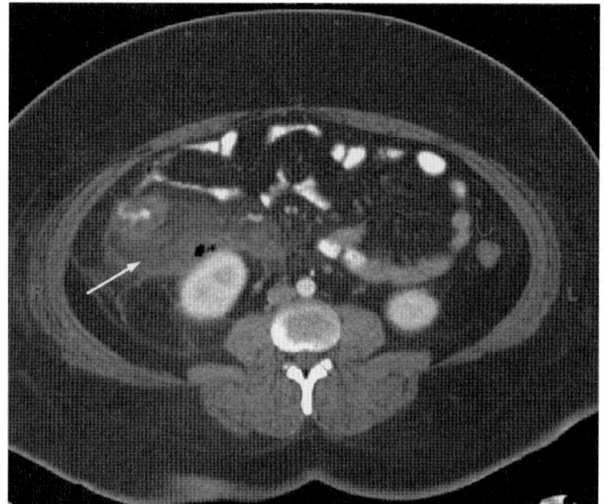

FIGURE 26-1
CT with oral and intravenous contrast of acute appendicitis. There is thickening of the wall of the appendix and periappendiceal stranding (*arrow*).

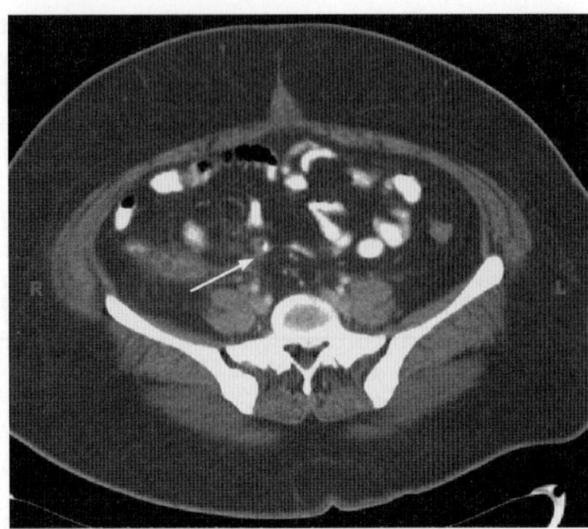

FIGURE 26-2
Appendiceal fecalith (*arrow*).

a 30% incidence of perforation in patients over 70. Elderly patients often present initially with a slightly painful mass (a primary appendiceal abscess) or with adhesive intestinal obstruction 5 or 6 days after a previously undetected perforated appendix.

Appendicitis occurs about once in every 500–2000 pregnancies and is the most common extrauterine condition requiring abdominal operation. The diagnosis may be missed or delayed because of the frequent occurrence of mild abdominal discomfort and nausea and vomiting during pregnancy and because of the gradual shift of the appendix from the right lower quadrant to the right upper quadrant during the second and third trimester of pregnancy. Appendicitis tends to be most common during the second trimester. The diagnosis is best made with ultrasound, which has an 80% accuracy; however, if perforation has already occurred, the accuracy of ultrasound decreases to 30%. Early intervention is warranted because the incidence of fetal loss with a normal appendix is 1.5%. With perforation, the incidence of fetal loss is 20–35%.

DIFFERENTIAL DIAGNOSIS

Acute appendicitis has been labeled the *masquerader*, and the diagnosis is often more difficult to make in young females. Obtaining a good history, including sexual activity and the presence of a vaginal discharge, will help differentiate acute appendicitis from pelvic inflammatory disease (PID). The presence of a malodorous vaginal discharge and gram-negative intracellular diplococci are pathognomonic for PID. Pain on movement of the cervix is also more specific for PID but may occur in appendicitis if perforation has occurred or if the appendix lies adjacent to the uterus or adnexa. *Rupture of a graafian follicle* (mittelschmerz) occurs at midcycle and will produce pain and tenderness more diffuse and usually of a less severe degree than in appendicitis. *Rupture of a corpus luteum cyst* is identical clinically to rupture of a graafian follicle but develops about the time of menstruation. The presence of an adnexal mass, evidence of blood loss, and a positive pregnancy test help differentiate *ruptured tubal pregnancy*. *Twisted ovarian cyst* and *endometriosis* are occasionally difficult to distinguish from appendicitis. In all these female conditions, ultrasonography and laparoscopy may be of great value.

Acute mesenteric lymphadenitis and *acute gastroenteritis* are the diagnoses usually given when enlarged, slightly reddened lymph nodes at the root of the mesentery and a normal appendix are encountered at operation in a patient who usually has right lower quadrant tenderness. Retrospectively, these patients may have had a higher temperature, diarrhea, more diffuse pain and abdominal tenderness, and a lymphocytosis. Between cramps, the abdomen is completely relaxed. Children seem to be affected more frequently than adults. Some of these patients have infection with *Y. pseudotuberculosis* or *Y. enterocolitica*, in which case the diagnosis can be established by culture of the mesenteric nodes or by serologic titers (Chap. 60). In *Salmonella* gastroenteritis, the abdominal findings are similar, although the pain may be more severe and more localized, and fever and chills are common. The occurrence of similar symptoms among other members of the family may be helpful. *Regional enteritis* (Crohn's disease) is usually associated with a more prolonged history, often with previous exacerbations regarded as episodes of gastroenteritis unless the diagnosis has been established previously. Often an inflammatory mass is palpable. In addition, acute cholecystitis, perforated ulcer, acute pancreatitis, acute diverticulitis, strangulating intestinal obstruction, ureteral calculus, and pyelonephritis may present diagnostic difficulties.

℞ Treatment: ACUTE APPENDICITIS

If the diagnosis is in question, 4–6 h of observation with serial abdominal exams is always more beneficial than harmful. Antibiotics should not be administered when the diagnosis is in question, since they will only mask the perforation. The treatment of presumed acute appendicitis is early operation and appendectomy as soon as the patient can be prepared. Appendectomy is frequently accomplished laparoscopically and is associated with less postoperative narcotic use and earlier discharge. It is acceptable to have a 15–20% incidence of a normal appendix at the time of appendectomy to avoid perforation. The use of early laparoscopy instead of close clinical observation has not shown a clinical benefit in the management of patients with nonspecific abdominal pain.

A different approach is indicated if a palpable mass is found 3–5 days after the onset of symptoms. This finding usually represents the presence of a phlegmon or abscess, and complications from attempted surgical excision are frequent. Such patients treated with broad-spectrum antibiotics, drainage of abscesses >3 cm, parenteral fluids, and bowel rest usually show resolution of symptoms within 1 week. *Interval appendectomy* can be performed safely 6–12 weeks later. A randomized clinical trial has demonstrated that antibiotics alone can effectively treat acute, nonperforated appendicitis in 86% of male patients. However, antibiotics alone were associated with a higher recurrence rate than surgical intervention. If the mass enlarges or the patient becomes more toxic, the abscess should be drained. Perforation is associated with generalized peritonitis and its complications, including subphrenic, pelvic, or other abscesses, and can be avoided by early diagnosis. The mortality rate for nonperforated appendicitis is 0.1%, little more than the risk of general anesthesia; for perforated appendicitis, mortality is 3% (and can reach 15% in the elderly).

ACUTE PERITONITIS

Peritonitis is an inflammation of the peritoneum; it may be localized or diffuse in location, acute or chronic in natural history, infectious or aseptic in pathogenesis. Acute peritonitis is most often infectious and is usually related to a perforated viscus (and called *secondary peritonitis*). When no intraabdominal source is identified, infectious peritonitis is called *primary* or *spontaneous*. Acute peritonitis is associated with decreased intestinal motor activity, resulting in distention of the intestinal lumen with gas and fluid. The accumulation of fluid in the bowel together with the lack of oral intake leads to rapid intravascular volume depletion with effects on cardiac, renal, and other systems.

ETIOLOGY

Infectious agents gain access to the peritoneal cavity through a perforated viscus, a penetrating wound of the abdominal wall, or external introduction of a foreign object that is or becomes infected (for example, a chronic peritoneal dialysis catheter). In the absence of immune compromise, host defenses are capable of eradicating small contaminations. The conditions that most commonly result in the introduction of bacteria into the peritoneum are ruptured appendix, ruptured diverticulum, perforated peptic ulcer, incarcerated hernia, gangrenous gall bladder, volvulus, bowel infarction, cancer, inflammatory bowel disease, or intestinal obstruction. However, a wide range of mechanisms may play a role (Table 26-2). Bacterial peritonitis can also occur in the apparent absence of an intraperitoneal source of bacteria (primary or spontaneous bacterial peritonitis). This condition occurs in the setting of ascites and liver cirrhosis in 90% of the cases, usually in patients with ascites with low protein concentration (<1 g/L). Bacterial peritonitis is discussed in detail in Chap. 24.

Aseptic peritonitis may be due to peritoneal irritation by abnormal presence of physiologic fluids (e.g., gastric juice, bile, pancreatic enzymes, blood, or urine) or sterile foreign bodies (e.g., surgical sponges or instruments, starch from surgical gloves) in the peritoneal cavity or as a complication of rare systemic diseases such as lupus erythematosus, porphyria, or familial Mediterranean fever. Chemical irritation of the peritoneum is greatest for acidic gastric juice and pancreatic enzymes. In chemical peritonitis, a major risk of secondary bacterial infection exists.

TABLE 26-2

CONDITIONS LEADING TO SECONDARY BACTERIAL PERITONITIS

Perforations of bowel	Perforations or leaking of other organs
Trauma, blunt or penetrating	Pancreas—pancreatitis
Inflammation	Gall bladder—cholecystitis
Appendicitis	Urinary bladder—trauma, rupture
Diverticulitis	Liver—bile leak after biopsy
Peptic ulcer disease	Fallopian tubes—salpingitis
Inflammatory bowel disease	Bleeding into the peritoneal cavity
Iatrogenic	**Disruption of integrity of peritoneal cavity**
Endoscopic perforation	Trauma
Anastomotic leaks	Continuous ambulatory peritoneal dialysis (indwelling catheter)
Catheter perforation	Intraperitoneal chemotherapy
Vascular	Perinephric abscess
Embolus	Iatrogenic—postoperative, foreign body
Ischemia	
Obstructions	
Adhesions	
Strangulated hernias	
Volvulus	
Intussusception	
Neoplasms	
Ingested foreign body, toothpick, fish bone	

CLINICAL FEATURES

The cardinal manifestations of peritonitis are acute abdominal pain and tenderness, usually with fever. The location of the pain depends on the underlying cause and whether the inflammation is localized or generalized. Localized peritonitis is most common in uncomplicated appendicitis and diverticulitis, and physical findings are limited to the area of inflammation. Generalized peritonitis is associated with widespread inflammation and diffuse abdominal tenderness and rebound. Rigidity of the abdominal wall is common in both localized and generalized peritonitis. Bowel sounds are usually absent. Tachycardia, hypotension, and signs of dehydration are common. Leukocytosis and marked acidosis are common laboratory findings. Plain abdominal films may show dilation of large and small bowel with edema of the bowel wall. Free air under the diaphragm is associated with a perforated viscus. CT and/or ultrasonography can identify the presence of free fluid or an abscess. When ascites is present, diagnostic paracentesis with cell count (>250 neutrophils/μL is usual in peritonitis), protein and lactate dehydrogenase levels, and culture is essential. In elderly and immunosuppressed patients, signs of peritoneal irritation may be more difficult to detect.

THERAPY AND PROGNOSIS

Treatment relies on rehydration, correction of electrolyte abnormalities, antibiotics, and surgical correction of the underlying defect. Mortality rates are <10% for uncomplicated peritonitis associated with a perforated ulcer or ruptured appendix or diverticulum in an otherwise healthy person. Mortality rates of ≥40% have been reported for elderly people, those with underlying illnesses, and when peritonitis has been present for >48 h.

FURTHER READINGS

ANDERSON RE: The natural history and traditional management of appendicitis revisited: Spontaneous resolution and predominance of prehospital perforations imply that a correct diagnosis is more important than an early diagnosis. World J Surg 31:86, 2007

CHEADLE WG, SPAIN DA: The continuing challenge of intraabdominal infection. Am J Surg 186(Suppl 1):15, 2003

FLUM DR et al: Has misdiagnosis of appendicitis decreased over time? A population-based analysis. JAMA 286:1748, 2001

GANGULI S et al: Right lower quadrant pain: Value of the nonvisualized appendix in patients at multidetector CT. Radiology 214:175, 2006

GRONROOS JM, GRONROOS P: Leucocyte count and C-reactive protein in the diagnosis of acute appendicitis. Br J Surg 86:501, 1999

MORINO M et al: Acute non-specific abdominal pain: A randomized controlled study comparing early laparoscopy vs. clinical observation. Ann Surg 241:881, 2006

RAMAN SS et al: Effect of CT on false positive diagnosis of appendicitis and perforation. N Engl J Med 358:972, 2008

STYRUD J et al: Appendectomy vs. antibiotic treatment in acute appendectomy: A prospective multicenter randomized controlled trial. World J Surg 30:1033, 2006

VAN RULER O et al: Comparison of on-demand vs planned relaparotomy strategy in patients with severe peritonitis: A randomized trial. JAMA 298:865, 2007

CHAPTER 27

URINARY TRACT INFECTIONS, PYELONEPHRITIS, AND PROSTATITIS

Walter E. Stamm

DEFINITIONS

Acute infections of the urinary tract fall into two general anatomic categories: lower tract infection (urethritis and cystitis) and upper tract infection (acute pyelonephritis, prostatitis, and intrarenal and perinephric abscesses). Infections at various sites may occur together or independently and may either be asymptomatic or present as one of the clinical syndromes described in this chapter. Infections of the urethra and bladder are often considered superficial (or mucosal) infections, whereas prostatitis, pyelonephritis, and renal suppuration signify tissue invasion.

From a microbiologic perspective, urinary tract infection (UTI) exists when pathogenic microorganisms are detected in the urine, urethra, bladder, kidney, or prostate. In most instances, growth of $\geq 10^5$ organisms per milliliter from a properly collected midstream "clean-catch" urine sample indicates infection. However, significant bacteriuria is lacking in some cases of true UTI. Especially in symptomatic patients, fewer bacteria (10^2–10^4/mL) may signify infection. In urine specimens obtained by suprapubic aspiration or "in-and-out" catheterization and in samples from a patient with an indwelling catheter, colony counts of 10^2–10^4/mL generally indicate infection. Conversely, colony counts of $>10^5$/mL in midstream urine are occasionally due to specimen contamination, which is especially likely when multiple bacterial species are found.

Infections that recur after antibiotic therapy can be due to the persistence of the originally infecting strain (as judged by species, antibiogram, serotype, and molecular type) or to reinfection with a new strain. "Same-strain" recurrent infections that become evident within 2 weeks of cessation of therapy can be the result of unresolved renal or prostatic infection (termed *relapse*) or of persistent vaginal or intestinal colonization leading to rapid reinfection of the bladder.

Symptoms of dysuria, urgency, and frequency that are unaccompanied by significant bacteriuria have been termed the *acute urethral syndrome*. Although widely used, this term lacks anatomic precision because many cases so designated are actually bladder infections. Moreover, since the pathogen can usually be identified, the term *syndrome*—implying unknown causation—is inappropriate.

Chronic pyelonephritis refers to chronic interstitial nephritis believed to result from bacterial infection of the kidney. Many noninfectious diseases also cause an interstitial nephritis that is indistinguishable pathologically from chronic pyelonephritis.

ACUTE UTIS: URETHRITIS, CYSTITIS, AND PYELONEPHRITIS

EPIDEMIOLOGY

Epidemiologically, UTIs are subdivided into catheter-associated (or nosocomial) infections and non–catheter-associated (or community-acquired) infections. Infections in either category may be symptomatic or asymptomatic. Acute community-acquired UTIs are very common and account for more than 7 million office visits annually in the United States. In the female population, these infections occur in 1–3% of schoolgirls and then increase markedly in incidence with the onset of sexual activity in adolescence. The vast majority of acute symptomatic infections involve young women; a prospective study demonstrated an annual incidence of 0.5–0.7 infections per patient-year in this group. In the male population, acute symptomatic UTIs occur in the first year of life (often in association with urologic abnormalities); thereafter, UTIs are unusual in male patients under the age of 50. The development of asymptomatic bacteriuria parallels that of symptomatic infection and is rare among men under 50 but common among women between 20 and 50. Asymptomatic bacteriuria is more common among elderly men and women, with rates as high as 40–50% in some studies. The incidence of acute uncomplicated pyelonephritis among community-dwelling women 18–49 years of age is 28 cases per 10,000 women.

ETIOLOGY

Many microorganisms can infect the urinary tract, but by far the most common agents are the gram-negative bacilli (Chap. 51). *Escherichia coli* causes ~80% of acute infections (both cystitis and pyelonephritis) in patients without catheters, urologic abnormalities, or calculi. Other gram-negative rods, especially *Proteus* and *Klebsiella* spp. and occasionally *Enterobacter* spp., account for a smaller proportion of uncomplicated infections. These organisms, along with *Serratia* spp. (Chap. 51) and *Pseudomonas* spp. (Chap. 53), assume increasing importance in recurrent infections and in infections associated with urologic manipulation, calculi, or obstruction. They play a major role in nosocomial, catheter-associated infections (see below). *Proteus* spp. (through the production of urease) and *Klebsiella* spp. (through the production of extracellular slime and polysaccharides) predispose to stone formation and are isolated more frequently from patients with calculi.

Gram-positive cocci play a lesser role in UTIs. However, *Staphylococcus saprophyticus* (Chap. 35)—a novobiocin-resistant, coagulase-negative species—accounts for 10–15% of acute symptomatic UTIs in young female patients. Enterococci occasionally cause acute uncomplicated cystitis in women. More commonly, enterococci (Chap. 36) and *Staphylococcus aureus* (Chap. 35) cause infections in patients with renal stones or with previous instrumentation or surgery. Isolation of *S. aureus* from the urine should arouse suspicion of bacteremic infection of the kidney. *Staphylococcus epidermidis* (Chap. 35) is a common cause of catheter-associated UTI.

About one-third of women with dysuria and frequency have either an insignificant number of bacteria in midstream urine cultures or completely sterile cultures and have been previously defined as having the urethral syndrome. About three-quarters of these women have pyuria, whereas one-quarter have no pyuria and little objective evidence of infection. In the women with pyuria, two groups of pathogens account for most infections. Low counts (10^2–10^4/mL) of typical bacterial uropathogens such as *E. coli*, *S. saprophyticus*, *Klebsiella*, or *Proteus* are found in midstream urine specimens from most of these women. These bacteria are probably the causative agents in these infections because they can usually be isolated from a suprapubic aspirate, are associated with pyuria, and respond to appropriate antimicrobial therapy. In other women with acute urinary symptoms, pyuria, and urine that is sterile (even when obtained by suprapubic aspiration), sexually transmitted urethritis-producing agents such as *Chlamydia trachomatis* (Chap. 77), *Neisseria gonorrhoeae* (Chap. 45), and herpes simplex virus (HSV; Chap. 80) are etiologically important. These agents are found most frequently in young, sexually active women with new sexual partners.

The causative role of several more unusual bacterial and nonbacterial pathogens in UTIs remains poorly defined. *Ureaplasma urealyticum* (Chap. 76) has frequently been isolated from the urethra and urine of patients with acute dysuria and frequency but is also found in specimens from many patients without urinary symptoms. Ureaplasmas and *Mycoplasma genitalium* (Chap. 76) probably account for some cases of urethritis and cystitis. *U. urealyticum* and *Mycoplasma hominis* have been isolated from prostatic and renal tissues of patients with acute prostatitis and pyelonephritis, respectively, and are probably responsible for some of these infections as well. Adenoviruses cause acute hemorrhagic cystitis in children and in some young adults, often in epidemics. Although other viruses can be isolated from urine (e.g., cytomegalovirus), they are thought not to cause acute UTI. Colonization of the urine of catheterized or diabetic patients by *Candida* and other fungal species is common and sometimes progresses to symptomatic invasive infection (Chap. 107). Mycobacterial infection of the genitourinary tract is discussed in Chap. 66.

PATHOGENESIS AND SOURCES OF INFECTION

The urinary tract should be viewed as a single anatomic unit that is united by a continuous column of urine extending from the urethra to the kidney. In the vast majority of UTIs, bacteria gain access to the bladder via the urethra. Ascent of bacteria from the bladder may follow and is probably the pathway for most renal parenchymal infections.

The vaginal introitus and distal urethra are normally colonized by diphtheroids, streptococcal species, lactobacilli, and staphylococcal species, but not by the enteric gram-negative bacilli that commonly cause UTIs. In females prone to the development of cystitis, however, enteric gram-negative organisms residing in the bowel colonize the introitus, the periurethral skin, and the distal urethra before and during episodes of bacteriuria. The factors that predispose to periurethral colonization with gram-negative bacilli remain poorly understood, but alteration of the normal vaginal flora by antibiotics, other genital infections, or contraceptives (especially spermicide) appears to play an important role. Loss of the normally dominant H_2O_2-producing lactobacilli from the vaginal flora appears to facilitate colonization by *E. coli*. Small numbers of periurethral bacteria probably gain entry to the bladder frequently, and this process is facilitated in some cases by urethral massage during intercourse. Whether bladder infection ensues depends on interacting effects of strain pathogenicity, inoculum size, and local and systemic host defense mechanisms. Recent data from both animal models and human studies indicate that *E. coli* sometimes invades the bladder epithelium, forming intracellular colonies (biofilms) that may persist and become a source of recurrent infection.

Under normal circumstances, bacteria placed in the bladder are rapidly cleared, partly through the flushing and dilutional effects of voiding, but also as a result of the antibacterial properties of urine and the bladder mucosa. Owing mostly to a high urea concentration and high osmolarity, the bladder urine of many healthy persons inhibits or kills bacteria. Prostatic secretions possess antibacterial properties as well. Bladder epithelial cells secrete cytokines and chemokines—primarily interleukin (IL) 6 and IL-8—upon interaction with bacteria, causing polymorphonuclear leukocytes to enter the bladder epithelium and the urine soon after infection arises and play a role in clearing bacteriuria. The role of locally produced antibody remains unclear.

Hematogenous pyelonephritis occurs most often in debilitated patients who are either chronically ill or receiving immunosuppressive therapy. Metastatic staphylococcal or candidal infections of the kidney may follow bacteremia or fungemia, spreading from distant foci of infection in the bone, skin, or vasculature or elsewhere.

CONDITIONS AFFECTING PATHOGENESIS

Gender and Sexual Activity

The female urethra appears to be particularly prone to colonization with colonic gram-negative bacilli because of its proximity to the anus, its short length (~4 cm), and its termination beneath the labia. Sexual intercourse causes the introduction of bacteria into the bladder and is temporally associated with the onset of cystitis; it thus appears to be important in the pathogenesis of UTIs in both pre- and postmenopausal women. Voiding after intercourse reduces the risk of cystitis, probably because it promotes the clearance of bacteria introduced during intercourse. Use of spermicidal compounds with a diaphragm or cervical cap or use of spermicide-coated condoms dramatically alters the normal introital bacterial flora and has been associated with marked increases in vaginal colonization with *E. coli* and in the risk of both cystitis and acute pyelonephritis. In healthy, community-dwelling postmenopausal women, the risk of UTI (both cystitis and pyelonephritis) is increased by a history of recent sexual activity, recent UTI, diabetes mellitus, and incontinence.

In male patients who are <50 years old and who have no history of heterosexual or homosexual insertive rectal intercourse, UTI is exceedingly uncommon, and this diagnosis should be questioned in the absence of clear documentation. An important factor predisposing to bacteriuria in men is urethral obstruction due to prostatic hypertrophy. Insertive rectal intercourse is also associated with an increased risk of cystitis in men. Men (and women) who are infected with HIV and who have CD4+ T-cell counts of <200/μL are at increased risk of both bacteriuria and symptomatic UTI. Finally, lack of circumcision has been identified as a risk factor for UTI in both male neonates and young men.

Pregnancy

UTIs are detected in 2–8% of pregnant women. Symptomatic upper tract infections, in particular, are unusually common during pregnancy; fully 20–30% of pregnant women with asymptomatic bacteriuria subsequently develop pyelonephritis. This predisposition to upper tract infection during pregnancy results from decreased ureteral tone, decreased ureteral peristalsis, and temporary incompetence of the vesicoureteral valves. Bladder catheterization during or after delivery causes additional infections. Increased incidences of low birth weight, premature delivery, and neonatal death result from UTIs (particularly upper tract infections) during pregnancy.

Obstruction

Any impediment to the free flow of urine—tumor, stricture, stone, or prostatic hypertrophy—results in hydronephrosis and a greatly increased frequency of UTI. Infection superimposed on urinary tract obstruction may lead to rapid destruction of renal tissue. It is of utmost importance, therefore, when infection is present, to identify and repair obstructive lesions. On the other hand, when an obstruction is minor and is not progressive or associated with infection, great caution should be exercised in attempting surgical correction. The introduction of infection in such cases may be more damaging than an uncorrected minor obstruction that does not significantly impair renal function.

Neurogenic Bladder Dysfunction

Interference with bladder enervation, as in spinal cord injury, tabes dorsalis, multiple sclerosis, diabetes, and other diseases, may be associated with UTI. The infection may be initiated by the use of catheters for bladder drainage and is favored by the prolonged stasis of urine in the bladder. An additional factor often operative in these cases is bone demineralization due to immobilization, which causes hypercalciuria, calculus formation, and obstructive uropathy.

Vesicoureteral Reflux

Defined as reflux of urine from the bladder cavity up into the ureters and sometimes into the renal pelvis, vesicoureteral reflux occurs during voiding or with elevation of pressure in the bladder. In practice, this condition is detected as retrograde movement of radiopaque or radioactive material during a voiding cystourethrogram.

An anatomically impaired vesicoureteral junction facilitates reflux of bacteria and thus upper tract infection. However, since—even in the healthy urinary system—a fluid connection between the bladder and the kidneys always exists, some retrograde movement of bacteria probably takes place during infection but is not detected by radiologic techniques.

Vesicoureteral reflux is common among children with anatomic abnormalities of the urinary tract or with anatomically normal but infected urinary tracts. In the latter group, reflux disappears with advancing age and is probably attributable to factors other than UTI. Long-term follow-up of children with UTI who have reflux has established that renal damage correlates with marked reflux, not with infection. Thus it appears reasonable to search for reflux in children with unexplained failure of renal growth or with renal scarring, because UTI per se is an insufficient explanation for these abnormalities. On the other hand, it is doubtful that all children who have recurrent UTIs but whose urinary tract appears normal on pyelography should be subjected to voiding cystoureterography merely for the detection of the rare patient with marked reflux not revealed by intravenous pyelography.

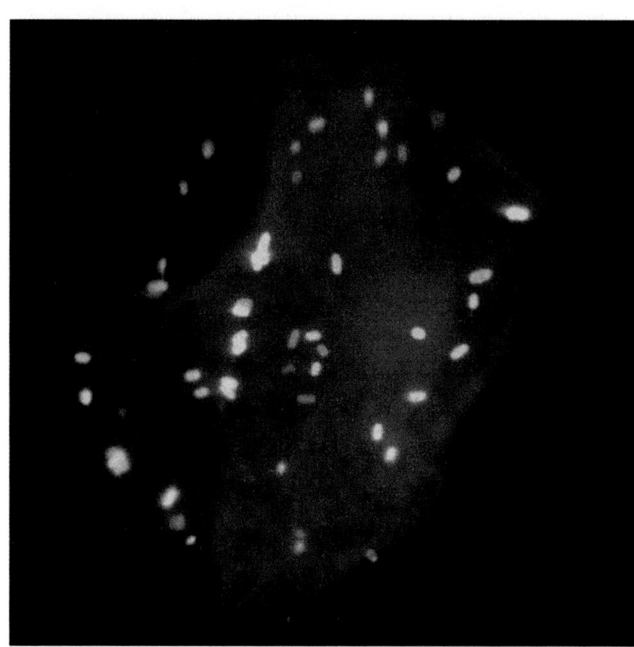

FIGURE 27-1
Adherence of fluorescein-labeled uropathogenic *Escherichia coli* to a uroepithelial cell.

Bacterial Virulence Factors

Not all strains of *E. coli* are equally capable of infecting the intact urinary tract. Bacterial virulence factors markedly influence the likelihood that a given strain, once introduced into the bladder, will cause UTI. Most *E. coli* strains that cause symptomatic UTIs in noncatheterized patients belong to a small number of specific O, K, and H serogroups. These uropathogenic clones have accumulated a number of virulence genes that are often closely linked on the bacterial chromosome in "pathogenicity islands." Bacterial adherence to uroepithelial cells is a critical first step in the initiation of infection (Fig. 27-1). For both *E. coli* and *Proteus* spp., fimbriae (hairlike proteinaceous surface appendages) mediate bacterial attachment to specific receptors on epithelial cells, which in turn initiates important events in the mucosal epithelial cell, including secretion of IL-6 and IL-8 (with subsequent chemotaxis of leukocytes to the bladder mucosa) and induction of apoptosis and epithelial cell desquamation. Besides fimbriae, uropathogenic *E. coli* strains usually produce cytotoxins, hemolysin, and aerobactin (a siderophore for scavenging iron) and are resistant to the bactericidal action of human serum. Nearly all *E. coli* strains causing acute pyelonephritis and most of those causing acute cystitis are uropathogenic strains possessing pathogenicity islands. In contrast, infections in patients with structural or functional abnormalities of the urinary tract are generally caused by bacterial strains that lack these uropathogenic properties; the implication is that these properties are not needed for infection of the compromised urinary tract.

Genetic Factors

Increasing evidence suggests that host genetic factors influence susceptibility to UTI. A maternal history of UTI is more often found among women who have experienced recurrent UTIs than among controls. The number and type of receptors on uroepithelial cells to which bacteria may attach are, at least in part, genetically determined. Many of these structures are components of blood group antigens and are present on both erythrocytes and uroepithelial cells. For example, P fimbriae mediate attachment of *E. coli* to P-positive erythrocytes and are found on nearly all strains causing acute uncomplicated pyelonephritis. Conversely, P blood group–negative individuals, who lack these receptors, are at decreased risk of pyelonephritis. Furthermore, nonsecretors of blood group antigens are at increased risk of recurrent UTI; this predisposition may relate to a different profile of genetically determined glycolipids on uroepithelial cells. Mutations in host genes integral to the immune response (e.g., Toll-like receptors, interferon γ receptors) may also affect susceptibility to UTI.

CLINICAL PRESENTATION

Localization of Infection

Unfortunately, available methods of distinguishing renal parenchymal infection from cystitis are neither reliable nor convenient enough for routine clinical use. Fever or an elevated C-reactive protein level often accompanies acute pyelonephritis and is found in rare cases of cystitis, but also occurs in infections other than pyelonephritis.

Cystitis

Patients with cystitis usually report dysuria, frequency, urgency, and suprapubic pain. The urine often becomes grossly cloudy and malodorous and is bloody in ~30% of cases. White cells and bacteria can be detected by examination of unspun urine in most cases. However, some women with cystitis have only 10^2–10^4 bacteria per milliliter of urine, and in these instances bacteria cannot be seen in a Gram-stained preparation of unspun urine. Physical examination generally reveals only tenderness of the urethra or the suprapubic area. If a genital lesion or a vaginal discharge is evident, especially in conjunction with $<10^5$ bacteria per milliliter on urine culture, then pathogens that may cause urethritis, vaginitis, or cervicitis (e.g., *C. trachomatis*, *N. gonorrhoeae*, *Trichomonas*, *Candida*, and HSV) should be considered. Prominent systemic manifestations, such as a temperature of >38.3°C (>101°F), nausea, and vomiting, usually indicate concomitant renal infection, as does costovertebral angle tenderness. However, the absence of these findings does not ensure that infection is limited to the bladder and urethra.

Acute Pyelonephritis

Symptoms of acute pyelonephritis generally develop rapidly over a few hours or a day and include fever, shaking chills, nausea, vomiting, abdominal pain, and diarrhea. Symptoms of cystitis are sometimes present. Besides fever, tachycardia, and generalized muscle tenderness, physical examination generally reveals marked tenderness on deep pressure in one or both costovertebral angles or on deep abdominal palpation. The range of illness severity is broad. Some patients have mild disease; in others, signs and symptoms of gram-negative sepsis predominate. Most patients have significant leukocytosis and bacteria detectable in Gram-stained unspun urine. Leukocyte casts are present in the urine of some patients, and the detection of these casts is pathognomonic. Hematuria may be demonstrated during the acute phase of the disease; if it persists after acute manifestations of infection have subsided, a stone, a tumor, or tuberculosis should be considered.

Except in individuals with papillary necrosis, abscess formation, or urinary obstruction, the manifestations of acute pyelonephritis usually respond to appropriate therapy within 48–72 h. However, despite the absence of symptoms, bacteriuria or pyuria may persist. In severe pyelonephritis, fever subsides more slowly and may not disappear for several days, even after appropriate antibiotic treatment has been instituted. Persistence of fever or of symptoms and signs beyond 72 h suggests the need for urologic imaging.

Urethritis

Of women with acute dysuria, frequency, and pyuria, ~30% have midstream urine cultures with either no growth or insignificant bacterial growth. Clinically, these women cannot always be readily distinguished from those with cystitis. In this situation, a distinction should be made between women infected with sexually transmitted pathogens (e.g., *C. trachomatis*, *N. gonorrhoeae*, or HSV) and those with low-count *E. coli* or *S. saprophyticus* infection of the urethra and bladder. Chlamydial or gonococcal infection should be suspected in women with a gradual onset of illness, no hematuria, no suprapubic pain, and >7 days of symptoms. The additional history of a recent sex-partner change, especially if the partner has recently had chlamydial or gonococcal urethritis, should heighten the suspicion of a sexually transmitted infection, as should the finding of mucopurulent cervicitis (Chap. 28). Gross hematuria, suprapubic pain, an abrupt onset of illness, a duration of illness of <3 days, and a history of UTIs favor the diagnosis of *E. coli* UTI.

Catheter-Associated UTIs

(See also Chap. 13) Bacteriuria develops in at least 10–15% of hospitalized patients with short-term indwelling urethral catheters. The risk of infection is ~3–5% per day of catheterization. *E. coli*, *Proteus*, *Pseudomonas*, *Klebsiella*, *Serratia*, staphylococci, enterococci, and *Candida* usually cause these infections. Many infecting strains display markedly broader antimicrobial resistance profiles than do organisms that cause community-acquired UTIs. Factors associated with an increased risk of catheter-associated UTI include female sex, prolonged catheterization, severe underlying illness, disconnection of the catheter and drainage tube, other types of faulty catheter care, and lack of systemic antimicrobial therapy.

Infection occurs when bacteria reach the bladder by one of two routes: migration through the column of urine in the catheter lumen (intraluminal route) or up the mucous sheath outside the catheter (periurethral route). Hospital-acquired pathogens can reach the patient's catheter or urine-collecting system on the hands of hospital personnel, in contaminated solutions or irrigants, and via contaminated instruments or disinfectants. Bacteria usually enter the catheter system at the catheter–collecting tube junction or at the drainage bag portal. The organisms then ascend intraluminally into the bladder within 24–72 h. Alternatively, the patient's own bowel flora may colonize the perineal skin and periurethral area and reach the bladder by ascending along the external surface of the catheter. Studies have shown the importance of bacterial attachment to and growth on the device's surfaces in the pathogenesis of catheter-associated UTI. Bacterial growth in biofilms on the catheter eventually produces encrustations consisting of bacteria, bacterial glycocalyces, host urinary proteins, and urinary salts. These encrustations provide a refuge for bacteria and may protect them from antimicrobial agents and phagocytes.

Clinically, catheter-associated infections usually cause minimal symptoms without fever and often resolve after withdrawal of the catheter. The frequency of upper tract infection associated with catheter-induced bacteriuria is unknown. Gram-negative bacteremia, which follows catheter-associated bacteriuria in 1–2% of cases, is the most significant recognized complication of catheter-induced UTIs. The catheterized urinary tract has repeatedly been shown to be the most common source of gram-negative bacteremia in hospitalized patients, generally accounting for ~30% of cases.

In patients catheterized for <2 weeks, catheter-associated UTIs can sometimes be prevented by use of a sterile closed collecting system, by attention to aseptic technique during catheter insertion and care, and by measures to minimize cross-infection. Other preventive approaches, including short courses of systemic antimicrobial therapy, topical application of periurethral antimicrobial ointments, use of preconnected catheter–drainage tube units, and addition of antimicrobial drugs to the drainage bag, have all been protective in at least one controlled trial but are not recommended for general use. The use of catheters impregnated with antimicrobial agents reduces the incidence of asymptomatic bacteriuria in patients catheterized for <2 weeks. Despite precautions, the majority of patients catheterized for >2 weeks eventually develop bacteriuria. For example, because of spinal cord injury, incontinence, or other factors, some patients in hospitals or nursing homes require long-term or semipermanent bladder catheterization. Measures intended to prevent infection have been largely unsuccessful in these chronically catheterized patients, essentially all of whom develop bacteriuria. If feasible, intermittent catheterization by a nurse or by the patient appears to reduce the incidence of bacteriuria and associated complications in such patients. Treatment should be provided when symptomatic infections arise, but treatment of asymptomatic bacteriuria in such patients has no apparent benefit.

DIAGNOSTIC TESTING

Determination of the number and type of bacteria in the urine is an extremely important diagnostic procedure. In symptomatic patients, bacteria are usually present in the urine in large numbers ($\geq 10^5$/mL). Since the large number of bacteria in the bladder urine is due in part to bacterial multiplication in the bladder cavity, samples of urine from the ureters or renal pelvis may contain $<10^5$ bacteria per milliliter and yet indicate infection. Similarly, the presence of bacteriuria of any degree in suprapubic aspirates or of $\geq 10^2$ bacteria per milliliter of urine obtained by catheterization usually indicates infection. In some circumstances (antibiotic treatment, high urea concentration, high osmolarity, low pH), urine inhibits bacterial multiplication, resulting in relatively low bacterial colony counts despite infection. For this reason, antiseptic solutions should not be used to wash the periurethral area before collection of the urine specimen. Water diuresis or recent voiding also reduces bacterial counts in urine.

Microscopy of urine from symptomatic patients can be of great diagnostic value. Microscopic bacteriuria, which is best assessed with Gram-stained uncentrifuged urine, is found in >90% of specimens from patients whose infections are associated with colony counts of at least 10^5/mL, and this finding is very specific. However, bacteria cannot usually be detected microscopically in infections with lower colony counts (10^2–10^4/mL). The detection of bacteria by urinary microscopy thus constitutes firm evidence of infection, but the absence of microscopically detectable bacteria does not exclude the diagnosis. When carefully sought by chamber-count microscopy, pyuria is a highly sensitive indicator of UTI in symptomatic patients. Pyuria is demonstrated in nearly all acute bacterial UTIs, and its absence calls the diagnosis into question. The leukocyte esterase "dipstick" method is less sensitive than microscopy in identifying pyuria but is a useful alternative when microscopy is not feasible. Pyuria in the absence of bacteriuria (sterile pyuria) may indicate infection with unusual agents such as *C. trachomatis*, *U. urealyticum*, or *Mycobacterium tuberculosis* or with fungi. Alternatively, sterile pyuria may be documented in noninfectious urologic conditions such as calculi, anatomic abnormality, nephrocalcinosis, vesicoureteral reflux, interstitial nephritis, or polycystic disease.

Although many authorities have recommended that urine culture and antimicrobial susceptibility testing be performed for any patient with a suspected UTI, it is more practical and cost-effective to manage women who have symptoms characteristic of acute uncomplicated cystitis without an initial urine culture. Two approaches to presumptive therapy have generally been used. In the first, treatment is initiated solely on the basis of a typical history and/or typical findings on physical examination. In the second, women with symptoms and signs of acute cystitis and without complicating factors are managed with urinary microscopy (or, alternatively, with a leukocyte esterase test). A positive result for pyuria and/or bacteriuria provides enough evidence of infection to omit urine culture and susceptibility testing and treat the patient empirically. Urine should be cultured, however, when a woman's symptoms and urine-examination findings leave the diagnosis of cystitis in question. Pretherapy cultures and susceptibility testing are also essential in the management of all patients with suspected upper tract infections and of those with complicating factors (including all men). In these situations, any of a variety of pathogens may be involved, and antibiotic therapy is best tailored to the individual organism.

UROLOGIC EVALUATION

Very few women with recurrent UTIs have correctable lesions discovered at cystoscopy or upon IV pyelography, and these procedures should not be undertaken routinely in such cases. Urologic evaluation should be performed for selected female patients—namely, women with relapsing infection, a history of childhood infections, stones or painless hematuria, or recurrent pyelonephritis. Most male patients with UTI should be considered to have complicated infection and thus should be evaluated urologically. Possible exceptions include young men who have cystitis associated with sexual activity, who are uncircumcised, or who have AIDS. Men or women presenting with acute infection and signs or symptoms suggestive of an obstruction or stones should undergo prompt urologic evaluation, generally by means of ultrasound.

℞ Treatment: URINARY TRACT INFECTIONS

The following principles underlie the treatment of UTIs:

1. Except in acute uncomplicated cystitis in women, a quantitative urine culture or a comparable alternative diagnostic test should be performed to confirm infection before empirical treatment is begun, and antimicrobial sensitivity testing should be used to direct therapy.

2. Factors predisposing to infection, such as obstruction and calculi, should be identified and corrected if possible.
3. Relief of clinical symptoms does not always indicate bacteriologic cure.
4. Each course of treatment should be classified after its completion as a failure (symptoms and/or bacteriuria not eradicated during therapy or in the immediate posttreatment culture) or a cure (resolution of symptoms and elimination of bacteriuria). Recurrent infections should be classified as same-strain or different-strain and as early (occurring within 2 weeks of the end of therapy) or late.
5. In general, uncomplicated infections confined to the lower urinary tract respond to short courses of therapy, whereas upper tract infections require longer treatment. After therapy, early recurrences due to the same strain may result from an unresolved upper tract focus of infection, but often (especially after short-course therapy for cystitis) result from persistent vaginal colonization. Recurrences >2 weeks after the cessation of therapy nearly always represent reinfection with a new strain or with the previously infecting strain that has persisted in the vaginal and rectal flora.
6. Despite increasing resistance, community-acquired infections (especially initial infections) are usually due to relatively antibiotic-sensitive strains.
7. In patients with repeated infections, instrumentation, or recent hospitalization, the presence of antibiotic-resistant strains should be suspected. Although many antimicrobial agents reach high concentrations in urine, in vitro resistance usually predicts a substantially higher failure rate.

The anatomic location of a UTI greatly influences the success or failure of a therapeutic regimen. Bladder bacteriuria (cystitis) can usually be eliminated with short courses or even single doses of antimicrobial agents. In the past, it was demonstrated that as little as a single 500-mg dose of intramuscular kanamycin eliminated bladder bacteriuria in most cases. With upper tract infections, however, single-dose therapy fails in the majority of cases, and 7- to 14-day courses are generally needed. Longer periods of treatment (2–6 weeks) aimed at eradicating a persistent focus of infection may be necessary in some cases.

ACUTE UNCOMPLICATED CYSTITIS Taken together, *E. coli* and *S. saprophyticus* cause >90–95% of cases of acute uncomplicated cystitis. Although resistance patterns vary geographically (both globally and within the United States), resistance has increased in many areas. Nevertheless, most strains are sensitive to several antibiotics. In most parts of the United States, more than one-quarter of *E. coli* strains causing acute cystitis are resistant to amoxicillin, sulfa drugs, and cephalexin; resistance to trimethoprim (TMP) and trimethoprim-sulfamethoxazole (TMP-SMX) is now approaching these levels in many areas. Substantially higher rates of resistance to TMP-SMX have been documented in some other countries, as has resistance to fluoroquinolones. Thus knowledge of local resistance patterns is needed to guide empirical therapy.

Many have advocated single-dose treatment for acute cystitis. The advantages include less expense, ensured compliance, fewer side effects, and perhaps less intense pressure favoring the selection of resistant organisms in the intestinal, vaginal, or perineal flora. However, more frequent recurrences develop shortly after single-dose therapy than after 3-day treatment, and single-dose therapy does not eradicate vaginal colonization with *E. coli* as effectively as do longer regimens. A 3-day course of TMP-SMX, TMP, norfloxacin, ciprofloxacin, or levofloxacin appears to preserve the low rate of side effects of single-dose therapy while improving efficacy (**Table 27-1**); thus 3-day regimens of these drugs are currently preferred for acute cystitis. In areas where TMP-SMX resistance exceeds 20%, either a fluoroquinolone or nitrofurantoin can be used (Table 27-1). Resistance to these agents among strains causing cystitis remains low. A 3-day regimen of amoxicillin/clavulanate was found to be significantly less effective than a 3-day regimen of ciprofloxacin in treating uncomplicated UTIs in women. Neither single-dose nor 3-day therapy should be used for women with symptoms or signs of pyelonephritis, urologic abnormalities or stones, or previous infections due to antibiotic-resistant organisms. Male patients with UTI often have urologic abnormalities or prostatic involvement and hence are not candidates for single-dose or 3-day therapy. For empirical therapy, they should generally receive a 7- to 14-day course of a fluoroquinolone (Table 27-1).

ACUTE URETHRITIS The choice of treatment for women with acute urethritis depends on the etiologic agent involved. In chlamydial infection, azithromycin (1 g in a single oral dose) or doxycycline (100 mg twice daily by mouth for 7 days) should be used. Women with acute dysuria and frequency, negative urine cultures, and no pyuria usually do not respond to antimicrobial agents.

ACUTE UNCOMPLICATED PYELONEPHRITIS In women, most cases of acute uncomplicated pyelonephritis without accompanying clinical evidence of calculi or urologic disease are due to *E. coli*. Although the optimal route and duration of therapy have not been established, a 7- to 14-day course of a fluoroquinolone is usually adequate. Neither ampicillin nor TMP-SMX should be used as initial therapy because >25% of *E. coli* strains causing pyelonephritis are now resistant to these drugs in vitro. For at least the first few days of treatment, antibiotics should probably be given intravenously to most patients, but patients with mild symptoms can be treated for 7–14 days with an oral antibiotic (usually ciprofloxacin or levofloxacin), with or without an initial single parenteral dose (Table 27-1). Patients who fail to respond to treatment within 72 h or who relapse after therapy should be evaluated for unrecognized suppurative foci, calculi, or urologic disease.

COMPLICATED URINARY TRACT INFECTIONS Complicated UTIs (those arising in a setting of catheteri-

TABLE 27-1

TREATMENT REGIMENS FOR BACTERIAL URINARY TRACT INFECTIONS

CONDITION	CHARACTERISTIC PATHOGENS	MITIGATING CIRCUMSTANCES	RECOMMENDED EMPIRICAL TREATMENT[a]
Acute uncomplicated cystitis in women	*Escherichia coli*, *Staphylococcus saprophyticus*, *Proteus mirabilis*, *Klebsiella pneumoniae*	None	3-Day regimens: oral TMP-SMX, TMP, quinolone; 7-day regimen: macrocrystalline nitrofurantoin[b]
		Diabetes, symptoms for >7 d, recent UTI, use of diaphragm, age >65 years	Consider 7-day regimen: oral TMP-SMX, TMP, quinolone[b]
		Pregnancy	Consider 7-day regimen: oral amoxicillin, macrocrystalline nitrofurantoin, cefpodoxime proxetil, or TMP-SMX[b]
Acute uncomplicated pyelonephritis in women	*E. coli*, *P. mirabilis*, *S. saprophyticus*	Mild to moderate illness, no nausea or vomiting; outpatient therapy	Oral[c] quinolone for 7–14 d (initial dose given IV if desired); or single-dose ceftriaxone (1 g) or gentamicin (3–5 mg/kg) IV followed by oral TMP-SMX[c] for 14 d
		Severe illness or possible urosepsis: hospitalization required	Parenteral[d] quinolone, gentamicin (± ampicillin), ceftriaxone, or aztreonam until defervescence; then oral[c] quinolone, cephalosporin, or TMP-SMX for 14 d
Complicated UTI in men and women	*E. coli*, *Proteus*, *Klebsiella*, *Pseudomonas*, *Serratia*, enterococci, staphylococci	Mild to moderate illness, no nausea or vomiting: outpatient therapy	Oral[c] quinolone for 10–14 d
		Severe illness or possible urosepsis: hospitalization required	Parenteral[d] ampicillin and gentamicin, quinolone, ceftriaxone, aztreonam, ticarcillin/clavulanate, or imipenem-cilastatin until defervescence; then oral[c] quinolone or TMP-SMX for 10–21 d

[a]Treatments listed are those to be prescribed before the etiologic agent is known; Gram's staining can be helpful in the selection of empirical therapy. Such therapy can be modified once the infecting agent has been identified. Fluoroquinolones should not be used in pregnancy. TMP-SMX, although not approved for use in pregnancy, has been widely used. Gentamicin should be used with caution in pregnancy because of its possible toxicity to eighth-nerve development in the fetus.

[b]Multiday oral regimens for cystitis are as follows: TMP-SMX, 160/800 mg q12h; TMP, 100 mg q12h; norfloxacin, 400 mg q12h; ciprofloxacin, 250 mg q12h; ofloxacin, 200 mg q12h; levofloxacin, 250 mg/d; lomefloxacin, 400 mg/d; enoxacin, 400 mg q12h; macrocrystalline nitrofurantoin, 100 mg qid; amoxicillin, 250 mg q8h; cefpodoxime proxetil, 100 mg q12h.

[c]Oral regimens for pyelonephritis and complicated UTI are as follows: TMP-SMX, 160/800 mg q12h; ciprofloxacin, 500 mg q12h; ofloxacin, 200–300 mg q12h; lomefloxacin, 400 mg/d; enoxacin, 400 mg q12h; levofloxacin, 200 mg q12h; amoxicillin, 500 mg q8h; cefpodoxime proxetil, 200 mg q12h.

[d]Parenteral regimens are as follows: ciprofloxacin, 400 mg q12h; ofloxacin, 400 mg q12h; levofloxacin, 500 mg/d; gentamicin, 1 mg/kg q8h; ceftriaxone, 1–2 g/d; ampicillin, 1 g q6h; imipenem-cilastatin, 250–500 mg q6–8h; ticarcillin/clavulanate, 3.2 g q8h; aztreonam, 1 g q8–12h.

Note: UTI, urinary tract infection; TMP, trimethoprim; TMP-SMX, trimethoprim-sulfamethoxazole.

zation, instrumentation, anatomic or functional urologic abnormalities, stones, obstruction, immunosuppression, renal disease, or diabetes) are typically due to hospital-acquired bacteria, including *E. coli*, *Klebsiella*, *Proteus*, *Serratia*, *Pseudomonas*, enterococci, and staphylococci. Many of the infecting strains are antibiotic-resistant. Empirical antibiotic therapy ideally provides broad-spectrum coverage against these pathogens. In patients with minimal or mild symptoms, oral therapy with a fluoroquinolone, such as ciprofloxacin or levofloxacin, can be administered until culture results and antibiotic sensitivities are known. In patients with more severe illness, including acute pyelonephritis or suspected urosepsis, hospitalization and parenteral therapy should be undertaken. In patients with diabetes, severe outcomes are more common and should be anticipated; they include renal suppurative foci, papillary necrosis, emphysematous infection, and unusual infecting agents. Commonly used empirical regimens include imipenem alone, an extended-spectrum penicillin or cephalosporin plus an aminoglycoside, and (when the involvement of enterococci is unlikely) ceftriaxone or ceftazidime. When information on the antimicrobial sensitivity pattern of the infecting strain becomes available, a more specific antimicrobial regimen can be selected. Therapy should generally be administered for 10–21 days, with the exact duration depending on the severity of the infection and the susceptibility of the infecting strain. Follow-up cultures should be performed 2–4 weeks after cessation of therapy to demonstrate cure.

ASYMPTOMATIC BACTERIURIA The need for treatment as well as the optimal type and duration of treatment for catheterized patients with asymptomatic bacteriuria have not been established. Removal of the catheter in conjunction with a short course of antibiotics to which the organism is susceptible probably constitutes the best course of action and nearly always eradicates bacteriuria. Treatment of asymptomatic catheter-associated bacteriuria may be of greatest benefit to elderly women, who most often develop symptoms if left untreated. If the catheter cannot be removed, antibiotic therapy usually proves unsuccessful and may in fact result in infection with a more resistant strain. In this situation, the bacteriuria should be ignored unless the patient develops symptoms or is at high risk of developing bacteremia. In these cases, use of systemic antibiotics or urinary bladder antiseptics may reduce the degree of bacteriuria and the likelihood of bacteremia.

Asymptomatic bacteriuria in noncatheterized patients is common, especially among the elderly, but has not been linked to adverse outcomes in most circumstances other than pregnancy (see below). Thus antimicrobial therapy is unnecessary and may in fact promote the emergence of resistant strains in most patients with asymptomatic bacteriuria. High-risk patients with neutropenia, renal transplants, obstruction, or other complicating conditions may require treatment when asymptomatic bacteriuria occurs. Seven days of therapy with an oral agent to which the organism is sensitive should be given initially. If bacteriuria persists, it can be monitored without further treatment in most patients. Longer-term therapy (4–6 weeks) may be necessary in high-risk patients with persistent asymptomatic bacteriuria.

TREATMENT DURING PREGNANCY In pregnancy, acute cystitis can be managed with 7 days of treatment with amoxicillin, nitrofurantoin, or a cephalosporin. All pregnant women should be screened for asymptomatic bacteriuria during the first trimester and, if bacteriuric, should be treated with one of the regimens listed in Table 27-1. After treatment, a culture should be performed to ensure cure, and cultures should be repeated monthly thereafter until delivery. Acute pyelonephritis in pregnancy should be managed with hospitalization and parenteral antibiotic therapy, generally with a cephalosporin or an extended-spectrum penicillin. Continuous low-dose prophylaxis with nitrofurantoin should be given to women who have recurrent infections during pregnancy.

PROGNOSIS

In uncomplicated cystitis or pyelonephritis, treatment ordinarily results in complete resolution of symptoms. Lower tract infections in women are of concern mainly because they cause discomfort, morbidity, loss of time from work, and substantial health care costs. Cystitis may also result in upper tract infection or in bacteremia (especially during instrumentation), but little evidence suggests that renal impairment follows. When repeated episodes of cystitis occur, they are more commonly reinfections rather than relapses.

Acute uncomplicated pyelonephritis in adults rarely progresses to renal functional impairment and chronic renal disease. Repeated upper tract infections often represent relapse rather than reinfection, and renal calculi or an underlying urologic abnormality should be vigorously sought. If neither is found, 6 weeks of chemotherapy may be useful in eradicating an unresolved focus of infection.

Repeated symptomatic UTIs in children and in adults with obstructive uropathy, neurogenic bladder, structural renal disease, or diabetes progress to renal scarring and chronic renal disease with unusual frequency. Asymptomatic bacteriuria in these groups as well as in adults without urologic disease or obstruction predisposes to increased numbers of episodes of symptomatic infection, but does not result in renal impairment in most instances.

PREVENTION

Women who experience frequent symptomatic UTIs (≥3 per year on average) are candidates for long-term administration of low-dose antibiotics directed at preventing recurrences. Such women should be advised to avoid spermicide use and to void soon after intercourse. Daily or thrice-weekly administration of a single dose of TMP-SMX (80/400 mg), TMP alone (100 mg), or nitrofurantoin (50 mg) has been particularly effective. Fluoroquinolones have also been used for prophylaxis. Prophylaxis should be initiated only after bacteriuria has been eradicated with a full-dose treatment regimen. The same prophylactic regimens can be used after sexual intercourse to prevent episodes of symptomatic infection in women in whom UTIs are temporally related to intercourse. Postmenopausal women who are not taking oral estrogen replacement therapy can effectively manage recurrent UTIs with topical intravaginal estrogen cream. Other patients for whom prophylaxis appears to have some merit include men with chronic prostatitis; patients undergoing prostatectomy, both during the operation and in the postoperative period; and pregnant women with asymptomatic bacteriuria. All pregnant women should be screened for bacteriuria in the first trimester and should be treated if bacteriuria is detected.

PAPILLARY NECROSIS

When infection of the renal pyramids develops in association with vascular diseases of the kidney or with urinary tract obstruction, renal papillary necrosis is likely to result. Patients with diabetes, sickle cell disease, chronic alcoholism, and vascular disease seem peculiarly susceptible to this complication. Hematuria, pain in the flank or abdomen, and chills and fever are the most common presenting symptoms. Acute renal failure with oliguria or anuria sometimes develops. Rarely, sloughing of a pyramid may take place without symptoms in a patient with chronic UTI, and the diagnosis is made when the necrotic tissue is passed in the urine or identified as a "ring shadow" on pyelography. If renal function deteriorates suddenly in a diabetic individual or a patient with chronic obstruction, the diagnosis of renal papillary necrosis should be entertained, even in the absence of fever or pain. Renal papillary necrosis is often bilateral; when it is unilateral, however, nephrectomy may be a life-saving approach to the management of overwhelming infection.

EMPHYSEMATOUS PYELONEPHRITIS AND CYSTITIS

These unusual clinical entities almost always occur in diabetic patients, often in concert with urinary obstruction and chronic infection. Emphysematous pyelonephritis is usually characterized by a rapidly progressive clinical course, with high fever, leukocytosis, renal parenchymal necrosis, and accumulation of fermentative gases in the kidney and perinephric tissues. Most patients also have pyuria and glucosuria. *E. coli* causes most cases, but occasionally other Enterobacteriaceae are isolated. Gas in tissues is often seen on plain films and is best confirmed and localized by CT. Surgical resection of the involved tissue in addition to systemic antimicrobial therapy is usually needed to prevent a fatal outcome in emphysematous pyelonephritis.

Emphysematous cystitis also occurs primarily in diabetic patients, usually in association with *E. coli* or other facultative gram-negative rods and often in relation to bladder outlet obstruction. Patients with this condition generally are less severely ill and have less rapidly progressive disease than those with emphysematous pyelonephritis. The patient typically reports abdominal pain, dysuria, frequency, and (in some cases) pneumaturia. CT shows gas within both the bladder lumen and the bladder wall. Generally, conservative therapy with systemic antimicrobial agents and relief of outlet obstruction are effective, but some patients do not respond to these measures and require cystectomy.

RENAL AND PERINEPHRIC ABSCESS

See Chap. 24.

PROSTATITIS

The term *prostatitis* has been used for various inflammatory conditions affecting the prostate, including acute and chronic infections with specific bacteria and, more commonly, instances in which signs and symptoms of prostatic inflammation are present, but no specific organisms can be detected. Patients with acute bacterial prostatitis can usually be identified readily on the basis of typical symptoms and signs, pyuria, and bacteriuria. To classify a patient with suspected chronic prostatitis correctly, a midstream urine specimen, a prostatic expressate, and a postmassage urine specimen should be quantitatively cultured and evaluated for numbers of leukocytes. On the basis of these studies and other considerations, patients with suspected chronic prostatitis can be categorized as having chronic bacterial prostatitis or chronic pelvic pain syndrome, with or without inflammation (Table 27-2).

ACUTE BACTERIAL PROSTATITIS

When it occurs spontaneously, this disease generally affects young men; however, it may also be associated with an indwelling urethral catheter in older men. It is characterized by fever, chills, dysuria, and a tense or boggy, extremely tender prostate. Although prostatic massage usually produces purulent secretions with a large number of bacteria on culture, vigorous massage may cause bacteremia and should be avoided. The etiologic agent can usually be identified by Gram's staining and culture of urine. In cases not associated with catheters, the infection

TABLE 27-2

CLASSIFICATION OF PROSTATITIS

CLASSIFICATION	CLINICAL PRESENTATION	PROSTATE	EPS	ETIOLOGIC AGENT	ANTIBIOTICS
Acute bacterial prostatitis	Acute onset of fever, chills, dysuria, urgency	Tender, tense, boggy	PMNs, bacteria	*Escherichia coli*, other uropathogens	Fluoroquinolone, other (see text)
Chronic bacterial prostatitis	Recurrent UTIs, obstructive symptoms, perineal pain	Normal	PMNs, bacteria	*E. coli*, other uropathogens	Fluoroquinolone, other (see text)
Chronic pelvic pain syndrome					
Inflammatory	Perineal and low-back pain, obstructive symptoms, recent NGU	Normal	↑PMNs	*Ureaplasma*? *Mycoplasma*? *Chlamydia*?	4–6 weeks of oral macrolide, tetracycline, other (see text)
Noninflammatory	Same as above	Normal	No PMNs	Unknown	None

Note: EPS, expressed prostatic secretion; NGU, nongonococcal urethritis; PMNs, polymorphonuclear leukocytes.

is generally due to common gram-negative urinary tract pathogens (*E. coli* or *Klebsiella*). Initially, an intravenous fluoroquinolone is the preferred antibiotic regimen; alternatively, a third-generation cephalosporin or an aminoglycoside can be administered. The response to antibiotics in acute bacterial prostatitis is usually prompt, perhaps because drugs penetrate readily into the acutely inflamed prostate. In catheter-associated cases, the spectrum of etiologic agents is broader, including hospital-acquired gram-negative rods and enterococci. The urinary Gram's stain may be particularly helpful in such cases. Imipenem, an aminoglycoside, a fluoroquinolone, or a third-generation cephalosporin should be used for initial empirical therapy. The long-term prognosis is good, although in some instances acute infection may result in abscess formation, epididymoorchitis, seminal vesiculitis, septicemia, or residual chronic bacterial prostatitis. Since the advent of antibiotics, the frequency of acute bacterial prostatitis has diminished markedly.

CHRONIC BACTERIAL PROSTATITIS

This entity is now infrequent but should be considered in men with a history of recurrent bacteriuria. Symptoms are often lacking between episodes, and the prostate usually feels normal on palpation. Obstructive symptoms or perineal pain develops in some patients. Intermittently, infection spreads to the bladder, producing frequency, urgency, and dysuria. A pattern of relapsing infection in a middle-aged man strongly suggests chronic bacterial prostatitis. Classically, the diagnosis is established by culture of *E. coli*, *Klebsiella*, *Proteus*, or other uropathogenic bacteria from the expressed prostatic secretion or postmassage urine in higher quantities than are found in midstream urine. Antibiotics promptly relieve the symptoms associated with acute exacerbations but are less effective in eradicating the focus of chronic infection in the prostate. This relative ineffectiveness for long-term cure is due in part to the poor penetration of most antibiotics into the prostate. In this respect, fluoroquinolones are considerably more successful than other antimicrobial agents, but even they must generally be given for at least 12 weeks to be effective. Patients with frequent episodes of acute cystitis in whom attempts at curative therapy fail can be managed with prolonged suppressive courses of low-dose antimicrobial agents (usually a sulfonamide, TMP, or nitrofurantoin). Total prostatectomy obviously results in the cure of chronic prostatitis but is associated with considerable morbidity. Transurethral prostatectomy is safer but cures only one-third of patients.

CHRONIC PELVIC PAIN SYNDROME (FORMERLY NONBACTERIAL PROSTATITIS)

Patients who present with symptoms of prostatitis (intermittent perineal and low-back pain, obstructive voiding symptoms), few signs on examination, no bacterial growth in cultures, and no history of recurrent episodes of bacterial prostatitis are classified as having chronic pelvic pain syndrome (CPPS). Patients with CPPS are divided into inflammatory and noninflammatory subgroups based on the presence or absence of prostatic inflammation. Prostatic inflammation can be considered present when the expressed prostatic secretion and postmassage urine contain at least tenfold more leukocytes than midstream urine or when the expressed prostatic secretion contains ≥1000 leukocytes per microliter.

The likely etiology of CPPS associated with inflammation is an infectious agent, but the agent has not yet been identified. Evidence for a causative role of both *U. urealyticum* and *C. trachomatis* has been presented but is not conclusive. Since most cases of inflammatory CPPS occur in young, sexually active men and since many cases follow an episode of nonspecific urethritis, the causative agent may well be sexually transmitted. The effectiveness of antimicrobial agents in this condition is uncertain. Some patients benefit from a 4- to 6-week course of treatment with erythromycin, doxycycline, TMP-SMX, or a fluoroquinolone, but controlled trials are lacking. Patients who have symptoms and signs of prostatitis but who have no evidence of prostatic inflammation (normal leukocyte counts) and negative urine cultures are classified as having noninflammatory CPPS. Despite their symptoms, these patients most likely do not have prostatic infection and should not be given antimicrobial agents.

FURTHER READINGS

BENWAY BM, MOON TD: Bacterial prostatitis. Urol Clin North Am 35:23, 2008

FIHN SD et al: Clinical practice: Acute uncomplicated urinary tract infection in women. N Engl J Med 349:259, 2003

GUPTA K et al: Increasing antimicrobial resistance and the management of uncomplicated community-acquired urinary tract infections. Ann Intern Med 135:41, 2001

HOOTON TM et al: Amoxicillin-clavulanate vs ciprofloxacin for the treatment of uncomplicated cystitis in women. A randomized trial. JAMA 293:949, 2005

——— et al: A prospective study of risk factors for symptomatic urinary tract infection in young women. N Engl J Med 335:468, 1996

JOHNSON JR et al: Systematic review. Antimicrobial urinary catheters to prevent catheter-associated UTI in hospitalized patients. Ann Intern Med 144:116, 2006

LEE SW et al: Acupuncture versus sham acupuncture for chronic prostatitis/chronic pelvic pain. Am J Med 121:79.e1, 2008

LUNDSTEDT AC et al: Inherited susceptibility to acute pyelonephritis: A family study of urinary tract infection. J Infect Dis 195:1227, 2007

MCISAAC WJ et al: Validation of a decision aid to assist physicians in reducing unnecessary antibiotic drug use for acute cystitis. Arch Intern Med 167:2201, 2007

PONTARI MA: Chronic prostatitis/chronic pelvic pain syndrome. Urol Clin North Am 35:81, 2008

SCHOLES D et al: Risk factors associated with acute pyelonephritis in healthy women. Ann Intern Med 142:20, 2005

STAMM WE, SCHAEFFER AJ (eds): *The State of the Art in the Management of Urinary Tract Infections*. Am J Med 113(Suppl 1A):1S, 2002

TALAN DA et al: Comparison of ciprofloxacin (7 days) and trimethoprim-sulfamethoxazole (14 days) for acute uncomplicated pyelonephritis in women. JAMA 283:1583, 2000

WARREN JW et al: Guidelines for antimicrobial therapy of uncomplicated acute bacterial cystitis and acute pyelonephritis in women. Clin Infect Dis 29:745, 1999

CHAPTER 28

SEXUALLY TRANSMITTED INFECTIONS: OVERVIEW AND CLINICAL APPROACH

King K. Holmes

CLASSIFICATION AND EPIDEMIOLOGY

Worldwide, most adults acquire at least one sexually transmitted infection (STI), and many remain at risk for complications. Each year, for example, an estimated 6.2 million persons in the United States acquire a new genital human papillomavirus (HPV) infection, and many of these individuals are at risk for genital neoplasias. Certain STIs, such as syphilis, gonorrhea, HIV infection, hepatitis B, and chancroid, are most concentrated within "core populations" characterized by high rates of partner change, multiple concurrent partners, or "dense," highly connected sexual networks—e.g., involving prostitutes and their clients, some homosexual men, and persons involved in the use of illicit drugs, particularly crack cocaine and methamphetamine. Other STIs are distributed more evenly throughout societies. For example, chlamydial infections, genital infections with HPV, and genital herpes can spread widely, even in relatively low-risk populations.

In general, the product of three factors determines the initial rate of spread of any STI within a population: rate of sexual exposure of susceptible to infectious people, efficiency of transmission per exposure, and duration of infectivity of those infected. Accordingly, efforts to prevent and control STIs aim to decrease the rate of sexual exposure of susceptibles to infected persons (e.g., through individual counseling and efforts to change the norms of sexual behavior), to decrease the duration of infectivity (through early diagnosis and curative or suppressive treatment), and to decrease the efficiency of transmission (e.g., through promotion of condom use and safer sexual practices and recently through male circumcision).

In all societies, STIs rank among the most common of all infectious diseases, with >30 infections now classified as predominantly sexually transmitted or as frequently sexually transmissible (Table 28-1). In developing countries, with three-quarters of the world's population and 90% of the world's STIs, such factors as population growth (especially in adolescent and young-adult age groups), rural-to-urban migration, wars, and poverty create exceptional vulnerability to disease resulting from risky sexual behaviors. During the 1990s, in China, Russia, the other states of the former Soviet Union, and South Africa, internal social structures changed rapidly as borders opened to the West, unleashing enormous new epidemics of HIV infection and other STIs. HIV has become the leading cause of death in some developing countries, and HPV and hepatitis B virus (HBV) remain important causes of cervical and hepatocellular carcinoma, respectively—two of the most common malignancies in the developing world. Sexually transmitted herpes simplex virus (HSV) infections now cause most genital ulcer disease throughout the world and an increasing proportion of cases of genital herpes in developing countries with generalized HIV epidemics, where the positive feedback loop between HSV and HIV transmission is a growing, intractable problem. Randomized trials of the efficacy of therapy against HSV-2 in preventing the acquisition or transmission of HIV infection will be completed in 2007–2008, and the outcome will help shape future efforts to prevent HIV infection. Globally, five curable STIs—gonorrhea, chlamydial infection, syphilis, chancroid, and trichomoniasis—caused ~350 million new infections annually in the mid-1990s. Up to 50% of women of reproductive age in developing countries have bacterial vaginosis (arguably acquired sexually). All six of these curable infections have been associated with increased risk of HIV transmission or acquisition.

In the United States, the prevalence of antibody to HSV-2 has begun to fall only recently (since the late 1990s), especially among adolescents and young adults; the decline is presumably due to delayed sexual debut, increased condom use, and lower rates of multiple (≥4) sex partners, as is well documented in the U.S. Youth Risk Behavior Surveillance System (YRBSS). Genital HPV remains the most common sexually transmitted pathogen in this country, infecting 60% of a cohort of initially HPV-negative, sexually active Washington state college women within 5 years in a study conducted from 1990 to 2000.

In industrialized countries, fear of HIV infection since the mid-1980s, coupled with widespread behavioral interventions and better-organized systems of care for the curable STIs, has helped curb the transmission of the latter diseases. Nonetheless, foci of hyperendemic transmission persist in the southeastern United States and in most large U.S. cities. Rates of gonorrhea and syphilis remain higher in the United States than in any other Western industrialized country. The remarkable resurgence of gonorrhea and syphilis among homosexual and bisexual men

TABLE 28-1

SEXUALLY TRANSMITTED AND SEXUALLY TRANSMISSIBLE MICROORGANISMS

BACTERIA	VIRUSES	OTHER[a]
Transmitted in Adults Predominantly by Sexual Intercourse		
Neisseria gonorrhoeae	HIV (types 1 and 2)	*Trichomonas vaginalis*
Chlamydia trachomatis	Human T-cell lymphotropic virus type I	*Phthirus pubis*
Treponema pallidum	Herpes simplex virus type 2	
Haemophilus ducreyi	Human papillomavirus (multiple genotypes)	
Calymmatobacterium granulomatis	Hepatitis B virus[b]	
Ureaplasma urealyticum	Molluscum contagiosum virus	
Sexual Transmission Repeatedly Described but Not Well Defined or Not the Predominant Mode		
Mycoplasma hominis	Cytomegalovirus	*Candida albicans*
Mycoplasma genitalium	Human T-cell lymphotropic virus type II	*Sarcoptes scabiei*
Gardnerella vaginalis and other vaginal bacteria	(?) Hepatitis C, D viruses	
	Herpes simplex virus type 1	
Group B *Streptococcus*	(?) Epstein-Barr virus	
Mobiluncus spp.	Human herpesvirus type 8	
Helicobacter cinaedi		
Helicobacter fennelliae		
Transmitted by Sexual Contact Involving Oral-Fecal Exposure; of Declining Importance in Homosexual Men		
Shigella spp.	Hepatitis A virus	*Giardia lamblia*
Campylobacter spp.		*Entamoeba histolytica*

[a]Includes protozoa, ectoparasites, and fungi.
[b]Among U.S. patients for whom a risk factor can be ascertained, most hepatitis B virus infections are transmitted sexually or by injection drug use.

in many parts of the United States and Europe since the 1990s reflects increased risk-taking after the advent of potent antiretroviral therapy and has been accompanied by increasing HIV transmission in this group.

In the United States, the Centers for Disease Control and Prevention (CDC) has compiled reported rates of STIs since 1941. The incidence of reported gonorrhea peaked at 468 cases per 100,000 population in the mid-1970s, fell to a low of 112 cases per 100,000 in 2004, and rose slightly in 2005. Because of increased testing and more sensitive tests, the incidence of reported *Chlamydia trachomatis* infection has been increasing steadily since reporting began in 1984, reaching 333 cases per 100,000 in 2005. The incidence of primary and secondary syphilis per 100,000 peaked at 71 cases in 1946, fell rapidly to 3.9 cases in 1956, ranged from ~10 to 15 cases through 1987 (with markedly increased rates among homosexual men and African Americans), and then fell to a nadir of 2.1 cases in 2000–2001 (with rates falling most rapidly among heterosexual African Americans). Unfortunately, since 1996, with the introduction of highly active antiretroviral therapy and the increased use of "serosorting" (i.e., the avoidance by some homosexual men of unprotected sex with HIV-serodiscordant partners but not with HIV-seroconcordant partners, a strategy that provides no protection against STIs other than HIV infection), gonorrhea, syphilis, and chlamydial infection have had a remarkable resurgence among homosexual men in North America and Europe, and an outbreak of a rare type of chlamydial infection (lymphogranuloma venereum; LGV) that had virtually disappeared during the AIDS era has occurred.

MANAGEMENT OF COMMON SEXUALLY TRANSMITTED DISEASE (STD) SYNDROMES

Although other chapters discuss management of specific STIs, delineating treatment based on diagnosis of a specific infection, most patients are actually managed (at least initially) on the basis of presenting symptoms and signs and associated risk factors, even in industrialized countries. Table 28-2 lists some of the most common clinical STD syndromes and their microbial etiologies. Strategies for their management are outlined below. Chapters 89 and 90 address the management of infections with human retroviruses.

STD care and management begin with risk assessment and proceed to clinical assessment, diagnostic testing or screening, treatment, and prevention. Indeed, the routine care of any patient begins with risk assessment (e.g., for risk of heart disease, cancer). STD/HIV risk assessment is important in primary care, urgent care, and emergency care settings as well as in specialty clinics providing adolescent, prenatal, and family planning services. STD/HIV risk assessment guides interpretation of symptoms that could reflect an STD, decisions on screening or prophylactic/preventive treatment, risk reduction counseling and intervention (e.g., hepatitis B vaccination), and notification of partners of patients with known infections. Consideration of routine demographic data (e.g., gender, age, marital status, area of residence) is a simple first step in STD/HIV risk assessment. For example, national guidelines now

TABLE 28-2

MAJOR STD SYNDROMES AND SEXUALLY TRANSMITTED MICROBIAL ETIOLOGIES

SYNDROME	ST MICROBIAL ETIOLOGIES
AIDS	HIV types 1 and 2
Urethritis: males	*Neisseria gonorrhoeae*, *Chlamydia trachomatis*, *Mycoplasma genitalium*, *Ureaplasma urealyticum* (?subspecies *urealyticum)*, *Trichomonas vaginalis*, HSV
Epididymitis	*C. trachomatis*, *N. gonorrhoeae*
Lower genital tract infections: females	
Cystitis/urethritis	*C. trachomatis*, *N. gonorrhoeae*, HSV
Mucopurulent cervicitis	*C. trachomatis*, *N. gonorrhoeae*, *M. genitalium*
Vulvitis	*Candida albicans*, HSV
Vulvovaginitis	*C. albicans*, *T. vaginalis*
Bacterial vaginosis (BV)	BV-associated bacteria (see text)
Acute pelvic inflammatory disease	*N. gonorrhoeae*, *C. trachomatis*, BV-associated bacteria, *M. genitalium,* group B streptococci
Infertility	*N. gonorrhoeae*, *C. trachomatis*, BV-associated bacteria
Ulcerative lesions of the genitalia	HSV-1, HSV-2, *Treponema pallidum*, *Haemophilus ducreyi*, *C. trachomatis* (LGV strains), *Calymmatobacterium granulomatis*
Complications of pregnancy/puerperium	Several agents implicated
Intestinal infections	
Proctitis	*C. trachomatis*, *N. gonorrhoeae*, HSV, *T. pallidum*
Proctocolitis or enterocolitis	*Campylobacter* spp., *Shigella* spp., *Entamoeba histolytica*, other enteric pathogens
Enteritis	*Giardia lamblia*
Acute arthritis with urogenital infection or viremia	*N. gonorrhoeae* (e.g., DGI), *C. trachomatis* (e.g., Reiter's syndrome), HBV
Genital and anal warts	HPV (30 genital types)
Mononucleosis syndrome	CMV, HIV, EBV
Hepatitis	Hepatitis viruses, *T. pallidum*, CMV, EBV
Neoplasias	
Squamous cell dysplasias and cancers of the cervix, anus, vulva, vagina, or penis	HPV (especially types 16, 18, 31, 45)
Kaposi's sarcoma, body-cavity lymphomas	HHV-8
T-cell leukemia	HTLV-I
Hepatocellular carcinoma	HBV
Tropical spastic paraparesis	HTLV-I
Scabies	*Sarcoptes scabiei*
Pubic lice	*Phthirus pubis*

Note: HSV, herpes simplex virus; LGV, lymphogranuloma venereum; DGI, disseminated gonococcal infection; HPV, human papillomavirus; CMV, cytomegalovirus; EBV, Epstein-Barr virus; HBV, hepatitis B virus; HTLV, human T-cell lymphotropic virus; HHV-8, human herpesvirus type 8.

recommend routine screening of sexually active females ≤25 years of age for *C. trachomatis* infection. Table 28-3 provides a set of 10 STD/HIV risk-assessment questions that clinicians can pose verbally or that health care systems can adapt (with yes/no responses) into a routine self-administered questionnaire for use in clinics. The initial framing statement gives permission to discuss taboo topics.

Risk assessment is followed by clinical assessment (elicitation of information on specific current symptoms and signs of STDs). Confirmatory diagnostic tests (for persons with symptoms or signs) or screening tests (for those without symptoms or signs) may involve microscopic examination, culture, antigen detection tests, genetic probe or amplification tests, or serology. Initial syndrome-based treatment should cover the most likely causes. For certain syndromes, results of rapid tests can narrow the spectrum of this initial therapy (e.g., wet mount of vaginal fluid for women with vaginal discharge, Gram's stain of urethral discharge for men with urethral discharge, rapid plasma reagin test for genital ulcer). After the institution of treatment, STD management proceeds to the "4 C's" of prevention and control: *c*ontact tracing (see "Prevention and Control of STIs" later in the chapter), ensuring *c*ompliance with therapy, and *c*ounseling on risk reduction, including *c*ondom promotion and provision.

TABLE 28-3

TEN-QUESTION STD/HIV RISK ASSESSMENT

Framing Statement:
In order to provide the best care for you today and to understand your risk for certain infections, it is necessary for us to talk about your sexual behavior.

Screening Questions:
(1) Do you have any reason to think you might have a sexually transmitted disease? If so, what reason?
(2) For all adolescents <18 years old: Have you begun having any kind of sex yet?

STD History:
(3) Have you ever had any sexually transmitted diseases or any genital infections? If so, which ones?

Sexual Preference:
(4) Have you had sex with men, women, or both?

Injection Drug Use:
(5) Have you ever injected yourself ("shot up") with drugs? (If yes, have you ever shared needles or injection equipment?)
(6) Have you ever had sex with a gay or bisexual man or with anyone who had ever injected drugs?

Characteristics of Partner(s):
(7) Has your sex partner(s) had any sexually transmitted infections? If so, which ones?

STD Symptoms Checklist:
(8) Have you recently developed any of these symptoms?

For Men	For Women
(a) Discharge of pus (drip) from the penis	(a) Abnormal vaginal discharge (increased amount, abnormal odor, abnormal yellow color)
(b) Genital sores (ulcers) or rash	(b) Genital sores (ulcers), rash, or itching

Sexual Practices, Past 2 Months (for patients answering yes to any of the above questions, to guide examination and testing):
(9) Now I'd like to ask what parts of your body may have been sexually exposed to an STD (e.g., your penis, mouth, vagina, anus)?

Query About Interest in STD Screening Tests (for patients answering no to all of the above questions):
(10) Would you like to be tested for HIV or any other STDs today? (If yes, clinician can explore which STD and why.)

Source: Adapted from JR Curtis, KK Holmes, in KK Holmes et al (eds): *Sexually Transmitted Diseases*, 3d ed. New York, McGraw-Hill, 1999.

URETHRITIS IN MEN

Urethritis in men produces urethral discharge, dysuria, or both, usually without frequency of urination. Causes include *Neisseria gonorrhoeae, C. trachomatis, Mycoplasma genitalium, Ureaplasma urealyticum, Trichomonas vaginalis,* HSV, and perhaps adenovirus.

Until recently, *C. trachomatis* caused ~30–40% of cases of nongonococcal urethritis (NGU); however, the proportion of cases due to this organism may have declined in some populations served by effective chlamydial-control programs, and older men with urethritis appear less likely to have chlamydial infection. HSV and *T. vaginalis* each cause a small proportion of NGU cases in the United States. Recently, multiple studies have consistently implicated *M. genitalium* as a probable cause of many *Chlamydia*-negative cases. Fewer studies than in the past have implicated *Ureaplasma*; the ureaplasmas have been differentiated into *U. urealyticum* and *U. parvum*, and a few studies suggest that *U. urealyticum*—but not *U. parvum*—is associated with NGU. Coliform bacteria can cause urethritis in men who practice insertive anal intercourse. The initial diagnosis of urethritis in men currently includes specific tests only for *N. gonorrhoeae* and *C. trachomatis*. The following summarizes the approach to the patient with suspected urethritis:

1. *Establish the presence of urethritis.* If proximal-to-distal "milking" of the urethra does not express a purulent or mucopurulent discharge, even after the patient has not voided for several hours (or preferably overnight), a Gram's-stained smear of overt discharge or of an anterior urethral specimen obtained by passage of a small urethrogenital swab 2–3 cm into the urethra usually reveals ≥5 neutrophils per 1000 × field in areas containing cells; in gonococcal infection, such a smear usually reveals gram-negative intracellular diplococci as well. Alternatively, the centrifuged sediment of the first 20–30 mL of voided urine—ideally collected as the first morning specimen—can be examined for inflammatory cells, either by microscopy showing ≥10 leukocytes per high-power field or by the leukocyte esterase test. Patients with symptoms who lack objective evidence of urethritis may have functional rather than organic problems and generally do not benefit from repeated courses of antibiotics.
2. *Evaluate for complications or alternative diagnoses.* A brief history and examination will exclude epididymitis and systemic complications, such as disseminated gonococcal infection (DGI) and Reiter's syndrome. Although digital examination of the prostate gland seldom contributes to the evaluation of sexually active young men with urethritis, men with dysuria who lack evidence of urethritis as well as sexually inactive men with urethritis should undergo prostate palpation, urinalysis, and urine culture to exclude bacterial prostatitis and cystitis.
3. *Evaluate for gonococcal and chlamydial infection.* An absence of typical gram-negative diplococci on Gram's-stained smear of urethral exudate containing inflammatory cells warrants a preliminary diagnosis of NGU and should lead to testing of the urethral specimen for *C. trachomatis*. However, an increasing proportion of men with symptoms and/or signs of urethritis are simultaneously assessed for infection with *N. gonorrhoeae* and *C. trachomatis* by "multiplex" nucleic acid amplification tests (NAATs) of early-morning first-voided urine. Culture or NAAT for *N. gonorrhoeae* may be positive when Gram's staining is negative; certain strains of *N. gonorrhoeae* can result in negative urethral Gram's stains in up to 30% of cases of urethritis. Results of tests for gonococcal and chlamydial infection predict the patient's prognosis (with greater risk for recurrent

TABLE 28-4

MANAGEMENT OF URETHRAL DISCHARGE IN MEN

Usual causes	Usual initial evaluation
Chlamydia trachomatis	Demonstration of urethral discharge or pyuria
Neisseria gonorrhoeae	Exclusion of local or systemic complications
Mycoplasma genitalium	Urethral Gram's stain to confirm urethritis, detect gram-negative diplococci
Ureaplasma urealyticum	Test for *N. gonorrhoeae*, *C. trachomatis*
Trichomonas vaginalis	
Herpes simplex virus	

Initial Treatment for Patient and Partners

Treat gonorrhea (unless excluded):	plus	Treat chlamydial infection:
Ceftriaxone, 125 mg IM; *or* Cefpodoxime, 400 mg PO; *or* Cefixime, 400 mg PO[a]		Azithromycin, 1 g PO; *or* Doxycycline, 100 mg bid for 7 days

Management of Recurrence

Confirm objective evidence of urethritis. If patient was reexposed to untreated or new partner, repeat treatment of patient and partner.

If patient was not reexposed, consider infection with *T. vaginalis*[b] or doxycycline-resistant *M. genitalium* or *Ureaplasma*, and consider treatment with metronidazole, azithromycin, or both.

[a]Updates on the availability of cefixime can be obtained from the Centers for Disease Control and Prevention or state health departments.
[b]In men, the diagnosis of *T. vaginalis* infection requires culture (or nucleic acid amplification test, where available) of early-morning first-voided urine sediment or of a urethral swab specimen obtained before voiding.

NGU if neither chlamydiae nor gonococci are found than if either is detected) and can guide both the counseling given to the patient and the management of the patient's sexual partner(s).

4. *Treat urethritis promptly, while test results are pending.*

Table 28-4 summarizes the steps in management of sexually active men with urethral discharge and/or dysuria.

℞ Treatment: URETHRITIS IN MEN

In practice, if Gram's stain does not reveal gonococci, urethritis is treated with a regimen effective for NGU, such as azithromycin (1.0 g PO in a single dose) or doxycycline (100 mg PO bid for 7 days). Both are effective, although azithromycin may give better results in *M. genitalium* infection. If gonococci are demonstrated by Gram's stain or if no diagnostic tests are performed to exclude gonorrhea definitively, treatment should include a single-dose regimen for gonorrhea (Chap. 45) plus azithromycin or doxycycline treatment for *C. trachomatis*, which frequently occurs as a urethral co-infection in men with gonococcal urethritis. Sexual partners should be tested for gonorrhea and chlamydial infection and should receive the same regimen given to the male index case. Patients with confirmed persistence or recurrence of urethritis after treatment should be re-treated with the initial regimen if they did not comply with the original treatment or were reexposed to an untreated partner. Otherwise, an intraurethral swab specimen and a first-voided urine sample should be tested for *T. vaginalis* (currently best done by culture, although NAATs appear to be more sensitive and are likely to become commercially available in the future). If compliance with initial treatment is confirmed and reexposure excluded, the recommended treatment is with metronidazole or tinidazole (2 g PO in a single dose) plus azithromycin (1 g PO in a single dose); the azithromycin component is especially important if this drug has not been given during initial therapy.

EPIDIDYMITIS

Acute epididymitis, almost always unilateral, produces pain, swelling, and tenderness of the epididymis, with or without symptoms or signs of urethritis. This condition must be differentiated from testicular torsion, tumor, and trauma. Torsion, a surgical emergency, usually occurs in the second or third decade of life and produces a sudden onset of pain, elevation of the testicle within the scrotal sac, rotation of the epididymis from a posterior to an anterior position, and absence of blood flow on Doppler examination or ^{99m}Tc scan. Persistence of symptoms after a course of therapy for epididymitis suggests the possibility of testicular tumor or of a chronic granulomatous disease, such as tuberculosis. In sexually active men under age 35, acute epididymitis is caused most frequently by *C. trachomatis* and less commonly by *N. gonorrhoeae* and is usually associated with overt or subclinical urethritis. Acute epididymitis occurring in older men or after urinary tract instrumentation is usually caused by urinary pathogens. Similarly, epididymitis in men who have practiced insertive rectal intercourse is often caused by Enterobacteriaceae. These men usually have no urethritis but do have bacteriuria.

℞ Treatment: EPIDIDYMITIS

Ceftriaxone (250 mg as a single dose IM) followed by doxycycline (100 mg PO twice daily for 10 days) constitutes effective treatment for epididymitis caused by *N. gonorrhoeae* or *C. trachomatis.* Fluoroquinolones are no longer recommended for treatment of gonorrhea in the United States because of the emergence of resistant strains of *N. gonorrhoeae,* especially (but not only) among homosexual men (Fig. 28-1). Levofloxacin (500 mg PO once daily for 10 days) is also effective for syndrome-based initial treatment of epididymitis when infection with Enterobacteriaceae is suspected; however, this regimen should probably be combined with effective therapy for possible gonococcal or chlamydial infection unless bacteriuria with Enterobacteriaceae is confirmed.

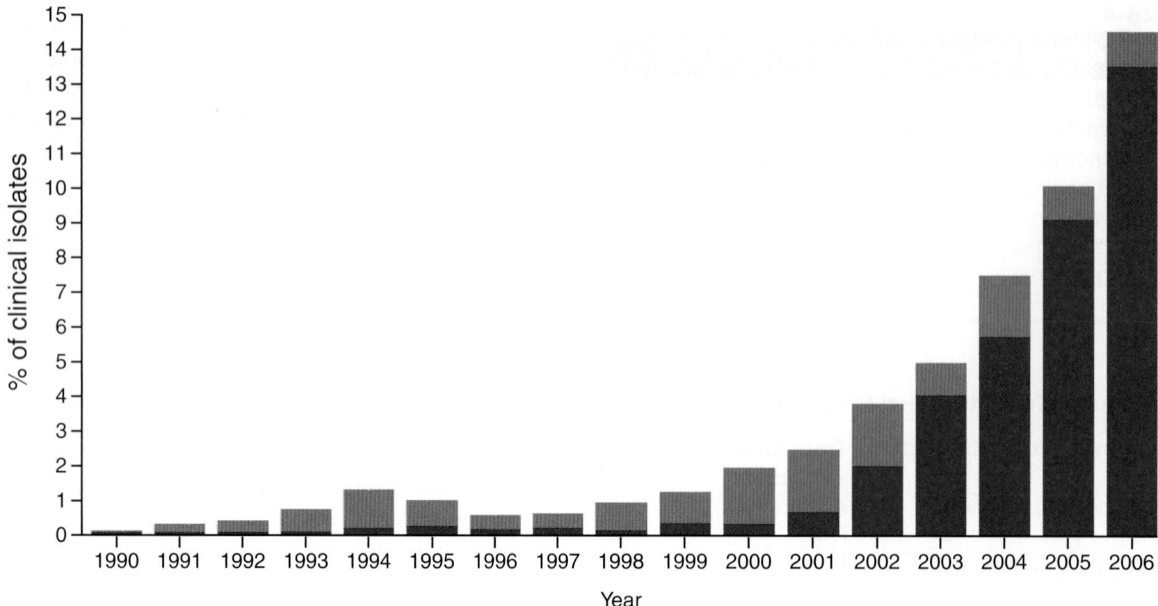

FIGURE 28-1

Percentage of *N. gonorrhoeae* isolates with intermediate resistance or resistance to ciprofloxacin, by year: Gonococcal Isolate Surveillance Project, United States, 1990–2006. Data for 2006 are preliminary (January–June only). ■ Intermediate resistance [ciprofloxacin minimum inhibitory concentrations (MICs) of 0.125–0.500 μg/mL]. ■ Resistance (ciprofloxacin MICs of ≥1.0 μg/mL). (*From Centers for Disease Control and Prevention: MMWR 56:332, 2007.*)

URETHRITIS AND THE URETHRAL SYNDROME IN WOMEN

C. trachomatis, *N. gonorrhoeae*, and occasionally HSV cause symptomatic urethritis—known as the urethral syndrome in women—that is characterized by "internal" dysuria (usually without urinary urgency or frequency), pyuria, and an absence of *Escherichia coli* and other uropathogens in urine at counts of $\geq 10^2$/mL. In contrast, the dysuria associated with vulvar herpes or vulvovaginal candidiasis (and perhaps with trichomoniasis) is often described as "external," being caused by painful contact of urine with the inflamed or ulcerated labia or introitus. Acute onset, association with urinary urgency or frequency, hematuria, or suprapubic bladder tenderness suggests bacterial cystitis. Among women with symptoms of acute bacterial cystitis, costovertebral pain and tenderness or fever suggests acute pyelonephritis. The management of bacterial urinary tract infection (UTI) is discussed in Chap. 27.

Signs of vulvovaginitis, coupled with symptoms of external dysuria, suggest vulvar infection (e.g., with HSV or *Candida albicans*). Among dysuric women without signs of vulvovaginitis, bacterial UTI must be differentiated from the urethral syndrome by assessment of risk, evaluation of the pattern of symptoms and signs, and specific microbiologic testing. An STI etiology of the urethral syndrome is suggested by young age, more than one current sexual partner, a new partner within the past month, a partner with urethritis, or coexisting mucopurulent cervicitis (see below). The finding of a single urinary pathogen, such as *E. coli* or *Staphylococcus saprophyticus*, at a concentration of $\geq 10^2$/mL in a properly collected specimen of midstream urine from a dysuric woman with pyuria indicates probable bacterial UTI, whereas pyuria with $<10^2$ conventional uropathogens per milliliter of urine ("sterile" pyuria) suggests acute urethral syndrome due to *C. trachomatis* or *N. gonorrhoeae*. Gonorrhea and chlamydial infection should be sought by specific tests (e.g., NAATs on the first 10 mL of voided urine). Among dysuric women with sterile pyuria caused by infection with *N. gonorrhoeae* or *C. trachomatis*, appropriate treatment alleviates dysuria.

VULVOVAGINAL INFECTIONS

Abnormal Vaginal Discharge

If directly questioned about vaginal discharge during routine health checkups, many women acknowledge having nonspecific symptoms of vaginal discharge that do not correlate with objective signs of inflammation or with actual infection. However, unsolicited reporting of abnormal vaginal discharge does suggest bacterial vaginosis or trichomoniasis. Specifically, an abnormally increased amount or an abnormal odor of the discharge is associated with one or both of these conditions. Cervical infection with *N. gonorrhoeae* or *C. trachomatis* does not appear to cause an increased amount or abnormal odor of discharge, but cervicitis, like trichomoniasis, can include the production of an increased number of neutrophils in vaginal fluid, resulting in a yellow color. Vulvar conditions such as genital herpes or vulvovaginal candidiasis can cause vulvar pruritus, burning, irritation, or lesions as well as external dysuria (as urine passes over the inflamed vulva) or vulvar dyspareunia.

Certain vulvovaginal infections may have serious sequelae. Trichomoniasis, bacterial vaginosis, and vulvovaginal candidiasis have all been associated with increased risk of acquisition of HIV infection. Vaginal trichomoniasis and bacterial vaginosis early in pregnancy independently predict premature onset of labor. Bacterial vaginosis can also lead to anaerobic bacterial infection of the endometrium and salpinges. Vaginitis may be an early and prominent feature of toxic shock syndrome, and recurrent or chronic vulvovaginal candidiasis develops with increased frequency among women with systemic illnesses, such as diabetes mellitus or HIV-related immunosuppression (although only a very small proportion of women with recurrent vulvovaginal candidiasis in industrialized countries actually have a serious predisposing illness).

Thus vulvovaginal symptoms or signs warrant careful evaluation, including pelvic examination, simple rapid diagnostic tests, and appropriate therapy specific for the anatomic site and type of infection. Unfortunately, a survey in the United States indicated that clinicians seldom perform the tests required to establish the cause of such symptoms. Further, comparison of telephone and office management of vulvovaginal symptoms has documented the inaccuracy of the former, and comparison of evaluations by nurse-midwives with those by physician-practitioners showed that the practitioners' clinical evaluations correlated poorly both with the nurses' evaluations and with diagnostic tests. The diagnosis and treatment of the three most common types of vaginal infection are summarized in Table 28-5.

Inspection of the vulva and perineum may reveal tender genital ulcerations (typically due to HSV infection, occasionally due to chancroid) or fissures (typically due to vulvovaginal candidiasis) or discharge visible at the introitus before insertion of a speculum (suggestive of bacterial vaginosis or trichomoniasis). Speculum examination permits the clinician to discern whether the discharge in fact looks abnormal and whether any abnormal discharge in the vagina emanates from the cervical os (mucoid and, if abnormal, yellow) or from the vagina (not mucoid, since the vaginal epithelium does not produce mucus). Symptoms or signs of abnormal vaginal discharge should prompt testing of vaginal fluid for pH, for a fishy odor when mixed with 10% KOH, and for certain microscopic features when mixed with saline (motile trichomonads and/or "clue cells") and with 10% KOH (pseudohyphae or hyphae indicative of vulvovaginal candidiasis). Additional objective laboratory tests useful for establishing the cause of abnormal vaginal discharge include Gram's staining to detect alterations in the vaginal flora; card tests for bacterial vaginosis, as described below; and a DNA probe test (the Affirm test) to detect *T. vaginalis* and *C. albicans* as well as the increased concentrations of *Gardnerella vaginalis* associated with bacterial vaginosis.

℞ Treatment: VAGINAL DISCHARGE

Patterns of treatment for vaginal discharge vary widely. In developing countries, where clinics or pharmacies often dispense treatment based on symptoms alone without examination or testing, oral treatment with metronidazole—either as a 2-g single dose or as a 7-day regimen—provides reasonable coverage against both trichomoniasis and bacterial vaginosis, the usual causes of symptoms of vaginal discharge; metronidazole treatment of sex partners prevents reinfection of women with trichomoniasis, even though it does not help prevent the recurrence of bacterial vaginosis. Guidelines promulgated during the 1990s by the World Health Organization suggested treatment for cervical infection and for vulvovaginal candidiasis in women with symptoms of abnormal vaginal discharge; in retrospect, these recommendations were faulty, since these conditions seldom produce such symptoms.

In industrialized countries, clinicians treating symptoms and signs of abnormal vaginal discharge should at least differentiate between bacterial vaginosis and trichomoniasis, because optimal management of patients and partners differs for these two conditions (as discussed briefly below).

Vaginal Trichomoniasis

(See also Chap. 122) Symptomatic trichomoniasis characteristically produces a profuse, yellow, purulent, homogeneous vaginal discharge and vulvar irritation, often with visible inflammation of the vaginal and vulvar epithelium and petechial lesions on the cervix (the so-called strawberry cervix, usually evident only by colposcopy). The pH of vaginal fluid usually rises to ≥5.0. In women with typical symptoms and signs of trichomoniasis, microscopic examination of vaginal discharge mixed with saline reveals motile trichomonads in most culture-positive cases. However, in the absence of symptoms or signs, culture is often required for detection of the organism. NAAT for *T. vaginalis* is as sensitive as or more sensitive than culture, and NAAT of urine has disclosed surprisingly high prevalences of this pathogen among men at several STD clinics in the United States. Treatment of asymptomatic as well as symptomatic cases reduces rates of transmission and prevents later development of symptoms.

℞ Treatment: VAGINAL TRICHOMONIASIS

Only nitroimidazoles (e.g., metronidazole and tinidazole) consistently cure trichomoniasis. A single 2-g oral dose of metronidazole is effective and much less expensive than the alternatives. Tinidazole has a longer half-life than metronidazole and is useful in treating trichomoniasis that fails to respond to metronidazole. Treatment of male sexual partners—often facilitated by dispensing metronidazole to the female patient to give to her partner(s), with a warning about avoiding the concurrent use of alcohol—significantly reduces both the risk of reinfection and the reservoir of infection; treating the partner is the standard of care. Treatment with 0.75% metronidazole gel intravaginally, although moderately effective for bacterial vaginosis, is not reliable for vaginal trichomoniasis. Systemic use of metronidazole is not recommended during the first trimester of pregnancy but is considered safe thereafter. In a large randomized trial,

TABLE 28-5

DIAGNOSTIC FEATURES AND MANAGEMENT OF VAGINAL INFECTION

FEATURE	NORMAL VAGINAL EXAMINATION	VULVOVAGINAL CANDIDIASIS	TRICHOMONAL VAGINITIS	BACTERIAL VAGINOSIS
Etiology	Uninfected; lactobacilli predominant	*Candida albicans*	*Trichomonas vaginalis*	Associated with *Gardnerella vaginalis*, various anaerobic and/or noncultured bacteria, and mycoplasmas
Typical symptoms	None	Vulvar itching and/or irritation	Profuse purulent discharge; vulvar itching	Malodorous, slightly increased discharge
Discharge				
Amount	Variable; usually scant	Scant	Often profuse	Moderate
Color[a]	Clear or slightly white	White	White or yellow	White or gray
Consistency	Nonhomogeneous, floccular	Clumped; adherent plaques	Homogeneous	Homogeneous, low viscosity; uniformly coats vaginal walls
Inflammation of vulvar or vaginal epithelium	None	Erythema of vaginal epithelium, introitus; vulvar dermatitis, fissures common	Erythema of vaginal and vulvar epithelium; colpitis macularis	None
pH of vaginal fluid[b]	Usually ≤4.5	Usually ≤4.5	Usually ≥5.0	Usually >4.5
Amine ("fishy") odor with 10% KOH	None	None	May be present	Present
Microscopy[c]	Normal epithelial cells; lactobacilli predominant	Leukocytes, epithelial cells; mycelia or pseudomycelia in up to 80% of *C. albicans* culture-positive persons with typical symptoms	Leukocytes; motile trichomonads seen in 80–90% of symptomatic patients, less often in the absence of symptoms	Clue cells; few leukocytes; no lactobacilli or only a few outnumbered by profuse mixed flora, nearly always including *G. vaginalis* plus anaerobic species on Gram's stain (Nugent's score ≥7)
Other laboratory findings		Isolation of *Candida* spp.	Isolation of *T. vaginalis* or positive NAAT[d]	
Usual treatment	None	Azole cream, tablet, or suppository—e.g., miconazole 100-mg vaginal suppository or clotrimazole 100-mg vaginal tablet, once daily for 7 days Fluconazole, 150 mg orally (single dose)	Metronidazole or tinidazole, 2 g orally (single dose) Metronidazole, 500 mg PO bid for 7 days	Metronidazole, 500 mg PO bid for 7 days Clindamycin, 2% cream, one full applicator vaginally each night for 7 days
Usual management of sexual partner	None	None; topical treatment if candidal dermatitis of penis is detected	Examination for STD; treatment with metronidazole, 2 g PO (single dose)	Examination for STD; no treatment if normal

[a]Color of discharge is best determined by examination against the white background of a swab.
[b]pH determination is not useful if blood is present.
[c]To detect fungal elements, vaginal fluid is digested with 10% KOH before microscopic examination; to examine for other features, fluid is mixed (1:1) with physiologic saline. Gram's stain is also excellent for detecting yeasts (less predictive of vulvovaginitis) and pseudomycelia or mycelia (strongly predictive of vulvovaginitis) and for distinguishing normal flora from the mixed flora seen in bacterial vaginosis, but it is less sensitive than the saline preparation for detection of *T. vaginalis*.
[d]NAAT, nucleic acid amplification test (where available).

metronidazole treatment of trichomoniasis during pregnancy did not reduce—and in fact actually increased—the frequency of perinatal morbidity.

Bacterial Vaginosis

This syndrome (formerly termed *nonspecific vaginitis, Haemophilus vaginitis, anaerobic vaginitis*, or *Gardnerella-associated vaginal discharge*) is characterized by symptoms of vaginal malodor and a slightly to moderately increased white discharge, which appears homogeneous, is low in viscosity, and evenly coats the vaginal mucosa. An interesting observation is that new genital HPV infection in young women is associated with increased subsequent risk of developing bacterial vaginosis. Other risk factors include multiple sexual partners and recent intercourse with a new partner, but metronidazole treatment of male partners has not reduced the rate of recurrence among affected women.

Among women with bacterial vaginosis, culture of vaginal fluid has shown markedly increased prevalences and concentrations of *G. vaginalis, Mycoplasma hominis*, and several anaerobic bacteria [e.g., *Mobiluncus* spp., *Prevotella* spp. (formerly *Bacteroides* spp.), and some *Peptostreptococcus* spp.] as well as an absence of hydrogen peroxide–producing *Lactobacillus* spp., which constitute most of the normal vaginal flora and perhaps help protect against certain cervical and vaginal infections. The use of broad-range polymerase chain reaction (PCR) amplification of 16S rDNA in vaginal fluid, with subsequent identification of specific bacterial species by various methods, has documented an even greater and unexpected bacterial diversity, including several unique species not previously cultivated [e.g., three species in the order Clostridiales that appear to be specific for bacterial vaginosis (Fig. 28-2)]. Also detected are DNA sequences related to *Atopobium vaginae*, an organism that is strongly associated with bacterial vaginosis, is resistant to metronidazole, and is associated with recurrent bacterial vaginosis after metronidazole treatment. Other species newly implicated in bacterial vaginosis include *Lactobacillus iners, Megasphaera, Leptotrichia, Eggerthella*, and *Dialister*.

Bacterial vaginosis is conventionally diagnosed clinically with the Amsel criteria, which include any three of the following four clinical abnormalities: (1) objective signs of increased white homogeneous vaginal discharge; (2) a vaginal discharge pH of >4.5; (3) liberation of a distinct fishy odor (attributable to volatile amines such as trimethylamine) immediately after vaginal secretions are mixed with a 10% solution of KOH; and (4) microscopic demonstration of "clue cells" (vaginal epithelial cells coated with coccobacillary organisms, which have a granular appearance and indistinct borders; Fig. 28-3) on a wet mount prepared by mixing vaginal secretions with normal saline in a ratio of ~1:1.

℞ Treatment: BACTERIAL VAGINOSIS

The standard dosage of metronidazole for the treatment of bacterial vaginosis is 500 mg PO twice daily for 7 days. The single 2-g oral dose of metronidazole recommended for trichomoniasis produces somewhat lower short-term cure rates. Intravaginal treatment with 2% clindamycin cream [one full applicator (5 g containing 100 mg of clindamycin phosphate) each night for 7 nights] or with 0.75% metronidazole gel [one full applicator (5 g containing 37.5 mg of metronidazole) twice daily for 5 days] is also approved for use in the

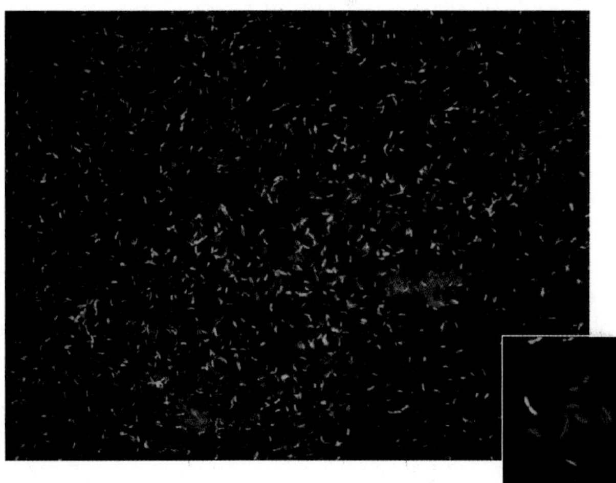

FIGURE 28-2
Broad-range PCR amplification of 16S rDNA in vaginal fluid from a woman with bacterial vaginosis shows a field of bacteria hybridizing with probes for bacterial vaginosis–associated bacterium 1 (BVAB1, visible as a thin, curved green rod) and for *Mobiluncus* (red). The inset shows that *Mobiluncus* (red) is larger than BVAB1 (green), but that the two have a similar morphology (curved rod). (*Reprinted with permission from DN Fredricks et al.*)

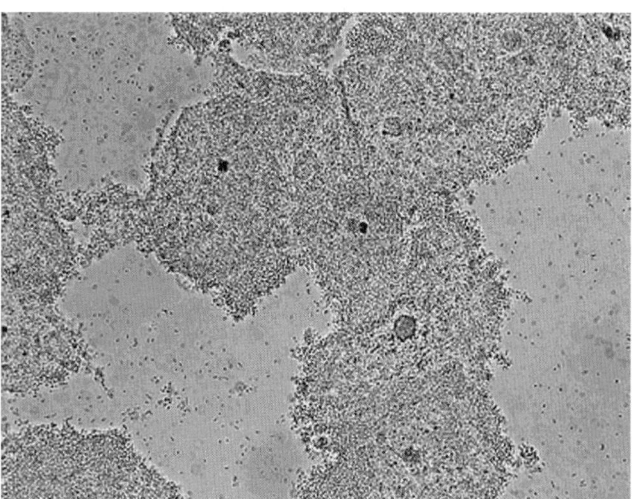

FIGURE 28-3
Wet mount of vaginal fluid showing typical clue cells from a woman with bacterial vaginosis. Note the obscured epithelial cell margins and the granular appearance attributable to many adherent bacteria (×400). [*Photograph provided by Lorna K. Rabe, reprinted with permission from S Hillier et al, in KK Holmes et al (eds). Sexually Transmitted Diseases, 4th ed. New York, McGraw-Hill, 2008.*]

United States and does not elicit systemic adverse reactions. Oral clindamycin (300 mg bid for 7 days) and clindamycin ovules (100 g intravaginally once at bedtime for 3 days) have also been approved. Unfortunately, long-term recurrence (i.e., several months later) is distressingly common after either oral or intravaginal treatment. A randomized trial comparing this intravaginal gel containing 37.5 mg of metronidazole with a suppository containing 500 mg of metronidazole plus nystatin (the latter not marketed in the United States) showed significantly higher rates of recurrent bacterial vaginosis with the 37.5-mg regimen; this result suggests that higher metronidazole dosages may be important in topical intravaginal therapy. Treatment of male partners with metronidazole does not prevent recurrence of bacterial vaginosis.

A randomized trial of orally ingested lactobacilli found reduced rates of recurrent bacterial vaginosis; however, this result has not yet been either confirmed or refuted. A randomized multicenter trial in the United States found no benefit of repeated intravaginal inoculation of a vaginal peroxide-producing *Lactobacillus* species after treatment of bacterial vaginosis with metronidazole. A meta-analysis of 18 studies concluded that bacterial vaginosis during pregnancy substantially increased the risk of preterm delivery and of spontaneous abortion. However, most studies of topical intravaginal treatment of bacterial vaginosis with clindamycin during pregnancy have not reduced adverse pregnancy outcomes. Numerous trials of oral metronidazole treatment during pregnancy have given inconsistent results, and a 2007 Cochrane review concluded that antenatal treatment of women with bacterial vaginosis—even those with previous preterm delivery—did not reduce the risk of preterm delivery.

Vulvovaginal Pruritus, Burning, or Irritation

Vulvovaginal candidiasis produces vulvar pruritus, burning, or irritation, generally without symptoms of increased vaginal discharge or malodor. Genital herpes can produce similar symptoms, with lesions sometimes difficult to distinguish from the fissures and inflammation caused by candidiasis. Signs of vulvovaginal candidiasis include vulvar erythema, edema, fissures, and tenderness. With candidiasis, a white scanty vaginal discharge sometimes takes the form of white thrush-like plaques or cottage cheese–like curds adhering loosely to the vaginal mucosa. *C. albicans* accounts for nearly all cases of symptomatic vulvovaginal candidiasis, which probably arise from endogenous strains of *C. albicans* that have colonized the vagina or the intestinal tract. Complicated vulvovaginal candidiasis includes cases that recur four or more times per year; are unusually severe; are caused by non-*albicans Candida* spp.; or occur in women with uncontrolled diabetes, debilitation, immunosuppression, or pregnancy.

The diagnosis of vulvovaginal candidiasis usually involves the demonstration of pseudohyphae or hyphae by microscopic examination of vaginal fluid mixed with saline or 10% KOH or subjected to Gram's staining. Microscopic examination is less sensitive than culture but correlates better with symptoms.

Treatment: ℞ VULVOVAGINAL PRURITUS, BURNING, OR IRRITATION

Symptoms and signs of vulvovaginal candidiasis warrant treatment, usually intravaginal administration of any of several imidazole antibiotics (e.g., miconazole or clotrimazole) for 3–7 days (Table 28-5). Over-the-counter marketing of such preparations has reduced the cost of care and made treatment more convenient for many women with recurrent yeast vulvovaginitis. However, most women who purchase these preparations do not have vulvovaginal candidiasis, whereas many do have other vaginal infections that require different treatment. Therefore, only women with classic symptoms of vulvar pruritus and a history of previous episodes of yeast vulvovaginitis documented by an experienced clinician should self-treat. Short-course topical intravaginal azole drugs are effective for the treatment of uncomplicated vulvovaginal candidiasis (e.g., clotrimazole, two 100-mg vaginal tablets daily for 3 days; or miconazole, a 1200-mg vaginal suppository as a single dose). Single-dose oral treatment with fluconazole (150 mg) is also effective and is preferred by many patients. Management of complicated cases (see above) and those that do not respond to the usual intravaginal or single-dose oral therapy often involves prolonged or periodic oral therapy; this situation is discussed extensively in the 2006 STD treatment guidelines published by the CDC. Treatment of sexual partners is not routinely indicated.

Other Causes of Vaginal Discharge or Vaginitis

In the ulcerative vaginitis associated with staphylococcal toxic shock syndrome, *Staphylococcus aureus* should be promptly identified in vaginal fluid by Gram's stain and by culture. In desquamative inflammatory vaginitis, smears of vaginal fluid reveal neutrophils, massive vaginal epithelial-cell exfoliation with increased numbers of parabasal cells, and gram-positive cocci; this syndrome may respond to treatment with 2% clindamycin cream. Additional causes of vaginitis and vulvovaginal symptoms include retained foreign bodies (e.g., tampons), cervical caps, vaginal spermicides, vaginal antiseptic preparations or douches, vaginal epithelial atrophy (in postmenopausal women or during prolonged breast-feeding in the postpartum period), allergic reactions to latex condoms, vaginal aphthae associated with HIV infection or Behçet's syndrome, and vestibulitis (a poorly understood syndrome).

MUCOPURULENT CERVICITIS

Mucopurulent cervicitis (MPC) refers to inflammation of the columnar epithelium and subepithelium of the endocervix and of any contiguous columnar epithelium that lies exposed in an ectopic position on the exocervix. MPC in women represents the "silent partner" of urethritis in men, being equally common and often caused by the same agents (*N. gonorrhoeae*, *C. trachomatis*, or—as shown by case-control studies—*M. genitalium*); however,

MPC is more difficult than urethritis to recognize. As the most common manifestation of these serious bacterial infections in women, MPC can be a harbinger or sign of upper genital tract infection, also known as *pelvic inflammatory disease* (PID; see below). In pregnant women, MPC can lead to obstetric complications. In a prospective study in Seattle of 167 consecutive patients with MPC [defined on the basis of yellow endocervical mucopus or ≥30 polymorphonuclear leukocytes (PMNs)/1000 × microscopic field] who were seen at STD clinics during the 1980s, slightly more than one-third of cervicovaginal specimens tested for *C. trachomatis*, *N. gonorrhoeae*, *M. genitalium*, HSV, and *T. vaginalis* revealed no identifiable etiology (Fig. 28-4).

The diagnosis of MPC rests on the detection of yellow mucopurulent discharge from the cervical os or of increased numbers of PMNs in Gram's-stained or Papanicolaou-stained smears of endocervical mucus. MPC due to *C. trachomatis* can also produce edematous cervical ectopy (see below) and endocervical bleeding upon gentle swabbing. Unlike the endocervicitis produced by gonococcal or chlamydial infection, cervicitis caused by HSV produces ulcerative lesions on the stratified squamous epithelium of the exocervix as well as on the columnar epithelium. Yellow cervical mucus on a white swab removed from the endocervix indicates the presence of PMNs. The mucus should be rolled thinly on a slide for Gram's staining. The presence of ≥20 PMNs/1000 × microscopic field within strands of cervical mucus not contaminated by vaginal squamous epithelial cells or vaginal bacteria indicates endocervicitis (Fig. 28-5). Detection of intracellular gram-negative diplococci in carefully collected endocervical mucus is quite specific but ≤50% sensitive for gonorrhea. Therefore, specific and sensitive tests for *N. gonorrhoeae* as well as for *C. trachomatis* (e.g., NAATs) are also indicated in the evaluation of MPC.

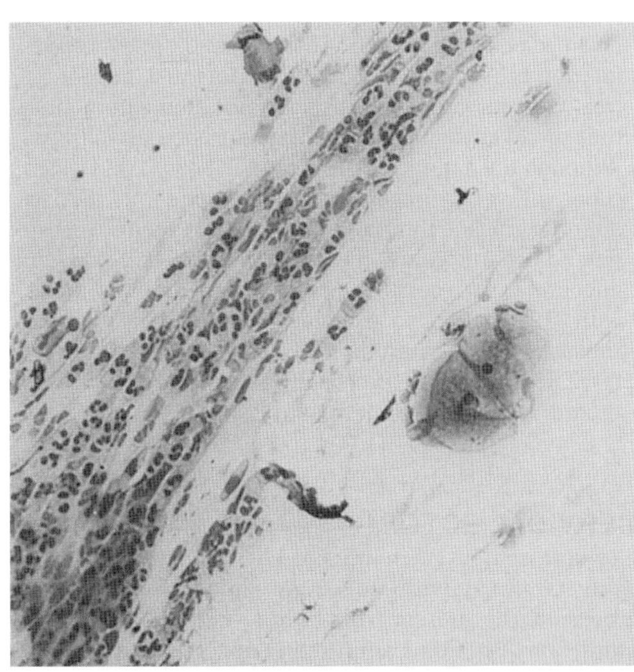

FIGURE 28-5
Gram's stain of cervical mucus, showing a strand of cervical mucus containing many polymorphonuclear leukocytes. This picture is typical of mucopurulent cervicitis. Note that leukocytes are not seen in areas of the slide containing vaginal epithelial cells, adjacent to the mucus strands.

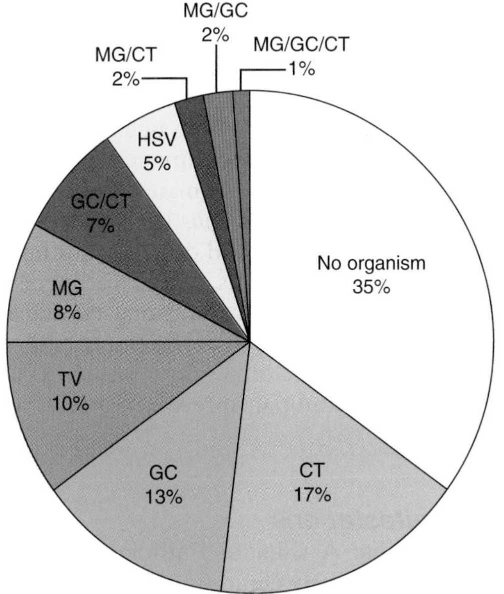

FIGURE 28-4
Organisms detected among female STD clinic patients with mucopurulent cervicitis (*n* = 167). GC, gonococcus; CT, *Chlamydia trachomatis*; MG, *Mycoplasma genitalium*; TV, *Trichomonas vaginalis*; HSV, herpes simplex virus. (*Courtesy of Dr. Lisa Manhart; with permission.*)

℞ Treatment: MUCOPURULENT CERVICITIS

Although the above criteria for MPC are neither highly specific nor highly predictive of gonococcal or chlamydial infection in some settings, the 2006 CDC guidelines call for consideration of empirical treatment for MPC, pending test results, in certain patients. Treatment with antibiotics active against *C. trachomatis* should be provided for women at increased risk for this common STI (risk factors: age <25 years, new or multiple sex partners, and unprotected sex), especially if follow-up cannot be ensured and if a relatively insensitive diagnostic test (not a NAAT) is used. Concurrent therapy for gonorrhea is indicated if the prevalence of this infection is high (>5%) in the relevant patient population (e.g., young adults, a clinic with documented high prevalence). In this situation, therapy should include a single-dose regimen effective for gonorrhea plus treatment for chlamydial infection, as outlined in Table 28-4 for the treatment of urethritis. In settings where gonorrhea is much less common than chlamydial infection, initial therapy for chlamydial infection alone suffices, pending test results for gonorrhea. The etiology and potential benefit of treatment for endocervicitis not associated with gonorrhea or chlamydial infection have not been established. Although the antimicrobial susceptibility of *M. genitalium* is not yet well defined, the organism frequently persists after doxycycline therapy, and it currently seems reasonable to use azithromycin to treat possible *M. genitalium* infection in such cases. The sexual partner(s) of a woman with MPC should be examined and given a regimen similar to that chosen for the woman unless results of tests for gonorrhea or chlamydial infection in either partner warrant different therapy or no therapy.

CERVICAL ECTOPY

Cervical ectopy, often mislabeled "cervical erosion," is easily confused with infectious endocervicitis. Ectopy represents the presence of the one-cell-thick columnar epithelium extending from the endocervix out onto the visible ectocervix. In ectopy, the cervical os may contain clear or slightly cloudy mucus but usually not yellow mucopus. Colposcopy shows intact epithelium. Normally found during adolescence and early adulthood, ectopy gradually recedes through the second and third decades of life, as squamous metaplasia replaces the ectopic columnar epithelium. Oral contraceptive use favors the persistence or reappearance of ectopy, while smoking apparently accelerates squamous metaplasia. Cauterization of ectopy is not warranted. Ectopy may render the cervix more susceptible to infection with *N. gonorrhoeae*, *C. trachomatis*, or HIV.

PELVIC INFLAMMATORY DISEASE

The term *pelvic inflammatory disease* usually refers to infection that ascends from the cervix or vagina to involve the endometrium and/or fallopian tubes. Infection can extend beyond the reproductive tract to cause pelvic peritonitis, generalized peritonitis, perihepatitis, perisplenitis, or pelvic abscess. Rarely in young women, infection not related to STI extends secondarily to the pelvic organs (1) from adjacent foci of inflammation (e.g., appendicitis, regional ileitis, or diverticulitis), (2) as a result of hematogenous dissemination (e.g., of tuberculosis), or (3) as a complication of certain tropical diseases (e.g., schistosomiasis). Intrauterine infection can be primary (spontaneously occurring and usually sexually transmitted) or secondary to invasive intrauterine surgical procedures [e.g., dilatation and curettage, termination of pregnancy, insertion of an intrauterine device (IUD), or hysterosalpingography] or to parturition.

Etiology

The agents most often implicated in acute PID include the primary causes of endocervicitis (e.g., *N. gonorrhoeae* and *C. trachomatis*) and organisms that can be regarded as components of an altered vaginal flora. In general, PID is most often caused by *N. gonorrhoeae* where there is a high incidence of gonorrhea—e.g., in developing countries and in indigent inner-city populations in the United States. In recent case-control studies, *M. genitalium* has also been significantly associated with histopathologic diagnoses of endometritis and with salpingitis.

Anaerobic and facultative organisms (especially *Prevotella* species, peptostreptococci, *E. coli*, *Haemophilus influenzae*, and group B streptococci) as well as genital mycoplasmas have been isolated from the peritoneal fluid or fallopian tubes in a varying proportion (typically one-fourth to one-third) of women with PID studied in the United States. The difficulty of determining the exact microbial etiology of an individual case of PID—short of using invasive procedures for specimen collection—has implications for the approach to empirical antimicrobial treatment of this infection.

Epidemiology

In the United States, the estimated annual number of initial visits to physicians' offices for PID by women 15–44 years of age fell from an average of 400,000 during the 1980s to 250,000 in 1999 and then to 176,000 in 2005. Hospitalizations for acute PID in the United States also declined steadily throughout the 1980s and early 1990s but have remained fairly constant at 70,000–100,000 per year since 1995. Important risk factors for acute PID include the presence of endocervical infection or bacterial vaginosis, a history of salpingitis or of recent vaginal douching, and the use of an IUD (especially among nulliparous women, during the first few months after IUD insertion, and among women with multiple sex partners). Certain other iatrogenic factors, such as dilatation and curettage or cesarean section, can increase the risk of PID, especially among women with endocervical gonococcal or chlamydial infection or bacterial vaginosis. Symptoms of *N. gonorrhoeae*–associated and *C. trachomatis*–associated PID often begin during or soon after the menstrual period; this timing suggests that menstruation is a risk factor for ascending infection from the cervix and vagina. Experimental inoculation of the fallopian tubes of lower primates has shown that repeated exposure to *C. trachomatis* leads to the greatest degree of tissue inflammation and damage; thus immunopathology probably contributes to the pathogenesis of chlamydial salpingitis. Women using oral contraceptives appear to be at decreased risk of symptomatic PID, and tubal sterilization reduces the risk of salpingitis by preventing intraluminal spread of infection into the tubes.

Clinical Manifestations

Endometritis: A Clinical Pathologic Syndrome

A study of women with clinically suspected PID who were undergoing both endometrial biopsy and laparoscopy showed that those with endometritis alone differed from those who also had salpingitis in significantly less often having lower quadrant, adnexal, or cervical motion or abdominal rebound tenderness; fever; or elevated C-reactive protein levels. In addition, women with endometritis alone differed from those with neither endometritis nor salpingitis in more often having gonorrhea, chlamydial infection, and risk factors such as douching or IUD use. Thus women with endometritis alone were intermediate between those with neither endometritis nor salpingitis and those with salpingitis with respect to risk factors, clinical manifestations, cervical infection prevalence, and elevated C-reactive protein level. Women with endometritis alone are at lower risk of subsequent tubal occlusion and resulting infertility than are those with salpingitis.

Salpingitis

Symptoms of nontuberculous salpingitis classically evolve from a yellow or malodorous vaginal discharge caused by MPC and/or bacterial vaginosis to midline abdominal pain and abnormal vaginal bleeding caused by endometritis and then to bilateral lower abdominal and pelvic pain caused by salpingitis, with nausea, vomiting, and increased abdominal tenderness if peritonitis develops.

The abdominal pain in nontuberculous salpingitis is usually described as dull or aching. In some cases, pain is lacking or atypical, but active inflammatory changes are found in the course of an unrelated evaluation or procedure, such as a laparoscopic evaluation for infertility. Abnormal uterine bleeding precedes or coincides with the onset of pain in ~40% of women with PID, symptoms of urethritis (dysuria) occur in 20%, and symptoms of proctitis (anorectal pain, tenesmus, and rectal discharge or bleeding) are occasionally seen in women with gonococcal or chlamydial infection.

Speculum examination shows evidence of MPC (yellow endocervical discharge, easily induced endocervical bleeding) in the majority of women with gonococcal or chlamydial PID. Cervical motion tenderness is produced by stretching of the adnexal attachments on the side toward which the cervix is pushed. Bimanual examination reveals uterine fundal tenderness due to endometritis and abnormal adnexal tenderness due to salpingitis that is usually, but not necessarily, bilateral. Adnexal swelling is palpable in about one-half of women with acute salpingitis, but evaluation of the adnexae in a patient with marked tenderness is not reliable. The initial temperature is >38°C in only about one-third of patients with acute salpingitis. Laboratory findings include elevation of the erythrocyte sedimentation rate (ESR) in 75% of patients with acute salpingitis and elevation of the peripheral white blood cell count in up to 60%.

Unlike nontuberculous salpingitis, genital tuberculosis often occurs in older women, many of whom are postmenopausal. Presenting symptoms include abnormal vaginal bleeding, pain (including dysmenorrhea), and infertility. About one-quarter of these women have had adnexal masses. Endometrial biopsy shows tuberculous granulomas and provides optimal specimens for culture.

Perihepatitis and Periappendicitis

Pleuritic upper abdominal pain and tenderness (usually localized to the right upper quadrant) develop in 3–10% of women with acute PID. Symptoms of perihepatitis arise during or after the onset of symptoms of PID and may overshadow lower abdominal symptoms, thereby leading to a mistaken diagnosis of cholecystitis. In perhaps 5% of cases of acute salpingitis, early laparoscopy reveals perihepatic inflammation ranging from edema and erythema of the liver capsule to exudate with fibrinous adhesions between the visceral and parietal peritoneum. When treatment is delayed and laparoscopy is performed late, dense "violin-string" adhesions can be seen over the liver; chronic exertional or positional right upper quadrant pain ensues when traction is placed on the adhesions. Although perihepatitis, also known as the *Fitz-Hugh–Curtis syndrome*, was for many years specifically attributed to gonococcal salpingitis, most cases are now attributed to chlamydial salpingitis. In patients with chlamydial salpingitis, serum titers of microimmunofluorescent antibody to *C. trachomatis* are typically much higher when perihepatitis is present than when it is absent.

Physical findings include right upper quadrant tenderness and usually include adnexal tenderness and cervicitis, even in patients whose symptoms do not suggest salpingitis. Results of liver function tests and right upper quadrant ultrasonography are nearly always normal. The presence of MPC and pelvic tenderness in a young woman with subacute pleuritic right upper quadrant pain and normal ultrasonography of the gallbladder points to a diagnosis of perihepatitis.

Periappendicitis (appendiceal serositis without involvement of the intestinal mucosa) has been found in ~5% of patients undergoing appendectomy for suspected appendicitis and can occur as a complication of gonococcal or chlamydial salpingitis.

Among women with salpingitis, HIV infection is associated with increased severity of salpingitis and with tuboovarian abscess requiring hospitalization and surgical drainage. Nonetheless, among women with HIV infection and salpingitis, the clinical response to conventional antimicrobial therapy (coupled with drainage of tuboovarian abscess, when found) has usually been satisfactory.

Diagnosis

Treatment appropriate for PID must not be withheld from patients who have an equivocal diagnosis; it is better to err on the side of overdiagnosis and overtreatment. On the other hand, it is essential to differentiate between salpingitis and other pelvic pathology, particularly surgical emergencies such as appendicitis and ectopic pregnancy.

Nothing short of laparoscopy definitively identifies salpingitis, but routine laparoscopy to confirm suspected salpingitis is generally impractical. Most patients with acute PID have lower abdominal pain of <3 weeks' duration, pelvic tenderness on bimanual pelvic examination, and evidence of lower genital tract infection (e.g., MPC). Approximately 60% of such patients have salpingitis at laparoscopy, and perhaps 10–20% have endometritis alone. Among the patients with these findings, a rectal temperature >38°C, a palpable adnexal mass, and elevation of the ESR to >15 mm/h also raise the probability of salpingitis, which has been found at laparoscopy in 68% of patients with one of these additional findings, 90% of patients with two, and 96% of patients with three. However, only 17% of all patients with laparoscopy-confirmed salpingitis have had all three additional findings.

In a woman with pelvic pain and tenderness, increased numbers of PMNs (30 per 1000 × microscopic field in strands of cervical mucus) or leukocytes outnumbering epithelial cells in vaginal fluid (in the absence of trichomonal vaginitis, which also produces PMNs in vaginal discharge) increase the predictive value of a clinical diagnosis of acute PID, as do onset with menses, history of recent abnormal menstrual bleeding, presence of an IUD, history of salpingitis, and sexual exposure to a male with urethritis. Appendicitis or another disorder of the gut is favored by the early onset of anorexia, nausea, or vomiting; the onset of pain later than day 14 of the menstrual cycle; or unilateral pain limited to the right or left lower quadrant. Whenever the diagnosis of PID is being considered, serum assays for human β-chorionic gonadotropin should be performed; these tests are usually positive with ectopic pregnancy. Ultrasonography and MRI can be useful for the identification of tuboovarian or pelvic abscess. MRI of the tubes can also show increased tubal diameter, intratubal fluid, or tubal wall thickening in cases of salpingitis.

The primary and uncontested value of laparoscopy in women with lower abdominal pain is for the exclusion of other surgical problems. Some of the most common or serious problems that may be confused with salpingitis (e.g., acute appendicitis, ectopic pregnancy, corpus luteum bleeding, ovarian tumor) are unilateral. Unilateral pain or pelvic mass, although not incompatible with PID, is a strong indication for laparoscopy unless the clinical picture warrants laparotomy instead. Atypical clinical findings, such as the absence of lower genital tract infection, a missed menstrual period, a positive pregnancy test, or failure to respond to appropriate therapy, are other common indications for laparoscopy. Endometrial biopsy is relatively sensitive and specific for the diagnosis of endometritis, which correlates well with the presence of salpingitis.

Endocervical swab specimens should be examined by Gram's staining for PMNs and gram-negative diplococci and by NAATs for *N. gonorrhoeae* and *C. trachomatis*. The clinical diagnosis of PID made by expert gynecologists is confirmed by laparoscopy or endometrial biopsy in ~90% of women who also have cultures positive for *N. gonorrhoeae* or *C. trachomatis*. Even among women with no symptoms suggestive of acute PID who were attending an STD clinic or a gynecology clinic in Pittsburgh, endometritis was significantly associated with endocervical gonorrhea or chlamydial infection or with bacterial vaginosis, being detected in 26%, 27%, and 15% of women with these conditions, respectively.

℞ Treatment: PELVIC INFLAMMATORY DISEASE

The 2006 CDC guidelines recommend initiation of empirical treatment for PID in sexually active young women and other women at risk for PID if they are experiencing pelvic or lower abdominal pain, if no other cause for the pain can be identified, and if pelvic examination reveals one or more of the following criteria for PID: cervical motion tenderness, uterine tenderness, or adnexal tenderness.

Women with suspected PID can be treated as either outpatients or inpatients. In the multicenter Pelvic Inflammatory Disease Evaluation and Clinical Health (PEACH) trial, 831 women with mild to moderately severe symptoms and signs of PID were randomized to receive either inpatient treatment with IV cefoxitin and doxycycline or outpatient treatment with a single IM dose of cefoxitin plus oral doxycycline. Short-term clinical and microbiologic outcomes and long-term outcomes were equivalent in the two groups. Nonetheless, hospitalization should be considered when (1) the diagnosis is uncertain and surgical emergencies such as appendicitis and ectopic pregnancy cannot be excluded, (2) the patient is pregnant, (3) pelvic abscess is suspected, (4) severe illness or nausea and vomiting preclude outpatient management, (5) the patient has HIV infection, (6) the patient is assessed as unable to follow or tolerate an outpatient regimen, or (7) the patient has failed to respond to outpatient therapy. Some experts also prefer to hospitalize adolescents with PID for initial therapy, although younger women do as well as older women on outpatient therapy.

Recommended combination regimens for ambulatory or parenteral management of PID are presented in Table 28-6. Women managed as outpatients should receive a combined regimen with broad activity, such as ceftriaxone to cover possible gonococcal infection followed by doxycycline to cover possible chlamydial infection. Metronidazole can be added, if tolerated, to enhance activity against anaerobes. Neither doxycycline nor the fluoroquinolones provide reliable coverage for gonococcal infection today. Although the 2006 CDC guidelines for ambulatory treatment of PID included the option of using an oral fluoroquinolone, with or without metronidazole, for 14 days, these guidelines are already outdated because of emerging gonococcal resistance to the fluoroquinolones. Although few methodologically sound clinical trials (especially with prolonged follow-up) have been conducted, one meta-analysis suggested a benefit of providing good coverage against anaerobes.

For hospitalized patients, the following two parenteral regimens have given nearly identical results in a multicenter randomized trial:

1. Doxycycline (100 mg twice daily, given IV or PO) plus cefotetan (2.0 g IV every 12 h) or cefoxitin (2.0 g IV every 6 h). Administration of these drugs should be continued by the IV route for at least 48 h after the patient's condition improves and then followed with oral doxycycline (100 mg twice daily) to complete 14 days of therapy.
2. Clindamycin (900 mg IV every 8 h) plus gentamicin (2.0 mg/kg IV or IM, followed by 1.5 mg/kg every 8 h) in patients with normal renal function. Once-daily

TABLE 28-6

COMBINATION ANTIMICROBIAL REGIMENS RECOMMENDED FOR OUTPATIENT TREATMENT OR FOR PARENTERAL TREATMENT OF PID

OUTPATIENT REGIMENS	PARENTERAL REGIMENS
Regimen A Ofloxacin 400 mg PO bid for 14 days *or* Levofloxacin 500 mg PO once daily for 14 days *plus*[a] Metronidazole 500 mg PO bid for 14 days **Regimen B** Ceftriaxone 250 mg IM once *plus* Doxycycline 100 mg PO bid for 14 days *plus*[a] Metronidazole 500 mg PO bid for 14 days	Initiate parenteral therapy with either of the following regimens; continue parenteral therapy until 48 h after clinical improvement; then change to outpatient therapy, as described in the text. **Regimen A** Cefotetan 2 g IV q12h *or* Cefoxitin 2 g IV q6h *plus* Doxycycline 100 mg IV or PO q12h **Regimen B** Clindamycin 900 mg IV q8h *plus* Gentamicin, loading dose of 2 mg/kg IV or IM, then maintenance dose of 1.5 mg/kg q8h

[a]The addition of metronidazole is recommended by some experts.
Source: Adapted from Centers for Disease Control and Prevention: MMWR Recomm Rep 55(RR-11):1, 2006.

dosing of gentamicin (with combination of the total daily dose into a single daily dose) has not been evaluated in PID but has been efficacious in other serious infections and could be substituted.

Treatment with these drugs should be continued for at least 48 h after the patient's condition improves and then followed with oral doxycycline (100 mg twice daily) or clindamycin (450 mg four times daily) to complete 14 days of therapy. In cases with tuboovarian abscess, clindamycin rather than doxycycline for continued therapy provides better coverage for anaerobic infection.

FOLLOW-UP Hospitalized patients should show substantial clinical improvement within 3–5 days. Women treated as outpatients should be clinically reevaluated within 72 h. A follow-up telephone survey of women seen in an emergency room and given a prescription for 10 days of oral doxycycline for PID found that 28% never filled the prescription and 41% stopped taking the medication early (after an average of 4.1 days), often because of persistent symptoms, lack of symptoms, or side effects. Women not responding favorably to ambulatory therapy should be hospitalized for parenteral therapy and further diagnostic evaluations, including a consideration of laparoscopy. Male sex partners should be evaluated and treated empirically for gonorrhea and chlamydial infection. After completion of treatment, tests for persistent or recurrent infection with *N. gonorrhoeae* or *C. trachomatis* should be performed if symptoms persist or recur or if the patient has not complied with therapy or has been reexposed to an untreated sex partner.

SURGERY Surgery is necessary for the treatment of salpingitis only in the face of life-threatening infection (such as rupture or threatened rupture of a tuboovarian abscess) or for drainage of an abscess. Conservative surgical procedures are usually sufficient. Pelvic abscesses can often be drained by posterior colpotomy, and peritoneal lavage can be used for generalized peritonitis.

Prognosis

Late sequelae include infertility due to bilateral tubal occlusion, ectopic pregnancy due to tubal scarring without occlusion, chronic pelvic pain, and recurrent salpingitis. The overall postsalpingitis risk of infertility due to tubal occlusion in a large study in Sweden was 11% after one episode of salpingitis, 23% after two episodes, and 54% after three or more episodes. A University of Washington study found a sevenfold increase in the risk of ectopic pregnancy and an eightfold increase in the rate of hysterectomy after PID.

Prevention

A randomized controlled trial designed to determine whether selective screening for chlamydial infection reduced the risk of subsequent PID showed that women randomized to undergo screening had a 56% lower rate of PID over the following year than did women receiving the usual care without screening. This report helped prompt U.S. national guidelines for risk-based chlamydial screening of young women to reduce the incidence of PID and the prevalence of post-PID sequelae, while also reducing sexual transmission of *C. trachomatis*.

ULCERATIVE GENITAL OR PERIANAL LESIONS

Genital ulceration reflects a set of important STIs, most of which sharply increase the risk of sexual acquisition and shedding of HIV. In a 1996 study of genital ulcers in 10 of the U.S. cities with the highest rates of primary syphilis, PCR testing of ulcer specimens demonstrated HSV in 62% of patients, *Treponema pallidum* in 13%, and *Haemophilus ducreyi* in 12–20%. Today, genital herpes probably represents an even higher proportion of genital ulcers in the United States and other industrialized countries.

In Asia and Africa, chancroid (Fig. 28-6) was once considered the most common type of genital ulcer, followed in frequency by primary syphilis and then genital herpes. With increased efforts to control chancroid and syphilis, together with more frequent recurrences or persistence of genital herpes attributable

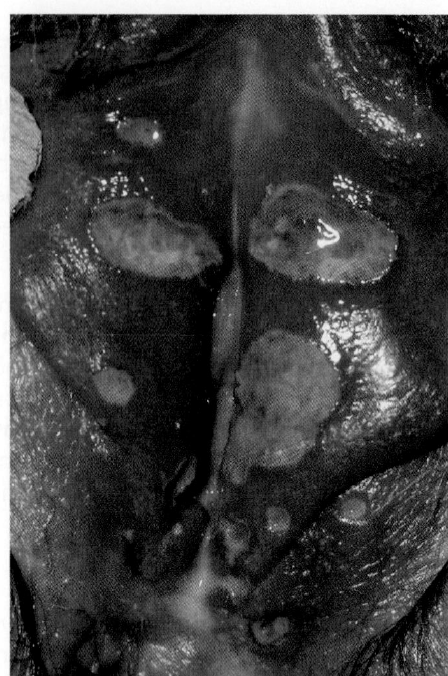

FIGURE 28-6
Chancroid: multiple, painful, punched-out ulcers with undermined borders on the labia occurring after autoinoculation.

to HIV infection, PCR testing of genital ulcers now clearly implicates genital herpes as the most common cause of genital ulceration in most developing countries. LGV (Fig. 28-7) and donovanosis (granuloma inguinale) continue to cause genital ulceration in developing countries. LGV virtually disappeared in industrialized countries during the first 20 years of the HIV pandemic, but outbreaks are again occurring in Europe (including the United Kingdom), in North America, and in Australia. In these outbreaks, LGV is usually causing anal and rectal disease in homosexual men, very often in association with HIV and/or hepatitis C virus infections. Other causes of genital ulcer include (1) candidiasis and traumatized genital warts—both readily recognized; (2) lesions due to genital involvement by more widespread dermatoses; and (3) cutaneous manifestations of systemic diseases, such as genital mucosal ulceration in Stevens-Johnson syndrome or Behçet's disease.

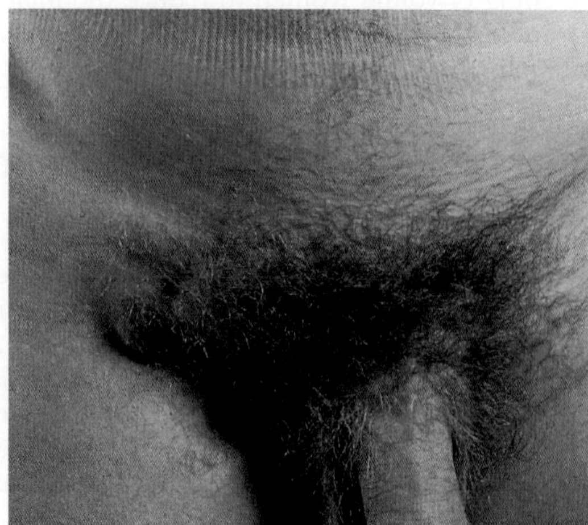

FIGURE 28-7
Lymphogranuloma venereum: striking tender lymphadenopathy occurring at the femoral and inguinal lymph nodes, separated by a groove made by Poupart's ligament. This "sign-of-the-groove" is not considered specific for LGV; for example, lymphomas may present with this sign.

Diagnosis

Although most genital ulcerations cannot be diagnosed confidently on clinical grounds alone, clinical findings plus epidemiologic considerations (Table 28-7) can usually guide initial management (Table 28-8) pending results of further tests. Clinicians should order a rapid serologic test for syphilis in all cases of genital ulcer and a dark-field or direct immunofluorescence test (or PCR test, where available) for *T. pallidum* in all lesions except those highly characteristic of infection with HSV (i.e., those with herpetic vesicles). All patients presenting with genital ulceration should be counseled and tested for HIV infection.

Typical vesicles or pustules or a cluster of painful ulcers preceded by vesiculopustular lesions suggests genital herpes. These typical clinical manifestations make detection of the virus optional; however, many patients want confirmation of the diagnosis, and differentiation of HSV-1 from HSV-2 has prognostic implications, since the latter causes more frequent genital recurrences.

Painless, nontender, indurated ulcers with firm, nontender inguinal adenopathy suggest primary syphilis. If dark-field examination and a rapid serologic test for syphilis are initially negative and the patient will comply with follow-up and sexual abstinence, the performance of two more dark-field examinations on successive days before treatment is begun will improve the sensitivity of the diagnosis of syphilis, and repeated serologic testing for syphilis 1 or 2 weeks after treatment of seronegative primary syphilis usually demonstrates seroconversion.

"Atypical" or clinically trivial ulcers may be more common manifestations of genital herpes than classic vesiculopustular lesions. Specific tests for HSV in such lesions are therefore indicated (Chap. 80). Type-specific serologic tests for serum antibody to HSV-2, now commercially available, may give negative results, especially when patients present early with the initial episode of genital herpes or when HSV-1 is the cause of genital herpes (as is often the case today). Furthermore, a positive test for antibody to HSV-2 does not prove that the current lesions are herpetic, since nearly one-fourth of the general population of the United States (and no doubt a higher proportion of those at risk for other STIs) becomes seropositive for HSV-2 during early adulthood. Although even type-specific tests for HSV-2 that are commercially available in the United States are not 100% specific, a positive HSV-2 serology does enable the clinician to tell the patient that he or she has probably had genital herpes, should learn to recognize symptoms, should avoid sex during recurrences, and should consider use of condoms or suppressive antiviral therapy, both of which can reduce transmission to a sexual partner.

TABLE 28-7

CLINICAL FEATURES OF GENITAL ULCERS

FEATURE	SYPHILIS	HERPES	CHANCROID	LYMPHOGRANULOMA VENEREUM	DONOVANOSIS
Incubation period	9–90 days	2–7 days	1–14 days	3 days–6 weeks	1–4 weeks (up to 6 months)
Early primary lesions	Papule	Vesicle	Pustule	Papule, pustule, or vesicle	Papule
No. of lesions	Usually one	Multiple	Usually multiple, may coalesce	Usually one; often not detected, despite lymphadenopathy	Variable
Diameter	5–15 mm	1–2 mm	Variable	2–10 mm	Variable
Edges	Sharply demarcated, elevated, round, or oval	Erythematous	Undermined, ragged, irregular	Elevated, round, or oval	Elevated, irregular
Depth	Superficial or deep	Superficial	Excavated	Superficial or deep	Elevated
Base	Smooth, nonpurulent, relatively nonvascular	Serous, erythematous, nonvascular	Purulent, bleeds easily	Variable, nonvascular	Red and velvety, bleeds readily
Induration	Firm	None	Soft	Occasionally firm	Firm
Pain	Uncommon	Frequently tender	Usually very tender	Variable	Uncommon
Lymphadenopathy	Firm, nontender, bilateral	Firm, tender, often bilateral with initial episode	Tender, may suppurate, loculated, usually unilateral	Tender, may suppurate, loculated, usually unilateral	None; pseudobuboes

Source: From RM Ballard, in KK Holmes et al (eds): *Sexually Transmitted Diseases*, 4th ed. New York, McGraw-Hill, 2008.

Demonstration of *H. ducreyi* by culture (or by PCR test, when available) is most useful when ulcers are painful and purulent, especially if inguinal lymphadenopathy with fluctuance or overlying erythema is noted; if chancroid is prevalent in the community; or if the patient has recently had a sexual exposure elsewhere in a chancroid-endemic area (e.g., a developing country). Enlarged, fluctuant lymph nodes should be aspirated for culture or PCR tests to detect *H. ducreyi* as well as for Gram's staining and culture to rule out the presence of other pyogenic bacteria.

When genital ulcers persist beyond the natural history of initial episodes of herpes (2–3 weeks) or of chancroid or syphilis (up to 6 weeks) and do not resolve with syndrome-based antimicrobial therapy, then—in addition to the usual tests for herpes, syphilis, and chancroid—biopsy is indicated to exclude donovanosis, carcinoma, and other nonvenereal dermatoses. HIV serology should also be undertaken, since chronic, persistent genital herpes is common in AIDS.

℞ Treatment: ULCERATIVE GENITAL OR PERIANAL LESIONS

Immediate syndrome-based treatment for acute genital ulcerations (after collection of all necessary diagnostic specimens at the first visit) is often appropriate before all test results become available, because patients with typical initial or recurrent episodes of genital or anorectal herpes can benefit from prompt oral antiviral therapy (Chap. 80); because early treatment of sexually transmitted causes of genital ulcers decreases further transmission; and because some patients do not return for test results and treatment. The patient with nonvesicular ulcerative lesions who may not return for follow-up or may not discontinue sexual activity should receive initial treatment for syphilis, together with empirical therapy for chancroid if there has been an exposure in an area where chancroid occurs or if regional lymph node suppuration is evident. In resource-poor settings lacking ready access to diagnostic tests, this approach to syndromic treatment for syphilis and chancroid has helped bring these two diseases under control. Finally, empirical antimicrobial therapy may be indicated if ulcers persist and the diagnosis remains unclear after a week of observation despite attempts to diagnose herpes, syphilis, and chancroid.

PROCTITIS, PROCTOCOLITIS, ENTEROCOLITIS, AND ENTERITIS

Sexually acquired *proctitis*, with inflammation limited to the rectal mucosa (the distal 10–12 cm), results from direct rectal inoculation of typical STD pathogens. In contrast,

TABLE 28-8

INITIAL MANAGEMENT OF GENITAL OR PERIANAL ULCER

Usual causes
- Herpes simplex virus (HSV)
- *Treponema pallidum* (primary syphilis)
- *Haemophilus ducreyi* (chancroid)

Usual initial laboratory evaluation
- Dark-field exam, direct FA, or PCR for *T. pallidum*; RPR or VDRL test for syphilis (if negative but primary syphilis suspected, repeat in 1 week); culture, direct FA, ELISA, or PCR for HSV; consider HSV-2-specific serology. In chancroid-endemic area: PCR or culture for *H. ducreyi*

Initial Treatment

Herpes confirmed or suspected (history or sign of vesicles):
- Treat for genital herpes with acyclovir, valacyclovir, or famciclovir

Syphilis confirmed (dark-field, FA, or PCR showing *T. pallidum*, or RPR reactive):
- Benzathine penicillin 2.4 million units IM once to patient, recent (e.g., within 3 months) seronegative partner(s), and all seropositive partners

Chancroid confirmed or suspected (diagnostic test positive, or HSV and syphilis excluded, and lesion persists):
- Ciprofloxacin 500 mg PO as single dose *or*
- Ceftriaxone 250 mg IM as single dose *or*
- Azithromycin 1 g PO as single dose

Note: FA, fluorescent antibody; PCR, polymerase chain reaction; RPR, rapid plasma reagin; ELISA, enzyme-linked immunosorbent assay; HSV, herpes simplex virus; VDRL, Venereal Disease Research Laboratory.

inflammation extending from the rectum to the colon (*proctocolitis*), involving both the small and the large bowel (*enterocolitis*), or involving the small bowel alone (*enteritis*) can result from ingestion of typical intestinal pathogens through oral-anal exposure during sexual contact. Anorectal pain and mucopurulent, bloody rectal discharge suggest proctitis or proctocolitis. Proctitis commonly produces tenesmus (causing frequent attempts to defecate, but not true diarrhea) and constipation, whereas proctocolitis and enterocolitis more often cause true diarrhea. In all three conditions, anoscopy usually shows mucosal exudate and easily induced mucosal bleeding (i.e., a positive "wipe test"), sometimes with petechiae or mucosal ulcers. Exudate should be sampled for Gram's staining and other microbiologic studies. Sigmoidoscopy or colonoscopy shows inflammation limited to the rectum in proctitis or disease extending at least up into the sigmoid colon in proctocolitis.

The AIDS era brought an extraordinary shift in the clinical and etiologic spectrum of intestinal infections among homosexual men. The number of cases of the acute intestinal STIs described above fell as high-risk sexual behaviors became less common in this group. At the same time, the number of AIDS-related opportunistic intestinal infections increased rapidly, many associated with chronic or recurrent symptoms. The incidence of these infections has since fallen with increasingly effective antiretroviral therapy. Two species initially isolated in association with intestinal symptoms in homosexual men are now known as *Helicobacter cinaedi* and *Helicobacter fennelliae*, and both have subsequently been isolated from the blood of HIV-infected men with a syndrome of multifocal dermatitis and arthritis.

Acquisition of HSV, *N. gonorrhoeae*, or *C. trachomatis* (now again including LGV strains of *C. trachomatis*) during receptive anorectal intercourse causes most cases of infectious proctitis in women and homosexual men. Primary and secondary syphilis can also produce anal or anorectal lesions, with or without symptoms. Gonococcal or chlamydial proctitis typically involves the most distal rectal mucosa and the anal crypts and is clinically mild, without systemic manifestations. In contrast, primary proctitis due to HSV and proctocolitis due to the strains of *C. trachomatis* that cause LGV usually produce severe anorectal pain and often cause fever. Perianal ulcers and inguinal lymphadenopathy, most commonly due to HSV, can also occur in LGV or syphilis. Sacral nerve root radiculopathies, usually presenting as urinary retention, laxity of the anal sphincter, or constipation, may complicate primary herpetic proctitis. In LGV, rectal biopsy typically shows crypt abscesses, granulomas, and giant cells—findings resembling those in Crohn's disease; such findings should always prompt rectal culture and serology for LGV, which is a curable infection. Syphilis can also produce rectal granulomas, usually in association with infiltration by plasma cells or other mononuclear cells. Syphilis, LGV, and HSV infection involving the rectum can produce perirectal adenopathy that is sometimes mistaken for malignancy; syphilis, LGV, HSV infection, and chancroid involving the anus can produce inguinal adenopathy, because anal lymphatics drain to inguinal lymph nodes.

Diarrhea and abdominal bloating or cramping pain without anorectal symptoms and with normal findings on anoscopy and sigmoidoscopy occur with inflammation of the small intestine (enteritis) or with proximal colitis. In homosexual men without HIV infection, enteritis is often attributable to *Giardia lamblia*. Sexually acquired proctocolitis is most often due to *Campylobacter* or *Shigella* spp.

Treatment: ℞ PROCTITIS, PROCTOCOLITIS, ENTEROCOLITIS, AND ENTERITIS

Acute proctitis in persons who have practiced receptive anorectal intercourse is usually sexually acquired. Such patients should undergo anoscopy to detect rectal ulcers or vesicles and petechiae after swabbing of the rectal mucosa, to examine rectal exudates for PMNs and gram-negative diplococci, and to obtain rectal swab specimens for testing for rectal gonorrhea, chlamydial infection, herpes, and syphilis. Pending test results, patients with proctitis should receive empirical syndromic treatment—e.g., with ceftriaxone (a single IM dose of 125 mg for gonorrhea) plus doxycycline (100 mg PO twice daily for 7 days for possible chlamydial infection) plus treatment for herpes or syphilis if indicated.

PREVENTION AND CONTROL OF STIs

Prevention and control of STIs require the following:

1. Reduction of the average rate of sexual exposure to STIs through alteration of sexual risk behaviors and behavioral norms among both susceptible and infected persons in all population groups. The necessary changes include reduction in the total number of sexual partners and the number of concurrent sexual partners.
2. Reduction of the efficiency of transmission through the promotion of safer sexual practices, the use of condoms during casual or commercial sex, vaccination against HBV and HPV infection, male circumcision, and a growing number of other approaches (e.g., early detection and treatment of other STIs to reduce the efficiency of sexual transmission of HIV). We now know from longitudinal studies over the past decade that consistent condom use is associated with significant protection of both males and females against all STIs that have been examined, including HIV, HPV, and HSV infections as well as gonorrhea and chlamydial infection. The only exceptions are probably sexually transmitted *Phthirus pubis* and *Sarcoptes scabiei* infestations.
3. Shortening of the duration of infectivity of STIs through early detection and curative or suppressive treatment of patients and their sexual partners.

Financial and time constraints imposed by managed-care practice patterns, along with the reluctance of some clinicians to ask questions about stigmatized sexual behaviors, often curtail screening and prevention services. As outlined in Fig. 28-8, the success of clinicians' efforts to detect and treat STIs depends in part on societal efforts to teach young people how to recognize symptoms of STIs, to motivate those with symptoms to seek care promptly, and to make high-quality, appropriate care accessible, affordable, and acceptable, especially to the young indigent patients most likely to acquire an STI.

Since many infected individuals develop no symptoms or fail to recognize and report symptoms, clinicians should routinely perform an STI risk assessment for teenagers and young adults as a guide to selective screening. U.S. Preventive Services Task Force Guidelines recommend screening sexually active female patients ≤25 years of age for *C. trachomatis* whenever they present for health care (at least once a year); older women should be tested if they have more than one sexual partner, have begun a new sexual relationship since the previous test, or have another STI diagnosed. In the United States, widespread selective

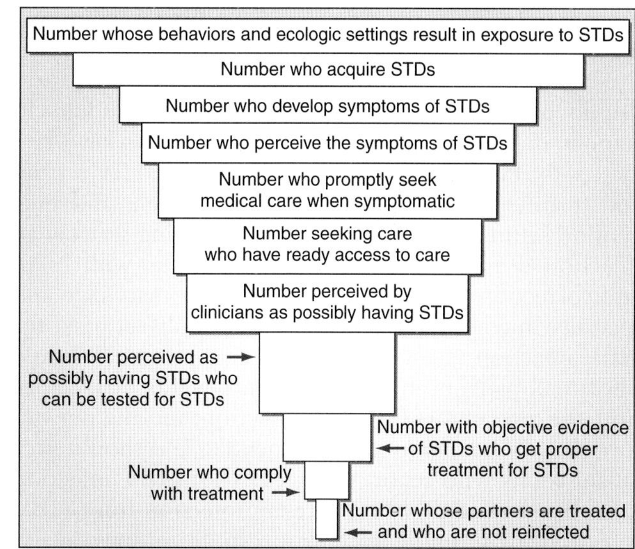

FIGURE 28-8
Critical control points for preventive and clinical interventions against sexually transmitted diseases (STDs). [*Adapted from HT Waller and MA Piot: Bull World Health Organ 41:75, 1969 and 43:1, 1970; and from "Resource allocation model for public health planning—a case study of tuberculosis control," Bull World Health Organ 84(Suppl), 1973.*]

screening of young women for cervical *C. trachomatis* infection in some regions has been associated with a 50–60% drop in prevalence, and such screening also protects the individual woman from PID. Sensitive urine-based genetic amplification tests permit expansion of screening to men, teenage boys, and girls in settings where examination is not planned or is impractical (e.g., during pre-participation sports examinations or during initial medical evaluation of adolescent girls).

Although gonorrhea is now substantially less common than chlamydial infection in industrialized countries, screening tests for *N. gonorrhoeae* are still appropriate for women and teenage girls attending STD clinics and for sexually active teens and young women from areas of high gonorrhea prevalence. Multiplex NAATs that combine screening for *N. gonorrhoeae* and *C. trachomatis* in a single low-cost assay now facilitate the prevention and control of both infections in populations at high risk.

All patients with newly detected STIs or at high risk for STIs according to routine risk assessment as well as all pregnant women should be encouraged to undergo serologic testing for syphilis and HIV infection, with appropriate HIV counseling before and after testing. Randomized trials have shown that risk-reduction counseling of patients with STIs significantly lowers subsequent risk of acquiring an STI; such counseling should now be considered a standard component of STI management. Preimmunization serologic testing for antibody to HBV is indicated for unvaccinated persons who are known to be at high risk, such as homosexually active men and injection drug users. In most young persons, however, it is more cost-effective to vaccinate against HBV without serologic screening. In 2006, the Advisory Committee on Immunization Practices (ACIP) of the CDC recommended the following: (1) Universal hepatitis B vaccination should be implemented for all unvaccinated adults in settings in which a high proportion of adults have risk factors for HBV infection (e.g., STD clinics, HIV testing and treatment facilities, drug-abuse treatment and prevention settings, health care settings targeting services to injection drug users or men who have sex with men, and correctional facilities). (2) In other primary care and specialty medical settings in which adults at risk for HBV infection receive care, health care providers should inform all patients about the health benefits of vaccination, the risk factors for HBV infection, and the persons for whom vaccination is recommended and should vaccinate adults who report risk factors for HBV infection as well as any adult who requests protection from HBV infection. To promote vaccination in all settings, health care providers should implement standing orders to identify adults recommended for hepatitis B vaccination, should administer HBV vaccination as part of routine clinical services, should not require acknowledgment of an HBV infection risk factor for adult vaccination, and should use available reimbursement mechanisms to remove financial barriers to hepatitis B vaccination.

In 2007, the ACIP recommended routine immunization of 9- to 26-year-old girls and women with the quadrivalent HPV vaccine (against HPV types 6, 11, 16, and 18) approved by the U.S. Food and Drug Administration; the optimal age for recommended vaccination is 11–12 years because of the very high risk of HPV infection after sexual debut.

Partner notification is the process of identifying and informing partners of infected patients about possible exposure to an STI and of examining, testing, and treating partners as appropriate. In a series of 22 reports concerning partner notification during the 1990s, index patients with gonorrhea or chlamydial infection named a mean of 0.75–1.6 partners, of whom one-fourth to one-third were infected; those with syphilis named 1.8–6.3 partners, with one-third to one-half infected; and those with HIV infection named 0.76–5.31 partners, with up to one-fourth infected. Persons who transmit infection or who have recently been infected and are still in the incubation period usually have no symptoms or only mild symptoms and seek medical attention only when notified of their exposure. Therefore, the clinician must encourage patients to participate in partner notification, must ensure that exposed persons are notified, and must guarantee confidentiality to all involved. In the United States, local health departments often offer assistance in partner notification, treatment, and/or counseling. It seems both feasible and most useful to notify those partners exposed within the patient's likely period of infectiousness, which is often considered the preceding 1 month for gonorrhea, 1–2 months for chlamydial infection, and up to 3 months for early syphilis.

Persons with a new-onset STI always have a *source* contact who gave them the infection; in addition, they may have a *secondary* (*spread* or *exposed*) contact with whom they had sex after becoming infected. The identification and treatment of these two types of contacts have different objectives. Treatment of the source contact (often a casual contact) benefits the community by preventing further transmission; treatment of the recently exposed secondary contact (typically a spouse or another steady sexual partner) prevents both the development of serious complications (such as PID) in the partner and reinfection of the index patient. A survey of a random sample of U.S. physicians found that most instructed patients to abstain from sex during treatment, to use condoms, and to inform their sex partners after being diagnosed with gonorrhea, chlamydial infection, or syphilis; physicians sometimes gave the patients drugs for their partners. However, follow-up of the partners by physicians was infrequent. A randomized trial compared patients' delivery of therapy to partners exposed to gonorrhea or chlamydial infection with conventional notification and advice to partners to seek evaluation for STD; patients' delivery of partners' therapy (PDPT), also known as *expedited partner therapy* (EPT), significantly reduced combined rates of reinfection of the index patient with *N. gonorrhoeae* or *Chlamydia*. State-by-state variations in regulations governing this approach have not been well defined, but the 2006 CDC STD treatment guidelines and the EPT final report of 2006 (*http://www.cdc.gov/std/treatment/EPTFinalReport2006.pdf*) describe its potential use. Currently, EPT is commonly used by many practicing physicians; it is not feasible in some settings and lacks clear legal sanctioning in some states.

In summary, clinicians and public health agencies share responsibility for the prevention and control of STIs. In the managed-care era, the role of primary care clinicians has become increasingly important in prevention as well as in diagnosis and treatment.

FURTHER READINGS

Centers for Disease Control and Prevention: Sexually transmitted diseases treatment guidelines, 2006. MMWR Recomm Rep 55(RR-11):1, 2006 (Erratum in MMWR Recomm Rep 55(36):997, 2006)

Centers for Disease Control and Prevention: Update to CDC's sexually transmitted diseases treatment guidelines, 2006: Fluoroquinolones no longer recommended for treatment of gonococcal infections. MMWR Morb Mortal Wkly Rep 56:332, 2007

Datta SD et al: Gonorrhea and chlamydia in the United States among persons 14 to 39 years of age, 1999 to 2002. Ann Intern Med 147:89, 2007

Fredricks DN et al: Molecular identification of bacteria associated with bacterial vaginosis. N Engl J Med 353:1899, 2005

Future II Group: Quadrivalent vaccine against human papillomavirus to prevent high-grade cervical lesions. N Engl J Med 356:1915, 2007

Golden MR et al: Effect of expedited treatment of sex partners on recurrent or persistent gonorrhea or chlamydial infection. N Engl J Med 352:676, 2005

Gupta R et al: Genital herpes. Lancet 370:2127, 2007

Holmes KK et al (eds): *Sexually Transmitted Diseases*, 4th ed. New York, McGraw-Hill, 2008

MANHART LE, HOLMES KK: Randomized controlled trials of individual-level, population-level, and multilevel interventions for preventing sexually transmitted infections: What has worked? J Infect Dis 191(Suppl 1):S7, 2005

MARKOWITZ LE et al: Quadrivalent human papillomavirus vaccine: Recommendations of the Advisory Committee on Immunization Practices (ACIP). MMWR Recomm Rep 56(RR-2):1, 2007

MAST EE et al: A comprehensive immunization strategy to eliminate transmission of hepatitis B virus infection in the United States: Recommendations of the Advisory Committee on Immunization Practices (ACIP) Part II: Immunization of adults. MMWR Recomm Rep 55(RR-16):1, 2006

MEYERS DS et al: Screening for chlamydial infection: An evidence update for the U.S. Preventive Services Task Force. Ann Intern Med 147:135, 2007

NAGOT N et al: Reduction of HIV-1 RNA levels with therapy to suppress herpes simplex virus. N Engl J Med 356:790, 2007

TRELLE S et al: Improved effectiveness of partner notification for patients with sexually transmitted infections: Systematic review. BMJ 334:354, 2007

TRIGG BG et al: Sexually transmitted infections and pelvic inflammatory disease in women. Med Clin North Am 92:1083, 2008

WANG SA et al: Antimicrobial resistance for *Neisseria gonorrhoeae* in the United States, 1988 to 2003: The spread of fluoroquinolone resistance. Ann Intern Med 147:81, 2007

WORKOWSKI KA: Sexually transmitted disease treatment guidelines. Clin Infect Dis 44(Suppl 3):S1, 2007

WORLD HEALTH ORGANIZATION: Sexually transmitted diseases diagnostics initiative. Geneva, WHO, 2001 *(http://www.who.int/std_diagnostics/news/SDI_founding_members.htm)*

CHAPTER 29

MENINGITIS, ENCEPHALITIS, BRAIN ABSCESS, AND EMPYEMA

Karen L. Roos ■ Kenneth L. Tyler

Acute infections of the nervous system are among the most important problems in medicine because early recognition, efficient decision making, and rapid institution of therapy can be lifesaving. These distinct clinical syndromes include acute bacterial meningitis, viral meningitis, encephalitis, focal infections such as brain abscess and subdural empyema, and infectious thrombophlebitis. Each may present with a nonspecific prodrome of fever and headache, which in a previously healthy individual may initially be thought to be benign, until (with the exception of viral meningitis) altered consciousness, focal neurologic signs, or seizures appear. Key goals of early management are to emergently distinguish between these conditions, identify the responsible pathogen, and initiate appropriate antimicrobial therapy.

Approach to the Patient:
SUSPECTED CENTRAL NERVOUS SYSTEM INFECTIONS

(Fig. 29-1) The first task is to identify whether an infection predominantly involves the subarachnoid space (*meningitis*) or whether there is evidence of either generalized or focal involvement of brain tissue in the cerebral hemispheres, cerebellum, or brainstem. When

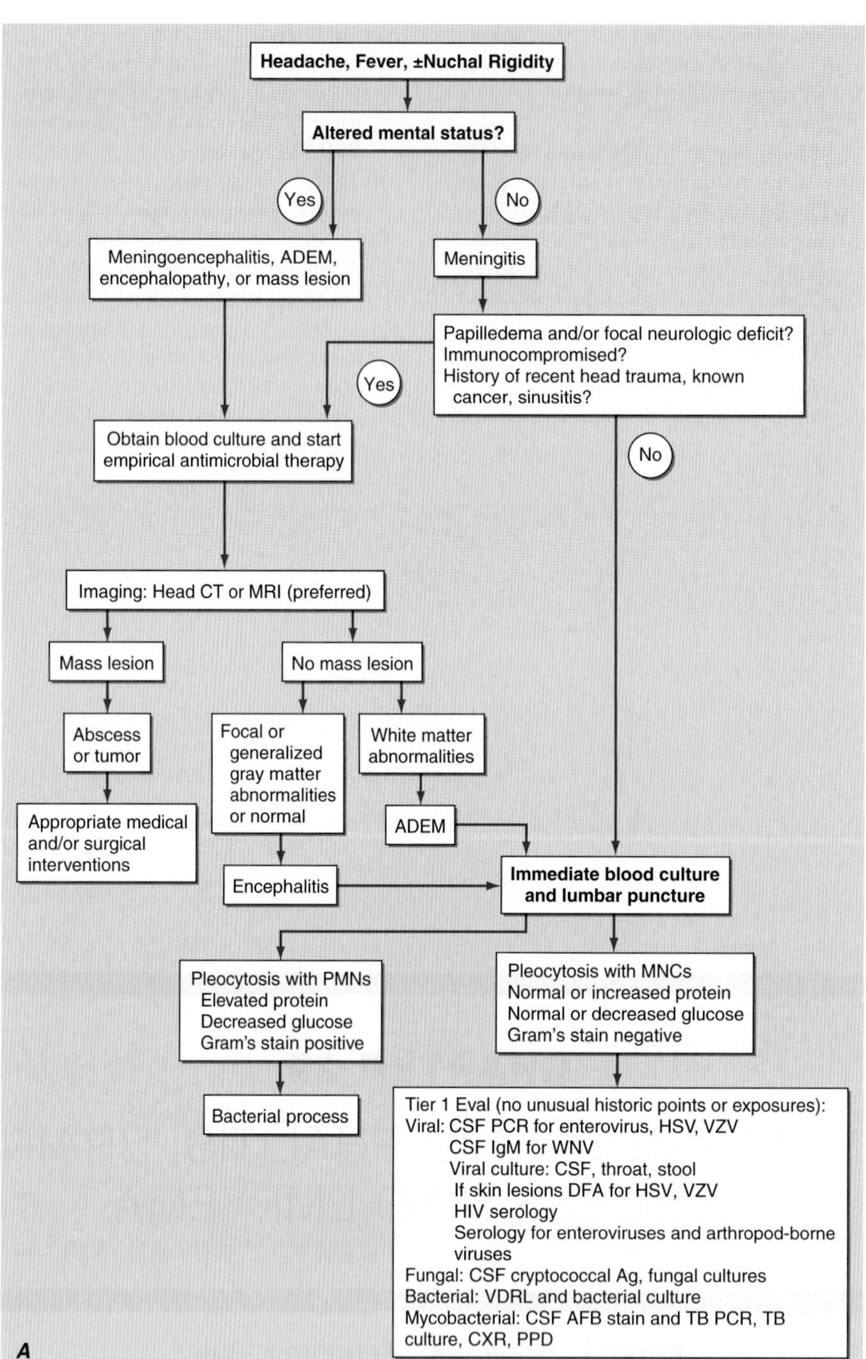

FIGURE 29-1

The management of patients with suspected CNS infection. ADEM, acute disseminated encephalomyelitis; CT, computed tomography; MRI, magnetic resonance imaging; PMNs, polymorphonuclear leukocytes; MNCs, mononuclear cells; CSF, cerebrospinal fluid; PCR, polymerase chain reaction; HSV, herpes simplex virus; VZV, varicella-zoster virus; WNV, West Nile virus; DFA, direct fluorescent antibody; Ag, antigen; VDRL, Venereal Disease Research Laboratory; AFB, acid-fast bacillus; TB, tuberculosis; CXR, chest x-ray; PPD, purified protein derivative; EBV, Epstein-Barr virus; CTFV, Colorado tick fever virus; HHV, human herpesvirus; LCMV, lymphocytic choriomeningitis virus.

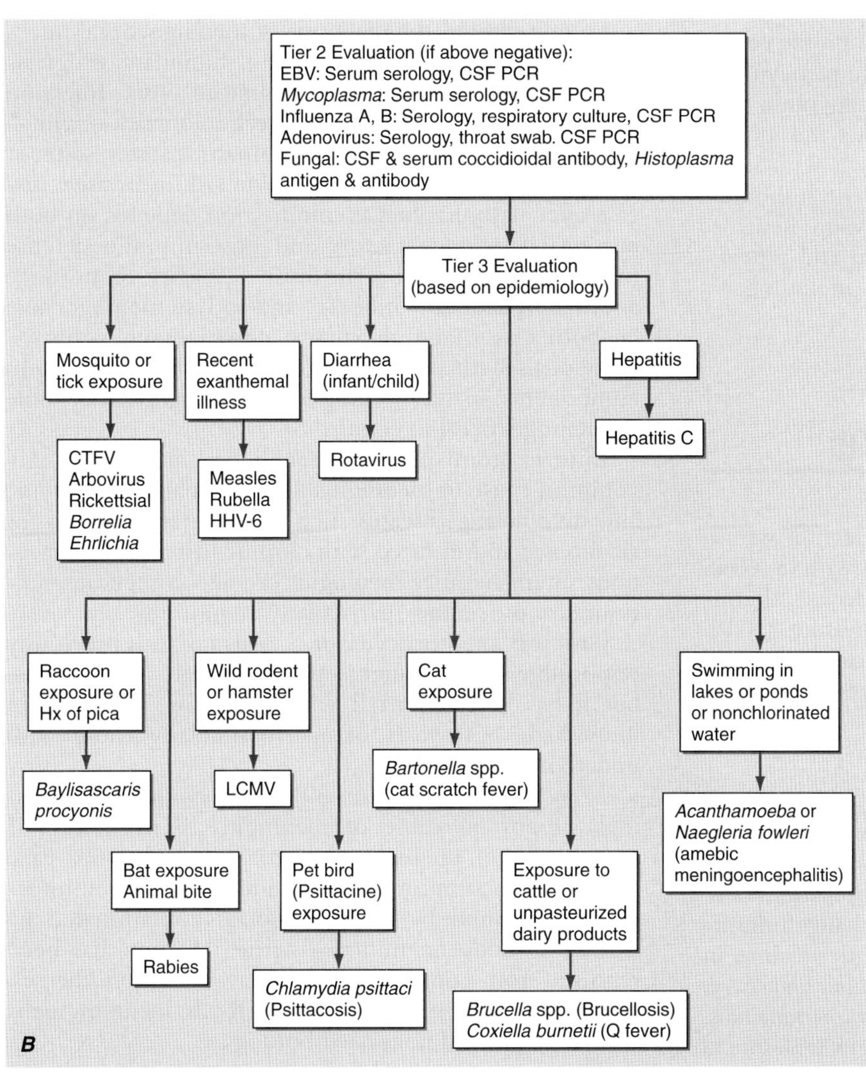

FIGURE 29-1 (*CONTINUED*)

brain tissue is directly injured by a viral infection, the disease is referred to as *encephalitis*, whereas focal bacterial, fungal, or parasitic infections involving brain tissue are classified as either *cerebritis* or *abscess*, depending on the presence or absence of a capsule.

Nuchal rigidity ("stiff neck") is the pathognomonic sign of meningeal irritation and is present when the neck resists passive flexion. Kernig's and Brudzinski's signs are also classic signs of meningeal irritation. *Kernig's sign* is elicited with the patient in the supine position. The thigh is flexed on the abdomen, with the knee flexed; attempts to passively extend the knee elicit pain when meningeal irritation is present. *Brudzinski's sign* is elicited with the patient in the supine position and is positive when passive flexion of the neck results in spontaneous flexion of the hips and knees. Although commonly tested on physical examinations, the sensitivity and specificity of Kernig's and Brudzinski's signs are uncertain. Both may be absent or reduced in very young or elderly patients, immunocompromised individuals, or patients with a severely depressed mental status. The high prevalence of cervical spine disease in older individuals may result in false-positive tests for nuchal rigidity.

Initial management can be guided by several considerations: (1) Empirical therapy should be initiated promptly whenever bacterial meningitis is a significant diagnostic consideration. (2) All patients who have had recent head trauma, are immunocompromised, have known malignant lesions or central nervous system (CNS) neoplasms, or have focal neurologic findings that include papilledema or a depressed level of consciousness should undergo CT or MRI of the brain prior to lumbar puncture (LP). In these cases empirical antibiotic therapy should not be delayed pending test results but should be administered before neuroimaging and LP. (3) A significantly depressed level of consciousness (e.g., somnolence, coma), seizures, or focal neurologic deficits do not occur in viral (*aseptic*) meningitis; patients with these symptoms should be hospitalized for further evaluation and treated empirically for bacterial and viral meningoencephalitis. (4) Immunocompetent patients with a normal level of consciousness, no prior antimicrobial treatment, and a cerebrospinal fluid (CSF) profile consistent with viral meningitis (lymphocytic pleocytosis and a normal glucose concentration) can often be treated as outpatients if appropriate contact and monitoring can be ensured. Failure of a patient with suspected viral meningitis to improve within 48 h should prompt a reevaluation including follow-up neurologic and general medical examination and repeat imaging and laboratory studies, often including a second LP.

ACUTE BACTERIAL MENINGITIS

DEFINITION

Bacterial meningitis is an acute purulent infection within the subarachnoid space. It is associated with a CNS inflammatory reaction that may result in decreased consciousness, seizures, raised intracranial pressure (ICP), and stroke. The meninges, the subarachnoid space, and the brain parenchyma are all frequently involved in the inflammatory reaction (*meningoencephalitis*).

EPIDEMIOLOGY

Bacterial meningitis is the most common form of suppurative CNS infection, with an annual incidence in the United States of >2.5 cases/100,000 population. The epidemiology of bacterial meningitis has changed significantly in recent years, reflecting a dramatic decline in the incidence of meningitis due to *Haemophilus influenzae*, and a smaller decline in that due to *Neisseria meningitidis*, following the introduction and increasingly widespread use of vaccines for both these organisms. Currently, the organisms most commonly responsible for community-acquired bacterial meningitis are *Streptococcus pneumoniae* (~50%), *N. meningitidis* (~25%), group B streptococci (~15%), and *Listeria monocytogenes* (~10%). *H. influenzae* now accounts for <10% of cases of bacterial meningitis in most series.

ETIOLOGY

S. pneumoniae (Chap. 34) is the most common cause of meningitis in adults >20 years of age, accounting for nearly half the reported cases (1.1 per 100,000 persons per year). There are a number of predisposing conditions that increase the risk of pneumococcal meningitis, the most important of which is pneumococcal pneumonia. Additional risk factors include coexisting acute or chronic pneumococcal sinusitis or otitis media, alcoholism, diabetes, splenectomy, hypogammaglobulinemia, complement deficiency, and head trauma with basilar skull fracture and CSF rhinorrhea. Mortality remains ~20% despite antibiotic therapy.

N. meningitidis (Chap. 44) accounts for 25% of all cases of bacterial meningitis (0.6 cases per 100,000 persons per year) and for up to 60% of cases in children and young adults between the ages of 2 and 20. The presence of petechial or purpuric skin lesions can provide an important clue to the diagnosis of meningococcal infection. In some patients the disease is fulminant, progressing to death within hours of symptom onset. Infection may be initiated by nasopharyngeal colonization, which can result in either an asymptomatic carrier state or invasive meningococcal disease. The risk of invasive disease after nasopharyngeal colonization depends on both bacterial virulence factors and host immune defense mechanisms, including the host's capacity to produce antimeningococcal antibodies and to lyse meningococci by both classic and alternative complement pathways. Individuals with deficiencies of any of the complement components, including properdin, are highly susceptible to meningococcal infections.

Enteric gram-negative bacilli are an increasingly common cause of meningitis in individuals with chronic and debilitating diseases such as diabetes, cirrhosis, or alcoholism and in those with chronic urinary tract infections. Gram-negative meningitis can also complicate neurosurgical procedures, particularly craniotomy.

Group B streptococcus, or *S. agalactiae*, was previously responsible for meningitis predominantly in neonates, but it has been reported with increasing frequency in individuals >50 years of age, particularly those with underlying diseases.

L. monocytogenes (Chap. 39) has become an increasingly important cause of meningitis in neonates (<1 month of age), pregnant women, individuals >60 years, and immunocompromised individuals of all ages. Infection is acquired by ingesting foods contaminated by *Listeria*. Foodborne human listerial infection has been reported from contaminated coleslaw, milk, soft cheeses, and several types of "ready-to-eat" foods, including delicatessen meat and uncooked hotdogs.

The frequency of *H. influenzae* type b meningitis in children has declined dramatically since the introduction of the Hib conjugate vaccine, although rare cases of Hib meningitis in vaccinated children have been reported. More frequently, *H. influenzae* causes meningitis in unvaccinated children and adults.

Staphylococcus aureus and coagulase-negative staphylococci (Chap. 35) are important causes of meningitis that occurs after invasive neurosurgical procedures, particularly shunting procedures for hydrocephalus, or as a complication of the use of subcutaneous Ommaya reservoirs for administration of intrathecal chemotherapy.

PATHOPHYSIOLOGY

The most common bacteria that cause meningitis, *S. pneumoniae* and *N. meningitidis*, initially colonize the nasopharynx by attaching to nasopharyngeal epithelial cells. Bacteria are transported across epithelial cells in membrane-bound vacuoles to the intravascular space or invade the intravascular space by creating separations in the apical tight junctions of columnar epithelial cells. Once in the bloodstream, bacteria are able to avoid phagocytosis by neutrophils and classic complement–mediated bactericidal activity because of the presence of a polysaccharide capsule. Bloodborne bacteria can reach the intraventricular choroid plexus, directly infect choroid plexus epithelial cells, and gain access to the CSF. Some bacteria, such as *S. pneumoniae*, can adhere to cerebral capillary endothelial cells and subsequently migrate through or between these cells to reach the CSF. Bacteria are able to multiply rapidly within CSF because of the absence of effective host immune defenses. Normal CSF contains few white blood cells (WBCs) and relatively small amounts of complement proteins and immunoglobulins. The paucity of the latter two prevents effective opsonization of bacteria, an essential prerequisite for bacterial phagocytosis by neutrophils. Phagocytosis of bacteria is further impaired by the fluid nature of CSF, which is less conducive to phagocytosis than a solid tissue substrate.

A critical event in the pathogenesis of bacterial meningitis is the inflammatory reaction induced by the invading bacteria. Many of the neurologic manifestations and complications of bacterial meningitis result from the immune response to the invading pathogen rather than from direct bacteria-induced tissue injury. As a result, neurologic injury can progress even after the CSF has been sterilized by antibiotic therapy.

The lysis of bacteria with the subsequent release of cell-wall components into the subarachnoid space is the initial step in the induction of the inflammatory response and the formation of a purulent exudate in the subarachnoid space (Fig. 29-2). Bacterial cell-wall components, such as the lipopolysaccharide (LPS) molecules of gram-negative bacteria and teichoic acid and peptidoglycans of *S. pneumoniae*, induce meningeal inflammation by stimulating the production of inflammatory cytokines and chemokines by microglia, astrocytes, monocytes, microvascular endothelial cells, and CSF leukocytes. In experimental models of meningitis, cytokines including tumor necrosis factor (TNF) and interleukin 1 (IL-1) are present in CSF within 1–2 h of intracisternal inoculation of LPS. This cytokine response is quickly followed by an increase in CSF protein concentration and leukocytosis. Chemokines (cytokines that induce chemotactic migration in leukocytes) and a variety of other proinflammatory cytokines are also produced and secreted by leukocytes and tissue cells that are stimulated by IL-1 and TNF. In addition, bacteremia and the inflammatory cytokines induce the production of excitatory amino acids, reactive oxygen and nitrogen species (free oxygen radicals, nitric oxide, and peroxynitrite), and other mediators that can induce death of brain cells.

Much of the pathophysiology of bacterial meningitis is a direct consequence of elevated levels of CSF cytokines

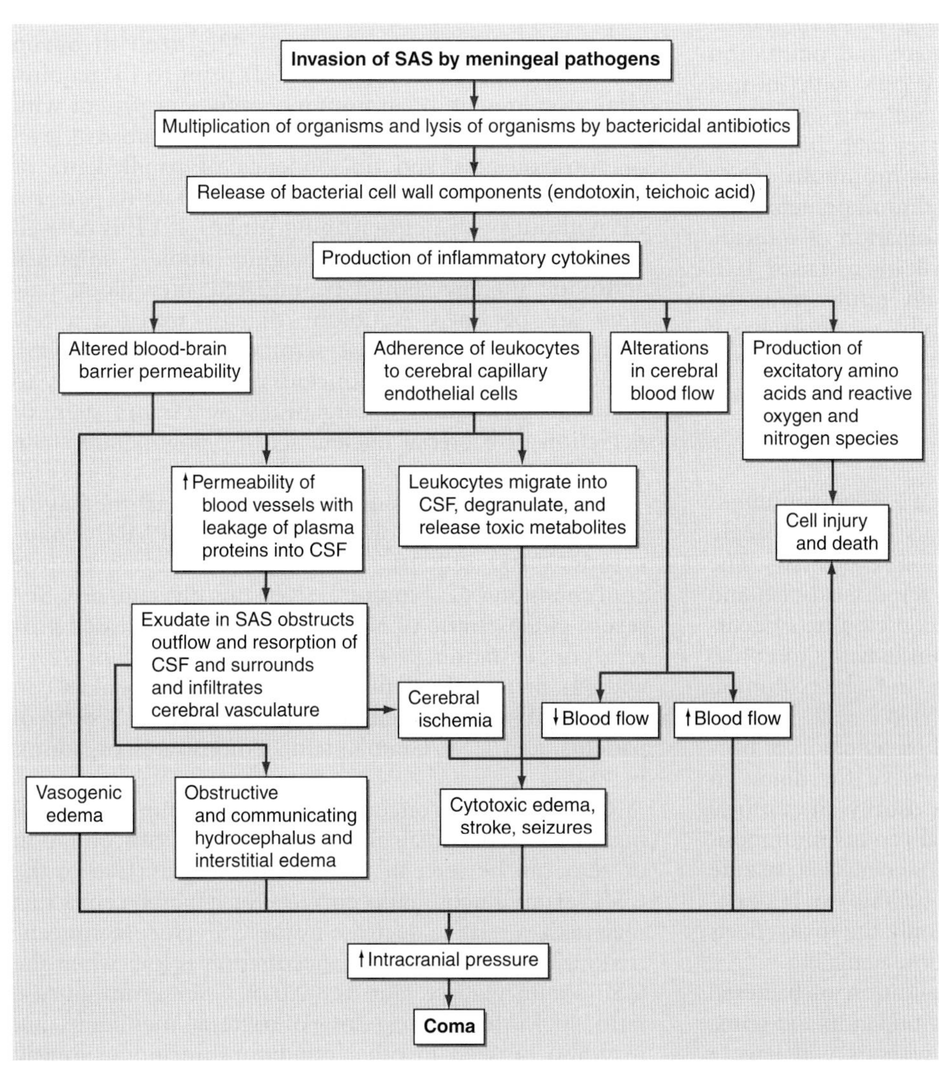

FIGURE 29-2

The pathophysiology of the neurologic complications of bacterial meningitis. SAS, subarachnoid space; CSF, cerebrospinal fluid.

and chemokines. TNF and IL-1 act synergistically to increase the permeability of the blood-brain barrier, resulting in induction of vasogenic edema and the leakage of serum proteins into the subarachnoid space (Fig. 29-2). The subarachnoid exudate of proteinaceous material and leukocytes obstructs the flow of CSF through the ventricular system and diminishes the resorptive capacity of the arachnoid granulations in the dural sinuses, leading to obstructive and communicating hydrocephalus and concomitant interstitial edema.

Inflammatory cytokines upregulate the expression of selectins on cerebral capillary endothelial cells and leukocytes, promoting leukocyte adherence to vascular endothelial cells and subsequent migration into the CSF. The adherence of leukocytes to capillary endothelial cells increases the permeability of blood vessels, allowing for the leakage of plasma proteins into the CSF, which adds to the inflammatory exudate. Neutrophil degranulation results in the release of toxic metabolites that contribute to cytotoxic edema, cell injury, and death. Contrary to previous beliefs, CSF leukocytes probably do little to contribute to the clearance of CSF bacterial infection.

During the very early stages of meningitis, there is an increase in cerebral blood flow, soon followed by a decrease in cerebral blood flow and a loss of cerebrovascular autoregulation. Narrowing of the large arteries at the base of the brain due to encroachment by the purulent exudate in the subarachnoid space and infiltration of the arterial wall by inflammatory cells with intimal thickening (*vasculitis*) also occur and may result in ischemia and infarction, obstruction of branches of the middle cerebral artery by thrombosis, thrombosis of the major cerebral venous sinuses, and thrombophlebitis of the cerebral cortical veins. The combination of interstitial, vasogenic, and cytotoxic edema leads to raised ICP and coma. Cerebral herniation usually results from the effects of cerebral edema, either focal or generalized; hydrocephalus and dural sinus or cortical vein thrombosis may also play a role.

CLINICAL PRESENTATION

Meningitis can present as either an acute fulminant illness that progresses rapidly in a few hours or as a subacute infection that progressively worsens over several days. The classic clinical triad of meningitis is fever, headache, and nuchal rigidity. A decreased level of consciousness occurs in >75% of patients and can vary from lethargy to coma. Nausea, vomiting, and photophobia are also common complaints.

Seizures occur as part of the initial presentation of bacterial meningitis or during the course of the illness in 20–40% of patients. Focal seizures are usually due to focal arterial ischemia or infarction, cortical venous thrombosis with hemorrhage, or focal edema. Generalized seizure activity and status epilepticus may be due to hyponatremia, cerebral anoxia, or, less commonly, the toxic effects of antimicrobial agents such as high-dose penicillin.

Raised ICP is an expected complication of bacterial meningitis and the major cause of obtundation and coma in this disease. More than 90% of patients will have a CSF opening pressure >180 mmH_2O, and 20% have opening pressures >400 mmH_2O. Signs of increased ICP include a deteriorating or reduced level of consciousness, papilledema, dilated poorly reactive pupils, sixth nerve palsies, decerebrate posturing, and Cushing's reflex (bradycardia, hypertension, and irregular respirations). The most disastrous complication of increased ICP is cerebral herniation. The incidence of herniation in patients with bacterial meningitis has been reported to occur in as few as 1% to as many as 8% of cases.

Specific clinical features may provide clues to the diagnosis of individual organisms and are discussed in more detail in specific chapters devoted to individual pathogens. The most important of these clues is the rash of meningococcemia, which begins as a diffuse erythematous maculopapular rash resembling a viral exanthem; however, the skin lesions of meningococcemia rapidly become petechial. Petechiae are found on the trunk and lower extremities, in the mucous membranes and conjunctiva, and occasionally on the palms and soles.

DIAGNOSIS

When bacterial meningitis is suspected, blood cultures should be immediately obtained and empirical antimicrobial therapy initiated without delay (Table 29-1). The diagnosis of bacterial meningitis is made by examination of the CSF (Table 29-2). The need to obtain neuroimaging studies (CT or MRI) prior to LP requires clinical judgment. In an immunocompetent patient with no known history of recent head trauma, a normal level of consciousness, and no evidence of papilledema or focal neurologic deficits, it is considered safe to perform LP without prior neuroimaging studies. If LP is delayed in order to obtain neuroimaging studies, empirical antibiotic therapy should be initiated after blood cultures are obtained. Antibiotic therapy initiated a few hours before LP will not significantly alter the CSF WBC count or glucose concentration, nor is it likely to prevent visualization of organisms by Gram's stain or detection of bacterial nucleic acid by polymerase chain reaction (PCR) assay.

The classic CSF abnormalities in bacterial meningitis (Table 29-2) are (1) polymorphonuclear (PMN) leukocytosis (>100 cells/μL in 90%), (2) decreased glucose concentration [<2.2 mmol/L (<40 mg/dL) and/or CSF/serum glucose ratio of <0.4 in ~60%], (3) increased protein concentration [>0.45 g/L (>45 mg/dL) in 90%], and (4) increased opening pressure (>180 mmH_2O in 90%). CSF bacterial cultures are positive in >80% of patients, and CSF Gram's stain demonstrates organisms in >60%.

CSF glucose concentrations <2.2 mmol/L (<40 mg/dL) are abnormal, and a CSF glucose concentration of zero can be seen in bacterial meningitis. Use of the CSF/serum glucose ratio corrects for hyperglycemia that may mask a relative decrease in the CSF glucose concentration. The CSF glucose concentration is low when the CSF/serum glucose ratio is <0.6. A CSF/serum glucose ratio <0.4 is highly suggestive of bacterial meningitis, but may also be seen in other conditions, including fungal,

TABLE 29-1

ANTIBIOTICS USED IN EMPIRICAL THERAPY OF BACTERIAL MENINGITIS AND FOCAL CNS INFECTIONS[a]

INDICATION	ANTIBIOTIC
Preterm infants to infants <1 month	Ampicillin + cefotaxime
Infants 1–3 mos	Ampicillin + cefotaxime or ceftriaxone
Immunocompetent children >3 mos and adults <55	Cefotaxime or ceftriaxone + vancomycin
Adults >55 and adults of any age with alcoholism or other debilitating illnesses	Ampicillin + cefotaxime or ceftriaxone + vancomycin
Hospital-acquired meningitis, posttraumatic or postneurosurgery meningitis, neutropenic patients, or patients with impaired cell-mediated immunity	Ampicillin + ceftazidime + vancomycin

ANTIMICROBIAL AGENT	TOTAL DAILY DOSE AND DOSING INTERVAL: CHILD (>1 MONTH)	ADULT
Ampicillin	200 (mg/kg)/d, q4h	12 g/d, q4h
Cefepime	150 (mg/kg)/d, q8h	6 g/d, q8h
Cefotaxime	200 (mg/kg)/d, q6h	12 g/d, q4h
Ceftriaxone	100 (mg/kg)/d, q12h	4 g/d, q12h
Ceftazidime	150 (mg/kg)/d, q8h	6 g/d, q8h
Gentamicin	7.5 (mg/kg)/d, q8h[b]	7.5 (mg/kg)/d, q8h
Meropenem	120 (mg/kg)/d, q8h	3 g/d, q8h
Metronidazole	30 (mg/kg)/d, q6h	1500–2000 mg/d, q6h
Nafcillin	100–200 (mg/kg)/d, q6h	9–12 g/d, q4h
Penicillin G	400,000 (U/kg)/d, q4h	20–24 million U/d, q4h
Vancomycin	60 (mg/kg)/d, q6h	2 g/d, q12h[b]

[a]All antibiotics are administered intravenously; doses indicated assume normal renal and hepatic function.

[b]Doses should be adjusted based on serum peak and trough levels: gentamicin therapeutic level: peak: 5–8 μg/mL; trough: <2 μg/mL; vancomycin therapeutic level: peak: 25–40 μg/mL; trough: 5–15 μg/mL.

tuberculous, and carcinomatous meningitis. It takes from 30 min to several hours for the concentration of CSF glucose to reach equilibrium with blood glucose levels; therefore, administration of 50 mL of 50% glucose (D50) before LP, as commonly occurs in emergency room settings, is unlikely to alter CSF glucose concentration significantly unless more than a few hours have elapsed between glucose administration and LP.

A broad-range PCR can detect small numbers of viable and nonviable organisms in CSF and is expected to be useful for making a diagnosis of bacterial meningitis in patients who have been pretreated with oral or

TABLE 29-2

CEREBROSPINAL FLUID (CSF) ABNORMALITIES IN BACTERIAL MENINGITIS

Opening pressure	>180 mmH_2O
White blood cells	10/μL to 10,000/μL; neutrophils predominate
Red blood cells	Absent in nontraumatic tap
Glucose	<2.2 mmol/L (<40 mg/dL)
CSF/serum glucose	<0.4
Protein	>0.45 g/L (>45 mg/dL)
Gram's stain	Positive in >60%
Culture	Positive in >80%
Latex agglutination	May be positive in patients with meningitis due to *S. pneumoniae*, *N. meningitidis*, *H. influenzae* type b, *E. coli*, group B streptococci
Limulus lysate	Positive in cases of gram-negative meningitis
PCR	Detects bacterial DNA

Note: PCR, polymerase chain reaction.

parenteral antibiotics and in whom Gram's stain and CSF culture are negative. When the broad-range PCR is positive, a PCR that uses specific bacterial primers to detect the nucleic acid of *S. pneumoniae, N. meningitidis, Escherichia coli, L. monocytogenes, H. influenzae*, and *S. agalactiae* can be obtained based on the clinical suspicion of the meningeal pathogen. The latex agglutination (LA) test for the detection of bacterial antigens of *S. pneumoniae*, *N. meningitidis*, *H. influenzae* type b, group B streptococcus, and *E. coli* K1 strains in the CSF has been useful for making a diagnosis of bacterial meningitis but is being replaced by the CSF bacterial PCR assay. The CSF LA test has a *specificity* of 95–100% for *S. pneumoniae* and *N. meningitidis*, so a positive test is virtually diagnostic of bacterial meningitis caused by these organisms. However, the *sensitivity* of the CSF LA test is only 70–100% for detection of *S. pneumoniae* and 33–70% for detection of *N. meningitidis* antigens, so a negative test does not exclude infection by these organisms. The Limulus amebocyte lysate assay is a rapid diagnostic test for the detection of gram-negative endotoxin in CSF and thus for making a diagnosis of gram-negative bacterial meningitis. The test has a specificity of 85–100% and a sensitivity approaching 100%. Thus a positive Limulus amebocyte lysate assay occurs in virtually all patients with gram-negative bacterial meningitis, but false positives may occur.

Almost all patients with bacterial meningitis will have neuroimaging studies performed during the course of their illness. MRI is preferred over CT because of its superiority in demonstrating areas of cerebral edema and ischemia. In patients with bacterial meningitis, diffuse meningeal enhancement is often seen after the administration of gadolinium. Meningeal enhancement is not diagnostic of meningitis but occurs in any CNS disease associated with increased blood-brain barrier permeability.

Petechial skin lesions, if present, should be biopsied. The rash of meningococcemia results from the dermal seeding of organisms with vascular endothelial damage, and biopsy may reveal the organism on Gram's stain.

DIFFERENTIAL DIAGNOSIS

Viral meningoencephalitis, and particularly herpes simplex virus (HSV) encephalitis, can mimic the clinical presentation of bacterial meningitis (see "Encephalitis" later in the chapter). HSV encephalitis typically presents with headache, fever, altered consciousness, focal neurologic deficits (e.g., dysphasia, hemiparesis), and focal or generalized seizures. The findings on CSF studies, neuroimaging, and electroencephalogram (EEG) distinguish HSV encephalitis from bacterial meningitis. The typical CSF profile with viral CNS infections is a lymphocytic pleocytosis with a normal glucose concentration, in contrast to PMN pleocytosis and hypoglycorrhachia characteristic of bacterial meningitis. MRI abnormalities (other than meningeal enhancement) are not seen in uncomplicated bacterial meningitis. By contrast, in HSV encephalitis, on T2-weighted and fluid-attenuated inversion recovery (FLAIR) MRI images, high signal intensity lesions are seen in the orbitofrontal, anterior, and medial temporal lobes in the majority of patients within 48 h of symptom onset. Some patients with HSV encephalitis have a distinctive periodic pattern on EEG (see below).

Rickettsial disease can resemble bacterial meningitis (Chap. 75). Rocky Mountain spotted fever (RMSF) is transmitted by a tick bite and caused by the bacteria *Rickettsia rickettsii*. The disease may present acutely with high fever, prostration, myalgia, headache, nausea, and vomiting. Most patients develop a characteristic rash within 96 h of the onset of symptoms. The rash is initially a diffuse erythematous maculopapular rash that may be difficult to distinguish from that of meningococcemia. It progresses to a petechial rash, then to a purpuric rash and, if untreated, to skin necrosis or gangrene. The color of the lesions changes from bright red to very dark red, then yellowish-green to black. The rash typically begins in the wrist and ankles and then spreads distally and proximally within a matter of a few hours, involving the palms and soles. Diagnosis is made by immunofluorescent staining of skin biopsy specimens. Ehrlichioses are also transmitted by a tick bite. These are small gram-negative coccobacilli of which two species cause human disease. *Anaplasma phagocytophilum* causes human granulocytic ehrlichiosis (anaplasmosis), and *Ehrlichia chaffeensis* causes human monocytic ehrlichiosis. The clinical and laboratory manifestations of the infections are similar. Patients present with fever, headache, nausea, and vomiting. Twenty percent of patients have a maculopapular or petechial rash. There is laboratory evidence of leukopenia, thrombocytopenia and anemia, and mild to moderate elevations in alanine aminotransferases, alkaline phosphatase, and lactate dehydrogenase. Patients with RMSF and those with ehrlichial infections may have an altered level of consciousness ranging from mild lethargy to coma, confusion, focal neurologic signs, cranial nerve palsies, hyperreflexia, and seizures.

Focal suppurative CNS infections (see below), including subdural and epidural empyema and brain abscess, should also be considered, especially when focal neurologic findings are present. MRI should be performed promptly in all patients with suspected meningitis who have focal features, both to detect the intracranial infection and to search for associated areas of infection in the sinuses or mastoid bones.

A number of noninfectious CNS disorders can mimic bacterial meningitis. Subarachnoid hemorrhage (SAH) is generally the major consideration. Other possibilities include chemical meningitis due to rupture of tumor contents into the CSF (e.g., from a cystic glioma or craniopharyngioma epidermoid or dermoid cyst); drug-induced hypersensitivity meningitis; carcinomatous or lymphomatous meningitis; meningitis associated with inflammatory disorders such as sarcoid, systemic lupus erythematosus (SLE), and Behçet's syndrome; pituitary apoplexy; and uveomeningitic syndromes (Vogt-Koyanagi-Harada syndrome).

On occasion, subacutely evolving meningitis (Chap. 30) may be considered in the differential diagnosis of acute meningitis. The principal causes include *Mycobacterium tuberculosis* (Chap. 66), *Cryptococcus neoformans* (Chap. 106), *Histoplasma capsulatum* (Chap. 103), *Coccidioides immitis* (Chap. 104), and *Treponema pallidum* (Chap. 70).

℞ Treatment: ACUTE BACTERIAL MENINGITIS

EMPIRICAL ANTIMICROBIAL THERAPY (Table 29-1) Bacterial meningitis is a medical emergency. The goal is to begin antibiotic therapy within 60 min of a patient's arrival in the emergency room. Empirical antimicrobial therapy is initiated in patients with suspected bacterial meningitis before the results of CSF Gram's stain and culture are known. *S. pneumoniae* (Chap. 34) and *N. meningitidis* (Chap. 44) are the most common etiologic organisms of community-acquired bacterial meningitis. Due to the emergence of penicillin- and cephalosporin-resistant *S. pneumoniae*, empirical therapy of community-acquired suspected bacterial meningitis in children and adults should include a combination of dexamethasone, a third- generation cephalosporin (e.g., ceftriaxone or cefotaxime) and vancomycin, plus acyclovir, as HSV encephalitis is the leading disease in the differential diagnosis, and doxycycline during tick season to treat tick-borne bacterial infections. Ceftriaxone or cefotaxime provides good coverage for susceptible *S. pneumoniae*, group B streptococci, and *H. influenzae* and adequate coverage for *N. meningitidis*. Cefepime is a broad-spectrum fourth-generation cephalosporin with in vitro activity similar to that of cefotaxime or ceftriaxone against *S. pneumoniae* and *N. meningitidis* and greater activity against *Enterobacter* species and *Pseudomonas aeruginosa*. In clinical trials, cefepime has been demonstrated to be equivalent to cefotaxime in the treatment of penicillin-sensitive pneumococcal and meningococcal meningitis, and it has been used successfully in some patients with meningitis due to

Enterobacter species and *P. aeruginosa*. Ampicillin should be added to the empirical regimen for coverage of *L. monocytogenes* in individuals <3 months of age, those >55, or those with suspected impaired cell-mediated immunity because of chronic illness, organ transplantation, pregnancy, malignancy, or immunosuppressive therapy. In hospital-acquired meningitis, and particularly meningitis after neurosurgical procedures, staphylococci and gram-negative organisms including *P. aeruginosa* are the most common etiologic organisms. In these patients, empirical therapy should include a combination of vancomycin and ceftazidime, cefepime, or meropenem. Ceftazidime, cefepime, or meropenem should be substituted for ceftriaxone or cefotaxime in neurosurgical patients and in neutropenic patients, as ceftriaxone and cefotaxime do not provide adequate activity against CNS infection with *P. aeruginosa*. Meropenem is a carbapenem antibiotic that is highly active in vitro against *L. monocytogenes*, has been demonstrated to be effective in cases of meningitis caused by *P. aeruginosa*, and shows good activity against penicillin-resistant pneumococci. In experimental pneumococcal meningitis, meropenem was comparable to ceftriaxone and inferior to vancomycin in sterilizing CSF cultures. The number of patients with bacterial meningitis enrolled in clinical trials of meropenem has not been sufficient to definitively assess the efficacy of this antibiotic.

TABLE 29-3

ANTIMICROBIAL THERAPY OF CNS BACTERIAL INFECTIONS BASED ON PATHOGEN[a]

ORGANISM	ANTIBIOTIC
Neisseria meningitidis	
Penicillin-sensitive	Penicillin G or ampicillin
Penicillin-resistant	Ceftriaxone or cefotaxime
Streptococcus pneumoniae	
Penicillin-sensitive	Penicillin G
Penicillin-intermediate	Ceftriaxone or cefotaxime
Penicillin-resistant	(Ceftriaxone or cefotaxime) + vancomycin
Gram-negative bacilli (except *Pseudomonas* spp.)	Ceftriaxone or cefotaxime
Pseudomonas aeruginosa	Ceftazidime or cefepime or meropenem
Staphylococcus spp.	
Methicillin-sensitive	Nafcillin
Methicillin-resistant	Vancomycin
Listeria monocytogenes	Ampicillin + gentamicin
Haemophilus influenzae	Ceftriaxone or cefotaxime
Streptococcus agalactiae	Penicillin G or ampicillin
Bacteroides fragilis	Metronidazole
Fusobacterium spp.	Metronidazole

[a]Doses are as indicated in Table 29-1.

SPECIFIC ANTIMICROBIAL THERAPY

Meningococcal Meningitis (Table 29-3) Although ceftriaxone and cefotaxime provide adequate empirical coverage for *N. meningitidis*, penicillin G remains the antibiotic of choice for meningococcal meningitis caused by susceptible strains. Isolates of *N. meningitidis* with moderate resistance to penicillin have been identified, but patients infected with these strains have still been successfully treated with penicillin. CSF isolates of *N. meningitidis* should be tested for penicillin and ampicillin susceptibility, and if resistance is found, cefotaxime or ceftriaxone should be substituted for penicillin. A 7-day course of intravenous antibiotic therapy is adequate for uncomplicated meningococcal meningitis. The index case and all close contacts should receive chemoprophylaxis with a 2-day regimen of rifampin (600 mg every 12 h for 2 days in adults and 10 mg/kg every 12 h for 2 days in children >1 year). Rifampin is not recommended in pregnant women. Alternatively, adults can be treated with one dose of ciprofloxacin (750 mg), one dose of azithromycin (500 mg), or one intramuscular dose of ceftriaxone (250 mg). Close contacts are defined as those individuals who have had contact with oropharyngeal secretions, either through kissing or by sharing toys, beverages, or cigarettes.

Pneumococcal Meningitis Antimicrobial therapy of pneumococcal meningitis is initiated with a cephalosporin (ceftriaxone, cefotaxime, or cefepime) and vancomycin. All CSF isolates of *S. pneumoniae* should be tested for sensitivity to penicillin and the cephalosporins. Once the results of antimicrobial susceptibility tests are known, therapy can be modified accordingly (Table 29-3). For *S. pneumoniae* meningitis, an isolate of *S. pneumoniae* is considered to be susceptible to penicillin with a minimal inhibitory concentration (MIC) <0.06 μg/mL, to have intermediate resistance when the MIC is 0.1–1.0 μg/mL, and to be highly resistant when the MIC >1.0 μg/mL. Isolates of *S. pneumoniae* that have cephalosporin MICs ≤0.5 μg/mL are considered sensitive to the cephalosporins (cefotaxime, ceftriaxone, cefepime). Those with MICs of 1 μg/mL are considered to have intermediate resistance, and those with MICs ≥2 μg/mL are considered resistant. For meningitis due to pneumococci with cefotaxime or ceftriaxone MICs ≤0.5 μg/mL, treatment with cefotaxime or ceftriaxone is usually adequate. If the MIC >1 μg/mL, vancomycin is the antibiotic of choice. Rifampin can be added to vancomycin for its synergistic effect but is inadequate as monotherapy because resistance develops rapidly when it is used alone.

A 2-week course of intravenous antimicrobial therapy is recommended for pneumococcal meningitis.

Patients with *S. pneumoniae* meningitis should have a repeat LP performed 24–36 h after the initiation of antimicrobial therapy to document sterilization of the CSF. Failure to sterilize the CSF after 24–36 h of antibiotic therapy should be considered presumptive evidence of antibiotic resistance. Patients with penicillin- and cephalosporin-resistant strains of *S. pneumoniae* who do not respond to intravenous vancomycin alone may benefit from the addition of intraventricular vancomycin.

The intraventricular route of administration is preferred over the intrathecal route because adequate concentrations of vancomycin in the cerebral ventricles are not always achieved with intrathecal administration.

***Listeria* Meningitis** Meningitis due to *L. monocytogenes* is treated with ampicillin for at least 3 weeks (Table 29-3). Gentamicin is often added (2 mg/kg loading dose, then 7.5 mg/kg per day given every 8 h and adjusted for serum levels and renal function). The combination of trimethoprim [10–20 (mg/kg)/d] and sulfamethoxazole [50–100 (mg/kg)/d] given every 6 h may provide an alternative in penicillin-allergic patients.

Staphylococcal Meningitis Meningitis due to susceptible strains of *S. aureus* or coagulase-negative staphylococci is treated with nafcillin (Table 29-3). Vancomycin is the drug of choice for methicillin-resistant staphylococci and for patients allergic to penicillin. In these patients, the CSF should be monitored during therapy. If the CSF is not sterilized after 48 h of intravenous vancomycin therapy, then either intraventricular or intrathecal vancomycin, 20 mg once daily, can be added.

Gram-Negative Bacillary Meningitis The third-generation cephalosporins—cefotaxime, ceftriaxone, and ceftazidime—are equally efficacious for the treatment of gram-negative bacillary meningitis, with the exception of meningitis due to *P. aeruginosa*, which should be treated with ceftazidime, cefepime, or meropenem (Table 29-3). A 3-week course of intravenous antibiotic therapy is recommended for meningitis due to gram-negative bacilli.

ADJUNCTIVE THERAPY The release of bacterial cell-wall components by bactericidal antibiotics leads to the production of the inflammatory cytokines IL-1 and TNF in the subarachnoid space. Dexamethasone exerts its beneficial effect by inhibiting the synthesis of IL-1 and TNF at the level of mRNA, decreasing CSF outflow resistance, and stabilizing the blood-brain barrier. The rationale for giving dexamethasone 20 min before antibiotic therapy is that dexamethasone inhibits the production of TNF by macrophages and microglia only if it is administered before these cells are activated by endotoxin. Dexamethasone does not alter TNF production once it has been induced. The results of clinical trials of dexamethasone therapy in children, predominantly with meningitis due to *H. influenzae* and *S. pneumoniae*, have demonstrated its efficacy in decreasing meningeal inflammation and neurologic sequelae such as the incidence of sensorineural hearing loss.

A prospective European trial of adjunctive therapy for acute bacterial meningitis in 301 adults found that dexamethasone reduced the number of unfavorable outcomes (15% vs 25%, $p = .03$) including death (7% vs 15%, $p = .04$). The benefits were most striking in patients with pneumococcal meningitis. Dexamethasone (10 mg intravenously) was administered 15–20 min before the first dose of an antimicrobial agent, and the same dose was repeated every 6 h for 4 days. These results were confirmed in a second trial of dexamethasone in adults with pneumococcal meningitis. Therapy with dexamethasone should ideally be started 20 min before, or not later than concurrent with, the first dose of antibiotics. It is unlikely to be of significant benefit if started >6 h after antimicrobial therapy has been initiated. Dexamethasone may decrease the penetration of vancomycin into CSF, and it delays the sterilization of CSF in experimental models of *S. pneumoniae* meningitis. As a result, its potential benefit should be carefully weighed when vancomycin is the antibiotic of choice. Alternatively, vancomycin can be administered by the intraventricular route.

INCREASED INTRACRANIAL PRESSURE Emergency treatment of increased ICP includes elevation of the patient's head to 30°–45°, intubation and hyperventilation (Pa_{CO_2} 25–30 mmHg), and mannitol. Patients with increased ICP should be managed in an intensive care unit; accurate ICP measurements are best obtained with an ICP monitoring device.

PROGNOSIS

Mortality is 3–7% for meningitis caused by *H. influenzae*, *N. meningitidis*, or group B streptococci; 15% for that due to *L. monocytogenes*; and 20% for *S. pneumoniae*. In general, the risk of death from bacterial meningitis increases with (1) decreased level of consciousness on admission, (2) onset of seizures within 24 h of admission, (3) signs of increased ICP, (4) young age (infancy) and age >50, (5) the presence of comorbid conditions including shock and/or the need for mechanical ventilation, and (6) delay in the initiation of treatment. Decreased CSF glucose concentration [<2.2 mmol/L (<40 mg/dL)] and markedly increased CSF protein concentration [>3 g/L (>300 mg/dL)] have been predictive of increased mortality and poorer outcomes in some series. Moderate or severe sequelae occur in ~25% of survivors, although the exact incidence varies with the infecting organism. Common sequelae include decreased intellectual function, memory impairment, seizures, hearing loss and dizziness, and gait disturbances.

ACUTE VIRAL MENINGITIS

CLINICAL MANIFESTATIONS

Patients with viral meningitis usually present with headache, fever, and signs of meningeal irritation coupled with an inflammatory CSF profile (see below). The headache of viral meningitis is usually frontal or retroorbital and is often associated with photophobia and pain on moving the eyes. Nuchal rigidity is present in most cases but may be mild and present only near the limit of neck anteflexion. Constitutional signs can include malaise, myalgia, anorexia, nausea and vomiting, abdominal pain, and/or diarrhea. Patients often have mild lethargy or drowsiness; however, profound alterations in consciousness, such as stupor, coma, or marked confusion, are unusual in viral meningitis and suggest the presence of encephalitis or other alternative diagnoses. Similarly, seizures or focal neurologic signs or symptoms or neuroimaging abnormalities indicative of brain parenchymal involvement are not typical of viral meningitis and suggest the presence of encephalitis or another CNS infectious or inflammatory process.

ETIOLOGY

Using a variety of diagnostic techniques, including CSF PCR, culture, and serology, a specific viral cause can be found in 75–90% of cases of viral meningitis. The most important agents are enteroviruses, HSV type 2 (HSV-2), and arboviruses (Table 29-4). CSF cultures are positive in 30–70% of patients, the frequency of isolation depending on the specific viral agent. Approximately two-thirds of culture-negative cases of aseptic meningitis have a specific viral etiology identified by CSF PCR testing (see below).

EPIDEMIOLOGY

Viral meningitis is not a nationally reportable disease; however, it has been estimated that the incidence is ~75,000 cases per year. In temperate climates, there is a substantial increase in cases during the summer and early fall months, reflecting the seasonal predominance of enterovirus and arthropod-borne virus (arbovirus) infections, with a peak monthly incidence of about 1 reported case per 100,000 population.

TABLE 29-4

VIRUSES CAUSING ACUTE MENINGITIS AND ENCEPHALITIS IN NORTH AMERICA

Acute Meningitis	
Common	**Less Common**
Enteroviruses (coxsackieviruses, echoviruses, and human enteroviruses 68–71)	Varicella-zoster virus
Herpes simplex virus 2	Epstein-Barr virus
Arthropod-borne viruses	Lymphocytic choriomeningitis virus
HIV	
Acute Encephalitis	
Common	**Less Common**
Herpesviruses	Rabies
Herpes simplex virus 1	Eastern equine encephalitis virus
Varicella-zoster virus	Western equine encephalitis virus
Epstein-Barr virus	Powassan virus
Arthropod-borne viruses	Cytomegalovirus[a]
La Crosse virus	Enteroviruses[a]
West Nile virus	Colorado tick fever
St. Louis encephalitis virus	Mumps

[a]Immunocompromised host.

LABORATORY DIAGNOSIS

CSF Examination

The most important laboratory test in the diagnosis of viral meningitis is examination of the CSF. The typical profile is a lymphocytic pleocytosis (25–500 cells/μL), a normal or slightly elevated protein concentration [0.2–0.8 g/L (20–80 mg/dL)], a normal glucose concentration, and a normal or mildly elevated opening pressure (100–350 mmH_2O). Organisms are *not* seen on Gram's or acid-fast stained smears or India ink preparations of CSF. Rarely, PMNs may predominate in the first 48 h of illness, especially with infections due to echovirus 9, eastern equine encephalitis (EEE) virus, or mumps. A pleocytosis of polymorphonuclear neutrophils also occurs in 45% of patients with West Nile virus (WNV) meningitis and can persist for a week or longer before shifting to a lymphocytic pleocytosis. Despite these exceptions, the presence of a CSF PMN pleocytosis in a patient with suspected viral meningitis should always prompt consideration of alternative diagnoses, including bacterial meningitis or parameningeal infections. The total CSF cell count in viral meningitis is typically 25–500/μL, although cell counts of several thousand/μL are occasionally seen, especially with infections due to lymphocytic choriomeningitis virus (LCMV) and mumps virus. The CSF glucose concentration is typically normal in viral infections, although it may be decreased in 10–30% of cases due to mumps or LCMV. Rare instances of decreased CSF glucose concentration occur in cases of meningitis due to echoviruses and other enteroviruses, HSV-2, and varicella-zoster virus (VZV). As a rule, a lymphocytic pleocytosis with a low glucose concentration should suggest fungal or tuberculous meningitis, *Listeria* meningoencephalitis, or noninfectious disorders (e.g., sarcoid, neoplastic meningitis).

A number of tests measuring levels of various CSF proteins, enzymes, and mediators—including C-reactive protein, lactic acid, lactate dehydrogenase, neopterin, quinolinate, IL-1β, IL-6, soluble IL-2 receptor, β_2-microglobulin, and TNF—have been proposed as potential discriminators between viral and bacterial meningitis or as markers of specific types of viral infection (e.g., infection with HIV), but they remain of uncertain sensitivity and specificity and are not widely used for diagnostic purposes.

Polymerase Chain Reaction Amplification of Viral Nucleic Acid

Amplification of viral-specific DNA or RNA from CSF using PCR amplification has become the single most important method for diagnosing CNS viral infections. In both enteroviral and HSV infections of the CNS, PCR has become the diagnostic procedure of choice and is substantially more sensitive than viral cultures. HSV PCR is also an important diagnostic test in patients with recurrent episodes of "aseptic" meningitis, many of whom have amplifiable HSV DNA in CSF despite negative viral cultures. CSF PCR is also used routinely to diagnose CNS viral infections caused by cytomegalovirus (CMV), Epstein-Barr virus (EBV), VZV, and human herpesvirus 6 (HHV-6). CSF PCR tests are available for WNV but are not as sensitive as CSF IgM. PCR is also useful in the diagnosis of CNS infection caused by *Mycoplasma pneumoniae,* which can mimic viral meningitis and encephalitis.

Viral Culture

The sensitivity of CSF cultures for the diagnosis of viral meningitis and encephalitis, in contrast to its utility in bacterial infections, is generally poor. In addition to CSF, specific viruses may also be isolated from throat swabs, stool, blood, and urine. Enteroviruses and adenoviruses may be found in feces; arboviruses, some enteroviruses, and LCMV in blood; mumps and CMV in urine; and enteroviruses, mumps, and adenoviruses in throat washings. During enteroviral infections, viral shedding in stool may persist for several weeks. The presence of enterovirus in stool is not diagnostic and may result from residual shedding from a previous enteroviral infection; it also occurs in some asymptomatic individuals during enteroviral epidemics.

Serologic Studies

For some viruses, including many arboviruses such as WNV, serologic studies remain a crucial diagnostic tool. Serum antibody determination is less useful for viruses with high seroprevalence rates in the general population such as HSV, VZV, CMV, and EBV. For viruses with low seroprevalence rates, diagnosis of acute viral infection can be made by documenting seroconversion between acute-phase and convalescent sera (typically obtained after 2–4 weeks) or by demonstrating the presence of virus-specific IgM antibodies. Documentation of synthesis of virus-specific antibodies in CSF, as shown by an increased IgG index or the presence of CSF IgM antibodies, is more useful than serum serology alone and can provide presumptive evidence of CNS infection. Although serum and CSF IgM antibodies generally persist for only a few months after acute infection, there are exceptions to this rule. For example, WNV IgM has been shown to persist in some patients for >1 year after acute infection. Unfortunately, the delay between onset of infection and the host's generation of a virus-specific antibody response often means that serologic data are useful mainly for the retrospective establishment of a specific diagnosis, rather than in aiding acute diagnosis or management.

CSF oligoclonal gamma globulin bands occur in association with a number of viral infections. The associated antibodies are often directed against viral proteins. Oligoclonal bands occur commonly in certain noninfectious neurologic diseases (e.g., multiple sclerosis) and may be found in nonviral infections (e.g., neurosyphilis, Lyme neuroborreliosis).

Other Laboratory Studies

All patients with suspected viral meningitis should have a complete blood count and differential, liver and renal function tests, erythrocyte sedimentation rate (ESR) and C-reactive protein, electrolytes, glucose, creatine kinase, aldolase, amylase, and lipase. Neuroimaging studies (MRI, CT) are not necessary in patients with uncomplicated viral meningitis but should be performed in patients with altered consciousness, seizures, focal neurologic signs or symptoms, or atypical CSF profiles.

DIFFERENTIAL DIAGNOSIS

The most important issue in the differential diagnosis of viral meningitis is to consider diseases that can mimic viral meningitis, including (1) untreated or partially treated bacterial meningitis; (2) early stages of meningitis caused by fungi, mycobacteria, or *Treponema pallidum* (neurosyphilis), in which a lymphocytic pleocytosis is common, cultures may be slow growing or negative, and hypoglycorrhachia may not be present early; (3) meningitis caused by agents such as *Mycoplasma, Listeria* spp., *Brucella* spp., *Coxiella* spp., *Leptospira* spp., and *Rickettsia* spp.; (4) parameningeal infections; (5) neoplastic meningitis; and (6) meningitis secondary to noninfectious inflammatory diseases, including hypersensitivity meningitis, SLE and other rheumatologic diseases, sarcoidosis, Behçet's syndrome, and the uveomeningitic syndromes.

SPECIFIC VIRAL ETIOLOGIES

Enteroviruses (Chap. 94) are the most common cause of viral meningitis, accounting for >75% of cases in which a specific etiology can be identified. CSF reverse transcriptase PCR (RT-PCR) is the diagnostic procedure of choice and is both sensitive (>95%) and specific (>100%). Enteroviruses are the most likely cause of viral meningitis in the summer months, especially in children (<15 years), although cases occur at reduced frequency year round. Although the incidence of enteroviral meningitis declines with increasing age, some outbreaks have preferentially affected older children and adults. Meningitis outside the neonatal period is usually benign. Patients present with sudden onset of fever, headache, nuchal rigidity, and often constitutional signs, including vomiting, anorexia, diarrhea, cough, pharyngitis, and myalgias. The physical examination should include a careful search for stigmata of enterovirus infection, including exanthemata, hand-foot-mouth disease, herpangina, pleurodynia, myopericarditis, and hemorrhagic conjunctivitis. The CSF profile is typically a lymphocytic pleocytosis (100–1000 cells/μL) with normal glucose and normal or mildly elevated protein concentration. In rare cases, PMNs may predominate during the first 48 h of illness. Treatment is supportive, and patients usually recover without sequelae. Chronic and severe infections can occur in neonates and in individuals with hypo- or agammaglobulinemia.

Arbovirus infections (Chap. 99) occur predominantly in the summer and early fall. Arboviral meningitis should be considered when clusters of meningitis and encephalitis cases occur in a restricted geographic region during the summer or early fall. In WNV epidemics, avian deaths may serve as sentinel infections for subsequent human disease. A history of tick exposure or travel or residence in the appropriate geographic area should suggest the possibility of Colorado tick fever virus or Powassan virus infection, although nonviral tick-borne diseases, including RMSF and Lyme neuroborreliosis, may present similarly. Arbovirus meningoencephalitis is typically associated with a CSF lymphocytic pleocytosis, normal glucose concentration, and normal or mildly elevated protein concentration. However, 40–45% of patients with WNV meningoencephalitis have CSF neutrophilia, which can persist for a week or more. The rarity of hypoglycorrhachia in WNV infection as well as the absence of positive Gram's stains and the negative cultures helps distinguish these patients from those with bacterial meningitis. The presence of increased numbers of plasmacytoid cells or Mollaret-like large mononuclear cells in the CSF may be a clue to the diagnosis of WNV infection. Definitive diagnosis of arboviral meningoencephalitis is based on demonstration of viral-specific IgM in CSF or seroconversion. CSF PCR tests are available for some viruses in selected diagnostic laboratories and at the Centers for Disease Control and Prevention (CDC), but in the case of WNV, sensitivity (~70%) of CSF PCR is less than that of CSF serology.

HSV-2 meningitis (Chap. 80) occurs in ~25% of women and 11% of men at the time of an initial (primary) episode of genital herpes. Of these patients, 20% go on to have recurrent attacks of meningitis. HSV-2 has been increasingly recognized as a major cause of viral meningitis in adults, and overall it is probably second in importance to enteroviruses as a cause of viral meningitis. Diagnosis of HSV meningitis is usually by HSV CSF PCR as cultures may be negative, especially in patients with recurrent meningitis. Demonstration of intrathecal synthesis of HSV-specific antibody may also be useful in diagnosis, although antibody tests are less sensitive and less specific than PCR and may not become positive until after the first week of infection. In contrast to HSV encephalitis in adults in which >90% of cases are due to HSV-1, the overwhelming majority of HSV meningitis is due to HSV-2. Although a history of or the presence of HSV genital lesions is an important diagnostic clue, many patients with HSV meningitis give no history and have no evidence of active genital herpes at the time of presentation. Most cases of recurrent viral or "aseptic" meningitis, including cases previously diagnosed as Mollaret's meningitis, are likely due to HSV.

VZV meningitis should be suspected in the presence of concurrent chickenpox or shingles. However, it is important to recognize that in some series, up to 40% of VZV meningitis cases have been reported to occur in the absence of rash. The frequency of VZV as a cause of meningitis is extremely variable, ranging from as low as 3% to as high as 20% in different series. Diagnosis is usually based on CSF PCR, although the sensitivity of this test may not be as high as for the other herpesviruses. In patients with negative CSF PCR results, the diagnosis of VZV CNS infection can be made by the demonstration of VZV-specific intrathecal antibody synthesis and/or the presence of VZV CSF IgM antibodies, or by positive CSF cultures.

EBV infections may also produce aseptic meningitis, with or without associated infectious mononucleosis. The presence of atypical lymphocytes in the CSF or peripheral blood is suggestive of EBV infection but may occasionally be seen with other viral infections. EBV is almost never cultured from CSF. Serum and CSF serology can help establish the presence of acute infection, which is characterized by IgM viral capsid antibodies (VCAs), antibodies to early antigens (EA), and the absence of antibodies to EBV-associated nuclear antigen (EBNA). CSF PCR is another important diagnostic test, although positive results may reflect viral reactivation associated with other infectious or inflammatory processes.

HIV meningitis should be suspected in any patient presenting with a viral meningitis with known or suspected risk factors for HIV infection. Meningitis may occur after primary infection with HIV in 5–10% of cases and less commonly at later stages of illness. Cranial nerve palsies, most commonly involving cranial nerves V, VII, or VIII, are more common in HIV meningitis than in other viral infections. Diagnosis can be confirmed by detection of HIV genome in blood or CSF. Seroconversion may be delayed, and patients with negative HIV serologies who are suspected of having HIV meningitis should be monitored for delayed seroconversion. For further discussion of HIV infection, see Chap. 90.

Mumps (Chap. 97) should be considered when meningitis occurs in the late winter or early spring, especially in males (male/female ratio 3:1). With the widespread use of the live attenuated mumps vaccine in the United States since 1967, the incidence of mumps meningitis has fallen by >95%. The presence of parotitis, orchitis, oophoritis, pancreatitis, or elevations in serum lipase and amylase are suggestive of mumps meningitis; however, their absence does not exclude the diagnosis. Clinical meningitis occurs in up to 30% of patients with mumps parotitis, and CSF pleocytosis occurs in >50%. Mumps infection confers lifelong immunity, so a documented history of previous infection excludes this diagnosis. Patients with meningitis have a CSF pleocytosis that can exceed 1000 cells/μL in 25%. Lymphocytes predominate in 75%, although CSF neutrophilia occurs in 25%. Hypoglycorrhachia occurs in 10–30% of patients and may be a clue to the diagnosis when present. Diagnosis is typically made by culture of virus from CSF or by detecting IgM antibodies or seroconversion. CSF PCR is available in some diagnostic and research laboratories. Rare cases of vaccine-associated meningitis occur, with a frequency of 10–100/100,000 doses typically 2–4 weeks after vaccination.

LCMV infection (Chap. 99) should be considered when aseptic meningitis occurs in the late fall or winter and in individuals with a history of exposure to house mice (*Mus musculus*), pet or laboratory rodents (e.g., hamsters, rats, mice), or their excreta. Some patients have an associated rash, pulmonary infiltrates, alopecia, parotitis, orchitis, or myopericarditis. Laboratory clues to the diagnosis of LCMV, in addition to the clinical findings noted above, may include the presence of leukopenia, thrombocytopenia, or abnormal liver function tests. Some cases present with a marked CSF pleocytosis (>1000 cells/μL) and hypoglycorrhachia (<30%). Diagnosis is based on serology and/or culture of virus from CSF.

℞ Treatment: ACUTE VIRAL MENINGITIS

Treatment of almost all cases of viral meningitis is primarily symptomatic and includes use of analgesics, antipyretics, and antiemetics. Fluid and electrolyte status should be monitored. Patients with suspected bacterial meningitis should receive appropriate empirical therapy pending culture results (see above). Hospitalization may not be required in immunocompetent patients with presumed viral meningitis and no focal signs or symptoms, no significant alteration in consciousness, and a classic CSF profile (lymphocytic pleocytosis, normal glucose, negative Gram's stain) if adequate provision for monitoring at home and medical follow-up can be ensured. Immunocompromised patients; patients with significant alteration in consciousness, seizures, or the presence of focal signs and symptoms suggesting the possibility of encephalitis or parenchymal brain involvement; and those patients who have an atypical CSF profile should be hospitalized. Oral or intravenous acyclovir may be of benefit in patients with meningitis caused by HSV-1 or -2 and in cases of severe EBV or VZV infection. Data concerning treatment of HSV, EBV, and VZV meningitis are extremely limited. Seriously ill patients should probably receive intravenous acyclovir (15–30 mg/kg per day in three divided doses), which can be followed by an oral drug such as acyclovir (800 mg, five times daily), famciclovir (500 mg tid), or valacyclovir (1000 mg tid) for a total course of 7–14 days. Patients who are less ill can be treated with oral drugs alone. Patients with HIV meningitis should receive highly active antiretroviral therapy (Chap. 90).

Patients with viral meningitis who are known to have deficient humoral immunity (e.g., X-linked agammaglobulinemia) and who are not already receiving either intramuscular gamma globulin or intravenous immunoglobulin (IVIg) should be treated with these agents. Intraventricular administration of immunoglobulin through an Ommaya reservoir has been tried in some patients with chronic enteroviral meningitis who have not responded to intramuscular or intravenous immunoglobulin.

An investigational drug, pleconaril, has shown efficacy against a variety of enteroviral infections and has good oral bioavailability and excellent CNS penetration. Clinical trials in patients with enteroviral meningitis indicated that pleconaril decreased the duration of symptoms compared with placebo. Most cases of enteroviral CNS infection are benign and self-limited and do not require specific antiviral therapy. However, pleconaril treatment might benefit patients with chronic CNS enteroviral infections in the setting of agammaglobulinemia or those who develop poliomyelitis as a complication of polio vaccine administration. Unfortunately, the availability of pleconaril for compassionate-use purposes is currently uncertain.

Vaccination is an effective method of preventing the development of meningitis and other neurologic complications associated with poliovirus, mumps, and measles infection. A live attenuated VZV vaccine (Varivax) is available in the United States. Clinical studies indicate an effectiveness rate of 70–90% for this vaccine, but a booster may be required to maintain immunity. An inactivated varicella vaccine is available for transplant recipients.

PROGNOSIS

In adults, the prognosis for full recovery from viral meningitis is excellent. Rare patients complain of persisting headache, mild mental impairment, incoordination, or generalized asthenia for weeks to months. The outcome in infants and neonates (<1 year) is less certain; intellectual impairment, learning disabilities, hearing loss, and other lasting sequelae have been reported in some studies.

VIRAL ENCEPHALITIS

DEFINITION

In contrast to viral meningitis, where the infectious process and associated inflammatory response are limited largely to the meninges, in encephalitis the brain parenchyma is also involved. Many patients with encephalitis also have evidence of associated meningitis (meningoencephalitis) and, in some cases, involvement of the spinal cord or nerve roots (encephalomyelitis, encephalomyeloradiculitis).

CLINICAL MANIFESTATIONS

In addition to the acute febrile illness with evidence of meningeal involvement characteristic of meningitis, the patient with encephalitis commonly has an altered level of consciousness (confusion, behavioral abnormalities) or a depressed level of consciousness, ranging from mild lethargy to coma, and evidence of either focal or diffuse neurologic signs and symptoms. Patients with encephalitis may have hallucinations, agitation, personality change, behavioral disorders, and, at times, a frankly psychotic state. Focal or generalized seizures occur in many patients with encephalitis. Virtually every possible type of focal neurologic disturbance has been reported in viral encephalitis; the signs and symptoms reflect the sites of infection and inflammation. The most commonly encountered focal findings are aphasia, ataxia, upper or lower motor neuron patterns of weakness, involuntary movements (e.g., myoclonic jerks, tremor), and cranial nerve deficits (e.g., ocular palsies, facial weakness). Involvement of the hypothalamic-pituitary axis may result in temperature dysregulation, diabetes insipidus, or the development of the syndrome of inappropriate secretion of antidiuretic hormone (SIADH). Despite the clear neuropathologic evidence that viruses differ in the regions of the CNS they injure, it is often impossible to distinguish reliably on clinical grounds alone one type of viral encephalitis (e.g., that caused by HSV) from others (see "Differential Diagnosis" later in the chapter).

ETIOLOGY

In the United States, there are ~20,000 reported cases of encephalitis per year, although the actual number of cases is likely to be significantly larger. Hundreds of viruses are capable of causing encephalitis, although only a limited subset is responsible for most cases in which a specific cause is identified (Table 29-4). The same organisms responsible for aseptic meningitis are also responsible for encephalitis, although the relative frequencies with which specific organisms cause these two patterns of infection often differ. The most important viruses causing sporadic cases of encephalitis in immunocompetent adults are herpesviruses (HSV, VZV, EBV). Epidemics of encephalitis are caused by arboviruses, which belong to several different viral taxonomic groups including *Alphaviruses* (e.g., EEE virus, western equine encephalitis virus), *Flaviviruses* (e.g., WNV, St. Louis encephalitis virus, Japanese encephalitis virus, Powassan virus), and *Bunyaviruses* (e.g., California encephalitis virus serogroup, LaCrosse virus). Historically, the largest number of cases of arbovirus encephalitis in the United States has been due to St. Louis encephalitis virus and the California encephalitis virus serogroup. However, since 2002, WNV has been responsible for the majority of arbovirus meningitis and encephalitis cases in the United States. The 2003 epidemic was the largest epidemic of arboviral neuroinvasive disease (encephalitis + meningitis) ever recorded in the United States, with 2860 cases and 264 deaths. Since 2003, WNV has accounted for ~1100–1300 cases of neuroinvasive disease per year and 100–120 deaths in the United States. New causes of viral CNS infections are constantly appearing, as evidenced by the recent outbreak of cases of encephalitis in Southeast Asia caused by Nipah virus, a newly identified member of the Paramyxovirus family, and of meningitis in Europe caused by Toscana virus, an arbovirus belonging to the Bunyavirus family.

LABORATORY DIAGNOSIS

CSF Examination

CSF examination should be performed in all patients with suspected viral encephalitis unless contraindicated by the presence of severely increased ICP. The characteristic CSF profile is indistinguishable from that of viral meningitis and typically consists of a lymphocytic pleocytosis, a mildly elevated protein concentration, and a normal glucose concentration. A CSF pleocytosis (>5 cells/μL) occurs in >95% of patients with documented viral encephalitis. In rare cases, a pleocytosis may be absent on the initial LP but present on subsequent LPs. Patients who are severely immunocompromised by HIV infection, glucocorticoid or other immunosuppressant drugs, chemotherapy, or lymphoreticular malignancies may fail to mount a CSF inflammatory response. CSF cell counts exceed 500/μL in only about 10% of patients with encephalitis. Infections with certain arboviruses (e.g., EEE virus or California encephalitis virus), mumps, and LCMV may occasionally result in cell counts >1000/μL, but this degree of pleocytosis should suggest the possibility of nonviral infections or other inflammatory processes. Atypical lymphocytes in the CSF may be seen in EBV infection and less commonly with other viruses, including CMV, HSV, and enteroviruses. Increased numbers of plasmacytoid or Mollaret-like large mononuclear cells have been reported in WNV encephalitis. Polymorphonuclear pleocytosis occurs in ~40% of patients with WNV encephalitis. Large numbers of CSF PMNs may be present in patients with encephalitis due to EEE virus, echovirus 9, and, more rarely, other enteroviruses. However, persisting CSF neutrophilia should prompt consideration of bacterial infection, leptospirosis, amebic infection, and noninfectious processes such as acute hemorrhagic leukoencephalitis. About 20% of patients with encephalitis will have a significant number of red blood cells (>500/μL) in the CSF in a nontraumatic tap. The pathologic correlate of this finding may be a hemorrhagic encephalitis of the type seen with HSV; however, CSF red blood cells occur with similar frequency and in similar numbers in patients with nonherpetic focal encephalitides. A decreased CSF glucose concentration is distinctly unusual in viral encephalitis and should suggest the possibility of bacterial, fungal, tuberculous, parasitic, leptospiral, syphilitic, sarcoid, or neoplastic meningitis. Rare patients with mumps, LCMV, or advanced HSV encephalitis may have low CSF glucose concentrations.

CSF PCR

CSF PCR has become the primary diagnostic test for CNS infections caused by CMV, EBV, VZV, HHV-6, and enteroviruses (see "Viral Meningitis" earlier in the chapter). The sensitivity and specificity of CSF PCRs varies with the virus being tested. The sensitivity (~96%) and specificity (~99%) of HSV CSF PCR is equivalent to or exceeds that of brain biopsy. It is important to recognize that HSV CSF PCR results need to be interpreted after considering the likelihood of disease in the patient being tested, the timing of the test in relationship to onset of symptoms, and the prior use of antiviral therapy. A negative HSV CSF PCR test performed by a qualified laboratory at the appropriate time during illness in a patient with a high likelihood of HSV encephalitis based on clinical and laboratory abnormalities significantly reduces the likelihood of HSV encephalitis, but does not exclude it. For example, in a patient with a pretest probability of 35% of having HSV encephalitis, a negative HSV CSF PCR reduces the posttest probability to ~2%, and for a patient with a pretest probability of 60%, a negative test reduces the posttest probability to ~6%. In both situations, a positive test makes the diagnosis almost certain (98–99%). There have been several recent reports of initially negative HSV CSF PCR tests that were obtained early (≤72 h) after symptom onset and that became positive when repeated 1–3 days later. The frequency of positive HSV CSF PCRs in patients with herpes encephalitis also decreases as a function of the duration of illness, with only ~20% of cases remaining positive after ≥14 days. PCR results are generally not affected by ≤1 week of antiviral therapy. In one study, 98% of CSF specimens remained PCR-positive during the first week of initiation of antiviral therapy, but the numbers fell to ~50% by 8–14 days and to ~21% by >15 days after initiation of antiviral therapy.

The sensitivity and specificity of CSF PCR tests for viruses other than herpes simplex have not been definitively characterized. Enteroviral CSF PCR appears to have a sensitivity and specificity of >95%. The specificity of EBV CSF PCR has not been established. Positive EBV CSF PCRs associated with positive tests for other pathogens have been reported and may reflect reactivation of EBV latent in lymphocytes that enter the CNS as a result of an unrelated infectious or inflammatory process. In patients with CNS infection due to VZV, CSF antibody and PCR studies should be considered complementary, as patients may have evidence of intrathecal synthesis of VZV-specific antibodies and negative CSF PCRs. In the case of WNV infection, CSF PCR appears to be less sensitive (~70% sensitivity) than detection of WNV-specific CSF IgM, although PCR testing remains useful in immunocompromised patients who may not mount an effective anti-WNV antibody response.

CSF Culture

Attempts to culture viruses from the CSF in cases of encephalitis are often disappointing. Cultures are negative in >95% of cases of HSV-1 encephalitis.

Serologic Studies and Antigen Detection

The basic approach to the serodiagnosis of viral encephalitis is identical to that discussed earlier for viral meningitis. In patients with HSV encephalitis, both antibodies to HSV-1 glycoproteins and glycoprotein antigens have been detected in the CSF. Optimal detection of both HSV antibodies and antigen typically occurs after the first week of illness, limiting the utility of these tests in acute diagnosis. Nonetheless, HSV CSF antibody testing is of value in selected patients whose illness is >1 week in duration and who are CSF PCR–negative for HSV. Demonstration of WNV IgM antibodies is diagnostic of WNV encephalitis as IgM antibodies do not cross the blood-brain barrier, and their presence in CSF is therefore indicative of intrathecal synthesis. Timing of antibody collection may be important, as the rate of CSF WNV IgM seropositivity increases by ~10% per day during the first week after illness onset.

MRI, CT, EEG

Patients with suspected encephalitis almost invariably undergo neuroimaging studies and often EEG. These tests help identify or exclude alternative diagnoses and assist in the differentiation between a focal, as opposed to a diffuse, encephalitic process. Focal findings in a patient with encephalitis should always raise the possibility of HSV encephalitis. Examples of focal findings include: (1) areas of increased signal intensity in the frontotemporal, cingulate, or insular regions of the brain on T2-weighted, FLAIR, or diffusion-weighted MRI images (Fig. 29-3); (2) focal areas of low absorption, mass effect, and contrast enhancement on CT; or (3) periodic focal temporal lobe spikes on a background of slow or low-amplitude ("flattened") activity on EEG. Approximately 10% of patients with PCR-documented HSV encephalitis will have a normal MRI, although nearly 80% will have abnormalities in the temporal lobe, and an additional 10% in extratemporal regions. The lesions are typically hyperintense on T2-weighted images. CT is less sensitive than MRI and is normal in up to 33% of patients. The addition of FLAIR and diffusion-weighted images to the standard MRI sequences enhances sensitivity. EEG abnormalities occur in >90% of PCR-documented cases of HSV encephalitis; they typically involve the temporal lobes but are often nonspecific. Some patients with HSV encephalitis have a distinctive EEG pattern consisting of periodic, stereotyped, sharp-and-slow complexes originating in one or both temporal lobes and repeating at regular intervals of 2–3 s. The periodic complexes are typically noted between the 2nd and 15th day of the illness and are present in two-thirds of pathologically proven cases of HSV encephalitis.

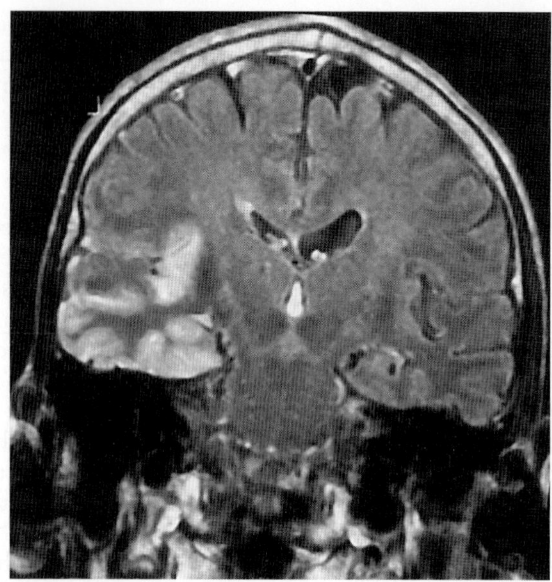

FIGURE 29-3
Coronal FLAIR magnetic resonance image from a patient with herpes simplex encephalitis. Note the area of increased signal in the right temporal lobe (left side of image) confined predominantly to the gray matter. This patient had predominantly unilateral disease; bilateral lesions are more common but may be quite asymmetric in their intensity.

Significant MRI abnormalities are found in only ~50% of patients with WNV encephalitis, a frequency less than that of patients with HSV encephalitis. When present, abnormalities often involve deep brain structures, including the thalamus, basal ganglia, and brainstem, rather than the cortex and may only be apparent on FLAIR images. EEGs typically show generalized slowing that may be more anteriorly prominent rather than the temporally predominant pattern of sharp or periodic discharges more characteristic of HSV encephalitis. Patients with VZV encephalitis may show multifocal areas of hemorrhagic and ischemic infarction reflecting the tendency of this virus to produce a CNS vasculopathy rather than a true encephalitis. Immunocompromised adult patients with CMV often have enlarged ventricles with areas of increased T2 signal on MRI outlining the ventricles and sub-ependymal enhancement on T1-weighted postcontrast images. Table 29-5 highlights specific diagnostic test results in encephalitis that can be useful in clinical decision making.

Brain Biopsy

Brain biopsy is now generally reserved for patients in whom CSF PCR studies fail to lead to a specific diagnosis, who have focal abnormalities on MRI, and who continue to show progressive clinical deterioration despite treatment with acyclovir and supportive therapy.

TABLE 29-5

USE OF DIAGNOSTIC TESTS IN ENCEPHALITIS

The best test for WNV encephalitis is the *CSF IgM antibody test*. The prevalence of positive CSF IgM tests increases by about 10%/day after illness onset and reaches 70–80% by the end of the first week. Serum WNV IgM can provide evidence for recent WNV infection, but in the absence of other findings does not establish the diagnosis of neuroinvasive disease (meningitis, encephalitis, acute flaccid paralysis).

Approximately 80% of patients with proven HSV encephalitis have *MRI* abnormalities involving the temporal lobes. This percentage likely increases to >90% when FLAIR and DWI MR sequences are also utilized. The absence of temporal lobe lesions on MR reduces the likelihood of HSV encephalitis and should prompt consideration of other diagnostic possibilities.

The *CSF HSV PCR* test may be negative in the first 72 h of symptoms of HSV encephalitis. A repeat study should be considered in patients with an initial early negative PCR in whom diagnostic suspicion of HSV encephalitis remains high and no alternative diagnosis has yet been established.

Detection of *intrathecal synthesis* (increased CSF/serum HSV antibody ratio corrected for breakdown of the blood-brain barrier) of *HSV-specific antibody* may be useful in diagnosis of HSV encephalitis in patients in whom only late (>1 week post-onset) CSF specimens are available and PCR studies are negative. Serum serology alone is of no value in diagnosis of HSV encephalitis due to the high seroprevalence rate in the general population.

Negative *CSF viral cultures* are of no value in excluding the diagnosis of HSV or EBV encephalitis.

VZV CSF IgM antibodies may be present in patients with a negative VZV CSF PCR. Both tests should be performed in patients with suspected VZV CNS disease.

The specificity of *EBV CSF PCR* for diagnosis of CNS infection is unknown. Positive tests may occur in patients with a CSF pleocytosis due to other causes. Detection of EBV CSF IgM or intrathecal synthesis of antibody to VCA supports the diagnosis of EBV encephalitis. Serological studies consistent with acute EBV infection (e.g., IgM VCA, presence of antibodies against EA but not against EBNA) can help support the diagnosis.

Note: CSF, cerebrospinal fluid; IgM, immunoglobulin M; WNV, West Nile virus; HSV, herpes simplex virus; MRI, magnetic resonance imaging; FLAIR, fluid attenuated inversion recovery; DWI, diffusion-weighted imaging; PCR, polymerase chain reaction; EBV, Epstein-Barr virus; VZV, varicella-zoster virus; CNS, central nervous system; VCA, viral capsid antibody; EA, early antigen; EBNA, EBV-associated nuclear antigen.

DIFFERENTIAL DIAGNOSIS

Infection by a variety of other organisms can mimic viral encephalitis. In studies of biopsy-proven HSV encephalitis, common infectious mimics of focal viral encephalitis included mycobacteria, fungi, rickettsia, *Listeria* and other bacteria (including *Bartonella* sp.), and *Mycoplasma*.

Infection caused by the ameba *Naegleria fowleri* can also cause acute meningoencephalitis (primary amebic meningoencephalitis), whereas that caused by *Acanthamoeba* and *Balamuthia* more typically produces subacute or chronic granulomatous amebic meningoencephalitis. *Naegleria* thrive in warm, iron-rich pools of water, including those found in drains, canals, and both natural and human-made outdoor pools. Infection has typically occurred in immunocompetent children with a history of swimming in potentially infected water. The CSF, in contrast to the typical profile seen in viral encephalitis, often resembles that of bacterial meningitis with a neutrophilic pleocytosis and hypoglycorrhachia. Motile trophozoites can be seen in a wet mount of warm, fresh CSF. No effective treatment has been identified, and mortality approaches 100%.

Encephalitis can be caused by the raccoon pinworm *Baylisascaris procyonis*. Clues to the diagnosis include a history of raccoon exposure and especially of playing in or eating dirt potentially contaminated with raccoon feces. Most patients are children, and many have an associated eosinophilia.

Once nonviral causes of encephalitis have been excluded, the major diagnostic challenge is to distinguish HSV from other viruses that cause encephalitis. This distinction is particularly important because in virtually every other instance the therapy is supportive, whereas specific and effective antiviral therapy is available for HSV, and its efficacy is enhanced when it is instituted early in the course of infection. HSV encephalitis should be considered when clinical features suggesting involvement of the inferomedial frontotemporal regions of the brain are present, including prominent olfactory or gustatory hallucinations, anosmia, unusual or bizarre behavior or personality alterations, or memory disturbance. HSV encephalitis should always be suspected in patients with focal findings on clinical examination, neuroimaging studies, or EEG. The diagnostic procedure of choice in these patients is CSF PCR analysis for HSV. A positive CSF PCR establishes the diagnosis, and a negative test dramatically reduces the likelihood of HSV encephalitis (see above).

The anatomic distribution of lesions may provide an additional clue to diagnosis. Patients with rapidly progressive encephalitis and prominent brainstem signs, symptoms, or neuroimaging abnormalities may be infected by flaviviruses (WNV, St. Louis encephalitis virus, Japanese encephalitis virus), HSV, rabies, or *L. monocytogenes*. Significant involvement of deep gray matter structures, including the basal ganglia and thalamus, should also suggest possible flavivirus infection. These patients may present clinically with prominent movement disorders (tremor, myoclonus) or parkinsonian features. Patients with WNV infection can also present with a poliomyelitis-like acute flaccid paralysis, as can patients infected with enterovirus 71 and, less commonly, other enteroviruses. Acute flaccid paralysis is characterized by the acute onset of a lower motor neuron type of weakness with flaccid tone, reduced or absent reflexes, and relatively preserved sensation. Despite an aggressive World Health Organization poliovirus eradication initiative, >1200 cases of wild-type poliovirus-induced poliomyelitis have been reported worldwide in 2006, with 88% occurring in Nigeria and India and >20 cases each from Somalia, Afghanistan, and Namibia. There have been recent small outbreaks of poliomyelitis associated with vaccine strains of virus that have reverted to virulence through mutation or recombination with circulating wild-type enteroviruses in Hispaniola, China, the Philippines, and Madagascar.

Epidemiologic factors may provide important clues to the diagnosis of viral meningitis or encephalitis. Particular attention should be paid to the season of the year, the geographic location and travel history, and possible exposure to animal bites or scratches, rodents, and ticks. Although transmission from the bite of an infected dog remains the most common cause of rabies worldwide, in the United States very few cases of dog rabies occur, and the most common risk factor is exposure to bats—although a clear history of a bite or scratch is often lacking. The classic clinical presentation of encephalitic (furious) rabies is of fever, fluctuating consciousness, and autonomic hyperactivity. Phobic spasms of the larynx, pharynx, neck muscles, and diaphragm can be triggered by attempts to swallow water (*hydrophobia*) or by inspiration (*aerophobia*). Patients may also present with paralytic (dumb) rabies characterized by acute ascending paralysis. Rabies due to the bite of a bat has a different clinical presentation than classic rabies. Patients present with focal neurologic deficits, myoclonus, seizures, and hallucinations; phobic spasms are not a typical feature. Patients with rabies have a CSF lymphocytic pleocytosis and may show areas of increased T2 signal abnormality in the brainstem, hippocampus, and hypothalamus. Diagnosis can be made by finding rabies virus antigen in brain tissue or in the neural innervation of hair follicles at the nape of the neck. PCR amplification of viral nucleic acid from CSF and saliva or tears may also enable diagnosis. Serology is frequently negative in both serum and CSF in the first week after onset of infection, which limits its acute diagnostic utility. No specific therapy is available, and cases are almost invariably fatal, with isolated survivors having devastating neurologic sequelae.

State public health authorities provide a valuable resource concerning isolation of particular agents in individual regions. Regular updates concerning the number, type, and distribution of cases of arboviral encephalitis can be found on the CDC and U.S. Geological Survey (USGS) websites (*http://www.cdc.gov* and *http://diseasemaps.usgs.gov*).

The major noninfectious etiologies that should be included in the differential diagnosis of acute encephalitis are nonvasculitic autoimmune meningoencephalitis, which may or may not be associated with serum antithyroid microsomal and antithyroglobulin antibodies; limbic encephalitis associated with antineuronal antibodies; limbic encephalopathy not associated with cancer; acute disseminated encephalomyelitis and related fulminant demyelinating disorders; and lymphoma. Finally, Creutzfeldt-Jakob disease (Chap. 101) can rarely present in an explosive fashion mimicking viral encephalitis.

℞ Treatment: VIRAL ENCEPHALITIS

Specific antiviral therapy should be initiated when appropriate. Vital functions, including respiration and blood pressure, should be monitored continuously and supported as required. In the initial stages of encephalitis, many patients will require care in an intensive care unit. Basic management and supportive therapy should include careful monitoring of ICP, fluid restriction, avoidance of hypotonic intravenous solutions, and suppression of fever. Seizures should be treated with standard anticonvulsant regimens, and prophylactic therapy should be considered in view of the high frequency of seizures in severe cases of encephalitis. As with all seriously ill, immobilized patients with altered levels of consciousness, encephalitis patients are at risk for aspiration pneumonia, stasis ulcers and decubiti, contractures, deep venous thrombosis and its complications, and infections of indwelling lines and catheters.

Acyclovir is of benefit in the treatment of HSV and should be started empirically in patients with suspected viral encephalitis, especially if focal features are present, while awaiting viral diagnostic studies. Treatment should be discontinued in patients found not to have HSV encephalitis, with the possible exception of patients with severe encephalitis due to VZV or EBV. HSV, VZV, and EBV all encode an enzyme, deoxypyrimidine (thymidine) kinase, that phosphorylates acyclovir to produce acyclovir-5′-monophosphate. Host cell enzymes then phosphorylate this compound to form a triphosphate derivative. It is the triphosphate that acts as an antiviral agent by inhibiting viral DNA polymerase and by causing premature termination of nascent viral DNA chains. The specificity of action depends on the fact that uninfected cells do not phosphorylate significant amounts of acyclovir to acyclovir-5′-monophosphate. A second level of specificity is provided by the fact that the acyclovir triphosphate is a more potent inhibitor of viral DNA polymerase than of the analogous host cell enzymes.

Adults should receive a dose of 10 mg/kg of acyclovir intravenously every 8 h (30 mg/kg per day total dose) for a minimum of 14 days. CSF PCR can be repeated at the completion of the 14-day course, with PCR-positive patients receiving an additional 7 days of treatment, followed by a repeat CSF PCR test. Neonatal HSV CNS infection is less responsive to acyclovir therapy than HSV encephalitis in adults; it is recommended that neonates with HSV encephalitis receive 20 mg/kg of acyclovir every 8 h (60 mg/kg per day total dose) for a minimum of 21 days.

Before intravenous administration, acyclovir should be diluted to a concentration ≤7 mg/mL. (A 70-kg person would receive a dose of 700 mg, which would be diluted in a volume of 100 mL.) Each dose should be infused slowly over 1 h rather than by rapid or bolus infusion, to minimize the risk of renal dysfunction. Care should be taken to avoid extravasation or intramuscular or subcutaneous administration. The alkaline pH of acyclovir can cause local inflammation and phlebitis (9%). Dose adjustment is required in patients with impaired renal glomerular filtration. Penetration into CSF is excellent, with average drug levels ~50% of serum levels. Complications of therapy include elevations in blood urea nitrogen and creatinine levels (5%), thrombocytopenia (6%), gastrointestinal toxicity (nausea, vomiting, diarrhea) (7%), and neurotoxicity (lethargy or obtundation, disorientation, confusion, agitation, hallucinations, tremors, seizures) (1%). Acyclovir resistance may be mediated by changes in either the viral deoxypyrimidine kinase or DNA polymerase. To date, acyclovir-resistant isolates have not been a significant clinical problem in immunocompetent individuals. However, there have been reports of clinically virulent acyclovir-resistant HSV isolates from sites outside the CNS in immunocompromised individuals, including those with AIDS.

Oral antiviral drugs with efficacy against HSV, VZV, and EBV, including acyclovir, famciclovir, and valacyclovir, have not been evaluated in the treatment of encephalitis either as primary therapy or as supplemental therapy after completion of a course of parenteral acyclovir. A National Institute of Allergy and Infectious Disease (NIAID)/National Institute of Neurological Disorders and Stroke–sponsored phase III trial of supplemental oral valacyclovir therapy (2 g tid for 3 months) after the initial 14- to 21-day course of therapy with parenteral acyclovir is ongoing in patients with HSV encephalitis; this may help clarify the role of extended oral antiviral therapy.

Ganciclovir and foscarnet, either alone or in combination, are often utilized in the treatment of CMV-related CNS infections, although their efficacy remains unproven. Cidofovir (see below) may provide an alternative in patients who fail to respond to ganciclovir and foscarnet, although data concerning its use in CMV CNS infections is extremely limited.

Ganciclovir is a synthetic nucleoside analogue of 2′-deoxyguanosine. The drug is preferentially phosphorylated by virus-induced cellular kinases. Ganciclovir triphosphate acts as a competitive inhibitor of the CMV DNA polymerase, and its incorporation into nascent viral DNA results in premature chain termination. After intravenous administration, CSF concentrations of ganciclovir are 25–70% of coincident plasma levels. The usual dose for treatment of severe neurologic illnesses is 5 mg/kg every 12 h given intravenously at a constant rate over 1 h. Induction therapy is followed by maintenance therapy of 5 mg/kg every day for an indefinite period. Induction therapy should be continued until patients show a decline in CSF pleocytosis and a reduction in CSF CMV DNA copy number on quantitative PCR testing (where available). Doses should be adjusted in patients with renal insufficiency. Treatment is often limited by the development of granulocytopenia and thrombocytopenia (20–25%), which may require reduction in or discontinuation of therapy. Gastrointestinal side effects, including nausea, vomiting, diarrhea, and abdominal pain, occur in ~20% of patients. Some patients treated with ganciclovir for CMV retinitis have developed retinal detachment, but the causal relationship to ganciclovir treatment is unclear. Valganciclovir is an orally bioavailable prodrug that can generate high serum levels of ganciclovir, although studies of its efficacy in treating CMV CNS infections are limited.

Foscarnet is a pyrophosphate analogue that inhibits viral DNA polymerases by binding to the pyrophosphate-binding site. After intravenous infusion, CSF concentrations range from 15 to 100% of coincident plasma levels. The usual dose for serious CMV-related neurologic illness is 60 mg/kg every 8 h administered by constant infusion over 1 h. Induction therapy for 14–21 days is followed by maintenance therapy (60–120 mg/kg per day). Induction therapy may need to be extended in patients who fail to show a decline in CSF pleocytosis and a reduction in CSF CMV DNA copy number on quantitative PCR tests (where available). Approximately one-third of patients develop renal impairment during treatment, which is reversible after discontinuation of therapy in most, but not all, cases. This is often associated with elevations in serum creatinine and proteinuria and is less frequent in patients who are adequately hydrated. Many patients experience fatigue and nausea. Reduction in serum calcium, magnesium, and potassium occur in ~15% of patients and may be associated with tetany, cardiac rhythm disturbances, or seizures.

Cidofovir is a nucleotide analogue that is effective in treating CMV retinitis and equivalent or better than ganciclovir in some experimental models of murine CMV encephalitis, although data concerning its efficacy in human CMV CNS disease are limited. The usual dose is 5 mg/kg intravenously once weekly for 2 weeks, then biweekly for two or more additional doses, depending on clinical response. Patients must be prehydrated with normal saline (e.g., 1 L over 1–2 h) before each dose and treated with probenecid (e.g., 1 g 3 h before cidofovir and 1 g 2 and 8 h after cidofovir). Nephrotoxicity is common; the dose should be reduced if renal function deteriorates.

Intravenous ribavirin (15–25 mg/kg per day in divided doses given every 8 h) has been reported to be of benefit in isolated cases of severe encephalitis due to California encephalitis (LaCrosse) virus. Ribavirin might be of benefit for the rare patients, typically infants or young children, with severe adenovirus or rotavirus encephalitis and in patients with encephalitis due to LCMV or other arenaviruses. However, clinical trials are lacking. Hemolysis, with resulting anemia, has been the major side effect limiting therapy.

No specific antiviral therapy of proven efficacy is currently available for treatment of WNV encephalitis. Patients have been treated with α-interferon, ribavirin, WNV-specific antisense oligonucleotides, and an Israeli IVIg preparation that contains high-titer anti-WNV antibody (Omr-IgG-am). WNV chimeric vaccines, in which WNV envelope and premembrane proteins are inserted into the background of another flavivirus, are already undergoing human clinical testing for safety and immunogenicity. Both chimeric and killed inactivated WNV vaccines have been found to be safe and effective in preventing equine WNV infection, and several effective flavivirus vaccines are already in human use, creating optimism that a safe and effective human WNV vaccine can also be developed.

SEQUELAE

There is considerable variation in the incidence and severity of sequelae in patients surviving viral encephalitis. In the case of EEE virus infection, nearly 80% of survivors have severe neurologic sequelae. At the other extreme are infections due to EBV, California encephalitis virus, and Venezuelan equine encephalitis virus, where severe sequelae are unusual. For example, approximately 5–15% of children infected with LaCrosse virus have a residual seizure disorder, and 1% have persistent hemiparesis. Detailed information about sequelae in patients with HSV encephalitis treated with acyclovir is available from the NIAID-CASG trials. Of 32 acyclovir-treated patients, 26 survived (81%). Of the 26 survivors, 12 (46%) had no or only minor sequelae, 3 (12%) were moderately impaired (gainfully employed but not functioning at their previous level), and 11 (42%) were severely impaired (requiring continuous supportive care). The incidence and severity of sequelae were directly related to the age of the patient and the level of consciousness at the time of initiation of therapy. Patients with severe neurologic impairment (Glasgow coma score 6) at initiation of therapy either died or survived with severe sequelae. Young patients (<30 years) with good neurologic function at initiation of therapy did substantially better (100% survival, 62% with no or mild sequelae) compared with their older counterparts (>30 years; 64% survival, 57% no or mild sequelae). Some recent studies using quantitative HSV CSF PCR tests indicate that clinical outcome after treatment also correlates with the amount of HSV DNA present in CSF at the time of presentation. Many patients with WNV infection have acute sequelae, including cognitive impairment; weakness; and hyper- or hypokinetic movement disorders, including tremor, myoclonus, and parkinsonism. Improvement in these symptoms may occur over the subsequent 6–12 months, although detailed clinical studies of the duration and severity of WNV sequelae are not yet available.

SUBACUTE MENINGITIS

CLINICAL MANIFESTATIONS

Patients with subacute meningitis typically have an unrelenting headache, stiff neck, low-grade fever, and lethargy for days to several weeks before they present for evaluation. Cranial nerve abnormalities and night sweats may be present. This syndrome overlaps that of chronic meningitis, discussed in detail in Chap. 30.

ETIOLOGY

Common causative organisms include *M. tuberculosis*, *C. neoformans*, *H. capsulatum*, *C. immitis*, and *T. pallidum*. Initial infection with *M. tuberculosis* is acquired by inhalation of aerosolized droplet nuclei. Tuberculous meningitis in adults does not develop acutely from hematogenous spread of tubercle bacilli to the meninges. Rather, millet seed–size (miliary) tubercles form in the parenchyma of the brain during hematogenous dissemination of tubercle bacilli in the course of primary infection. These tubercles enlarge and are usually caseating. The propensity for a caseous lesion to produce meningitis is determined by its proximity to the subarachnoid space (SAS) and the rate at which fibrous encapsulation develops. Subependymal caseous foci cause meningitis via discharge of bacilli and tuberculous antigens into the SAS. Mycobacterial antigens produce an intense inflammatory reaction that leads to the production of a thick exudate that fills the basilar cisterns and surrounds the cranial nerves and major blood vessels at the base of the brain.

Fungal infections are typically acquired by the inhalation of airborne fungal spores. The initial pulmonary infection may be asymptomatic or present with fever, cough, sputum production, and chest pain. The pulmonary infection is often self-limited. A localized pulmonary fungal infection can then remain dormant in the lungs until there is an abnormality in cell-mediated immunity that allows the fungus to reactivate and disseminate to the CNS. The most common pathogen causing fungal meningitis is *C. neoformans*. This fungus is found worldwide in soil and bird excreta. *H. capsulatum* is endemic to the Ohio and Mississippi River valleys of the central United States and to parts of Central and South America. *C. immitis* is endemic to the desert areas of the southwest United States, northern Mexico, and Argentina.

Syphilis is a sexually transmitted disease that is manifest by the appearance of a painless chancre at the site of inoculation. *T. pallidum* invades the CNS early in the course of syphilis. Cranial nerves VII and VIII are most frequently involved.

LABORATORY DIAGNOSIS

The classic CSF abnormalities in tuberculous meningitis are as follows: (1) elevated opening pressure, (2) lymphocytic pleocytosis (10–500 cells/μL), (3) elevated protein concentration in the range of 1–5 g/L (10–500 mg/dL), and (4) decreased glucose concentration in the range of 1.1–2.2 mmol/L (20–40 mg/dL). *The combination of unrelenting headache, stiff neck, fatigue, night sweats, and fever with a CSF lymphocytic pleocytosis and a mildly decreased glucose concentration is highly suspicious for tuberculous meningitis.* The last tube of fluid collected at LP is the best tube to send for a smear for acid-fast bacilli (AFB). If there is a pellicle in the CSF or a cobweb-like clot on the surface of the fluid, AFB can best be demonstrated in a smear of the clot or pellicle. Positive smears are typically reported in only 10–40% of cases of tuberculous meningitis in adults. Cultures of CSF take 4–8 weeks to identify the organism and are positive in ~50% of adults. Culture remains the "gold standard" to make the diagnosis of tuberculous meningitis. PCR for the detection of *M. tuberculosis* DNA has a sensitivity of 70–80% but is limited at the present time by a high rate of false-positive results.

The characteristic CSF abnormalities in fungal meningitis are a mononuclear or lymphocytic pleocytosis, an increased protein concentration, and a decreased glucose concentration. There may be eosinophils in the CSF in *C. immitis* meningitis. Large volumes of CSF are often required to demonstrate the organism on India ink smear or grow the organism in culture. If spinal fluid examined by LP on two separate occasions fails to yield an organism, CSF should be obtained by high-cervical or cisternal puncture.

The cryptococcal polysaccharide antigen test is a highly sensitive and specific test for cryptococcal meningitis. A reactive CSF cryptococcal antigen test establishes the diagnosis. The detection of the histoplasma polysaccharide antigen in CSF establishes the diagnosis of a fungal meningitis but is not specific for meningitis due to *H. capsulatum*. It may be falsely positive in coccidioidal meningitis. The CSF complement fixation antibody test is reported to have a specificity of 100% and a sensitivity of 75% for coccidioidal meningitis.

The diagnosis of syphilitic meningitis is made when a reactive serum treponemal test [fluorescent treponemal antibody absorption test (FTA-ABS) or microhemagglutination-*T. pallidum* (MHA-TP)] is associated with a CSF lymphocytic or mononuclear pleocytosis and an elevated protein concentration, or when the CSF VDRL (Venereal Disease Research Laboratory) is positive. A reactive CSF FTA-ABS is not definitive evidence of neurosyphilis. The CSF FTA-ABS can be falsely positive from blood contamination. A negative CSF VDRL does not rule out neurosyphilis. A negative CSF FTA-ABS or MHA-TP rules out neurosyphilis.

℞ Treatment: SUBACUTE MENINGITIS

Empirical therapy of tuberculous meningitis is often initiated on the basis of a high index of suspicion without adequate laboratory support. Initial therapy is a combination of isoniazid (300 mg/d), rifampin (10 mg/kg per day), pyrazinamide (30 mg/kg per day in divided doses), ethambutol (15–25 mg/kg per day in divided doses), and pyridoxine (50 mg/d). If the clinical response is good, pyrazinamide and ethambutol can be discontinued after 8 weeks and isoniazid and rifampin continued alone for the next 6–12 months. A 6-month course of therapy is acceptable, but therapy should be prolonged for 9–12 months in patients who have an inadequate resolution of symptoms of meningitis or who have positive mycobacterial cultures of CSF during the course of therapy. Dexamethasone therapy is recommended for patients who develop hydrocephalus.

Meningitis due to *C. neoformans* is treated with amphotericin B (0.7 mg/kg IV per day) or AmBisome (5 mg/kg per day), plus flucytosine (100 mg/kg per day in four divided doses) for 2 weeks or until CSF culture is sterile. This treatment is followed by an 8–10-week course of fluconazole (400–800 mg/d PO). If the CSF culture is sterile after 10 weeks of acute therapy, the dose of fluconazole is decreased to 200 mg/d for 6 months to a year. Patients with HIV infection may require indefinite maintenance therapy. Meningitis due to *H. capsulatum* is treated with amphotericin B (0.7–1.0 mg/kg per day) for 4–12 weeks. A total dose of 30 mg/kg is recommended. Therapy with amphotericin B is not discontinued until fungal cultures are sterile. After completing a course of amphotericin B, maintenance therapy with itraconazole 200 mg twice daily is initiated and continued for at least 6 months to a year. *C. immitis* meningitis is treated with either high-dose fluconazole (1000 mg daily) as monotherapy or intravenous amphotericin B (0.5–0.7 mg/kg per day) for >4 weeks. Intrathecal amphotericin B (0.25–0.75 mg/d three times weekly) may be required to eradicate the infection. Lifelong therapy with fluconazole (200–400 mg daily) is recommended to prevent relapse. AmBisome (5 mg/kg per day) or amphotericin B lipid complex (5 mg/kg per day) can be substituted for amphotericin B in patients who have or who develop significant renal dysfunction. The most common complication of fungal meningitis is hydrocephalus. Patients who develop hydrocephalus should receive a CSF diversion device. A ventriculostomy can be used until CSF fungal cultures are sterile, at which time the ventriculostomy is replaced by a ventriculoperitoneal shunt.

Syphilitic meningitis is treated with aqueous penicillin G in a dose of 3–4 million units intravenously every 4 h for 10–14 days. An alternative regimen is 2.4 million units of procaine penicillin G intramuscularly daily with 500 mg of oral probenecid four times daily for 10–14 days. Either regimen is followed with 2.4 million units of benzathine penicillin G intramuscularly once a week for 3 weeks. The standard criterion for treatment success is reexamination of the CSF. The CSF should be reexamined at 6-month intervals for 2 years. The cell count is expected to normalize within 12 months, and the VDRL titer to decrease by two dilutions or revert to nonreactive within 2 years of completion of therapy. Failure of the CSF pleocytosis to resolve or an increase in the CSF VDRL titer by two or more dilutions requires retreatment.

CHRONIC ENCEPHALITIS

PROGRESSIVE MULTIFOCAL LEUKOENCEPHALOPATHY

Clinical Features and Pathology

Progressive multifocal leukoencephalopathy (PML) is a progressive disorder characterized pathologically by multifocal areas of demyelination of varying size distributed throughout the brain but sparing the spinal cord and optic nerves. In addition to demyelination, there are characteristic cytologic alterations in both astrocytes and oligodendrocytes. Astrocytes are enlarged and contain hyperchromatic, deformed, and bizarre nuclei and frequent mitotic figures. Oligodendrocytes have enlarged, densely staining nuclei that contain viral inclusions formed by crystalline arrays of JC virus (JCV) particles. Patients often present with visual deficits (45%), typically a homonymous hemianopia; mental impairment (38%) (dementia, confusion, personality change); weakness, including hemi- or monoparesis; and ataxia. Seizures occur in ~20% of patients, predominantly in those with lesions abutting the cortex.

Almost all patients have an underlying immunosuppressive disorder. In recent series, the most common associated conditions were AIDS (80%), hematologic malignancies (13%), transplant recipients (5%), and chronic inflammatory diseases (2%). It has been estimated that up to 5% of AIDS patients will develop PML. There have been three cases of PML occurring in patients being treated for multiple sclerosis and inflammatory bowel disease with natalizumab, a humanized monoclonal antibody that inhibits lymphocyte trafficking into CNS and bowel mucosa by binding to α_4 integrins. Risk in these patients has been estimated at 1 PML case per 1000 treated patients after a mean of 18 months of therapy. The basic clinical and diagnostic features are similar in AIDS and non-AIDS–associated PML.

Diagnostic Studies

The diagnosis of PML is frequently suggested by MRI. MRI reveals multifocal asymmetric, coalescing white matter lesions located periventricularly, in the centrum semiovale, in the parietal-occipital region, and in the cerebellum. These lesions have increased signal on T2 and FLAIR images and decreased signal on T1-weighted images. PML lesions are classically nonenhancing (90%) but may rarely show ring enhancement, especially in more immunocompetent patients. PML lesions are not typically associated with edema or mass effect. CT scans, which are less sensitive than MRI for the diagnosis of PML, often show hypodense nonenhancing white matter lesions.

The CSF is typically normal, although mild elevation in protein and/or IgG may be found. Pleocytosis occurs in <25% of cases, is predominantly mononuclear, and rarely exceeds 25 cells/μL. PCR amplification of JCV DNA from CSF has become an important diagnostic tool. The presence of a positive CSF PCR for JCV DNA in association with typical MRI lesions in the appropriate clinical setting is diagnostic of PML, reflecting the assay's relatively high specificity (92–100%); however, sensitivity is variable. In HIV-negative patients and HIV-positive patients not receiving highly active antiviral therapy (HAART), sensitivity is likely 70–90%. In HAART-treated patients, sensitivity may be closer to 60%, reflecting the lower JCV CSF viral load in this relatively more immunocompetent group. Studies with quantitative JCV CSF PCR indicate that patients with low JCV loads (<100 copies/μL) have a generally better prognosis than those with higher viral loads. Patients with negative CSF PCR studies may require brain biopsy for definitive diagnosis. In biopsy or necropsy specimens of brain, JCV antigen and nucleic acid can be detected by immunocytochemistry, in situ hybridization, or PCR amplification. Detection of JCV antigen or genomic material should only be considered diagnostic of PML if accompanied by characteristic pathologic changes, since both antigen and genomic material have been found in the brains of normal patients.

Serologic studies are of no utility in diagnosis due to high basal seroprevalence level (>80%).

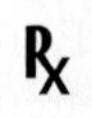

Treatment: PROGRESSIVE MULTIFOCAL LEUKOENCEPHALOPATHY

No effective therapy for PML is available. Intravenous and/or intrathecal cytarabine were not shown to be of benefit in a randomized controlled trial in HIV-associated PML. Another randomized controlled trial of cidofovir in HIV-associated PML also failed to show significant benefit. Some patients with HIV-associated PML have shown disease stabilization and, in rare cases, improvement associated with improvement in their immune status after institution of HAART. In HIV-positive patients treated with HAART, 1-year survival is ~50%, although up to 80% of survivors may have significant neurologic sequelae. HIV-positive patients with higher CD4 counts (>300 mm^3) and low or nondetectable HIV viral loads have a better prognosis than those with lower CD4 counts and higher viral loads.

SUBACUTE SCLEROSING PANENCEPHALITIS (SSPE)

SSPE is a rare chronic, progressive demyelinating disease of the CNS associated with a chronic nonpermissive infection of brain tissue with measles virus. The frequency has been estimated at 1 in 100,000–500,000 measles cases. An average of five cases per year are reported in the United States. The incidence has declined dramatically since the introduction of a measles vaccine. Most patients give a history of primary measles infection at an early age (2 years), which is followed after a latent interval of 6–8 years by the development of progressive neurologic disorder. Some 85% of patients are between 5 and 15 years old at diagnosis. Initial manifestations include poor school performance and mood and personality changes. Typical signs of a CNS viral infection, including fever and headache, do not occur. As the disease progresses, patients develop progressive intellectual deterioration, focal and/or generalized seizures, myoclonus, ataxia, and visual disturbances. In the late stage of the illness, patients are unresponsive, quadriparetic, and spastic, with hyperactive tendon reflexes and extensor plantar responses.

Diagnostic Studies

MRI is often normal early, although areas of increased T2 signal develop in the white matter of the brain and brainstem as disease progresses. The EEG may initially show only nonspecific slowing, but with disease progression, patients develop a characteristic periodic pattern with bursts of high-voltage, sharp, slow waves every 3–8 s, followed by periods of attenuated ("flat") background. The CSF is acellular with a normal or mildly elevated protein concentration and a markedly elevated gamma globulin level (>20% of total CSF protein). CSF antimeasles antibody levels are invariably elevated, and oligoclonal antimeasles antibodies are often present. Measles virus can be cultured from brain tissue using special cocultivation techniques. Viral antigen can be identified immunocytochemically, and viral genome can be detected by in situ hybridization or PCR amplification.

℞ Treatment: SUBACUTE SCLEROSING PANENCEPHALITIS

No definitive therapy for SSPE is available. Treatment with isoprinosine (Inosiplex, 100 mg/kg per day), alone or in combination with intrathecal or intraventricular alpha interferon, has been reported to prolong survival and produce clinical improvement in some patients but has never been subjected to a controlled clinical trial.

PROGRESSIVE RUBELLA PANENCEPHALITIS

This is an extremely rare disorder that primarily affects males with congenital rubella syndrome, although isolated cases have been reported after childhood rubella. After a latent period of 8–19 years, patients develop progressive neurologic deterioration. The manifestations are similar to those seen in SSPE. CSF shows a mild lymphocytic pleocytosis, slightly elevated protein concentration, markedly increased gamma globulin, and rubella virus–specific oligoclonal bands. No therapy is available. Universal prevention of both congenital and childhood rubella through the use of the available live attenuated rubella vaccine would be expected to eliminate the disease.

BRAIN ABSCESS

DEFINITION

A brain abscess is a focal, suppurative infection within the brain parenchyma, typically surrounded by a vascularized capsule. The term *cerebritis* is often employed to describe a nonencapsulated brain abscess.

EPIDEMIOLOGY

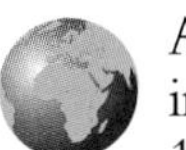

A bacterial brain abscess is a relatively uncommon intracranial infection, with an incidence of ~0.3–1.3/100,000 persons per year. Predisposing conditions include otitis media and mastoiditis, paranasal sinusitis, pyogenic infections in the chest or other body sites, penetrating head trauma or neurosurgical procedures, and dental infections. In immunocompetent individuals, the most important pathogens are *Streptococcus* spp. [anaerobic, aerobic, and viridans (40%)], Enterobacteriaceae [*Proteus* spp., *E. coli* sp., *Klebsiella* spp. (25%)], anaerobes [e.g., *Bacteroides* spp., *Fusobacterium* spp. (30%)], and staphylococci (10%). In immunocompromised hosts with underlying HIV infection, organ transplantation, cancer, or immunosuppressive therapy, most brain abscesses are caused by *Nocardia* spp., *Toxoplasma gondii*, *Aspergillus* spp., *Candida* spp., and *C. neoformans*. In Latin America and in immigrants from Latin America, the most common cause of brain abscess is *Taenia solium* (neurocysticercosis). In India and the Far East, mycobacterial infection (tuberculoma) remains a major cause of focal CNS mass lesions.

ETIOLOGY

A brain abscess may develop (1) by direct spread from a contiguous cranial site of infection, such as paranasal sinusitis, otitis media, mastoiditis, or dental infection; (2) after head trauma or a neurosurgical procedure; or (3) as a result of hematogenous spread from a remote site of infection. In up to 25% of cases, no obvious primary source of infection is apparent (cryptogenic brain abscess).

Approximately one-third of brain abscesses are associated with otitis media and mastoiditis, often with an associated cholesteatoma. Otogenic abscesses occur predominantly in the temporal lobe (55–75%) and cerebellum (20–30%). In some series, up to 90% of cerebellar abscesses are otogenic. Common organisms include streptococci, *Bacteroides* spp., *Pseudomonas* spp., *Haemophilus* spp., and Enterobacteriaceae. Abscesses that develop as a result of direct spread of infection from the frontal, ethmoidal, or sphenoidal sinuses and those that occur due to dental infections are usually located in the frontal lobes. Approximately 10% of brain abscesses are associated with paranasal sinusitis, and this association is particularly strong in young males in their second and third decades of life. The most common pathogens in brain abscesses associated with paranasal sinusitis are streptococci (especially *S. milleri*), *Haemophilus* spp., *Bacteroides* spp., *Pseudomonas* spp., and *S. aureus*. Dental infections are associated with ~2% of brain abscesses, although it is often suggested that many "cryptogenic" abscesses are in fact due to dental infections. The most common pathogens in this setting are streptococci, staphylococci, *Bacteroides* spp., and *Fusobacterium* spp.

Hematogenous abscesses account for ~25% of brain abscesses. Hematogenous abscesses are often multiple, and multiple abscesses often (50%) have a hematogenous origin. These abscesses show a predilection for the territory of the middle cerebral artery (i.e., posterior frontal or parietal lobes). Hematogenous abscesses are often located at the junction of the gray and white matter and are often poorly encapsulated. The microbiology of hematogenous abscesses is dependent on the primary source of infection. For example, brain abscesses that develop as a complication of infective endocarditis are often due to viridans streptococci or *S. aureus*. Abscesses associated with pyogenic lung infections such as lung abscess or bronchiectasis are often due to streptococci, staphylococci, *Bacteroides* spp., *Fusobacterium* spp., or Enterobacteriaceae. Abscesses that follow penetrating head trauma or neurosurgical procedures are frequently due to methicillin-resistant *S. aureus* (MRSA), *S. epidermidis*, Enterobacteriaceae, *Pseudomonas* spp., and *Clostridium* spp. Enterobacteriaceae and *P. aeruginosa* are important causes of abscesses associated with urinary sepsis. Congenital cardiac malformations that produce a right-to-left shunt, such as tetralogy of Fallot, patent ductus arteriosus, and atrial and ventricular septal defects, allow bloodborne bacteria to bypass the pulmonary capillary bed and reach the brain. Similar phenomena can occur with pulmonary arteriovenous malformations. The decreased arterial oxygenation and saturation from the right-to-left shunt and polycythemia may cause focal areas of cerebral ischemia, thus providing a nidus for microorganisms that bypassed the pulmonary circulation to multiply and form an abscess. Streptococci are the most common pathogens in this setting.

PATHOGENESIS AND HISTOPATHOLOGY

Results of experimental models of brain abscess formation suggest that for bacterial invasion of brain parenchyma to occur, there must be preexisting or concomitant areas of ischemia, necrosis, or hypoxia in brain tissue. The intact brain parenchyma is relatively resistant to infection. Once bacteria have established infection, brain abscess frequently evolves through a series of stages, influenced by the nature of the infecting organism and by the immunocompetence of the host. The early cerebritis stage (days 1–3) is characterized by a perivascular infiltration of inflammatory cells, which surround a central core of coagulative necrosis. Marked edema surrounds the lesion at this stage. In the late cerebritis stage (days 4–9), pus formation leads to enlargement of the necrotic center, which is surrounded at its border by an inflammatory infiltrate of macrophages and fibroblasts. A thin capsule of fibroblasts and reticular fibers gradually develops, and the surrounding area of cerebral edema becomes more distinct than in the previous stage. The third stage, early capsule formation (days 10–13), is characterized by the formation of a capsule that is better developed on the cortical than on the ventricular side of the lesion. This stage correlates with the appearance of a ring-enhancing capsule on neuroimaging studies. The final stage, late capsule formation (day 14 and beyond), is defined by a well-formed necrotic center surrounded by a dense collagenous capsule. The surrounding area of cerebral edema has regressed, but marked gliosis with large numbers of reactive astrocytes has developed outside the capsule. This gliotic process may contribute to the development of seizures as a sequelae of brain abscess.

CLINICAL PRESENTATION

A brain abscess typically presents as an expanding intracranial mass lesion rather than as an infectious process. Although the evolution of signs and symptoms is extremely variable, ranging from hours to weeks or even months, most patients present to the hospital 11–12 days after onset of symptoms. The classic clinical triad of headache, fever, and a focal neurologic deficit is present in <50% of cases. The most common symptom in patients with a brain abscess is headache, occurring in >75% of patients. The headache is often characterized as a constant, dull, aching sensation, either hemicranial or generalized, and it becomes progressively more severe and refractory to therapy. Fever is present in only 50% of patients at the time of diagnosis, and its absence should not exclude the diagnosis. The new onset of focal or generalized seizure activity is a presenting sign in 15–35% of patients. Focal neurologic deficits including hemiparesis, aphasia, or visual field defects are part of the initial presentation in >60% of patients.

The clinical presentation of a brain abscess depends on its location, the nature of the primary infection if present, and the level of the ICP. Hemiparesis is the most common localizing sign of a frontal lobe abscess. A temporal lobe abscess may present with a disturbance of language (dysphasia) or an upper homonymous quadrantanopia. Nystagmus and ataxia are signs of a cerebellar abscess. Signs of raised ICP—papilledema, nausea and vomiting, and drowsiness or confusion—can be the dominant presentation of some abscesses, particularly those in the cerebellum. Meningismus is not present unless the abscess has ruptured into the ventricle or the infection has spread to the subarachnoid space.

DIAGNOSIS

Diagnosis is made by neuroimaging studies. MRI (Fig. 29-4) is better than CT for demonstrating abscesses in the early (cerebritis) stages and is superior to CT for identifying abscesses in the posterior fossa. Cerebritis appears on MRI as an area of low-signal intensity on T1-weighted images with irregular postgadolinium enhancement and as an area of increased signal intensity on T2-weighted images. Cerebritis is often not visualized by CT scan but, when present, appears as an area of hypodensity. On a contrast-enhanced CT scan, a mature brain abscess appears as a focal area of hypodensity surrounded by ring enhancement with surrounding edema (hypodensity). On contrast-enhanced T1-weighted MRI, a mature brain abscess has a capsule that enhances surrounding a hypodense center and surrounded by a hypodense area of edema. On T2-weighted MRI, there is a hyperintense central area of pus surrounded by a well-defined hypointense capsule and a hyperintense surrounding area of edema. It is important to recognize that the CT and MR appearance, particularly of the capsule, may be altered by treatment with glucocorticoids. The distinction between a brain abscess and other focal CNS lesions such as primary or metastatic tumors may be facilitated by the use of diffusion-weighted imaging sequences on which brain abscesses typically show increased signal and low apparent diffusion coefficient.

Microbiologic diagnosis of the etiologic agent is most accurately determined by Gram's stain and culture of abscess material obtained by stereotactic needle aspiration. Aerobic

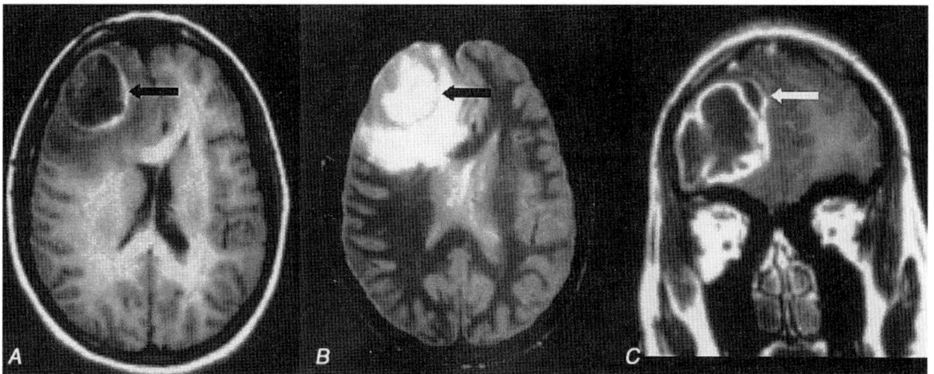

FIGURE 29-4

Pneumococcal brain abscess. Note that the abscess wall has hyperintense signal on the axial T1-weighted MRI (***A***, *black arrow*), hypointense signal on the axial proton density images (***B***, *black arrow*), and enhances prominently after gadolinium administration on the coronal T1-weighted image (***C***). The abscess is surrounded by a large amount of vasogenic edema and has a small "daughter" abscess (***C***, *white arrow*). (*Courtesy of Joseph Lurito, MD; with permission.*)

and anaerobic bacterial cultures and mycobacterial and fungal cultures should be obtained. Up to 10% of patients will also have positive blood cultures. LP should not be performed in patients with known or suspected focal intracranial infections such as abscess or empyema; CSF analysis contributes nothing to diagnosis or therapy, and LP increases the risk of herniation.

Additional laboratory studies may provide clues to the diagnosis of brain abscess in patients with a CNS mass lesion. About 50% of patients have a peripheral leukocytosis, 60% an elevated ESR, and 80% an elevated C-reactive protein. Blood cultures are positive in ~10% of cases overall but may be positive in >85% of patients with abscesses due to *Listeria*.

DIFFERENTIAL DIAGNOSIS

Conditions that can cause headache, fever, focal neurologic signs, and seizure activity include brain abscess, subdural empyema, bacterial meningitis, viral meningoencephalitis, superior sagittal sinus thrombosis, and acute disseminated encephalomyelitis. When fever is absent, primary and metastatic brain tumors become the major differential diagnosis. Less commonly, cerebral infarction or hematoma can have an MRI or CT appearance resembling brain abscess.

℞ Treatment: BRAIN ABSCESS

Optimal therapy of brain abscesses involves a combination of high-dose parenteral antibiotics and neurosurgical drainage. Empirical therapy of community-acquired brain abscess in an immunocompetent patient typically includes a third-generation cephalosporin (e.g., cefotaxime or ceftriaxone) and metronidazole (see Table 29-1 for antibiotic dosages). In patients with penetrating head trauma or recent neurosurgical procedures, treatment should include ceftazidime as the third-generation cephalosporin to enhance coverage of *Pseudomonas* spp. and vancomycin for coverage of staphylococci. Meropenem plus vancomycin also provides good coverage in this setting.

Aspiration and drainage of the abscess under stereotactic guidance are beneficial for both diagnosis and therapy. Empirical antibiotic coverage should be modified based on the results of Gram's stain and culture of the abscess contents. Complete excision of a bacterial abscess via craniotomy or craniectomy is generally reserved for multiloculated abscesses or those in which stereotactic aspiration is unsuccessful.

Medical therapy alone is not optimal for treatment of brain abscess and should be reserved for patients whose abscesses are neurosurgically inaccessible, for patients with small (<2–3 cm) or nonencapsulated abscesses (cerebritis), and patients whose condition is too tenuous to allow performance of a neurosurgical procedure. All patients should receive a minimum of 6–8 weeks of parenteral antibiotic therapy. The role, if any, of supplemental oral antibiotic therapy after completion of a standard course of parenteral therapy has never been adequately studied.

In addition to surgical drainage and antibiotic therapy, patients should receive prophylactic anticonvulsant therapy because of the high risk (~35%) of focal or generalized seizures. Anticonvulsant therapy is continued for at least 3 months after resolution of the abscess, and decisions regarding withdrawal are then based on the EEG. If the EEG is abnormal, anticonvulsant therapy should be continued. If the EEG is normal, anticonvulsant therapy can be slowly withdrawn, with close follow-up and repeat EEG after the medication has been discontinued.

Glucocorticoids should not be given routinely to patients with brain abscesses. Intravenous dexamethasone therapy (10 mg every 6 h) is usually reserved for patients with substantial periabscess edema and associated mass effect and increased ICP. Dexamethasone should be tapered as rapidly as possible to avoid delaying the natural process of encapsulation of the abscess.

Serial MRI or CT scans should be obtained on a monthly or twice-monthly basis to document resolution of the abscess. More frequent studies (e.g., weekly) are probably warranted in the subset of patients who are receiving antibiotic therapy alone. A small amount of enhancement may remain for months after the abscess has been successfully treated.

PROGNOSIS

The mortality of brain abscess has declined in parallel with the development of enhanced neuroimaging techniques, improved neurosurgical procedures for stereotactic aspiration, and improved antibiotics. In modern series, the mortality is typically <15%. Significant sequelae, including seizures, persisting weakness, aphasia, or mental impairment, occur in ≥20% of survivors.

NONBACTERIAL CAUSES OF INFECTIOUS FOCAL CNS LESIONS

ETIOLOGY

Neurocysticercosis is the most common parasitic disease of the CNS worldwide. Humans acquire cysticercosis by the ingestion of food contaminated with the eggs of the parasite *T. solium*. Toxoplasmosis is a parasitic disease caused by *T. gondii* and acquired from the ingestion of undercooked meat and from handling cat feces.

CLINICAL PRESENTATION

The most common manifestation of neurocysticercosis is new-onset partial seizures with or without secondary generalization. Cysticerci may develop in the brain parenchyma and cause seizures or focal neurologic deficits. When present in the subarachnoid or ventricular spaces, cysticerci can produce increased ICP by interference with CSF flow. Spinal cysticerci can mimic the presentation of intraspinal tumors. When the cysticerci first lodge in the brain, they frequently cause little in the way of an inflammatory response. As the cysticercal cyst degenerates, it elicits an inflammatory response that may present clinically as a seizure. Eventually the cyst dies, a process that may take several years and is typically associated with resolution of the inflammatory response and, often, abatement of seizures.

Primary *toxoplasma* infection is often asymptomatic. However, during this phase parasites may spread to the CNS, where they become latent. Reactivation of CNS infection is almost exclusively associated with immunocompromised hosts, particularly those with HIV infection. During this phase patients present with headache, fever, seizures, and focal neurologic deficits.

DIAGNOSIS

The lesions of neurocysticercosis are readily visualized by MRI or CT scans. Lesions with viable parasites appear as cystic lesions. The scolex can often be visualized on MRI. Lesions may appear as contrast-enhancing lesions surrounded by edema. A very early sign of cyst death is hypointensity of the vesicular fluid on T2-weighted images when compared with CSF. Parenchymal brain calcifications are the most common finding and evidence that the parasite is no longer viable. MRI findings of toxoplasmosis consist of multiple lesions in the deep white matter, the thalamus, and basal ganglia and at the gray-white junction in the cerebral hemispheres. With contrast administration, the majority of the lesions enhance in a ringed, nodular, or homogeneous pattern and are surrounded by edema. In the presence of the characteristic neuroimaging abnormalities of *T. gondii* infection, serum IgG antibody to *T. gondii* should be obtained and, when positive, the patient should be treated.

℞ Treatment: INFECTIOUS FOCAL CNS LESIONS

Anticonvulsant therapy is initiated when the patient with neurocysticercosis presents with a seizure. There is controversy about whether or not antihelminthic therapy should be given to all patients. Such therapy does not necessarily reduce the risk of seizure recurrence. Cysticerci appearing as cystic lesions or as enhancing lesions in the brain parenchyma or in the subarachnoid space at the convexity of the cerebral hemispheres should be treated with anticysticidal therapy. Cysticidal drugs accelerate the destruction of the parasites, resulting in a faster resolution of the infection. Albendazole and praziquantel are used in the treatment of neurocysticercosis. Approximately 85% of parenchymal cysts are destroyed by a single course of albendazole, and ~75% are destroyed by a single course of praziquantel. The dose of albendazole is 15 mg/kg per day in two doses for 8 days. The dose of praziquantel is 50 mg/kg per day for 15 days, although a number of other dosage regimens are also frequently cited. Antiepileptic therapy can be stopped once the follow-up CT scan shows resolution of the lesion. Long-term antiepileptic therapy is recommended when seizures occur after resolution of edema and resorption or calcification of the degenerating cyst.

CNS toxoplasmosis is treated with a combination of sulfadiazine, 1.5–2.0 g orally qid, plus pyrimethamine, 100 mg orally to load then 75–100 mg orally qd, plus folinic acid, 10–15 mg orally qd. Folinic acid is added to the regimen to prevent megaloblastic anemia. Therapy is continued until there is no evidence of active disease on neuroimaging studies, which typically takes at least 6 weeks, and then the dose of sulfadiazine is reduced to 2–4 g/d and pyrimethamine to 50 mg/d. Clindamycin plus pyrimethamine is an alternative therapy for patients who cannot tolerate sulfadiazine, but the combination of pyrimethamine and sulfadiazine is more effective.

SUBDURAL EMPYEMA

A subdural empyema (SDE) is a collection of pus between the dura and arachnoid membranes (Fig. 29-5).

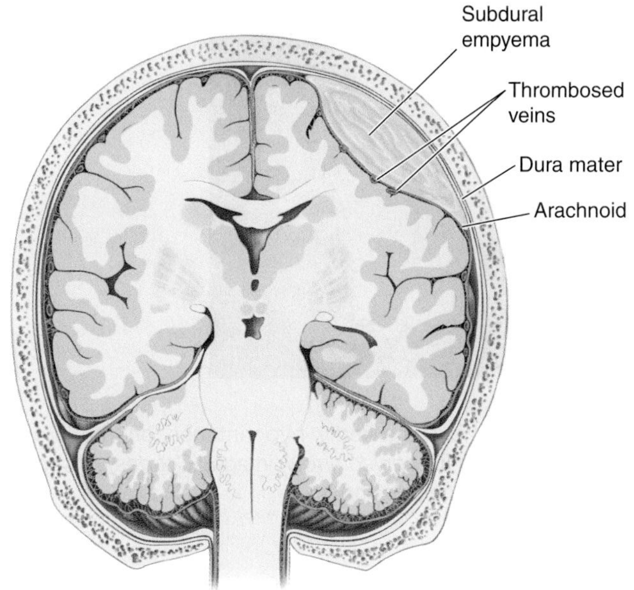

FIGURE 29-5
Subdural empyema.

EPIDEMIOLOGY

SDE is a rare disorder that accounts for 15–25% of focal suppurative CNS infections. Sinusitis is the most common predisposing condition and typically involves the frontal sinuses, either alone or in combination with the ethmoid and maxillary sinuses. Sinusitis-associated empyema has a striking predilection for young males, possibly reflecting sex-related differences in sinus anatomy and development. It has been suggested that SDE may complicate 1–2% of cases of frontal sinusitis severe enough to require hospitalization. As a consequence of this epidemiology, SDE shows an ~3:1 male:female predominance, with 70% of cases occurring in the second and third decades of life. SDE may also develop as a complication of head trauma or neurosurgery. Secondary infection of a subdural effusion may also result in empyema, although secondary infection of hematomas, in the absence of a prior neurosurgical procedure, is rare.

ETIOLOGY

Aerobic and anaerobic streptococci, staphylococci, Enterobacteriaceae, and anaerobic bacteria are the most common causative organisms of sinusitis-associated SDE. Staphylococci and gram-negative bacilli are often the etiologic organisms when SDE follows neurosurgical procedures or head trauma. Up to one-third of cases are culture-negative, possibly reflecting difficulty in obtaining adequate anaerobic cultures.

PATHOPHYSIOLOGY

Sinusitis-associated SDE develops as a result of either retrograde spread of infection from septic thrombophlebitis of the mucosal veins draining the sinuses or contiguous spread of infection to the brain from osteomyelitis in the posterior wall of the frontal or other sinuses. SDE may also develop from direct introduction of bacteria into the subdural space as a complication of a neurosurgical procedure. The evolution of SDE can be extremely rapid because the subdural space is a large compartment that offers few mechanical barriers to the spread of infection. In patients with sinusitis-associated SDE, suppuration typically begins in the upper and anterior portions of one cerebral hemisphere and then extends posteriorly. SDE is often associated with other intracranial infections, including epidural empyema (40%), cortical thrombophlebitis (35%), and intracranial abscess or cerebritis (>25%). Cortical venous infarction produces necrosis of underlying cerebral cortex and subcortical white matter, with focal neurologic deficits and seizures (see below).

CLINICAL PRESENTATION

A patient with SDE typically presents with fever and a progressively worsening headache. The diagnosis of SDE should always be suspected in a patient with known sinusitis who presents with new CNS signs or symptoms. Patients with underlying sinusitis frequently have symptoms related to this infection. As the infection progresses, focal neurologic deficits, seizures, nuchal rigidity, and signs of increased ICP commonly occur. Headache is the most common complaint at the time of presentation; initially it is localized to the side of the subdural infection, but then it becomes more severe and generalized. Contralateral hemiparesis or hemiplegia is the most common focal neurologic deficit and can occur from the direct effects of the SDE on the cortex or as a consequence of venous infarction. Seizures begin as partial motor seizures that then become secondarily generalized. Seizures may be due to the direct irritative effect of the SDE on the underlying cortex or result from cortical venous infarction (see above). In untreated SDE, the increasing mass effect and increase in ICP cause progressive deterioration in consciousness, leading ultimately to coma.

DIAGNOSIS

MRI (Fig. 29-6) is superior to CT in identifying SDE and any associated intracranial infections. The administration of gadolinium greatly improves diagnosis by enhancing the rim of the empyema and allowing the empyema to be clearly delineated from the underlying brain parenchyma. Cranial MRI is also extremely valuable in identifying sinusitis, other focal CNS infections, cortical venous infarction, cerebral edema, and cerebritis. CT may show a crescent-shaped hypodense lesion over one or both hemispheres or in the interhemispheric fissure. Frequently the degree of mass effect, exemplified by midline shift, ventricular compression, and sulcal effacement, is far out of proportion to the mass of the SDE.

CSF examination should be avoided in patients with known or suspected SDE, as it adds no useful information and is associated with the risk of cerebral herniation.

DIFFERENTIAL DIAGNOSIS

The differential diagnosis of the combination of headache, fever, focal neurologic signs, and seizure activity that

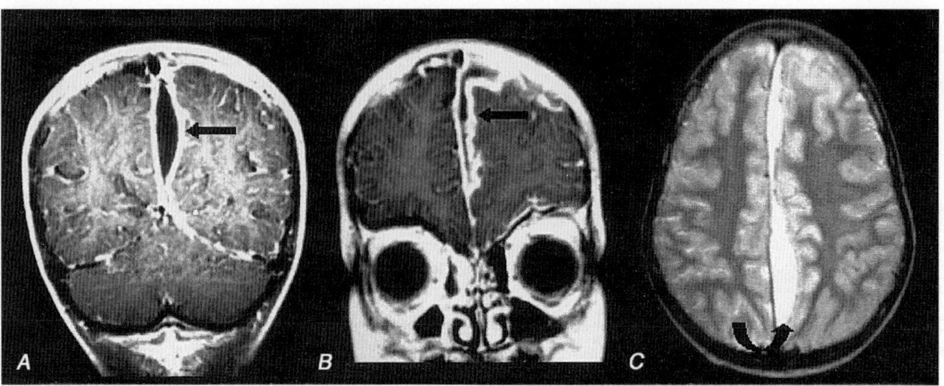

FIGURE 29-6
Subdural empyema. There is marked enhancement of the dura and leptomeninges (***A***, ***B***, *straight arrows*) along the left medial hemisphere. The pus is hypointense on T1-weighted images (***A***, ***B***) but markedly hyperintense on the proton density–weighted (***C***, *curved arrow*) image. (*Courtesy of Joseph Lurito, MD; with permission.*)

progresses rapidly to an altered level of consciousness includes subdural hematoma, bacterial meningitis, viral encephalitis, brain abscess, superior sagittal sinus thrombosis, and acute disseminated encephalomyelitis. The presence of nuchal rigidity is unusual with brain abscess or epidural empyema and should suggest the possibility of SDE when associated with significant focal neurologic signs and fever. Patients with bacterial meningitis also have nuchal rigidity but do not typically have focal deficits of the severity seen with SDE.

℞ Treatment: SUBDURAL EMPYEMA

SDE is a medical emergency. Emergent neurosurgical evacuation of the empyema, either through burr-hole drainage or craniotomy, is the definitive step in the management of this infection. Empirical antimicrobial therapy should include a combination of a third-generation cephalosporin (e.g., cefotaxime or ceftriaxone), vancomycin, and metronidazole (see Table 29-1 for dosages). Parenteral antibiotic therapy should be continued for a minimum of 4 weeks. Specific diagnosis of the etiologic organisms is made based on Gram's stain and culture of fluid obtained via either burr holes or craniotomy; the initial empirical antibiotic coverage can be modified accordingly.

PROGNOSIS

Prognosis is influenced by the level of consciousness of the patient at the time of hospital presentation, the size of the empyema, and the speed with which therapy is instituted. Long-term neurologic sequelae, which include seizures and hemiparesis, occur in up to 50% of cases.

EPIDURAL ABSCESS

Cranial epidural abscess is a suppurative infection occurring in the potential space between the inner skull table and dura (Fig. 29-7).

ETIOLOGY AND PATHOPHYSIOLOGY

Epidural abscess is less common than either brain abscess or SDE and accounts for <2% of focal suppurative CNS infections. A cranial epidural abscess develops as a complication of a craniotomy or compound skull fracture or as a result of spread of infection from the frontal sinuses, middle ear, mastoid, or orbit. An epidural abscess may develop contiguous to an area of osteomyelitis, when craniotomy is complicated by infection of the wound or bone flap, or as a result of direct infection of the epidural space. Infection in the frontal sinus, middle ear, mastoid, or orbit can reach the epidural space through retrograde spread of infection from septic thrombophlebitis in the emissary veins that drain these areas or by way of direct spread of infection through areas of osteomyelitis. Unlike the subdural space, the epidural space is really a potential rather than an actual compartment. The dura is normally tightly adherent to the inner skull table, and infection must dissect the dura away from the skull table as it spreads. As a result, epidural abscesses are often smaller than SDEs. Cranial epidural abscesses, unlike brain abscesses, only rarely result from hematogenous spread of infection from extracranial primary sites. The bacteriology of a

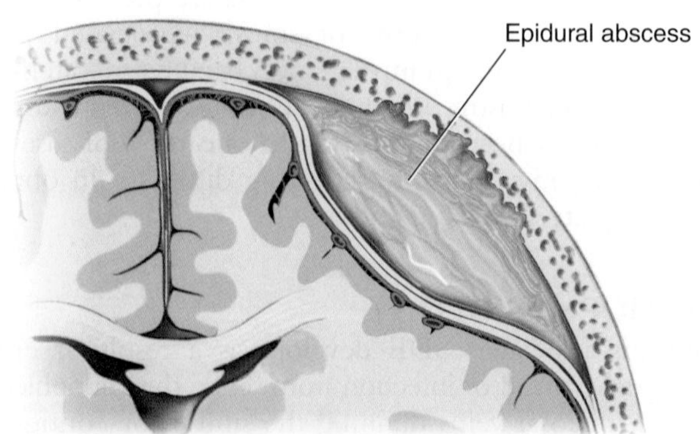

FIGURE 29-7
Cranial epidural abscess is a collection of pus between the dura and the inner table of the skull.

cranial epidural abscess is similar to that of SDE (see above). The etiologic organisms of an epidural abscess that arises from frontal sinusitis, middle ear infections, or mastoiditis are usually streptococci or anaerobic organisms. Staphylococci or gram-negative organisms are the usual cause of an epidural abscess that develops as a complication of craniotomy or compound skull fracture.

CLINICAL PRESENTATION

Patients present with fever (60%), headache (40%), nuchal rigidity (35%), seizures (10%), and focal deficits (5%). Periorbital edema and Potts puffy tumor, reflecting underlying associated frontal bone osteomyelitis, are present in ~40%. In patients with a recent neurosurgical procedure, wound infection is invariably present, but other symptoms may be subtle and can include altered mental status (45%), fever (35%), and headache (20%). The diagnosis should also be considered when fever and headache follow recent head trauma or occur in the setting of frontal sinusitis, mastoiditis, or otitis media.

DIAGNOSIS

Cranial MRI is the procedure of choice to demonstrate a cranial epidural abscess. The sensitivity of CT is limited by the presence of signal artifacts arising from the bone of the inner skull table. The CT appearance of an epidural empyema is that of a lens or crescent-shaped hypodense extraaxial lesion. On MRI, an epidural empyema appears as a lentiform or crescent-shaped fluid collection that is hyperintense compared with CSF on T2-weighted images. On T1-weighted images, the fluid collection has a signal intensity that is intermediate between that of brain tissue and CSF. After the administration of gadolinium, a significant enhancement of the dura is seen on T1-weighted images. In distinction to subdural empyema, signs of mass effect or other parenchymal abnormalities are uncommon.

℞ Treatment: EPIDURAL ABSCESS

Immediate neurosurgical drainage is indicated. Empirical antimicrobial therapy, pending the results of Gram's stain and culture of the purulent material obtained at surgery, should include a combination of a third-generation cephalosporin, vancomycin, and metronidazole (Table 29-1). Ceftazidime or meropenem should be substituted for ceftriaxone or cefotaxime in neurosurgical patients. When the organism has been identified, antimicrobial therapy can be modified accordingly. Antibiotics should be continued for at least 3 weeks after surgical drainage.

PROGNOSIS

Mortality is <5% in modern series, and full recovery is the rule in most survivors.

SUPPURATIVE THROMBOPHLEBITIS

DEFINITION

Suppurative intracranial thrombophlebitis is septic venous thrombosis of cortical veins and sinuses. This may occur as a complication of bacterial meningitis; SDE; epidural abscess; or infection in the skin of the face, paranasal sinuses, middle ear, or mastoid.

ANATOMY AND PATHOPHYSIOLOGY

The cerebral veins and venous sinuses have no valves; therefore, blood within them can flow in either direction. The superior sagittal sinus is the largest of the venous sinuses (Fig. 29-8). It receives blood from the frontal, parietal, and occipital superior cerebral veins and the diploic veins, which communicate with the meningeal veins. Bacterial meningitis is a common predisposing condition for septic thrombosis of the superior sagittal sinus. The diploic veins, which drain into the superior sagittal sinus, provide a route for the spread of infection from the meninges, especially in cases where there is purulent exudate near areas of the superior sagittal sinus. Infection can also spread to the superior sagittal sinus from nearby SDE or epidural abscess. Dehydration from vomiting, hypercoagulable states, and immunologic abnormalities, including the presence of circulating antiphospholipid antibodies, also contribute to cerebral venous sinus thrombosis. Thrombosis may extend from one sinus to another, and at autopsy thrombi of different histologic ages can often be detected in several sinuses. Thrombosis of the superior sagittal sinus is often associated with thrombosis of superior cortical veins and small parenchymal hemorrhages.

The superior sagittal sinus drains into the transverse sinuses (Fig. 29-8). The transverse sinuses also receive venous drainage from small veins from both the middle ear and mastoid cells. The transverse sinus becomes the sigmoid sinus before draining into the internal jugular vein. Septic transverse/sigmoid sinus thrombosis can be a complication of acute and chronic otitis media or mastoiditis. Infection

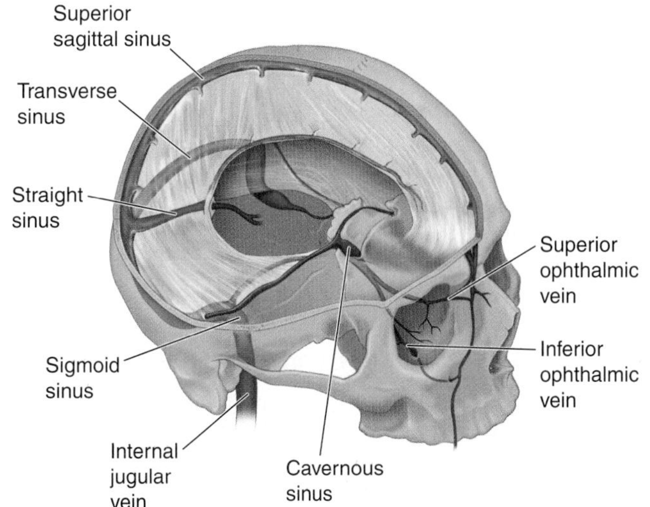

FIGURE 29-8
Anatomy of the cerebral venous sinuses.

spreads from the mastoid air cells to the transverse sinus via the emissary veins or by direct invasion. The cavernous sinuses are inferior to the superior sagittal sinus at the base of the skull. The cavernous sinuses receive blood from the facial veins via the superior and inferior ophthalmic veins. Bacteria in the facial veins enter the cavernous sinus via these veins. Bacteria in the sphenoid and ethmoid sinuses can spread to the cavernous sinuses via the small emissary veins. The sphenoid and ethmoid sinuses are the most common sites of primary infection resulting in septic cavernous sinus thrombosis.

CLINICAL MANIFESTATIONS

Septic thrombosis of the superior sagittal sinus presents with headache, fever, nausea and vomiting, confusion, and focal or generalized seizures. There may be a rapid development of stupor and coma. Weakness of the lower extremities with bilateral Babinski signs or hemiparesis is often present. When superior sagittal sinus thrombosis occurs as a complication of bacterial meningitis, nuchal rigidity and Kernig's and Brudzinski's signs may be present.

The oculomotor nerve, the trochlear nerve, the abducens nerve, the ophthalmic and maxillary branches of the trigeminal nerve, and the internal carotid artery all pass through the cavernous sinus. The symptoms of *septic cavernous sinus thrombosis* are fever, headache, frontal and retroorbital pain, and diplopia. The classic signs are ptosis, proptosis, chemosis, and extraocular dysmotility due to deficits of cranial nerves III, IV, and VI; hyperesthesia of the ophthalmic and maxillary divisions of the fifth cranial nerve and a decreased corneal reflex may be detected. There may be evidence of dilated, tortuous retinal veins and papilledema.

Headache and earache are the most frequent symptoms of *transverse sinus thrombosis*. A transverse sinus thrombosis may also present with otitis media, sixth nerve palsy, and retroorbital or facial pain (*Gradenigo's syndrome*). Sigmoid sinus and internal jugular vein thrombosis may present with neck pain.

DIAGNOSIS

The diagnosis of septic venous sinus thrombosis is suggested by an absent flow void within the affected venous sinus on MRI and confirmed by magnetic resonance venography, CT angiogram, or the venous phase of cerebral angiography. The diagnosis of thrombophlebitis of intracerebral and meningeal veins is suggested by the presence of intracerebral hemorrhage but requires cerebral angiography for definitive diagnosis.

Rx Treatment: SUPPURATIVE THROMBOPHLEBITIS

Septic venous sinus thrombosis is treated with antibiotics, hydration, and removal of infected tissue and thrombus in septic lateral or cavernous sinus thrombosis. The choice of antimicrobial therapy is based on the bacteria responsible for the predisposing or associated condition. Optimal duration of therapy is unknown, but antibiotics are usually continued for 6 weeks or until there is radiographic evidence of resolution of thrombosis. Anticoagulation with dose-adjusted heparin has been reported to be beneficial in patients with aseptic venous sinus thrombosis; it is also used in the treatment of septic venous sinus thrombosis complicating bacterial meningitis in patients who are worsening despite antimicrobial therapy and intravenous fluids. The presence of a small intracerebral hemorrhage from septic thrombophlebitis is not an absolute contraindication to heparin therapy. Successful management of aseptic venous sinus thrombosis has been reported with catheter-directed urokinase therapy and with a combination of intrathrombus recombinant tissue plasminogen activator and intravenous heparin, but there has not been enough experience with these therapies in septic venous sinus thrombosis to make recommendations regarding their use.

FURTHER READINGS

Bartt RE: Multiple sclerosis, natalizumab therapy, and progressive multifocal leukoencephalopathy. Curr Opin Neurol 19:341, 2006

Cabellos C et al: Community-acquired bacterial meningitis in elderly patients: Experience over 30 years. Medicine (Baltimore) 88:115, 2009

De Gans J, van de Beek D: Dexamethasone in adults with bacterial meningitis. N Engl J Med 347:1549, 2002

Glaser CA et al: In search of encephalitis etiologies: Diagnostic challenges from the California Encephalitis project, 1998–2000. Clin Infect Dis 36:731, 2003

Halperin JJ et al: Practice Parameter: Treatment of nervous system Lyme disease (an evidence-based review). Report of the Quality Standards Subcommittee of the American Academy of Neurology. Neurology 69:91, 2007 (Erratum: Neurology 70:1223, 2008)

Lu CH et al: Bacterial brain abscess: Microbiological features, epidemiological trends and therapeutic outcomes. QJM 95:501, 2002

Read WL: Community-acquired bacterial meningitis. N Engl J Med 354:1429, 2006

Rosenstein NE et al: Meningococcal disease. N Engl J Med 344:1378, 2001

Scarborough M et al: Corticosteroids for bacterial meningitis in adults in sub-Saharan Africa. N Engl J Med 357:2441, 2007

Solomon T et al: West Nile encephalitis. BMJ 326:865, 2003

Stephens DS et al: Epidemic meningitis, meningococcaemia, and Neisseria meningitidis. Lancet 369:2196, 2007

Tunkel AR et al: Practice guidelines for the management of bacterial meningitis. Clin Infect Dis 39:1267, 2004

Whitley RJ: Herpes simplex encephalitis: Adolescents and adults. Antiviral Res 71:141, 2006

CHAPTER 30

CHRONIC AND RECURRENT MENINGITIS

Walter J. Koroshetz ■ Morton N. Swartz

Chronic inflammation of the meninges (pia, arachnoid, and dura) can produce profound neurologic disability and may be fatal if not successfully treated. The condition is most commonly diagnosed when a characteristic neurologic syndrome exists for >4 weeks and is associated with a persistent inflammatory response in the cerebrospinal fluid (CSF) (white blood cell count >5/μL). The causes are varied, and appropriate treatment depends on identification of the etiology. Five categories of disease account for most cases of chronic meningitis: (1) meningeal infections, (2) malignancy, (3) noninfectious inflammatory disorders, (4) chemical meningitis, and (5) parameningeal infections.

CLINICAL PATHOPHYSIOLOGY

Neurologic manifestations of chronic meningitis (Table 30-1) are determined by the anatomic location of the inflammation and its consequences. Persistent headache with or without stiff neck, hydrocephalus, cranial neuropathies, radiculopathies, and cognitive or personality changes are the cardinal features. These can occur alone or in combination. When they appear in combination, widespread dissemination of the inflammatory process along CSF pathways has occurred. In some cases, the presence of an underlying systemic illness points to a specific agent or class of agents as the probable cause. The diagnosis of chronic meningitis is usually made when the clinical presentation prompts the astute physician to examine the CSF for signs of inflammation. CSF is produced by the choroid plexus of the cerebral ventricles, exits through narrow foramina into the subarachnoid space surrounding the brain and spinal cord, circulates around the base of the brain and over the cerebral hemispheres, and is resorbed by arachnoid villi projecting into the superior sagittal sinus. CSF flow provides a pathway for rapid spread of infectious and other infiltrative processes over the brain, spinal cord, and cranial and spinal nerve roots. Spread from the subarachnoid space into brain parenchyma may occur via the arachnoid cuffs that surround blood vessels that penetrate brain tissue (Virchow-Robin spaces).

Intracranial Meningitis

Nociceptive fibers of the meninges are stimulated by the inflammatory process, resulting in headache or neck or back pain. Obstruction of CSF pathways at the foramina or arachnoid villi may produce *hydrocephalus* and symptoms of raised intracranial pressure (ICP), including headache, vomiting, apathy or drowsiness, gait instability, papilledema, visual loss, impaired upgaze, or palsy of the sixth cranial nerve (CN). Cognitive and behavioral changes during the course of chronic meningitis may also result from vascular damage, which may similarly produce seizures, stroke, or myelopathy. Inflammatory deposits seeded via the CSF circulation are often prominent around the brainstem and cranial nerves and along the undersurface of the frontal and temporal lobes. Such cases, termed *basal meningitis*, often present as multiple cranial neuropathies, with visual loss (CN II), facial weakness (CN VII), hearing loss (CN VIII), diplopia (CNs III, IV, and VI), sensory or motor abnormalities of the oropharynx (CNs IX, X, and XII), decreased olfaction (CN I), or facial sensory loss and masseter weakness (CN V).

Spinal Meningitis

Injury may occur to motor and sensory roots as they traverse the subarachnoid space and penetrate the meninges. These cases present as multiple radiculopathies with combinations of radicular pain, sensory loss, motor weakness, and sphincter dysfunction. Meningeal inflammation can encircle the cord, resulting in myelopathy. Patients with slowly progressive involvement of multiple cranial nerves and/or spinal nerve roots are likely to have chronic meningitis. Electrophysiologic testing (electromyography, nerve conduction studies, and evoked response testing) may be helpful in determining whether there is involvement of cranial and spinal nerve roots.

Systemic Manifestations

In some patients, evidence of systemic disease provides clues to the underlying cause of chronic meningitis. A careful history and physical examination are essential before embarking on a diagnostic workup, which may be costly, prolonged, and associated with risk from invasive procedures. A complete history of travel, sexual practice, and exposure to infectious agents should be sought. Infectious causes are often associated with fever, malaise, anorexia, and signs of localized or disseminated infection outside the nervous system. Infectious causes are of major concern in the immunosuppressed patient, especially in patients with AIDS, in whom chronic meningitis may present without headache or fever. Noninfectious

TABLE 30-1

SYMPTOMS AND SIGNS OF CHRONIC MENINGITIS

SYMPTOM	SIGN
Chronic headache	+/– Papilledema
Neck or back pain	Brudzinski's or Kernig's sign of meningeal irritation
Change in personality	Altered mental status—drowsiness, inattention, disorientation, memory loss, frontal release signs (grasp, suck, snout), perseveration
Facial weakness	Peripheral seventh CN palsy
Double vision	Palsy of CNs III, IV, VI
Visual loss	Papilledema, optic atrophy
Hearing loss	Eighth CN palsy
Arm or leg weakness	Myelopathy or radiculopathy
Numbness in arms or legs	Myelopathy or radiculopathy
Sphincter dysfunction	Myelopathy or radiculopathy
	Frontal lobe dysfunction (hydrocephalus)
Clumsiness	Ataxia

Note: CN, cranial nerve.

inflammatory disorders often produce systemic manifestations, but meningitis may be the initial manifestation. Carcinomatous meningitis may or may not be accompanied by clinical evidence of the primary neoplasm.

Approach to the Patient: CHRONIC MENINGITIS

The occurrence of chronic headache, hydrocephalus, cranial neuropathy, radiculopathy, and/or cognitive decline in a patient should prompt consideration of a lumbar puncture for evidence of meningeal inflammation. On occasion the diagnosis is made when an imaging study (CT or MRI) shows contrast enhancement of the meninges, which is always abnormal, with the exception of dural enhancement after lumbar puncture, neurosurgical procedures, or spontaneous CSF leakage. Once chronic meningitis is confirmed by CSF examination, effort is focused on identifying the cause (Tables 30-2 and 30-3) by (1) further analysis of the CSF, (2) diagnosis of an underlying systemic infection or noninfectious inflammatory condition, or (3) pathologic examination of meningeal biopsy specimens.

Two clinical forms of chronic meningitis exist. In the first, the symptoms are chronic and persistent, whereas in the second, there are recurrent, discrete episodes of illness. In the latter group, all symptoms, signs, and CSF parameters of meningeal inflammation resolve completely between episodes without specific therapy. In such patients, the likely etiologies include herpes simplex virus (HSV) type 2; chemical meningitis due to leakage into CSF of contents from an epidermoid tumor, craniopharyngioma, or cholesteatoma; primary inflammatory conditions, including Vogt-Koyanagi-Harada syndrome, Behçet's syndrome, systemic lupus erythematosus (SLE); and drug hypersensitivity with repeated administration of the offending agent.

The epidemiologic history is of considerable importance and may provide direction for selection of laboratory studies. Pertinent features include a history of tuberculosis or exposure to a likely case; past travel to areas endemic for fungal infections (the San Joaquin Valley in California and southwestern states for coccidioidomycosis, midwestern states for histoplasmosis, southeastern states for blastomycosis); travel to the Mediterranean region or ingestion of imported unpasteurized dairy products (*Brucella*); time spent in wooded areas endemic for Lyme disease; exposure to sexually transmitted disease (syphilis); exposure of an immunocompromised host to pigeons and their droppings (*Cryptococcus*); gardening (*Sporothrix schenckii*); ingestion of poorly cooked meat or contact with a household cat (*Toxoplasma gondii*); residence in Thailand or Japan (*Gnathostoma spinigerum*), Latin America (*Paracoccidioides brasiliensis*), or the South Pacific (*Angiostrongylus cantonensis*); rural residence and raccoon exposure (*Baylisascaris procyonis*); and residence in Latin America, the Philippines, or Southeast Asia when eosinophilic meningitis is present (*Taenia solium*).

The presence of focal cerebral signs in a patient with chronic meningitis suggests the possibility of a brain abscess or other parameningeal infection; identification of a potential source of infection (chronic draining ear, sinusitis, right-to-left cardiac or pulmonary shunt, chronic pleuropulmonary infection) supports this diagnosis. In some cases, diagnosis may be established by recognition and biopsy of unusual skin lesions (Behçet's syndrome, cryptococcosis, blastomycosis, SLE, Lyme disease, IV drug use, sporotrichosis, trypanosomiasis) or enlarged lymph nodes (lymphoma, tuberculosis, sarcoid, infection with HIV, secondary syphilis, or Whipple's disease). A careful ophthalmologic examination may reveal uveitis [Vogt-Koyanagi-Harada syndrome, sarcoid, or central nervous system (CNS) lymphoma], keratoconjunctivitis sicca (Sjögren's syndrome), or iridocyclitis (Behçet's syndrome) and is essential to assess visual loss from papilledema. Aphthous oral lesions, genital ulcers, and hypopyon suggest Behçet's syndrome. Hepatosplenomegaly suggests lymphoma, sarcoid, tuberculosis, or brucellosis. Herpetic lesions in the genital area or on the thighs suggests HSV-2 infection. A breast nodule, a suspicious pigmented skin lesion, focal bone pain, or an abdominal mass directs attention to possible carcinomatous meningitis.

IMAGING Once the clinical syndrome is recognized as a potential manifestation of chronic meningitis, proper analysis of the CSF is essential. However, if the possibility of raised ICP exists, a brain imaging study

TABLE 30-2

INFECTIOUS CAUSES OF CHRONIC MENINGITIS

CAUSATIVE AGENT	CSF FORMULA	HELPFUL DIAGNOSTIC TESTS	RISK FACTORS AND SYSTEMIC MANIFESTATIONS
Common Bacterial Causes			
Partially treated suppurative meningitis	Mononuclear or mixed mononuclear-polymorphonuclear cells	CSF culture and Gram's stain	History consistent with acute bacterial meningitis and incomplete treatment
Parameningeal infection	Mononuclear or mixed polymorphonuclear-mononuclear cells	Contrast-enhanced CT or MRI to detect parenchymal, subdural, epidural, or sinus infection	Otitis media, pleuropulmonary infection, right-to-left cardiopulmonary shunt for brain abscess; focal neurologic signs; neck, back, ear, or sinus tenderness
Mycobacterium tuberculosis	Mononuclear cells except polymorphonuclear cells in early infection (commonly <500 WBC/μL); low CSF glucose, high protein	Tuberculin skin test may be negative; AFB culture of CSF (sputum, urine, gastric contents if indicated); tuberculostearic acid detection in CSF; identify tubercle bacillus on acid-fast stain of CSF or protein pellicle; PCR	Exposure history; previous tuberculous illness; immunosuppressed or AIDS; young children; fever, meningismus, night sweats, miliary TB on x-ray or liver biopsy; stroke due to arteritis
Lyme disease (Bannwarth's syndrome) *Borrelia burgdorferi*	Mononuclear cells; elevated protein	Serum Lyme antibody titer; Western blot confirmation; (patients with syphilis may have false-positive Lyme titer)	History of tick bite or appropriate exposure history; erythema chronicum migrans skin rash; arthritis, radiculopathy, Bell's palsy, meningoencephalitis–multiple sclerosis–like syndrome
Syphilis (secondary, tertiary) *Treponema pallidum*	Mononuclear cells; elevated protein	CSF VDRL; serum VDRL (or RPR); FTA or MHA-TP; serum VDRL may be negative in tertiary syphilis	Appropriate exposure history; HIV seropositive individuals at increased risk of aggressive infection; "dementia"; cerebral infarction due to endarteritis
Uncommon Bacterial Causes			
Actinomyces	Polymorphonuclear cells	Anaerobic culture	Parameningeal abscess or sinus tract (oral or dental focus); pneumonitis
Nocardia	Polymorphonuclear; occasionally mononuclear cells; often low glucose	Isolation may require weeks; weakly acid fast	Associated brain abscess may be present
Brucella	Mononuclear cells (rarely polymorphonuclear); elevated protein; often low glucose	CSF antibody detection; serum antibody detection	Intake of unpasteurized dairy products; exposure to goats, sheep, cows; fever, arthralgia, myalgia, vertebral osteomyelitis
Whipple's disease *Tropheryma whipplei*	Mononuclear cells	Biopsy of small bowel or lymph node; CSF PCR for *T. whippelii*; brain and meningeal biopsy (with PAS stain and EM examination)	Diarrhea, weight loss, arthralgias, fever, dementia, ataxia, paresis, ophthalmoplegia, oculomasticatory myoclonus
Rare Bacterial Causes			
Leptospirosis (occasionally if left untreated may last 3–4 weeks)			

(*Continued*)

TABLE 30-2 (CONTINUED)

INFECTIOUS CAUSES OF CHRONIC MENINGITIS

CAUSATIVE AGENT	CSF FORMULA	HELPFUL DIAGNOSTIC TESTS	RISK FACTORS AND SYSTEMIC MANIFESTATIONS
Fungal Causes			
Cryptococcus neoformans	Mononuclear cells; count not elevated in some patients with AIDS	India ink or fungal wet mount of CSF (budding yeast); blood and urine cultures; antigen detection in CSF	AIDS and immune suppression; pigeon exposure; skin and other organ involvement due to disseminated infection
Coccidioides immitis	Mononuclear cells (sometimes 10–20% eosinophils); often low glucose	Antibody detection in CSF and serum	Exposure history—southwestern United States; increased virulence in dark-skinned races
Candida sp.	Polymorphonuclear or mononuclear	Fungal stain and culture of CSF	IV drug abuse; post surgery; prolonged intravenous therapy; disseminated candidiasis
Histoplasma capsulatum	Mononuclear cells; low glucose	Fungal stain and culture of large volumes of CSF; antigen detection in CSF, serum, and urine; antibody detection in serum, CSF	Exposure history—Ohio and central Mississippi River Valley; AIDS; mucosal lesions
Blastomyces dermatitidis	Mononuclear cells	Fungal stain and culture of CSF; biopsy and culture of skin, lung lesions; antibody detection in serum	Midwestern and southeastern United States; usually systemic infection; abscesses, draining sinus, ulcers
Aspergillus sp.	Mononuclear or polymorphonuclear	CSF culture	Sinusitis; granulocytopenia or immunosuppression
Sporothrix schenckii	Mononuclear cells	Antibody detection in CSF and serum; CSF culture	Traumatic inoculation; IV drug use; ulcerated skin lesion
Rare Fungal Causes			
Xylohypha (formerly *Cladosporium*) trichoides and other dark-walled (dematiaceous) fungi such as *Curvularia*, *Drechslera*; *Mucor*, *Pseudoallescheria boydii*			
Protozoal Causes			
Toxoplasma gondii	Mononuclear cells	Biopsy or response to empirical therapy in clinically appropriate context (including presence of antibody in serum)	Usually with intracerebral abscesses; common in HIV seropositive patients
Trypanosomiasis *Trypanosoma gambiense*, *T. rhodesiense*	Mononuclear cells, elevated protein	Elevated CSF IgM; identification of trypanosomes in CSF and blood smear	Endemic in Africa; chancre, lymphadenopathy; prominent sleep disorder
Rare Protozoal Causes			
Acanthamoeba sp. causing granulomatous amebic encephalitis and meningoencephalitis in immunocompromised and debilitated individuals			
Helminthic Causes			
Cysticercosis (infection with cysts of *Taenia solium*)	Mononuclear cells; may have eosinophils; glucose level may be low	Indirect hemagglutination assay in CSF; ELISA immunoblotting in serum	Usually with multiple cysts in basal meninges and hydrocephalus; cerebral cysts, muscle calcification

(*Continued*)

TABLE 30-2 (*CONTINUED*)

INFECTIOUS CAUSES OF CHRONIC MENINGITIS

CAUSATIVE AGENT	CSF FORMULA	HELPFUL DIAGNOSTIC TESTS	RISK FACTORS AND SYSTEMIC MANIFESTATIONS
Helminthic Causes (*Continued*)			
Gnathostoma spinigerum	Eosinophils, mononuclear cells	Peripheral eosinophilia	History of eating raw fish; common in Thailand and Japan; subarachnoid hemorrhage; painful radiculopathy
Angiostrongylus cantonensis	Eosinophils, mononuclear cells	Recovery of worms from CSF	History of eating raw shellfish; common in tropical Pacific regions; often benign
Baylisascaris procyonis (raccoon ascarid)	Eosinophils, mononuclear cells		Infection follows accidental ingestion of *B. procyonis* eggs from raccoon feces; fatal meningoencephalitis
Rare Helminthic Causes			
Trichinella spiralis (trichinosis); *Echinococcus* cysts; *Schistosoma* sp. The former may produce a lymphocytic pleocytosis whereas the latter two may produce an eosinophilic response in CSF associated with cerebral cysts (*Echinococcus*) or granulomatous lesions of brain or spinal cord			
Viral Causes			
Mumps	Mononuclear cells	Antibody in serum	No prior mumps or immunization; may produce meningoencephalitis; may persist for 3–4 weeks
Lymphocytic choriomeningitis	Mononuclear cells	Antibody in serum	Contact with rodents or their excreta; may persist for 3–4 weeks
Echovirus	Mononuclear cells; may have low glucose	Virus isolation from CSF	Congenital hypogammaglobulinemia; history of recurrent meningitis
HIV (acute retroviral syndrome)	Mononuclear cells	p24 antigen in serum and CSF; high level of HIV viremia	HIV risk factors; rash, fever, lymphadenopathy; lymphopenia in peripheral blood; syndrome may persist long enough to be considered as "chronic meningitis"; or chronic meningitis may develop in later stages (AIDS) due to HIV
Herpes simplex (HSV)	Mononuclear cells	PCR for HSV, CMV DNA; CSF antibody for HSV, EBV	Recurrent meningitis due to HSV-2 (rarely HSV-1) often associated with genital recurrences; EBV associated with myeloradiculopathy, CMV with polyradiculopathy

Note: AFB, acid-fast bacillus; CMV, cytomegalovirus; CSF, cerebrospinal fluid; CT, computed tomography; EBV, Epstein-Barr virus; ELISA, enzyme-linked immunosorbent assay; EM, electron microscopy; FTA, fluorescent treponemal antibody absorption test; HSV, herpes simplex virus; MHA-TP, microhemagglutination assay–*T. pallidum*; MRI, magnetic resonance imaging; PAS, periodic acid–Schiff; PCR, polymerase chain reaction; RPR, rapid plasma reagin test; TB, tuberculosis; VDRL, Venereal Disease Research Laboratory test.

TABLE 30-3

NONINFECTIOUS CAUSES OF CHRONIC MENINGITIS

CAUSATIVE AGENTS	CSF FORMULA	HELPFUL DIAGNOSTIC TESTS	RISK FACTORS AND SYSTEMIC MANIFESTATIONS
Malignancy	Mononuclear cells, elevated protein, low glucose	Repeated cytologic examination of large volumes of CSF; CSF exam by polarizing microscopy; clonal lymphocyte markers; deposits on nerve roots or meninges seen on myelogram or contrast-enhanced MRI; meningeal biopsy	Metastatic cancer of breast, lung, stomach, or pancreas; melanoma, lymphoma, leukemia; meningeal gliomatosis; meningeal sarcoma; cerebral dysgerminoma; meningeal melanoma or B-cell lymphoma
Chemical compounds (may cause recurrent meningitis)	Mononuclear or PMNs, low glucose, elevated protein; xanthochromia from subarachnoid hemorrhage in week before presentation with "meningitis"	Contrast-enhanced CT scan or MRI Cerebral angiogram to detect aneurysm	History of recent injection into the subarachnoid space; history of sudden onset of headache; recent resection of acoustic neuroma or craniopharyngioma; epidermoid tumor of brain or spine, sometimes with dermoid sinus tract; pituitary apoplexy
Primary inflammation			
CNS sarcoidosis	Mononuclear cells; elevated protein; often low glucose	Serum and CSF angiotensin-converting enzyme levels; biopsy of extraneural affected tissues or brain lesion/meningeal biopsy	CN palsy, especially of CN VII; hypothalamic dysfunction, especially diabetes insipidus; abnormal chest radiograph; peripheral neuropathy or myopathy
Vogt-Koyanagi-Harada syndrome (recurrent meningitis)	Mononuclear cells		Recurrent meningoencephalitis with uveitis, retinal detachment, alopecia, lightening of eyebrows and lashes, dysacousia, cataracts, glaucoma
Isolated granulomatous angiitis of the nervous system	Mononuclear cells, elevated protein	Angiography or meningeal biopsy	Subacute dementia; multiple cerebral infarctions; recent zoster ophthalmicus
Systemic lupus erythematosus	Mononuclear or PMNs	Anti-DNA antibody, antinuclear antibodies	Encephalopathy; seizures; stroke; transverse myelopathy; rash; arthritis
Behçet's syndrome (recurrent meningitis)	Mononuclear or PMNs, elevated protein		Oral and genital aphthous ulcers; iridocyclitis; retinal hemorrhages; pathergic lesions at site of skin puncture
Chronic benign lymphocytic meningitis	Mononuclear cells		Recovery in 2–6 months, diagnosis by exclusion
Mollaret's meningitis (recurrent meningitis)	Large endothelial cells and PMNs in first hours, followed by mononuclear cells	PCR for herpes; MRI/CT to rule out epidermoid tumor or dural cyst	Recurrent meningitis; exclude HSV-2; rare cases due to HSV-1; occasional case associated with dural cyst
Drug hypersensitivity	PMNs; occasionally mononuclear cells or eosinophils		Exposure to ibuprofen, sulfonamides, isoniazid, tolmetin, ciprofloxacin, phenazopyridine; improvement after discontinuation of drug; recurrent episodes with recurrent exposure
Wegener's granulomatosis	Mononuclear cells	Chest and sinus radiographs; urinalysis; ANCA antibodies in serum	Associated sinus, pulmonary, or renal lesions; CN palsies; skin lesions; peripheral neuropathy
Other: multiple sclerosis, Sjögren's syndrome, neonatal onset multisystemic inflammatory disease (NOMID), and rarer forms of vasculitis (e.g., Cogan's syndrome)			

Note: ANCA, anti-neutrophil cytoplasmic antibodies; CN, cranial nerve; CSF, cerebrospinal fluid; CT, computed tomography; HSV, herpes simplex virus; MRI, magnetic resonance imaging; PCR, polymerase chain reaction; PMNs, polymorphonuclear cells.

should be performed before lumbar puncture. If ICP is elevated because of a mass lesion, brain swelling, or a block in ventricular CSF outflow (obstructive hydrocephalus), then lumbar puncture carries the potential risk of brain herniation. Obstructive hydrocephalus usually requires direct ventricular drainage of CSF. In patients with open CSF flow pathways, elevated ICP can still occur due to impaired resorption of CSF by arachnoid villi. In such patients, lumbar puncture is usually safe, but repetitive or continuous lumbar drainage may be necessary to prevent relatively sudden death from raised ICP. In some patients, especially those with cryptococcal meningitis, fatal levels of raised ICP can occur without enlarged ventricles.

Contrast-enhanced MRI or CT studies of the brain and spinal cord can identify meningeal enhancement, parameningeal infections (including brain abscess), encasement of the spinal cord (malignancy or inflammation and infection), or nodular deposits on the meninges or nerve roots (malignancy or sarcoidosis) (Fig. 30-1). Imaging studies are also useful to localize areas of meningeal disease before meningeal biopsy.

Cerebral angiography may be indicated in patients with chronic meningitis and stroke to identify cerebral arteritis (granulomatous angiitis, other inflammatory arteritides, or infectious arteritis).

CEREBROSPINAL FLUID ANALYSIS The CSF pressure should be measured and samples sent for bacterial, fungal, and tuberculous culture; Venereal Disease Research Laboratory (VDRL) test; cell count and differential; Gram's stain; and measurement of glucose and protein. Wet mount for fungus and parasites, India ink preparation and culture, culture for fastidious bacteria and fungi, assays for cryptococcal antigen and oligoclonal immunoglobulin bands, and cytology should be performed. Other specific CSF tests (Tables 30-2 and 30-3) or blood tests and cultures should be ordered as indicated on the basis of the history, physical examination, or preliminary CSF results (i.e., eosinophilic, mononuclear, or polymorphonuclear meningitis). Rapid diagnosis may be facilitated by serologic tests and polymerase chain reaction (PCR) testing to identify DNA sequences in the CSF that are specific for the suspected pathogen.

In most categories of chronic (not recurrent) meningitis, mononuclear cells predominate in the CSF. When neutrophils predominate after 3 weeks of illness, the principal etiologic considerations are *Nocardia asteroides*, *Actinomyces israelii*, *Brucella*, *Mycobacterium tuberculosis* (5–10% of early cases only), various fungi (*Blastomyces dermatitidis*, *Candida albicans*, *Histoplasma capsulatum*, *Aspergillus* spp., *Pseudallescheria boydii*, *Cladophialophora bantiana*), and noninfectious causes (SLE, exogenous chemical meningitis). When eosinophils predominate or are present in limited numbers in a primarily mononuclear cell response in the CSF, the differential diagnosis includes parasitic diseases (*A. cantonensis*, *G. spinigerum*, *B. procyonis*, or *Toxocara canis* infection, cysticercosis, schistosomiasis, echinococcal disease, *T. gondii* infection), fungal infections (6–20% eosinophils along with a predominantly lymphocyte pleocytosis, particularly with coccidioidal meningitis), neoplastic disease (lymphoma, leukemia, metastatic carcinoma), or other inflammatory processes (sarcoidosis, hypereosinophilic syndrome).

It is often necessary to broaden the number of diagnostic tests if the initial workup does not reveal the cause. In addition, repeated samples of large volumes of CSF may be required to diagnose certain infectious and malignant causes of chronic meningitis. For instance, lymphomatous or carcinomatous meningitis may be diagnosed by examination of sections cut from a cell block formed by spinning down the sediment from a large volume of CSF. The diagnosis of fungal meningitis may require large volumes of CSF for culture of sediment. If standard lumbar puncture is unrewarding, a cervical cisternal tap to sample CSF near to the basal meninges may be fruitful.

LABORATORY INVESTIGATION In addition to the CSF examination, an attempt should be made to uncover pertinent underlying illnesses. Tuberculin skin test, chest radiograph, urine analysis and culture, blood count and differential, renal and liver function tests, alkaline phosphatase, sedimentation rate, antinuclear antibody, anti-Ro, anti-La antibody, and serum angiotensin- converting enzyme level are often indicated. Liver or bone marrow biopsy may be diagnostic in some cases of miliary tuberculosis, disseminated fungal infection, sarcoidosis, or metastatic malignancy. Abnormalities discovered on chest radiograph or chest CT can be pursued by bronchoscopy or transthoracic needle biopsy.

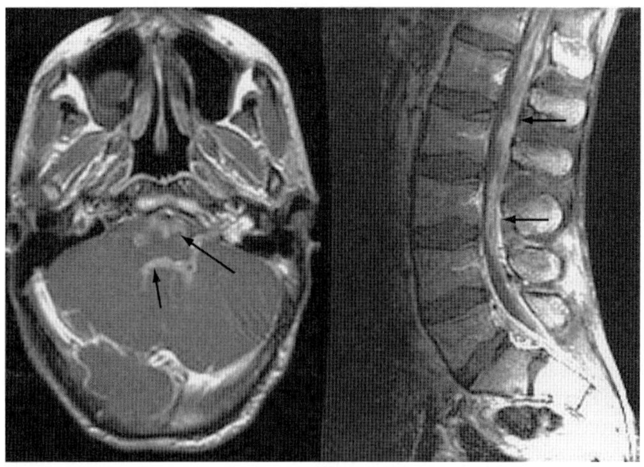

FIGURE 30-1

Primary central nervous system lymphoma. A 24-year-old man, immunosuppressed due to intestinal lymphangiectasia, developed multiple cranial neuropathies. CSF findings consisted of 100 lymphocytes/μL and a protein of 2.5 g/L (250 mg/dL); cytology and cultures were negative. Gadolinium-enhanced T1 MRI revealed diffuse, multifocal meningeal enhancement surrounding the brainstem (***A***), spinal cord, and cauda equina (***B***).

MENINGEAL BIOPSY A meningeal biopsy should be strongly considered in patients who are severely disabled, who need chronic ventricular decompression, or whose illness is progressing rapidly. The activities of the surgeon, pathologist, microbiologist, and cytologist should be coordinated so that a large enough sample is obtained and the appropriate cultures and histologic and molecular studies, including electron-microscopic and PCR studies, are performed. The diagnostic yield of meningeal biopsy can be increased by targeting regions that enhance with contrast on MRI or CT. With current microsurgical techniques, most areas of the basal meninges can be accessed for biopsy via a limited craniotomy. In a series from the Mayo Clinic reported by Cheng et al., MRI demonstrated meningeal enhancement in 47% of patients undergoing meningeal biopsy. Biopsy of an enhancing region was diagnostic in 80% of cases; biopsy of nonenhancing regions was diagnostic in only 9%; sarcoid (31%) and metastatic adenocarcinoma (25%) were the most common conditions identified. Tuberculosis is the most common condition identified in many reports from outside the United States.

APPROACH TO THE ENIGMATIC CASE In approximately one-third of cases, the diagnosis is not known despite careful evaluation of CSF and potential extraneural sites of disease. A number of the organisms that cause chronic meningitis may take weeks to be identified by cultures. In enigmatic cases, several options are available, determined by the extent of the clinical deficits and rate of progression. It is prudent to wait until cultures are finalized if the patient is asymptomatic or symptoms are mild and not progressive. Unfortunately, in many cases progressive neurologic deterioration occurs, and rapid treatment is required. Ventricular-peritoneal shunts may be placed to relieve hydrocephalus, but the risk of disseminating the undiagnosed inflammatory process into the abdomen must be considered.

Empirical Treatment Diagnosis of the causative agent is essential because effective therapies exist for many etiologies of chronic meningitis, but if the condition is left untreated, progressive damage to the CNS and cranial nerves and roots is likely to occur. Occasionally, empirical therapy must be initiated when all attempts at diagnosis fail. In general, empirical therapy in the United States consists of antimycobacterial agents, amphotericin for fungal infection, or glucocorticoids for noninfectious inflammatory causes. It is important to direct empirical therapy of lymphocytic meningitis at tuberculosis, particularly if the condition is associated with hypoglycorrhachia and sixth and other CN palsies, since untreated disease is fatal in 4–8 weeks. In the Mayo Clinic series, the most useful empirical therapy was administration of glucocorticoids rather than antituberculous therapy. Carcinomatous or lymphomatous meningitis may be difficult to diagnose initially, but the diagnosis becomes evident with time.

THE IMMUNOSUPPRESSED PATIENT

Chronic meningitis is not uncommon in the course of HIV infection. Pleocytosis and mild meningeal signs often occur at the onset of HIV infection, and occasionally low-grade meningitis persists. Toxoplasmosis commonly presents as intracranial abscesses and may also be associated with meningitis. Other important causes of chronic meningitis in AIDS include infection with *Cryptococcus*, *Nocardia*, *Candida*, or other fungi; syphilis; and lymphoma (Fig. 30-1). Toxoplasmosis, cryptococcosis, nocardiosis, and other fungal infections are important etiologic considerations in individuals with immunodeficiency states other than AIDS, including those due to immunosuppressive medications. Because of the increased risk of chronic meningitis and the attenuation of clinical signs of meningeal irritation in immunosuppressed individuals, CSF examination should be performed for any persistent headache or unexplained change in mental state.

FURTHER READINGS

Caws M et al: Role of IS6110-targeted PCR, culture, biochemical, clinical, and immunological criteria for diagnosis of tuberculous meningitis. J Clin Microbiol 38(9):3150, 2000

Gilden DH et al: Herpesvirus infections of the nervous system. Nat Clin Pract Neurol 3:82, 2007

Gleissner B, Chamberlain MC: Neoplastic meningitis. Lancet Neurol 5:443, 2006

Halperin JJ et al: Practice parameter: Treatment of nervous system Lyme disease (an evidence-based review): Report of the Quality Standards Subcomittee of the American Academy of Neurology. Neurology 69:91, 2007

Lan SH et al: Cerebral infarction in chronic meningitis: A comparison of tuberculous meningitis and cryptococcal meningitis. Q J Med 94(5):247, 2001

Liliang PC et al: Use of ventriculoperitoneal shunts to treat uncontrollable intracranial hypertension in patients who have cryptococcal meningitis without hydrocephalus. Clin Infect Dis 34(12):E64, 2002

Thurtell MJ et al: Tuberculous cranial pachymeningitis. Neurology 68:298, 2007

CHAPTER 31

CHRONIC FATIGUE SYNDROME

Stephen E. Straus†

DEFINITION

Chronic fatigue syndrome (CFS) is the current name for a disorder characterized by debilitating fatigue and several associated physical, constitutional, and neuropsychological complaints (Table 31-1). This syndrome is not new; in the past, patients diagnosed with conditions such as the vapors, neurasthenia, effort syndrome, chronic brucellosis, epidemic neuromyasthenia, myalgic encephalomyelitis, hypoglycemia, multiple chemical sensitivity syndrome, chronic candidiasis, chronic mononucleosis, chronic Epstein-Barr virus (EBV) infection, and postviral fatigue syndrome may have had what is now called CFS. A subset of ill veterans of military campaigns suffer from CFS. The U.S. Centers for Disease Control and Prevention (CDC) has developed diagnostic criteria for CFS based upon symptoms and the exclusion of other illnesses (Table 31-2).

EPIDEMIOLOGY

Patients with CFS are twice as likely to be women as men and are generally 25–45 years old, although cases in childhood and in later life have been described.

Cases are recognized in many developed countries. Most arise sporadically, but many clusters have also been reported. Famous outbreaks of CFS occurred in Los Angeles County Hospital in 1934; in Akureyri, Iceland, in 1948; in the Royal Free Hospital, London, in 1955; and in Incline Village, Nevada, in 1985. Although these clustered cases suggest a common environmental or infectious cause, none has been identified.

Estimates of the prevalence of CFS have depended on the case definition used and the method of study. Chronic fatigue itself is a common symptom, occurring in as many as 20% of patients attending general medical clinics; CFS is far less common. Community-based studies find that 100–300 individuals per 100,000 population in the United States meet the current CDC case definition.

PATHOGENESIS

The diverse names for the syndrome reflect the many and controversial hypotheses about its etiology. Several common themes underlie attempts to understand the disorder: (1) it is often postinfectious; (2) it is associated with mild immunologic disturbances and sedentary behavior during childhood; and (3) it is commonly accompanied by neuropsychological complaints, somatic preoccupation, and/or depression.

Many studies over the past quarter century sought to link CFS to acute and/or persisting infections with EBV, cytomegalovirus, human herpesvirus type 6, retroviruses, enteroviruses, *Candida albicans*, *Mycoplasma* spp., or *Coxiella burnetii*, among other microbial pathogens. Compared with findings in age-matched control subjects, the titers of antibodies to some microorganisms are elevated in CFS patients. Reports that viral antigens and nucleic acids could be specifically identified in patients with CFS, however, have not been confirmed. One study from the United Kingdom failed to detect any association between acute infections and subsequent prolonged fatigue. Another study found that chronic fatigue did not develop after typical upper respiratory infections but did in some individuals after infectious mononucleosis. Thus, although antecedent infections are associated with CFS, a direct microbial causality is unproven and unlikely.

Changes in numerous immune parameters of uncertain functional significance have been reported in CFS. Modest elevations in titers of antinuclear antibodies, reductions in immunoglobulin subclasses, deficiencies in mitogen-driven lymphocyte proliferation, reductions in natural killer cell activity, disturbances in cytokine production, and shifts in lymphocyte subsets have been described. None of these immune findings appear in most patients, nor do any correlate with the severity of CFS. Comparison of monozygotic twin pairs discordant for CFS showed no substantive immunologic differences between affected and unaffected individuals. In theory, symptoms of CFS could result from excessive production of a cytokine, such as interleukin 1, that induces asthenia and other flulike symptoms; however, compelling data in support of this hypothesis are lacking. A recently published population-based study from Wichita, Kansas, reported differences in gene expression patterns and in candidate gene polymorphisms between CFS patients and controls; these results are controversial and await confirmation.

In some but not the more recent studies, patients with CFS commonly manifested sensitivity to sustained

†Deceased.

TABLE 31-1

SPECIFIC SYMPTOMS REPORTED BY PATIENTS WITH CHRONIC FATIGUE SYNDROME

SYMPTOM	PERCENTAGE
Fatigue	100
Difficulty concentrating	90
Headache	90
Sore throat	85
Tender lymph nodes	80
Muscle aches	80
Joint aches	75
Feverishness	75
Difficulty sleeping	70
Psychiatric problems	65
Allergies	55
Abdominal cramps	40
Weight loss	20
Rash	10
Rapid pulse	10
Weight gain	5
Chest pain	5
Night sweats	5

Source: From SE Straus: J Infect Diseases 157:405, 1988; with permission.

upright posture or tilting, resulting in hypotension and syncope, so as to suggest a form of dysautonomia.

Disturbances in hypothalamic-pituitary-adrenal function have been identified in several controlled studies of CFS, with some evidence for normalization in patients whose fatigue abates. These neuroendocrine abnormalities could contribute to the impaired energy and depressed mood of patients.

Mild to moderate depression is present in one-half to two-thirds of patients. Much of this depression may be reactive, but its prevalence exceeds that seen in other chronic medical illnesses. Some propose that CFS is fundamentally a psychiatric disorder and that the various neuroendocrine and immune disturbances arise secondarily.

TABLE 31-2

CDC CRITERIA FOR DIAGNOSIS OF CHRONIC FATIGUE SYNDROME

A case of chronic fatigue syndrome is defined by the presence of:

1. Clinically evaluated, unexplained, persistent or relapsing fatigue that is of new or definite onset, is not the result of ongoing exertion, is not alleviated by rest, and results in substantial reduction of previous levels of occupational, educational, social, or personal activities; and
2. Four or more of the following symptoms that persist or recur during 6 or more consecutive months of illness and that do not predate the fatigue:
   - Self-reported impairment in short-term memory or concentration
   - Sore throat
   - Tender cervical or axillary nodes
   - Muscle pain
   - Multijoint pain without redness or swelling
   - Headaches of a new pattern or severity
   - Unrefreshing sleep
   - Postexertional malaise lasting ≥24 h

Note: CDC, U.S. Centers for Disease Control and Prevention.
Source: Adapted from K Fukuda et al: Ann Intern Med 121:953, 1994; with permission.

MANIFESTATIONS

Typically, CFS arises suddenly in a previously active individual. An otherwise unremarkable flulike illness or some other acute stress leaves unbearable exhaustion in its wake. Other symptoms, such as headache, sore throat, tender lymph nodes, muscle and joint aches, and frequent feverishness, lead to the belief that an infection persists, and medical attention is sought. Over weeks to months, despite reassurances that "nothing serious is wrong," the symptoms persist and other features of the syndrome become evident—disturbed sleep, difficulty in concentration, and depression (Table 31-1).

Depending on the dominant symptoms and the beliefs of the patient, additional consultations may be sought from allergists, rheumatologists, infectious disease specialists, psychiatrists, ecologic therapists, homeopaths, or other professionals, frequently with unsatisfactory results. Once the pattern of illness is established, the symptoms may fluctuate somewhat. Many patients report that CFS symptoms, including cognitive problems, are exacerbated by intensive physical or other stressors, yet recent prospective studies have not confirmed this impression.

Most patients remain capable of meeting family, work, or community obligations despite their symptoms; discretionary activities are abandoned first. Some feel unable to engage in any gainful employment. A minority of individuals require help with the activities of daily living. Econometric analyses conducted by the CDC have confirmed that CFS exacts a significant toll on household and workforce productivity.

Ultimately, isolation, frustration, and pathetic resignation can mark the protracted course of illness. Patients may become angry at physicians for failing to acknowledge or resolve their plight. Fortunately, CFS does not appear to progress. On the contrary, many patients experience gradual improvement, and a minority recover fully.

DIAGNOSIS

A thorough history, physical examination, and judicious use of laboratory tests are required to exclude other causes of the patient's symptoms. Prominent abnormalities argue strongly in favor of alternative diagnoses. No laboratory test, however, can diagnose this condition or measure its severity. In most cases, elaborate, expensive workups are not helpful. Early claims that MRI or single-photon emission CT can identify abnormalities in the brain of CFS patients have not withstood further study. The dilemma for patient and clinician alike is that

CFS has no pathognomonic features and remains a constellation of symptoms and a diagnosis of exclusion. Often the patient presents with features that also meet criteria for other subjective disorders, such as fibromyalgia and irritable bowel syndrome. Questions have been raised regarding the relative merits of rendering a diagnosis of CFS. Being diagnosed can provide validation of a patient's perceived symptoms, but may also perpetuate or exacerbate them. Refusal to label a patient as having CFS, however, can deny the patient the opportunity to undertake treatments that are of proven merit.

Treatment: CHRONIC FATIGUE SYNDROME

After other illnesses have been excluded, there are several points to address in the long-term care of a patient with chronic fatigue.

The patient should be educated about the illness and what is known of its pathogenesis; potential impact on the physical, psychological, and social dimensions of life; and prognosis. Periodic reassessment is appropriate to identify a possible underlying process that is late in declaring itself and to address intercurrent symptoms that should not be simply dismissed as additional subjective complaints.

Many symptoms of CFS respond to treatment. Nonsteroidal anti-inflammatory drugs alleviate headache, diffuse pain, and feverishness. Allergic rhinitis and sinusitis are common; when present, antihistamines or decongestants may be helpful. Although the patient may be averse to psychiatric diagnoses, depression and anxiety are often prominent and should be treated. Expert psychiatric assessment is sometimes advisable. Nonsedating antidepressants improve mood and disordered sleep and may attenuate the fatigue. Even modest improvements in symptoms can make an important difference in the patient's degree of self-sufficiency and ability to appreciate life's pleasures.

Practical advice should be given regarding lifestyle. Sleep disturbances are common; consumption of heavy meals, alcohol, and caffeine at night can make sleep even more elusive, compounding fatigue. Total rest leads to further deconditioning and the self-image of being an invalid, whereas overexertion may worsen exhaustion and lead to total avoidance of exercise. A carefully graded exercise regimen should be encouraged and has been proven to relieve symptoms and enhance exercise tolerance.

Controlled therapeutic trials have established that acyclovir, fludrocortisone, galantamine, modafinil, and IV immunoglobulin, among other agents, offer no significant benefit in CFS. Low doses of hydrocortisone provide modest benefit but may lead to adrenal suppression. Countless anecdotes circulate regarding other traditional and nontraditional therapies. It is important to guide patients away from those therapeutic modalities that are toxic, expensive, or unreasonable.

The physician should promote the patient's efforts to recover. Several controlled trials conducted in the United Kingdom, in Australia, and in the Netherlands showed cognitive-behavioral therapy to be helpful in adolescents and adults with CFS. This approach aims to dispel misguided beliefs and fears about CFS that can contribute to inactivity and despair. For CFS, as for many other conditions, a comprehensive approach to physical, psychological, and social aspects of well-being is in order.

FURTHER READINGS

Baker R, Shaw EJ: Diagnosis and management of chronic fatigue syndrome or myalgic encephalomyelitis (or encephalopathy): Summary of NICE guidance. BMJ 335:446, 2007

Prins JB et al: Chronic fatigue syndrome. Lancet 367:346, 2006

Vernon SD, Reeves WC: The challenge of integrating high-content data: Epidemiological, clinical and laboratory data collected during an in-hospital study of chronic fatigue syndrome. Pharmacogenomics 7:341, 2006

White P et al: Chronic fatigue syndrome or myalgic encephalomyelitis. BMJ 335:411, 2007

CHAPTER 32

INFECTIOUS COMPLICATIONS OF BURNS AND BITES

Lawrence C. Madoff ■ Florencia Pereyra

The skin is an essential component of the nonspecific immune system, protecting the host from potential pathogens in the environment. Breaches in this protective barrier thus represent a form of immunocompromise that predisposes the patient to infection. Thermal burns may cause massive destruction of the integument as well as derangements in humoral and cellular immunity, permitting the development of infection caused by environmental opportunists and components of the host's skin flora. Bites and scratches from animals and humans allow the inoculation of microorganisms past the skin's protective barrier into deeper, susceptible host tissues.

BURNS

EPIDEMIOLOGY

Over the past decade, the estimated incidence of burn injuries in the United States has steadily declined; still, however, >1 million burn injuries are brought to medical attention each year. Although many burn injuries are minor and require little or no intervention, 50,000 persons are hospitalized for these injuries, and 20,000 have major burns involving at least 25% of the total body surface area. The majority of burn patients are men. Infants account for ~10% of all reported cases. Scalds, structural fires, and flammable liquids and gases are the major causes of burns, but electrical, chemical, and smoking-related sources are also important. Burns predispose to infection by damaging the protective barrier function of the skin, thus facilitating the entry of pathogenic microorganisms, and by inducing systemic immunosuppression. It is therefore not surprising that multiorgan failure and infectious complications are the major causes of morbidity and death in serious burn injury and that as many as 10,000 patients in the United States die of burn-related infections each year.

PATHOPHYSIOLOGY

Loss of the cutaneous barrier facilitates entry of the patient's own flora and of organisms from the hospital environment into the burn wound. Initially, the wound is colonized with gram-positive bacteria from the surrounding tissue, but the number of bacteria grows rapidly beneath the burn eschar, reaching ~8.4×10^3 cfu/g on day 4 after the burn. The avascularity of the eschar, along with the impairment of local immune responses, favors further bacterial colonization and proliferation. By day 7, the wound is colonized with other microbes, including gram-positive bacteria, gram-negative bacteria, and yeasts derived from the gastrointestinal and upper respiratory flora. Invasive infection—localized and/or systemic—occurs when these bacteria penetrate viable tissue. In addition, a role for biofilms has been recognized in experimental animal models of burn-wound infection. (Biofilms are surface-associated communities of bacteria, often embedded in a matrix, that allow the microbes to persist and to resist the effects of host immunity and antimicrobial agents.)

Streptococci and staphylococci were the predominant causes of burn-wound infection in the preantibiotic era and remain important pathogens at present. With the advent of antimicrobial agents, *Pseudomonas aeruginosa* became a major problem in burn-wound management. Less common anaerobic bacteria are typically found in infections of electrical burns or when open wound dressings are used. As antibiotics more effective against *Pseudomonas* have become available, fungi (particularly *Candida albicans*, *Aspergillus* spp., and the agents of mucormycosis) have emerged as increasingly important pathogens in burn-wound patients. Herpes simplex virus (HSV) infection has also been found in burn wounds, especially those on the face.

The cascade of events that follow a severe burn injury and that lead to multiorgan system failure and death are thought to represent a two-step process: The burn injury itself, with ensuing hypovolemia and tissue hypoxia, is followed by invasive infection arising from large amounts of devitalized tissue. The frequency of infection parallels the extent and severity of the burn injury. Severe burn injuries cause a state of immunosuppression that affects innate and adaptive immune responses. The substantial impact of immunocompromise on infection is due to effects on both the cellular and the humoral arms of the immune system. For example, decreases in the number and activity of circulating helper T cells, increases in suppressor T cells, decreases in production and release of monocytes and macrophages, and diminution in levels of immunoglobulin follow major burns. Neutrophil and complement functions have also been shown to be impaired after burns. The increased levels of multiple cytokines detected in burn patients are compatible with the widely held belief that the inflammatory response becomes dysregulated in these individuals; bacterial cell products play a potent role in inducing proinflammatory mediators that contribute to this uncontrolled systemic inflammatory response. Increased permeability of the gut wall to bacteria and their components (e.g., endotoxin) also contributes to immune dysregulation and sepsis. Thus the burn patient is predisposed to infection at remote sites (see below) as well as at the sites of burn injury. Another contributor to secondary immunosuppression after burn injuries is the endocrine system; increasing levels of vasopressin, aldosterone, cortisol, glucagon, growth hormone, catecholamines, and other hormones that directly affect lymphocyte proliferation, secretion of proinflammatory cytokines, natural killer cell activity, and suppressive T cells are seen.

CLINICAL MANIFESTATIONS

Since clinical indications of wound infection are difficult to interpret, wounds must be monitored carefully for changes that may reflect infection. A margin of erythema frequently surrounds the sites of burns and by itself is not usually indicative of infection. Signs of infection include the conversion of a partial-thickness to a full-thickness burn, color changes (e.g., the appearance of a dark brown or black discoloration of the wound), the new appearance of erythema or violaceous edema in normal tissue at the wound margins, the sudden separation of the eschar from subcutaneous tissues, and the degeneration of the wound with the appearance of a new eschar.

Early surgical excision of devitalized tissue is now widely used, and burn-wound infections can be classified in relation to the excision site as (1) burn-wound impetigo (infection characterized by loss of epithelium from a previously reepithelialized surface, as seen in a

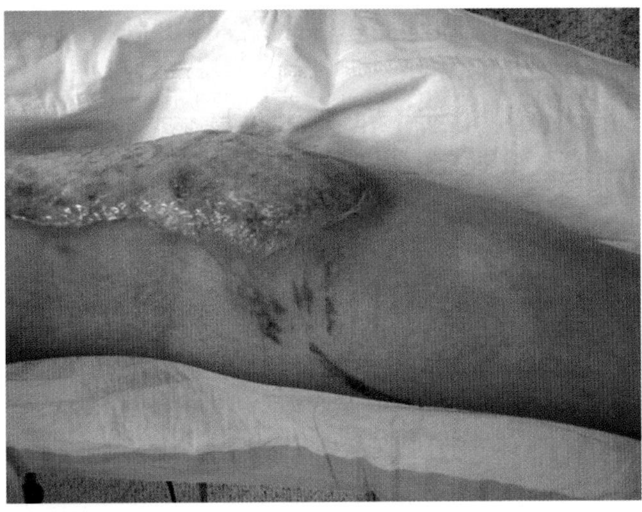

FIGURE 32-1
Cellulitis complicating a burn wound of the arm and demonstrating extension of the infection to adjacent healthy tissue. *(Courtesy of Dr. Robert L. Sheridan, Massachusetts General Hospital, Boston; with permission.)*

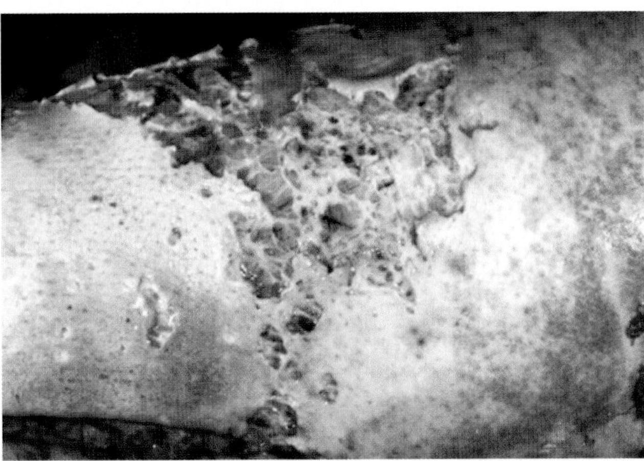

FIGURE 32-3
A burn wound infected with *Pseudomonas aeruginosa*, with liquefaction of tissue. Note the green discoloration at the wound margins, which is suggestive of *Pseudomonas* infection. *(Courtesy of Dr. Robert L. Sheridan, Massachusetts General Hospital, Boston; with permission.)*

partial-thickness burn that is allowed to close by secondary intention, a grafted burn, or a healed skin donor site); (2) burn-related surgical wound infection (purulent infection of excised burn and donor sites that have not yet epithelialized, accompanied by positive cultures); (3) burn-wound cellulitis (extension of infection to surrounding healthy tissue; Fig. 32-1); and (4) invasive infection in unexcised burn wounds (infection that is secondary to a partial- or full-thickness burn wound and is manifested by separation of the eschar or by violaceous, dark brown, or black discoloration of the eschar; Fig. 32-2). The appearance of a green discoloration of the wound or subcutaneous fat (Fig. 32-3) or the development of ecthyma gangrenosum at a remote site points to a diagnosis of invasive *P. aeruginosa* infection.

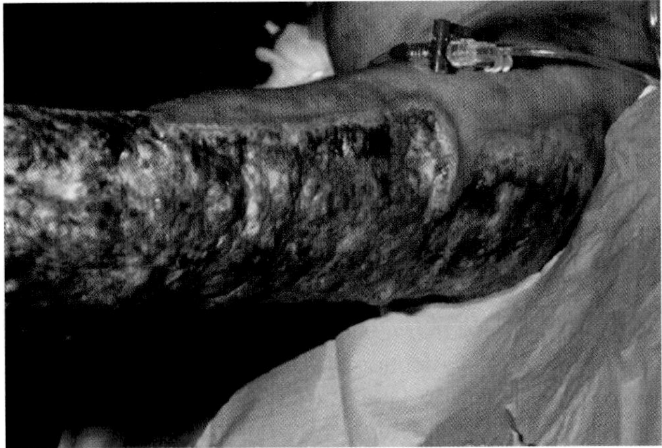

FIGURE 32-2
A severe upper-extremity burn infected with *Pseudomonas aeruginosa*. The wound requires additional debridement. Note the dark brown to black discoloration of the eschar. *(Courtesy of Dr. Robert L. Sheridan, Massachusetts General Hospital, Boston; with permission.)*

Changes in body temperature, hypotension, tachycardia, altered mentation, neutropenia or neutrophilia, thrombocytopenia, and renal failure may result from invasive burn wounds and sepsis. However, because profound alterations in homeostasis occur as a consequence of burns per se and because inflammation without infection is a normal component of these injuries, the assessment of these changes is complicated. Alterations in body temperature, for example, are attributable to thermoregulatory dysfunction; tachycardia and hyperventilation accompany the metabolic changes induced by extensive burn injury and are not necessarily indicative of bacterial sepsis.

Given the difficulty of evaluating burn wounds solely on the basis of clinical observation and laboratory data, wound biopsies are necessary for definitive diagnosis of infection. The timing of these biopsies can be guided by clinical changes, but in some centers, burn wounds are routinely biopsied at regular intervals. The biopsy specimen is examined for histologic evidence of bacterial invasion, and quantitative microbiologic cultures are performed. The presence of $>10^5$ viable bacteria per gram of tissue is highly suggestive of invasive infection and of a dramatically increased risk of sepsis. Histopathologic evidence of invasion of viable tissue by microorganisms is a more definitive indicator of infection. A blood culture positive for the same organism seen in large quantities in biopsied tissue is a reliable indicator of burn sepsis. Surface cultures may provide some indication of the microorganisms present in the hospital environment but are not indicative of the etiology of infection. This noninvasive technique might be of use in determining the flora present in excised burn areas or in areas where the skin is too thin for biopsy (e.g., over the ears, eyes, or digits).

In addition to infection of the burn wound itself, a number of other infections due to the immunosuppression caused by extensive burns and the manipulations necessary for clinical care put burn patients at risk. Pneumonia, now the most common infectious complication among hospitalized burn patients, is most often nosocomially acquired via the respiratory route; among the risk factors associated with secondary pneumonia are inhalation injury, intubation, full-thickness chest wall burns, immobility, and uncontrolled wound sepsis with hematogenous spread. Septic pulmonary emboli may also occur. Suppurative thrombophlebitis may complicate the vascular catheterization necessary for fluid and nutritional support in burns. Endocarditis, urinary tract infection, bacterial chondritis (particularly in patients with burned ears), and intraabdominal infection also complicate serious burn injury.

℞ Treatment: BURN-WOUND INFECTIONS

The ultimate goal of burn-wound management is closure and healing of the wound. Early surgical excision of burned tissue, with extensive debridement of necrotic tissue and grafting of skin or skin substitutes, greatly decreases mortality rates associated with severe burns. In addition, the four widely used topical antimicrobial agents—silver sulfadiazine cream, mafenide acetate cream, silver nitrate cream, and nanocrystalline silver dressings—dramatically decrease the bacterial burden of burn wounds and reduce the incidence of burn-wound infection; these agents are routinely applied to partial- and full-thickness burns. The bactericidal properties of silver are related to its effect on respiratory enzymes on bacterial cell walls; its interaction with structural proteins causes keratinocyte and fibroblast toxicity that can delay wound healing if silver-based compounds are used indiscriminately. All four agents are broadly active against many bacteria and some fungi and are useful before bacterial colonization is established. Silver sulfadiazine is often used initially, but its value can be limited by bacterial resistance, poor wound penetration, or toxicity (leukopenia). Mafenide acetate has broader activity against gram-negative bacteria. The cream penetrates eschars and thus can prevent or treat infection beneath them; its use without dressings allows regular examination of the wound area. The foremost disadvantages of mafenide acetate are that it can inhibit carbonic anhydrase, resulting in metabolic acidosis, and that it elicits hypersensitivity reactions in up to 7% of patients. This agent is most often used when gram-negative bacteria invade the burn wound and when treatment with silver sulfadiazine fails. The activity of mafenide acetate against gram-positive bacteria is limited. Nanocrystalline silver dressings provide broader antimicrobial coverage than any other available topical preparation, exhibiting activity against methicillin-resistant *Staphylococcus aureus* (MRSA) and vancomycin-resistant enterococci (VRE), moderate ability to penetrate eschars, and limited toxicity. In addition, this approach provides controlled and prolonged release of nanocrystalline silver into the wound, limiting the number of dressing changes and therefore reducing the risk of nosocomial infections as well as the cost of treatment. Mupirocin, a topical antimicrobial agent used to eradicate nasal colonization with MRSA, is increasingly being used in burn units where MRSA is prevalent. The efficacy of mupirocin in reducing burn-wound bacterial counts and preventing systemic infections is comparable to that of silver sulfadiazine.

In recent years, rates of fungal infection have increased in burn patients. When superficial fungal infection occurs, nystatin may be mixed with silver sulfadiazine or mafenide acetate as topical therapy. A small study found that nystatin powder (6 million units/g) was effective for treatment of superficial and deep burn-wound infections caused by *Aspergillus* or *Fusarium* spp. In addition to these products, moisture-retention ointments with antimicrobial properties can promote rapid autolysis, debridement, and moist healing of partial-thickness wounds.

When invasive wound infection is diagnosed, topical therapy should be changed to mafenide acetate. Subeschar clysis (the direct instillation of an antibiotic, often piperacillin, into wound tissues under the eschar) is a useful adjunct to surgical and systemic antimicrobial therapy. Systemic treatment with antibiotics active against the pathogens present in the wound should be instituted. In the absence of culture data, treatment should be broad in spectrum, covering organisms commonly encountered in that particular burn unit. Such coverage is usually achieved with an antibiotic active against gram-positive pathogens (e.g., oxacillin, 2 g IV every 4 h) and with a drug active against *P. aeruginosa* and other gram-negative rods (e.g., mezlocillin, 3 g IV every 4 h; and gentamicin, 5 mg/kg IV per day). In penicillin-allergic patients, vancomycin (1 g IV every 12 h) may be substituted for oxacillin (and is efficacious against MRSA), and ciprofloxacin (400 mg IV every 12 h) may be substituted for mezlocillin. Patients with burn wounds frequently have alterations in metabolism and renal clearance mechanisms that mandate the monitoring of serum antibiotic levels; the levels achieved with standard doses are often subtherapeutic.

Treatment of infections caused by emerging resistant pathogens remains a challenge in the care of burn patients. MRSA, resistant enterococci, multidrug-resistant gram-negative rods, and Enterobacteriaceae producing extended-spectrum β-lactamases have been associated with burn-wound infections and identified in burn-unit outbreaks. Strict infection-control practices (including microbiologic surveillance in burn units) and appropriate antimicrobial therapy remain important measures in reducing rates of infection due to resistant organisms.

In general, prophylactic systemic antibiotics have no role in the management of burn wounds and can in fact lead to colonization with resistant microorganisms. In some studies, antibiotic prophylaxis has been associated with increased secondary infections of the upper and lower respiratory tract and the urinary tract as well as with prolonged hospitalization. An exception involves cases requiring burn-wound manipulation. Since procedures such as debridement, excision, or grafting frequently result in bacteremia, prophylactic systemic antibiotics are administered at the time of wound manipulation; the specific agents used should be chosen on the basis of data obtained by wound culture or data on the hospital's resident flora.

The use of oral antibiotics for selective digestive decontamination (SDD) to decrease bacterial colonization and the risk of burn-wound infection is controversial and has not been widely adopted. In a randomized, double-blind, placebo-controlled trial in patients with burns involving >20% of the total body surface area, SDD was associated with reduced mortality rates in the burn intensive care unit and in the hospital and also with a reduced incidence of pneumonia. The effects of SDD on the normal anaerobic bowel flora must be taken into consideration before this approach is used.

All burn-injury patients should undergo tetanus booster immunization if they have completed primary immunization but have not received a booster dose in the past 5 years. Patients without prior immunization should receive tetanus immune globulin and undergo primary immunization.

BITES AND SCRATCHES

Each year in the United States, millions of animal bite wounds are sustained. The vast majority are inflicted by pet dogs and cats, which number >100 million; the annual incidence of dog and cat bites has been reported as 300 bites per 100,000 population. Other bite wounds are a consequence of encounters with animals in the wild or in occupational settings. Although many of these wounds require minimal or no therapy, a significant number result in infection, which may be life-threatening. The microbiology of bite-wound infections in general reflects the oropharyngeal flora of the biting animal, although organisms from the soil, the skin of the animal and victim, and the animal's feces may also be involved.

DOG BITES

In the United States, dogs bite >4.7 million people each year and are responsible for 80% of all animal-bite wounds, an estimated 15–20% of which become infected. Each year, 800,000 Americans seek medical attention for dog bites; of those injured, 386,000 require treatment in an emergency department, with >1000 emergency department visits each day and about a dozen deaths per year. Most dog bites are provoked and are inflicted by the victim's pet or by a dog known to the victim. These bites frequently occur during efforts to break up a dogfight. Children are more likely than adults to sustain canine bites, with the highest incidence of 6 bites per 1000 population among boys 5–9 years old. Victims are more often male than female, and bites most often involve an upper extremity. Among children <4 years old, two-thirds of all these injuries involve the head or neck. Infection typically manifests 8–24 h after the bite as pain at the site of injury with cellulitis accompanied by purulent, sometimes foul-smelling discharge. Septic arthritis and osteomyelitis may develop if a canine tooth penetrates synovium or bone. Systemic manifestations (e.g., fever, lymphadenopathy, and lymphangitis) may also occur. The microbiology of dog bite-wound infections is usually mixed and includes β-hemolytic streptococci, *Pasteurella* spp., *Staphylococcus* spp., *Eikenella corrodens*, and *Capnocytophaga canimorsus* (formerly designated DF-2). Many wounds also include anaerobic bacteria such as *Actinomyces*, *Fusobacterium*, *Prevotella*, and *Porphyromonas* spp.

Although most infections resulting from dog bite injuries are localized to the area of injury, many of the microorganisms involved are capable of causing systemic infection, including bacteremia, meningitis, brain abscess, endocarditis, and chorioamnionitis. These infections are particularly likely in hosts with edema or compromised lymphatic drainage in the involved extremity (e.g., after a bite on the arm in a woman who has undergone radical or modified radical mastectomy) and in patients who are immunocompromised by medication or disease (e.g., glucocorticoid use, systemic lupus erythematosus, acute leukemia, or hepatic cirrhosis). In addition, dog bites and scratches may result in systemic illnesses such as rabies (Chap. 98) and tetanus (Chap. 40).

Infection with *C. canimorsus* after dog bite wounds may result in fulminant sepsis, disseminated intravascular coagulation, and renal failure, particularly in hosts who have impaired hepatic function, who have undergone splenectomy, or who are immunosuppressed. This organism is a thin gram-negative rod that is difficult to culture on most solid media but grows in a variety of liquid media. The bacteria are occasionally seen within polymorphonuclear leukocytes on Wright-stained smears of peripheral blood from septic patients. Tularemia (Chap. 59) has also been reported to follow dog bites.

CAT BITES

Although less common than dog bites, cat bites and scratches result in infection in more than half of all cases. Because the narrow, sharp feline incisors penetrate deeply into tissue, cat bites are more likely than dog bites to cause septic arthritis and osteomyelitis; the development of these conditions is particularly likely when punctures are located over or near a joint, especially in the hand. Women sustain cat bites more frequently than do men. These bites most often involve the hands and arms. Both bites and scratches from cats are prone to infection from organisms in the cat's oropharynx. *Pasteurella multocida*, a normal component of the feline oral flora, is a small gram-negative coccobacillus implicated in the majority of cat bite-wound infections. Like that of dog bite-wound infections, however, the microflora of cat bite-wound infections is usually mixed. Other microorganisms causing infection after cat bites are similar to those causing dog bite-wound infections.

The same risk factors for systemic infection after dog bite wounds apply to cat bite wounds. *Pasteurella* infections tend to advance rapidly, often within hours, causing severe inflammation accompanied by purulent drainage; *Pasteurella* may also be spread by respiratory droplets from animals, resulting in pneumonia or bacteremia. Like dog bite wounds, cat bite wounds may result in the transmission of rabies or in the development of tetanus. Infection with *Bartonella henselae* causes cat-scratch disease (Chap. 61) and is an important late consequence of cat bites and scratches. Tularemia (Chap. 59) has also been reported to follow cat bites.

OTHER ANIMAL BITES

Infections have been attributed to bites from many animal species. Often these bites are sustained as a consequence of occupational exposure (farmers, laboratory workers, veterinarians) or recreational exposure (hunters and trappers, wilderness campers, owners of exotic pets). Generally, the microflora of bite wounds reflects the oral flora of the biting animal. Most members of the cat family, including feral cats, harbor *P. multocida*. Bite wounds from aquatic animals such as alligators or piranhas may contain *Aeromonas hydrophila*. Venomous snakebites result in severe inflammatory responses and tissue necrosis—conditions that render these injuries prone to infection. The snake's oral flora includes many species of aerobes and anaerobes, such as *P. aeruginosa*, *Proteus* spp., *Staphylococcus epidermidis*, *Bacteroides fragilis*, and *Clostridium* spp. Bites from nonhuman primates are highly susceptible to infection with pathogens similar to those isolated from human bites (see below). Bites from Old World monkeys (*Macaca*) may also result in the transmission of B virus (*Herpesvirus simiae*, Cercopithecine herpesvirus), a cause of serious infection of the human central nervous system. Bites of seals, walruses, and polar bears may cause a chronic suppurative infection known as *seal finger*, which is probably due to one or more species of *Mycoplasma* colonizing these animals.

Small rodents, including rats, mice, and gerbils, as well as animals that prey on rodents may transmit *Streptobacillus moniliformis* (a microaerophilic, pleomorphic gram-negative rod) or *Spirillum minor* (a spirochete), which cause a clinical illness known as *rat-bite fever*. The vast majority of cases in the United States are streptobacillary, whereas *Spirillum* infection occurs mainly in Asia.

In the United States, the risk of rodent bites is usually greatest among laboratory workers or inhabitants of rodent-infested dwellings (particularly children). Rat-bite fever is distinguished from acute bite-wound infection by its typical manifestation after the initial wound has healed. Streptobacillary disease follows an incubation period of 3–10 days. Fever, chills, myalgias, headache, and severe migratory arthralgias are usually followed by a maculopapular rash, which characteristically involves the palms and soles and may become confluent or purpuric. Complications include endocarditis, myocarditis, meningitis, pneumonia, and abscesses in many organs. *Haverhill fever* is an *S. moniliformis* infection acquired from contaminated milk or drinking water and has similar manifestations. Streptobacillary rat-bite fever was frequently fatal in the preantibiotic era. The differential diagnosis includes Rocky Mountain spotted fever, Lyme disease, leptospirosis, and secondary syphilis. The diagnosis is made by direct observation of the causative organisms in tissue or blood, by culture of the organisms on enriched media, or by serologic testing with specific agglutinins.

Spirillum infection (referred to in Japan as *sodoku*) causes pain and purple swelling at the site of the initial bite, with associated lymphangitis and regional lymphadenopathy, after an incubation period of 1–4 weeks. The systemic illness includes fever, chills, and headache. The original lesion may eventually progress to an eschar. The infection is diagnosed by direct visualization of the spirochetes in blood or tissue or by animal inoculation.

Finally, NO-1 (CDC nonoxidizer group 1) is a recently identified bacterium associated with dog- and cat-bite wounds. Infections in which NO-1 has been isolated have tended to manifest locally (i.e., as abscess and cellulitis). These infections have occurred in healthy persons with no underlying illness and in some instances have progressed from localized to systemic illnesses. The phenotypic characteristics of NO-1 are similar to those of asaccharolytic *Acinetobacter* species; i.e., NO-1 is oxidase-, indole-, and urease-negative. To date, all strains identified have been shown to be susceptible to aminoglycosides, β-lactam antibiotics, tetracyclines, quinolones, and sulfonamides.

HUMAN BITES

Human bites may be self-inflicted; may be sustained by medical personnel caring for patients; or may take place during fights, domestic abuse, or sexual activity. Human bite wounds become infected more frequently (~10–15% of the time) than do bites inflicted by other animals. These infections reflect the diverse oral microflora of humans, which includes multiple species of aerobic and anaerobic bacteria. Common aerobic isolates include viridans streptococci, *Staphylococcus aureus*, *E. corrodens* (which is particularly common in clenched-fist injury; see below), and *Haemophilus influenzae*. Anaerobic species, including *Fusobacterium nucleatum* and *Prevotella*, *Porphyromonas*, and *Peptostreptococcus* spp., are isolated from 50% of human-bite wound infections; many of these isolates produce β-lactamases. The oral flora of hospitalized and debilitated patients often includes Enterobacteriaceae in addition to the usual organisms. Hepatitis B, hepatitis C, HSV infection, syphilis, tuberculosis, actinomycosis, and tetanus have been reported to be transmitted by human bites; it is biologically possible to transmit HIV through human bites, although this event is quite unlikely.

Human bites are categorized as "occlusional" injuries, which are inflicted by actual biting, and "clenched-fist" injuries, which are sustained when the fist of one individual strikes the teeth of another, causing traumatic laceration of the hand. For several reasons, clenched-fist injuries, which are more common than occlusional injuries, result in particularly serious infections. The deep spaces of the hand, including the bones, joints, and tendons, are frequently inoculated with organisms in the course of such injuries. The clenched position of the fist during injury, followed by extension of the hand, may further promote the introduction of bacteria as contaminated tendons retract beneath the skin's surface. Moreover, medical attention is often sought only after frank infection develops.

Approach to the Patient: ANIMAL OR HUMAN BITES

A careful history should be elicited, including the type of biting animal, the type of attack (provoked or unprovoked), and the amount of time elapsed since injury. Local and regional authorities should be contacted to determine whether an individual species could be rabid and/or to locate and observe the biting animal when rabies prophylaxis may be indicated (Chap. 98). Suspicious human bite wounds should provoke careful questioning regarding domestic or child abuse. Details on antibiotic allergies, immunosuppression, splenectomy, liver disease, mastectomy, and immunization history should be obtained. The wound should be inspected carefully for evidence of infection, including redness, exudate, and foul odor. The type of wound (puncture, laceration, or scratch), the depth of penetration, and the possible involvement of joints, tendons, nerves, and bones should be assessed. It is often useful to include a diagram or photograph of the wound in the medical record. In addition, a general physical examination should be conducted and should include an assessment of vital signs as well as an evaluation for evidence of lymphangitis, lymphadenopathy, dermatologic lesions, and functional limitations. Injuries to the hand warrant consultation with a hand surgeon for the assessment of tendon, nerve, and muscular damage. Radiographs should be obtained when the bone may have been penetrated or a tooth fragment may be present. Culture and Gram's staining of all infected wounds are essential; anaerobic cultures should be undertaken if abscesses, devitalized tissue, or foul-smelling exudate is present. A small-tipped swab may be used to culture deep punctures or small lacerations. It is also reasonable to culture samples from uninfected wounds due to bites inflicted by animals other than dogs and cats, since the microorganisms causing disease are less predictable in these cases. The white blood cell count should be determined and blood cultured if systemic infection is suspected.

℞ Treatment: BITE-WOUND INFECTIONS

WOUND MANAGEMENT Wound closure is controversial in bite injuries. Many authorities prefer not to attempt primary closure of wounds that are or may become infected, preferring to irrigate these wounds copiously, debride devitalized tissue, remove foreign bodies, and approximate the wound edges. Delayed primary closure may be undertaken after the risk of infection is over. Small uninfected wounds may be allowed to close by secondary intention. Puncture wounds due to cat bites should be left unsutured because of the high rate at which they become infected. Facial wounds are usually sutured after thorough cleaning and irrigation because of the importance of a good cosmetic result in this area and because anatomic factors such as an excellent blood supply and the absence of dependent edema lessen the risk of infection.

ANTIBIOTIC THERAPY

Established Infection Antibiotics should be administered in all established bite-wound infections and should be chosen in light of the most likely potential pathogens, as indicated by the biting species and by Gram's stain and culture results (Table 32-1). For dog and cat bites, antibiotics should be effective against *S. aureus*, *Pasteurella* spp., *C. canimorsus*, streptococci, and oral anaerobes. For human bites, agents with activity against *S. aureus*, *H. influenzae*, and β-lactamase–positive oral anaerobes should be used. The combination of an extended-spectrum penicillin with a β-lactamase inhibitor (amoxicillin/clavulanic acid, ticarcillin/clavulanic acid, ampicillin/sulbactam) appears to offer the most reliable coverage for these pathogens. Second-generation cephalosporins (cefuroxime, cefoxitin) also offer substantial coverage. The choice of antibiotics for penicillin-allergic patients (particularly those in whom immediate-type hypersensitivity makes the use of cephalosporins hazardous) is more difficult and is based primarily on in vitro sensitivity since data on clinical efficacy are inadequate. The combination of an antibiotic active against gram-positive cocci and anaerobes (such as clindamycin) with trimethoprim-sulfamethoxazole or a fluoroquinolone, which is active against many of the other potential pathogens, would appear reasonable. In vitro data suggest that azithromycin alone provides coverage against most commonly isolated bite-wound pathogens.

Antibiotics are generally given for 10–14 days, but the response to therapy must be carefully monitored. Failure to respond should prompt a consideration of diagnostic alternatives and surgical evaluation for possible drainage or debridement. Complications such as osteomyelitis or septic arthritis mandate a longer duration of therapy.

Management of *C. canimorsus* sepsis requires a 2-week course of IV penicillin G (2 million units IV every 4 h) and supportive measures. Alternative agents for the treatment of *C. canimorsus* infection include cephalosporins and fluoroquinolones. Serious infection with *P. multocida* (e.g., pneumonia, sepsis, or meningitis) should also be treated with IV penicillin G. Alternative agents include second- or third-generation cephalosporins or ciprofloxacin.

Bites by venomous snakes may not require antibiotic treatment. Because it is often difficult to distinguish signs of infection from tissue damage caused by the envenomation, many authorities continue to recommend treatment directed against the snake's oral flora—i.e., the administration of broadly active agents such as ceftriaxone (1–2 g IV every 12–24 h) or ampicillin/sulbactam (1.5–3.0 g IV every 6 h).

TABLE 32-1

MANAGEMENT OF WOUND INFECTIONS AFTER ANIMAL AND HUMAN BITES

BITING SPECIES	COMMONLY ISOLATED PATHOGENS	PREFERRED ANTIBIOTIC(S)[a]	ALTERNATIVE IN PENICILLIN-ALLERGIC PATIENT	PROPHYLAXIS ADVISED FOR EARLY UNINFECTED WOUNDS	OTHER CONSIDERATIONS
Dog	*Staphylococcus aureus*, *Pasteurella multocida*, anaerobes, *Capnocytophaga canimorsus*	Amoxicillin/ clavulanate (250–500 mg PO tid) or ampicillin/ sulbactam (1.5–3.0 g IV q6h)	Clindamycin (150–300 mg PO qid) plus either TMP-SMX (1 DS tablet PO bid) or ciprofloxacin (500 mg PO bid)	Sometimes[b]	Consider rabies prophylaxis.
Cat	*P. multocida*, *S. aureus*, anaerobes	Amoxicillin/ clavulanate or ampicillin/ sulbactam, as above	Clindamycin plus TMP-SMX as above or a fluoroquinolone	Usually	Consider rabies prophylaxis. Carefully evaluate for joint/bone penetration.
Human, occlusional	Viridans streptococci, *S. aureus*, *Haemophilus influenzae*, anaerobes	Amoxicillin/ clavulanate or ampicillin/ sulbactam, as above	Erythromycin (500 mg PO qid) or a fluoroquinolone	Always	
Human, clenched-fist	As for occlusional plus *Eikenella corrodens*	Ampicillin/ sulbactam as above or imipenem (500 mg q6h)	Cefoxitin[c]	Always	Examine for tendon, nerve, or joint involvement.
Monkey	As for human bite	As for human bite	As for human bite	Always	For macaque monkeys, consider B virus prophylaxis with acyclovir.
Snake	*Pseudomonas aeruginosa*, *Proteus* spp., *Bacteroides fragilis*, *Clostridium* spp.	Ampicillin/ sulbactam as above	Clindamycin plus TMP-SMX as above or a fluoroquinolone	Sometimes, especially with venomous snakes	Antivenin for venomous snake bite
Rodent	*Streptobacillus moniliformis*, *Leptospira* spp., *P. multocida*	Penicillin VK (500 mg PO qid)	Doxycycline (100 mg PO bid)	Sometimes	

[a]Antibiotic choices should be based on culture data when available. These are suggestions for empirical therapy and need to be tailored to individual circumstances and local conditions. IV regimens should be used for hospitalized patients. A single IV dose of antibiotics may be given to patients who will be discharged after initial management.
[b]Prophylactic antibiotics are suggested for severe or extensive wounds, facial wounds, and crush injuries; when bone or joint may be involved; and when comorbidity is present (see text).
[c]May be hazardous in patients with immediate-type hypersensitivity reaction to penicillin.
Note: TMP-SMX, trimethoprim-sulfamethoxazole; DS, double-strength.

Seal finger appears to respond to doxycycline (100 mg twice daily for an interval guided by the response to therapy).

Presumptive or Prophylactic Therapy The use of antibiotics in patients presenting early after bite injury (within 8 h) is controversial. Although symptomatic infection frequently will not yet have manifested at this point, many early wounds will harbor pathogens, and many will become infected. Studies of antibiotic prophylaxis for wound infections are limited and have often included only small numbers of cases in which various types of wounds have been managed according to various protocols. A meta-analysis of eight randomized trials of prophylactic antibiotics in patients with dog bite wounds demonstrated a reduction in the rate of infection by 50% with prophylaxis. However, in the absence of sound clinical trials, many clinicians base the decision to treat bite wounds with empirical antibiotics on the species of the biting animal; the location, severity, and extent of the bite wound; and the existence of comorbid conditions in the host. All human and monkey bite wounds should be treated presumptively because of the high rate of infection. Most cat bite wounds, particularly those involving the hand, should be treated. Other factors favoring treatment for bite wounds include severe injury, as in crush wounds; potential bone or joint involvement; involvement of the hands or genital region; host immunocompromise, including that due to liver disease or splenectomy; and prior mastectomy on the side of an involved upper extremity. When prophylactic antibiotics are administered, they are usually given for 3–5 days.

Rabies and Tetanus Prophylaxis Rabies prophylaxis, consisting of both passive administration of rabies immune globulin (with as much of the dose as possible infiltrated into and around the wound) and active immunization with rabies vaccine, should be given in consultation with local and regional public health authorities for many wild animal (and some domestic animal) bites and scratches as well as for certain nonbite exposures (Chap. 98). Rabies is endemic in a variety of animals, including dogs and cats in many areas of the world. Many local health authorities require the reporting of all animal bites. A tetanus booster immunization should be given if the patient has undergone primary immunization but has not received a booster dose in the past 5 years. Patients who have not previously completed primary immunization should be immunized and should also receive tetanus immune globulin. Elevation of the site of injury is an important adjunct to antimicrobial therapy. Immobilization of the infected area, especially the hand, is also beneficial.

FURTHER READINGS

Baker AS et al: Isolation of *Mycoplasma* species from a patient with seal finger. Clin Infect Dis 27:1168, 1998

Centers for Disease Control and Prevention: Nonfatal dog bite–related injuries treated in hospital emergency departments—United States, 2001. MMWR 52:605, 2003

Cummings P: Antibiotics to prevent infection in patients with dog bite wounds: A meta-analysis of randomized trials. Ann Emerg Med 23:535, 1994

de La Cal M et al: Survival benefit in critically ill burned patients receiving selective decontamination of the digestive tract: A randomized, placebo-controlled, double-blind trial. Ann Surg 241:424, 2005

Fallouji MA: Traumatic love bites. Br J Surg 77:100, 1990

Fleisher GR: The management of bite wounds. N Engl J Med 340:138, 1999

Goldstein EJ: Bite wounds and infection. Clin Infect Dis 14:633, 1992

Holmes GP et al: Guidelines for the prevention and treatment of B-virus infections in exposed persons. The B Virus Working Group. Clin Infect Dis 20:421, 1995

Kaye ET: Topical antibacterial agents. Infect Dis Clin North Am 14:321, 2000

Kullberg BJ et al: Purpura fulminans and symmetrical peripheral gangrene caused by *Capnocytophaga canimorsus* (formerly DF-2) septicemia—a complication of dog bite. Medicine (Baltimore) 70:287, 1991

McManus WF et al: Subeschar antibiotic infusion in the treatment of burn wound infection. J Trauma 20:1021, 1980

Pruitt BJ et al: The changing epidemiology of infection in burn patients. World J Surg 16:57, 1992

Sheridan RL et al: Cutaneous herpetic infections complicating burns. Burns 26:621, 2000

Sing A et al: Methicillin-resistant *Staphylococcus aureus* in a family and its pet cat. N Engl J Med 358:1200, 2008

Steer JA et al: Quantitative microbiology in the management of burn patients. I. Correlation between quantitative and qualitative burn wound biopsy culture and surface alginate swab culture. Burns 22:173, 1996

——— et al: Quantitative microbiology in the management of burn patients. II. Relationship between bacterial counts obtained by burn wound biopsy culture and surface alginate swab culture, with clinical outcome following burn surgery and change of dressings. Burns 22:177, 1996

Talan DA et al: Bacteriological analysis of infected dog and cat bites. N Engl J Med 340:85, 1999

Tan JS: Human zoonotic infections transmitted by dogs and cats. Arch Intern Med 157:1933, 1977

Weber DJ et al: Infections resulting from animal bites. Infect Dis Clin North Am 5:663, 1991

Weiss HB et al: Incidence of dog bite injuries treated in emergency departments. JAMA 279:51, 1998

Youn YK et al: The role of mediators in the response to thermal injury. World J Surg 16:30, 1992

Yurt RW: Burns, in *Principles and Practice of Infectious Diseases*, 5th ed, G Mandell et al (eds). New York, Churchill Livingstone, 2000, pp 3198–3206

SECTION IV

BACTERIAL INFECTIONS

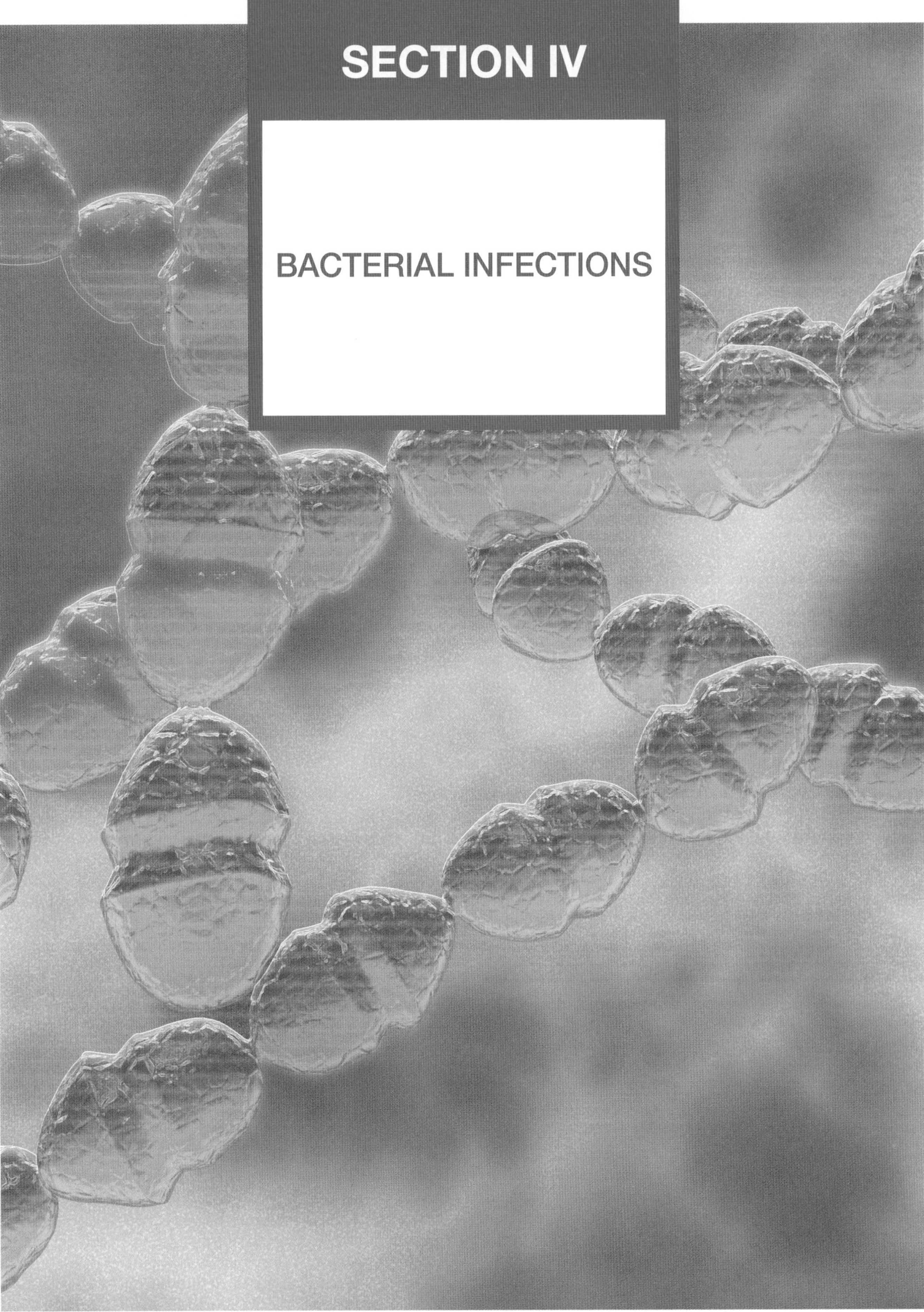

CHAPTER 33

TREATMENT AND PROPHYLAXIS OF BACTERIAL INFECTIONS

Gordon L. Archer ■ Ronald E. Polk

The development of vaccines and drugs that prevent and cure bacterial infections was one of the twentieth century's major contributions to human longevity and quality of life. Antibacterial agents are among the most commonly prescribed drugs of any kind worldwide. Used appropriately, these drugs are lifesaving. However, their indiscriminate use drives up the cost of health care, leads to a plethora of side effects and drug interactions, and fosters the emergence of bacterial resistance, rendering previously valuable drugs useless. The rational use of antibacterial agents depends on an understanding of (1) the drugs' mechanisms of action, spectrum of activity, pharmacokinetics, pharmacodynamics, toxicities, and interactions; (2) mechanisms underlying bacterial resistance; and (3) strategies that can be used by clinicians to limit resistance. In addition, patient-associated parameters, such as infection site, other drugs being taken, allergies, and immune and excretory status, are critically important to appropriate therapeutic decisions. This chapter provides specific data required for making an informed choice of antibacterial agent.

MECHANISMS OF ACTION

Antibacterial agents, like all antimicrobial drugs, are directed against unique targets not present in mammalian cells. The goal is to limit toxicity to the host and maximize chemotherapeutic activity affecting invading microbes only. *Bactericidal drugs* kill the bacteria that are within their spectrum of activity; *bacteriostatic drugs* only inhibit bacterial growth. Although bacteriostatic activity is adequate for the treatment of most infections, bactericidal activity may be necessary for cure in patients with altered immune systems (e.g., neutropenia), protected infectious foci (e.g., endocarditis or meningitis), or specific infections (e.g., complicated *Staphylococcus aureus* bacteremia). The mechanisms of action of the antibacterial agents to be discussed in this section are summarized in Table 33-1 and are depicted in Fig. 33-1.

INHIBITION OF CELL-WALL SYNTHESIS

One major difference between bacterial and mammalian cells is the presence in bacteria of a rigid wall external to the cell membrane. The wall protects bacterial cells from osmotic rupture, which would result from the cell's usual marked hyperosmolarity (by up to 20 atm) relative to the host environment. The structure conferring cell-wall rigidity and resistance to osmotic lysis in both gram-positive and gram-negative bacteria is peptidoglycan, a large, covalently linked sacculus that surrounds the bacterium. In gram-positive bacteria, peptidoglycan is the only layered structure external to the cell membrane and is thick (20–80 nm); in gram-negative bacteria, there is an outer membrane external to a very thin (1-nm) peptidoglycan layer.

Chemotherapeutic agents directed at any stage of the synthesis, export, assembly, or cross-linking of peptidoglycan lead to inhibition of bacterial cell growth and, in most cases, to cell death. Peptidoglycan is composed of (1) a backbone of two alternating sugars, *N*-acetylglucosamine and *N*-acetylmuramic acid; (2) a chain of four amino acids that extends down from the backbone (stem peptides); and (3) a peptide bridge that cross-links the peptide chains. Peptidoglycan is formed by the addition of subunits (a sugar with its five attached amino acids) that are assembled in the cytoplasm and transported through the cytoplasmic membrane to the cell surface. Subsequent cross-linking is driven by cleavage of the terminal stem-peptide amino acid.

Virtually all the antibiotics that inhibit bacterial cell-wall synthesis are bactericidal. That is, they eventually result in the cell's death due to osmotic lysis. However, much of the loss of cell-wall integrity after treatment with cell wall–active agents is due to the bacteria's own cell-wall remodeling enzymes (autolysins) that cleave peptidoglycan bonds in the normal course of cell growth. In the presence of antibacterial agents that inhibit cell-wall growth, autolysis proceeds without normal cell-wall repair; weakness and eventual cellular lysis occur.

Antibacterial agents act to inhibit cell-wall synthesis in several ways, as described below.

TABLE 33-1

MECHANISMS OF ACTION OF AND RESISTANCE TO MAJOR CLASSES OF ANTIBACTERIAL AGENTS

LETTER FOR FIG. 33-1	ANTIBACTERIAL AGENT[a]	MAJOR CELLULAR TARGET	MECHANISM OF ACTION	MAJOR MECHANISMS OF RESISTANCE
A	β-Lactams (penicillins and cephalosporins)	Cell wall	Inhibit cell-wall cross-linking	1. Drug inactivation (β-lactamase) 2. Insensitivity of target (altered penicillin-binding proteins) 3. Decreased permeability (altered gram-negative outer-membrane porins) 4. Active efflux
B	Vancomycin	Cell wall	Interferes with addition of new cell-wall subunits (muramyl pentapeptides)	Alteration of target (substitution of terminal amino acid of peptidoglycan subunit)
	Bacitracin	Cell wall	Prevents addition of cell-wall subunits by inhibiting recycling of membrane lipid carrier	Not defined
C	Macrolides (erythromycin)	Protein synthesis	Bind to 50S ribosomal subunit	1. Alteration of target (ribosomal methylation and mutation of 23S rRNA) 2. Active efflux
	Lincosamides (clindamycin)	Protein synthesis	Bind to 50S ribosomal subunit	Alteration of target (ribosomal methylation)
D	Chloramphenicol	Protein synthesis	Binds to 50S ribosomal subunit	1. Drug inactivation (chloramphenicol acetyltransferase) 2. Active efflux
E	Tetracycline	Protein synthesis	Binds to 30S ribosomal subunit	1. Decreased intracellular drug accumulation (active efflux) 2. Insensitivity of target
F	Aminoglycosides (gentamicin)	Protein synthesis	Bind to 30S ribosomal subunit	1. Drug inactivation (aminoglycoside-modifying enzyme) 2. Decreased permeability through gram-negative outer membrane 3. Active efflux
G	Mupirocin	Protein synthesis	Inhibits isoleucine tRNA synthetase	Mutation of gene for target protein or acquisition of new gene for drug-insensitive target
H	Quinupristin/ dalfopristin (Synercid)	Protein synthesis	Binds to 50S ribosomal subunit	1. Alteration of target (ribosomal methylation: dalfopristin) 2. Active efflux (quinupristin) 3. Drug inactivation (quinupristin and dalfopristin)
I	Linezolid	Protein synthesis	Bind to 50S ribosomal subunit	Alteration of target (mutation of 23S rRNA)
J	Sulfonamides and trimethoprim	Cell metabolism	Competitively inhibit enzymes involved in two steps of folic acid biosynthesis	Production of insensitive targets [dihydropteroate synthetase (sulfonamides) and dihydrofolate reductase (trimethoprim)] that bypass metabolic block
K	Rifampin	Nucleic acid synthesis	Inhibits DNA-dependent RNA polymerase	Insensitivity of target (mutation of polymerase gene)

(Continued)

TABLE 33-1 (*CONTINUED*)

MECHANISMS OF ACTION OF AND RESISTANCE TO MAJOR CLASSES OF ANTIBACTERIAL AGENTS

LETTER FOR FIG. 33-1	ANTIBACTERIAL AGENT[a]	MAJOR CELLULAR TARGET	MECHANISM OF ACTION	MAJOR MECHANISMS OF RESISTANCE
L	Metronidazole	Nucleic acid synthesis	Intracellularly generates short-lived reactive intermediates that damage DNA by electron transfer system	Not defined
M	Quinolones (ciprofloxacin)	DNA synthesis	Inhibit DNA gyrase (A subunit) and topoisomerase IV	1. Insensitivity of target (mutation of gyrase genes) 2. Decreased intracellular drug accumulation (active efflux)
	Novobiocin	DNA synthesis	Inhibits DNA gyrase (B subunit)	Not defined
N	Polymyxins (polymyxin B)	Cell membrane	Disrupt membrane permeability by charge alteration	Not defined
	Gramicidin	Cell membrane	Forms pores	Not defined
O	Daptomycin	Cell membrane	Forms channels that disrupt membrane potential	Not defined

[a]Compounds in parentheses are major representatives for the class.

Bacitracin

Bacitracin, a cyclic peptide antibiotic, inhibits the conversion to its active form of the lipid carrier that moves the water-soluble cytoplasmic peptidoglycan subunits through the cell membrane to the cell exterior.

Glycopeptides

Glycopeptides (vancomycin and teicoplanin) are high-molecular-weight antibiotics that bind to the terminal D-alanine–D-alanine component of the stem peptide while the subunits are external to the cell membrane but still linked to the lipid carrier. This binding sterically inhibits the addition of subunits to the peptidoglycan backbone.

β-Lactam Antibiotics

β-Lactam antibiotics (penicillins, cephalosporins, carbapenems, and monobactams; Table 33-2) are characterized by a four-membered β-lactam ring and prevent the cross-linking reaction called *transpeptidation*. The energy for attaching a peptide cross-bridge from the stem peptide of one peptidoglycan subunit to another is derived from the cleavage of a terminal D-alanine residue from the subunit stem peptide. The cross-bridge amino acid is then attached to the penultimate D-alanine by transpeptidase enzymes. The β-lactam ring of the antibiotic forms an irreversible covalent acyl bond with the transpeptidase enzyme (probably because of the antibiotic's steric similarity to the enzyme's D-alanine–D-alanine target), preventing the cross-linking reaction. Transpeptidases and similar enzymes involved in cross-linking are called *penicillin-binding proteins* (PBPs) because they all have active sites that bind β-lactam antibiotics.

INHIBITION OF PROTEIN SYNTHESIS

Most of the antibacterial agents that inhibit protein synthesis interact with the bacterial ribosome. The difference between the composition of bacterial and mammalian ribosomes gives these compounds their selectivity.

Aminoglycosides

Aminoglycosides (gentamicin, kanamycin, tobramycin, streptomycin, neomycin, and amikacin) are a group of structurally related compounds containing three linked hexose sugars. They exert a bactericidal effect by binding irreversibly to the 30S subunit of the bacterial ribosome and blocking initiation of protein synthesis. Uptake of aminoglycosides and their penetration through the cell membrane constitute an aerobic, energy-dependent process. Thus aminoglycoside activity is markedly reduced in an anaerobic environment. *Spectinomycin*, an aminocyclitol antibiotic, also acts on the 30S ribosomal subunit but has a different mechanism of action from the aminoglycosides and is bacteriostatic rather than bactericidal.

Macrolides, Ketolides, and Lincosamides

Macrolide antibiotics (erythromycin, clarithromycin, and azithromycin) consist of a large lactone ring to which sugars are attached. *Ketolide antibiotics*, including telithromycin, replace the cladinose sugar on the macrolactone ring with a ketone group. These drugs bind specifically to the 50S portion of the bacterial ribosome and inhibit protein chain elongation. Although structurally unrelated to the macrolides, *lincosamides* (clindamycin and lincomycin) bind to a site on the 50S ribosome nearly identical to the binding site for macrolides.

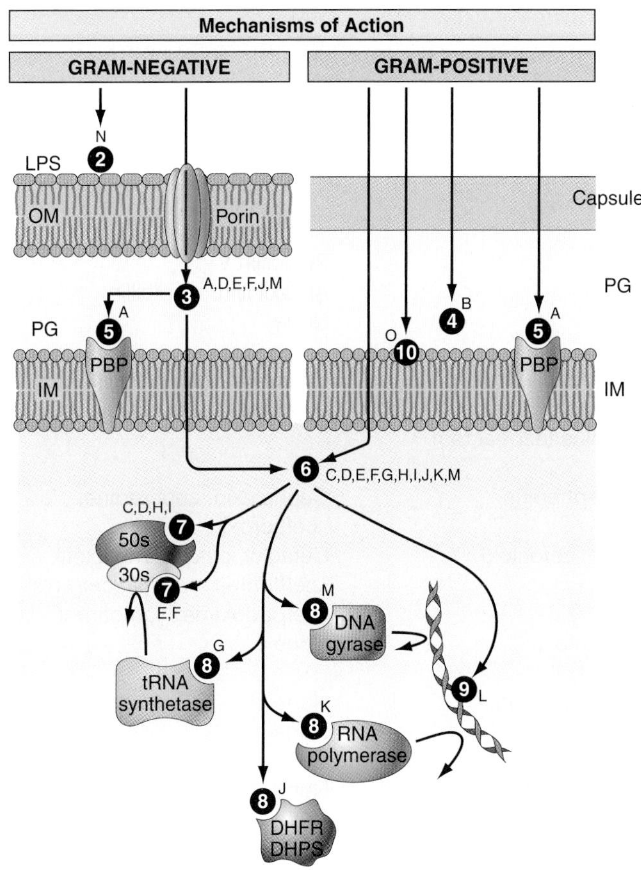

Mechanisms of Resistance

GRAM-NEGATIVE GRAM-POSITIVE

2 Detergent action on lipid gram ⊖ outer membrane.

3 Penetration of hydrophilic drugs through porin channels in gram ⊖ outer membrane.

4 Free diffusion through gram ⊕ cell envelope with binding to cell wall PG **or**

5 Binding to cell membrane PBP. Drug confined to space external to IM.

6 Diffusion or transport of drugs with intracellular target through IM.

7 Binding to ribosomal target for protein synthesis inhibition.

8 Antibiotic interaction with target protein leading to metabolic (DHFR, DHPS), protein synthetic (tRNA synthetase), or nucleic acid (DNA gyrase, RNA polymerase) abnormalities.

9 Direct interaction of reactive intermediates with nucleic acid.

10 Insertion into cell membrane, disrupting membrane potential.

1 **Intrinsic resistance:** Inability of antibiotic to penetrate gram ⊖ envelope (e.g., vancomycin).

3 Mutant porin channels **decrease** antimicrobial **penetration**.

4 **Production of insensitive target** by acquired gene mediating production of altered peptidoglycan.

5a **Production of β-lactam-insensitive PBP target** by mutation of gene or acquisition of new gene.

5b **Inactivation** of β-lactam antibiotic by β-lactamases in periplasm (gram ⊖) or surrounding medium (gram ⊕).

6 **Active efflux** of drugs from cytoplasm or from gram ⊖ periplasm.

7a Decreased ribosomal binding due to **target site alteration**.

7b **Inactivation** of drug by chemical modification leading to decreased ribosomal interaction.

8 Mutation of target gene or acquisition of new gene producing a **drug-insensitive target** protein.

FIGURE 33-1

Mechanisms of action of and resistance to antibacterial agents. Black lines trace the routes of drug interaction with bacterial cells, from entry to target site. The letters in each figure indicate specific antibacterial agents or classes of agents, as shown in Table 33-1. The numbers correspond to mechanisms listed beneath each panel. 50s and 30s, large and small ribosome subunits; Ac, acetylation; Ad, adenylation; DHFR, dihydrofolate reductase; DHPS, dihydropteroate synthetase; IM, inner (cytoplasmic) membrane; LPS, lipopolysaccharide; OM, outer membrane; P, phosphorylation; PBP, penicillin-binding protein; PG, peptidoglycan.

Streptogramins

Streptogramins [quinupristin (streptogramin B) and dalfopristin (streptogramin A)], which are supplied as a combination in Synercid, are peptide macrolactones that also bind to the 50S ribosomal subunit and block protein synthesis. Streptogramin B binds to a ribosomal site similar to the binding site for macrolides and lincosamides, whereas streptogramin A binds to a different ribosomal site, blocking the late phase of protein synthesis. The two streptogramins act synergistically to kill bacteria if the strain is susceptible to both components.

TABLE 33-2

CLASSIFICATION OF β-LACTAM ANTIBIOTICS

CLASS	ROUTE OF ADMINISTRATION: PARENTERAL	ORAL
Penicillins		
β-Lactamase–susceptible		
Narrow-spectrum	Penicillin G	Penicillin V
Enteric-active	Ampicillin	Amoxicillin, ampicillin
Enteric-active and antipseudomonal	Ticarcillin, piperacillin	None
β-Lactamase–resistant		
Antistaphylococcal	Oxacillin, nafcillin	Cloxacillin, dicloxacillin
Combined with β-lactamase inhibitors	Ticarcillin plus clavulanic acid, ampicillin plus sulbactam, piperacillin plus tazobactam	Amoxicillin plus clavulanic acid
Cephalosporins		
First-generation	Cefazolin, cephalothin, cephapirin	Cephalexin, cephradine, cefadroxil
Second-generation		
Haemophilus-active	Cefamandole, cefuroxime, cefonicid, ceforanide	Cefaclor, cefuroxime axetil, ceftibuten, cefdinir, cefprozil, cefpodoxime,[a] loracarbef
Bacteroides-active	Cefoxitin, cefotetan, cefmetazole	None
Third-generation		
Extended-spectrum	Ceftriaxone, cefotaxime, ceftizoxime	None
Extended-spectrum and antipseudomonal	Ceftazidime, cefepime	None
Carbapenems	Imipenem-cilastatin, meropenem, ertapenem	None
Monobactams	Aztreonam	None

[a]Some sources classify cefpodoxime as a third-generation oral agent because of a marginally broader spectrum.

Chloramphenicol

Chloramphenicol consists of a single aromatic ring and a short side chain. This antibiotic binds reversibly to the 50S portion of the bacterial ribosome at a site close to but not identical with the binding sites for the macrolides and lincosamides, inhibiting peptide bond formation.

Linezolid

Linezolid is the only commercially available drug in the oxazolidinone class. Linezolid binds to the 50S ribosomal subunit and blocks the initiation of protein synthesis.

Tetracyclines and Glycylcyclines

Tetracyclines (tetracycline, doxycycline, and minocycline) and glycylcyclines (tigecycline) consist of four aromatic rings with various substituent groups. They interact reversibly with the bacterial 30S ribosomal subunit, blocking the binding of aminoacyl tRNA to the mRNA-ribosome complex. This mechanism is markedly different from that of the aminoglycosides, which also bind to the 30S subunit.

Mupirocin

Mupirocin (pseudomonic acid) inhibits isoleucine tRNA synthetase by competing with bacterial isoleucine for its binding site on the enzyme and depleting cellular stores of isoleucine-charged tRNA.

INHIBITION OF BACTERIAL METABOLISM

The *antimetabolites* are all synthetic compounds that interfere with bacterial synthesis of folic acid. Products of the folic acid synthesis pathway function as coenzymes for the one-carbon transfer reactions that are essential for the synthesis of thymidine, all purines, and several amino acids. Inhibition of folate synthesis leads to cessation of bacterial cell growth and, in some cases, to bacterial cell death. The principal antibacterial antimetabolites are sulfonamides (sulfisoxazole, sulfadiazine, and sulfamethoxazole) and trimethoprim.

Sulfonamides

Sulfonamides are structural analogues of *p*-aminobenzoic acid (PABA), one of the three structural components of folic acid (the other two being pteridine and glutamate). The first step in the synthesis of folic acid is the addition of PABA to pteridine by the enzyme dihydropteroic acid synthetase. Sulfonamides compete with PABA as substrates for the enzyme. The selective effect of sulfonamides is due to the fact that bacteria synthesize folic acid, whereas mammalian cells cannot synthesize the cofactor and must use exogenous supplies. However, the activity of sulfonamides can be greatly reduced by the presence of excess PABA or by the exogenous addition of end products of one-carbon transfer reactions (e.g., thymidine and purines). High concentrations of the latter substances may be present in some infections as a result of tissue and white cell breakdown, compromising sulfonamide activity.

Trimethoprim

Trimethoprim is a diaminopyrimidine, a structural analogue of the pteridine moiety of folic acid. Trimethoprim is a competitive inhibitor of dihydrofolate reductase; this enzyme is responsible for reduction of dihydrofolic acid to tetrahydrofolic acid—the essential final component in the folic acid synthesis pathway. Like that of the sulfonamides, the activity of trimethoprim is compromised in the presence of exogenous thymine or thymidine.

INHIBITION OF NUCLEIC ACID SYNTHESIS OR ACTIVITY

Numerous antibacterial compounds have disparate effects on nucleic acids.

Quinolones

The quinolones, including nalidixic acid and its fluorinated derivatives (ciprofloxacin, levofloxacin, and moxifloxacin), are synthetic compounds that inhibit the activity of the A subunit of the bacterial enzyme DNA gyrase as well as topoisomerase IV. DNA gyrase and topoisomerases are responsible for negative supercoiling of DNA—an essential conformation for DNA replication in the intact cell. Inhibition of the activity of DNA gyrase and topoisomerase IV is lethal to bacterial cells. The antibiotic *novobiocin* also interferes with the activity of DNA gyrase, but it interferes with the B subunit.

Rifampin

Rifampin, used primarily against *Mycobacterium tuberculosis*, is also active against a variety of other bacteria. Rifampin binds tightly to the B subunit of bacterial DNA-dependent RNA polymerase, thus inhibiting transcription of DNA into RNA. Mammalian-cell RNA polymerase is not sensitive to this compound.

Nitrofurantoin

Nitrofurantoin, a synthetic compound, causes DNA damage. The nitrofurans, compounds containing a single five-membered ring, are reduced by a bacterial enzyme to highly reactive, short-lived intermediates that are thought to cause DNA strand breakage, either directly or indirectly.

Metronidazole

Metronidazole, a synthetic imidazole, is active only against anaerobic bacteria and protozoa. The reduction of metronidazole's nitro group by the bacterial anaerobic electron-transport system produces a transient series of reactive intermediates that are thought to cause DNA damage.

ALTERATION OF CELL-MEMBRANE PERMEABILITY

Polymyxins

The polymyxins [polymyxin B and colistin (polymyxin E)] are cyclic, basic polypeptides. They behave as cationic, surface-active compounds that disrupt the permeability of both the outer and the cytoplasmic membranes of gram-negative bacteria.

Gramicidin A

Gramicidin A is a polypeptide of 15 amino acids that acts as an ionophore, forming pores or channels in lipid bilayers.

Daptomycin

Insertion of daptomycin, a new bactericidal lipopeptide antibiotic, into the cell membrane of gram-positive bacteria forms a channel that causes depolarization of the membrane by efflux of intracellular ions, resulting in cell death.

MECHANISMS OF RESISTANCE

Some bacteria exhibit *intrinsic resistance* to certain classes of antibacterial agents (e.g., obligate anaerobic bacteria to aminoglycosides and gram-negative bacteria to vancomycin). In addition, bacteria that are ordinarily susceptible to antibacterial agents can acquire resistance. *Acquired resistance* is a major limitation to effective antibacterial chemotherapy. Resistance can develop by mutation of resident genes or by acquisition of new genes. New genes mediating resistance are usually spread from cell to cell by way of mobile genetic elements such as plasmids, transposons, and bacteriophages. The resistant bacterial populations flourish in areas of high antimicrobial use, where they enjoy a selective advantage over susceptible populations.

The major mechanisms used by bacteria to resist the action of antimicrobial agents are inactivation of the compound, alteration or overproduction of the antibacterial target through mutation of the target protein's gene, acquisition of a new gene that encodes a drug-insensitive target, decreased permeability of the cell envelope to the agent, failure to convert an inactive prodrug to its active derivative, and active efflux of the compound from the periplasm or interior of the cell. Specific mechanisms of bacterial resistance to the major antibacterial agents are outlined below, summarized in Table 33-1, and depicted in Fig. 33-1.

β-LACTAM ANTIBIOTICS

Bacteria develop resistance to β-lactam antibiotics by a variety of mechanisms. Most common is the destruction of the drug by β-lactamases. The β-lactamases of gram-negative bacteria are confined to the periplasm, between the inner and outer membranes, whereas gram-positive bacteria secrete their β-lactamases into the surrounding medium. These enzymes have a higher affinity for the antibiotic than the antibiotic has for its target. Binding results in hydrolysis of the β-lactam ring. Genes encoding β-lactamases have been found in both chromosomal and extrachromosomal locations and in both gram-positive and gram-negative bacteria; these genes are often on mobile genetic elements. Many "advanced-generation" β-lactam antibiotics, such as ceftriaxone and cefepime, are stable in the presence of plasmid-mediated β-lactamases and are active against bacteria resistant to earlier-generation β-lactam antibiotics. However, extended-spectrum β-lactamases (ESBLs), either acquired on mobile genetic elements by gram-negative bacteria (e.g., *Klebsiella pneumoniae* and *Escherichia coli*) or present as stable chromosomal genes in other gram-negative species (e.g., *Enterobacter* spp.), have broad substrate specificity, hydrolyzing virtually all penicillins and cephalosporins. One strategy that has been devised for circumventing resistance mediated by β-lactamases is to combine the β-lactam agent with an inhibitor that avidly binds the inactivating enzyme, preventing its attack on the antibiotic. Unfortunately, the inhibitors (e.g., clavulanic acid, sulbactam, and tazobactam) do not bind all chromosomal β-lactamases (e.g., that of *Enterobacter*) and thus cannot be depended on to prevent the inactivation of β-lactam antibiotics by such enzymes. No β-lactam antibiotic or inhibitor has been produced that can resist all of the many β-lactamases that have been identified.

A second mechanism of bacterial resistance to β-lactam antibiotics is an alteration in PBP targets so that the PBPs have a markedly reduced affinity for the drug. Although this alteration may occur by mutation of existing genes, the acquisition of new PBP genes (as in staphylococcal resistance to methicillin) or of new pieces of PBP genes (as in streptococcal, gonococcal, and meningococcal resistance to penicillin) is more important.

A final resistance mechanism is the coupling, in gram-negative bacteria, of a decrease in outer-membrane permeability with rapid efflux of the antibiotic from the periplasm to the cell exterior. Mutations of genes encoding outer-membrane protein channels called *porins* decrease the entry of β-lactam antibiotics into the cell, while additional proteins form channels that actively pump β-lactams out of the cell. Resistance of Enterobacteriaceae to some cephalosporins and resistance of *Pseudomonas* spp. to cephalosporins and piperacillin are the best examples of this mechanism.

VANCOMYCIN

Clinically important resistance to vancomycin was first described among enterococci in France in 1988. Vancomycin-resistant enterococci (VRE) have subsequently become disseminated worldwide. The genes encoding resistance are carried on plasmids that can transfer themselves from cell to cell and on transposons that can jump from plasmids to chromosomes. Resistance is mediated by enzymes that substitute D-lactate for D-alanine on the peptidoglycan stem peptide so that there is no longer an appropriate target for vancomycin binding. This alteration does not appear to affect cell-wall integrity, however. This type of acquired vancomycin resistance was confined for 14 years to enterococci—more specifically, to *Enterococcus faecium* rather than the more common pathogen *E. faecalis*. However, since 2002, *S. aureus* isolates that are highly resistant to vancomycin have been recovered from four patients in the United States. All of the isolates contain *vanA*, the gene that mediates vancomycin resistance in enterococci. In addition, since 1996, a few isolates of both *S. aureus* and *Staphylococcus epidermidis* that display a four- to eightfold reduction in susceptibility to vancomycin have been found worldwide, and many more isolates may contain subpopulations with reduced vancomycin susceptibility. These isolates have not acquired the genes that mediate vancomycin resistance in enterococci but are mutant bacteria with markedly thickened cell walls. These mutants were apparently selected in patients who were undergoing prolonged vancomycin therapy. The failure of vancomycin therapy in some patients infected with *S. aureus* or *S. epidermidis* strains exhibiting only intermediate susceptibility to this drug is thought to have resulted from this resistance.

AMINOGLYCOSIDES

The most common aminoglycoside resistance mechanism is inactivation of the antibiotic. Aminoglycoside-modifying enzymes, usually encoded on plasmids, transfer phosphate, adenyl, or acetyl residues from intracellular molecules to hydroxyl or amino side groups on the antibiotic. The modified antibiotic is less active because of diminished binding to its ribosomal target. Modifying enzymes that can inactivate any of the available aminoglycosides have been found in both gram-positive and gram-negative bacteria. A second aminoglycoside resistance mechanism, which has been identified predominantly in clinical isolates of *Pseudomonas aeruginosa*, is decreased antibiotic uptake, presumably due to alterations in the bacterial outer membrane.

MACROLIDES, KETOLIDES, LINCOSAMIDES, AND STREPTOGRAMINS

Resistance in gram-positive bacteria, which are the usual target organisms for macrolides, ketolides, lincosamides, and streptogramins, can be due to the production of an enzyme—most commonly plasmid-encoded—that methylates ribosomal RNA, interfering with binding of the antibiotics to their target. Methylation mediates resistance to erythromycin, clarithromycin, azithromycin, clindamycin, and streptogramin B. Resistance to streptogramin B converts quinupristin/dalfopristin from a bactericidal to a bacteriostatic antibiotic. Streptococci can also actively cause the efflux of macrolides, and staphylococci can cause the efflux of macrolides, clindamycin, and streptogramin A. Ketolides such as telithromycin retain activity against most isolates of *Streptococcus pneumoniae* that are resistant to macrolides. In addition, staphylococci can inactivate streptogramin A by acetylation and streptogramin B by either acetylation or hydrolysis. Finally, mutations in 23S ribosomal RNA that alter the binding of macrolides to their targets have been found in both staphylococci and streptococci.

CHLORAMPHENICOL

Most bacteria resistant to chloramphenicol produce a plasmid-encoded enzyme, chloramphenicol acetyltransferase, that inactivates the compound by acetylation.

TETRACYCLINES AND TIGECYCLINE

The most common mechanism of tetracycline resistance in gram-negative bacteria is a plasmid-encoded active-efflux pump that is inserted into the cytoplasmic membrane and extrudes antibiotic from the cell. Resistance in gram-positive bacteria is due either to active efflux or to ribosomal alterations that diminish binding of the antibiotic to its target. Genes involved in ribosomal protection are found on mobile genetic elements. A new parenteral tetracycline derivative (a glycylcycline), tigecycline, is active against tetracycline-resistant bacteria because it is not removed by efflux and can bind to altered ribosomes.

MUPIROCIN

Although the topical compound mupirocin was introduced into clinical use relatively recently, resistance is already becoming widespread in some areas. The mechanism appears to be either mutation of the target isoleucine tRNA synthetase so that it is no longer inhibited by the antibiotic or plasmid-encoded production of a form of the target enzyme that binds mupirocin poorly.

TRIMETHOPRIM AND SULFONAMIDES

The most prevalent mechanism of resistance to trimethoprim and the sulfonamides in both gram-positive and gram-negative bacteria is the acquisition of plasmid-encoded genes that produce a new, drug-insensitive target—specifically, an insensitive dihydrofolate reductase for trimethoprim and an altered dihydropteroate synthetase for sulfonamides.

QUINOLONES

The most common mechanism of resistance to quinolones is the development of one or more mutations in target DNA gyrases and topoisomerase IV that prevent the antibacterial agent from interfering with the enzymes' activity. Some gram-negative bacteria develop mutations that both decrease outer-membrane porin permeability and cause active drug efflux from the cytoplasm. Mutations that result in active quinolone efflux are also found in gram-positive bacteria.

RIFAMPIN

Bacteria rapidly become resistant to rifampin by developing mutations in the B subunit of RNA polymerase that render the enzyme unable to bind the antibiotic. The rapid selection of resistant mutants is the major limitation to the use of this antibiotic against otherwise-susceptible staphylococci and requires that the drug be used in combination with another antistaphylococcal agent.

LINEZOLID

Enterococci, streptococci, and staphylococci become resistant to linezolid in vitro by mutation of the 23S rRNA binding site. Clinical isolates of *E. faecium* and *E. faecalis* acquire resistance to linezolid readily by this mechanism, often during therapy, but linezolid-resistant staphylococcal and streptococcal isolates are rare.

MULTIPLE ANTIBIOTIC RESISTANCE

The acquisition by one bacterium of resistance to multiple antibacterial agents is becoming increasingly common. The two major mechanisms are the acquisition of multiple unrelated resistance genes and the development of mutations in a single gene or gene complex that mediate resistance to a series of unrelated compounds. The construction of multiresistant strains by acquisition of multiple genes occurs by sequential steps of gene transfer and environmental selection in areas of high-level antimicrobial use. In contrast, mutations in a single gene can conceivably be selected in a single step. Bacteria that are multiresistant by virtue of the acquisition of new genes include hospital-associated strains of gram-negative bacteria, enterococci, and staphylococci and community-acquired strains of salmonellae, gonococci, and pneumococci. Mutations that confer resistance to multiple unrelated antimicrobial agents occur in the genes encoding outer-membrane porins and efflux proteins of gram-negative bacteria. These mutations decrease bacterial intracellular and periplasmic accumulation of β-lactams, quinolones, tetracyclines, chloramphenicol, and aminoglycosides. Multiresistant bacterial isolates pose increasing problems in U.S. hospitals; strains resistant to all available antibacterial chemotherapy have already been identified.

PHARMACOKINETICS OF ANTIBIOTICS

The *pharmacokinetic profile* of an antibacterial agent refers to concentrations in serum and tissue versus time and reflects the processes of absorption, distribution, metabolism, and excretion. Important characteristics include peak and trough serum concentrations and mathematically derived parameters such as half-life, clearance, and distribution volume. Pharmacokinetic information is useful for estimating the appropriate antibacterial dose and frequency of administration, for adjusting dosages in patients with impaired excretory capacity, and for comparing one drug with another. In contrast, the *pharmacodynamic profile* of an antibiotic refers to the relationship between the pharmacokinetics of the antibiotic and its minimal inhibitory concentrations (MICs) for bacteria (see "Principles of Antibacterial Chemotherapy" later in the chapter).

ABSORPTION

Antibiotic *absorption* refers to the rate and extent of a drug's systemic bioavailability after oral, IM, or IV administration.

Oral Administration

Most patients with infection are treated with oral antibacterial agents in the outpatient setting. Advantages of oral therapy over parenteral therapy include lower cost, generally fewer adverse effects (including complications of indwelling lines), and greater acceptance by patients. The percentage of an orally administered antibacterial agent that is absorbed (i.e., its *bioavailability*) ranges from as little as 10–20% (erythromycin and penicillin G) to nearly 100% [amoxicillin, clindamycin, metronidazole, doxycycline, trimethoprim-sulfamethoxazole (TMP-SMX), linezolid, and most fluoroquinolones]. These differences in bioavailability are not clinically important as long as drug concentrations at the site of infection are sufficient to inhibit or kill the pathogen. However, therapeutic efficacy may be compromised when absorption is reduced as a result of physiologic or pathologic conditions (such as the presence of food for some drugs or the shunting of blood away from the gastrointestinal tract in patients with hypotension), drug interactions (such as that of quinolones and metal cations), or noncompliance. The oral route is usually used for patients with relatively mild infections in whom absorption is not thought to be compromised by the preceding conditions. In addition, the oral route can often be used in more severely ill patients after they have responded to parenteral therapy.

Intramuscular Administration

Although the IM route of administration usually results in 100% bioavailability, it is not as widely used in the United States as the oral and IV routes, in part because of the pain often associated with IM injections and the relative ease of IV access in the hospitalized patient. IM injection may be suitable for specific indications requiring an "immediate" and reliable effect (e.g., with long-acting forms of penicillin, including benzathine and procaine, and with single doses of ceftriaxone for acute otitis media or uncomplicated gonococcal infection).

Intravenous Administration

The IV route is appropriate when oral antibacterial agents are not effective against a particular pathogen, when bioavailability is uncertain, or when larger doses are required than are feasible with the oral route. After IV administration, bioavailability is 100%; serum concentrations are maximal at the end of the infusion. For many patients in whom long-term antimicrobial therapy is required and oral therapy is not feasible, outpatient parenteral antibiotic therapy (OPAT), including the use of convenient portable pumps, may be cost-effective and safe. Alternatively, some oral antibacterial drugs (e.g., fluoroquinolones) are sufficiently active against Enterobacteriaceae to provide potency equal to that of parenteral therapy; oral use of such drugs may allow the patient to return home from the hospital earlier or to avoid hospitalization entirely.

DISTRIBUTION

To be effective, concentrations of an antibacterial agent must exceed the pathogen's MIC. Serum antibiotic concentrations usually exceed the MIC for susceptible bacteria, but since most infections are extravascular, the antibiotic must also distribute to the site of the infection. Concentrations of most antibacterial agents in interstitial fluid are similar to free-drug concentrations in serum. However, when the infection is located in a "protected" site where penetration is poor, such as cerebrospinal fluid (CSF), the eye, the prostate, or infected cardiac vegetations, high parenteral doses or local administration for prolonged periods may be required for cure. In addition, even though an antibacterial agent may penetrate to the site of infection, its activity may be antagonized by factors in the local environment, such as an unfavorable pH or inactivation by cellular degradation products. For example, since the activity of aminoglycosides is reduced at acidic pH, the acidic environment in many infected tissues may be partly responsible for the relatively poor efficacy of aminoglycoside monotherapy. In addition, the abscess milieu reduces the penetration and local activity of many antibacterial compounds, so that surgical drainage may be required for cure.

Most bacteria that cause human infections are located extracellularly. Intracellular pathogens such as *Legionella*, *Chlamydia*, *Brucella*, and *Salmonella* may persist or cause relapse if the antibacterial agent does not enter the cell. In general, β-lactams, vancomycin, and aminoglycosides penetrate cells poorly, whereas macrolides, ketolides, tetracyclines, metronidazole, chloramphenicol, rifampin, TMP-SMX, and quinolones penetrate cells well.

METABOLISM AND ELIMINATION

Like other drugs, antibacterial agents are disposed of by hepatic elimination (metabolism or biliary elimination), by renal excretion of the unchanged or metabolized form, or by a combination of the two processes. For most of the antibacterial drugs, metabolism leads to loss of in vitro activity, although some agents, such as cefotaxime, rifampin, and clarithromycin, have bioactive metabolites that may contribute to their overall efficacy.

The most practical application of information on the mode of excretion of an antibacterial agent is in adjusting dosage when elimination capability is impaired (Table 33-3). Direct, nonidiosyncratic toxicity from antibacterial drugs may result from failure to reduce the dosage given to patients with impaired elimination. For agents that are primarily cleared intact by glomerular filtration, drug clearance is correlated with creatinine clearance, and estimates of the latter can be used to guide dosage. For drugs whose elimination is primarily hepatic, no simple marker is useful for dosage adjustment in patients with liver disease. However, in patients with severe hepatic disease, residual metabolic capability is usually sufficient to preclude accumulation and toxic effects.

PRINCIPLES OF ANTIBACTERIAL CHEMOTHERAPY

The choice of an antibacterial compound for a particular patient and a specific infection involves more than just a knowledge of the agent's pharmacokinetic profile and in

TABLE 33-3

ANTIBACTERIAL DRUG DOSE ADJUSTMENTS IN PATIENTS WITH RENAL IMPAIRMENT

ANTIBIOTIC	MAJOR ROUTE OF EXCRETION	DOSAGE ADJUSTMENT WITH RENAL IMPAIRMENT
Aminoglycosides	Renal	Yes
Azithromycin	Biliary	No
Cefazolin	Renal	Yes
Cefepime	Renal	Yes
Ceftazidime	Renal	Yes
Ceftriaxone	Renal/biliary	Modest reduction in severe renal impairment
Ciprofloxacin	Renal/biliary	Only in severe renal insufficiency
Clarithromycin	Renal/biliary	Only in severe renal insufficiency
Daptomycin	Renal	Yes
Erythromycin	Biliary	Only when given in high IV doses
Levofloxacin	Renal	Yes
Linezolid	Metabolism	No
Metronidazole	Biliary	No
Nafcillin	Biliary	No
Penicillin G	Renal	Yes (when given in high IV doses)
Piperacillin	Renal	Only with Cl_{cr} of <40 mL/min
Quinupristin/dalfopristin	Metabolism	No
Ticarcillin	Renal	Yes
Tigecycline	Biliary	No
TMP-SMX	Renal/biliary	Only in severe renal insufficiency
Vancomycin	Renal	Yes

Note: Cl_{cr}, creatinine clearance rate; TMP-SMX, trimethoprim-sulfamethoxazole.

vitro activity. The basic tenets of chemotherapy, to be elaborated below, include the following: When appropriate, material containing the infecting organism(s) should be obtained before the start of treatment so that presumptive identification can be made by microscopic examination of stained specimens and the organism can be grown for definitive identification and susceptibility testing. Awareness of local susceptibility patterns is useful when the patient is treated empirically. Once the organism is identified and its susceptibility to antibacterial agents is determined, the regimen with the narrowest effective spectrum should be chosen. The choice of antibacterial agent is guided by the pharmacokinetic and adverse-reaction profile of active compounds, the site of infection, the immune status of the host, and evidence of efficacy from well-performed clinical trials. If all other factors are equal, the least expensive antibacterial regimen should be chosen.

SUSCEPTIBILITY OF BACTERIA TO ANTIBACTERIAL DRUGS IN VITRO

Determination of the susceptibility of the patient's infecting organism to a panel of appropriate antibacterial agents is an essential first step in devising a chemotherapeutic regimen. Susceptibility testing is designed to estimate the susceptibility of a bacterial isolate to an antibacterial drug under standardized conditions. These conditions favor rapidly growing aerobic or facultative organisms and assess bacteriostasis only. Specialized testing is required for the assessment of bactericidal antimicrobial activity; for the detection of resistance among such fastidious organisms as obligate anaerobes, *Haemophilus* spp., and pneumococci; and for the determination of resistance phenotypes with variable expression, such as resistance to methicillin or oxacillin among staphylococci. Antimicrobial susceptibility testing is important when susceptibility is unpredictable, most often as a result of increasing acquired resistance among bacteria infecting hospitalized patients.

PHARMACODYNAMICS: RELATIONSHIP OF PHARMACOKINETICS AND IN VITRO SUSCEPTIBILITY TO CLINICAL RESPONSE

Bacteria have often been considered *susceptible* to an antibacterial drug if the achievable peak serum concentration exceeds the MIC by approximately fourfold. The *breakpoint* is the concentration of the antibiotic that separates susceptible from resistant bacteria (Fig. 33-2). When a majority of the isolates of a given bacterial species are inhibited at concentrations below the breakpoint, the species is considered to be within the spectrum of the antibiotic.

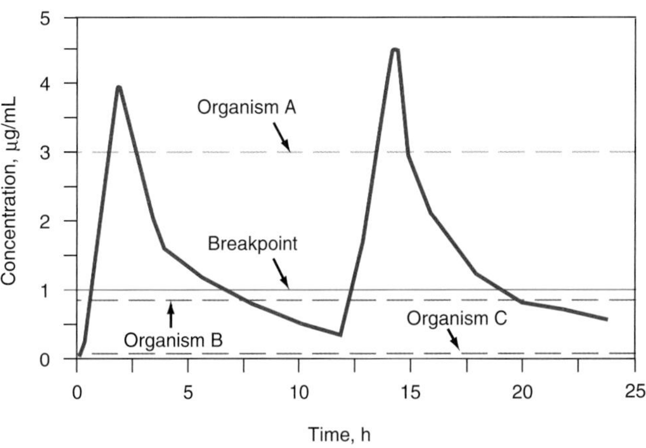

FIGURE 33-2

Relationship between pharmacokinetics of an antibiotic and susceptibility. Organism A is resistant, organism B is moderately susceptible, and organism C is very susceptible. Pharmacodynamic indices include the ratio of the peak serum concentration to MIC (C_{max}/MIC), the ratio of the area under the serum concentration vs time curve to MIC (AUC/MIC), and the time that serum concentrations exceed the MIC (t > MIC).

The pharmacodynamic profile of an antibiotic refers to the quantitative relationships between the time course of antibiotic concentrations in serum and tissue, in vitro susceptibility (MIC), and microbial response (inhibition of growth or rate of killing). Three pharmacodynamic parameters quantify these relationships: the ratio of the area under the plasma concentration vs time curve to MIC (AUC/MIC), the ratio of the maximal serum concentration to the MIC (C_{max}/MIC), and the time during a dosing interval that plasma concentrations exceed the MIC (t > MIC). The pharmacodynamic profile of an antibiotic class is characterized as either *concentration dependent* (fluoroquinolones, aminoglycosides), such that an increase in antibiotic concentration leads to a more rapid rate of bacterial death, or *time dependent* (β-lactams), such that the reduction in bacterial density is proportional to the time that concentrations exceed the MIC. For concentration-dependent antibiotics, the C_{max}/MIC or AUC/MIC ratio correlates best with the reduction in microbial density in vitro and in animal investigations. Dosing strategies attempt to maximize these ratios by the administration of a large dose relative to the MIC for anticipated pathogens, often at long intervals (relative to the serum half-life). Once-daily dosing of aminoglycoside antibiotics is the most practical consequence of these relationships. In contrast, dosage strategies for time-dependent antibiotics emphasize the administration of doses sufficient to maintain serum concentrations above the MIC for a critical portion of the dose interval. Response to β-lactam antibiotics, measured as the decline in bacterial density at the site of infection, is maximal when serum and tissue concentrations are maintained above the MIC for 30–50% of the dose interval. For example, the use of high-dose amoxicillin (90–100 mg/kg per day) in the treatment of acute otitis media increases not only the penetration of amoxicillin into the inner ear, but also the duration of time that concentrations exceed the MIC for pneumococci. This approach provides effective therapy in most patients, including those whose pneumococcal isolates are penicillin resistant. The clinical implications of these pharmacodynamic relationships are in the early stages of investigation; their elucidation should eventually result in more rational antibacterial dosage regimens. Table 33-4 summarizes the pharmacodynamic properties of the major antibiotic classes.

TABLE 33-4

PHARMACODYNAMIC INDICES OF MAJOR ANTIMICROBIAL CLASSES

PARAMETER PREDICTING RESPONSE	DRUG OR DRUG CLASS
Time above the MIC	Penicillins, cephalosporins, carbapenems, aztreonam
24-h AUC/MIC	Aminoglycosides, fluoroquinolones, tetracyclines, vancomycin, macrolides, clindamycin, quinupristin/dalfopristin, tigecycline, daptomycin
Peak to MIC	Aminoglycosides, fluoroquinolones

Note: MIC, minimal inhibitory concentration; AUC, area under the concentration curve.

STATUS OF THE HOST

Various host factors must be considered in the devising of antibacterial chemotherapy. The host's antibacterial *immune function* is of importance, particularly as it relates to opsonophagocytic function. Since the major host defense against acute, overwhelming bacterial infection is the polymorphonuclear leukocyte, patients with neutropenia must be treated aggressively and empirically with bactericidal drugs for suspected infection (Chap. 11). Likewise, patients who have deficient humoral immunity (e.g., those with chronic lymphocytic leukemia and multiple myeloma) and individuals with surgical or functional asplenia (e.g., those with sickle cell disease) should be treated empirically for infections with encapsulated organisms, especially the pneumococcus.

Pregnancy increases the risk of toxicity of certain antibacterial drugs for the mother (e.g., hepatic toxicity of tetracycline), affects drug disposition and pharmacokinetics, and—because of the risk of fetal toxicity—severely limits the choice of agents for treating infections. Certain antibacterial agents are contraindicated in pregnancy either because their safety has not been established (categories B and C) or because they are known to be toxic (categories D and X). Table 33-5 summarizes drug safety in pregnancy.

In patients with *concomitant viral infections*, the incidence of adverse reactions to antibacterial drugs may be unusually high. For example, persons with infectious mononucleosis and those infected with HIV experience skin reactions more often to penicillins and folic acid synthesis inhibitors such as TMP-SMX, respectively.

In addition, the patient's age, sex, racial heritage, genetic background, and excretory status all determine the incidence and type of side effects that can be expected with certain antibacterial agents.

SITE OF INFECTION

The location of the infected site may play a major role in the choice and dose of antimicrobial drug. Patients with suspected *meningitis* should receive drugs that can cross the blood-CSF barrier; in addition, because of the relative paucity of phagocytes and opsonins at the site of infection, the agents should be bactericidal. Chloramphenicol, an older drug but occasionally useful in the treatment of meningitis, is bactericidal for common organisms causing meningitis (i.e., meningococci, pneumococci, and *Haemophilus influenzae*, but *not* enteric gram-negative bacilli), is highly lipid-soluble, and enters the CSF well. However, β-lactam drugs, the mainstay of

TABLE 33-5

ANTIBACTERIAL DRUGS IN PREGNANCY

ANTIBACTERIAL DRUG	TOXICITY IN PREGNANCY	RECOMMENDATION
Aminoglycosides	Possible 8th-nerve toxicity	Caution[a]
Chloramphenicol	Gray syndrome in newborn	Caution at term
Fluoroquinolones	Arthropathy in immature animals	Caution
Clarithromycin	Teratogenicity in animals	Contraindicated
Ertapenem	Decreased weight in animals	Caution
Erythromycin estolate	Cholestatic hepatitis	Contraindicated
Imipenem/cilastatin	Toxicity in some pregnant animals	Caution
Linezolid	Embryonic and fetal toxicity in rats	Caution
Meropenem	Unknown	Caution
Metronidazole	None known, but carcinogenic in rats	Caution
Nitrofurantoin	Hemolytic anemia in newborns	Caution; contraindicated at term
Quinupristin/dalfopristin	Unknown	Caution
Sulfonamides	Hemolysis in newborn with G6PD deficiency; kernicterus in newborn	Caution; contraindicated at term
Tetracyclines/tigecycline	Tooth discoloration, inhibition of bone growth in fetus; hepatotoxicity	Contraindicated
Vancomycin	Unknown	Caution

[a]Use only for strong clinical indication in the absence of a suitable alternative.
Note: G6PD, glucose-6-phosphate dehydrogenase.

therapy for most of these infections, do not normally reach high levels in CSF. Their efficacy is based on the increased permeability of the blood-brain and blood-CSF barriers to hydrophilic molecules during inflammation and the extreme susceptibility of most infectious organisms to even small amounts of β-lactam drug.

The vegetation, which is the major site of infection in *bacterial endocarditis*, is also a focus that is protected from normal host-defense mechanisms. Antibacterial therapy needs to be bactericidal, with the selected agent administered parenterally over a long period and at a dose that produces serum levels at least eight times higher than the minimal bactericidal concentration (MBC) for the infecting organism. Likewise, *osteomyelitis* involves a site that is resistant to opsonophagocytic removal of infecting bacteria; furthermore, avascular bone (sequestrum) represents a foreign body that thwarts normal host-defense mechanisms. *Chronic prostatitis* is exceedingly difficult to cure because most antibiotics do not penetrate through the capillaries serving the prostate, especially when acute inflammation is absent. *Intraocular infections*, especially endophthalmitis, are difficult to treat because retinal capillaries lacking fenestration hinder drug penetration into the vitreous from blood. Inflammation does little to disrupt this barrier. Thus direct injection into the vitreous is necessary in many cases. Antibiotic penetration into *abscesses* is usually poor, and local conditions (e.g., low pH or the presence of enzymes that hydrolyze the drug) may further antagonize antibacterial activity.

In contrast, *urinary tract infections* (UTIs), when confined to the bladder, are relatively easy to cure, in part because of the higher concentration of most antibiotics in urine than in blood. Since blood is the usual reference fluid in defining susceptibility (Fig. 33-2), even organisms found to be resistant to achievable serum concentrations may be susceptible to achievable urine concentrations. For drugs that are used only for the treatment of UTIs, such as the urinary tract antiseptics nitrofurantoin and methenamine salts, achievable urine concentrations are used to determine susceptibility. Nitrofurantoin is often active against VRE and is a less expensive alternative to linezolid for the treatment of lower UTIs.

COMBINATION CHEMOTHERAPY

One of the tenets of antibacterial chemotherapy is that if the infecting bacterium has been identified, the most specific chemotherapy possible should be used. The use of a single agent with a narrow spectrum of activity against the pathogen diminishes the alteration of normal flora and thus limits the overgrowth of resistant nosocomial organisms (e.g., *Candida albicans*, enterococci, *Clostridium difficile*, or methicillin-resistant staphylococci), avoids the potential toxicity of multiple-drug regimens, and reduces cost. However, certain circumstances call for the use of more than one antibacterial agent. These are summarized below.

1. *Prevention of the emergence of resistant mutants.* Spontaneous mutations occur at a detectable frequency in certain genes encoding the target proteins for some antibacterial agents. The use of these agents can eliminate the susceptible population, select out resistant mutants at the site of infection, and result in the failure of chemotherapy. Resistant mutants are usually selected when the MIC of the antibacterial agent for the infecting bacterium is close to achievable levels in

serum or tissues and/or when the site of infection limits the access or activity of the agent. Among the most common examples are rifampin for staphylococci, imipenem for *Pseudomonas*, and fluoroquinolones for staphylococci and *Pseudomonas*. Small-colony variants of staphylococci resistant to aminoglycosides also emerge during monotherapy with these antibiotics. A second antibacterial agent with a mechanism of action different from that of the first is added to prevent the emergence of these resistant mutants (e.g., imipenem plus an aminoglycoside or a fluoroquinolone for systemic *Pseudomonas* infections). However, since resistant mutants have emerged after combination chemotherapy, this approach clearly is not uniformly successful.

2. *Synergistic or additive activity*. Synergistic or additive activity involves a lowering of the MIC or MBC of each or all of the drugs tested in combination against a specific bacterium. In *synergy*, each agent is more active when combined with a second drug than it would be alone, and the drugs' combined activity is therefore greater than the sum of the individual activities of each drug. In an *additive relationship*, the combined activity of the drugs is equal to the sum of their individual activities. Among the best examples of a synergistic or additive effect, confirmed both in vitro and by animal studies, are the enhanced bactericidal activities of certain β-lactam/aminoglycoside combinations against enterococci, viridans streptococci, and *P. aeruginosa*. The synergistic or additive activity of these combinations has also been demonstrated against selected isolates of enteric gram-negative bacteria and staphylococci. The combination of trimethoprim and sulfamethoxazole has synergistic or additive activity against many enteric gram-negative bacteria. Most other antimicrobial combinations display indifferent activity (i.e., the combination is no *better* than the more active of the two agents alone), and some combinations (e.g., penicillin plus tetracycline against pneumococci) may be antagonistic (i.e., the combination is *worse* than either drug alone).
3. *Therapy directed against multiple potential pathogens*. For certain infections, either a mixture of pathogens is suspected or the patient is desperately ill with an as-yet-unidentified infection (see "Empirical Therapy" next in the chapter). In these situations, the most important of the likely infecting bacteria must be covered by therapy until culture and susceptibility results become available. Examples of the former infections are intraabdominal or brain abscesses and infections of limbs in diabetic patients with microvascular disease. The latter situations include fevers in neutropenic patients, acute pneumonia from aspiration of oral flora by hospitalized patients, and septic shock or sepsis syndrome.

EMPIRICAL THERAPY

In many situations, antibacterial therapy is begun before a specific bacterial pathogen has been identified. The choice of agent is guided by the results of studies identifying the usual pathogens at that site or in that clinical setting, by pharmacodynamic considerations, and by the resistance profile of the expected pathogens in a particular hospital or geographic area. Situations in which empirical therapy is appropriate include the following:

1. *Life-threatening infection*. Any suspected bacterial infection in a patient with a life-threatening illness should be treated presumptively. Therapy is usually begun with more than one agent and is later tailored to a specific pathogen if one is eventually identified. Early therapy with an effective antimicrobial regimen has consistently been demonstrated to improve survival rates.
2. *Treatment of community-acquired infections.* In many situations, it is appropriate to treat non–life-threatening infections without obtaining cultures. These situations include outpatient infections such as community-acquired upper and lower respiratory tract infections, cystitis, cellulitis or local wound infection, urethritis, and prostatitis. However, if any of these infections recurs or fails to respond to initial therapy, every effort should be made to obtain cultures to guide retreatment.

CHOICE OF ANTIBACTERIAL THERAPY

Infections for which specific antibacterial agents are among the drugs of choice are detailed in Table 33-6. No attempt has been made to include all of the potential situations in which antibacterial agents may be used. A more detailed discussion of specific bacteria and infections that they cause can be found elsewhere in this volume.

The choice of antibacterial therapy increasingly involves an assessment of the acquired resistance of major microbial pathogens to the antimicrobial agents available to treat them. Resistance rates are dynamic (Table 33-6), both increasing and decreasing in response to the environmental pressure applied by antimicrobial use. For example, a threefold increase in fluoroquinolone use in the community between 1995 and 2002 was associated with increasing rates of quinolone resistance in community-acquired strains of *S. pneumoniae*, *E. coli*, *Neisseria gonorrhoeae*, and *K. pneumoniae*. Fluoroquinolone resistance has also emerged rapidly among nosocomial isolates of *S. aureus* and *Pseudomonas* spp. as hospital use of this drug class has increased. In contrast, staphylococcal resistance to tetracyclines has decreased as the use of these antibiotics has declined. It is important to note that, in many cases, wide variations in worldwide antimicrobial-resistance trends may not be reflected in the values recorded at U.S. hospitals. Therefore, the most important factor in choosing initial therapy for an infection in which the susceptibility of the specific pathogen(s) is not known is information on local resistance rates. This information can be obtained from local clinical microbiology laboratories, state health departments, or publications of the Centers for Disease Control and Prevention (e.g., *Emerging Infectious Diseases* and *Morbidity and Mortality Weekly Report*).

TABLE 33-6

INFECTIONS FOR WHICH SPECIFIC ANTIBACTERIAL AGENTS ARE AMONG THE DRUGS OF CHOICE

AGENT	INFECTIONS	COMMON PATHOGEN(S) (RESISTANCE RATE, %)[a]
Penicillin G	Syphilis, yaws, leptospirosis, groups A and B streptococcal infections, pneumococcal infections, actinomycosis, oral and periodontal infections, meningococcal meningitis and meningococcemia, viridans streptococcal endocarditis, clostridial myonecrosis, tetanus, anthrax, rat-bite fever, *Pasteurella multocida* infections, and erysipeloid (*Erysipelothrix rhusiopathiae*)	*Neisseria meningitidis*[b] (intermediate,[c] 15–30; resistant, 0; geographic variation) Viridans streptococci (intermediate, 15–30; resistant, 5–10) *Streptococcus pneumoniae* (intermediate, 23; resistant, 17)
Ampicillin, amoxicillin	Salmonellosis, acute otitis media, *Haemophilus influenzae* meningitis and epiglottitis, *Listeria monocytogenes* meningitis, *Enterococcus faecalis* UTI	*Escherichia coli* (37) *H. influenzae* (35) *Salmonella* spp.[b] (30–50; geographic variation) *Enterococcus* spp. (24)
Nafcillin, oxacillin	*Staphylococcus aureus* (non-MRSA) bacteremia and endocarditis	*S. aureus* (46; MRSA) *Staphylococcus epidermidis* (78; MRSE)
Piperacillin plus tazobactam	Intraabdominal infections (facultative enteric gram-negative bacilli plus obligate anaerobes); infections caused by mixed flora (aspiration pneumonia, diabetic foot ulcers); infections caused by *Pseudomonas aeruginosa*	*P. aeruginosa* (6)
Cefazolin	*E. coli* UTI, surgical prophylaxis, *S. aureus* (non-MRSA) bacteremia and endocarditis	*E. coli* (7) *S. aureus* (46; MRSA)
Cefoxitin, cefotetan	Intraabdominal infections and pelvic inflammatory disease	*Bacteroides fragilis* (12)
Ceftriaxone	Gonococcal infections, pneumococcal meningitis, viridans streptococcal endocarditis, salmonellosis and typhoid fever, hospital-acquired infections caused by nonpseudomonal facultative gram-negative enteric bacilli	*S. pneumoniae* (intermediate, 16; resistant, 0) *E. coli* and *Klebsiella pneumoniae* (1; ESBL producers)
Ceftazidime, cefepime	Hospital-acquired infections caused by facultative gram-negative enteric bacilli and *Pseudomonas*	*P. aeruginosa* (16) (See ceftriaxone for ESBL producers)
Imipenem, meropenem	Intraabdominal infections, hospital-acquired infections (non-MRSA), infections caused by *Enterobacter* spp. and ESBL-producing gram-negative bacilli	*P. aeruginosa* (6) *Acinetobacter* spp. (35)
Aztreonam	Hospital-acquired infections caused by facultative gram-negative bacilli and *Pseudomonas* in penicillin-allergic patients	*P. aeruginosa* (16)
Vancomycin	Bacteremia, endocarditis, and other serious infections due to MRSA; pneumococcal meningitis; antibiotic-associated pseudomembranous colitis[d]	*Enterococcus* spp. (24)
Daptomycin	VRE infections; MRSA bacteremia	UNK
Gentamicin, amikacin, tobramycin	Combined with a penicillin for staphylococcal, enterococcal, or viridans streptococcal endocarditis; combined with a β-lactam antibiotic for gram-negative bacteremia; pyelonephritis	Gentamicin: *E. coli* (6) *P. aeruginosa* (17) *Acinetobacter* spp. (32)
Erythromycin, clarithromycin, azithromycin	*Legionella*, *Campylobacter*, and *Mycoplasma* infections; CAP; group A streptococcal pharyngitis in penicillin-allergic patients; bacillary angiomatosis (*Bartonella henselae*); gastric infections due to *Helicobacter pylori*; *Mycobacterium avium-intracellulare* infections	*S. pneumoniae* (28) *Streptococcus pyogenes*[b] (0–10; geographic variation) *H. pylori*[b] (2–20; geographic variation)
Clindamycin	Severe, invasive group A streptococcal infections; infections caused by obligate anaerobes; infections caused by susceptible staphylococci	*S. aureus* (nosocomial = 58; CA-MRSA = 10[b])

(*Continued*)

TABLE 33-6 (*CONTINUED*)

INFECTIONS FOR WHICH SPECIFIC ANTIBACTERIAL AGENTS ARE AMONG THE DRUGS OF CHOICE

AGENT	INFECTIONS	COMMON PATHOGEN(S) (RESISTANCE RATE, %)[a]
Doxycycline, minocycline	Acute bacterial exacerbations of chronic bronchitis, granuloma inguinale, brucellosis (with streptomycin), tularemia, glanders, melioidosis, spirochetal infections caused by *Borrelia* (Lyme disease and relapsing fever; doxycycline), infections caused by *Vibrio vulnificus*, some *Aeromonas* infections, infections due to *Stenotrophomonas* (minocycline), plague, ehrlichiosis, chlamydial infections (doxycycline), granulomatous skin infections due to *Mycobacterium marinum* (minocycline), rickettsial infections, mild CAP, skin and soft tissue infections caused by gram-positive cocci (CA-MRSA infections, leptospirosis, syphilis, actinomycosis in the penicillin-allergic patient)	*S. pneumoniae* (17) MRSA (5)
Trimethoprim-sulfamethoxazole	Community-acquired UTI; *S. aureus* skin and soft tissue infections (CA-MRSA)	*E. coli* (19) MRSA (3)
Sulfonamides	Nocardial infections, leprosy (dapsone, a sulfone), and toxoplasmosis (sulfadiazine)	UNK
Ciprofloxacin, levofloxacin, moxifloxacin	CAP (levofloxacin and moxifloxacin); UTI; bacterial gastroenteritis; hospital-acquired gram-negative enteric infections; *Pseudomonas* infections (ciprofloxacin and levofloxacin)	*S. pneumoniae* (1) *E. coli* (13) *P. aeruginosa* (23) *Salmonella* spp. (10–50; geographic variation) *Neisseria gonorrhoeae*[e]
Rifampin	Staphylococcal foreign body infections, in combination with other antistaphylococcal agents; *Legionella* pneumonia	Staphylococci rapidly develop resistance during rifampin monotherapy.
Metronidazole	Obligate anaerobic gram-negative bacteria (*Bacteroides* spp.): abscess in lung, brain, or abdomen; bacterial vaginosis; antibiotic-associated *Clostridium difficile* disease	UNK
Linezolid	VRE; staphylococcal skin and soft tissue infection (CA-MRSA)	UNK
Polymyxin E (colistin)	Hospital-acquired infection due to gram-negative bacilli resistant to all other chemotherapy: *P. aeruginosa*, *Acinetobacter* spp., *Stenotrophomonas maltophilia*	UNK
Quinupristin/ dalfopristin	VRE	Vancomycin-resistant *E. faecalis*[b] (100) Vancomycin-resistant *E. faecium* (10)
Mupirocin	Topical application to nares to eradicate *S. aureus* carriage	UNK

[a]Unless otherwise noted, resistance rates are based on all isolates tested in 2005 in the clinical microbiology laboratory at Virginia Commonwealth University Medical Center. The rates are consistent with those reported by the National Nosocomial Infections Surveillance System (Am J Infect Control 32:470,2004).
[b]Data from recent literature sources.
[c]Intermediate resistance.
[d]Drug is given orally for this indication.
[e]Resistance rates vary geographically. Fluoroquinolones are now considered drugs of choice only for gonococcal isolates whose susceptibility is documented by laboratory testing.
Note: CA-MRSA, community-acquired methicillin-resistant *S. aureus;* CAP, community-acquired pneumonia; MRSA, methicillin-resistant *S. aureus;* MRSE, methicillin-resistant *S. epidermidis;* UTI, urinary tract infection; VRE, vancomycin-resistant enterococci; ESBL, extended-spectrum β-lactamase; UNK, resistance rates unknown.

ADVERSE REACTIONS

Adverse drug reactions are frequently classified by mechanism as either *dose-related* ("toxic") or *unpredictable*. Unpredictable reactions are either idiosyncratic or allergic. Dose-related reactions include aminoglycoside-induced nephrotoxicity, linezolid-induced thrombocytopenia, penicillin-induced seizures, and vancomycin-induced anaphylactoid reactions. Many of these reactions can be avoided by reducing dosage in patients with impaired renal function, limiting the duration of therapy, or reducing the rate of administration. Adverse reactions to antibacterial agents are a common cause of morbidity, requiring alteration in therapy and additional expense, and they occasionally result in death. The elderly, often those with the more severe infections, may be especially prone to certain adverse reactions. The most clinically relevant adverse reactions to common antibacterial drugs are listed in Table 33-7.

DRUG INTERACTIONS

Antimicrobial drugs are a common cause of drug-drug interactions. Table 33-8 lists the most common and best-documented interactions of antibacterial agents with other drugs and characterizes the clinical relevance of these interactions. Coadministration of drugs paired in the tables does not necessarily result in clinically important adverse consequences. Recognition of the potential for an interaction before the administration of an antibacterial agent is crucial to the rational use of these drugs, since adverse consequences can often be prevented if the interaction is anticipated. Table 33-8 is intended only to heighten awareness of the potential for an interaction. Additional sources should be consulted to identify appropriate options.

MACROLIDES AND KETOLIDES

Erythromycin, clarithromycin, and telithromycin inhibit CYP3A4, the hepatic P450 enzyme that metabolizes many drugs, including cyclosporine, certain statins (lovastatin, simvastatin), theophylline, carbamazepine, warfarin, certain antineoplastic agents (e.g., vincristine, irinotecan), and ergot alkaloids. In ~10% of patients receiving digoxin, concentrations increase significantly when erythromycin or telithromycin is coadministered, and this increase may lead to digoxin toxicity. Azithromycin has little effect on the metabolism of other drugs.

Many drugs (e.g., azole antifungal drugs, diltiazem, verapamil, and nefazodone) can also increase absorption or inhibit erythromycin metabolism. These effects are associated with prolongation of the QT interval and a fivefold increase in mortality rate. This example serves as a reminder that the true significance of drug-drug interactions may be subtle yet profound and that close attention to the evolving safety literature is important.

QUINUPRISTIN/DALFOPRISTIN

Quinupristin/dalfopristin is an inhibitor of CYP3A4. Its interactions with other drugs should be similar to those of erythromycin.

LINEZOLID

Linezolid is a monoamine oxidase inhibitor. Its concomitant administration with sympathomimetics (e.g., phenylpropanolamine) and with foods with high concentrations of tyramine should be avoided. Many case reports describe serotonin syndrome after coadministration of linezolid with selective serotonin reuptake inhibitors.

TETRACYCLINES

The most important interaction involving tetracyclines is reduced absorption when these drugs are coadministered with divalent and trivalent cations, such as antacids, iron compounds, or dairy products. Food also adversely affects absorption of most tetracyclines. Inducers of hepatic isoenzymes, such as phenytoin and rifampin, increase the clearance of doxycycline; although the clinical significance of this effect is unknown, use of an alternative antibiotic may be appropriate.

SULFONAMIDES

Sulfonamides, including TMP-SMX, increase the hypoprothrombinemic effect of warfarin by inhibition of its metabolism or by protein-binding displacement.

FLUOROQUINOLONES

There are two clinically important drug interactions involving fluoroquinolones. First, like tetracyclines, all fluoroquinolones are chelated by divalent and trivalent cations, with a consequential significant reduction in absorption. Second, ciprofloxacin inhibits the hepatic enzyme that metabolizes theophylline. Scattered case reports suggest that quinolones can also potentiate the effects of warfarin, but this effect has not been observed in most controlled trials.

RIFAMPIN

Rifampin is an excellent inducer of many cytochrome P450 enzymes and increases the hepatic clearance of a large number of drugs, including the following (with the indicated predictable outcomes): HIV-1 protease inhibitors (loss of viral suppression), oral contraceptives (pregnancy), warfarin (decreased prothrombin times), cyclosporine and prednisone (organ rejection or exacerbations of any underlying inflammatory condition), and verapamil and diltiazem (increased dosage requirements). Before rifampin is prescribed for any patient, a review of concomitant drug therapy is essential.

METRONIDAZOLE

Metronidazole can cause a disulfiram-like syndrome when alcohol is ingested. Thus patients taking metronidazole should be instructed to avoid alcohol. Inhibition of the metabolism of warfarin by metronidazole leads to significant rises in prothrombin times.

PROPHYLAXIS OF BACTERIAL INFECTIONS

Antibacterial agents are occasionally indicated for use in patients who have no evidence of infection but who have been or are expected to be exposed to bacterial pathogens under circumstances that constitute a major risk of infection. The basic tenets of antimicrobial

TABLE 33-7

MOST CLINICALLY RELEVANT ADVERSE REACTIONS TO COMMON ANTIBACTERIAL DRUGS

DRUG	ADVERSE EVENT	COMMENTS
β-Lactams	Allergies in ~1–4% of treatment courses	Cephalosporins cause allergy in 2–4% of penicillin-allergic patients. Aztreonam is safe in β-lactam–allergic patients.
	Nonallergic skin reactions	Ampicillin "rash" is common among patients with Epstein-Barr virus infection.
	Diarrhea, including *Clostridium difficile* colitis (Chap. 43)	—
Vancomycin	Anaphylactoid reaction ("red man syndrome")	Give as a 1- to 2-h infusion.
	Nephrotoxicity, ototoxicity, allergy, neutropenia	Rare
Aminoglycosides	Nephrotoxicity (generally reversible)	Greatest with prolonged therapy in the elderly or with preexisting renal insufficiency. Monitor serum creatinine every 2–3 days.
	Ototoxicity (often irreversible)	Risk factors similar to those for nephrotoxicity; both vestibular and hearing toxicities
Macrolides/ ketolides	Gastrointestinal distress	Most common with erythromycin
	Ototoxicity	High-dose IV erythromycin
	Cardiac toxicity	QTc prolongation and torsades de pointes, especially when inhibitors of erythromycin metabolism are given simultaneously
	Hepatic toxicity (telithromycin)	Warning added to prescribing information (July 2006)
	Respiratory failure in patients with myasthenia gravis (telithromycin)	Warning added to prescribing information (July 2006)
Clindamycin	Diarrhea, including *C. difficile* colitis	—
Sulfonamides	Allergic reactions	Rashes (more common in HIV-infected patients); serious dermal reactions, including erythema multiforme, Stevens-Johnson syndrome, toxic epidermal necrolysis
	Hematologic reactions	Uncommon; include agranulocytosis and granulocytopenia (more common in HIV-infected patients), hemolytic and megaloblastic anemia, thrombocytopenia
	Renal insufficiency	Crystalluria with sulfadiazine therapy
Fluoroquinolones	Diarrhea, including *C. difficile* colitis	—
	Contraindicated for general use in patients <18 years old and pregnant women	Appear safe in treatment of pulmonary infections in children with cystic fibrosis
	Central nervous system adverse effects (e.g., insomnia)	—
	Miscellaneous: allergies, tendon rupture, dysglycemias, QTc prolongation	Rare
Rifampin	Hepatotoxicity	Rare
	Orange discoloration of urine and body fluids	Common
	Miscellaneous: flulike symptoms, hemolysis, renal insufficiency	Uncommon; usually related to intermittent administration
Metronidazole	Metallic taste	Common
Tetracyclines/ glycylcyclines	Gastrointestinal distress	Up to 20% with tigecycline
	Esophageal ulceration	Doxycycline (take in A.M. with fluids)
Linezolid	Myelosuppression	Follows long-term treatment
	Ocular and peripheral neuritis	Follow long-term treatment
Daptomycin	Distal muscle pain or weakness	Weekly creatine phosphokinase measurements, especially in patients also receiving statins

TABLE 33-8

INTERACTIONS OF ANTIBACTERIAL AGENTS WITH OTHER DRUGS

ANTIBIOTIC	INTERACTS WITH	POTENTIAL CONSEQUENCE (CLINICAL SIGNIFICANCE[a])
Erythromycin/clarithromycin/ telithromycin	Theophylline	Theophylline toxicity (1)
	Carbamazepine	CNS depression (1)
	Digoxin	Digoxin toxicity (2)
	Triazolam/midazolam	CNS depression (2)
	Ergotamine	Ergotism (1)
	Warfarin	Bleeding (2)
	Cyclosporine/tacrolimus	Nephrotoxicity (1)
	Cisapride	Cardiac arrhythmias (1)
	Statins[b]	Rhabdomyolysis (2)
	Valproate	Valproate toxicity (2)
	Vincristine/vinblastine	Excess neurotoxicity (2)
Quinupristin/dalfopristin	Similar to erythromycin[c]	
Fluoroquinolones	Theophylline	Theophylline toxicity (2)[d]
	Antacids/sucralfate/iron	Subtherapeutic antibiotic levels (1)
Tetracycline	Antacids/sucralfate/iron	Subtherapeutic antibiotic levels (1)
Trimethoprim-sulfamethoxazole	Phenytoin	Phenytoin toxicity (2)
	Oral hypoglycemics	Hypoglycemia (2)
	Warfarin	Bleeding (1)
	Digoxin	Digoxin toxicity (2)
Metronidazole	Ethanol	Disulfiram-like reactions (2)
	Fluorouracil	Bone marrow suppression (1)
	Warfarin	Bleeding (2)
Rifampin	Warfarin	Clot formation (1)
	Oral contraceptives	Pregnancy (1)
	Cyclosporine/tacrolimus	Rejection (1)
	HIV-1 protease inhibitors	Increased viral load, resistance (1)
	Nonnucleoside reverse-transcriptase inhibitors	Increased viral load, resistance (1)
	Glucocorticoids	Loss of steroid effect (1)
	Methadone	Narcotic withdrawal symptoms (1)
	Digoxin	Subtherapeutic digoxin levels (1)
	Itraconazole	Subtherapeutic itraconazole levels (1)
	Phenytoin	Loss of seizure control (1)
	Statins	Hypercholesterolemia (1)
	Diltiazem	Subtherapeutic diltiazem levels (1)
	Verapamil	Subtherapeutic verapamil levels (1)

[a]1 = a well-documented interaction with clinically important consequences; 2 = an interaction of uncertain frequency but of potential clinical importance.

[b]Lovastatin and simvastatin are most affected; pravastatin and atorvastatin are less prone to clinically important effects.

[c]The macrolide antibiotics and quinupristin/dalfopristin inhibit the same human metabolic enzyme, CYP3A4, and similar interactions are anticipated.

[d]Ciprofloxacin only. Levofloxacin and moxifloxacin do not inhibit theophylline metabolism.

Note: New interactions are commonly reported after marketing. Consult the most recent prescribing information for updates.

CNS, central nervous system.

prophylaxis are as follows: (1) The risk or potential severity of infection should outweigh the risk of side effects from the antibacterial agent. (2) The antibacterial agent should be given for the shortest period necessary to prevent target infections. (3) The antibacterial agent should be given before the expected period of risk (e.g., within 1 h of incision before elective surgery) or as soon as possible after contact with an infected individual (e.g., prophylaxis for meningococcal meningitis).

Table 33-9 lists the major indications for antibacterial prophylaxis in adults. The table includes only those indications that are widely accepted, supported by well-designed studies, or recommended by expert panels. Prophylaxis is also used but is less widely accepted for

TABLE 33-9

PROPHYLAXIS OF BACTERIAL INFECTIONS IN ADULTS

CONDITION	ANTIBACTERIAL AGENT	TIMING OR DURATION OF PROPHYLAXIS
Nonsurgical		
Cardiac lesions susceptible to bacterial endocarditis	Amoxicillin[a]	Before and after procedures causing bacteremia
Recurrent *S. aureus* infections	Mupirocin	5 days (intranasal)
Contact with patient with meningococcal meningitis	Rifampin	2 days
	Fluoroquinolone	Single dose
Bite wounds[b]	Penicillin V or amoxicillin/clavulanic acid	3–5 days
Recurrent cystitis	Trimethoprim-sulfamethoxazole or a fluoroquinolone or nitrofurantoin	3 times per week for up to 1 year or after sexual intercourse
Surgical		
Clean (cardiac, vascular, neurologic, or orthopedic surgery)	Cefazolin (vancomycin)[c]	Before and during procedure
Ocular	Topical combinations and subconjunctival cefazolin	During and at end of procedure
Clean-contaminated (head and neck, high-risk gastroduodenal or biliary tract surgery; high-risk cesarean section; hysterectomy)	Cefazolin (or clindamycin for head and neck)	Before and during procedure
Clean-contaminated (vaginal or abdominal hysterectomy)	Cefazolin or cefoxitin or cefotetan	Before and during procedure
Clean-contaminated (high-risk genitourinary surgery)	Fluoroquinolone	Before and during procedure
Clean-contaminated (colorectal surgery or appendectomy)	Cefoxitin or cefotetan (add oral neomycin + erythromycin for colorectal)	Before and during procedure
Dirty[b] (ruptured viscus)	Cefoxitin or cefotetan ± gentamicin, clindamycin + gentamicin, or another appropriate regimen directed at anaerobes and gram-negative aerobes	Before and for 3–5 days after procedure
Dirty[b] (traumatic wound)	Cefazolin	Before and for 3–5 days after trauma

[a]Gentamicin should be added to the amoxicillin regimen for high-risk gastrointestinal and genitourinary procedures; vancomycin should be used in penicillin-allergic patients.
[b]In these cases, use of antibacterial agents actually constitutes treatment of infection rather than prophylaxis.
[c]Vancomycin is recommended only in institutions that have a high incidence of infection with methicillin-resistant staphylococci.

recurrent cellulitis in conjunction with lymphedema, recurrent pneumococcal meningitis in conjunction with deficiencies in humoral immunity or CSF leaks, traveler's diarrhea, gram-negative sepsis in conjunction with neutropenia, and spontaneous bacterial peritonitis in conjunction with ascites. The use of antibacterial agents in children to prevent rheumatic fever and otitis media under certain circumstances is also common practice.

The major use of antibacterial prophylaxis is to prevent infections after surgical procedures. Antibacterial agents are administered just before the surgical procedure—and, for long operations, during the procedure as well—to ensure high drug concentrations in serum and tissues during surgery. The objective is to eradicate bacteria originating from the air of the operating suite, the skin of the surgical team, or the patient's own flora that may contaminate the wound. In all but colorectal surgical procedures, prophylaxis is predominantly directed against staphylococci and cefazolin is the drug most commonly recommended. Prophylaxis is intended to prevent wound infection or infection of implanted devices, not all infections that may occur during the postoperative period (e.g., UTIs or pneumonia). Prolonged prophylaxis (beyond 24 h) merely alters the normal flora and favors infections with organisms resistant to the antibacterial agents used. A focus on appropriate surgical prophylaxis by the Centers for Medicare and Medicaid Services, coupled with national efforts by surgical societies, appears to be having a favorable impact on the appropriate use of antimicrobial drugs in the surgical setting, although additional improvements are needed.

DURATION OF THERAPY AND TREATMENT FAILURE

Until recently, there was little incentive to establish the most appropriate duration of treatment; patients were instructed to take a 7- or 10-day course of treatment for most common infections. A number of recent investigations have evaluated shorter durations of therapy, especially in patients with community-acquired pneumonia. Table 33-10 lists common bacterial infections for which treatment duration guidelines have been established or for which there is sufficient clinical experience to establish treatment durations. The ultimate test of cure for a bacterial infection is the absence of relapse when therapy is discontinued. *Relapse* is defined as a recurrence of infection with the identical organism that caused the first infection. In general, therefore, the duration of therapy should be long enough to prevent relapse yet not excessive. Extension of therapy beyond the limit of effectiveness may increase the medication's side effects and encourage the selection of resistant bacteria. The art of treating bacterial infections lies in the ability to determine the appropriate duration of therapy for infections that are not covered by established guidelines. Re-treatment of infections for which therapy has failed usually requires a prolonged course (>4 weeks) with combinations of antibacterial agents.

TABLE 33-10

DURATION OF THERAPY FOR BACTERIAL INFECTIONS

DURATION OF THERAPY	INFECTIONS
Single dose	Gonococcal urethritis, streptococcal pharyngitis (penicillin G benzathine), primary and secondary syphilis (penicillin G benzathine)
3 days	Cystitis in young women, community- or travel-acquired diarrhea
3–10 days	Community-acquired pneumonia (3–5 days), community-acquired meningitis (pneumococcal or meningococcal), antibiotic-associated diarrhea (10 days), *Giardia* enteritis, cellulitis, epididymitis
2 weeks	*Helicobacter pylori*–associated peptic ulcer, neurosyphilis (penicillin IV), penicillin-susceptible viridans streptococcal endocarditis (penicillin plus aminoglycoside), disseminated gonococcal infection with arthritis, acute pyelonephritis, uncomplicated *S. aureus* catheter-associated bacteremia
3 weeks	Lyme disease, septic arthritis (nongonococcal)
4 weeks	Acute and chronic prostatitis, infective endocarditis (penicillin-resistant streptococcal)
>4 weeks	Acute and chronic osteomyelitis, *S. aureus* endocarditis, foreign-body infections (prosthetic-valve and joint infections), relapsing pseudomembranous colitis

MECHANISMS TO OPTIMIZE ANTIMICROBIAL USE

Antibiotic use is often not "rational," and it is easy to understand why. The diagnosis of bacterial infection is often uncertain, and patients may expect or demand antimicrobial agents in this tenuous situation. There is a bewildering array of drugs, each with claims of superiority over the competition. The rates of resistance for many bacterial pathogens are ever-changing, and even experts may not agree on the clinical significance of resistance in some pathogens. Investigations consistently report that ~50% of antibiotic use is in some way "inappropriate." Aside from the monetary cost of using unnecessary or overly expensive antibiotics, there are the more serious costs associated with excess morbidity from superinfections such as *C. difficile* disease, adverse drug reactions, drug interactions, and selection of resistant organisms. Although these costs are not yet well quantified, they add substantially to the overall costs of medical care.

At a time when fewer new antimicrobial drugs are entering the worldwide market than in the past, much has been written about the continued rise in rates of resistant microorganisms and its causes. The message seems clear: the use of existing and new antimicrobial agents must be more judicious and infection control more effective if we are to slow or reverse trends in resistance. The phrase *antimicrobial stewardship* is used to describe the new attitude toward antibacterial agents that must be adopted to preserve their usefulness. Appropriate stewardship requires that these drugs be used only when necessary, at the most appropriate dosage, and for the most appropriate duration. Increasing attention is being given to the relationships between differences in antibiotic consumption and differences in rates of resistance in different countries. Although some newer antibacterial drugs undeniably represent important advances in therapy, many offer no advantage over older, less expensive agents. With rare exceptions, newer drugs are usually found to be no more effective than the comparison antibiotic in controlled trials, despite the "high prevalence of resistance" often touted to market the advantage of the new antibiotic over older therapies.

The following suggestions are intended to provide guidance through the antibiotic maze. First, objective evaluation of the merits of newer and older drugs is available. Online references such as the Johns Hopkins website (*www.hopkins-abxguide.org*) offer current and practical information regarding antimicrobial drugs and treatment regimens. Evidence-based practice guidelines for most infections are available from the Infectious Diseases Society of America (*www.idsociety.org*). Second, clinicians should become comfortable using a few drugs recommended by independent experts and professional organizations and should resist the temptation to use a new drug unless the merits are clear. A new antibacterial agent with a "broader spectrum and greater potency" or a "higher serum concentration-to-MIC ratio" will not necessarily be more clinically efficacious. Third, clinicians should become familiar with local bacterial susceptibility profiles. It may not be necessary to use a new drug with "improved activity against *P. aeruginosa*" if that pathogen is rarely encountered or if it retains full susceptibility to older drugs. Fourth, a skeptical attitude toward manufacturers' claims is still appropriate. For example, rising rates of penicillin resistance in *S. pneumoniae* have been used to promote the use of broader-spectrum drugs, notably the fluoroquinolones. However, except in patients with meningitis, amoxicillin is still effective for infections caused by these "penicillin-resistant" strains. Finally, with regard to inpatient treatment with antibacterial drugs, a number of efforts to improve use are under study. The strategy of antibiotic "cycling" or rotation has not proved effective, but other strategies, such as heterogeneity or diversity of antibiotic use, may hold promise. Adoption of other evidence-based strategies to improve antimicrobial use may be the best way to retain the utility of existing compounds. For example, appropriate empirical treatment of the seriously ill patient with one or more broad-spectrum agents is important for improving survival rates, but therapy may often be simplified by switching to a narrower-spectrum agent or even an oral drug once the results of cultures and susceptibility tests become available. Although there is an understandable temptation not to alter effective therapy, switching to a more specific agent once the patient's clinical condition has improved does not compromise outcome. A promising and active area of research includes the use of shorter courses of antimicrobial therapy. Many antibiotics that once were given for 7–10 days can be given for 3–5 days with no loss of efficacy and no increase in relapse rates (Table 33-10). Adoption of new guidelines for shorter-course therapy will not undermine the care of patients, many unnecessary complications and expenses will be avoided, and the useful life of these valuable drugs will perhaps be extended.

FURTHER READINGS

BARTLETT JG, PERL TM: The new *Clostridium difficile*—What does it mean? N Engl J Med 353:2503, 2005

COSGROVE SE, CARMELI Y: The impact of antimicrobial resistance on health and economic outcomes. Clin Infect Dis 36:1433, 2003

FISHMAN N: Antimicrobial stewardship. Am J Med 119:S53, 2006

GRUCHALLA RS, PIRMOHAMED M: Antibiotic allergy. N Engl J Med 354:601, 2006

JACOBY GA, MUNOZ-PRICE LS: The new β-lactamases. N Engl J Med 352:380, 2005

KOLLEF M: Appropriate empirical antibacterial therapy for nosocomial infections: Getting it right the first time. Drugs 63:2157, 2003

NAHUM GG et al: Antibiotic use in pregnancy and lactation: What is and is not known about teratogenic and toxic risks. Obstet Gynecol 107:1120, 2006

PETERSON LR: Penicillins for treatment of pneumococcal pneumonia: Does in vitro resistance really matter? Clin Infect Dis 42:224, 2006

POLK HC JR: Continuing refinements in surgical antibiotic prophylaxis. Arch Surg 140:1066, 2005

RAY WA et al: Oral erythromycin and the risk of sudden death from cardiac causes. N Engl J Med 351:1089, 2004

PART 2 DISEASES CAUSED BY GRAM-POSITIVE BACTERIA

CHAPTER 34

PNEUMOCOCCAL INFECTIONS

Daniel M. Musher

Streptococcus pneumoniae (the pneumococcus) was recognized as a major cause of pneumonia in the 1880s. Although the name *Diplococcus pneumoniae* was originally assigned to the pneumococcus, the organism was renamed *Streptococcus pneumoniae* because, like other streptococci, it grows in chains in liquid medium. Widespread vaccination has reduced the incidence of pneumococcal infection, but this organism remains the principal bacterial cause of otitis media, acute purulent rhinosinusitis, pneumonia, and meningitis.

MICROBIOLOGY

Pneumococci are identified in the clinical laboratory as catalase-negative, gram-positive cocci that grow in pairs or chains and cause α-hemolysis on blood agar. More than 98% of pneumococcal isolates are susceptible to ethylhydrocupreine (optochin), and virtually all pneumococcal colonies are dissolved by bile salts.

Peptidoglycan and teichoic acid are the principal constituents of the pneumococcal cell wall, whose integrity depends on the presence of numerous peptide side chains cross-linked by the activity of enzymes such as trans- and carboxypeptidases. α-Lactam antibiotics inactivate these enzymes by covalently binding their active site. Unique to *S. pneumoniae* and present in all strains is C-substance ("cell-wall" substance), a polysaccharide consisting of teichoic acid with a phosphorylcholine residue. Surface-exposed choline residues serve as a site of attachment for potential virulence factors, such as pneumococcal surface protein A (PspA) and pneumococcal surface adhesin A (PsaA), which may prevent phagocytosis. Except for strains that cause conjunctivitis, nearly every clinical isolate of *S. pneumoniae* has a polysaccharide capsule, a structure that renders the bacteria virulent by preventing phagocytosis. All strains produce pneumolysin, a toxin that may cause many of the manifestations of pneumococcal infection.

There are 90 serologically distinct capsules of *S. pneumoniae*. Serotyping remains clinically relevant because the activity of available vaccines is based on stimulating antibody to specific capsular polysaccharides.

EPIDEMIOLOGY

S. pneumoniae colonizes the nasopharynx and, on any single occasion, can be isolated from 5–10% of healthy adults and from 20–40% of healthy children. Once adults are colonized, organisms are likely to persist for 4–6 weeks but may be present for as long as 6 months. Pneumococci spread from one individual to another by direct or droplet transmission as a result of close contact; transmission may be enhanced by crowding or poor ventilation. Day-care centers have been a site of spread, especially of penicillin-resistant strains of serotypes 6B, 14, 19F, and 23F. Outbreaks of pneumococcal disease occur among adults in crowded living conditions—e.g., in military barracks, prisons, and shelters for the homeless—as well as among susceptible populations in settings such as nursing homes. The risk of pneumococcal pneumonia is generally not increased by contact in schools or workplaces (including hospitals).

The incidence data provided below were obtained before widespread administration of pneumococcal conjugate vaccine to infants and children. (For the impact of widespread vaccination, see "Prevention" later in the chapter.) In the absence of vaccination (which alters natural history), invasive pneumococcal disease is, by far, most prevalent among children <2 years old. The incidence is low among older children and adults <65 years of age but then rises in older adults. The fatality rate is also highest at the extremes of age. One surveillance study in the late 1980s found incidences of pneumococcal bacteremia among infants, young adults, and persons ≥70 years of age to be 160, 5, and 70 cases per 100,000 population, respectively. Most cases of pneumococcal bacteremia in adults are due to pneumonia, and there are 3–4 cases of nonbacteremic pneumonia for every bacteremic case. Thus an estimated 20 cases of pneumococcal pneumonia per 100,000 young adults and 280 cases per 100,000 persons over the age of 70 occur annually. The disease is more frequent among men than among women. The incidence of pneumococcal bacteremia among adults exhibits a distinct midwinter peak and a striking dip in summer; in children, the incidence is relatively constant throughout the year except for a marked dip in midsummer. For reasons that are unclear but probably multifactorial, Native Americans, Native Alaskans, and African Americans are more susceptible to invasive pneumococcal disease than are Caucasians. Natives of the Pacific Rim region are likewise more susceptible.

PATHOGENETIC MECHANISMS

Infection results when pneumococci colonizing the nasopharynx are carried into anatomically contiguous areas (e.g., the eustachian tubes, the nasal sinuses) and bacterial clearance is hindered (e.g., by mucosal edema due to allergy or viral infection). Clearly, the resistance of pneumococci to phagocytosis is central to their capacity to cause infection. Pneumonia ensues when organisms are inhaled or aspirated into the bronchioles or alveoli and are not cleared—especially, for example, if mucus production is increased and/or ciliary action is damaged by viral infection or by cigarette smoke or other toxic substances. Viral infection may also inhibit clearance by upregulating pneumocyte receptors that bind pneumococci.

In normally sterile sites, such as the sinuses or the lungs, pneumococci activate complement, stimulating the production of cytokines that attract polymorphonuclear leukocytes (PMNs). The polysaccharide capsule, however, renders the pneumococci resistant to phagocytosis. In the absence of anticapsular antibody, a large bacterial inoculum and/or a compromise of phagocytic function allows the initiation of infection. Infection of the meninges, joints, bones, and peritoneal cavity may result from pneumococcal spread through the bloodstream, usually from a respiratory tract focus of infection. Unencapsulated pneumococci virtually never cause invasive disease, although they can cause conjunctivitis.

Symptoms of disease are largely attributable to the inflammatory response, which may cause pain by increasing pressure (as in sinusitis or otitis media) or may interfere with vital bodily functions by preventing oxygenation of blood (as in pneumonia) or by inhibiting blood flow (as in vasculitis due to meningitis). Cell-wall constituents of *S. pneumoniae*, especially peptidoglycan, activate complement by the alternative pathway; the reaction between cell-wall structures and antibody (present in all humans) also activates the classic complement pathway. The result is the release of C5a, a potent attractant for PMNs, into the surrounding medium. Peptidoglycan can also directly stimulate the release of proinflammatory cytokines such as interleukin (IL) 1β, tumor necrosis factor (TNF) α, and IL-6. All pneumococci generate pneumolysin, a toxin that damages ciliary cells and PMNs and also activates the classic complement pathway. Injection of pneumolysin into the lungs of experimental animals produces the histologic features of pneumonia; in mice, immunization with this substance or challenge with genetically engineered mutants that do not produce it is associated with a significant reduction in virulence.

HOST DEFENSE MECHANISMS

Mechanisms of host defense may be nonimmunologic or immunologic. Immunologic mechanisms may be natural (innate) or specific (humoral).

Nonimmunologic Mechanisms

Nonimmunologic mechanisms that protect against pneumonia include filtration of air as it passes through the nasopharynx, the glottal reflex, laryngeal closure, the cough reflex, clearance of organisms from the lower airways by ciliated cells, and ingestion by pulmonary macrophages and PMNs of small bacterial inocula that manage to reach alveolar spaces. Respiratory virus infection, chronic pulmonary disease, or heart failure compromises these mechanisms, predisposing to the development of pneumococcal pneumonia.

Immunologic Mechanisms

Innate Immunity

Innate immune mechanisms participate in clearance of pneumococci from the nasopharynx as well as in phagocytosis by PMNs and macrophages via the microbial pattern recognition receptor Toll-like receptor 2 (TLR2).

Humoral Immunity

Immunologically specific humoral mechanisms provide the best protection against pneumococcal infection. Most healthy adults have antibody to constituents of *S. pneumoniae*, such as PspA, PsaA, and the cell wall; however, there is no convincing evidence for an opsonic role of these antibodies, especially at their usual concentrations. Most healthy adults lack IgG antibody to the majority of pneumococcal capsular polysaccharides. Antibody appears after colonization, infection, or vaccination. In the first few weeks after colonization, nonspecific mechanisms probably protect the host from infection. Thereafter, newly developed anticapsular antibody provides a high degree of specific protection. Adults who are at risk of aspirating pharyngeal contents and/or who have diminished mechanisms of lower airway clearance are at risk of developing pneumonia before antibody is produced. Persons with a diminished capacity to form antibody probably remain susceptible as long as they are colonized.

The risk of serious pneumococcal infection is greatly increased in persons with conditions that compromise IgG synthesis and/or the phagocytic function of PMNs and macrophages. Most patients hospitalized for pneumococcal pneumonia have one or more of these conditions (Table 34-1). Once a pneumococcal infection has been initiated, the absence of a spleen predisposes to fulminant disease. The liver can remove opsonized (antibody-coated) pneumococci from the circulation; in the absence of antibody, however, only the slow passage of blood through the splenic sinuses and prolonged contact with reticuloendothelial cells in the cords of Billroth can result in bacterial clearance. Patients without spleens tend to develop overwhelming pneumococcal disease that rapidly progresses to death.

TABLE 34-1

CONDITIONS THAT COMMONLY PREDISPOSE TO PNEUMOCOCCAL INFECTION

Increased risk of exposure	Defective complement function
Day-care centers	Defective bacterial clearance[a]
Military training camps	Congenital asplenia, hyposplenia
Prisons	Splenectomy
Shelters for the homeless	Sickle cell disease
Respiratory infection, inflammation	Multifactorial conditions
Influenza, other viral respiratory infections	Infancy and aging
Air pollution	Chronic disease
Allergies	Prior hospitalization
Cigarette smoking	Alcoholism
Chronic obstructive pulmonary disease	Malnutrition
Other causes of chronic pulmonary inflammation or obstruction	HIV infection
Anatomical disruption of meninges (dural tear)	Chronic lung disease
Defective antibody formation	Glucocorticoid treatment
Common variable hypogammaglobulinemia	Cirrhosis of the liver
Selective IgG subclass deficiency	Renal insufficiency
Multiple myeloma	Diabetes mellitus
Chronic lymphocytic leukemia	Anemia
Lymphoma	Coronary artery disease
	Fatigue, stress, and/or exposure to cold

[a]The absence of a spleen predisposes to more fulminant infection (see text).

SPECIFIC INFECTIONS CAUSED BY *S. PNEUMONIAE*

S. pneumoniae causes infections of the middle ear, sinuses, trachea, bronchi, and lungs (Table 34-2) by direct spread from the nasopharyngeal site of colonization. Infections of the central nervous system (CNS), heart valves, bones, joints, and peritoneal cavity usually arise by hematogenous spread. Peritoneal infection may also result from ascent via the fallopian tubes. The CNS may also be infected by drainage from nasopharyngeal lymphatics or veins or by contiguous spread of organisms (e.g., through a tear in the dura). Primary pneumococcal bacteremia—i.e., the presence of pneumococci in the blood with no apparent source—occurs commonly in children <2 years of age and

TABLE 34-2

MOST COMMON INFECTIONS CAUSED BY *STREPTOCOCCUS PNEUMONIAE* IN ADULTS

SITE	INFECTIONS
Respiratory tract	Otitis media Acute sinusitis Tracheobronchitis Pneumonia Empyema
Central nervous system	Meningitis Brain abscess
Cardiac	Endocarditis Pericarditis
Soft tissue/skeletal	Septic arthritis Osteomyelitis Cellulitis
Other	Peritonitis Endometritis Primary bacteremia

accounts for a small percentage of all cases of pneumococcal bacteremia in adults; if no therapy is given, a source and/or a secondary site of infection may become apparent. Pleural infection results either from direct extension of pneumonia to the visceral pleura or from hematogenous bacterial spread from a pulmonary or extrapulmonary focus to the pleural space; the route usually cannot be determined in any individual case. Infections listed after meningitis in Table 34-2 are uncommon or rare.

Otitis Media and Sinusitis

Otitis media and acute rhinosinusitis are similar in terms of pathogenesis. Bacteria are trapped in a normally sterile site when drainage is impaired, often as a result of viral infection, allergies, or exposure to pollutants (including cigarette smoke). In both disease states, *S. pneumoniae* is the most common or second most common isolate (after nontypable *Haemophilus influenzae*) from cultures of the infected site.

Pneumonia

The distinctive symptoms and signs of pneumonia, whether due to the pneumococcus or to other bacteria, are (1) cough and sputum production, which reflect bacterial proliferation and the resulting inflammatory response in the alveoli; (2) fever; and (3) radiographic detection of an infiltrate.

Predisposing Conditions

Pneumococcal pneumonia is most common at the extremes of age. Despite the undisputed role of *S. pneumoniae* as a major pathogenic bacterium for humans, the great majority of adults with pneumococcal pneumonia have underlying diseases that predispose them to infection. Otherwise-healthy military recruits involved in outbreaks of infection may be an exception to this rule; however, many of these individuals have been under extreme physical and/or psychological stress and/or have had an antecedent viral-type illness that may have reduced their normal host resistance. Infections with respiratory viruses, especially influenza virus, predispose to pneumococcal pneumonia. Other common predisposing conditions are alcoholism, malnutrition, chronic pulmonary disease of any kind (including asthma), cigarette smoking, HIV infection, diabetes mellitus, cirrhosis of the liver, anemia, prior hospitalization for any reason, renal insufficiency, and coronary artery disease (with or without recognized congestive heart failure). In elderly subjects, the predisposition is generally multifactorial.

Presenting Symptoms

Patients often present with a clear exacerbation of a preexisting respiratory condition. They may have felt unwell for several days, with coryza or a nonproductive cough and low-grade fever, but they feel distinctly worse at the time of onset of pneumonia. Coughing, often productive of purulent sputum, becomes prominent. The temperature may rise to 38.9°–39.4°C (102°–103°F), although a substantial proportion of patients are afebrile at admission. In a small proportion of cases, the onset of disease follows a hyperacute pattern in which the patient suddenly has a single episode of shaking chills followed by sustained fever and a cough productive of blood-tinged sputum. In the elderly, the onset of disease may be especially insidious and may not suggest pneumonia at all. Such persons may have minimal cough, no sputum production, and no fever, instead appearing tired or confused. Nausea and vomiting or diarrhea occurs in up to 20% of cases of pneumococcal pneumonia. Symptoms of a new cardiac arrhythmia, myocardial ischemia, or an actual infarction occur in 10% of patients at a veterans' hospital who are admitted for pneumonia, and these manifestations may even predominate. The pneumonia may precipitate cardiogenic or noncardiogenic pulmonary edema. Pleuritic chest pain may result from extension of the inflammatory process to the visceral pleura; persistence of this pain, especially after the first day or two of treatment, raises concern about empyema (see "Complications" later in the chapter). Clearly, the range of symptoms is sufficiently broad that no characteristic presentation distinguishes pneumococcal pneumonia from other types of bacterial pneumonia or from some types of nonbacterial pneumonia.

Physical Findings

Patients with pneumococcal pneumonia usually appear ill and have a grayish, anxious appearance that differs from that of persons with viral or mycoplasmal pneumonia. Temperature, pulse, and respiratory rate are typically elevated. Elderly patients may have only a slight temperature elevation or may be afebrile. Hypothermia may be documented instead of fever and is associated with increased morbidity and mortality. Pleuritic chest pain may cause diminished respiratory excursion (splinting) on the affected side. Dullness to percussion is noted in about half of cases, and vocal fremitus is increased over the area of consolidation. Breath sounds may be bronchial or tubular, and crackles are heard in most cases if enough air is being moved to generate them. Flatness to percussion at the lung base, absent fremitus, and lack of the expected degree of diaphragmatic motion suggest the presence of pleural fluid, which raises the possibility of empyema. The finding of a heart murmur—certainly if new—raises concern about endocarditis, a rare but serious complication. Hypoxia or the generalized response to pneumonia may cause the patient to be confused, but the appearance of confusion should also raise concern about meningitis. Obtundation or neck stiffness should lead to an immediate consideration of this complication.

Radiographic Findings

In patients sick enough to be hospitalized, pneumococcal pneumonia is limited to one lung segment in one-fourth of cases and to one lobe in another one-fourth, with multilobar disease in the remaining one-half. Air-space consolidation is the predominant finding and is detected in 80% of cases (Fig. 34-1). Air bronchogram (visualization of the air-filled bronchus against a background of alveolar consolidation) is evident in fewer than half of cases and is more common in bacteremic than in nonbacteremic disease. Rarely, pneumococcal pneumonia leads to a lung abscess. Although some pleural fluid may actually be present in half of cases, ≤20% of patients have a sufficient volume of fluid to allow aspiration, and in only a minority of these patients is empyema documented.

General Laboratory Findings

Anemia (hemoglobin level, <10 g/dL) is documented in 25% of cases. The peripheral-blood white blood cell (WBC) count exceeds 12,000/μL in the great majority of patients with pneumococcal pneumonia. A low WBC count (<6000/μL) is found in 5–10% of persons hospitalized for pneumococcal pneumonia and is strongly associated with fatal disease. The serum bilirubin level is modestly elevated in one-third of cases; hypoxia, inflammatory changes in the liver, and breakdown of red blood cells in the lung are all thought to contribute to this increase. A serum albumin level of <2.5 g/dL in 30% of cases may indicate predisposing malnutrition or may be the result of sepsis. About 20% of patients have serum sodium concentrations of ≤130 meq/L, and another 20% have serum creatinine concentrations of ≥2 mg/dL. Abnormalities of pleural fluid in empyema are reviewed in Chap. 17.

Differential Diagnosis

S. pneumoniae is the most common cause of so-called community-acquired pneumonia, but patients who present with this syndrome may actually have infection due to a broad array of microorganisms. The extensive list includes (but is not limited to) the following: *H. influenzae* or *Moraxella catarrhalis* in persons with little to predispose them other than chronic or acute inflammation of the airways; *Staphylococcus aureus,* especially in persons who take glucocorticoids, who have influenza, or who have major anatomic disruption of the airways; *Streptococcus pyogenes*; *Neisseria meningitidis*; anaerobic and microaerophilic bacteria in persons who may have aspirated oropharyngeal contents; *Legionella*; *Pasteurella multocida* in dog or cat owners; gram-negative bacilli, especially in persons who have severely damaged lungs and are taking glucocorticoids; viruses, especially influenza virus (in season), adenovirus, or

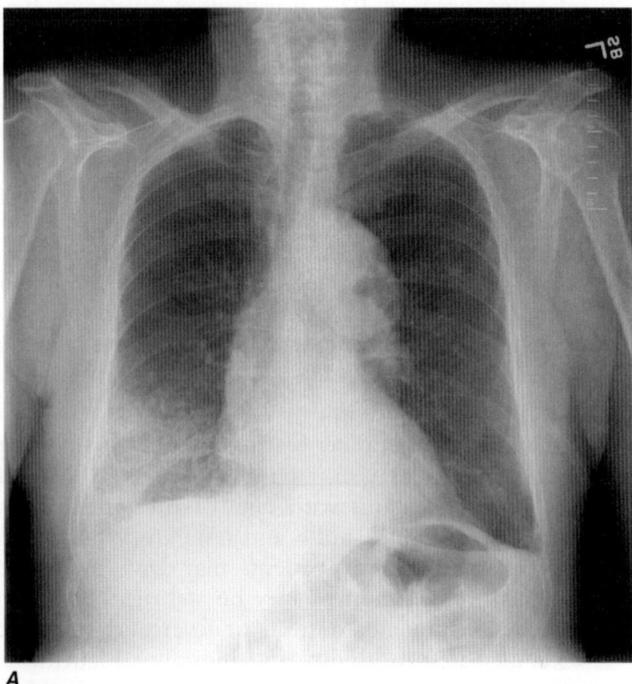
A

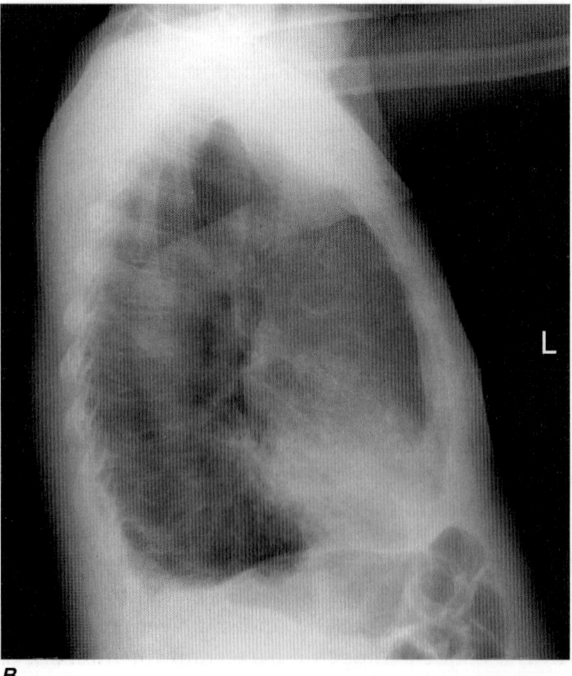

B

FIGURE 34-1

A retrocardiac infiltrate in a patient with pneumococcal pneumonia. Right-lower-lobe consolidation is apparent in posterior-anterior ***(A)*** and lateral ***(B)*** views of the chest.

TABLE 34-3

CAUSES OF A PNEUMONIA SYNDROME LEADING TO HOSPITALIZATION OF ADULTS IN HOUSTON, TEXAS[a]

COMMON	LESS COMMON
Streptococcus pneumoniae	*Moraxella catarrhalis*
Haemophilus influenzae	*Staphylococcus aureus*
Lung cancer	Pulmonary infarction
Mycobacterium tuberculosis	*Klebsiella pneumoniae*
Pneumocystis	*Cryptococcus, Histoplasma*
Influenza (seasonal)	Respiratory syncytial virus
	Microaerophilic and anaerobic mouth flora
	Pseudomonas aeruginosa
	Legionella species
	Nontuberculous mycobacteria
	Chlamydophila pneumoniae
	Nocardia species
	Hamman-Rich syndrome, others

[a]Pneumonia was defined as a syndrome consisting of fever, increased cough, sputum production, and an abnormal pulmonary shadow on chest x-ray.

respiratory syncytial virus; *Mycobacterium tuberculosis*; fungi, including *Pneumocystis* (depending on epidemiologic factors and HIV infection status); *Mycoplasma*; *Chlamydia pneumoniae*, especially in older adults; and *Chlamydia psittaci* in bird owners. Many older men with lung cancer present with pneumonia, as do persons who have acute-onset inflammatory pulmonary conditions of uncertain etiology or those with pulmonary embolus and infarction. The breadth of this list vividly illustrates the deficiency of empirical therapy for community-acquired pneumonia (Table 34-3). Many of these diseases require evaluation, and the increasing availability of specific therapy makes a precise etiologic diagnosis desirable.

Diagnostic Microbiology

In patients with community-acquired pneumonia, a pneumococcal etiology is strongly suggested by the microscopic demonstration of large numbers of PMNs and slightly elongated gram-positive cocci in pairs and chains in the sputum. A sample such as the one shown in Fig. 34-2 is highly specific for pneumococcal infection of the lower airways. In the absence of such microscopic findings, the identification of pneumococci by culture is less specific, possibly reflecting colonization of the upper airways. Prior treatment with antibiotics can rapidly clear pneumococci from sputum. These factors need to be considered when sputum cultures from patients who appear to have pneumococcal pneumonia are said to yield only "normal mouth flora" and when the medical literature describes what appear to be poor results of sputum culture. A study of sputum Gram's stain and culture in patients with proven (bacteremic) pneumococcal pneumonia showed that about half of patients could not provide a sputum sample, provided a sample of poor quality, or had received antibiotics for >18 h; results in the remaining cases showed >80% sensitivity of microscopic examination of a Gram-stained sputum sample and 90% sensitivity of a sputum culture. Blood cultures yield *S. pneumoniae* in ~25% of patients hospitalized for pneumococcal pneumonia.

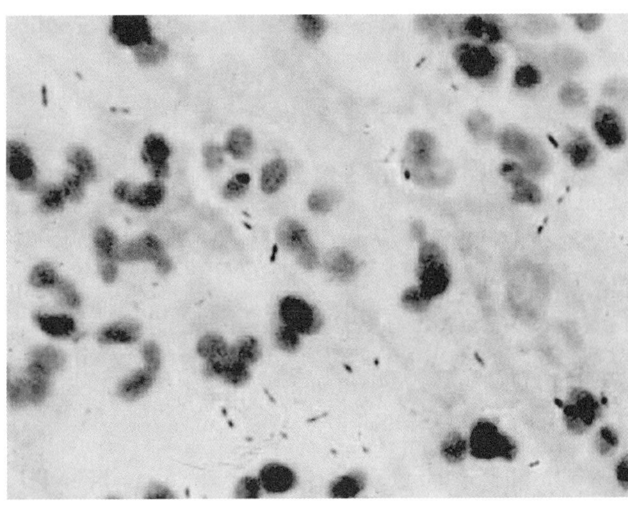

FIGURE 34-2
Gram-stained sputum from a patient with pneumococcal pneumonia shows polymorphonuclear cells with no epithelial cells, indicating the origin of the sample in inflammatory exudate without contamination by saliva. Slightly pleomorphic gram-positive coccobacilli appear, generally in pairs. Displacement of stained proteinaceous background material outlines a capsule surrounding some of the organisms. When obtained from a patient with pneumonia, a sample like this one is highly specific in identifying the pneumococcus as the etiologic agent.

Complications

Empyema is the most common complication of pneumococcal pneumonia, occurring in ~2% of cases. Some fluid appears in the pleural space in a substantial proportion of cases of pneumococcal pneumonia, but this parapneumonic effusion usually reflects an inflammatory response to infection that has been contained within the lung, and its presence is self-limited. When bacteria reach the pleural space—either hematogenously or as a result of contiguous spread, possibly across lymphatics of the visceral pleura—empyema results. The finding of frank pus, bacteria (by microscopic examination), or fluid with a pH of ≤7.1 indicates the need for aggressive and complete drainage, preferably by prompt insertion of a chest tube, with verification by CT that fluid has been removed. Failure to drain most or all of the fluid indicates the need for additional treatment, including placement of other tube(s) (thoracostomy) or thoracotomy. Empyema is likely if fluid is present and fever and leukocytosis (even low-grade) persist after 4–5 days of appropriate antibiotic treatment for pneumococcal pneumonia. At this stage, thoracotomy is often needed for cure. Aggressive drainage is likely to reduce morbidity and mortality from empyema.

Meningitis

Except during outbreaks of meningococcal infection, *S. pneumoniae* is the most common cause of bacterial meningitis in adults. Because of the remarkable success of *H. influenzae* type b vaccine, *S. pneumoniae* now predominates among cases in infants and toddlers as well (but not among those in newborns); nevertheless, the incidence of pneumococcal meningitis among children has been dramatically reduced by use of the pediatric pneumococcal conjugate vaccine (see "Prevention" later in the chapter).

No distinctive clinical or laboratory features differentiate pneumococcal meningitis from other bacterial meningitides. Patients note the sudden onset of fever, headache, and stiffness or pain in the neck. Without treatment, there is a progression over 24–48 h to confusion and then obtundation. On physical examination, the patient looks acutely ill and has a rigid neck. In such cases, lumbar puncture should not be delayed for CT of the head unless papilledema or focal neurologic signs are evident. Typical findings in cerebrospinal fluid (CSF) consist of an increased WBC count (500–10,000 cells/μL) with ≥85% PMNs, an elevated protein level (100–500 mg/dL), and a decreased glucose level (<30 mg/dL). If antibiotics have not been given, large numbers of pneumococci are seen in Gram-stained CSF in virtually all cases, and specific therapy can be administered, although, because of its similar appearance, *Listeria* may be misidentified as the pneumococcus. If an effective antibiotic has already been given, the number of bacteria may be greatly decreased and microscopic examination of a Gram-stained specimen may yield negative results. In this situation, immunologic methods may detect pneumococcal capsule in the CSF in up to two-thirds of cases.

Other Syndromes

The appearance of pneumococcal infection at other, ordinarily sterile body sites indicates hematogenous spread, usually during frank pneumonia or, in a small proportion of cases, from an inapparent focus of infection. A case of pneumococcal endocarditis is seen every few years at large tertiary-care hospitals. Purulent pericarditis, occurring as a separate entity or together with endocarditis, is even rarer. The name *Austrian's syndrome* is given to the concurrence of pneumococcal pneumonia, endocarditis, and meningitis. Septic arthritis can arise spontaneously in a natural or prosthetic joint or as a complication of rheumatoid arthritis. Osteomyelitis in adults tends to involve vertebral bones. Pneumococcal peritonitis occurs by one of three pathogenetic pathways: (1) hematogenous spread when ascites or other preexisting peritoneal disease is present; (2) local spread from a perforated viscus (usually appendicitis or perforated ulcer); or (3) transit via the fallopian tubes. Salpingitis may be recognized with or without accompanying peritonitis. Epidural and brain abscesses arise as a complication of sinusitis or mastoiditis. Cellulitis is also uncommon, developing most often in persons who have connective tissue diseases or HIV infection. The appearance of any of these unusual pneumococcal infections may suggest that tests for HIV infection should be undertaken. Finally, for reasons that are unclear, unencapsulated (but not encapsulated) pneumococci may cause sporadic or epidemic conjunctivitis.

℞ Treatment: PNEUMOCOCCAL INFECTIONS

ANTIBIOTIC SUSCEPTIBILITY β-Lactam antibiotics, the cornerstone of therapy for serious pneumococcal infection, bind covalently to the active site and thereby block the action of enzymes (endo-, trans-, and carboxypeptidases) needed for cell-wall synthesis. Because these enzymes were identified by their reaction with radiolabeled penicillin, they are called *penicillin-binding proteins.* Until the late 1970s, virtually all clinical isolates of *S. pneumoniae* were susceptible to penicillin (i.e., were inhibited in vitro by concentrations of <0.06 μg/mL). Since then, an increasing number of isolates have shown some degree of resistance to penicillin. Resistance results when spontaneous mutation or acquisition of new genetic material alters penicillin-binding proteins in a manner that reduces their affinity for penicillin, thereby necessitating a higher concentration of penicillin for their saturation. The genetic information that renders pneumococci resistant to penicillin is acquired from oral streptococci and is transmitted along with genes that convey resistance to other antibiotics as well. Selection of antibiotic-resistant strains worldwide—especially in countries where antibiotics are available without prescription and in loci of high antibiotic use, such as day-care centers—greatly contributes to the prevalence of multidrug resistance.

At present, ~20% of pneumococcal isolates in the United States exhibit intermediate resistance to penicillin [minimal inhibitory concentration (MIC) 0.1–1.0 μg/mL], and 15% are resistant (MIC ≥2.0 μg/mL; Fig. 34-3). The rate of resistance is lower in countries that, by tradition, are conservative in their antibiotic use (e.g., Holland and Germany) and higher in countries where usage is more liberal (e.g., France). In Hong Kong and Korea, resistance rates approach 80%. These definitions of resistance, however, were based on drug levels achievable in CSF during treatment of meningitis, whereas levels reached in the bloodstream, lungs, and sinuses are actually much higher. Thus the MIC needs to be interpreted in light of the infection being treated. Pneumonia caused by a penicillin-resistant strain is likely to respond to conventional doses of β-lactam antibiotics, whereas meningitis may not. The recently revised definition of amoxicillin resistance (susceptible, MIC ≤2 μg/mL; intermediately resistant, MIC = 4 μg/mL; and resistant, MIC ≥8 μg/mL) is based on susceptibility to serum levels, with the assumption that no physician would knowingly treat meningitis with this oral medication. Pneumonia due to a pneumococcal strain with intermediate amoxicillin resistance is still likely to respond to treatment with this drug, whereas

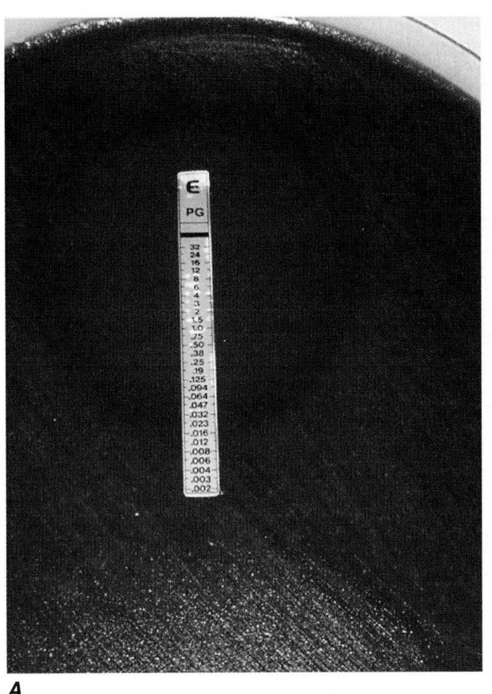

A

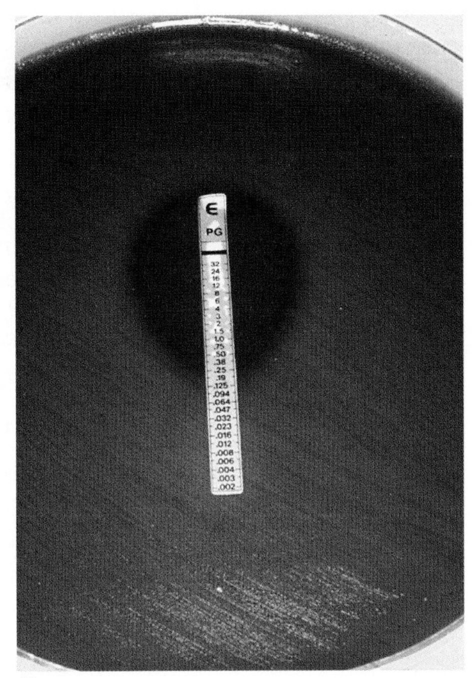

B

FIGURE 34-3

The e-strip method currently used by most laboratories to determine the susceptibility of *S. pneumoniae* to antibiotics. After the plate is streaked with a suspension of pneumococci, a strip impregnated with graded concentrations of the antibiotic under study (penicillin in the example shown) is placed on the surface, and the plate is incubated overnight at 37°C. The organism on ***A*** is inhibited by a penicillin concentration of 0.016 μg/mL and is fully susceptible to this drug. The organism on ***B*** is inhibited only by a penicillin concentration of 0.25 μg/mL and is intermediately resistant to this agent.

that due to a resistant strain may not. On the assumption that antibiotic concentrations in middle-ear fluid or sinus cavities approach those in serum, similar inferences can be made about the treatment of otitis or sinusitis.

Penicillin-susceptible pneumococci are susceptible to all commonly used cephalosporins. Penicillin-intermediate strains tend to be resistant to all first- and many second-generation cephalosporins (of which cefuroxime retains the best efficacy), but most are susceptible to certain third-generation cephalosporins, including cefotaxime, ceftriaxone, cefepime, and the oral cefpodoxime. One-half of highly penicillin-resistant pneumococci are also resistant to cefotaxime, ceftriaxone, and cefepime, and nearly all are resistant to cefpodoxime. Just as in the case of penicillin, susceptibility to cefotaxime and ceftriaxone is defined on the basis of achievable CSF levels. Thus pneumonia caused by intermediately resistant strains (MIC = 2 μg/mL) still responds well to usual doses of these drugs, and pneumonia due to a resistant organism (MIC ≥4 μg/mL) is likely to respond. Meningitis due to intermediately resistant strains may not respond, and meningitis due to a resistant strain is likely not to respond to treatment with cefotaxime or ceftriaxone.

About one-quarter of all pneumococcal isolates in the United States are resistant to erythromycin and the newer macrolides, including azithromycin and clarithromycin, with much higher rates of resistance among penicillin-resistant strains. This resistance will certainly affect empirical therapy for bronchitis, sinusitis, and pneumonia. In the United States, the majority of macrolide-resistant pneumococci bear the so-called M phenotype (erythromycin MIC = 1–8 μg/mL) and are susceptible to clindamycin. In this case, resistance is mediated by an efflux pump mechanism; to some extent, M-type resistance can be overcome by clinically achievable levels of macrolides. In Europe, most macrolide resistance is due to a mutation in *ermB*, which confers high-level resistance not only to macrolides but also to clindamycin; >90% of pneumococcal isolates in the United States are susceptible to clindamycin. Rates of doxycycline resistance are similar to those observed for macrolides. One-third of pneumococcal isolates are resistant to trimethoprim-sulfamethoxazole. The newer fluoroquinolones remain effective against pneumococci; the rate of resistance is generally <2–3% in the United States but is higher elsewhere and may be much higher in closed environments where these drugs are heavily prescribed, such as nursing homes and assisted-living facilities. Ketolides (such as telithromycin) appear to be uniformly effective against pneumococci, as does vancomycin.

ANTIBIOTIC REGIMENS

Otitis Media (Table 34-4) Current treatment recommendations for otitis media are based on the following points: (1) Acute otitis media is the most common diagnosis leading to an antibiotic prescription in the

TABLE 34-4

REGIMENS FOR THE TREATMENT OF PNEUMOCOCCAL OTITIS MEDIA OR SINUSITIS[a]

REGIMEN	DRUG, DOSE	DURATION	COMMENTS
First-line	Amoxicillin, 1 g q8h[b]	Otitis: 3–5 days after clinical response, not to exceed 7 days total (see text) Sinusitis: 7–10 days after clinical response, not to exceed 2 weeks total	If this regimen fails, try a second-line regimen.
Second-line	Amoxicillin, 1 g q8h, plus clavulanic acid, 125 mg q8h[c] *or* Fluoroquinolone[d] *or* Telithromycin, 800 mg/d	Same as above	If this regimen fails, try the third-line regimen.
Third-line	Ceftriaxone, 1 g qd	Otitis: 3–5 days Sinusitis: Longer	If this regimen fails, consider complications. Consult an otolaryngologist and/or infectious disease specialist.

[a]Except as noted, doses are for adults. Treatment for otitis media or sinusitis is empirical, since aspiration of the involved area to establish an etiologic diagnosis is rarely undertaken, except under the conditions of a research protocol.
[b]Dose for infants and toddlers: 80–90 mg/kg per day in 2 or 3 divided doses.
[c]Give half as amoxicillin alone (500 mg) and half as amoxicillin (500 mg)/clavulanic acid (125 mg).
[d]Moxifloxacin, 400 mg/d; or levofloxacin, 500 mg/d.

United States. (2) The diagnosis is often based on inadequate evidence for true middle-ear infection. (3) In proven cases, *S. pneumoniae* and *H. influenzae* are the most likely causes. (4) Because penetration into a closed space may be reduced, high serum levels of an effective antibiotic are required to treat otitis caused by intermediately or fully resistant pneumococci. (5) *S. pneumoniae* is more likely than *Haemophilus* and much more likely than *Moraxella* to cause progression to serious complications without specific therapy. (6) Antibiotics that are effective against pneumococci and yet resist β-lactamases tend to be very expensive compared with amoxicillin.

As a result of these considerations, the American Academies of Pediatrics and Family Practice recommend that clinicians apply due diligence in diagnosing otitis. In children 6 months to 2 years of age with nonsevere illness and an uncertain diagnosis and in children >2 years of age with nonsevere illness (even if the diagnosis seems certain), symptom-based therapy and observation may be used instead of antimicrobial therapy. When parents of children with otitis are given a prescription for an antibiotic but are instructed not to fill it unless the disease progresses, no antibiotic is given in many cases, yet rates of patient satisfaction are high. If otitis media is clearly diagnosed, high-dose amoxicillin is recommended (Table 34-4). If this regimen fails, highly penicillin-resistant pneumococci or β-lactamase–producing *Haemophilus* or *Moraxella* may be responsible; amoxicillin may be given at the same total dosage but with one-half of the dose in the form of amoxicillin/clavulanic acid. If this regimen fails, three doses of ceftriaxone at daily intervals are likely to be curative. A quinolone or ketolide may also be tried in adults. Patients must be monitored closely for a response. An otolaryngology consultation is recommended if all these treatments fail. Despite the detection (by molecular analysis) of pneumococcal DNA in middle-ear fluid, chronic serous otitis ("glue ear") is probably not due to active infection and does not require antibiotic therapy. Treatment for otitis is recommended for a total of 10 days in children <2 years of age but for only 5 days in children ≥2 years old who do not have complicated infections. A recent study reported identical rates of clinical and bacteriologic cure with a 10-day course of amoxicillin and a single dose of azithromycin (30 mg/kg).

Acute Sinusitis (Table 34-4) Just as the pathogenesis and microbial etiology of acute rhinosinusitis are similar to those of otitis media, so are the principles of diagnosis and treatment. The diagnosis is often empirical, and the less rigorously it is made, the more irrelevant antibiotics are likely to be. The estimated efficacy rate for amoxicillin/clavulanic acid, fluoroquinolones, and ceftriaxone (available for parenteral use only) is 90–92%, as opposed to 83–88% for amoxicillin, trimethoprim-sulfamethoxazole, and oral second- or third-generation cephalosporins and 71–81% for macrolides and doxycycline. Treatment should be given for longer periods than are recommended for otitis media (perhaps 10–14 days), but the optimal duration is uncertain.

Pneumonia (Table 34-5) This section will deal primarily with the treatment of pneumococcal pneumonia. The

TABLE 34-5

REGIMENS FOR THE TREATMENT OF PNEUMOCOCCAL PNEUMONIA IN ADULTS[a]

ROUTE, DRUG	DOSE, SCHEDULE[b]
Oral Therapy	
Amoxicillin	1 g q8h
Quinolone, e.g., levofloxacin	500 mg q24h
Telithromycin	800 mg q24h
Parenteral Therapy	
Penicillin[c]	3–4 mU q4h
Ampicillin	1–2 g q6h
Ceftriaxone	1 g q12–24h
Cefotaxime	1–2 g q6–8h
Quinolone	400 mg q24h
Imipenem	500 mg q6h
Vancomycin[d]	500 mg q6h

[a]These regimens are recommended for treatment after a presumptive diagnosis of pneumococcal pneumonia is made on the basis of examination of a Gram-stained sputum sample or as a replacement for broader spectrum empirical therapy after a diagnosis of pneumococcal pneumonia is proven by culture. When a valid sputum specimen cannot be obtained, concern about other likely pathogens should prompt the selection of more all-inclusive therapeutic regimens. Readers are referred to guidelines for empirical treatment of community-acquired pneumonia.

[b]Therapy should continue for 5 days after defervescence, not to exceed 7–10 days total. A switch from parenteral to oral drug administration may be made as soon as the patient can tolerate oral medications.

[c]This regimen is listed more for historic than for practical reasons. The spectrum is overly narrow, although perfectly acceptable if a Gram-stained sputum specimen shows only pneumococci. However, the need for frequent administration, mandated by the short half-life of penicillin, renders this regimen impractical.

[d]Not proven to be effective by the extensive clinical experience that applies to the other regimens.

broader issue of empirical therapy for community-acquired pneumonia is covered elsewhere (Chap. 17). Unless epidemiologic, clinical, and radiologic findings strongly favor another etiology, empirical therapy for pneumonia must include an agent that will be effective against *S. pneumoniae*, which remains the most likely causative agent of community-acquired pneumonia.

Outpatient Therapy Amoxicillin (1 g three times daily) effectively treats virtually all cases of pneumococcal pneumonia. Neither cefuroxime nor cefpodoxime offers any advantages over amoxicillin, and they are far more expensive. Telithromycin is likely to be equally effective. Moxifloxacin is also highly likely to be effective in the United States except in patients who come from a closed population where these drugs are used widely or who have themselves been treated recently with a quinolone. Clindamycin is effective in 90% of cases and doxycycline, azithromycin, or clarithromycin in 80%. Treatment failure resulting in bacteremic disease due to macrolide-resistant isolates has been amply documented in patients treated empirically with azithromycin. As noted above, rates of resistance to all these antibiotics are lower in some countries and much higher in others; high-dose amoxicillin remains the best option worldwide.

Inpatient Therapy Pneumococcal pneumonia is readily treatable with β-lactam antibiotics. The conventional dosages shown in Table 34-5 are acceptable against intermediately resistant strains and against many or most fully resistant isolates. Recommended agents include ceftriaxone and cefotaxime. Ampicillin is also widely used, usually in the form of ampicillin/sulbactam. The likely efficacy of newer quinolones such as moxifloxacin, macrolides such as azithromycin, and clindamycin is discussed above. On the basis of in vitro considerations, vancomycin is likely to be uniformly effective against pneumococci; this drug or a quinolone should be used together with a third-generation cephalosporin for initial therapy in a patient who is likely to be infected with a highly antibiotic-resistant strain. Patients who have had a severe allergic reaction to penicillins or cephalosporins may be treated with a carbapenem (e.g., imipenem-cilastatin), a quinolone, or vancomycin. The failure of a patient to respond promptly should at least prompt consideration of drug resistance. Evidence for loculated infections (such as empyema) and/or other causes of fever should be sought and addressed appropriately.

Duration of Therapy The optimal duration of treatment for pneumococcal pneumonia is uncertain. Pneumococci begin to disappear from the sputum within several hours after the first dose of an effective antibiotic, and a single dose of procaine penicillin, which produces an effective antimicrobial level for 24 h, was curative in otherwise-healthy young adults in an era when all isolates were susceptible. Early in the antibiotic era, most physicians treated pneumococcal pneumonia for 5–7 days. In the absence of data suggesting a need for longer treatment, younger physicians tend to treat the infection for 10–14 days. In the opinion of this author, a few days of close observation and parenteral therapy followed by an oral antibiotic—with the entire course of treatment continuing for no more than 5 days after the patient becomes afebrile—may be the best approach for treating pneumococcal pneumonia, even in the presence of bacteremia. Cases with a second focus of infection (e.g., empyema or septic arthritis) require longer therapy.

Meningitis (Table 34-6) Pneumococcal meningitis should be treated initially with ceftriaxone plus vancomycin. Equivalent doses of cefotaxime or cefepime may be used in place of ceftriaxone. The cephalosporin will be effective against most—but not all—isolates and will readily penetrate the blood-brain barrier; all isolates will be susceptible to vancomycin, but this drug has a somewhat unpredictable capacity to cross the blood-brain barrier. If the isolate is shown to be susceptible or intermediately resistant, treatment can be continued with ceftriaxone, and vancomycin can be discontinued. If the organism is resistant, treatment with both drugs should be continued. A very few studies of

TABLE 34-6

TREATMENT OF PNEUMOCOCCAL MENINGITIS

CIRCUMSTANCE	APPROPRIATE COURSE[a]
Diagnosis of pneumococcal meningitis; antibiotic susceptibility unknown	Treat with ceftriaxone, 2 g q12h, plus vancomycin, 500 mg q6h, until antibiotic susceptibility of organism is known.
Susceptibility results available	Continue treatment with ceftriaxone alone if organism is susceptible or intermediate; continue both ceftriaxone and vancomycin if organism is resistant.
Life-threatening penicillin allergy	Treat with imipenem, 500 mg q6h, rather than a β-lactam antibiotic.

[a]Treatment should be administered for 5–7 days after defervescence or for a total of 10 days.

TABLE 34-7

PROTECTIVE EFFICACY OF POLYVALENT PNEUMOCOCCAL POLYSACCHARIDE VACCINE[a]

AGE, YEARS	NO. OF SUBJECT PAIRS	YEARS SINCE LAST VACCINATION <3	3–5	>5
<55	125	93	89	85
55–64	149	88	82	75
65–74	213	80	71	58
75–84	188	67	53	32
≥85	133	46	22	−13

[a]Results of a case-control study involving all cases of invasive pneumococcal disease in Connecticut during 7 years (1984–1990). Vaccinated subjects were matched with controls, and the rate of invasive pneumococcal disease was related to age and time since vaccination. The data, showing protective efficacy, suggest that, within 5 years of vaccination, protection rates decline with age—i.e., from ~90% in persons <65 years of age to <50% in persons ≥85 years old. Protection also declines with increasing time from vaccination to infection, and this decline is more prominent in older patients.

Source: Data adapted from ED Shapiro et al: N Engl J Med 325:1453, 1991; with permission.

experimental animals suggest benefits of the addition of rifampin, but in vitro studies indicate antagonism between this drug and ceftriaxone or vancomycin; in the absence of data to support the practice in humans, this author does not recommend that rifampin be added. Imipenem may be used in place of the cephalosporin in patients who have had life-threatening allergic reactions to β-lactam antibiotics. The total duration of therapy for pneumococcal meningitis is 10 days. A recent study demonstrated clear benefit from the addition of glucocorticoids (Chap. 29).

Endocarditis Pneumococcal endocarditis is associated with rapid destruction of heart valves. Pending results of susceptibility studies, treatment should be initiated with ceftriaxone or cefotaxime; if the prevalence of highly resistant strains increases, it might be prudent to add vancomycin until results of susceptibility studies are available. In vitro, aminoglycosides are somewhat synergistic and rifampin or quinolones are antagonistic with β-lactams against pneumococci; there is no clear evidence from in vivo studies that adding any of these antibiotics to the regimen is beneficial.

OTHER THERAPEUTIC MODALITIES Addition of drotrecogin, an activated protein C preparation, may be beneficial in treating patients with severe pneumococcal sepsis. Glucocorticoids and agents that block the action of TNF-α, IL-1, or platelet-activating factor have conferred no benefit.

PREVENTION

Capsular Polysaccharide Vaccine

The pneumococcal capsular polysaccharide vaccine administered to adults since the early 1980s contains 25 μg per dose of capsular polysaccharide from each of the 23 most prevalent serotypes of *S. pneumoniae*. Vaccination stimulates antibody to most serotypes in most recipients. One case-control study showed a protection rate of 85% lasting ≥5 years in adults <55 years old (Table 34-7). The level and duration of protection decreased with advancing age. Other studies have suggested an overall protection rate in the adult population of 50–70%. In high-risk subgroups (e.g., debilitated elderly persons and individuals with severe chronic lung disease), vaccine has not been shown conclusively to be effective. Persons who most need the vaccine because of poor IgG responses (e.g., those with lymphoma or AIDS) are likely not to respond at all. Nevertheless, the Advisory Committee on Immunization Practices of the Centers for Disease Control and Prevention has broadened its recommendations for pneumococcal vaccination to include all persons >2 years of age who are at substantially increased risk of developing pneumococcal infection and/or having a serious complication of such an infection. Perhaps most in need of vaccination are persons with anatomic or functional asplenia, who are at risk for overwhelming, life-threatening infections. Others who might fall within these recommendations are persons who (1) are over the age of 65; (2) have a CSF leak, diabetes mellitus, alcoholism, cirrhosis, chronic renal insufficiency, chronic pulmonary disease, or advanced cardiovascular disease; (3) have an immunocompromising condition associated with increased risk of pneumococcal disease (e.g., multiple myeloma, lymphoma, Hodgkin's disease, HIV infection, organ transplantation, or chronic glucocorticoid use); (4) are genetically at increased risk (e.g., Native Americans and Native Alaskans); or (5) live in environments where outbreaks are particularly likely to occur (e.g., nursing homes).

Recommendations regarding revaccination seem somewhat inconsistent. A single revaccination is advocated for persons over the age of 65 if >5 years have elapsed since the first vaccination. Since antibody levels decline and there is no anamnestic response, it seems more reasonable simply to recommend revaccination at 5-year intervals, especially in persons over the age of 65, who tend to have almost no adverse reaction to vaccination, and in splenectomized patients, who are most in need.

Protein-Conjugate Pneumococcal Vaccine

Pneumococcal polysaccharide vaccine is not useful in children <2 years of age, whose immune system does not respond well to polysaccharide antigens. Conjugating the polysaccharide to a protein yields an immunogen that is effective in infants and young children. Initial studies of a protein-conjugate pneumococcal vaccine consisting of capsular material from the seven serotypes most likely to cause disease in children (Prevnar) showed a 98% reduction in rates of bacteremia and meningitis and a 67% reduction in rates of otitis media due to vaccine serotypes. Since it was marketed in 2000, widespread use of this vaccine has caused a dramatic decline in the incidence of invasive pneumococcal disease among infants and children (Fig. 34-4). Colonization rates have also greatly decreased. In an Alaskan village, rates of carriage of vaccine strains decreased in children from 55 to 10% and in adults from 15 to 5%. Studies of protein conjugate vaccines that contain antigen from more than seven common infecting serotypes are nearing completion, with favorable results.

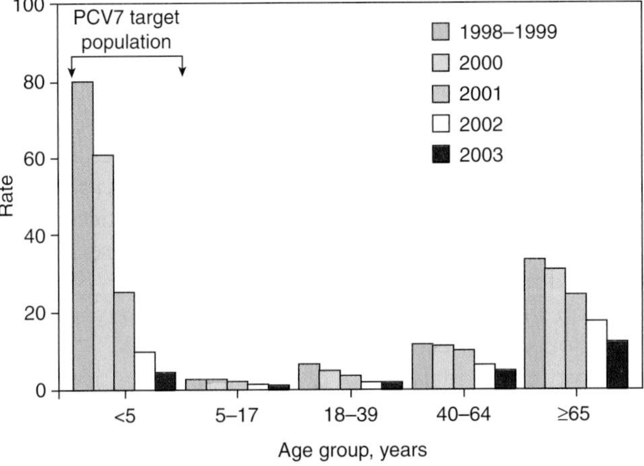

FIGURE 34-4

The rate of invasive pneumococcal disease per 100,000 population (*vertical axis*) is presented for each year since 2000 (*bars*) for different age groups (*horizontal axis*). Invasive pneumococcal disease is more common at the extremes of age. The incidence in all age groups has fallen steadily during the past 5 years. The observed reductions reflect direct effects and indirect ("herd") effects of widespread use of the 7-valent pneumococcal protein-conjugate vaccine (PCV7; see text). *(Adapted from Centers for Disease Control and Prevention, MMWR 54:893, 2005.)*

The incidence of invasive pneumococcal disease has also declined among unvaccinated children and among adults, to whom this vaccine is not even offered (Fig. 34-4). This decrease illustrates the "herd effect"—i.e., the impact of widespread vaccination on unvaccinated members of the population—and is probably attributable to the effects of the conjugate vaccine on nasopharyngeal carriage of vaccine serotypes. Another effect of the widespread use of this vaccine is the decreasing proportion of all pneumococcal disease that is due to antibiotic-resistant isolates, a trend that reflects the targeting of antibiotic-resistant strains by the vaccine. An unwanted effect of vaccination has been an increase in infections caused by serotypes that are not included in the vaccine (*replacement serotypes*), which, in fact, are increasingly expressing antibiotic resistance. Still, as noted above, the overall incidence of pneumococcal disease in all segments of the population has steadily declined. For further information, the reader is referred to the American Academy of Pediatrics *Red Book Online* (*http://aapredbook.aappublications.org*).

FURTHER READINGS

Alanee SR et al: Association of serotypes of *Streptococcus pneumoniae* with disease severity and outcome in adults: An international study. Clin Infect Dis 45:46, 2007

Albrich WC et al: Changing characteristics of invasive pneumococcal disease in metropolitan Atlanta, Georgia, after introduction of a 7-valent pneumococcal conjugate vaccine. Clin Infect Dis 44:1569, 2007

American Academy of Pediatrics and American Academy of Family Physicians Clinical Practice Guideline: Diagnosis and management of acute otitis media. Pediatrics 113:1451, 2004

Centers for Disease Control and Prevention: Direct and indirect effects of routine vaccination of children with 7-valent conjugate vaccine on incidence of invasive pneumococcal disease—United States 1998-2003. MMWR 54:893, 2005

Fedson DS, Musher DM: Pneumococcal vaccine, in *Vaccines,* 4th ed, SA Plotkin, EA Mortimer Jr (eds). Philadelphia, Saunders, 2003

Karlowsky JA et al: Factors associated with relative rates of antimicrobial resistance among *Streptococcus pneumoniae* in the United States: Results from the TRUST Surveillance Program (1998-2002). Clin Infect Dis 36:963, 2003

Lexau CA et al: Changing epidemiology of invasive pneumococcal disease among older adults in the era of pediatric pneumococcal conjugate vaccine. JAMA 294:2043, 2005

Mandell LA et al: Infectious Diseases Society of America/American Thoracic Society consensus guidelines on the management of community-acquired pneumonia in adults. Clin Infect Dis 44(Suppl 2):S27, 2007

——— et al: Update of practice guidelines for the management of community-acquired pneumonia in immunocompetent adults. Clin Infect Dis 37:1405, 2003

Musher DM: Pneumococcal vaccine—direct and indirect ("herd") effects (editorial). N Engl J Med 354:1522, 2006

———: *Streptococcus pneumoniae,* in *Principles and Practice of Infectious Diseases,* 6th ed, GL Mandell et al (eds). New York, Churchill Livingstone, 2004

——— et al: A fresh look at the definition of susceptibility of *Streptococcus pneumoniae* to beta-lactam antibiotics. Arch Intern Med 161:2538, 2001

Tuomanen EI et al (eds): *The Pneumococcus*. Washington, DC, ASM Press, 2004

CHAPTER 35

STAPHYLOCOCCAL INFECTIONS

Franklin D. Lowy

Staphylococcus aureus, the most virulent of the many staphylococcal species, has demonstrated its versatility by remaining a major cause of morbidity and mortality despite the availability of numerous effective antistaphylococcal antibiotics. *S. aureus* is a pluripotent pathogen, causing disease through both toxin-mediated and non–toxin-mediated mechanisms. This organism is responsible for both nosocomial and community-based infections that range from relatively minor skin and soft tissue infections to life-threatening systemic infections.

The "other" staphylococci, collectively designated *coagulase-negative staphylococci* (CoNS), are considerably less virulent than *S. aureus* but remain important pathogens in infections associated with prosthetic devices.

MICROBIOLOGY AND TAXONOMY

Staphylococci, gram-positive cocci in the family Micrococcaceae, form grapelike clusters on Gram's stain (Fig. 35-1). These organisms are catalase-positive (unlike streptococcal species), nonmotile, aerobic, and facultatively anaerobic. They are capable of prolonged survival on environmental surfaces in varying conditions.

More than 30 staphylococcal species are pathogenic. A simple strategy for identification of the more clinically important species is outlined in Fig. 35-2. Automated diagnostic systems, kits for biochemical characterization, and DNA-based assays are available for distinguishing among species. With few exceptions, *S. aureus* is distinguished from other staphylococcal species by its production of coagulase, a surface enzyme that converts fibrinogen to fibrin. Latex kits designed to detect both protein A and clumping factor also distinguish *S. aureus* from other staphylococcal species. *S. aureus* ferments mannitol, is positive for protein A, and produces DNAse. On blood agar plates, *S. aureus* tends to form golden β-hemolytic colonies; in contrast, CoNS produce small white nonhemolytic colonies.

Determining whether multiple isolates (especially of CoNS) from a particular patient are the same or different is often an important factor in distinguishing contaminants from genuine pathogens. Determining whether multiple isolates from different patients are the same or different is relevant when there is concern that a nosocomial outbreak may have been due to a common point source (e.g., a contaminated medical instrument). Biochemical tests, often performed in conjunction with antimicrobial susceptibility testing, have been used as a relatively simple means of distinguishing among staphylococcal species or strains. More discriminating molecular typing methods, such as pulsed-field gel electrophoresis and sequence-based techniques, have also been used for this purpose.

S. AUREUS INFECTIONS

EPIDEMIOLOGY

S. aureus is a part of the normal human flora; ~25–50% of healthy persons may be persistently or transiently colonized. The rate of colonization is higher among patients with insulin-dependent diabetes, HIV-infected patients, patients undergoing hemodialysis, and individuals with skin damage. The anterior nares are the most frequent site of human colonization, although the skin (especially when damaged), vagina, axilla, perineum, and oropharynx may also be colonized. These colonization sites serve as a reservoir of strains for future infections, and persons colonized with *S. aureus* are at greater risk of subsequent infection than are uncolonized individuals.

Overall, *S. aureus* is a leading cause of nosocomial infections. It is the most common cause of surgical wound infections and is second only to CoNS as a cause of primary bacteremia. Increasingly, nosocomial isolates are resistant to multiple drugs. In the community, *S. aureus* remains an important cause of skin and soft tissue infections, respiratory infections, and (among injection drug users) infective endocarditis. The increasing prevalence of home infusion therapy is another cause of community-acquired staphylococcal infections.

Most individuals who develop *S. aureus* infections are infected with their own colonizing strains. However, *S. aureus* may also be acquired from other people or from environmental exposures. Transmission most frequently results from transient colonization of the hands of hospital personnel, who then transfer strains from one patient to another. Spread of staphylococci in aerosols of respiratory or nasal secretions from heavily colonized individuals has also been reported.

In the past 10 years, numerous outbreaks of community-based infection caused by methicillin-resistant *S. aureus* (MRSA) in individuals with no prior medical exposure have been reported. These outbreaks have taken place in both rural and urban

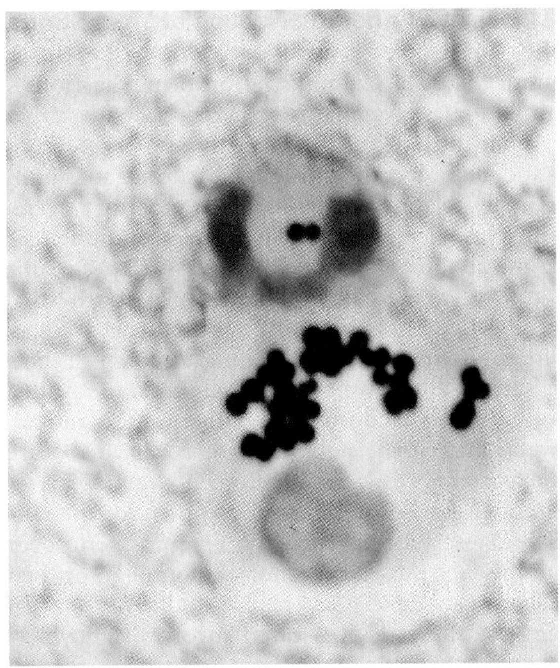

FIGURE 35-1
Gram's stain of *S. aureus* in a sputum sample with polymorphonuclear leukocytes. (*Reprinted with permission from FD Lowy: Staphylococcus aureus infections. N Engl J Med 339:520, 1998. © 1998 Massachusetts Medical Society. All rights reserved.*)

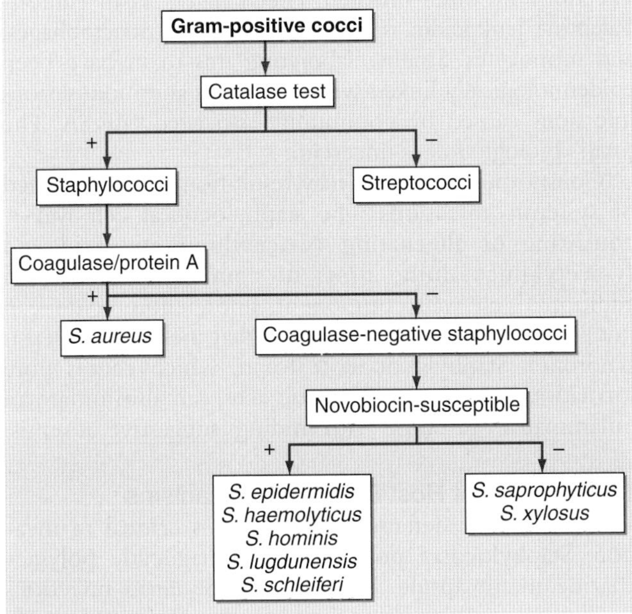

FIGURE 35-2
Biochemical characterization of staphylococci: algorithm of biochemical tests used to discriminate among the clinically important staphylococci. Additional tests are necessary to identify all of the different species.

settings in widely separated regions throughout the world. The reports document a dramatic change in the epidemiology of MRSA infections. The outbreaks have occurred among such diverse groups as prisoners, athletes, Native Americans, and drug users. Risk factors common to these outbreaks include poor hygienic conditions, close contact, contaminated material, and damaged skin. The community-associated infections have been caused by a limited number of MRSA strains. In the United States, strain USA300 has been the predominant clone and is also responsible for an increasing number of nosocomial infections. Of concern has been the apparent capacity of community-acquired MRSA strains to cause serious disease in immunocompetent individuals. This ability may be due to the presence of different toxin-producing genes in these strains.

PATHOGENESIS

General Concepts

S. aureus is a pyogenic pathogen known for its capacity to induce abscess formation at sites of both local and metastatic infections. This classic pathologic response to *S. aureus* defines the framework within which the infection will progress. The bacteria elicit an inflammatory response characterized by an initial intense polymorphonuclear leukocyte (PMN) response and the subsequent infiltration of macrophages and fibroblasts. Either the host cellular response (including the deposition of fibrin and collagen) contains the infection, or infection spreads to the adjoining tissue or the bloodstream.

In toxin-mediated staphylococcal disease, infection is not invariably present. For example, once toxin has been elaborated into food, staphylococcal food poisoning can develop in the absence of viable bacteria. In staphylococcal toxic shock syndrome (TSS), conditions allowing toxin elaboration at colonization sites (e.g., the presence of a superabsorbent tampon) suffice for initiation of clinical illness.

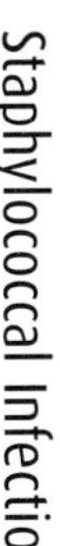

The S. Aureus *Genome*

The entire genome has been sequenced for numerous strains of *S. aureus*. Among the interesting revelations are (1) a high degree of nucleotide sequence similarity among the different strains; (2) acquisition of a relatively large amount of genetic information by horizontal transfer from other bacterial species; and (3) the presence of unique "pathogenicity" or "genomic" islands—mobile genetic elements that contain clusters of enterotoxin and exotoxin genes or antimicrobial resistance determinants. Among the genes in these islands are those carrying *mecA*, the gene responsible for methicillin resistance. Methicillin resistance–containing islands have been designated *staphylococcal cassette chromosome mecs* (SCC*mecs*) and range in size from ~20 to 60 kb. To date, five SCC*mecs* have been identified. Type 4 and type 5 SCC*mecs* have been associated with community-acquired MRSA strains.

A limited number of MRSA clones have been responsible for most community and hospital-associated infections worldwide. A comparison of these strains with those from earlier outbreaks (e.g., the phage 80/81 strains from the 1950s) has revealed preservation of the nucleotide sequence over time. This observation suggests that these strains possess determinants facilitating survival and spread.

Regulation of Virulence Gene Expression

In both toxin-mediated and non–toxin-mediated diseases due to *S. aureus*, the expression of virulence determinants associated with infection depends on a series of regulatory genes [e.g., accessory gene regulator (*agr*) and staphylococcal accessory regulator (*sar*)] that coordinately control the expression of many virulence genes. The regulatory gene *agr* is part of a quorum-sensing signal transduction pathway that senses and responds to bacterial density. Staphylococcal surface proteins are synthesized during the bacterial exponential growth phase in vitro. In contrast, many secreted proteins, such as α toxin, the enterotoxins, and assorted enzymes, are released during the postexponential growth phase.

It has been hypothesized that these regulatory genes serve a similar function in vivo. Successful invasion requires the sequential expression of these different bacterial elements. Bacterial adhesins are needed to initiate colonization of host tissue surfaces. The subsequent release of various enzymes enables the colony to obtain nutritional support and permits bacteria to spread to adjacent tissues. Studies with mutant strains in which these regulatory genes are inactivated show reduced virulence in several animal models of *S. aureus* infection.

Pathogenesis of Invasive S. Aureus Infection

Staphylococci are opportunists. For these organisms to invade the host and cause infection, some or all of the following steps are necessary: inoculation and local colonization of tissue surfaces, invasion, evasion of the host response, and metastatic spread. The initiation of staphylococcal infection requires a breach in cutaneous or mucosal barriers. Colonizing strains or strains transferred from other individuals are inoculated into damaged skin, a wound, or the bloodstream.

Recurrences of *S. aureus* infections are common, apparently because of the capacity of these pathogens to survive, to persist in a quiescent state in various tissues, and then to cause recrudescent infections when suitable conditions arise.

Nasal Colonization

The anterior nares is the principal site of staphylococcal colonization in humans. Colonization appears to involve the attachment of *S. aureus* to both nasal mucin and keratinized epithelial cells of the anterior nares. Other factors that may contribute to colonization include the influence of other resident nasal flora and their bacterial density, nasal mucosal damage (e.g., that resulting from inhalational drug use), and the antimicrobial properties of nasal secretions.

Inoculation and Colonization of Tissue Surfaces

Staphylococci may be introduced into tissue as a result of minor abrasions, administration of medications such as insulin, or establishment of IV access with catheters. After their introduction into a tissue site, bacteria replicate and colonize the host tissue surface. A family of structurally related *S. aureus* surface proteins referred to as MSCRAMMs (microbial surface components recognizing adhesive matrix molecules) plays an important role as a mediator of adherence to these sites. MSCRAMMs such as clumping factor and collagen-binding protein enable the bacteria to colonize different tissue surfaces; these proteins contribute to the pathogenesis of invasive infections such as endocarditis and arthritis by facilitating the adherence of *S. aureus* to surfaces with exposed fibrinogen or collagen.

Although CoNS are classically known for their ability to elaborate a biofilm and colonize prosthetic devices, *S. aureus* also possesses genes responsible for biofilm formation, such as the intercellular adhesion (*ica*) locus. Binding to these devices often involves staphylococcal adherence to serum constituents that have coated the device surface. As a result, *S. aureus* is frequently isolated from biomedical-device infections.

Invasion

After colonization, staphylococci replicate at the initial site of infection, elaborating enzymes that include serine proteases, hyaluronidases, thermonucleases, and lipases. These enzymes facilitate bacterial survival and local spread across tissue surfaces, although their precise role in infections is not well defined. The lipases may facilitate survival in lipid-rich areas such as the hair follicles, where *S. aureus* infections are often initiated. The *S. aureus* toxin Panton-Valentine leukocidin is cytolytic to PMNs, macrophages, and monocytes. Strains elaborating this toxin have been epidemiologically linked with cutaneous and more serious infections caused by community-associated MRSA. The toxin's biologic role is uncertain.

Constitutional findings may result from either localized or systemic infections. The staphylococcal cell wall—consisting of alternating *N*-acetylmuramic acid and *N*-acetylglucosamine units in combination with an additional cell wall component, lipoteichoic acid—can initiate an inflammatory response that includes the sepsis syndrome. Staphylococcal α toxin, which causes pore formation in various eukaryotic cells, can also initiate an inflammatory response with findings suggestive of sepsis.

Evasion of Host Defense Mechanisms

Evasion of host defense mechanisms is critical to invasion. Staphylococci possess an antiphagocytic polysaccharide microcapsule. Most human *S. aureus* infections are due to capsular types 5 and 8. The *S. aureus* capsule also plays a role in the induction of abscess formation. The capsular polysaccharides are characterized by a zwitterionic charge pattern (the presence of both negatively and positively charged molecules) that is critical to abscess formation. Protein A, an MSCRAMM unique to *S. aureus*, acts as an Fc receptor. It binds the Fc portion of IgG subclasses 1, 2, and 4, preventing opsonophagocytosis by PMNs. Both chemotaxis inhibitory protein of staphylococci (CHIPS, a secreted protein) and extracellular adherence protein (EAP, a surface protein) interfere with PMN migration to infection sites. The arginine catabolic mobile element (ACME), a cluster of genes unique to the USA300 clone, also may facilitate evasion.

An additional mechanism of *S. aureus* evasion is its capacity for intracellular survival. Both professional and nonprofessional phagocytes internalize staphylococci. Internalization by endothelial cells may provide a sanctuary that protects bacteria against the host's defenses. It also results in cellular changes, such as the expression of integrins and Fc receptors that may contribute to systemic manifestations of disease, including sepsis and vasculitis.

The intracellular environment favors the phenotypic expression of *S. aureus* small-colony variants. These menadione and hemin auxotrophic mutants are generally deficient in α toxin and can persist within endothelial cells. Small-colony variants are often selected after aminoglycoside therapy and are more commonly found in sites of persistent infections (e.g., chronic bone infections) and in respiratory secretions from patients with cystic fibrosis. These variants represent another mechanism for prolonged staphylococcal survival that may enhance the likelihood of recurrences. Finally, *S. aureus* can survive within PMNs and may use these cells to spread and to seed other tissue sites.

Host Response to S. Aureus *Infection*

The primary host response to *S. aureus* infection is the recruitment of PMNs. These cells are attracted to infection sites by bacterial components, such as formylated peptides or peptidoglycan, as well as by the cytokines tumor necrosis factor (TNF) and interleukins (ILs) 1 and 6, which are released by activated macrophages and endothelial cells.

Although most individuals have antistaphylococcal antibodies, it is not clear that the antibody levels are qualitatively or quantitatively sufficient to protect against infection. Anticapsular and anti-MSCRAMM antibodies facilitate opsonization in vitro and have been protective against infection in several animal models.

Groups at Increased Risk of Infection

Some diseases appear to entail multiple risk factors for *S. aureus* infection; diabetes, for example, combines an increased rate of *S. aureus* colonization and the use of injectable insulin with the possibility of impaired leukocyte function. Individuals with congenital or acquired qualitative or quantitative PMN defects are at increased risk of *S. aureus* infections; these include neutropenic patients (e.g., those receiving chemotherapeutic agents), individuals with defective intracellular staphylococcal killing (e.g., chronic granulomatous disease), and persons with Job's syndrome or Chédiak-Higashi syndrome. Other groups at risk include individuals with skin abnormalities and those with prosthetic devices.

Pathogenesis of Toxin-Mediated Disease

S. aureus produces three types of toxin: cytotoxins, pyrogenic-toxin superantigens, and exfoliative toxins. Both epidemiologic and animal data suggest that antitoxin antibodies are protective against illness in TSS, staphylococcal food poisoning, and staphylococcal scalded-skin syndrome (SSSS). Illness develops after toxin synthesis and absorption and the subsequent toxin-initiated host response.

Enterotoxin and Toxic Shock Syndrome Toxin 1 (TSST-1)

The pyrogenic toxin superantigens are a family of small-molecular-size, structurally similar proteins that are responsible for two diseases: TSS and food poisoning. TSS results from the ability of enterotoxins and TSST-1 to function as T-cell mitogens. In the normal process of antigen presentation, the antigen is first processed within the cell, and peptides are then presented in the major histocompatibility complex (MHC) class II groove, initiating a measured T-cell response. In contrast, enterotoxins bind directly to the invariant region of MHC—outside the MHC class II groove. The enterotoxins can then bind T-cell receptors via the vβ chain, resulting in a dramatic overexpansion of T-cell clones (up to 20% of the total T-cell population).

The consequence of this T-cell expansion is a "cytokine storm," with the release of inflammatory mediators that include interferon (IFN) γ, IL-1, IL-6, TNF-α, and TNF-β. The resulting multisystem disease produces a constellation of findings that mimic those in endotoxin shock; however, the pathogenic mechanisms differ. It has been hypothesized that a contributing factor to TSS is the release of endotoxin from the gastrointestinal tract, which may synergistically enhance the toxin's effects.

A different region of the enterotoxin molecule is responsible for the symptoms of food poisoning. The enterotoxins are heat stable and can survive conditions that kill the bacteria. Illness results from the ingestion of preformed toxin. As a result, the incubation period is short (1–6 h). The toxin stimulates the vagus nerve and the vomiting center of the brain. It also appears to stimulate intestinal peristaltic activity.

Exfoliative Toxins and the Staphylococcal Scalded-Skin Syndrome

The exfoliative toxins are responsible for SSSS. The toxins that produce disease in humans are of two serotypes: ETA and ETB. These toxins disrupt the desmosomes that link adjoining cells. Although the mechanism of this disruption remains uncertain, studies suggest that the toxins possess serine protease activity, which—through undefined mechanisms—triggers exfoliation. The result is a split in the epidermis at the granular level, and this event is responsible for the superficial desquamation of the skin that typifies this illness.

Diagnosis

Staphylococcal infections are readily diagnosed by Gram's stain (Fig. 35-1) and microscopic examination of abscess contents or of infected tissue. Routine culture of infected material usually yields positive results, and blood cultures are sometimes positive even when infections are localized to extravascular sites. Polymerase chain reaction (PCR)–based assays have been applied to the rapid diagnosis of *S. aureus* infection and are increasingly used in clinical microbiology laboratories. To date, serologic assays have not proved useful for the diagnosis of staphylococcal infections. Determining whether patients with documented *S. aureus* bacteremia also have infective endocarditis or a metastatic focus of infection remains a diagnostic challenge (see "Bacteremia, Sepsis, and Infective Endocarditis" later in the chapter).

CLINICAL SYNDROMES

(See Table 35-1)

TABLE 35-1

COMMON ILLNESSES CAUSED BY *STAPHYLOCOCCUS AUREUS*
Skin and Soft Tissue Infections
Folliculitis
Furuncle, carbuncle
Cellulitis
Impetigo
Mastitis
Surgical wound infections
Hidradenitis suppurativa
Musculoskeletal Infections
Septic arthritis
Osteomyelitis
Pyomyositis
Psoas abscess
Respiratory Tract Infections
Ventilator-associated or nosocomial pneumonia
Septic pulmonary emboli
Postviral pneumonia (e.g., influenza)
Empyema
Bacteremia and Its Complications
Sepsis, septic shock
Metastatic foci of infection (kidney, joints, bone, lung)
Infective endocarditis
Infective Endocarditis
Injection drug use–associated
Native-valve
Prosthetic-valve
Nosocomial
Device-Related Infections
(e.g., intravascular catheters, prosthetic joints)
Toxin-Mediated Illnesses
Toxic shock syndrome
Food poisoning
Staphylococcal scalded-skin syndrome
Invasive Infections Associated with Community-Acquired MRSA
Necrotizing fasciitis
Waterhouse-Friderichsen syndrome
Necrotizing pneumonia
Purpura fulminans

Skin and Soft Tissue Infections

S. aureus causes a variety of cutaneous infections. Common predisposing factors include skin disease, skin damage (e.g., insect bites, minor trauma), injections (e.g., in diabetes, injection drug use), and poor personal hygiene. These infections are characterized by the formation of pus-containing blisters, which often begin in hair follicles and spread to adjoining tissues. *Folliculitis* is a superficial infection that involves the hair follicle, with a central area of purulence (pus) surrounded by induration and erythema. *Furuncles* (boils) are more extensive, painful lesions that tend to occur in hairy, moist regions of the body and extend from the hair follicle to become a true abscess with an area of central purulence. *Carbuncles* are most often located in the lower neck and are even more severe and painful, resulting from the coalescence of other lesions that extend to a deeper layer of the subcutaneous tissue. In general, furuncles and carbuncles are readily apparent, with pus often expressible or discharging from the abscess.

Mastitis develops in 1–3% of nursing mothers. The infection, which generally presents within 2–3 weeks after delivery, is characterized by findings that range from cellulitis to abscess formation. Systemic signs, such as fever and chills, are often present in more severe cases.

Other cutaneous *S. aureus* infections include impetigo, cellulitis, and hidradenitis suppurativa (recurrent follicular infections in regions such as the axilla). *S. aureus* is one of the most common causes of surgical wound infection.

It should be noted that many of these syndromes may also be due to group A streptococci or, less commonly, to other streptococcal species.

Musculoskeletal Infections

S. aureus is among the most common causes of bone infections—both those resulting from hematogenous dissemination and those arising from contiguous spread from a soft tissue site.

Hematogenous osteomyelitis in children most often involves the long bones. Infections present as fever and bone pain or with a child's reluctance to bear weight. The white blood cell count and erythrocyte sedimentation rate are often elevated. Blood cultures are positive in ~50% of cases. When necessary, bone biopsies for culture and histopathologic examination are usually diagnostic. Routine x-rays may be normal for up to 14 days after the onset of symptoms. ^{99m}Tc-phosphonate scanning often detects early evidence of infection. MRI is more sensitive than other techniques in establishing a radiologic diagnosis.

In adults, hematogenous osteomyelitis involving the long bones is less common. However, *vertebral osteomyelitis* is among the more common clinical presentations. Vertebral bone infections are most often seen in patients with endocarditis, those undergoing hemodialysis, diabetics, and injection drug users. These infections may present as intense back pain and fever, but may also be clinically occult, presenting as chronic back pain and low-grade fever. *S. aureus* is the most common cause of

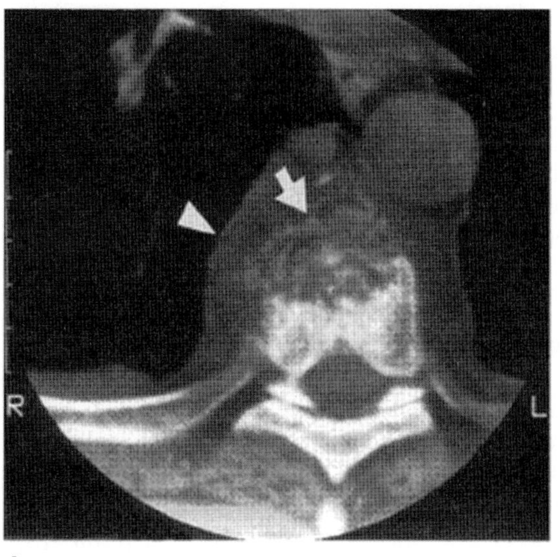

A

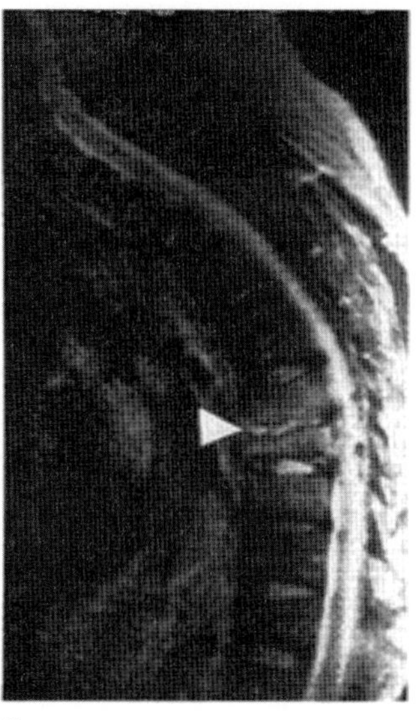

B

FIGURE 35-3

S. aureus **vertebral osteomyelitis involving the thoracic disk between T8 and T9 in a 63-year-old man.** ***A.*** The lower end plate is damaged (*arrow*), and there is an adjacent paraspinal mass (*arrowhead*). ***B.*** Sagittal T2-weighted MRI of the spine, illustrating anterior wedging of the body of T8. (*Reprinted with permission from MA Artinian et al: Images in clinical medicine. Vertebral osteomyelitis. N Engl J Med 329:399, 1993.* *© 1993 Massachusetts Medical Society. All rights reserved.*)

epidural abscess, a complication that can result in neurologic compromise. Patients complain of difficulty voiding or walking and of radicular pain in addition to the symptoms associated with their osteomyelitis. Surgical intervention in this setting often constitutes a medical emergency. MRI most reliably establishes the diagnosis (Fig. 35-3).

Bone infections that result from contiguous spread tend to develop from soft tissue infections, such as those associated with diabetic or vascular ulcers, surgery, or trauma. Exposure of bone, a draining fistulous tract, failure to heal, or continued drainage suggests involvement of underlying bone. Bone involvement is established by bone culture and histopathologic examination (revealing, for example, evidence of PMN infiltration). Contamination of culture material from adjacent tissue can make the diagnosis of osteomyelitis difficult in the absence of pathologic confirmation. In addition, it is sometimes hard to distinguish radiologically between osteomyelitis and overlying soft tissue infection with underlying osteitis.

In both children and adults, *S. aureus* is the most common cause of *septic arthritis* in native joints. This infection is rapidly progressive and may be associated with extensive joint destruction if left untreated. It presents as intense pain on motion of the affected joint, swelling, and fever. Aspiration of the joint reveals turbid fluid, with >50,000 PMNs/μL and gram-positive cocci in clusters on Gram's stain (Fig. 35-1). In adults, arthritis may result from trauma, surgery, or hematogenous dissemination. The most commonly involved joints include the knees, shoulders, hips, and phalanges. Infection frequently develops in joints previously damaged by osteoarthritis or rheumatoid arthritis. Iatrogenic infections resulting from aspiration or injection of agents into the joint also occur. In these settings, the patient experiences increased pain and swelling in the involved joint in association with fever.

Pyomyositis is an unusual infection of skeletal muscles that is seen primarily in tropical climates but also occurs in immunocompromised and HIV-infected patients. Pyomyositis presents as fever, swelling, and pain overlying the involved muscle. Aspiration of fluid from the involved tissue reveals pus. Although a history of trauma may be associated with the infection, its pathogenesis is poorly understood.

Respiratory Tract Infections

Respiratory tract infections caused by *S. aureus* occur in selected clinical settings. *S. aureus* is a cause of serious infections in newborns and infants; these infections present as shortness of breath, fever, and respiratory failure. Chest x-ray may reveal pneumatoceles (shaggy, thin-walled cavities). Pneumothorax and empyema are recognized complications of this infection.

In adults, nosocomial *S. aureus* pulmonary infections are commonly seen in intubated patients in intensive care units. The clinical presentation is no different from that encountered in pulmonary infections of other bacterial etiologies. Patients produce increased volumes of purulent sputum and develop respiratory distress, fever, and new pulmonary infiltrates. Distinguishing bacterial pneumonia from respiratory failure of other causes or new pulmonary infiltrates in critically ill patients is often difficult and relies on a constellation of clinical, radiologic, and laboratory findings.

Community-acquired respiratory tract infections due to *S. aureus* most commonly follow viral infections or septic pulmonary emboli (e.g., in injection drug users). Influenza is the most common cause of the former type of presentation. Patients may present with fever, bloody sputum production, and midlung-field pneumatoceles or multiple, patchy pulmonary infiltrates. Diagnosis is made by sputum Gram's stain and culture. Blood cultures, although useful, are usually negative.

Bacteremia, Sepsis, and Infective Endocarditis

S. aureus bacteremia may be complicated by sepsis, endocarditis, vasculitis, or metastatic seeding (establishment of suppurative collections at other tissue sites). The frequency of metastatic seeding during bacteremia has been estimated to be as high as 31%. Among the more commonly seeded tissue sites are bones, joints, kidneys, and lungs.

Recognition of these complications by clinical and laboratory diagnostic methods alone is often difficult. Comorbid conditions that are frequently seen in association with *S. aureus* bacteremia and that increase the risk of complications include diabetes, HIV infection, and renal insufficiency. Other host factors associated with an increased risk of complications include presentation with community-acquired *S. aureus* bacteremia (except in injection drug users), lack of an identifiable primary focus, and the presence of prosthetic devices or material.

Clinically, *S. aureus* sepsis presents in a manner similar to that documented for sepsis due to other bacteria. The well-described progression of hemodynamic changes—beginning with respiratory alkalosis and clinical findings of hypotension and fever—is commonly seen. The microbiologic diagnosis is established by positive blood cultures.

The overall incidence of *S. aureus* endocarditis has increased over the past 20 years. *S. aureus* is now the leading cause of endocarditis worldwide, accounting for 25–35% of cases. This increase is due, at least in part, to the increased use of intravascular devices; transesophageal echocardiography (TEE) studies found an infective endocarditis incidence of 25% among patients with *S. aureus* bacteremia and intravascular catheters. Other factors associated with an increased risk of endocarditis are injection drug use, hemodialysis, the presence of intravascular prosthetic devices, and immunosuppression. Despite the availability of effective antibiotics, mortality rates from these infections continue to range from 20 to 40%, depending on both the host and the nature of the infection. Complications of *S. aureus* endocarditis include cardiac valvular insufficiency, peripheral emboli, metastatic seeding, and central nervous system (CNS) involvement.

S. aureus is now a leading cause of endocarditis in many countries. *S. aureus* endocarditis is encountered in four clinical settings: (1) right-sided endocarditis in association with injection drug use, (2) left-sided native-valve endocarditis, (3) prosthetic-valve endocarditis, and (4) nosocomial endocarditis. In each of these settings, the diagnosis is established by recognition of clinical stigmata suggestive of endocarditis. These findings include cardiac manifestations, such as new or changing cardiac valvular murmurs; cutaneous evidence, such as vasculitic lesions, Osler's nodes, or Janeway lesions; evidence of right- or left-sided embolic disease; and a history suggesting a risk for *S. aureus* bacteremia. In the absence of antecedent antibiotic therapy, blood cultures are almost uniformly positive. Transthoracic echocardiography, although less sensitive than TEE, is less invasive and often establishes the presence of valvular vegetations.

Acute right-sided tricuspid valvular *S. aureus* endocarditis is most often seen in injection drug users. The classic presentation includes a high fever, a toxic clinical appearance, pleuritic chest pain, and the production of purulent (sometimes bloody) sputum. Chest x-rays reveal evidence of septic pulmonary emboli (small, peripheral, circular lesions that may cavitate with time). A high percentage of affected patients have no history of antecedent valvular damage. At the outset of their illness, patients may present with fever alone, without cardiac or other localizing findings. As a result, a high index of clinical suspicion is essential to the diagnosis.

Individuals with antecedent cardiac valvular damage more commonly present with left-sided native-valve endocarditis involving the previously affected valve. These patients tend to be older than those with right-sided endocarditis, their prognosis is worse, and their incidence of complications (including peripheral emboli, cardiac decompensation, and metastatic seeding) is higher.

S. aureus is one of the more common causes of prosthetic-valve endocarditis. This infection is especially fulminant in the early postoperative period and is associated with a high mortality rate. In most instances, medical therapy alone is not sufficient and urgent valve replacement is necessary. Patients are prone to develop valvular insufficiency or myocardial abscesses originating from the region of valve implantation.

The increased frequency of nosocomial endocarditis (15–30% of cases, depending on the series) reflects in part the increased use of intravascular devices. This form of endocarditis is most commonly caused by *S. aureus*. Because patients often are critically ill, are receiving antibiotics for various other indications, and have comorbid conditions, the diagnosis is not easily recognized.

Urinary Tract Infections

Urinary tract infections (UTIs) are infrequently caused by *S. aureus*. In contrast with that of most other urinary pathogens, the presence of *S. aureus* in the urine suggests hematogenous dissemination. Ascending *S. aureus* infections occasionally result from instrumentation of the genitourinary tract.

Prosthetic Device–Related Infections

S. aureus accounts for a large proportion of prosthetic device–related infections. These infections often involve intravascular catheters, prosthetic valves, orthopedic devices, peritoneal or intraventricular catheters, left-ventricular-assist devices, and vascular grafts. In contrast with the more indolent presentation of CoNS infections, *S. aureus* device-related infections often present more acutely, with both localized and systemic manifestations. The latter infections also tend to progress more rapidly. It is relatively common for a pyogenic collection to be present at the device site. Aspiration of these collections and performance of blood cultures are important components in establishing a diagnosis. *S. aureus* infections tend to occur more commonly soon after implantation unless the device is used for access (e.g., intravascular or hemodialysis catheters). In the latter instance, infections can occur at any time. As in most prosthetic-device infections, successful therapy usually involves removal of the device. Left in place, the device is a potential nidus for either persistent or recurrent infections.

Infections Associated with Community-Acquired MRSA

The many unusual clinical presentations encountered in patients with community-associated MRSA infections include necrotizing fasciitis, necrotizing pneumonia, and sepsis with Waterhouse-Friderichsen syndrome or purpura fulminans. These life-threatening infections reflect the increased virulence of MRSA strains.

Toxin-Mediated Diseases

Toxic Shock Syndrome

TSS was first recognized as a disease in children in 1978. The disease gained attention in the early 1980s, when a nationwide outbreak occurred among young, otherwise healthy, menstruating women. Epidemiologic investigation demonstrated that these cases were associated with menstruation and the use of a highly absorbent tampon that had recently been introduced to the market. Subsequent studies established the role of TSST-1 in these illnesses. Withdrawal of the tampon from the market resulted in a rapid decline in the incidence of this disease. However, menstrual and nonmenstrual cases continue to be reported.

The clinical presentation is similar in menstrual and nonmenstrual TSS, although the nature of the risk clearly differs. Evidence of clinical *S. aureus* infection is not a prerequisite. TSS results from the elaboration of an enterotoxin or the structurally related enterotoxin-like TSST-1. More than 90% of menstrual cases are caused by TSST-1, whereas a high percentage of nonmenstrual cases are caused by enterotoxins.

TSS begins with relatively nonspecific flulike symptoms. In menstrual cases, the onset usually comes 2 or 3 days after the start of menstruation. Patients present with fever, hypotension, and erythroderma of variable intensity. Mucosal involvement is common (e.g., conjunctival hyperemia). The illness can rapidly progress to symptoms that include vomiting, diarrhea, confusion, myalgias, and abdominal pain. These symptoms reflect the multisystemic nature of the disease, with involvement of the liver, kidneys, gastrointestinal tract, and/or CNS. Desquamation of the skin occurs during convalescence, usually 1–2 weeks after the onset of illness. Laboratory findings may include azotemia, leukocytosis, hypoalbuminemia, thrombocytopenia, and liver function abnormalities.

TABLE 35-2

CASE DEFINITION OF *S. AUREUS* TOXIC SHOCK SYNDROME

1. Fever: temperature of ≥38.9°C (≥102°F)
2. Hypotension: systolic blood pressure of ≤90 mmHg, or orthostatic hypotension (orthostatic drop in diastolic blood pressure by ≥15 mmHg, orthostatic syncope, or orthostatic dizziness)
3. Diffuse macular rash with subsequent desquamation in 1–2 weeks after onset (including the palms and soles)
4. Multisystem involvement
   a. Hepatic: bilirubin or aminotransferase levels ≥2 times normal
   b. Hematologic: platelet count ≤100,000/μL
   c. Renal: blood urea nitrogen or serum creatinine level ≥2 times the normal upper limit
   d. Mucous membranes: vaginal, oropharyngeal, or conjunctival hyperemia
   e. Gastrointestinal: vomiting or diarrhea at onset of illness
   f. Muscular: severe myalgias or serum creatine phosphokinase level ≥2 times the upper limit
   g. Central nervous system: disorientation or alteration in consciousness without focal neurologic signs and in the absence of fever and hypotension
5. Negative serologic or other tests for measles, leptospirosis, and Rocky Mountain spotted fever, as well as negative blood or cerebrospinal fluid cultures for organisms other than *S. aureus*

Source: M Wharton et al: Case definitions for public health surveillance. MMWR 39:1, 1990; with permission.

Diagnosis of TSS still depends on a constellation of findings rather than one specific finding (Table 35-2). Part of the case definition is the absence of laboratory evidence of other illnesses that are often included in the differential (e.g., Rocky Mountain spotted fever, rubeola, leptospirosis). Other diagnoses to be considered are drug toxicities, viral exanthems, sepsis, and Kawasaki's disease. Illness occurs only in persons who lack antibody to TSST-1. Recurrences are possible if antibody fails to develop after the illness.

Food Poisoning

S. aureus is among the most common causes of food-borne outbreaks of infection in the United States. *S. aureus* food poisoning results from the inoculation of toxin-producing *S. aureus* into food by colonized food handlers. Toxin is then elaborated in such growth-promoting food as custards, potato salad, or processed meats. Even if the bacteria are killed by warming, the heat-stable toxin is not destroyed. The onset of illness is rapid, occurring within 1–6 h of ingestion. The illness is characterized by nausea and vomiting, although diarrhea, hypotension, and dehydration may also occur. The differential diagnosis includes diarrhea of other etiologies, especially that caused by similar toxins (e.g., the toxins elaborated by *Bacillus cereus*). The rapidity of onset, the absence of fever, and the epidemic nature of the presentation arouse suspicion of food poisoning. Symptoms generally resolve within 8–10 h. The diagnosis can be established by the demonstration of bacteria or the documentation of enterotoxin in the implicated food. Treatment is entirely supportive.

Staphylococcal Scalded-Skin Syndrome

SSSS most often affects newborns and children. The illness may vary from localized blister formation to exfoliation of much of the skin surface. The skin is usually fragile and often tender, with thin-walled, fluid-filled bullae. Gentle pressure results in rupture of the lesions, leaving denuded underlying skin (Nikolsky's sign; Fig. 35-4). The mucous membranes are usually spared. In more generalized infection, there are often constitutional symptoms, including fever, lethargy, and irritability with poor feeding. Significant amounts of fluid can be lost in more extensive cases. Illness usually follows localized infection at one of a number of possible sites. SSSS is much less common among adults but can follow infections caused by exfoliative toxin–producing strains.

PREVENTION

Prevention of the spread of *S. aureus* infections in the hospital setting involves hand washing and careful attention to appropriate isolation procedures. Through strict isolation practices, some Scandinavian countries have been remarkably successful at preventing the introduction and dissemination of MRSA in hospitals. Other countries, such as the United States and Great Britain, have been less successful.

The use of topical antimicrobial agents (e.g., mupirocin) to eliminate nasal colonization with *S. aureus* and to prevent subsequent infection has been investigated in a number of clinical settings. Elimination of nasal carriage of *S. aureus* has reduced the incidence of infections among patients undergoing hemodialysis and peritoneal dialysis. The prophylactic efficacy of topical mupirocin applied to the nares has been extensively investigated. Although mupirocin eliminates nasal colonization with *S. aureus*, clinical trials to date have failed to demonstrate a subsequent reduction in the incidence of staphylococcal infections.

A capsular polysaccharide–protein conjugate vaccine and antibodies to the ligand-binding domains of several MSCRAMMs (e.g., clumping factor) are under investigation. Although in vivo studies have been promising in either preventing or reducing the incidence of infections, none of these vaccines have yet been successful for either prophylaxis or therapy.

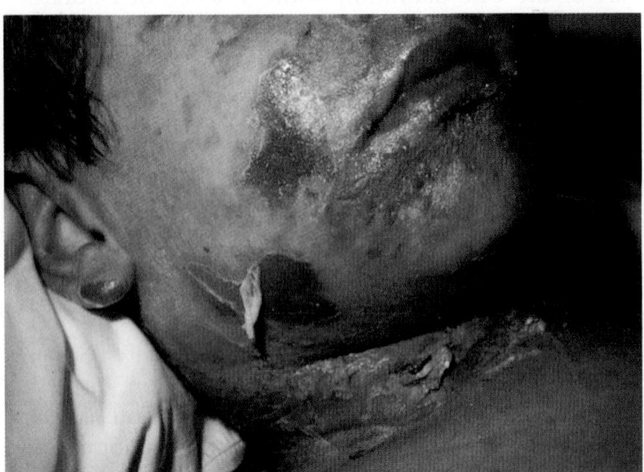

FIGURE 35-4

Evidence of staphylococcal scalded-skin syndrome in a 6-year-old boy. Nikolsky's sign, with separation of the superficial layer of the outer epidermal layer, is visible. *(Reprinted with permission from LA Schenfeld et al: Images in clinical medicine. Staphylococcal scalded skin syndrome. N Engl J Med 342:1178, 2000. © 2000 Massachusetts Medical Society. All rights reserved.)*

COAGULASE-NEGATIVE STAPHYLOCOCCAL INFECTIONS

CoNS, although considerably less virulent than *S. aureus*, are among the most common causes of prosthetic-device infections. Approximately half of the identified CoNS species have been associated with human infections. Of these species, *S. epidermidis* is the most common human pathogen overall; this component of the normal human flora is found on the skin (where it is the most abundant bacterial species) as well as in the oropharynx and vagina. *S. saprophyticus*, a novobiocin-resistant species, is a pathogen in UTIs.

PATHOGENESIS

Among CoNS, *S. epidermidis* is the species most commonly associated with prosthetic-device infections. Infection is a two-step process, with initial adhesion to the device followed by colonization. *S. epidermidis* is uniquely adapted to colonize these devices by its capacity to elaborate the extracellular polysaccharide (glycocalyx or slime) that facilitates formation of a protective biofilm on the device surface.

Implanted prosthetic material is often coated with host serum or tissue constituents such as fibrinogen or fibronectin. These molecules serve as potential bridging ligands, facilitating bacterial attachment to the device surface. A number of surface-associated proteins, such as autolysin (AtlE), fibrinogen-binding protein, and accumulation-associated protein (AAP), may play a role in attachment to either modified or unmodified prosthetic surfaces. The polysaccharide intercellular adhesin facilitates subsequent staphylococcal colonization and accumulation on the device surface. In *S. epidermidis*, *ica* genes are more commonly found in strains associated with device infections than in strains associated with colonization of mucosal surfaces. Biofilm appears to act as a barrier protecting bacteria from host defense mechanisms as well as from antibiotics, while providing a suitable environment for bacterial survival. Poly-γ-DL-glutamic acid is secreted by *S. epidermidis* and promotes protection against neutrophil phagocytosis.

Two additional staphylococcal species, *S. lugdunensis* and *S. schleiferi*, produce more serious infections (native-valve endocarditis and osteomyelitis) than do other CoNS. The basis for this enhanced virulence is not known, although both species appear to share more virulence determinants with *S. aureus* (e.g., clumping factor and lipase) than do other CoNS.

The capacity of *S. saprophyticus* to cause UTIs in young women appears to be related to its enhanced capacity to adhere to uroepithelial cells. A 160-kDa hemagglutinin/adhesin may contribute to this affinity.

DIAGNOSIS

Although the detection of CoNS at sites of infection or in the bloodstream is not difficult by standard microbiologic culture methods, interpretation of these results is frequently problematic. Since these organisms are present in large numbers on the skin, they often contaminate cultures. It has been estimated that only 10–25% of blood cultures positive for CoNS reflect true bacteremia. Similar problems arise with cultures of other sites. Among the clinical findings suggestive of true bacteremia are fever, evidence of local infection (e.g., erythema or purulent drainage at the IV catheter site), leukocytosis, and systemic signs of sepsis. Laboratory findings suggestive of true bacteremia include multiple isolations of the same strain (i.e., the same species with the same antibiogram or a closely related DNA fingerprint) from separate cultures, growth of the strain within 48 h, and bacterial growth in both aerobic and anaerobic bottles.

CLINICAL SYNDROMES

CoNS cause diverse prosthetic device–related infections, including those that involve prosthetic cardiac valves and joints, vascular grafts, intravascular devices, and CNS shunts. In all of these settings, the clinical presentation is similar. The signs of localized infection are often subtle, the rate of disease progression is slow, and the systemic findings are often limited. Signs of infection, such as purulent drainage, pain at the site, or loosening of prosthetic implants, are sometimes evident. Fever is frequently but not always present, and there may be mild leukocytosis.

Infections that are not associated with prosthetic devices are infrequent, although native-valve endocarditis due to CoNS has accounted for ~5% of cases in some reviews. *S. lugdunensis* appears to be a more aggressive pathogen in this setting, causing greater mortality and rapid valvular destruction with abscess formation.

℞ Treatment: STAPHYLOCOCCAL INFECTIONS

GENERAL PRINCIPLES OF THERAPY Surgical incision and drainage of all suppurative collections constitute the most important therapeutic intervention for staphylococcal infections. The emergence of MRSA in the community has increased the importance of culturing all collections in order to identify pathogens and to determine antimicrobial susceptibility. Prosthetic-device infections are unlikely to be successfully managed unless the device is removed. In the limited number of situations in which removal is not possible or the infection is due to CoNS, an initial attempt at medical therapy without device removal may be warranted. Because of the well-recognized risk of complications associated with *S. aureus* bacteremia, therapy is generally prolonged (4–8 weeks) unless the patient is identified as being one of the small percentage of individuals who are at low risk for complications—e.g., immunocompetent patients and patients whose *S. aureus* infection is associated with a removable focus (such as an IV catheter) and whose device is promptly removed.

DURATION OF ANTIMICROBIAL THERAPY Debate continues regarding the duration of therapy for bacteremic *S. aureus* infections. No carefully controlled, prospective study has addressed this question. A meta-analysis reviewing studies relevant to this issue concluded that insufficient information was available to determine which patients were candidates for short-course therapy (2 weeks rather than 4–8 weeks).

Among the findings associated with an increased risk of complicated bacteremia are persistently positive blood cultures 48–96 h after institution of therapy, acquisition of the infection in the community, a removable focus of infection (i.e., an intravascular catheter) that is not removed, and cutaneous or embolic manifestations of infection. In those immunocompetent patients for whom short-course therapy is planned, TEE to rule out endocarditis is warranted since neither clinical nor laboratory findings are adequate to detect cardiac involvement. In addition, an aggressive radiologic investigation to identify potential metastatic collections is indicated. All symptomatic sites must be carefully evaluated.

CHOICE OF ANTIMICROBIAL AGENTS The choice of antimicrobial agents to treat both coagulase-positive staphylococcal and CoNS infections has become increasingly problematic because of the prevalence of multidrug-resistant strains. Staphylococcal resistance has increased to most antibiotic families, including β-lactams, aminoglycosides, fluoroquinolones, and (to a lesser extent) glycopeptides. This trend is more apparent with CoNS: >80% of nosocomial isolates are resistant to methicillin, and these MRSA strains are usually resistant to most other antibiotics as well. Because the selection of antimicrobial agents for the treatment of *S. aureus* infections is similar to that for CoNS infections, treatment options for these pathogens are discussed together and are summarized in Table 35-3.

As a result of the widespread dissemination of plasmids containing the enzyme penicillinase, few strains of staphylococci (<5%) remain susceptible to penicillin. However, against susceptible strains, penicillin remains the drug of choice. Penicillin-resistant isolates are treated with semisynthetic penicillinase-resistant penicillins (SPRPs), such as oxacillin or nafcillin. Methicillin, the first of the

TABLE 35-3

ANTIMICROBIAL THERAPY FOR SERIOUS STAPHYLOCOCCAL INFECTIONS[a]

SENSITIVITY/ RESISTANCE OF ISOLATE	DRUG OF CHOICE	ALTERNATIVE(S)	COMMENTS
Sensitive to penicillin	Penicillin G (4 mU q4h)	Nafcillin (2 g q4h) or oxacillin (2 g q4h), cefazolin (2 g q8h), vancomycin (1 g q12h[b])	Fewer than 5% of isolates are sensitive to penicillin.
Sensitive to methicillin	Nafcillin or oxacillin (2 g q4h)	Cefazolin (2 g q8h[b]), vancomycin (1 g q12h[b])	Patients with penicillin allergy can be treated with a cephalosporin if the allergy does not involve an anaphylactic or accelerated reaction; vancomycin is the alternative. Desensitization to β-lactams may be indicated in selected cases of serious infection where maximal bactericidal activity is needed (e.g., prosthetic-valve endocarditis[d]). Type A β-lactamase may rapidly hydrolyze cefazolin and reduce its efficacy in endocarditis.
Resistant to methicillin	Vancomycin (1 g q12h[b])	TMP-SMX (TMP, 5 mg/kg q12h[b]), minocycline or doxycycline (100 mg PO q12h[b]), ciprofloxacin (400 mg q12h[b]), levofloxacin (500 mg q24h[b]), quinupristin/dalfopristin (7.5 mg/kg q8h), linezolid (600 mg q12h *except*: 400 mg q12h for uncomplicated skin infections); daptomycin (4–6 mg/kg q24h[b,c]) for bacteremia, endocarditis, and complicated skin infections; tigecycline (100 mg IV once, then 50 mg q12h) for skin and soft tissue infections; investigational drugs: oritavancin, dalbavancin, telavancin	Sensitivity testing is necessary before an alternative drug is used. Adjunctive drugs (those that should be used only in combination with other antimicrobial agents) include gentamicin (1 mg/kg q8h[b]), rifampin (300 mg PO q8h), and fusidic acid (500 mg q8h; not readily available in the United States). Quinupristin/dalfopristin is bactericidal against methicillin-resistant isolates unless the strain is resistant to erythromycin or clindamycin. The newer quinolones may retain in vitro activity against ciprofloxacin-resistant isolates; resistance may develop during therapy. The efficacy of adjunctive therapy is not well established in many settings. Both linezolid and quinupristin/dalfopristin have had in vitro activity against most VISA and VRSA strains. See footnote for treatment of prosthetic-valve endocarditis.[d]
Resistant to methicillin with intermediate or complete resistance to vancomycin[e]	Uncertain	Same as for methicillin-resistant strains; check antibiotic susceptibilities.	Same as for methicillin-resistant strains; check antibiotic susceptibilities.
Not yet known (i.e., empirical therapy)	Vancomycin (1 g q12h)	—	Empirical therapy is given when the susceptibility of the isolate is not known. Vancomycin with or without an aminoglycoside is recommended for suspected community- or hospital-acquired *S. aureus* infections because of the increased frequency of methicillin-resistant strains in the community.

[a]Recommended dosages are for adults with normal renal and hepatic function. The route of administration is intravenous unless otherwise indicated.

[b]The dosage must be adjusted in patients with reduced creatinine clearance.

[c]Daptomycin cannot be used for pneumonia.

[d]For the treatment of prosthetic-valve endocarditis, the addition of gentamicin (1 mg/kg q8h) and rifampin (300 mg PO q8h) is recommended, with adjustment of the gentamicin dosage if the creatinine clearance rate is reduced.

[e]Vancomycin-resistant *S. aureus* isolates from clinical infections have been reported.

Note: TMP-SMX, trimethoprim-sulfamethoxazole; VISA, vancomycin-intermediate *S. aureus*; VRSA, vancomycin-resistant *S. aureus*.

Source: Modified with permission of the *New England Journal of Medicine* (Lowy, 1998). © 1998 Massachusetts Medical Society. All rights reserved.

SPRPs, is now used infrequently. Cephalosporins are alternative therapeutic agents for these infections. Second- and third-generation cephalosporins do not have a therapeutic advantage over first-generation cephalosporins for the treatment of staphylococcal infections. The carbapenem imipenem has excellent activity against methicillin-sensitive *S. aureus* (MSSA), but not MRSA.

The isolation of MRSA was reported within 1 year of the introduction of methicillin. The prevalence of MRSA has since increased steadily. In many hospitals, 40–50% of *S. aureus* isolates are now resistant to methicillin. Resistance to methicillin indicates resistance to all SPRPs, as well as all cephalosporins. Many MRSA isolates are also resistant to other antimicrobial families, including aminoglycosides, quinolones, and macrolides.

Production of a novel penicillin-binding protein (PBP 2a or 2′) is responsible for methicillin resistance. This protein is synthesized by the *mecA* gene, which (as stated above) is part of a large mobile genetic element—a pathogenicity or genomic island—called SCC*mec*. It is hypothesized that acquisition of this genetic material resulted from horizontal transfer from a related staphylococcal species, such as *S. sciuri*. Phenotypic expression of methicillin resistance may be constitutive (i.e., expressed in all organisms in a population) or heterogeneous (i.e., displayed by only a proportion of the total organism population). Detection of methicillin resistance in the clinical microbiology laboratory can be difficult if the strain expresses heterogeneous resistance. Therefore, susceptibility studies are routinely performed at reduced temperatures (≤35°C for 24 h), with increased concentrations of salt in the medium to enhance the expression of resistance. In addition to PCR-based techniques, a number of rapid methods for the detection of methicillin resistance have been developed.

Vancomycin remains the drug of choice for the treatment of MRSA infections. Because it is less bactericidal than the β-lactams, it should be used only after careful consideration in patients with a history of β-lactam allergies. In 1997, an *S. aureus* strain with reduced susceptibility to vancomycin (VISA) was reported from Japan. Subsequently, additional clinical isolates of VISA were reported from geographically disparate locations. These strains were all resistant to methicillin and many other antimicrobial agents. The VISA strains appear to evolve (under vancomycin selective pressure) from strains that are susceptible to vancomycin but are heterogeneous, with a small proportion of the bacterial population expressing the resistance phenotype. The mechanism of VISA resistance is due to an abnormal cell wall. Vancomycin is trapped by the abnormal peptidoglycan cross-linking and is unable to gain access to its target site.

In 2002, the first clinical isolate of fully vancomycin-resistant *S. aureus* was reported. Resistance in this and three subsequently reported clinical isolates was due to the presence of *vanA*, the gene responsible for expression of vancomycin resistance in enterococci. This observation suggested that resistance was acquired as a result of horizontal conjugal transfer from a vancomycin-resistant strain of *Enterococcus faecalis*. Several patients had both MRSA and vancomycin-resistant enterococci cultured from infection sites. The isolates remained susceptible to chloramphenicol, linezolid, minocycline, quinupristin/dalfopristin, and trimethoprim-sulfamethoxazole (TMP-SMX). The *vanA* gene is responsible for the synthesis of the dipeptide D-Ala-D-Lac in place of D-Ala-D-Ala. Vancomycin cannot bind to the altered peptide.

Alternatives to the β-lactams and vancomycin have less antistaphylococcal activity. Although the quinolones have reasonable in vitro activity against staphylococci, the frequency of fluoroquinolone resistance has increased progressively, especially among methicillin-resistant isolates. MSSA strains have remained more susceptible to the fluoroquinolones than have methicillin-resistant strains. Of particular concern in MRSA is the possible emergence of quinolone resistance during therapy. Resistance to the quinolones is most commonly chromosomal and results from mutations of the topoisomerase IV or DNA gyrase genes, although multidrug efflux pumps may also contribute. Although the newer quinolones exhibit increased in vitro activity against staphylococci, it is uncertain whether this increase translates into enhanced in vivo activity. Other antibiotics, such as minocycline and TMP-SMX, have been successfully used to treat MRSA infections in the face of vancomycin toxicity or intolerance.

Among the newer antistaphylococcal agents, the parenteral streptogramin quinupristin/dalfopristin displays bactericidal activity against all staphylococci, including VISA strains. This drug has been used successfully to treat serious MRSA infections. In cases of erythromycin or clindamycin resistance, quinupristin/dalfopristin is bacteriostatic against staphylococci.

Linezolid—the first member of a new drug family, the oxazolidinones—is bacteriostatic against staphylococci, has been well tolerated, and offers the advantage of comparable bioavailability after oral or parenteral administration. Cross-resistance with other inhibitors of protein synthesis has not been reported. Resistance to linezolid, although limited, has been reported. The efficacy of linezolid in the treatment of deep-seated infections such as osteomyelitis has not yet been established. There are insufficient data on the efficacy of either quinupristin/dalfopristin or linezolid for the treatment of infective endocarditis. Daptomycin, a new parenteral bactericidal agent with antistaphylococcal activity, is approved for the treatment of bacteremias (including right-sided endocarditis) and complicated skin infections. It is not effective in respiratory infections. This drug has a novel mechanism of action: it disrupts the cytoplasmic membrane. Staphylococcal resistance to daptomycin has been reported. Tigecycline, a broad-spectrum minocycline analogue, has bacteriostatic activity against MRSA and is approved for use in skin and soft tissue infections as well as intraabdominal infections caused by *S. aureus*. A number of additional antistaphylococcal agents (e.g., dalbavancin, oritavancin, and ceftobiprole) are undergoing clinical trials.

Combinations of antistaphylococcal agents are sometimes used to enhance bactericidal activity in the treatment of serious infections such as endocarditis or osteomyelitis. In selected instances (e.g., right-sided endocarditis), drug combinations are also used to shorten the duration of therapy. Among the antimicrobial agents used in combinations are rifampin, aminoglycosides (e.g., gentamicin), and fusidic acid (which is not readily available in the United States). Although these agents are not effective singly because of the frequent emergence of resistance, they have proved useful in combination with other agents because of their bactericidal activity against staphylococci.

In vitro studies have demonstrated synergy against staphylococci with the following combinations: (1) β-lactams and aminoglycosides; (2) vancomycin and gentamicin; (3) vancomycin, gentamicin, and rifampin (against CoNS); and (4) vancomycin and rifampin. In several instances, these in vitro observations have been supported by studies in the experimental animal model of endocarditis. There is limited information on combinations including newer agents such as daptomycin and tigecycline.

ANTIMICROBIAL THERAPY FOR SELECTED SETTINGS For uncomplicated skin and soft tissue infections, the use of oral antistaphylococcal agents is usually successful. For other infections, parenteral therapy is indicated.

S. aureus endocarditis is usually an acute, life-threatening infection. Thus prompt collection of blood for cultures must be followed immediately by empirical antimicrobial therapy. For *S. aureus* native-valve endocarditis, a combination of antimicrobial agents is often used. In a large prospective study, an SPRP combined with an aminoglycoside did not alter clinical outcome but did reduce the duration of *S. aureus* bacteremia. As a result, many clinicians begin therapy for life-threatening infections with a 3- to 5-day course of a β-lactam and an aminoglycoside (gentamicin, 1 mg/kg IV every 8 h). If a MRSA strain is isolated, vancomycin (30 mg/kg every 24 h, given in two equal doses up to a total of 2 g) is recommended. Patients are generally treated for 6 weeks.

In prosthetic-valve endocarditis, surgery in addition to antibiotic therapy is often necessary. The combination of a β-lactam agent—or, if the isolate is β-lactam-resistant, vancomycin (30 mg/kg every 24 h, given in two equal doses up to a total of 2 g)—with an aminoglycoside (gentamicin, 1 mg/kg IV every 8 h) and rifampin (300 mg orally or IV every 8 h) is recommended. This combination is used to avoid the possible emergence of rifampin resistance during therapy if only two drugs are used.

For hematogenous osteomyelitis or septic arthritis in children, a 4-week course of therapy is usually adequate. In adults, treatment is often more prolonged. For chronic forms of osteomyelitis, surgical debridement is necessary in combination with antimicrobial therapy. For joint infections, a critical component of therapy is the repeated aspiration or arthroscopy of the affected joint to prevent damage from leukocytes. The combination of rifampin with ciprofloxacin has been used successfully to treat prosthetic-joint infections, especially when the device cannot be removed. The efficacy of this combination may reflect enhanced activity against staphylococci in biofilms, as well as the attainment of effective intracellular concentrations.

The choice of empirical therapy for staphylococcal infections depends in part on susceptibility data for the local geographic area. Increasingly, vancomycin (in combination with an aminoglycoside or rifampin for serious infections) is the drug of choice for both community- and hospital-acquired infections.

The increase in community-based MRSA skin and soft tissue infections has drawn attention to the need for initiation of appropriate empirical therapy. Oral agents that have been effective against these isolates include clindamycin, TMP-SMX, doxycycline, and linezolid. The antimicrobial susceptibility of isolates in different geographic regions has varied.

THERAPY FOR TOXIC SHOCK SYNDROME Supportive therapy with reversal of hypotension is the mainstay of therapy for TSS. Both fluids and pressors may be necessary. Tampons or other packing material should be promptly removed. The role of antibiotics is less clear. Some investigators recommend a combination of clindamycin and a semisynthetic penicillin. Clindamycin is advocated because, as a protein synthesis inhibitor, it reduces toxin synthesis in vitro. A semisynthetic penicillin is suggested to eliminate any potential focus of infection, as well as to eradicate persistent carriage that might increase the likelihood of recurrent illness. Anecdotal reports document the successful use of IV immunoglobulin to treat TSS. The role of glucocorticoids in the treatment of this disease is uncertain at present.

THERAPY FOR OTHER TOXIN-MEDIATED DISEASES Therapy for staphylococcal food poisoning is entirely supportive. For SSSS, antistaphylococcal therapy targets the primary site of infection.

FURTHER READINGS

Chu VH et al: Emergence of coagulase-negative staphylococci as a cause of native valve endocarditis. Clin Infect Dis 46:232, 2008

Diep BA et al: Complete genome sequence of USA300, an epidemic clone of community-acquired methicillin-resistant *Staphylococcus aureus*. Lancet 367:731, 2006

Fowler VG Jr et al: *Staphylococcus aureus* endocarditis: A consequence of medical progress. JAMA 293:3012, 2005

——— et al: Role of echocardiography in evaluation of patients with *Staphylococcus aureus* bacteremia: Experience in 103 patients. J Am Coll Cardiol 30:1072, 1997

Fridkin SK et al: Methicillin-resistant *Staphylococcus aureus* disease in three communities. N Engl J Med 352:1436, 2005

Grundmann H et al: Emergence and resurgence of methicillin-resistant *Staphylococcus aureus* as a public-health threat. Lancet 368:874, 2006

Harbarth S et al: Universal screening for methicillin-resistant Staphylococcus aureus at hospital admission and nosocomial infection in surgical patients. JAMA 299:1149, 2008

Lowy FD: Antimicrobial resistance: The example of *Staphylococcus aureus*. J Clin Invest 111:1265, 2003

McCormick JK et al: Toxic shock syndrome and bacterial superantigens: An update. Annu Rev Microbiol 55:77, 2001

MORAN GJ et al: Methicillin-resistant *S. aureus* infections among patients in the emergency department. N Engl J Med 355:666, 2006

MYLOTTE JM, TAYARA A: *Staphylococcus aureus* bacteremia: Predictors of 30-day mortality in a large cohort. Clin Infect Dis 31:1170, 2000

PERLROTH J et al: Adjunctive use of rifampin for the treatment of *Staphylococcus aureus* infections: A systematic review of the literature. Arch Intern Med 168:805, 2008

ROBICSEK A et al: Universal surveillance for methicillin-resistant *Staphylococcus aureus* in 3 affiliated hospitals. Ann Intern Med 148:409, 2008

SEYBOLD U et al: Emergence of community-associated methicillin-resistant *Staphylococcus aureus* USA300 genotype as a major cause of health care–associated blood stream infections. Clin Infect Dis 42:647, 2006

CHAPTER 36

STREPTOCOCCAL AND ENTEROCOCCAL INFECTIONS

Michael R. Wessels

Many varieties of streptococci are found as part of the normal flora colonizing the human respiratory, gastrointestinal, and genitourinary tracts. Several species are important causes of human disease. Group A *Streptococcus* (GAS, *S. pyogenes*) is responsible for streptococcal pharyngitis, one of the most common bacterial infections of school-age children, and for the postinfectious syndromes of acute rheumatic fever (ARF) and poststreptococcal glomerulonephritis (PSGN). Group B *Streptococcus* (GBS, *S. agalactiae*) is the leading cause of bacterial sepsis and meningitis in newborns and a major cause of endometritis and fever in parturient women. Enterococci are important causes of urinary tract infection, nosocomial bacteremia, and endocarditis. Viridans streptococci are the most common cause of bacterial endocarditis.

Streptococci are gram-positive, spherical to ovoid bacteria that characteristically form chains when grown in liquid media. Most streptococci that cause human infections are facultative anaerobes, although some are strict anaerobes. Streptococci are relatively fastidious organisms, requiring enriched media for growth in the laboratory. Clinicians and clinical microbiologists identify streptococci by several classification systems, including hemolytic pattern, Lancefield group, species name, and common or trivial name. Many streptococci associated with human infection produce a zone of complete (β) hemolysis around the bacterial colony when cultured on blood agar. The β-hemolytic streptococci can be classified by the Lancefield system, a serologic grouping based on the reaction of specific antisera with bacterial cell-wall carbohydrate antigens. With rare exceptions, organisms belonging to Lancefield groups A, B, C, and G are all β-hemolytic, and each is associated with characteristic patterns of human infection. Other streptococci produce a zone of partial (α) hemolysis, often imparting a greenish appearance to the agar. These α-hemolytic streptococci are further identified by biochemical testing and include *S. pneumoniae* (Chap. 34), an important cause of pneumonia, meningitis, and other infections, and several species referred to collectively as the *viridans streptococci*, which are part of the normal oral flora and are important agents of subacute bacterial endocarditis. Finally, some streptococci are nonhemolytic, a pattern sometimes called *γ hemolysis*. The classification of the major streptococcal groups causing human infections is outlined in Table 36-1. Among the organisms classified serologically as group D streptococci, the enterococci are now considered a separate genus on the basis of DNA homology studies. Thus species previously designated as *S. faecalis* and *S. faecium* have been renamed *Enterococcus faecalis* and *E. faecium*, respectively.

GROUP A STREPTOCOCCI

Lancefield's group A consists of a single species, *S. pyogenes*. As its species name implies, this organism is associated with a variety of suppurative infections. In addition, GAS can trigger the postinfectious syndromes of ARF (which is uniquely associated with *S. pyogenes* infection; Chap. 37) and PSGN.

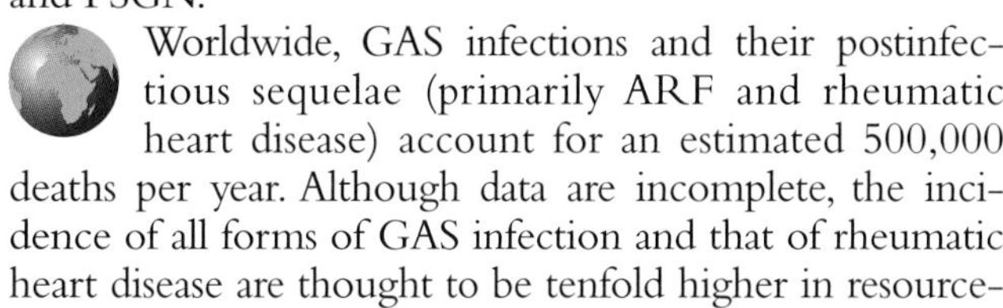

Worldwide, GAS infections and their postinfectious sequelae (primarily ARF and rheumatic heart disease) account for an estimated 500,000 deaths per year. Although data are incomplete, the incidence of all forms of GAS infection and that of rheumatic heart disease are thought to be tenfold higher in resource-limited countries than in developed countries (Fig. 36-1).

PATHOGENESIS

GAS elaborates a number of cell-surface components and extracellular products important in both the pathogenesis of infection and the human immune response.

TABLE 36-1

CLASSIFICATION OF STREPTOCOCCI

LANCEFIELD'S GROUP	REPRESENTATIVE SPECIES	HEMOLYTIC PATTERN	TYPICAL INFECTIONS
A	*S. pyogenes*	β	Pharyngitis, impetigo, cellulitis, scarlet fever
B	*S. agalactiae*	β	Neonatal sepsis and meningitis, puerperal infection, urinary tract infection, diabetic ulcer infection, endocarditis
C, G	*S. dysgalactiae* subsp. *equisimilis*	β	Cellulitis, bacteremia, endocarditis
D	Enterococci: *E. faecalis*; *E. faecium*	Usually nonhemolytic	Urinary tract infection, nosocomial bacteremia, endocarditis
	Nonenterococci: *S. bovis*	Usually nonhemolytic	Bacteremia, endocarditis
Variable or nongroupable	Viridans streptococci: *S. sanguis*; *S. mitis*	α	Endocarditis, dental abscess, brain abscess
	Intermedius or *milleri* group: *S. intermedius*, *S. anginosus*, *S. constellatus*	Variable	Brain abscess, visceral abscess
	Anaerobic streptococci: *Peptostreptococcus magnus*	Usually nonhemolytic	Sinusitis, pneumonia, empyema, brain abscess, liver abscess

The cell wall contains a carbohydrate antigen that may be released by acid treatment. The reaction of such acid extracts with group A–specific antiserum is the basis for definitive identification of a streptococcal strain as *S. pyogenes*. The major surface protein of GAS is M protein, which occurs in more than 100 antigenically distinct types and is the basis for the serotyping of strains with specific antisera. The M protein molecules are fibrillar structures anchored in the cell wall of the organism that extend as hairlike projections away from the cell surface. The amino acid sequence of the distal or amino-terminal portion of the M protein molecule is quite variable, accounting for the antigenic variation of the different M types, whereas more proximal regions of the protein are relatively conserved. A newer technique for assignment of M type to GAS isolates uses the polymerase chain reaction to amplify the variable region of the M protein gene. DNA sequence analysis of the amplified gene segment can be compared with an extensive database [developed at the Centers for Disease Control and

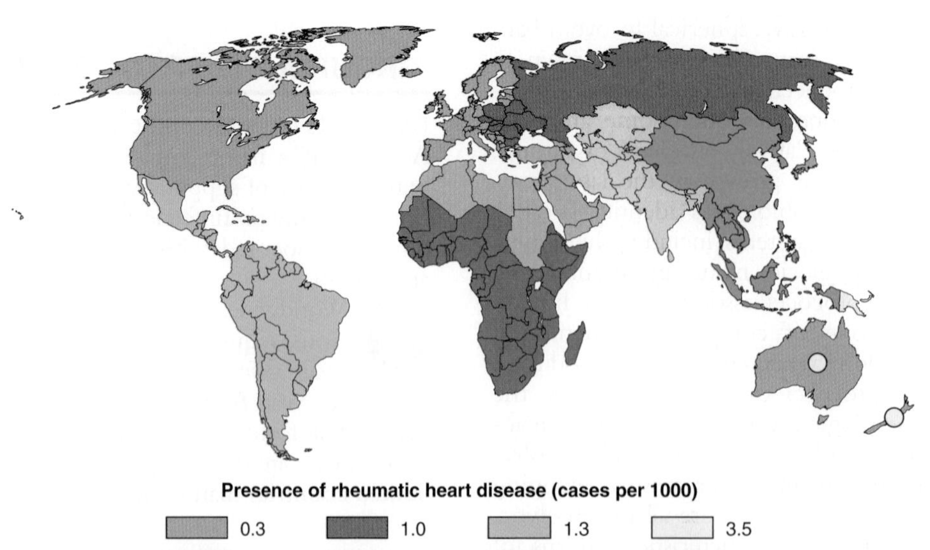

FIGURE 36-1

Prevalence of rheumatic heart disease in children 5–14 years old. The circles within Australia and New Zealand represent indigenous populations (and also Pacific Islanders in New Zealand). (*From Carapetis et al, 2005, with permission.*)

Prevention (CDC)] for assignment of M type. This method eliminates the need for typing sera, which are available in only a few reference laboratories. The presence of M protein on a GAS isolate correlates with its capacity to resist phagocytic killing in fresh human blood. This phenomenon appears to be due, at least in part, to the binding of plasma fibrinogen to M protein molecules on the streptococcal surface, which interferes with complement activation and deposition of opsonic complement fragments on the bacterial cell. This resistance to phagocytosis may be overcome by M protein–specific antibodies; thus individuals with antibodies to a given M type acquired as a result of prior infection are protected against subsequent infection with organisms of the same M type, but not against that with different M types.

GAS also elaborates, to varying degrees, a polysaccharide capsule composed of hyaluronic acid. The production of large amounts of capsule by certain strains lends a characteristic mucoid appearance to the colonies. The capsular polysaccharide plays an important role in protecting GAS from ingestion and killing by phagocytes. In contrast to M protein, the hyaluronic acid capsule is a weak immunogen, and antibodies to hyaluronate have not been shown to be important in protective immunity. The presumed explanation is the apparent structural identity between streptococcal hyaluronic acid and the hyaluronic acid of mammalian connective tissues. The capsular polysaccharide may also play a role in GAS colonization of the pharynx by binding to CD44, a hyaluronic acid–binding protein expressed on human pharyngeal epithelial cells.

GAS produces a large number of extracellular products that may be important in local and systemic toxicity and in the spread of infection through tissues. These products include streptolysins S and O, toxins that damage cell membranes and account for the hemolysis produced by the organisms; streptokinase; DNases; protease; and pyrogenic exotoxins A, B, and C. The pyrogenic exotoxins, previously known as erythrogenic toxins, cause the rash of scarlet fever. Since the mid-1980s, pyrogenic exotoxin–producing strains of GAS have been linked to unusually severe invasive infections, including necrotizing fasciitis and the streptococcal toxic shock syndrome. Several extracellular products stimulate specific antibody responses useful for serodiagnosis of recent streptococcal infection. Tests for these antibodies are used primarily for detection of preceding streptococcal infection in cases of suspected ARF or PSGN.

CLINICAL MANIFESTATIONS

Pharyngitis

Although seen in patients of all ages, GAS pharyngitis is one of the most common bacterial infections of childhood, accounting for 20–40% of all cases of exudative pharyngitis in children; it is rare among those under the age of 3. Younger children may manifest streptococcal infection with a syndrome of fever, malaise, and lymphadenopathy without exudative pharyngitis. Infection is acquired through contact with another individual carrying the organism. Respiratory droplets are the usual mechanism of spread, although other routes, including food-borne outbreaks, have been well described.

The incubation period is 1–4 days. Symptoms include sore throat, fever and chills, malaise, and sometimes abdominal complaints and vomiting, particularly in children. Both symptoms and signs are quite variable, ranging from mild throat discomfort with minimal physical findings to high fever and severe sore throat associated with intense erythema and swelling of the pharyngeal mucosa and the presence of purulent exudate over the posterior pharyngeal wall and tonsillar pillars. Enlarged, tender anterior cervical lymph nodes commonly accompany exudative pharyngitis.

The differential diagnosis of streptococcal pharyngitis includes the many other bacterial and viral etiologies (Table 36-2). Streptococcal infection is an unlikely cause when symptoms and signs suggestive of viral infection are prominent (conjunctivitis, coryza, cough, hoarseness, or discrete ulcerative lesions of the buccal or pharyngeal mucosa). Because of the range of clinical presentations of streptococcal pharyngitis and the large number of other agents that can produce the same clinical picture, diagnosis of streptococcal pharyngitis on clinical grounds alone is not reliable.

The throat culture remains the diagnostic gold standard. Culture of a throat specimen that is properly collected (i.e., by vigorous rubbing of a sterile swab over both tonsillar pillars) and properly processed is the most sensitive and specific means of definitive diagnosis. A rapid diagnostic kit for latex agglutination or enzyme immunoassay of swab specimens is a useful adjunct to throat culture. Although precise figures on sensitivity and specificity vary, rapid diagnostic kits generally are >95% specific. Thus a positive result can be relied upon for definitive diagnosis and eliminates the need for throat culture. However, because rapid diagnostic tests are less sensitive than throat culture (relative sensitivity in comparative studies, 55–90%), a negative result should be confirmed by throat culture.

℞ Treatment: GAS PHARYNGITIS

In the usual course of uncomplicated streptococcal pharyngitis, symptoms resolve after 3–5 days. The course is shortened little by treatment, which is given primarily to prevent suppurative complications and ARF. Prevention of ARF depends on eradication of the organism from the pharynx, not simply on resolution of symptoms, and requires 10 days of penicillin treatment (Table 36-3). Erythromycin may be substituted for penicillin in cases of penicillin allergy. Once-daily azithromycin is a more convenient but expensive alternative; a 5-day course is approved, but only limited data support equivalent efficacy to a standard 10-day course.

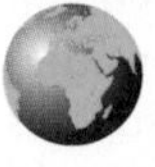

Resistance to erythromycin and other macrolides is common among isolates from several countries, including Spain, Italy, Finland, Japan, and Korea.

TABLE 36-2

INFECTIOUS ETIOLOGIES OF ACUTE PHARYNGITIS

ORGANISM	ASSOCIATED CLINICAL SYNDROME(S)
Viruses	
Rhinovirus	Common cold
Coronavirus	Common cold
Adenovirus	Pharyngoconjunctival fever
Influenza virus	Influenza
Parainfluenza virus	Cold, croup
Coxsackievirus	Herpangina, hand-foot-and-mouth disease
Herpes simplex virus	Gingivostomatitis (primary infection)
Epstein-Barr virus	Infectious mononucleosis
Cytomegalovirus	Mononucleosis-like syndrome
HIV	Acute (primary) infection syndrome
Bacteria	
Group A streptococci	Pharyngitis, scarlet fever
Group C or G streptococci	Pharyngitis
Mixed anaerobes	Vincent's angina
Arcanobacterium haemolyticum	Pharyngitis, scarlatiniform rash
Neisseria gonorrhoeae	Pharyngitis
Treponema pallidum	Secondary syphilis
Francisella tularensis	Pharyngeal tularemia
Corynebacterium diphtheriae	Diphtheria
Yersinia enterocolitica	Pharyngitis, enterocolitis
Yersinia pestis	Plague
Chlamydiae	
Chlamydophila pneumoniae	Bronchitis, pneumonia
Chlamydophila psittaci	Psittacosis
Mycoplasmas	
Mycoplasma pneumoniae	Bronchitis, pneumonia

Macrolide resistance may be becoming more prevalent elsewhere with the increasing use of this class of antibiotics. In areas with resistance rates exceeding 5–10%, macrolides should be avoided unless results of susceptibility testing are known. Follow-up culture after treatment is no longer routinely recommended but may be warranted in selected cases, such as those involving patients or families with frequent streptococcal infections or those occurring in situations in which the risk of ARF is thought to be high (e.g., when cases of ARF have recently been reported in the community).

Complications

Suppurative complications of streptococcal pharyngitis have become uncommon with the widespread use of antibiotics for most symptomatic cases. These complications result from the spread of infection from the pharyngeal mucosa to deeper tissues by direct extension or by the hematogenous or lymphatic route and may include cervical lymphadenitis, peritonsillar or retropharyngeal abscess, sinusitis, otitis media, meningitis, bacteremia, endocarditis, and pneumonia. Local complications, such as peritonsillar or parapharyngeal abscess formation, should be considered in a patient with unusually severe or prolonged symptoms or localized pain associated with high fever and a toxic appearance. Nonsuppurative complications include ARF (Chap. 37) and PSGN, both of which are thought to result from immune responses to streptococcal infection. Penicillin treatment of streptococcal pharyngitis has been shown to reduce the likelihood of ARF, but not that of PSGN.

Bacteriologic Treatment Failure and the Asymptomatic Carrier State

Surveillance cultures have shown that up to 20% of individuals in certain populations may have asymptomatic pharyngeal colonization with GAS. There are no definitive guidelines for management of these asymptomatic carriers or of asymptomatic patients who still have a positive throat culture after a full course of treatment for symptomatic pharyngitis. A reasonable course of action is to give a single 10-day course of penicillin for symptomatic pharyngitis and, if positive cultures persist, not to re-treat unless symptoms recur. Studies of the natural history of streptococcal carriage and infection have shown that the risk both of developing ARF and of transmitting infection to others is substantially

TABLE 36-3

TREATMENT OF GROUP A STREPTOCOCCAL INFECTIONS

INFECTION	TREATMENT[a]
Pharyngitis	Benzathine penicillin G, 1.2 mU IM; *or* penicillin V, 250 mg PO tid or 500 mg PO bid × 10 days (Children <27 kg: Benzathine penicillin G, 600,000 units IM; *or* penicillin V, 250 mg PO bid or tid × 10 days)
Impetigo	Same as pharyngitis
Erysipelas/cellulitis	Severe: Penicillin G, 1–2 mU IV q4h Mild to moderate: Procaine penicillin, 1.2 mU IM bid
Necrotizing fasciitis/myositis	Surgical debridement; *plus* penicillin G, 2–4 mU IV q4h; *plus* clindamycin,[b] 600–900 mg q8h
Pneumonia/empyema	Penicillin G, 2–4 mU IV q4h; *plus* drainage of empyema
Streptococcal toxic shock syndrome	Penicillin G, 2–4 mU IV q4h; *plus* clindamycin,[b] 600–900 mg q8h; *plus* intravenous immunoglobulin,[b] 2 g/kg as a single dose

[a]Penicillin allergy: Erythromycin (10 mg/kg PO qid up to a maximum of 250 mg per dose) may be substituted for oral penicillin. Alternative agents for parenteral therapy include first-generation cephalosporins—if the nature of the allergy is not an immediate hypersensitivity reaction (anaphylaxis or urticaria) or another potentially life-threatening manifestation (e.g., severe rash and fever)—or vancomycin.

[b]Efficacy unproven, but recommended by several experts. See text for discussion.

lower among asymptomatic carriers than among individuals with symptomatic pharyngitis. Therefore, overly aggressive attempts to eradicate carriage probably are not justified under most circumstances. An exception is the situation in which an asymptomatic carrier is a potential source of infection to others. Outbreaks of food-borne infection and nosocomial puerperal infection have been traced to asymptomatic carriers who may harbor the organisms in the throat, vagina, or anus or on the skin.

℞ Treatment: ASYMPTOMATIC PHARYNGEAL COLONIZATION WITH GAS

When a carrier is transmitting infection to others, attempts to eradicate carriage are warranted. Data are limited on the best regimen to clear GAS after penicillin alone has failed. The combination of penicillin V (500 mg four times daily for 10 days) and rifampin (600 mg twice daily for the last 4 days) has been used to eliminate pharyngeal carriage. A 10-day course of oral vancomycin (250 mg four times daily) and rifampin (600 mg twice daily) has eradicated rectal colonization.

Scarlet Fever

Scarlet fever consists of streptococcal infection, usually pharyngitis, accompanied by a characteristic rash (Fig. 36-2). The rash arises from the effects of one of three toxins, currently designated streptococcal pyrogenic exotoxins A, B, and C and previously known as erythrogenic or scarlet fever toxins. In the past, scarlet fever was thought to reflect infection of an individual lacking toxin-specific immunity with a toxin-producing strain of GAS. Susceptibility to scarlet fever was correlated with results of the Dick test, in which a small amount of erythrogenic toxin injected intradermally produced local erythema in susceptible individuals but elicited no reaction in those with specific immunity. Subsequent studies have suggested that development of the scarlet fever rash may reflect a hypersensitivity reaction requiring prior exposure to the toxin. For reasons that are not clear, scarlet fever has become less common in recent years, although strains of GAS that produce pyrogenic exotoxins continue to be prevalent in the population.

The symptoms of scarlet fever are the same as those of pharyngitis alone. The rash typically begins on the first or second day of illness over the upper trunk, spreading to involve the extremities but sparing the palms and soles.

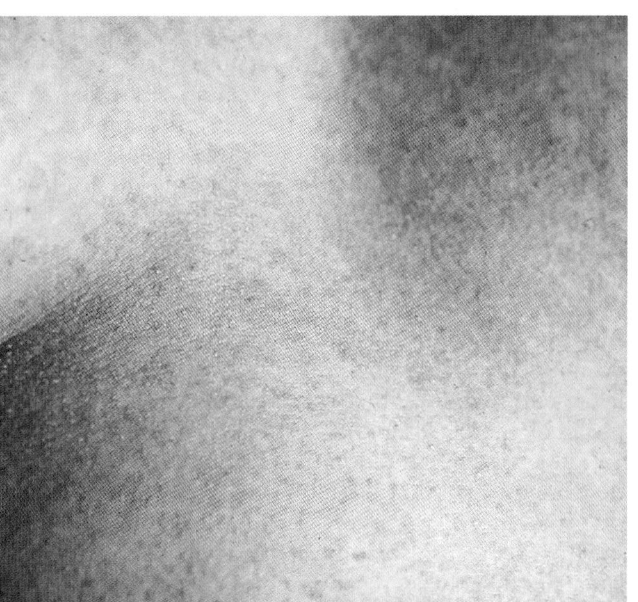

FIGURE 36-2

Scarlet fever exanthem. Finely punctate erythema has become confluent (scarlatiniform); petechiae can occur and have a linear configuration within the exanthem in body folds (Pastia's lines). (*From Fitzpatrick, Johnson, Wolff: Color Atlas and Synopsis of Clinical Dermatology, 4th ed, New York, McGraw-Hill, 2001, with permission.*)

The rash is made up of minute papules, giving a characteristic "sandpaper" feel to the skin. Associated findings include circumoral pallor, "strawberry tongue" (enlarged papillae on a coated tongue, which later may become denuded), and accentuation of the rash in skin folds (Pastia's lines). Subsidence of the rash in 6–9 days is followed after several days by desquamation of the palms and soles. The differential diagnosis of scarlet fever includes other causes of fever and generalized rash, such as measles and other viral exanthems, Kawasaki's disease, toxic shock syndrome, and systemic allergic reactions (e.g., drug eruptions).

Skin and Soft Tissue Infections

GAS—and occasionally other streptococcal species—causes a variety of infections involving the skin, subcutaneous tissues, muscles, and fascia. Although several clinical syndromes offer a useful means for classification of these infections, not all cases fit exactly into one category. The classic syndromes are general guides to predicting the level of tissue involvement in a particular patient, the probable clinical course, and the likelihood that surgical intervention or aggressive life support will be required.

Impetigo (Pyoderma)

Impetigo, a superficial infection of the skin, is caused primarily by GAS and occasionally by other streptococci or *Staphylococcus aureus*. Impetigo is seen most often in young children, tends to occur during warmer months, and is more common in semitropical or tropical climates than in cooler regions. Infection is more common among children living under conditions of poor hygiene. Prospective studies have shown that colonization of unbroken skin with GAS precedes clinical infection. Minor trauma, such as a scratch or an insect bite, may then serve to inoculate organisms into the skin. Impetigo is best prevented, therefore, by attention to adequate hygiene. The usual sites of involvement are the face (particularly around the nose and mouth) and the legs, although lesions may occur at other locations. Individual lesions begin as red papules, which evolve quickly into vesicular and then pustular lesions that break down and coalesce to form characteristic honeycomb-like crusts (Fig. 36-3). Lesions are generally not painful, and patients do not appear ill. Fever is not a feature of impetigo and, if present, suggests either infection extending to deeper tissues or another diagnosis.

The classic presentation of impetigo usually poses little diagnostic difficulty. Cultures of impetiginous lesions often yield *S. aureus* as well as GAS. In almost all cases, streptococci are isolated initially and staphylococci appear later, presumably as secondary colonizing flora. In the past, penicillin was nearly always effective against these infections. However, an increasing frequency of penicillin treatment failure suggests that *S. aureus* may have become more prominent as a cause of impetigo. *Bullous impetigo* due to *S. aureus* is distinguished from typical streptococcal infection by more extensive, bullous lesions that break down and leave thin paper-like crusts instead of the thick amber crusts of streptococcal impetigo.

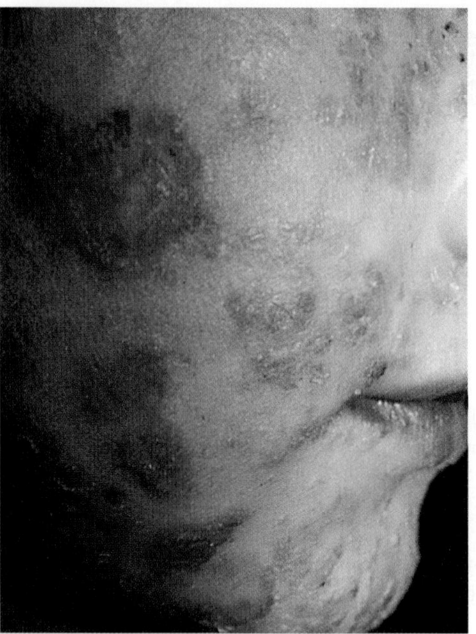

FIGURE 36-3
Impetigo contagiosa is a superficial streptococcal or *Staphylococcus aureus* infection consisting of honey-colored crusts and erythematous weeping erosions. Occasionally, bullous lesions may be seen. (*Courtesy of Mary Spraker, MD; with permission.*)

Other skin lesions that may be confused with impetigo include herpetic lesions—either those of orolabial herpes simplex or those of chickenpox or zoster. Herpetic lesions can generally be distinguished by their appearance as more discrete, grouped vesicles and by a positive Tzanck test. In difficult cases, cultures of vesicular fluid should yield GAS in impetigo and the responsible virus in *Herpesvirus* infections.

℞ Treatment: STREPTOCOCCAL IMPETIGO

Treatment of streptococcal impetigo is the same as that for streptococcal pharyngitis (Table 36-3). In view of evidence that *S. aureus* has become a relatively frequent cause of impetigo, empirical regimens should cover both streptococci and *S. aureus*. For example, either dicloxacillin or cephalexin can be given at a dose of 250 mg four times daily for 10 days. Topical mupirocin ointment is also effective. ARF is not a sequela to streptococcal skin infections, although PSGN may follow either skin or throat infection. The reason for this difference is not known. One hypothesis is that the immune response necessary for development of ARF occurs only after infection of the pharyngeal mucosa. In addition, the strains of GAS that cause pharyngitis are generally of different M protein types than those associated with skin infections; thus the strains that cause pharyngitis may have rheumatogenic potential, whereas the skin-infecting strains may not.

Cellulitis

Inoculation of organisms into the skin may lead to *cellulitis*: infection involving the skin and subcutaneous tissues. The portal of entry may be a traumatic or surgical wound, an insect bite, or any other break in skin integrity. Often, no entry site is apparent.

One form of streptococcal cellulitis, *erysipelas*, is characterized by a bright red appearance of the involved skin, which forms a plateau sharply demarcated from surrounding normal skin (Fig. 36-4). The lesion is warm to the touch, may be tender, and appears shiny and swollen. The skin often has a *peau d'orange* texture, which is thought to reflect involvement of superficial lymphatics; superficial blebs or bullae may form, usually 2–3 days after onset. The lesion typically develops over a few hours and is associated with fever and chills. Erysipelas tends to occur on the malar area of the face (often with extension over the bridge of the nose to the contralateral malar region) and the lower extremities. After one episode, recurrence at the same site—sometimes years later—is not uncommon.

Classic cases of erysipelas, with typical features, are almost always due to β-hemolytic streptococci, usually GAS and occasionally group C or G. Often, however, the appearance of streptococcal cellulitis is not sufficiently distinctive to permit a specific diagnosis on clinical grounds. The area involved may not be typical for erysipelas, the lesion may be less intensely red than usual and may fade into surrounding skin, and/or the patient may appear only mildly ill. In such cases, it is prudent to broaden the spectrum of empirical antimicrobial therapy to include other pathogens, particularly *S. aureus*, that can produce cellulitis with the same appearance. Staphylococcal infection should be suspected if cellulitis develops around a wound or an ulcer.

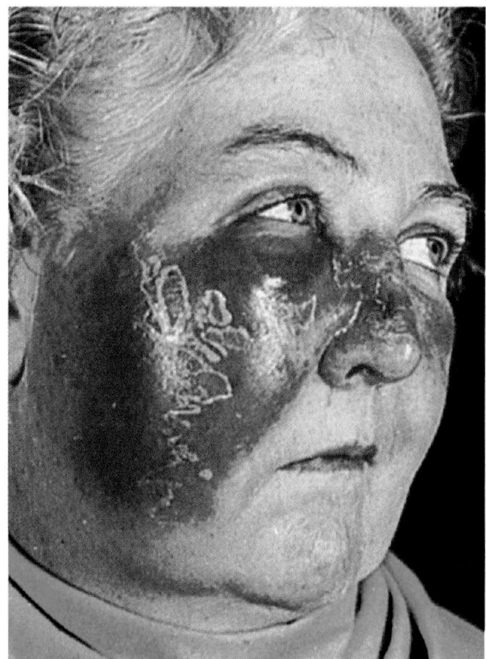

FIGURE 36-4
Erysipelas is a streptococcal infection of the superficial dermis and consists of well-demarcated, erythematous, edematous, warm plaques.

Streptococcal cellulitis tends to develop at anatomic sites in which normal lymphatic drainage has been disrupted, such as sites of prior cellulitis, the arm ipsilateral to a mastectomy and axillary lymph node dissection, a lower extremity previously involved in deep venous thrombosis or chronic lymphedema, or the leg from which a saphenous vein has been harvested for coronary artery bypass grafting. The organism may enter via a dermal breach some distance from the eventual site of clinical cellulitis. For example, some patients with recurrent leg cellulitis after saphenous vein removal stop having recurrent episodes only after treatment of tinea pedis on the affected extremity. Fissures in the skin presumably serve as a portal of entry for streptococci, which then produce infection more proximally in the leg at the site of previous injury. Streptococcal cellulitis may also involve recent surgical wounds. GAS is among the few bacterial pathogens that typically produce signs of wound infection and surrounding cellulitis within the first 24 h after surgery. These wound infections are usually associated with a thin exudate and may spread rapidly, either as cellulitis in the skin and subcutaneous tissue or as a deeper tissue infection (see below). Streptococcal wound infection or localized cellulitis may also be associated with *lymphangitis*, manifested by red streaks extending proximally along superficial lymphatics from the infection site.

℞ Treatment: STREPTOCOCCAL CELLULITIS

See Table 36-3 and Chap. 21.

Deep Soft-Tissue Infections

Necrotizing fasciitis (*hemolytic streptococcal gangrene*) involves the superficial and/or deep fascia investing the muscles of an extremity or the trunk. The source of the infection is either the skin, with organisms introduced into tissue through trauma (sometimes trivial), or the bowel flora, with organisms released during abdominal surgery or from an occult enteric source, such as a diverticular or appendiceal abscess. The inoculation site may be inapparent and is often some distance from the site of clinical involvement; e.g., the introduction of organisms via minor trauma to the hand may be associated with clinical infection of the tissues overlying the shoulder or chest. Cases associated with the bowel flora are usually polymicrobial, involving a mixture of anaerobic bacteria (such as *Bacteroides fragilis* or anaerobic streptococci) and facultative organisms (usually gram-negative bacilli). Cases unrelated to contamination from bowel organisms are most commonly caused by GAS alone or in combination with other organisms (most often *S. aureus*). Overall, GAS is implicated in ~60% of cases of necrotizing fasciitis. The onset of symptoms is usually quite acute and is marked by severe pain at the site of involvement, malaise, fever, chills, and a toxic appearance. The physical findings, particularly early on, may not be striking, with only minimal erythema of the overlying skin. Pain and tenderness are usually severe. In contrast, in more superficial cellulitis, the skin appearance is more abnormal, but pain and tenderness are only mild or moderate. As the infection progresses (often over several hours), the severity and extent of symptoms worsen, and skin changes become more evident, with the appearance of dusky or mottled erythema and edema. The marked tenderness of the involved area may evolve into anesthesia as the spreading inflammatory process produces infarction of cutaneous nerves.

Although myositis is more commonly due to *S. aureus* infection, GAS occasionally produces abscesses in skeletal muscles (*streptococcal myositis*), with little or no involvement of the surrounding fascia or overlying skin. The presentation is usually subacute, but a fulminant form has been described in association with severe systemic toxicity, bacteremia, and a high mortality rate. The fulminant form may reflect the same basic disease process seen in necrotizing fasciitis, but with the necrotizing inflammatory process extending into the muscles themselves rather than remaining limited to the fascial layers.

℞ Treatment: DEEP SOFT-TISSUE INFECTIONS

Once necrotizing fasciitis is suspected, early surgical exploration is both diagnostically and therapeutically indicated. Surgery reveals necrosis and inflammatory fluid tracking along the fascial planes above and between muscle groups, without involvement of the muscles themselves. The process usually extends beyond the area of clinical involvement, and extensive debridement is required. Drainage and debridement are central to the management of necrotizing fasciitis; antibiotic treatment is a useful adjunct (Table 36-3), but surgery is life-saving.

Treatment for streptococcal myositis consists of surgical drainage—usually by an open procedure that permits evaluation of the extent of infection and ensures adequate debridement of involved tissues—and high-dose penicillin (Table 36-3).

Pneumonia and Empyema

GAS is an occasional cause of pneumonia, generally in previously healthy individuals. The onset of symptoms may be abrupt or gradual. Pleuritic chest pain, fever, chills, and dyspnea are the characteristic manifestations. Cough is usually present but may not be prominent. Approximately one-half of patients with GAS pneumonia have an accompanying pleural effusion. In contrast to the sterile parapneumonic effusions typical of pneumococcal pneumonia, those complicating streptococcal pneumonia are almost always infected. The empyema fluid is usually visible by chest radiography on initial presentation, and its volume may increase rapidly. These pleural collections should be drained early, as they tend to become loculated rapidly, resulting in a chronic fibrotic reaction that may require thoracotomy for removal.

Bacteremia, Puerperal Sepsis, and Streptococcal Toxic Shock Syndrome

GAS bacteremia is usually associated with an identifiable local infection. Bacteremia occurs rarely with otherwise uncomplicated pharyngitis, occasionally with cellulitis or pneumonia, and relatively frequently with necrotizing fasciitis. Bacteremia without an identified source raises the possibility of endocarditis, an occult abscess, or osteomyelitis. A variety of focal infections may arise secondarily from streptococcal bacteremia, including endocarditis, meningitis, septic arthritis, osteomyelitis, peritonitis, and visceral abscesses.

GAS is occasionally implicated in infectious complications of childbirth, usually endometritis and associated bacteremia. In the preantibiotic era, puerperal sepsis was commonly caused by GAS; currently, it is more often caused by GBS. Several nosocomial outbreaks of puerperal GAS infection have been traced to an asymptomatic carrier, usually someone present at delivery. The site of carriage may be the skin, throat, anus, or vagina.

Beginning in the late 1980s, several reports described patients with GAS infections associated with shock and multisystem organ failure. This syndrome was called the streptococcal toxic shock syndrome (TSS) because it shares certain features with staphylococcal TSS. In 1993, a case definition for streptococcal TSS was formulated (Table 36-4). The general features of the illness include fever, hypotension, renal impairment, and respiratory distress syndrome. Various types of rash have been described, but rash usually does not develop. Laboratory abnormalities include a marked shift to the left in the white blood cell differential, with many immature granulocytes; hypocalcemia; hypoalbuminemia; and thrombocytopenia, which usually becomes more pronounced on the second

TABLE 36-4

PROPOSED CASE DEFINITION FOR THE STREPTOCOCCAL TOXIC SHOCK SYNDROME[a]

I. Isolation of group A streptococci (*Streptococcus pyogenes*)
   A. From a normally sterile site
   B. From a nonsterile site
II. Clinical signs of severity
   A. Hypotension *and*
   B. ≥2 of the following signs
      1. Renal impairment
      2. Coagulopathy
      3. Liver function impairment
      4. Adult respiratory distress syndrome
      5. A generalized erythematous macular rash that may desquamate
      6. Soft tissue necrosis, including necrotizing fasciitis or myositis; *or* gangrene

[a]An illness fulfilling criteria IA, IIA, and IIB is defined as a *definite* case. An illness fulfilling criteria IB, IIA, and IIB is defined as a *probable* case if no other etiology for the illness is identified.

Source: Modified from Working Group on Severe Streptococcal Infections: JAMA 269:390, 1993.

or third day of illness. In contrast to patients with staphylococcal TSS, the majority with streptococcal TSS are bacteremic. The most common associated infection is a soft tissue infection—necrotizing fasciitis, myositis, or cellulitis—although a variety of other associated local infections have been described, including pneumonia, peritonitis, osteomyelitis, and myometritis. Streptococcal TSS is associated with a mortality rate of ≥30%, with most deaths secondary to shock and respiratory failure. Because of its rapidly progressive and lethal course, early recognition of the syndrome is essential. Patients should receive aggressive supportive care (fluid resuscitation, pressors, and mechanical ventilation) in addition to antimicrobial therapy and, in cases associated with necrotizing fasciitis, surgical debridement. Exactly why certain patients develop this fulminant syndrome is not known. Early studies of the streptococcal strains isolated from these patients demonstrated a strong association with the production of pyrogenic exotoxin A. This association has been inconsistent in subsequent case series. Pyrogenic exotoxin A and several other streptococcal exotoxins act as superantigens to trigger release of inflammatory cytokines from T lymphocytes. Fever, shock, and organ dysfunction in streptococcal TSS may reflect, in part, the systemic effects of superantigen-mediated cytokine release.

Treatment: ℞ STREPTOCOCCAL TOXIC SHOCK SYNDROME

In light of the possible role of pyrogenic exotoxins or other streptococcal toxins in streptococcal TSS, treatment with clindamycin has been advocated by some authorities (Table 36-3), who argue that, through its direct action on protein synthesis, clindamycin is more effective in rapidly terminating toxin production than penicillin—a cell-wall agent. Support for this view comes from studies of an experimental model of streptococcal myositis, in which mice given clindamycin had a higher rate of survival than those given penicillin. Comparable data on the treatment of human infections are not available. Although clindamycin resistance in GAS is uncommon (<2% among U.S. isolates), it has been documented. Thus, if clindamycin is used for initial treatment of a critically ill patient, penicillin should be given as well until the antibiotic susceptibility of the streptococcal isolate is known.

Intravenous immunoglobulin has been used as adjunctive therapy for streptococcal TSS (Table 36-3). Pooled immunoglobulin preparations contain antibodies capable of neutralizing the effects of streptococcal toxins. Anecdotal reports and case series have suggested favorable clinical responses to intravenous immunoglobulin, but no prospective controlled trials have been reported.

PREVENTION

No vaccine against GAS is commercially available. A formulation that consists of recombinant peptides containing epitopes of 26 M-protein types has undergone phase I and II testing in volunteers. Early results indicate that the vaccine is well tolerated and elicits type-specific antibody responses.

Household contacts of individuals with invasive GAS infection (e.g., bacteremia, necrotizing fasciitis, or streptococcal TSS) are at greater risk of invasive infection than the general population. Asymptomatic pharyngeal colonization with GAS has been detected in up to 25% of persons with >4 h/d of same-room exposure to an index case. However, antibiotic prophylaxis is not routinely recommended for contacts of patients with invasive disease since such an approach (if effective) would require treatment of hundreds of contacts to prevent a single case.

STREPTOCOCCI OF GROUPS C AND G

Group C and group G streptococci are β-hemolytic bacteria that occasionally cause human infections similar to those caused by GAS. Strains that form small colonies on blood agar (<0.5 mm) are generally members of the *S. milleri* (*S. intermedius, S. anginosus*) group (see "Viridans Streptococci" later in the chapter). Large-colony group C and G streptococci of human origin are now considered a single species, *S. dysgalactiae* subsp. *equisimilis*. They have been associated with pharyngitis, cellulitis and soft-tissue infections, pneumonia, bacteremia, endocarditis, and septic arthritis. Puerperal sepsis, meningitis, epidural abscess, intraabdominal abscess, urinary tract infection, and neonatal sepsis have also been reported. Group C or G streptococcal bacteremia most often affects elderly or chronically ill patients and, in the absence of obvious local infection, is likely to reflect endocarditis. Septic arthritis, sometimes involving multiple joints, may complicate endocarditis or develop in its absence. Distinct streptococcal species of Lancefield's group C cause infections in domesticated animals, especially horses and cattle; some human infections are acquired through contact with animals or consumption of unpasteurized milk. These zoonotic organisms include *S. equi* subsp. *zooepidemicus* and *S. equi* subsp. *equi*.

Treatment: ℞ GROUP C OR G STREPTOCOCCAL INFECTION

Penicillin is the drug of choice for treatment of group C or G streptococcal infections. Antibiotic treatment is the same as for similar syndromes due to GAS (Table 36-3). Patients with bacteremia or septic arthritis should receive intravenous penicillin (2–4 mU every 4 h). All group C and G streptococci are sensitive to penicillin; nearly all are inhibited in vitro by concentrations of ≤0.03 μg/mL. Occasional isolates exhibit tolerance: although inhibited by low concentrations of penicillin, they are killed only by significantly higher concentrations. The clinical significance of tolerance is unknown. Because of the poor clinical response of some patients to penicillin alone, the addition of gentamicin (1 mg/kg every 8 h for patients with normal renal function) is recommended by some authorities for treatment of endocarditis or septic arthritis due to group C or G streptococci; however, combination therapy has not been shown to be superior to penicillin treatment alone. Patients with joint infections often require repeated aspiration or open drainage and debridement for cure; the response to treatment may be slow, particularly in debilitated patients and those with involvement of multiple joints. Infection of prosthetic joints almost always requires prosthesis removal in addition to antibiotic therapy.

GROUP B STREPTOCOCCI

Identified first as a cause of mastitis in cows, streptococci belonging to Lancefield's group B have since been recognized as a major cause of sepsis and meningitis in human neonates. GBS is also a frequent cause of peripartum fever in women and an occasional cause of serious infection in nonpregnant adults. Since the widespread institution of prenatal screening for GBS in the 1990s, the incidence of neonatal infection per 1000 live births has fallen from ~2–3 cases to ~1 case. During the same period, GBS infection in adults with underlying chronic illnesses has become more common; adults now account for a larger proportion of invasive GBS infections than do newborns. Lancefield's group B consists of a single species, *S. agalactiae*, which is definitively identified with specific antiserum to the group B cell wall–associated carbohydrate antigen. A streptococcal isolate can be classified presumptively as GBS on the basis of biochemical tests, including hydrolysis of sodium hippurate (in which 99% of isolates are positive), hydrolysis of bile esculin agar (in which 99–100% are negative), bacitracin susceptibility (in which 92% are resistant), and production of CAMP factor (in which 98–100% are positive). CAMP factor is a phospholipase produced by GBS that causes synergistic hemolysis with β lysin produced by certain strains of *S. aureus*. Its presence can be demonstrated by cross-streaking of the test isolate and an appropriate staphylococcal strain on a blood agar plate. GBS organisms causing human infections are encapsulated by one of nine antigenically distinct polysaccharides. The capsular polysaccharide is an important virulence factor. Antibodies to the capsular polysaccharide afford protection against GBS of the same (but not of a different) capsular type.

INFECTION IN NEONATES

Two general types of GBS infection in infants are defined by the age of the patient at presentation. *Early-onset infections* occur within the first week of life, with a median age of 20 h at onset. Approximately half of these infants have signs of GBS disease at birth. The infection is acquired during or shortly before birth from the colonized maternal genital tract. Surveillance studies have shown that 5–40% of women are vaginal or rectal carriers of GBS. Approximately 50% of infants delivered vaginally by carrier mothers become colonized, although only 1–2% of those colonized develop clinically evident infection. Prematurity and maternal risk factors (prolonged labor, obstetric complications, and maternal fever) are often involved. The presentation of early-onset infection is the same as that of other forms of neonatal sepsis. Typical findings include respiratory distress, lethargy, and hypotension. Essentially all infants with early-onset disease are bacteremic, one-third to one-half have pneumonia and/or respiratory distress syndrome, and one-third have meningitis.

Late-onset infections occur in infants 1 week to 3 months old (mean age at onset, 3–4 weeks). The infecting organism may be acquired during delivery (as in early-onset cases) or during later contact with a colonized mother, nursery personnel, or another source. Meningitis is the most common manifestation of late-onset infection and in most cases is associated with a strain of capsular type III. Infants present with fever, lethargy or irritability, poor feeding, and seizures. The various other types of late-onset infection include bacteremia without an identified source, osteomyelitis, septic arthritis, and facial cellulitis associated with submandibular or preauricular adenitis.

Treatment: ℞ GROUP B STREPTOCOCCAL INFECTION IN NEONATES

Penicillin is the agent of choice for all GBS infections. Empirical broad-spectrum therapy for suspected bacterial sepsis, consisting of ampicillin and gentamicin, is generally administered until culture results become available. If cultures yield GBS, many pediatricians continue to administer gentamicin, along with ampicillin or penicillin, for a few days until clinical improvement becomes evident. Infants with bacteremia or soft-tissue infection should receive penicillin at a dosage of 200,000 units/kg per day in divided doses; those with meningitis should receive 400,000 units/kg per day. Meningitis should be treated for at least 14 days because of the risk of relapse with shorter courses.

Prevention

The incidence of GBS infection is unusually high among infants of women with risk factors: preterm delivery, early rupture of membranes (>24 h before delivery), prolonged labor, fever, or chorioamnionitis. Because the usual source of the organisms infecting a neonate is the mother's birth canal, efforts have been made to prevent GBS infections by the identification of high-risk carrier mothers and their treatment with various forms of antibiotic or immunoprophylaxis. Prophylactic administration of ampicillin or penicillin to such patients during delivery reduces the risk of infection in the newborn. This approach has been hampered by logistical difficulties in identifying colonized women before delivery; the results of vaginal cultures early in pregnancy are poor predictors of carrier status at delivery. The CDC recommends screening for anogenital colonization at 35–37 weeks of pregnancy by a swab culture of the lower vagina and anorectum; intrapartum chemoprophylaxis is recommended for culture-positive women and for women who, regardless of culture status, have previously given birth to an infant with GBS infection or have a history of GBS bacteriuria during pregnancy. Women whose culture status is unknown and who develop premature labor (<37 weeks), prolonged rupture of membranes (>18 h), or intrapartum fever should also receive intrapartum chemoprophylaxis. The recommended regimen for chemoprophylaxis is 5 million units of penicillin G followed by 2.5 million units every 4 h until delivery. Cefazolin is an alternative for women with a history of penicillin allergy who are thought not to be at high risk for anaphylaxis. For women with a history of immediate hypersensitivity, clindamycin or erythromycin may be substituted, but only if the colonizing isolate has been demonstrated to be susceptible. If susceptibility testing results are not available or indicate resistance, vancomycin should be used in this situation.

Treatment of all pregnant women who are colonized or have risk factors for neonatal infection will result in exposure of 15–25% of pregnant women and newborns to antibiotics, with the attendant risks of allergic reactions and selection for resistant organisms. Although still in the developmental stages, a GBS vaccine may ultimately offer a better solution to prevention. Because transplacental passage of maternal antibodies produces protective antibody levels in newborns, efforts are underway to develop a vaccine against GBS that can be given to childbearing-age women before or during pregnancy. Results of phase 1 clinical trials of GBS capsular polysaccharide–protein conjugate vaccines suggest that a multivalent conjugate vaccine would be safe and highly immunogenic.

INFECTION IN ADULTS

The majority of GBS infections in otherwise healthy adults are related to pregnancy and parturition. Peripartum fever, the most common manifestation, is sometimes accompanied by symptoms and signs of endometritis or chorioamnionitis (abdominal distention and uterine or adnexal tenderness). Blood and vaginal swab cultures are often positive. Bacteremia is usually transitory but occasionally results in meningitis or endocarditis. Infections in adults that are not associated with the peripartum period generally involve individuals who are elderly or have an underlying chronic illness, such as diabetes mellitus or a malignancy. Among the infections that develop with some frequency in adults are cellulitis and soft tissue infection (including infected diabetic skin ulcers), urinary tract infection, pneumonia, endocarditis, and septic arthritis. Other reported infections include meningitis, osteomyelitis, and intraabdominal or pelvic abscesses. Relapse or recurrence of invasive infection weeks to months after a first episode is documented in ~4% of cases.

Rx Treatment: GROUP B STREPTOCOCCAL INFECTION IN ADULTS

GBS is less sensitive to penicillin than GAS, requiring somewhat higher doses. Adults with serious localized infections (pneumonia, pyelonephritis, abscess) should receive doses of ~12 million units of penicillin G daily; patients with endocarditis or meningitis should receive 18–24 million units per day in divided doses. Vancomycin is an acceptable alternative for penicillin-allergic patients.

ENTEROCOCCI AND NONENTEROCOCCAL GROUP D STREPTOCOCCI

ENTEROCOCCI

Lancefield's group D includes the enterococci—organisms now classified in a separate genus from other streptococci—and nonenterococcal group D streptococci. Enterococci are distinguished from nonenterococcal group D streptococci by their ability to grow in the presence of 6.5% sodium chloride and by the results of other biochemical tests. The enterococcal species that are significant pathogens for humans are *E. faecalis* and *E. faecium*. Less commonly, similar infections are caused by *E. casseliflavus*, *E. durans*, *E. gallinarum*, or other enterococcal species. These organisms tend to affect patients who are elderly or debilitated, whose mucosal or epithelial barriers have been disrupted, or whose normal flora has been altered by antibiotic treatment. Urinary tract infections due to enterococci are quite common, particularly among patients who have received antibiotic treatment or undergone urinary tract instrumentation. Enterococci are a common cause of nosocomial bacteremia in patients with intravascular catheters and account for 10–20% of cases of bacterial endocarditis on both native and prosthetic valves. The presentation of enterococcal endocarditis is usually subacute but may be acute, with rapidly progressive valve destruction. Enterococci are frequently cultured from bile and are involved in infectious complications of biliary surgery and in liver abscesses. Moreover, enterococci are often isolated from polymicrobial infections arising from the bowel flora (e.g., intraabdominal abscesses), from abdominal surgical wounds, and from diabetic foot ulcers. Although such mixed infections are frequently cured by antimicrobials not active against enterococci, specific therapy directed against enterococci is warranted when these organisms predominate or are isolated from blood cultures.

Rx Treatment: ENTEROCOCCAL INFECTION

Unlike streptococci, enterococci are not reliably killed by penicillin or ampicillin alone at concentrations achieved clinically in the blood or tissues. Ampicillin reaches sufficiently high urinary concentrations to constitute adequate monotherapy for uncomplicated urinary tract infections. Because in vitro testing has shown evidence of synergistic killing of most enterococcal strains by the combination of penicillin or ampicillin with an aminoglycoside, combined therapy is recommended for enterococcal endocarditis and meningitis; the regimen is penicillin (3–4 million units every 4 h) or ampicillin (2 g every 4 h) plus moderate-dose gentamicin (1 mg/kg every 8 h for patients with normal renal function). Enterococcal endocarditis should be treated for at least 4 weeks and for 6 weeks if symptoms have been present for ≥3 months or if the infection involves a prosthetic valve. For nonendocarditis bacteremia and other serious enterococcal infections, it is not known whether the efficacy of a single β-lactam agent is improved by the addition of gentamicin, but many infectious disease specialists use combination therapy for such infections, especially in critically ill patients. Vancomycin, in combination with gentamicin, may be substituted for penicillin in allergic patients. Enterococci are resistant to all cephalosporins.

Antimicrobial susceptibility testing should be performed routinely on enterococcal isolates from serious infections, with therapy adjusted according to the results (Table 36-5). Most enterococci are resistant to streptomycin, which should not be used unless in vitro testing indicates susceptibility. Although less widespread than streptomycin resistance, high-level resistance to gentamicin—with a minimum inhibitory concentration (MIC) of >2000 μg/mL—is common. Gentamicin-resistant enterococci should be tested for streptomycin susceptibility, which they occasionally exhibit. If the isolate is resistant to all aminoglycosides, treatment with penicillin or ampicillin alone may be successful. Prolonged administration (i.e., for at least 6 weeks) of high-dose ampicillin (e.g., 12 g/d) is recommended for endocarditis due to these highly resistant enterococci.

Enterococci may be resistant to penicillins via two distinct mechanisms. The first is β-lactamase production (mediating resistance to penicillin and ampicillin), which has been reported for *E. faecalis* isolates from several locations in the United States and other countries. Because the amount of β-lactamase produced may be insufficient for detection by routine antibiotic susceptibility testing, isolates from serious infections should be screened specifically for β-lactamase production with a chromogenic cephalosporin or another method. For the treatment of β-lactamase–producing strains, vancomycin, ampicillin/sulbactam, amoxicillin/clavulanate, imipenem, or meropenem may be used in combination with gentamicin.

The second mechanism of penicillin resistance is not mediated by β-lactamase and may be due to altered penicillin-binding proteins. This intrinsic penicillin resistance is common among *E. faecium* isolates, which routinely are more resistant to β-lactam antibiotics than are isolates of *E. faecalis*. Moderately resistant enterococci (MICs of penicillin and ampicillin, 16–64 μg/mL) may be susceptible to high-dose penicillin or ampicillin plus gentamicin, but strains with MICs of ≥200 μg/mL must be considered resistant to clinically achievable levels of β-lactam antibiotics, including imipenem and meropenem. Vancomycin plus gentamicin is the recommended regimen for infections due to enterococci with high-level intrinsic resistance to β-lactams.

Vancomycin-resistant enterococci (VRE), first reported from clinical sources in the late 1980s, have become common in many hospitals. Three major vancomycin resistance phenotypes have been described: VanA, VanB, and VanC. The VanA phenotype is associated with high-level resistance to vancomycin and to teicoplanin, a related glycopeptide antibiotic not currently available in the United States. VanB and VanC strains are resistant to vancomycin but susceptible to teicoplanin, although teicoplanin resistance may develop during treatment in VanB strains. For enterococci resistant to both vancomycin and β-lactams, no established therapies provide uniformly bactericidal activity. Two newer agents active against VRE are quinupristin/dalfopristin and linezolid, which were approved for use in the United States in 1999 and 2000, respectively. Quinupristin/dalfopristin is a streptogramin combination with in vitro bacteriostatic activity against *E. faecium*, including VRE, but not against *E. faecalis* or other enterococcal species. Disadvantages of quinupristin/dalfopristin are its limited spectrum of activity against enterococcal species and its relatively frequent side effects of phlebitis and myalgia. Linezolid is an oxazolidinone antibiotic with good bacteriostatic activity against nearly all enterococci, including VRE. Limited clinical experience suggests that linezolid is at least as efficacious as quinupristin/dalfopristin, and linezolid is usually preferred because of its broader activity against all enterococci and the availability of both parenteral and oral formulations. Bone marrow toxicity (especially thrombocytopenia) and peripheral neuropathy are potential side effects. Two other antibiotics are active in vitro against VRE (both *E. faecalis* and *E. faecium*), although neither has been approved for treatment of these infections: daptomycin, a cyclic lipopeptide, and tigecycline, a glycylcycline related to tetracycline.

TABLE 36-5

TREATMENT OPTIONS FOR ANTIBIOTIC-RESISTANT ENTEROCOCCAL INFECTIONS

RESISTANCE PATTERN	RECOMMENDED THERAPY
β-Lactamase production	Gentamicin plus ampicillin/sulbactam, amoxicillin/clavulanate, imipenem, or vancomycin
β-Lactam resistance, but no β-lactamase production	Gentamicin plus vancomycin
High-level gentamicin resistance	Streptomycin-sensitive isolate: Streptomycin plus ampicillin or vancomycin Streptomycin-resistant isolate: No proven therapy (continuous-infusion ampicillin, prolonged treatment)
Vancomycin resistance	Ampicillin plus gentamicin
Vancomycin and β-lactam resistance	No uniformly bactericidal drugs; linezolid (all enterococci) or quinupristin/dalfopristin (*E. faecium* only)

OTHER GROUP D STREPTOCOCCI

The main nonenterococcal group D streptococcal species that causes human infections is *S. bovis*. *S. bovis* endocarditis is often associated with neoplasms of the gastrointestinal tract—most frequently, a colon carcinoma or polyp—but is also reported in association with other bowel lesions. When occult gastrointestinal lesions are carefully sought, abnormalities are found in ≥60% of patients with *S. bovis* endocarditis. In contrast to the enterococci, nonenterococcal group D streptococci like *S. bovis* are reliably killed by penicillin as a single agent, and penicillin is the agent of choice for *S. bovis* infections.

VIRIDANS AND OTHER STREPTOCOCCI

VIRIDANS STREPTOCOCCI

Consisting of multiple species of α-hemolytic streptococci, the viridans streptococci are a heterogeneous group of organisms that are important agents of bacterial endocarditis (Chap. 19). Several species of viridans streptococci, including *S. salivarius*, *S. mitis*, *S. sanguis*, and *S. mutans*, are part of the normal flora of the mouth, where they live in close association with the teeth and gingiva. Some species contribute to the development of dental caries.

Previously known as *S. morbillorum*, *Gemella morbillorum* has been placed in a separate genus, along with *G. haemolysans*, on the basis of genetic-relatedness studies. These species resemble viridans streptococci with respect to habitat in the human host and associated infections.

The transient viridans streptococcal bacteremia induced by eating, tooth-brushing, flossing, and other sources of minor trauma, together with adherence to biologic surfaces, is thought to account for the predilection of these organisms to cause endocarditis (see Fig. 19-1). Viridans streptococci are also isolated, often as part of a mixed flora, from sites of sinusitis, brain abscess, and liver abscess.

Viridans streptococcal bacteremia occurs relatively frequently in neutropenic patients, particularly after bone marrow transplantation or high-dose chemotherapy for cancer. Some of these patients develop a sepsis syndrome with high fever and shock. Risk factors for viridans streptococcal bacteremia include chemotherapy with high-dose cytarabine, prior treatment with trimethoprim-sulfamethoxazole or a fluoroquinolone, treatment with antacids or histamine antagonists, mucositis, and profound neutropenia.

The *S. milleri* group (also referred to as the *S. intermedius* or *S. anginosus* group) includes three species that cause human disease: *S. intermedius*, *S. anginosus*, and *S. constellatus*. These organisms are often considered viridans streptococci, although they differ somewhat from other viridans streptococci in both their hemolytic pattern (they may be α-, β-, or nonhemolytic) and the disease syndromes they cause. This group commonly produces suppurative infections, particularly abscesses of brain and abdominal viscera, and infections related to the oral cavity or respiratory tract, such as peritonsillar abscess, lung abscess, and empyema.

Treatment: ℞ INFECTION WITH VIRIDANS STREPTOCOCCI

Isolates from neutropenic patients with bacteremia are often resistant to penicillin; thus these patients should be treated presumptively with vancomycin until the results of susceptibility testing become available. Viridans streptococci isolated in other clinical settings usually are sensitive to penicillin.

ABIOTROPHIA SPECIES (NUTRITIONALLY VARIANT STREPTOCOCCI)

Occasional isolates cultured from the blood of patients with endocarditis fail to grow when subcultured on solid media. These *nutritionally variant streptococci* require supplemental thiol compounds or active forms of vitamin B_6 (pyridoxal or pyridoxamine) for growth in the laboratory. The nutritionally variant streptococci are generally grouped with the viridans streptococci because they cause similar types of infections. However, they have been reclassified on the basis of 16S ribosomal RNA sequence comparisons into a separate genus, *Abiotrophia*, with two species: *A. defectivus* and *A. adjacens*.

Treatment: ℞ INFECTION WITH NUTRITIONALLY VARIANT STREPTOCOCCI

Treatment failure and relapse appear to be more common in cases of endocarditis due to nutritionally variant streptococci than in those due to the usual viridans streptococci. Thus the addition of gentamicin (1 mg/kg every 8 h for patients with normal renal function) to the penicillin regimen is recommended for endocarditis due to the nutritionally variant organisms.

OTHER STREPTOCOCCI

S. suis is an important pathogen in swine and has been reported to cause meningitis in humans, usually in individuals with occupational exposure to pigs. Strains of *S. suis* associated with human infections have generally reacted with Lancefield's group R typing serum and sometimes with group D typing serum as well. Isolates may be α- or β-hemolytic and are sensitive to penicillin. *S. iniae*, a pathogen of fish, has been associated with infections in humans who have handled live or freshly killed fish. Cellulitis of the hand is the most common form of human infection, although bacteremia and endocarditis have been reported. *Anaerobic streptococci*, or *peptostreptococci*, are part of the normal flora of the oral cavity, bowel, and vagina. Infections caused by the anaerobic streptococci are discussed in Chap. 65.

BADDOUR LM et al: Infective endocarditis: Diagnosis, antimicrobial therapy, and management of complications: A statement for healthcare professionals from the Committee on Rheumatic Fever, Endocarditis, and Kawasaki Disease, Council on Cardiovascular Disease in the Young, and the Councils on Clinical Cardiology, Stroke, and Cardiovascular Surgery and Anesthesia, American Heart Association: Endorsed by the Infectious Diseases Society of America. Circulation 111:e394, 2005

BISNO AL et al: Practice guidelines for the diagnosis and management of group A streptococcal pharyngitis. Clin Infect Dis 35:113, 2002

———, STEVENS DL: Streptococcal infections of skin and soft tissues. N Engl J Med 334:240, 1996

CARAPETIS JR et al: The global burden of group A streptococcal diseases. Lancet Infect Dis 5:685, 2005

CENTERS FOR DISEASE CONTROL AND PREVENTION: Prevention of perinatal group B streptococcal disease. MMWR 51(RR-11):1, 2002

GASSAS A et al: Predictors of viridans streptococcal shock syndrome in bacteremic children with cancer and stem-cell transplant recipients. J Clin Oncol 22:1222, 2004

GAVALDÀ J et al: Brief communication: Treatment of *Enterococcus faecalis* endocarditis with ampicillin plus ceftriaxone. Ann Intern Med 146:574, 2007

GIBBS RS et al: Perinatal infections due to group B streptococci. Obstet Gynecol 104:1062, 2004

JACKSON LA et al: Risk factors for group B streptococcal disease in adults. Ann Intern Med 123:415, 1995

KAUFFMAN CA: Therapeutic and preventative options for the management of vancomycin-resistant enterococcal infections. J Antimicrob Chemother 51(Suppl3):iii23, 2003

KAUL R et al: Intravenous immunoglobulin therapy for streptococcal toxic shock syndrome—a comparative observational study. The Canadian Streptococcal Study Group. Clin Infect Dis 28:800, 1999

PFOH E et al: Burden and economic cost of group A streptococcal pharyngitis. Pediatrics 121:229, 2008

PHARES CR et al: Epidemiology of invasive group B streptococcal disease in the United States, 1999–2005. JAMA 299:2056, 2008

ROGERS S et al: Strain prevalence, rather than innate virulence potential, is the major factor responsible for an increase in serious group A streptococcus infections. J Infect Dis 195:1625, 2007

THE PREVENTION OF INVASIVE GROUP A STREPTOCOCCAL INFECTIONS WORKSHOP PARTICIPANTS: Prevention of invasive group A streptococcal disease among household contacts of case patients and among postpartum and postsurgical patients: Recommendations from the Centers for Disease Control and Prevention. Clin Infect Dis 35:950, 2002

WILSON W et al: Prevention of infective endocarditis: Guidelines from the American Heart Association. A guideline from the American Heart Association Rheumatic Fever, Endocarditis, and Kawasaki Disease Committee, Council on Cardiovascular Disease in the Young, and the Council on Clinical Cardiology, Council on Cardiovascular Surgery and Anesthesia, and the Quality of Care and Outcomes Research Interdisciplinary Working Group. J Am Dent Assoc 138:739, 2007

CHAPTER 37

ACUTE RHEUMATIC FEVER

Jonathan R. Carapetis

Acute rheumatic fever (ARF) is a multisystem disease resulting from an autoimmune reaction to infection with group A streptococci. Although many parts of the body may be affected, almost all of the manifestations resolve completely. The exception is cardiac valvular damage [rheumatic heart disease (RHD)], which may persist after the other features have disappeared.

ARF and RHD are diseases of poverty. They were common in all countries until the early twentieth century, when their incidence began to decline in industrialized nations. This decline was largely attributable to improved living conditions—particularly less crowded housing and better hygiene—which resulted in reduced transmission of group A streptococci. The introduction of antibiotics and improved systems of medical care had a supplemental effect. Recurrent outbreaks of ARF began in the 1980s in the Rocky Mountain states of the United States, where elevated rates persist.

The virtual disappearance of ARF and reduction in the incidence of RHD in industrialized countries during the twentieth century unfortunately was not replicated in developing countries, where these diseases continue unabated. RHD is the most common cause of heart disease in children in developing countries and is a major cause of mortality and morbidity in adults as well. It was recently estimated that between 15 and 19 million people worldwide are affected by RHD, with approximately one-quarter of a million deaths occurring each year. Some 95% of ARF cases and RHD deaths now occur in developing countries.

Although ARF and RHD are relatively common in all developing countries, they occur at particularly elevated

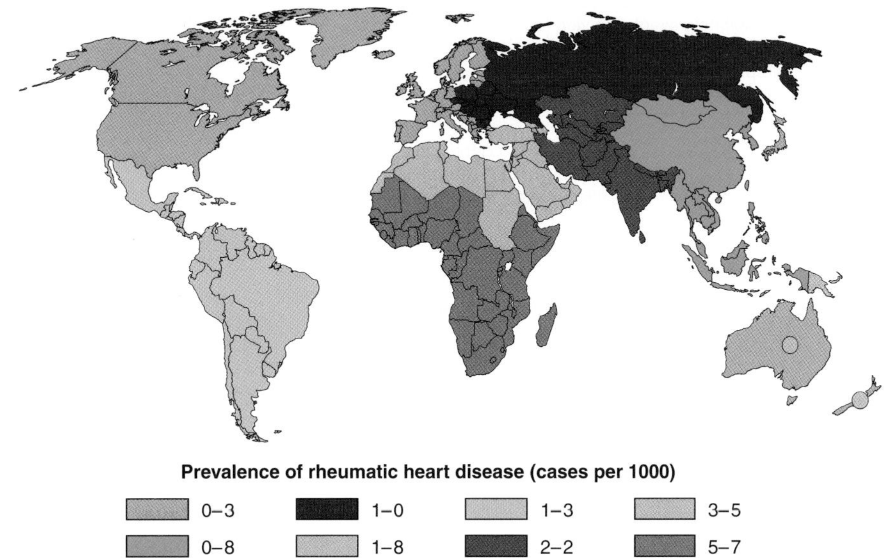

FIGURE 37-1

Prevalence of rheumatic heart disease in children aged 5–14 years. Circles within Australia and New Zealand represent indigenous populations, and also Pacific Islanders in New Zealand. (*Reprinted with permission from JR Carapetis et al: Lancet Infect Dis.*)

rates in certain regions. These "hot spots" are Sub-Saharan Africa, Pacific nations, Australasia, and the Indian subcontinent (Fig. 37-1).

EPIDEMIOLOGY

ARF is mainly a disease of children aged 5–14 years. Initial episodes become less common in older adolescents and young adults and are rare in persons aged >30 years. By contrast, recurrent episodes of ARF remain relatively common in adolescents and young adults. This pattern contrasts with the prevalence of RHD, which peaks between 25 and 40 years. There is no clear gender association for ARF, but RHD more commonly affects females, sometimes up to twice as frequently as males.

PATHOGENESIS

Organism Factors

Based on currently available evidence, ARF is exclusively caused by infection of the upper respiratory tract with group A streptococci. It is now thought that any strain of group A streptococcus has the potential to cause ARF. Potential role of skin infection and of groups C and G streptococci are currently being investigated. It has been postulated that a series of preceding streptococcal infections is needed to "prime" the immune system before the final infection that directly causes disease.

Host Factors

Approximately 3–6% of any population may be susceptible to ARF, and this proportion does not vary dramatically between populations. Findings of familial clustering of cases and concordance in monozygotic twins—particularly for chorea—confirm that susceptibility to ARF is an inherited characteristic. Particular HLA class II alleles appear to be strongly associated with susceptibility. Associations have also been described with high levels of circulating mannose-binding lectin and polymorphisms of transforming growth factor β_1 gene and immunoglobulin genes. High-level expression of a particular alloantigen present on B cells, D8-17, has been found in patients with a history of ARF in many populations, with intermediate-level expression in first-degree family members, suggesting that this may be a marker of inherited susceptibility.

The Immune Response

When a susceptible host encounters a group A streptococcus, an autoimmune reaction results, which leads to damage to human tissues as a result of cross-reactivity between epitopes on the organism and the host (Fig. 37-2).

Epitopes present in the cell wall, cell membrane, and the A, B, and C repeat regions of the streptococcal M protein are immunologically similar to molecules in human myosin, tropomyosin, keratin, actin, laminin, vimentin, and *N*-acetylglucosamine. This molecular mimicry is the basis for the autoimmune response that leads to ARF. It has been hypothesized that human molecules—particularly epitopes in cardiac myosin—result in T-cell sensitization. These T cells are then recalled after subsequent exposure to group A streptococci bearing immunologically similar epitopes.

However, myosin cross-reactivity with M protein does not explain the valvular damage that is the hallmark of rheumatic carditis, given that myosin is not present in valvular tissue. The link may be laminin, another α-helical coiled-coil protein like myosin and M protein, which

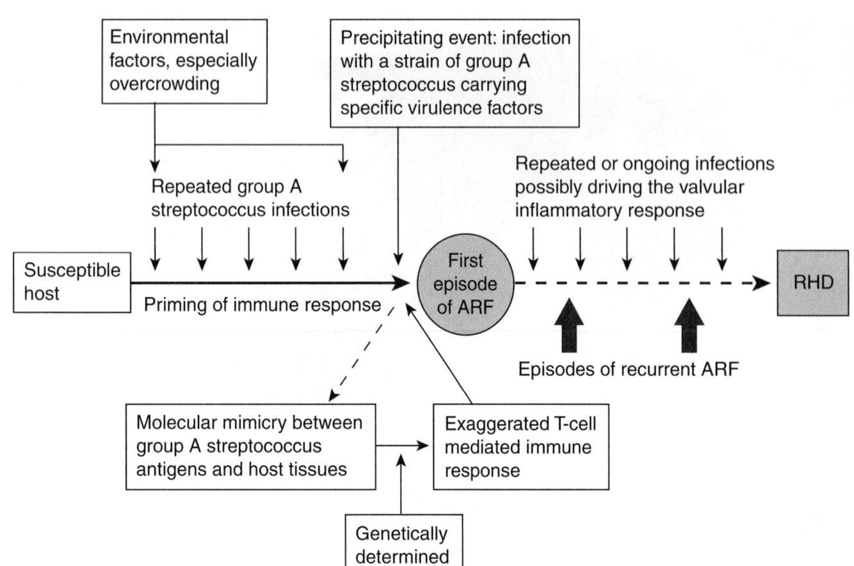

FIGURE 37-2

Pathogenetic pathway for acute rheumatic fever and rheumatic heart disease. *(Reprinted with permission from Lancet 366:155, 2005.)*

is found in cardiac endothelium and is recognized by anti-myosin, anti-M protein T cells. Moreover, antibodies to cardiac valve tissue cross-react with the *N*-acetylglucosamine of group A streptococcal carbohydrate, and there is some evidence that these antibodies may be responsible for valvular damage.

CLINICAL FEATURES

There is a latent period of ~3 weeks (1–5 weeks) between the precipitating group A streptococcal infection and the appearance of the clinical features of ARF. The exceptions are chorea and indolent carditis, which may follow prolonged latent periods lasting up to 6 months. Although many patients report a prior sore throat, the preceding group A streptococcal infection is commonly subclinical; in these cases it can only be confirmed using streptococcal antibody testing. The most common clinical presentation of ARF is polyarthritis and fever. Polyarthritis is present in 60–75% of cases and carditis in 50–60%. The prevalence of chorea in ARF varies substantially between populations, ranging from <2 to 30%. Erythema marginatum and subcutaneous nodules are now rare, being found in <5% of cases.

Heart Involvement

Up to 60% of patients with ARF progress to RHD. The endocardium, pericardium, or myocardium may be affected. Valvular damage is the hallmark of rheumatic carditis. The mitral valve is almost always affected, sometimes together with the aortic valve; isolated aortic valve involvement is rare. Early valvular damage leads to regurgitation. Over ensuing years, usually as a result of recurrent episodes, leaflet thickening, scarring, calcification, and valvular stenosis may develop. Pericarditis most commonly causes a friction rub or a small effusion on echocardiography and may occasionally cause pleuritic central chest pain. Myocardial involvement is almost never responsible in itself for cardiac failure. Therefore, the characteristic manifestation of carditis in previously unaffected individuals is mitral regurgitation, sometimes accompanied by aortic regurgitation. Myocardial inflammation may affect electrical conduction pathways, leading to P-R interval prolongation (first-degree AV block or rarely higher-level block) and softening of the first heart sound.

Joint Involvement

To qualify as a major manifestation, joint involvement in ARF must be arthritic, i.e., objective evidence of inflammation, with hot, swollen, red and/or tender joints and involvement of more than one joint (i.e., polyarthritis). The typical arthritis is migratory, moving from one joint to another over a period of hours. ARF almost always affects the large joints—most commonly the knees, ankles, hips, and elbows—and is asymmetric. The pain is severe and usually disabling until anti-inflammatory medication is commenced.

Less severe joint involvement is also relatively common but qualifies only as a minor manifestation. Arthralgia without objective joint inflammation usually affects large joints in the same migratory pattern as polyarthritis. In some populations, aseptic monoarthritis may be a presenting feature of ARF. This may occur because of early commencement of anti-inflammatory medication before the typical migratory pattern is established.

The joint manifestations of ARF are highly responsive to salicylates and other nonsteroidal anti-inflammatory drugs (NSAIDs). Indeed, joint involvement that persists more than 1 or 2 days after starting salicylates is unlikely to be due to ARF. Conversely, if salicylates are commenced early in the illness, before fever and migratory polyarthritis have become manifest, it may be difficult to make a diagnosis of ARF. For this reason, salicylates and other NSAIDs should be withheld—and pain managed with acetaminophen or codeine—until the diagnosis is confirmed.

Chorea

Sydenham's chorea commonly occurs in the absence of other manifestations, follows a prolonged latent period after group A streptococcal infection, and is found mainly in females. The choreiform movements affect particularly the head (causing characteristic darting movements of the tongue) and the upper limbs. They may be generalized or restricted to one side of the body (hemi-chorea). The chorea varies in severity. In mild cases it may be evident only on careful examination, whereas in the most severe cases the affected individuals are unable to perform activities of daily living and are at risk of injuring themselves. Chorea eventually resolves completely, usually within 6 weeks.

Skin Manifestations

The classic rash of ARF is *erythema marginatum* (Chap. 8), which begins as pink macules that clear centrally, leaving a serpiginous, spreading edge. The rash is evanescent, appearing and disappearing before the examiner's eyes. It occurs usually on the trunk, sometimes on the limbs, but almost never on the face.

Subcutaneous nodules occur as painless, small (0.5–2 cm), mobile lumps beneath the skin overlying bony prominences, particularly of the hands, feet, elbows, occiput, and occasionally the vertebrae. They are a delayed manifestation, appearing 2–3 weeks after the onset of disease, last for just a few days up to 3 weeks, and are commonly associated with carditis.

Other Features

Fever occurs in most cases of ARF, although rarely in cases of pure chorea. Although high-grade fever (≥39°C) is the rule, lower-grade temperature elevations are not uncommon. Elevated acute-phase reactants are also present in most cases. C-reactive protein (CRP) and erythrocyte sedimentation rate (ESR) are often dramatically elevated. Occasionally the peripheral leukocyte count is mildly elevated.

Evidence of a Preceding Group A Streptococcal Infection

With the exception of chorea and low-grade carditis, both of which may become manifest many months later, evidence of a preceding group A streptococcal infection is essential in making the diagnosis of ARF. Because most cases do not have a positive throat swab culture or rapid antigen test, serologic evidence is usually needed. The most common serologic tests are the anti-streptolysin O (ASO) and anti-DNase B (ADB) titers. Where possible, age-specific reference ranges should be determined in a local population of healthy people without a recent group A streptococcal infection.

Other Post-Streptococcal Syndromes That May Be Confused with Rheumatic Fever

Post-streptococcal reactive arthritis (PSRA) is differentiated from ARF on the basis of: (1) small-joint involvement that is often symmetric; (2) a short latent period after streptococcal infection (usually <1 week); (3) occasional causation by non-group A β-hemolytic streptococcal infection; (4) slower responsiveness to salicylates; and (5) the absence of other features of ARF, particularly carditis.

Pediatric Autoimmune Neuropsychiatric Disorders Associated with Streptococcal infection (PANDAS) is a term that links a range of tic disorders and obsessive-compulsive symptoms with group A streptococcal infections. People with PANDAS are said not to be at risk of carditis, unlike patients with Sydenham's chorea. The diagnoses of PANDAS and PSRA should rarely be made in populations with a high incidence of ARF.

Confirming the Diagnosis

Because there is no definitive test, the diagnosis of ARF relies on the presence of a combination of typical clinical features together with evidence of the precipitating group A streptococcal infection and the exclusion of other diagnoses. This uncertainty led Dr. T. Duckett Jones in 1944 to develop a set of criteria (subsequently known as the *Jones criteria*) to aid in the diagnosis. An expert panel convened by the World Health Organization (WHO) clarified the use of the Jones criteria in ARF recurrences (Table 37-1). These criteria include a preceding streptococcal type A infection as well as some combination of major and minor manifestations.

℞ Treatment: ACUTE RHEUMATIC FEVER

Patients with possible ARF should be followed closely to ensure that the diagnosis is confirmed, treatment of heart failure and other symptoms is undertaken, and preventive measures including commencement of secondary prophylaxis, inclusion on an ARF registry, and health education are commenced. Echocardiography should be performed on all possible cases to aid in making the diagnosis and to determine the severity at baseline of any carditis. Other tests that should be performed are listed in Table 37-2.

There is no treatment for ARF that has been proven to alter the likelihood of developing, or the severity of, RHD. With the exception of treatment of heart failure, which may be life-saving in cases of severe carditis, the treatment of ARF is symptomatic.

ANTIBIOTICS All patients with ARF should receive antibiotics sufficient to treat the precipitating group A streptococcal infection (Chap. 36). Penicillin is the drug of choice and can be given orally (as penicillin, 500 mg PO twice daily for 10 days) or as a single dose of 1.2 million units IM benzathine penicillin G. Erythromycin, 250 mg bid, may be used for patients with penicillin allergy. Because long-term secondary prophylaxis will be needed—and penicillin is the drug of choice for this—reported penicillin allergy should be confirmed, preferably in consultation with an allergist.

TABLE 37-1

2002–2003 WORLD HEALTH ORGANIZATION CRITERIA FOR THE DIAGNOSIS OF RHEUMATIC FEVER AND RHEUMATIC HEART DISEASE (BASED ON THE 1992 REVISED JONES CRITERIA)

DIAGNOSTIC CATEGORIES	CRITERIA
Primary episode of rheumatic fever[a]	Two major or one major and two minor manifestations plus evidence of preceding group A streptococcal infection
Recurrent attack of rheumatic fever in a patient without established rheumatic heart disease	Two major or one major and two minor manifestations plus evidence of preceding group A streptococcal infection
Recurrent attack of rheumatic fever in a patient with established rheumatic heart disease[b]	Two minor manifestations plus evidence of preceding group A streptococcal infection[c]
Rheumatic chorea	Other major manifestations or evidence of group A streptococcal infection not required
Insidious onset rheumatic carditis[b]	Do not require any other criteria to be diagnosed as having rheumatic heart disease
Chronic valve lesions of rheumatic heart disease (patients presenting for the first time with pure mitral stenosis or mixed mitral valve disease and/or aortic valve disease)[d]	
Major manifestations	Carditis Polyarthritis Chorea Erythema marginatum Subcutaneous nodules
Minor manifestations	Clinical: fever, polyarthralgia Laboratory: elevated erythrocyte sedimentation rate or leukocyte count[e] Electrocardiogram: prolonged P-R interval
Supporting evidence of a preceding streptococcal infection within the last 45 days	Elevated or rising anti-streptolysin O or other streptococcal antibody, *or* A positive throat culture, *or* Rapid antigen test for group A streptococcus, *or* Recent scarlet fever[e]

[a]Patients may present with polyarthritis (or with only polyarthralgia or monoarthritis) and with several (three or more) other minor manifestations, together with evidence of recent group A streptococcal infection. Some of these cases may later turn out to be rheumatic fever. It is prudent to consider them as cases of "probable rheumatic fever" (once other diagnoses are excluded) and advise regular secondary prophylaxis. Such patients require close follow-up and regular examination of the heart. This cautious approach is particularly suitable for patients in vulnerable age groups in high incidence settings.
[b]Infective endocarditis should be excluded.
[c]Some patients with recurrent attacks may not fulfill these criteria.
[d]Congenital heart disease should be excluded.
[e]1992 Revised Jones criteria do not include elevated leukocyte count as a laboratory minor manifestation (but do include elevated C-reactive protein), and do not include recent scarlet fever as supporting evidence of a recent streptococcal infection.
Source: Reprinted with permission from WHO Expert Consultation on Rheumatic Fever and Rheumatic Heart Disease (2001: Geneva, Switzerland): *Rheumatic Fever and Rheumatic Heart Disease: Report of a WHO Expert Consultation* (WHO Tech Rep Ser, 923). Geneva, World Health Organization, 2004.

SALICYLATES AND NSAIDS These may be used for the treatment of arthritis, arthralgia, and fever, once the diagnosis is confirmed. They are of no value in the treatment of carditis or chorea. Aspirin is the drug of choice. An initial dose of 80–100 mg/kg per day in children (4–8 g/d in adults) in 4–5 divided doses is often needed for the first few days up to 2 weeks. A lower dose should be used if symptoms of salicylate toxicity emerge, such as nausea, vomiting, or tinnitus. When the acute symptoms are substantially resolved, the dose can be reduced to 60–70 mg/kg per day for a further 2–4 weeks. Fever, joint manifestations, and elevated acute-phase reactants sometimes recur up to 3 weeks after the medication is discontinued. This does not indicate a recurrence and can be managed by recommencing salicylates for a brief period. Although less well studied, naproxen at a dose of 10–20 mg/kg per day has been reported to lead to good symptomatic response.

CONGESTIVE HEART FAILURE

Glucocorticoids The use of glucocorticoids in ARF remains controversial. Two meta-analyses have failed to demonstrate a benefit of glucocorticoids compared with placebo or salicylates in improving the short- or longer term outcome of carditis. However, the studies included in these meta-analyses all took place >40 years ago and did not use medications in common usage today. Many

TABLE 37-2

RECOMMENDED TESTS IN CASES OF POSSIBLE ACUTE RHEUMATIC FEVER

Recommended for all cases
White blood cell count
Erythrocyte sedimentation rate
C-reactive protein
Blood cultures if febrile
Electrocardiogram (repeat in 2 weeks and 2 months if prolonged P-R interval or other rhythm abnormality)
Chest x-ray if clinical or echocardiographic evidence of carditis
Echocardiogram (consider repeating after 1 month if negative)
Throat swab (preferably before giving antibiotics)—culture for group A streptococcus
Anti-streptococcal serology: both anti-streptolysin O and anti-DNase B titres, if available (repeat 10–14 days later if 1st test not confirmatory)
Tests for alternative diagnoses, depending on clinical features
Repeated blood cultures if possible endocarditis
Joint aspirate (microscopy and culture) for possible septic arthritis
Copper, ceruloplasmin, antinuclear antibody, drug screen for choreiform movements
Serology and autoimmune markers for arboviral, autoimmune or reactive arthritis

Source: Reprinted with permission from National Heart Foundation of Australia.

clinicians treat cases of severe carditis (causing heart failure) with glucocorticoids in the belief that they may reduce the acute inflammation and result in more rapid resolution of failure. However, the potential benefits of this treatment should be balanced against the possible adverse effects, including gastrointestinal bleeding and fluid retention. If used, prednisone or prednisolone are recommended at doses of 1–2 mg/kg per day (maximum, 80 mg). Intravenous methylprednisolone may be used in very severe carditis. Glucocorticoids are often only required for a few days or up to a maximum of 3 weeks.

BED REST Traditional recommendations for long-term bed rest, once the cornerstone of management, are no longer widely practiced. Instead, bed rest should be prescribed as needed while arthritis and arthralgia are present, and for patients with heart failure. Once symptoms are well controlled, gradual mobilization can commence as tolerated.

CHOREA Medications to control the abnormal movements do not alter the duration or outcome of chorea. Milder cases can usually be managed by providing a calm environment. In patients with severe chorea, carbamazepine or sodium valproate are preferred to haloperidol. A response may not be seen for 1–2 weeks, and a successful response may only be to reduce rather than resolve the abnormal movements. Medication should be continued for 1–2 weeks after symptoms subside.

INTRAVENOUS IMMUNOGLOBULIN (IVIg) Small studies have suggested that IVIg may lead to more rapid resolution of chorea but has shown no benefit on the short- or long-term outcome of carditis in ARF without chorea. In the absence of better data, IVIg is *not* recommended, except in cases of severe chorea refractory to other treatments.

PROGNOSIS

Untreated, ARF lasts on average 12 weeks. With treatment, patients are usually discharged from hospital within 1–2 weeks. Inflammatory markers should be monitored every 1–2 weeks until they have normalized (usually within 4–6 weeks), and an echocardiogram should be performed after 1 month to determine whether there has been progression of carditis. Cases with more severe carditis need close clinical and echocardiographic monitoring in the longer term.

Once the acute episode has resolved, the priority in management is to ensure long-term clinical follow-up and adherence to a regimen of secondary prophylaxis. Patients should be entered onto the local ARF registry (if present) and contact made with primary care practitioners to ensure a plan for follow-up and administration of secondary prophylaxis before the patient is discharged. Patients and their families should also be educated about their disease, emphasizing the importance of adherence to secondary prophylaxis. If carditis is present, they should also be informed of the need for antibiotic prophylaxis against endocarditis for dental and surgical procedures.

PREVENTION

Primary Prevention

Ideally, primary prevention would entail elimination of the major risk factors for streptococcal infection, particularly overcrowded housing and inadequate hygiene infrastructure. This is difficult to achieve in most places where ARF is common.

Therefore, the mainstay of primary prevention for ARF remains primary prophylaxis, i.e., the timely and complete treatment of group A streptococcal sore throat with antibiotics. If commenced within 9 days of sore throat onset, a course of 10 days of penicillin V (500 mg bid PO in adults) or a single IM injection of 1.2 million units of benzathine penicillin G will prevent almost all cases of ARF that would otherwise have developed. This important strategy relies on individuals presenting for medical care when they have a sore throat, the availability of trained health and microbiology staff along with the materials and infrastructure to take throat swabs, and a reliable supply of penicillin. Unfortunately, many of these elements are not available in developing countries. Moreover, the majority of cases of ARF do not follow a sore throat sufficiently severe for the patient to seek medical attention.

TABLE 37-3

SUGGESTED DURATION OF SECONDARY PROPHYLAXIS[a]

CATEGORY OF PATIENT	DURATION OF PROPHYLAXIS
Patient without proven carditis	For 5 years after the last attack or 18 years of age (whichever is longer)
Patient with carditis (mild mitral regurgitation or healed carditis)	For 10 years after the last attack, or 25 years of age (whichever is longer)
More severe valvular disease	Lifelong
Valvular surgery	Lifelong

[a]These are only recommendations and must be modified by individual circumstances as warranted.

Source: Reprinted with permission from WHO Expert Consultation on Rheumatic Fever and Rheumatic Heart Disease (2001: Geneva, Switzerland): *Rheumatic Fever and Rheumatic Heart Disease: Report of a WHO Expert Consultation* (WHO Tech Rep Ser, 923). Geneva, World Health Organization, 2004.

Secondary Prevention

The mainstay of controlling ARF and RHD is secondary prevention. Because patients with ARF are at dramatically higher risk than the general population of developing a further episode of ARF after a group A streptococcal infection, they should receive long-term penicillin prophylaxis to prevent recurrences. The best antibiotic for secondary prophylaxis is benzathine penicillin G (1.2 million units, or 600,000 units if <30 kg) delivered every 4 weeks or more frequently (e.g., every 3 weeks or even every 2 weeks) to persons considered to be at particularly high risk. Oral penicillin V (250 mg) can be given twice-daily instead but is somewhat less effective than benzathine penicillin G. Penicillin allergic patients can receive erythromycin (250 mg) twice daily.

The duration of secondary prophylaxis is determined by many factors, in particular the duration since the last episode of ARF (recurrences become less likely with increasing time), age (recurrences are less likely with increasing age), and the severity of RHD (if severe, it may be prudent to avoid even a very small risk of recurrence because of the potentially serious consequences) (Table 37-3). Secondary prophylaxis is best delivered as part of a coordinated RHD control program, based around a registry of patients. Registries improve the ability to follow patients and identify those who default from prophylaxis and institute strategies to improve adherence.

FURTHER READINGS

Bryant PA et al: Some of the people, some of the time: Susceptibility to acute rheumatic fever. Circulation 119:742, 2009

Carapetis JR et al: Acute rheumatic fever. Lancet 366:155, 2005

——— et al: The global burden of group A streptococcal diseases. Lancet Infect Dis 5:685, 2005

Cilliers AM: Rheumatic fever and its management. BMJ 333:1153, 2006

Guilherme L et al: Molecular mimicry in the autoimmune pathogenesis of rheumatic heart disease. Autoimmunity 39:31, 2006

National Heart Foundation of Australia: *Diagnosis and Management of Acute Rheumatic Fever and Rheumatic Heart Disease in Australia: Complete Evidence-Based Review and Guideline.* Melbourne, National Heart Foundation of Australia, 2006

Special Writing Group of the Committee on Rheumatic Fever, Endocarditis and Kawasaki Disease of the American Heart Association: Guidelines for the diagnosis of acute rheumatic fever: Jones criteria, 1992 update. JAMA 268:2069, 1992

Tibazarwa KB et al: Incidence of acute rheumatic fever in the world: A systematic review of population-based studies. Heart 94:1534, 2008

CHAPTER 38

DIPHTHERIA AND OTHER INFECTIONS CAUSED BY CORYNEBACTERIA AND RELATED SPECIES

William R. Bishai ■ John R. Murphy

DIPHTHERIA

Diphtheria is a nasopharyngeal and skin infection caused by *Corynebacterium diphtheriae*. Toxigenic strains of *C. diphtheriae* produce a protein toxin that causes systemic toxicity, myocarditis, and polyneuropathy. The toxin is associated with the formation of pseudomembranes in the pharynx during respiratory diphtheria. Although toxigenic strains most frequently cause pharyngeal diphtheria, nontoxigenic strains commonly cause cutaneous disease. In the United States and Europe, diphtheria has been controlled in recent years with effective vaccination, although sporadic outbreaks have occurred. Diphtheria is still common in the Caribbean, Latin America, and the Indian subcontinent, where mass immunization programs are not enforced. Large epidemics have occurred in the independent states formerly encompassed by the Soviet Union. Additional outbreaks have been reported in Algeria, China, and Ecuador.

ETIOLOGY

C. diphtheriae is a gram-positive, unencapsulated, nonmotile, nonsporulating bacillus. *C. diphtheriae* organisms have a characteristic club-shaped bacillary appearance and typically form clusters of parallel rays (palisades) that are referred to as *Chinese characters*. In the specific laboratory media recommended for the cultivation of *C. diphtheriae*, tellurite, colistin, or nalidixic acid is responsible for selective isolation of the organism in the presence of other autochthonous pharyngeal microbes. Human isolates of *C. diphtheriae* may display nontoxigenic (tox^-) or toxigenic (tox^+) phenotypes. Corynebacteriophage beta carries the structural gene (*tox*) encoding diphtheria toxin, and a family of closely related corynebacteriophages are responsible for toxigenic conversion of tox^- *C. diphtheriae* to the tox^+ phenotype. Moreover, lysogenic conversion from a nontoxigenic to a toxigenic phenotype has been shown to occur in situ. Growth of toxigenic strains of *C. diphtheriae* under iron-limiting conditions leads to the optimal expression of diphtheria toxin, and these conditions are believed to be a mechanism of pathogenesis during human infection.

EPIDEMIOLOGY

C. diphtheriae is transmitted via the aerosol route, primarily during close contact. There are no significant reservoirs other than humans. The incubation period for respiratory diphtheria is 2–5 days; however, disease can develop as long as 10 days after exposure. Before the vaccine era, most individuals over the age of 10 were immune to *C. diphtheriae*; infants were protected by maternal IgG antibodies but became susceptible after ~6 months of age. Thus the disease was seen primarily in children and nonimmune young adults. In temperate regions, respiratory diphtheria occurs year-round but is most common during winter months.

The development of diphtheria antitoxin and diphtheria toxoid vaccine led to the near-elimination of diphtheria in Western countries. The annual peak incidence rate was 191 cases per 100,000 population in the United States in 1921; in contrast, since 1980, the annual figure for the United States as a whole has been <5 cases. Nevertheless, pockets of colonization have persisted in North America, particularly in South Dakota, Ontario, and Washington state. Immunity induced by vaccination during childhood gradually decreases in adulthood. An estimated 30% of men 60–69 years old have antitoxin titers below the protective level. In addition to older age and lack of vaccination, risk factors for diphtheria outbreaks include alcoholism, low socioeconomic status, crowded living conditions, and Native American ethnic background. An outbreak that occurred in Seattle in 1972–1982 included 1100 cases, primarily manifesting as cutaneous disease. During the 1990s in the states of the former Soviet Union, a much larger diphtheria epidemic caused >150,000 cases and >5000 deaths. Clonally related toxigenic *C. diphtheriae* strains of the ET8 complex were associated with this outbreak. Given that the ET8 complex expressed a toxin against which the prevalent diphtheria toxoid vaccine was effective, the epidemic was attributed to failure of the public health infrastructure to effectively vaccinate the population. Beginning in 1998, the epidemic was controlled by mass vaccination programs. During the epidemic, the incidence rate was high among individuals from >15 years of age up to 50 years of age. Socioeconomic instability, migration, deteriorating public health programs, frequent vaccine shortages, delays in implementation of vaccination and of treatment in response to cases, and lack of public education and awareness were contributing factors in that outbreak.

Cutaneous diphtheria is usually a secondary infection that follows a primary skin lesion due to trauma, allergy, or autoimmunity. Most often, isolates from cases of cutaneous disease lack the *tox* gene and therefore do not express diphtheria toxin. In tropical regions, cutaneous diphtheria is more common than respiratory diphtheria. In contrast to respiratory disease, cutaneous diphtheria is not a reportable disease in United States.

Nontoxigenic strains of *C. diphtheriae* have also been associated with pharyngitis in Europe. Outbreaks have occurred among homosexual men and IV drug users.

PATHOGENESIS AND IMMUNOLOGY

Diphtheria toxin, produced by toxigenic strains of *C. diphtheriae*, is the primary virulence factor in clinical disease. The toxin is synthesized in precursor form; is released as a 535-amino-acid, single-chain protein; and has an LD_{50} of ~100 ng/kg of body weight. The toxin is produced in the pseudomembranous lesion and is taken up into the bloodstream, through which it is distributed to all organ systems. Once bound to its cell surface receptor (a heparin-binding, epidermal growth factor–like precursor), the toxin is internalized by receptor-mediated endocytosis and enters the cytosol from an acidified early endosomal compartment. In vitro, the toxin may be separated into two chains after digestion with serine proteases: the N-terminal A fragment and the C-terminal B fragment. Delivery of the A fragment into the eukaryotic cell cytosol results in irreversible inhibition of protein synthesis by NAD+-dependent ADP ribosylation of elongation factor 2. The eventual result is the death of the cell.

In 1926, Ramon at the Institut Pasteur found that formalinization of diphtheria toxin resulted in the production of diphtheria toxoid, which was nontoxic but highly immunogenic. Subsequent studies showed that immunization with diphtheria toxoid elicited antibodies that neutralized the toxin and prevented most manifestations of diphtheria. In the 1930s, mass immunization of children and susceptible adults commenced in the United States and Europe.

Individuals with an antitoxin titer of >0.01 unit/mL are at low risk of diphtheria disease. In populations where a majority of individuals have protective antitoxin titers, the carrier rate for toxigenic strains of *C. diphtheriae* decreases and the overall risk of diphtheria among susceptible individuals is reduced. Nevertheless, individuals with nonprotective titers may contract diphtheria through either travel or exposure to individuals who have recently returned from regions where the disease is endemic.

Characteristic pathologic findings of diphtheria include mucosal ulcers with a pseudomembranous coating composed of an inner band of fibrin and a luminal band of neutrophils. Initially white and firmly adherent, in advanced diphtheria the pseudomembranes turn gray and even green or black as necrosis progresses. Mucosal ulcers result from toxin-induced necrosis of the epithelium accompanied by edema, hyperemia, and vascular congestion of the submucosal base. A fibrinosuppurative exudate from the ulcer develops into the pseudomembrane. Ulcers and pseudomembranes in severe respiratory diphtheria may extend from the pharynx into medium-sized bronchial airways. Expanding and sloughing membranes may result in fatal airway obstruction.

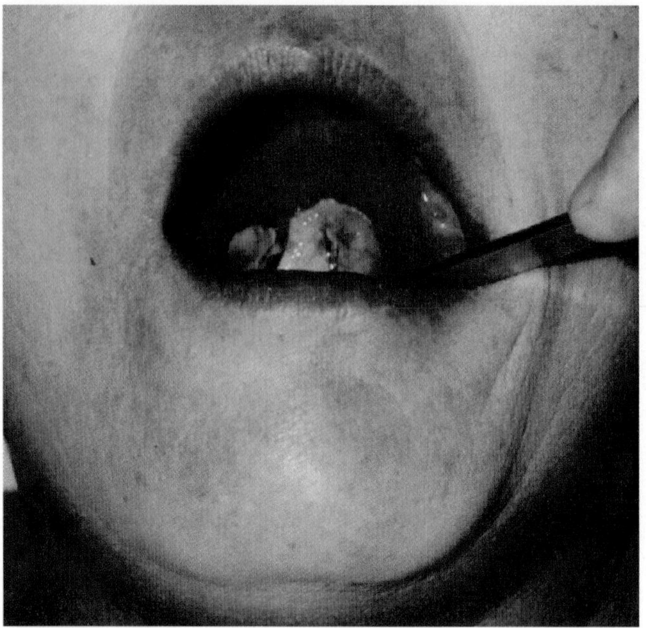

FIGURE 38-1
Respiratory diphtheria due to toxigenic *C. diphtheriae* producing exudative pharyngitis in a 47-year-old woman with neck edema and a pseudomembrane extending from the uvula to the pharyngeal wall. The characteristic white pseudomembrane is caused by diphtheria toxin–mediated necrosis of the respiratory epithelial layer, producing fibrinous coagulative exudate. Submucosal edema adds to airway narrowing. The pharyngitis is acute in onset, and respiratory obstruction from the pseudomembrane may occur in severe cases. Inoculation of pseudomembrane fragments or submembranous swabs onto Löffler's or tellurite selective medium reveals C. diphtheriae. (*Photograph by P. Strebel, MD, used with permission. From Kadirova et al.*)

Approach to the Patient: DIPHTHERIA

Although diphtheria is rare in the United States and other developed countries, this diagnosis should be considered in patients who have severe pharyngitis, particularly with difficulty swallowing, respiratory compromise, or signs of systemic disease, including myocarditis or generalized weakness. In the differential diagnosis, the leading causes of pharyngitis that should be considered are respiratory viruses (rhinoviruses, influenza viruses, parainfluenza viruses, coronaviruses, and adenoviruses; ~25% of cases), group A streptococci (15–30%), group C streptococci (~5%), atypical bacteria such as *Mycoplasma pneumoniae* and *Chlamydophila pneumoniae* (15–20% in some series), and other viruses such as herpes simplex virus (~4%) and Epstein-Barr virus (EBV; <1% in infectious mononucleosis). Less common causes are acute HIV infection, infection with *Neisseria gonorrhoeae*, fusobacterial infection (e.g., Lemierre's syndrome), and thrush due to *Candida albicans* or other *Candida* species. The presence of a pharyngeal pseudomembrane or an extensive exudate should prompt consideration of diphtheria (Fig. 38-1).

CLINICAL MANIFESTATIONS

Respiratory Diphtheria

The clinical diagnosis of diphtheria is based on the constellation of sore throat; adherent tonsillar, pharyngeal, or nasal pseudomembranous lesions; and low-grade fever. In addition, diagnosis requires the isolation of *C. diphtheriae* or the histopathologic isolation of compatible gram-positive organisms. The Centers for Disease Control and Prevention (CDC) recognizes confirmed respiratory diphtheria (laboratory proven or epidemiologically linked to a culture-confirmed case) and probable respiratory diphtheria (clinically compatible but not laboratory proven or epidemiologically linked). Carriers are defined as individuals who have positive cultures for *C. diphtheriae* and either are asymptomatic or have symptoms but lack pseudomembranes. Most patients seek medical care for initial manifestations of sore throat and fever. Occasionally, weakness, dysphagia, headache, and voice change are the initial manifestations. Neck edema and difficulty breathing are seen in more advanced cases and carry a poor prognosis.

The systemic manifestations of diphtheria stem from the effects of diphtheria toxin and include weakness as a result of neurotoxicity and cardiac arrhythmias or congestive heart failure due to myocarditis. The pseudomembranous lesion is most often located in the tonsillopharyngeal region. Less commonly, the lesions are detected in the larynx, nares, and trachea or bronchial passages. Large pseudomembranes are associated with severe disease and a poor prognosis. A few patients develop massive swelling of the tonsils and present with "bull-neck" diphtheria, which results from massive edema of the submandibular and paratracheal region

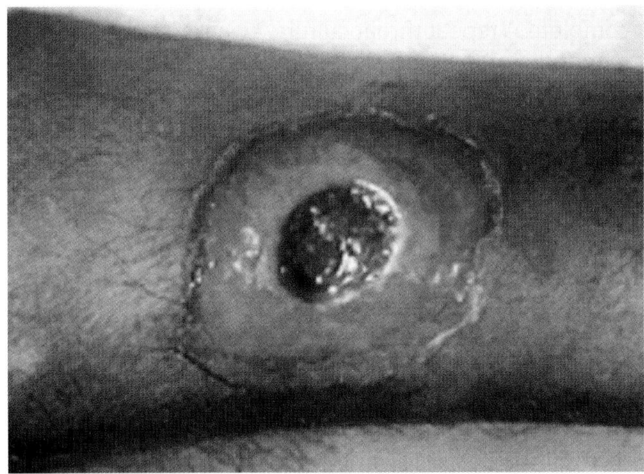

FIGURE 38-2
Cutaneous diphtheria due to nontoxigenic *C. diphtheriae* on the lower extremity. (*From the Centers for Disease Control and Prevention.*)

and is further characterized by foul breath, thick speech, and stridorous breathing. The diphtheritic pseudomembrane is gray or whitish and sharply demarcated. Unlike the exudative lesion associated with streptococcal pharyngitis, the pseudomembrane in diphtheria is tightly adherent to the underlying tissues. Attempts to dislodge the membrane may cause bleeding. Hoarseness suggests laryngeal diphtheria, in which laryngoscopy may be diagnostically helpful.

Cutaneous Diphtheria

This is a variable dermatosis most often characterized by punched-out ulcerative lesions with necrotic sloughing or pseudomembrane formation (Fig. 38-2). The diagnosis requires cultivation of *C. diphtheriae* from lesions, which most commonly occur on the extremities. Patients usually seek medical attention because of nonhealing or enlarging skin ulcers, which may be associated with a preexisting wound or dermatoses such as eczema, psoriasis, and venous stasis disease. The lesions rarely exceed 5 cm.

Other Clinical Manifestations

C. diphtheriae causes rare cases of endocarditis and septic arthritis, most often in patients with preexisting risk factors such as cardiac valvular disease, injection drug use, or cirrhosis.

COMPLICATIONS

Airway obstruction poses a significant early risk in patients presenting with advanced diphtheria. Pseudomembranes may slough and obstruct the airway or may advance to the larynx or into the tracheobronchial tree. Children are particularly prone to obstruction because of their small airways.

Polyneuropathy and myocarditis are late toxic manifestations of diphtheria. During the outbreak in the Kyrgyz Republic in 1995, myocarditis was seen in 22% and neuropathy in 5% of hospitalized patients. The mortality rate was 7% among patients with myocarditis as opposed to 2% among those without myocardial manifestations. The median time to death in hospitalized patients was 4.5 days. Myocarditis is typically associated with dysrhythmia of the conduction tract and dilated cardiomyopathy.

Neurologic manifestations may appear during the first or second week of illness, typically beginning with dysphagia and nasal dysarthria and progressing to other signs of cranial nerve involvement, including weakness of the tongue and facial numbness. Ciliary paralysis, which is typical, manifests as blurred vision due to paralysis of pupillary accommodation, with a preserved light reflex. Cranial neuropathy may be followed by respiratory and abdominal muscle weakness requiring artificial ventilation. Several weeks later—sometimes as cranial neuropathy is improving—a generalized sensorimotor polyneuropathy may appear, with prominent autonomic manifestations (including hypotension) in some cases. The clinical syndrome and the findings on lumbar puncture of raised levels of protein without pleocytosis in cerebrospinal fluid resemble Guillain-Barré syndrome. Pathologically, diphtheria neuropathy is a noninflammatory demyelinating disorder mediated by the exotoxin. Gradual improvement is the rule in patients who survive the acute phase.

Other complications of diphtheria include pneumonia, renal failure, encephalitis, cerebral infarction, and pulmonary embolism. Serum sickness can result from treatment with diphtheria antitoxin (see "Diphtheria Treatment" later in the chapter).

DIAGNOSIS

The diagnosis of diphtheria is based on clinical signs and symptoms plus laboratory confirmation. Respiratory diphtheria should be considered in patients with sore throat, pharyngeal exudates, and fever. Other symptoms may include hoarseness, stridor, or palatal paralysis. The presence of a pseudomembrane should prompt consideration of diphtheria. Once a clinical diagnosis of diphtheria is made, diphtheria antitoxin should be administered as soon as possible.

Laboratory diagnosis is based either on cultivation of *C. diphtheriae* or toxigenic *C. ulcerans* from the site of infection or on the demonstration of local lesions with characteristic histopathology. *C. pseudodiphtheriticum*, a nontoxigenic organism, is a common component of the normal throat flora and does not pose a significant risk. Throat samples should be submitted to the laboratory for culture with the notation that diphtheria is being considered. This information should prompt cultivation on special selective medium and subsequent biochemical testing to differentiate *C. diphtheriae* from other nasopharyngeal commensal corynebacteria. All laboratory isolates of *C. diphtheriae*, including nontoxigenic strains, should be submitted to the CDC.

A diagnosis of cutaneous diphtheria requires laboratory confirmation since the lesions are not characteristic and are clinically indistinguishable from other dermatoses. Diphtheritic ulcers occasionally—but not consistently—have a punched-out appearance (Fig. 38-2). Patients in whom cutaneous diphtheria is identified should have the nasopharynx cultured for *C. diphtheriae*. The laboratory media for cutaneous diphtheria are the same as those used for respiratory diphtheria: Löffler's or Tinsdale's selective medium in addition to nonselective medium such as blood agar. As has been mentioned, respiratory diphtheria remains a notifiable disease in the United States, whereas cutaneous diphtheria is not.

℞ Treatment: DIPHTHERIA

DIPHTHERIA ANTITOXIN Prompt administration of diphtheria antitoxin is critical in the management of respiratory diphtheria. The antitoxin—a horse antiserum—is effective in reducing the extent of local disease as well as the risk of complications of myocarditis and neuropathy. Rapid institution of antitoxin therapy is also associated with a significant reduction in mortality risk. Because diphtheria antitoxin cannot neutralize cell-bound toxin, prompt initiation is important. This product, which is no longer made commercially in the United States, is available from the CDC under an investigational new drug protocol and may be obtained by calling the Bacterial Vaccine Preventable Disease Branch of the National Immunization Program at 404-639-3670 between 8:00 A.M. and 4:30 P.M. U.S. Eastern time or at 770-488-7100 at other hours; the relevant website is *http://www.cdc.gov/vaccines/vpd-vac/diphtheria/dat/dat-main.htm.* The current protocol for the use of antitoxin includes a test dose to rule out immediate-type hypersensitivity. Patients who exhibit hypersensitivity require desensitization before a full therapeutic dose of antitoxin is administered.

ANTIMICROBIAL THERAPY Antibiotics are used in the management of diphtheria primarily to prevent transmission to other susceptible contacts. Recommended options for the treatment of patients with respiratory diphtheria are as follows: (1) procaine penicillin G at a dosage of 600,000 units (for children, 12,500–25,000 U/kg) IM every 12 h until the patient can swallow comfortably, after which oral penicillin V is given at 125–250 mg four times daily to complete a 14-day course; or (2) erythromycin at a dosage of 500 mg IV every 6 h (for children, 40–50 mg/kg per day IV in two or four divided doses) until the patient can swallow comfortably, after which 500 mg is given PO four times daily to complete a 14-day course.

A clinical study in Vietnam found that penicillin was associated with a more rapid resolution of fever and a lower rate of bacterial resistance than erythromycin; however, relapses were more common with penicillin. Erythromycin therapy targets protein synthesis and thus offers the presumed benefit of stopping toxin synthesis more quickly than a cell wall–active β-lactam agent. Alternative agents for patients who are allergic to penicillin or cannot take erythromycin include rifampin and clindamycin. Eradication of *C. diphtheriae* should be documented at least 1 day after antimicrobial therapy is complete. A repeat throat culture 2 weeks later is recommended. For patients in whom the organism is not eradicated after a 14-day course of erythromycin or penicillin, an additional 10-day course followed by repeat culture is recommended.

Cutaneous diphtheria should be treated as described above for respiratory disease. Individuals infected with toxigenic strains should receive antitoxin. It is important to treat the underlying cause of the dermatoses in addition to the superinfection with *C. diphtheriae.*

Patients who recover from respiratory or cutaneous diphtheria should have antitoxin levels measured. If diphtheria antitoxin has been administered, this test should be performed 6 months later. Patients who recover from respiratory or cutaneous diphtheria should receive the appropriate vaccine (see "Prevention" later in the chapter) to ensure the development of protective antibody titers, which does not occur in all cases.

MANAGEMENT Patients in whom diphtheria is suspected should be hospitalized in respiratory isolation rooms, with close monitoring of cardiac and respiratory function. A cardiac workup is recommended to assess the possibility of myocarditis. In patients with extensive pseudomembranes, consultation with an anesthesiologist or an ear, nose, and throat specialist is recommended because of the possibility that tracheostomy or intubation will be required. In some settings, pseudomembranes can be removed surgically. Treatment with glucocorticoids has not been shown to reduce the risk of myocarditis or polyneuropathy.

PROGNOSIS

Fatal pseudomembranous diphtheria typically occurs in patients with nonprotective antibody titers and in unimmunized patients. The pseudomembrane may increase in size from the time it is first noted. Risk factors for death include bullneck diphtheria, myocarditis with ventricular tachycardia, atrial fibrillation, complete heart block, an age of >60 years or <6 months, alcoholism, extensive pseudomembrane elongation, and laryngeal, tracheal, or bronchial involvement. Another important predictor of fatal outcome is the interval between local disease development and antitoxin administration. Cutaneous diphtheria has a low mortality rate and is rarely associated with myocarditis or peripheral neuropathy.

PREVENTION

Vaccination

Sustained campaigns for vaccination of children and adequate boosting vaccination of adults are responsible for the exceedingly low incidence of diphtheria in most developed nations. At present, diphtheria toxoid vaccine is coadministered with tetanus (with or without acellular pertussis) vaccine. DTaP (full-level diphtheria and tetanus toxoids and acellular pertussis vaccine, adsorbed) is the currently recommended vaccine for children up to the age of 7; DTaP replaced DTP (diphtheria and tetanus toxoids and whole-cell pertussis vaccine) in 1997. Tdap is a tetanus toxoid, reduced diphtheria toxoid, and acellular pertussis vaccine formulated for adolescents and adults. Tdap was licensed for use in the United States in 2005 and is the recommended booster vaccine for children 11–12 years old and the recommended catch-up vaccine for children 7–10 and 13–18 years old. As of 2006, it is recommended that (1) adults 19–64 years old receive a single dose of Tdap if their last dose of Td (tetanus and reduced-dose diphtheria toxoids, adsorbed) was >10 years earlier and (2) intervals of <10 years be implemented for Tdap vaccination of health care workers, adults anticipating contact with infants, and adults not previously vaccinated for pertussis. Adults who have received acellular pertussis vaccines should continue to receive decennial Td booster vaccinations.

The vaccination schedule is detailed in Chap. 3.

Prophylaxis of Contacts

Close contacts of diphtheria cases should undergo throat culture to determine whether they are carriers. After samples for throat culture are obtained, antimicrobial prophylaxis should be considered for all close contacts, even those who are culture-negative. The options are 7–10 days of oral erythromycin or one dose of IM benzathine penicillin G (1.2 million units for persons ≥6 years old or 600,000 units for children <6 years old).

Contacts of diphtheria cases who have an uncertain immunization status should receive the appropriate diphtheria toxoid–containing vaccine. Tdap (rather than Td) is now recommended as the booster vaccine of choice for adults who have not recently received an acellular pertussis–containing vaccine. Carriers of *C. diphtheriae* in the community should be treated and vaccinated when identified.

NONDIPHTHERIAL CORYNEBACTERIA AND RELATED SPECIES

Nondiphtherial corynebacteria, which are also referred to as *diphtheroids* or *coryneforms*, are a widely diverse collection of bacteria that are taxonomically lumped together on the basis of their 16S rDNA signature nucleotides. The diversity of this group is exemplified by the wide range in guanine-plus-cytosine content (45–70%). Although frequently considered colonizers or contaminants, the nondiphtherial corynebacteria have been associated with invasive disease, particularly in immunocompromised patients. Specifically, for example, these organisms have been implicated in bacteremia, particularly in association with catheterization, endocarditis, prosthetic valve infection, meningitis, neurosurgical shunt infection, brain abscess, peritonitis (often in the setting of chronic ambulatory peritoneal dialysis), osteomyelitis, septic arthritis, urinary tract infection, empyema, and pneumonia. Patients infected with nondiphtherial corynebacteria usually have significant medical comorbidity or immunosuppression. Several of these organisms, including *C. jeikeium* and *C. urealyticum*, are associated with resistance to multiple antibiotics. The related organism *Rhodococcus equi* is associated with necrotizing pneumonia and granulomatous infection, particularly in immunocompromised individuals. Other related species that can cause infections in humans are *Actinomyces* (formerly *Corynebacterium*) *pyogenes* and *Arcanobacterium* (formerly *Corynebacterium*) *haemolyticum*.

MICROBIOLOGY AND LABORATORY DIAGNOSIS

These organisms are non–acid-fast, catalase-positive, aerobic or facultatively anaerobic bacilli. Their colonial morphologies vary widely; some species are small and α-hemolytic (similar to lactobacilli), whereas others form large white colonies (similar to yeasts). Many nondiphtherial coryneforms require special medium (e.g., Löffler's, Tinsdale's, or telluride medium) for growth.

EPIDEMIOLOGY

Humans are the natural reservoirs for several nondiphtherial coryneforms, including *C. xerosis*, *C. pseudodiphtheriticum*, *C. striatum*, *C. minutissimum*, *C. jeikeium*, *C. urealyticum*, and *A. haemolyticum*. Animal reservoirs are responsible for carriage of *A. pyogenes*, *C. ulcerans*, and *C. pseudotuberculosis*. Soil is the natural reservoir for *R. equi*.

C. pseudodiphtheriticum is part of the normal flora of the human pharynx and skin. *C. xerosis* is found on the skin, nasopharynx, and conjunctiva; *C. auris* in the external auditory canal; and *C. striatum* in the anterior nares and on the skin. *C. jeikeium* and *C. urealyticum* are found in the axilla, groin, and perineum, particularly in hospitalized patients. *C. ulcerans* and *C. pseudotuberculosis* infections have been associated with the consumption of raw milk from infected cattle.

Specific Nondiphtherial Coryneforms

C. Ulcerans

This organism causes a diphtheria-like illness and produces both diphtheria toxin and a dermonecrotic toxin. *C. ulcerans* is a commensal in horses and cattle and has been isolated from cow's milk. The organism causes exudative pharyngitis, primarily during summer months, in rural areas, and among individuals exposed to cattle. In contrast to diphtheria, *C. ulcerans* infection is considered a zoonosis, and person-to-person transmission has not been firmly established. Nevertheless, treatment with antitoxin and antibiotics should be initiated when respiratory *C. ulcerans* is identified, and a contact investigation (including throat cultures to determine the need for antimicrobial prophylaxis and vaccination with the appropriate diphtheria toxoid–containing vaccine for unimmunized human contacts) should be conducted. The organism grows on Löffler's, Tinsdale's, and telluride media as well as blood agar. In addition to exudative pharyngitis, cutaneous disease due to *C. ulcerans* has been reported. *C. ulcerans* is susceptible to a wide panel of antibiotics. Erythromycin and macrolides appear to be the first-line agents.

C. Pseudotuberculosis (ovis)

Infections caused by *C. pseudotuberculosis* are rare and are reported almost exclusively from Australia. *C. pseudotuberculosis* causes suppurative granulomatous lymphadenitis and an eosinophilic pneumonia syndrome among individuals who handle horses, cattle, goats, and deer or who drink unpasteurized milk. The organism is an important veterinary pathogen, causing suppurative lymphadenitis, abscesses, and pneumonia, but is rarely a human pathogen. Successful treatment with erythromycin or tetracycline has been reported, with surgery also performed when indicated.

C. Jeikeium (Group JK)

After a 1976 survey of diseases caused by nondiphtherial corynebacteria, CDC Group JK was recognized as an important opportunistic pathogen among neutropenic patients and later emerged in HIV-infected patients as an AIDS-associated opportunistic infection. This led to the organism's reclassification as a separate species, *C. jeikeium*. The predominant syndrome associated with *C. jeikeium* is sepsis, which can occur in conjunction with pneumonia, endocarditis, meningitis, osteomyelitis, or epidural abscess. Risk factors for *C. jeikeium* infection include hematologic malignancy, neutropenia from comorbid conditions, prolonged hospitalization, exposure to multiple antibiotics, and skin disruption. There is evidence that *C. jeikeium* is part of the normal flora of the inguinal, axillary, genital, and perirectal areas in hospitalized patients.

Broad-spectrum antimicrobial therapy appears to select for colonization. Originally described in the United States, *C. jeikeium* has also been reported in Europe. The gram-positive coccobacilli, which slightly resemble streptococci, grow as small, gray to white, glistening, nonhemolytic colonies on blood agar. *C. jeikeium* lacks urease and nitrate reductase and does not ferment most carbohydrates. It is resistant to most antibiotics tested except for vancomycin. Effective therapy involves removal of the source of infection, be it a catheter, a prosthetic joint, or a prosthetic valve. There have been efforts to prevent *C. jeikeium* infection by use of antibacterial soap in the care of high-risk patients in intensive care settings.

C. Urealyticum (Group D2)

Identified as a urease-positive nondiphtherial *Corynebacterium* in 1972, *C. urealyticum* is an opportunistic cause of sepsis and urinary tract infection. This organism appears to be the etiologic agent of a severe urinary tract syndrome known as *alkaline-encrusted cystitis*: a chronic inflammatory bladder infection associated with deposition of ammonium magnesium phosphate on the surface and walls of ulcerating lesions in the bladder. In addition, *C. urealyticum* has been associated with pneumonia, peritonitis, endocarditis, osteomyelitis, and wound infection. It is similar to *C. jeikeium* in its resistance to most antibiotics except vancomycin, which has been used successfully in the treatment of severe infections.

C. Minutissimum

Erythrasma is a cutaneous infection producing reddish-brown, macular, scaly, pruritic intertriginous patches. The dermatologic presentation under the Wood's lamp is of coral-red fluorescence. *C. minutissimum* appears to be a common cause of erythrasma, although there is evidence for a polymicrobial etiology in certain settings. In addition, this fluorescent microbe has been associated with bacteremia in patients with hematologic malignancy. Erythrasma responds to topical erythromycin, clarithromycin, clindamycin, or fusidic acid, although more severe infections may require oral macrolide therapy.

Other Nondiphtherial Corynebacteria

C. xerosis is a human commensal found in the conjunctiva, nasopharynx, and skin. This nontoxigenic organism is occasionally identified as a source of invasive infection in immunocompromised or postoperative patients and prosthetic joint recipients. *C. striatum* is found in the anterior nares and on the skin, face, and upper torso of normal individuals. Also nontoxigenic, this organism has been associated with invasive opportunistic infections in severely ill or immunocompromised patients. *C. amycolatum* is a new species isolated from human skin and is identified on the basis of a unique 16S ribosomal RNA sequence associated with opportunistic infection. *C. glucuronolyticum* is a new nonlipophilic species that causes male genitourinary tract infections such as prostatitis and urethritis. These infections may be successfully treated with a wide variety of antibacterial agents, including β-lactams, rifampin, aminoglycosides, or vancomycin; however, the organism appears to be resistant to fluoroquinolones, macrolides, and tetracyclines. *C. imitans* has been identified in Eastern Europe as a nontoxigenic cause of pharyngitis. *C. auris* has been isolated from children with otitis media and is susceptible to fluoroquinolones, rifampin, tetracycline, and vancomycin but resistant to penicillin G and variably susceptible to macrolides. *C. pseudodiphtheriticum* (*C. hofmannii*) is a nontoxigenic component of the normal human flora. Human infections—particularly endocarditis of either prosthetic or native valves and invasive pneumonia—have been identified only rarely. Although *C. pseudodiphtheriticum* may be isolated from the nasopharynx of patients with suspected diphtheria, it is part of the normal flora and does not produce diphtheria toxin. *C. propinquum*, a close relative of *C. pseudodiphtheriticum*, is part of CDC Group ANF-3 and is isolated from human respiratory tract specimens and blood. *C. afermentans* subspecies *lipophilum* belongs to CDC Group ANF-1 and has been isolated from human blood and abscess infections. *C. accolens* has been isolated from wound drainage, throat swabs, and sputum and is typically identified as a satellite of staphylococcal organisms; it has been associated with endocarditis. *C. bovis* is a veterinary commensal that has not been clearly identified as a cause of human disease. *C. aquaticum* is a water-associated organism that is occasionally isolated from patients using medical devices (e.g., for chronic ambulatory peritoneal dialysis or venous access).

Rhodococcus

Rhodococcus species are phylogenetically related to the corynebacteria. These gram-positive coccobacilli have been associated with tuberculosis-like infections in humans with granulomatous pathology. Although *R. equi* is best known, other species have been identified, including *R.* (also *Gordonia*) *bronchialis, R.* (also *Tsukamurella*) *aurantiacus, R. luteus, R. erythropolis, R. rhodochrous*, and *R. rubropertinctus. R. equi* has been recognized as a cause of pneumonia in horses since the 1920s; it causes related infections in cattle, sheep, and swine. *R. equi* is found in soil as an environmental microbe. The organisms vary in length; appear as spherical to long, curved, clubbed rods; and produce large, irregular mucoid colonies. *R. equi* does not ferment carbohydrates or liquefy gelatin and is often acid fast. An intracellular pathogen of macrophages, *R. equi* can cause granulomatous necrosis and caseation. The organism has been identified most commonly in pulmonary infections, but infections of brain, bone, and skin have also been reported. Most commonly, *R. equi* disease manifests as nodular cavitary pneumonia of the upper lobe—a picture similar to that seen in tuberculosis or nocardiosis. Most patients are immunocompromised, often with HIV infection. Subcutaneous nodular lesions have also been identified. The involvement of *R. equi* should be considered in any patient presenting with a tuberculosis-like syndrome. Infection due to *R. equi* has been treated successfully with antibiotics that penetrate intracellularly, including macrolides, clindamycin, rifampin, and trimethoprim-sulfamethoxazole. β-Lactam antibiotics have not been useful. The organism is routinely susceptible to vancomycin, which is considered the drug of choice.

Actinomyces Pyogenes

A cause of seasonal leg ulcers in humans in rural Thailand, *A. pyogenes* is a well-known pathogen of cattle, sheep, goats, and pigs. A few human cases of sepsis, endocarditis, septic arthritis, pneumonia, meningitis, and empyema have been reported. The agent is susceptible to β-lactams, tetracycline, aminoglycosides, and fluoroquinolones.

Arcanobacterium Haemolyticum

A. haemolyticum was identified as an agent of wound infections in U.S. soldiers in the South Pacific during World War II. This organism appears to be a commensal of the human nasopharynx and skin but has been implicated as a cause of pharyngitis and chronic skin ulcers. In contrast to the much more common pharyngitis caused by *Streptococcus pyogenes, A. haemolyticum* pharyngitis is associated with a scarlatiniform rash on the trunk and proximal extremities in about half of cases; this illness is occasionally confused with toxic shock syndrome. Because *A. haemolyticum* pharyngitis primarily affects teenagers, it has been postulated that the rash-pharyngitis syndrome may represent copathogenicity or synergy with EBV or opportunistic secondary infection complicating EBV infection. *A. haemolyticum* has also been reported as a cause of bacteremia, soft tissue infection, osteomyelitis, and cavitary pneumonia, predominantly in the setting of underlying diabetes mellitus. The organism is susceptible to β-lactams, macrolides, fluoroquinolones, clindamycin, vancomycin, and doxycycline. Penicillin resistance has been reported.

FURTHER READINGS

Centers for Disease Control and Prevention: Availability of diphtheria antitoxin through an investigational new drug protocol. MMWR 53:413, 2004

———: Vaccine preventable deaths and the Global Immunization Vision and Strategy, 2006–2015. MMWR 55:511, 2006

Dittmann S et al: Successful control of epidemic diphtheria in the states of the former Union of Soviet Socialist Republics: Lessons learned. J Infect Dis 181(Suppl 1):S10, 2000

Holmes RK: Biology and molecular epidemiology of diphtheria toxin and the tox gene. J Infect Dis 181(Suppl 1):S156, 2000

Kadirova R et al: Clinical characteristics and management of 676 hospitalized diphtheria cases, Kyrgyz Republic, 1995. J Infect Dis 181(Suppl 1):S110, 2000

Kretsinger K et al: Preventing tetanus, diphtheria, and pertussis among adults: Use of tetanus toxoid, reduced diphtheria toxoid, and acellular pertussis vaccine; recommendations of the Advisory Committee on Immunization Practices (ACIP) and recommendation of ACIP, supported by the Healthcare Infection Control Practices Advisory Committee (HICPAC), for use of Tdap among health-care personnel. MMWR Recomm Rep 55(RR-17): 1, 2006

MacGregor RR: *Corynebacterium diphtheriae*, in *Principles and Practice of Infectious Diseases*, 6th ed, GL Mandell et al (eds). Philadelphia, Elsevier Churchill Livingstone, 2005, pp 2457–2465

McNeil SA et al: Comparison of the safety and immunogenicity of concomitant and sequential administration of an adult formulation tetanus and diphtheria toxoids adsorbed combined with acellular pertussis (Tdap) vaccine and trivalent inactivated influenza vaccine in adults. Vaccine 25:3464, 2007; Epub 2007 Jan 9.

Meyer DK, Reboli AC: Other coryneform bacteria and *Rhodococcus*, in *Principles and Practice of Infectious Diseases*, 6th ed, GL Mandell et al (eds). Philadelphia, Elsevier Churchill Livingstone, 2005, pp 2465–2478

Mookadam F et al: *Corynebacterium jeikeium* endocarditis: A systematic overview spanning four decades. Eur J Clin Microbiol Infect Dis 25:349, 2006

Pichichero ME et al: Combined tetanus, diphtheria, and 5-component pertussis vaccine for use in adolescents and adults. JAMA 293:3003, 2005

CHAPTER 39

INFECTIONS CAUSED BY *LISTERIA MONOCYTOGENES*

Elizabeth L. Hohmann ■ Daniel A. Portnoy

Listeria monocytogenes is a food-borne pathogen that can cause serious infections, particularly in pregnant women and immunocompromised individuals. A ubiquitous saprophytic environmental bacterium, *L. monocytogenes* is also a pathogen with a broad host range. Humans are probably accidental hosts for this microorganism. *L. monocytogenes* is of interest not only to clinicians, but also to basic scientists as a model intracellular pathogen that is used to study basic mechanisms of microbial pathogenesis and host immunity.

MICROBIOLOGY

L. monocytogenes is a facultatively anaerobic, nonsporulating, gram-positive rod that grows over a broad temperature range, including refrigeration temperatures. This organism is motile during growth at low temperatures, but much less so at 37°C. The vast majority of cases of human listerial disease can be traced to serotypes 1/2a, 1/2b, and 4. *L. monocytogenes* is weakly β-hemolytic on blood agar, and (as detailed below) its β-hemolysin is an essential determinant of its pathogenicity.

PATHOGENESIS

Infections with *L. monocytogenes* follow ingestion of contaminated food that contains the bacteria at high concentrations. The conversion from environmental saprophyte to a pathogen involves the coordinate regulation of bacterial determinants of pathogenesis that mediate entry into cells, intracellular growth, and cell-to-cell spread. One essential determinant of *L. monocytogenes* pathogenesis is the transcriptional activator PrfA, which activates the majority of genes required for cell entry and intracellular parasitism. Many of the organism's pathogenic strategies can be examined experimentally in tissue culture models of infection; such a model is presented in Fig. 39-1. Like other enteric pathogens, *L. monocytogenes* induces its own internalization by cells that are not normally phagocytic. Its entry into cells is mediated by host surface proteins classified as internalins. Internalin-mediated entry is important in the crossing of intestinal, blood-brain, and fetoplacental barriers, although how *L. monocytogenes* traffics from the intestine to the brain or fetus is only beginning to be investigated. In a pregnant guinea pig model of infection, *L. monocytogenes* was shown to traffic from maternal organs to the placenta; surprisingly, however, it also trafficked from the placenta back to maternal organs.

Perhaps the most important determinant of the pathogenesis of *L. monocytogenes* is its β-hemolysin, listeriolysin O (LLO). LLO is a pore-forming, cholesterol-dependent cytolysin. (Related cytolysins include streptolysin O, pneumolysin, and perfringolysin O, all of which are produced by extracellular pathogens.) LLO is largely responsible for mediating the rupture of the phagosomal membrane that forms after phagocytosis of *L. monocytogenes*. LLO probably acts by inserting itself into an acidifying phagosome, thereby preventing the vesicle's maturation. In addition, LLO acts as a translocation pore for one or both of the *L. monocytogenes* phospholipases that also contribute to vacuolar lysis. LLO synthesis and activity are controlled at multiple levels to ensure that its lytic activity is limited to acidic vacuoles and does not affect the cytosol. Mutations in LLO that influence its synthesis, cytosolic half-life, or pH optimum cause premature toxicity to infected cells. There is an inverse relationship between toxicity and virulence—i.e., the more cytotoxic the strain, the less virulent it is in animals.

Once in the cytosol, *L. monocytogenes* grows rapidly, with intracellular doubling times equivalent to those in rich media. One of the PrfA-regulated genes encodes a hexose-phosphate transporter that facilitates the growth of cytosolic bacteria on phosphorylated glucose derivatives of host origin.

Shortly after exposure to the mammalian-cell cytosol, *L. monocytogenes* produces ActA, another PrfA-regulated surface protein that mediates the nucleation of host actin filaments to propel the bacteria intra- and intercellularly. ActA mimics host proteins of the Wiskott-Aldrich syndrome protein (WASP) family by promoting the actin nucleation properties of the Arp2/3 complex. Thus *L. monocytogenes* can enter the cytosol of almost any eukaryotic cell or cell extract and can exploit a conserved and essential actin-based motility system. Other pathogens as diverse as certain *Shigella*, *Mycobacterium*, *Rickettsia*, and *Burkholderia* spp. use a related pathogenic strategy that allows cell-to-cell spread without exposure to the extracellular milieu.

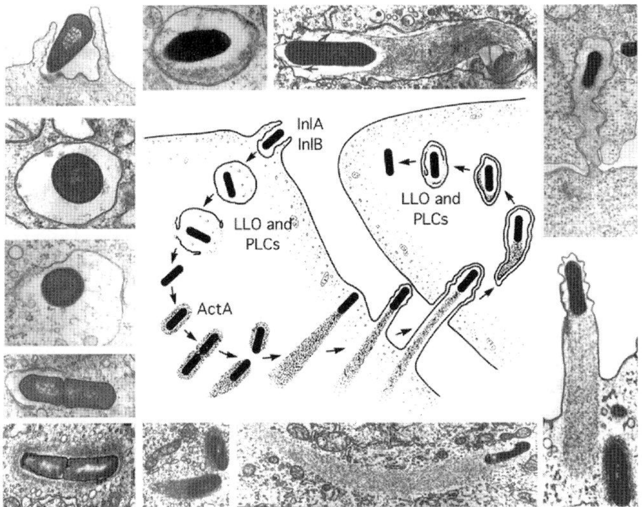

FIGURE 39-1

Stages in the intracellular life cycle of *Listeria monocytogenes*. The central diagram depicts cell entry, escape from a vacuole, actin nucleation, actin-based motility, and cell-to-cell spread. Surrounding the diagram are representative electron micrographs from which it was derived. ActA, surface protein mediating nucleation of host actin filaments to propel bacteria intra- and intercellularly; LLO, listeriolysin O; PLCs, phospholipases C; Inl, internalin. See text for further details. (*Adapted with permission from LG Tilney and DA Portnoy: Actin filaments and the growth, movement, and spread of the intracellular bacterial parasite, Listeria monocytogenes. J Cell Biol 109:1597, 1989. © Rockefeller University Press.*)

IMMUNE RESPONSE

The innate and acquired immune responses to *L. monocytogenes* have been studied extensively in mice. Shortly after IV injection, most bacteria are found in Kupffer cells in the liver, with some organisms in splenic macrophages. Listeriae that survive the bactericidal activity of initially infected macrophages grow in the cytosol and spread from cell to cell. In the liver, the result is infection of hepatocytes. Neutrophils are crucial to host defense during the first 24 h of infection, whereas influx of activated macrophages from the bone marrow is critical subsequently. Mice that survive sublethal infection clear the infection within a week, with consequent sterile immunity. Knockout mice have been used to show that interferon γ and tumor necrosis factor (TNF) are essential in controlling infection. Although innate immunity is sufficient to control infection, the acquired immune response is required for sterile immunity. Immunity is cell-mediated; antibody plays no measurable role. The critical effector cells are cytotoxic (CD8+) T cells that recognize and lyse infected cells. The bacteria grow and spread from cell to cell. The host recognizes and lyses infected cells, and extracellular bacteria are killed by circulating activated phagocytes. A hallmark of the *L. monocytogenes* model is that killed vaccines do not provide protective immunity. The explanation for this fundamental observation is multifactorial, involving the generation of appropriate cytokines and the compartmentalization of bacterial proteins for antigen processing and presentation.

EPIDEMIOLOGY

L. monocytogenes usually enters the body via the gastrointestinal tract in foods. Listeriosis is most often sporadic, although outbreaks do occur. Recent annual incidences in the United States range from 2 to 9 cases per 1 million population. No epidemiologic or clinical evidence supports human-to-human transmission (other than vertical transmission from mother to fetus) or waterborne infection. In line with its survival and multiplication at refrigeration temperatures, *L. monocytogenes* is commonly found in processed and unprocessed foods of animal and plant origin, especially soft cheeses, delicatessen meats, hot dogs, milk, and cold salads. Because food supplies are increasingly centralized and normal hosts tolerate the organism well, outbreaks may not be immediately apparent; pulsed-field gel electrophoresis has proved useful in linking cases to specific foods. FoodNet, an active U.S. surveillance program, has demonstrated decreases in listeriosis incidence, although recent data from some European countries show a stable or increased number of cases, perhaps because of enhanced active surveillance. The U.S. Food and Drug Administration has a zero-tolerance policy for *L. monocytogenes* in ready-to-eat foods.

DIAGNOSIS

Symptoms of listerial infection overlap greatly with those of other infectious diseases. Timely diagnosis requires that the illness be considered in groups at risk: pregnant women; elderly persons; neonates; individuals immunocompromised by organ transplants, cancer, or treatment with TNF antagonists or glucocorticoids; and patients with a variety of chronic medical conditions, including alcoholism, diabetes, renal disease, rheumatologic illness, and iron overload. Meningitis in older adults (especially with parenchymal brain involvement or subcortical brain abscess) or a local outbreak of culture-negative febrile gastroenteritis should trigger consideration of *L. monocytogenes* infection. Listeriosis occasionally affects healthy, young, nonpregnant individuals. HIV-infected patients are at risk; however, listeriosis seems to be prevented by trimethoprim-sulfamethoxazole (TMP-SMX) prophylaxis targeting other AIDS-related infections. The diagnosis is typically made by culture of blood, cerebrospinal fluid (CSF), or amniotic fluid. *L. monocytogenes* may be confused with "diphtheroids" or pneumococci in gram-stained CSF or may be gram-variable and confused with *Haemophilus* spp. Serologic tests and polymerase chain reaction assays are not clinically useful diagnostic tools at present.

CLINICAL MANIFESTATIONS

Listerial infections present as several clinical syndromes, of which meningitis and septicemia are most common. Monocytosis is seen in infected rabbits but is not a hallmark of human infection.

Gastroenteritis

Appreciated only since the outbreaks of the late 1980s, listerial gastroenteritis typically develops within 48 h of ingestion of a large inoculum of bacteria in contaminated foods such as milk, deli meats, and salads. Attack rates are high (50–100%). *L. monocytogenes* is neither sought nor found in routine fecal cultures, but its involvement should be considered in outbreaks when cultures for other likely pathogens are negative. Manifestations include fever, diarrhea, headache, and constitutional symptoms. The largest reported outbreak occurred in an Italian school system and included 1566 individuals; ~20% of patients were hospitalized, but only one person had a positive blood culture. Isolated gastrointestinal illness does not require antibiotic treatment. Surveillance studies show that 0.1–5% of healthy asymptomatic adults may have stool cultures positive for the organism.

Bacteremia

L. monocytogenes septicemia presents with fever, chills, and myalgias/arthralgias and cannot be differentiated from septicemia involving other organisms. Meningeal symptoms, focal neurologic findings, or mental status changes may suggest the diagnosis. Bacteremia is documented in 70–90% of cancer patients with listeriosis. A nonspecific flulike illness with fever is a common presentation in pregnant women. Endocarditis of prosthetic and native valves is an uncommon complication, with reported fatality rates of 35–50% in case series. A lumbar puncture is often prudent, although not necessary, in pregnant women without central nervous system (CNS) symptoms.

Meningitis

L. monocytogenes causes ~5–10% of all cases of community-acquired bacterial meningitis in adults in the United States. Case-fatality rates are reported to be 15–26% and do not appear to have changed over time. This diagnosis should be considered in all older or chronically ill adults with "aseptic" meningitis. The presentation is more frequently subacute (with illness developing over several days) than in meningitis of other bacterial etiologies, and nuchal rigidity and meningeal signs are less common. Photophobia is infrequent. Focal findings and seizures are common in some but not all series. The CSF profile in listerial meningitis most often shows white blood cell (WBC) counts in the range of 100–5000/μL (rarely higher); 75% of patients have WBC counts below 1000/μL, usually with a neutrophil predominance more modest than that in other bacterial meningitides. Low glucose levels and positive results on Gram's staining are found ~30–40% of the time.

Meningoencephalitis and Focal CNS Infection

L. monocytogenes can directly invade the brain parenchyma, producing either cerebritis or focal abscess. Approximately 10% of cases of CNS infection are macroscopic abscesses resulting from bacteremic seeding; the affected patients often have positive blood cultures. Concurrent meningitis can exist, but the CSF may appear normal. Abscesses can be misdiagnosed as metastatic or primary tumors and, in rare instances, occur in the cerebellum and the spinal cord. Invasion of the brainstem results in a characteristic severe rhombencephalitis, usually in otherwise healthy older adults. The presentation may be biphasic, with a prodrome of fever and headache followed by asymmetric cranial nerve deficits, cerebellar signs, and hemiparetic and hemisensory deficits. Respiratory failure can occur. The subacute course and the often minimally abnormal CSF findings may delay the diagnosis, which may be suggested by MRI images showing ring-enhancing lesions after gadolinium contrast and hyperintense lesions on diffusion-weighted imaging. MRI is superior to CT for the diagnosis of these infections.

Other Focal Infections

Focal infections of visceral organs; the eye; the pleural, peritoneal, and pericardial spaces; and the bones and joints have all been reported.

Infection in Pregnancy and Neonatal Infection

Listeriosis in pregnancy is a severe and important infection. The usual presentation is a nonspecific acute or subacute febrile illness with myalgias, arthralgias, backache, and headache. Pregnant women with listeriosis are usually bacteremic. This syndrome should prompt blood cultures, especially in the absence of another reasonable explanation. Involvement of the CNS is rare in the absence of other risk factors. Preterm delivery is a common complication, and the diagnosis may be made only postpartum. As many as 70–90% of fetuses from infected women can become infected. Prepartum treatment of bacteremic women enhances the chances of delivery of a healthy infant. Women usually do well after delivery: maternal deaths are very rare, even when the diagnosis is made late in pregnancy or postpartum. Overall mortality rates for fetuses infected in utero approach 50% in some series; among live-born neonates treated with antibiotics, mortality rates are much lower (~20%). *Granulomatosis infantiseptica* is an overwhelming listerial fetal infection with miliary microabscesses and granulomas, most often in the skin, liver, and spleen. Less severe neonatal infection acquired in utero presents at birth. "Late-onset" neonatal illness typically develops ~10 days after delivery but can occur up to a month postpartum. Mothers of infants with late-onset disease are not ill.

Rx Treatment: INFECTIONS CAUSED BY *LISTERIA MONOCYTOGENES*

No clinical trials have compared antimicrobial agents for the treatment of *L. monocytogenes* infections. Data obtained in studies conducted in vitro and in animals as well as observational clinical data indicate that ampicillin is the drug of choice, although penicillin is also highly active. Adults should receive IV ampicillin at high doses (2 g every 4 h), and most experts recommend the addition of gentamicin for synergy (1.0–1.7 mg/kg every 8 h). TMP-SMX, given IV, is the best alternative for the penicillin-allergic patient (15–20 mg of TMP/kg per day in divided doses every 6–8 h). The dosages recommended cover CNS infection and bacteremia (see below for duration); dosages must be reduced for patients with renal insufficiency. One small nonrandomized study supports a combination of ampicillin and TMP-SMX. Case reports document success with vancomycin, tetracycline, and erythromycin, although there are also reports of clinical failure with all three agents. Imipenem and the newer quinolones are possible alternative agents that have been efficacious in animal models, but clinical experience is very limited. Cephalosporins are *not* effective and should not be used. Neonates should receive ampicillin and gentamicin at doses based on weight.

The duration of therapy depends on the syndrome: 2 weeks for bacteremia, 3 weeks for meningitis, 6–8 weeks for brain abscess/encephalitis, and 4–6 weeks for endocarditis in both neonates and adults. Early-onset neonatal disease may be more severe and should be treated for >2 weeks.

COMPLICATIONS AND PROGNOSIS

About 50–70% of individuals who are promptly diagnosed and treated recover fully, but permanent neurologic sequelae are common in patients with brain abscess or rhombencephalitis. Of 100 live-born treated neonates in one series, 60% recovered fully, 24% died, and 13% had long-term neurologic or other complications.

PREVENTION

Healthy persons should take standard precautions to prevent food-borne illness: fully cooking meats, washing fresh vegetables, carefully cleaning utensils, and avoiding unpasteurized dairy products. In addition, persons at risk for listeriosis, including pregnant women, should avoid soft cheeses (although hard cheeses and yogurt are not problematic) and should avoid or thoroughly reheat ready-to-eat and delicatessen foods, even though the absolute risk they pose is relatively low.

FURTHER READINGS

Bakardjiev AI et al: *Listeria monocytogenes* traffics from maternal organs to the placenta and back. PLoS Pathog 2:e66, 2006

Bortolussi R: Listeriosis: A primer. CMAJ 179:795, 2008

Bortolussi R, Mailman TM: Listeriosis, in *Infectious Disease of the Fetus and Newborn Infant*, 6th ed, S Remington et al (eds). Philadelphia, Elsevier Saunders, 2005, p 465

Cabellos C et al: Community-acquired bacterial meningitis in elderly patients: Experience over 30 years. Medicine (Baltimore) 88:115, 2009

Hamon M et al: *Listeria monocytogenes*: A multifaceted model. Nat Rev Microbiol 4:423, 2006

Mylonakis E et al: Listeriosis during pregnancy: A case series and review of 222 cases. Medicine (Baltimore) 81:260, 2002

Ooi ST, Lorber B: Gastroenteritis due to *Listeria monocytogenes*. Clin Infect Dis 40:1327, 2005

Portnoy DA (section ed): The listeriae, in *Gram-Positive Pathogens*, 2d edition, VA Fischetti et al (eds). Washington, DC, ASM Press, 2006, Section 4

Tweten RK: Cholesterol-dependent cytolysins, a family of versatile pore-forming toxins. Infect Immun 73:6199, 2005

www.cdc.gov/foodnet/

CHAPTER 40

TETANUS

Elias Abrutyn†

DEFINITION

Tetanus is a neurologic disorder, characterized by increased muscle tone and spasms, that is caused by tetanospasmin, a powerful protein toxin elaborated by *Clostridium tetani*. Tetanus occurs in several clinical forms, including generalized, neonatal, and localized disease.

ETIOLOGIC AGENT

C. tetani is an anaerobic, motile, gram-positive rod that forms an oval, colorless, terminal spore and thus assumes a shape resembling a tennis racket or drumstick. The organism is found worldwide in soil, in the inanimate environment, in animal feces, and occasionally in human

†Deceased. A contributor to *Harrison's Principles of Internal Medicine* since the 12th edition, Dr. Abrutyn passed away on February 22, 2007.

feces. Spores may survive for years in some environments and are resistant to various disinfectants and to boiling for 20 min. Vegetative cells, however, are easily inactivated and are susceptible to several antibiotics, including metronidazole and penicillin.

Tetanospasmin is formed in vegetative cells under plasmid control. With autolysis, the single-chain toxin is released and cleaved to form a heterodimer consisting of a heavy chain (100 kDa), which mediates binding to and entry into nerve cells, and a light chain (50 kDa), which blocks neurotransmitter release. The genome of *C. tetani* has been sequenced. The amino acid structures of the two most powerful toxins known, botulinum toxin and tetanus toxin, are partially homologous.

EPIDEMIOLOGY

Tetanus occurs sporadically and almost always affects unimmunized persons; partially immunized persons and fully immunized individuals who fail to maintain adequate immunity with booster doses of vaccine may be affected as well.

Although tetanus is entirely preventable by immunization, the burden of disease worldwide is great. Tetanus is a notifiable disease in many countries, but reporting is known to be inaccurate and incomplete, particularly in developing countries. As a result, the World Health Organization considers the number of reported cases to be an underestimate and periodically undertakes case/death estimates to assess the burden of disease. In 2002 (the last year for which data were available as of this writing), the *estimated* number of tetanus-related deaths in all age groups was 213,000, of which 180,000 (85%) were attributable to neonatal tetanus. In contrast, only 18,781 tetanus cases in total and 11,762 neonatal cases were actually *reported* for that year.

Tetanus is common in areas where soil is cultivated, in rural areas, in warm climates, during summer months, and among males. In countries without a comprehensive immunization program, tetanus occurs predominantly in neonates and other young children. It is noteworthy that international programs to eliminate neonatal tetanus have been in place for some time. In the United States and other nations with successful immunization programs, neonatal tetanus is rare (only three cases were reported in the United States during 1990–2004), and the disease affects other age groups (Fig. 40-1) and groups inadequately covered by immunization (such as nonwhites). The success of immunization in the United States is depicted in Fig. 40-2. Since 1976, fewer than 100 cases have been reported yearly. At present, the risk of tetanus in this country is highest among the elderly. A large-scale national serologic survey performed in 1988–1994 showed that 72% of Americans ≥6 years old had protective antibody levels. In contrast, only 30% of persons >70 years old were protected.

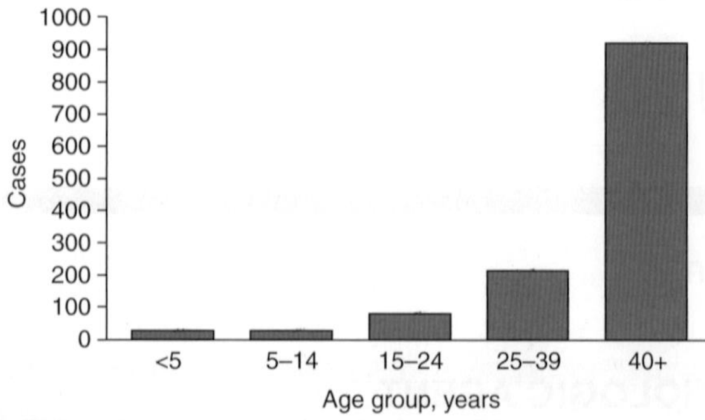

FIGURE 40-1
Tetanus: reported cases in the United States, by age group, 1980–2003; $N = 1277$. (*From Centers for Disease Control and Prevention, National Immunization Program. Tetanus and Tetanus Toxoid: Epidemiology and Prevention of Vaccine-Preventable Diseases. www.cdc.gov/nip/ed/vpd2006/Slides/chap06-tetanus9.ppt. Revised January 2006. Accessed 1/30/2007.*)

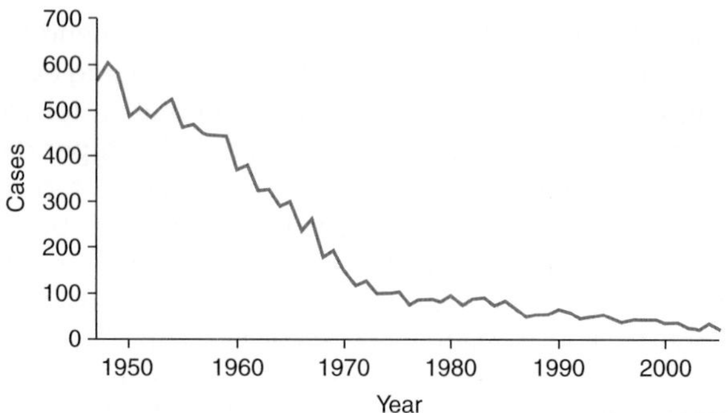

FIGURE 40-2
Impact of tetanus immunization in the United States, 1947–2005 (2005, provisional total). Tetanus vaccine became part of the routine childhood immunization schedule in the late 1940s. (*From Centers for Disease Control and Prevention, National Immunization Program. Tetanus and Tetanus Toxoid: Epidemiology and Prevention of Vaccine-Preventable Diseases. www.cdc.gov/nip/ed/vpd2006/Slides/chap06-tetanus9.ppt. Revised January 2006. Accessed 1/30/2007.*)

In the United States, most cases of tetanus follow an acute injury (puncture wound, laceration, abrasion, or other trauma). Tetanus may be acquired indoors or during outdoor activities (e.g., farming, gardening). The implicated injury may be major, but can be so trivial that medical attention is not sought. In some cases, no injury or portal of entry can be identified. The disease may complicate chronic conditions such as skin ulcers, abscesses, and gangrene. Tetanus has also been associated with burns, frostbite, middle-ear infection, surgery, abortion, childbirth, body piercing, and drug abuse (notably "skin popping"). Recurrent tetanus has been reported.

PATHOGENESIS

Contamination of wounds with spores of *C. tetani* is probably a frequent occurrence. Germination and toxin production, however, take place only in wounds with low oxidation-reduction potential, such as those with devitalized tissue, foreign bodies, or active infection. *C. tetani* does not itself evoke inflammation, and the portal of entry retains a benign appearance unless coinfection with other organisms is present.

Toxin released in the wound binds to peripheral motor neuron terminals, enters the axon, and is transported to the nerve-cell body in the brainstem and spinal cord by retrograde intraneuronal transport. The toxin then migrates across the synapse to presynaptic terminals, where it blocks release of the inhibitory neurotransmitters glycine and γ-aminobutyric acid (GABA) from vesicles (see Fig. 41-1). The blocking of neurotransmitter release by tetanospasmin, a zinc metalloprotease, involves cleavage of synaptobrevin, a protein essential to proper function of the synaptic vesicle release apparatus. With diminished inhibition, the resting firing rate of the α motor neuron increases, producing rigidity. With lessened activity of reflexes that limit polysynaptic spread of impulses (a glycinergic activity), agonists and antagonists may be recruited rather than inhibited, with the consequent production of spasms. Toxin may also affect preganglionic sympathetic neurons in the lateral gray matter of the spinal cord and parasympathetic centers. Loss of inhibition of preganglionic sympathetic neurons may produce sympathetic hyperactivity and high circulating catecholamine levels. Tetanospasmin, like botulinum toxin, may block neurotransmitter release at the neuromuscular junction and produce weakness or paralysis, but this effect is clinically evident only in cephalic tetanus. Recovery requires sprouting of new nerve terminals.

In local tetanus, only the nerves supplying the affected muscles are involved. Generalized tetanus occurs when toxin released in the wound enters the lymphatics and bloodstream and is spread widely to distant nerve terminals; the blood-brain barrier blocks direct entry into the central nervous system. If it is assumed that intraneuronal transport times are equal for all nerves, short nerves are affected before long nerves: this fact explains the sequential involvement of nerves of the head, trunk, and extremities in generalized tetanus.

CLINICAL MANIFESTATIONS

Generalized tetanus, the most common form of the disease, is characterized by increased muscle tone and generalized spasms. The median time of onset after injury is 7 days; 15% of cases occur within 3 days and 10% after 14 days.

Typically, the patient first notices increased tone in the masseter muscles (trismus, or lockjaw). Dysphagia or stiffness or pain in the neck, shoulder, and back muscles appears concurrently or soon thereafter. The subsequent involvement of other muscles produces a rigid abdomen and stiff proximal limb muscles; the hands and feet are relatively spared. Sustained contraction of the facial muscles results in a grimace or sneer (risus sardonicus), and contraction of the back muscles produces an arched back (opisthotonos). Some patients develop paroxysmal, violent, painful, generalized muscle spasms that may cause cyanosis and threaten ventilation. These spasms occur repetitively and may be spontaneous or provoked by even the slightest stimulation. A constant threat during generalized spasms is reduced ventilation or apnea or laryngospasm. The severity of illness may be mild (muscle rigidity and few or no spasms), moderate (trismus, dysphagia, rigidity, and spasms), or severe (frequent explosive paroxysms). The patient may be febrile, although many patients have no fever; mentation is unimpaired. Deep tendon reflexes may be increased. Dysphagia or ileus may preclude oral feeding.

Autonomic dysfunction commonly complicates severe cases and is characterized by labile or sustained hypertension, tachycardia, dysrhythmia, hyperpyrexia, profuse sweating, peripheral vasoconstriction, and increased plasma and urinary catecholamine levels. Periods of bradycardia and hypotension may also be documented. Sudden cardiac arrest sometimes occurs, but its basis is unknown. Other complications include aspiration pneumonia, fractures, muscle rupture, deep-vein thrombophlebitis, pulmonary emboli, decubitus ulcer, and rhabdomyolysis.

Neonatal tetanus usually occurs as the generalized form and is usually fatal if left untreated. It develops in children born to inadequately immunized mothers, frequently after unsterile treatment of the umbilical cord stump. Its onset generally comes during the first 2 weeks of life.

Local tetanus is an uncommon form in which manifestations are restricted to muscles near the wound. The prognosis is excellent. *Cephalic tetanus*, a rare form of local tetanus, follows head injury or ear infection and involves one or more facial cranial nerves. The incubation period is a few days and mortality is high.

DIAGNOSIS

The diagnosis of tetanus is based entirely on clinical findings. Tetanus is unlikely if a reliable history indicates the completion of a primary vaccination series and the receipt of appropriate booster doses. Wounds should be cultured in suspected cases. However, *C. tetani* can be isolated from wounds of patients without tetanus and frequently cannot be recovered from wounds of those with tetanus. The leukocyte count may be elevated. Cerebrospinal fluid examination yields normal results. Electromyograms may show continuous discharge of motor units and shortening or absence of the silent interval normally seen after an action potential. Nonspecific changes may be evident on the electrocardiogram. Muscle enzyme levels may be raised. Serum antitoxin levels of ≥0.1 IU/mL (as measured by enzyme-linked immunosorbent assay) are considered protective and make tetanus unlikely, although cases in patients with protective antitoxin levels have been reported.

The differential diagnosis includes conditions also producing trismus, such as alveolar abscess, strychnine poisoning, dystonic drug reactions (e.g., phenothiazines and metoclopramide), and hypocalcemic tetany. In addition, meningitis/encephalitis, rabies, and an acute intraabdominal process (because of the rigid abdomen) might be considered. Markedly increased tone in central muscles (face, neck, chest, back, and abdomen), with superimposed generalized spasms and relative sparing of the hands and feet, strongly suggests tetanus.

℞ Treatment: TETANUS

GENERAL MEASURES The goals of therapy are to eliminate the source of toxin, neutralize unbound toxin, and prevent muscle spasms while monitoring the patient's condition and providing support—especially respiratory support—until recovery. Patients should be admitted to a quiet room in an intensive care unit, where observation and cardiopulmonary monitoring can be maintained continuously, but stimulation can be minimized. Protection of the airway is vital. Wounds should be explored, carefully cleansed, and thoroughly debrided.

ANTIBIOTIC THERAPY Although of unproven value, antibiotic therapy is administered to eradicate vegetative cells—the source of toxin. The use of penicillin (10–12 million units IV, given daily for 10 days) has been recommended, but metronidazole (500 mg every 6 h or 1 g every 12 h) is preferred by some experts on the basis of this drug's excellent antimicrobial activity and the absence of the GABA-antagonistic activity seen with penicillin. The drug of choice remains unclear: one nonrandomized clinical trial found a survival benefit with metronidazole, but another study failed to find a difference among benzathine penicillin, benzyl penicillin, and metronidazole. Clindamycin and erythromycin are alternatives for the treatment of penicillin-allergic patients. Additional specific antimicrobial therapy should be given for active infection with other organisms.

ANTITOXIN Given to neutralize circulating toxin and unbound toxin in the wound, antitoxin effectively lowers mortality; toxin already bound to neural tissue is unaffected. Human tetanus immune globulin (TIG) is the preparation of choice and should be given promptly. The dose is 3000–6000 units IM, usually in divided doses because the volume is large. The optimal dose is not known, however, and results from one study indicated that a 500-unit dose was as effective as higher doses. Pooled IVIg may be an alternative to TIG, but the specific antitoxin concentration in this formulation is not standardized. The value of administering antitoxin before wound manipulation or of injecting a dose proximal to the wound or infiltrating the wound is unclear. Additional doses are unnecessary because the half-life of antitoxin is long. Antibody does not penetrate the blood-brain barrier. Intrathecal administration should be considered experimental. Equine tetanus antitoxin (TAT) is not available in the United States but is used elsewhere. It is cheaper than human antitoxin, but the half-life is shorter, and its administration commonly elicits a hypersensitivity reaction and serum sickness.

CONTROL OF MUSCLE SPASMS Many agents, alone and in combination, have been used to treat the muscle spasms of tetanus, which are painful and can threaten ventilation by causing laryngospasm or sustained contraction of ventilatory muscles.

In some developing countries, cost, availability, and the ability to provide ventilatory support are important factors in the choice of therapy. The ideal therapeutic regimen would abolish spasmodic activity without causing oversedation and hypoventilation. Diazepam, a benzodiazepine and GABA agonist, is in wide use. The dose is titrated, and large doses (≥250 mg/d) may be required. Lorazepam, with a longer duration of action, and midazolam, with a short half-life, are other options. Barbiturates and chlorpromazine are considered second-line agents. Therapeutic paralysis with a nondepolarizing neuromuscular blocking agent and mechanical ventilation may be used for spasms unresponsive to medication or spasms that threaten ventilation. However, prolonged paralysis after discontinuation of therapy has been described. Other agents include propofol, which is expensive; dantrolene and intrathecal baclofen, which may allow shortening of the duration of therapeutic paralysis; succinylcholine, which has been associated with hyperkalemia; and magnesium sulfate. A recent double-blind, randomized, placebo-controlled clinical trial of magnesium sulfate in severe tetanus did not find a reduction in the need for ventilation or in mortality rate; however, use of midazolam and pipecuronium for treatment of muscle spasms and of verapamil for treatment of cardiovascular instability was reduced.

RESPIRATORY CARE Intubation or tracheostomy, with or without mechanical ventilation, may be required for hypoventilation due to oversedation or laryngospasm or for the avoidance of aspiration by patients with trismus, disordered swallowing, or dysphagia. The need for these procedures should be anticipated, and they should be undertaken electively and early.

AUTONOMIC DYSFUNCTION The optimal therapy for sympathetic overactivity has not been defined. Agents that have been considered include labetalol (an α- and β-adrenergic blocking agent that is recommended by some experts but that reportedly has caused sudden death), esmolol administered by continuous infusion (a beta blocker whose short half-life may be advantageous in the event of severe hypertension from unopposed α-adrenergic activity), clonidine (a central-acting antiadrenergic drug), verapamil, and morphine sulfate. Parenteral magnesium sulfate and continuous spinal or epidural anesthesia have been used but may be more difficult to administer and monitor. The relative efficacy of these modalities has yet to be determined. Hypotension or bradycardia may require volume expansion, use of vasopressors or chronotropic agents, or pacemaker insertion.

VACCINE Patients recovering from tetanus should be actively immunized (see below) because immunity is not induced by the small amount of toxin required to produce disease.

ADDITIONAL MEASURES Like all patients receiving ventilatory support, patients with tetanus require attention to hydration; nutrition; physiotherapy; prophylactic anticoagulation; bowel, bladder, and renal function; decubitus ulcer prevention; and treatment of intercurrent infection.

PREVENTION

Active Immunization

All partially immunized and unimmunized adults should receive vaccine, as should those recovering from tetanus. The primary series for adults consists of three doses: the first and second doses are given 4–8 weeks apart, and the third dose is given 6–12 months after the second. A booster dose is required every 10 years and may be given at mid-decade ages—35, 45, and so on. Combined tetanus and diphtheria toxoid, adsorbed (Td, for adult use)—rather than single-antigen tetanus toxoid—is preferred for persons >7 years of age. Adsorbed vaccine is preferred because it produces more persistent antibody titers than fluid vaccine. Two combined tetanus/diphtheria/attenuated pertussis vaccines have recently been approved: one (ADACEL) for adults 19–64 years of age and the other (BOOSTRIX) for adolescents 11–18 years of age. The Advisory Committee on Immunization Practices has recommended a single dose of Tdap (ADACEL) for adults 19–64 years old who have not received Tdap.

Wound Management

Proper wound management requires consideration of the need for (1) passive immunization with TIG and (2) active immunization with vaccine (Tdap or Td; Table 40-1). The dose of TIG for passive immunization of persons with wounds of average severity (250 units IM) produces a protective serum antibody level for at least 4–6 weeks; the appropriate dose of TAT, an equine-derived product, is 3000–6000 units. Vaccine and antibody should be administered at separate sites with separate syringes.

Neonatal Tetanus

Preventive measures include maternal vaccination, even during pregnancy; efforts to increase the proportion of births that take place in the hospital; and the provision of training for nonmedical birth attendants.

TABLE 40-1

GUIDE TO TETANUS PROPHYLAXIS AND ROUTINE WOUND MANAGEMENT

HISTORY OF ADSORBED TETANUS TOXOID (DOSES)	CLEAN MINOR WOUND		ALL OTHER WOUNDS[a]	
	Tdap OR Td[b]	TIG	Tdap OR Td[b]	TIG
Unknown or <3	Yes	No	Yes	Yes
≥3	No[c]	No	No[d]	No

[a]Such as, but not limited to, wounds contaminated with dirt, feces, soil, and saliva; puncture wounds; avulsions; and wounds from missile or crushing injuries, burns, and frostbite.
[b]Tdap is preferred to Td for adults 19–64 years old who have never received Tdap. Td is preferred for adults who have received Tdap previously and is used when Tdap is not available. Td is also recommended for persons >64 years old. If TT and TIG are both used, TT adsorbed rather than TT for booster use only (fluid vaccine) should be used.
[c]Yes, if ≥10 years have elapsed since the last TT-containing vaccine dose.
[d]Yes, if ≥5 years have elapsed since the last TT-containing vaccine dose.
Note: Tdap, tetanus toxoid, reduced diphtheria toxoid, and acellular pertussis vaccine, adsorbed; DT, diphtheria and tetanus vaccine; DTP, diphtheria, tetanus, and pertussis vaccine; Td, tetanus-diphtheria toxoid, adsorbed; TIG, tetanus immune globulin; TT, tetanus toxoid.
Source: Modified from Centers for Disease Control and Prevention, 2006.

PROGNOSIS

The application of methods to monitor and support oxygenation has markedly improved the prognosis in tetanus. Mortality rates as low as 10% have been reported from units accustomed to handling such cases. In the United States in 2003, there were 20 cases and 2 deaths; no cases were in patients <18 years old, and 19 cases were ascribed to inadequate immunization. The outcome is poor in neonates and the elderly and in patients with a short incubation period, a short interval from the onset of symptoms to admission, or a short period from the onset of symptoms to the first spasm (period of onset). Outcome is also related to the extent of prior vaccination.

The course of tetanus extends over 4–6 weeks, and patients may require prolonged ventilator support. Increased tone and minor spasms can last for months, but recovery is usually complete.

FURTHER READINGS

Abrutyn E, Berlin JA: Intrathecal therapy of tetanus: A meta-analysis. JAMA 266:2262, 1991

Ahmadsyah I, Salim A: Treatment of tetanus: An open study to compare the efficacy of procaine penicillin and metronidazole. BMJ 291:648, 1985

Amanna IJ et al: Duration of humoral immunity to common viral and vaccine antigens. N Engl J Med 357:1903, 2007

BLECK TP: *Clostridium tetani* (tetanus), in *Principles and Practice of Infectious Diseases,* 5th ed, GL Mandell et al (eds). New York, Churchill Livingstone, 2000, pp 2537–2543

CENTERS FOR DISEASE CONTROL AND PREVENTION: Preventing tetanus, diphtheria, and pertussis among adults: Use of tetanus toxoid, reduced diphtheria toxoid and acellular pertussis vaccine: Recommendations of the Advisory Committee on Immunization Practices (ACIP) and recommendation of ACIP, supported by the Healthcare Infection Control Practices Advisory Committee (HICPAC), for use of Tdap among health-care personnel. MMWR 55(RR17):1, 2006

CENTERS FOR DISEASE CONTROL AND PREVENTION: Tetanus—Puerto Rico, 2002. MMWR 51:613, 2002

———: Tetanus surveillance—United States, 1998–2000. Surveillance summaries, June 20, 2003. MMWR 52(SS-3):1, 2003

COOK TM et al: Tetanus: A review of the literature. Br J Anaesth 87:477, 2001

HSU SS et al: Tetanus in the emergency department: A current review. J Emerg Med 20:357, 2001

MCQUILLAN CM et al: Serologic immunity to diphtheria and tetanus in the United States. Ann Intern Med 136:660, 2002

ROUSH SW et al: Historical comparisons of morbidity and mortality for vaccine-preventable diseases in the United States. JAMA 298:2155, 2007

THWAITES CL et al: Magnesium sulphate for the treatment of severe tetanus: A randomized controlled trial. Lancet 368:1436, 2006

CHAPTER 41

BOTULISM

Elias Abrutyn†

DEFINITION

Botulism is a paralytic disease caused by potent protein neurotoxins elaborated by *Clostridium botulinum*. Illness begins with cranial nerve involvement and proceeds caudally to involve the extremities. Cases may be classified as (1) *food-borne botulism*, from ingestion of preformed toxin in food contaminated with *C. botulinum*; (2) *wound botulism*, from toxin produced in wounds contaminated with the organism; and (3) *intestinal botulism*, from ingestion of spores and production of toxin in the intestine of infants (infant botulism) or adults. Botulinum toxin, because of its extraordinary potency, has long been considered a threat as an agent of bioterrorism or biologic warfare that could be acquired by inhalation or ingestion (Chap. 6). Iatrogenic botulism can follow cosmetic or therapeutic use of toxin.

ETIOLOGIC AGENT

C. botulinum, a species encompassing a heterogeneous group of anaerobic gram-positive organisms that form subterminal spores, is found in soil and marine environments throughout the world and elaborates the most potent bacterial toxin known. Organisms of types A through G have been distinguished by the antigenic specificities of their toxins; a classification system based on physiologic characteristics has also been described. Rare strains of other clostridial species—*C. butyricum* and *C. baratii*—have been found to produce toxin. *C. botulinum* strains with proteolytic activity can digest food and produce a spoiled appearance; nonproteolytic types leave the appearance of food unchanged.

Of the eight distinct toxin types described (A, B, C_1, C_2, D, E, F, and G), all except C_2 are neurotoxins; C_2 is a cytotoxin of unknown clinical significance. Botulinum neurotoxin, whether ingested, inhaled, or produced in the intestine or a wound, enters the vascular system and is transported to peripheral cholinergic nerve terminals, including neuromuscular junctions, postganglionic parasympathetic nerve endings, and peripheral ganglia. The central nervous system is not involved. Steps in neurotoxin activity include binding, internalization in endocytic vesicles, translocation to the cytosol, and proteolysis resulting in a blockage of the release of the neurotransmitter acetylcholine (Fig. 41-1). Cure follows sprouting of new nerve terminals.

Toxin types A, B, E, and (rarely) F cause disease in humans; type G (from *C. argentinense*) has been associated with sudden death, but not with neuroparalytic illness, in a few patients in Switzerland; and types C and D cause disease in animals.

EPIDEMIOLOGY

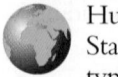

Human botulism occurs worldwide. In the United States, the geographic distribution of cases by toxin type parallels the distribution of organism types found in the environment. Type A predominates west of the Rocky Mountains; type B is generally distributed

†Deceased. A contributor to *Harrison's Principles of Internal Medicine* since the 12th edition, Dr. Abrutyn passed away on February 22, 2007.

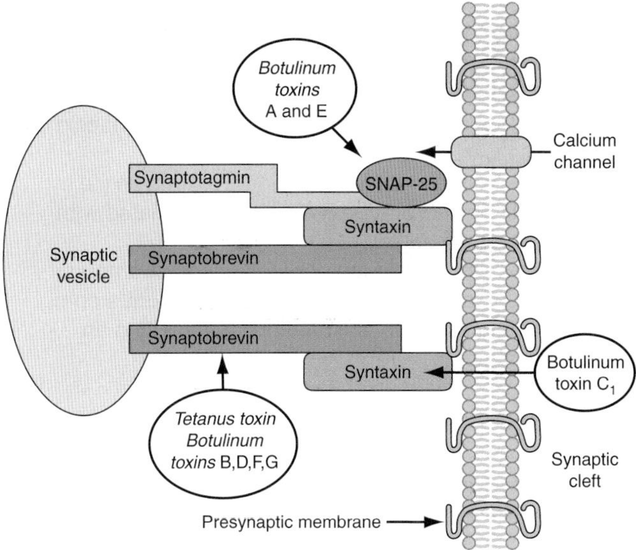

FIGURE 41-1

The synaptic vesicle release apparatus and the sites of action of botulinum toxins. Toxin acts to block neurotransmitter release from the synaptic vesicle into the synaptic cleft. The site of action of tetanus toxin is also shown. [*From TP Bleck et al: In WM Scheld et al (eds): Infections of the Central Nervous System, 2d ed. New York, Raven Press, 1997; with permission.*]

but is more common in the East; and type E is found in the Pacific Northwest, Alaska, and the Great Lakes area.

Food-borne botulism in the United States is associated primarily with home-canned food (particularly vegetables, fruit, and condiments) and less commonly with meat and fish. Type E outbreaks are frequently associated with fish products. Commercial products occasionally cause outbreaks, some of which are attributable to improper handling after purchase. Outbreaks in restaurants, schools, and private homes have been traced to uncommon sources (commercial potpies, beef stew, turkey loaf, sautéed onions, baked potatoes, preserved green olives, bamboo shoots, and chopped garlic in oil). Food-borne botulism can occur when (1) food to be preserved is contaminated with spores, (2) preservation does not inactivate the spores but kills other putrefactive bacteria that might inhibit growth of *C. botulinum* and provides anaerobic conditions at a pH and temperature that allow germination and toxin production, and (3) food is not heated to a temperature that destroys toxin before being eaten.

CLINICAL MANIFESTATIONS

Food-Borne Botulism

After ingestion of food containing toxin, illness varies from a mild condition for which no medical advice is sought to very severe disease that can result in death within 24 h. The incubation period is usually 18–36 h but, depending on toxin dose, can range from a few hours to several days. Symmetric descending paralysis is characteristic and can lead to respiratory failure and death. Cranial nerve involvement, which almost always marks the onset of symptoms, usually produces diplopia, dysarthria, dysphonia, and/or dysphagia. Weakness progresses, often rapidly, from the head to involve the neck, arms, thorax, and legs; occasionally, weakness is asymmetric. Nausea, vomiting, and abdominal pain may precede or follow the onset of paralysis. Dizziness, blurred vision, dry mouth, and very dry, occasionally sore throat are common. Patients are generally alert and oriented, but they may be drowsy, agitated, and anxious. Typically, they have no fever. Ptosis is frequent; the pupillary reflexes may be depressed, and fixed or dilated pupils are noted in half of patients. The gag reflex may be suppressed, and deep tendon reflexes may be normal or decreased. Sensory findings are usually absent. Paralytic ileus, severe constipation, and urinary retention are common.

Wound Botulism

Wound botulism occurs when the spores contaminating a wound germinate and form vegetative organisms that produce toxin. This rare condition resembles food-borne illness except that the incubation period is longer, averaging about 10 days, and gastrointestinal symptoms are lacking. Wound botulism has been documented after traumatic injury involving contamination with soil; in injection drug users, for whom black-tar heroin use has been identified as a risk factor; and after cesarean delivery. The illness has occurred even after antibiotics have been given to prevent wound infection. When present, fever is probably attributable to concurrent infection with other bacteria. The wound may appear benign.

Intestinal Botulism

In intestinal botulism, toxin is produced in and absorbed from the intestine after the germination of ingested spores. Intestinal botulism in infants (infant botulism) is the most common form of botulism. The severity ranges from mild illness with failure to thrive to fulminant severe paralysis with respiratory failure. Infant botulism may be one cause of sudden infant death. The identification of contaminated honey as one source of spores has led to the recommendation that honey not be fed to children <12 months of age. Most cases, however, cannot be attributed to a particular food source. The factors permitting intestinal colonization with *C. botulinum* are not fully defined, but cases usually involve infants <6 months of age; susceptibility may decrease as the normal intestinal flora develops. Intestinal botulism involving adults is uncommon. The patient may have a history of gastrointestinal disease, gastrointestinal surgery, or recent antibiotic therapy. Toxin and organisms may be identified in the stool.

Bioterrorism and Biologic Warfare

(See also Chap. 6) Botulinum toxin could be dispersed as an aerosol (producing inhalational botulism) or as a contaminant in material to be ingested (producing food-borne botulism). Inhalational botulism resembles food-borne illness, but gastrointestinal symptoms are absent. Botulism follows adsorption of toxin from mucosal surfaces (gut, lung) and wounds, but the toxin does not penetrate intact skin. As a toxin-mediated illness, botulism is noncommunicable, and standard isolation precautions are sufficient. Features suggestive of an outbreak due to deliberate release of botulinum toxin are shown in Table 41-1.

TABLE 41-1

FEATURES OF OUTBREAKS SUGGESTING DELIBERATE RELEASE OF BOTULINUM TOXIN[a]

- Outbreak of a large number of cases of acute flaccid paralysis with prominent bulbar palsies
- Outbreak with an unusual botulinum toxin type (i.e., type C, D, F, or G or type E toxin not associated with food of aquatic origin)
- Outbreak with a common geographic factor among cases (e.g., airport, work location) but without a common dietary exposure (i.e., features suggesting an aerosol attack)
- Multiple simultaneous outbreaks with no common source

[a]A careful travel and activity history, as well as a dietary history, should be taken in any suspected botulism outbreak. Patients should also be asked whether they know of other persons with similar symptoms.

Source: Reproduced with permission of the publisher from Arnon et al, 2002.

DIAGNOSIS

A diagnosis of botulism must be considered in patients with symmetric descending paralysis who are afebrile and mentally intact. The bulbar musculature is involved initially, but sensory findings are absent and, early on, deep tendon reflexes remain intact. The differential diagnosis of botulism and distinguishing features are listed in Table 41-2. Depending on season and other epidemiologic factors, West Nile virus infection may also be a consideration.

TABLE 41-2

SELECTED MIMICS THAT MAY LEAD TO MISDIAGNOSIS OF BOTULISM

CONDITION	FEATURES DISTINGUISHING CONDITION FROM BOTULISM
Common Misdiagnoses	
Guillain-Barré syndrome[a] and its variants, especially Miller-Fisher variant	History of antecedent infection; paresthesias; often ascending paralysis; early areflexia; eventual CSF protein increase; EMG findings
Myasthenia gravis[a]	Recurrent paralysis; EMG findings; sustained response to anticholinesterase
Stroke[a]	Paralysis often asymmetric; abnormal CNS image
Intoxication with depressants (e.g., acute alcohol intoxication), organophosphates, carbon monoxide, or nerve gas	History of exposure; excessive drug levels detected in body fluids
Lambert-Eaton syndrome	Increased strength with sustained contraction; evidence of lung carcinoma; EMG findings similar to botulism
Tick paralysis	Paresthesias; ascending paralysis; tick attached to skin
Other Misdiagnoses	
Poliomyelitis	Antecedent febrile illness; asymmetric paralysis; CSF pleocytosis
CNS infections, especially of the brainstem	Mental status changes; CSF and EEG abnormalities
CNS tumor	Paralysis often asymmetric; abnormal CNS image
Streptococcal pharyngitis[b]	Absence of bulbar palsies; positive rapid antigen test result or throat culture
Psychiatric illness[a]	Normal EMG in conversion paralysis
Viral syndrome[a]	Absence of bulbar palsies and flaccid paralysis
Inflammatory myopathy[a]	Elevated creatine kinase level
Diabetic complications[a]	Sensory neuropathy; few cranial nerve palsies
Hyperemesis gravidarum[a]	Absence of bulbar palsies and acute flaccid paralysis
Hypothyroidism[a]	Abnormal thyroid function tests
Laryngeal trauma[a]	Absence of flaccid paralysis; dysphonia without flaccid paralysis
Overexertion[a]	Absence of bulbar palsies and acute flaccid paralysis

[a]Misdiagnoses made in a large outbreak of botulism (St. Louis ME et al: Botulism from chopped garlic: Delayed recognition of a major outbreak. Ann Intern Med 108:363, 1988).

[b]Pharyngeal erythema can occur in botulism.

Note: CNS, central nervous system; CSF, cerebrospinal fluid; EEG, electroencephalogram; EMG, electromyogram.

Source: Reproduced with permission of the publisher from Arnon et al, 2002.

The demonstration of toxin in serum by bioassay in mice is definitive, but this test may give negative results, particularly in wound and infant botulism. It is performed only by specific laboratories, which can be identified through regional public health authorities. Other assays are being developed and remain experimental. The demonstration of *C. botulinum* or its toxin in vomitus, gastric fluid, or stool is strongly suggestive of the diagnosis because intestinal carriage is rare. Isolation of the organism from food without toxin is insufficient grounds for the diagnosis. Wound cultures yielding the organism are suggestive of botulism. The edrophonium chloride (Tensilon) test for myasthenia gravis may be falsely positive in botulism but is usually less dramatically positive than in the former condition. Nerve conduction velocity is normal, but compound muscle action potentials on routine nerve stimulation studies are decreased with a supramaximal stimulus, and facilitation is evident after repetitive stimulation at high frequency. Single-fiber electromyography may be helpful. The white blood cell count and erythrocyte sedimentation rate are normal.

℞ Treatment: BOTULISM

Patients should be hospitalized and monitored closely, both clinically and by spirometry, pulse oximetry, and measurement of arterial blood gases for incipient respiratory failure. Intubation and mechanical ventilation should be strongly considered when the vital capacity is <30% of predicted, especially when paralysis is progressing rapidly and hypoxemia with absolute or relative hypercarbia is documented. Serial measurements of the maximal static inspiratory pressure may be useful in predicting respiratory failure.

In food-borne illness, equine antitoxin should be administered as soon as possible after specimens are obtained for laboratory analysis. Treatment should not await laboratory analyses, which may take days. The previous trivalent antitoxin preparation (types A, B, and E) is no longer available. Instead, a bivalent preparation containing toxin types A and B and an investigational monovalent type E preparation can be obtained. The bivalent preparation is administered routinely; monovalent type E antitoxin is given in addition when exposure to type E toxin is suspected (after seafood ingestion, for example). In the United States, antitoxin as well as help with clinical management and laboratory confirmation are available at *any* time from state health departments or from the Centers for Disease Control and Prevention (CDC; emergency number, 770-488-7100). A limited supply of an investigational heptavalent antitoxin (types A through G) is maintained by the U.S. military for emergency use.

After testing for hypersensitivity to horse serum, antitoxin is given as recommended by the CDC; repeated doses are not considered necessary. Anaphylaxis and serum sickness are risks inherent in use of the equine product, and desensitization of allergic patients may be required. If there is no ileus, cathartics and enemas may be used to purge the gut of toxin; emetics or gastric lavage can also be used if the time since ingestion is brief (only a few hours). Neither the use of antibiotics to eliminate an intestinal source of possible continued toxin production nor the administration of guanidine hydrochloride and other drugs to reverse paralysis is of proven value.

Treatment of infant botulism requires supportive care and administration of human botulism immune globulin, which can be obtained by calling the California Department of Health Services at 510-231-7600 or by following the instructions at *www.infantbotulism.org*. Neither equine antitoxin nor antibiotics have been shown to be beneficial. In wound botulism, equine antitoxin is administered. The wound should be thoroughly explored and debrided, and an antibiotic such as penicillin should be given to eradicate *C. botulinum* from the site, even though the benefit of this therapy is unproven. Results of wound cultures should guide the use of other antibiotics.

Botulinum toxins are being employed for a variety of cosmetic and therapeutic purposes, and new uses are being evaluated. Generalized botulism-like weakness complicating therapy (iatrogenic botulism) has been reported but is rare.

PROGNOSIS

Type A disease is generally more severe than type B, and mortality rates from botulism are higher among patients older than age 60 than among younger patients. With improved respiratory and intensive care, the case-fatality rate in food-borne illness has been reduced to ~7.5% and is low in infant botulism as well. Artificial respiratory support may be required for months in severe cases. Some patients experience residual weakness and autonomic dysfunction for as long as a year after disease onset.

PREVENTION

A pentavalent vaccine (types A through E) is available for use in highly exposed individuals. Spores are highly resistant to heat but can be inactivated by exposure to high temperature (116–121°C) and pressure, as in steam sterilizers or pressure cookers used in accordance with the manufacturer's instructions. Toxin is heat-labile and can be inactivated by exposure to a temperature of 85°C for 5 min. Newly identified cases should be reported immediately to public health authorities.

FURTHER READINGS

ARNON SS et al: Human botulism immune globulin for the treatment of infant botulism. N Engl J Med 354:462, 2006

——— et al: Botulinum toxin as a biological weapon, in *Bioterrorism: Guidelines for Medical and Public Health Management*, DA Henderson et al (eds). Chicago, AMA Press, 2002, pp 141–165

CAWTHORNE A et al: Botulism and preserved green olives. Emerg Infect Dis 11:781, 2005

Caya JG et al: *Clostridium botulinum* and the clinical laboratorian: A detailed review of botulism, including biological warfare ramifications of botulinum toxin. Arch Pathol Lab Med 128:653, 2004

Centers for Disease Control and Prevention: Botulism from home-canned bamboo shoots—Nan Province, Thailand. MMWR 55:389, 2006

Chertow DS et al: Botulism in 4 adults following cosmetic injections with an unlicensed highly concentrated botulinum preparation. JAMA 206:2476, 2006

Cooper JG et al: *Clostridium botulinum*: An increasing complication of heroin misuse. Eur J Emerg Med 12:251, 2005

Fagan RP et al: Persistence of botulinum toxin in patients' serum: Alaska, 1959–2007. J Infect Dis 199:1029, 2009

Gupta A et al: Adult botulism type F in the United States, 1981-2002. Neurology 65:1694, 2005

Koepke R et al: Global occurrence of infant botulism, 1976–2006. Pediatrics 122:e73, 2008

Lindström M, Korkeala H: Laboratory diagnostics of botulism. Clin Microbiol Rev 19:298, 2006

Montecucco C, Molgo J: Botulinal neurotoxins: Revival of an old killer. Curr Opin Pharmacol 5:274, 2005

Sobel J: Botulism. Clin Infect Dis 41:1167, 2005

CHAPTER 42

GAS GANGRENE AND OTHER CLOSTRIDIAL INFECTIONS

Dennis L. Kasper ■ Lawrence C. Madoff

DEFINITION

Bacteria of the genus *Clostridium* are gram-positive, spore-forming, obligate anaerobes that are ubiquitous in nature. There are >60 recognized species of clostridia, many of which are generally considered saprophytic. Some of these species are pathogenic for humans and animals, particularly under conditions of lowered oxidation-reduction potential. Infections associated with these organisms range from localized wound contamination to overwhelming systemic disease. The four major disease categories for which clostridia are responsible are intestinal disorders, suppurative deep-tissue infections, skin and soft tissue infections, and bacteremia. Toxins play a major role in some of these syndromes.

Colitis caused by *C. difficile* is discussed in Chap. 43.

ETIOLOGY

In humans, clostridia normally reside in the gastrointestinal tract and in the female genital tract, although they occasionally are isolated from the skin or the mouth. Of the known clostridial species, at least 30 have been isolated from human infections. Like several other pathogenic anaerobic bacterial species, clostridia are quite aerotolerant, but they do not grow on artificial media in the presence of oxygen. Clostridia characteristically produce abundant gas in artificial media and form subterminal endospores. *C. perfringens*, one of the most clinically important species, is encapsulated and nonmotile and rarely sporulates in artificial media; the spores can usually be destroyed by boiling.

C. tetani and *C. botulinum* are discussed in detail in Chaps. 40 and 41, respectively.

Clostridia are present in the normal colonic flora at concentrations of 10^9–10^{10}/g. Of the ≥30 species that normally colonize humans, *C. ramosum* is the most abundant and is followed in frequency by *C. perfringens*. These organisms are universally present in soil at concentrations of up to 10^4/g. *C. perfringens* strains are classified (on the basis of their production of several lethal toxins) into five types, designated A through E. Type A predominates in fecal flora of humans as well as in soil, whereas the habitats of types B through E are thought to be the intestinal tracts of other animals. Although clostridia are gram-positive organisms, many species may appear to be gram-negative in clinical specimens or stationary-phase cultures. Therefore, the results of Gram's staining of cultures or clinical material should be interpreted with great care.

C. perfringens is the most common of the clostridial species isolated from tissue infections and bacteremias; next in frequency are *C. novyi* and *C. septicum*. In the category of enteric infections, *C. difficile* is an important cause of antibiotic-associated colitis, and *C. perfringens* is associated with food poisoning (type A) and enteritis necroticans (type C).

PATHOGENESIS

Despite the isolation of clostridial species from many serious traumatic wounds, the prevalence of severe infections due to these organisms is low. Two factors that appear to be essential to the development of severe disease are tissue necrosis and a low oxidation-reduction potential. *C. perfringens* requires ~14 amino acids and at least 6 additional growth factors for optimal growth.

These nutrients are not found in appreciable concentrations in normal body fluids but are present in necrotic tissue. When *C. perfringens* grows in necrotic tissue, a zone of tissue damage due to the toxins elaborated by the organism allows progressive growth. In contrast, when only a few bacteria leak into the bloodstream from a small defect in the intestinal wall, the organisms do not have the opportunity to multiply rapidly because blood as a medium for growth is relatively deficient in certain amino acids and growth factors. Therefore, in a patient without tissue necrosis, bacteremia is usually benign.

C. perfringens possesses at least 17 possible virulence factors, including 12 active tissue toxins and enterotoxins. The enterotoxins include four major lethal toxins: α, β, ε, and ι. The α toxin is a phospholipase C (lecithinase) that splits lecithin into phosphorylcholine and diglyceride. It has been associated with gas gangrene and is known to be hemolytic, to destroy platelets and polymorphonuclear leukocytes (PMNs), and to cause widespread capillary damage. When injected IV, it causes massive intravascular hemolysis and damages liver mitochondria. The α toxin may be important in the initiation of muscle infections that can progress to gas gangrene. Experimentally, the higher the concentration of α toxin in the culture fluid, the smaller the dose of *C. perfringens* required to produce infection. The protective effect of antiserum is directly proportional to its content of α antitoxin. Studies suggest that θ toxin, a thiol-activated cytolysin that is also called *perfringolysin O* and is related to other cholesterol-dependent cytolysins such as listeriolysin and streptolysin O, may play an important role in pathogenesis by promoting vascular leukostasis, endothelial cell injury, and regional tissue hypoxia. The resulting perfusion defects extend the anaerobic environment and contribute to rapidly advancing tissue destruction. A characteristic pathologic finding in gas gangrene is the near absence of PMNs despite extensive tissue destruction. Experimental data indicate that both α and θ toxins are essential in the leukocyte aggregation that occurs at the margins of tissue injury instead of the expected infiltration of these cells into the area of damage. Genetically altered strains induce less leukocyte aggregation when α toxin is absent and none when θ toxin is missing. The other major toxins—β, ε, and ι—are known to increase capillary permeability.

CLINICAL MANIFESTATIONS

Intestinal Disorders

Food Poisoning

C. perfringens, primarily type A, is the second or third most common cause of food poisoning in the United States (Chap. 25). The responsible toxin is thought to be a cytotoxin produced by >75% of strains isolated from cases of food-borne disease. The cytotoxin binds to a receptor on the small-bowel brush border and induces a calcium ion–dependent alteration in permeability. The associated loss of ions alters intracellular metabolism, resulting in cell death. Outbreaks generally have resulted from problems in the cooling and storage of food cooked in bulk. The food sources primarily involved are meat, meat products, and poultry. Generally, the implicated meats have been cooked, allowed to cool, and then recooked the following day, often in a stew or hash. Strains of *C. perfringens* that contaminate meat manage to survive initial cooking. During reheating, the organisms sporulate and germinate. The disease is associated with an attack rate that is often as high as 70%. Symptoms of food poisoning from type A strains develop 8–24 h after ingestion of foods heavily contaminated with the organism. The primary symptoms include epigastric pain, nausea, and watery diarrhea usually lasting 12–24 h. Fever and vomiting are uncommon. Molecular methods including ribotyping and pulsed-field gel electrophoresis have been used to detect fecal cytotoxin in outbreaks of food poisoning caused by *C. perfringens*.

C. perfringens has also been implicated in a more severe form of diarrhea than that of classic food poisoning. This more severe disease tends to occur in the elderly and has been associated with antibiotic use in hospitalized populations. In this form of disease, diarrhea is generally more profuse, of longer duration, and accompanied by abdominal pain. Blood and mucus have been detected in the feces of the affected patients. In one hospital-based study of a cluster of cases, widespread environmental contamination with *C. perfringens* spores was documented.

Enteritis Necroticans

Necrotizing enteritis (enteritis necroticans or *pigbel*) is caused by β toxin produced by type C strains of *C. perfringens* after ingestion of a high-protein meal in conjunction with trypsin inhibitors (e.g., in sweet potatoes) by a susceptible host who has limited intestinal proteolytic activity. This disease has been reported among children and adults in New Guinea. A similar disease, *darmbrand*, was epidemic in Germany after World War II. Clinical features of pigbel include acute abdominal pain, bloody diarrhea, vomiting, shock, and peritonitis; 40% of patients die. Pathologic studies reveal an acute ulcerative process of the bowel restricted to the small intestine. The mucosa is lifted off the submucosa, with the formation of large denuded areas. Pseudomembranes composed of sloughed epithelium are common, and gas may dissect into the submucosa. The source of the organisms may be the patient's own intestinal flora; cultures of ingested pork have failed to yield the organism. Antibodies to the β toxin of *C. perfringens* have been of considerable benefit in changing the course of established disease. In a large-scale trial, children immunized with *C. perfringens* β toxoid were protected.

Neutropenic Enterocolitis (Typhlitis)

See Chaps. 11 and 65.

Suppurative Deep-Tissue Infections

Clostridia are frequently recovered from various suppurative conditions in conjunction with other anaerobic and aerobic bacteria, but can also be the only organisms isolated. These suppurative conditions, which exist with severe local inflammation but usually without the characteristic systemic signs induced by clostridial toxins, include intraabdominal sepsis, empyema, pelvic abscess, subcutaneous abscess, frostbite with gas gangrene, infection of a stump in an amputee, brain abscess, prostatic abscess, perianal abscess, conjunctivitis, infection of a renal cell carcinoma, and infection of an aortic graft.

Clostridia are isolated from approximately two-thirds of patients with intraabdominal infections resulting from intestinal perforation. *C. ramosum*, *C. perfringens*, and *C. bifermentans* are the most commonly isolated species. The presence of clostridial species does not affect the clinical presentation or outcome of these infections (Chap. 65).

An association has been made between malignancy and the isolation of *C. septicum* in the absence of a grossly contaminated deep traumatic wound; in this situation, *C. septicum* may cause spontaneous nontraumatic myonecrosis (Fig. 42-1). A major site for such a malignancy is the gastrointestinal tract, particularly the colon. An association with leukemia or with other solid tumors has also been noted, and one case of fatal myonecrosis has been reported in a patient with ovarian cancer. Some of these patients present with *C. septicum* bacteremia; these cases have a fulminant clinical course (discussed below). Others develop localized suppurative infection in the abdomen or the abdominal wall without bacteremia. Presumably, this infection arises from a silent perforation that leads to intraabdominal abscess formation.

Clostridia have been isolated from suppurative infections of the female genital tract, particularly tuboovarian

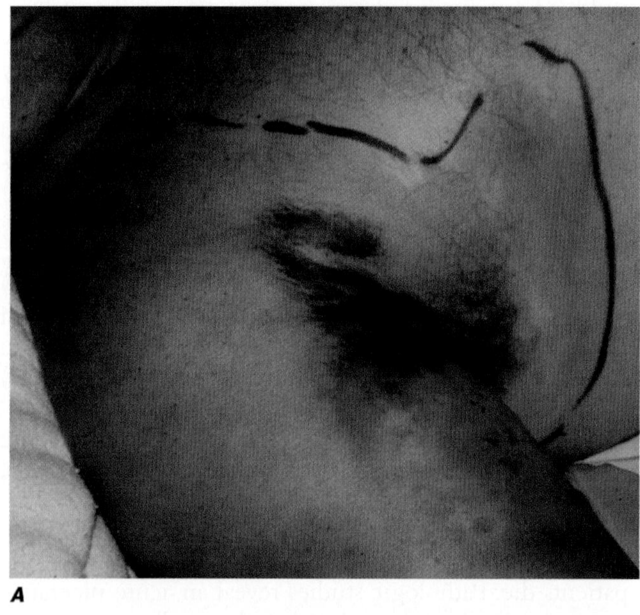

A

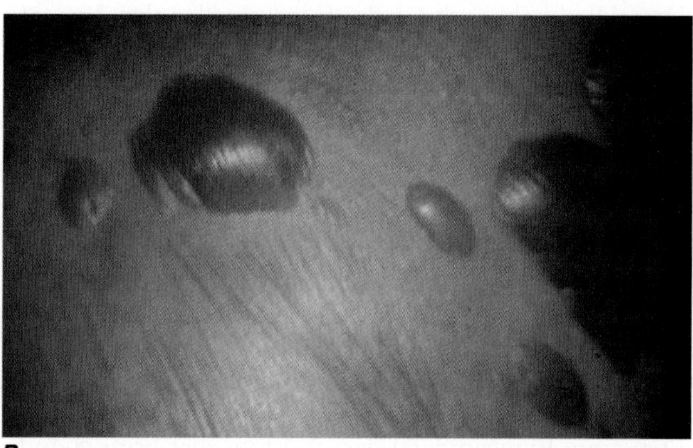

B

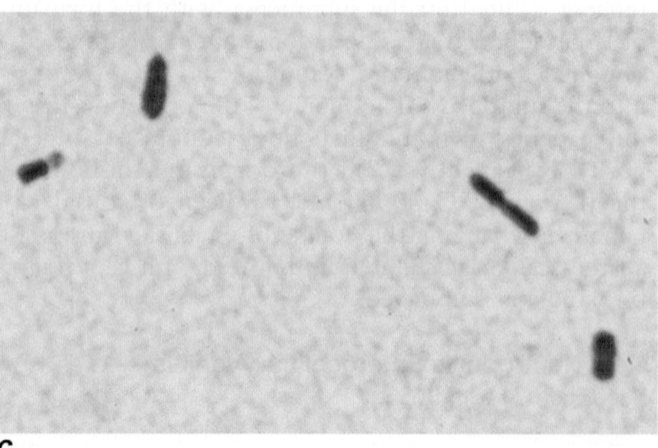

C

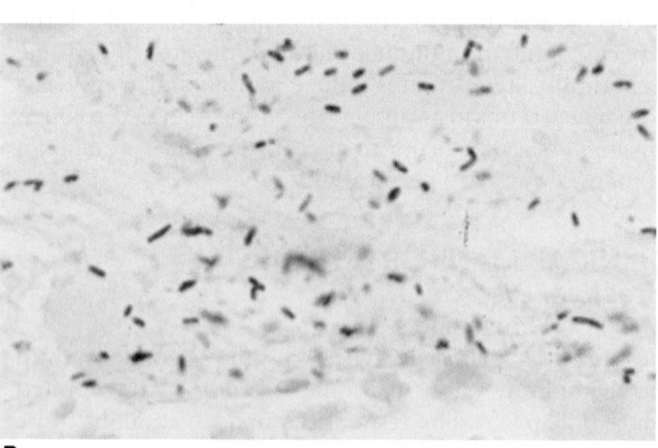

D

FIGURE 42-1

Spontaneous nontraumatic clostridial myonecrosis (gas gangrene). A man in his 50s presented with severe pain in the right upper extremity. Over several hours, he developed progressive swelling and discoloration in that extremity (***A***), with hemorrhagic ecchymoses and bullae (***B***). Gram's stain of aspirate from bullous lesions revealed gram-positive bacilli (***C***). The patient underwent amputation of the extremity. Tissue Gram's stain (***D***) also showed gram-positive bacilli, and surgical cultures grew *C. septicum*. Subsequent evaluation of the patient led to the diagnosis of invasive colonic carcinoma. *(Images used with permission of Stephen Calderwood, MD, and www.idimages.org.)*

and pelvic abscesses. The major species involved has been *C. perfringens*. Most of these suppurative infections are mild, with no evidence of uterine gangrene. *C. perfringens* has been isolated from as many as 20% of diseased gallbladders at surgery. One clinical syndrome, *emphysematous cholecystitis*, is caused by clostridial species at least 50% of the time. In this syndrome, gas forms in the biliary radicles and the wall of the gallbladder. Emphysematous cholecystitis is seen most often in diabetic patients. Although the mortality rate in this entity is higher than in more common forms of cholecystitis, there is no evidence of myonecrosis.

Clostridia are among the many organisms found in empyema fluid or isolated by transtracheal aspiration from patients with lung abscesses. There is no unique clinical clue to the presence of clostridia (as opposed to other organisms) in these infections. *C. perfringens* has been reported as a cause of empyema arising from aspiration pneumonia, pulmonary emboli, and infarction. However, the majority of cases of clostridial empyema are secondary to trauma.

Skin and Soft Tissue Infections

Various categories of traumatic wound infections due to clostridia have been described: simple contamination, anaerobic cellulitis, fasciitis with or without systemic manifestations, and anaerobic myonecrosis.

Simple Contamination

Clostridia are cultured most often from wounds in the absence of clinical signs of sepsis. As many as 30% of battle wounds are contaminated by clostridia without signs of suppuration, and 16% of penetrating abdominal wounds yield clostridia on culture despite treatment with cephalothin and kanamycin. In cases of trauma, clostridia are isolated with equal frequency from suppurative and well-healing wounds. Thus the diagnosis of clostridial infection should be based on clinical rather than bacteriologic criteria.

Localized Infection of the Skin and Soft Tissue without Systemic Signs

This condition, originally referred to as *anaerobic cellulitis*, is a localized infection involving the skin and soft tissue and is due to clostridia alone or with other bacteria. There are no systemic signs of toxicity, although the infection may invade locally, producing necrosis. These infections tend to be relatively indolent, spreading slowly to contiguous areas. Localized infections are relatively free of pain and edema. Perhaps because of the lack of edema, gas that is limited to the wound and the immediately surrounding tissue may be more evident than in gas gangrene. In these localized infections, gas is never found intramuscularly. Cellulitis, perirectal abscesses, and diabetic foot ulcers are typical infections from which clostridial species can be isolated. If inadequately treated, these localized infections advance by extension through subcutaneous tissue and fascial planes into muscle and may produce severe systemic disease with signs of toxemia.

A localized form of suppurative myositis has been described in heroin addicts. These patients develop local pain and tenderness in discrete areas (particularly the thigh and forearm), with the subsequent appearance of fluctuance and crepitance that require surgical drainage. The unusual aspect of these infections is that they remain localized without systemic signs of toxicity. Moreover, the affected local areas are not necessarily sites of trauma or heroin injection. Pathologic examination reveals subcutaneous abscesses, purulent myositis, and fasciitis from which clostridia are recovered in pure culture; on occasion, mixed infections involving aerobes and anaerobes are found. Wound botulism has been reported in association with the injection of black tar heroin.

Spreading Cellulitis and Fasciitis with Systemic Toxicity

This condition involves diffuse spreading cellulitis and fasciitis, without myonecrosis and with only mild inflammation in muscle. Patients present with the abrupt onset of a syndrome that progresses rapidly (within hours) through the fascial planes. In cases with suppuration and gas in soft tissues as well as overwhelming toxemia, the infection is rapidly fatal. On physical examination, there is subcutaneous crepitation but little localized pain. Surgery is of no proven value because there are no discretely involved tissues amenable to resection, as may be the case in myonecrosis. However, in rapidly advancing fasciitis, incision of the affected area is still the cornerstone of therapy. The initial local lesion may be quite innocuous and arises from an area involved by tumor or other infection and not by injury. The systemic toxic effects include hemolysis and injury of capillary membranes. Usually, this infection is fatal within 48 h, despite intensive therapy involving antitoxin and exchange transfusion. This syndrome is seen most commonly in patients with carcinoma, especially of the sigmoid or the cecum. Presumably, the tumor invades the fascia, and colonic contents leak into the abdominal wall. Patients present with extreme toxicity and occasionally with total-body crepitation. The syndrome differs from necrotizing fasciitis caused by other organisms in three respects: (1) rapid mortality, (2) rapid tissue invasion, and (3) the systemic effects of the toxin, typified by massive hemolysis.

Gas Gangrene (Clostridial Myonecrosis)

Gas gangrene is characterized by rapid and extensive necrosis of muscle accompanied by gas formation and systemic toxicity and occurs when bacteria invade healthy muscle from adjacent traumatized muscle or soft tissue. The infection originates in a wound contaminated with clostridia. Although >30% of deep wounds are infected with clostridia, the incidence of clostridial myonecrosis is quite low. These infections occur in both military and civilian settings. An essential factor in the genesis of gas gangrene appears to be trauma, particularly involving deep muscle laceration. The entity of clostridial myonecrosis is relatively uncommon after simple, through-and-through bullet wounds without shattering of bone and is relatively common after shrapnel fragmentation wounds, particularly when deep muscle is involved. In civilian cases, gas gangrene can follow trauma, surgery, or IM injection. The trauma need not be severe; however, the wound must be deep, necrotic, and without communication to the surface. Indeed, seeding of muscle tissue by *C. septicum* from a gastrointestinal source—often a malignancy—may lead to spontaneous nontraumatic clostridial myonecrosis (Fig. 42-1).

The incubation period of gas gangrene is usually short: almost always <3 days and frequently <24 h. Some 80% of cases are caused by *C. perfringens,* whereas *C. novyi*, *C. septicum*, and *C. histolyticum* cause most of the remaining cases. Typically, gas gangrene begins with the sudden onset of pain in the region of the wound, which helps to differentiate it from spreading cellulitis. Once established, the pain increases steadily in severity but remains localized to the infected area and spreads only if the infection spreads. Soon after pain develops, local swelling and edema—accompanied by a thin, often hemorrhagic exudate—appear. Patients frequently develop marked tachycardia, but elevation in temperature may be only minimal. Gas usually is not obvious at this early stage and may be completely absent. Frothiness of the wound exudate may be noted. The skin is tense, white, often marbled with blue, and cooler than normal. The symptoms progress rapidly; swelling, edema, and toxemia increase, and a profuse serous discharge, which may have a peculiar sweetish smell, appears. Gram's staining of the wound exudate shows many gram-positive rods with relatively few inflammatory cells (Fig. 42-1*C*).

At surgery, muscle may appear pale because of the intensity of edema, but it does not contract when probed with a scalpel. When dissected, the muscle is beefy red and nonviable and can progress to become black, friable, and gangrenous. It is important to establish a diagnosis early, preferably by frozen-section biopsy of muscle.

Despite hypotension, renal failure, and (often) body crepitation, patients with myonecrosis frequently have a heightened awareness of their surroundings until just before death, when they lapse into toxic delirium and coma. In untreated cases, as the local wounds progress, the skin becomes bronzed; bullae appear, become filled with dark red fluid, and are accompanied by dark patches of cutaneous gangrene. Gas appears in later phases but may not be as obvious as in anaerobic cellulitis. Jaundice is rare in wound gas gangrene (in contrast to uterine infections) and, when it does appear, is almost invariably associated with hemoglobinuria, hemoglobinemia, and septicemia. Cases of clostridial myonecrosis without a history of trauma have been reported. These patients have bullous lesions and crepitation of the skin; they present with a rapidly worsening course that includes myonecrosis, especially of the extremities.

Bacteremia and Clostridial Sepsis

The relatively common entity of transient clostridial bacteremia can arise in any hospitalized patient but is most common with a predisposing focus in the gastrointestinal tract, biliary tract, or uterus. Fever frequently resolves within 24–48 h without therapy. Despite the finding of clostridial bacteremia after septic abortions and the frequent isolation of clostridia from the lochia, most of the patients involved do not have evidence of sepsis. In one series of 60 patients with clostridial bacteremia, half had an infected site that could be associated with the bacteremia, whereas the other half had a totally unrelated illness, such as tuberculous pneumonia, meningitis, or benign gastroenteritis. By the time blood culture reports are returned, patients frequently are completely well and sometimes have been discharged. Therefore, when a blood culture is positive for clostridia, the patient must be assessed clinically rather than simply treated on the basis of the culture result.

Clostridial sepsis is an uncommon but almost invariably fatal illness after clostridial infection—primarily that of the uterus, colon, or biliary tract. This entity must be differentiated from transient clostridial bacteremia, which is much more common. *C. perfringens* causes the majority of cases of both sepsis and transient bacteremia. *C. septicum*, *C. sordellii*, and *C. novyi* account for most of the remainder of cases. *C. sordellii* sepsis with toxic shock syndrome has been associated with pregnancy and more recently with medically induced abortion. Clostridia account for 1–2.5% of all positive blood cultures in major hospital centers.

The majority of cases of clostridial sepsis originate from the female genital tract and follow septic abortion. Introduction of a foreign body is a common antecedent event. In the uterus, residual necrotic fetal and placental tissues and traumatized endometrium may allow the growth of clostridia. Only a small fraction of cases of septic abortion (1%) are followed by serious sepsis. In these instances, sepsis, fever, and chills begin 1–3 days after the attempted abortion. The initial signs are malaise, headache, severe myalgias, abdominal pain, nausea, vomiting, and occasionally diarrhea. Frequently, a bloody or brown vaginal discharge is noted. Patients may rapidly develop oliguria, hypotension, jaundice, and hemoglobinuria. The hemolysis, which is secondary to *C. perfringens* α toxin, causes a characteristic bronzing of the skin. As in myonecrosis, the mental status of severely ill patients is characterized by increased alertness and apprehension. Local examination of the pelvis reveals foul cervical discharge, occasionally with gas. Frequently, laceration marks around the cervix or perforation of the cervical segment is evident. If the infection involves the myometrium or has spread to the adnexa, extreme tenderness, guarding, and an adnexal mass may be found.

Laboratory studies in patients with sepsis reveal an elevated white blood cell count and may show pink, hemoglobin-tinged plasma. Anemia is proportional to the degree of hemolysis, and the hematocrit may be extremely low. Platelet counts may be reduced, and there is often evidence of disseminated intravascular coagulation (DIC). Oliguria or anuria, increasingly refractory hypotension, and hemorrhage and bruising may develop.

Clostridia may enter the bloodstream from the gastrointestinal or biliary tract. This occurrence is associated with ulcerative lesions or obstruction of the small or large intestine, necrotic or infiltrating malignancy, bowel surgery, or various abdominal catastrophes. The patient may present with an acute febrile illness, with chills and fever but no other signs of localized infection. Intravascular hemolysis occurs in as many as half of such cases. Biliary or gastrointestinal symptoms, if present, may be the only clue to the etiology. Positive blood cultures provide the definitive clue to the diagnosis.

Patients with malignant disease can also develop rapidly fatal clostridial sepsis, particularly from a gastrointestinal focus. The most common species in this setting is *C. septicum*. Characteristic signs and symptoms include fever, tachycardia, hypotension, abdominal pain or tenderness, nausea, vomiting, and (preterminally) coma. The tachycardia may be out of proportion to the fever. Only ~20–30% of patients develop hemolysis. A striking feature of this syndrome is the rapidity of death, which frequently occurs in <12 h.

DIAGNOSIS

The diagnosis of clostridial disease, in association with positive cultures, must be based primarily on clinical findings. Because of the presence of clostridia in many wounds, their mere isolation from any site, including the blood, does not necessarily indicate severe disease. Smears of wound exudates, uterine scrapings, or cervical discharge may show abundant large gram-positive rods as well as other organisms. Cultures should be placed in selective media and incubated anaerobically for identification of clostridia. The diagnosis of clostridial myonecrosis can be established by frozen-section biopsy of muscle.

The urine of patients with severe clostridial sepsis may contain protein and casts, and some patients may develop severe uremia. Profound alterations of circulating erythrocytes are seen in severely toxemic patients. Patients have hemolytic anemia, which develops extremely rapidly, along with hemoglobinemia, hemoglobinuria, and elevated levels of serum bilirubin. Spherocytosis, increased osmotic and mechanical red blood cell fragility, erythrophagocytosis, and methemoglobinemia have been described. DIC may develop in patients with severe infection. In patients with severe sepsis, Wright's or Gram's staining of a smear of peripheral blood or buffy coat may demonstrate clostridia.

X-ray examination sometimes provides an important clue to the diagnosis by revealing gas in muscles, subcutaneous tissue, or the uterus. However, the finding of gas is not pathognomonic for clostridial infection. Other anaerobic bacteria, frequently mixed with aerobic organisms, may produce gas.

℞ Treatment: CLOSTRIDIAL INFECTIONS

(Table 42-1) Traumatic wounds should be thoroughly cleansed and debrided. Traditionally, the antibiotic of choice for severe clostridial infection has been penicillin G (20 million units per day in adults). Penicillin G treatment of gas gangrene has become more controversial because of increasing resistance to this drug and data obtained from animal models of infection. In a mouse model of gas gangrene, antibiotics inhibiting toxin synthesis appeared to be preferable to cell wall–active drugs; clindamycin treatment enhanced survival more than therapy with penicillin; and the combination of clindamycin and penicillin was superior to penicillin alone. For severe clostridial sepsis, clindamycin may be used at a dose of 600 mg every 6 h in combination with

TABLE 42-1

TREATMENT OF CLOSTRIDIAL INFECTIONS[a]

CONDITION	ANTIBIOTIC TREATMENT	PENICILLIN ALLERGY	ADJUNCTIVE TREATMENT/NOTE
Contamination	None	—	—
Gas gangrene	Penicillin, 3–4 million units IV q4h, *plus* Clindamycin, 600 mg IV q6h	Chloramphenicol, metronidazole, imipenem, doxycycline (see text)[b]	Surgical debridement with wide excision is essential. Consider hyperbaric oxygen.
Clostridial sepsis	Penicillin, 3–4 million units IV q4h, *plus* Clindamycin, 600 mg IV q6h	Chloramphenicol, metronidazole, imipenem, doxycycline (see text)[b]	Transient bacteremia may be clinically insignificant.
Suppurative deep-tissue infections (e.g., abdominal wall, gynecologic)	Penicillin, 3–4 million units IV q4h, *plus* Gentamicin, 5 mg/kg IV q24h, *or* A third-generation cephalosporin (e.g., ceftriaxone, 2 g IV q12h)	As above, plus gentamicin or a quinolone	Empirical therapy should be given. Therapy should be based on Gram's stain and culture results when available.

[a]Treatment recommendations for *C. difficile* colitis, tetanus, and botulism are found in Chaps. 43, 40, and 41, respectively.
[b]Perform sensitivity testing; consider desensitization.

high-dose penicillin (3–4 million units every 4 h). Although no clinical trials validate this choice, it is gaining acceptance in the infectious disease community.

In cases of penicillin sensitivity or allergy, other antibiotics should be considered, but all should be tested for in vitro activity because of the occasional isolation of resistant strains. Clostridia are frequently, but not universally, susceptible in vitro to cefoxitin, carbenicillin, chloramphenicol, clindamycin, metronidazole, doxycycline, imipenem, minocycline, tetracycline, third-generation cephalosporins, and vancomycin. For severe clostridial infections, sensitivity testing should be done before an antimicrobial agent with unpredictable activity is used. Simple contamination of a wound with clostridia should not be treated with antibiotics. Localized skin and soft tissue infection can be managed by debridement rather than with systemic antibiotics. Drugs are required when the process extends into adjacent tissue or when fever and systemic signs of sepsis are present. Surgery is a mainstay of therapy for gas gangrene. Amputation is often required for rapidly spreading infection involving a limb, as the process frequently fails to respond to antibiotics. Hysterectomy is required for uterine myonecrosis. Abdominal wall myonecrosis usually continues despite initial aggressive surgery and antibiotic therapy and requires repeated surgical debridement of all involved muscle.

Suppurative infections should be treated with antibiotics. Frequently, broad-spectrum antibiotics must be used because of the mixed flora involved in these infections. Aminoglycosides can be used for the aerobic gram-negative bacteria involved in mixed infections.

The use of a polyvalent gas gangrene antitoxin is still recommended by some authorities. At present, no such antitoxin is produced in the United States, and most centers have discontinued its use in the management of patients with suspected gas gangrene or clostridial postabortion sepsis because of questionable efficacy and the substantial risk of hypersensitivity to horse serum, from which the antitoxin is derived.

The use of hyperbaric oxygen in the treatment of gas gangrene is also controversial. Studies in humans are not well designed to answer questions on efficacy, but several knowledgeable authors believe that hyperbaric oxygen therapy has contributed to dramatic clinical improvement. Such therapy may, however, be associated with untoward effects due to oxygen toxicity and high atmospheric pressure. Some centers without hyperbaric chambers have reported acceptable mortality rates; thus expert surgical and medical management and control of complications are probably the most important factors in the treatment of gas gangrene. Fasciotomy should not be delayed for hyperbaric oxygen therapy.

ACKNOWLEDGMENT

The authors acknowledge the contributions of Dori F. Zaleznik, MD, to this chapter in earlier editions of Harrison's Principles of Internal Medicine.

FURTHER READINGS

ANAYA DA et al: Necrotizing soft-tissue infection: Diagnosis and management. Clin Infect Dis 44:705, 2007

ARONOFF DM et al: Misoprostol impairs female reproductive tract innate immunity against *Clostridium sordellii*. J Immunol 180:8222, 2008

BORRIELLO SP: Clostridial disease of the gut. Clin Infect Dis 20:S242, 1995

CENTERS FOR DISEASE CONTROL AND PREVENTION: *Clostridium sordellii* toxic shock syndrome after medical abortion with mifepristone and intravaginal misoprostol—United States and Canada, 2001–2005. MMWR 54:724, 2005

LORBER B: Gas gangrene and other *Clostridium*-associated diseases, in *Principles and Practice of Infectious Diseases*, 6th ed, GL Mandell et al (eds). Philadelphia, Elsevier Churchill Livingstone, 2005, pp 2828–2838

MURRAY-LILLIBRIDGE K et al: Epidemiological findings and medical, legal, and public health challenges of an investigation of severe soft tissue infections and deaths among injecting drug users—Ireland, 2000. Epidemiol Infect 134:894, 2006

PRINSSEN HM et al: *Clostridium septicum* myonecrosis and ovarian cancer: A case report and review of literature. Gynecol Oncol 72:116, 1999

ROOD JI: Virulence genes of *Clostridium perfringens*. Annu Rev Microbiol 52:333, 1998

STEVENS DL, BRYANT AE: The role of clostridial toxins in the pathogenesis of gas gangrene. Clin Infect Dis 35:S93, 2002

WANG C et al: Hyperbaric oxygen for treating wounds: A systematic review of the literature. Arch Surg 138:272, 2003

CHAPTER 43

CLOSTRIDIUM DIFFICILE–ASSOCIATED DISEASE, INCLUDING PSEUDOMEMBRANOUS COLITIS

Dale N. Gerding ■ Stuart Johnson

DEFINITION

Clostridium difficile–associated disease (CDAD) is a unique colon infection that is acquired almost exclusively in association with antimicrobial use and the consequent disruption of the normal colonic flora. The most commonly diagnosed diarrheal illness acquired in the hospital, CDAD results from the ingestion of spores of *C. difficile* that vegetate, multiply, and secrete toxins, causing diarrhea and pseudomembranous colitis (PMC).

ETIOLOGY AND EPIDEMIOLOGY

C. difficile is an obligately anaerobic, gram-positive, spore-forming bacillus whose spores are found widely in nature, particularly in the environment of hospitals and chronic-care facilities. CDAD occurs most frequently in hospitals and nursing homes where the level of antimicrobial use is high and the environment is contaminated by *C. difficile* spores.

Clindamycin, ampicillin, and cephalosporins were the first antibiotics associated with CDAD. The second- and third-generation cephalosporins, particularly cefotaxime, ceftriaxone, cefuroxime, and ceftazidime, are agents frequently responsible for this condition, and the fluoroquinolones (ciprofloxacin, levofloxacin, gatifloxacin, and moxifloxacin) are the most recent drug class to be implicated in hospital outbreaks. Penicillin/β-lactamase-inhibitor combinations such as ticarcillin/clavulanate and piperacillin/tazobactam pose significantly less risk. However, all antibiotics, including vancomycin and metronidazole (the agents most commonly used to treat CDAD), have been found to carry a risk of subsequent CDAD. Rare cases are reported in patients without prior antibiotic exposure.

C. difficile is acquired exogenously, most frequently in the hospital, and is carried in the stool of symptomatic and asymptomatic patients. The rate of fecal colonization is often ≥20% among adult patients hospitalized for >1 week; in contrast, the rate is 1–3% among community residents. The risk of *C. difficile* acquisition increases in proportion to length of hospital stay. Asymptomatic fecal carriage of *C. difficile* in healthy neonates is very common, with rates often exceeding 50% during the first 6 months of life, but associated disease in this population is rare. Spores of *C. difficile* are found on environmental surfaces (where the organism can persist for months) and on the hands of hospital personnel who fail to practice good hand hygiene. Hospital epidemics of CDAD have been attributed to a single *C. difficile* strain and to multiple strains present simultaneously. Other identified risk factors for CDAD include older age, greater severity of underlying illness, gastrointestinal surgery, use of electronic rectal thermometers, enteral tube feeding, and antacid treatment. Use of proton pump inhibitors may be a risk factor.

PATHOLOGY AND PATHOGENESIS

Spores of toxigenic *C. difficile* are ingested, survive gastric acidity, germinate in the small bowel, and colonize the lower intestinal tract, where they elaborate two large toxins: toxin A, an enterotoxin, and toxin B, a cytotoxin. These toxins initiate processes resulting in the disruption of epithelial-cell barrier function, diarrhea, and pseudomembrane formation. Toxin A is a potent neutrophil chemoattractant, and both toxins glucosylate the GTP-binding proteins of the Rho subfamily that regulate the actin cell cytoskeleton. Disruption of the cytoskeleton results in loss of cell shape, adherence, and tight junctions, with consequent fluid leakage. A third toxin, binary toxin CDT, was previously found in only ~6% of strains but is present in all isolates of the newly recognized epidemic strain (see "Global Considerations" next in the chapter); this toxin is related to *C. perfringens* iota toxin. Its role in the pathogenesis of CDAD has not yet been defined.

The pseudomembranes of PMC are confined to the colonic mucosa and initially appear as 1- to 2-mm whitish-yellow plaques. The intervening mucosa appears unremarkable, but, as the disease progresses, the pseudomembranes coalesce to form larger plaques and become confluent over the entire colon wall (Fig. 43-1). The whole colon is usually involved, but 10% of patients have rectal sparing. Viewed microscopically, the pseudomembranes have a mucosal attachment point and contain necrotic leukocytes, fibrin, mucus, and cellular debris. The epithelium is eroded and necrotic in focal areas, with neutrophil infiltration of the mucosa.

Patients colonized with *C. difficile* were initially thought to be at high risk for CDAD. However, four prospective studies have shown that colonized patients actually have a decreased risk of subsequent CDAD. At least three events are proposed as essential for the development of CDAD

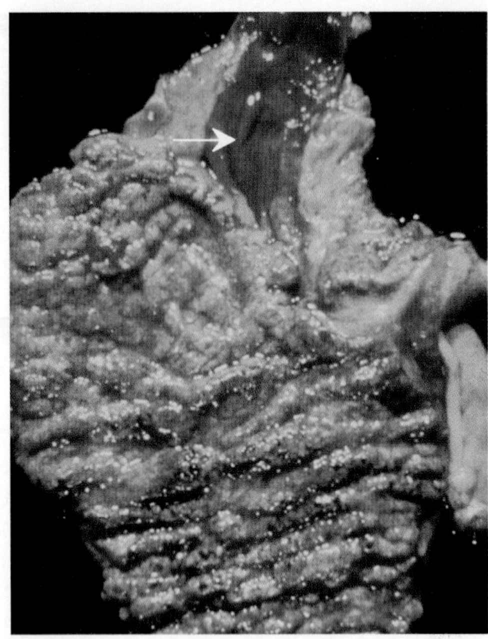

FIGURE 43-1
Autopsy specimen showing confluent pseudomembranes covering the cecum of a patient with pseudomembranous colitis. Note the sparing of the terminal ileum (*arrow*).

(Fig. 43-2). Exposure to antimicrobial agents is the first event and establishes susceptibility to *C. difficile* infection. The second event is exposure to toxigenic *C. difficile*. Given that the majority of patients do not develop CDAD after the first two events, a third event is clearly essential for its occurrence. Candidate third events include exposure to a *C. difficile* strain of particular virulence, exposure to antimicrobial agents especially likely to cause CDAD, and an inadequate host immune response. The host anamnestic serum IgG antibody response to toxin A of *C. difficile* is the most likely third event that determines which patients develop diarrhea and which patients remain asymptomatic. The majority of humans first develop antibody to *C. difficile* toxins when colonized asymptomatically during the first year of life. Infants are thought not to develop symptomatic CDAD because they lack suitable mucosal toxin receptors that develop later in life. In adulthood, serum levels of IgG antibody to toxin A increase more in response to infection in individuals who become asymptomatic carriers than in those who develop CDAD. For persons who develop CDAD, increasing levels of antitoxin A during treatment correlate with a lower risk of recurrence of CDAD.

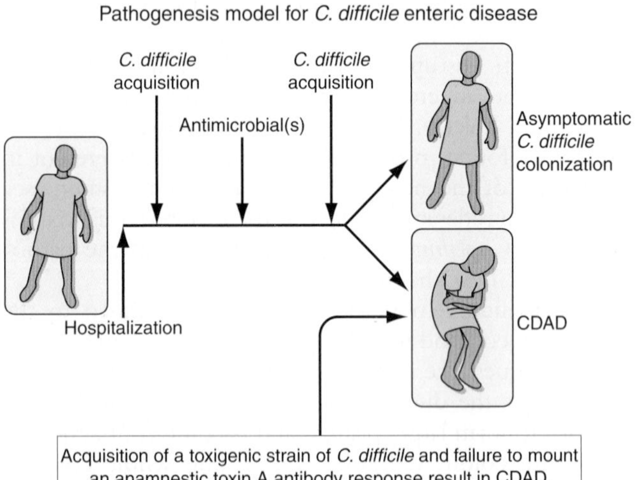

Pathogenesis model for *C. difficile* enteric disease
C. difficile acquisition
C. difficile acquisition
Antimicrobial(s)
Asymptomatic *C. difficile* colonization
Hospitalization
CDAD
Acquisition of a toxigenic strain of *C. difficile* and failure to mount an anamnestic toxin A antibody response result in CDAD.

FIGURE 43-2
Pathogenesis model for hospital-acquired *Clostridium difficile*–associated diarrhea (CDAD). At least three events are integral to *C. difficile* pathogenesis. Exposure to antibiotics establishes susceptibility to infection. Once susceptible, the patient may acquire nontoxigenic (nonpathogenic) or toxigenic strains of *C. difficile* as a second event. Acquisition of toxigenic *C. difficile* may be followed by asymptomatic colonization or CDAD, depending on one or more additional events, including an inadequate host anamnestic IgG response to *C. difficile* toxin A.

GLOBAL CONSIDERATIONS

Rates and severity of CDAD in the United States, Canada, and Europe have increased markedly since the year 2000. Rates in U.S. hospitals tripled between 2000 and 2005. Hospitals in Montreal, Quebec, have reported rates four times higher than the 1997 baseline, with directly attributable mortality of 6.9% (increased from 1.5% previously). An epidemic strain, variously known as toxinotype III, REA type BI, PCR ribotype 027, and pulsed-field type NAP1, is thought to account for much of the increase in incidence and has been found in the United States, Canada, and Europe. The epidemic organism is characterized by (1) an ability to produce 16–23 times as much toxin A and toxin B as control strains in vitro; (2) the presence of a third toxin (binary toxin CDT); and (3) high-level resistance to all fluoroquinolones.

CLINICAL MANIFESTATIONS

Diarrhea is the most common manifestation caused by *C. difficile*. Stools are almost never grossly bloody and range from soft and unformed to watery or mucoid in consistency, with a characteristic odor. Patients may have as many as 20 bowel movements per day. Clinical and laboratory findings include fever in 28% of cases, abdominal pain in 22%, and leukocytosis in 50%. When adynamic ileus (which is seen on x-ray in ~20% of cases) results in cessation of stool passage, the diagnosis of CDAD is frequently overlooked. A clue to the presence of unsuspected CDAD in these patients is unexplained leukocytosis, with ≥15,000 cells/μL. Such patients are at high risk for complications of *C. difficile* infection, particularly toxic megacolon and sepsis.

C. difficile diarrhea recurs after treatment in ~15–30% of cases, and this figure may be increasing. Recurrences may represent either relapses due to the same strain or reinfections with a new strain. Recurrence of clinical CDAD is likely to be a result of continued disruption of the normal fecal flora by the antibiotic used to treat CDAD.

DIAGNOSIS

The diagnosis of CDAD is based on a combination of clinical criteria: (1) diarrhea (≥3 unformed stools per 24 h for ≥2 days), with no other recognized cause; plus (2) toxin A or B detected in the stool, toxin-producing *C. difficile* detected by stool culture, or pseudomembranes seen in the colon. PMC is a more advanced form of CDAD and is visualized at endoscopy in only ~50% of patients with diarrhea who have a positive stool culture and toxin assay for *C. difficile* (Table 43-1). Endoscopy is a rapid diagnostic tool in seriously ill patients with suspected PMC and an acute abdomen, but a negative result in this examination does not rule out CDAD.

Despite the array of tests available for *C. difficile* and its toxins (Table 43-1), no single test has high sensitivity, high specificity, and rapid turnaround. The turnaround time for reporting of a positive result in the cell cytotoxicity test can be shortened to <24 h if cell cultures are examined at intervals as short as 4 h. However, this approach is labor intensive, and observation for 48 h is required for a conclusive test result. Most laboratory tests for toxins lack sensitivity. However, testing of multiple additional stool specimens is not recommended. Empirical treatment is appropriate if CDAD is strongly suspected on clinical grounds. Testing of asymptomatic patients is not recommended except for epidemiologic study purposes. In particular, so-called tests of cure after treatment are not recommended because many patients continue to harbor the organism and toxin after diarrhea has ceased and test results do not always predict recurrence of CDAD. Thus these results should not be used to restrict placement of patients in long-term care or nursing home facilities.

Rx Treatment: *CLOSTRIDIUM DIFFICILE*-ASSOCIATED DISEASE

PRIMARY CDAD When possible, discontinuation of any ongoing antimicrobial administration is recommended as the first step in treatment of CDAD. Earlier studies indicated that 15–23% of patients respond to this simple measure. However, with the advent of the current epidemic strain and the associated rapid clinical deterioration of some patients, prompt initiation of specific CDAD treatment has become the standard. General treatment guidelines include hydration and the avoidance of antiperistaltic agents and opiates, which may mask symptoms and possibly worsen disease. Nevertheless, antiperistaltic agents have been used safely with vancomycin or metronidazole for mild to moderate CDAD.

Although limited prospective randomized clinical trials showed no statistical differences among treatment agents for cessation of diarrhea (the primary outcome endpoint; Table 43-2), later observational studies suggest that response rates to metronidazole may have decreased. The clinical response rate for bacitracin is

TABLE 43-1

RELATIVE SENSITIVITY AND SPECIFICITY OF DIAGNOSTIC TESTS FOR *CLOSTRIDIUM DIFFICILE*-ASSOCIATED DISEASE (CDAD)

TYPE OF TEST	RELATIVE SENSITIVITY[a]	RELATIVE SPECIFICITY[a]	COMMENT
Stool culture for *C. difficile*	++++	+++	Most sensitive test; specificity is ++++ if the *C. difficile* isolate tests positive for toxin; with clinical data, is diagnostic of CDAD
Cell culture cytotoxin test on stool	+++	++++	With clinical data, is diagnostic of CDAD; highly specific but not as sensitive as stool culture
Enzyme immunoassay for toxin A or toxins A and B in stool	++ to +++	+++	With clinical data, is diagnostic of CDAD; rapid results, but not as sensitive as stool culture or cell culture cytotoxin test
Latex test for *C. difficile* antigen in stool	++	+++	Detects glutamate dehydrogenase found in toxigenic and nontoxigenic strains of *C. difficile* and other stool organisms; less sensitive and specific than other tests; rapid results
Colonoscopy or sigmoidoscopy	+	++++	Highly specific if pseudomembranes are seen; insensitive compared with other tests

[a] According to both clinical and test-based criteria.
Note: ++++, >90%; +++, 71–90%; ++, 51–70%; +, ~50%.

TABLE 43-2

EXPECTED TREATMENT OUTCOMES BASED ON RANDOMIZED COMPARATIVE TRIALS OF ORAL THERAPY FOR *CLOSTRIDIUM DIFFICILE*-ASSOCIATED DISEASE

TREATMENT	DOSE AND DURATION	RESOLUTION OF DIARRHEA, %	RECURRENCE, %
Placebo or discontinuation of offending antibiotics	None	21	Unknown
Metronidazole	250 mg qid × 10 d	95	5
	250 mg qid × 10 d[a]	82	30
	500 mg tid × 10 d	94	17
Vancomycin	500 mg tid × 10 d	94	17
	500 mg qid × 10 d	100	15
	125 mg qid × 10 d[a]	91	19
	125 mg qid × 7 d	86	33
	125 mg qid × 5 d	75	Unknown
Teicoplanin	400 mg bid × 10 d	96	7
	100 mg bid × 10 d	96	8
Nitazoxanide	500 mg bid × 10 d[a]	89	22
Fusidic acid	500 mg tid × 10 d	93	28
Bacitracin	25,000 U qid × 10 d	80	42

[a]Data from randomized trials reported in 2006.

10–20% lower than that for vancomycin; therefore, bacitracin use for first-line therapy is discouraged. All drugs, particularly vancomycin, should be given orally if possible. When IV metronidazole is administered, fecal bactericidal drug concentrations are achieved during acute diarrhea, and CDAD treatment has been successful; however, in the presence of adynamic ileus, IV metronidazole treatment of PMC has failed. In previous randomized trials, diarrhea response rates to oral therapy with vancomycin or metronidazole were ≥94%, but two recent observational studies found that metronidazole response rates had declined to 74% and 78%. Although the mean time to resolution of diarrhea is 2–4 days, the response to metronidazole may be much slower. Treatment should not be deemed a failure until a drug has been given for at least 6 days. On the basis of data for shorter courses of vancomycin (Table 43-2), it is recommended that metronidazole and vancomycin be given for at least 10 days, although no controlled comparisons are available. Although metronidazole is not approved for this indication by the U.S. Food and Drug Administration (FDA), most patients with mild to moderate illness respond to 500 mg given by mouth three times a day for 10 days; extension of the treatment period may be needed for slow responders. Because of the recent increase in metronidazole failures, patients treated with this drug should be monitored carefully for progressive defervescence (if fever is present), alleviation of abdominal pain and tenderness, decreases in the number of daily bowel movements, and decreases in the white blood cell (WBC) count. Clinical deterioration, with worsening signs and symptoms, or an unexplained increase in the WBC count during treatment are indications for a switch to vancomycin (usual dose, 125 mg orally four times a day). Although the use of vancomycin is discouraged for treatment of mildly to moderately ill patients, it is appropriate to use this agent for the initial treatment of patients who appear seriously ill, particularly if they have a high WBC count (>15,000/μL); controlled clinical outcome data on vancomycin use against the epidemic strain are not available. A randomized prospective trial of the antiparasitic drug nitazoxanide showed that (although not approved by the FDA for this indication) it was at least as effective as metronidazole for the treatment of CDAD, providing a potential alternative to vancomycin and metronidazole.

RECURRENT CDAD Overall, ~15–30% of patients experience recurrences of CDAD, either as relapses caused by the original organism or as reinfections after treatment (Table 43-2). Recurrence rates are higher among patients ≥65 years old and among patients who remain in the hospital after the initial episode of CDAD. Patients who have a first recurrence of CDAD have a high rate of second recurrence (33–65%). In the first recurrence, re-treatment with metronidazole is comparable to treatment with vancomycin. Recurrent disease, once thought to be relatively mild, has been documented to pose a significant (11%) risk of serious complications (shock, megacolon, perforation, colectomy, or death within 30 days). There is no standard treatment for multiple recurrences, but long or repeated metronidazole courses should be avoided because of potential neurotoxicity. Approaches include the administration of vancomycin followed by the yeast *Saccharomyces boulardii*; the administration of vancomycin followed by synthetic fecal bacterial enema; and the intentional colonization of the patient with a nontoxigenic strain of *C. difficile*. None of these biotherapeutic approaches has been approved by the FDA for use in the United States. Other strategies include (1) the use of vancomycin in tapering doses or with pulse dosing every other day for 4–6 weeks and (2) sequential treatment with vancomycin (125 mg four times daily) followed by rifaximin (400 mg twice daily) for 14 days. IV immunoglobulin, which has also been used with some success, presumably provides antibodies to *C. difficile* toxins.

FULMINANT CDAD Fulminant (rapidly progressive and severe) CDAD presents the most difficult treatment challenge. Patients with fulminant disease often do not have diarrhea, and their illness mimics an acute surgical abdomen. Sepsis (hypotension, fever, tachycardia, leukocytosis) may result from severe CDAD. An acute abdomen (with or without toxic megacolon) may include signs of obstruction, ileus, colon-wall thickening, and ascites on abdominal CT, often with peripheral-blood leukocytosis (≥20,000 cells/μL). Whether or not the patient has diarrhea, the differential diagnosis of an acute abdomen, sepsis, or toxic megacolon should include CDAD if the patient has received antibiotics in the past 2 months. Cautious sigmoidoscopy or colonoscopy to visualize PMC and an abdominal CT examination are the best diagnostic tests in patients without diarrhea.

Medical management of fulminant CDAD is suboptimal because of the difficulty of delivering metronidazole or vancomycin to the colon by the oral route in the presence of ileus. Vancomycin (given via nasogastric tube and by retention enema) plus IV metronidazole have been used in uncontrolled studies with some success, but surgical colectomy may be life-saving if there is no response to medical management. The incidence of fulminant CDAD requiring colectomy appears to be increasing in the evolving epidemic.

PROGNOSIS

The mortality rate attributed to CDAD, previously found to be 0.6–3.5%, has reached 6.9% in recent outbreaks and is progressively higher with increasing age. Most patients recover, but recurrences are common.

PREVENTION AND CONTROL

Strategies for the prevention of CDAD are of two types: those aimed at preventing transmission of the organism to the patient and those aimed at reducing the risk of CDAD if the organism is transmitted. Transmission of *C. difficile* in clinical practice has been prevented by gloving of personnel, elimination of the use of contaminated electronic thermometers, and use of hypochlorite (bleach) solution for environmental decontamination of patients' rooms. Hand hygiene is critical; hand washing is recommended in CDAD outbreaks because alcohol hand gels are not sporicidal. CDAD outbreaks have been best controlled by restricting the use of specific antibiotics, such as clindamycin and second- and third-generation cephalosporins. Outbreaks of CDAD due to clindamycin-resistant strains have resolved promptly when clindamycin use was restricted.

FURTHER READINGS

Hubert B et al: A portrait of the geographic dissemination of the *Clostridium difficile* North American pulsed-field type 1 strain and the epidemiology of *C. difficile*–associated disease in Quebec. Clin Infect Dis 44:238, 2007

Johnson S et al: Interruption of recurrent *Clostridium difficile*–associated diarrhea episodes by serial therapy with vancomycin and rifaximin. Clin Infect Dis 44:846, 2007

Kyne L et al: Association between antibody response to toxin A and protection against recurrent *Clostridium difficile* diarrhea. Lancet 357:189, 2001

——— et al: Asymptomatic carriage of *Clostridium difficile* and serum levels of IgG antibody against toxin A. N Engl J Med 342:390, 2000

Loo VG et al: A predominantly clonal multi-institutional outbreak of *Clostridium difficile*–associated diarrhea with high morbidity and mortality. N Engl J Med 353:2442, 2005

McDonald LC et al: *Clostridium difficile* infection in patients discharged from US short-stay hospitals, 1996-2003. Emerg Infect Dis 12:409, 2006

——— et al: An epidemic, toxin gene–variant strain of *Clostridium difficile*. N Engl J Med 353:2433, 2005

McFarland LV: Alternative treatments for *Clostridium difficile* disease: What really works? J Med Microbiol 54:101, 2005

Miller MA: Clinical management of *Clostridium difficile*–associated disease. Clin Infect Dis 45(Suppl 2):S122, 2007

Pepin J et al: The management and outcomes of a first recurrence of *Clostridium difficile* associated disease in Quebec. Clin Infect Dis 42:758, 2006

Zar FA et al: A comparison of vancomycin and metronidazole for the treatment of *Clostridium difficile*–associated diarrhea, stratified by disease severity. Clin Infect Dis 45:302, 2007

CHAPTER 44

MENINGOCOCCAL INFECTIONS

Lee M. Wetzler

DEFINITION

Neisseria meningitidis is the etiologic agent of two life-threatening diseases: meningococcal meningitis and fulminant meningococcemia. More rarely, meningococci cause pneumonia, septic arthritis, pericarditis, urethritis, and conjunctivitis. Most cases are potentially preventable by vaccination.

ETIOLOGIC AGENT

Meningococci are gram-negative aerobic diplococci. Unlike the other neisseriae, they have a polysaccharide capsule. They are transmitted among humans—their only known habitat—via respiratory secretions. Colonization of the nasopharynx or pharynx is much more common than invasive disease.

MICROBIOLOGY AND CLASSIFICATION

On the basis of genome sequencing, *N. meningitidis* is categorized as a β-proteobacterium related to *Bordetella*, *Burkholderia*, *Kingella*, and *Methylomonas* and—more distantly—to *Vibrio*, *Haemophilus*, and *Escherichia coli*. Meningococci are traditionally classified by serologic typing systems based on structural differences in capsule (serogroup), major outer-membrane protein (OMP) porin (PorB, serotype), minor porin (PorA, serosubtype), and lipooligosaccharide (LOS, immunotype). Thus, for example, the meningococcal strain designation B:2b:P1.5: L3,7,9 reflects the serogroup (B), serotype (2b), serosubtype (P1.5), and immunotype (L3,7,9). Meningococci are also differentiated from the other Neisseriaceae by their pattern of sugar fermentation. *N. gonorrhoeae* ferments only glucose; *N. meningitidis* ferments glucose and maltose; and *N. lactamica* ferments glucose, maltose, and lactose.

Meningococci are classified into serogroups according to the antigenicity of their capsular polysaccharides, which reflects structural differences in these carbohydrates. Five serogroups (A, B, C, Y, and W-135; see below) are responsible for >90% of cases of meningococcal disease worldwide. One limitation of serogroup classification based on polysaccharide capsular structure is that the genes for capsule biosynthesis can be transferred from one strain to another, with consequent changes in the capsule structure of the recipient strain and therefore in its serogroup. Meningococcal serotypes and subtypes are defined by antigenic differences in specific OMPs. Thus other methods for tracking meningococcal strains have become increasingly useful. Multilocus enzyme electrophoresis classifies bacteria into electrophoretic types (ETs), and variations in ET are not based on antigenic variations or alterations in outer-membrane component structures. Other techniques for establishing strain identity or nonidentity—i.e., pulsed-field gel electrophoresis of large DNA fragments and amplification of bacterial genomic sequences by polymerase chain reaction (PCR)—are based on the genetic makeup of the strain. These techniques are used for identification of the strains associated with outbreaks of disease. For example, the virulent III-1 clonal complex of serogroup A was first recognized in Nepal in 1983–1984; it spread to Mecca, then to Sub-Saharan Africa, and subsequently to temperate Africa. The serogroup B ET-5 complex was first identified in Norway in the 1970s and later caused outbreaks in Europe, Cuba, and South and North America (most recently, in the Pacific Northwest). Serogroup C ET-24 (the ET-37 complex) has caused sporadic cases and outbreaks in Canada and the United States; in some analyses, it has been associated with high rates of mortality and morbidity.

EPIDEMIOLOGY

Meningococcal disease occurs worldwide as isolated (sporadic) cases, institution- or community-based outbreaks, and large epidemics. Despite effective antibiotics and partially effective vaccines, *N. meningitidis* is still a leading global cause of meningitis and rapidly fatal sepsis, often in otherwise-healthy individuals.

N. meningitidis is unique among the major bacterial agents of meningitis in that it causes epidemic as well as endemic (sporadic) disease. In all, 300,000–500,000 cases of meningococcal disease occur worldwide each year—numbers that frequently are increased by large epidemics. The annual incidence of meningococcal disease is 1–2 cases per 100,000 population for sporadic disease, 5–10 cases per 100,000 for hypersporadic disease (localized outbreaks and case clusters), and 10–>1000 cases per 100,000 for pandemic and epidemic disease (e.g., serogroup A epidemics).

Serogroup A strains, which caused most of the large epidemics of meningococcal disease during the first half of the twentieth century, are now associated with recurring epidemics in Sub-Saharan Africa (the African meningitis belt) and other locales in the developing world. In the largest meningococcal epidemic recorded, >300,000 cases and 30,000 deaths due to serogroup A *N. meningitidis* occurred in Sub-Saharan Africa in 1996–1997. Serogroups B and C cause most cases of sporadic and epidemic meningococcal disease in industrialized countries. Since 1980, large serogroup B epidemics and/or outbreaks of serogroup A or C meningococcal disease have also occurred in Europe, the United States, Canada, China, Nepal, Mongolia, New Zealand, Cuba, Brazil, Chile, Saudi Arabia, and South Africa. In the United States and Canada during the 1990s, serogroup B was the most common cause of sporadic disease, whereas serogroup C was a more frequent cause of outbreaks. Serogroup Y has recently been isolated from almost one-third of cases of meningococcal disease in the United States. In general, patients with serogroup Y disease are older and more likely to be African American or to have a chronic underlying illness than are patients with disease caused by other serogroups. Serogroups Y and W-135 are isolated more often than the other serogroups from patients with pneumonia. In 2000, 2001, and 2002, worldwide epidemics of serogroup W-135 meningococcal disease occurred in association with the Muslim pilgrimage to Mecca (the Hajj) and in the meningitis belt of Sub-Saharan Africa.

In the United States, the attack rate for sporadic meningococcal disease is ~1 case per 100,000 persons per year. Disease attack rates are highest among infants 3–9 months of age (10–15 cases per 100,000 infants per year). Attack rates are higher among children than among adults, and there is a second peak of incidence among teenagers, in whom outbreaks have often been tied to residence in barracks, dormitories, or other crowded conditions. This observation has prompted the recommendation that meningococcal polysaccharide-based vaccines (see below) be administered to incoming college freshmen to prevent outbreaks at colleges. Although the age-specific incidence is much lower among adults (<1 case per 100,000 persons per year), one-third to one-half of all cases of sporadic meningococcal disease occur in individuals ≥18 years of age. Peak disease incidence coincides with the winter peak of respiratory viral illnesses. During epidemics, disease incidence increases disproportionately among teenagers and young adults. In Sub-Saharan Africa, epidemic outbreaks occur with the dry season and the coming of the dry dusty winds of the harmattan.

Meningococcal disease occurs more commonly among the household contacts of primary cases than in the general population. The secondary attack rate is 400–1000 per 100,000 household members. School-based clusters of cases have also been described; the attack rate among school contacts of cases has been estimated at 2–4 cases per 100,000 exposed individuals. In outbreaks on college campuses, attack rates have been highest among students living in dormitories. Most secondary cases occur within 2 weeks of the primary case, although some cases may develop as long as several months later. Secondary cases account for <2% of all cases reported each year in the United States.

Meningococcal colonization of the nasopharynx (asymptomatic carriage) can persist for months. In nonepidemic periods, ~10% of healthy individuals are colonized, as are up to 30% of persons living in relatively crowded conditions (e.g., in military barracks or college dormitories). Factors that predispose individuals to colonization with *N. meningitidis* include residence in the same household with a person who has meningococcal disease or is a carrier, household or institutional crowding, active or passive exposure to tobacco smoke, and a recent history of a viral upper respiratory infection. These factors have also been associated with an increased risk of meningococcal disease.

PATHOGENESIS

(Fig. 44-1) Meningococci that colonize the upper respiratory tract are internalized by nonciliated mucosal cells and may traverse them to enter the submucosa, from which they can make their way into the bloodstream. Although meningococcal colonization of healthy humans is common, bloodstream infection is an infrequent event that is not essential for the organisms' survival and spread. The production of human disease has no obvious evolutionary advantage for either pathogen or host. Although some strains of *N. meningitidis* are thought to cause more severe disease in humans than do other strains, the basis for this difference is not understood. Meningococci may undergo important phenotypic changes when they adapt to growth in vivo; presumed virulence traits include the antiphagocytic capsular polysaccharide, an ability to sialylate LOS so that it mimics host-cell carbohydrate moieties and inhibits complement deposition, the secretion of IgA protease, and mechanisms for iron acquisition. However, there is little evidence that alteration in meningococcal components, putative toxins, or other secreted substances affects virulence. Moreover, the ET-5 strain of serogroup B *N. meningitidis* has been associated with high case-fatality rates in some populations but not in others. These points suggest that host factors, as opposed to bacterial components, are the main mediators of immune resistance and disease pathogenesis.

A meningococcal organism that enters the bloodstream from the nasopharynx and survives host defenses generally has one of two fates. If multiplication occurs slowly, the bacteria eventually may seed local sites, such

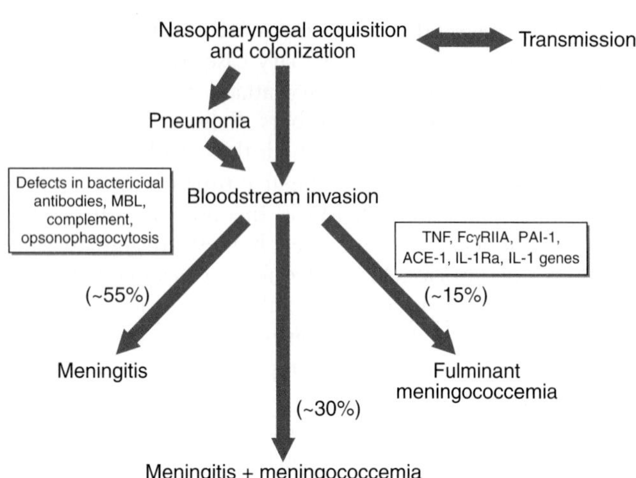

FIGURE 44-1

Meningococcal disease pathogenesis, susceptibility, and severity. After human-to-human transmission, environmental factors (smoking, co-infections), polymorphisms in innate immunity or other genes, and absence of mucosal antibodies may confer susceptibility to meningococcal invasion from the nasopharynx into the bloodstream. In individuals who lack bactericidal antibodies, terminal or alternative pathway complement-deficiency states and other genetic polymorphisms may influence the severity of the ensuing host response and the clinical presentation. Although each of these gene associations has been reported, most of them require confirmation in different ethnic groups. MBL, mannose-binding lectin; TNF, tumor necrosis factor; FcγRIIA, FCγRIIA R131 allele; PAI-1, plasminogen activator inhibitor 1; ACE-1, angiotensin-converting enzyme 1; IL, interleukin; IL-1Ra, interleukin 1 receptor antagonist.

as the meninges and/or (rarely) the joints or the pericardium. More rapid multiplication in the bloodstream is associated with the clinical features of meningococcemia [i.e., petechiae, purpura, disseminated intravascular coagulation (DIC), and shock], which usually causes symptoms before local sites become infected. Thus compartmentalization of bacterial growth and host inflammation either in the blood or at a local site (usually the meninges) can occur.

Outer-Membrane Components Associated with Virulence

Meningococcal strains are characterized by the expression of capsular polysaccharide and other outer-membrane structures, including LOS (endotoxin). Outer-membrane blebbing, meningococcal autolysis, molecular mimicry, genome plasticity, horizontal DNA exchange, and phase and/or antigenic variation are all important in meningococcal virulence.

Capsule

The polysaccharide capsule is a major—if not *the* major—virulence factor of *N. meningitidis*. As stated above, meningococci isolated from the blood or cerebrospinal fluid (CSF) of patients with invasive meningococcal disease most often express capsules of serogroups A, B, C, Y, and W-135. Isolates from asymptomatic nasopharyngeal carriers are nongroupable or express B, Y, X, Z, or 29E capsular serogroups. Capsules impart antiphagocytic and antibactericidal properties to the meningococcus and thus enhance meningococcal survival during invasion of the bloodstream or CSF. Capsules also provide protective properties (e.g., preventing desiccation and phagocytic killing) and antiadherent properties; these properties promote meningococcal transmission, spread, and survival externally and within intracellular compartments such as phagocytic vacuoles.

Except in serogroup A, the major meningococcal capsular polysaccharides associated with invasive disease are composed of polymers of sialic acid (*N*-acetyl neuraminic acid, NANA) derivatives. The serogroup B capsule is composed of (α2→8)-linked NANA, the serogroup C capsule of (α2→9)-linked NANA, the serogroup Y capsule of alternating D-glucose and NANA, and the serogroup W-135 capsule of D-galactose and NANA. The differences in sialic acid capsule composition are derived from the distinct polysialyltransferases encoded by the fourth gene of the capsule biosynthesis operon, which is also used as a basis for capsule-specific PCR diagnosis. A four-gene operon encoding the capsule transport apparatus (ctr) is conserved among different serogroups and is also used in PCR diagnosis. The serogroup A capsule is composed of repeating units of (α)-linked *N*-acetyl-mannosamine-1-phosphate and is encoded by a four-gene biosynthesis cassette unique for this serogroup.

Outer-Membrane Proteins

Meningococci isolated from sites of colonization or invasive disease are piliated. Pili are complex outer-membrane, protein-based organelles that facilitate adhesion—the first step in meningococcal–host cell interactions. Meningococci express two major OMP porins, PorA and PorB. Human opsonins and bactericidal antibodies induced during meningococcal disease have been shown to recognize PorA and PorB. Vaccines based on PorA-containing outer-membrane vesicles are under development. Another OMP, Opc, is involved in cell attachment and is also a target of bactericidal antibodies. Meningococci encounter iron-restricted environments during infection. The majority of host iron is presented intracellularly as hemoglobin and extracellularly as human transferrin and lactoferrin. Meningococci have evolved systems for acquisition of these iron-carrying molecules.

Lipooligosaccharide

Meningococcal LOS is structurally related to the lipopolysaccharide (LPS) expressed by many gram-negative bacilli. However, LOS does not have repeating O-antigen subunits of sugars. The lipid A moiety of LOS, which has been classically termed *endotoxin* (as opposed to the bacterial exotoxins), is the portion that mediates the induction of inflammatory cytokines often seen in disease. The effect of lipid A is due to an interaction with the innate immune receptor Toll-like receptor 4 (TLR4) in association with the membrane protein MD2. TLR4 and MD2 are found mainly on macrophages/monocytes, dendritic cells, and other phagocytes.

Rates of morbidity and mortality associated with meningococcal bacteremia and meningitis have been directly correlated with the amount of circulating meningococcal endotoxin. Whether this measure is an indication of overall bacterial load or is a direct pathogenic mechanism of disease is debatable. The ability of signaling through TLR4 by the lipid A moiety of LOS to induce production of inflammatory and proinflammatory cytokines from various immune cells suggests a direct relationship. However, other meningococcal outer-membrane components—e.g., meningococcal porins and lipoproteins (including the H8 lipoprotein)—induce immune cell activation via other TLRs, especially TLR2. A recently derived LOS$^-$ meningococcal mutant was still able to induce significant production of proinflammatory cytokines [especially tumor necrosis factor α (TNF-α), interleukin (IL) 6, and IL-1β] by macrophages and cytokines. This observation suggests a potential role for these components in induction of meningococcal sepsis.

Other Virulence Mechanisms

The outer-membrane components of *N. meningitidis* (e.g., pili, LOS, Opa proteins, Opc, capsule) vary in expression or structure at high frequencies (10^{-2}–10^{-4} per cell per generation). Variation is the result of genetic switches that turn expression of a component on or off, regulate the amount of a component, or alter the structure of a component. Genetic events leading to phase and structural variation allow immune escape and create variability in the structures that are important in pathogenesis (on and off expression of attachment ligands, protection against serum killing, invasion determinants). The serogroup B capsule provides an example of how meningococci downregulate the human immune response through the expression of host-like antigens. The (α2→8)-linked polysialic acid capsule of serogroup B meningococci is identical to structures on the human neural cell adhesion molecule N-CAM. Meningococci are also characterized by frequent vesiculation (blebbing) of the outer membrane, and the amount of blebbing may vary between strains. Blebs may contribute to the rapid initiation of the inflammatory and clotting cascades. They may also be related to the natural autolysis of meningococci that results in DNA release and facilitates genetic transformation.

Association of Virulence Mechanisms with Specific Meningococcal Infections

Specific disease manifestations of meningococcal infections have specific virulence and pathogenic mechanisms, as described below for fulminant meningococcemia and meningitis.

Fulminant Meningococcemia

Purpura Fulminans

Fulminant meningococcemia is perhaps the most rapidly lethal form of septic shock experienced by humans. It differs from most other forms of septic shock by the prominence of hemorrhagic skin lesions (petechiae, purpura) and the consistent development of DIC.

The dominant proinflammatory molecule in the meningococcal cell wall is the endotoxin or LOS, and the outer membrane that contains it is poorly tethered to the underlying peptidoglycan. This structural peculiarity seems to account for the fact that meningococci shed LOS-containing membrane blebs as they grow. The bacteria can multiply to very high concentrations in the blood. The concentrations of endotoxin detected in the blood of patients with fulminant meningococcemia are 10- to 1000-fold higher than those found in the blood of patients with bacteremia due to other gram-negative bacteria. The bacteria and endotoxin-containing blebs stimulate monocytes, neutrophils, and endothelial cells, which then release cytokines and other mediators that can activate many distant targets, including other leukocytes, platelets, and endothelial cells. In addition, meningococci can invade the vascular endothelium. When activated, the endothelium produces molecules that can be procoagulant as well as adhesive for leukocytes.

Patients with fulminant meningococcemia usually have extremely high blood levels of both proinflammatory mediators—i.e., TNF-α, IL-1, interferon γ (IFN-γ), and IL-8—and anti-inflammatory mediators—i.e., IL-1 receptor antagonist (IL-1Ra), soluble IL-1 receptors, soluble TNF-α receptors, and IL-10. The plasma of patients with meningococcal shock can decrease the responses of normal leukocytes to stimuli such as LOS; the implication is that anti-inflammatory mediators predominate in the blood late in infection.

Procoagulant, antifibrinolytic forces are also active in the blood of patients with fulminant meningococcemia (Fig. 44-2). Monocytes express large amounts of tissue

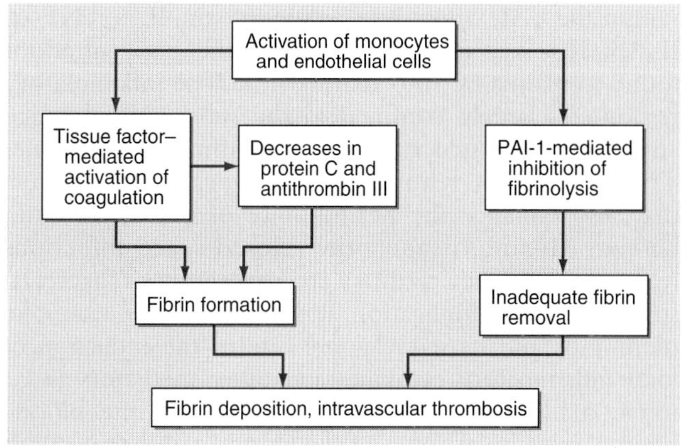

FIGURE 44-2
The pathogenesis of fibrin deposition in patients with fulminant meningococcemia. PAI-1, plasminogen activator inhibitor 1. (*Adapted from M Levi et al: Eur J Clin Invest 27:3, 1997.*)

factor. Fibrinopeptide A and thrombin-antithrombin levels are high, reflecting active clotting, whereas antithrombin and fibrinogen levels are low. Although the tissue factor–regulated ("extrinsic") arm of coagulation predominates, the contact system (factors XII and XI, prekallikrein, high-molecular-weight kininogen) is also activated. Striking deficiencies of antithrombin and proteins C and S can occur; studies have found a strong negative correlation between protein C activity and both the size of purpuric skin lesions and the mortality rate. Plasminogen levels are decreased, whereas plasmin-antiplasmin complexes and plasminogen activator inhibitor 1 (PAI-1) levels in the blood are very high. PAI-1 levels have been correlated with mortality risk.

Fibrin deposition is therefore favored both by the procoagulant tendency (promoted through activation of tissue factor and deficiencies of proteins C and S and antithrombin) and by an antifibrinolytic tendency (favored by excessive PAI-1). Both platelets and leukocytes doubtless contribute to the formation of microthrombi and to the vascular injury that ensues. Thrombosis of small- to mid-sized arteries can produce peripheral necrosis and gangrene, necessitating limb or digit amputation.

Meningitis

Meningococcal bacteremia can result in the seeding of the meninges, pericardium, and large joints. Up to one-third of patients with meningococcal disease present with meningitis or other closed-space infections without signs of sepsis. How meningococci traverse the blood-brain barrier and enter the CSF or reach other closed sites is unclear. Meningococci have been shown to invade endothelial cells both experimentally and in vivo. The choroid plexus is also a potential site of meningococcal entry into the CSF. Meningococcal pili may bind CD46, a complement-regulatory protein that is expressed by the choroid plexus and meningeal epithelia. Upon meningococcal entry into the CSF, a vigorous local inflammatory response ensues, probably triggered by endotoxin-containing meningococcal membranes. Both bacterial growth and the inflammatory response occur within the CSF, where levels of endotoxin, IL-6, TNF-α, IL-1β, IL-1Ra, and IL-10 exceed the concentrations found in plasma by 100- to 1000-fold. The inflammatory response is largely confined to the subarachnoid space and contiguous structures. The inflammatory cytokines TNF-α and IL-1 released in meningococcal bacteremia may also enhance the permeability of the blood-brain barrier. Meningitis and other closed-space infections (e.g., arthritis, pericarditis) are the result of bacterial survival and multiplication at these sites. For example, meningitis and its sequelae are due to the induction of local inflammatory cytokines and other mediators (e.g., nitric oxide), leukocyte infiltration across the blood-brain barrier, breakdown of the blood-brain barrier with edema, release of metalloproteases, induction of cellular apoptosis, coagulation of vessels, and ischemia.

Patients who develop meningitis without meningococcemia may be individuals in whom meningococci do not grow rapidly in or have been cleared from the blood, may have antibodies or phagocytes that slow meningococcal growth, or may lack the (unknown) factors that allow *N. meningitidis* to multiply rapidly in vivo. If disease is recognized early, the prognosis of patients with meningococcal meningitis is substantially better than that of patients with fulminant meningococcemia.

HOST DEFENSE MECHANISMS

Preventing meningococcal growth in blood requires bactericidal and opsonic antibodies, complement, and phagocytes (Fig. 44-3). The major bactericidal antibodies are IgM and IgG, which (except for serogroup B) bind to the capsular polysaccharide. Immunity to meningococci is therefore serogroup specific. Antibodies to other surface (subcapsular) antigens may confer cross-serogroup protection. PorA, PorB, Opc, and LOS appear to be major targets of cross-reactivity and of serogroup B bactericidal antibodies. Infants are protected from meningococcal disease during the first months of life by passively transferred maternal IgG antibodies. As maternal antibody levels wane, the attack rate increases, peaking at 3–9 months of age. Disease incidence declines as protective antibodies are induced by colonization with nonpathogenic bacteria that have cross-reactive antigens. In addition to *N. lactamica*, which frequently colonizes young children, some enteric bacteria have antigens that cross-react with those of meningococci. One theory relates the occurrence of some cases of meningococcal disease to the presence of high levels of IgA antibodies to meningococci, since these antibodies can block the bactericidal activity of IgM.

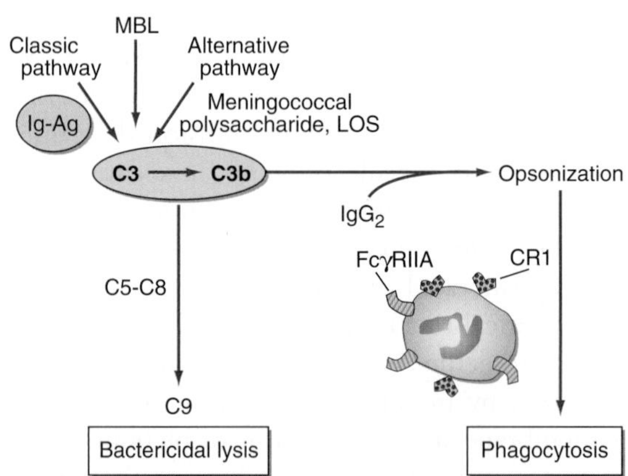

FIGURE 44-3

Protection from meningococcal disease involves both antimeningococcal immunoglobulins and complement. Activation of complement by antimeningococcal IgM or IgG promotes bacterial lysis via the membrane attack complex (C5–C9), whereas C3b [produced by alternative, mannose-binding lectin (MBL), or classic pathway activation] and antimeningococcal IgG_2 cooperate to produce effective opsonophagocytosis. A neutrophil defect in binding IgG_2 (the FcγRIIA R131 allele) has been associated with more severe meningococcal disease. CR1, complement receptor 1; LOS, lipooligosaccharide.

Complement is required for bactericidal activity and for efficient opsonophagocytosis. Individuals deficient in any of the late complement components (C5–C9) cannot assemble the membrane-attack complex (MAC) needed to kill *Neisseria*. Although the incidence of meningococcal disease is higher among those with late-complement–component deficiencies, these persons typically develop less severe disease than complement-sufficient individuals, do so at an older age, and tend to have disease due to uncommon serogroups (W-135, X, Y, Z, and 29E). Although only one-half of individuals with known late-complement-component deficiency ever experience meningococcal disease, some affected persons have several episodes. Deficiency of each of the terminal complement components is inherited in an autosomal recessive fashion. Properdin deficiency, in contrast, is X-linked; some affected males develop overwhelming meningococcal disease, an observation indicating that the alternative complement pathway is also needed for antimeningococcal host defense. Disease onset in properdin-deficient individuals typically occurs in the teens or twenties. There is also recent evidence that inherited differences in the mannose-binding lectin (MBL) pathway of complement activation may influence the risk of acquiring meningococcal disease in childhood. Alleles that decrease MBL synthesis have been associated with increased risk in the few studies reported to date.

Activation of the classic pathway of complement by antigen-antibody complexes or of the alternative pathway by LOS or capsular polysaccharide is important for producing and maintaining C3b (Fig. 44-3). Without C3b, neither bactericidal lysis nor phagocytosis can proceed effectively. When C3b is generated, meningococcal growth is probably checked by the MAC's bactericidal activity (induction of bacterial lysis) and by robust phagocytosis and opsonophagocytic killing of the bacterium due to complement deposition. Most IgG antibodies to the meningococcal polysaccharide are of the IgG_2 isotype; a phagocytic cell defect (the FcγRIIA R131 allele) that impairs the phagocytosis of IgG_2-coated particles has been associated with more severe meningococcal disease. This allele has also been associated with a more severe clinical course in patients with late-complement–component deficiency; thus effective phagocytosis may contribute to the relatively mild meningococcal disease usually observed in these individuals.

The results of studies of gene polymorphism–disease associations are summarized in Figs. 44-1 and 44-3. In individuals who lack bactericidal antibodies, protection from acquiring meningococcal bacteremia may be provided, at least in part, by innate immune mechanisms such as the MBL pathway for activating complement, complement factor C4b, and the TLR4 pathway for LOS recognition. Other genes may influence meningococcal survival in vivo [FcγIIA (CD32)], whereas still others seem to regulate the host inflammatory (IL-1β, IL-1Ra, TNF-α, angiotensin-converting enzyme) and clotting (PAI-1) responses to invading meningococci. Although many of these associations await confirmation in other populations of patients, in sum they point to important genetic influences on the acquisition and severity of meningococcal disease. This conclusion is supported by the overrepresentation of ABO blood group nonsecretors among patients with meningococcal disease and by the striking variability in meningococcal disease incidence among different racial groups.

CLINICAL MANIFESTATIONS

Upper Respiratory Tract Infections

Although many patients who develop meningococcal meningitis or meningococcemia report having had throat soreness or other upper respiratory symptoms during the preceding week, it is uncertain whether these symptoms are due to infection with meningococci. Meningococcal pharyngitis is rarely diagnosed. Adult patients with *N. meningitidis* bacteremia more often have clinically apparent disease of the respiratory tract (pneumonia, sinusitis, tracheobronchitis, conjunctivitis) than do younger patients.

Meningococcemia

Patients with meningococcal disease may have both meningococcemia and meningitis. These conditions have a wide clinical spectrum, with many overlapping features.

Approximately 10–30% of patients with meningococcal disease have meningococcemia without clinically apparent meningitis. Although meningococcal bacteremia may occasionally be transient and asymptomatic, in most individuals it is associated with fever, chills, nausea, vomiting, and myalgias. Prostration is common. The most distinctive feature is rash. Erythematous macules rapidly become petechial and, in severe cases, purpuric. Although the lesions are typically found on the trunk and lower extremities, they may also occur on the face, arms, and mucous membranes. The petechiae may coalesce into hemorrhagic bullae or may undergo necrosis and ulcerate. Patients with severe coagulopathy may develop ischemic extremities or digits, often with a sharp line of demarcation between normal and ischemic tissue.

In many patients with fulminant meningococcemia, the CSF may be normal and the CSF culture negative. Indeed, the absence of meningitis in a patient with meningococcemia is a poor prognostic sign; it suggests that the bacteria have multiplied so rapidly in the blood that meningeal seeding has not yet occurred or had time to elicit inflammation in the CSF. Most of these patients also lack evidence of an acute-phase response; i.e., the erythrocyte sedimentation rate is normal, and the C-reactive protein concentration in blood is low.

The *Waterhouse-Friderichsen syndrome* is a dramatic example of DIC-induced microthrombosis, hemorrhage, and tissue injury. Although overt adrenal failure is infrequently documented in patients with fulminant meningococcemia, patients may have partial adrenal insufficiency and be unable to mount the normal hypercortisolemic response to severe stress or cosyntropin stimulation. Almost all patients who die from fulminant meningococcemia have adrenal hemorrhages at autopsy.

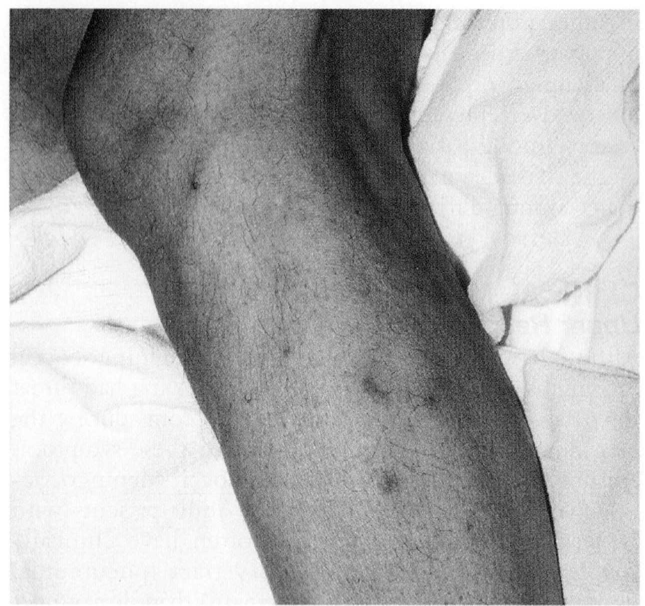

FIGURE 44-4
Erythematous papular lesions are seen on the leg of this patient with chronic meningococcemia. *(Courtesy of Kenneth M. Kaye, MD, and Elaine T. Kaye, MD; with permission).*

Chronic meningococcemia (Fig. 44-4) is a rare syndrome of episodic fever, rash, and arthralgias that can last for weeks to months. The rash may be maculopapular; it is occasionally petechial. Splenomegaly may develop. If untreated or if treated with glucocorticoids, chronic meningococcemia may evolve into meningitis, fulminant meningococcemia, or (rarely) endocarditis.

Meningitis

(See also Chap. 29) Common presenting symptoms of patients with meningococcal meningitis include nausea and vomiting, headache, neck stiffness, lethargy, and confusion. The symptoms and signs of meningococcal meningitis cannot be distinguished from those elicited by other meningeal pathogens. Many patients with meningococcal meningitis have concurrent meningococcemia, however, and petechial or purpuric skin lesions may suggest the correct diagnosis. CSF findings are consistent with those of purulent meningitis: hypoglycorrhachia, an elevated protein concentration, and a neutrophilic leukocytosis. A Gram's stain of CSF is usually positive (see "Diagnosis" later in the chapter); when this finding is unaccompanied by CSF leukocytosis, the prognosis for normal recovery is often poor.

Other Manifestations

Arthritis occurs in ~10% of patients with meningococcal disease. When arthritis develops during the first few days of the patient's illness, it usually reflects direct meningococcal invasion of the joint. Arthritis that begins later in the course is thought to be due to immune complex deposition. Primary meningococcal pneumonia occurs principally in adults, often in military populations, and is often due to serogroup Y. Although meningococcal pericarditis is occasionally seen, endocarditis due to *N. meningitidis* is now exceedingly rare. Primary meningococcal conjunctivitis can be complicated by meningococcemia; systemic therapy is therefore warranted when this condition is diagnosed. Meningococcal urethritis has been reported in individuals who practice oral sex.

Complications

Patients with meningococcal meningitis may develop cranial nerve palsies, cortical venous thrombophlebitis, and cerebral edema. Children may develop subdural effusions. Permanent sequelae can include mental retardation, deafness, and hemiparesis. The major long-term morbidity of fulminant meningococcemia is the loss of skin, limbs, or digits that results from ischemic necrosis and infarction.

DIAGNOSIS

Few clinical clues help the physician distinguish the patient with early meningococcal disease from patients with other acute systemic infections. The most useful clinical finding is the petechial or purpuric rash, but it must be differentiated from the petechial lesions seen with gonococcemia (see Fig. 45-2), Rocky Mountain spotted fever (see Fig. 75-1), hypersensitivity vasculitis, endemic typhus, and some viral infections. In one case series, one-half of the adults with meningococcal bacteremia had neither meningitis nor a rash.

The definitive diagnosis is established by recovering *N. meningitidis*, its antigens, or its DNA from normally sterile body fluids (e.g., blood, CSF, or synovial fluid) or from skin lesions. Meningococci grow best on Mueller-Hinton or chocolate blood agar at 35°C in an atmosphere that contains 5–10% CO_2. Specimens should be plated without delay. *N. meningitidis* bacteria are oxidase-positive, gram-negative diplococci that typically utilize maltose and glucose.

A Gram's stain of CSF reveals intra- or extracellular organisms in ~85% of patients with meningococcal meningitis. The latex agglutination test for meningococcal polysaccharides in the CSF is less sensitive. PCR amplification of DNA in buffy coat or CSF samples is more sensitive than either of these tests; like the latex agglutination test, PCR is unaffected by prior antibiotic therapy, as neither method requires viable organisms.

Throat or nasopharyngeal specimens should be cultured on Thayer-Martin medium, which suppresses the competing oral flora. Throat or nasopharyngeal cultures are recommended only for research or epidemiologic purposes, since a positive result merely confirms the carrier state and does not establish the existence of systemic disease.

℞ Treatment: MENINGOCOCCAL INFECTIONS

(Table 44-1) A third-generation cephalosporin, such as cefotaxime or ceftriaxone, is preferred for initial therapy. One of these cephalosporins in combination with other

TABLE 44-1

ANTIBIOTIC TREATMENT, CHEMOPROPHYLAXIS, AND VACCINATIONS FOR INVASIVE MENINGOCOCCAL DISEASE

Antibiotic Treatment[a]

1. Ceftriaxone 2 g IV q12h (100 mg/kg per day) or cefotaxime 2 g IV q4h
2. For penicillin-sensitive *N. meningitidis*: Penicillin G 18–24 million units per day in divided doses q4h (250,000 units/kg per day)
3. Chloramphenicol 75–100 mg/kg per day in divided doses q6h
4. Meropenem 1.0 g (children, 40 mg) IV q8h
5. In an outbreak setting in developing countries: Long-acting chloramphenicol in oil suspension (Tifomycin), single dose
   - Adults: 3.0 g (6 mL)
   - Children 1–15 years old: 100 mg/kg
   - Children <1 year old: 50 mg/kg

Chemoprophylaxis[b]

Rifampin (oral)
- Adults: 600 mg bid for 2 days
- Children ≥1 month old: 10 mg/kg bid for 2 days
- Children <1 month old: 5 mg/kg bid for 2 days

Ciprofloxacin (oral)
- Adults: 500 mg, 1 dose

Ofloxacin (oral)
- Adults: 400 mg, 1 dose

Ceftriaxone (IM)
- Adults: 250 mg, 1 dose
- Children <15 years old: 125 mg, 1 dose

Azithromycin (oral)
- 500 mg, 1 dose

Vaccination[c]

A, C, Y, W-135 vaccine (Menomune, Aventis Pasteur) or A, C vaccine
Single 0.5-mL subcutaneous injection
New C; A, C; and A, C, Y, W-135 meningococcal conjugate vaccines[d]

[a]Patients with meningococcal meningitis should receive antimicrobial therapy for at least 5 days.
[b]Use is recommended for close contacts of cases or if ceftriaxone is not used for primary treatment.
[c]At present, use is generally limited to the control of epidemics and to individuals with increased risk of meningococcal disease. Vaccine efficacy wanes after 3–5 years, and vaccine is not effective in recipients <2 years of age.
[d]These vaccines appear to provide immunity in young children, a prolonged immune response, and herd immunity (decreased transmission and colonization).

agents may cover other bacteria (such as *Streptococcus pneumoniae* and *Haemophilus influenzae*) that can cause the same syndromes (Chap. 29). Penicillin G remains an acceptable alternative for confirmed invasive meningococcal disease in most countries. However, the prevalence of meningococci with reduced susceptibility to penicillin has been increasing, and high-level penicillin resistance has been reported. Other options include meropenem. In the patient who is allergic to β-lactam drugs, chloramphenicol is a suitable alternative; chloramphenicol-resistant meningococci have been reported from Vietnam and France. The newer fluoroquinolones gatifloxacin, moxifloxacin, and gemifloxacin have excellent in vitro activity against *N. meningitidis*, with measurable central nervous system (CNS) penetration, and appear promising in animal models. Patients with meningococcal meningitis should be given antimicrobial therapy for at least 5 days. Although glucocorticoid therapy for meningitis in adults is controversial, many experts administer dexamethasone, beginning if possible before antibiotic therapy is initiated; the schedule is 10 mg IV given 15–20 min before the first antibiotic dose and then every 6 h for 4 days. The data regarding steroid use to diminish CNS inflammation are strongest for *H. influenzae* and *S. pneumoniae* meningitis, especially in children.

Patients with fulminant meningococcemia often experience diffuse leakage of fluid into extravascular spaces, shock, and multiple-organ dysfunction (Chap 15). Myocardial depression may be prominent. Supportive therapy, although never studied in randomized, placebo-controlled trials, is recommended. Standard measures include vigorous fluid resuscitation (often requiring several liters over the first 24 h), elective ventilation, and pressors. Some authorities recommend early hemodialysis or hemofiltration. Fresh-frozen plasma is often given to patients who are bleeding extensively or who have severely deranged clotting parameters. Many European experts have administered antithrombin III to such patients. Patients with fulminant meningococcemia in whom shock persists despite vigorous fluid resuscitation should receive supplemental glucocorticoid treatment (hydrocortisone, 1 mg/kg every 6 h) pending tests of adrenal reserve.

Although it has not been formally tested in patients with fulminant meningococcemia, activated protein C (drotrecogin alfa, Xigris) is approved for use in patients with severe sepsis and dysfunction of more than one organ (APACHE II score >25). Because of the pathophysiology, patients with meningococcemia may represent a group most likely to benefit from administration of activated protein C. The recommended dose is 24 μg/kg per hour, given as a continuous IV infusion for 96 h. Drotrecogin alfa is contraindicated when the peripheral-blood platelet count is <50,000/μL, however, and when there is active bleeding or a high risk of bleeding. Clotting parameters should be monitored closely while the drug is being infused; its administration should be discontinued 4–6 h before the performance of an invasive procedure. Drotrecogin alfa should not be used in patients with meningitis pending further evidence that it does not induce intracranial bleeding when the meninges are inflamed.

PROGNOSIS

When patients are first evaluated, the clinical features most strongly associated with a fatal outcome are shock, a purpuric or ecchymotic rash, a low or normal blood leukocyte count, an age of ≥60 years, and coma. The absence of meningitis, the presence of thrombocytopenia, low blood concentrations of antithrombin or proteins S and C, high blood levels of PAI-1, and a low erythrocyte sedimentation rate (or C-reactive protein level) have also been associated with increased mortality risk from meningococcal disease. It is possible that when meningitis symptoms are lacking, the patient may delay seeking medical therapy; this scenario could account for the increased mortality risk in asymptomatic meningitis. In contrast, the receipt of antibiotics before hospital admission has been associated with lower mortality rates in some studies.

PREVENTION

Meningococcal Polysaccharide Vaccines

A single injection of quadrivalent meningococcal polysaccharide vaccine (serogroups A, C, W-135, and Y) immunizes ~80–95% of immunocompetent adults (Table 44-1). Children ≥3 months of age can be vaccinated to prevent serogroup A disease, but multiple doses are required; the vaccine is otherwise ineffective in children <2 years old. The duration of vaccine-induced immunity in adults is probably <5 years. There is currently no vaccine for serogroup B; its polysaccharide is a sialic acid homopolymer that is poorly immunogenic in humans. In addition to individuals with late-complement–component or properdin deficiency, persons with sickle cell anemia, asplenia, or splenectomy should receive the quadrivalent vaccine. Vaccination is also recommended for military recruits, pilgrims on the Hajj, and individuals traveling to Sub-Saharan Africa during the dry months (June to December) or to other areas with epidemic meningococcal disease. The Advisory Committee on Immunization Practices of the Centers for Disease Control and Prevention (CDC) recommends vaccination of incoming college freshmen who will live in dormitories. In general, the vaccine should be given only to persons >2 years of age.

New meningococcal capsular oligosaccharide and polysaccharide conjugate vaccines (C; A and C; A, C, Y, and W-135) are being developed; some are currently undergoing clinical trials, and some are now in use in Europe and Canada. These vaccines are based on the approach used for the highly successful *H. influenzae* type b conjugate vaccines. Covalent linkage of the polysaccharide to a carrier protein converts the polysaccharide to a thymus-dependent antigen enhancing IgG anticapsular antibodies and memory B cells. Because levels of antibody in mucosal secretions are much higher after the administration of a conjugate vaccine than after vaccination with an unconjugated preparation, a major benefit of these vaccines may be the introduction of herd immunity. Memory response to meningococcal polysaccharide also appears to be an important effect of the conjugate vaccines. Meningococcal conjugate vaccines are not yet licensed in the United States. However, in the United Kingdom, serogroup C conjugate vaccines introduced in 2000 have had a marked impact on the incidence of serogroup C disease in the population vaccinated. If conjugate meningococcal vaccines prove to be capable of providing durable antibody or memory responses (particularly in infants and young children), their integration into the routine childhood immunization schedule would appear warranted. Vaccines for serogroup B meningococcal disease remain elusive; none of the group B vaccines studied in clinical trials has proven to be broadly effective, but these products have a role in the control of serogroup B epidemics. The identification of new meningococcal protective antigens and the development of better meningococcal vaccines are areas of continued research and hold promise for the prevention of diseases due to *N. meningitidis*.

In one new approach, *reverse vaccinology*, the sequenced genome of *N. meningitidis* is used to identify previously unrecognized OMPs that are common to all meningococcal strains and serogroups and that may be universal vaccinogen candidates. Thus far, a few promising candidates have been identified and are ready to undergo clinical trials.

Screening tests for complement-component deficiency should be conducted in patients who have a family history of meningococcal or disseminated gonococcal disease, especially in areas without epidemic or endemic meningococcal disease; in patients who have a recurrence; in patients whose first case occurs at ≥15 years of age; in patients with cases caused by serogroups other than A, B, or C; and in family members of patients found to have a complement deficiency.

Antimicrobial Chemoprophylaxis

The attack rate for meningococcal disease among household or other close contacts of cases is >400-fold greater than that in the population as a whole. Close contacts of cases should receive chemoprophylaxis with rifampin, ciprofloxacin, ofloxacin, or azithromycin (Table 44-1). A single IM injection of ceftriaxone is also effective. Close contacts include persons who live in the same household, day-care center contacts, and anyone directly exposed to a patient's oral secretions. Casual contacts are not at increased risk. Chemoprophylaxis should be administered as soon as possible after the case is identified. Patients with meningococcal disease who have been treated with antibiotics other than ceftriaxone need some type of prophylaxis in order to eliminate meningococcal colonization in the oropharynx.

Isolation Precautions

The CDC recommends that patients with meningococcal disease who are hospitalized be placed in respiratory isolation for the first 24 h.

Outbreak Control

An organization- or community-based outbreak of meningococcal disease is defined as the occurrence of three or more cases within ≤3 months in persons who have a common affiliation or reside in the same area but who are not close contacts of one another; in addition, the primary disease attack rate must exceed 10 cases per 100,000 persons, and the case strains of *N. meningitidis* must be of the same molecular type. Mass vaccination should be considered when such outbreaks occur, and mass chemoprophylaxis may be used to control school- or other institution-based outbreaks. Consultation with public health authorities is recommended when such campaigns are contemplated.

ACKNOWLEDGMENT

The substantial contributions of David S. Stephens, MD, and Robert S. Munford, MD, to this chapter in previous editions of Harrison's Principles of Internal Medicine are gratefully acknowledged.

FURTHER READINGS

BILUKHA O et al: Use of meningococcal vaccines in the United States. Pediatr Infect Dis J 26:371, 2007

BORG J et al: Outcomes of meningococcal disease in adolescence: Prospective, matched-cohort study. Pediatrics 123:e502, 2009

GARDNER P: Clinical practice. Prevention of meningococcal disease. N Engl J Med 355:1466, 2006 (Erratum: N Engl J Med 356:536, 2007)

GIULIANI MM et al: A universal vaccine for serogroup B meningococcus. Proc Natl Acad Sci USA 103:10834, 2006

HECKENBERG SG et al: Clinical features, outcome, and meningococcal genotype in 258 adults with meningococcal meningitis: A prospective cohort study. Medicine (Baltimore) 87:185, 2008

SCHNEIDER MC et al: Interactions between *Neisseria meningitidis* and the complement system. Trends Microbiol 15:233, 2007

SMIRNOVA I et al: Assay of locus-specific genetic load implicates rare Toll-like receptor 4 mutations in meningococcal susceptibility. Proc Natl Acad Sci USA 100:6075, 2003

SNAPE MD et al: Immunogenicity of a tetravalent meningococcal glycoconjugate vaccine in infants: A randomized controlled trial. JAMA 299:173, 2008

——— et al: Meningococcal polysaccharide-protein conjugate vaccines. Lancet Infect Dis 5:21, 2005

SNYDER LA et al: The majority of genes in the pathogenic *Neisseria* species are present in non-pathogenic *Neisseria lactamica*, including those designated as 'virulence genes.' BMC Genomics 7:128, 2006

STEPHENS DS et al: Epidemic meningitis, meningococcaemia, and *Neisseria meningitidis*. Lancet 369:2196, 2007

THOMPSON MJ et al: Clinical recognition of meningococcal disease in children and adolescents. Lancet 367:397, 2006

WU HM et al: Emergence of ciprofloxacin-resistant *Neisseria meningitidis* in North America. N Engl J Med 360:886, 2009

ZIMMER SM et al: Serogroup B meningococcal vaccines. Curr Opin Invest Drugs 7:733, 2006

CHAPTER 45

GONOCOCCAL INFECTIONS

Sanjay Ram ■ Peter A. Rice

DEFINITION

Gonorrhea is a sexually transmitted infection (STI) of epithelium and commonly manifests as cervicitis, urethritis, proctitis, and conjunctivitis. If untreated, infections at these sites can lead to local complications such as endometritis, salpingitis, tuboovarian abscess, bartholinitis, peritonitis, and perihepatitis in female patients; periurethritis and epididymitis in male patients; and ophthalmia neonatorum in newborns. Disseminated gonococcemia is an uncommon event whose manifestations include skin lesions, tenosynovitis, arthritis, and (in rare cases) endocarditis or meningitis.

MICROBIOLOGY

Neisseria gonorrhoeae is a gram-negative, nonmotile, non–spore-forming organism that grows singly and in pairs (i.e., as monococci and diplococci, respectively). Exclusively a human pathogen, the gonococcus contains, on average, three genome copies per coccal unit; this polyploidy permits a high level of antigenic variation and the survival of the organism in its host. Gonococci, like all other *Neisseria* species, are oxidase positive. They are distinguished from other neisseriae by their ability to grow on selective media and to utilize glucose but not maltose, sucrose, or lactose.

EPIDEMIOLOGY

The incidence of gonorrhea has declined significantly in the United States, but there were still ~325,000 newly reported cases in 2006. Gonorrhea remains a major public health problem worldwide, is a significant cause of morbidity in developing countries, and may play a role in enhancing transmission of HIV.

Gonorrhea predominantly affects young, nonwhite, unmarried, less educated members of urban populations. The number of reported cases probably represents half of the true number of cases—a discrepancy resulting from underreporting, self-treatment, and nonspecific treatment without a laboratory-proven diagnosis. The number of reported cases of gonorrhea in the United States rose from ~250,000 in the early 1960s to a high of 1.01 million in 1978. The peak recorded incidence of gonorrhea in modern times was reported in 1975, with 468 cases per 100,000 population in the United States. This peak was attributable to the interaction of several variables, including improved accuracy of diagnosis, changes in patterns of contraceptive use, and changes in sexual behavior. The incidence of the disease has since gradually declined and is currently estimated at 120 cases per 100,000, a figure that is still the highest among industrialized countries. A further decline in the overall incidence of gonorrhea in the United States over the past two decades may reflect increased condom use resulting from public health efforts to curtail HIV transmission. At present, the attack rate in the United States is highest among 15- to 19-year-old women and 20- to 24-year-old men; 40% of all reported cases occur in the preceding two groups together. From the standpoint of ethnicity, rates are highest among African Americans and lowest among persons of Asian or Pacific Island descent.

The incidence of gonorrhea is higher in developing countries than in industrialized nations. The exact incidence of any of the STIs is difficult to ascertain in developing countries because of limited surveillance and variable diagnostic criteria. Studies in Africa have clearly demonstrated that nonulcerative STIs such as gonorrhea (in addition to ulcerative STIs) are an independent risk factor for the transmission of HIV (Chap. 90).

Gonorrhea is transmitted from males to females more efficiently than in the opposite direction. The rate of transmission to a woman during a single unprotected sexual encounter with an infected man is ~40–60%. Oropharyngeal gonorrhea occurs in ~20% of women who practice fellatio with infected partners. Transmission in either direction by cunnilingus is rare.

In any population, there exists a small minority of individuals who have high rates of new-partner acquisition. These "core-group members" or "high-frequency transmitters" are vital in sustaining STI transmission at the population level. Another instrumental factor in sustaining gonorrhea in the population is the large number of infected individuals who are asymptomatic or have minor symptoms that are ignored. These persons, unlike symptomatic individuals, may not cease sexual activity and therefore continue to transmit the infection. This situation underscores the importance of contact tracing and empirical treatment of the sex partners of index cases.

PATHOGENESIS, IMMUNOLOGY, AND ANTIMICROBIAL RESISTANCE

Outer-Membrane Proteins

Pili

Fresh clinical isolates of *N. gonorrhoeae* initially form piliated (fimbriated) colonies distinguishable on translucent agar. Pilus expression is rapidly switched off with unselected subculture because of rearrangements in pilus genes. This change is a basis for antigenic variation of gonococci. Piliated strains adhere better to cells derived from human mucosal surfaces and are more virulent in organ culture models and human inoculation experiments than nonpiliated variants. In a fallopian tube explant model, pili mediate gonococcal attachment to nonciliated columnar epithelial cells. This event initiates gonococcal phagocytosis and transport through these cells to intercellular spaces near the basement membrane or directly into the subepithelial tissue. CD46 (membrane cofactor protein) is present on urogenital epithelial cells in both men and women and has been determined to be a receptor for PilC; this subunit is located at the tip of the pilus molecule and is critical in mediating adherence. Pili are also essential for genetic competence and transformation of *N. gonorrhoeae*, which permit horizontal transfer of genetic material between different gonococcal lineages in vivo.

Opacity-Associated Protein

Another gonococcal surface protein that is important in adherence to epithelial cells is opacity-associated protein (Opa, formerly called protein II). Opa contributes to intergonococcal adhesion, which is responsible for the opaque nature of gonococcal colonies on translucent agar and the organism's adherence to a variety of eukaryotic cells, including polymorphonuclear leukocytes (PMNs). Certain Opa variants promote invasion of epithelial cells, and this effect has been linked with the ability of Opa to bind vitronectin, glycosaminoglycans, and several members of the carcinoembryonic antigen–related cell adhesion molecule (CEACAM) receptor family. *N. gonorrhoeae* Opa proteins that bind CEACAM 1, which is expressed by primary CD4+ T lymphocytes, suppress the activation and proliferation of these lymphocytes. This phenomenon may serve to explain the transient decrease in CD4+ T-lymphocyte counts associated with gonococcal infection.

Porin

Porin (previously designated protein I) is the most abundant gonococcal surface protein, accounting for >50% of the organism's total outer-membrane protein. Porin molecules exist as trimers that provide anion-transporting aqueous channels through the otherwise-hydrophobic outer membrane. Porin shows stable interstrain antigenic variation and forms the basis for gonococcal serotyping. Two main serotypes have been identified: PorB.1A strains are often associated with disseminated gonococcal infection (DGI), whereas PorB.1B strains usually cause local genital infections only. DGI strains are generally resistant to the killing action of normal human serum and do not incite a significant local inflammatory response; therefore, they may not cause symptoms at genital sites. These characteristics may be related to the ability of PorB.1A strains to bind to complement-inhibitory molecules, resulting in a diminished inflammatory response. Porin can translocate to the cytoplasmic membrane of host cells—a process that could initiate gonococcal endocytosis and invasion.

Other Outer-Membrane Proteins

Other notable outer-membrane proteins include H.8, a lipoprotein that is present in high concentration on the surface of all gonococcal strains and is an excellent target for antibody-based diagnostic testing. Transferrin-binding proteins (Tbp1 and Tbp2) and lactoferrin-binding protein are required for scavenging iron from transferrin and lactoferrin in vivo. Transferrin and iron have been shown to enhance the attachment of iron-deprived *N. gonorrhoeae* to human endometrial cells. IgA1 protease is produced by *N. gonorrhoeae* and may protect the organism from the action of mucosal IgA.

Lipooligosaccharide

Gonococcal lipooligosaccharide (LOS) consists of a lipid A and a core oligosaccharide that lacks the repeating O-carbohydrate antigenic side chain seen in other gram-negative bacteria (Chap. 2). Gonococcal LOS possesses marked endotoxic activity and contributes to the local cytotoxic effect in a fallopian tube model. LOS core sugars undergo a high degree of phase variation under different conditions of growth; this variation reflects genetic regulation and expression of glycotransferase genes that dictate the carbohydrate structure of LOS. These phenotypic changes may affect interactions of *N. gonorrhoeae* with elements of the humoral immune system (antibodies and complement) and may also influence direct binding of organisms to both professional phagocytes and nonprofessional phagocytes (epithelial cells). For example, gonococci that are sialylated at their LOS sites bind complement factor H and inhibit the alternative pathway of complement. LOS sialylation may also decrease nonopsonic Opa-mediated association with neutrophils and inhibit the oxidative burst in PMNs. The unsialylated terminal lactosamine residue of LOS binds to an asialoglycoprotein receptor on male epithelial cells, which facilitates binding and subsequent gonococcal invasion of these cells.

Host Factors

In addition to gonococcal structures that interact with epithelial cells, host factors seem to be important in mediating entry of gonococci into nonphagocytic cells. Activation of phosphatidylcholine-specific phospholipase C and acidic sphingomyelinase by *N. gonorrhoeae*, which results in the release of diacylglycerol and ceramide, is a requirement for the entry of *N. gonorrhoeae* into epithelial cells. Ceramide accumulation within cells leads to apoptosis, which may disrupt epithelial integrity and facilitate entry of gonococci into subepithelial tissue. Release of chemotactic factors as a result of complement activation contributes to inflammation, as does the toxic effect of LOS in provoking the release of inflammatory cytokines.

The importance of humoral immunity in host defenses against neisserial infections is best illustrated by the predisposition of persons deficient in terminal complement components (C5 through C9) to recurrent bacteremic gonococcal infections and to recurrent meningococcal meningitis or meningococcemia. Gonococcal porin induces T-cell–proliferative responses in persons with urogenital gonococcal disease. A significant increase in porin-specific interleukin (IL) 4–producing CD4+ as well as CD8+ T lymphocytes is seen in individuals with mucosal gonococcal disease. A portion of these lymphocytes that show a porin-specific T_H2-type response could traffic to mucosal surfaces and play a role in immune protection against the disease. Few data clearly indicate that protective immunity is acquired from a previous gonococcal infection, although bactericidal and opsonophagocytic antibodies to porin and LOS may offer partial protection. On the other hand, women who are infected and acquire high levels of antibody to another outer-membrane protein, Rmp (reduction modifiable protein, formerly called protein III), may be especially likely to become reinfected with *N. gonorrhoeae* because Rmp antibodies block the effect of bactericidal antibodies to porin and LOS. Rmp shows little, if any, interstrain antigenic variation; therefore, Rmp antibodies potentially may block antibody-mediated killing of all gonococci. The mechanism of blocking has not been fully characterized, but Rmp antibodies noncompetitively inhibit binding of porin and LOS antibodies because of the proximity of these structures in the gonococcal outer membrane. In male volunteers who have no history of gonorrhea, the net effect of these events may influence the outcome of experimental challenge with *N. gonorrhoeae*. Because Rmp bears extensive homology to enterobacterial OmpA and meningococcal class 4 proteins, it is possible that these blocking antibodies result from prior exposure to cross-reacting proteins from these species and also play a role in first-time infection with *N. gonorrhoeae*.

Gonococcal Resistance to Antimicrobial Agents

It is no surprise that *N. gonorrhoeae*, with its remarkable capacity to alter its antigenic structure and adapt to changes in the microenvironment, has become resistant to numerous antibiotics. The first effective agents against gonorrhea were the sulfonamides, which were introduced in the 1930s and became ineffective within a decade. Penicillin was then employed as the drug of choice for the treatment of gonorrhea. By 1965, 42% of gonococcal isolates had developed low-level resistance to penicillin G. Resistance due to the production of penicillinase arose later.

Gonococci become fully resistant to antibiotics either by chromosomal mutations or by acquisition of R factors (plasmids). Two types of chromosomal mutations have been described. The first type, which is drug specific, is a single-step mutation leading to high-level resistance. The second type involves mutations at several chromosomal loci that combine to determine the level as well as the pattern of resistance. Strains with mutations in chromosomal genes were first observed in the late 1950s. As recently as 2004, chromosomal mutations accounted for resistance to penicillin, tetracycline, or both in ~12% of strains surveyed in the United States.

β-Lactamase (penicillinase)–producing strains of *N. gonorrhoeae* (PPNG) carrying plasmids with the Pc^r determinant had rapidly spread worldwide by the early 1980s. *N. gonorrhoeae* strains with plasmid-borne tetracycline resistance (TRNG) can mobilize some β-lactamase plasmids, and PPNG and TRNG occur together, sometimes along with strains exhibiting chromosomally mediated resistance (CMRNG). Penicillin, ampicillin, and tetracycline are no longer reliable for the treatment of gonorrhea and should not be used. Third-generation cephalosporins have remained highly effective as single-dose therapy for gonorrhea. Even though the minimal inhibitory concentrations (MICs) of ceftriaxone for certain strains may reach 0.015–0.125 mg/L (higher than the MICs of 0.0001–0.008 mg/L for fully susceptible strains), these levels are greatly exceeded in the blood, the urethra, and the cervix when the routinely recommended ceftriaxone and cefixime regimens are administered (see below). These regimens almost always result in an effective cure.

Quinolone-containing regimens were also recommended for treatment of gonococcal infections; the fluoroquinolones offered the advantage of antichlamydial activity when administered for 7 days. However, quinolone-resistant *N. gonorrhoeae* (QRNG) appeared soon after these agents were first used to treat gonorrhea; in the United States, quinolone-containing regimens are no longer routinely recommended for the treatment of gonorrhea.

QRNG is particularly common in the Pacific Islands (including Hawaii) and Asia, where, in certain areas, all gonococcal strains are now resistant to quinolones. At present, QRNG is also common in parts of Europe and the Middle East. In the United States, QRNG has been identified in midwestern and eastern areas as well as in states on the Pacific coast, where resistant strains were first seen. Alterations in DNA gyrase and topoisomerase IV have been implicated as mechanisms of fluoroquinolone resistance.

Resistance to spectinomycin, which has been used in the past as an alternative agent, has been reported. Since this agent is usually not associated with resistance to other antibiotics, spectinomycin can be reserved for use against multiresistant strains of *N. gonorrhoeae*. Nevertheless, outbreaks caused by strains resistant to spectinomycin have been documented in Korea and England when the drug has been used for primary treatment of gonorrhea.

CLINICAL MANIFESTATIONS

Gonococcal Infections in Males

Acute urethritis is the most common clinical manifestation of gonorrhea in males. The usual incubation period after exposure is 2–7 days, although the interval can be longer and some men remain asymptomatic. Strains of the PorB.1A serotype tend to cause a greater proportion of cases of mild and asymptomatic urethritis than do PorB.1B strains. Urethral discharge and dysuria, usually without urinary frequency or urgency, are the major symptoms. The discharge initially is scant and mucoid but becomes profuse and purulent within a day or two. Gram's stain of the urethral discharge may reveal PMNs and gram-negative intracellular monococci and diplococci (Fig. 45-1). The clinical manifestations of gonococcal urethritis are usually more severe and overt than those of nongonococcal urethritis, including urethritis caused by *Chlamydia trachomatis* (Chap. 77); however, exceptions are common, and it is often impossible to differentiate the causes of urethritis on clinical grounds alone. The majority of cases of urethritis seen in the United States today are not caused by *N. gonorrhoeae* and/or *C. trachomatis*. Although a number of other organisms may be responsible, most cases do not have a specific etiologic agent identified.

Most symptomatic men with gonorrhea seek treatment and cease to be infectious. The remaining men, who are largely asymptomatic, accumulate in number over time and constitute about two-thirds of all infected men at any point in time. Together with men incubating the organism (who shed the organism but are

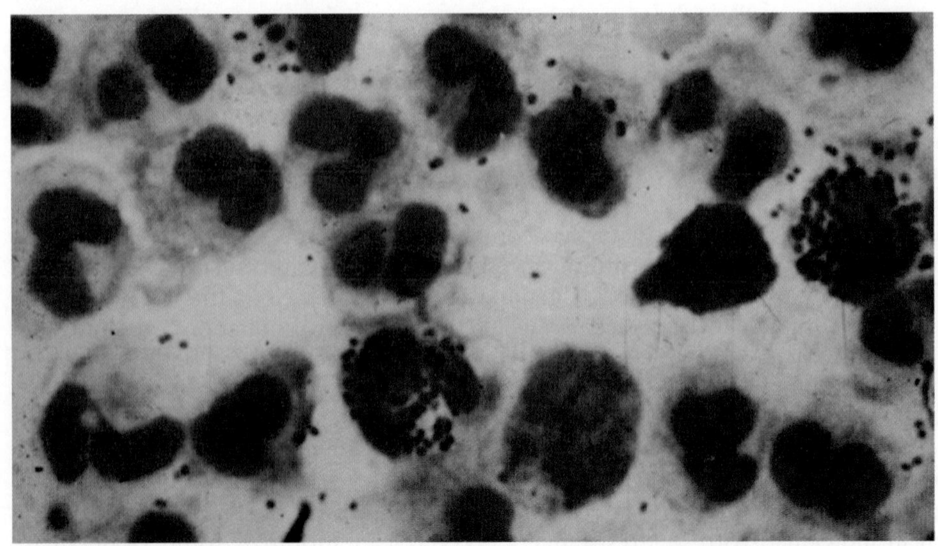

FIGURE 45-1
Gram's stain of urethral discharge from a male patient with gonorrhea shows gram-negative intracellular monococci and diplococci. (*From the Public Health Agency of Canada.*)

asymptomatic), they serve as the source of spread of infection. Before the antibiotic era, symptoms of urethritis persisted for ~8 weeks. Epididymitis is now an uncommon complication, and gonococcal prostatitis occurs rarely, if at all. Other unusual local complications of gonococcal urethritis include edema of the penis due to dorsal lymphangitis or thrombophlebitis, submucous inflammatory "soft" infiltration of the urethral wall, periurethral abscess or fistulae, inflammation or abscess of Cowper's gland, and seminal vesiculitis. Balanitis may develop in uncircumcised men.

Gonococcal Infections in Females

Gonococcal Cervicitis

Mucopurulent cervicitis is the most common STI diagnosis in American women and may be caused by *N. gonorrhoeae*, *C. trachomatis*, and other organisms. Cervicitis may coexist with candidal or trichomonal vaginitis. *N. gonorrhoeae* primarily infects the columnar epithelium of the cervical os. Bartholin's glands occasionally become infected.

Women infected with *N. gonorrhoeae* usually develop symptoms. However, the women who either remain asymptomatic or have only minor symptoms may delay in seeking medical attention. These minor symptoms may include scant vaginal discharge issuing from the inflamed cervix (without vaginitis or vaginosis per se) and dysuria (often without urgency or frequency) that may be associated with gonococcal urethritis. Although the incubation period of gonorrhea is less well defined in women than in men, symptoms usually develop within 10 days of infection and are more acute and intense than those of chlamydial cervicitis.

The physical examination may reveal a mucopurulent discharge (mucopus) issuing from the cervical os. Because Gram's stain is not sensitive for the diagnosis of gonorrhea in women, specimens should be submitted for culture or a nonculture assay (see below). Edematous and friable cervical ectopy as well as endocervical bleeding induced by gentle swabbing are more often seen in chlamydial infection. Gonococcal infection may extend deep enough to produce dyspareunia and lower abdominal or back pain. In such cases, it is imperative to consider a diagnosis of pelvic inflammatory disease (PID) and to administer treatment for that disease (Chaps. 28 and 77).

N. gonorrhoeae may be recovered from the urethra and rectum of women with cervicitis, but these are rarely the only infected sites. Urethritis in women may produce symptoms of internal dysuria, which is often attributed to "cystitis." Pyuria in the absence of bacteriuria seen on Gram's stain of unspun urine, accompanied by urine cultures that fail to yield $>10^5$ colonies of bacteria usually associated with urinary tract infection, signifies the possibility of urethritis due to *C. trachomatis*. Urethral infection with *N. gonorrhoeae* may also occur in this context, but in this instance, urethral cultures are usually positive.

Gonococcal Vaginitis

The vaginal mucosa of healthy women is lined by stratified squamous epithelium and is rarely infected by *N. gonorrhoeae*. However, gonococcal vaginitis can occur in anestrogenic women (e.g., prepubertal girls and postmenopausal women), in whom the vaginal stratified squamous epithelium is often thinned down to the basilar layer, which can be infected by *N. gonorrhoeae*. The intense inflammation of the vagina makes the physical (speculum and bimanual) examination extremely painful. The vaginal mucosa is red and edematous, and an abundant purulent discharge is present. Infection in the urethra and in Skene's and Bartholin's glands often accompanies gonococcal vaginitis. Inflamed cervical erosion or abscesses in nabothian cysts may also occur. Coexisting cervicitis may result in pus in the cervical os.

Anorectal Gonorrhea

Because the female anatomy permits the spread of cervical exudate to the rectum, *N. gonorrhoeae* is sometimes recovered from the rectum of women with uncomplicated gonococcal cervicitis. The rectum is the sole site of infection in only 5% of women with gonorrhea. Such women are usually asymptomatic but occasionally have acute proctitis manifested by anorectal pain or pruritus, tenesmus, purulent rectal discharge, and rectal bleeding. Among men who have sex with men (MSM), the frequency of gonococcal infection, including rectal infection, fell by ≥90% throughout the United States in the early 1980s, but a resurgence of gonorrhea among MSM has been documented in several cities since the 1990s. Gonococcal isolates from the rectum of MSM tend to be more resistant to antimicrobial agents than are gonococcal isolates from other sites. Gonococcal isolates with a mutation in *mtrR* (multiple transferable resistance repressor) or in the promoter region of the gene that encodes for this transcriptional repressor develop increased resistance to antimicrobial hydrophobic agents such as bile acids and fatty acids in feces and thus are found with increased frequency in MSM. This situation may have been responsible for higher rates of failure of treatment for rectal gonorrhea with older regimens consisting of penicillin or tetracyclines.

Pharyngeal Gonorrhea

Pharyngeal gonorrhea is usually mild or asymptomatic, although symptomatic pharyngitis does occasionally occur with cervical lymphadenitis. The mode of acquisition is oral-genital sexual exposure, with fellatio being a more efficient means of transmission than cunnilingus. Most cases resolve spontaneously, and transmission from the pharynx to sexual contacts is rare. Pharyngeal infection almost always coexists with genital infection. Swabs from the pharynx should be plated directly onto gonococcal selective media. Pharyngeal colonization with *Neisseria meningitidis* needs to be differentiated from that with other *Neisseria* species.

Ocular Gonorrhea in Adults

Ocular gonorrhea in an adult usually results from autoinoculation from an infected genital site. As in genital infection, the manifestations range from severe to occasionally mild or asymptomatic disease. The variability in clinical manifestations may be attributable to differences in the ability of the infecting strain to elicit an inflammatory response. Infection may result in a markedly swollen eyelid, severe hyperemia and chemosis, and a profuse purulent discharge. The massively inflamed conjunctiva may be draped over the cornea and limbus. Lytic enzymes from the infiltrating PMNs occasionally cause corneal ulceration and rarely cause perforation.

Prompt recognition and treatment of this condition are of paramount importance. Gram's stain and culture of the purulent discharge establish the diagnosis. Genital cultures should also be performed.

Gonorrhea in Pregnant Women, Neonates, and Children

Gonorrhea in pregnancy can have serious consequences for both the mother and the infant. Recognition of gonorrhea early in pregnancy also identifies a population at risk for other STIs, particularly chlamydial infection and syphilis. The risks of salpingitis and PID—conditions associated with a high rate of fetal loss—are highest during the first trimester. Pharyngeal infection, most often asymptomatic, may be more common during pregnancy because of altered sexual practices. Prolonged rupture of the membranes, premature delivery, chorioamnionitis, funisitis (infection of the umbilical cord stump), and sepsis in the infant (with *N. gonorrhoeae* detected in the newborn's gastric aspirate during delivery) are common complications of maternal gonococcal infection at term. Other microorganisms and conditions, including *Mycoplasma hominis*, *Ureaplasma urealyticum*, *C. trachomatis*, and bacterial vaginosis, have been associated with similar complications.

The most common form of gonorrhea in neonates is ophthalmia neonatorum, which results from exposure to infected cervical secretions during parturition. Ocular neonatal instillation of a prophylactic agent (e.g., 1% silver nitrate eyedrops or ophthalmic preparations containing erythromycin or tetracycline) prevents ophthalmia neonatorum but is not effective for its treatment, which requires systemic antibiotics. The clinical manifestations are acute and usually begin 2–5 days after birth. An initial nonspecific conjunctivitis with a serosanguineous discharge is followed by tense edema of both eyelids, chemosis, and a profuse, thick, purulent discharge. Corneal ulcerations that result in nebulae or perforation may lead to anterior synechiae, anterior staphyloma, panophthalmitis, and blindness. Infections described at other mucosal sites in infants, including vaginitis, rhinitis, and anorectal infection, are likely to be asymptomatic. Pharyngeal colonization has been demonstrated in 35% of infants with gonococcal ophthalmia, and coughing is the most prominent symptom in these cases. Septic arthritis (see below) is the most common manifestation of systemic infection or DGI in the newborn. The onset usually comes at 3–21 days of age, and polyarticular involvement is common. Sepsis, meningitis, and pneumonia are seen in rare instances.

Any STI in children beyond the neonatal period raises the possibility of sexual abuse. Gonococcal vulvovaginitis is the most common manifestation of gonococcal infection in children beyond infancy. Anorectal and pharyngeal infections are common in these children and are frequently asymptomatic. The urethra, Bartholin's and Skene's glands, and the upper genital tract are rarely involved. All children with gonococcal infection should also be evaluated for chlamydial infection, syphilis, and possibly HIV infection.

Gonococcal Arthritis (DGI)

DGI or gonococcal arthritis results from gonococcal bacteremia. In the 1970s, DGI occurred in ~0.5–3% of persons with untreated gonococcal mucosal infection. The lower incidence of DGI at present is probably attributable to a decline in the prevalence of particular strains that are likely to disseminate. DGI strains resist the bactericidal action of human serum and generally do not incite inflammation at genital sites, probably because of limited generation of chemotactic factors. Strains recovered from DGI cases in the 1970s were often of the PorB.1A serotype, were highly susceptible to penicillin, and had special growth requirements (i.e., the AHU auxotype) that made the organism more fastidious and more difficult to isolate.

Menstruation is a risk factor for dissemination, and approximately two-thirds of cases of DGI are in women. In about half of affected women, symptoms of DGI begin within 7 days of onset of menses. Complement deficiencies, especially of the components involved in the assembly of the membrane attack complex (C5 through C9), predispose to neisserial bacteremia, and persons with more than one episode of DGI should be screened with an assay for total hemolytic complement activity.

The clinical manifestations of DGI have sometimes been classified into two stages: a bacteremic stage, which is less common today, and a joint-localized stage with suppurative arthritis. A clear-cut progression usually is not evident. Patients in the bacteremic stage have higher temperatures, and their fever is more frequently accompanied by chills. Painful joints are common and often occur in conjunction with tenosynovitis and skin lesions. Polyarthralgias usually include the knees, elbows, and more distal joints; the axial skeleton is generally spared. Skin lesions are seen in ~75% of patients and include papules and pustules, often with a hemorrhagic component (Fig. 45-2). Other manifestations of noninfectious dermatitis, such as nodular lesions, urticaria, and erythema multiforme, have been described. These lesions are usually on the extremities and number between 5 and 40. The differential diagnosis of the bacteremic stage of DGI includes reactive arthritis, acute rheumatoid arthritis, sarcoidosis, erythema nodosum, drug-induced arthritis, and viral infections (e.g., hepatitis B and acute HIV infection). The distribution of joint symptoms in reactive

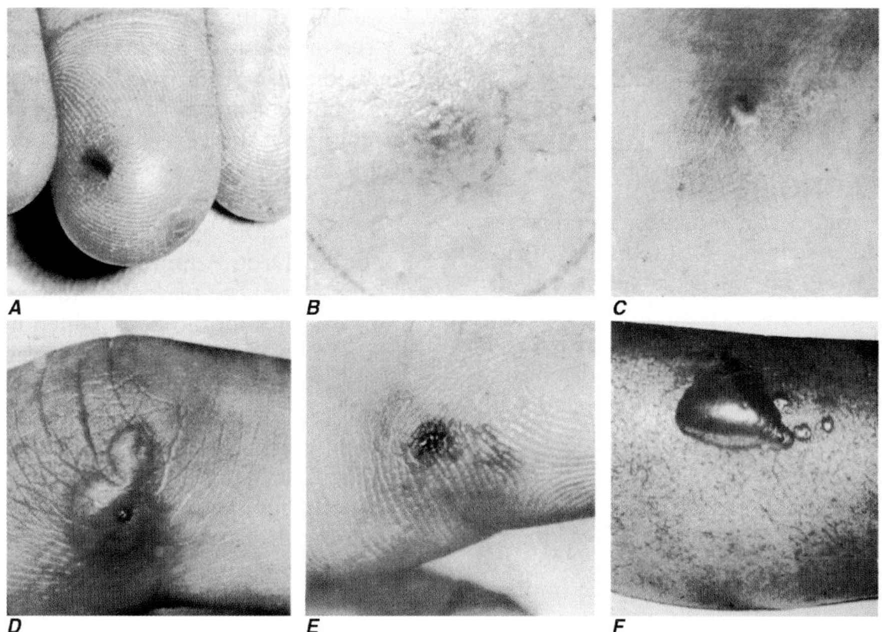

FIGURE 45-2

Characteristic skin lesions in patients with proven gonococcal bacteremia. The lesions are in various stages of evolution. ***A.*** Very early petechia on finger. ***B.*** Early papular lesion, 7 mm in diameter, on lower leg. ***C.*** Pustule with central eschar resulting from early petechial lesion. ***D.*** Pustular lesion on finger. ***E.*** Mature lesion with central necrosis (black) on hemorrhagic base. ***F.*** Bullae on anterior tibial surface. (*Reprinted with permission from KK Holmes et al: Disseminated gonococcal infection. Ann Intern Med 74:979, 1971.*)

arthritis differs from that in DGI (Fig. 45-3), as do the skin and genital manifestations.

Suppurative arthritis involves one or two joints, most often (in decreasing order of frequency) the knees, wrists, ankles, and elbows; other joints are occasionally involved. Most patients who develop gonococcal septic arthritis do so without prior polyarthralgias or skin lesions; in the absence of symptomatic genital infection, this disease cannot be distinguished from septic arthritis caused by other pathogens. The differential diagnosis of acute arthritis in young adults is discussed in Chap. 23. Rarely, osteomyelitis complicates septic arthritis involving small joints of the hand.

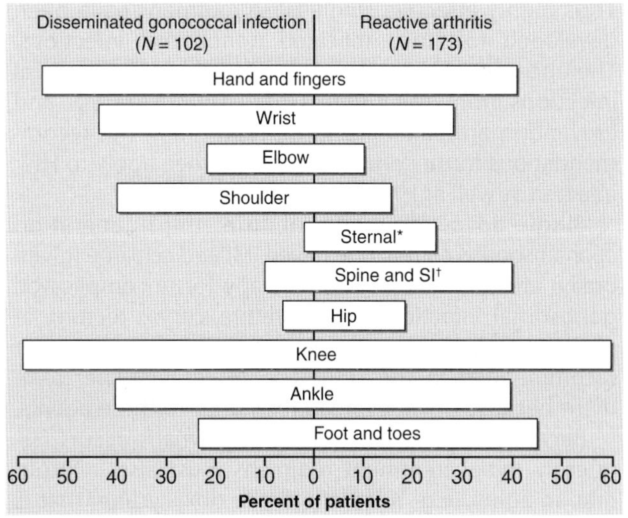

FIGURE 45-3

Distributions of joints with arthritis in 102 patients with disseminated gonococcal infection and 173 patients with reactive arthritis. *Includes the sternoclavicular joints. †SI, sacroiliac joint. (*Reprinted with permission from M Kousa et al: Frequent association of chlamydial infection with Reiter's syndrome. Sex Transm Dis 5:57, 1978.*)

Gonococcal endocarditis, although rare today, was a relatively common complication of DGI in the preantibiotic era, causing about one-quarter of reported cases of endocarditis. Another unusual complication of DGI is meningitis.

Gonococcal Infections in HIV-Infected Persons

The association between gonorrhea and the acquisition of HIV has been demonstrated in several well-controlled studies, mainly in Kenya and Zaire. The nonulcerative STIs enhance the transmission of HIV by three- to fivefold, possibly because of increased viral shedding by persons with urethritis or cervicitis (Chap. 90). HIV has been detected by polymerase chain reaction (PCR) more commonly in ejaculates from HIV-positive men with gonococcal urethritis than in those from HIV-positive men with nongonococcal urethritis. PCR positivity diminishes twofold after appropriate therapy for urethritis. Not only does gonorrhea enhance the transmission of HIV; it may also increase the individual's risk for acquisition of HIV. A proposed mechanism is the significantly greater number of CD4+ T lymphocytes and dendritic cells that can be infected by HIV in endocervical secretions of women with nonulcerative STIs than in those of women with ulcerative STIs.

LABORATORY DIAGNOSIS

A rapid diagnosis of gonococcal infection in men may be obtained by Gram's staining of urethral exudates (Fig. 45-1). The detection of gram-negative intracellular monococci and diplococci is usually highly specific and sensitive in diagnosing gonococcal urethritis in symptomatic males but is only ~50% sensitive in diagnosing gonococcal cervicitis. Samples should be collected with Dacron or rayon swabs. Part of the sample should be inoculated onto a plate of modified Thayer-Martin or other gonococcal selective medium for culture. It is important to process all samples immediately because gonococci do not tolerate drying. If plates cannot be incubated immediately, they can be held safely for several hours at room temperature in candle extinction jars before incubation. If processing is to occur within 6 h, transport of specimens may be facilitated by the use of nonnutritive swab transport systems such as Stuart or Amies medium. For longer holding periods (e.g., when specimens for culture are to be mailed), culture media with self-contained CO_2-generating systems (such as the JEMBEC or Gono-Pak systems) may be used. Specimens should also be obtained for the diagnosis of chlamydial infection.

PMNs are often seen in the endocervix on a Gram's stain, and an abnormally increased number (≥30 PMNs per field in five 1000× oil-immersion microscopic fields) establishes the presence of an inflammatory discharge. Unfortunately, the presence or absence of gram-negative intracellular monococci or diplococci in cervical smears does not accurately predict which patients have gonorrhea, and the diagnosis in this setting should be made by culture or another suitable nonculture diagnostic method. The sensitivity of a single endocervical culture is ~80–90%. If a history of rectal sex is elicited, a rectal wall swab (uncontaminated with feces) should be cultured. A presumptive diagnosis of gonorrhea cannot be made on the basis of gram-negative diplococci in smears from the pharynx, where other *Neisseria* species are components of the normal flora.

Nucleic acid probe tests are sometimes substituted for culture for the direct detection of *N. gonorrhoeae* in urogenital specimens. A common assay employs a nonisotopic chemiluminescent DNA probe that hybridizes specifically with gonococcal 16S ribosomal RNA; this assay is as sensitive as conventional culture techniques. A disadvantage of non-culture-based assays is that *N. gonorrhoeae* cannot be grown from the transport systems. Thus a culture-confirmatory test and formal antimicrobial susceptibility testing, if needed, cannot be performed. Nucleic acid amplification tests (NAATs), including Roche Amplicor, Gen-Probe APTIMA Combo2 (which also detects *Chlamydia*), and BD ProbeTec ET, offer an advantage: urine samples can be tested with a sensitivity similar to that obtained when urethral or cervical swab samples are assessed by culture and other non-NAATs.

Because of the legal implications, the preferred method for the diagnosis of gonococcal infection in children is a standardized culture. Two positive NAATs, each targeting a different nucleic acid sequence, may be substituted for culture of the cervix or the urethra as legal evidence of infection; however, cervical specimens are not recommended for prepubertal girls. Nonculture tests for gonococcal infection have not been approved by the U.S. Food and Drug Administration for use with specimens obtained from the pharynx and rectum of infected children. Cultures should be obtained from the pharynx and anus of both girls and boys, the vagina of girls, and the urethra of boys. For boys with a urethral discharge, a meatal specimen of the discharge is adequate for culture. Presumptive colonies of *N. gonorrhoeae* should be identified definitively by at least two independent methods.

Blood should be cultured in suspected cases of DGI. The use of Isolator blood culture tubes may enhance the yield. The probability of positive blood cultures decreases after 48 h of illness. Synovial fluid should be inoculated into blood culture broth medium and plated onto chocolate agar rather than selective medium because this fluid is not likely to be contaminated with commensal bacteria. Gonococci are infrequently recovered from early joint effusions containing <20,000 leukocytes/μL, but may be recovered from effusions containing >80,000 leukocytes/μL. The organisms are seldom recovered from blood and synovial fluid of the same patient.

℞ Treatment: GONOCOCCAL INFECTIONS

Treatment failure can lead to continued transmission and the emergence of antibiotic resistance. The importance of adequate treatment with a regimen that the patient will adhere to cannot be overemphasized. Thus highly effective single-dose regimens have been developed for uncomplicated gonococcal infections. The updated 2006 treatment guidelines for gonococcal infections from the Centers for Disease Control and Prevention are summarized in Table 45-1; the recommendations for uncomplicated gonorrhea apply to HIV-infected as well as HIV-uninfected patients.

Single-dose regimens of the third-generation cephalosporins ceftriaxone (given IM) and cefixime (given orally) are the mainstays of therapy for uncomplicated gonococcal infection of the urethra, cervix, rectum, or pharynx. Quinolone-containing regimens are no longer recommended in the United States as first-line treatment because of widespread resistance to these agents.

Because co-infection with *C. trachomatis* occurs frequently, initial treatment regimens must also incorporate an agent (e.g., azithromycin or doxycycline) that is effective against chlamydial infection. Pregnant women with gonorrhea, who should not take doxycycline, should receive concurrent treatment with a macrolide antibiotic for possible chlamydial infection. A single 1-g dose of azithromycin, which is effective therapy for uncomplicated chlamydial infections, results in an unacceptably low cure rate (93%) for gonococcal infections

TABLE 45-1

RECOMMENDED TREATMENT FOR GONOCOCCAL INFECTIONS: 2006 GUIDELINES OF THE CENTERS FOR DISEASE CONTROL AND PREVENTION (UPDATED IN 2007)

DIAGNOSIS	TREATMENT OF CHOICE
Uncomplicated gonococcal infection of the cervix, urethra, pharynx, or rectum[a]	
First-line regimens	Ceftriaxone (125 mg IM, single dose) *or* Cefixime (400 mg PO, single dose) *plus* Treatment for *Chlamydia* if chlamydial infection is not ruled out: Azithromycin (1 g PO, single dose) *or* Doxycycline (100 mg PO bid for 7 days)
Alternative regimens	Ceftizoxime (500 mg IM, single dose) *or* Cefotaxime (500 mg IM, single dose) *or* Spectinomycin (2 g IM, single dose)[b,c] *or* Cefotetan (1 g IM, single dose) plus probenecid (1 g PO, single dose)[b] *or* Cefoxitin (2 g IM, single dose) plus probenecid (1 g PO, single dose)[b]
Epididymitis	See Chap. 28
Pelvic inflammatory disease	See Chap. 28
Gonococcal conjunctivitis in an adult	Ceftriaxone (1 g IM, single dose)[d]
Ophthalmia neonatorum[e]	Ceftriaxone (25–50 mg/kg IV, single dose, not to exceed 125 mg)
Disseminated gonococcal infection[f]	
Initial therapy[g]	
Patient tolerant of β-lactam drugs	Ceftriaxone (1 g IM or IV q24h; recommended) *or* Cefotaxime (1 g IV q8h) *or* Ceftizoxime (1 g IV q8h)
Patients allergic to β-lactam drugs	Spectinomycin (2 g IM q12h)[c]
Continuation therapy	Cefixime (400 mg PO bid)
Meningitis or endocarditis	See text[h]

[a]True failure of treatment with a recommended regimen is rare and should prompt an evaluation for reinfection or consideration of an alternative diagnosis.
[b]Spectinomycin, cefotetan, and cefoxitin, which are alternative agents, currently are unavailable or in short supply in the United States.
[c]Spectinomycin may be ineffective for the treatment of pharyngeal gonorrhea.
[d]Plus lavage of the infected eye with saline solution (once).
[e]Prophylactic regimens are discussed in the text.
[f]Hospitalization is indicated if the diagnosis is uncertain, if the patient has frank arthritis with an effusion, or if the patient cannot be relied on to adhere to treatment.
[g]All initial regimens should be continued for 24–48 h after clinical improvement begins, at which time therapy may be switched to one of the continuation regimens to complete a full week of antimicrobial treatment. Treatment for chlamydial infection (as above) should be given if this infection has not been ruled out.
[h]Hospitalization is indicated to exclude suspected meningitis or endocarditis.

and should not be used alone. Spectinomycin has been an alternative regimen for the treatment of uncomplicated gonococcal infections in penicillin-allergic persons. However, spectinomycin is not available in the United States at this time. A single 2-g dose of azithromycin is effective against sensitive strains, but this drug is expensive, causes gastrointestinal distress, and is not recommended for routine or first-line treatment of gonorrhea.

Persons with uncomplicated infections who receive a recommended regimen do not need a test of cure. Cultures for *N. gonorrhoeae* should be performed if symptoms persist after therapy with an established regimen, and any gonococci isolated should be tested for antimicrobial susceptibility.

Symptomatic gonococcal pharyngitis is more difficult to eradicate than genital infection. Persons who cannot tolerate cephalosporins and those in whom quinolones are contraindicated may be treated with spectinomycin if it is available, but this agent results in a cure rate of ≤52%. Persons given spectinomycin should have a pharyngeal sample cultured 3–5 days after treatment as a test of cure. A single 2-g dose of azithromycin may be used in areas where rates of resistance to azithromycin are low.

Treatments for gonococcal epididymitis and PID are discussed in Chap. 28. Ocular gonococcal infections in older children and adults should be managed with a single dose of ceftriaxone combined with saline irrigation of the conjunctivae (both undertaken expeditiously), and patients should undergo a careful ophthalmologic evaluation that includes a slit-lamp examination.

DGI may require higher dosages and longer durations of therapy (Table 45-1). Hospitalization is indicated if the diagnosis is uncertain, if the patient has localized joint disease that requires aspiration, or if the patient cannot be relied on to comply with treatment. Open drainage is necessary only occasionally—e.g., for management of hip infections that may be difficult to drain percutaneously. Nonsteroidal anti-inflammatory agents may be indicated to alleviate pain and hasten improvement of affected joints. Gonococcal meningitis and endocarditis should be treated in the hospital with high-dose IV ceftriaxone (1–2 g every 12 h); therapy should continue for 10–14 days for meningitis and for at least 4 weeks for endocarditis. All persons who experience more than one episode of DGI should be evaluated for complement deficiency.

PREVENTION AND CONTROL

Condoms, if properly used, provide effective protection against the transmission and acquisition of gonorrhea as well as other infections that are transmitted to and from genital mucosal surfaces. Spermicidal preparations used with a diaphragm or cervical sponges impregnated with nonoxynol 9 offer some protection against gonorrhea and chlamydial infection. However, the frequent use of preparations that contain nonoxynol 9 is associated with mucosal disruption that paradoxically may enhance the risk of HIV infection in the event of exposure. All patients should be instructed to refer sex partners for evaluation and treatment. All sex partners of persons with gonorrhea should be evaluated and treated for *N. gonorrhoeae* and *C. trachomatis* infections if their last contact with the patient took place within 60 days before the onset of symptoms or the diagnosis of infection in the patient. If the patient's last sexual encounter was >60 days before onset of symptoms or diagnosis, the patient's most recent sex partner should be treated. Partner-delivered medications or prescriptions for medications to treat gonorrhea and chlamydial infection diminish the likelihood of reinfection (or relapse) in the infected patient. In states where it is legal, this approach is an option for partner management. Patients should be instructed to abstain from sexual intercourse until therapy is completed and until they and their sex partners no longer have symptoms. Greater emphasis must be placed on prevention by public health education, individual patient counseling, and behavior modification. Sexually active persons, especially adolescents, should be offered screening for STIs. For males, an NAAT on urine or a urethral swab may be used for screening. Preventing the spread of gonorrhea may help reduce the transmission of HIV. No effective vaccine for gonorrhea is yet available, but efforts to test several candidates are underway.

ACKNOWLEDGMENT

The authors acknowledge the contributions of Dr. King K. Holmes and Dr. Stephen A. Morse to the chapter on this subject in earlier editions of Harrison's Principles of Internal Medicine.

FURTHER READINGS

Centers for Disease Control and Prevention: Gonococcal Isolate Surveillance Project (GISP); *www.cdc.gov/std/GISP/*

———: Update to CDC's sexually transmitted disease treatment guidelines 2006: Fluoroquinolones no longer recommended for treatment of gonococcal infections. MMWR 56(14):332, 2007

Datta SD et al: Gonorrhea and chlamydia in the United States among persons 14 to 39 years of age, 1999 to 2002. Ann Intern Med 147:89, 2007

Gaydos CA: Nucleic acid amplification tests for gonorrhea and *Chlamydia*: Practice and applications. Infect Dis Clin North Am 19:367, 2005

Golden MR et al: Effect of expedited treatment of sex partners on recurrent or persistent gonorrhea or chlamydial infections. N Engl J Med 352:676, 2005

Hook EW III, Holmes KK: Gonococcal infections. Ann Intern Med 102:229, 1985

Laga M et al: Non-ulcerative sexually transmitted diseases as risk factors for HIV-1 transmission in women: Results from a cohort study. AIDS 7:95, 1993

Newman LM et al: Update on the management of gonorrhea in adults in the United States. Clin Infect Dis 44(Suppl 3):S84, 2007

O'Brien JP et al: Disseminated gonococcal infection: A prospective analysis of 49 patients and a review of pathophysiology and immune mechanisms. Medicine (Baltimore) 62:395, 1983

Wang SA et al: Antimicrobial resistance for *Neisseria gonorrhoeae* in the United States, 1988 to 2003: The spread of fluoroquinolone resistance. Ann Intern Med 147:81, 2007

CHAPTER 46

MORAXELLA INFECTIONS

Daniel M. Musher

MORAXELLA CATARRHALIS

The gram-negative coccus *Moraxella catarrhalis* is a component of the normal bacterial flora of the upper airways and has been increasingly recognized as a cause of otitis media, sinusitis, and bronchopulmonary infection. Over the past several decades, this organism has been variously designated as *Micrococcus catarrhalis, Neisseria catarrhalis, and Branhamella catarrhalis.*

BACTERIOLOGY AND IMMUNITY

On Gram's staining, *M. catarrhalis* organisms appear as gram-negative cocci, sometimes occurring in pairs and having the side-by-side kidney-bean configuration of *Neisseria* (Fig. 46-1). These cocci tend to retain crystal violet during the decolorizing step and may be confused with *Staphylococcus aureus*. *Moraxella* colonies grow well on blood or chocolate agar but may be overlooked because of their resemblance to the *Neisseria* spp. that are major components of the normal pharyngeal flora. *Moraxella* is readily distinguishable from *Neisseria* spp. by biochemical tests.

Strains of *M. catarrhalis* show a surprising degree of homogeneity in terms of their outer-membrane proteins. Antibody to some of these proteins is generally present in serum of children >4 years old; however, colonizing or disease-causing isolates may survive in serum despite this naturally present antibody and complement. Bactericidal antibody emerges after natural infection and may be directed against one or more conserved outer-membrane proteins—a property of potential value in vaccine development. The presence of certain outer-membrane proteins is associated with virulence in mice, and antibody to these proteins may be protective. Antibody to lipooligosaccharide may also provide some degree of protection. These and other bacterial constituents are under investigation for use as vaccines.

EPIDEMIOLOGY

With repeated cultures and the use of selective media, *M. catarrhalis* can be isolated from the upper respiratory tract or saliva of >50% of healthy children and 3–7% of healthy adults. When conventional microbiologic techniques are used, *Moraxella* can be isolated from sputum of ~10% of persons who have chronic bronchitis and ~25% of those who have bronchiectasis in the absence of acute infection. Investigators in both the northern and southern hemispheres have reported a striking seasonal variation in the isolation of this organism from clinical specimens, with a peak in late winter/early spring and a nadir in late summer/early fall. Direct contact has not been shown to contribute to community-acquired infection, but nosocomial spread of infection has been documented occasionally.

CLINICAL MANIFESTATIONS

Otitis Media and Sinusitis

M. catarrhalis is the third most common bacterial isolate from middle-ear fluid of children with otitis media, being surpassed only by *Streptococcus pneumoniae* and nontypable *Haemophilus influenzae*. This organism is also a prominent isolate from sinus cavities in acute and chronic sinusitis.

Purulent Tracheobronchitis and Pneumonia

M. catarrhalis causes acute exacerbations of chronic bronchitis (increased production and/or purulence of sputum, which may be accompanied by fever and leukocytosis) and pneumonia. Acquisition of a new bacterial strain is often responsible. The great majority of infected persons are >50 years old and have a long history of cigarette smoking and underlying chronic obstructive pulmonary disease (COPD); many have lung cancer as well. In one study, 76% of affected persons had COPD (severe in many cases), and one-third of those with COPD had lung cancer; most patients also had clinical evidence of malnutrition. In one extensive series of cases, *M. catarrhalis* pneumonia did not occur in otherwise-healthy hosts. Recent prospective studies implicate this organism in ~10% of exacerbations of chronic bronchitis.

Symptoms of *M. catarrhalis* infection have been regarded as modest in severity. Both cough and the amount and purulence of sputum are usually increased above baseline. Chills are reported in one-quarter of patients, pleuritic pain in one-third, and malaise in 40%. Most patients have peak temperatures of <38.3°C (<101°F), and peripheral white blood cell counts are <10,000/μL in nearly one-quarter of cases. Microscopic examination of a high-quality sputum specimen after Gram's staining regularly reveals profuse organisms, and quantitative culture yields ~2 × 10^8 colony-forming units per milliliter. The radiologic appearance is variable; in one study, 43% of subjects

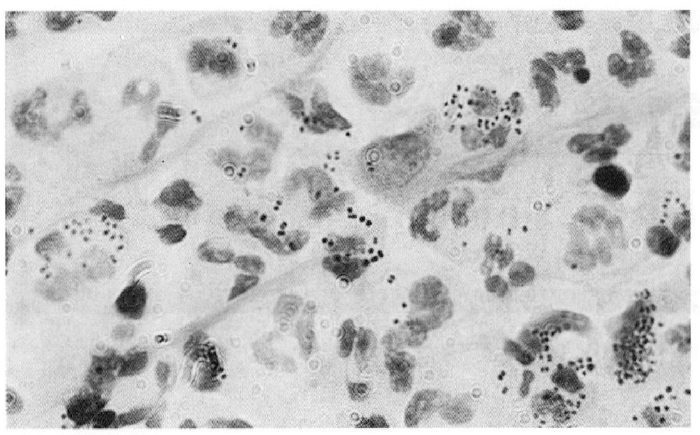

FIGURE 46-1

Gram-stained sputum from a patient with acute purulent tracheobronchitis. Many polymorphonuclear neutrophils and a few macrophages are seen along with many gram-negative cocci (*Moraxella catarrhalis*), a few of which appear as pairs. Nearly all organisms are cell associated and probably have been taken up by phagocytes, consistent with the notion that *Moraxella* is a lower-grade pathogen than organisms that are found extracellularly in sputum specimens (e.g., *Streptococcus pneumoniae*).

had segmental or lobar infiltrates, and the remainder had a mixed pattern of subsegmental, segmental, interstitial, and diffuse involvement. These clinical, laboratory, and radiographic findings do not differ from those of pneumococcal or *Haemophilus* pneumonia in an older patient population. However, a far lesser degree of bloodstream invasion occurs in *M. catarrhalis* infection; in one series, none of 25 patients with *M. catarrhalis* pneumonia had bacteremia. Nevertheless, pneumonia due to *M. catarrhalis* is a marker for severe underlying disease: nearly half of patients die within 3 months of onset.

Other Syndromes

Local extension causing empyema is very uncommon, and—as might be inferred from the low rate of bacteremia—metastatic complications of *M. catarrhalis* pneumonia, such as septic arthritis, are exceedingly rare. As of 1995, 58 cases of bacteremic infection due to *M. catarrhalis* had been reported, mainly in children <10 years old or adults >60 years old; most of these patients had severe underlying lung disease and/or were immunocompromised. The syndromes reported have included bacteremia with no apparent focus, pneumonia, endocarditis, and meningitis. A petechial or purpuric rash, reminiscent of that observed in meningococcal sepsis and associated with disseminated intravascular coagulation, has been described in a few cases.

DIAGNOSIS

Microscopic examination of Gram-stained sputum yields characteristic findings (Fig. 46-1). The presence of many polymorphonuclear leukocytes without epithelial cells indicates that the sputum sample is of good quality; since most patients with *Moraxella* infection have chronic lung disease, it is usually not difficult to obtain an acceptable specimen. Large numbers of *Moraxella* organisms are seen as gram-negative cocci, often lining up side by side and thus resembling pairs of kidneys.

℞ Treatment: *MORAXELLA* INFECTIONS

M. catarrhalis is widely susceptible to most antibiotics used to treat lower respiratory tract infection (Table 46-1). Penicillin resistance first appeared in isolated strains in the mid-1970s and is now found in 94% of clinical isolates. This resistance is mediated by two closely related β-lactamases, BRO-1 and BRO-2. These enzymes are active against penicillin, ampicillin, and amoxicillin but less so against cephalosporins, especially third-generation cephalosporins; they also bind avidly to clavulanic acid and sulbactam. Thus a β-lactam/β-lactamase inhibitor combination such as amoxicillin/clavulanate offers excellent treatment. Second- and third-generation cephalosporins are effective alternatives. Isolates in the United States are also nearly uniformly susceptible to fluoroquinolones, newer macrolides, ketolides, and doxycycline; ~90% are susceptible to trimethoprim-sulfamethoxazole. A 5-day course of therapy has been shown to cure respiratory infection, although a longer course is required in sinusitis.

Treatment of sinusitis or otitis media is empirical, as appropriate specimens are usually obtained only in

TABLE 46-1

THERAPY FOR INFECTION CAUSED BY *MORAXELLA CATARRHALIS*

DRUG(S)	DOSE AND DURATION
Oral Therapy for Lower Respiratory Infection[a]	
Trimethoprim-sulfamethoxazole	160/800 mg qd for 5–7 days
Doxycycline	200 mg/d for 5–7 days
Azithromycin	500 mg/d for 5 days
Telithromycin	800 mg/d for 5–7 days
Amoxicillin/clavulanic acid	500 mg tid for 7 days
Ciprofloxacin	500 mg bid for 5 days
Cefuroxime	250–500 mg bid for 10 days
Cefpodoxime	200 mg bid for 10–14 days
Parenteral Therapy for Lower Respiratory Infection in Hospitalized Patients[b]	
Ampicillin/sulbactam	1.5/0.5 g q6h
Ceftriaxone	1 g/d
Cefotaxime	1 g q8h
Azithromycin	500 mg/d

[a]The same dosages apply for sinusitis, but some authorities treat for 10 days with macrolides, tetracyclines, and quinolones and for 14 days with β-lactam agents.

[b]After the patient's condition has stabilized, the regimen may be changed to oral medications at the indicated doses and durations.

TABLE 46-2

MORAXELLA* SPECIES OTHER THAN *M. CATARRHALIS

MORAXELLA SPECIES	NUMBER OF ISOLATES	COMMON SITES/ CLINICAL ASSOCIATION	NUMBER (PERCENT) FOR EACH SITE
M. osloensis[a]	199	Blood	44 (22)
		CSF	18 (9)
		Urine	17 (9)
		Respiratory tract	24 (12)
M. nonliquefaciens	356	Blood	27 (8)
		CSF	6 (2)
		Respiratory tract	196 (55)
M. canis	74	Dog-bite wound	53 (72)
M-6	47	Blood, bone	15 (32)
M. lacunata	33	Conjunctivitis, keratitis	23 (70)
M. urethralis	28	Urine	16 (57)
		Genital tract	3 (11)
M. phenylpyruvica	73	Blood	19 (26)
		CSF	8 (11)
		Urine	12 (16)
M. atlantae	44	Blood	20 (45)
		CSF	5 (11)

[a]Some of these isolates would now be distinguished as a new species, *Moraxella lincolnii*.
Note: CSF, cerebrospinal fluid.
Source: Adapted from a summary of CDC experience (Graham et al).

research studies. In the treatment of pneumonia during the period between the identification of gram-negative cocci in a Gram-stained specimen and the final identification of the organisms by culture, the severity of the condition and the potential presence of other infecting organisms should guide antibiotic selection. For example, an exacerbation of bronchitis caused by *M. catarrhalis* might be treated with doxycycline or an advanced macrolide. However, the microscopic identification of this organism in a patient with pneumonia may still lead to a preference for initial therapy (at least until culture results become available) with ampicillin/sulbactam, a third-generation cephalosporin, or a quinolone because of the possibility that resistant pneumococci are also present but have been overlooked by Gram's stain.

OTHER *MORAXELLA* SPECIES

Other *Moraxella* species are occasional causes of a wide range of infections, including bronchitis, pneumonia, empyema, endocarditis, meningitis, conjunctivitis, endophthalmitis, urinary tract infection, septic arthritis, and wound infection. In a report on all *Moraxella* isolates submitted to the Centers for Disease Control and Prevention between 1953 and 1980, certain clinical associations were apparent (Table 46-2). *M. osloensis* and *M. nonliquefaciens*, the most commonly isolated species, were cultured from various normally sterile body sites, including blood, cerebrospinal fluid, and joints. *M. osloensis* was the *Moraxella* species most frequently isolated from blood; *M. nonliquefaciens* tended to be isolated from the ears, nose, or throat (47%) or the sputum (8%) and has since been implicated as a cause of conjunctivitis and keratitis. *M. urethralis* was isolated most often from urine and the genital tract and probably represents the *Moraxella* species implicated previously in urethritis. More than half of isolates of *M. phenylpyruvica* and *M. atlantae* were obtained from normally sterile sites. One study found *Moraxella* spp., including *M. catarrhalis*, in 35% of infected cat-bite wounds and in 10% of infected dog-bite wounds. The clinical features of infections due to *Moraxella* spp. other than *M. catarrhalis* and the nature of the hosts in which they occur have not been fully characterized.

FURTHER READINGS

Bisgaard H et al: Childhood asthma after bacterial colonization of the airway in neonates. N Engl J Med 357:1487, 2007

Graham DR et al: Infections caused by *Moraxella, Moraxella urethralis, Moraxella*-like groups M-5 and M-6, and *Kingella kingae* in the United States, 1953–1980. Rev Infect Dis 12:423, 1990

Ioannidis JPA et al: Spectrum and significance of bacteremia due to *Moraxella catarrhalis*. Clin Infect Dis 21:390, 1995

Maayan H et al: Infective endocarditis due to *Moraxella lacunata:* Report of 4 patients and review of published cases of *Moraxella* endocarditis. Scand J Infect Dis 36:878, 2005

Murphy TF et al: *Moraxella catarrhalis* in chronic obstructive pulmonary disease: Burden of disease and immune response. Am J Respir Crit Care Med 172:195, 2005

Sethi S et al: New strains of bacteria and exacerbations of chronic obstructive pulmonary disease. N Engl J Med 347:465, 2002

Talan DA et al: Bacteriologic analysis of infected dog and cat bites. N Engl J Med 340:85, 1999

Verduin CM et al: *Moraxella catarrhalis*: From emerging to established pathogen. Clin Microbiol Rev 15:125, 2002

CHAPTER 47

HAEMOPHILUS INFECTIONS

Timothy F. Murphy

HAEMOPHILUS INFLUENZAE

MICROBIOLOGY

Haemophilus influenzae was first recognized in 1892 by Pfeiffer, who erroneously concluded that the bacterium was the cause of influenza. The bacterium is a small (1- by 0.3-μm) gram-negative organism of variable shape; hence it is often described as a pleomorphic coccobacillus. In clinical specimens such as cerebrospinal fluid (CSF) and sputum, it frequently stains only faintly with phenosafranin and therefore can easily be overlooked.

H. influenzae grows both aerobically and anaerobically. Its aerobic growth requires two factors: hemin (X factor) and nicotinamide adenine dinucleotide (V factor). These requirements are used in the clinical laboratory to identify the bacterium. Caution must be used to distinguish *H. influenzae* from *H. haemolyticus*, a respiratory tract commensal that has identical growth requirements. *H. haemolyticus* has classically been distinguished from *H. influenzae* by hemolysis on horse blood agar. However, a significant proportion of isolates of *H. haemolyticus* have recently been recognized as nonhemolytic. Analysis of 16S ribosomal sequences is one reliable method to distinguish these two species.

Six major serotypes of *H. influenzae* have been identified; designated *a* through *f*, they are based on antigenically distinct polysaccharide capsules. In addition, some strains lack a polysaccharide capsule and are referred to as *nontypable* strains. Type b and nontypable strains are the most relevant strains clinically (Table 47-1), although encapsulated strains other than type b can cause disease. *H. influenzae* was the first free-living organism to have its entire genome sequenced.

The antigenically distinct type b capsule is a linear polymer composed of ribosyl-ribitol phosphate. Strains of *H. influenzae* type b (Hib) cause disease primarily in infants and children <6 years of age. Nontypable strains are primarily mucosal pathogens but occasionally cause invasive disease.

EPIDEMIOLOGY AND TRANSMISSION

H. influenzae, an exclusively human pathogen, is spread by airborne droplets or by direct contact with secretions or fomites. Nontypable strains colonize the upper respiratory tract of up to three-fourths of healthy adults. Colonization with nontypable *H. influenzae* is a dynamic process; new strains are acquired and other strains are replaced periodically.

The widespread use of Hib conjugate vaccines in many industrialized countries has resulted in striking decreases in the rate of nasopharyngeal colonization by Hib and in the incidence of Hib infection (Fig. 47-1). However, the majority of the world's children remain unimmunized. Worldwide, invasive Hib disease occurs predominantly in unimmunized children and in those who have not completed the primary immunization series.

Certain groups have a higher incidence of invasive Hib disease than the general population. The incidence of meningitis due to Hib has been three to four times higher among black children than among white children in several studies. In some Native American groups, the incidence of invasive Hib disease is 10 times higher than that in the general population. Although this increased incidence has not yet been accounted for, several factors may be relevant, including age at exposure to the bacterium, socioeconomic conditions, and genetic differences in the ability to mount an immune response.

PATHOGENESIS

Hib strains cause systemic disease by invasion and hematogenous spread from the respiratory tract to distant sites such as the meninges, bones, and joints. The type b polysaccharide capsule is an important virulence factor affecting the bacterium's ability to avoid opsonization and cause systemic disease.

Nontypable strains cause disease by local invasion of mucosal surfaces. Otitis media results when bacteria reach the middle ear by way of the eustachian tube. Adults with chronic bronchitis experience recurrent lower respiratory tract infection due to nontypable strains. In addition, persistent nontypable *H. influenzae* colonization of the lower airways of adults with chronic obstructive pulmonary disease (COPD) contributes to the airway inflammation that is a hallmark of the disease. The incidence of invasive disease caused by nontypable strains is low.

IMMUNE RESPONSE

Antibody to the capsule is important in protection from infection by Hib strains. The level of (maternally acquired) serum antibody to the capsular polysaccharide, which is a polymer of polyribitol ribose phosphate (PRP), declines from birth to 6 months of age and, in the absence of

TABLE 47-1

CHARACTERISTICS OF TYPE b AND NONTYPABLE STRAINS OF *HAEMOPHILUS INFLUENZAE*

FEATURE	TYPE b STRAINS	NONTYPABLE STRAINS
Capsule	Ribosyl-ribitol phosphate	Unencapsulated
Pathogenesis	Invasive infections due to hematogenous spread	Mucosal infections due to contiguous spread
Clinical manifestations	Meningitis and invasive infections in incompletely immunized infants and children	Otitis media in infants and children; lower respiratory tract infections in adults with chronic bronchitis
Evolutionary history	Basically clonal	Genetically diverse
Vaccine	Highly effective conjugate vaccines	None available; under development

vaccination, remains low until ~2 or 3 years of age. The age at the antibody nadir correlates with that of the peak incidence of type b disease. Antibody to PRP then appears partly as a result of exposure to Hib or cross-reacting antigens. Systemic Hib disease is unusual after the age of 6 years because of the presence of protective antibody. Vaccines in which PRP is conjugated to protein carrier molecules have been developed and are now used widely. These vaccines generate an antibody response to PRP in infants and effectively prevent invasive infections in infants and children.

Since nontypable strains lack a capsule, the immune response to infection is directed at noncapsular antigens. These antigens have generated considerable interest as immune targets and potential vaccine components. The human immune response to nontypable strains appears to be strain-specific, accounting in part for the propensity of these strains to cause recurrent otitis media and recurrent exacerbations of chronic bronchitis in immunocompetent hosts.

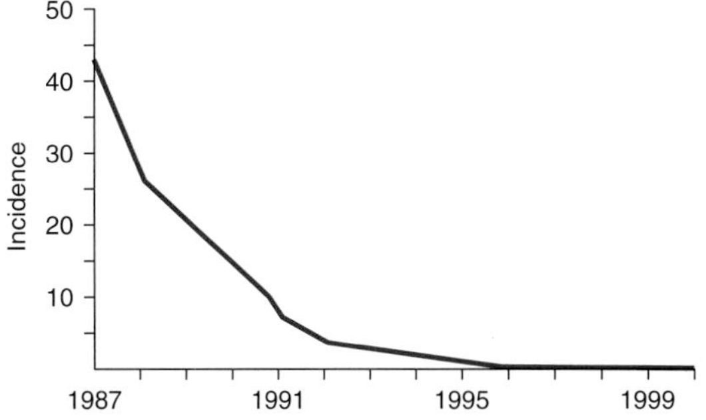

FIGURE 47-1

Estimated incidence (rate per 100,000) of invasive disease due to *Haemophilus influenzae* type b among children <5 years of age: 1987–2000. (*Data from the Centers for Disease Control and Prevention.*)

CLINICAL MANIFESTATIONS

Hib

The most serious manifestation of infection with Hib is *meningitis* (Chap. 29). The age of peak incidence varies somewhat among populations, depending in part on the use of vaccine, but this infection primarily affects infants <2 years of age. The clinical manifestations of Hib meningitis are similar to those of meningitis caused by other bacterial pathogens. Fever and altered central nervous system function are the most common features at presentation. Nuchal rigidity may or may not be evident. Subdural effusion, the most common complication, is suspected when, despite 2 or 3 days of appropriate antibiotic therapy, the infant has seizures, hemiparesis, or continued obtundation. The overall mortality rate from Hib meningitis is ~5%, and the morbidity rate is high. Of survivors, 6% have permanent sensorineural hearing loss, and about one-fourth have a significant handicap of some type. If more subtle handicaps are sought, up to half of survivors are found to have some neurologic sequelae, such as partial hearing loss and delayed language development.

Epiglottitis (Chap. 16) is a life-threatening Hib infection involving cellulitis of the epiglottis and supraglottic tissues. It can lead to acute upper airway obstruction. Its unique epidemiologic features are its occurrence in an older age group (2–7 years old) than other Hib infections and its absence among Navajo Indians and Alaskan Eskimos. Sore throat and fever rapidly progress to dysphagia, drooling, and airway obstruction. Epiglottitis also occurs in adults.

Cellulitis (Chap. 21) due to Hib occurs in young children. The most common location is on the head or neck, and the involved area sometimes takes on a characteristic bluish-red color. Most patients have bacteremia, and 10% have an additional focus of infection.

Hib causes *pneumonia* in infants. The infection is clinically indistinguishable from other types of bacterial pneumonia (e.g., pneumococcal pneumonia) except that Hib is more likely to involve the pleura.

Several less common invasive conditions can be important clinical manifestations of Hib infection in children. These include osteomyelitis, septic arthritis, pericarditis, orbital cellulitis, endophthalmitis, urinary tract infection, abscesses, and bacteremia without an identifiable focus. As has been mentioned, Hib infections are unusual among patients >6 years old.

Nontypable H. Influenzae

Nontypable *H. influenzae* is a common cause of community-acquired bacterial pneumonia in adults. Nontypable *H. influenzae* pneumonia is especially common among patients with COPD or AIDS. The clinical features of

H. influenzae pneumonia are similar to those of other types of bacterial pneumonia (including pneumococcal pneumonia). Patients present with fever, cough, and purulent sputum, usually of several days' duration. Chest radiography reveals alveolar infiltrates in a patchy or lobar distribution. Gram-stained sputum contains a predominance of small, pleomorphic, coccobacillary gram-negative bacteria.

Exacerbations of COPD caused by nontypable *H. influenzae* are characterized by increased cough, sputum production, and shortness of breath. Fever is low-grade, and no infiltrates are evident on chest x-ray.

Nontypable *H. influenzae* is one of the three most common causes of childhood otitis media (the other two being *Streptococcus pneumoniae* and *Moraxella catarrhalis*) (Chap. 16). Infants are febrile and irritable, whereas older children report ear pain. Symptoms of viral upper respiratory infection often precede otitis media. The diagnosis is made by pneumatic otoscopy. An etiologic diagnosis, although not routinely sought, can be established by tympanocentesis and culture of middle-ear fluid. The increasing use of pneumococcal polysaccharide conjugate vaccines in infants is resulting in a relative increase in the proportion of otitis media cases that are caused by *H. influenzae*.

Nontypable *H. influenzae* also causes puerperal sepsis and is an important cause of neonatal bacteremia. These nontypable strains, which are closely related to *H. haemolyticus*, tend to be of biotype IV and cause invasive disease after colonizing the female genital tract.

Nontypable *H. influenzae* causes sinusitis (Chap. 16) in adults and children. In addition, the bacterium is a less common cause of various invasive infections that are reported primarily as small-series descriptions and case reports. These infections include empyema, adult epiglottitis, pericarditis, cellulitis, septic arthritis, osteomyelitis, endocarditis, cholecystitis, intraabdominal infections, urinary tract infections, mastoiditis, aortic graft infection, and bacteremia without a detectable focus.

DIAGNOSIS

The most reliable method for establishing a diagnosis of Hib infection is recovery of the organism in culture. The CSF of a patient in whom meningitis is suspected should be subjected to Gram's staining and culture. The presence of gram-negative coccobacilli in Gram-stained CSF is strong evidence for Hib meningitis. Recovery of the organism from CSF confirms the diagnosis. Cultures of other normally sterile body fluids, such as blood, joint fluid, pleural fluid, pericardial fluid, and subdural effusion, are confirmatory in other infections.

Detection of PRP is an important adjunct to culture in rapid diagnosis of Hib meningitis. Immunoelectrophoresis, latex agglutination, coagglutination, and enzyme-linked immunosorbent assay are effective in detecting PRP. These assays are particularly helpful when patients have received prior antimicrobial therapy and thus are especially likely to have negative cultures.

Before the early 1980s, nontypable strains of *H. influenzae* were frequently misidentified as Hib because of their autoagglutination when serotypes were determined in agglutination assays. Since nontypable *H. influenzae* is primarily a mucosal pathogen, it is a component of a mixed flora; this situation makes etiologic diagnosis challenging. Nontypable *H. influenzae* infection is strongly suggested by the predominance of gram-negative coccobacilli among abundant polymorphonuclear leukocytes in a Gram-stained sputum specimen from a patient in whom pneumonia or tracheobronchitis is suspected. A sputum culture is helpful when interpreted along with the results of Gram's staining. Although bacteremia is detectable in a small proportion of patients with pneumonia due to nontypable *H. influenzae*, most such patients have negative blood cultures.

A diagnosis of otitis media is based on the detection by pneumatic otoscopy of fluid in the middle ear. An etiologic diagnosis requires tympanocentesis but is not routinely sought. An invasive procedure is also required to determine the etiology of sinusitis; thus treatment is often empirical once the diagnosis is suspected in light of clinical symptoms and sinus radiographs.

℞ Treatment: *HAEMOPHILUS INFLUENZAE*

Initial therapy for meningitis due to Hib should consist of a cephalosporin such as ceftriaxone or cefotaxime. For children, the dosage of ceftriaxone is 75–100 mg/kg daily given in two doses 12 h apart. The pediatric dosage of cefotaxime is 200 mg/kg daily given in four doses 6 h apart. Adult dosages are 2 g every 12 h for ceftriaxone and 2 g every 4–6 h for cefotaxime. An alternative regimen for initial therapy is ampicillin (200–300 mg/kg daily in four divided doses) plus chloramphenicol (75–100 mg/kg daily in four divided doses). Therapy should continue for a total of 1–2 weeks.

Administration of glucocorticoids to patients with Hib meningitis reduces the incidence of neurologic sequelae. The presumed mechanism is reduction of the inflammation induced by bacterial cell-wall mediators of inflammation when cells are killed by antimicrobial agents. Dexamethasone (0.6 mg/kg per day intravenously in four divided doses for 2 days) is recommended for the treatment of Hib meningitis in children >2 months of age.

Invasive infections other than meningitis are treated with the same antimicrobial agents. For epiglottitis, the dosage of ceftriaxone is 50 mg/kg daily, and the dosage of cefotaxime is 150 mg/kg daily, given in three divided doses 8 h apart. Epiglottitis constitutes a medical emergency, and maintenance of an airway is critical. The duration of therapy is determined by the clinical response. A course of 1–2 weeks is usually appropriate.

Many infections caused by nontypable strains of *H. influenzae*, such as otitis media, sinusitis, and exacerbations of COPD, can be treated with oral antimicrobial agents. Approximately 20–35% of nontypable strains produce β-lactamase (with the exact proportion depending on geographic location), and these strains are resistant to ampicillin. Several agents have excellent activity against nontypable *H. influenzae*, including amoxicillin/clavulanic acid, various extended-spectrum cephalosporins, the macrolides azithromycin and clarithromycin, and the new ketolide telithromycin. Fluoroquinolones are highly active against *H. influenzae* and are useful in adults with exacerbations of COPD. However, fluoroquinolones are not currently recommended for the treatment of children or pregnant women because of possible effects on articular cartilage.

In addition to β-lactamase production, alteration of penicillin-binding proteins—a second mechanism of ampicillin resistance—has been detected in isolates of *H. influenzae*. Although rare in the United States, these β-lactamase-negative ampicillin-resistant strains are increasing in prevalence in Europe and Japan. Continued monitoring of the evolving antimicrobial susceptibility patterns of *H. influenzae* will be important.

PREVENTION

Vaccination

(See also Chap. 3) The development of conjugate vaccines that prevent invasive infections with Hib in infants and children has been a dramatic success. Three such vaccines are licensed in the United States. In addition to eliciting protective antibody, these vaccines prevent disease by reducing rates of pharyngeal colonization with Hib.

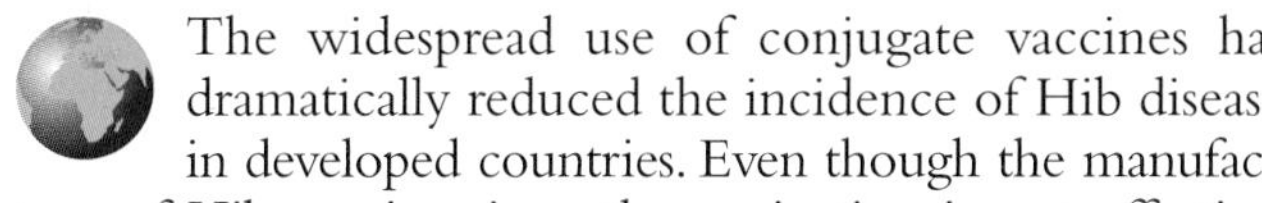

The widespread use of conjugate vaccines has dramatically reduced the incidence of Hib disease in developed countries. Even though the manufacture of Hib vaccines is costly, vaccination is cost-effective. The Global Alliance for Vaccines and Immunizations has recognized the underuse of Hib conjugate vaccines. The disease burden has been reduced in developing countries that have implemented routine vaccination (e.g., The Gambia, Chile). An important obstacle to more widespread vaccination is the lack of data on the epidemiology and burden of Hib disease in many developing countries.

All children should be immunized with a Hib conjugate vaccine, receiving the first dose at ~2 months of age, the rest of the primary series at 2–6 months of age, and a booster dose at 12–15 months of age. Specific recommendations vary for the different conjugate vaccines. The reader is referred to the recommendations of the American Academy of Pediatrics (Chap. 3 and *www.cispimmunize.org*). Currently, no vaccines are available for the prevention of disease caused by nontypable *H. influenzae*.

Chemoprophylaxis

The risk of secondary disease is greater than normal among household contacts of patients with Hib disease. Therefore, all children and adults (except pregnant women) in households with at least one incompletely immunized contact <4 years of age should receive prophylaxis with oral rifampin. When two or more cases of invasive Hib disease have occurred within 60 days at a child-care facility attended by incompletely vaccinated children, administration of rifampin to all attendees and personnel is indicated, as is recommended for household contacts. Chemoprophylaxis is not indicated in nursery and child-care contacts of a single index case. The reader is referred to the recommendations of the American Academy of Pediatrics.

HAEMOPHILUS INFLUENZAE BIOGROUP AEGYPTIUS

H. influenzae biogroup aegyptius was formerly called *Haemophilus aegyptius* because of phenotypic characteristics distinct from those of *H. influenzae*. However, later studies involving DNA hybridization and DNA transformation demonstrated that *H. aegyptius* and *H. influenzae* are members of the same species.

H. influenzae biogroup aegyptius has long been associated with conjunctivitis. Moreover, this strain is now known to be the cause of Brazilian purpuric fever (BPF), which was first recognized in 1984 in the rural Brazilian town of Promissão. The sharing of many phenotypic and genotypic characteristics by the various strains of *H. influenzae* biogroup aegyptius that cause BPF indicates that these strains represent a clone of *H. influenzae* that has acquired specific virulence factors, several of which are associated with a pathogenicity island. The age of peak incidence of BPF is 1–4 years, with a range of 3 months to 8 years. The illness can occur sporadically or in outbreaks. Typically, after an episode of purulent conjunctivitis, high fever occurs in association with vomiting and abdominal pain. Within 12–48 h after onset, the patient develops petechiae, purpura, and peripheral necrosis and experiences vascular collapse. The characteristic laboratory features are thrombocytopenia, prolonged prothrombin time, uniformly unrevealing CSF findings, and blood cultures positive for *H. influenzae* biogroup aegyptius. Initial reports cited high mortality (70%), but subsequent studies have indicated that milder forms of the illness exist. Most patients have resolved or resolving purulent conjunctivitis, and culture of the conjunctiva is positive in approximately one-third of cases. BPF has been seen in several towns in Brazil and on two occasions in Australia.

HAEMOPHILUS DUCREYI

Haemophilus ducreyi is the etiologic agent of chancroid (Chap. 28), a sexually transmitted disease characterized by genital ulceration and inguinal adenitis. *H. ducreyi* poses a significant health problem in developing countries. Although this infection is less common in the United States, its incidence has increased dramatically in the past several years. In addition to being a cause of morbidity in itself, chancroid is associated with HIV infection because of the role played by genital ulceration in HIV transmission.

MICROBIOLOGY

H. ducreyi is a highly fastidious coccobacillary gram-negative bacterium whose growth requires X factor (hemin). Although, in light of this requirement, the bacterium has been classified in the genus *Haemophilus*, DNA homology and chemotaxonomic studies have established substantial differences between *H. ducreyi* and other *Haemophilus* species. Taxonomic reclassification of the organism is likely in the future but awaits further study.

The histology of the genital ulcer of chancroid is characterized by perivascular and interstitial infiltrates of macrophages and of CD4+ and CD8+ T lymphocytes. The appearance is consistent with a delayed-type hypersensitivity, cell-mediated immune response. The presence of CD4+ T cells and macrophages in the ulcer may explain, in part, the facilitation of HIV transmission in patients with chancroid.

EPIDEMIOLOGY AND PREVALENCE

Chancroid is a common cause of genital ulcers in developing countries. In the United States, chancroid is now endemic in some regions, and several large outbreaks have occurred since 1981. Recurring epidemiologic themes have been apparent in these outbreaks: (1) transmission has been predominantly heterosexual; (2) males have outnumbered females by ratios of 3:1 to 25:1; (3) prostitutes have been important in transmission of the infection; and (4) chancroid has been strongly associated with illicit drug use.

CLINICAL MANIFESTATIONS

Infection is acquired as the result of a break in the epithelium during sexual contact with an infected individual. After an incubation period of 4–7 days, the initial lesion—a papule with surrounding erythema—appears. In 2 or 3 days, the papule evolves into a pustule, which spontaneously ruptures and forms a sharply circumscribed ulcer that is generally not indurated (Fig. 47-2).

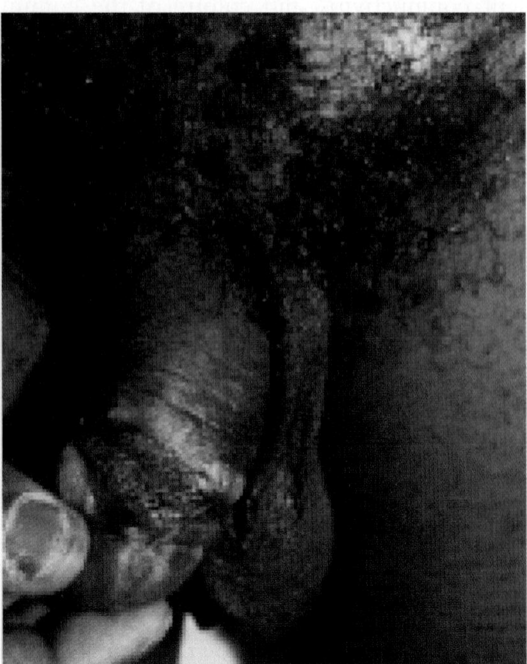

FIGURE 47-2
Chancroid with characteristic penile ulcers and associated left inguinal adenitis (bubo).

The ulcers are painful and bleed easily; little or no inflammation of the surrounding skin is evident. Approximately half of patients develop enlarged, tender inguinal lymph nodes, which frequently become fluctuant and spontaneously rupture. Patients usually seek medical care after 1–3 weeks of painful symptoms.

The presentation of chancroid does not usually include all of the typical clinical features and is sometimes atypical. Multiple ulcers can coalesce to form giant ulcers. Ulcers can appear and then resolve, with inguinal adenitis (Fig. 47-2) and suppuration following 1–3 weeks later; this clinical picture can be confused with that of lymphogranuloma venereum (Chap. 77). Multiple small ulcers can resemble folliculitis. Other differential diagnostic considerations include the various infections causing genital ulceration, such as primary syphilis, condyloma latum of secondary syphilis, genital herpes, and donovanosis. In rare cases, chancroid lesions become secondarily infected with bacteria; the result is extensive inflammation.

DIAGNOSIS

Clinical diagnosis of chancroid is often inaccurate, and laboratory confirmation should be attempted in suspected cases. Gram's staining of a swab of the lesion may reveal a predominance of characteristic gram-negative coccobacilli, but the presence of other bacteria often makes it difficult to interpret this result. An accurate diagnosis of chancroid relies on culture of *H. ducreyi* from the lesion. In addition, aspiration and culture of suppurative lymph nodes should be considered. Since the organism can be difficult to grow, the use of selective and supplemented media is necessary. A multiplex polymerase chain reaction assay has been developed for simultaneous amplification of DNA targets from *H. ducreyi*, *Treponema pallidum*, and herpes simplex virus types 1 and 2. When this assay becomes commercially available, it will be a useful diagnostic tool to identify the etiology of genital ulcers.

℞ Treatment: *HAEMOPHILUS DUCREYI*

The treatment regimen recommended by the Centers for Disease Control and Prevention is a single 1-g oral dose of azithromycin. Alternative regimens include ceftriaxone (250 mg intramuscularly in a single dose), ciprofloxacin (500 mg orally bid for 3 days), or erythromycin base (500 mg orally tid for 7 days). Isolates from patients who do not respond promptly to treatment should be tested for antimicrobial susceptibility. In patients with HIV infection, healing may be slow, and longer courses of treatment may be necessary. Clinical treatment failure in HIV-seropositive patients may reflect co-infection, especially with herpes simplex virus. Contacts of patients with chancroid should be identified and treated, whether or not symptoms are present, if they had sexual contact with the patient during the 10 days preceding the patient's onse of symptoms.

FURTHER READINGS

BISGAARD H et al: Childhood asthma after bacterial colonization of the airway in neonates. N Engl J Med 357:1487, 2007

BONG CT et al: *Haemophilus ducreyi*: Clinical features, epidemiology, and prospects for disease control. Microbes Infect 4:1141, 2002

CASEY JR, PICHICHERO ME: Changes in frequency and pathogens causing acute otitis media in 1995–2003. Pediatr Infect Dis J 23:824, 2004

COMMITTEE ON INFECTIOUS DISEASES: *Haemophilus influenzae* infections, in *2003 Red Book, Report of the Committee on Infectious Diseases*, 26th ed, LK Pickering et al (eds). Elk Grove Village, IL, American Academy of Pediatrics, 2003

DOMINGUEZ SR, DAUM RS: Toward global *Haemophilus influenzae* type b immunization. Clin Infect Dis 37:1600, 2003

HEILMANN KP et al: Decreasing prevalence of beta-lactamase production among respiratory tract isolates of *Haemophilus influenzae* in the United States. Antimicrob Agents Chemother 49:2561, 2005

KELLY DF et al: *Haemophilus influenzae* type b conjugate vaccines. Immunology 113:163, 2004

LIEBOWITZ E et al: *Haemophilus influenzae*: A significant pathogen in acute otitis media. Pediatr Infect Dis J 23:1142, 2004

MCGILLIVARY G et al: Cloning and sequencing of a genomic island found in the Brazilian purpuric fever clone of *Haemophilus influenzae* biogroup aegyptius. Infect Immun 73:1927, 2005

MURPHY TF: Respiratory infections caused by non-typeable *Haemophilus influenzae*. Curr Opin Infect Dis 16:129, 2003

——— et al: Persistent colonization by *Haemophilus influenzae* in chronic obstructive pulmonary disease. Am J Respir Crit Care Med 170:266, 2004

SETHI S et al: Strain-specific immune response to *Haemophilus influenzae* in chronic obstructive pulmonary disease. Am J Respir Crit Care Med 169:448, 2004

CHAPTER 48

INFECTIONS DUE TO THE HACEK GROUP AND MISCELLANEOUS GRAM-NEGATIVE BACTERIA

Tamar F. Barlam ■ Dennis L. Kasper

THE HACEK GROUP

HACEK organisms are a group of fastidious, slow-growing, gram-negative bacteria whose growth requires an atmosphere of carbon dioxide. Species belonging to this group include several ***H**aemophilus* species, ***A**ctinobacillus actinomycetemcomitans*, ***C**ardiobacterium hominis*, ***E**ikenella corrodens*, and ***K**ingella kingae*. HACEK bacteria normally reside in the oral cavity and have been associated with local infections in the mouth. They are also known to cause severe systemic infections—most often bacterial endocarditis, which can develop on either native or prosthetic valves (Chap. 19).

HACEK ENDOCARDITIS

In large series, up to 3% of cases of infective endocarditis are attributable to HACEK organisms, most often *A. actinomycetemcomitans, Haemophilus* species, and *C. hominis.* The clinical course of HACEK endocarditis tends to be subacute; however, embolization is common. The overall prevalence of major emboli associated with HACEK endocarditis ranges from 28 to 71% in different series. On echocardiography, valvular vegetations are seen in up to 85% of patients. The vegetations are frequently large, although vegetation size has not been directly correlated with the risk of embolization. Cultures of blood from patients with suspected HACEK endocarditis may require up to 30 days to become positive, and the microbiology laboratory should be alerted when a HACEK organism is being considered. However, most cultures that ultimately yield a HACEK organism become positive within the first week, especially with improved culture systems such as BACTEC. In addition, polymerase chain reaction techniques are facilitating the diagnosis of HACEK infections. Because of the organisms' slow growth, antimicrobial testing may be difficult, and β-lactamase production may not be detected. E-test methodology may increase the accuracy of susceptibility testing.

Haemophilus *Species*

Haemophilus species are differentiated by their in vitro growth requirements for X factor (hemin) and V factor (nicotinamide adenine dinucleotide). *H. aphrophilus* requires only X factor for growth, whereas species designated *para-* require only V factor. *H. aphrophilus* and *H. parainfluenzae* are the most common *Haemophilus* species isolated from cases of HACEK endocarditis; *H. paraphrophilus* is less common. Invasive infection typically occurs in patients with a history of cardiac valvular disease, often in the setting of a recent dental procedure. Sixty percent of these patients have been ill for <2 months before presentation, and 19–50% develop congestive heart failure. Mortality rates as high as 30–50% have been reported in older series; however, more recent studies have documented mortality rates of <5%. *H. aphrophilus* also causes invasive bone and joint infections, and *H. parainfluenzae* has been isolated from other infections such as meningitis; brain, dental, and liver abscess; pneumonia; and septicemia.

Actinobacillus Actinomycetemcomitans

A. actinomycetemcomitans can be isolated from soft tissue infections and abscesses in association with *Actinomyces israelii*. Typically, patients who develop endocarditis with *A. actinomycetemcomitans* have severe periodontal disease or have recently undergone dental procedures in the setting of underlying cardiac valvular damage. The disease is insidious; patients may be sick for several months before diagnosis. Frequent complications include embolic phenomena, congestive heart failure, and renal failure. *A. actinomycetemcomitans* has been isolated from patients with brain abscess, meningitis, endophthalmitis, parotitis, osteomyelitis, urinary tract infection, pneumonia, and empyema, among other infections.

Cardiobacterium Hominis

C. hominis primarily causes endocarditis in patients with underlying valvular heart disease or with prosthetic valves. This organism most frequently affects the aortic valve. Many patients have signs and symptoms of long-standing infection before diagnosis, with evidence of arterial embolization, vasculitis, cerebrovascular accidents, immune complex glomerulonephritis, or arthritis at presentation. Embolization, mycotic aneurysms, and congestive heart failure are common complications.

Eikenella Corrodens

E. corrodens is most frequently recovered from sites of infection in conjunction with other bacterial species. Clinical sources of *E. corrodens* include sites of human bite wounds (clenched-fist injuries), endocarditis, soft tissue infections, osteomyelitis, respiratory infections, chorioamnionitis, gynecologic infections associated with intrauterine devices, meningitis and brain abscesses, and visceral abscesses.

Kingella Kingae

Because of improved microbiologic methodology, isolation of *K. kingae* is increasingly common. Inoculation of clinical specimens (e.g., synovial fluid) into aerobic blood culture bottles enhances recovery of this organism. In recent series, *K. kingae* has been the third most common cause of septic arthritis in children <24 months of age; staphylococcal and streptococcal species remain most prevalent. Invasive *K. kingae* infections with bacteremia are associated with upper respiratory tract infections and stomatitis. Both *K. kingae* colonization and primary herpes—a major cause of stomatitis—peak in children 6–48 months of age. *K. kingae* bacteremia can present with a petechial rash similar to that seen in *Neisseria meningitidis* sepsis.

Infective endocarditis, unlike other infections with *K. kingae*, occurs in older children and adults. The majority of patients have preexisting valvular disease. There is a high incidence of complications, including arterial emboli, cerebrovascular accidents, tricuspid insufficiency, and congestive heart failure with cardiovascular collapse.

Rx Treatment: ENDOCARDITIS CAUSED BY HACEK ORGANISMS

See Table 48-1. Native-valve endocarditis should be treated for 4 weeks with antibiotics, whereas prosthetic-valve endocarditis requires 6 weeks of therapy. The cure

TABLE 48-1

TREATMENT OF ENDOCARDITIS CAUSED BY HACEK GROUP ORGANISMS[a]

ORGANISM	INITIAL THERAPY	ALTERNATIVE AGENTS	COMMENTS
Haemophilus species, *Actinobacillus actinomycetemcomitans*	Ceftriaxone (2 g/d)	Ampicillin/sulbactam (3 g of ampicillin q6h) **or** fluoroquinolones[b]	Ampicillin ± an aminoglycoside can be used if the organism does not produce β-lactamase.[c]
Cardiobacterium hominis	Penicillin (16–18 mU/d in 6 divided doses) or ampicillin (2 g q4h)	Ceftriaxone (2 g/d) **or** ampicillin/sulbactam (3 g of ampicillin q6h)	An aminoglycoside (gentamicin, 3 mg/kg per day in 3 divided doses) may be added, but its value has not been proven. The organism is usually pansensitive, but high-level penicillin resistance has been reported.
Eikenella corrodens	Ampicillin (2 g q4h)	Ceftriaxone (2 g/d) **or** fluoroquinolones[b]	The organism is typically resistant to clindamycin, metronidazole, and aminoglycosides.
Kingella kingae	Ceftriaxone (2 g/d) or ampicillin/sulbactam (3 g of ampicillin q6h)	Fluoroquinolones[b]	The prevalence of β-lactamase-producing strains is increasing. Efficacy for invasive infections is best demonstrated for first-line treatments.

[a]Susceptibility testing should be performed in all cases to guide therapy.
[b]Fluoroquinolones are not recommended for treatment of children <17 years of age.
[c]European guidelines for endocarditis recommend the addition of gentamicin (3 mg/kg per day in 3 divided doses for 2–4 weeks).

rates for HACEK prosthetic-valve endocarditis appear to be high. Unlike prosthetic-valve endocarditis caused by other gram-negative organisms, HACEK endocarditis is often cured with antibiotic treatment alone—i.e., without surgical intervention.

OTHER GRAM-NEGATIVE BACTERIA

Achromobacter Xylosoxidans

A. xylosoxidans (previously *Alcaligenes xylosoxidans*) is probably part of the endogenous intestinal flora and has been isolated from water sources. Immunocompromised hosts, including patients with cancer and postchemotherapy neutropenia, cirrhosis, and chronic renal failure, are at increased risk. Nosocomial outbreaks of *A. xylosoxidans* infection have been attributed to contaminated fluids, and clinical illness has been associated with isolates from many sites, including blood (often in the setting of intravascular devices). Community-acquired bacteremia with *A. xylosoxidans* usually occurs in the setting of pneumonia. Metastatic skin lesions are present in one-fifth of cases. The reported mortality rate is 67%—a figure similar to rates for other bacteremic gram-negative pneumonias.

℞ Treatment: *ACHROMOBACTER XYLOSOXIDANS* INFECTIONS

Treatment is based on in vitro susceptibility testing of all clinically relevant isolates.

Aeromonas *Species*

More than 85% of *Aeromonas* infections are caused by *A. hydrophila*, *A. caviae*, and *A. veronii* biovar *sobria*. *Aeromonas* proliferates in potable and fresh water and in soil. It remains controversial whether *Aeromonas* is a cause of bacterial gastroenteritis; asymptomatic colonization of the intestinal tract with *Aeromonas* occurs frequently. However, rare cases of hemolytic-uremic syndrome after bloody diarrhea have been shown to be secondary to the presence of *Aeromonas*.

Aeromonas causes sepsis and bacteremia in infants with multiple medical problems and in immunocompromised hosts, particularly those with cancer or hepatobiliary disease. *Aeromonas* infection and sepsis can occur in patients with trauma (including severe trauma with myonecrosis) and in burn patients exposed to *Aeromonas* by environmental (freshwater or soil) contamination of their wounds. Reported mortality rates range from 25% among immunocompromised adults with sepsis to >90% among patients with myonecrosis. *Aeromonas* can produce ecthyma gangrenosum (hemorrhagic vesicles surrounded by a rim of erythema with central necrosis and ulceration) resembling the lesions seen in *Pseudomonas aeruginosa* infection. *Aeromonas* causes nosocomial infections related to catheters, surgical incisions, or use of leeches. Other manifestations include meningitis, peritonitis, pneumonia, and ocular infections.

℞ Treatment: *AEROMONAS* INFECTIONS

Aeromonas species are generally susceptible to fluoroquinolones (e.g., ciprofloxacin at a dosage of 500 mg every 12 h PO or 400 mg every 12 h IV), trimethoprim-sulfamethoxazole (TMP-SMX; trimethoprim dosage, 10 mg/kg per day in 3 or 4 divided doses), third-generation cephalosporins, and aminoglycosides. Because *Aeromonas* can produce various β-lactamases, including carbapenemases, susceptibility testing must be used to guide therapy.

Capnocytophaga *Species*

This genus of fastidious, fusiform, gram-negative coccobacilli is facultatively anaerobic and requires an atmosphere enriched in carbon dioxide for optimal growth. *C. ochracea*, *C. gingivalis*, and *C. sputigena* have been associated with sepsis in immunocompromised hosts, particularly neutropenic patients with hematologic malignancy, and probably play a role in localized juvenile periodontitis in the immunocompetent host. These species have been isolated from many other sites as well, usually as part of a polymicrobial infection.

C. canimorsus and *C. cynodegmi* are endogenous to the canine mouth (Chap. 32). Patients infected with these species frequently have a history of dog bites or of exposure to dogs without scratches or bites. Asplenia, glucocorticoid therapy, and alcohol abuse are predisposing conditions that can be associated with fulminant infections. *C. canimorsus* causes a wide range of infections, including severe sepsis with shock and disseminated intravascular coagulation, meningitis, endocarditis, cellulitis, and septic arthritis.

℞ Treatment: *CAPNOCYTOPHAGA* INFECTIONS

Because of increasing β-lactamase production, clindamycin (600–900 mg every 6–8 h) or drug combinations including a penicillin derivative plus a β-lactamase inhibitor—such as ampicillin/sulbactam (1.5–3.0 g of ampicillin every 6 h)—are currently recommended for empirical treatment of infections caused by *C. ochracea*, *C. gingivalis*, and *C. sputigena*. Infections with *C. canimorsus* should be treated with penicillin (12–18 million units every 4 h). This regimen or ampicillin/sulbactam should be given prophylactically to asplenic patients sustaining dog-bite injuries. *C. canimorsus* is also susceptible to clindamycin, imipenem, fluoroquinolones, and third-generation cephalosporins.

Chryseobacterium *Species (Formerly* Flavobacterium)

C. meningosepticum is an important cause of nosocomial infections, including outbreaks due to contaminated fluids (e.g., disinfectants and aerosolized antibiotics) and sporadic infections due to indwelling devices, feeding tubes, and other fluid-associated apparatuses. Patients with nosocomial *C. meningosepticum* infection usually have underlying immunosuppression (e.g., related to malignancy). *C. meningosepticum* has been reported to cause meningitis (primarily in neonates), sepsis, endocarditis, bacteremia, soft tissue infections, and pneumonia. *C. indologenes* has caused bacteremia, sepsis, and pneumonia, typically in immunocompromised patients with indwelling devices.

℞ Treatment: *CHRYSEOBACTERIUM* INFECTIONS

Chryseobacteria are often susceptible to fluoroquinolones, TMP-SMX, imipenem, and third- or fourth-generation cephalosporins, but susceptibility testing should be performed.

Pasteurella Multocida

P. multocida is a bipolar-staining, gram-negative coccobacillus that colonizes the respiratory and gastrointestinal tracts of domestic animals; oropharyngeal colonization rates are 70–90% in cats and 50–65% in dogs. *P. multocida* can be transmitted to humans through bites or scratches, via the respiratory tract from contact with contaminated dust or infectious droplets, or via deposition of the organism on injured skin or mucosal surfaces during licking. Most human infections affect skin and soft tissue; almost two-thirds of these infections are caused by cats. Patients at the extremes of age or with serious underlying disorders (e.g., cirrhosis) are at increased risk for systemic manifestations, including meningitis, peritonitis, osteomyelitis, endocarditis, and septic shock, but cases have also occurred in healthy individuals. If inhaled, *P. multocida* can cause acute respiratory tract infection, particularly in patients with underlying sinus and pulmonary disease.

℞ Treatment: *PASTEURELLA MULTOCIDA* INFECTIONS

P. multocida is susceptible to penicillin, ampicillin, ampicillin/sulbactam, second- and third-generation cephalosporins, tetracyclines, and fluoroquinolones. β-lactamase-producing strains have been reported.

MISCELLANEOUS ORGANISMS

Agrobacterium radiobacter (tumefaciens) has usually been associated with infection in the presence of medical devices, including intravascular catheter–related infections, prosthetic-joint and prosthetic-valve infections, and peritonitis caused by dialysis catheters. Most cases occur in immunocompromised hosts, especially individuals with malignancy or HIV infection. Strains are usually susceptible to fluoroquinolones, third-generation cephalosporins, imipenem, TMP-SMX, and aminoglycosides.

Chromobacterium violaceum, although rarely a human pathogen, reportedly has been responsible for life-threatening infections with severe sepsis and metastatic abscesses, particularly in children with defective neutrophil function (e.g., those with chronic granulomatous disease). *C. violaceum* is generally susceptible to ciprofloxacin (500 mg every 12 h PO or 400 mg every 12 h IV), TMP-SMX, and gentamicin.

Plesiomonas shigelloides is a freshwater organism that causes acute diarrhea (Chap. 25) and occasionally serious extraintestinal disease, most commonly in immunocompromised hosts. *Ochrobactrum anthropi* causes infections related to central venous catheters in compromised hosts; other invasive infections have been described. Other organisms include *Weeksella* species; various CDC groups, such as EF4 and Ve-2; Flavimonas species; *Sphingobacterium* species; *Protomonas* species; *Oligella urethralis*; and *Shewanella putrefaciens*. The reader is advised to consult subspecialty texts and references for further guidance on these organisms.

FURTHER READINGS

BADDOUR LM et al: Infective endocarditis: Diagnosis, antimicrobial therapy, and management of complications: A statement for healthcare professionals from the Committee on Rheumatic Fever, Endocarditis, and Kawasaki Disease, Council on Cardiovascular Disease in the Young, and the Councils on Clinical Cardiology, Stroke, and Cardiovascular Surgery and Anesthesia, American Heart Association: Endorsed by the Infectious Diseases Society of America. Circulation 111:e394, 2005

BROUQUI P, RAOULT D: Endocarditis due to rare and fastidious bacteria. Clin Microbiol Rev 14:177, 2001

CHOMETON S et al: Specific real-time polymerase chain reaction places *Kingella kingae* as the most common cause of osteoarticular infections in young children. Pediatr Infect Dis J 26:377, 2007

ELLIOTT TSJ et al: Guidelines for the antibiotic treatment of endocarditis in adults: Report of the Working Party of the British Society for Antimicrobial Chemotherapy. J Antimicrob Chemother 54:971, 2004

GOLDBERG MH, KATZ J: Infective endocarditis caused by fastidious oro-pharyngeal HACEK micro-organisms. J Oral Maxillofac Surg 64:969, 2006

JOLIVET-GOUGEON A et al: Antimicrobial treatment of *Capnocytophaga* infections. Int J Antimicrob Agents 29:367, 2007

HUANG ST et al: Clinical characteristics of invasive *Haemophilus aphrophilus* infections. J Microbiol Immunol Infect 38:271, 2005

MARTINO R et al: Bacteremia caused by *Capnocytophaga* species in patients with neutropenia and cancer: Results of a multicenter study. Clin Infect Dis 33:E20, 2001

PATUREL L et al: *Actinobacillus actinomycetemcomitans* endocarditis. Clin Microbiol Infect 10:98, 2004

PETTI CA et al: Utility of extended blood culture incubation for isolation of *Haemophilus, Actinobacillus, Cardiobacterium, Eikenella,* and *Kingella* organisms: A retrospective multicenter evaluation. J Clin Microbiol 44:257, 2006

SHIE SS et al: Characteristics of *Achromobacter xylosoxidans* bacteremia in northern Taiwan. J Microbiol Immunol Infect 38:277, 2005

UDAKA T et al: *Eikenella corrodens* in head and neck infections. J Infect 54:343, 2007

CHAPTER 49

LEGIONELLA INFECTION

Miguel Sabria ■ Victor L. Yu

Legionellosis refers to the two clinical syndromes caused by bacteria of the genus *Legionella*. *Pontiac fever* is an acute, febrile, self-limited illness that has been serologically linked to *Legionella* species, whereas *Legionnaires' disease* is the designation for pneumonia caused by these species. Legionnaires' disease was first recognized in 1976, when an outbreak of pneumonia took place at a hotel in Philadelphia during the American Legion Convention. The causative agent proved to be a newly discovered bacterium, *Legionella pneumophila*, that was isolated from lung specimens obtained from the victims at autopsy.

MICROBIOLOGY

The family Legionellaceae comprises more than 49 species with more than 64 serogroups. The species *L. pneumophila* causes 80–90% of human infections and includes at least 16 serogroups; serogroups 1, 4, and 6 are most commonly implicated in human infections. To date, 18 species other than *L. pneumophila* have been associated with human infections, among which *L. micdadei* (Pittsburgh pneumonia agent), *L. bozemanii*, *L. dumoffii*, and *L. longbeachae* are the most common.

Members of the Legionellaceae are aerobic gram-negative bacilli that do not grow on routine microbiologic media. Buffered charcoal yeast extract (BCYE) agar is the medium used to grow *Legionella*. Antibiotics added to the medium suppress the growth of competing flora from nonsterile sites, and dyes color the colonies and assist in identification.

The direct fluorescent antibody (DFA) test can definitively identify a number of individual species. In the case of *L. pneumophila*, the serogroup-specific antigen and antibodies detected by immunofluorescence are directed primarily at the lipopolysaccharide, a prominent outer-membrane component. Both polyclonal and monoclonal DFA reagents are commercially available. The monoclonal reagent is less cross-reactive but is specific for *L. pneumophila*.

ECOLOGY AND TRANSMISSION

The natural habitats for *L. pneumophila* are aquatic bodies, including lakes and streams. *L. longbeachae* has been isolated from soil. Legionellae can survive under a wide range of environmental conditions; for example, the organisms can live for years in refrigerated water samples. Natural bodies of water contain only small numbers of legionellae. However, once the organisms enter human-constructed aquatic reservoirs (such as water-distribution systems), they can grow and proliferate. Factors known to enhance colonization by and amplification of legionellae include warm temperatures (25°–42°C), stagnation, and scale and sediment. *L. pneumophila* can form microcolonies within biofilms; its eradication from water-distribution systems requires disinfectants that can penetrate the biofilm. The presence of symbiotic microorganisms, including algae, amebas, ciliated protozoa, and other water-dwelling bacteria, promotes the growth of *L. pneumophila*. Legionellae can invade and multiply within free-living protozoa.

The source of *Legionella* is water. Community-acquired Legionnaires' disease has been linked to colonization of residential and industrial water supplies. Potable-water distribution systems in hospitals, long-term care facilities, hotels, and large buildings have been implicated. Sporadic community-acquired cases have been linked to residential water systems.

Cooling towers and evaporative condensers have been overestimated as sources of *Legionella*. Early investigations that implicated cooling towers antedated the discovery that the organism could also exist in potable-water distribution systems. It is now known that, in many outbreaks attributed to cooling towers, cases of Legionnaires' disease continued to occur despite disinfection of the cooling towers; the potable water supply was the actual source. Koch's postulates have never been fulfilled for cooling tower–associated outbreaks as they have been for hospital-acquired Legionnaires' disease. Nevertheless, cooling towers are occasionally identified in community-acquired outbreaks.

L. longbeachae infections have been linked to potting soil.

Multiple modes of transmission of *Legionella* to humans exist, including aerosolization, aspiration, and direct instillation into the lungs during respiratory tract manipulations. Aspiration is now known to be the predominant mode of transmission, but it is unclear whether *Legionella* enters the lungs via oropharyngeal colonization or directly via the drinking of contaminated water. Oropharyngeal colonization has been demonstrated in patients undergoing transplantation. Nasogastric tubes have been linked to hospital-acquired Legionnaires' disease; microaspiration of contaminated water was the hypothesized mode of transmission. Surgery with general anesthesia is a known risk factor that is consistent with aspiration. Especially compelling is the reported 30% incidence of postoperative *Legionella* pneumonia among patients undergoing head and neck surgery at a hospital with a contaminated water supply; aspiration is a recognized sequela in such cases. Studies of patients with hospital-acquired Legionnaires' disease have shown that these individuals underwent endotracheal intubation significantly more often and for a significantly longer duration than patients with hospital-acquired pneumonia of other etiologies.

Aerosolization of *Legionella* by devices filled with tap water, including whirlpools, nebulizers, and humidifiers, has been implicated. An ultrasonic mist machine in the produce section of a grocery store was the source in a community outbreak. Pontiac fever has been linked to *Legionella*-containing aerosols from water-using machinery, a cooling tower, air-conditioners, and whirlpools.

EPIDEMIOLOGY

The incidence of Legionnaires' disease depends on the degree of contamination of the aquatic reservoir, the immune status of the persons exposed to water from that reservoir, the intensity of exposure, and the availability of specialized laboratory tests on which the correct diagnosis can be based.

Numerous prospective studies have ranked *Legionella* among the top four microbial causes of community-acquired pneumonia (with *Streptococcus pneumoniae*, *Haemophilus influenzae*, and *Chlamydophila pneumoniae* usually ranked first, second, and third, respectively), accounting for 2–9% of cases. On the basis of a multihospital study of community-acquired pneumonia in Ohio, the Centers for Disease Control and Prevention (CDC) estimated that as many as 18,000 cases of sporadic community-acquired Legionnaires' disease occur annually in the United States and that only 3% of these cases are correctly diagnosed. *Legionella* is responsible for 10–50% of cases of nosocomial pneumonia when a hospital's water system is colonized with the organisms. The incidence of hospital-acquired Legionnaires' disease depends on the degree of contamination of the water system as defined by the rate of positivity of distal water sites (not as defined quantitatively by the number of colony-forming units per milliliter).

Risk factors for Legionnaires' disease include cigarette smoking; chronic lung disease; advanced age; prior hospitalization, with discharge within 10 days before onset of pneumonia symptoms; and immunosuppression. Immunosuppressive conditions that predispose to Legionnaires' disease include transplantation, HIV infection, and treatment with glucocorticoids or tumor necrosis factor α. However, in a large prospective study of community-acquired pneumonia, 28% of patients with Legionnaires' disease did not have these classic risk factors. Surgery is a prominent predisposing factor in hospital-acquired infection, with transplant recipients at highest risk. Hospital-acquired cases are now being recognized among neonates and immunosuppressed children.

Pontiac fever occurs in epidemics. The high attack rate (>90%) reflects airborne transmission.

PATHOGENESIS AND IMMUNITY

Legionella enters the lungs through aspiration or direct inhalation. Attachment to host cells is mediated by bacterial type IV pili, heat-shock proteins, and the major outer-membrane protein. *Legionella* binds to complement CR1 and CR3 integrin receptors on the surface of the host cell. Because the organisms possess pili that may mediate adherence to respiratory tract epithelial cells, conditions that impair mucociliary clearance, including cigarette smoking, lung disease, or alcoholism, predispose to Legionnaires' disease.

Cell-mediated immunity is the primary mechanism of host defense against *Legionella*, as it is against other intracellular pathogens. Thus Legionnaires' disease is more common and its manifestations are more severe among patients with depressed cell-mediated immunity. The disease also occurs with unusual frequency among patients with hairy cell leukemia, which is characterized by monocyte deficiency and dysfunction.

Alveolar macrophages readily phagocytose *Legionella*. The attachment of the bacteria to phagocytes is mediated via Fc receptors and complement receptors, which attach to the bacterial major outer-membrane protein. Binding to these receptors promotes phagocytosis but fails to trigger an oxidative burst. The *L. pneumophila* phagosome resists acidification and evades fusion with late endocytic compartments and lysosomes. Although many legionellae are killed, some proliferate intracellularly until the cells rupture; the bacteria are then phagocytosed again by newly recruited phagocytes, and the cycle begins anew.

The role of neutrophils in immunity appears to be minimal: neutropenic patients are not predisposed to Legionnaires' disease. Although *L. pneumophila* is susceptible to oxygen-dependent microbiologic systems in vitro, it resists killing by neutrophils.

The humoral immune system is active against *Legionella*. Type-specific IgM and IgG antibodies are measurable within weeks of infection. In vitro, antibodies promote killing of *Legionella* by phagocytes (neutrophils, monocytes, and alveolar macrophages). Immunized animals develop a specific antibody response, with subsequent resistance to *Legionella* challenge. However, antibodies neither enhance lysis by complement nor inhibit intracellular multiplication within phagocytes.

Some *L. pneumophila* strains are clearly more virulent than others, although the precise factors mediating virulence remain uncertain. For example, although multiple strains may colonize water-distribution systems, only a few cause disease in patients exposed to water from these systems. At least one surface epitope of *L. pneumophila* serogroup 1 is associated with virulence. Monoclonal antibody subtype mAb2 has been linked to virulence. *L. pneumophila* serogroup 6 is more commonly involved in hospital-acquired Legionnaires' disease and is more likely to be associated with a poor outcome.

The genome of *L. pneumophila* has been sequenced. A broad range of membrane transporters within the genome are thought to optimize the use of nutrients in water and soil. Genes responsible for establishment of an intracellular growth site in human alveolar macrophages and replication in symbiotic microorganisms have been identified.

CLINICAL AND LABORATORY FEATURES

Pontiac Fever

Pontiac fever is an acute, self-limiting, flulike illness with an incubation period of 24–48 h. Pneumonia does not develop. Malaise, fatigue, and myalgias are the most common symptoms, occurring in 97% of cases. Fever (usually with chills) develops in 80–90% of cases and headache in 80%. Other symptoms (seen in <50% of cases) include arthralgias, nausea, cough, abdominal pain, and diarrhea. Modest leukocytosis with a neutrophilic predominance is sometimes detected. Without antibiotic therapy, complete recovery takes place in only a few days; a few patients may experience lassitude for many weeks thereafter. The diagnosis is established by antibody seroconversion.

Legionnaires' Disease (Pneumonia)

Legionnaires' disease is often included in the differential diagnosis of "atypical pneumonia," along with infection due to *C. pneumoniae*, *Chlamydophila psittaci*, *Mycoplasma pneumoniae*, *Coxiella burnetii*, and some viruses. The clinical similarities among these types of pneumonia include a relatively nonproductive cough and a low incidence of grossly purulent sputum. However, the clinical manifestations of Legionnaires' disease are usually more severe than those of most "atypical" pneumonias, and the course and prognosis of *Legionella* pneumonia more closely resemble those of bacteremic pneumococcal pneumonia than those of pneumonia due to other "atypical" pathogens. Patients with community-acquired Legionnaires' disease are significantly more likely than patients with pneumonia of other etiologies to be admitted to an intensive care unit on presentation.

The incubation period for Legionnaires' disease is usually 2–10 days, although longer incubation periods have been documented. The symptoms and signs may range from a mild cough and a slight fever to stupor with widespread pulmonary infiltrates and multisystem failure. Nonspecific symptoms—malaise, fatigue, anorexia, and headache—are seen early in the illness. Myalgias and arthralgias are uncommon but are prominent in a few patients. Upper respiratory symptoms, including coryza, are rare.

The mild cough of Legionnaires' disease is only slightly productive. Sometimes the sputum is streaked with blood. Chest pain—either pleuritic or nonpleuritic—can be a prominent feature and, when coupled with hemoptysis, can lead to an incorrect diagnosis of pulmonary embolism. Shortness of breath is reported by one-third to one-half of patients.

Gastrointestinal difficulties are often pronounced; abdominal pain, nausea, and vomiting affect 10–20% of patients. Diarrhea (watery rather than bloody) is reported in 25–50% of cases. The most common neurologic abnormalities are confusion or changes in mental status; however, the multitudinous neurologic symptoms reported range from headache and lethargy to encephalopathy.

Patients with Legionnaires' disease virtually always have fever. Temperatures in excess of 40.5°C (104.9°F) were recorded in 20% of the cases in one series. Relative bradycardia has been overemphasized as a useful diagnostic finding; it occurs primarily in older patients with severe pneumonia. Chest examination reveals rales early in the course and evidence of consolidations as the disease progresses. Abdominal examination may reveal generalized or local tenderness.

TABLE 49-1

CLINICAL CLUES SUGGESTIVE OF LEGIONNAIRES' DISEASE
Diarrhea
High fever (>40°C; >104°F)
Numerous neutrophils but no organisms revealed by Gram's staining of respiratory secretions
Hyponatremia (serum sodium level <131 mg/dL)
Failure to respond to β-lactam drugs (penicillins or cephalosporins) and aminoglycoside antibiotics
Occurrence of illness in an environment in which the potable water supply is known to be contaminated with *Legionella*
Onset of symptoms within 10 days after discharge from the hospital

Although the clinical manifestations often considered classic for Legionnaires' disease (Table 49-1) may suggest the diagnosis, prospective comparative studies have shown that clinical manifestations are generally nonspecific and that Legionnaires' disease is not readily distinguishable from pneumonia of other etiologies. In a review of 13 studies of community-acquired pneumonia, clinical manifestations that occurred significantly more often in Legionnaires' disease included diarrhea, neurologic findings (including confusion), and a temperature of >39°C. Hyponatremia, elevated values in liver function tests, and hematuria also occurred more frequently in Legionnaires' disease. Other laboratory abnormalities include creatine phosphokinase elevation, hypophosphatemia, serum creatinine elevation, and proteinuria.

Extrapulmonary Legionellosis

Since the portal of entry for *Legionella* is the lung in virtually all cases, extrapulmonary manifestations usually result from bloodborne dissemination from the lung. In a prospective survey of patients with Legionnaires' disease diagnosed by isolation of the organism from sputum, *Legionella* was isolated from the blood by a special culture method in 38% of cases.

Legionella has been identified in lymph nodes, spleen, liver, or kidneys in autopsied cases. The most common extrapulmonary site of legionellosis is the heart; numerous reports have described myocarditis, pericarditis, postcardiotomy syndrome, and prosthetic-valve endocarditis. Most cases have been hospital-acquired. In some patients

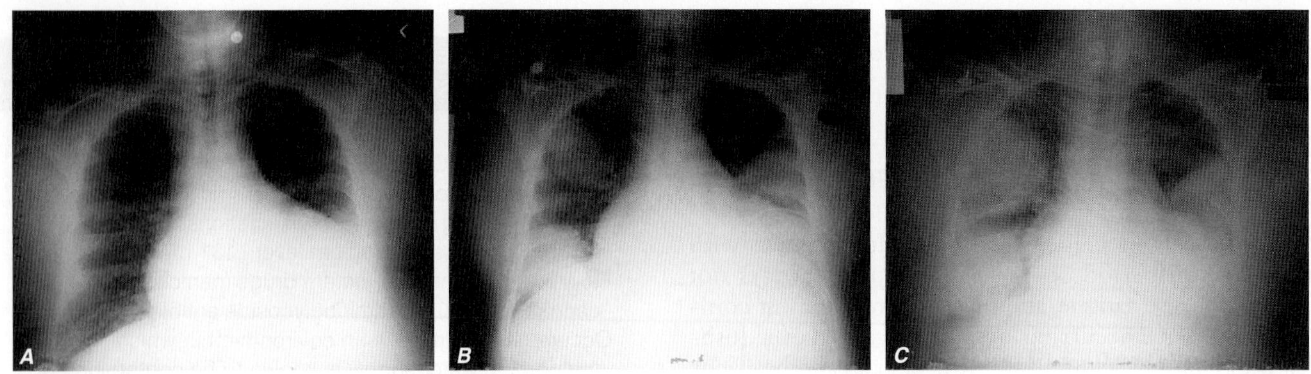

FIGURE 49-1

Chest radiographic findings in a 52-year-old man who presented with pneumonia subsequently diagnosed as Legionnaires' disease. The patient was a cigarette smoker with chronic obstructive pulmonary disease and alcoholic cardiomyopathy; he had received glucocorticoids. *L. pneumophila* was identified by DFA staining and culture of sputum. ***A.*** Baseline chest radiograph showing long-standing cardiomegaly. ***B.*** Admission chest radiograph showing new rounded opacities. ***C.*** Chest radiograph taken 3 days after admission, during treatment with erythromycin.

without overt evidence of pneumonia, the organisms may gain entry through a postoperative sternal wound exposed to contaminated tap water or through a mediastinal-tube insertion site. Sinusitis, peritonitis, pyelonephritis, skin and soft tissue infection, septic arthritis, and pancreatitis have been seen predominantly in immunosuppressed patients.

Chest Radiography

Virtually all patients with Legionnaires' disease have abnormal chest radiographs showing pulmonary infiltrates at the time of clinical presentation. In a few cases of hospital-acquired disease, fever and respiratory tract symptoms have preceded the radiographic appearance of the infiltrate. Findings on chest radiography are useful for assessing the severity of illness in that they identify multilobar involvement and permit monitoring of disease progression. However, these findings are nonspecific and do not serve to distinguish Legionnaires' disease from pneumonias of other etiologies. Pleural effusion is evident in 28–63% of patients on hospital admission. In immunosuppressed patients, especially those receiving glucocorticoids, distinctive rounded nodular opacities may be seen; these lesions may expand and cavitate (Fig. 49-1). Likewise, abscesses can occur in immunosuppressed hosts. The progression of infiltrates and pleural effusion on chest radiography despite appropriate antibiotic therapy within the first week is common, and radiographic improvement lags behind clinical improvement by several days. Complete clearing of infiltrates requires 1–4 months.

DIAGNOSIS

Because clinical manifestations are nonspecific, the diagnosis of Legionnaires' disease requires special microbiologic tests (Table 49-2). The sensitivity of bronchoscopy specimens is approximately the same as that of sputum samples for culture on selective media; if sputum is not available, bronchoscopy specimens may yield the organism. Bronchoalveolar lavage fluid gives higher yields than bronchial wash specimens. Thoracentesis should be performed if pleural effusion is found, and the fluid should be evaluated by DFA staining, culture, and the antigen assay designed for use with urine (see "Urinary Antigen" later in the chapter).

Staining

Gram's staining of material from normally sterile sites, such as pleural fluid or lung tissue, occasionally suggests the diagnosis; efforts to detect *Legionella* in sputum by Gram's staining typically reveal numerous leukocytes but no organisms. When they are visualized, the organisms appear as small, pleomorphic, faint, gram-negative bacilli. *L. micdadei* organisms can be detected as weakly or partially acid-fast bacilli in clinical specimens. Modified

TABLE 49-2

UTILITY OF SPECIAL LABORATORY TESTS FOR THE DIAGNOSIS OF LEGIONNAIRES' DISEASE

TEST	SENSITIVITY, %	SPECIFICITY, %
Culture		
Sputum[a]	80	100
Transtracheal aspirate	90	100
Direct fluorescent antibody staining of sputum	50–70	96–99
Urinary antigen testing[b]	70	100
Antibody serology[c]	40–60	96–99

[a]Use of multiple selective media with dyes.
[b]Serogroup 1 only.
[c]IgG and IgM testing of both acute- and convalescent-phase sera. A single titer of ≥1:256 is considered presumptive, whereas fourfold seroconversion is considered definitive.

acid-fast staining substitutes 1% sulfuric acid for the traditional 3% hydrochloric acid; the less aggressive decolorizer increases the yield of *L. micdadei*. *Legionella*-infected patients have occasionally been treated empirically with antituberculosis medications because of false-positive acid-fast smears.

The DFA test is rapid and highly specific but is less sensitive than culture because large numbers of organisms are required for microscopic visualization. This test is more likely to be positive in advanced than in early disease.

Culture

The definitive method for diagnosis of *Legionella* infection is isolation of the organism from respiratory secretions or other specimens. Multiple selective BCYE media containing dyes are required for maximal sensitivity. Colonies grow slowly, requiring 3–5 days to become grossly visible. When culture plates are overgrown with other microflora, pretreatment of the specimen with acid or heat can markedly improve the yield. *L. pneumophila* is often isolated from sputum that is not grossly or microscopically purulent; sputum containing more than 25 epithelial cells per high-power field (a finding that classically suggests contamination) may still yield *L. pneumophila*.

Antibody Detection

Antibody testing of both acute- and convalescent-phase sera is necessary. A fourfold rise in titer is diagnostic; 12 weeks are often required for the detection of an antibody response. A single titer of 1:128 in a patient with pneumonia constitutes circumstantial evidence for Legionnaires' disease. Serology is of use primarily in epidemiologic studies. The specificity of serology for *Legionella* species other than *L. pneumophila* is uncertain; there is cross-reactivity with *Legionella* spp. and some gram-negative bacilli.

Urinary Antigen

The assay for *Legionella* soluble antigen in urine is rapid, relatively inexpensive, easy to perform, second only to culture in terms of sensitivity, and highly specific. Several enzyme immunoassays and a rapid immunochromatographic assay are commercially available. Like the urinary antigen assay, the rapid immunochromatographic assay is relatively inexpensive and easy to perform. The use of urinary antigen testing in every clinical laboratory is recommended. The urinary antigen test is available only for *L. pneumophila* serogroup 1, which causes ~80% of *Legionella* infections. Cross-reactivity with other *L. pneumophila* serogroups and other *Legionella* species has been detected in up to 22% of urine samples from patients with culture-proven cases. Antigen in urine is detectable 3 days after the onset of clinical disease and disappears over 2 months; positivity can be prolonged when patients receive glucocorticoids. The test is not affected by antibiotic administration.

Molecular Methods

Polymerase chain reaction (PCR) with DNA probes is theoretically more sensitive and specific than other methods. A molecular probe is undergoing evaluation. PCR has proven somewhat useful in the identification of *Legionella* from environmental water specimens. In PCR (unlike culture), epidemiologic links cannot be made since the infecting pathogen is not available for molecular subtyping.

PATHOLOGY

The consistent pathologic features of Legionnaires' disease are confined to the lungs. Multifocal pneumonia, with patchy lobular inflammation and extensive multilobar consolidation, has been observed. Visible abscesses with central necrosis were seen in 20% of autopsied cases in one study. On histologic examination, fibrinopurulent pneumonia with intensive alveolitis and bronchiolitis is evident. The DFA stain is not only specific, but is also the most sensitive option for visualization of the organism in tissues. Polyvalent but not monoclonal DFA stain can be used for formalinized specimens. Culture is the preferred method for diagnosis based on clinical specimens.

℞ Treatment: *LEGIONELLA* INFECTION

Because *Legionella* is an intracellular pathogen, antibiotics that can reach intracellular concentrations exceeding the minimal inhibitory concentration are most likely to be clinically efficacious. The dosages for various drugs used in the treatment of Legionella infection are listed in Table 49-3.

The newer macrolides (especially azithromycin) and respiratory tract quinolones are now the antibiotics of choice and are effective as monotherapy. Compared with erythromycin, the newer macrolides have superior in vitro activity, display greater intracellular activity, reach higher concentrations in respiratory secretions and in lung tissue, and have fewer adverse effects. The pharmacokinetics of the newer macrolides and quinolones also allow once- or twice-daily dosing. Quinolones are the preferred antibiotics for transplant recipients because both macrolides and rifampin interact pharmacologically with cyclosporine and tacrolimus. Retrospective uncontrolled studies have shown that complications of pneumonia are fewer and clinical response is more rapid in patients receiving quinolones than in those receiving macrolides. Ketolides (telithromycin) are highly active in vitro and in intracellular models, but clinical experience is less extensive than that with macrolides and quinolones. Alternative agents include tetracycline and its analogues doxycycline and minocycline. Tigecycline is active in vitro, but clinical experience is lacking. Anecdotal reports have described both successes and failures with trimethoprim-sulfamethoxazole, imipenem, and clindamycin. For severely ill patients with extensive pulmonary infiltrates, a two-drug combination of a newer macrolide or a quinolone with rifampin can be considered for initial treatment.

TABLE 49-3

ANTIBIOTIC THERAPY FOR *LEGIONELLA* INFECTION

ANTIMICROBIAL AGENT	DOSAGE[a]
Macrolides	
Azithromycin	500 mg[b] PO or IV[c] q24h
Clarithromycin	500 mg PO or IV[c] q12h
Quinolones	
Levofloxacin	750 mg IV q24h
	500 mg[b] PO q24h
Ciprofloxacin	400 mg IV q8h
	750 mg PO q12h
Moxifloxacin	400 mg[b] PO q24h
Ketolide	
Telithromycin	800 mg PO q24h
Tetracyclines	
Doxycycline	100 mg[b] PO or IV q12h
Minocycline	100 mg[b] PO or IV q12h
Tetracycline	500 mg PO or IV q6h
Tigecycline	100-mg IV load, then 50 mg IV q12h[d]
Others	
Trimethoprim-sulfamethoxazole	160/800 mg IV q8h 160/800 mg PO q12h
Rifampin[e]	100–600 mg PO or IV q12h

[a]Dosages are derived from clinical experience.
[b]The authors recommend doubling the first dose.
[c]The IV formulation is not available in some countries.
[d]Undergoing evaluation.
[e]Rifampin should be used only in combination with a macrolide or a quinolone.

Initial therapy should be given by the IV route. A clinical response usually occurs within 3–5 days, after which oral therapy can be substituted. The total duration of therapy in the immunocompetent host is 10–14 days; a longer course (3 weeks) may be appropriate for immunosuppressed patients and those with advanced disease. For azithromycin, with its long half-life, a 5- to 10-day course is sufficient.

Pontiac fever requires only symptom-based treatment, not antimicrobial therapy.

PROGNOSIS

Mortality rates for Legionnaires' disease vary with the patient's underlying disease and its severity, the patient's immune status, the severity of pneumonia, and the timing of administration of appropriate antimicrobial therapy. Mortality rates are highest (80%) among immunosuppressed patients who do not receive appropriate antimicrobial therapy early in the course of illness. With appropriate and timely antibiotic treatment, mortality rates from community-acquired Legionnaires' disease among immunocompetent patients range from 0 to 11%; without treatment, the figure may be as high as 31%. In a study of survivors of an outbreak of community-acquired Legionnaires' disease, sequelae of fatigue, neurologic symptoms, and weakness were found in 63–75% of patients 17 months after receipt of antibiotics.

PREVENTION

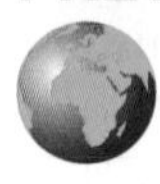

Routine environmental culture of hospital water supplies is recommended as an approach to the prevention of hospital-acquired Legionnaires' disease. Guidelines mandating this proactive approach have been adopted in Denmark, France, Germany, Italy, the Netherlands, and Taiwan. The CDC has thus far avoided this issue, but routine-culture guidelines from U.S. health departments have been adopted in Pittsburgh (PA), New York, and Maryland. Positive cultures from the water supply mandate the use of specialized laboratory tests (especially culture on selective media and the urinary antigen test) for patients with hospital-acquired pneumonia. Studies have shown that neither a high degree of outward cleanliness of the water system nor routine application of maintenance measures decreases the frequency or intensity of *Legionella* contamination. Thus engineering guidelines and building codes, although routinely advocated as preventive measures, have little impact on the presence of *Legionella*.

Disinfection of the water supply is now feasible. Two methods have proven reliable and cost-effective. The superheat-and-flush method requires heating of the water so that the distal-outlet temperature is 70–80°C and flushing of the distal outlets with hot water for at least 30 min. This method is ideal for emergency situations. A commercial copper and silver ionization method has proved effective in numerous hospitals. Carbon dioxide and monochloramine are undergoing evaluation, and preliminary results are promising. Tap water filters have been effective for high-risk patient areas, such as transplantation units. Hyperchlorination is no longer recommended because of its expense, carcinogenicity, corrosive effects on piping, and unreliable efficacy.

FURTHER READINGS

GREENBERG D et al: Problem pathogens: Paediatric legionellosis—implications for improved diagnosis. Lancet Infect Dis 6:529, 2006

JACOBSON KL et al: *Legionella* pneumonia in cancer patients. Medicine (Baltimore) 87:152, 2008

LETTINGA KD et al: Health-related quality of life and posttraumatic stress disorder among survivors of an outbreak of Legionnaires' disease. Clin Infect Dis 35:11, 2002

MODOL J et al: Hospital-acquired Legionnaires' disease in a university hospital: Impact of the copper-silver ionization system. Clin Infect Dis 44:263, 2007

MUDER R, YU VL: Infection due to *Legionella* species other than *L. pneumophila*. Clin Infect Dis 35:990, 2002

MULAZIMOGLU L, YU VL: Can Legionnaires' disease be diagnosed by clinical criteria? A critical review. Chest 120:1049, 2001

PEDRO-BOTET ML et al: Legionnaires' disease contracted from patient homes: The coming of the third plague? Eur J Clin Microbiol Infect Dis 21:699, 2002

Roig J, Pedro-Botet ML: *Legionella* spp: Community acquired and nosocomial infections. Curr Opin Infect Dis 16:45, 2003

Sabria M et al: Fluoroquinolones vs macrolides in the treatment of Legionnaires' disease. Chest 128:1401, 2005

———, Yu VL: Hospital-acquired legionellosis: Solutions for preventable infection. Lancet Infect Dis 2:368, 2002

Squier CL et al: A proactive approach to prevention of healthcare-acquired Legionnaires' disease: The Allegheny County (Pittsburgh) experience. Am J Infect Control 33:360, 2005

Tubach F et al: Emergence of *L. pneumophila* pneumonia in patients receiving tumor necrosis factor-α antagonists. Clin Infect Dis 43:e95, 2006

CHAPTER 50

PERTUSSIS AND OTHER *BORDETELLA* INFECTIONS

Scott A. Halperin

Pertussis is an acute infection of the respiratory tract caused by *Bordetella pertussis*. The name *pertussis* means "violent cough," which aptly describes the most consistent and prominent feature of the illness. The inspiratory sound made at the end of an episode of paroxysmal coughing gives rise to the common name for the illness, "whooping cough"; however, this feature is variable: it is uncommon among infants ≤6 months of age and is frequently absent in older children and adults. The Chinese name for pertussis is "the 100-day cough," which accurately describes the clinical course of the illness. The identification of *B. pertussis* was first reported by Bordet and Gengou in 1906, and vaccines were produced over the following two decades.

MICROBIOLOGY

Of the nine identified species in the genus *Bordetella*, only three are of major medical significance. *B. pertussis* infects only humans and is the most important *Bordetella* species causing human disease. *B. parapertussis* causes an illness in humans that is similar to pertussis but is typically milder; co-infections with *B. parapertussis* and *B. pertussis* have been documented. *B. bronchiseptica* is an important pathogen of domestic animals that causes kennel cough in dogs, atrophic rhinitis and pneumonia in pigs, and pneumonia in cats. Both respiratory infection and opportunistic infection are occasionally reported in humans. Two additional species, *B. hinzii* and *B. holmesii*, are unusual causes of bacteremia; both have been isolated from patients with sepsis, most often from those who are immunocompromised.

Bordetella species are gram-negative pleomorphic aerobic bacilli that share common genotypic characteristics. *B. pertussis* and *B. parapertussis* are the most similar of the species, but *B. parapertussis* does not express the gene coding for pertussis toxin. *B. pertussis* is a slow-growing fastidious organism that requires selective medium and forms small glistening bifurcated colonies. Suspicious colonies are presumptively identified as *B. pertussis* by direct fluorescent antibody testing or by agglutination with species-specific antiserum. *B. pertussis* is further differentiated from other *Bordetella* species by biochemical and motility characteristics.

B. pertussis produces a wide array of toxins and biologically active products that are important in its pathogenesis and in immunity. Most of these virulence factors are under the control of a single genetic locus that regulates their production, resulting in antigenic modulation and phase variation. Although these processes occur both in vitro and in vivo, their importance in the pathobiology of the organism is unknown; they may play a role in intracellular persistence and person-to-person spread. The organism's most important virulence factor is *pertussis toxin*, which is composed of a B oligomer–binding subunit and an enzymatically active A protomer that ADP-ribosylates a guanine nucleotide-binding regulatory protein (G protein) in target cells, producing a variety of biologic effects. Pertussis toxin has important mitogenic activity, affects the circulation of lymphocytes, and serves as an adhesin for bacterial binding to respiratory ciliated cells. Other important virulence factors and adhesins are *filamentous hemagglutinin*, a component of the cell wall, and *pertactin*, an outer-membrane protein. *Fimbriae*, bacterial appendages that play a role in bacterial attachment, are the major antigens against which agglutinating antibodies are directed. These agglutinating antibodies have historically been the primary means of serotyping *B. pertussis* strains. Other virulence factors include tracheal cytotoxin, which causes respiratory epithelial damage; adenylate cyclase toxin, which impairs host immune-cell function; dermonecrotic toxin, which may contribute to respiratory mucosal damage; and lipooligosaccharide, which has properties similar to those of other gram-negative bacterial endotoxins.

EPIDEMIOLOGY

Pertussis is a highly communicable disease, with attack rates of 80–100% among unimmunized household contacts and 20% within households in well-immunized

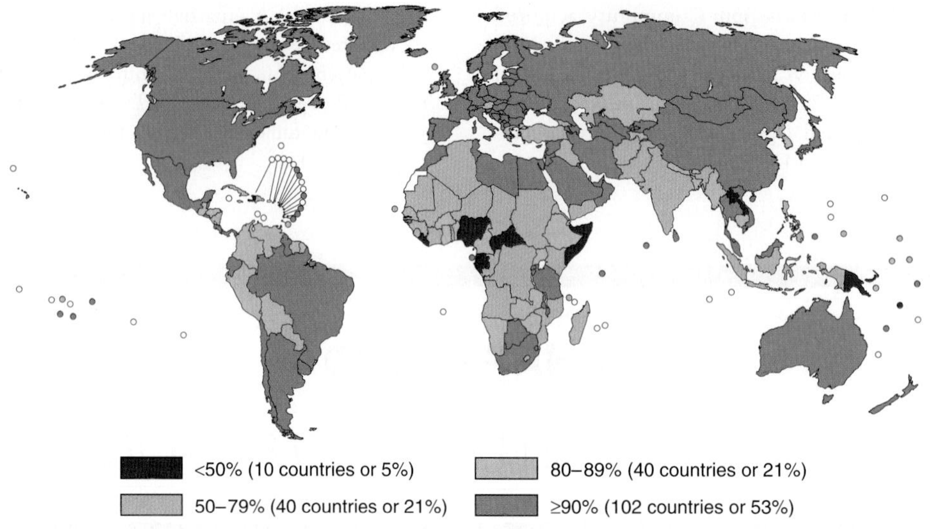

FIGURE 50-1

Immunization coverage with DTP3 vaccines (diphtheria toxoid, tetanus toxoid, and pertussis, 3 doses) in infants, 2004. *(Reprinted with permission of the World Health Organization. Source: WHO/IVB database, 2005. This map does not imply the expression of any opinion whatsoever on the part of the World Health Organization concerning the legal status of any country, territory, city, or area of its authorities or concerning the delimitation of its frontiers or boundaries.)*

populations. The infection has a worldwide distribution, with cyclical outbreaks every 3–5 years (a pattern that has persisted despite widespread immunization). Pertussis occurs in all months; however, in North America, its activity peaks in summer and autumn.

In developing countries, pertussis remains an important cause of infant morbidity and death. The reported incidence of pertussis worldwide has decreased as a result of improved vaccine coverage. However, coverage rates are still <50% in many developing nations (Fig. 50-1); the World Health Organization (WHO) estimates that 90% of the burden of pertussis is in the developing world. In addition, overreporting of immunization coverage and underreporting of disease result in substantial underestimation of the global burden of pertussis (Fig. 50-2). The WHO estimates that more than 17.6 million people worldwide were infected by *B. pertussis* in 2003, with 279,000 deaths from pertussis among children.

Before the institution of widespread immunization programs in the developed world, pertussis was one of the most common infectious causes of morbidity and death. In the United States before the 1940s, between 115,000 and 270,000 cases of pertussis were reported annually, with an average yearly rate of 150 cases per 100,000 population. With universal childhood immunization, the number of reported cases fell by >95%, and mortality rates decreased even more dramatically. Only 1010 cases of pertussis were reported in 1976. Since that time, however, rates have slowly increased. In 2003, more than 11,600 cases of pertussis were reported in the United States.

Although thought of as a disease of childhood, pertussis can affect people of all ages and is increasingly being identified as a cause of prolonged coughing illness in adolescents and adults. In unimmunized populations, pertussis incidence peaks during the preschool years, and well over half of children have the disease before reaching adulthood. In highly immunized populations such as those in North America, the peak incidence is among infants <1 year of age who have not completed the three-dose primary immunization series. Recent trends, however, show an increasing incidence of pertussis among adolescents and adults. In the United States between 2001 and 2003, 23% of patients were <1 year of age, 33% were adolescents, and 23% were adults. The figures for adolescents

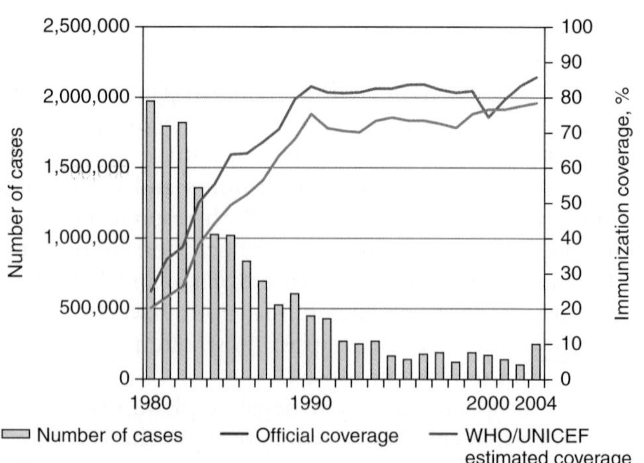

FIGURE 50-2

Global annual reported pertussis incidence and rate of coverage with DTP3 (diphtheria toxoid, tetanus toxoid, and pertussis vaccine, 3 doses), 1980–2004. *(Reprinted with permission of the World Health Organization. Source: WHO/IVB database, 2005.)*

and adults are probably underestimates because of a greater degree of underrecognition and underreporting in these age groups. A number of studies of prolonged coughing illness suggest that pertussis may be the etiologic agent in 12–30% of adults with cough that does not improve within 2 weeks. In one study of the efficacy of an acellular pertussis vaccine in adolescents and adults, the incidence of pertussis in the placebo group was 3.7–4.5 cases per 1000 person-years. Although this prospective cohort study yielded a lower estimate than the studies of cough illness, its results still translate to 600,000–800,000 cases of pertussis annually among adults in the United States. Severe morbidity and high mortality rates, however, are restricted almost entirely to infants. In Canada, there were 10 deaths from pertussis between 1991 and 1998; all those who died were infants ≤6 months of age. Although school-age children are the source of infection for most households, adults are the likely source for high-risk infants and may serve as the reservoir of infection between epidemic years.

PATHOGENESIS

Infection with *B. pertussis* is initiated by attachment of the organism to the ciliated epithelial cells of the nasopharynx. Attachment is mediated by surface adhesins (e.g., pertactin and filamentous hemagglutinin), which bind to the integrin family of cell-surface proteins, probably in conjunction with pertussis toxin. The role of fimbriae in adhesion and in maintenance of infection has not been fully delineated. At the site of attachment, the organism multiplies, producing a variety of other toxins that cause local mucosal damage (tracheal cytotoxin, dermonecrotic toxin). Impairment of host defense by *B. pertussis* is mediated by pertussis toxin and adenylate cyclase toxin. There is local cellular invasion, with intracellular bacterial persistence; however, systemic dissemination does not occur. Systemic manifestations (lymphocytosis) result from the effects of the toxins.

The pathogenesis of the clinical manifestations of pertussis is poorly understood. It is not known what causes the hallmark paroxysmal cough. A pivotal role for pertussis toxin has been proposed. Proponents of this position point to the efficacy of preventing clinical symptoms with a vaccine containing only pertussis toxoid. Detractors counter that pertussis toxin is not the critical factor because paroxysmal cough also occurs in patients infected with *B. parapertussis*, which does not produce pertussis toxin. It is thought that neurologic events in pertussis, such as seizures and encephalopathy, are due to hypoxia from coughing paroxysms or apnea rather than to the effects of specific bacterial products. *B. pertussis* pneumonia, which occurs in up to 10% of infants with pertussis, is usually a diffuse bilateral primary infection. In older children and adults with pertussis, pneumonia is often due to secondary bacterial infection with streptococci or staphylococci.

IMMUNITY

Both humoral and cell-mediated immunity are thought to be important in pertussis. Antibodies to pertussis toxin, filamentous hemagglutinin, pertactin, and fimbriae are all protective in animal models. Pertussis agglutinins were correlated with protection in early studies of whole-cell pertussis vaccines. Serologic correlates of protection conferred by acellular pertussis vaccines have not been established, although antibody to pertactin, fimbriae, and (to a lesser degree) pertussis toxin correlated best with protection in two efficacy trials. The duration of immunity after whole-cell pertussis vaccination is short-lived, with little protection remaining after 10–12 years. After a three-dose infant primary series of acellular pertussis vaccine, protection persists for at least 5–6 years; the duration of immunity after a four- or five-dose schedule is not yet known. Although immunity after natural infection has been said to be lifelong, seroepidemiologic evidence suggests that it may not be and that subsequent episodes of clinical pertussis are prevented by intermittent subclinical infection.

CLINICAL MANIFESTATIONS

Pertussis is a prolonged coughing illness with clinical manifestations that vary by age (Table 50-1). Although not uncommon among adolescents and adults, classic

TABLE 50-1

CLINICAL FEATURES OF PERTUSSIS, BY AGE GROUP AND DIAGNOSTIC STATUS

	PERCENTAGE OF PATIENTS		
	ADOLESCENTS AND ADULTS		
FEATURE	LABORATORY CONFIRMATION	NO LABORATORY CONFIRMATION	CHILDREN
Cough	95–100	95–100	95–100
Prolonged	60–80	60–80	60–95
Paroxysmal	60–90	50–90	80–95
Sleep-disturbing	50–80	50–80	90–100
Whoop	10–40	5–30	40–80
Posttussive vomiting	20–50	5–30	80–90

pertussis is most often seen in preschool and school-age children. After an incubation period averaging 7–10 days, an illness develops that is indistinguishable from the common cold and is characterized by coryza, lacrimation, mild cough, low-grade fever, and malaise. After 1–2 weeks, this *catarrhal phase* evolves into the *paroxysmal phase*: the cough becomes more frequent and spasmodic with repetitive bursts of 5–10 coughs, often within a single expiration. Posttussive vomiting is frequent, with a mucous plug occasionally expelled at the end of an episode. The episode may be terminated by an audible whoop, which occurs upon rapid inspiration against a closed glottis at the end of a paroxysm. During a spasm, there may be impressive neck-vein distension, bulging eyes, tongue protrusion, and cyanosis. Paroxysms may be precipitated by noise, eating, or physical contact. Between attacks, the patient's appearance is normal, but increasing fatigue is evident. The frequency of paroxysmal episodes varies widely, from several per hour to 5–10 per day. Episodes are often worse at night and interfere with sleep. Weight loss is not uncommon as a result of the illness's interference with eating. Most complications occur during the paroxysmal stage. Fever is uncommon and suggests bacterial superinfection.

After 2–4 weeks, the coughing episodes become less frequent and less severe—changes heralding the onset of the *convalescent phase*. This phase can last 1–3 months and is characterized by gradual resolution of coughing episodes. For 6–12 months, intercurrent viral infections may be associated with a recrudescence of paroxysmal cough.

Not all individuals who develop pertussis have classic disease. The clinical manifestations in adolescents and adults are more often atypical. In a German study of pertussis in adults, more than two-thirds had paroxysmal cough and more than one-third had whoop. Adult illness in North America differs from this experience: the cough may be severe and prolonged but is less frequently paroxysmal, and a whoop is uncommon. Vomiting with cough is the best predictor of pertussis as the cause of prolonged cough in adults. Other predictive features are a cough at night and exposure to other individuals with a prolonged coughing illness.

COMPLICATIONS

Complications are frequently associated with pertussis and are more common among infants than among older children or adults. Subconjunctival hemorrhages, abdominal and inguinal hernias, pneumothoraces, and facial and truncal petechiae can result from increased intrathoracic pressure generated by severe fits of coughing. Weight loss can follow decreased caloric intake. In a series of more than 1100 children <2 years of age who were hospitalized with pertussis, 27.1% had apnea, 9.4% had pneumonia, 2.6% had seizures, and 0.4% had encephalopathy; 10 children (0.9%) died. Pneumonia is reported in <5% of adolescents and adults and increases in frequency after 50 years of age. In contrast to the primary *B. pertussis* pneumonia that develops in infants, pneumonia in adolescents and adults with pertussis is usually caused by a secondary infection with encapsulated organisms such as *Streptococcus pneumoniae* or *Haemophilus influenzae*. Pneumothorax, severe weight loss, inguinal hernia, rib fracture, carotid artery aneurysm, and cough syncope have all been reported in adolescents and adults with pertussis.

DIAGNOSIS

If the classic symptoms of pertussis are present, clinical diagnosis is not difficult. However, particularly in older children and adults, it is difficult to differentiate infections caused by *B. pertussis* and *B. parapertussis* from other respiratory tract infections on clinical grounds. Therefore, laboratory confirmation should be attempted in all cases. Lymphocytosis—an absolute lymphocyte count of $>10 \times 10^9$/L—is common among young children (in whom it is unusual with other infections) but not among adolescents and adults. Culture of nasopharyngeal secretions remains the gold standard of diagnosis, although DNA detection by polymerase chain reaction (PCR) is replacing culture in many laboratories because of increased sensitivity and quicker results. The best specimen is collected by nasopharyngeal aspiration, in which a fine flexible plastic catheter attached to a 10-mL syringe is passed into the nasopharynx and withdrawn while gentle suction is applied. Since *B. pertussis* is highly sensitive to drying, secretions for culture should be inoculated without delay onto appropriate medium (Bordet-Gengou or Regan-Lowe), or the catheter should be flushed with a phosphate-buffered saline solution for culture and/or PCR. An alternative to the aspirate is a Dacron or rayon nasopharyngeal swab; again, inoculation of culture plates should be immediate or an appropriate transport medium (e.g., Regan-Lowe charcoal medium) should be used. Results of PCR can be available within hours; cultures become positive by day 5 of incubation. *B. pertussis* and *B. parapertussis* can be differentiated by agglutination with specific antisera or by direct immunofluorescence.

Nasopharyngeal cultures in untreated pertussis remain positive for a mean of 3 weeks after the onset of illness; these cultures become negative within 5 days of the institution of appropriate antimicrobial therapy. The duration of a positive PCR in untreated pertussis or after therapy is not known but exceeds that of positive cultures. Since much of the period during which the organism can be recovered from the nasopharynx falls into the catarrhal phase, when the etiology of the infection is not suspected, there is only a small window of opportunity for culture-proven diagnosis. Cultures from infants and young children are more frequently positive than those from older children and adults; this difference may reflect earlier presentation of the former age group for medical care. Direct fluorescent antibody tests of nasopharyngeal secretions for direct diagnosis may still be available in some laboratories but should not be used because of poor sensitivity and specificity.

As a result of the difficulties with laboratory diagnosis of pertussis in adolescents, adults, and patients who have been symptomatic for >4 weeks, increasing attention is being given to serologic diagnosis. Enzyme immunoassays detecting IgA and IgG antibodies to pertussis toxin, filamentous hemagglutinin, pertactin, and fimbriae have been developed and assessed for reproducibility. Two- or fourfold increases in antibody titer are suggestive of pertussis, although cross-reactivity of some antigens (such as filamentous hemagglutinin and pertactin) among *Bordetella* species makes it difficult to depend diagnostically on seroconversion involving a single type of antibody. Late presentation for medical care and prior immunization also complicate serologic diagnosis because the first sample obtained may in fact be a convalescent-phase specimen. Criteria for serologic diagnosis based on a single serum specimen compared with established population values are gaining acceptance, and serology will likely become more widely available for the diagnosis of pertussis.

DIFFERENTIAL DIAGNOSIS

A child presenting with paroxysmal cough, posttussive vomiting, and whoop is likely to have an infection caused by *B. pertussis* or *B. parapertussis*; lymphocytosis increases the likelihood of a *B. pertussis* etiology. Viruses such as respiratory syncytial virus and adenovirus have been isolated from patients with clinical pertussis but probably represent co-infection. In adolescents and adults, who often do not have paroxysmal cough or whoop, the differential diagnosis of a prolonged coughing illness is more extensive. Pertussis should be suspected in anyone with a cough that does not improve within 14 days, a paroxysmal cough of any duration, or any respiratory symptoms after contact with a laboratory-confirmed case of pertussis. Other etiologies to consider include infections caused by *Mycoplasma pneumoniae*, *Chlamydophila pneumoniae*, adenovirus, influenza virus, and other respiratory viruses. Use of angiotensin-converting enzyme (ACE) inhibitors, reactive airway disease, and gastroesophageal reflux disease are well-described noninfectious causes of prolonged cough in adults.

℞ Treatment: PERTUSSIS

ANTIBIOTICS The purpose of antibiotic therapy for pertussis is to eradicate the infecting bacteria from the nasopharynx; therapy does not substantially alter the clinical course unless given early in the catarrhal phase. Macrolide antibiotics are the drugs of choice for treatment of pertussis (Table 50-2); macrolide-resistant *B. pertussis* strains have been reported but are rare. Trimethoprim-sulfamethoxazole is recommended as an alternative for individuals allergic to macrolides.

SUPPORTIVE CARE Young infants have the highest rates of complication and death from pertussis; therefore, most infants (and older children with severe disease) should be hospitalized. A quiet environment may decrease the stimulation that can trigger paroxysmal episodes. Use of β-adrenergic agonists and/or glucocorticoids has been advocated by some authorities but has not been proven to be effective. Cough suppressants are not effective and play no role in the management of pertussis.

INFECTION CONTROL MEASURES Hospitalized patients with pertussis should be placed in respiratory isolation, with the use of precautions appropriate for pathogens spread by large respiratory droplets. Isolation should continue for 5 days after initiation of erythromycin therapy or for 3 weeks (i.e., until nasopharyngeal cultures are consistently negative) when the patient cannot tolerate antimicrobial therapy.

PREVENTION

Chemoprophylaxis

Because the risk of transmission of *B. pertussis* within households is high, chemoprophylaxis is widely recommended for household contacts of pertussis cases. The effectiveness of chemoprophylaxis, although unproven, is supported by several epidemiologic studies of institutional and community outbreaks. In the only randomized placebo-controlled study, erythromycin estolate (50 mg/kg per day in three divided doses; maximum dose, 1 g/d) was effective in reducing the incidence of bacteriologically confirmed pertussis by 67%; however, there was no decrease in the incidence of clinical disease. Despite these disappointing results, many authorities continue to recommend chemoprophylaxis, particularly in households with members at high risk of severe disease (children <1 year of age). Data are not available on use of the newer macrolides for chemoprophylaxis, but these drugs are commonly used because of their increased tolerability and their effectiveness.

TABLE 50-2

ANTIMICROBIAL THERAPY FOR PERTUSSIS

DRUG	ADULT DAILY DOSE	FREQUENCY	DURATION (DAYS)	COMMENTS
Erythromycin estolate	1–2 g	3 divided doses	7–14	Frequent gastrointestinal side effects
Clarithromycin	500 mg	2 divided doses	7	
Azithromycin	500 mg on day 1, 250 mg subsequently	1 daily dose	5	
Trimethoprim-sulfamethoxazole	160 mg of trimethoprim, 800 mg of sulfamethoxazole	2 divided doses	14	For patients allergic to macrolides; data on effectiveness limited

Immunization

(See also Chap. 3) The mainstay of pertussis prevention is active immunization. Pertussis vaccine, now available for >80 years, became widely used in North America after 1940; the reported number of pertussis cases has since fallen by >90%. Whole-cell pertussis vaccines are prepared through the heating, chemical inactivation, and purification of whole *B. pertussis* organisms. Although effective (average efficacy estimate, 85%; range for different products, 30–100%), whole-cell pertussis vaccines are associated with adverse events—both common (fever; injection-site pain, erythema, and swelling; irritability) and uncommon (febrile seizures, hypotonic hyporesponsive episodes). Alleged associations of whole-cell pertussis vaccine with encephalopathy, sudden infant death syndrome, and autism, although not substantiated, have spawned an active anti-immunization lobby. The development of acellular pertussis vaccines, which are effective but less reactogenic, has greatly alleviated concerns about the inclusion of pertussis vaccine in the combined infant immunization series. Although whole-cell vaccines are still used extensively in the developing world, acellular pertussis vaccines are used exclusively for childhood immunization in much of the developed world. In North America, acellular pertussis vaccines are given as a three-dose primary series at 2, 4, and 6 months of age, with a reinforcing dose at 15–18 months of age and a booster dose at 4–6 years of age.

Although a wide variety of acellular pertussis vaccines were developed, only a few are still widely marketed; all contain pertussis toxoid and filamentous hemagglutinin. One acellular pertussis vaccine also contains pertactin, and another contains pertactin and two types of fimbriae. In light of analyses of phase 3 efficacy studies, most experts have concluded that two-component acellular pertussis vaccines are more effective than monocomponent vaccines and that the addition of pertactin increases efficacy still more. The further addition of fimbriae appears to enhance protective efficacy against milder disease. In two studies, protection conferred by pertussis vaccines correlated best with the production of antibody to pertactin, fimbriae, and pertussis toxin.

The development of acellular pertussis vaccines has sparked interest in the potential for pertussis control in adolescents and adults and in the possibility that pertussis control in those groups will enhance the protection of infants too young to be immunized. Whole-cell pertussis vaccine is contraindicated in individuals ≥7 years of age because of their poor toleration of possible adverse events. However, adult formulations of acellular pertussis vaccines have been shown to be safe, immunogenic, and efficacious in clinical trials in adolescents and adults and are now recommended for routine immunization of these groups in several countries, including the United States.

FURTHER READINGS

Altunaiji S et al: Antibiotics for whooping cough (pertussis). Cochrane Database Syst Rev Jul 18;(3):CD004404, 2007

De Serres G et al: Morbidity of pertussis in adolescents and adults. J Infect Dis 182:174, 2000

Halperin SA et al: A randomized, placebo-controlled trial of erythromycin estolate chemoprophylaxis for household contacts of children with culture-positive *Bordetella pertussis* infection. Pediatrics 104:e42, 1999

——— et al: Epidemiological features of pertussis in hospitalized patients in Canada, 1991–1997: Report of the Immunization Monitoring Program—Active (IMPACT). Clin Infect Dis 28:1238, 1999

Lee GM et al: Pertussis in adolescents and adults: Should we vaccinate? Pediatrics 115:1675, 2005

Mattoo S, Cherry JD: Molecular pathogenesis, epidemiology, and clinical manifestations of respiratory infections due to *Bordetella pertussis* and other *Bordetella* subspecies. Clin Microbiol Rev 18:326, 2005

Murphy TV et al: Prevention of pertussis, tetanus, and diphtheria among pregnant and postpartum women and their infants recommendations of the Advisory Committee on Immunization Practices (ACIP). MMWR Recomm Rep 57:1, 2008

Riffelmann M et al: Pertussis PCR Consensus Group. Nucleic acid amplification tests for diagnosis of *Bordetella* infections. J Clin Microbiol 43:4925, 2005

Skowronski DM et al: The changing age and seasonal profile of pertussis in Canada. J Infect Dis 185:1448, 2002

Tan T et al: Epidemiology of pertussis. Pediatr Infect Dis J 24(Suppl):S10, 2005

Ward JI et al: APERT Study Group. Efficacy of an acellular pertussis vaccine among adolescents and adults. N Engl J Med 353:1555, 2005

Yih WK et al: The increasing incidence of pertussis in Massachusetts adolescents and adults, 1989–1998. J Infect Dis 182:1409, 2000

CHAPTER 51

DISEASES CAUSED BY GRAM-NEGATIVE ENTERIC BACILLI

Thomas A. Russo ■ James R. Johnson

GENERAL FEATURES AND PRINCIPLES

EPIDEMIOLOGY

Escherichia coli, Klebsiella, Proteus, Enterobacter, Serratia, Citrobacter, Morganella, Providencia, Edwardsiella, and *Acinetobacter* are components of the normal animal and human colonic flora and/or of the flora of a variety of environmental habitats, including long-term care facilities (LTCFs) and hospitals. As a result, except for certain pathotypes of intestinal pathogenic *E. coli*, these genera are global pathogens. In healthy humans, *E. coli* is the predominant species of gram-negative bacilli (GNB) in the colonic flora. GNB (primarily *E. coli, Klebsiella,* and *Proteus*) only transiently colonize the oropharynx and skin of healthy individuals. In contrast, in LTCF and hospital settings, a variety of GNB emerge as the dominant flora of both mucosal and skin surfaces, particularly in association with antimicrobial use, severe illness, and extended length of stay. This colonization may lead to subsequent infection; for example, oropharyngeal colonization may lead to pneumonia.

STRUCTURE AND FUNCTION

GNB possess an extracytoplasmic outer membrane, a feature shared generally among gram-negative bacteria. This outer membrane consists of a lipid bilayer with associated proteins, lipoproteins, and polysaccharides [capsule, lipopolysaccharide (LPS)]. The outer membrane interfaces with the bacterial environment, including the human host. A variety of components of the outer membrane are critical determinants in pathogenesis and antimicrobial resistance.

PATHOGENESIS

Multiple bacterial virulence factors are required for the pathogenesis of infections caused by GNB. Possession of specialized virulence genes defines pathogens and enables them to infect the host efficiently. It is becoming clear that hosts and their cognate pathogens have been co-adapting throughout evolutionary history, and it has been speculated that infection is just one point on the spectrum of evolved relationships between microbes and hosts. At one end of this spectrum is a commensal/symbiotic interaction (e.g., mitochondria—formerly bacteria—within eukaryotic cells); at the other end is a lethal outcome, producing a "dead-end relationship" (e.g., Ebola virus). During the host-pathogen "chess match" over time, various and redundant strategies have emerged in both the pathogens and their hosts that enable these partners to maintain their coexistence (Table 51-1).

Extraintestinal pathogenic strains of *E. coli* (ExPEC) and the other genera discussed in this chapter cause infection outside the bowel. All are extracellular pathogens and therefore share certain pathogenic features. Innate immunity (including the activities of complement, antimicrobial peptides, and professional phagocytes) and humoral immunity are the principal host-defense components. Both susceptibility to and severity of infection are increased with dysfunction or deficiencies of these components (Chap. 1). In contrast, the virulence traits of intestinal pathogenic *E. coli*—i.e., the distinctive strains that can cause diarrheal disease—are for the most part different from those of extraintestinal pathogenic *E. coli* and other GNB that cause extraintestinal infections. This difference reflects site-specific differences in host environments and defense mechanisms.

A given extraintestinal pathogen usually possesses multiple adhesins for binding to a variety of host cells (e.g., in *E. coli*: type 1 fimbriae, Sfa/Foc fimbriae, P pili). Nutrient acquisition (e.g., of iron via siderophores) requires many genes that are necessary but not sufficient for pathogenesis. The ability to resist the bactericidal activity of complement and phagocytes in the absence of antibody (e.g., as conferred by capsule or O antigen of LPS) is one of the defining traits of an extracellular pathogen. Tissue damage (e.g., as mediated by hemolysin in the case of *E. coli*) may facilitate spread. Without doubt, many important virulence genes await identification, and our understanding of many aspects of the pathogenesis of infections due to GNB is in its infancy (Chap. 2).

The ability to induce septic shock is another defining feature of these genera. GNB are the most common causes of this potentially lethal syndrome. The lipid A moiety of LPS (via interaction with host Toll-like receptor 4) and probably other bacterial factors as well stimulate a proinflammatory host response that, if overly exuberant, results in shock (Chap. 15).

Many antigenic variants (serotypes) exist in most genera of GNB. For example, there are >150 O-specific antigens and >80 capsular antigens in *E. coli*. This antigenic

TABLE 51-1

INTERACTIONS OF EXTRAINTESTINAL PATHOGENIC *E. COLI* WITH THE HUMAN HOST: A PARADIGM FOR EXTRACELLULAR, EXTRAINTESTINAL GRAM-NEGATIVE BACTERIAL PATHOGENS

BACTERIAL GOAL	HOST OBSTACLE	BACTERIAL SOLUTION
Extraintestinal attachment	Flow of urine, mucociliary blanket	Multiple adhesins (e.g., type 1 fimbriae, Sfa/Foc, P pili)
Nutrient acquisition for growth	Nutrient sequestration (e.g., iron via intracellular storage and extracellular scavenging via lactoferrin and transferrin)	Cellular lysis (e.g., hemolysin); multiple mechanisms for competing for extracellular iron (e.g., siderophores) and other nutrients
Initial avoidance of host bactericidal activity	Complement, phagocytic cells, antimicrobial peptides	Capsular polysaccharide, lipopolysaccharide
Transmission	?	Irritant tissue damage resulting in increased excretion (e.g., toxins such as hemolysin)
Late avoidance of host bactericidal activity	Acquired immunity (e.g., specific antibodies), treatment with antibiotics	? Cell entry, acquisition of antimicrobial resistance

variability, which permits immune evasion and allows recurrent infection by different strains of the same species, has impeded vaccine development (Chap. 3).

INFECTIOUS SYNDROMES

Although certain strains of *E. coli* have evolved to be strictly intestinal pathogens, causing gastroenteritis by a variety of unique pathogenic mechanisms, extraintestinal infections are the predominant presentation of disease caused by enteric GNB. Depending on both the host and the pathogen, nearly every organ or body cavity can be infected with GNB. *E. coli* and—to a lesser degree—*Klebsiella* and *Proteus* account for most extraintestinal infections due to GNB and are the most virulent pathogens of this group. However, the other genera are becoming increasingly important, particularly among LTCF residents and hospitalized patients. This expanding role is due in large part to the intrinsic or acquired antimicrobial resistance of these organisms and the increasing number of individuals with alterations or disruptions of host defenses. The mortality rate is significant in many GNB infections and correlates with the severity of illness. Especially problematic are pneumonia and bacteremia (arising from any source) when complicated by organ failure (severe sepsis) and/or shock; associated mortality rates are 20–50%.

DIAGNOSIS

Isolation of GNB from ordinarily sterile anatomic sites almost always implies infection, whereas their isolation from nonsterile sites, particularly from open soft-tissue wounds and the respiratory tract, requires clinical correlation to differentiate colonization from infection. Tentative laboratory identification based on lactose fermentation and indole production (described for each genus below), which usually is possible before final identification of the organism and determination of its antimicrobial susceptibilities, may guide empirical antimicrobial therapy.

Treatment: ℞ INFECTIONS CAUSED BY GRAM-NEGATIVE ENTERIC BACILLI

(See also Chap. 33) Accumulating evidence indicates that initiation of appropriate empirical antimicrobial therapy early in the course of GNB infections (particularly serious infections) leads to improved outcomes. Familiarity with evolving patterns of antimicrobial resistance in enteric GNB is necessary in the selection of appropriate empirical therapy. The antimicrobial resistance profiles of GNB vary by species, geographic location, regional antimicrobial use, and hospital site [e.g., intensive care units (ICUs) vs wards]. At present, the most reliably active agents against enteric GNB are the carbapenems (e.g., imipenem), the aminoglycoside amikacin, the fourth-generation cephalosporin cefepime, and piperacillin-tazobactam.

β-Lactamases, which inactivate β-lactam agents, are the most important mediators of resistance to these drugs in GNB. Decreased permeability and/or active efflux of β-lactam agents, although less common, may occur alone or in combination with β-lactamase-mediated resistance. *Broad-spectrum* β-lactamases, which mediate resistance to many penicillins and first-generation cephalosporins, are frequently expressed in enteric GNB. These enzymes are inhibited by agents such as clavulanate. *Extended-spectrum* β-lactamases (ESBLs) confer resistance to the same drugs as broad-spectrum β-lactamases as well as to third-generation cephalosporins, aztreonam, and (in some instances) fourth-generation cephalosporins.

The acquisition of ESBL-encoding genes via transferable plasmids is increasing in GNB worldwide, with rates varying greatly even among hospitals in a given region. To date, ESBLs are most prevalent in *Klebsiella pneumoniae*, *K. oxytoca*, and *E. coli* but also occur (and are probably underrecognized) in *Enterobacter*,

Citrobacter, Proteus, Serratia, and other enteric GNB. At present, the regional prevalence of ESBL-producing GNB declines in rank order as follows: Latin America > Western Pacific > Europe > United States and Canada. ESBL-producing GNB are most prevalent in hospitals (ICUs > wards) but recently have emerged in the community. Hospital outbreaks due to ESBL-producing strains have been associated with extensive use of third-generation cephalosporins, particularly ceftazidime. The carbapenems are the most reliably active β-lactam agents against ESBL-expressing strains. GNB that express ESBLs may also possess porin mutations that result in decreased uptake of cephalosporins and β-lactam/β-lactamase inhibitor combinations. Thus ESBL-producing isolates should be considered resistant to all penicillins, cephalosporins, and aztreonam.

AmpC β-lactamases confer resistance to the same substrates as ESBLs plus the cephamycins, a subset of the second-generation cephalosporins. AmpC enzymes resist inhibition by β-lactamase inhibitors. Constitutive chromosomal AmpC β-lactamases are present in nearly all strains of *Enterobacter, Serratia, Citrobacter, Proteus vulgaris, Providencia, Morganella*, and *Acinetobacter*, resulting in resistance to aminopenicillins, cefazolin, and cefoxitin. In addition, some strains of *E. coli, K. pneumoniae*, and other Enterobacteriaceae have acquired plasmids containing AmpC β-lactamase genes. The fourth-generation cephalosporin cefepime is stable to AmpC β-lactamases and is an appropriate treatment option if the concomitant presence of an ESBL can be excluded.

Carbapenemases confer resistance to the same drugs as ESBLs plus cephamycins and carbapenems. At present, carbapenemase-producing enteric GNB are uncommon. In the United States, strains of *Klebsiella* and *Enterobacter* that possess carbapenemases on transferable plasmids and exhibit resistance to fluoroquinolones and aminoglycosides have been found. Tigecycline (a glycylcycline, a new antimicrobial class) and the polymyxins (agents of last resort, given their potential toxicities) are the most active drugs in vitro, but their clinical efficacy has not been demonstrated.

Resistance to fluoroquinolones usually is due to alterations of the target site (DNA gyrase and/or topoisomerase IV), with or without decreased permeability, active efflux, or protection of the target site. Resistance to fluoroquinolones is increasingly prevalent among GNB; 20–80% of ESBL-producing enteric GNB are also resistant to fluoroquinolones. At present, this drug class should be considered unreliable as empirical therapy for infections due to GNB in critically ill patients.

Not all clinical laboratories screen for ESBLs, screening protocols are limited, and no recommended tests identify AmpC β-lactamases or carbapenemases. For these reasons, these resistance mechanisms are underreported, and it is important to assess the clinical response to treatment in addition to in vitro susceptibility data.

Given the increasing prevalence of multidrug resistance in enteric GNB, it is reasonable—pending susceptibility results—to combine agents for empirical treatment of GNB infections in critically ill patients. Although supporting clinical evidence is limited, combination therapy may increase antimicrobial efficacy and/or diminish the emergence of resistance in some circumstances. In addition, drainage of abscesses and removal of infected foreign bodies are often required for cure.

GNB are commonly involved in polymicrobial infections, in which the role of each specific pathogen is uncertain (Chap. 65). Although some GNB are more pathogenic than others, it is usually prudent, if possible, to design an antimicrobial regimen active against all of the GNB identified, since each is capable of pathogenicity in its own right.

PREVENTION

(See also Chap. 13) Diligent adherence to hand-hygiene protocols by health care personnel and avoidance of inappropriate antimicrobial use are key measures in preventing infection and the further development of antimicrobial resistance. Likewise, avoidance of the use of indwelling devices that predispose to infections due to GNB (e.g., urinary and intravascular catheters, endotracheal tubes) decreases infection risk.

ESCHERICHIA COLI INFECTIONS

COMMENSAL STRAINS

For the most part, commensal *E. coli* variants, which constitute the bulk of the normal facultative intestinal flora in most humans, confer benefits to the host (e.g., resistance to colonization with pathogenic organisms). These strains generally lack the specialized virulence traits that enable extraintestinal and intestinal pathogenic *E. coli* strains to cause disease outside and within the gastrointestinal tract, respectively. However, even commensal *E. coli* strains can be involved in extraintestinal infections in the presence of an aggravating factor, such as a foreign body (e.g., a urinary catheter), host compromise (e.g., local anatomic or functional abnormalities such as urinary or biliary tract obstruction or systemic immunocompromise), or an inoculum that is large or contains a mixture of bacterial species (e.g., fecal contamination of the peritoneal cavity).

EXTRAINTESTINAL PATHOGENIC (ExPEC) STRAINS

The majority of *E. coli* isolates from symptomatic infections of the urinary tract, bloodstream, cerebrospinal fluid, respiratory tract, and peritoneum (spontaneous bacterial peritonitis) can be differentiated from commensal and intestinal pathogenic strains of *E. coli* by virtue of their distinctive virulence factor profiles (Tables 51-1 and 51-2) and phylogenetic background. ExPEC strains can also cause surgical wound infection, osteomyelitis, and myositis, but the number of cases evaluated to date is too small for a reliable assessment of proportions.

Like commensal *E. coli* (but in contrast to intestinal pathogenic *E. coli*), ExPEC strains are often found in the normal intestinal flora and do not cause gastroenteritis

TABLE 51-2

INTESTINAL PATHOGENIC *E. COLI*

PATHOTYPE[a]	EPIDEMIOLOGY	CLINICAL SYNDROME[b]	DEFINING MOLECULAR TRAIT	RESPONSIBLE GENETIC ELEMENT[c]
STEC	Food, water, person-to-person; all ages, industrialized countries	Hemorrhagic colitis, hemolytic-uremic syndrome	Shiga toxin	Lambda-like Stx1- or Stx2-encoding bacteriophage
ETEC	Food, water; young children in and travelers to developing countries	Traveler's diarrhea	Heat-stable and -labile enterotoxins, colonization factors	Virulence plasmid(s)
EPEC	Person-to-person; young children and neonates in developing countries	Watery diarrhea	Localized adherence, attaching and effacing lesion on intestinal epithelium	EPEC adherence factor plasmid pathogenicity island (locus for enterocyte effacement)
EIEC	Food, water; children in and travelers to developing countries	Dysentery	Invasion of colonic epithelial cells, intracellular multiplication, cell-to-cell spread	Multiple genes contained primarily in large virulence plasmid
EAEC	? Food, water; children in and travelers to developing countries; all ages, industrialized countries	Traveler's diarrhea, acute diarrhea, persistent diarrhea	Aggregative/diffuse adherence, virulence factors regulated by AggR	Chromosomal or plasmid-associated adherence and toxin genes

[a]STEC, Shiga toxin–producing *E. coli;* ETEC, enterotoxigenic *E. coli;* EPEC, enteropathogenic *E. coli;* EIEC, enteroinvasive *E. coli;* EAEC, enteroaggregative *E. coli.*
[b]Classic syndromes; see text for details on spectrum of disease.
[c]Pathogenesis is multigenic, including genes in addition to those listed.

in humans. Although acquisition of an ExPEC strain by the host is a prerequisite for ExPEC infection, it is not the rate-limiting step, which instead is entry of an ExPEC strain from its site of colonization (e.g., the colon, vagina, or oropharynx) into a normally sterile extraintestinal site (e.g., the urinary tract, peritoneal cavity, or lungs). ExPEC strains have acquired genes encoding diverse extraintestinal virulence factors that enable the bacteria to cause infections outside the gastrointestinal tract in both normal and compromised hosts (Table 51-1). These virulence genes are, for the most part, distinct from those that enable intestinal pathogenic strains to cause diarrheal disease. All age groups, all types of hosts, and nearly all organs and anatomic sites are susceptible to infection by ExPEC. Previously healthy hosts infected with ExPEC can become severely ill or die; however, adverse outcomes are more prevalent in the presence of comorbid illnesses and host defense abnormalities. *E. coli* is the most common enteric gram-negative species to cause extraintestinal infection in ambulatory, LTCF, and hospital settings. The diversity and the medical and economic impact of ExPEC infections are evident from consideration of the following specific syndromes.

Extraintestinal Infectious Syndromes

Urinary Tract Infection (UTI)

The urinary tract is the site most frequently infected by ExPEC. An exceedingly common infection among ambulatory patients, UTI accounts for 1% of ambulatory care visits in the United States and is second only to lower respiratory tract infection among infections responsible for hospitalization. UTIs are best considered by clinical syndrome (e.g., uncomplicated cystitis, pyelonephritis, and catheter-associated UTIs) and within the context of specific hosts (e.g., premenopausal women, compromised hosts; Chap. 27). *E. coli* is the single most common pathogen for all UTI syndrome/host group combinations. Each year in the United States, *E. coli* causes 85–95% of an estimated 6–8 million episodes of uncomplicated cystitis in premenopausal women, with an estimated $1 billion in direct health care costs. Furthermore, 20% of women with an initial cystitis episode develop frequent recurrences (from 0.3 to >20 per year).

Uncomplicated cystitis, the most common acute UTI syndrome, is characterized by dysuria, frequency, and suprapubic pain. Fever and/or back pain suggests progression to pyelonephritis. Fever may take 5–7 days to resolve completely in appropriately treated patients with pyelonephritis. Persistently elevated or increasing fever and neutrophil counts should prompt evaluation for intrarenal or perinephric abscess and/or obstruction. Renal parenchymal damage and loss of renal function during pyelonephritis occur primarily with urinary obstruction. Pregnant women are at unusually high risk for developing pyelonephritis, which can adversely affect the outcome of pregnancy. As a result, prenatal screening for and treatment of asymptomatic bacteriuria are standard.

Prostatic infection is a potential complication of UTI in men. The diagnosis and treatment of UTI, as detailed in Chap. 27, should be tailored to the individual host, the nature and site of infection, and local patterns of antimicrobial susceptibility.

Abdominal and Pelvic Infection

The abdomen/pelvis is the second most common site of extraintestinal infection due to *E. coli*. A wide variety of clinical syndromes occur in this location, including acute peritonitis secondary to fecal contamination, spontaneous bacterial peritonitis, dialysis-associated peritonitis, diverticulitis, appendicitis, intraperitoneal or visceral abscesses (hepatic, pancreatic, splenic), infected pancreatic pseudocysts, and septic cholangitis and/or cholecystitis. In intraabdominal infections, *E. coli* can be isolated either alone or (as is often the case) along with other facultative and/or anaerobic members of the intestinal flora (Chap. 24).

Pneumonia

E. coli is not usually considered a cause of pneumonia (Chap. 17). Indeed, enteric GNB account for only 2–5% of cases of community-acquired pneumonia (CAP), in part because these organisms only transiently colonize the oropharynx of a minority of healthy individuals. However, rates of oral colonization with *E. coli* and other GNB increase with the severity of illness and with antibiotic use. Thus GNB are a common cause of pneumonia among residents of LTCFs and are the most common cause (60–70% of cases) of hospital-acquired pneumonia (Chap. 13), particularly among postoperative and intensive care patients. Pulmonary infection is usually acquired by small-volume aspiration but occasionally occurs via hematogenous spread, in which case multifocal nodular infiltrates can be seen. Tissue necrosis, probably due to cytotoxins produced by GNB, is common. Despite significant institutional variation, *E. coli* is generally the third or fourth most commonly isolated gram-negative bacillus in hospital-acquired pneumonia, accounting for 5–8% of episodes in both U.S.-based and European-based studies. Regardless of the host, pneumonia due to enteric GNB is a serious disease, with high crude and attributable mortality rates (20–60% and 10–20%, respectively).

Meningitis

(See also Chap. 29) *E. coli* is one of the two leading causes of neonatal meningitis (the other being group B *Streptococcus*). Most of the responsible strains possess the K1 capsular antigen. After the first month of life, *E. coli* meningitis is uncommon, occurring predominantly in the setting of disruption of the meninges from craniotomy or trauma or in the presence of cirrhosis. In patients with cirrhosis, the meninges are presumably seeded as a result of poor hepatic clearance of portal vein bacteremia.

Cellulitis/Musculoskeletal Infection

E. coli contributes frequently to infection of decubitus ulcers and occasionally to infection of ulcers and wounds of the lower extremity in diabetic patients and other hosts with neurovascular compromise. Osteomyelitis secondary to contiguous spread can occur in these settings. In addition, *E. coli* occasionally causes cellulitis or infections of burn sites or surgical wounds, particularly when the infection originates close to the perineum. Hematogenously acquired osteomyelitis, particularly of vertebral bodies, is more commonly caused by *E. coli* than is generally appreciated; this organism accounts for up to 10% of cases in some series (Chap. 22). *E. coli* occasionally causes orthopedic device–associated infection or septic arthritis and rarely causes hematogenous myositis. Upper-leg myositis or fasciitis due to *E. coli* should prompt an evaluation for an abdominal source with contiguous spread.

Endovascular Infection

Despite being one of the most common causes of bacteremia, *E. coli* rarely seeds native or prosthetic heart valves. When the organism does seed native valves, it usually does so in the setting of prior valve disease. *E. coli* infections of aneurysms and vascular grafts are quite uncommon.

Miscellaneous Infections

E. coli can cause infection in nearly every organ and anatomic site. It occasionally causes postoperative mediastinitis or complicated sinusitis and uncommonly causes endophthalmitis or brain abscess.

Bacteremia

E. coli bacteremia can arise from primary infection at any extraintestinal site. In addition, primary *E. coli* bacteremia can arise from percutaneous intravascular devices or transrectal prostate biopsy or can result from the increased intestinal mucosal permeability seen in neonates and in the settings of neutropenia and chemotherapy-induced mucositis, trauma, and burns. Roughly equal proportions of *E. coli* bacteremia cases originate in the community and in the hospital. In most studies, *E. coli* and *Staphylococcus aureus* are the two most common blood isolates of clinical significance; *E. coli*, which is isolated in 17–37% of cases, is the gram-negative bacillus most often isolated from the blood in the ambulatory setting and in most LTCF and hospital settings. Isolation of *E. coli* from the blood is almost always clinically significant and typically is accompanied by the sepsis syndrome, severe sepsis (sepsis-induced dysfunction of at least one organ or system), or septic shock (Chap. 15). Calculations based on a conservative estimate for the proportional contribution of *E. coli* to severe sepsis (i.e., 17% of all cases) translate into an estimated 40,000 deaths among the affected patients in the United States in 2001.

The urinary tract is the most common source of *E. coli* bacteremia, accounting for one-half to two-thirds of episodes. Bacteremia from a urinary tract source is particularly common in patients with pyelonephritis, urinary tract obstruction, or instrumentation in the presence of infected urine. The abdomen is the second most common source, accounting for 25% of episodes. Although biliary obstruction (stones, tumor) and overt bowel disruption are responsible for many of these cases, some abdominal sources (e.g., abscesses) are remarkably silent clinically and require identification via imaging studies (e.g., CT). Therefore, the physician should be cautious in designating the urinary tract as the source of *E. coli* bacteremia in the absence of characteristic signs and symptoms of UTI. Soft tissue, bone, pulmonary, and intravascular catheter infections are other sources of *E. coli* bacteremia.

Diagnosis

Strains of *E. coli* that cause extraintestinal infections usually grow both aerobically and anaerobically within 24 h on standard diagnostic media and are easily identified by the clinical microbiology laboratory according to routine biochemical criteria. More than 90% of ExPEC strains are rapid lactose fermenters and are indole positive.

℞ Treatment: EXTRAINTESTINAL *E. COLI* INFECTIONS

In the past, most *E. coli* isolates were highly susceptible to a broad range of antimicrobial agents. Unfortunately, this situation has changed. In general, the frequency of ampicillin resistance precludes its empirical use, even in community-acquired infections. The prevalence of resistance to first-generation cephalosporins and trimethoprim-sulfamethoxazole (TMP-SMX) is increasing among community-acquired strains in the United States (with current rates of 10–40%) and is even higher outside North America. Until recently, TMP-SMX was the drug of choice for the treatment of uncomplicated cystitis in many locales. Although continued empirical use of TMP-SMX will predictably result in ever-diminishing cure rates, a wholesale switch to alternative agents (e.g., fluoroquinolones) will just as predictably accelerate the widespread emergence of resistance to these antimicrobial classes, as is already occurring in some areas. Resistance to fluoroquinolones has increased steadily over the last decade; in 2002–2005, prevalence rates were 5–20% in North America and even higher in other regions. The prevalence of resistance is higher in settings where fluoroquinolone prophylaxis is used extensively (e.g., in patients with leukemia, transplant recipients, and patients with cirrhosis) and among isolates from LTCFs and hospitals. Among quinolone-resistant strains, a significant (30–40%) prevalence of co-resistance to amoxicillin/clavulanic acid and piperacillin has been reported. The prevalence of co-resistance to more advanced cephalosporins (second-, third-, and fourth-generation), monobactams (e.g., aztreonam), piperacillin-tazobactam, and the non-amikacin aminoglycosides is increasing but is still generally <10%. Carbapenems (e.g., imipenem) and amikacin are the most predictably active agents. Although relevant clinical experience is limited, tigecycline and polymyxin B (the agent of last resort because of its potential toxicities) are highly active in vitro.

INTESTINAL PATHOGENIC STRAINS

Certain strains of *E. coli* are capable of causing diarrheal disease. Other important intestinal pathogens are discussed in Chaps. 25, 42, and 54–57. At least in the industrialized world, intestinal pathogenic strains of *E. coli* are rarely encountered in the fecal flora of healthy persons and instead appear to be essentially obligate pathogens. These strains have evolved a special ability to cause enteritis, enterocolitis, and colitis when ingested in sufficient quantities by a naive host. At least five distinct pathotypes of intestinal pathogenic *E. coli* exist: (1) Shiga toxin–producing *E. coli* (STEC)/enterohemorrhagic *E. coli* (EHEC), (2) enterotoxigenic *E. coli* (ETEC), (3) enteropathogenic *E. coli* (EPEC), (4) enteroinvasive *E. coli* (EIEC), and (5) enteroaggregative *E. coli* (EAEC). Diffusely adherent *E. coli* (DAEC) and cytodetaching *E. coli* are additional putative pathotypes. Transmission occurs predominantly via contaminated food and water for ETEC, STEC, EIEC, and probably EAEC and by person-to-person spread for EPEC (and occasionally STEC/EHEC). Gastric acidity confers some protection against infection; therefore, persons with decreased stomach acid levels are especially susceptible. Humans are the major reservoir (except for STEC/EHEC); host range appears to be dictated by species-specific attachment factors. Although there is some overlap, each pathotype possesses a unique combination of virulence traits that results in a distinctive intestinal pathogenic mechanism (Table 51-2). These strains are largely incapable of causing disease outside the intestinal tract. Except in the case of STEC/EHEC and perhaps EAEC, disease due to this group of pathogens occurs primarily in developing countries.

Shiga Toxin–Producing and Enterohemorrhagic E. coli

STEC/EHEC strains constitute an emerging group of pathogens that can cause hemorrhagic colitis and the hemolytic-uremic syndrome (HUS). Several large outbreaks resulting from the consumption of undercooked ground beef and other foods (e.g., fresh spinach) have received significant media attention. O157:H7 is the most prominent serotype, but serogroups O6, O26, O55, O91, O103, O111, O113, and OX3 have also been associated with these syndromes. The ability of STEC/EHEC to produce Shiga toxin (Stx2 and/or Stx1) or related toxins is a critical factor in the expression of clinical disease. *Shigella dysenteriae* strains that produce the closely related Shiga toxin Stx can cause the same syndrome. Stx2 appears to be more important than Stx1 in the development of HUS. All Shiga toxins studied to date are multimers composing one enzymatically active A subunit and five identical B subunits that mediate binding to globoceramides. The A subunit cleaves an adenine from the host cell's 28S rRNA, thereby irreversibly inhibiting ribosomal function. Therefore, Shiga toxins belong to the class of toxins known as *ribosome-inactivating proteins*.

Additional factors, such as acid tolerance and adherence, are necessary for full pathogenicity among STEC strains. Most disease-causing isolates possess the genomic locus for enterocyte effacement (LEE). This pathogenicity island was first described in EPEC strains and contains genes that mediate adherence to intestinal epithelial cells. EHEC strains make up the subgroup of STEC strains that possess *stx*$_1$ and/or *stx*$_2$ as well as LEE.

Domesticated ruminant animals, particularly cattle and young calves, serve as the major reservoir for STEC/EHEC. Ground beef—the most common food source of STEC/EHEC strains—is often contaminated during processing. Furthermore, manure from cattle or other animals that is used as fertilizer can contaminate produce (potatoes, lettuce, spinach, sprouts, fallen apples), and fecal runoff from this source can contaminate water. It is estimated that $<10^3$ CFU of STEC/EHEC can cause disease. Therefore, not only can low levels of food or environmental contamination (e.g., in water swallowed while swimming) result in disease, but person-to-person transmission (e.g., at day-care centers and in institutions) is an important route for secondary spread. Laboratory-associated infections also take place. Illness due to this group of pathogens occurs both as outbreaks and as sporadic cases, with a peak incidence in the summer months.

In contrast to other intestinal pathotypes, STEC/EHEC causes infections more frequently in industrialized countries than in developing regions. O157:H7 strains are the fourth most commonly reported cause of bacterial diarrhea in the United States (after *Campylobacter*, *Salmonella*, and *Shigella*). Colonization of the colon and perhaps the ileum results in symptoms after an incubation period of 3 or 4 days. Colonic edema and an initial secretory diarrhea may develop into the STEC/EHEC hallmark syndrome of grossly bloody diarrhea (as detected by history or examination) in >90% of cases. Significant abdominal pain and fecal leukocytes are common (70% of cases), whereas fever is not; a lack of fever often results in diagnostic consideration of noninfectious conditions (e.g., intussusception and inflammatory or ischemic bowel disease). Occasionally, infections caused by *Clostridium difficile*, *Campylobacter*, and *Salmonella* present in a similar fashion. STEC/EHEC disease is usually self-limited, lasting 5–10 days. This infection can be complicated by HUS, which occurs 2–14 days after diarrhea in 2–8% of cases and most often affects very young or elderly patients. It is estimated that >50% of all cases of HUS in the United States are caused by STEC/EHEC. This complication is probably mediated by the systemic translocation of Shiga toxins. Erythrocytes may serve as carriers of Stx to endothelial cells located in the small vessels of the kidney and brain. The subsequent development of thrombotic microangiopathy (perhaps with direct toxin-mediated effects on various nonendothelial cells) commonly produces some combination of fever, thrombocytopenia, renal failure, and encephalopathy. Although the mortality rate with dialysis support is <10%, residual renal and neurologic dysfunction may persist.

Enterotoxigenic E. coli

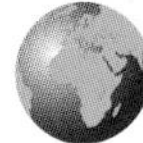

In tropical or developing countries, ETEC is a major cause of endemic diarrhea. After weaning, children in these locales commonly experience several episodes of ETEC infection during the first 3 years of life. The incidence of disease diminishes with age, a pattern that correlates with the development of mucosal immunity to colonization factors (i.e., adhesins). In industrialized countries, infection usually follows travel to endemic areas. ETEC is the most common agent of traveler's diarrhea, causing 25–75% of cases. The incidence of infection is decreased by prudent avoidance of potentially contaminated fluids and foods (Chap. 4). ETEC infection is uncommon in the United States, but outbreaks secondary to consumption of food products imported from endemic areas have occurred. A large inoculum (10^6–10^{10} CFU) is needed to produce disease. After ingestion of contaminated water or food (particularly items that are poorly cooked, unpeeled, or unrefrigerated), colonization factor–mediated intestinal adherence occurs over 12–72 h.

Disease is mediated primarily by a heat-labile toxin (LT-1) and/or a heat-stable toxin (STa) that causes net fluid secretion via activation of adenylate cyclase (LT-1) and/or guanylate cyclase (STa) in the jejunum and ileum. The result is watery diarrhea accompanied by cramps. LT-1 consists of an A and a B subunit and is structurally and functionally similar to cholera toxin. Strong binding of the B subunit to the GM$_1$ ganglioside on intestinal epithelial cells leads to the intracellular translocation of the A subunit, which functions as an ADP-ribosyltransferase. Mature STa is an 18- or 19-amino-acid secreted peptide whose biologic activity is mediated by binding to the guanylate cyclase C found in the brush-border membrane of enterocytes; this binding results in increased intracellular concentrations of cyclic GMP. Characteristically absent are histopathologic changes within the small bowel; mucus, blood, and inflammatory cells in stool; and fever. The disease spectrum ranges from a mild illness to a life-threatening cholera-like syndrome. Although symptoms are usually self-limited (typically lasting for 3 days), infection may result in significant morbidity and mortality when access to health care is limited and when small and/or undernourished children are affected.

Enteropathogenic E. coli

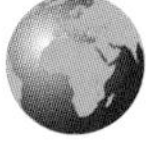

EPEC causes disease primarily in young children, including neonates. The first *E. coli* pathotype recognized as an agent of diarrheal disease, EPEC was responsible for outbreaks of infantile diarrhea (including some outbreaks in hospital nurseries) in industrialized countries in the 1940s and 1950s. At present, EPEC infection is an uncommon cause of diarrhea in developed countries but is an important cause of diarrhea (both sporadic and epidemic) among infants in developing countries. Breast-feeding diminishes the incidence of EPEC infection. Rapid person-to-person spread may occur. Upon colonization of the small bowel, symptoms develop after a brief incubation period (1 or 2 days). Initial localized adherence leads to a characteristic effacement of microvilli, with the formation of cuplike, actin-rich pedestals. The actual mechanism(s) of diarrhea production are an area of ongoing investigation. Diarrheal stool often contains mucus but not blood. Although usually self-limited (lasting 5–15 days), EPEC diarrhea may persist for weeks.

Enteroinvasive E. coli

EIEC, a relatively uncommon cause of diarrhea, is rarely identified in the United States, although a few food-related outbreaks have been described. In developing countries, sporadic disease is infrequently recognized in children and travelers. EIEC shares many genetic and clinical features with *Shigella*; however, unlike *Shigella*, EIEC produces disease only at a large inoculum (10^8–10^{10} CFU), with onset generally following an incubation period of 1–3 days. Initially, enterotoxins are believed to induce secretory small-bowel diarrhea. Subsequently, colonization and invasion of the colonic mucosa, followed by replication therein and cell-to-cell spread, result in the development of inflammatory colitis characterized by fever, abdominal pain, tenesmus, and scant stool containing mucus, blood, and inflammatory cells. Symptoms are usually self-limited (7–10 days).

Enteroaggregative and Diffusely Adherent E. coli

EAEC has been described primarily in developing countries and in young children. However, a recent study indicates that it may be a relatively common cause of diarrhea in all age groups in industrialized countries. EAEC has also been recognized increasingly as an important cause of traveler's diarrhea. A large inoculum is required for infection, which manifests as watery, sometimes prolonged diarrhea. In vitro, the organisms exhibit a diffuse or "stacked-brick" pattern of adherence to epithelial cells. Virulence factors that probably contribute to disease are regulated in part by the transcriptional activator AggR and include the aggregative adherence fimbriae (AAF/I-III) and the enterotoxins Pet, EAST-1, Shet1, and Shet2. Some but not all strains of DAEC are capable of causing diarrheal disease, primarily in children 2–6 years of age in some developing countries. The Afa/Dr adhesins may contribute to the pathogenesis of infection.

Diagnosis

A practical approach to the evaluation of diarrhea is to distinguish noninflammatory from inflammatory cases (Chap. 25). ETEC, EPEC, and DAEC are uncommon causes of noninflammatory diarrhea in the United States; EAEC has recently been described as a cause of diarrhea in this country. The diagnosis of these infections requires specialized assays that are not routinely available and whose use is rarely indicated since the diseases are self-limited. ETEC causes the majority and EAEC a minority of cases of noninflammatory traveler's diarrhea. Definitive diagnosis generally is not necessary. Empirical antimicrobial (or symptom-based) treatment, along with rehydration therapy, is a reasonable approach. If diarrhea persists despite treatment, *Giardia* or *Cryptosporidium* (or, in immunocompromised hosts, certain other microbial agents) should be sought. The diagnosis of infection with EIEC, a rare cause of inflammatory diarrhea in the United States, also requires specialized assays. However, evaluation for STEC/EHEC infection, particularly when bloody diarrhea is reported or observed, is appropriate. Although screening for *E. coli* strains that do not ferment sorbitol, with subsequent serotyping for O157, is the most common method currently used to detect STEC/EHEC, testing for Shiga toxins or toxin genes is more sensitive, specific, and rapid. The latter approach offers another advantage as well: it detects both non-O157 STEC/EHEC and sorbitol-fermenting strains of O157:H7, which otherwise are difficult to identify. DNA-based, enzyme-linked immunosorbent, and cytotoxicity assays are in various stages of development and are likely to emerge as the diagnostic standards.

℞ Treatment: INTESTINAL *E. COLI* INFECTIONS

The mainstay of treatment for all diarrheal syndromes is replacement of water and electrolytes (Chap. 25). The use of prophylactic antibiotics to prevent traveler's diarrhea generally should be discouraged, especially in light of high rates of antimicrobial resistance. However, in selected patients (e.g., those who cannot afford a brief illness or have an increased susceptibility to infection), the use of rifaximin, which is nonabsorbable and well tolerated, is reasonable. When stools are free of mucus and blood, early patient-initiated treatment of traveler's diarrhea with a quinolone or azithromycin decreases the duration of illness, and the use of loperamide may halt symptoms within a few hours (Chap. 25). Although dysentery caused by EIEC is self-limited, treatment hastens the resolution of symptoms, particularly in severe cases. Antimicrobial therapy for STEC/EHEC infection (the presence of which is suggested by bloody diarrhea without fever) should be avoided, since antibiotics may increase the incidence of HUS (possibly via increased production/release of Stx).

KLEBSIELLA INFECTIONS

K. pneumoniae is the most important *Klebsiella* species from a medical standpoint, causing community-acquired, LTCF-acquired, and nosocomial infections. *K. oxytoca* is primarily a pathogen in LTCF and hospital settings. The *K. pneumoniae* subspecies *rhinoscleromatis* and *ozaenae* are usually isolated from patients in tropical climates. *Klebsiella* species are broadly prevalent in the environment and colonize mucosal surfaces of mammals. In healthy humans, *K. pneumoniae* colonization rates are 5–35% in the colon and 1–5% in the oropharynx; the skin is usually colonized only transiently. In LTCFs and hospitals, colonization occurs with *K. oxytoca* as well, and carriage rates are significant among both staff and patients. Person-to-person spread is the predominant mode of acquisition. Classically, *Klebsiella* is associated with CAP, primarily among alcoholics. However, most *Klebsiella* infections now occur in LTCFs and hospitals. *Klebsiella* causes a spectrum of extraintestinal infections similar to that caused by *E. coli*. However, extraintestinal infections due to *Klebsiella* occur at a lower incidence at all sites except the respiratory tract, possibly because of differences in colonization rates and site-specific virulence traits. Antibiotic-resistant strains have been responsible for a number of outbreaks of nosocomial infection in ICUs and neonatal nurseries. The most common clinical syndromes are pneumonia, UTI, abdominal infection, surgical site infection, soft tissue infection, and subsequent bacteremia. *K. pneumoniae* subspecies *rhinoscleromatis* is the causative agent of rhinoscleroma—a granulomatous, slowly progressive (over months to years) infection of the upper respiratory mucosa that causes necrosis and occasional obstruction of the nasal passages. *K. pneumoniae* subspecies *ozaenae* has been implicated in chronic atrophic rhinitis and in rare cases of invasive disease in compromised hosts.

INFECTIOUS SYNDROMES

Pneumonia

K. pneumoniae causes only a small proportion of cases of CAP (Chap. 17). CAP due to *K. pneumoniae* occurs primarily in hosts with underlying conditions (e.g., alcoholism, diabetes, or chronic lung disease). As in all pneumonias due to enteric GNB, production of purulent sputum and evidence of airspace disease are typically encountered. Presentation with earlier, less extensive infection is more common than the classically described lobar infiltrate with a bulging fissure. Pulmonary necrosis, pleural effusion, and empyema can occur with disease progression. Pulmonary infection is especially common among residents of LTCFs and hospitalized patients because of increased rates of oropharyngeal colonization. Mechanical ventilation is an important risk factor.

UTI

K. pneumoniae accounts for only 1–2% of UTI episodes among otherwise healthy adults, but for 5–17% of episodes of complicated UTI, including infections associated with indwelling bladder catheters.

Abdominal Infection

Klebsiella causes a spectrum of abdominal infections similar to that caused by *E. coli* but is less frequently isolated from these infections. Recently, however, the incidence of hepatic abscesses caused by *Klebsiella* (the majority due to strains with the K1 capsular serotype) has increased in Taiwan and elsewhere. Diabetes appears to be an important risk factor. Associated bacteremia is common, resulting in metastatic complications (e.g., endophthalmitis and pulmonary, renal, and CNS abscesses).

Other Infections

Klebsiella cellulitis or soft tissue infection most frequently affects devitalized tissue (e.g., decubitus and diabetic ulcers, burn sites) and immunocompromised hosts. *Klebsiella* causes some cases of surgical site infection, hematogenously derived endophthalmitis (especially that associated with hepatic abscess), and nosocomial sinusitis, as well as occasional cases of osteomyelitis contiguous to soft tissue infection, temperate myositis, and meningitis (in the neonatal period or after neurosurgery).

Bacteremia

Klebsiella infection at any site can produce bacteremia. Infections of the urinary tract, respiratory tract, and abdomen (especially hepatic abscess) each account for 15–30% of *Klebsiella* bacteremias. Intravascular device–related infections account for another 5–15% of episodes and surgical site and miscellaneous infections for the rest. *Klebsiella* is a cause of sepsis in neonates and of bacteremia in neutropenic patients. Like enteric GNB in general, *Klebsiella* rarely causes endocarditis or endovascular infection.

DIAGNOSIS

Klebsiellae are readily isolated and identified in the laboratory. These organisms usually ferment lactose, although the subspecies *rhinoscleromatis* and *ozaenae* are nonfermenters and are indole negative.

Rx Treatment: *KLEBSIELLA* INFECTIONS

K. pneumoniae and *K. oxytoca* have antibiotic resistance profiles that are largely similar. These species are intrinsically resistant to ampicillin and ticarcillin. Data from the National Nosocomial Infections Surveillance System (NNIS) indicated that 20.6% of ICU patients were infected with strains resistant to third-generation cephalosporins in 2003—a 47% increase over figures for 1998–2002. Even higher rates have been reported outside North America. This increasing resistance is mediated primarily by plasmid-encoded ESBLs. In addition, these plasmids usually encode resistance to aminoglycosides, tetracyclines, and TMP-SMX. Resistance to β-lactam/β-lactamase inhibitor combinations and second-generation cephalosporins independent of ESBL-containing plasmids has also been described with increasing frequency. The prevalence of quinolone resistance is 15–20% overall and 50% in ESBL-containing strains. Given both the undesirability of treating the latter strains with penicillins or cephalosporins and the quinolone resistance often associated with ESBLs, empirical treatment of serious or health care–associated *Klebsiella* infections with amikacin, carbapenems, or tigecycline (to which resistance rates are generally <10% in North America) is prudent. However, clinical experience with tigecycline is limited, and this approach assumes the continued low prevalence of carbapenemases. Polymyxin B can be considered for use against highly resistant strains but is an agent of last resort because of its potential toxicities.

PROTEUS INFECTIONS

P. mirabilis causes 90% of *Proteus* infections, which occur in the community, LTCFs, and hospitals. *P. vulgaris* and *P. penneri* are associated primarily with infections acquired in LTCFs or hospitals. *Proteus* species are part of the colonic flora of a wide variety of mammals, birds, fish, and reptiles. The ability of these GNB to generate histamine from contaminated fish has implicated them in the pathogenesis of scombroid (fish) poisoning. *P. mirabilis* colonizes healthy humans (prevalence, 50%), whereas *P. vulgaris* and *P. penneri* are isolated primarily from individuals with underlying disease. The urinary tract is by far the most common site of *Proteus* infection, with adhesins, flagella, IgA protease, and urease representing the principal urovirulence factors. *Proteus* less commonly causes infection at a variety of other extraintestinal sites.

INFECTIOUS SYNDROMES

UTI

Most *Proteus* infections arise from the urinary tract. *P. mirabilis* causes only 1–2% of cases of UTI in healthy women, and *Proteus* species collectively cause only 5% of cases of hospital-acquired UTI. However, *Proteus* is responsible for 10–15% of cases of complicated UTI, primarily those associated with catheterization; in the setting of long-term catheterization, the prevalence of *Proteus* UTI is 20–45%. This high prevalence is due in part to bacterial production of urease, which hydrolyzes urea to ammonia and results in alkalization of the urine. Alkalization of urine, in turn, leads to precipitation of organic and inorganic compounds, with the formation of struvite and carbonate-apatite crystals, the formation of biofilms on catheters, and/or the development of calculi. *Proteus* becomes associated with the stones and biofilms; thereafter, it usually can be eradicated only by the removal of the stones or the catheter. Over time, staghorn calculi may form and lead to obstruction and renal failure. Thus urine samples with unexplained alkalinity should be cultured for *Proteus*, and identification of a *Proteus* species should prompt an evaluation for urolithiasis.

Other Infections

Proteus occasionally causes pneumonia (primarily in LTCF residents or hospitalized patients), nosocomial sinusitis, intraabdominal abscesses, biliary tract infection, surgical site infection, soft tissue infection (especially decubitus and diabetic ulcers), and osteomyelitis (primarily contiguous); in rare cases, it causes temperate myositis. In addition, *Proteus* occasionally causes neonatal meningitis (with the umbilicus often implicated as the source); this disease is often complicated by the development of a cerebral abscess. Otogenic brain abscess also occurs.

Bacteremia

The majority of *Proteus* bacteremias originate from the urinary tract; however, any of the less common sites of infection as well as intravascular devices are also potential sources. Endovascular infection is rare. *Proteus* species are occasional agents of sepsis in neonates and of bacteremia in neutropenic patients.

DIAGNOSIS

Proteus is readily isolated and identified in the laboratory. Most strains are lactose negative, produce H_2S, and demonstrate characteristic swarming motility on agar plates. *P. mirabilis* is indole negative, whereas *P. vulgaris* and *P. penneri* are indole positive.

℞ Treatment: *PROTEUS* INFECTIONS

P. mirabilis is usually susceptible to most antimicrobial agents except tetracycline, polymyxin B, and tigecycline. Resistance to ampicillin and first-generation cephalosporins has been acquired by 10–50% of strains. Overall, 10–15% of *P. mirabilis* isolates are resistant to quinolones; 5% of isolates in the United States now produce ESBLs. *P. vulgaris* and *P. penneri* exhibit more extensive drug resistance than does *P. mirabilis*. Resistance to ampicillin and first-generation cephalosporins is the rule, and 30–40% of isolates are resistant to quinolones. Derepression of an inducible chromosomal AmpC β-lactamase (not present in *P. mirabilis*) occurs in up to 30% of isolates. Imipenem, fourth-generation cephalosporins (e.g., cefepime), amikacin, and TMP-SMX display excellent activity against *Proteus* species (90–100% of isolates susceptible).

ENTEROBACTER INFECTIONS

E. cloacae and *E. aerogenes* are responsible for most *Enterobacter* infections (65–75% and 15–25%, respectively); *E. sakazakii* and *E. gergoviae* are less commonly isolated (1% and <1% of *Enterobacter* isolates, respectively). Enterobacters cause primarily hospital-acquired and other health care–related infections. The organisms are widely prevalent in foods, environmental sources (including equipment at health care facilities), and a wide variety of animals. Few healthy humans are colonized, but the percentage increases significantly in the setting of LTCF residence or hospitalization. Although colonization is an important prelude to infection, direct introduction via IV lines (e.g., contaminated IV fluids or pressure monitors) also occurs. Significant antibiotic resistance has developed in *Enterobacter* species and has contributed to the emergence of the organisms as prominent nosocomial pathogens. Individuals who have previously received antibiotic treatment, have comorbid disease, and are being treated in ICUs are at greatest risk for infection. *Enterobacter* causes a spectrum of extraintestinal infections similar to that described for other GNB.

INFECTIOUS SYNDROMES

Pneumonia, UTI (particularly catheter-related), intravascular device–related infection, surgical site infection, and abdominal infection (primarily postoperative or related to devices such as biliary stents) are the most common syndromes encountered. Nosocomial sinusitis, meningitis related to neurosurgical procedures (including use of pressure monitors), osteomyelitis, and endophthalmitis after eye surgery are less frequent. *E. sakazakii* is associated with neonatal meningitis/sepsis (particularly in premature infants); contaminated formula has been implicated as a source of this infection, which is often complicated by brain abscess or ventriculitis. Bacteremia can result from infection at any of these sites. In *Enterobacter* bacteremia of unclear origin, the contamination of IV fluids or medications, blood components or plasma derivatives, catheter-flushing fluids, pressure monitors, and dialysis equipment should be considered, particularly in an outbreak setting. *Enterobacter* can also cause bacteremia in neutropenic patients. *Enterobacter* endocarditis is rare, occurring primarily in association with illicit IV drug use or prosthetic valves.

DIAGNOSIS

Enterobacter is readily isolated and identified in the laboratory. Most strains are lactose positive and indole negative.

℞ Treatment: *ENTEROBACTER* INFECTIONS

Significant antimicrobial resistance exists among *Enterobacter* strains. Ampicillin and the first- and second-generation cephalosporins have little or no activity. The extensive use of third-generation cephalosporins has resulted in the selection of strains that are derepressed for production of AmpC β-lactamase, which confers resistance to third-generation cephalosporins, monobactams (e.g., aztreonam), and (frequently) β-lactam/β-lactamase inhibitor combinations. Resistance may emerge during therapy; in one study, the emergence of resistance was documented in 20% of patients. Resistance should be considered a possibility when clinical deterioration follows initial improvement, and third-generation cephalosporins should be avoided in the treatment of serious *Enterobacter* infections. NNIS data for 2003 identified resistance to third-generation cephalosporins in 31% of ICU isolates. Cefepime is stable, even in the presence of AmpC β-lactamases; thus it is a suitable option for treatment of *Enterobacter* infections in the absence of a coexistent ESBL. However, the prevalence of ESBL production in *Enterobacter* (particularly in *E. cloacae*) has been increasing and is now 5–30%. Such strains are challenging to treat. Fortunately, in the United States, imipenem, amikacin, and quinolones have generally retained excellent activity (90–99% of isolates susceptible). Although clinical experience is limited, tigecycline is highly active in vitro.

SERRATIA INFECTIONS

S. marcescens causes the majority of *Serratia* infections (>90%), and *S. liquefaciens* is isolated occasionally. Serratiae are found primarily in the environment (including in health care institutions), particularly in moist foci. Although serratiae have been isolated from a variety of animals, healthy humans are rarely colonized. In LTCFs or hospitals, reservoirs for the organisms include health care personnel, food, milk (neonatal units), sinks, respiratory equipment, pressure monitors, IV solutions, multiply accessed medication vials, blood products (e.g., platelets), lotions, irrigation solutions, and even disinfectants. Infection results from either direct inoculation (e.g., via IV fluid) or colonization (primarily of the respiratory tract) and subsequent infection. Sporadic infection is most common, but epidemics and common-source outbreaks occasionally occur. The spectrum of extraintestinal infections caused by *Serratia* is similar to that for other GNB. *Serratia* species account for 1–3% of hospital-acquired infections.

INFECTIOUS SYNDROMES

The respiratory tract, the genitourinary tract, intravascular devices, and surgical wounds are the most common sites of *Serratia* infection and sources of *Serratia* bacteremia. Soft tissue infections (including myositis), osteomyelitis, abdominal and biliary tract infection (postprocedural), contact lens–associated keratitis, endophthalmitis, septic arthritis (primarily from intraarticular injections), and infusion-related bacteremias occur less commonly. Serratiae are uncommon causes of neonatal or postsurgical meningitis and of bacteremia in neutropenic patients. Endocarditis is rare.

DIAGNOSIS

Serratiae are readily cultured and identified by the laboratory and are usually lactose and indole negative. Some *S. marcescens* strains are red-pigmented.

℞ Treatment: *SERRATIA* INFECTIONS

Most *Serratia* strains (>80%) are resistant to ampicillin, first-generation cephalosporins, and polymyxin B. Derepression of inducible chromosomal AmpC β-lactamases may be preexistent or may develop during therapy. Both in the United States and globally, the prevalence of ESBL-producing isolates is <5%. In general, >90% of *Serratia* isolates are susceptible to other GNB-appropriate antibiotics.

CITROBACTER INFECTIONS

C. freundii and *C. koseri* cause most human *Citrobacter* infections, which are epidemiologically and clinically similar to *Enterobacter* infections. *Citrobacter* species are commonly present in water, food, soil, and certain animals. *Citrobacter* is part of the normal fecal flora in a minority of healthy humans, but colonization rates increase in LTCFs and hospitals—the settings in which nearly all infections occur. *Citrobacter* species account for 1–2% of nosocomial infections. The affected hosts are usually immunocompromised or have comorbid disease. *Citrobacter* causes extraintestinal infections similar to those described for other GNB.

INFECTIOUS SYNDROMES

The urinary tract accounts for 40–50% of *Citrobacter* infections. Less commonly involved sites include the biliary tree (particularly with stones or obstruction), the respiratory tract, surgical sites, soft tissue (e.g., decubitus ulcers), the peritoneum, and intravascular devices. Osteomyelitis (usually from a contiguous focus), neurosurgery-related infection, and myositis occur rarely. *Citrobacter* (particularly *C. koseri*) also uncommonly causes neonatal meningitis, with brain abscess complicating 50–80% of cases. Bacteremia is most often due to UTI, biliary or abdominal infection, or intravascular device infection. *Citrobacter* uncommonly causes bacteremia in neutropenic patients. Endocarditis and endovascular infections are rare.

DIAGNOSIS

Citrobacter species are readily isolated and identified; 35–50% of isolates are lactose positive. *C. freundii* is indole negative, whereas *C. koseri* is indole positive.

Treatment: *CITROBACTER* INFECTIONS

C. freundii is more resistant to antibiotics than is *C. koseri.* Ampicillin and the first- and second-generation cephalosporins display poor activity. *Citrobacter* species possess inducible AmpC β-lactamases; derepression may be preexistent or may develop during therapy. Resistance to antipseudomonal penicillins, aztreonam, quinolones, gentamicin, and third-generation cephalosporins is variable but increasing. Combination with β-lactamase inhibitors usually does not increase the susceptibility of *Citrobacter* to β-lactam agents. The prevalence of ESBL-producing isolates is <5%. Imipenem, amikacin, cefepime, tigecycline (with which there is limited clinical experience), and polymyxin B (the agent of last resort because of potential toxicities) are most active, with >90% of strains susceptible.

MORGANELLA AND *PROVIDENCIA* INFECTIONS

M. morganii, *P. stuartii*, and (less frequently) *P. rettgeri* are the members of their respective genera that cause human infections. In terms of epidemiologic associations, pathogenic properties, and clinical manifestations, these organisms are largely similar to *Proteus* species; however, *Morganella* and *Providencia* occur almost exclusively among LTCF residents; to a lesser degree, they affect hospitalized patients.

INFECTIOUS SYNDROMES

These species are primarily urinary tract pathogens, causing UTIs that are most often associated with long-term (>30-day) catheterization. Such infections often lead to biofilm formation and catheter encrustation (sometimes causing catheter obstruction) or to the development of struvite bladder or renal stones (sometimes causing renal obstruction and serving as foci for relapse). Other, less common infectious syndromes include surgical site infection, soft tissue infection (primarily involving decubitus and diabetic ulcers), burn site infection, pneumonia (particularly ventilator-associated), intravascular device infection, and intraabdominal infection. Rarely, the other extraintestinal infections described for GNB also occur. Bacteremia is uncommon; although any infected site can serve as the source, the urinary tract accounts for most cases, and the next most common sources are surgical sites and soft tissues.

DIAGNOSIS

M. morganii and *Providencia* are readily isolated and identified. Nearly all isolates are indole positive but are unable to ferment lactose.

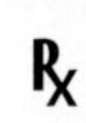

Treatment: *MORGANELLA* AND *PROVIDENCIA* INFECTIONS

Morganella and *Providencia* may be extensively resistant to antibiotics. Most isolates are resistant to ampicillin, first-generation cephalosporins, tigecycline, and polymyxin B; 40% are resistant to quinolones. *Morganella* and *Providencia* possess inducible AmpC β-lactamases; derepression may be preexistent or may develop during therapy. Resistance to antipseudomonal penicillins, aztreonam, gentamicin, TMP-SMX, and the second- and third-generation cephalosporins is emerging but variable. The β-lactamase inhibitor tazobactam increases susceptibility to β-lactam agents, but sulbactam and clavulanic acid do not. Imipenem, amikacin, and cefepime are the most active agents (>90% of isolates susceptible). Removal of an infected catheter or stone may be critical for eradication of UTI.

EDWARDSIELLA INFECTIONS

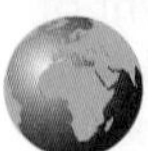

E. tarda is the only member of the genus *Edwardsiella* that is associated with human disease. This organism is found predominantly in freshwater and marine environments and among the animals associated with these settings. Human acquisition occurs primarily during interaction with these reservoirs. *E. tarda* infection is rare in the United States; recently reported cases are mostly from Southeast Asia. This pathogen shares clinical features with both *Salmonella* species and *Vibrio vulnificus.*

INFECTIOUS SYNDROMES

Gastroenteritis is the predominant infectious syndrome (50–80% of infections). Self-limiting watery diarrhea is most common, but severe colitis also occurs. The most common extraintestinal infection is wound infection due to direct inoculation, which is often associated with freshwater-, marine-, or snake-related injuries. Other infectious syndromes result from invasion of the gastrointestinal tract and subsequent bacteremia. Most afflicted hosts have comorbidities (e.g., hepatobiliary disease or iron overload, cancer, or diabetes mellitus). A primary bacteremic syndrome, sometimes complicated by meningitis, has a 40% case-fatality rate. Visceral (primarily hepatic) and intraperitoneal abscesses also occur.

DIAGNOSIS

Although *E. tarda* can readily be isolated and identified, most laboratories do not routinely seek to identify it in stool samples.

Treatment: *EDWARDSIELLA* INFECTIONS

E. tarda is susceptible to most antimicrobial agents appropriate for use against GNB. Gastroenteritis is generally self-limiting, but treatment with a quinolone may hasten resolution. In the setting of severe sepsis, quinolones, third- or fourth-generation cephalosporins, imipenem, and amikacin—either alone or in combination—are the safest choices pending susceptibility information.

ACINETOBACTER INFECTIONS

The *A. baumannii-calcoaceticus* complex is responsible for most *Acinetobacter* infections. *Acinetobacter* is highly prevalent in the environment, being found in most water and soil samples. Whereas *Acinetobacter* has only occasionally been cultured from the moist skin of healthy humans, colonization of the skin and the respiratory and gastrointestinal tracts is common among residents of LTCFs and hospitalized patients. It is not surprising that the overwhelming majority of *Acinetobacter* infections are acquired in LTCFs and hospitals, where the sources for acquisition include health care personnel, medical equipment, food, and the environment. The spectrum of extraintestinal infections caused by *Acinetobacter* is similar to that caused by other GNB. *Acinetobacter* species account for 1–3% of hospital-acquired infections and primarily affect immunocompromised hosts and patients with comorbid disease, especially patients in ICUs. In some centers, the incidence of *Acinetobacter* infections, particularly those due to antibiotic-resistant strains, is increasing significantly. Both sporadic and epidemic infections occur, usually after the first week of hospitalization. Until recently, *A. baumannii* was best known as an agent of nosocomial infections. However, *A. baumannii* can also cause severe community-acquired pneumonia and diverse infections after battlefield injuries.

INFECTIOUS SYNDROMES

The respiratory tract (particularly in mechanically ventilated patients) and intravascular devices are the favored sites of infection. *A. baumannii* uncommonly causes severe CAP, usually in compromised hosts (e.g., alcoholic patients), with the preponderance of cases reported from warm, humid geographic locales. Infections of the catheterized urinary tract, postoperative sites, burn sites, biliary stents, and sinuses (with tube-related ostial obstruction) are less common, as are neurosurgical infections, which may be associated with devices such as pressure monitors. Infections of soft tissue and bone have been common among soldiers with battlefield injuries. Uncommon infections include ophthalmic infection and peritonitis associated with continuous ambulatory peritoneal dialysis. The respiratory tract and intravascular devices are the most common sources of bacteremia.

DIAGNOSIS

On Gram's stain, *Acinetobacter* organisms usually appear as short GNB or coccobacilli. They are strictly aerobic, nonfermenting, and oxidase negative and are readily isolated and identified.

Treatment: *ACINETOBACTER* INFECTIONS

Many strains of *Acinetobacter* are extensively resistant to antimicrobial agents. Empirical combination therapy is prudent pending susceptibility studies. Ampicillin, aztreonam, and the first- and second-generation cephalosporins exhibit little or no activity. The prevalences of resistance to antipseudomonal penicillins, quinolones, third-generation cephalosporins, and gentamicin are 20–90%. Ampicillin/sulbactam, rifampin, tetracyclines, imipenem/cilastatin, tigecycline, and amikacin are often active; however, resistance to all of these agents has been reported. Colistin and polymyxin B have been used with some success against extensively resistant isolates, but probably should be considered a last resort because of their potential toxicities.

INFECTIONS CAUSED BY MISCELLANEOUS GENERA

Species of *Hafnia, Kluyvera, Cedecea, Pantoea, Ewingella, and Photorhabdus* are occasionally isolated from diverse clinical specimens, including blood, sputum, cerebrospinal fluid, joint fluid, bile, and wounds. These organisms are rare and usually opportunistic human pathogens.

FURTHER READINGS

Drudy D et al: *Enterobacter sakazakii*: An emerging pathogen in powdered infant formula. Clin Infect Dis 42:996, 2006

Fang CT et al: *Klebsiella pneumoniae* genotype K1: An emerging pathogen that causes septic ocular or central nervous system complications from pyogenic liver abscess. Clin Infect Dis 45:284, 2007

Fournier PE, Richet H: The epidemiology and control of *Acinetobacter baumannii* in health care facilities. Clin Infect Dis 44:1577, 2007

Hejazi A, Falkiner FR: *Serratia marcescens*. J Med Microbiol 46:903, 1997

Högenauer C et al: *Klebsiella oxytoca* as a causative organism of antibiotic-associated hemorrhagic colitis. N Engl J Med 355:2418, 2006

Kaper J et al: Pathogenic *Escherichia coli*. Nat Rev Microbiol 2:123, 2004

Kim B et al: Bacteraemia due to the tribe Proteeae: A review of 132 cases during a decade (1991-2000). Scand J Infect Dis 35:98, 2003

Lederman E, Crum N: Pyogenic liver abscess with a focus on Klebsiella pneumoniae as a primary pathogen: An emerging disease with unique clinical characteristics. Am J Gastroenterol 100:322, 2005

Munoz-Price LS, Weinstein RA: *Acinetobacter* infection. N Engl J Med 358:1271, 2008

Murray CK, Hospenthal DR: Treatment of multidrug resistant Acinetobacter. Curr Opin Infect Dis 18:502, 2005

Paterson DL: Resistance in gram-negative bacteria: Enterobacteriaceae. Am J Infect Control 34:S20, 2006

Russo TA, Johnson JR: Medical and economic impact of extraintestinal infections due to *Escherichia coli*: Focus on an increasingly important endemic problem. Microbes Infect 5:449, 2003

Scott P et al: An outbreak of multidrug-resistant *Acinetobacter baumannii-calcoaceticus* complex infection in the US military health care system associated with military operations in Iraq. Clin Infect Dis 44:1577, 2007

Shih CC et al: Bacteremia due to *Citrobacter* species: Significance of primary intraabdominal infection. Clin Infect Dis 23:543, 1996

Slaven EM et al: Myonecrosis caused by *Edwardsiella tarda:* A case report and case series of extraintestinal *E. tarda* infections. Clin Infect Dis 32:1430, 2001

CHAPTER 52

HELICOBACTER PYLORI INFECTIONS

John C. Atherton ■ Martin J. Blaser

DEFINITION

Helicobacter pylori, which persistently colonizes the stomachs of ~50% of the world's human population, is the main risk factor for peptic ulceration as well as for gastric adenocarcinoma and gastric MALT (mucosa-associated lymphoid tissue) lymphoma. Treatment for *H. pylori* has revolutionized the management of peptic ulcer disease, providing a permanent cure in many cases. The prevention of *H. pylori* colonization could potentially represent primary prevention of gastric malignancy and peptic ulceration. However, controversial but increasing evidence indicates that *H. pylori* may in fact offer some protection against recently emergent diseases—most notably gastroesophageal reflux disease (GERD) and its complications (e.g., esophageal adenocarcinoma). Thus clearance of *H. pylori* from human populations may not be without negative repercussions.

ETIOLOGIC AGENT

H. pylori is a gram-negative bacillus that has naturally colonized humans for at least tens of thousands of years. It is noninvasive and lives in gastric mucus, with a small proportion of the bacteria adherent to the mucosa. Its spiral shape and flagella render *H. pylori* motile in the mucus environment. This organism has several acid-resistance mechanisms, most notably a highly expressed urease that catalyzes urea hydrolysis to produce buffering ammonia. *H. pylori* is microaerophilic (requiring low levels of oxygen), is slow-growing, and requires complex growth media in vitro. Publication of several complete genomic sequences of *H. pylori* since 1997 has led to significant advances in the understanding of the organism's biology.

A very small proportion of gastric *Helicobacter* infections are due to species other than *H. pylori*, which probably are acquired most often as zoonoses. Whether these non-*pylori* gastric helicobacters cause disease remains controversial. In immunocompromised hosts, several nongastric (intestinal) *Helicobacter* species can cause disease with clinical features resembling those of *Campylobacter* infections; these species are covered in Chap. 56.

EPIDEMIOLOGY

The prevalence of *H. pylori* among adults is ~30% in the United States and other developed countries as opposed to >80% in most developing countries. In the United States, prevalence varies with age: ~50% of 60-year-old persons and ~20% of 30-year-old persons are colonized. *H. pylori* is usually acquired in childhood. The age association is due mostly to a birth-cohort effect whereby current 60-year-olds were more commonly colonized as children than current 30-year-olds. Spontaneous acquisition or loss of *H. pylori* in adulthood is uncommon. Other strong risk factors for *H. pylori* colonization are markers of crowding and poor hygiene in childhood. The very low incidence among children in developed countries at present is probably due, at least in part, to improved living standards and increased use of antibiotics.

Humans are the only important reservoir of *H. pylori*. Children may acquire the organism from their parents (more often from the mother) or from other children. Whether transmission usually takes place by the fecal-oral or the oral-oral route is unknown, but *H. pylori* is easily cultured from vomitus and gastroesophageal refluxate and is less easily cultured from stool.

PATHOLOGY AND PATHOGENESIS

H. pylori colonization induces a tissue response in the stomach; termed *chronic superficial gastritis*, this response includes infiltration of the mucosa by both mononuclear and polymorphonuclear cells. (The term *gastritis* should be used specifically to describe histologic features; it has also been used to describe endoscopic appearances and even symptoms, which do not correlate with microscopic findings or even with the presence of *H. pylori*.) Although *H. pylori* is capable of numerous adaptations that prevent excessive stimulation of the immune system, colonization is accompanied by a considerable persistent immune response, including the production of both local and systemic antibodies as well as cell-mediated responses. However, these responses are ineffective in clearing the bacterium. This inefficient clearing appears to be due in part to *H. pylori*'s downregulation of the immune system, which fosters its own persistence.

Most *H. pylori*–colonized persons do not develop clinical sequelae. That some persons develop overt disease whereas others do not is related to a combination of factors: bacterial strain differences, host susceptibility to disease, and environmental factors. Several *H. pylori* virulence factors are more common among strains that are associated with disease than among those that are not. The *cag* pathogenicity island (PaI) is a group of genes that encodes a secretion system through which a specific protein, CagA, is translocated into epithelial cells. CagA affects host cell signal transduction, inducing proliferative and cytoskeletal changes. The secretion system also induces a proinflammatory cytokine response, which results in enhanced inflammation. Patients with peptic ulcer disease or gastric adenocarcinoma are more likely than persons without these conditions to be colonized by *cag* PaI-positive strains. The secreted *H. pylori* protein VacA occurs in several forms. Strains with the more active forms are more commonly isolated from patients with peptic ulcer disease or gastric carcinoma than from persons without these conditions. BabA and SabA, adhesins expressed by only some strains, are associated with increased gastric inflammation and with increased risk of peptic ulceration and gastric adenocarcinoma. Other *H. pylori* factors that may affect disease risk are still being described.

The best-characterized host determinants of disease are genetic polymorphisms leading to enhanced *H. pylori*–stimulated secretion of proinflammatory cytokines such as interleukin 1β. *H. pylori*–positive individuals with these polymorphisms are at increased risk of hypochlorhydria and gastric adenocarcinoma. In addition, environmental cofactors are important in pathogenesis. Smoking increases the risks of ulcers and cancer in *H. pylori*–positive individuals. Diets high in salt and preserved foods increase cancer risk, whereas diets high in antioxidants and vitamin C are protective.

The pattern of gastric inflammation is associated with disease risk: antral-predominant gastritis is most closely linked with duodenal ulceration, whereas pangastritis is linked with gastric ulceration and adenocarcinoma. This difference probably explains why patients with duodenal ulceration rarely develop gastric adenocarcinoma later in life, despite being colonized by *H. pylori*.

How gastric colonization causes duodenal ulceration is now becoming clearer. *H. pylori*–induced gastritis diminishes the number of somatostatin-producing D cells. Since somatostatin inhibits gastrin release, gastrin levels are higher than in *H. pylori*–negative persons. These increased gastrin levels lead to increased meal-stimulated acid secretion in the gastric corpus, which is only mildly inflamed in antral-predominant gastritis. In turn, increased acid secretion eventually induces protective gastric metaplasia in the duodenum; the duodenum can then become colonized by *H. pylori*, inflamed, and ulcerated.

The pathogenesis of gastric ulceration and that of gastric adenocarcinoma are less well understood, although both conditions arise in association with pan- or corpus-predominant gastritis. The hormonal changes described above still occur, but the inflamed acid-producing gastric corpus produces less acid, with consequent relative hypochlorhydria, despite the hypergastrinemia. Gastric ulcers usually occur at the junction of antral and corpus-type mucosa, and this region is particularly inflamed. Gastric cancer probably stems from progressive DNA damage and the survival of abnormal epithelial cell clones. The DNA damage is thought to be due principally to reactive oxygen and nitrogen species arising from inflammatory cells and perhaps from other bacteria that survive in hypochlorhydric stomachs. Longitudinal analyses of gastric biopsy specimens taken years apart from the same patient show that the common *intestinal* type of gastric adenocarcinoma follows the stepwise changes from simple gastritis to gastric atrophy, intestinal metaplasia, and dysplasia. A second, *diffuse* type of gastric adenocarcinoma may arise directly from simple chronic gastritis.

CLINICAL MANIFESTATIONS

Essentially all *H. pylori*–colonized persons have gastric tissue responses, but fewer than 15% develop associated illnesses such as peptic ulceration, gastric adenocarcinoma, or gastric lymphoma (Fig. 52-1).

Worldwide, >80% of duodenal ulcers and >60% of gastric ulcers are related to *H. pylori* colonization, although the proportion of ulcers due to aspirin and nonsteroidal anti-inflammatory drugs (NSAIDs) is increasing, especially in developed countries. The main lines of evidence for an ulcer-promoting role for *H. pylori* are (1) that the presence of the organism is a risk factor for the development of ulcers, (2) that non–NSAID-induced ulcers rarely develop in the absence of *H. pylori*, (3) that eradication of *H. pylori* markedly reduces rates of ulcer relapse, and (4) that experimental *H. pylori* infection of gerbils causes gastric ulceration.

Prospective nested case-control studies have shown that *H. pylori* colonization is a risk factor for adenocarcinomas of the distal (noncardia) stomach. Long-term

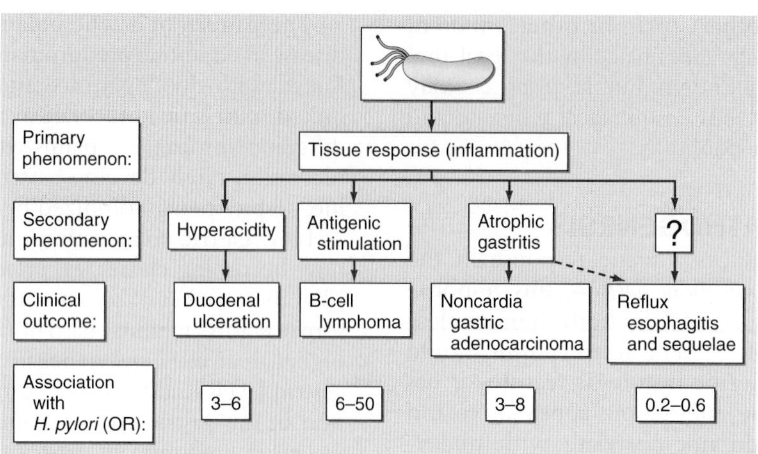

FIGURE 52-1

Schematic representation of the relationships between colonization with *Helicobacter pylori* and diseases of the upper gastrointestinal tract among persons in developed countries. Essentially all persons colonized with *H. pylori* develop a host response, which is generally termed *chronic gastritis.* The nature of the interaction of the host with the particular bacterial population determines the clinical outcome. *H. pylori* colonization increases the lifetime risk of peptic ulcer disease, noncardia gastric cancer, and B-cell non-Hodgkin's gastric lymphoma [odds ratios (ORs) for all, >3]. In contrast, a growing body of evidence indicates that *H. pylori* colonization (especially with *cagA*⁺ strains) protects against adenocarcinoma of the esophagus (and the sometimes related gastric cardia) and premalignant lesions such as Barrett's esophagus (OR, <1). Although the incidences of peptic ulcer disease (cases not due to nonsteroidal anti-inflammatory drugs) and noncardia gastric cancer are declining in developed countries, the incidence of adenocarcinoma of the esophagus is rapidly increasing. [*Adapted from Blaser MJ: Hypothesis: The changing relationships of Helicobacter pylori and humans: Implications for health and disease. J Infect Dis 179:1523, 1999, with permission.*]

experimental infection of gerbils also may result in gastric adenocarcinoma. Moreover, the presence of *H. pylori* is strongly associated with primary gastric lymphoma, although this condition is less common. Many low-grade gastric B-cell lymphomas arising from MALT are driven by T-cell stimulation, which in turn is driven by *H. pylori* antigen stimulation; *H. pylori* antigen–driven tumors may regress either fully or partially after *H. pylori* eradication.

Many patients have upper gastrointestinal symptoms but have normal results in upper gastrointestinal endoscopy (so-called functional or nonulcer dyspepsia). Because *H. pylori* is common, some of these patients will be positive for the organism. *H. pylori* eradication leads to symptom resolution only a little (<10%) more commonly than does placebo treatment. Whether such patients have peptic ulcers in remission at the time of endoscopy or whether a small subgroup of patients with true functional dyspepsia respond to *H. pylori* treatment is unclear.

Much interest has focused on a possible protective role for *H. pylori* against GERD and adenocarcinoma of the esophagus and gastric cardia. The main lines of evidence for this role are (1) that there is a temporal relationship between a falling prevalence of *H. pylori* colonization and a rising incidence of these conditions, and (2) that, in most studies, the prevalence of *H. pylori* colonization (especially with proinflammatory *cagA*⁺ strains) is significantly lower among patients with these esophageal diseases than among control subjects. The mechanism underlying this protective effect appears to include *H. pylori*–induced hypochlorhydria. Since, at the individual level, GERD symptoms may decrease, worsen, or remain unchanged after treatment targeting *H. pylori*, concerns about GERD should not affect decisions about *H. pylori* treatment when a definite indication exists.

H. pylori has an increasingly recognized role in other gastric pathologies. It may be one initial precipitant of autoimmune gastritis and pernicious anemia and also may predispose some patients to iron deficiency through hypochlorhydria and reduced iron absorption. In addition, several extragastrointestinal pathologies have been linked with *H. pylori* colonization, although evidence of causality is less strong. Several small studies have documented improvement or resolution of idiopathic thrombocytopenic purpura after treatment for *H. pylori* colonization. A potentially important but even more controversial association is with ischemic heart disease and cerebrovascular disease. However, the strength of these associations is reduced if confounding factors are taken into account, and most authorities consider the associations to be noncausal.

DIAGNOSIS

Tests for *H. pylori* can be divided into two groups: invasive tests, which require upper gastrointestinal endoscopy and are based on the analysis of gastric biopsy specimens, and noninvasive tests (Table 52-1). Endoscopy often is not performed in the initial management of young dyspeptic patients without "alarm" symptoms, but is commonly used to exclude malignancy in older patients. If endoscopy is performed, the most convenient biopsy-based test is the biopsy urease test, in which one large or

TABLE 52-1

TESTS COMMONLY USED TO DETECT *HELICOBACTER PYLORI*

TEST	ADVANTAGES	DISADVANTAGES
Invasive (Based on Endoscopic Biopsy)		
Biopsy urease test	Quick, simple	Some commercial tests not fully sensitive before 24 h
Histology	May give additional histologic information	Sensitivity dependent on experience and use of special stains
Culture	Permits determination of antibiotic susceptibility	Sensitivity dependent on experience
Noninvasive		
Serology	Inexpensive and convenient	Cannot be used for early follow-up; some commercial kits inaccurate
^{13}C or ^{14}C urea breath test	Inexpensive and simpler than endoscopy; useful for follow-up after treatment	Low-dose irradiation in ^{14}C test (although ^{14}C is rarely used)
Stool antigen test	Inexpensive and convenient; useful for follow-up after treatment; may be useful in children	New test; role not fully established; appears less accurate than urea breath test, particularly when used to assess treatment success

two small antral biopsy specimens are placed into a gel containing urea and an indicator. The presence of *H. pylori* urease elicits a color change, which often occurs within minutes but can require up to 24 h. Histologic examination of biopsy specimens for *H. pylori* is also accurate, provided that a special stain (e.g., a modified Giemsa or silver stain) permitting optimal visualization of the organism is used. If biopsy specimens are obtained from both antrum and corpus, histologic study yields additional information, including the degree and pattern of inflammation, atrophy, metaplasia, and dysplasia. Microbiologic culture is most specific but may be insensitive because of difficulty with *H. pylori* isolation. Once the organism is cultured, its identity as *H. pylori* can be confirmed by its typical appearance on Gram's stain and its positive reactions in oxidase, catalase, and urease tests. Moreover, the organism's susceptibility to antibiotics can be determined; this information can be clinically useful in difficult cases. The occasional biopsy specimens containing the less common non-*pylori* gastric helicobacters give only weakly positive results in the biopsy urease test. Positive identification of these bacteria requires visualization of the characteristic long, tight spirals in histologic sections.

Noninvasive *H. pylori* testing is the norm if gastric cancer does not need to be excluded by endoscopy. The most consistently accurate test is the urea breath test. In this simple test, the patient drinks a labeled urea solution and then blows into a tube. The urea is labeled with either the nonradioactive isotope ^{13}C or a minute dose of the radioactive isotope ^{14}C. If *H. pylori* urease is present, the urea is hydrolyzed and labeled carbon dioxide is detected in breath samples. The stool antigen test, another simple assay, is more convenient and potentially less expensive than the urea breath test but has been slightly less accurate in some comparative studies. The simplest tests for ascertaining *H. pylori* status are serologic assays measuring specific IgG levels in serum by enzyme-linked immunosorbent assay or immunoblot. The best of these tests are as accurate as other diagnostic methods, but many commercial tests—especially rapid office tests—do not perform well.

The urea breath test, the stool antigen test, and biopsy-based tests can all be used to assess the success of treatment (Fig. 52-2). However, because these tests are dependent on *H. pylori* load, their use <4 weeks after treatment may lead to false-negative results. Furthermore, these tests are unreliable if performed within 4 weeks of intercurrent treatment with antibiotics or bismuth compounds or within 2 weeks of the discontinuation of proton pump inhibitor (PPI) treatment. In the assessment of treatment success, noninvasive tests are normally preferred; however, after gastric ulceration, endoscopy should be repeated to ensure healing and to exclude gastric carcinoma by further histologic sampling.

Serologic tests are not used to monitor treatment success, as the gradual drop in titer of *H. pylori*–specific antibodies is too slow to be of practical use.

℞ Treatment: *H. PYLORI* INFECTIONS

The most clear-cut indications for treatment are *H. pylori*–related duodenal or gastric ulceration or low-grade gastric B-cell lymphoma. *H. pylori* should be eradicated in patients with documented ulcer disease, whether or not the ulcers are currently active, to reduce the likelihood of relapse (Fig. 52-2). Many guidelines now recommend *H. pylori* treatment in uninvestigated simple dyspepsia after noninvasive diagnosis; others also recommend treatment in functional dyspepsia, in case the patient is one of the perhaps 5–10% to benefit (beyond placebo effects) from such treatment. People with a strong family history of gastric cancer should be treated to eradicate *H. pylori* in the hope that their risk will be reduced. For several reasons, widespread community screening for and treatment of *H. pylori* as primary prophylaxis for gastric cancer and peptic ulcers are not currently recommended. To begin with, it is unclear whether treatment for *H. pylori* reduces the risk of cancer from that in persons who have never acquired the organism. The largest study to date (performed in China) showed no such risk

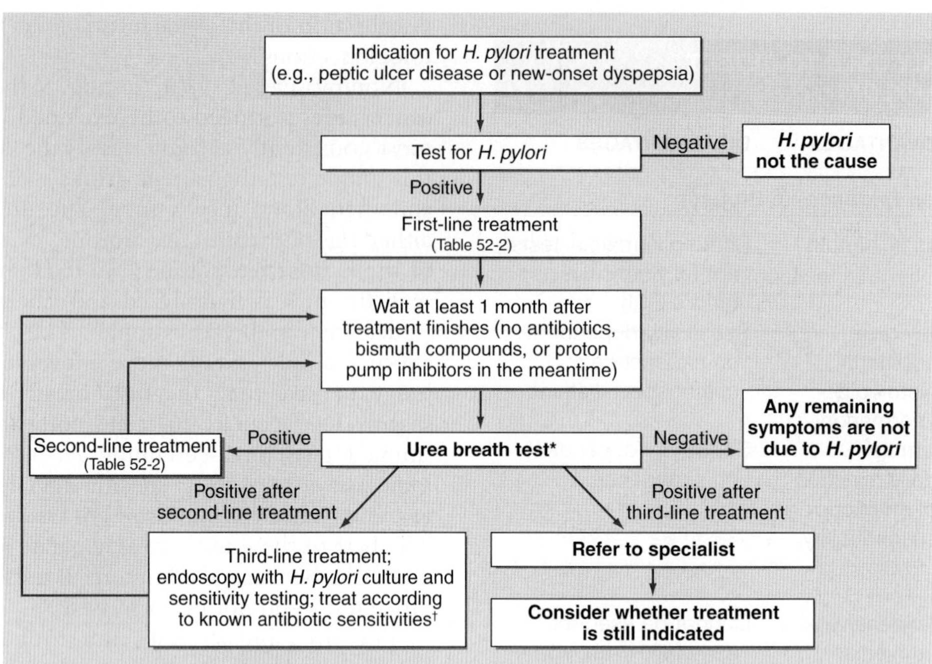

FIGURE 52-2

Algorithm for the management of *Helicobacter pylori* infection. *Occasionally, an endoscopy and a biopsy-based test are used instead of a urea breath test in follow-up after treatment. The main indication for these invasive tests is gastric ulceration; in this condition, as opposed to duodenal ulceration, it is important to check healing and to exclude underlying gastric adenocarcinoma. †Some authorities now use empirical third-line regimens, several of which have been described.

reduction during the 7 years of follow-up. Moreover, treatment has side effects that can be severe in rare cases. Antibiotic resistance may arise in *H. pylori* or other incidentally carried bacteria. Otherwise healthy people may become anxious, especially if treatment is unsuccessful. Finally, it is possible that treatment for *H. pylori* will provoke or exacerbate GERD.

Although *H. pylori* is susceptible to a wide range of antibiotics in vitro, monotherapy has been disappointing in vivo, probably because of inadequate antibiotic delivery to the colonization niche. Failure of monotherapy has prompted the development of multidrug regimens, the most successful of which are triple and quadruple combinations that produce *H. pylori* eradication rates of >90% in many trials and >75% in clinical practice. Current regimens consist of a PPI or ranitidine bismuth citrate and two or three antimicrobial agents given for 7–14 days (Table 52-2).

The two most important factors in successful *H. pylori* treatment are the patient's close compliance with the regimen and the use of drugs to which *H. pylori* has not acquired resistance. Treatment failure after minor lapses in compliance is common and often leads to acquired resistance to metronidazole or clarithromycin. To stress the importance of compliance, written instructions should be given to the patient, and minor side effects of the regimen should be explained. Resistance to metronidazole and clarithromycin is of growing concern. Clarithromycin resistance is less prevalent but, if present, usually results in treatment failure. Metronidazole-resistant strains of *H. pylori* are more common, but these strains still may be cleared by metronidazole-containing regimens. Assessment of antibiotic susceptibilities before treatment would be optimal but is not usually undertaken because endoscopy and mucosal biopsy are necessary to obtain *H. pylori* for culture and because most microbiology laboratories are inexperienced in *H. pylori* culture. In the absence of susceptibility information, a history of the patient's antibiotic use should be obtained, and, even if only distant exposure is identified (e.g., previous metronidazole consumption for giardiasis or trichomoniasis), use of the agent should be avoided if possible. If initial *H. pylori* treatment fails, two strategies are commonly used (Fig. 52-2). One is re-treatment with a quadruple-drug regimen (Table 52-2). The second is endoscopy, biopsy, and culture plus treatment based on documented antibiotic sensitivities. If re-treatment fails, susceptibility testing should usually be performed, although empirical third-line therapies have been described.

Clearance of non-*pylori* gastric helicobacters can follow the use of bismuth compounds alone or of triple-drug regimens. However, in the absence of trials, it is unclear whether this outcome represents successful treatment or natural clearance of the bacterium.

PREVENTION

Carriage of *H. pylori* has considerable public health significance in developed countries, where it is associated with peptic ulcer disease and gastric adenocarcinoma, and in developing countries, where gastric adenocarcinoma is an even more common cause of cancer death

TABLE 52-2

RECOMMENDED TREATMENT REGIMENS FOR *HELICOBACTER PYLORI*

REGIMEN, DURATION	DRUG 1	DRUG 2	DRUG 3	DRUG 4
First-Line Treatment				
Regimen 1: OCA (7–14 days)[a]	Omeprazole[b] (20 mg bid)	Clarithromycin (500 mg bid)	Amoxicillin (1 g bid)	—
Regimen 2: OCM (7–14 days)	Omeprazole[b] (20 mg bid)	Clarithromycin (500 mg bid)	Metronidazole (500 mg bid)	—
Second-Line Treatment[c]				
Regimen 3: OBTM (14 days)[d]	Omeprazole[b] (20 mg bid)	Bismuth subsalicylate (2 tabs qid)	Tetracycline HCl (500 mg qid)	Metronidazole (500 mg tid)

[a]Meta-analyses show that a 14-day course of therapy is slightly superior to a 7-day course. However, the success rate for 7-day therapy is so high in northern Europe (>80%) that 7-day treatment is recommended in most guidelines.

[b]Omeprazole may be replaced with any proton pump inhibitor at an equivalent dosage or, in Regimens 1 and 2, with ranitidine bismuth citrate (400 mg).

[c]An alternative to this second-line therapy is to culture *H. pylori* and to be guided by antibiotic susceptibility data. Patients in whom second-line therapy fails should undergo endoscopy for *H. pylori* culture and antibiotic susceptibility testing.

[d]Data supporting this regimen come mainly from Europe and are based on the use of bismuth subcitrate and metronidazole (400 mg tid).

late in life. However, given that *H. pylori* has co-evolved with its human host over millennia, preventing or eliminating colonization on a population basis may have distinct disadvantages. For example, absence of *H. pylori* has been reported to increase the risk of diarrheal diseases and of GERD and its complications, including esophageal adenocarcinoma. Recently, we have speculated that the disappearance of *H. pylori* is associated with an increased risk of other emerging diseases reflecting aspects of the current Western lifestyle, such as asthma, obesity, and type 2 diabetes mellitus. If mass prevention were contemplated, vaccination would be the most obvious method, and experimental immunization of animals has given promising results. However, in the United States and other developed countries, rates of *H. pylori* carriage, peptic ulceration, and gastric adenocarcinoma are falling, whereas rates of esophageal reflux disease and its sequelae are increasing. Thus prevention of colonization in these countries may be unnecessary or even unwise.

FURTHER READINGS

Agarwal K, Agarwal S: *Helicobacter pylori* vaccine: from past to future. Mayo Clin Proc 83:169, 2008

Blaser MJ: Who are we? Indigenous microbes and the ecology of human diseases. EMBO Rep 7:956, 2006

———, Atherton JC: *Helicobacter pylori* persistence: Biology and disease. J Clin Invest 113:321, 2004

Chen Y, Blaser MJ: Inverse associations of *Helicobacter pylori* with asthma and allergies. Arch Intern Med 167:821, 2007

Chey WD et al: American College of Gastroenterology Guideline on the Management of *Helicobacter pylori* Infection. Am J Gastroenterol 102:1808, 2007

Franco AT et al: Activation of beta-catenin by carcinogenic *Helicobacter pylori*. Proc Natl Acad Sci USA 102:10646, 2005

Fuccio L et al: Meta-analysis: Duration of first-line proton-pump inhibitor based triple therapy for *Helicobacter pylori* eradication. Ann Intern Med 147:553, 2007

Hansson LE et al: The risk of stomach cancer in patients with gastric or duodenal ulcer disease. N Engl J Med 335:242, 1996

Kamangar F et al: Opposing risks of gastric cardia and noncardia gastric adenocarcinomas associated with *Helicobacter pylori* seropositivity. J Natl Cancer Inst 98:1445, 2006

Linz B et al: An African origin for the intimate association between humans and *Helicobacter pylori*. Nature 445:915, 2007

Marshall BJ, Warren JR: Unidentified curved bacilli in the stomach of patients with gastritis and peptic ulceration. Lancet 1:1311, 1984

Odenbreit S et al: Translocation of *Helicobacter pylori* CagA into gastric epithelial cells by type IV secretion. Science 287:1497, 2000

Parsonnet J et al: *Helicobacter pylori* infection and gastric lymphoma. N Engl J Med 330:1267, 1994

Rieder G et al: *Helicobacter pylori* cag-type IV secretion system facilitates corpus colonization to induce precancerous conditions in Mongolian gerbils. Gastroenterology 128:1229, 2005

Tomb JF et al: The complete genome sequence of the gastric pathogen *Helicobacter pylori*. Nature 388:539, 1997

Vaira D et al: Sequential therapy versus standard triple-drug therapy for *Helicobacter pylori* eradication: A randomized trial. Ann Intern Med 146:556, 2007

Wong BC et al: *Helicobacter pylori* eradication to prevent gastric cancer in a high-risk region of China: A randomized controlled trial. JAMA 291:187, 2004

CHAPTER 53

INFECTIONS DUE TO *PSEUDOMONAS* SPECIES AND RELATED ORGANISMS

Reuben Ramphal

The pseudomonads are a heterogeneous group of gram-negative bacteria that have in common an inability to ferment lactose. Once classified in the genus *Pseudomonas*, the members of this group are now assigned to three medically important genera—*Pseudomonas, Burkholderia*, and *Stenotrophomonas*—whose biologic behaviors encompass both similarities and marked differences and whose genetic makeups differ in many respects. The pathogenicity of most pseudomonads is based on opportunism; the exceptions are the organisms that cause melioidosis (*B. pseudomallei*) and glanders (*B. mallei*).

P. aeruginosa, the major pathogen of the group, is mainly associated with infections in hospitalized patients and in patients with cystic fibrosis (CF). Cytotoxic chemotherapy, mechanical ventilation, and broad-spectrum antibiotic therapy probably paved the way for increasing colonization and infection by *P. aeruginosa*. Since the implementation of these advances in medical therapy, most conditions predisposing to *P. aeruginosa* infections have involved host compromise and/or broad-spectrum antibiotic use. Other members of the genus *Pseudomonas*—*P. putida, P. fluorescens*, and *P. stutzeri*—infect humans infrequently.

The genus *Burkholderia* comprises >40 species, of which *B. cepacia* is most frequently encountered in Western countries. Like *P. aeruginosa, B. cepacia* is both a nosocomial pathogen and a cause of infection in CF. The other medically important members of this genus are *B. pseudomallei* and *B. mallei,* which, as mentioned above, cause melioidosis and glanders, respectively.

The genus *Stenotrophomonas* contains one species of medical significance, *S. maltophilia* (previously classified in the genera *Pseudomonas* and *Xanthomonas*). This organism is strictly an opportunist that "overgrows" in the setting of potent broad-spectrum antibiotic use.

PSEUDOMONAS AERUGINOSA

EPIDEMIOLOGY

P. aeruginosa is found in most moist environments. Soil, plants, vegetables, tap water, and countertops can all be reservoirs for this microbe, which has simple nutritional needs. Given the ubiquity of *P. aeruginosa*, contact with the organism obviously is not sufficient for colonization or infection. Clinical and experimental observations suggest that *P. aeruginosa* infection often occurs concomitantly with host defense compromise, mucosal trauma, physiologic derangement, and antibiotic-mediated suppression of normal flora. Thus it comes as no surprise that the majority of *P. aeruginosa* infections occur in intensive care units (ICUs), where these factors frequently converge. It is believed that the organism is initially acquired from environmental sources, but patient-to-patient spread also occurs in clinics and families.

Burn patients once appeared to be unusually susceptible to *P. aeruginosa*. For example, in 1959–1963, *Pseudomonas* burn-wound sepsis was the principal cause of death in 60% of burn patients at the U.S. Army Institute of Surgical Research. For reasons that are unclear, however, *P. aeruginosa* infection in burn patients is no longer the major problem that it was during the 1950s and 1960s. Similarly, in the 1960s, *P. aeruginosa* appeared as a common pathogen in patients receiving cytotoxic chemotherapy at many institutions in the United States, subsequently diminishing in importance. Despite this subsidence, *P. aeruginosa* remains one of the most feared pathogens in this population because of its high mortality rate.

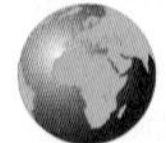

Moreover, in the Far East and some parts of Latin America, *P. aeruginosa* continues to be the most common cause of gram-negative bacteremia in neutropenic patients.

In contrast to the trends for burn patients and neutropenic patients in the United States, the incidence of *P. aeruginosa* infections among patients with CF has not changed. *P. aeruginosa* remains the most common contributing factor to respiratory failure in CF and is responsible for the majority of deaths among CF patients.

LABORATORY FEATURES

P. aeruginosa is a nonfastidious, motile gram-negative rod that grows on most common laboratory media, including blood and MacConkey agars. It is easily identified in the laboratory on primary-isolation agar plates by pigment production that confers a yellow to dark green or even bluish appearance. Colonies have a shiny "gun-metal" appearance and a characteristic fruity odor. Two of the identifying biochemical characteristics of *P. aeruginosa* are an inability to ferment lactose on MacConkey agar and a positive reaction in the oxidase test. Most strains are identified on the basis of these readily detectable laboratory features even before extensive biochemical testing is done. Some isolates from CF patients are easily identified by their mucoid appearance, which is due to the production of large amounts of the mucoid exopolysaccharide alginate.

PATHOGENESIS

Unraveling the mechanisms underlying disease caused by *P. aeruginosa* has proven challenging. Of the common gram-negative bacteria, no other species produces such a large number of putative virulence factors (Table 53-1). Yet *P. aeruginosa* rarely initiates an infectious process in the absence of host injury or compromise, and few of its putative virulence factors have been shown definitively to be involved in disease in humans. Despite its metabolic versatility and possession of multiple colonizing factors, *P. aeruginosa* exhibits no competitive advantage over enteric bacteria in the human gut; neither is it a normal inhabitant of the human gastrointestinal tract, despite the host's continuous environmental exposure to the organism.

Acute P. Aeruginosa *Infections*

Motility and Colonization

A general tenet of bacterial pathogenesis is that most bacteria must adhere to surfaces or colonize a host niche in order to initiate disease. Most pathogens examined thus far possess adherence factors called *adhesins*. *P. aeruginosa* is no exception. Among its many adhesins are its pili, which demonstrate adhesive properties for a variety of cells and adhere best to injured cell surfaces. In the organism's flagellum, the flagellin molecule binds to cells, and the flagellar cap attaches to mucins through the recognition of glycan chains. Nonflagellated *P. aeruginosa* mutants are less virulent or avirulent in some animal models; however, it is unclear whether this decreased virulence is due to the loss of adhesion or to the loss of other flagellar functions. Other *P. aeruginosa* adhesins include the outer core of the lipopolysaccharide (LPS) molecule, which binds to the cystic fibrosis transmembrane conductance regulator (CFTR) and aids in internalization of the organism, and the alginate coat of mucoid strains, which enhances adhesion to cells and mucins. In addition, membrane proteins and lectins have been proposed as colonization factors. It appears that the deletion of any given adhesin is not sufficient to abrogate the ability of *P. aeruginosa* to colonize surfaces.

TABLE 53-1

MAIN PUTATIVE VIRULENCE FACTORS OF *PSEUDOMONAS AERUGINOSA*

SUBSTANCE/ ORGANELLE	FUNCTION	VIRULENCE IN ANIMAL DISEASE
Pili	Adhesion to cells	?
Flagella	Adhesion, motility, inflammation	Yes
Lipopolysaccharide	Antiphagocytic activity, inflammation	Yes
Type III secretion system	Cytotoxic activity (ExoU)	Yes
Proteases	Proteolytic activity, cytotoxicity	?
Phospholipases	Cytotoxicity	?
Exotoxin A	Cytotoxicity	?

Evasion of Host Defenses

The transition from bacterial colonization to disease requires the evasion of host defenses by a substantial number of bacteria. *P. aeruginosa* appears to be well equipped for evasion. Attached bacteria inject four known toxins (ExoS, ExoU, ExoT, and ExoY) via a type III secretion system that allows the bacteria to evade phagocytic cells either by cytotoxicity or by inhibition of phagocytosis. Mutants with defects in this system fail to disseminate in some animal models of infection. Secreted toxins such as exotoxin A and leukocidin have the potential to kill phagocytic cells, and multiple secreted elastases may degrade host effector molecules released in response to infection.

Tissue Injury

Among gram-negative bacteria, *P. aeruginosa* probably produces the largest number of substances that are toxic to cells and thus may injure tissues. The type III toxins are capable of tissue injury. However, their delivery requires the adherence of the organism to cells. Thus the effects of these toxins are likely to be local or to depend on the presence of vast numbers of bacteria. On the other hand, secreted diffusible toxins can act freely wherever they come into contact with cells. Exotoxin A, four different elastases, at least two phospholipases, rhamnolipids, pyocyanin, and hydrocyanic acid are all produced by this organism and are all capable of inducing host injury.

Inflammatory Components

The inflammatory response to many products of *P. aeruginosa* is arguably the most important factor in disease causation. For example, injurious inflammatory responses to the lipid A component of the LPSs and to the flagellin are mediated through the Toll-like receptor (TLR) system (principally TLR4 and TLR5). These inflammatory responses are required for successful defense against *P. aeruginosa* (i.e., in their absence, animals are defenseless against *P. aeruginosa* infection), but florid responses are likely to result in disease. When the sepsis syndrome and septic shock develop in *P. aeruginosa* infection, they are probably the result of the host response to one or both of these substances. Another layer of complexity is added by the possibility that injury to cells by many of the described factors may cause cell death and the release of cellular components (e.g., heat-shock proteins) that may activate the TLR system.

Chronic P. Aeruginosa *Infections*

Chronic infection due to *P. aeruginosa* occurs mainly in the lungs in the setting of structural pulmonary diseases. The classic example is CF; others include bronchiectasis and chronic relapsing panbronchiolitis, a disease seen in Japan and some Pacific Islands. Hallmarks of these illnesses are altered mucociliary clearance leading to mucus stasis and mucus accumulation in the lungs. There is probably a common factor that selects for *P. aeruginosa* colonization in these lung diseases—perhaps the adhesiveness of *P. aeruginosa* for mucus, a phenomenon that is not noted for most other common gram-negative bacteria, and/or the ability of *P. aeruginosa* to evade host defenses in mucus. Furthermore, *P. aeruginosa* seems to change in ways that allow its prolonged survival in the lung without an early fatal outcome for the host. The strains found in CF patients exhibit minimal production of virulence factors. Some strains even lose the ability to produce pili and flagella, and most become complement-sensitive because of the loss of the O side chain of their LPS molecules. An example of the impact of these changes is found in the organism's discontinuation of the production of flagellin (probably its most strongly proinflammatory molecule) when it encounters purulent mucus. This response probably dampens the host's response, allowing the organism to survive in mucus. *P. aeruginosa* is also believed to lose the ability to secrete many of its injectable toxins during growth in mucus. Although the alginate coat is thought to play a role in the organism's survival, alginate is not essential, since nonmucoid strains are commonly found in chronic lung diseases other than CF. In short, virulence in chronic infections may be mediated mainly by the attenuated host inflammatory response, which slowly injures the lungs over decades.

CLINICAL MANIFESTATIONS

P. aeruginosa causes infections at almost all sites in the body. The infections encountered most commonly in hospitalized patients are described below.

Bacteremia

Crude mortality rates exceeding 50% have been reported among patients with *P. aeruginosa* bacteremia. Consequently, this clinical entity has been much feared, and its management has been attempted with the use of multiple antibiotics. Recent publications report attributable mortality rates of 28–44%, with the precise figure depending on the adequacy of treatment and the seriousness of the underlying disease. In the past, the patient with *P. aeruginosa* bacteremia classically was neutropenic or had a burn injury. Today, however, a minority of patients in these categories have bacteremic *P. aeruginosa* infections. Rather, *P. aeruginosa* bacteremia is seen most often in patients on ICUs.

The clinical presentation of *P. aeruginosa* bacteremia rarely differs from that of sepsis in general. Patients are usually febrile, but those who are most severely ill may be in shock or even hypothermic. The only point differentiating this entity from gram-negative sepsis of other causes may be the distinctive skin lesions (ecthyma gangrenosum) of *Pseudomonas* infection, which occur almost exclusively in markedly neutropenic patients and patients with AIDS. These small or large, painful, reddish, maculopapular lesions have a geographic margin; they are initially pink, then darken to purple, and finally become black and necrotic (Fig. 53-1). Histopathologic studies indicate that the lesions are due to vascular invasion and are teeming with bacteria. Although similar lesions may occur in aspergillosis and mucormycosis, their presence suggests *P. aeruginosa* bacteremia as the most likely diagnosis.

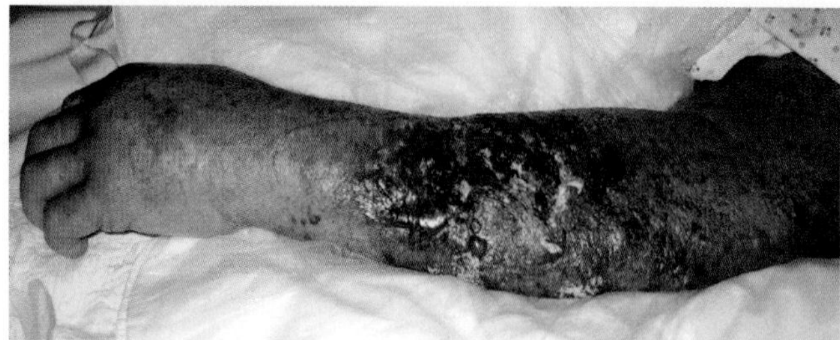

FIGURE 53-1
Ecthyma gangrenosum in a neutropenic patient 3 days after onset.

℞ Treatment: BACTEREMIA

(Table 53-2) Antimicrobial treatment of *P. aeruginosa* bacteremia has been controversial. Before 1971, the outcome of *Pseudomonas* bacteremia in febrile neutropenic patients treated with the available agents—gentamicin and the polymyxins—was dismal. Studies published around that time indicated that treatment with carbenicillin, with or without an aminoglycoside, significantly improved outcome. Concurrently, several retrospective analyses suggested that the use of two agents that were synergistic against gram-negative pathogens in vitro resulted in better outcomes in neutropenic patients. Thus combination therapy became the standard of care—first for *P. aeruginosa* bacteremia in febrile neutropenic patients and then for all *P. aeruginosa* infections in neutropenic or nonneutropenic patients.

With the introduction of newer antipseudomonal drugs, a number of studies have revisited the choice between combination treatment and monotherapy for *Pseudomonas* bacteremia. Although the majority of experts still favor combination therapy, most of these observational studies indicate that a single modern antipseudomonal β-lactam agent to which the isolate is sensitive is as efficacious as a combination. Even in patients at greatest risk of early death from *P. aeruginosa* bacteremia (i.e., those with fever and neutropenia), empirical antipseudomonal monotherapy is deemed to be as efficacious as empirical combination therapy by the practice guidelines of the Infectious Diseases Society of America. One firm conclusion is that monotherapy with an aminoglycoside is not optimal.

TABLE 53-2

ANTIBIOTIC TREATMENT OF INFECTIONS DUE TO *PSEUDOMONAS AERUGINOSA* AND RELATED SPECIES

INFECTION	ANTIBIOTICS AND DOSAGES	OTHER CONSIDERATIONS
Bacteremia		
Nonneutropenic host	Monotherapy: Ceftazidime (2 g q8h IV) or cefepime (2 g q12h IV) Combination therapy: Piperacillin/tazobactam (3.375 g q4h IV) or imipenem (500 mg q6h IV) or meropenem (1 g q8h IV) *plus* Amikacin (7.5 mg/kg q12h or 15 mg/kg q24h IV)	Add an aminoglycoside for patients in shock and in regions or hospitals where rates of resistance to the primary β-lactam agents are high. Tobramycin may be used instead of amikacin (susceptibility permitting).
Neutropenic host	Cefepime (2 g q8h IV) or all other agents in above dosages	
Endocarditis	Antibiotic regimens as for bacteremia for 6–8 weeks	Resistance during therapy is common. Surgery is required for relapse.
Pneumonia	Drugs and dosages as for bacteremia, except that the available carbapenems should not be the primary drugs because of high rates of resistance during therapy	IDSA guidelines recommend the addition of an aminoglycoside or ciprofloxacin. The duration of therapy is 10–14 days.
Bone infection, malignant otitis externa	Cefepime or ceftazidime at the same dosages as for bacteremia; aminoglycosides not a necessary component of therapy; ciprofloxacin (500–750 mg q12h PO) may be used	Duration of therapy varies with the drug used (e.g., 6 weeks for a β-lactam agent; at least 3 months for oral therapy except in puncture-wound osteomyelitis, for which the duration should be 2–4 weeks).
Central nervous system infection	Ceftazidime or cefepime (2 g q8h IV) or meropenem (1 g q8h IV)	Abscesses or other closed-space infections may require drainage. The duration of therapy is ≥2 weeks.
Eye infection		
Keratitis/ulcer	Topical therapy with tobramycin/ciprofloxacin/levofloxacin eyedrops	Use maximal strengths available or compounded by pharmacy.
Endophthalmitis	Ceftazidime or cefepime as for central nervous system infection *plus* Topical therapy	
Urinary tract infection	Ciprofloxacin (500 mg q12h PO) or levofloxacin (750 mg q24h) or any aminoglycoside (total daily dose given once daily)	Relapse may occur if an obstruction or a foreign body is present.
Multidrug-resistant *P. aeruginosa* infection	Colistin (100 mg q12h IV) for the shortest possible period to obtain a clinical response	Doses used have varied. Dosage adjustment is required in renal failure. Inhaled colistin may be added for pneumonia (100 mg q12h).
Stenotrophomonas maltophilia infection	TMP-SMX (1600/320 mg q12h IV for 14 days) Ticarcillin/clavulanate (3.1 g q4h IV for 14 days)	Resistance to all agents is increasing. Levofloxacin may be an alternative, but there is little published clinical experience with this agent.
Burkholderia cepacia infection	Meropenem (1 g q8h IV for 14 days) TMP-SMX (1600/320 mg q12h IV for 14 days)	Resistance to both agents is increasing. Do not use them in combination because of possible antagonism.
Melioidosis, glanders	Ceftazidime (2 g q6h for 2 weeks) or meropenem (1 g q8h for 2 weeks) or imipenem (500 mg q6h for 2 weeks) *followed by* TMP-SMX (1600/320 mg q12h PO for 3 months)	See "Further Readings" for more details on therapy and alternative agents.

Note: IDSA, Infectious Diseases Society of America; TMP-SMX, trimethoprim-sulfamethoxazole.

There are, of course, institutions and countries where rates of susceptibility of *P. aeruginosa* to first-line antibiotics are <80%. When a septic patient with a high probability of *P. aeruginosa* infection is encountered in such settings, empirical combination therapy should be administered until the pathogen is identified and susceptibility data become available. Thereafter, whether one or two agents should be continued remains a matter of individual preference.

Acute Pneumonia

Respiratory infections are the most common of all infections caused by *P. aeruginosa*. This organism appears first or second on most lists of the causes of ventilator-associated pneumonia (VAP). However, much debate centers on the actual role of *P. aeruginosa* in VAP. Many of the relevant data are based on cultures of sputum or endotracheal tube aspirates and may represent nonpathogenic colonization of the tracheobronchial tree, biofilms on the endotracheal tube, or simple tracheobronchitis.

Older reports of *P. aeruginosa* pneumonia described patients with an acute clinical syndrome of fever, chills, cough, and necrotizing pneumonia indistinguishable from other gram-negative bacterial pneumonias. The traditional accounts described a fulminant infection, with cyanosis, tachypnea, copious sputum, and systemic toxicity. Chest radiographs demonstrated bilateral pneumonia, often with nodular densities with or without cavities. This picture is now remarkably rare. Today, the typical patient is using a ventilator, has a slowly progressive infiltrate, and has been colonized with *P. aeruginosa* for days. Although some cases may progress rapidly over 48–72 h, they are the exceptions. Nodular densities are not commonly seen. However, infiltrates may go on to necrosis. Necrotizing pneumonia has also been seen in the community (e.g., after inhalation of hot-tub water contaminated with *P. aeruginosa*). The typical patient has fever, leukocytosis, and purulent sputum, and the chest radiograph shows a new infiltrate or the expansion of a preexisting infiltrate. Chest examination generally detects rales or dullness. Of course, such findings are quite common among ventilated patients in the ICU. A sputum Gram's stain showing mainly polymorphonuclear leukocytes (PMNs) in conjunction with a culture positive for *P. aeruginosa* in this setting suggests a diagnosis of acute *P. aeruginosa* pneumonia. The emerging consensus is that an invasive procedure (e.g., bronchoalveolar lavage or protected-brush sampling of the distal airways) should be used to obtain samples for quantitative lung cultures in order to substantiate the occurrence of *P. aeruginosa* pneumonia and prevent antibiotic overuse.

℞ Treatment: ACUTE PNEUMONIA

(Table 53-2) The results of therapy for *P. aeruginosa* pneumonia have been unsatisfactory. Reports suggest mortality rates of 40–80%, but how many of these deaths are attributable to underlying disease remains unknown. The drugs of choice for *P. aeruginosa* pneumonia are similar to those given for bacteremia. A potent antipseudomonal β-lactam drug is the mainstay of therapy. Failure rates were high when aminoglycosides were used as single agents, possibly because of binding to airway secretions. Thus a strong case cannot be made for the inclusion of the aminoglycoside component in regimens used against fully susceptible organisms, especially given the evidence that aminoglycosides are not optimally active in the lungs at concentrations normally reached after IV administration. Nonetheless, aminoglycosides are commonly used in clinical practice. Some experts suggest the combination of a β-lactam agent and an antipseudomonal fluoroquinolone instead.

Chronic Respiratory Tract Infections

P. aeruginosa is responsible for chronic infections of the airways associated with a number of underlying or predisposing conditions—most commonly CF in Caucasian populations. A state of chronic colonization beginning early in childhood is seen in some Asian populations with chronic or diffuse panbronchiolitis, a disease of unknown etiology. *P. aeruginosa* is one of the organisms that colonizes damaged bronchi in bronchiectasis, a disease secondary to multiple causes in which profound structural abnormalities of the airways result in mucus stasis.

℞ Treatment: CHRONIC RESPIRATORY TRACT INFECTIONS

Optimal management of chronic *P. aeruginosa* lung infection has not been determined, but it is customary to treat these patients on the basis of bacterial sensitivity. Patients respond clinically to antipseudomonal therapy, but the organism is rarely eradicated. Since eradication is unlikely, the aim of treatment for chronic infection is to quell exacerbations of inflammation. The regimens used are similar to those used for pneumonia, but an aminoglycoside is almost always added because resistance is common in chronic disease. It may be most appropriate to use an inhaled aminoglycoside preparation in order to maximize airway drug levels.

Endovascular Infections

Infective endocarditis due to *P. aeruginosa* is seen mainly in IV drug users whose native valves are involved. This organism has also been reported to cause prosthetic valve endocarditis. Sites of prior native-valve injury due to the injection of foreign material such as talc or fibers probably serve as niduses for bacterial attachment to the heart valve. The manifestations of *P. aeruginosa* endocarditis resemble those of other forms of acute endocarditis in IV drug users except that the disease is more indolent than *Staphylococcus aureus* endocarditis. Although most disease involves the right side of the heart, left-sided involvement is not rare, and multivalvular disease is common. Fever is a common manifestation, as is pulmonary involvement (due to septic emboli to the lungs). Hence patients may also experience chest pain and hemoptysis. Involvement of the left side of the heart may lead to signs of cardiac failure, systemic emboli, and local cardiac involvement with sinus of Valsalva's abscesses and conduction defects. Skin manifestations are rare in this disease, and ecthyma gangrenosum is not seen. The diagnosis is based on positive blood cultures along with clinical signs of endocarditis.

℞ Treatment: ENDOVASCULAR INFECTIONS

(Table 53-2) It has been customary to use synergistic antibiotic combinations in treating *P. aeruginosa* endocarditis because of the development of resistance during therapy with a single antipseudomonal β-lactam agent. Which combination therapy is preferable is unclear, as all combinations have failed. Cases of *P. aeruginosa* endocarditis that relapse during or fail to respond to therapy are often caused by resistant organisms and may require surgical therapy. Other considerations for valve replacement are similar to those in other forms of endocarditis (Chap. 19).

Bone and Joint Infections

Although *P. aeruginosa* is an infrequent cause of bone and joint infections, *Pseudomonas* bacteremia or infective endocarditis caused by the injection of contaminated illicit drugs has been well documented to result in vertebral osteomyelitis and sternoclavicular joint arthritis. The clinical presentation of vertebral *P. aeruginosa* osteomyelitis is more indolent than that of staphylococcal osteomyelitis. The duration of symptoms in IV drug users with vertebral osteomyelitis due to *P. aeruginosa* varies from weeks to months. Fever is not uniformly present; when present, it tends to be low grade. There may be mild tenderness at the site of involvement. Blood cultures are usually negative unless there is concomitant endocarditis. The erythrocyte sedimentation rate (ESR) is generally elevated. Vertebral osteomyelitis due to *P. aeruginosa* has also been reported in the elderly, in whom it originates from urinary tract infections (UTIs). The infection generally involves the lumbosacral area because of a shared venous drainage (Batson's plexus) between the lumbosacral spine and the pelvis. Sternoclavicular septic arthritis due to *P. aeruginosa* is seen almost exclusively in IV drug users. This disease may occur with or without endocarditis, and a primary site of infection often is not found. Plain radiographs show joint or bone involvement. Treatment of these forms of disease is generally successful.

Pseudomonas osteomyelitis of the foot most often follows puncture wounds through sneakers and mostly affects children. The main manifestation is pain in the foot, sometimes with superficial cellulitis around the puncture wound and tenderness on deep palpation of the wound. Multiple joints or bones of the foot may be involved. Systemic symptoms are generally absent, and blood cultures are usually negative. Radiographs may or may not be abnormal, but the bone scan is usually positive, as are MRI studies. Needle aspiration usually yields a diagnosis. Prompt surgery, with exploration of the nail puncture tract and debridement of the involved bones and cartilage, is generally recommended in addition to antibiotic therapy.

Central Nervous System (CNS) Infections

CNS infections due to *P. aeruginosa* are relatively rare. Involvement of the CNS is almost always secondary to a surgical procedure or head trauma. The entity seen most often is postoperative or posttraumatic meningitis. Subdural or epidural infection occasionally results from contamination of these areas. Embolic disease arising from endocarditis in IV drug users and leading to brain abscesses has also been described. The cerebrospinal fluid (CSF) profile of *P. aeruginosa* meningitis is no different from that of pyogenic meningitis of any other etiology.

℞ Treatment: CENTRAL NERVOUS SYSTEM INFECTIONS

(Table 53-2) Treatment of *Pseudomonas* meningitis is difficult; little information has been published, and no controlled trials in humans have been undertaken. However, the general principles involved in the treatment of meningitis apply, including the need for high doses of bactericidal antibiotics to attain high drug levels in the CSF. The agent with which there is the most published experience in *P. aeruginosa* meningitis is ceftazidime, but other antipseudomonal β-lactam drugs that reach high CSF concentrations, such as cefepime and meropenem, have also been used successfully. Other forms of *P. aeruginosa* CNS infection, such as brain abscesses and epidural and subdural empyema, generally require surgical drainage in addition to antibiotic therapy.

Eye Infections

Eye infections due to *P. aeruginosa* occur mainly as a result of direct inoculation into the tissue during trauma or surface injury by contact lenses. Keratitis and corneal ulcers are the most common types of eye disease and are often associated with contact lenses (especially the extended-wear variety). Keratitis can be slowly or rapidly progressive, but the classic description is disease progressing over 48 h to involve the entire cornea, with opacification and sometimes perforation. *P. aeruginosa* keratitis should be considered a medical emergency because of the rapidity with which it can progress to loss of sight. *P. aeruginosa* endophthalmitis secondary to bacteremia is the most devastating of *P. aeruginosa* eye infections. The disease is fulminant, with severe pain, chemosis, decreased visual acuity, anterior uveitis, vitreous involvement, and panophthalmitis.

Treatment: EYE INFECTIONS

(Table 53-2) The usual therapy for keratitis is the administration of topical antibiotics. Therapy for endophthalmitis includes the use of high-dose local and systemic antibiotics (to achieve higher drug concentrations in the eye) and vitrectomy.

Ear Infections

P. aeruginosa infections of the ears vary from mild swimmer's ear to serious life-threatening infections with neurologic sequelae. Swimmer's ear is common among children and results from infection of moist macerated skin of the external ear canal. Most cases resolve with treatment, but some patients develop chronic drainage. Swimmer's ear is managed with topical antibiotic agents (otic solutions). The most serious form of *Pseudomonas* infection involving the ear has been given various names: two of these designations, malignant otitis externa and necrotizing otitis externa, are now used for the same entity. This disease was originally described in elderly diabetic patients, in whom the majority of cases still occur. However, it has also been described in patients with AIDS and in elderly patients without underlying diabetes or immunocompromise. The usual presenting symptoms are decreased hearing and ear pain, which may be severe and lancinating. The pinna is usually painful, and the external canal may be tender. The ear canal almost always shows signs of inflammation, with granulation tissue and exudate. Tenderness anterior to the tragus may extend as far as the temporomandibular joint and mastoid process. A small minority of patients have systemic symptoms. Patients in whom the diagnosis is made late may present with cranial nerve palsies or even with cavernous venous sinus thrombosis. The ESR is invariably elevated (≥100 mm/h). The diagnosis is made on clinical grounds in severe cases; however, the "gold standard" is a positive technetium-99 bone scan in a patient with otitis externa due to *P. aeruginosa*. In diabetic patients, a positive bone scan constitutes presumptive evidence for this diagnosis and should prompt biopsy or empirical therapy.

Treatment: EAR INFECTIONS

(Table 53-2) Given the infection of the ear cartilage, sometimes with mastoid or petrous ridge involvement, patients with malignant (necrotizing) otitis externa are treated as for osteomyelitis.

Urinary Tract Infections

UTIs due to *P. aeruginosa* generally occur as a complication of a foreign body in the urinary tract, an obstruction in the genitourinary system, or urinary tract instrumentation or surgery. However, UTIs caused by *P. aeruginosa* have been described in pediatric outpatients without stones or evident obstruction.

Treatment: URINARY TRACT INFECTIONS

(Table 53-2) Most *P. aeruginosa* UTIs are considered complicated infections that must be treated longer than uncomplicated cystitis. In general, a 7- to 10-day course of treatment suffices, with up to 2 weeks of therapy in cases of pyelonephritis. Urinary catheters, stents, or stones should be removed to prevent relapse, which is common and may be due not to resistance but rather to factors such as a foreign body that has been left in place or an ongoing obstruction.

Skin and Soft Tissue Infections

Besides pyoderma gangrenosum in neutropenic patients (an entity described earlier in this chapter), folliculitis and other papular or vesicular lesions due to *P. aeruginosa* have been extensively described and are collectively referred to as *dermatitis*. Multiple outbreaks have been linked to whirlpools, spas, and swimming pools. To prevent such outbreaks, the growth of *P. aeruginosa* in the home and in recreational environments must be controlled by proper chlorination of water. Most cases of hot-tub folliculitis are self-limited, requiring only the avoidance of exposure to the contaminated source of water.

Toe-web infections occur especially often in the tropics, and the "green nail syndrome" is caused by *P. aeruginosa* paronychia, which results from frequent submersion of the hands in water. In the latter entity, the green discoloration results from diffusion of pyocyanin into the nail bed. *P. aeruginosa* remains a prominent cause of burn wound infections in some parts of the world. Its management is best left to specialists in burn wound care.

Infections in Febrile Neutropenic Patients

In febrile neutropenia, *P. aeruginosa* has historically been the organism against which empirical coverage is always essential. In the 1960s and early 1970s, *P. aeruginosa* infection occurred commonly in febrile neutropenic patients, with high associated mortality rates. Although in Western countries these infections are now less common, their importance has not diminished because of persistently high mortality rates. In other parts of the world as well, *P. aeruginosa* continues to be a significant problem in febrile neutropenia, causing a larger proportion of infections in febrile neutropenic patients than any other single organism. For example, *P. aeruginosa* was responsible for 28% of documented infections in 499 febrile neutropenic patients in one study from the Indian subcontinent and for 31% of these infections in another. In a large study of infections in leukemia patients from Japan, *P. aeruginosa* was the most frequently documented cause of bacterial infection. In studies performed in North America, northern Europe, and Australia, the incidence of *P. aeruginosa* bacteremia in febrile neutropenia was quite variable. In a review of 97 reports published in 1987–1994, the incidence was reported to be 1–2.5%

among febrile neutropenic patients given empirical therapy and 5–12% among microbiologically documented infections. The most common clinical syndromes encountered were bacteremia, pneumonia, and soft tissue infections manifesting mainly as ecthyma gangrenosum.

Rx Treatment: INFECTIONS IN FEBRILE NEUTROPENIC PATIENTS

(Table 53-2) Compared with rates three decades ago, improved rates of response to antibiotic therapy have been reported in many studies. A study of 127 patients demonstrated a reduction in the mortality rate from 71% to 25% with the introduction of ceftazidime and imipenem. Since neutrophils—the normal host defenses against this organism—are absent in febrile neutropenic patients, maximal doses of antipseudomonal β-lactam antibiotics should be used for the management of *P. aeruginosa* bacteremia in this setting.

Infections in Patients with AIDS

Both community- and hospital-acquired *P. aeruginosa* infections were documented in patients with AIDS before the advent of antiretroviral therapy. Since the introduction of protease inhibitors, *P. aeruginosa* infections in AIDS patients have been seen less frequently but still occur, particularly in the form of sinusitis. The clinical presentation of *Pseudomonas* infection (especially pneumonia and bacteremia) in AIDS patients is remarkable in that, although the illness may appear not to be severe, the infection may nonetheless be fatal. Patients with bacteremia may have only a low-grade fever and may present with ecthyma gangrenosum. Bacteremia may herald underlying disease at another site (often pneumonia or sinusitis). Pneumonia, with or without bacteremia, is perhaps the most common type of *P. aeruginosa* infection in AIDS patients. Patients with AIDS and *P. aeruginosa* pneumonia exhibit the classic clinical signs and symptoms of pneumonia, such as fever, productive cough, and chest pain. The infection may be lobar or multilobar and shows no predisposition for any particular location. The most striking feature is the high frequency of cavitary disease.

Rx Treatment: INFECTIONS IN AIDS PATIENTS

Therapy for any of these conditions in AIDS patients is no different from that in other patients. However, relapse is the rule unless the patient's CD4+ T-cell count rises to >50/μL or suppressive antibiotic therapy is given. In attempts to achieve cures and prevent relapses, therapy tends to be more prolonged than that in the immunocompetent patient.

Multidrug-Resistant Infections

(Table 53-2) *P. aeruginosa* is notorious for antibiotic resistance. During three decades, the impact of resistance was minimized by the rapid development of potent antipseudomonal agents. However, the situation has recently changed, with the worldwide selection of strains carrying determinants that mediate resistance to β-lactams, fluoroquinolones, and aminoglycosides. This situation has been compounded by the lack of development of new classes of antipseudomonal drugs for nearly two decades. Physicians now resort to drugs such as colistin and polymyxin, which were discarded decades ago. These alternative approaches to the management of multiresistant *P. aeruginosa* infections were first used some time ago in CF patients, who receive colistin (polymyxin E) IV and by aerosol despite its renal toxicity. Colistin is rapidly becoming the last-resort agent of choice, even in non-CF patients infected with multiresistant *P. aeruginosa*.

The clinical outcome of multidrug-resistant *P. aeruginosa* infections treated with colistin is difficult to judge from case reports, especially given the many drugs used in the complicated management of these patients. Although earlier reports described marginal efficacy and serious nephrotoxicity and neurotoxicity, recent reports have been more encouraging. Because colistin shows synergy with other antimicrobial agents in vitro, it may be possible to reduce the dosage—and thus the toxicity—of this drug when it is combined with drugs such as rifampin and β-lactams; however, no studies in humans or animals support this approach at this time.

OTHER PSEUDOMONADS

STENOTROPHOMONAS MALTOPHILIA

S. maltophilia is the only potential human pathogen among a genus of ubiquitous organisms found in the rhizosphere (i.e., the soil that surrounds the roots of plants). The organism is an opportunist that is acquired from the environment but is even more limited than *P. aeruginosa* in its ability to colonize patients or cause infections. Immunocompromise is not sufficient to permit these events; rather, major perturbations of the human flora are usually necessary for the establishment of *S. maltophilia*. Accordingly, most cases of human infection occur in the setting of very broad-spectrum antibiotic therapy with agents such as advanced cephalosporins and carbapenems, which eradicate the normal flora and other pathogens. The remarkable ability of *S. maltophilia* to resist virtually all classes of antibiotics is attributable to the possession of antibiotic efflux pumps and of two β-lactamases (L1 and L2) that mediate β-lactam resistance, including that to carbapenems. Fortunately, the virulence of *S. maltophilia* appears to be limited. Although a serine protease is present in some strains, virulence is probably a result of the host's inflammatory response to components of the organism such as LPS and flagellin. *S. maltophilia* is most commonly found in the respiratory tract of ventilated patients, where the distinction between its roles as a colonizer and as a pathogen is often difficult to make. However, *S. maltophilia* does cause pneumonia and bacteremia in such patients, and these infections have led to septic shock. Also common is central venous line–associated infection (with or without bacteremia), which has been reported most often in patients with cancer. *S. maltophilia* is a rare cause of ecthyma gangrenosum in neutropenic patients. It has been isolated from ~5% of CF patients but is not believed to be a significant pathogen in this setting.

℞ Treatment: *S. MALTOPHILIA*

The intrinsic resistance of *S. maltophilia* to most antibiotics renders infection difficult to treat. The antibiotics to which it is most often (although not uniformly) susceptible are trimethoprim-sulfamethoxazole (TMP-SMX), ticarcillin/clavulanate, and levofloxacin (Table 53-2). Consequently, a combination of TMP-SMX and ticarcillin/clavulanate is recommended for initial therapy. Catheters must be removed in the treatment of bacteremia to hasten cure and prevent relapses. The treatment of VAP due to *S. maltophilia* is much more difficult than that of bacteremia, with the frequent development of resistance during therapy.

BURKHOLDERIA CEPACIA

B. cepacia gained notoriety as the cause of a rapidly fatal syndrome of respiratory distress and septicemia (the cepacia syndrome) in CF patients. Previously, it had been recognized as an antibiotic-resistant nosocomial pathogen (then designated *P. cepacia*) in ICU patients. Patients with chronic granulomatous disease are also predisposed to *B. cepacia* lung disease. The organism has been reclassified into nine subgroups, only some of which are common in CF. *B. cepacia* is an environmental organism that inhabits moist environments and is found in the rhizosphere. This organism possesses multiple virulence factors that may play roles in disease as well as colonizing factors that are capable of binding to lung mucus—an ability that may explain the predilection of *B. cepacia* for the lungs in CF. *B. cepacia* secretes elastase and possesses components of an injectable toxin-secretion system like that of *P. aeruginosa*; its LPS is among the most potent of all LPSs in stimulating an inflammatory response in the lungs and may be the cause of the lung disease seen in the cepacia syndrome. The organism can penetrate epithelial surfaces by virtue of motility and inhibition of host innate immune defenses. Besides infecting the lungs in CF, *B. cepacia* appears as an airway colonizer during broad-spectrum antibiotic therapy and is a cause of VAP, catheter-associated infections, and wound infections.

℞ Treatment: *B. CEPACIA*

B. cepacia is intrinsically resistant to many antibiotics. Therefore, treatment must be tailored according to sensitivities. TMP-SMX, meropenem, and doxycycline are the most effective agents in vitro and may be started as first-line agents (Table 53-2). Some strains are susceptible to third-generation cephalosporins and fluoroquinolones, and these agents may be used against isolates known to be susceptible. Combination therapy for serious pulmonary infection (e.g., in CF) is suggested for multidrug-resistant strains; the combination of meropenem and TMP-SMX may be antagonistic, however. Resistance to all agents used has been reported during therapy.

BURKHOLDERIA PSEUDOMALLEI

B. pseudomallei is the causative agent of melioidosis, a disease of humans and animals that is geographically restricted to Southeast Asia and northern Australia, with occasional cases in countries such as India and China. This organism may be isolated from individuals returning directly from these endemic regions and from military personnel who have served in endemic regions and then returned home after stops in Europe. Symptoms of this illness may develop only at a later date because of the organism's ability to cause latent infections. *B. pseudomallei* is found in soil and water. Humans and animals are infected by inoculation, inhalation, or ingestion; only rarely is the organism transmitted from person to person. Humans are not colonized without being infected. Among the pseudomonads, *B. pseudomallei* is perhaps the most virulent. Host compromise is not an essential prerequisite for disease, although many patients have common underlying medical diseases (e.g., diabetes or renal failure). *B. pseudomallei* is a facultative intracellular organism whose replication in PMNs and macrophages may be aided by the possession of a polysaccharide capsule. The organism also possesses elements of a type III secretion system that plays a role in its intracellular survival. During infection, there is a florid inflammatory response whose role in disease is unclear.

B. pseudomallei causes a wide spectrum of disease, ranging from asymptomatic infection to abscesses, pneumonia, and disseminated disease. It is a significant cause of fatal community-acquired pneumonia and septicemia in endemic areas, with mortality rates as high as 44% reported in Thailand. Acute pulmonary infections are the most commonly diagnosed form of melioidosis. Pneumonia may be asymptomatic (with routine chest radiographs showing mainly upper-lobe infiltrates) or may present as severe necrotizing disease. *B. pseudomallei* also causes chronic pulmonary infections with systemic manifestations that mimic those of tuberculosis, including chronic cough, fever, hemoptysis, night sweats, and cavitary lung disease. Besides pneumonia, the other principal form of *B. pseudomallei* disease is skin ulceration with associated lymphangitis and regional lymphadenopathy. Spread from the lungs or skin, which is most often documented in debilitated individuals, gives rise to septicemic forms of melioidosis that carry a high mortality rate.

℞ Treatment: *B. PSEUDOMALLEI*

B. pseudomallei is susceptible to advanced penicillins and cephalosporins and to carbapenems. Treatment is divided into two stages: an intensive 2-week phase of therapy with ceftazidime or a carbapenem followed by at least 12 weeks of oral TMP-SMX to eradicate the organism and prevent relapse. The recognition of this bacterium as a potential agent of biologic warfare has stimulated interest in the development of a vaccine.

BURKHOLDERIA MALLEI

B. mallei causes the equine disease glanders in Africa, Asia, and South America. The organism was eradicated from Europe and North America decades ago. The last case seen in the United States occurred in 2001 in a laboratory worker; before that, *B. mallei* had last been seen in this country in 1949. In contrast to the other organisms discussed in this chapter, *B. mallei* is not an environmental organism and does not persist outside its equine hosts. Consequently, *B. mallei* infection is an occupational risk for handlers of horses, equine butchers, and veterinarians in areas of the world where it still exists. The polysaccharide capsule is a critical virulence determinant; diabetics are thought to be more susceptible to infection by this organism. The organism is transmitted from animals to humans by inoculation into the skin, where it causes local infection with nodules and lymphadenitis. Regional lymphadenopathy is common. Respiratory secretions from infected horses are extremely infectious. Inhalation results in clinical signs of typical pneumonia, but may also cause an acute febrile illness with ulceration of the trachea. The organism may disseminate from the skin or lungs to cause septicemia with signs of sepsis. The septicemic form is frequently associated with shock and a high mortality rate. The infection may also enter a chronic phase and present as disseminated abscesses. *B. mallei* infection may present as early as 1–2 days after inhalation or (in cutaneous disease) may not become evident for months.

℞ Treatment: *B. MALLEI*

The antibiotic susceptibility pattern of *B. mallei* is similar to that of *B. pseudomallei;* in addition, the organism is susceptible to the newer macrolides azithromycin and clarithromycin. *B. mallei* infection should be treated with the same drugs and for the same duration as melioidosis.

FURTHER READINGS

Chastre J et al: Comparison of 8 vs 15 days of antibiotic therapy for ventilator-associated pneumonia in adults: A randomized trial. JAMA 290:2588, 2003

Currie BJ: *Burkholderia pseudomallei* and *Burkholderia mallei*: Melioidosis and glanders, in *Principles and Practice of Infectious Diseases,* 6th ed, GL Mandell et al (eds). Philadelphia, Elsevier Churchill Livingstone, 2005, pp 2622–2632

Johnson MP, Ramphal R: Malignant external otitis: Report on therapy with ceftazidime and review of therapy and prognosis. Rev Infect Dis 12:173, 1990

Kallel H et al: Colistin as a salvage therapy for nosocomial infections caused by multidrug-resistant bacteria in the ICU. Int J Antimicrob Agents 28:366, 2006

Lodise TP Jr et al: Predictors of 30-day mortality among patients with *Pseudomonas aeruginosa* bloodstream infections: Impact of delayed appropriate antibiotic selection. Antimicrob Agents Chemother 51:3510, 2007

Maschmeyer G, Göbel UB: *Stenotrophomonas maltophilia* and *Burkholderia cepacia*, in *Principles and Practice of Infectious Diseases,* 6th ed, GL Mandell et al (eds). Philadelphia, Elsevier Churchill Livingstone, 2005, pp 2616–2622

Mendelson MH et al: *Pseudomonas aeruginosa* bacteremia in AIDS. Clin Infect Dis: 886, 1994

Micek ST et al: *Pseudomonas aeruginosa* bloodstream infection: Importance of appropriate antibiotic therapy. Antimicrob Agents Chemother 49:1306, 2005

Murray S et al: Impact of *Burkholderia* infection on lung transplantation in cystic fibrosis. Am J Respir Crit Care Med 178:363, 2008

Obritsch MD et al: Nosocomial infections due to multidrug resistant *Pseudomonas aeruginosa:* Epidemiology and treatment options. Pharmacotherapy 25:1353, 2006

Pier GB, Ramphal R et al: *Pseudomonas aeruginosa*, in *Principles and Practice of Infectious Diseases*, 6th ed, GL Mandell et al (eds). Philadelphia, Elsevier Churchill Livingstone, 2005, pp 2587–2615

St Denis M et al: Infection with *Burkholderia cepacia* complex bacteria and pulmonary exacerbations of cystic fibrosis. Chest 131: 1188, 2007

CHAPTER 54

SALMONELLOSIS

David A. Pegues ■ Samuel I. Miller

Bacteria of the genus *Salmonella* are highly adapted for growth in both humans and animals and cause a wide spectrum of disease. The growth of serotypes *S.* Typhi and *S.* Paratyphi is restricted to human hosts, in whom these organisms cause enteric (typhoid) fever. The remaining serotypes (nontyphoidal *Salmonella*, or NTS) can colonize the gastrointestinal tracts of a broad range of animals, including mammals, reptiles, birds, and insects. More than 200 serotypes are pathogenic to humans, in whom they often cause gastroenteritis and can be associated with localized infections and/or bacteremia.

ETIOLOGY

This large genus of gram-negative bacilli within the family Enterobacteriaceae consists of two species: *S. choleraesuis*, which contains six subspecies, and *S. bongori*. *S. choleraesuis* subspecies I contains almost all the serotypes pathogenic for humans. Because the designation *S. choleraesuis* refers to both a species and a serotype, the species designation *S. enterica* has been recommended and widely adopted. According to the current *Salmonella* nomenclature system, the full taxonomic designation *Salmonella enterica* subspecies *enterica* serotype Typhimurium can be shortened to *Salmonella* serotype Typhimurium, or simply *Salmonella* Typhimurium.

Members of the seven *Salmonella* subspecies are classified into >2400 serotypes (serovars) according to the somatic O antigen [lipopolysaccharide (LPS) cell-wall components], the surface Vi antigen (restricted to *S.* Typhi and *S.* Paratyphi C), and the flagellar H antigen. For simplicity, most *Salmonella* serotypes are named for the city where they were identified, and the serotype is often used as the species designation.

Salmonellae are gram-negative, non–spore-forming, facultatively anaerobic bacilli that measure 2–3 by 0.4–0.6 μm. The initial identification of salmonellae in the clinical microbiology laboratory is based on growth characteristics. Salmonellae, like other Enterobacteriaceae, produce acid on glucose fermentation, reduce nitrates, and do not produce cytochrome oxidase. In addition, all salmonellae except *S.* Gallinarum-Pullorum are motile by means of peritrichous flagella, and all but *S.* Typhi produce gas (H_2S) on sugar fermentation. Notably, only 1% of clinical isolates ferment lactose; a high level of suspicion must be maintained to detect these rare clinical lactose-fermenting isolates.

Although serotyping of all surface antigens can be used for formal identification, most laboratories perform a few simple agglutination reactions that define specific O-antigen serogroups, designated A, B, C_1, C_2, D, and E. Strains in these six serogroups cause ~99% of *Salmonella* infections in humans and warm-blooded animals. Molecular typing methods, including pulsed-field gel electrophoresis, are used in epidemiologic investigations to differentiate *Salmonella* strains of a common serotype.

PATHOGENESIS

All *Salmonella* infections begin with ingestion of organisms in contaminated food or water. The infectious dose is 10^3–10^6 colony-forming units. Conditions that decrease either stomach acidity (an age of <1 year, antacid ingestion, or achlorhydric disease) or intestinal integrity (inflammatory bowel disease, prior gastrointestinal surgery, or alteration of the intestinal flora by antibiotic administration) increase susceptibility to *Salmonella* infection.

Once salmonellae reach the small intestine, they penetrate the mucous layer of the gut and traverse the intestinal layer through phagocytic microfold (M) cells that reside within Peyer's patches. Salmonellae can trigger the formation of membrane ruffles in normally nonphagocytic epithelial cells. These ruffles reach out and enclose adherent bacteria within large vesicles by a process referred to as *bacteria-mediated endocytosis* (BME). BME is dependent on the direct delivery of *Salmonella* proteins into the cytoplasm of epithelial cells by a specialized bacterial secretion system (*type III secretion*). These bacterial proteins mediate alterations in the actin cytoskeleton that are required for *Salmonella* uptake.

After crossing the epithelial layer of the small intestine, *S.* Typhi and *S.* Paratyphi, which cause enteric (typhoid) fever, are phagocytosed by macrophages. These salmonellae survive the antimicrobial environment of the macrophage by sensing environmental signals that trigger alterations in regulatory systems of the phagocytosed bacteria. For example, PhoP/PhoQ (the best-characterized regulatory system) triggers the expression of outer-membrane proteins and mediates modifications in LPS so that the altered bacterial surface can resist microbicidal activities and potentially alter host cell signaling. In addition, salmonellae encode a second type III secretion system that directly delivers bacterial proteins across the phagosome membrane into the macrophage cytoplasm. This secretion system functions to remodel the *Salmonella*-containing vacuole, promoting bacterial survival and replication.

Once phagocytosed, salmonellae disseminate throughout the body in macrophages via the lymphatics and colonize reticuloendothelial tissues (liver, spleen, lymph nodes, and bone marrow). Patients have relatively few or no signs and symptoms during this initial incubation stage. Signs and symptoms, including fever and abdominal pain, probably result from secretion of cytokines by macrophages and epithelial cells in response to bacterial products that are recognized by innate immune receptors when a critical number of organisms have replicated. Over time, the development of hepatosplenomegaly is likely to be related to the recruitment of mononuclear cells and the development of a specific acquired cell-mediated immune response to *S.* typhi colonization. The recruitment of additional mononuclear cells and lymphocytes to Peyer's patches during the several weeks after initial colonization/infection can result in marked enlargement and necrosis of the Peyer's patches, which may be mediated by bacterial products that promote cell death as well as the inflammatory response.

In contrast to enteric fever, which is characterized by an infiltration of mononuclear cells into the small-bowel mucosa, NTS gastroenteritis is characterized by massive polymorphonuclear leukocyte (PMN) infiltration into both the large- and small-bowel mucosa. This response appears to depend on the induction of interleukin (IL) 8, a strong neutrophil chemotactic factor, which is secreted by intestinal cells as a result of *Salmonella* colonization and translocation of bacterial proteins into host cell cytoplasm. The degranulation and release of toxic substances by neutrophils may result in damage to the intestinal mucosa, causing the inflammatory diarrhea observed with nontyphoidal gastroenteritis.

ENTERIC (TYPHOID) FEVER

Typhoid fever is a systemic disease characterized by fever and abdominal pain and caused by dissemination of S. Typhi or S. Paratyphi. The disease was initially called *typhoid fever* because of its clinical similarity to typhus. However, in the early 1800s, typhoid fever was clearly defined pathologically as a unique illness on the basis of its association with enlarged Peyer's patches and mesenteric lymph nodes. In 1869, given the anatomic site of infection, the term *enteric fever* was proposed as an alternative designation to distinguish typhoid fever from typhus. However, to this day, the two designations are used interchangeably.

EPIDEMIOLOGY

In contrast to other *Salmonella* serotypes, the etiologic agents of enteric fever—S. Typhi and S. Paratyphi serotypes A, B, and C—have no known hosts other than humans. Most commonly, food-borne or waterborne transmission results from fecal contamination by ill or asymptomatic chronic carriers. Sexual transmission between male partners has been described. Health care workers occasionally acquire enteric fever after exposure to infected patients or during processing of clinical specimens and cultures.

With improvements in food handling and water/sewage treatment, enteric fever has become rare in developed nations. Worldwide, however, there were an estimated 22 million cases of enteric fever, with 200,000 deaths annually. The incidence is highest (>100 cases per 100,000 population per year) in south-central and Southeast Asia; medium (10–100 cases per 100,000) in the rest of Asia, Africa, Latin America, and Oceania (excluding Australia and New Zealand); and low in other parts of the world. A high incidence of enteric fever is correlated with poor sanitation and lack of access to clean drinking water. In endemic regions, enteric fever is more common in urban than rural areas and among young children and adolescents. Risk factors include contaminated water or ice, flooding, food and drinks purchased from street vendors, raw fruits and vegetables grown in fields fertilized with sewage, ill household contacts, lack of hand washing and toilet access, and evidence of prior *Helicobacter pylori* infection (an association probably related to chronically reduced gastric acidity). It is estimated that there is one case of paratyphoid fever for every four cases of typhoid fever, but the incidence of infection associated with S. Paratyphi A appears to be increasing, especially in India.

Multidrug-resistant (MDR) strains of S. Typhi emerged in 1989 in China and Southeast Asia and have since disseminated widely (Fig. 54-1). These strains contain plasmids encoding resistance to chloramphenicol, ampicillin, and trimethoprim—antibiotics long used to treat enteric fever. With the increased use of fluoroquinolones to treat MDR enteric fever, strains of S. Typhi and S. Paratyphi with reduced susceptibility to ciprofloxacin [minimal inhibitory concentration (MIC), 0.125–1.0 μg/mL] have emerged in India and Vietnam and have been associated with clinical treatment failure. Testing of isolates for resistance to the first-generation quinolone nalidixic acid detects most but not all strains with reduced susceptibility to ciprofloxacin.

The incidence of enteric fever among U.S. travelers is estimated at 3–30 cases per 100,000. Of 1393 cases reported to the Centers for Disease Control and Prevention (CDC) in 1994–1999, 74% were associated with recent international travel, most commonly to India (30%), Pakistan (13%), Mexico (12%), Bangladesh (8%), the Philippines (8%), and Haiti (5%). Likewise, of 356 cases reported in the United States in 2003, ~74% occurred in

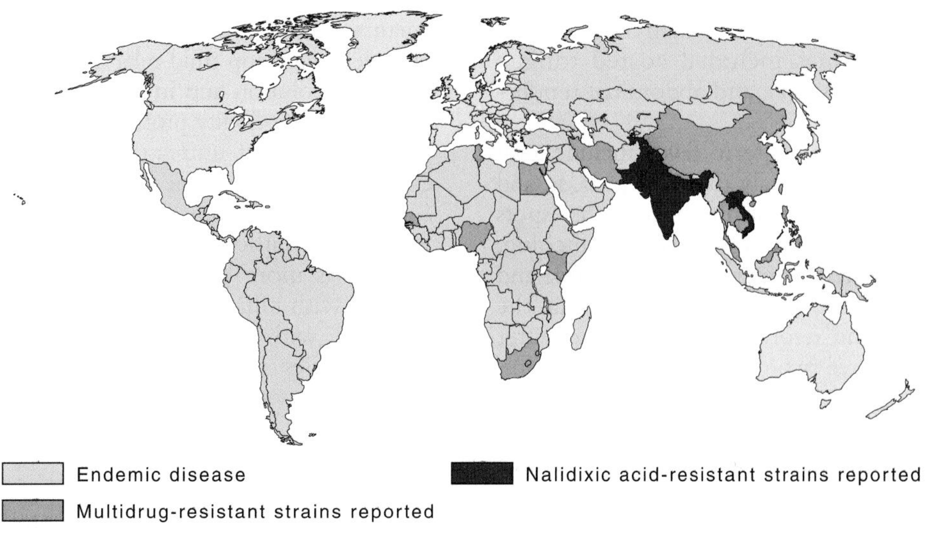

FIGURE 54-1
Global distribution of resistance to S. Typhi, 1990–2002. *(Reprinted with permission from Parry CM et al: Typhoid fever. N Engl J Med 347:1770, 2002. © 2002 Massachusetts Medical Society. All rights reserved.)*

persons who reported international travel during the preceding 6 weeks. Only 4% of travelers diagnosed with enteric fever gave a history of S. Typhi vaccination within the previous 5 years. Increased rates of MDR S. Typhi and S. Paratyphi have been reported among travelers. In 1996–1997, 80% of U.S. travelers with enteric fever acquired in Vietnam were infected with MDR S. Typhi strains. Of the 25–30% of reported cases of enteric fever in the United States that are domestically acquired, the majority are sporadic, but 7% have occurred in recognized outbreaks linked to contaminated food products and previously unrecognized chronic carriers. An increasing proportion of cases (currently ~80%) are associated with foreign-born U.S. residents visiting friends and relatives in their native countries.

FIGURE 54-2
"Rose spots," the rash of enteric fever due to *S.* Typhi or *S.* Paratyphi.

CLINICAL COURSE

Enteric fever is a misnomer, in that the hallmark features of this disease—fever and abdominal pain—are variable. Although fever is documented at presentation in >75% of cases, abdominal pain is reported in only 30–40%. Thus a high index of suspicion for this potentially fatal systemic illness is necessary when a person presents with fever and a history of recent travel to a developing country.

The incubation period for S. Typhi averages 10–14 days but ranges from 3 to 21 days, with the duration likely reflecting the inoculum size and the host's health and immune status. The most prominent symptom is prolonged fever (38.8°–40.5°C; 101.8°–104.9°F), which can continue for up to 4 weeks if untreated. S. Paratyphi A is thought to cause milder disease than S. Typhi, with predominantly gastrointestinal symptoms. However, a prospective study of 669 consecutive cases of enteric fever in Kathmandu, Nepal, found that the infections were clinically indistinguishable. In this series, symptoms reported on initial medical evaluation included headache (80%), chills (35–45%), cough (30%), sweating (20–25%), myalgias (20%), malaise (10%), and arthralgia (2–4%). Gastrointestinal symptoms included anorexia (55%), abdominal pain (30–40%), nausea (18–24%), vomiting (18%), and diarrhea (22–28%) more commonly than constipation (13–16%). Physical findings included coated tongue (51–56%), splenomegaly (5–6%), and abdominal tenderness (4–5%).

Early physical findings of enteric fever include rash ("rose spots"), hepatosplenomegaly (3–6%), epistaxis, and relative bradycardia at the peak of high fever. Rose spots (Fig. 54-2) make up a faint, salmon-colored, blanching, maculopapular rash located primarily on the trunk and chest. The rash is evident in ~30% of patients at the end of the first week and resolves without a trace after 2–5 days. Patients can have two or three crops of lesions, and *Salmonella* can be cultured from punch biopsies of these lesions. The faintness of the rash makes it difficult to detect in highly pigmented patients.

The development of severe disease (which occurs in ~10–15% of patients) depends on host factors (immunosuppression, antacid therapy, previous exposure, and vaccination), strain virulence and inoculum, and choice of antibiotic therapy. Gastrointestinal bleeding (10–20%) and intestinal perforation (1–3%) most commonly occur in the third and fourth weeks of illness and result from hyperplasia, ulceration, and necrosis of the ileocecal Peyer's patches at the initial site of *Salmonella* infiltration. Both complications are life-threatening and require immediate fluid resuscitation and surgical intervention, with broadened antibiotic coverage for polymicrobial peritonitis (Chap. 24) and treatment of gastrointestinal hemorrhages, including bowel resection. Neurologic manifestations occur in 2–40% of patients and include meningitis, Guillain-Barré syndrome, neuritis, and neuropsychiatric symptoms (described as "muttering delirium" or "coma vigil"), with picking at bedclothes or imaginary objects.

Rare complications whose incidences are reduced by prompt antibiotic treatment include disseminated intravascular coagulation, hematophagocytic syndrome, pancreatitis, hepatic and splenic abscesses and granulomas, endocarditis, pericarditis, myocarditis, orchitis, hepatitis, glomerulonephritis, pyelonephritis and hemolytic uremic syndrome, severe pneumonia, arthritis, osteomyelitis, and parotitis. Up to 10% of patients develop mild relapse, usually within 2–3 weeks of fever resolution and in association with the same strain type and susceptibility profile.

Up to 10% of untreated patients with typhoid fever excrete S. Typhi in the feces for up to 3 months, and 1–4% develop chronic asymptomatic carriage, shedding S. Typhi in either urine or stool for >1 year. Chronic carriage is more common among women, infants, and persons with biliary abnormalities or concurrent bladder infection with *Schistosoma haematobium*. The anatomic abnormalities associated with the latter conditions presumably allow prolonged colonization.

DIAGNOSIS

Since the clinical presentation of enteric fever is relatively nonspecific, the diagnosis needs to be considered in any febrile traveler returning from a developing country, especially the Indian subcontinent, the Philippines, or

Latin America. Other diagnoses that should be considered in these travelers include malaria, hepatitis, bacterial enteritis, dengue fever, rickettsial infections, leptospirosis, amebic liver abscesses, and acute HIV infection (Chap. 4). Other than a positive culture, no specific laboratory test is diagnostic for enteric fever. In 15–25% of cases, leukopenia and neutropenia are detectable. Leukocytosis is more common among children, during the first 10 days of illness, and in cases complicated by intestinal perforation or secondary infection. Other nonspecific laboratory findings include moderately elevated liver function tests and muscle enzyme levels.

The definitive diagnosis of enteric fever requires the isolation of *S.* Typhi or *S.* Paratyphi from blood, bone marrow, other sterile sites, rose spots, stool, or intestinal secretions. The yield of blood cultures is quite variable; sensitivity is as high as 90% during the first week of infection and decreases to 50% by the third week. A low yield in infected patients is related to low numbers of salmonellae (<15 organisms/mL) and/or to recent antibiotic treatment. Since almost all *S.* Typhi organisms in blood are associated with the mononuclear-cell/platelet fraction, centrifugation of blood and culture of the buffy coat can substantially reduce the time to isolation of the organism but does not increase sensitivity.

Unlike blood culture, bone marrow culture remains highly (90%) sensitive despite ≤5 days of antibiotic therapy. Culture of intestinal secretions (best obtained by a noninvasive duodenal string test) can be positive despite a negative bone marrow culture. If blood, bone marrow, and intestinal secretions are all cultured, the yield is >90%. Stool cultures, although negative in 60–70% of cases during the first week, can become positive during the third week of infection in untreated patients.

Several serologic tests, including the classic Widal's test for "febrile agglutinins," are available. None of these tests are sufficiently sensitive or specific to replace culture-based methods for the diagnosis of enteric fever in developed countries. Polymerase chain reaction and DNA probe assays to detect *S.* Typhi in blood are being developed.

℞ Treatment: ENTERIC (TYPHOID) FEVER

Prompt administration of appropriate antibiotic therapy prevents severe complications of enteric fever and results in a case-fatality rate of <1%. The initial choice of antibiotics depends on the susceptibility of the *S.* Typhi and *S.* Paratyphi strains in the area of residence or travel (Table 54-1). For treatment of drug-susceptible typhoid fever, fluoroquinolones are the most effective class of agents, with cure rates of ~98% and relapse and fecal carriage rates of <2%. Experience is most extensive with

TABLE 54-1

ANTIBIOTIC THERAPY FOR ENTERIC FEVER IN ADULTS

INDICATION	AGENT	DOSAGE (ROUTE)	DURATION, DAYS
Empirical Treatment			
	Ceftriaxone[a]	1–2 g/d (IV)	7–14
	Azithromycin	1 g/d (PO)	5
Fully Susceptible			
	Ciprofloxacin[b] (first line)	500 mg bid (PO) or 400 mg q12h (IV)	5–7
	Amoxicillin (second line)	1 g tid (PO) or 2 g q6h (IV)	14
	Chloramphenicol	25 mg/kg tid (PO or IV)	14–21
	Trimethoprim-sulfamethoxazole	160/800 mg bid (PO)	14
Multidrug-Resistant			
	Ciprofloxacin	500 mg bid (PO) or 400 mg q12h (IV)	5–7
	Ceftriaxone	2–3 g/d (IV)	7–14
	Azithromycin	1 g/d (PO)[c]	5
Nalidixic Acid–Resistant			
	Ceftriaxone	1–2 g/d (IV)	7–14
	Azithromycin	1 g/d (PO)	5
	High-dose ciprofloxacin	750 mg bid (PO) or 400 mg q8h (IV)	10–14

[a]Or another third-generation cephalosporin [e.g., cefotaxime, 2 g q8h (IV), or cefixime, 400 mg bid (PO)].
[b]Or ofloxacin, 400 mg bid (PO) for 2–5 days.
[c]Or 1 g on day 1 followed by 500 mg/d PO for 6 days.

ciprofloxacin. Short-course ofloxacin therapy is similarly successful against infection caused by nalidixic acid–susceptible strains. However, the increased incidence of nalidixic acid–resistant (NAR) *S.* Typhi in Asia, which is probably related to the widespread availability of fluoroquinolones over the counter, is now limiting the use of this drug class for empirical therapy. Patients infected with NAR *S.* Typhi strains should be treated with ceftriaxone, azithromycin, or high-dose ciprofloxacin. However, high-dose fluoroquinolone therapy for NAR enteric fever has been associated with delayed resolution of fever and high rates of fecal carriage during convalescence.

Ceftriaxone, cefotaxime, and (oral) cefixime are effective for treatment of MDR enteric fever, including NAR and fluoroquinolone-resistant strains. These agents clear fever in ~1 week, with failure rates of ~5–10%, fecal carriage rates of <3%, and relapse rates of 3–6%. Oral azithromycin results in defervescence in 4–6 days, with rates of relapse and convalescent stool carriage of <3%. Despite efficient in vitro killing of *Salmonella*, first- and second-generation cephalosporins as well as aminoglycosides are ineffective in treating clinical infections.

Patients with persistent vomiting, diarrhea, and/or abdominal distension should be hospitalized and given supportive therapy as well as a parenteral third-generation cephalosporin or fluoroquinolone, depending on the susceptibility profile. Therapy should be administered for at least 10 days or for 5 days after fever resolution.

In a randomized, prospective, double-blind study of critically ill patients with enteric fever (i.e., those with shock and obtundation) in Indonesia in the early 1980s, the administration of dexamethasone (3-mg initial dose followed by eight doses of 1 mg/kg every 6 h) with chloramphenicol was associated with a substantially lower mortality rate than treatment with chloramphenicol alone (10% vs 55%). Although this study has not been repeated in the "post-chloramphenicol era," severe enteric fever remains one of the few indications for glucocorticoid treatment of an acute bacterial infection.

The 1–5% of patients who develop chronic carriage of *Salmonella* can be treated for 4–6 weeks with an appropriate oral antibiotic. Treatment with oral amoxicillin, trimethoprim-sulfamethoxazole (TMP-SMX), ciprofloxacin, or norfloxacin is ~80% effective in eradicating chronic carriage of susceptible organisms. However, in cases of anatomic abnormality (e.g., biliary or kidney stones), eradication often requires both antibiotic therapy and surgical correction.

PREVENTION AND CONTROL

Theoretically, it is possible to eliminate the salmonellae that cause enteric fever since they survive only in human hosts and are spread by contaminated food and water. However, given the high prevalence of the disease in developing countries that lack adequate sewage disposal and water treatment, this goal is currently unrealistic. Thus travelers to developing countries should be advised to monitor their food and water intake carefully and to consider vaccination.

Two typhoid vaccines are commercially available: (1) Ty21a, an oral live attenuated *S.* Typhi vaccine (given on days 1, 3, 5, and 7, with a booster every 5 years); and (2) Vi CPS, a parenteral vaccine consisting of purified Vi polysaccharide from the bacterial capsule (given in one dose, with a booster every 2 years). The old parenteral whole-cell typhoid/paratyphoid A and B vaccine is no longer licensed, largely because of significant side effects (see below). An acetone-killed whole-cell vaccine is available only for use by the U.S. military. The minimal age for vaccination is 6 years for Ty21a and 2 years for Vi CPS. Currently, there is no licensed vaccine for paratyphoid fever.

A large-scale meta-analysis of vaccine trials comparing whole-cell vaccine, Ty21a, and Vi CPS in populations in endemic areas indicates that, although all three vaccines are similarly effective for the first year, the 3-year cumulative efficacy of the whole-cell vaccine (73%) exceeds that of both Ty21a (51%) and Vi CPS (55%). In addition, the heat-killed whole-cell vaccine maintains its efficacy for 5 years, whereas Ty21a and Vi CPS maintain their efficacy for 4 and 2 years, respectively. However, the whole-cell vaccine is associated with a much higher incidence of side effects (especially fever: 16% vs 1–2%) than the other two vaccines.

Vi CPS typhoid vaccine is poorly immunogenic in children <5 years of age because of T-cell–independent properties. In the recently developed Vi-rEPA vaccine, Vi is bound to a nontoxic recombinant protein that is identical to *Pseudomonas aeruginosa* exotoxin A. In 2- to 4-year-olds, two injections of Vi-rEPA induced higher T-cell responses and higher levels of serum IgG antibody to Vi than did Vi CPS in 5- to 14-year-olds. In a two-dose trial in 2- to 5-year-old children in Vietnam, Vi-rEPA provided 91% efficacy at 27 months and 88% efficacy at 43 months and was very well tolerated. Similar results were obtained in a trial in Cambodia. This vaccine is not yet commercially available in the United States. At least three new live vaccines are in clinical development and may prove more efficacious and longer-lasting than previous live vaccines.

Although data on typhoid vaccines in travelers are limited, some evidence suggests that efficacy rates may be substantially lower than those for local populations in endemic areas. Both the CDC and the World Health Organization recommend typhoid vaccination for travelers to typhoid-endemic countries. Recent analyses from the CDC found that 16% of travel-associated cases occurred among persons who stayed at their travel destination for ≤2 weeks. Thus vaccination should be strongly considered even for persons planning short-term travel to high-risk areas such as the Indian subcontinent. In the United States, persons who have intimate or household contact with a chronic carrier or laboratory workers who frequently deal with *S.* Typhi also should receive typhoid vaccine.

Enteric fever is a notifiable disease in the United States. Individual health departments have their own guidelines for allowing ill or colonized food handlers or health care workers to return to their jobs. The reporting system enables public health departments to identify potential source patients and to treat chronic carriers in order to prevent further outbreaks. In addition, since 1–4% of patients with *S.* Typhi infection become chronic carriers, it is important to monitor patients (especially child-care providers and food handlers) for chronic carriage and to treat this condition if indicated.

NONTYPHOIDAL SALMONELLOSIS

EPIDEMIOLOGY

During 1996–1999, there were an estimated 1.4 million cases of nontyphoidal salmonellosis in the United States, resulting in 168,000 physician office visits, 15,000 hospitalizations, and 400 deaths annually. In 2004, the incidence of NTS infection in this country was 14.7 per 100,000 persons—the highest rate among the nine food-borne enteric pathogens under active surveillance. Five serotypes accounted for 57% of U.S. infections in 2004: Typhimurium (20%), Enteritidis (15%), Newport (10%), Javiana (7%), and Heidelberg (5%).

The incidence of nontyphoidal salmonellosis is highest during the rainy season in tropical climates and during the warmer months in temperate climates, coinciding with the peak in food-borne outbreaks. Rates of morbidity and mortality associated with NTS are highest among the elderly, infants, and immunocompromised individuals, including those with hemoglobinopathies, HIV infection, or infections that cause blockade of the reticuloendothelial system (e.g., bartonellosis, malaria, schistosomiasis, and histoplasmosis).

Unlike *S.* Typhi and *S.* Paratyphi, whose only reservoir is humans, NTS can be acquired from multiple animal reservoirs. Transmission is most commonly associated with animal food products, especially eggs, poultry, undercooked ground meat, and dairy products and fresh produce contaminated with animal waste.

S. Enteritidis infection associated with chicken eggs emerged as a major cause of food-borne disease during the 1980s and 1990s. *S.* Enteritidis infection of the ovaries and upper oviduct tissue of hens results in contamination of egg contents before shell deposition. Infection is spread to egg-laying hens from breeding flocks and through contact with rodents and manure. Of the 360 outbreaks of *S.* Enteritidis with a confirmed source that were reported to the CDC in 1985–1998, 279 (78%) were associated with raw or undercooked eggs. After peaking at 3.9 cases per 100,000 U.S. population in 1995, the incidence of *S.* Enteritidis infection declined dramatically to 1.98 per 100,000 in 1999; this decrease probably reflected improved on-farm control measures, refrigeration, and education of consumers and food-service workers. Transmission via contaminated eggs can be prevented by cooking eggs until the yolk is solidified and through pasteurization of egg products.

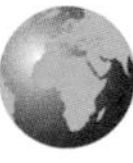

Centralization of food processing and widespread food distribution have contributed to the increased incidence of NTS in developing countries. Manufactured foods to which recent *Salmonella* outbreaks have been traced include pasteurized milk, infant formula, powdered milk products, and various processed foods. Large outbreaks have also been linked to fresh produce, including alfalfa sprouts, cantaloupe, fresh-squeezed orange juice, and tomatoes; these items become contaminated by manure or water at a single site and then are widely distributed.

An estimated 6% of sporadic *Salmonella* infections in the United States are attributed to contact with reptiles and amphibians, especially iguanas, snakes, turtles, and lizards. Reptile-associated *Salmonella* infection more commonly leads to hospitalization and more frequently involves infants than do other *Salmonella* infections. Other pets, including African hedgehogs, snakes, birds, rodents, baby chicks, ducklings, dogs, and cats, are also potential sources of NTS.

Increasing antibiotic resistance in NTS species is a global problem and has been linked to the widespread use of antimicrobial agents in food animals and especially in animal feed. In the early 1990s, *S.* Typhimurium definitive phage type 104 (DT104), characterized by resistance to ≥5 antibiotics (ampicillin, chloramphenicol, streptomycin, sulfonamides, and tetracyclines; R-type ACSSuT), emerged worldwide. From 1979–1980 to 2001, the prevalence of *S.* Typhimurium ACSSuT increased in the United States from 0.6% to 7% of all NTS isolates, and most (65%) of these ACSSuT isolates were phage type DT104. Acquisition is associated with exposure to ill farm animals and to various meat products, including uncooked or undercooked ground beef. In an analysis of U.S. surveillance data for 1996–2001, antibiotic-resistant NTS strains, especially *S.* Typhimurium DT104, were associated with an increased risk of bloodstream infection and hospitalization. NAR and trimethoprim-resistant DT104 strains are emerging, especially in the United Kingdom.

Because of increased resistance to conventional antibiotics such as ampicillin and TMP-SMX, extended-spectrum cephalosporins and fluoroquinolones have emerged as the agents of choice for the treatment of MDR NTS infections. With the increased use of these agents, the CDC reported that the prevalence of ceftriaxone-resistant NTS strains rose from 0 in 1995 to 0.5% in 1998. Of the ceftriaxone-resistant isolates, 77% were from children <18 years of age, in whom ceftriaxone is the antibiotic of choice for treatment of invasive infection. These strains contained plasmid-encoded AmpC β-lactamases that were probably acquired by horizontal genetic transfer from *Escherichia coli* strains in food-producing animals—an event linked to the widespread use of the veterinary cephalosporin ceftiofur.

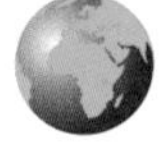

Resistance to nalidixic acid and fluoroquinolones also has begun to emerge and is most commonly associated with point mutations in the DNA gyrase genes *gyr*A and *gyr*B. Nalidixic acid resistance is a good predictor of reduced susceptibility to clinically useful fluoroquinolones. From 1994–1995 to 2000, the rate of NAR NTS isolates in the United States increased fivefold (from 0.5% to 2.5%). In Denmark, infection with

NAR *S.* Typhimurium DT104 has been linked to swine and associated with a threefold higher risk of invasive disease or death within 90 days. In Taiwan in 2000, a strain of ciprofloxacin-resistant (MIC, ≥4 μg/mL) *S.* Choleraesuis caused a large outbreak of invasive infections that was linked to the use of enrofloxacin in swine feed.

CLINICAL MANIFESTATIONS

Gastroenteritis

Infection with NTS most often results in gastroenteritis indistinguishable from that caused by other enteric pathogens. Nausea, vomiting, and diarrhea occur 6–48 h after the ingestion of contaminated food or water. Patients often experience abdominal cramping and fever (38–39°C; 100.5–102.2°F). Diarrheal stools are usually loose, nonbloody, and of moderate volume. However, large-volume watery stools, bloody stools, or symptoms of dysentery may occur. Rarely, NTS causes pseudoappendicitis or an illness that mimics inflammatory bowel disease.

Gastroenteritis caused by NTS is usually self-limited. Diarrhea resolves within 3–7 days and fever within 72 h. Stool cultures remain positive for 4–5 weeks after infection and—in rare cases of chronic carriage (<1%)—for >1 year. Antibiotic treatment usually is not recommended and in some studies has prolonged fecal carriage. Neonates, the elderly, and immunosuppressed patients (e.g., transplant recipients, HIV-infected persons) with NTS gastroenteritis are especially susceptible to dehydration and dissemination and may require hospitalization and antibiotic therapy. Acute NTS gastroenteritis was associated with a threefold increased risk of dyspepsia and irritable bowel syndrome at 1 year in a recent study from Spain.

Bacteremia and Endovascular Infections

Up to 5% of patients with NTS gastroenteritis develop bacteremia; of these, 5–10% develop localized infections. Bacteremia and metastatic infection are most common with *S.* Choleraesuis and *S.* Dublin and among infants, the elderly, and immunocompromised patients. NTS endovascular infection should be suspected in high-grade bacteremia, especially with preexisting valvular heart disease, atherosclerotic vascular disease, prosthetic vascular graft, or aortic aneurysm. Arteritis should be suspected in elderly patients with prolonged fever and back, chest, or abdominal pain developing after an episode of gastroenteritis. Endocarditis and arteritis are rare (<1% of cases) but are associated with potentially fatal complications, including valve perforation, endomyocardial abscess, infected mural thrombus, pericarditis, mycotic aneurysms, aneurysm rupture, aortoenteric fistula, and vertebral osteomyelitis.

Localized Infections

Intraabdominal Infections

Intraabdominal infections due to NTS are rare and usually manifest as hepatic or splenic abscesses or as cholecystitis. Risk factors include hepatobiliary anatomic abnormalities (e.g., gallstones), abdominal malignancy, and sickle cell disease (especially with splenic abscesses). Eradication of the infection often requires surgical correction of abnormalities and percutaneous drainage of abscesses.

Central Nervous System Infections

Meningitis most commonly develops in infants 1–4 months of age. It often results in severe sequelae (including seizures, hydrocephalus, brain infarction, and mental retardation), with death in up to 60% of cases. Other rare central nervous system infections include ventriculitis, subdural empyema, and brain abscesses.

Pulmonary Infections

NTS pulmonary infections usually present as lobar pneumonia, and complications include lung abscess, empyema, and bronchopleural fistula formation. The majority of cases occur in patients with lung cancer, structural lung disease, sickle cell disease, or glucocorticoid use.

Urinary and Genital Tract Infections

Urinary tract infections caused by NTS present as either cystitis or pyelonephritis. Risk factors include malignancy, urolithiasis, structural abnormalities, HIV infection, and renal transplantation. NTS genital infections are rare and include ovarian and testicular abscesses, prostatitis, and epididymitis. Like other focal infections, both genital and urinary tract infections can be complicated by abscess formation.

Bone, Joint, and Soft Tissue Infections

Salmonella osteomyelitis most commonly affects the femur, tibia, humerus, or lumbar vertebrae and is most often seen in association with sickle cell disease, hemoglobinopathies, or preexisting bone disease (e.g., fractures). Prolonged antibiotic treatment is recommended to decrease the risk of relapse and chronic osteomyelitis. Septic arthritis occurs in the same patient population as osteomyelitis and usually involves the knee, hip, or shoulder joints. Reactive arthritis (Reiter's syndrome) can follow NTS gastroenteritis and is seen most frequently in persons with the HLA-B27 histocompatibility antigen. NTS rarely can cause soft tissue infections, usually at sites of local trauma in immunosuppressed patients.

DIAGNOSIS

The diagnosis of NTS infection is based on the isolation of the organism from freshly passed stool or from blood or another ordinarily sterile body fluid. All salmonellae isolated in clinical laboratories should be sent to local public health departments for serotyping. Blood cultures should be done whenever a patient has prolonged or recurrent fever. Endovascular infection should be suspected if there is high-grade bacteremia (>50% of three or more blood cultures positive). Echocardiography, computed tomography, and indium-labeled white cell scanning are used to identify localized infection. When another localized infection is suspected, joint fluid, abscess drainage, or cerebrospinal fluid should be cultured, as clinically indicated.

℞ Treatment: NONTYPHOIDAL SALMONELLOSIS

Antibiotics should not be used routinely to treat uncomplicated NTS gastroenteritis. The symptoms are usually self-limited, and the duration of fever and diarrhea is not significantly decreased by antibiotic therapy. In addition, antibiotic treatment has been associated with increased rates of relapse and prolonged gastrointestinal carriage. Dehydration secondary to diarrhea should be treated with fluid and electrolyte replacement.

Preemptive antibiotic treatment (Table 54-2) should be considered for patients at increased risk for invasive NTS infection, including neonates (probably up to 3 months of age); persons >50 years of age with suspected atherosclerosis; and patients with immunosuppression, cardiac valvular or endovascular abnormalities, or significant joint disease. Treatment should consist of an oral or IV antibiotic administered for 48–72 h or until the patient becomes afebrile. Immunocompromised persons may require up to 7–14 days of therapy. The <1% of persons who develop chronic carriage of NTS should receive a prolonged antibiotic course, as described above for chronic carriage of *S.* Typhi.

Because of the increasing prevalence of antibiotic resistance, empirical therapy for life-threatening NTS bacteremia or focal NTS infection should include a third-generation cephalosporin or a fluoroquinolone (Table 54-2). If the bacteremia is low-grade (<50% of blood cultures positive), the patient should be treated for 7–14 days. Patients with AIDS and NTS bacteremia should receive 1–2 weeks of IV antibiotic therapy followed by 4 weeks of oral therapy with a fluoroquinolone. Patients whose infections relapse after this regimen should receive long-term suppressive therapy with a fluoroquinolone or TMP-SMX, as indicated by bacterial sensitivities.

TABLE 54-2

ANTIBIOTIC THERAPY FOR NONTYPHOIDAL *SALMONELLA* INFECTION IN ADULTS

INDICATION	AGENT	DOSAGE (ROUTE)	DURATION, DAYS
Preemptive Treatment[a]			
	Ciprofloxacin[b]	500 mg bid (PO)	2–3
Severe Gastroenteritis[c]			
	Ciprofloxacin	500 mg bid (PO) or 400 mg q12h (IV)	3–7
	Trimethoprim-sulfamethoxazole	160/800 mg bid (PO)	
	Amoxicillin	1 g tid (PO)	
	Ceftriaxone	1–2 g/d (IV)	
Bacteremia			
	Ceftriaxone[d]	2 g/d (IV)	7–14
	Ciprofloxacin	400 mg q12h (IV), then 500 mg bid (PO)	
Endocarditis or Arteritis			
	Ceftriaxone	2 g/d (IV)	42
	Ciprofloxacin	400 mg q8h (IV), then 750 mg bid (PO)	
	Ampicillin	2 g q4h (IV)	
Meningitis			
	Ceftriaxone	2 g q12 h (IV)	14–21
	Ampicillin	2 g q4h (IV)	
Other Localized Infection			
	Ceftriaxone	2 g/d (IV)	14–28
	Ciprofloxacin	500 mg bid (PO) or 400 mg q12h (IV)	
	Ampicillin	2 g q6h (IV)	

[a]Consider for neonates, persons >50 years of age with possible atherosclerotic vascular disease, and patients with immunosuppression, endovascular graft, or joint prosthesis.
[b]Or ofloxacin, 400 mg bid (PO).
[c]Consider on an individualized basis for patients with severe diarrhea and high fever who require hospitalization.
[d]Or cefotaxime, 2 g q8h (IV).

If the patient has endocarditis or arteritis, treatment for 6 weeks with an IV β-lactam antibiotic (such as ceftriaxone or ampicillin) is indicated. IV ciprofloxacin followed by prolonged oral therapy is an option, but published experience is limited. Early surgical resection of infected aneurysms or other infected endovascular sites is recommended. Patients with infected prosthetic vascular grafts that cannot be resected have been maintained successfully on chronic suppressive oral therapy. For extraintestinal nonvascular infections, a 2- to 4-week course of antibiotic therapy (depending on the infection site) is usually recommended. In chronic osteomyelitis, abscess, or urinary or hepatobiliary infection associated with anatomic abnormalities, surgical resection or drainage may be required in addition to prolonged antibiotic therapy for eradication of infection.

PREVENTION AND CONTROL

Despite widespread efforts to prevent or reduce bacterial contamination of animal-derived food products and to improve food-safety education and training, recent declines in the incidence of NTS in the United States have been modest compared with those of other food-borne pathogens. This observation probably reflects the complex epidemiology of NTS. Identifying effective risk-reduction strategies requires monitoring of every step of food production, from handling of raw animal or plant products to preparation of finished foods. Contaminated food can be made safe for consumption by pasteurization, irradiation, or proper cooking. All cases of NTS infection should be reported to local public health departments, since tracking and monitoring of these cases can identify the source(s) of infection and help authorities anticipate large outbreaks. Lastly, the prudent use of antimicrobial agents in both humans and animals is needed to limit the emergence of MDR *Salmonella*.

FURTHER READINGS

Centers for Disease Control and Prevention: Preliminary FoodNet data on the incidence of infection with pathogens transmitted commonly through food—10 states, 2008. MMWR Morb Mortal Wkly Rep 58:333, 2009

Cohen JI et al: Extra-intestinal manifestations of *Salmonella* infections. Medicine 66:349, 1987

Fraser A et al: Vaccines for preventing typhoid fever. Cochrane Database Syst Rev Jul 18(3):CD001261, 2007

Glynn MK et al: Emergence of multidrug-resistant *Salmonella enterica* serotype *typhimurium* DT104 infections in the United States. N Engl J Med 338:1333, 1998

Hoffman SL et al: Reduction in mortality in chloramphenicol-treated severe typhoid fever by high-dose dexamethasone. N Engl J Med 310:82, 1984

Lin FY et al: The efficacy of a *Salmonella typhi* Vi conjugate vaccine in two-to-five-year-old children. N Engl J Med 344:1263, 2001

Maskey AP et al: *Salmonella* enteric serovar Paratyphi A and *S. enterica* serovar Typhi cause indistinguishable clinical syndromes in Kathmandu, Nepal. Clin Infect Dis 42:1247, 2006

Ohl ME, Miller SI: *Salmonella*: A model for bacterial pathogenesis. Annu Rev Med 52:259, 2001

Steinberg EB et al: Typhoid fever in travelers: Who should be targeted for prevention. Clin Infect Dis 39:186, 2004

Su LH et al: Antimicrobial resistance in nontyphoid *Salmonella* serotypes: A global challenge. Clin Infect Dis 39:546, 2004

Varma JK et al: Antimicrobial-resistant nontyphoidal *Salmonella* is associated with excess bloodstream infections and hospitalizations. J Infect Dis 191:554, 2005

CHAPTER 55

SHIGELLOSIS

Philippe Sansonetti ■ Jean Bergounioux

The discovery of *Shigella* as the etiologic agent of dysentery—a clinical syndrome of fever, intestinal cramps, and frequent passage of small, bloody, mucopurulent stools—is attributed to the Japanese microbiologist Kiyoshi Shiga, who isolated the Shiga bacillus (now known as *Shigella dysenteriae* type 1) from patients' stools in 1897 during a large and devastating dysentery epidemic. *Shigella* cannot be distinguished from *Escherichia coli* by DNA hybridization and remains a separate species only on historical and clinical grounds.

DEFINITION

Shigella is a non–spore-forming, gram-negative bacterium that, unlike *E. coli*, is nonmotile and does not produce gas from sugars, decarboxylate lysine, or hydrolyze arginine. Some serovars produce indole, and occasional strains utilize sodium acetate. *S. dysenteriae*, *S. flexneri*, *S. boydii*, and *S. sonnei* (serogroups A, B, C, and D, respectively) can be differentiated on the basis of biochemical and serologic characteristics. Genome sequencing of *E. coli* K12, *S. flexneri* 2a, *S. sonnei*, *S. dysenteriae* type 1, and *S. boydii* has revealed that these species have ~93% of genes in common. The three major genomic "signatures" of *Shigella* are (1) a 215-kb virulence plasmid that carries most of the genes required for pathogenicity (particularly invasive capacity); (2) the lack or alteration of genetic sequences encoding products (e.g., lysine decarboxylase) that, if expressed, would attenuate pathogenicity; and (3) in *S. dysenteriae* type 1, the presence of genes encoding Shiga toxin, a potent cytotoxin.

EPIDEMIOLOGY

The human intestinal tract represents the major reservoir of *Shigella*, which is also found (albeit rarely) in the higher primates. Because excretion of shigellae is greatest in the acute phase of disease, the bacteria are transmitted most efficiently by the fecal-oral route. Most cases of shigellosis are caused by person-to-person transmission, although some outbreaks reflect contamination of water or food. *Shigella* can also be transmitted by flies and, given its capacity to survive in foodstuffs, can be a significant cause of food-borne infection. The high-level infectivity of *Shigella* is reflected by the very small inoculum required for experimental infection of volunteers [100 colony-forming units (CFU)], by the very high attack rates during outbreaks in day care centers (33–73%), and by the high rates of secondary cases among family members of sick children (26–33%). Shigellosis can also be transmitted sexually.

In a review published under the auspices of the World Health Organization (WHO), the total annual number of cases in 1966–1997 was estimated at 165 million, and 69% of these cases occurred in children <5 years of age. In this review, the annual number of deaths was calculated to range between 500,000 and 1.1 million. More recent data (2000–2004) from six Asian countries (Bangladesh, China, Pakistan, Indonesia, Vietnam, and Thailand) indicate that even though the incidence of shigellosis remains stable, mortality rates associated with this disease may have decreased significantly, possibly as a result of improved nutritional standards. However, extensive and essentially uncontrolled use of antibiotics has increased the risk of emergence of multidrug-resistant *Shigella* strains.

Throughout history, *Shigella* epidemics have often occurred in settings of human crowding under poor hygienic conditions—e.g., among soldiers in campaigning armies, inhabitants of besieged cities, groups on pilgrimages, and refugees in camps. Epidemics follow a cyclic pattern in areas such as the Indian subcontinent and Sub-Saharan Africa. These devastating epidemics, which are most often caused by *S. dysenteriae* type 1, are characterized by high attack rates and high mortality rates. In Bangladesh, for instance, an epidemic caused by *S. dysenteriae* type 1 was associated with a 42% increase in mortality rates among children 1–4 years of age. Apart from these epidemics, shigellosis is essentially an endemic disease, with 99% of cases occurring in the developing world and particularly high prevalences in the most impoverished areas, where personal and general hygiene are substandard. *S. flexneri* isolates predominate in less well-developed areas, whereas *S. sonnei* is more prevalent in economically emerging regions and in the industrialized world.

An often-overlooked complication of shigellosis is the short- and long-term impairment of the nutritional status of infected children in endemic areas. Combined with anorexia, the exudative enteropathy resulting from mucosal abrasions contributes to rapid exacerbation of the patient's nutritional status. Shigellosis is thus a major contributor to stunted growth among children in developing countries.

PATHOGENESIS AND PATHOLOGY

Shigella infection occurs through oral contamination. Direct fecal-oral transmission predominates since the organism is not well adapted to survive in the environment. Resistance to low-pH conditions allows shigellae to survive passage through the gastric barrier, an ability that may explain in part why a small inoculum (as few as 100 CFU) is sufficient to cause infection.

The watery diarrhea that usually precedes the dysenteric syndrome is attributable to active secretion and abnormal water reabsorption, a secretory effect at the jejunal level described in experimentally infected rhesus monkeys. This initial purge is probably due to the combined action of an enterotoxin (ShET-1) and mucosal inflammation. The dysenteric syndrome, manifested by bloody and mucopurulent stools, reflects invasion of the mucosa.

The pathogenesis of *Shigella* is essentially determined by a large virulence plasmid of 214 kb comprising ~100 genes, of which 25 encode a type III secretion system that inserts into the membrane of the host cell to allow effectors to transit from the bacterial cytoplasm to the cell cytoplasm (Fig. 55-1). Bacteria are thereby able to invade intestinal epithelial cells by inducing their own uptake after the initial crossing of the epithelial barrier through M cells (the specialized translocating epithelial cells in the follicle-associated epithelium that covers mucosal lymphoid nodules). The organisms induce apoptosis of subepithelial resident macrophages. Once inside the cytoplasm of intestinal epithelial cells, *Shigella* effectors trigger the cytoskeletal rearrangements necessary to direct uptake of the organism into the epithelial cell. The *Shigella*-containing vacuole is then quickly lysed, releasing bacteria into the cytosol.

Intracellular shigellae next use cytoskeletal components to propel themselves inside the infected cell; when the moving organism and the host cell membrane come into contact, cellular protrusions form and are engulfed by neighboring cells. This series of events permits bacterial cell-to-cell spread that is protected from immune effector mechanisms.

Cytokines released by a growing number of infected intestinal epithelial cells attract increased numbers of immune cells [particularly polymorphonuclear leukocytes (PMNs)] to the infected site, thus further destabilizing the epithelial barrier, exacerbating inflammation, and leading to the acute colitis that characterizes shigellosis. Recent evidence indicates that some of the type III

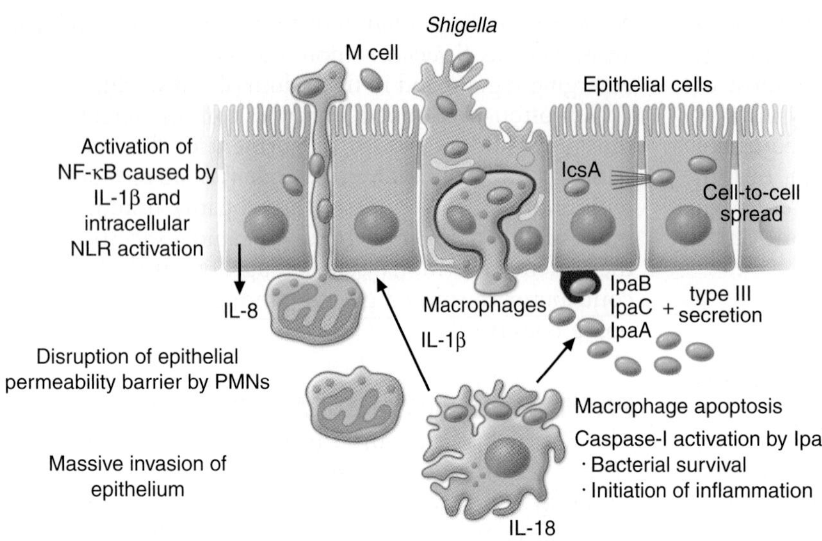

FIGURE 55-1
Invasive strategy of *Shigella flexneri*. IL, interleukin; NLR, nod-like receptor; PMN, polymorphonuclear leukocyte.

secretion system–injected effectors can control the extent of inflammation, thus facilitating bacterial survival.

Shiga toxin produced by *S. dysenteriae* type 1 increases disease severity. Shiga toxin and Shiga-like toxins belong to a group of A1-B5 protein toxins whose B subunit binds to the cell surface and whose catalytic A subunit expresses an RNA N-glycosidase on 28S ribosomal RNA. These events lead to inhibition of binding of the aminoacyl-tRNA to the 60S ribosomal subunit and thus to a general shutoff of cell protein biosynthesis. Shiga toxins are translocated from the bowel into the circulation. After binding to the receptor globotriaosylceramide on target cells in the kidney, toxin is internalized by receptor-mediated endocytosis and interacts with the subcellular machinery to inhibit protein synthesis. The consequent pathophysiologic changes may result in hemolytic-uremic syndrome (HUS; see below).

CLINICAL MANIFESTATIONS

The presentation and severity of shigellosis depend to some extent on the infecting species, but even more on the age and the immunologic and nutritional status of the host. Poverty and a poor hygienic environment are strongly related to the number and severity of diarrheal episodes, especially in children <5 years old.

Shigellosis typically evolves through four phases: incubation, watery diarrhea, dysentery, and the postinfectious phase. The incubation period usually lasts 1–4 days but may be as long as 8 days. Typical initial manifestations are transient fever, limited watery diarrhea, malaise, and anorexia. Signs and symptoms may range from mild abdominal discomfort to severe cramps, diarrhea, fever, vomiting, and tenesmus. The manifestations are usually exacerbated in children, with temperatures up to 40°–41°C and more severe anorexia and watery diarrhea. Unlike most diarrheal syndromes, dysenteric syndromes do not have dehydration as a major feature. This initial phase may represent the only clinical manifestation of shigellosis, especially in developed countries. Otherwise, dysentery follows within hours or days and is characterized by small volumes of bloody mucopurulent stools with increased tenesmus and abdominal cramps. At this stage, *Shigella* produces acute colitis involving mainly the distal colon and the rectum. Endoscopy demonstrates an edematous and hemorrhagic mucosa, with ulcerations and possibly overlying exudates resembling pseudomembranes. The extent of the lesions is correlated with the number and frequency of stools and with the degree of protein loss by exudative mechanisms. Most episodes are self-limited and resolve without treatment in 1 week. With appropriate treatment, recovery takes place within a few days to a week, with no sequelae.

Acute life-threatening complications are seen most often in children <5 years of age, particularly affecting malnourished children in developing countries. Risk factors for death include nonbloody diarrhea, moderate to severe dehydration, bacteremia, absence of fever, abdominal tenderness, and rectal prolapse. Major complications are predominantly intestinal (e.g., toxic megacolon, intestinal perforations, rectal prolapse) or metabolic (e.g., hypoglycemia, hyponatremia, dehydration). Bacteremia is rare and is reported most frequently in severely malnourished children, HIV-infected patients, and patients with defects in innate immunity. Alterations of consciousness, including seizures, delirium, and coma, may occur, especially in children <5 years old, and are associated with a poor prognosis; fever and severe metabolic alterations are more often the major causes of altered consciousness than is meningitis or Ekiri's syndrome (toxic encephalopathy associated with bizarre posturing, cerebral edema, and fatty degeneration of viscera), which has been reported in Japanese children. Pneumonia, vaginitis, and keratoconjunctivitis due to *Shigella* are rarely reported. In the absence of serious malnutrition, severe and very unusual clinical manifestations, such as meningitis, may be linked to disorders of immune function and require relevant investigations.

Two complications of particular importance are toxic megacolon and HUS. Toxic megacolon is a consequence of severe inflammation extending to the colonic smooth-muscle layer and causing paralysis and dilatation. The patient presents with abdominal distention and tenderness, with or without signs of localized or generalized peritonitis. The abdominal x-ray characteristically shows marked dilatation of the transverse colon (with the greatest distention in the ascending and descending colons), thumbprinting caused by mucosal inflammatory edema, and loss of the normal haustral pattern associated with pseudopolyps, often extending into the lumen. Pneumatosis coli is an occasional finding. If perforation occurs, radiographic signs of pneumoperitoneum may be apparent. Predisposing factors (e.g., hypokalemia and use of opioids, anticholinergics, loperamide, psyllium seeds, and antidepressants) should be sought.

Shiga toxin produced by *S. dysenteriae* type 1 has been linked to HUS in developing countries but rarely in industrialized countries. HUS is an early complication that most often develops after several days of diarrhea. Clinical examination shows pallor, asthenia, and irritability and, in some cases, bleeding of the nose and gums, oliguria, and increasing edema. HUS is a nonimmune (Coombs test–negative) hemolytic anemia defined by a diagnostic triad: microangiopathic hemolytic anemia [hemoglobin level typically <80 g/L (<8 g/dL)], thrombocytopenia (mild to moderate in severity; typically <60,000 platelets/μL), and acute renal failure due to thrombosis of the glomerular capillaries (with markedly elevated creatinine levels). Anemia is severe, with fragmented red blood cells (schizocytes) in the peripheral smear, high serum concentrations of lactate dehydrogenase and free circulating hemoglobin, and elevated reticulocyte counts. Acute renal failure occurs in 55–70% of cases; however, renal function recovers in most of these cases (up to 70% in various series). Leukemoid reactions, with leukocyte counts of 50,000/μL, are sometimes noted in association with HUS.

The postinfectious immunologic complication known as reactive arthritis (Reiter's syndrome) can develop weeks or months after shigellosis, especially in patients expressing the histocompatibility antigen HLA-B27. About 3% of patients infected with *S. flexneri* later develop Reiter's syndrome, with arthritis, ocular inflammation, and urethritis—a condition that can last for months or years and progress to difficult-to-treat chronic arthritis. Postinfectious arthropathy occurs only after infection with *S. flexneri* and not after infection with the other *Shigella* serotypes.

LABORATORY DIAGNOSIS

The differential diagnosis in patients with a dysenteric syndrome depends on the clinical and environmental context. In developing areas, infectious diarrhea caused by other invasive pathogenic bacteria (*Salmonella enteritidis, Campylobacter jejuni, Clostridium difficile, Yersinia enterocolitica*) or parasites (*Entamoeba histolytica*) should be considered. Only bacteriologic and parasitologic examinations of stool can truly differentiate among these pathogens. A first flare of inflammatory bowel disease, such as Crohn's disease or ulcerative colitis, should be considered in patients in industrialized countries. Despite similar symptoms, anamnesis discriminates between shigellosis, which usually follows recent travel in an endemic zone, and these other conditions.

Microscopic examination of stool smears shows the presence of erythrophagocytic trophozoites with very few PMNs in *E. histolytica* infection, whereas bacterial enteroinvasive infections (particularly shigellosis) are characterized by high PMN counts in each microscopic field. However, because shigellosis often manifests only as watery diarrhea, systematic attempts to isolate *Shigella* are necessary.

The "gold standard" for the diagnosis of *Shigella* infection remains the isolation and identification of the pathogen from fecal material. One major difficulty, particularly in endemic areas where laboratory facilities are not immediately available, is the fragility of *Shigella* and its common disappearance during transport, especially with rapid changes in temperature and pH. In the absence of a reliable enrichment medium, buffered glycerol saline or Cary-Blair medium can be used as a holding medium, but prompt inoculation onto isolation medium is essential. The probability of isolation is higher if the portion of stools that contains bloody and/or mucopurulent material is directly sampled. Rectal swabs can be used as they offer the highest rate of successful isolation during the acute phase of disease. Blood cultures are positive in <5% of cases and should be done only when a patient presents with a clinical picture of severe sepsis.

In addition to quick processing, the use of several media increases the likelihood of successful isolation: a nonselective medium such as bromocresol-purple agar lactose; a low-selectivity medium such as MacConkey or eosin-methylene blue; and a high-selectivity medium such as Hektoen, *Salmonella-Shigella*, or xylose-lysine-deoxycholate agar. After incubation on these media for 12–18 h at 37°C, shigellae appear as non–lactose-fermenting colonies that measure 0.5–1 mm in diameter and have a convex, translucent, smooth surface. Suspected colonies on nonselective or low-selectivity medium can be subcultured on a high-selectivity medium before being specifically identified or can be identified directly by standard commercial systems on the basis of four major characteristics: glucose positivity (usually without production of gas), lactose negativity, H_2S negativity, and lack of motility. The four *Shigella* serogroups (A–D) can then be differentiated by additional characteristics. This approach adds time and difficulty to the identification process, however; thus, after presumptive diagnosis, the use of serologic methods—e.g., slide agglutination, with group- and then type-specific antisera—should be considered. Group-specific antisera are widely available; in contrast, because of the large number of serotypes and subserotypes that must be considered, type-specific antisera are rare and more expensive and are often restricted to reference laboratories.

℞ Treatment: SHIGELLOSIS

ANTIBIOTIC SUSCEPTIBILITY OF *SHIGELLA* As an enteroinvasive disease, shigellosis requires antibiotic treatment. Since the mid-1960s, however, increasing resistance to multiple drugs has been a dominant factor in treatment decisions. Resistance rates are highly dependent on the geographic area. Clonal spread of particular strains and horizontal transfer of resistance determinants, particularly via plasmids and transposons, contribute to multidrug resistance. Quinolone resistance is essentially due to chromosomal mutations affecting DNA gyrase and topoisomerase IV. A review of the antibiotic resistance history of *Shigella* in India found that, after their introduction in the late 1980s, the second-generation quinolones norfloxacin, ciprofloxacin, and ofloxacin were highly effective in the treatment of shigellosis, including cases caused by multidrug-resistant strains of *S. dysenteriae* type 1. In contrast, investigations of recent outbreaks in India and Bangladesh have shown high levels of resistance (generally 5%) to norfloxacin, ciprofloxacin, and ofloxacin among certain isolates. The incidence of multidrug resistance parallels widespread uncontrolled use of antibiotics (particularly in developing areas), calls for the rational use of effective drugs, and underscores the need for alternative drugs to treat infections caused by resistant strains.

ANTIBIOTIC TREATMENT OF SHIGELLOSIS (Table 55-1) Because of the ready transmissibility of *Shigella*, current public health recommendations in the United States are that every case be treated with antibiotics. Ciprofloxacin is recommended as first-line treatment. A number of other drugs have been tested and shown to be effective, including ceftriaxone, azithromycin, pivmecillinam, and some fifth-generation quinolones. Although infections caused by non-*dysenteriae Shigella* in immunocompetent individuals are routinely treated with a 3-day course of antibiotics, it is recommended that *S. dysenteriae* infections be treated for 5 days and that *Shigella* infections in immunocompromised patients be treated for 7–10 days.

Treatment for shigellosis must be adapted to the clinical context, with the recognition that the most fragile patients are children <5 years old, who represent two-thirds of all cases worldwide. There are few data on the use of quinolones in children. The half-life of ciprofloxacin is longer in infants than in older individuals. The ciprofloxacin dose generally recommended for children is 30 mg/kg per day in two divided doses. Adults living in areas with high hygienic standards are likely to develop milder, shorter-duration disease, whereas infants in endemic areas can develop severe, sometimes fatal dysentery. In the former setting, treatment will remain minimal and bacteriologic proof of infection will often come after symptoms have resolved; in the latter setting, more aggressive measures, possibly including resuscitation, may be required.

REHYDRATION AND NUTRITION *Shigella* infection rarely causes significant dehydration. Cases requiring aggressive rehydration (particularly in industrialized countries) are uncommon. In developing countries,

TABLE 55-1

RECOMMENDED ANTIMICROBIAL THERAPY FOR SHIGELLOSIS

	TREATMENT SCHEDULE		
ANTIMICROBIAL AGENT	IN CHILDREN	IN ADULTS	LIMITATIONS
First line			
Ciprofloxacin	15 mg/kg 2 times per day for 3 days, PO	500 mg	
Second line			
Pivmecillinam	20 mg/kg 4 times per day for 5 days, PO	100 mg	Cost No pediatric formulation Frequent administration Resistance emerging
Ceftriaxone	50–100 mg/kg Once a day IM for 2–5 days	—	Efficacy not validated Must be injected
Azithromycin	6–20 mg/kg Once a day for 1–5 days, PO	1–1.5 g	Cost Efficacy not validated MIC near serum concentration Resistance emerges rapidly and spreads to other bacteria

Source: WHO Library Cataloguing-in-Publication Data: Guidelines for the control of shigellosis, including epidemics due to *Shigella dysenteriae* type 1 (*www.searo.who.int/LinkFiles/CAH_Publications_shigella.pdf*).

malnutrition remains the primary indicator for diarrhea-related death, highlighting the importance of nutrition in early management. Rehydration should be oral unless the patient is comatose or presents in shock. Because of the improved effectiveness of reduced-osmolarity oral rehydration solution (especially for children with acute noncholera diarrhea), the WHO and UNICEF now recommend a standard solution of 245 mOsm/L (sodium, 75 mmol/L; chloride, 65 mmol/L; glucose (anhydrous), 75 mmol/L; potassium, 20 mmol/L; citrate, 10 mmol/L). In shigellosis, as in acute infectious diarrhea of most etiologies (including cholera), the coupled transport of sodium to glucose or other solutes is largely unaffected, and oral rehydration therapy represents the easiest and most efficient form of rehydration, especially in severe cases.

Nutrition should be started as soon as possible after completion of initial rehydration. Early refeeding is safe, well tolerated, and clinically beneficial. Because breast-feeding reduces diarrheal losses and the need for oral rehydration in infants, it should be maintained in the absence of contraindications (e.g., maternal HIV infection).

NONSPECIFIC, SYMPTOM-BASED THERAPY Antimotility agents have been implicated in prolonged fever in volunteers with shigellosis. These agents are suspected of increasing the risk of toxic megacolon and are thought to have been responsible for HUS in children infected by Shiga toxin–producing strains of *E. coli*. For safety reasons, it is better to avoid antimotility agents in bloody diarrhea.

TREATMENT OF COMPLICATIONS There is no consensus regarding the best treatment for toxic megacolon. The patient should be assessed frequently by both medical and surgical teams. Anemia, dehydration, and electrolyte deficits (particularly hypokalemia) may aggravate colonic atony and should be actively treated. Nasogastric aspiration helps to deflate the colon. Parenteral nutrition has not been proved to be beneficial. Fever persisting beyond 48–72 h raises the possibility of local perforation or abscess. Most studies recommend colectomy if, after 48–72 h, colonic distention persists. However, some physicians recommend continuation of medical therapy for up to 7 days if the patient seems to be improving clinically despite persistent megacolon without free perforation. Intestinal perforation, either isolated or complicating toxic megacolon, requires surgical treatment and intensive medical support.

Rectal prolapse must be treated as soon as possible. With the health care provider using surgical gloves or a soft warm wet cloth and the patient in the knee-chest position, the prolapsed rectum is gently pushed back into place. If edema of the rectal mucosa is evident (rendering reintegration difficult), it can be osmotically reduced by applying gauze impregnated with a warm solution of saturated magnesium sulfate. Rectal prolapse often relapses but usually resolves along with the resolution of dysentery.

HUS must be treated by water restriction, including discontinuation of oral rehydration solution and potassium-rich alimentation. Hemofiltration is usually required.

PREVENTION

Hand washing after defecation or handling of children's feces and before handling of food is recommended. However, this protocol entails an average of 32 hand washes per day, with consumption of 20 L of water. If soap is too costly, ash or mud can be used, but access to water remains essential. Stool precautions, together with a cleaning protocol for medical staff as well as for patients, have proven useful in limiting the spread of infection during *Shigella* outbreaks. Ideally, patients should have a negative stool culture before their infection is considered cured. Recurrences are rare if treatment and prevention are correctly implemented.

Although several live attenuated oral and subunit parenteral vaccine candidates have been produced and are undergoing clinical trials, no vaccine against shigellosis is currently available. Especially given the rapid progression of antibiotic resistance in *Shigella*, a vaccine is urgently needed.

FURTHER READINGS

Bennish ML, Wojtyniak BJ: Mortality due to shigellosis: Community and hospital data. Rev Infect Dis 13(Suppl 4):S245, 1991

Centers for Disease Control and Prevention: Preliminary FoodNet data on the incidence of infection with pathogens transmitted commonly through food—10 States, 2008. MMWR Morb Mortal Wkly Rep 58:333, 2009

Cossart P, Sansonetti PJ: Bacterial invasion: The paradigms of enteroinvasive pathogens. Science 304:242, 2004

Kotloff KL et al: Overview of live vaccine strategies against *Shigella*, in *New Generation Vaccines*, 3d ed, MM Levine et al (eds). London, Informa Healthcare, 2004, pp 723–735

——— et al: Global burden of *Shigella* infections: Implications for vaccine development and implementation of control strategies. Bull World Health Organ 77:651, 1999

Niyogi SK: Shigellosis. J Microbiol 43:133, 2005

Phalipon A, Sansonetti PJ: Shigella's ways of manipulating the host intestinal innate and adaptive immune system: A tool box for survival? Immunol Cell Biol 85:119, 2007

von Seidlein L et al: A multicentre study of *Shigella* diarrhoea in six Asian countries: Disease burden, clinical manifestations, and microbiology. PLoS Med 3(9):e353, 2006

World Health Organization: Guidelines for the control of shigellosis, including epidemics due to *Shigella dysenteriae* type 1. WHO Library Cataloguing-in-Publication Data (*www.searo.who.int/LinkFiles/CAH_Publications_shigella.pdf*)

CHAPTER 56

INFECTIONS DUE TO *CAMPYLOBACTER* AND RELATED SPECIES

Martin J. Blaser

DEFINITION

Bacteria of the genus *Campylobacter* and of the related genera *Arcobacter* and *Helicobacter* (Chap. 52) cause a variety of inflammatory conditions. Although acute diarrheal illnesses are most common, these organisms may cause infections in virtually all parts of the body, especially in compromised hosts, and these infections may have late nonsuppurative sequelae. The designation *Campylobacter* comes from the Greek for "curved rod" and refers to the organism's vibrio-like morphology.

ETIOLOGY

Campylobacters are motile, non–spore-forming, curved, gram-negative rods. Originally known as *Vibrio fetus*, these bacilli were reclassified as a new genus in 1973, after their dissimilarity to other vibrios was recognized. More than 15 species have since been identified. These species are currently divided into three genera: *Campylobacter*, *Arcobacter*, and *Helicobacter*. Not all of the species are pathogens of humans. The human pathogens fall into two major groups: those that primarily cause diarrheal disease and those that cause extraintestinal infection. The principal diarrheal pathogen is *C. jejuni*, which accounts for 80–90% of all cases of recognized illness due to campylobacters and related genera. Other organisms that cause diarrheal disease include *C. coli*, *C. upsaliensis*, *C. lari*, *C. hyointestinalis*, *C. fetus*, *A. butzleri*, *A. cryaerophilus*, *H. cinaedi*, and *H. fennelliae*. The two *Helicobacter* species causing diarrheal disease, *H. cinaedi* and *H. fennelliae*, are intestinal rather than gastric organisms; in terms of the clinical features of the illnesses they cause, these species most closely resemble *Campylobacter* rather than *H. pylori* (Chap. 52) and thus are considered in this chapter.

The major species causing extraintestinal illnesses is *C. fetus*. However, any of the diarrheal agents listed above may cause systemic or localized infection as well. Neither aerobes nor strict anaerobes, these microaerophilic organisms are adapted for survival in the gastrointestinal mucous layer. This chapter focuses on *C. jejuni* and *C. fetus* as the major pathogens in and prototypes for their groups. The key features of infection are listed by species (excluding *C. jejuni*, described in detail in the text below) in Table 56-1.

EPIDEMIOLOGY

Campylobacters are found in the gastrointestinal tract of many animals used for food (including poultry, cattle, sheep, and swine) and many household pets (including birds, dogs, and cats). These microorganisms usually do not cause illness in their animal hosts. In most cases, campylobacters are transmitted to humans in raw or undercooked food products or through direct contact with infected animals. In the United States and other developed countries, ingestion of contaminated poultry that has not been sufficiently cooked is the most common mode of acquisition (30–70% of cases). Other modes include ingestion of raw (unpasteurized) milk or untreated water, contact with infected household pets, travel to developing countries (campylobacters being among the leading causes of traveler's diarrhea; Chaps. 4 and 25), oral-anal sexual contact, and (occasionally) contact with an index case who is incontinent of stool.

Campylobacter infections are common. Several studies indicate that, in the United States, diarrheal disease due to campylobacters is more common than that due to *Salmonella* and *Shigella* combined. Infections occur throughout the year, but their incidence peaks during summer and early autumn. Persons of all ages are affected; however, attack rates for *C. jejuni* are highest among young children and young adults, whereas those for *C. fetus* are highest at the extremes of age. Systemic infections due to *C. fetus* (and to other *Campylobacter* and related species) are most common among compromised hosts. Persons at increased risk include those with AIDS, hypogammaglobulinemia, neoplasia, liver disease, diabetes mellitus, and generalized atherosclerosis, as well as neonates and pregnant women. However, apparently healthy nonpregnant persons occasionally develop transient *Campylobacter* bacteremia as part of a gastrointestinal illness.

In developing countries, *C. jejuni* infections are hyperendemic, with the highest rates among children <2 years old. Infection rates fall with age, as does the illness-to-infection ratio. These observations suggest that frequent exposure to *C. jejuni* leads to the acquisition of immunity.

TABLE 56-1

CLINICAL FEATURES ASSOCIATED WITH INFECTION DUE TO "ATYPICAL" *CAMPYLOBACTER* AND RELATED SPECIES IMPLICATED AS CAUSES OF HUMAN ILLNESS

SPECIES	COMMON CLINICAL FEATURES	LESS COMMON CLINICAL FEATURES	ADDITIONAL INFORMATION
Campylobacter coli	Fever, diarrhea, abdominal pain	Bacteremia[a]	Clinically indistinguishable from *C. jejuni*
Campylobacter fetus	Bacteremia,[a] sepsis, meningitis, vascular infections	Diarrhea, relapsing fevers	Not usually isolated from media containing cephalothin or incubated at 42°C
Campylobacter upsaliensis	Watery diarrhea, low-grade fever, abdominal pain	Bacteremia, abscesses	Difficult to isolate because of cephalothin susceptibility
Campylobacter lari	Abdominal pain, diarrhea	Colitis, appendicitis	Seagulls frequently colonized; organism often transmitted to humans via contaminated water
Campylobacter hyointestinalis	Watery or bloody diarrhea, vomiting, abdominal pain	Bacteremia	Causes proliferative enteritis in swine
Helicobacter fennelliae	Chronic mild diarrhea, abdominal cramps, proctitis	Bacteremia[a]	Best treated with fluoroquinolones
Helicobacter cinaedi	Chronic mild diarrhea, abdominal cramps, proctitis	Bacteremia[a]	Best treated with fluoroquinolones; identified in healthy hamsters
Campylobacter jejuni subspecies *doylei*	Diarrhea	Chronic gastritis, bacteremia[b]	Uncertain role as human pathogen
Arcobacter cryaerophilus	Diarrhea	Bacteremia	Cultured under aerobic conditions
Arcobacter butzleri	Fever, diarrhea, abdominal pain, nausea	Bacteremia, appendicitis	Cultured under aerobic conditions; enzootic in nonhuman primates
Campylobacter sputorum	Pulmonary, perianal, groin, and axillary abscesses	Bacteremia	Three clinically relevant biovars: *C. sputorum* subspecies *sputorum*, *C. sputorum* subspecies *bubulus*, and *Campylobacter mucosalis*

[a]In immunocompromised hosts, especially HIV-infected persons.
[b]In children.
Source: Adapted from BM Allos, MJ Blaser: *Campylobacter jejuni* and the expanding spectrum of related infections. Clin Infect Dis 20:1092, 1995.

PATHOLOGY AND PATHOGENESIS

Many *C. jejuni* infections are subclinical, especially in hosts in developing countries who have had multiple prior infections and thus are partially immune. Most illnesses occur within 2–4 days (range, 1–7 days) of exposure to the organism in food or water. The sites of tissue injury include the jejunum, ileum, and colon. Biopsies show an acute nonspecific inflammatory reaction, with neutrophils, monocytes, and eosinophils in the lamina propria, as well as damage to the epithelium, including loss of mucus, glandular degeneration, and crypt abscesses. Biopsy findings may be consistent with Crohn's disease or ulcerative colitis, but these "idiopathic" chronic inflammatory diseases should not be diagnosed unless infectious colitis, *specifically including* that due to infection with *Campylobacter* species and related organisms, has been ruled out.

The high frequency of *C. jejuni* infections and their severity and recurrence among hypogammaglobulinemic patients suggest that antibodies are important in protective immunity. The pathogenesis of infection is uncertain. Both the motility of the strain and its capacity to adhere to host tissues appear to favor disease, but classic enterotoxins and cytotoxins (although described and including cytolethal distending toxin, or CDT) appear not to play substantial roles in tissue injury or disease production. The organisms have been visualized in the epithelium, albeit in low numbers. The documentation of a significant tissue response and occasionally of *C. jejuni* bacteremia further suggests that tissue invasion is clinically significant, and in vitro studies are consistent with this pathogenetic feature.

The pathogenesis of *C. fetus* infections is better defined. Virtually all clinical isolates of *C. fetus* possess a proteinaceous capsule-like structure (an S-layer) that renders the organisms resistant to complement-mediated killing and opsonization. As a result, *C. fetus* can cause bacteremia and can seed sites beyond the intestinal tract. The ability of the organism to switch the S-layer proteins expressed—a phenomenon that results in antigenic variability—may contribute to the chronicity and high rate of recurrence of *C. fetus* infections in compromised hosts.

CLINICAL MANIFESTATIONS

The clinical features of infections due to *Campylobacter* and the related *Arcobacter* and intestinal *Helicobacter* species causing enteric disease appear to be highly similar. *C. jejuni* can be considered the prototype, in part because it is by far the most common enteric pathogen. A prodrome of fever, headache, myalgia, and/or malaise often occurs 12–48 h before the onset of diarrheal symptoms. The most common signs and symptoms of the intestinal phase are diarrhea, abdominal pain, and fever. The degree of diarrhea varies from several loose stools to grossly bloody stools; most patients presenting for medical attention have ≥10 bowel movements on the worst day of illness. Abdominal pain usually consists of cramping and may be the most prominent symptom. Pain is usually generalized but may become localized; *C. jejuni* infection may cause pseudoappendicitis. Fever may be the only initial manifestation of *C. jejuni* infection, a situation mimicking the early stages of typhoid fever. Febrile young children may develop convulsions. *Campylobacter* enteritis is generally self-limited; however, symptoms persist for >1 week in 10–20% of patients seeking medical attention, and clinical relapses occur in 5–10% of untreated patients.

C. fetus may cause a diarrheal illness similar to that due to *C. jejuni*, especially in normal hosts. This organism may also cause either intermittent diarrhea or nonspecific abdominal pain without localizing signs. Sequelae are uncommon, and the outcome is benign. *C. fetus* may also cause a prolonged relapsing systemic illness (with fever, chills, and myalgias) that has no obvious primary source; this manifestation is especially common among compromised hosts. Secondary seeding of an organ (e.g., meninges, brain, bone, urinary tract, or soft tissue) complicates the course, which may be fulminant. *C. fetus* infections have a tropism for vascular sites: endocarditis, mycotic aneurysm, and septic thrombophlebitis may all occur. Infection during pregnancy often leads to fetal death. A variety of *Campylobacter* species and *H. cinaedi* can cause recurrent cellulitis with fever and bacteremia in immunocompromised hosts.

COMPLICATIONS

Except in infection with *C. fetus*, bacteremia is uncommon, developing most often in immunocompromised hosts and at the extremes of age. Three patterns of extraintestinal infection have been noted: (1) transient bacteremia in a normal host with enteritis (benign course, no specific treatment needed); (2) sustained bacteremia or focal infection in a normal host (bacteremia originating from enteritis, with patients responding well to antimicrobial therapy); and (3) sustained bacteremia or focal infection in a compromised host. Enteritis may not be clinically apparent. Antimicrobial therapy, possibly prolonged, is necessary for suppression or cure of the infection.

Campylobacter, Arcobacter, and intestinal *Helicobacter* infections in patients with AIDS or hypogammaglobulinemia may be severe, persistent, and extraintestinal; relapse after cessation of therapy is common. Hypogammaglobulinemic patients may also develop osteomyelitis and an erysipelas-like rash or cellulitis.

Local suppurative complications of infection include cholecystitis, pancreatitis, and cystitis; distant complications include meningitis, endocarditis, arthritis, peritonitis, cellulitis, and septic abortion. All these complications are rare, except in immunocompromised hosts. Hepatitis, interstitial nephritis, and the hemolytic-uremic syndrome occasionally complicate acute infection. Reactive arthritis and other rheumatologic complaints may develop several weeks after infection, especially in persons with the HLA-B27 phenotype. Guillain-Barré syndrome (or its Miller Fisher or cranial polyneuropathy variant) follows *Campylobacter* infections uncommonly—i.e., in 1 of every 1000–2000 cases or, for certain *C. jejuni* serotypes (such as O19), in 1 of every 100–200 cases. Despite the low frequency of this complication, it is now estimated that *Campylobacter* infections, because of their high incidence, may trigger 20–40% of all cases of Guillain-Barré syndrome. Immunoproliferative small-intestinal disease (*alpha chain disease*), a form of lymphoma that originates in small-intestinal mucosa-associated lymphoid tissue, has been associated with *C. jejuni*; antimicrobial therapy has led to marked clinical improvement.

DIAGNOSIS

In patients with *Campylobacter* enteritis, peripheral leukocyte counts reflect the severity of the inflammatory process. However, stools from nearly all *Campylobacter*-infected patients presenting for medical attention in the United States contain leukocytes or erythrocytes. Fecal smears should be treated with Gram's or Wright's stain and examined in all suspected cases. When the diagnosis of *Campylobacter* enteritis is suspected on the basis of findings indicating inflammatory diarrhea (fever, fecal leukocytes), clinicians can ask the laboratory to attempt the visualization of organisms with characteristic vibrioid morphology by direct microscopic examination of stools with Gram's staining or to use phase-contrast or dark-field microscopy to identify the organisms' characteristic "darting" motility. Confirmation of the diagnosis of *Campylobacter* infection is based on identification of an isolate from cultures of stool, blood, or another site. *Campylobacter*-specific media should be used to culture stools from all patients with inflammatory or bloody diarrhea. Since all *Campylobacter* species are fastidious, they will not be isolated unless selective media or other selective techniques are used. Not all media are equally useful for isolation of the broad array of campylobacters; therefore, failure to isolate campylobacters from stool does not entirely rule out their presence. The detection of the organisms in stool almost always implies infection; there is a brief period of postconvalescent fecal carriage and no commensalism in humans. In contrast, *C. sputorum* and related organisms found in the oral cavity are commensals with rare pathogenic significance. Because of low levels of metabolic activity in standard blood culture media, *Campylobacter* bacteremia may be difficult to detect unless laboratorians are looking for low-positive results in quantitative assays.

DIFFERENTIAL DIAGNOSIS

The symptoms of *Campylobacter* enteritis are not sufficiently unusual to distinguish this illness from that due to *Salmonella*, *Shigella*, *Yersinia*, and other pathogens. The combination of fever and fecal leukocytes or erythrocytes is indicative of inflammatory diarrhea, and definitive diagnosis is based on culture or demonstration of the characteristic organisms on stained fecal smears. Similarly, extraintestinal *Campylobacter* illness is diagnosed by culture. Infection due to *Campylobacter* should be suspected in the setting of septic abortion, and that due to *C. fetus* should be suspected specifically in the setting of septic thrombophlebitis. It is important to reiterate that (1) the presentation of *Campylobacter* enteritis may mimic that of ulcerative colitis or Crohn's disease, (2) *Campylobacter* enteritis is much more common than either of the latter (especially among young adults), and (3) biopsy may not distinguish among these entities. Thus a diagnosis of inflammatory bowel disease should not be made until *Campylobacter* infection has been ruled out, especially in persons with a history of foreign travel, significant animal contact, immunodeficiency, or exposure incurring a high risk of transmission.

℞ Treatment: INFECTIONS DUE TO *CAMPYLOBACTER* AND RELATED SPECIES

Fluid and electrolyte replacement is central to the treatment of diarrheal illnesses (Chap. 25). Even among patients presenting for medical attention with *Campylobacter* enteritis, not all clearly benefit from specific antimicrobial therapy. Indications for therapy include high fever, bloody diarrhea, severe diarrhea, persistence for >1 week, and worsening of symptoms. A 5- to 7-day course of erythromycin (250 mg orally four times daily or—for children—30–50 mg/kg per day, in divided doses) is the regimen of choice. Both clinical trials and in vitro susceptibility testing indicate that other macrolides, including clarithromycin and azithromycin, also are useful therapeutic agents. An alternative regimen for adults is ciprofloxacin (500 mg orally twice daily) or another fluoroquinolone for 5–7 days, but resistance to this class of agents as well as to tetracyclines has been increasing. Patients infected with antibiotic-resistant strains are at increased risk of adverse outcomes. Use of antimotility agents, which may prolong the duration of symptoms and have been associated with toxic megacolon and with death, is not recommended.

For systemic infections, treatment with gentamicin (1.7 mg/kg IV every 8 h after a loading dose of 2 mg/kg), imipenem (500 mg IV every 6 h), or chloramphenicol (50 mg/kg IV each day in three or four divided doses) should be started empirically, but susceptibility testing should then be performed. Ciprofloxacin and amoxicillin/clavulanate are alternative agents for susceptible strains. In the absence of immunocompromise or endovascular infections, therapy should be administered for 14 days. For immunocompromised patients with systemic infections due to *C. fetus* and for patients with endovascular infections, prolonged therapy (for up to 4 weeks) is usually necessary. For recurrent infections in immunocompromised hosts, lifelong therapy/prophylaxis is sometimes necessary.

PROGNOSIS

Nearly all patients recover fully from *Campylobacter* enteritis, either spontaneously or after antimicrobial therapy. Volume depletion probably contributes to the few deaths that are reported. As stated above, occasional patients develop reactive arthritis or Guillain-Barré syndrome or its variants. Systemic infection with *C. fetus* is much more often fatal than that due to related species; this higher mortality rate reflects in part the population affected. Prognosis depends on the rapidity with which appropriate therapy is begun. Otherwise-healthy hosts usually survive *C. fetus* infections without sequelae. Compromised hosts often have recurrent and/or life-threatening infections due to a variety of *Campylobacter* species.

FURTHER READINGS

Centers for Disease Control and Prevention: Preliminary FoodNet data on the incidence of infection with pathogens transmitted commonly through food—10 States, 2008. MMWR Morb Mortal Wkly Rep 58:333, 2009

Helms M et al: Adverse health events associated with antimicrobial drug resistance in *Campylobacter* species: A registry-based cohort study. J Infect Dis 191:1050, 2005

Lang DR et al (eds): Development of Guillain-Barré syndrome following *Campylobacter* infection. J Infect Dis 176(Suppl 2):S91, 1997

Lecuit M et al: Immunoproliferative small intestinal disease associated with *Campylobacter jejuni*. N Engl J Med 350:239, 2004

Mead PS et al: Food-related illness and death in the United States. Emerg Infect Dis 5:607, 1999

Nachamkin I, Blaser MJ (eds): *Campylobacter jejuni*, 2d ed. Washington, American Society for Microbiology, 2000

Smith KE et al: Quinolone-resistant *Campylobacter jejuni* infections in Minnesota, 1992–1998. Investigation Team. N Engl J Med 340: 1525, 1999

Ternhag A et al: A meta-analysis on the effects of antibiotic treatment on duration of symptoms caused by infection with *Campylobacter* species. Clin Infect Dis 44:696, 2007

CHAPTER 57

CHOLERA AND OTHER VIBRIOSES

Matthew K. Waldor ■ Gerald T. Keusch

Members of the genus *Vibrio* cause a number of important infectious syndromes. Classic among them is cholera, a devastating diarrheal disease caused by *V. cholerae* that has been responsible for seven global pandemics and much suffering over the past two centuries. Epidemic cholera remains a significant public health concern in the developing world today. Other vibrioses caused by other *Vibrio* species include syndromes of diarrhea, soft tissue infection, or primary sepsis. All *Vibrio* species are highly motile, facultatively anaerobic, curved gram-negative rods with one or more flagella. In nature, vibrios most commonly reside in tidal rivers and bays under conditions of moderate salinity. They proliferate in the summer months when water temperatures exceed 20°C. As might be expected, the illnesses they cause also increase in frequency during the warm months.

CHOLERA

DEFINITION

Cholera is an acute diarrheal disease that can, in a matter of hours, result in profound, rapidly progressive dehydration and death. Accordingly, cholera gravis (the severe form of cholera) is a much-feared disease, particularly in its epidemic presentation. Fortunately, prompt aggressive fluid repletion and supportive care can obviate the high mortality that cholera has historically wrought. Although the term *cholera* has occasionally been applied to any severely dehydrating secretory diarrheal illness, whether infectious in etiology or not, it has generally referred to disease caused by *V. cholerae* serogroup O1. In 1992, however, a new serogroup (O139) that causes epidemic cholera emerged on the Indian subcontinent and has since killed thousands of people.

MICROBIOLOGY AND EPIDEMIOLOGY

The species *V. cholerae* comprises a host of organisms classified on the basis of the carbohydrate determinants of their lipopolysaccharide (LPS) O antigens. Some 200 serogroups have now been recognized. They are divided into those that agglutinate in antisera to the O1 group antigen (*V. cholerae* O1) and those that do not (non-O1 *V. cholerae*). Although some non-O1 *V. cholerae* serogroups have occasionally caused sporadic outbreaks of diarrhea, serogroup O1 was, until the emergence of serogroup O139, the exclusive cause of epidemic cholera. Two biotypes of *V. cholerae* O1, classical and El Tor, are distinguished. Each biotype is further subdivided into two serotypes, termed *Inaba* and *Ogawa*.

The natural habitat of *V. cholerae* is coastal salt water and brackish estuaries, where the organism lives in close relation to plankton. Humans become infected incidentally but, once infected, can act as vehicles for spread. Ingestion of water contaminated by human feces is the most common means of acquisition of *V. cholerae*. Consumption of contaminated food can also contribute to spread. There is no known animal reservoir. Although the infectious dose is relatively high, it is markedly reduced in hypochlorhydric persons, in those using antacids, and when gastric acidity is buffered by a meal. Cholera is predominantly a pediatric disease in endemic areas, but it affects adults and children equally when newly introduced into a population. Children <2 years of age are less likely to develop severe cholera than are older children, perhaps because of passive immunity acquired from breast milk. In endemic areas, the disease is more common in the summer and fall months. For unexplained reasons, susceptibility to cholera is significantly influenced by ABO blood group status; persons with type O blood are at greatest risk, whereas those with type AB are at least risk.

Cholera is native to the Ganges delta in the Indian subcontinent. Since 1817, seven global pandemics have occurred. The current (seventh) pandemic—the first due to the El Tor biotype—began in Indonesia in 1961 and spread throughout Asia as *V. cholerae* El Tor displaced the endemic classical strain. In the early 1970s, El Tor cholera erupted in Africa, causing major epidemics before becoming a persistent endemic problem. Currently, >90% of cholera cases reported annually to the World Health Organization (WHO) are from Africa (Fig. 57-1). In the period 2000–2004, the annual worldwide number of cholera cases reported to the WHO remained stable at ~100,000. This number is certainly a significant underestimate, as several nations with endemic cholera do not report cholera cases to the WHO.

The recent history of cholera has been punctuated by severe outbreaks. Such outbreaks are often precipitated by war or other circumstances that lead to the breakdown of public health measures. Such was the case in the camps for Rwandan refugees set up in 1994 around Goma, Zaire. Since 1973, sporadic endemic infections due to

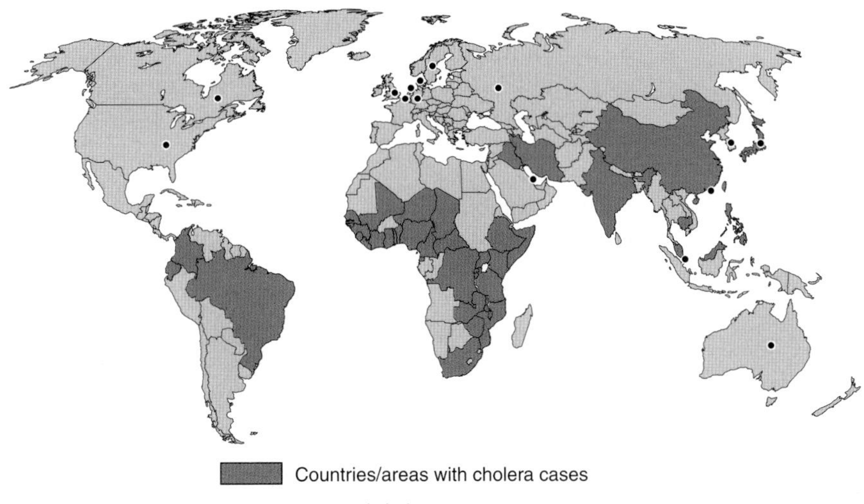

FIGURE 57-1
World distribution of cholera in 2004.
(Adapted from WHO: Cholera, 2004.)

V. cholerae O1 strains related to the seventh-pandemic strain have been recognized along the U.S. Gulf Coast of Louisiana and Texas. These infections are typically associated with the consumption of contaminated, locally harvested shellfish. Occasionally, cases in U.S. locations remote from the Gulf Coast have been linked to shipped-in Gulf Coast seafood.

It was not until 1991 that the current cholera pandemic reached Latin America. Beginning along the Peruvian coast in January 1991, the disease spread in an explosive epidemic to virtually all of South and Central America and to Mexico (Fig. 57-2). About 400,000 cases were reported in the first year of the outbreak, and >1 million had been reported by the end of 1994. Although the cumulative mortality rate has been <1%, the mortality rate approached 30% in the communities first affected, where a lack of familiarity with the disease led initially to the deployment of ineffective treatment. Intensive education of health care providers and of the community at large has enhanced awareness of the disease and its appropriate management and has greatly diminished mortality. As it did in Africa two decades earlier, the epidemic El Tor strain proved capable of establishing itself in inland waters rather than in its classic niche of coastal salt waters; the organism has already become endemic in many of the Latin American countries into which it was recently introduced. Cases linked to the Latin American epidemic have occurred (via importation of contaminated seafood) in the United States. Although secondary spread of this strain has not taken place in the United States, these events underscore the need for vigilance among health care professionals, even in locations remote from an epidemic.

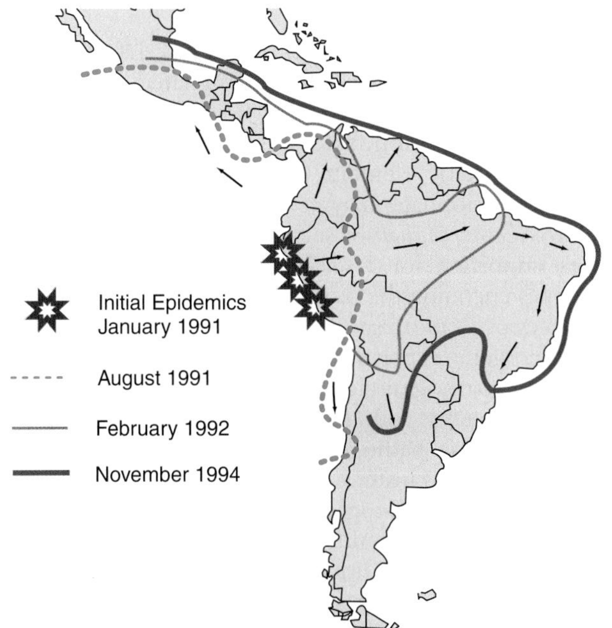

FIGURE 57-2
Spread of *Vibrio cholerae* O1 in the Americas, 1991–1994.
(Courtesy of Dr. Robert V. Tauxe, Centers for Disease Control and Prevention, Atlanta; with permission.)

In October 1992, a large-scale outbreak of clinical cholera occurred in southeastern India. The etiologic agent proved to be of a novel *V. cholerae* serogroup. This strain spread rapidly up and down the coast of the Bay of Bengal, reaching Bangladesh in December 1992. There alone, it caused more than 100,000 cases of cholera in the first 3 months of 1993. It subsequently spread across the Indian subcontinent and to neighboring countries, affecting Pakistan, Nepal, western China, Thailand, and Malaysia by the end of 1994 (Fig. 57-3). The organism has since been designated *V. cholerae* O139 Bengal in recognition of its novel O antigen and its geographic origin. The clinical manifestations and epidemiologic features of the disease caused by *V. cholerae* O139 Bengal are indistinguishable from those of O1 cholera. Immunity to the latter, however, is not protective against the former. Because naturally acquired immunity to *V. cholerae* O1 does not cross-protect against *V. cholerae* O139 Bengal, vaccines being developed against the former are unlikely to be effective against the latter.

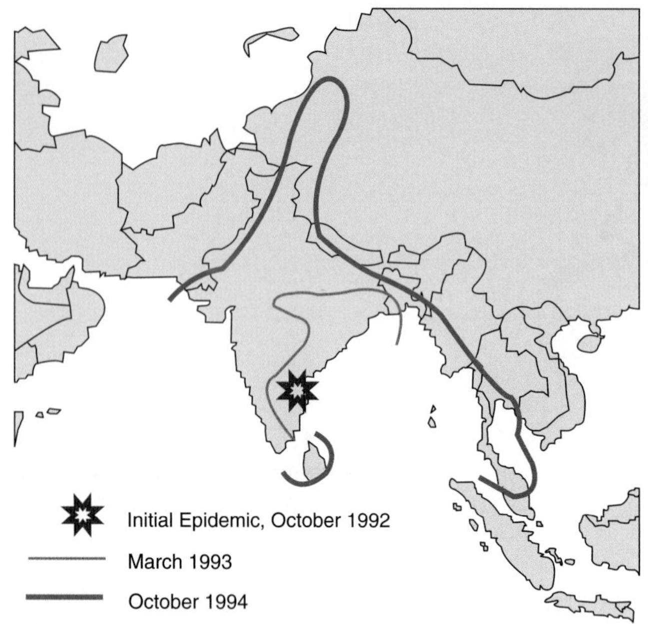

FIGURE 57-3

Spread of *Vibrio cholerae* O139 in the Indian subcontinent and elsewhere in Asia, 1992–1994. *(Courtesy of Dr. Robert V. Tauxe, CDC, Atlanta; with permission.)*

Some authorities believed that the emergence of *V. cholerae* O139 signaled the beginning of the eighth global cholera pandemic. Indeed, just as O1 El Tor replaced the classical biotype that preceded it, O139 Bengal in 1993 rapidly replaced O1 El Tor as the most common environmental isolate and the predominant cause of clinical cholera in the areas in which it had appeared. However, by the beginning of 1994, O1 El Tor had resumed its dominance in Bangladesh. *V. cholerae* O139 has not spread outside of Asia, and currently, in most regions of Southeast Asia, *V. cholerae* O1 remains dominant.

PATHOGENESIS

In the final analysis, cholera is a toxin-mediated disease. Its characteristic watery diarrhea is due to the action of cholera toxin, a potent protein enterotoxin elaborated by the organism after it colonizes the small intestine. For *V. cholerae* to colonize the small intestine and produce cholera toxin, it must first recognize, contend with, and traverse several hostile environments. The first of these is the acidic milieu of the stomach. To elude the bactericidal effects of gastric acidity, *V. cholerae* relies, at least in part, on a relatively large inoculum size (compared with that needed for colonization by *Shigella*, for instance). The organism must next traverse the mucous layer lining the small bowel. *V. cholerae* chemotaxis and motility and the action of a variety of proteases may allow the organism to traverse this gel covering the intestinal epithelium. The toxin-coregulated pilus (TCP), so named because its synthesis is regulated in parallel with that of cholera toxin, is essential for *V. cholerae* intestinal colonization. Cholera toxin, TCP, and several other virulence factors are coordinately regulated by ToxR. This protein modulates the expression of virulence genes in response to environmental signals via a cascade of regulatory proteins. Additional regulatory processes, including bacterial responses to the density of the bacterial population (in a phenomenon known as *quorum sensing*), control the virulence of *V. cholerae*.

Once established in the human small bowel, the organism produces cholera toxin, which consists of a monomeric enzymatic moiety (the A subunit) and a pentameric binding moiety (the B subunit). The B pentamer binds to G_{M1} ganglioside, a glycolipid on the surface of epithelial cells that serves as the toxin receptor and makes possible the delivery of the A subunit to its cytosolic target. The activated A subunit (A_1) irreversibly transfers ADP-ribose from nicotinamide adenine dinucleotide to its specific target protein, the GTP-binding regulatory component of adenylate cyclase. The ADP-ribosylated G protein upregulates the activity of adenylate cyclase; the result is the intracellular accumulation of high levels of cyclic AMP. In intestinal epithelial cells, cyclic AMP inhibits the absorptive sodium transport system in villus cells and activates the secretory chloride transport system in crypt cells, and these events lead to the accumulation of sodium chloride in the intestinal lumen. Since water moves passively to maintain osmolality, isotonic fluid accumulates in the lumen. When the volume of that fluid exceeds the capacity of the rest of the gut to resorb it, watery diarrhea results. Unless the wasted fluid and electrolytes are adequately replaced, shock (due to profound dehydration) and acidosis (due to loss of bicarbonate) follow. Although perturbation of the adenylate cyclase pathway is the primary mechanism by which cholera toxin causes excess fluid secretion, increasing evidence indicates that cholera toxin also enhances intestinal secretion via prostaglandins and/or neural histamine receptors.

The genes encoding cholera toxin (*ctxAB*) are part of the genome of a bacteriophage designated CTXΦ. The receptor for this phage on the *V. cholerae* surface is the intestinal colonization factor TCP. Since *ctxAB* is part of a mobile genetic element (CTXΦ), horizontal transfer of this bacteriophage may account for the emergence of new toxigenic *V. cholerae* serogroups. Many of the other genes important for *V. cholerae* pathogenicity, including the genes encoding the biosynthesis of TCP, those encoding accessory colonization factors, and those regulating virulence gene expression, are clustered together in the *V. cholerae* pathogenicity island. Similar clustering of virulence genes is found in other bacterial pathogens. It is believed that pathogenicity islands are acquired by horizontal gene transfer.

V. cholerae O139 Bengal is closely related to the O1 El Tor strains of the seventh pandemic and seems to have arisen from them by horizontal gene transfer. It shares the virulence attributes and general pathogenic mechanisms of O1 vibrios. *V. cholerae* O139 Bengal is in fact virtually identical to the seventh-pandemic strains of *V. cholerae* O1 El Tor except for two important differences: production of the novel O139 LPS and of an immunologically related O-antigen polysaccharide capsule. Encapsulation is not a feature of O1 strains and may explain the resistance of O139 strains to human serum in vitro as well as the occasional development of O139 bacteremia.

CLINICAL MANIFESTATIONS

After a 24- to 48-h incubation period, cholera begins with the sudden onset of painless watery diarrhea that may quickly become voluminous and is often followed shortly by vomiting. In severe cases, stool volume can exceed 250 mL/kg in the first 24 h. If fluids and electrolytes are not replaced, hypovolemic shock and death ensue. Fever is usually absent. Muscle cramps due to electrolyte disturbances are common. The stool has a characteristic appearance: a nonbilious, gray, slightly cloudy fluid with flecks of mucus, no blood, and a somewhat sweet, inoffensive odor. It has been called "rice-water" stool because of its resemblance to the water in which rice has been washed. Clinical symptoms parallel volume contraction: At losses of 3–5% of normal body weight, thirst develops; at 5–8%, postural hypotension, weakness, tachycardia, and decreased skin turgor are documented; and at >10%, oliguria, weak or absent pulses, sunken eyes (and, in infants, sunken fontanelles), wrinkled ("washerwoman") skin, somnolence, and coma are characteristic. Complications derive exclusively from the effects of volume and electrolyte depletion and include renal failure due to acute tubular necrosis. Thus, if the patient is adequately treated with fluid and electrolytes, complications are averted and the process is self-limited, resolving in a few days.

Laboratory data usually reveal an elevated hematocrit (due to hemoconcentration) in nonanemic patients; mild neutrophilic leukocytosis; elevated levels of blood urea nitrogen and creatinine consistent with prerenal azotemia; normal sodium, potassium, and chloride levels; a markedly reduced bicarbonate level (<15 mmol/L); and an elevated anion gap (due to increases in serum lactate, protein, and phosphate). Arterial pH is usually low (~7.2).

DIAGNOSIS

The clinical suspicion of cholera can be confirmed by the identification of *V. cholerae* in stool; however, the organism must be specifically sought. With experience, it can be detected directly by dark-field microscopy on a wet mount of fresh stool, and its serotype can be discerned by immobilization with specific antiserum. Laboratory isolation of the organism requires the use of a selective medium. The best of these is thiosulfate–citrate–bile salts–sucrose (TCBS) agar, on which the organism grows as a flat yellow colony. If a delay in sample processing is expected, Carey-Blair transport medium and/or alkaline-peptone water-enrichment medium should be inoculated as well. In endemic areas, there is little need for biochemical confirmation and characterization, although these tasks may be worthwhile in places where *V. cholerae* is an uncommon isolate. Standard microbiologic biochemical testing for Enterobacteriaceae will suffice for identification of *V. cholerae*. All vibrios are oxidase-positive.

The yield of stool cultures for the diagnosis of *V. cholerae* infection declines late in the course of the illness or when effective antibacterial therapy is initiated. Monoclonal antibody–based diagnostic kits and methods based on the polymerase chain reaction and on DNA probes have been developed for detection of *V. cholerae* O1 and O139.

℞ Treatment: CHOLERA

Cholera is simple to treat; only the rapid and adequate replacement of fluids, electrolytes, and base is required. The mortality rate for appropriately treated disease is usually <1%. However, analysis of a large outbreak of cholera among airline travelers from an endemic country to the United States revealed frequent misdiagnoses by U.S. health professionals and poor appreciation on their part of the principles of management. Fluid replacement may be given orally, but oral rehydration is not always feasible in the presence of significant vomiting. Oral rehydration takes advantage of the hexose-Na^+ cotransport mechanism to move Na^+ across the gut mucosa together with an actively transported molecule such as glucose. For the sake of simplicity, the WHO advises routine use of a single solution of oral rehydration salts (ORS) for diarrheal disease rather than encouraging attempts to choose among multiple formulations according to etiology (Table 57-1). If available, rice-based ORS is considered superior to standard ORS in the treatment of cholera.

For initial management of severely dehydrated patients, IV fluid replacement is preferable. Because profound acidosis (pH < 7.2) is common in this group, Ringer's lactate is the best choice among commercial products (Table 57-2). It must be used with additional potassium supplements, preferably given by mouth. The total fluid deficit in severely dehydrated patients (≥10% of body weight) can be replaced safely within the first 4 h of therapy, half within the first hour. Thereafter, oral therapy can usually be initiated, with the goal of maintaining fluid intake equal to fluid output. However, patients with continued large-volume diarrhea may require prolonged IV treatment to keep up with gastrointestinal fluid losses.

TABLE 57-1

COMPOSITION OF WORLD HEALTH ORGANIZATION ORAL REHYDRATION SOLUTION (ORS)[a,b]

CONSTITUENT	CONCENTRATION, mmol/L
Na^+	75
K^+	20
Cl^-	65
Citrate[c]	10
Glucose	75

[a]Contains (per package, to be added to 1 L of drinking water): NaCl, 2.6 g; $Na_3C_6H_5O_7 \cdot 2H_2O$, 2.9 g; KCl, 1.5 g; and glucose, 15 g.
[b]If prepackaged ORS is unavailable, a simple homemade alternative can be prepared by combining 5 g NaCl (about 1 level teaspoon) with either 50 g precooked rice cereal or 40 g sucrose in 1 L of drinking water. In that case, potassium must be supplied separately (e.g., in orange juice or coconut water).
[c]10 mmol citrate per liter, which supplies 30 mmol HCO_3/L.

TABLE 57-2

ELECTROLYTE COMPOSITION OF CHOLERA STOOL AND OF INTRAVENOUS REHYDRATION SOLUTION

	CONCENTRATION, mmol/L			
SUBSTANCE	**Na^+**	**K^+**	**Cl^-**	**BASE**
Stool				
Adult	135	15	90	30
Child	100	25	90	30
Ringer's lactate	130	4[a]	109	28

[a]Potassium supplements, preferably administered by mouth, are required to replace the usual potassium losses from stool.

Severe hypokalemia can develop but will respond to potassium given either IV or orally. In the absence of adequate staff to monitor the patient's progress, the oral route of rehydration and potassium replacement is safer than the IV route.

Although not necessary for cure, the use of an antibiotic to which the organism is susceptible diminishes the duration and volume of fluid loss and hastens clearance of the organism from the stool. Single-dose tetracycline (2 g) or doxycycline (300 mg) is effective in adults but is not recommended for children <8 years of age because of possible deposition in bone and developing teeth. Emerging drug resistance is an ever-present concern. For adults with cholera in areas where tetracycline resistance is prevalent, ciprofloxacin [either in a single dose (30 mg/kg, not to exceed a total dose of 1 g) or in a short course (15 mg/kg bid for 3 days, not to exceed a total daily dose of 1 g)], erythromycin (a total of 40 mg/kg daily in three divided doses for 3 days), or a single 1-g dose of azithromycin is a clinically effective substitute. These drugs are highly effective in reducing total stool output and are significantly better than trimethoprim-sulfamethoxazole. For children, furazolidone has been the recommended agent and trimethoprim-sulfamethoxazole the second choice. Because of cost and/or toxicity issues related to the other drugs, erythromycin is a good choice for pediatric cholera.

PREVENTION

Provision of safe water and facilities for sanitary disposal of feces, improved nutrition, and attention to food preparation and storage in the household can significantly reduce the incidence of cholera.

Much effort has been devoted to the development of an effective cholera vaccine over the past two decades, with a particular focus on oral vaccine strains. Traditional killed cholera vaccine given intramuscularly provides little protection to nonimmune subjects and predictably causes adverse effects, including pain at the injection site, malaise, and fever. The vaccine's limited efficacy is due, at least in part, to its failure to induce a local immune response at the intestinal mucosal surface.

Two types of oral cholera vaccines have been developed. The first is a killed whole-cell (WC) vaccine. Two formulations of the killed WC vaccine have been prepared: one that also contains the nontoxic B subunit of cholera toxin (WC/BS) and one composed solely of killed bacteria. In field trials in Bangladesh, both of the killed vaccines offered significant protection from cholera compared with placebo for the first 6 months after vaccination, with protection rates of ~58% for WC and 85% for WC/BS. Protective efficacy rates for both vaccines declined to ~50% by 3 years after vaccine administration. Immunity was relatively sustained in persons vaccinated at an age of >5 years but was not well sustained in younger vaccinees. The WC/BS vaccine proved effective in a trial conducted in a Sub-Saharan African population with a high prevalence of HIV infection. Killed oral vaccines also confer herd protection to unvaccinated individuals living in proximity to vaccinated individuals. Serious consideration should be given to the administration of the WC/BS vaccine in high-risk environments such as refugee camps. The WC/BS vaccine is available in Europe but not in the United States.

The second approach is a live attenuated vaccine strain developed, for example, by the isolation or creation of mutants lacking the genes encoding cholera toxin. Strain CVD 103-HgR, an oral live cholera vaccine licensed for immunization of travelers in Europe, is derived from a classical biotype strain of *V. cholerae* and contains a deletion of the cholera toxin A subunit gene. This strain has been extensively tested in volunteers; a single dose yielded a high degree of protection against experimental challenge with classical *V. cholerae* strains, with almost no side effects. Protective efficacy was not as great against challenge with El Tor *V. cholerae*. Unfortunately, in a large field trial in Indonesian children, this vaccine failed to induce protection against clinical cholera. Other live attenuated vaccine candidate strains have been prepared from El Tor and O139 *V. cholerae* and are now undergoing clinical trials. Because of the minimal efficacy of existing parenteral vaccines, cholera immunization is recommended for U.S. travelers only if it is mandated by the countries they plan to visit.

OTHER *VIBRIO* SPECIES

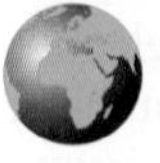

The genus *Vibrio* includes several human pathogens that do not cause cholera. Abundant in coastal waters throughout the world, noncholera vibrios can reach high concentrations in the tissues of filter-feeding mollusks. As a result, human infection commonly follows the ingestion of seawater or of raw or undercooked shellfish (Table 57-3). Most noncholera vibrios can be cultured on blood or MacConkey agar, which contains enough salt to support the growth of these halophilic species. In the microbiology laboratory, the species of noncholera vibrios are distinguished by standard biochemical tests. The most important of these organisms are *V. parahaemolyticus* and *V. vulnificus*.

The two major types of syndromes for which these species are responsible are gastrointestinal illness (due to

TABLE 57-3

FEATURES OF SELECTED NONCHOLERA VIBRIOSES

ORGANISM	VEHICLE OR ACTIVITY	HOST AT RISK	SYNDROME
V. parahaemolyticus	Shellfish, seawater	Normal	Gastroenteritis
	Seawater	Normal	Wound infection
Non-O1 *V. cholerae*	Shellfish, travel	Normal	Gastroenteritis
	Seawater	Normal	Wound infection, otitis media
V. vulnificus	Shellfish	Immunosuppressed[a]	Sepsis, secondary cellulitis
	Seawater	Normal	Wound infection, cellulitis
V. alginolyticus	Seawater	Normal	Wound infection, cellulitis, otitis
	Seawater	Burned, other immunosuppressed	Sepsis

[a]Especially with liver disease or hemochromatosis.

Source: Table 161-3 in *Harrison's Principles of Internal Medicine,* 14th edition.

V. parahaemolyticus, non-O1 *V. cholerae*, *V. mimicus*, *V. fluvialis*, *V. hollisae*, and *V. furnissii*) and soft tissue infections (due to *V. vulnificus*, *V. alginolyticus*, and *V. damselae*). *V. vulnificus* is also a cause of primary sepsis in some compromised individuals. *V. parahaemolyticus* causes rare cases of wound infection and otitis and very rare cases of sepsis.

SPECIES ASSOCIATED PRIMARILY WITH GASTROINTESTINAL ILLNESS

V. Parahaemolyticus

Widespread in marine environments, *V. parahaemolyticus* grows in saline concentrations up to 8–10%. This species was originally implicated in enteritis in Japan in 1953, accounting for 24% of reported cases in one study—a rate that presumably was due to the common practice of eating raw seafood in that country. *V. parahaemolyticus* has since been identified as a significant intestinal pathogen in many regions of the world. In the United States, common-source outbreaks of diarrhea caused by this organism have been linked to the consumption of undercooked or improperly handled seafood or of other foods contaminated by seawater. Since the mid-1990s, the incidence of *V. parahaemolyticus* infections has increased in several countries, including the United States. Serotypes O3:K6, O4:K68, and O1:K-untypable, which are genetically related to one another, account for this increase. The enteropathogenicity of *V. parahaemolyticus* is closely linked to its ability to cause hemolysis on Wagatsuma agar (i.e., the *Kanagawa phenomenon*). Although the mechanism by which the organism causes diarrhea remains unclear, the genome sequence of *V. parahaemolyticus* contains a pathogenicity island—a cluster of likely virulence-associated genes. *V. parahaemolyticus* should be considered a possible etiologic agent in all cases of diarrhea that can be linked epidemiologically to seafood consumption or to the sea itself.

Infections with *V. parahaemolyticus* can result in two distinct gastrointestinal presentations. The more common of the two presentations (including nearly all cases in North America) is characterized by watery diarrhea, usually occurring in conjunction with abdominal cramps, nausea, and vomiting and accompanied in ~25% of cases by fever and chills. After an incubation period of 4 h to 4 days, symptoms develop and persist for a median of 3 days. Dysentery, the less common presentation, is characterized by severe abdominal cramps, nausea, vomiting, and bloody or mucoid stools.

Most cases of *V. parahaemolyticus*–associated gastrointestinal illness, regardless of the presentation, are self-limited and require neither antimicrobial treatment nor hospitalization. Deaths are extremely rare. Severe infections are associated with underlying diseases, including diabetes, preexisting liver disease, iron-overload states, or immunosuppression. The occasional severe case should be treated with fluid replacement and antibiotics, as described above for cholera.

Non-O1 V. Cholerae

The heterogeneous non-O1 *V. cholerae* organisms cannot be distinguished from *V. cholerae* O1 by routine biochemical tests but do not agglutinate in O1 antiserum. Non-O1 strains have caused several well-studied food-borne outbreaks of gastroenteritis and have also been responsible for sporadic cases of otitis media, wound infection, and bacteremia. Like other vibrios, non-O1 *V. cholerae* organisms are widely distributed in marine environments. In most instances, recognized cases in the United States have been associated with the consumption of raw oysters or with recent travel, typically to Mexico. The broad clinical spectrum of diarrheal illness caused by these organisms is probably due to the group's heterogeneous virulence attributes. *V. cholerae* O139 Bengal, although technically a non-O1 vibrio, is not grouped with these pathogens because it can cause epidemic cholera.

In the United States, about half of all non-O1 *V. cholerae* isolates are from stool samples. The typical incubation period for gastroenteritis due to these organisms is <2 days, and the illness lasts for ~2–7 days. Patients' stools may be copious and watery or may be partly formed, less voluminous, and bloody or mucoid. Diarrhea can result in severe dehydration. Many cases include abdominal cramps, nausea, vomiting, and fever. Like those with cholera, patients who are seriously dehydrated should receive oral or IV fluids; the value of antibiotics is not clear.

Extraintestinal infections due to non-O1 *V. cholerae* commonly follow occupational or recreational exposure to seawater. Approximately 10% of non-O1 *V. cholerae* isolates come from cases of wound infection, 10% from cases of otitis media, and 20% from cases of bacteremia (which is particularly likely to develop in patients with liver disease). Extraintestinal infections should be treated with antibiotics. Information to guide antibiotic selection and dosing is limited, but most strains are sensitive in vitro to tetracycline, ciprofloxacin, and third-generation cephalosporins.

SPECIES ASSOCIATED PRIMARILY WITH SOFT TISSUE INFECTION OR BACTEREMIA

(See also Chap. 21)

V. Vulnificus

V. vulnificus is the most common cause of severe vibrio infections in the United States. Like most vibrios, this organism proliferates in the warm summer months and requires a saline environment for growth. In this country, infections in humans typically occur in coastal states between May and October and most commonly affect men >40 years of age. *V. vulnificus* has been linked to two distinct syndromes: primary sepsis, which usually occurs in patients with underlying liver disease, and primary wound infection, which generally affects people without underlying disease. Some authors have suggested that *V. vulnificus* also causes gastroenteritis independent of other clinical manifestations. *V. vulnificus* is endowed with a number of virulence attributes, including a capsule that confers resistance to phagocytosis and to the bactericidal activity of human serum as well as a cytolysin. Measured as the 50% lethal dose in mice, the organism's virulence is considerably increased under conditions of iron overload; this observation is consistent with the propensity of *V. vulnificus* to infect patients who have hemochromatosis.

Primary sepsis most often develops in patients who have cirrhosis or hemochromatosis. However, *V. vulnificus* bacteremia can also affect individuals who have hematopoietic disorders or chronic renal insufficiency, those who are using immunosuppressive medications or alcohol, or (in rare instances) those who have no known underlying disease. After a median incubation period of 16 h, the patient develops malaise, chills, fever, and prostration. One-third of patients develop hypotension, which is often apparent at admission. Cutaneous manifestations develop in most cases (usually within 36 h of onset) and characteristically involve the extremities (the lower more often than the upper). In a common sequence, erythematous patches are followed by ecchymoses, vesicles, and bullae. In fact, sepsis and bullous skin lesions suggest the diagnosis in appropriate settings. Necrosis and sloughing may also be evident. Laboratory studies reveal leukopenia more often than leukocytosis, thrombocytopenia, or elevated levels of fibrin split products. *V. vulnificus* can be cultured from blood or cutaneous lesions. The mortality rate approaches 50%, with most deaths due to uncontrolled sepsis. Accordingly, prompt treatment is critical and should include empirical antibiotic administration, aggressive debridement, and general supportive care. *V. vulnificus* is sensitive in vitro to a number of antibiotics, including tetracycline, fluoroquinolones, and third-generation cephalosporins. Data from animal models suggest that either a fluoroquinolone or the combination of minocycline and cefotaxime should be used in the treatment of *V. vulnificus* septicemia.

V. vulnificus can infect either a fresh or an old wound that comes into contact with seawater; the patient may or may not have underlying disease. After a short incubation period (4 h to 4 days; mean, 12 h), the disease begins with swelling, erythema, and (in many cases) intense pain around the wound. These signs and symptoms are followed by cellulitis, which spreads rapidly and is sometimes accompanied by vesicular, bullous, or necrotic lesions. Metastatic events are uncommon. Most patients have a fever and leukocytosis. *V. vulnificus* can be cultured from skin lesions and occasionally from the blood. Prompt antibiotic therapy and debridement are usually curative.

V. Alginolyticus

First identified as a pathogen of humans in 1973, *V. alginolyticus* occasionally causes eye, ear, and wound infections. This species is the most salt-tolerant of the vibrios and can grow in salt concentrations of >10%. Most clinical isolates come from superinfected wounds that presumably become contaminated at the beach. Although severity varies, *V. alginolyticus* infection tends not to be serious and generally responds well to antibiotic therapy and drainage. A few cases of otitis externa, otitis media, and conjunctivitis due to this pathogen have been described. Tetracycline treatment usually results in cure. *V. alginolyticus* is a rare cause of bacteremia in immunocompromised hosts.

ACKNOWLEDGMENT

The authors gratefully acknowledge the valuable contributions of Dr. Robert Deresiewicz, a coauthor of this chapter for the 14th edition of Harrison's Principles of Internal Medicine.

FURTHER READINGS

GRIFFITH DC et al: Review of reported cholera outbreaks worldwide, 1995–2005. Am J Trop Med Hyg 75:973, 2006

LUCAS MES et al: Effectiveness of mass oral cholera vaccination in Beira, Mozambique. N Engl J Med 352:757, 2005

SACK DA et al: Cholera. Lancet 363:223, 2004

SAHA D et al: Single-dose azithromycin for the treatment of cholera in adults. N Engl J Med 354:2452, 2006

TANG HJ et al: In vitro and in vivo activities of newer fluoroquinolones against *Vibrio vulnificus*. Antimicrob Agents Chemother 46:3580, 2002

WORLD HEALTH ORGANIZATION: *The Treatment of Diarrhoea: A Manual for Physicians and Other Senior Health Workers*. Geneva, World Health Organization, 2005 (*www.who.int/child-adolescent-health/New_Publications/CHILD_HEALTH/ISBN_92_4_159318_0.pdf*)

———: Cholera, 2004. Wkly Epidemiol Rec 80:261, 2005 (*www.who.int/wer*)

CHAPTER 58

BRUCELLOSIS

Michael J. Corbel ■ Nicholas J. Beeching

DEFINITION

Brucellosis is a bacterial zoonosis transmitted directly or indirectly to humans from infected animals, predominantly domesticated ruminants and swine. The disease is known colloquially as *undulant fever* because of its remittent character. Its distribution is worldwide apart from the few countries where it has been eradicated from the animal reservoir. Although brucellosis commonly presents as an acute febrile illness, its clinical manifestations vary widely, and definitive signs indicative of the diagnosis may be lacking. Thus the clinical diagnosis usually must be supported by the results of bacteriologic and/or serologic tests.

ETIOLOGIC AGENTS

Human brucellosis is caused by strains of *Brucella*, a bacterial genus that has been suggested, on genetic grounds, to comprise a single species, *Brucella melitensis,* with a number of biologic variants that exhibit particular host preferences. Recently, this view has been challenged on the basis of detailed differences in chromosomal structure and host preference. The traditional classification into nomen species is now favored both because of these differences and because this classification scheme closely reflects the epidemiologic patterns of the infection. The nomen system recognizes *B. melitensis*, which is the commonest cause of symptomatic disease in humans and for which the main sources are sheep, goats, and camels; *B. abortus,* which is usually acquired from cattle or buffalo: *B. suis,* which generally is acquired from swine but has one variant enzootic in reindeer and caribou and another in rodents; and *B. canis*, which is acquired most often from dogs. *B. ovis,* which causes reproductive disease in sheep, and *B. neotomae,* which is specific for desert rodents, have not been clearly implicated in human disease. Other brucellae have been isolated from marine mammals, and two new nomen species, *B. cetaceae* and *B. pinnipediae,* have been proposed. At least one case of laboratory-acquired human disease due to one of these proposed species has been described, and apparent cases of natural infection have been reported. As infections in marine mammals seem widespread, more cases of zoonotic infection may be identified.

All brucellae are small, gram-negative, unencapsulated, nonsporulating rods or coccobacilli. They grow aerobically on peptone-based medium incubated at 37°C; the growth of some types is improved by supplementary CO_2. In vivo, brucellae behave as facultative intracellular parasites. The organisms are sensitive to sunlight, ionizing radiation, and moderate heat; they are killed by boiling and pasteurization but are resistant to freezing and drying. Their resistance to drying renders brucellae stable in aerosol form, facilitating airborne transmission. The organisms can survive for up to 2 months in soft cheeses made from goat's or sheep's milk; for at least 6 weeks in dry soil contaminated with infected urine, vaginal discharge, or placental or fetal tissues; and for at least 6 months in damp soil or liquid manure kept under cool dark conditions. Brucellae are easily killed by a wide range of common disinfectants used under optimal conditions but are likely to be much more resistant at low temperatures or in the presence of heavy organic contamination.

EPIDEMIOLOGY

Brucellosis is a zoonosis whose occurrence is closely related to its prevalence in domesticated animals. The true global prevalence of human brucellosis is unknown because of the imprecision of diagnosis and the inadequacy of reporting and surveillance systems in many countries. Even in developed countries, the true incidence may be 10–20 times higher than the reported figures. Bovine brucellosis has been the target of control programs in many parts of the world and has been eradicated from the cattle populations of Australia, New Zealand, Bulgaria, Canada, Cyprus, Great Britain (including the Channel Islands), Japan, Luxembourg, Romania, the Scandinavian countries, Switzerland, and the Czech and Slovak Republics. Its incidence has been reduced to a low level in the United States and most Western European countries, with a varied picture in other parts of the world. There is evidence of a resurgence in Eastern Europe following economic changes in recent years, and new outbreaks have also occurred in Ireland. Efforts to eradicate *B. melitensis* infection from sheep and goat populations have been much less successful. These efforts have relied heavily on vaccination programs, which have tended to fluctuate with changing economic and political conditions. In some countries (e.g., Israel), *B. melitensis* has caused serious outbreaks in cattle. Infections with *B. melitensis* still pose a major public health problem in Mediterranean countries; in western, central, and southern Asia; and in parts of Africa and South and Central America.

Human brucellosis is usually associated with occupational or domestic exposure to infected animals or their products. Farmers, shepherds, goatherds, veterinarians, and employees in slaughterhouses and meat-processing plants in endemic areas are occupationally exposed to infection. Family members of individuals involved in animal husbandry may be at risk, although it is often difficult to differentiate food-borne infection from environmental contamination under these circumstances. Laboratory workers who handle cultures or infected samples are also at risk. Travelers and urban dwellers usually acquire the infection through consumption of contaminated foods. In countries that have eradicated the disease, new cases are most commonly acquired abroad. Dairy products, especially soft cheeses, unpasteurized milk, and ice cream, are the most frequently implicated sources of infection; raw meat and bone marrow may be sources under exceptional circumstances. Infections acquired through cosmetic treatments using materials of fetal origin have been reported. Person-to-person transmission is extremely rare, as is transfer of infection by blood or tissue donation. Although brucellosis is a chronic intracellular infection, there is no evidence for increased prevalence or severity among individuals with HIV infection or with immunodeficiency or immunosuppression of other etiologies.

Brucellosis may be acquired by ingestion, inhalation, or mucosal or percutaneous exposure. Accidental injection of the live vaccine strains of *B. abortus* (19 and RB51) and *B. melitensis* (Rev 1) can cause disease. *B. melitensis* and *B. suis* have been developed as biological weapons by several countries and could be exploited for bioterrorism (Chap. 6). This possibility should be borne in mind in the event of sudden unexplained outbreaks.

IMMUNITY AND PATHOGENESIS

Exposure to brucellosis elicits both humoral and cell-mediated immune responses. The mechanisms of protective immunity against human brucellosis are presumed to be similar to those documented in laboratory animals. The response to infection and its outcome are influenced by the virulence, phase, and species of the infecting strain. Differences have been reported between *B. abortus* and *B. suis* in the modes of cellular entry and subsequent compartmentalization and processing. Antibodies promote clearance of extracellular brucellae by bactericidal action and by facilitation of phagocytosis by polymorphonuclear and mononuclear phagocytes; however, antibodies alone cannot eradicate infection. Organisms taken up by macrophages and other cells can establish persistent intracellular infections. The key target cell is the macrophage, and bacterial mechanisms for suppressing intracellular killing and apoptosis result in very large intracellular populations. Opsonized bacteria are actively phagocytosed by neutrophilic granulocytes and by monocytes. In these and other cells, initial attachment takes place via specific receptors, including Fc, C3, fibronectin, and mannose-binding proteins. Opsonized—but not unopsonized—bacteria trigger an oxidative burst inside phagocytes. Unopsonized bacteria are internalized via similar receptors but at much lower efficiency. Smooth strains enter host cells via lipid rafts. Smooth lipopolysaccharide (LPS), β-cyclic glucan, and possibly an invasion-attachment protein (IalB) are involved in this process. Tumor necrosis factor α (TNF-α) produced early in the course of infection stimulates cytotoxic lymphocytes and activates macrophages, which can kill intracellular brucellae (probably mainly through production of reactive oxygen and nitrogen intermediates) and may clear infection. However, virulent *Brucella* cells can suppress the TNF-α response, and control of infection in this situation depends on macrophage activation and interferon γ (IFN-γ) responses. Cytokines such as interleukin (IL) 12 promote production of IFN-γ, which drives T_H1-type responses and stimulates macrophage activation. Inflammatory cytokines, including IL-4, IL-6, and IL-10, downregulate the protective response. As in other types of intracellular infection, it is assumed that initial replication of brucellae takes place within cells of the lymph nodes draining the point of entry. Subsequent hematogenous spread may result in chronic localizing infection at almost any site, although the reticuloendothelial system, musculoskeletal tissues, and genitourinary system are most frequently targeted. Both acute and chronic inflammatory responses develop in brucellosis, and the local tissue response may include granuloma formation with or without necrosis and caseation. Abscesses may also develop, especially in chronic localized infection.

The determinants of pathogenicity of *Brucella* have not been fully characterized, and the mechanisms underlying the manifestations of brucellosis are incompletely understood. The organism's survival strategy is centered on processes that permit survival within monocytic cells. The smooth *Brucella* LPS, which has an unusual O-chain and core-lipid composition, has relatively low endotoxin activity and plays a key role in pyrogenicity and in resistance to phagocytosis and serum killing in the nonimmune host. LPS is believed also to play a key role in suppressing phagosome-lysosome fusion and diverting the internalized bacteria into vacuoles located in endoplasmic reticulum, where intracellular replication takes place. Specific exotoxins have not been isolated, but a type IV secretion system (VirB) that regulates intracellular survival and trafficking has been identified. In *B. abortus* this system can be activated extracellularly, but in *B. suis* it is activated (by low pH) only during intracellular growth. Brucellae then produce acid-stable proteins that facilitate the organisms' survival in phagosomes and may enhance their resistance to reactive oxygen intermediates. Virulent brucellae are resistant to defensins and produce a Cu-Zn superoxide dismutase that increases their resistance to reactive oxygen intermediates.

CLINICAL FEATURES

Brucellosis almost invariably causes fever, which may be associated with profuse sweats, especially at night. In endemic areas, brucellosis may be difficult to distinguish from the many other causes of fever. However, two features recognized in the nineteenth century distinguish brucellosis from other tropical fevers, such as typhoid and malaria. (1) Left untreated, the fever of brucellosis shows an undulating pattern that persists for weeks before the commencement of an afebrile period that may be followed by relapse. (2) The fever of brucellosis is associated with musculoskeletal symptoms and signs in about one-half of all patients.

The clinical syndromes caused by the different nomen species are similar, although *B. melitensis* tends to be associated with a more acute and aggressive presentation and *B. suis* with focal abscess induction. *B. abortus* infections may be more insidious in onset and more likely to become chronic.

The incubation period varies from 1 week to several months, and the onset of fever and other symptoms may be abrupt or insidious. In addition to experiencing fever and sweats, patients become increasingly apathetic and fatigued, lose appetite and weight, and have nonspecific myalgia, headache, and chills. Overall, the presentation of brucellosis often fits one of three patterns: febrile illness that resembles typhoid but is less severe; fever and acute monoarthritis, typically of the hip or knee, in a young child; and long-lasting fever, misery, and low-back or hip pain in an older man. In an endemic area (e.g., much of the Middle East), a patient with fever and difficulty walking into the clinic would be regarded as having brucellosis until it was proved otherwise.

Diagnostic clues in the patient's history include travel to an endemic area, employment in a diagnostic microbiology laboratory, consumption of unpasteurized milk products (including soft cheeses), contact with animals, and—in an endemic setting—a history of similar illness in the family (documented in almost 50% of cases).

Focal features are present in the majority of patients. The most common are musculoskeletal pain and physical findings in the peripheral and axial skeleton (~40% of cases). Osteomyelitis more commonly involves the lumbar and low thoracic vertebrae than the cervical and high thoracic spine. Individual joints that are most commonly affected by septic arthritis are the knee, hip, sacroiliac, shoulder, and sternoclavicular joints; the pattern may be one of monoarthritis or polyarthritis. Osteomyelitis may also accompany septic arthritis.

In addition to the usual causes of vertebral osteomyelitis or septic arthritis, the most important differential diagnosis is tuberculosis. This point influences the therapeutic approach as well as the prognosis, given that several antimicrobial agents used to treat brucellosis are also used to treat tuberculosis. Septic arthritis in brucellosis progresses slowly, starting with small pericapsular erosions. In the vertebrae, anterior erosions of the superior end plate are typically the first features to become evident, with eventual involvement and sclerosis of the whole vertebra. Anterior osteophytes eventually develop, but vertebral destruction or impingement on the spinal cord is rare and usually suggests tuberculosis (Table 58-1).

Other systems may be involved in a manner that resembles typhoid. About one-quarter of patients have a dry cough, usually with few changes visible on the chest x-ray, although pneumonia, empyema, intrathoracic adenopathy, or lung abscess can occur. One-quarter of patients have hepatosplenomegaly, and 10–20% have significant lymphadenopathy; the differential diagnosis includes glandular fever–like illness such as that caused by Epstein-Barr virus, *Toxoplasma*, and cytomegalovirus; HIV infection; or tuberculosis. Up to 10% of men have acute epididymoorchitis, which must be distinguished from mumps and from surgical problems such as torsion. Prostatitis, inflammation of the seminal vesicles, salpingitis, and pyelonephritis all occur. There is an increased incidence of fetal loss among infected pregnant women, although teratogenicity has not been described and the tendency to cause abortions is much less pronounced in humans than in farm animals.

TABLE 58-1

RADIOLOGY OF THE SPINE: DIFFERENTIATION OF BRUCELLOSIS FROM TUBERCULOSIS

	BRUCELLOSIS	TUBERCULOSIS
Site	Lumbar and others	Dorsolumbar
Vertebrae	Multiple or contiguous	Contiguous
Diskitis	Late	Early
Body	Intact until late	Morphology lost early
Canal compression	Rare	Common
Epiphysitis	Anterosuperior (Pom's sign)	General: upper and lower disk regions, central, subperiosteal
Osteophyte	Anterolateral (parrot beak)	Unusual
Deformity	Wedging uncommon	Anterior wedge, gibbus
Recovery	Sclerosis, whole body	Variable
Paravertebral abscess	Small, well-localized	Common and discrete loss, transverse process
Psoas abscess	Rare	More likely

Neurologic involvement is common, with depression and lethargy whose severity may not be truly appreciated by either the patient or the physician until after treatment. A small proportion of patients develop lymphocytic meningoencephalitis that mimics neurotuberculosis or noninfectious conditions and that may be complicated by intracerebral abscess, a variety of cranial nerve deficits, or ruptured mycotic aneurysms.

Endocarditis occurs in ~1% of cases, most often affecting the aortic valve (natural or prosthetic). Any site in the body may be involved in metastatic abscess formation or inflammation; the female breast and the thyroid gland are affected particularly often. Nonspecific maculopapular rashes and other skin manifestations are uncommon and are rarely noticed by the patient even if they are present.

DIAGNOSIS

Because the clinical picture of brucellosis is not distinctive, the diagnosis must be based on a history of potential exposure, a presentation consistent with the disease, and supporting laboratory findings. Results of routine biochemical assays are usually within normal limits, although serum levels of hepatic enzymes and bilirubin may be elevated. Peripheral leukocyte counts are usually normal or low, with relative lymphocytosis. Mild anemia may be documented. Thrombocytopenia and disseminated intravascular coagulation with raised levels of fibrinogen degradation products can develop. The erythrocyte sedimentation rate and C-reactive protein levels are often normal but may be raised.

In body fluids such as cerebrospinal fluid (CSF) or joint fluid, lymphocytosis and low glucose levels are the norm. Elevated CSF levels of adenosine deaminase cannot be used to distinguish tubercular meningitis, as they may also be found in brucellosis. Biopsied samples of tissues such as lymph node or liver may show noncaseating granulomas (Fig. 58-1) without acid/alcohol-fast bacilli. The radiologic features of bony disease develop late and are much more subtle than those of tuberculosis or septic arthritis of other etiologies, with less bone and joint destruction. Isotope scanning is more sensitive than plain x-ray and continues to give positive results long after successful treatment.

Isolation of brucellae from blood, CSF, bone marrow, or joint fluid or from a tissue aspirate or biopsy sample is definitive, and attempts at isolation are usually successful in 50–70% of cases. Duplicate cultures should be incubated for up to 6 weeks (in air and 10% CO_2, respectively). Concentration and lysis of buffy coat cells before culture may increase the isolation rate. Cultures in modern nonradiometric or similar signaling systems (e.g., Bactec) usually become positive within 7–10 days but should be maintained for at least 3 weeks before the results are declared negative. All cultures should be handled under containment conditions appropriate for dangerous pathogens. *Brucella* spp. may be misidentified as *Agrobacterium, Ochrobactrum*, or *Psychrobacter (Moraxella) phenylpyruvicus* by the gallery identification strips commonly used in the diagnostic laboratory.

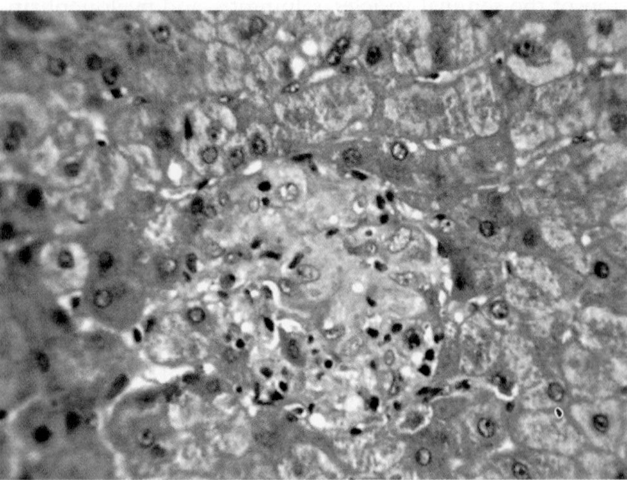

FIGURE 58-1
Liver biopsy specimen from a patient with brucellosis shows a noncaseating granuloma. *[From Mandell's Atlas of Infectious Diseases, Vol II, in DL Stevens (ed): Skin, Soft Tissue, Bone and Joint Infections, Fig. 5-9; with permission.]*

The peripheral blood–based polymerase chain reaction (PCR) has enormous potential to detect bacteremia, to predict relapse, and to exclude "chronic brucellosis." PCR is probably more sensitive and is certainly quicker than blood culture, and it does not carry the attendant biohazard risk posed by culture. Nucleic acid amplification techniques are now quite widely used, although no single standardized procedure has been adopted. Primers for the spacer region between the genes encoding the 16S and 23S ribosomal RNAs (*rrs-rrl),* the outer membrane protein Omp2, the insertion sequence *IS711*, and protein BCSP31 are sensitive and specific. Blood and other tissues are the most suitable samples for analysis.

Serologic examination often provides the only positive laboratory findings in brucellosis. In acute infection, IgM antibodies appear early and are followed by IgG and IgA. All these antibodies are active in agglutination tests, whether performed by tube, plate, or microagglutination methods. The majority of patients have detectable agglutinins at this stage. As the disease progresses, IgM levels decline, and the avidity and subclass distribution of IgG and IgA change. The result is reduced or undetectable agglutinin titers. However, the antibodies are detectable by alternative tests, including the complement fixation test, Coombs' antiglobulin test, and enzyme-linked immunosorbent assay. There is no clear cutoff value for a diagnostic titer. Rather, serology results must be interpreted in the context of exposure history and clinical presentation. In endemic areas or in settings of potential occupational exposure, agglutinin titers of 1:320–1:640 or higher are considered diagnostic; in nonendemic areas, a titer of ≥1:160 is considered significant. Repetition of tests after 2–4 weeks may demonstrate a rising titer.

In most centers, the standard agglutination test (SAT) is still the mainstay of serologic diagnosis, although some investigators rely on the rose bengal test, which has not been fully validated for human diagnostic use. Dipstick assays for anti-*Brucella* IgM are useful for the diagnosis of acute infection but are less sensitive for infection with symptoms of several months' duration. In an endemic setting, >90% of patients with acute bacteremia have SAT titers of at least 1:320.

Antibody to the *Brucella* LPS O chain—the dominant antigen—is detected by all the conventional tests that employ smooth *B. abortus* cells as antigen. Since *B. abortus* cross-reacts with *B. melitensis* and *B. suis*, there is no advantage in replicating the tests with these antigens. Cross-reactions also occur with the O chains of some other gram-negative bacteria, including *Escherichia coli* O157, *Francisella tularensis*, *Salmonella enterica* group N, *Stenotrophomonas maltophilia*, and *Vibrio cholerae*. Cross-reactions do not occur with the cell-surface antigens of rough *Brucella* strains such as *B. canis* or *B. ovis*; serologic tests for these nomen species must employ an antigen prepared from either one. Most protein antigens are shared by all *Brucella* strains, and some are also common to *Ochrobactrum* species. Immunoblotting against protein extracts has been advocated as a differential test, but no validated procedure is yet available.

℞ Treatment: BRUCELLOSIS

The broad aims of antimicrobial therapy are to treat current infection and relieve its symptoms and to prevent relapse. Focal disease presentations may require specific intervention in addition to more prolonged and tailored antibiotic therapy. In addition, tuberculosis must always be excluded, or—to prevent the emergence of resistance—therapy must be tailored to specifically exclude drugs active against tuberculosis (e.g., rifampin used alone) or to include a full antituberculous regimen.

Early experience with streptomycin monotherapy showed that relapse was common; thus dual therapy with tetracyclines became the norm. This is still the most effective combination, but alternatives may be used, with the options depending on local or national policy about the use of rifampin for the treatment of nonmycobacterial infection. Antimicrobial efficacy can usually be predicted by in vitro testing; however, the use of fluoroquinolones remains controversial despite the good in vitro activity and white cell penetration of most agents of this class. Low intravacuolar pH is probably a factor in the poor performance of these drugs.

For adults with acute nonfocal brucellosis (duration, <1 month), a 6-week course of therapy incorporating at least two antimicrobial agents is required. Complex or focal disease necessitates ≥3 months of therapy. Adherence to the therapeutic regimen is very important, and poor compliance underlies almost all cases of apparent treatment failure; such failure is rarely due to the emergence of drug resistance, although increasing resistance to trimethoprim-sulfamethoxazole (TMP-SMX) has been reported at one center. There is good retrospective evidence that a 3-week course of two agents is as effective as a 6-week course for treatment and prevention of relapse in children, but this point has not yet been proven in prospective studies.

The "gold standard" for the treatment of brucellosis in adults is IM streptomycin (0.75–1 g daily for 14–21 days) together with doxycycline (100 mg twice daily for 6 weeks). In both clinical trials and observational studies, relapse follows such treatment in 5–10% of patients. The usual alternative regimen (and the current World Health Organization recommendation) is rifampin (600–900 mg/d) plus doxycycline (100 mg twice daily) for 6 weeks. The relapse/failure rate is ~10% in trial conditions but rises to >20% in many nontrial situations, possibly because doxycycline levels are reduced and clearance rates increased by concomitant rifampin administration. Patients who cannot tolerate or receive tetracyclines (children, pregnant women) can be given high-dose TMP-SMX instead (2 or 3 standard-strength tablets twice daily for adults, depending on weight).

Evidence is beginning to accumulate that other aminoglycosides can be substituted for streptomycin—e.g., netilmicin or gentamicin given at a dosage of 5–6 mg/kg per day for at least 2 weeks. (Shorter courses have been associated with high failure rates in adults.) A 5- to 7-day course of therapy with gentamicin (and a 3-week course of TMP-SMX) is probably adequate for children with uncomplicated disease. Early experience with fluoroquinolone monotherapy was disappointing, but high-dose ofloxacin (400 mg twice daily) or ciprofloxacin (500 mg twice daily), given together with rifampin for 6 weeks, may become accepted as an alternative to the other 6-week regimens for adults.

Significant neurologic disease due to *Brucella* requires prolonged treatment (i.e., for 3–6 months), usually with ceftriaxone supplementation of a standard regimen. *Brucella* endocarditis is treated with at least three drugs (an aminoglycoside, a tetracycline, and rifampin), and many experts add ceftriaxone and/or a fluoroquinolone to reduce the need for valve replacement. Treatment is usually given for at least 6 months, and clinical endpoints for its discontinuation are often difficult to define. Surgery is still required for the majority of cases of infection of prosthetic heart valves and prosthetic joints.

There is no evidence base to guide prophylaxis after exposure to brucellae (e.g., in the laboratory), inadvertent immunization with live vaccine intended for use in animals, or deliberately released brucellae. Most authorities recommend the administration of rifampin plus doxycycline for 3 weeks after a low-risk exposure (e.g., a nonspecific laboratory accident) and for 6 weeks after a major exposure to aerosol or injected material. However, such regimens are poorly tolerated, and doxycycline monotherapy of the same duration may be substituted.

PROGNOSIS AND FOLLOW-UP

Relapse occurs in up to 30% of poorly compliant patients. Thus patients should ideally be followed clinically for up to 2 years to detect relapse, which responds to a prolonged course of the same therapy used originally. The general well-being and the body weight of the patient are more useful guides than serology to lack of relapse. IgG antibody levels detected by the SAT and its variants can remain in the diagnostic range for >2 years after successful treatment. Complement fixation titers usually fall to normal within 1 year of cure. Immunity is not solid; patients can be reinfected after repeated exposures. Fewer than 1% of patients die of brucellosis. When the outcome is fatal, death is usually a consequence of cardiac involvement; more rarely, it results from severe neurologic disease. Despite the low mortality rate, recovery from brucellosis is slow, and the illness can cause prolonged inactivity, with consequent domestic and economic losses.

The existence of a prolonged chronic brucellosis state after successful treatment remains controversial. Evaluation of patients in whom this state is considered (often those with work-related exposure to brucellae) includes careful exclusion of malingering, nonspecific chronic fatigue syndromes, and other causes of excessive sweating, such as alcohol abuse and obesity. In the future, the availability of more sensitive assays to detect *Brucella* antigen or DNA may help to identify patients with ongoing infection.

PREVENTION

Vaccines based on live attenuated *Brucella* strains, such as *B. abortus* strain 19BA or 104M, have been used in some countries to protect high-risk populations but have displayed only short-term efficacy and high reactogenicity. Subunit vaccines have been developed but are of uncertain value and cannot be recommended at present. Research in this area has been stimulated by interest in biodefense (Chap. 6) and may eventually yield new products, some of which may be based on the live attenuated WR 201 variant of *B. melitensis* strain 16M. The mainstay of veterinary prevention is a national commitment to testing and slaughter of infected herds/flocks (with compensation for owners), control of animal movement, and active immunization of animals. These measures are usually sufficient to control human disease as well. In their absence, pasteurization of all milk products before consumption is sufficient to prevent nonoccupational animal-to-human transmission. All cases of brucellosis in animals and humans should be reported to the appropriate public health authorities.

FURTHER READINGS

Almuneef M, Memish ZA: Prevalence of brucella antibodies after acute brucellosis. J Chemother 15:148, 2003

Corbel MJ, Banai M: Genus *Brucella* Meyer and Shaw 1920,173[AL], in *Bergey's Manual of Systematic Bacteriology*, 2d ed, vol 2: *The Proteobacteria*, DJ Bruner et al (eds). New York, Springer, 2006, pp 370–386

Gerberding JL et al: Case records of the Massachusetts General Hospital. Case 34-2008. A 58-year-old woman with neck pain and fever. N Engl J Med 359:1942, 2008

Hasanjani Roushan MR et al: Efficacy of gentamicin and doxycycline versus streptomycin plus doxycycline in the treatment of brucellosis in humans. Clin Infect Dis 42:1075, 2006

Khan MY et al: Brucellosis in pregnant women. Clin Infect Dis 32:1172, 2000

Maley MW et al: Prevention of laboratory-acquired brucellosis: Significant side effects of prophylaxis. Clin Infect Dis 42:433, 2006

Memish Z et al: *Brucella* bacteraemia: Clinical and laboratory observations in 160 patients. J Infect 40:59, 2000

Navarro E et al: Use of real time quantitative polymerase chain reaction to monitor the evolution of *Brucella melitensis* DNA load during therapy and post-therapy follow-up in patients with brucellosis. Clin Infect Dis 42:1266, 2006

Pappas G et al: New approaches to the antibiotic therapy of brucellosis. Int J Antimicrob Agents 26:101, 2005

——— et al: Brucellosis. N Engl J Med 352:2325, 2005

Saltoglu N et al: Efficacy of rifampicin plus doxycycline versus rifampicin plus quinolone in the treatment of brucellosis. Saudi Med J 23:921, 2002

Skalsky K et al: Treatment of human brucellosis: Systematic review and meta-analysis of randomised controlled trials. BMJ 336:701, 2008

CHAPTER 59

TULAREMIA

Richard F. Jacobs ■ Gordon E. Schutze

DEFINITION

Tularemia is a zoonosis caused by *Francisella tularensis*. Humans of any age, sex, or race are universally susceptible to this systemic infection. Tularemia is primarily a disease of wild animals and persists in contaminated environments, ectoparasites, and animal carriers. Human infection is incidental and usually results from interaction with biting or blood-sucking insects, contact with wild or domestic animals, ingestion of contaminated water or food, or inhalation of infective aerosols.

Tularemia is common in Arkansas, Oklahoma, and Missouri, where >50% of the cases in the United States occur. Increasing numbers of cases have been reported from the Scandinavian countries, eastern Europe, and Siberia. The illness is characterized by various clinical syndromes, the most common of which consists of an ulcerative lesion at the site of inoculation, with regional lymphadenopathy and lymphadenitis. Systemic manifestations, including pneumonia, typhoidal tularemia, and fever without localizing findings, pose a greater diagnostic challenge.

ETIOLOGY AND EPIDEMIOLOGY

With rare exceptions, tularemia is the only disease produced by *F. tularensis*—a small (0.2 μm by 0.2–0.7 μm), gram-negative, pleomorphic, nonmotile, non–spore-forming bacillus. Bipolar staining results in a coccoid appearance. The organism is a thinly encapsulated, nonpiliated strict aerobe that invades host cells. In nature,

F. tularensis is a hardy organism that persists for weeks or months in mud, water, and decaying animal carcasses. Dozens of biting and blood-sucking insects, especially ticks and tabanid flies, serve as vectors. Ticks and wild rabbits are the source for most of the human cases in the endemic areas of the southeastern and Rocky Mountain states. In Utah, Nevada, and California, tabanid flies are the most common vectors. Animal reservoirs include wild rabbits, squirrels, birds, sheep, beavers, muskrats, and domestic dogs and cats. Person-to-person transmission is rare or nonexistent. Tularemia is more common among men than among women.

The two main biovars of *F. tularensis*—*tularensis* (type A) and *holarctica* (type B)—are both found in the United States. Type A produces more serious disease in humans; without treatment, the associated fatality rate is ~5%. Type B produces a milder, often subclinical infection that is usually contracted from water or marine mammals. Although all strains appear serologically identical, individual strains may possess varying degrees of virulence. Currently, there are four proposed subspecies among which 16S RNA analyses show ≥99.8% similarity. *F. tularensis* does not produce an exotoxin, but an endotoxin similar to that of other gram-negative bacilli has been identified. The progression of illness depends on the organism's virulence, the inoculum size, the portal of entry, and the host's immune status.

Ticks pass *F. tularensis* to their offspring transovarially. The organism is found in tick feces but not in large quantities in tick salivary glands. In the United States, the disease is carried by *Dermacentor andersoni* (Rocky Mountain wood tick), *D. variabilis* (American dog tick), *D. occidentalis* (Pacific coast dog tick), and *Amblyomma americanum* (Lone Star tick). *F. tularensis* is transmitted frequently during blood meals taken by embedded ticks after hours of attachment. It is the taking of a blood meal through a fecally contaminated field that transmits the organism. Transmission of the organism by ticks and tabanid flies takes place mainly in the spring and summer. However, continued transmission in the winter by trapped or hunted animals has been documented. The organism is extremely infectious. Biosafety level 2 is recommended for clinical laboratory work with material whose contamination with *F. tularensis* is suspected, and biosafety level 3 is required for culture of the organism in large quantities. Issues related to the intentional spread of tularemia through ingestion or inhalation are discussed in Chap. 6.

PATHOGENESIS AND PATHOLOGY

The most common portal of entry for human infection is through skin or mucous membranes, either directly—through the bite of ticks, other arthropods, or other animals—or via inapparent abrasions. Inhalation or ingestion of *F. tularensis* also can result in infection. Although $>10^8$ organisms are usually required to produce infection via the oral route (oropharyngeal or gastrointestinal tularemia), fewer than 50 organisms will result in infection when injected into the skin (ulceroglandular/glandular tularemia) or inhaled (tularemia pneumonia). After inoculation into the skin, the organism multiplies locally; within 2–5 days (range, 1–10 days), it produces an erythematous, tender, or pruritic papule. The papule rapidly enlarges and forms an ulcer with a black base (chancriform lesion). The bacteria spread to regional lymph nodes, producing lymphadenopathy (buboes), and, with bacteremia, may spread to distant organs.

Tularemia is characterized by mononuclear cell infiltration with pyogranulomatous pathology. The histopathologic findings can be quite similar to those in tuberculosis, although tularemia develops more rapidly. As a facultatively intracellular bacterium, *F. tularensis* can parasitize both phagocytic and nonphagocytic host cells and can survive intracellularly for prolonged periods. In the acute phase of infection, the primary organs affected (skin, lymph nodes, liver, and spleen) include areas of focal necrosis, initially surrounded by polymorphonuclear leukocytes (PMNs). Subsequently, granulomas form, with epithelioid cells, lymphocytes, and multinucleated giant cells surrounded by areas of necrosis. These areas may resemble caseation necrosis but later coalesce to form abscesses.

Conjunctival inoculation can result in infection of the eye, with regional lymph node enlargement (preauricular lymphadenopathy, Parinaud's complex). Aerosolization and inhalation or hematogenous spread of organisms can result in pneumonia. In the lung, an inflammatory reaction develops, including foci of alveolar necrosis and cell infiltration (initially polymorphonuclear and later mononuclear) with granulomas. Chest roentgenograms usually reveal bilateral patchy infiltrates rather than large areas of consolidation. Pleural effusions are common and may contain blood. Lymphadenopathy occurs in regions draining infected organs. Therefore, in pulmonary infection, mediastinal adenopathy may be evident, whereas patients with oropharyngeal tularemia develop cervical lymphadenopathy. In gastrointestinal or typhoidal tularemia, mesenteric lymphadenopathy may follow the ingestion of large numbers of organisms. (The term *typhoidal tularemia* may be used to describe severe bacteremic disease, irrespective of the mode of transmission or portal of entry.) Meningitis has been reported as a primary or secondary manifestation of bacteremia. Patients may also present with fever and no localizing signs.

IMMUNOLOGY

Infection with *F. tularensis* stimulates the host to produce antibodies. However, this antibody response probably plays only a minor role in the containment of infection. In contrast, cell-mediated immunity, which develops over 2–4 weeks, plays a major role in containment and eradication. Macrophages, once activated, can kill *F. tularensis*. Recovery from infection generally renders the patient resistant to reinfection; this point is not completely understood.

Immunospecific protection against tularemia can be afforded either by natural infection or by vaccination with live attenuated strains of *F. tularensis*. Killed vaccines, on the other hand, induce no protection against virulent *F. tularensis*. After natural infection or vaccination, serum antibodies to surface-exposed carbohydrate antigens predominate, whereas T-cell determinants are located on membrane proteins beneath the bacterial capsule. T-cell responses are thought to be due to priming by the organism. The anamnestic T-cell response to *F. tularensis* seems to involve a multitude of microbial proteins, each with a distinct set of T-cell determinants. A predominant role for CD4+ T cells is supported by the results of experiments in mice, which indicated that resistance to infection was restricted at the level of the major histocompatibility complex (MHC) class II determinants. Humans primed to *F. tularensis* (like those primed to *Mycobacterium tuberculosis*) show a T_H1-like response. T-cell proliferation is associated with the production of interleukin (IL) 2 and interferon γ but with little or no production of IL-4. Recent evidence indicates that the percentage of γδ T cells expressing tumor necrosis factor α is decreased during the first 7–40 days after infection. This decrease may reflect the modulation of an inflammatory response. Investigations of neutrophils in tularemia suggest that PMNs are needed for defense against primary infection. PMNs may restrict the growth of *F. tularensis* before the organism becomes intracellular.

CLINICAL MANIFESTATIONS

Tularemia often starts with a sudden onset of fever, chills, headache, and generalized myalgias and arthralgias (Table 59-1). This onset takes place when the organism penetrates the skin, is ingested, or is inhaled. An incubation period of 2–10 days is followed by the formation of an ulcer at the site of penetration, with local inflammation. The ulcer may persist for several months as organisms are transported via the lymphatics to the regional lymph nodes. These nodes enlarge and may become necrotic and suppurative. If the organism enters the bloodstream, widespread dissemination as well as signs and symptoms of endotoxemia may result.

In the United States, most patients with tularemia (75–85%) acquire the infection by inoculation of the skin. In adults, the most common localized form is inguinal/femoral lymphadenopathy; in children, it is cervical lymphadenopathy. About 20% of patients develop a generalized maculopapular rash, which occasionally becomes pustular. Erythema nodosum occurs infrequently. The clinical manifestations of tularemia have been divided into various syndromes, which are listed in Table 59-2.

TABLE 59-1

CLINICAL PRESENTATION OF TULAREMIA

	RATE OF OCCURRENCE, %	
SIGN OR SYMPTOM	**CHILDREN**	**ADULTS**
Lymphadenopathy	96	65
Fever (≥38.3°C or ≥101°F)	87	21
Ulcer/eschar/papule	45	51
Myalgias/arthralgias	39	2
Headache	9	5
Cough	9	5
Pharyngitis	43	—
Diarrhea	43	—

Source: Adapted from RF Jacobs, JP Narain: Tularemia in adults and children: A changing presentation. *Pediatrics* 76:818, 1985; with permission.

TABLE 59-2

CLINICAL SYNDROMES OF TULAREMIA

	RATE OF OCCURRENCE, %	
SYNDROME	**CHILDREN**	**ADULTS**
Ulceroglandular	45	51
Glandular	25	12
Pulmonary (pneumonia)	14	18
Oropharyngeal	4	—
Oculoglandular	2	—
Typhoidal	2	12
Unclassified	6	11

Source: Adapted from RF Jacobs, JP Narain: Tularemia in adults and children: A changing presentation. *Pediatrics* 76:818, 1985; with permission.

Ulceroglandular/Glandular Tularemia

These two forms of tularemia account for ~75–85% of cases. The predominant form in children involves cervical or posterior auricular lymphadenopathy and is usually related to tick bites on the head and neck. In adults, the most common form is inguinal/femoral lymphadenopathy resulting from insect and tick exposures on the lower limbs. In cases related to wild game, the usual portal of entry for *F. tularensis* is either an injury sustained while skinning or cleaning an animal carcass or a bite (usually on the hand). Epitrochlear lymphadenopathy/lymphadenitis is common in patients with bite-related injuries.

In ulceroglandular tularemia, the ulcer is erythematous, indurated, and nonhealing, with a punched-out appearance that lasts 1–3 weeks. The papule may begin as an erythematous lesion that is tender or pruritic; it evolves over several days into an ulcer with sharply demarcated edges and a yellow exudate. The ulcer gradually develops a black base, and simultaneously the regional lymph nodes become tender and severely enlarged (Fig. 59-1). The affected lymph nodes may become fluctuant and drain spontaneously, but usually the condition resolves with effective treatment. Late suppuration of lymph nodes has been described in up to 25% of patients with ulceroglandular/glandular tularemia. Examination of material taken from these late fluctuant nodes after successful antimicrobial treatment reveals sterile necrotic tissue. In 5–10% of patients, the skin lesion may be inapparent, with lymphadenopathy plus systemic signs and symptoms the only physical findings (*glandular tularemia*). Conversely, a tick or deerfly bite on the trunk may result in an ulcer without evident lymphadenopathy.

Oculoglandular Tularemia

In ~1% of patients, the portal of entry for *F. tularensis* is the conjunctiva. Usually, the organism reaches the

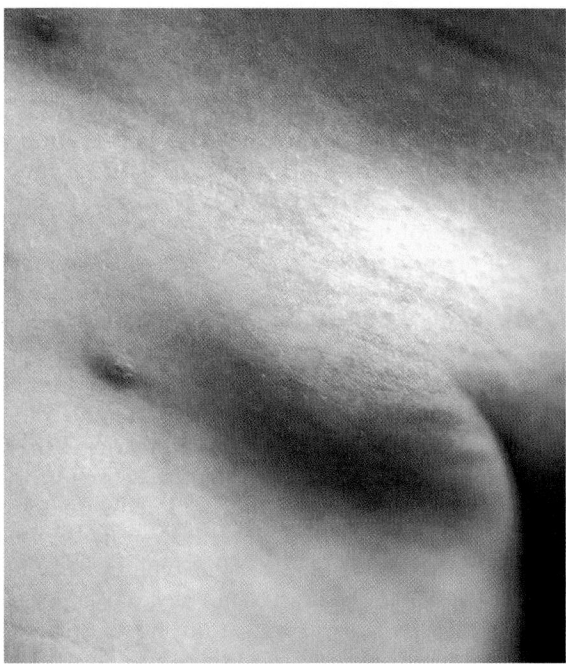

FIGURE 59-1
An 8-year-old boy with inguinal lymphadenitis and associated tick-bite site characteristic of ulceroglandular tularemia

conjunctiva through contact with contaminated fingers. The inflamed conjunctiva is painful, with numerous yellowish nodules and pinpoint ulcers. Purulent conjunctivitis with regional lymphadenopathy (preauricular, submandibular, or cervical) is evident. Because of debilitating pain, the patient may seek medical attention before regional lymphadenopathy develops. Painful preauricular lymphadenopathy is unique to tularemia and distinguishes it from cat-scratch disease, tuberculosis, sporotrichosis, and syphilis. Corneal perforation may occur.

Oropharyngeal and Gastrointestinal Tularemia

Rarely, tularemia follows ingestion of contaminated undercooked meat, oral inoculation of *F. tularensis* from the hands in association with the skinning and cleaning of animal carcasses, or consumption of contaminated food or water. Oral inoculation may result in acute, exudative, or membranous pharyngitis associated with cervical lymphadenopathy or in ulcerative intestinal lesions associated with mesenteric lymphadenopathy, diarrhea, abdominal pain, nausea, vomiting, and gastrointestinal bleeding. Infected tonsils become enlarged and develop a yellowish-white pseudomembrane, which can be confused with that of diphtheria. The clinical severity of gastrointestinal tularemia varies from mild, unexplained, persistent diarrhea with no other symptoms to a fulminant, fatal disease. In fatal cases, the extensive intestinal ulceration found at autopsy suggests an enormous inoculum.

Pulmonary Tularemia

Tularemia pneumonia presents as variable parenchymal infiltrates that are unresponsive to treatment with β-lactam antibiotics. Tularemia must be considered in the differential diagnosis of atypical pneumonia in a patient with a history of travel to an endemic area. The disease can result from inhalation of an infectious aerosol or can spread to the lungs and pleura after bloodstream dissemination. Inhalation-related pneumonia has been described in laboratory workers after exposure to contaminated materials and is associated with a relatively high mortality rate. Exposure to *F. tularensis* in aerosols from live domestic animals or dead wildlife (including birds) has been reported to cause pneumonia. Hematogenous dissemination to the lungs occurs in 10–15% of cases of ulceroglandular tularemia and in about half of cases of typhoidal tularemia. Previously, tularemia pneumonia was thought to be a disease of older patients, but as many as 10–15% of children with clinical manifestations of tularemia have parenchymal infiltrates detected by chest roentgenography. Patients with pneumonia usually have a nonproductive cough and may have dyspnea or pleuritic chest pain. Roentgenograms of the chest usually reveal bilateral patchy infiltrates (described as ovoid or lobar densities), lobar parenchymal infiltrates, and cavitary lesions. Pleural effusions may have a predominance of mononuclear leukocytes or PMNs and sometimes red blood cells. Empyema may develop. Blood cultures may be positive for *F. tularensis*.

Typhoidal Tularemia

The typhoidal presentation is now considered rare in the United States. The source of infection in typhoidal tularemia is usually associated with pharyngeal and/or gastrointestinal inoculation or bacteremic disease. Fever usually develops without apparent skin lesions or lymphadenopathy. Some patients have cervical and mesenteric lymphadenopathy. In the absence of a history of possible contact with a vector, diagnosis can be extremely difficult. Blood cultures may be positive and patients may present with classic sepsis or septic shock in this acute systemic form of the infection. Typhoidal tularemia is usually associated with a huge inoculum or with a preexisting compromising condition. High continuous fevers, signs of endotoxemia, and severe headache are common. The patient may be delirious and may develop prostration and shock. If presumptive antibiotic therapy in culture-negative cases does not include an aminoglycoside, the mortality rate can approach 30%.

Other Manifestations

F. tularensis infection has been associated with meningitis, pericarditis, hepatitis, peritonitis, endocarditis, osteomyelitis, and sepsis and septic shock with rhabdomyolysis and acute renal failure. In the rare cases of tularemia meningitis, a predominantly lymphocytic response is demonstrated in cerebrospinal fluid.

DIFFERENTIAL DIAGNOSIS

When patients in endemic areas present with fever, chronic ulcerative skin lesions, and large tender lymph nodes (Fig. 59-1), a diagnosis of tularemia should be made presumptively, and confirmatory diagnostic testing and appropriate therapy should be undertaken. When the possibility of tularemia is considered in a nonendemic area, an attempt should be made to identify contact with a potential animal vector. The level of suspicion should be especially high in hunters, trappers, game wardens, veterinarians, laboratory workers, and individuals exposed to an insect or another animal vector. However, up to 40% of patients with tularemia have no known history of epidemiologic contact with an animal vector.

The characteristic presentation of ulceroglandular tularemia does not pose a diagnostic problem, but a less classic progression of regional lymphadenopathy or glandular tularemia must be differentiated from other diseases (Table 59-3). The skin lesion of tularemia may resemble those seen in various other diseases but is generally accompanied by more impressive regional lymphadenopathy. In children, the differentiation of tularemia from cat-scratch disease is made more difficult by the chronic papulovesicular lesion associated with *Bartonella henselae* infection (Chap. 61). Oropharyngeal tularemia can resemble and must be differentiated from pharyngitis due to other bacteria or viruses. Tularemia pneumonia may resemble any atypical pneumonia. Typhoidal tularemia may resemble a variety of other infections.

LABORATORY DIAGNOSIS

Direct microscopic examination of polychromatically stained tissue smears or clinical specimens reveals *F. tularensis* organisms, singly and in groups, both intra- and extracellularly. Gram's staining of clinical or biopsy material is of little value, as the small, weakly staining, gram-negative, nonmotile, non–spore-forming bacteria are difficult to distinguish from the background. An indirect fluorescent antibody test with commercially available antisera can be useful, although false-positive results due to *Legionella* spp. have been reported.

The diagnosis of tularemia is most frequently confirmed by agglutination testing. Microagglutination and tube agglutination are the techniques most commonly used to detect antibody to *F. tularensis*. In the standard tube agglutination test, a single titer of ≥1:160 is interpreted as a presumptive positive result. A fourfold increase in titer between paired serum samples collected 2–3 weeks apart is considered diagnostic. False-negative serologic responses are obtained early in infection; up to 30% of patients infected for 3 weeks have sera that test negative. Late in infection, titers into the thousands are common, and titers of 1:20–1:80 may persist for years. Enzyme-linked immunosorbent assays have proved useful for the detection of both antibodies and antigens. Analysis of urine for *F. tularensis* antigen has yielded promising results in clinical trials, but facilities for this type of analysis are not widely available. A skin test for delayed hypersensitivity to *F. tularensis* turns positive during the first week of illness and remains positive for years. The skin-test antigen, which is not commercially available, can boost titers of agglutinating antibody.

Culture and isolation of *F. tularensis* are difficult. In one study, the organism was isolated in only 10% of more than 1000 human cases, 84% of which were confirmed by serology. The medium of choice is cysteine-glucose-blood agar. *F. tularensis* can be isolated directly from infected ulcer scrapings, lymph-node biopsy specimens, gastric washings, sputum, and blood cultures. Colonies are blue-gray, round, smooth, and slightly mucoid. On media containing blood, a small zone of α hemolysis usually surrounds the colony. Slide agglutination tests or direct fluorescent

TABLE 59-3

TULAREMIA: DIFFERENTIAL DIAGNOSIS, BY CLINICAL DISEASE CATEGORY

GLANDULAR	OROPHARYNGEAL	TYPHOIDAL	PNEUMONIA
Pyogenic bacterial infection[a]	Group A streptococcal pharyngitis	Typhoid fever	*Mycoplasma pneumoniae* pneumonia
Nontuberculous mycobacterial infection	*Arcanobacterium haemolyticum* pharyngitis	Other *Salmonella* bacteremias	*Chlamydophila pneumoniae* pneumonia
Sporotrichosis	Diphtheria	Rocky Mountain spotted fever	Psittacosis
Tuberculosis	Infectious mononucleosis	Human monocytotropic ehrlichiosis	*Legionella pneumophila* pneumonia
Syphilis	Various viral infections[b]	Human granulocytotropic ehrlichiosis	Q fever
Anthrax		Infectious mononucleosis	Histoplasmosis
Rat-bite fever		Brucellosis	Blastomycosis
Scrub typhus		Toxoplasmosis	Coccidioidomycosis
Plague		Tuberculosis	Various viral infections[d]
Lymphogranuloma venereum		Sarcoidosis	
Cat-scratch disease		Malignancy[c]	

[a]*Staphylococcus aureus, Streptococcus pyogenes.*
[b]Adenovirus, enteroviruses, parainfluenza virus, influenza virus A and B, respiratory syncytial virus.
[c]Hematologic and reticuloendothelial malignancies.
[d]Influenza virus A and B, parainfluenza virus, respiratory syncytial virus, adenovirus, enteroviruses, hantavirus.

antibody tests with commercially available antisera can be applied directly to culture suspensions for identification. Most clinical laboratories will not attempt to culture *F. tularensis* because of the infectivity of the organism from the culture media. Although tularemia is not spread from person to person, the organism can be inhaled from culture plates and infect unsuspecting laboratory workers. In most clinical laboratories, biosafety level 2 practices are recommended to handle clinical specimens thought to contain *F. tularensis*.

A variety of polymerase chain reaction (PCR) methods have been used to detect *F. tularensis* DNA in multiple clinical specimens. The majority of these methods target the genes encoding the outer-membrane proteins (e.g., *fopA* or *tul4*). A 16S rDNA sequence identification PCR is helpful when the patient's clinical information does not lead the clinician to suspect a diagnosis of tularemia.

℞ Treatment: TULAREMIA

F. tularensis cannot be subjected to standardized antimicrobial susceptibility testing because the organism will not grow on the media used. A wide variety of antibiotics, including all β-lactam antibiotics and the newer cephalosporins, are ineffective for the treatment of tularemia. Several studies indicated that third-generation cephalosporins were active against *F. tularensis* in vitro, but clinical case reports suggested a nearly universal failure rate of ceftriaxone in pediatric patients with tularemia. Although in vitro data indicate that imipenem may be active, therapy with imipenem, sulfanilamides, and macrolides is not presently recommended because of the lack of relevant clinical data. Fluoroquinolones have shown promise in terms of their relatively low toxicity and their potential for oral administration. With intracellular activity, fluoroquinolones have been used for successful treatment of tularemia and are candidates for primary or alternative therapy, pending clinical trials. The use of these agents should also be considered when patients are allergic or intolerant to other treatments. When used, ciprofloxacin should be given for a total of 10 days. Chloramphenicol and tetracycline have been used successfully for treatment of the acute stages of tularemia but have been associated with higher relapse rates (up to 20%) than conventionally used agents. Oral chloramphenicol is no longer available in the United States.

Gentamicin is considered the drug of choice for both adults and children. The dosage for adults is 5 mg/kg daily in two divided doses. The dosage for children is 2.5 mg/kg tid or 5 mg/kg bid. Gentamicin therapy is typically continued for 7–10 days; however, in mild to moderate cases of tularemia in which the patient becomes afebrile within the first 48–72 h of gentamicin treatment, a 5- to 7-day course has been successful.

If available (shortages have been reported over the past several years), streptomycin given intramuscularly also is effective. The dosage for adults is 2 g/d in two divided doses. For children, the dosage is 30 mg/kg daily in two divided doses (maximal daily dose, 2 g). After a clinical response is demonstrated at 3–5 days, the dose can be reduced to 10–15 mg/kg daily in two divided doses. The total duration of streptomycin therapy in both adults and children is usually 10 days.

Virtually all strains of *F. tularensis* are susceptible to streptomycin and gentamicin. In successfully treated patients, defervescence usually occurs within 2 days, but skin lesions and lymph nodes may take 1–2 weeks to heal. When therapy is not initiated within the first several days of illness, defervescence may be delayed. Relapses are uncommon with streptomycin or gentamicin therapy. Late lymph-node suppuration, however, occurs in ~40% of children, regardless of the treatment received. These nodes have typically been found to contain sterile necrotic tissue without evidence of active infection. Patients with fluctuant nodes should receive several days of antibiotic therapy before drainage to minimize the risk to hospital personnel. Unlike streptomycin and gentamicin, tobramycin is ineffective in the treatment of tularemia and should not be used.

PROGNOSIS

If tularemia goes untreated, symptoms usually last 1–4 weeks but may continue for months. The mortality rate from severe untreated infection (including all cases of untreated tularemia pneumonia and typhoidal tularemia) can be as high as 30%. However, the overall mortality rate for untreated tularemia is <8%. Mortality is <1% with appropriate treatment. Poor outcomes are often associated with long delays in diagnosis and treatment. Lifelong immunity usually follows tularemia.

PREVENTION

The prevention of tularemia is based on avoidance of exposure to biting and blood-sucking insects, especially ticks and deerflies. A vaccine made from live attenuated *F. tularensis* was developed in the United States and found to be effective. Because of difficulty with standardization, however, the vaccine is not currently licensed in the United States or Europe. A live attenuated vaccine is still available in some parts of the former Soviet Union. Prophylaxis of tularemia has not proved effective in patients with embedded ticks or insect bites. However, in patients who are known to have been exposed to large quantities of organisms (e.g., in the laboratory) and who have incubating infection with *F. tularensis*, early treatment can prevent the development of significant clinical disease.

FURTHER READINGS

BARNS SM et al: Detection of diverse new *Francisella*-like bacteria in environmental samples. Appl Environ Microbiol 71:5494, 2005

CENTERS FOR DISEASE CONTROL AND PREVENTION: Tularemia—United States, 1990–2000. MMWR 51:181, 2002

DE LA PUENTE-REDONDO VA et al: Comparison of different PCR approaches for typing of *Francisella tularensis* strains. J Clin Microbiol 38:1016, 2000

DENNIS DT et al: Tularemia as a biological weapon: Medical and public health management. JAMA 285:2763, 2001

ELIASSON H et al: The 2000 tularemia outbreak: A case-control study of risk factors in disease-endemic and emergent areas, Sweden. Emerg Infect Dis 8:956, 2002

HOFINGER DM et al: Tularemic meningitis in the United States. Arch Neurol 66:523, 2009

IKÄHEIMO I et al: In vitro antibiotic susceptibility of *Francisella tularensis* isolated from humans and animals. J Antimicrob Chemother 46:287, 2000

JOHANSSON A et al: In vitro susceptibility to quinolones of *Francisella tularensis* subspecies tularensis. Scand J Infect Dis 34:327, 2002

PETERSEN JM et al: Methods for the enhanced recovery of *Francisella tularensis* cultures. Appl Environ Microbiol 70:3733, 2004

TARNVIK A et al: Tularemia in Europe: An epidemiological overview. Scand J Infect Dis 36:350, 2004

VERSAGE JL et al: Development of a multitarget real-time TaqMan PCR assay for enhanced detection of *Francisella tularensis* in complex specimens. J Clin Microbiol 41:5492, 2003

CHAPTER 60

PLAGUE AND OTHER *YERSINIA* INFECTIONS

David T. Dennis ■ Grant L. Campbell

PLAGUE

DEFINITION

Plague is an acute febrile disease caused by infection with *Yersinia pestis*. Human cases are infrequent and are curable with antibiotics. Plague is, however, one of the most virulent and potentially lethal bacterial diseases known, and fatality rates remain high among patients who are not treated in the early stages of infection. Plague occurs in widely scattered foci in Asia, Africa, and the Americas (Fig. 60-1), where its usual hosts are various wild rodents and human-associated rats. Infection is transmitted to humans typically by flea bite and infrequently by direct contact with infected animal tissues or by airborne droplet. The principal clinical forms of plague are bubonic, septicemic, and pneumonic. Although most cases are now sporadic, occurring singly or in small clusters, the potential for outbreaks and epidemic spread remains. Because of its virulence and transmissibility, *Y. pestis* is considered an important potential agent of biological terrorism that requires special countermeasures to protect the public's health (Chap. 6).

ETIOLOGIC AGENT

Y. pestis is a gram-negative coccobacillus in the family Enterobacteriaceae. Genomic analysis suggests that it has only recently evolved from *Y. pseudotuberculosis*. *Y. pestis* is microaerophilic, nonmotile, nonsporulating, oxidase and urease negative, and biochemically unreactive. The organism is nonfastidious and infective for laboratory rodents. It grows well, if slowly, on routinely used microbiologic media (e.g., sheep blood agar, brain-heart infusion broth, and MacConkey agar). *Y. pestis* can multiply within a wide range of temperatures (–2°C to 45°C) and pH values (5.0–9.6), but optimal growth occurs at 28°C and at pH ~7.4. When stained with a polychromatic stain (e.g., Wayson or Giemsa), *Y. pestis* isolated from clinical specimens exhibits a characteristic bipolar appearance, resembling closed safety pins. The bacterium is nonencapsulated but, when grown at ≥30°C, produces a plasmid-expressed envelope glycoprotein, fraction 1 (F1) antigen—a virulence factor that serves as the principal immunodiagnostic marker of infection.

HISTORIC BACKGROUND

Plague's deadly epidemic potential is notorious and well documented. The Justinian pandemic (542–767 A.D.) is thought to have spread from central Africa to the Mediterranean littoral and thence to Asia Minor, causing an estimated 40 million deaths. The second pandemic began in central Asia, was carried to Sicily by ship from Constantinople in 1347, and within a few years swept through Europe and the British Isles; successive epidemics of lesser magnitude occurred over the next four centuries. At its height, the second plague pandemic killed as many as a quarter of the affected population and became known as the Black Death. In the third (modern) pandemic, epidemic plague appeared in Yunnan, China, in the latter half of the nineteenth century; established itself in Hong Kong in 1894; and spread by ship to Bombay in 1896 and subsequently to major port cities throughout the world, including San Francisco and several other West Coast and Gulf Coast ports in the United States. The plague bacillus was first cultured by Alexandre Yersin in Hong Kong in 1894. In 1898, Paul-Louis Simond, a French scientist sent to investigate epidemic bubonic plague in Bombay, identified the bacillus in the tissues of dead rats and proposed transmission by rat fleas. Waldemar Haffkine, also in Bombay at that time, developed a crude vaccine.

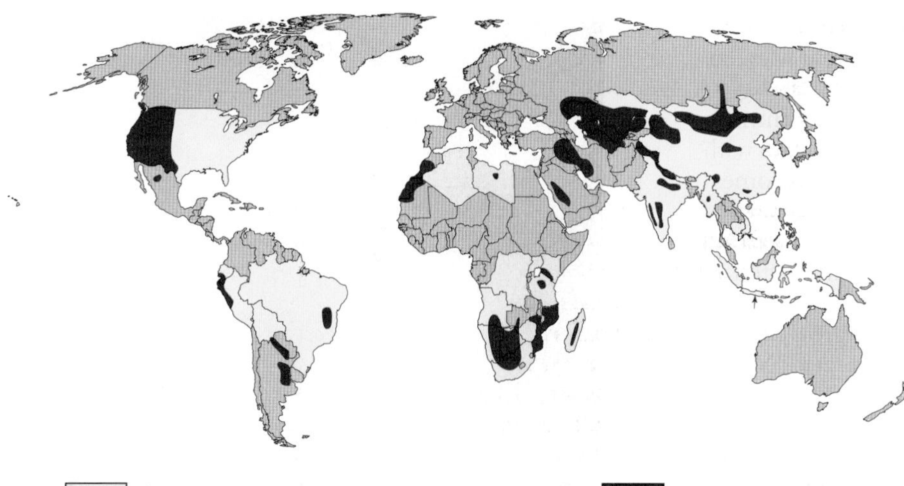

FIGURE 60-1
Approximate global distribution of *Yersinia pestis*. *(Compiled from WHO, CDC, and country sources.)*

By 1910, the oriental strain of *Y. pestis* had circled the globe and was established in rodent populations on all inhabited continents other than Australia. After 1920, however, the spread of plague was largely halted by international regulations that mandated control of rats in harbors and inspection and rat-proofing of ships. Before subsiding, the third pandemic had resulted in an estimated 26 million plague cases and >12 million deaths, the vast majority in India. By 1950, plague outbreaks around the world had become isolated, sporadic, and manageable with modern techniques of surveillance, flea and rat control, and antimicrobial treatment of patients. Plague has nearly disappeared from cities and now occurs mostly in rural and semirural areas, where it is maintained in various rodents and their fleas. In the United States, the last outbreak of urban plague occurred in Los Angeles in 1924 and 1925, and human cases since then have, with very few exceptions, resulted from exposures in rural areas of western states.

Plague remains one of three diseases subject to international health regulations (the other two being cholera and yellow fever). The alarm that plague is still able to evoke was highlighted by the public panic and exaggerated official responses to reported outbreaks of bubonic and pneumonic plague in India in 1994. Recently, there has been increasing concern that *Y. pestis* might be used as an agent of terrorism. The agent is available around the world, has been "weaponized" for airborne delivery, and would be expected to cause a high primary fatality rate as well as secondary spread among an affected population (Chap. 6).

EPIDEMIOLOGY

Y. pestis is maintained in well-established "silent" enzootic cycles involving relatively resistant wild rodents and their fleas in remote, lightly populated areas of Asia, Africa, and the Americas and in limited rural foci in extreme southeastern Europe near the Caspian Sea (Fig. 60-1). Humans and mammals other than rodents are incidental hosts. Outbreaks (epizootics) of plague in susceptible rodent populations may result in widespread rodent die-offs, an avid search by their fleas for new hosts, and an increased risk of spread of infection to humans. In the United States, the principal epizootic hosts are various ground squirrels, prairie dogs, and chipmunks; various burrowing rodents act as reservoir hosts in natural areas elsewhere in the world. *Y. pestis* occasionally spills over from wild rodents to rat species that inhabit cultivated fields and adjacent homes, villages, and towns. The organism can then be transported from towns to cities by these highly adaptable rats and their fleas.

Plague in populated areas is most likely to develop when sanitation is poor and rats are numerous—especially the common black or roof rat (*Rattus rattus*), its close relatives, and the larger brown sewer or Norway rat (*R. norvegicus*). The cosmopolitan oriental rat flea *Xenopsylla cheopis* and (in southern Africa and Brazil) the related species *X. brasiliensis* are efficient vectors of the plague bacillus from rat to rat and from rats to humans. *Y. pestis* multiplies to enormous numbers in the foregut (proventriculus) of these fleas, resulting in a bolus of organisms and clotted blood that blocks the passage of subsequent blood meals. This blockage occurs at temperatures of ≤28°C and depends on a single protease expressed by the plasminogen activator (*pla*) gene of a 9.5-kb plasmid of *Y. pestis*. Regurgitation by a "blocked" flea while it feeds facilitates transmission of the plague bacillus to the new host. Except for large outbreaks of pneumonic plague in Manchuria in the early part of the twentieth century, person-to-person respiratory transmission of plague has since occurred only sporadically and has been limited to clusters of close, direct contacts of pneumonic plague patients, such as household members and caregivers.

International health regulations require that national authorities immediately report plague cases to the World Health Organization (WHO). During 1989–2003, a total of 38,359 human cases of plague were reported to the WHO from 25 countries (a mean of 2557 cases per year). The reported case-fatality rate was 7%. More than 80% (31,273) of the total number of cases were reported from Africa, ~14% (5449) from Asia, and the rest (1637) from the Americas.

In the United States, 5–10 human plague cases typically are reported each year. Most cases occur in New Mexico, Arizona, Colorado, and California (*http://www.cdc.gov/ncidod/dvbid/plague/plagwest.htm*). The most common modes of transmission are flea bite and direct contact with infected animals, especially exposure to an infected domestic cat. The overall case-fatality rate is ~10%. Most cases of plague occur in the summer months, when rodents and their fleas are most active. The disease is acquired often in the environs of the patient's residential property and less often during work or recreation in natural areas remote from the patient's place of residence. The arid Native American reservations of New Mexico and Arizona are active plague foci, and Native Americans account for a disproportionately high percentage of plague cases.

Plague can be transmitted during the skinning and handling of carcasses of wild animals such as rabbits and hares, prairie dogs, wildcats, and coyotes. Such direct inoculation of mammal-adapted organisms expressing the F1 antigen is associated with primary septicemia and high mortality rates. Pharyngeal plague can result from the ingestion of undercooked contaminated meat; outbreaks of pharyngeal plague have been reported among persons eating undercooked camel and goat meat. Plague can also be acquired by inhalation of infective respiratory droplets and perhaps by manual transfer of infected fluids to the mouth during the handling of infected animal tissues.

Carnivores, including dogs and cats, can become infected with *Y. pestis* by eating infected rodents and possibly by being bitten by infective fleas. Although clinical plague commonly develops in infected cats, it rarely does so in infected dogs. Both dogs and cats may transport infected fleas from rodent-infested areas to the home environment.

PATHOGENESIS AND PATHOLOGY

Y. pestis is highly invasive and pathogenic. The mechanisms by which the organism causes disease are incompletely understood, but both chromosome- and plasmid-encoded gene products as well as altered cell-mediated immune responses are involved. Three plasmids encode for a variety of known or presumed virulence factors, including the F1 envelope antigen and various *Yersinia* outer-membrane proteins, which confer bacterial resistance to phagocytosis; the V antigen, which is essential for virulence and suppresses the synthesis of various proinflammatory cytokines (e.g., interferon γ and tumor necrosis factor α); pesticin, which interferes with iron uptake; a protease that activates plasminogen and degrades serum complement and is thought to enhance dissemination of *Y. pestis* after inoculation of the skin; a coagulase; and a fibrinolysin. A chromosomally encoded lipopolysaccharide endotoxin is important in sepsis, playing a role in triggering the systemic inflammatory response syndrome and its complications.

Y. pestis organisms inoculated through the skin or mucous membranes are typically carried to regional lymph nodes via lymphatic channels, although direct bloodstream inoculation and dissemination may take place. Mononuclear phagocytes, which can phagocytize *Y. pestis* organisms without destroying them, may play a role in dissemination of the infection to distant sites. Plague can involve almost any organ, and untreated plague generally results in widespread and massive tissue destruction. In the early stages, infected lymph nodes (*buboes*, Fig. 60-2) are characterized by edema and congestion without inflammatory infiltrates or apparent vascular injury. Fully developed buboes contain huge numbers of infectious plague organisms and show distorted or obliterated lymph node architecture with loss of vascular integrity, hemorrhage, necrosis, infiltration of polymorphonuclear neutrophils (PMNs), and extensive serosanguineous effusion. The effusion typically involves perinodal tissues. If several adjacent lymph nodes are involved, a boggy edematous mass can result.

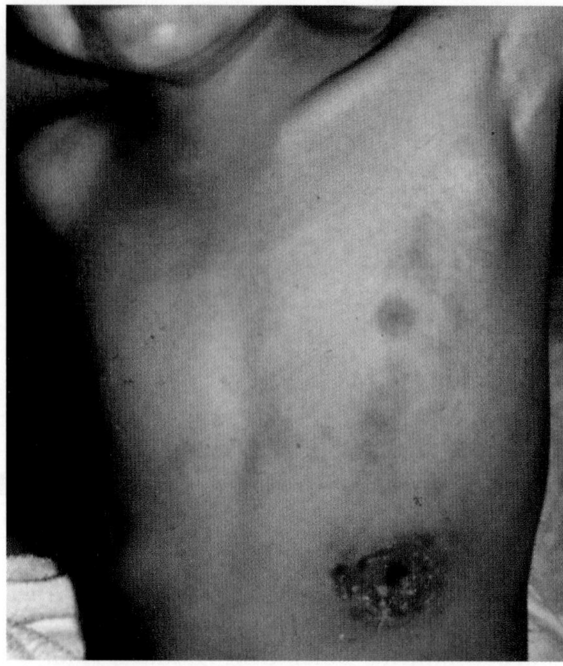

FIGURE 60-2
Plague patient in the southwestern United States with a left axillary bubo and an unusual plague ulcer and eschar at the site of the infective flea bite.

Primary septicemic plague consists of sepsis in the absence of a bubo; secondary septicemic plague is a complication of bubonic or pneumonic plague that occurs when local host defenses are breached. In fatal septicemic plague, multifocal hepatic and splenic necrosis is common. Diffuse interstitial myocarditis with cardiac dilatation is sometimes found. If disseminated intravascular coagulation (DIC) ensues, vascular necrosis may lead to widespread cutaneous, mucosal, and serosal ecchymoses and petechiae. Acral ischemia and resulting gangrene sometimes develop.

Primary plague pneumonia generally begins as a lobular process and then extends by confluence, becoming lobar and then multilobar (Fig. 60-3). Plague organisms are typically most numerous in the alveoli. Secondary plague pneumonia begins more diffusely, with organisms at first most numerous in the interstitium. In advanced cases of both primary and secondary plague pneumonia,

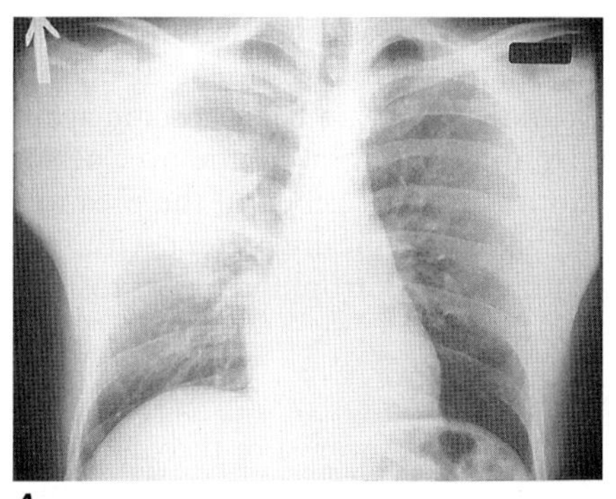

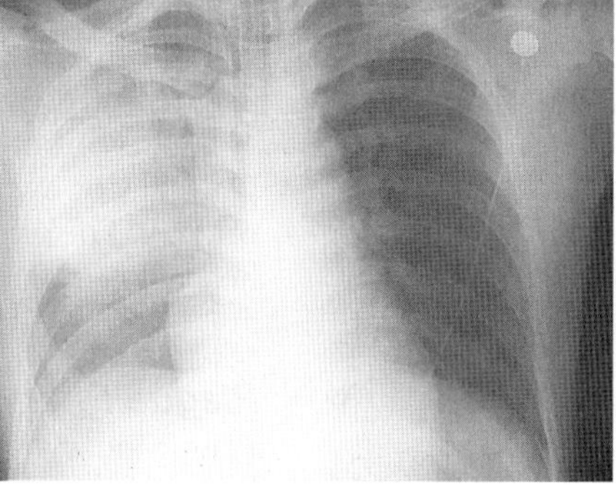

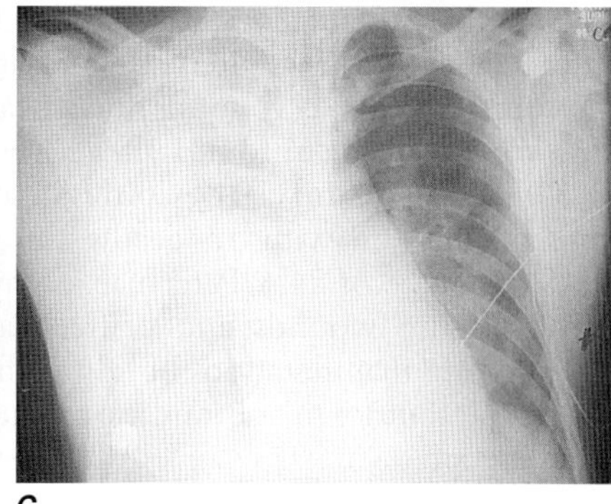

A B C

FIGURE 60-3

Sequential chest radiographs of a patient with fatal primary plague pneumonia. *A.* Upright posteroanterior film taken at admission to hospital emergency department on third day of illness, showing segmental consolidation of right upper lobe. ***B.*** Portable anteroposterior film taken 8 h after admission, showing extension of pneumonia to right middle and right lower lobes. ***C.*** Portable anteroposterior film taken 13 h after admission (when patient had clinical adult respiratory distress syndrome), showing diffuse infiltration throughout right lung and patchy infiltration of left lower lung. A cavity later developed at the site of initial right-upper-lobe consolidation.

affected lung tissue is characterized by edema, hemorrhagic necrosis, and infiltration by neutrophilic leukocytes.

CLINICAL MANIFESTATIONS

Plague is characterized by a rapid onset of fever and other systemic manifestations of gram-negative bacterial infection. If it is not quickly and correctly treated, plague can follow a toxic course, resulting in shock, multiple-organ failure, and death. In humans, the three principal forms of plague are bubonic, septicemic, and pneumonic. *Bubonic* plague, accounting in the United States for ~75% of cases, is almost always caused by the bite of an infected flea but occasionally results from direct contact with infectious materials. *Septicemic* and *pneumonic* plague can be either primary or secondary to metastatic spread. Unusual forms include plague meningitis, endophthalmitis, and lymphadenitis at multiple sites. Primary plague pharyngitis has been documented by culture of organisms from throat swabs and can result from respiratory exposure or ingestion of undercooked flesh of infected animals.

Bubonic Plague

Bubonic plague has a usual incubation period of 2–6 days. Patients experience chills; fever, with temperatures that rise within hours to ≥38°C; myalgias; arthralgias; headache; and a feeling of weakness. Soon—usually within 24 h—the patient notices tenderness and pain in one or more regional lymph nodes proximal to the site of inoculation of the plague bacillus (Fig. 60-2). Because fleas most often bite the legs, femoral and inguinal nodes are most commonly involved; axillary and cervical nodes are next most commonly affected. Within hours, the enlarging bubo becomes progressively painful and tender, sometimes exquisitely so. The patient usually guards against palpation and limits movement, pressure, and stretch around the bubo. The surrounding tissue often becomes edematous, sometimes markedly so, and the overlying skin may be erythematous, warm, and tense. Inspection of the skin surrounding or distal to the bubo sometimes reveals the site of a flea bite marked by a papule, pustule, or ulcer. The ulcer may be covered by an eschar (Fig. 60-2). A list of lymphadenitic conditions that could be confused with bubonic plague includes *Staphylococcus aureus* and group A β-hemolytic streptococcal infections, cat-scratch disease, tularemia, and—in filariasis-endemic areas—acute filarial lymphadenitis. The bubo of plague is distinguishable from lymphadenitis of most other causes, however, by its rapid onset, its extreme tenderness, the accompanying signs of toxemia, and the absence of cellulitis or obvious ascending lymphangitis. The pain and swelling of bubonic plague can be confused with a strangulated hernia or trauma.

Treated in the uncomplicated state with an appropriate antibiotic, bubonic plague usually responds quickly, with resolution of fever and alleviation of other systemic manifestations over 2–5 days. Buboes often remain enlarged and tender for a week or more after the initiation of treatment and can become fluctuant. Without effective antimicrobial treatment, patients with typical bubonic plague manifest an increasingly toxic state of fever, tachycardia, lethargy leading to prostration, agitation and confusion, and (occasionally) convulsions and delirium. Secondary plague sepsis may result in an alarmingly rapid and refractory cascade of DIC, bleeding, shock, and organ failure.

Septicemic Plague

Primary septicemia, which accounts for ~20% of cases in the United States, develops in the absence of a detectable bubo. The diagnosis often is not suspected until preliminary blood culture results are reported to be positive by the laboratory. *Y. pestis*, however, can also be cultured from the blood of most patients with bubonic plague, and bacteremia must be distinguished from septicemia, in which the patient is desperately ill and requires aggressive care. Septic patients often present with gastrointestinal symptoms of nausea, vomiting, diarrhea, and abdominal pain, which may confound the correct diagnosis. In the United States in 1947–2001, 55 cases of primary septicemic plague with 13 deaths were reported, for a case-fatality rate of 24%. Petechiae, ecchymoses, bleeding from puncture wounds and orifices, and gangrene of acral parts are manifestations of DIC; refractory hypotension, renal shutdown, obtundation, and other signs of shock are preterminal events. Adult respiratory distress syndrome (ARDS) can occur at any stage of septicemic plague. The differential diagnosis of septicemic plague includes sepsis of other gram-negative bacterial etiology, meningococcemia, and acute severe viral infections such as hantavirus illness.

Pneumonic Plague

Pneumonic plague is the most life-threatening form of the disease. Primary pneumonic plague accounts for ~5% of plague cases in the United States. The incubation period for primary pneumonic plague is usually 3–5 days (range, 1–7 days). The onset is most often sudden, with chills, fever, headache, myalgias, weakness, and dizziness. Pulmonary signs, including tachypnea and dyspnea, cough, sputum production, and chest pain, typically arise on the second day of illness and may be accompanied by hemoptysis, increasing respiratory distress, cardiopulmonary insufficiency, and circulatory collapse. In primary plague pneumonia, the sputum is most often watery or mucoid, frothy, and blood-tinged, but it may become frankly bloody. Pulmonary signs in primary pneumonic plague may indicate involvement of a single lobe in the early stage, with rapidly developing segmental consolidation before bronchopneumonic spread to other lobes of the same and opposite lungs (Fig. 60-3). Liquefaction necrosis and cavitation may occur early in areas of consolidation and may or may not leave significant residual scarring.

Secondary plague pneumonia, which occurs in 10–15% of bubonic plague cases in the United States, typically manifests first as diffuse interstitial pneumonitis in which sputum production is scant; because the sputum is more likely to be inspissated and tenacious in character than the sputum found in primary pneumonia, it may be less infectious. In the United States in 1947–2001, 46 cases of secondary pneumonic plague and 8 cases of primary pneumonic plague were described, with no known transmission to contacts and an overall case-fatality rate of 41%.

Plague Meningitis

Meningitis is an unusual manifestation of plague. In the United States, there were 17 meningitis cases among the 409 evaluable plague cases reported during 1947–2005. All cases of meningitis were complications of bubonic plague, and all but three patients survived. Although meningitis may be a part of the initial presentation of plague, its onset is often delayed and is a manifestation of insufficient treatment. Recent cases in the United States have occurred in association with treatment of bubonic plague with tetracyclines, which are bacteriostatic against *Y. pestis*. Chronic relapsing meningeal plague over periods of weeks or even months was described in the preantibiotic era. The affected patients typically present with fever, headache, meningismus, and neutrophilic pleocytosis.

Plague Pharyngitis

Plague pharyngitis presents as fever, sore throat, cervical lymphadenitis, and headache and is often indistinguishable clinically from pharyngitis and tonsillitis of other infectious etiologies, especially streptococcal pharyngitis. Plague pharyngitis can be difficult to distinguish from cervical bubonic plague arising from an infective flea bite on the head and neck region.

LABORATORY FINDINGS AND DIAGNOSIS

A high index of clinical suspicion and a thorough clinical and epidemiologic examination are required for timely diagnosis and treatment. When the diagnosis of plague is delayed or missed, a high case-fatality rate results; infected travelers who seek medical care after they have left endemic areas (peripatetic plague cases) are at especially high risk. When the diagnosis of plague is being considered, close communication between clinicians and the diagnostic laboratory and between the diagnostic laboratory and a qualified reference laboratory is essential. Tests for plague are highly reliable when conducted by laboratory personnel experienced with *Y. pestis*, but such expertise is usually limited to selected reference laboratories, including state health department laboratories in some plague-endemic states and the CDC plague laboratory (Fort Collins, CO; tel. 970-221-6400).

When plague is suspected, specimens should be collected promptly for laboratory studies, chest roentgenograms should be obtained, and specific antimicrobial therapy should be initiated pending confirmation. Appropriate diagnostic specimens for smear and culture include blood from all patients; lymph node aspirates from those with buboes; sputum samples, pharyngeal swabs, and lower respiratory secretions from those with suspected pneumonic plague; and cerebrospinal fluid (CSF) from those with meningeal signs. Since early buboes are often exquisitely tender and are seldom fluctuant or necrotic, they usually require aspiration under local anesthesia after the injection of 1–2 mL of normal saline (sterile but nonbacteriostatic) into the bubo with a 20- to 22-gauge needle. Typically, aspiration produces a scant amount of serosanguineous fluid.

Patients with plague typically have white blood cell (WBC) counts of 10,000–25,000/μL, with a predominance of PMNs and a left shift. Leukemoid reactions, with WBC counts as high as 100,000/μL, can occur. Modest thrombocytopenia is usually present, and fibrin-fibrinogen split products are often detected, even in patients without frank DIC. In plague pneumonia, stained respiratory secretions usually contain PMNs and characteristic bipolar-staining bacilli. In *Y. pestis* septicemia, visualization of the

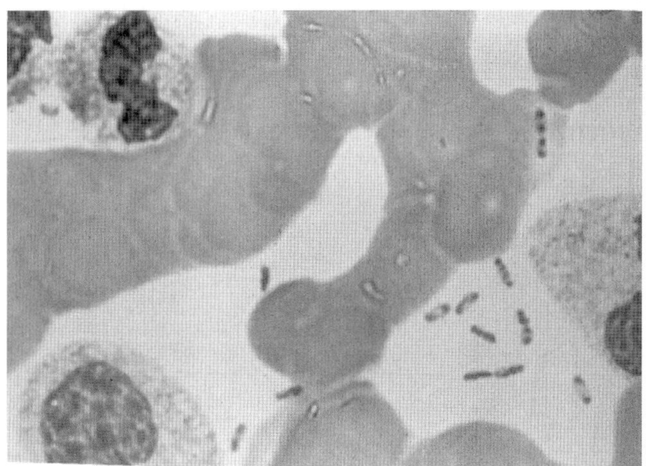

FIGURE 60-4

Peripheral blood smear from a patient with fatal plague septicemia and shock, showing characteristic bipolar-staining *Y. pestis* bacilli (Wright's stain, oil immersion).

characteristic bacilli in a routine blood smear or a buffy-coat smear is an uncommon but grave prognostic sign (Fig. 60-4). In patients with plague meningitis, PMN pleocytosis is typical, and the bacilli are usually visible in stained CSF smears.

A variety of appropriate culture media (including brain-heart infusion broth, sheep blood agar, and MacConkey agar) should be inoculated with a portion of each specimen. Moreover, for each specimen, at least one smear should be examined immediately with Wayson or Giemsa stain and at least one with Gram's stain; a smear should also be submitted to a reference laboratory for direct fluorescent antibody testing, antigen-capture enzyme-linked immunosorbent assay (ELISA), polymerase chain reaction (PCR) analysis, or testing by another rapid detection method (e.g., immunochromatographic hand-held assay). An acute-phase serum specimen should be tested for antibody to *Y. pestis*; whenever possible, a convalescent-phase serum specimen collected 3–4 weeks later should also be tested. When a patient dies and plague is suspected, appropriate autopsy tissues for culture, direct fluorescent antibody testing, and immunohistochemical staining include buboes, all solid organs (especially liver, spleen, and lung), and bone marrow. If culture of such specimens is to be attempted, they should be sent to the laboratory either fresh or frozen on dry ice, not in preservatives or fixatives. If necessary, Cary-Blair or a similar medium can be used to transport *Y. pestis*–infected tissues. Laboratory confirmation of plague depends on the isolation of *Y. pestis* from cultures of body fluids or tissues. Cultures of three blood samples taken over a 45-min period before treatment usually result in isolation of the bacterium. *Y. pestis* strains are readily distinguished from those of the closely related species *Y. pseudotuberculosis* by differences in biochemical profile, temperature-dependent susceptibility to lysis by a *Y. pestis*– specific bacteriophage, and motility. Automated bacteriologic test systems can be used to assist in the identification of isolates as *Y. pestis*, but *Y. pestis* can be misidentified (e.g., as *Y. pseudotuberculosis*) or overlooked if these systems are improperly programmed.

In the absence of *Y. pestis* isolation, plague cases can be confirmed either by the demonstration of seroconversion (a fourfold or greater titer rise) to *Y. pestis* F1 antigen in passive hemagglutination tests of acute- and convalescent-phase serum specimens or by detection of an antibody titer of >128 in a single serum sample from a patient with a plague-compatible illness who has not received plague vaccine. The specificity of a positive passive-hemagglutination test requires confirmation with the F1 antigen hemagglutination-inhibition test. A few plague patients seroconvert to F1 antigen as early as 5 days after the onset of illness; most seroconvert 1–2 weeks after onset; a few seroconvert >3 weeks after onset; and a few (<5%) fail to seroconvert at all. Early, specific antibiotic treatment may delay seroconversion by several weeks. After seroconversion, positive serologic titers diminish gradually over months to years. ELISAs for IgM and IgG antibodies to *Y. pestis* are replacing hemagglutination tests in some laboratories. Other new test methods include those mentioned above: antigen-capture ELISAs, PCR, and immunochromatographic hand-held assays for rapid identification of *Y. pestis* in aspirates, sputum, and other infected body fluids or tissues. The hand-held assays can be used at the bedside in the remote rural settings where most plague cases occur and could prove important in responding to bioterrorism (Chap. 6).

℞ Treatment: PLAGUE

Left untreated, plague is fatal in >50% of bubonic cases and in nearly all septicemic and pneumonic cases. The overall mortality rate for plague cases in the United States since 1950 has been ~14%; deaths are almost always due to delays in seeking treatment, misdiagnosis, delays in the institution of treatment, or incorrect treatment. Rapid diagnosis and appropriate antimicrobial therapy are essential.

Guidelines for the treatment of plague are given in Table 60-1. Although streptomycin is the drug of choice, gentamicin is increasingly used for the treatment of plague in the United States because of its ready availability; it is probably as effective as streptomycin and less toxic. Alternative antibiotics include the tetracyclines and chloramphenicol; these agents are usually given orally with initial loading doses but may be given intravenously to critically ill patients and to patients who cannot tolerate oral medication. Doxycycline is considered the tetracycline of choice. Penicillins, cephalosporins, and macrolides are suboptimal and should not be used. Trimethoprim-sulfamethoxazole (TMP-SMX) has been used successfully to treat bubonic plague but is not considered a first-line agent. Chloramphenicol may be indicated for the treatment of plague meningitis, pleuritis, endophthalmitis, and myocarditis because of its superior tissue penetration; it is used alone or in combination with streptomycin or another first-line agent. In general, antimicrobial treatment should

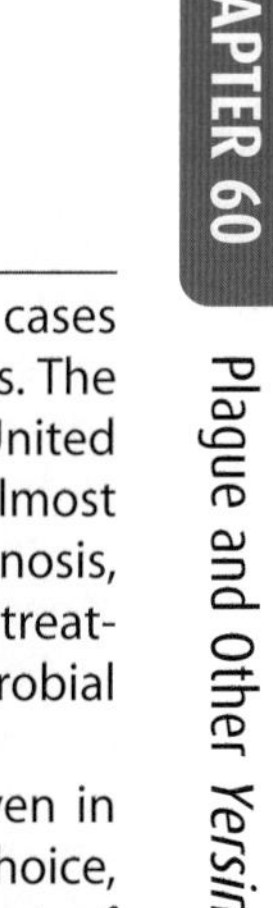

TABLE 60-1

GUIDELINES FOR THE TREATMENT OF PLAGUE

DRUG	DAILY DOSAGE	INTERVAL, h	ROUTE(S) OF ADMINISTRATION
Streptomycin			
Adults	2 g	12	IM
Children	30 mg/kg	12	IM
Gentamicin			
Adults	3–5 mg/kg[a]	8	IM or IV
Children	6.0–7.5 mg/kg	8	IM or IV
Infants/neonates	7.5 mg/kg	8	IM or IV
Tetracycline			
Adults	2 g	6	PO or IV
Children ≥8 y	25–50 mg/kg	6	PO or IV
Doxycycline			
Adults	200 mg	12 or 24	PO or IV
Children ≥8 y	4.4 mg/kg	12 or 24	PO or IV
Chloramphenicol			
Adults	50 mg/kg[b]	6	PO or IV
Children ≥1 y	50 mg/kg[b]	6	PO or IV

[a]Dosage should be reduced to 3 mg/kg daily as soon as clinically indicated.
[b]For meningitis, up to 100 (mg/kg)/d initially.

be continued for 7–10 days or for at least 3 days after the patient has become afebrile and has made a clinical recovery. Patients initially given IV antibiotics may be switched to oral regimens upon clinical improvement. Such improvement is usually evident 2–3 days after the start of treatment, even though fever may continue for several days. National bioterrorism-response protocols propose gentamicin, ciprofloxacin, and doxycycline as antimicrobial agents of first choice for treatment and postexposure prophylaxis in the event of an attack using *Y. pestis* (Chap. 6).

Complications of sepsis require intensive monitoring and close physiologic support, as outlined elsewhere (Chap. 15). Buboes may require surgical drainage. Abscessed nodes can cause recurrent fever in patients who have apparently recovered; the cause may be occult if intrathoracic or intraabdominal nodes are involved. Although *Y. pestis* is considered to be genetically stable, a multidrug-resistant strain was isolated from a plague patient in Madagascar. This strain exhibited resistance (mediated by a transferable plasmid) to principal first-line antibiotics used for treatment and prophylaxis of plague.

PREVENTION AND CONTROL

Persons at greatest risk for plague in the United States are individuals who live, work, and participate in outdoor recreational activities in areas of those western states in which plague is enzootic. Surveillance, education, and environmental management are the cornerstones of prevention and control. Personal protective measures include the avoidance of areas with known epizootic plague (in which warning signs may be posted) and of sick or dead animals; the use of repellents, insecticides, and protective clothing when at risk of exposure to rodents' fleas; and the wearing of gloves when handling animal carcasses. Short-term antibiotic prophylaxis (Table 60-2) is recommended for persons known to have had close contact with a patient with suspected or confirmed pneumonic plague. The recommended duration of postexposure prophylaxis is 5 days. Patients in whom respiratory plague is suspected should be managed under isolation, with use of respiratory-droplet precautions until pneumonia has been ruled out or until 48 h of effective antimicrobial therapy has been administered, after which standard infection-control precautions are adequate. Masks that block droplets are considered to be protective against respiratory transmission of plague and would be expected to be an important tool to prevent secondary plague spread in the event of bioterrorism (Chap. 6).

Rodent food (garbage, pet food) and habitats (brush piles, junk heaps, woodpiles) should be eliminated in residential and occupational environments; buildings and food stores should be rodent-proofed. The control of fleas with insecticides is a key public health measure in situations where epizootic plague activity places humans at high risk; this effort includes dusting and spraying of rodent burrows, rodent runs, and other sites where rodents and their fleas are found. In plague-endemic areas of the western United States, persons should keep their dogs and cats free of fleas and restrained. The decision to control plague by killing rodents should be left to public health authorities, and such a program should be carried out only in conjunction with effective flea control. Killing of rodents has no lasting benefit without environmental sanitation.

The previously used killed, whole-cell plague vaccine is no longer available in the United States. New and

TABLE 60-2

GUIDELINES FOR PLAGUE PROPHYLAXIS

DRUG	DAILY DOSAGE	INTERVAL, h	ROUTE(S) OF ADMINISTRATION
Tetracycline			
Adults	1–2 g	6 or 12	PO
Children ≥8 y	25–50 mg/kg	6 or 12	PO
Doxycycline			
Adults	100–200 mg	12 or 24	PO
Children ≥8 y	2–4 mg/kg	12 or 24	PO
Trimethoprim-sulfamethoxazole			
Adults	320 mg[a]	12	PO
Children ≥2 mo	8 mg/kg[a]	12	PO
Ciprofloxacin[b]			
Adults	1 g	12	PO
Children	40 mg/kg	12	PO

[a]Trimethoprim component.
[b]Recommended as an alternative to doxycycline in bioterrorism-response plans.

improved vaccines that use recombinant F1 and V antigens to induce protective antibodies are undergoing clinical trials. In the United States, the indications for use of these newer vaccines would probably be similar to those for the previously available killed vaccine, which was mostly limited to protecting laboratory personnel who routinely worked with *Y. pestis* and some persons whose vocations brought them into regular contact with wild rodents and their fleas in areas with enzootic or epizootic plague. In addition, a vaccine might be useful in protecting selected persons at risk from biowarfare or bioterrorism.

OTHER *YERSINIA* INFECTIONS

DEFINITION

Yersiniosis is an uncommon bacterial zoonosis caused primarily by infection with either of two enteropathogenic *Yersinia* species: *Y. enterocolitica* or *Y. pseudotuberculosis*. Reservoir hosts of these bacteria include swine and other wild and domestic animals, and transmission to humans is predominantly via the oral route. Both sporadic cases and common-source outbreaks occur. The most frequent acute clinical manifestations are (1) enteritis or enterocolitis with self-limited diarrhea (especially with *Y. enterocolitica*) and (2) mesenteric adenitis and terminal ileitis (especially with *Y. pseudotuberculosis*), which can be confused with acute appendicitis. Septicemia and metastatic focal infections are less common. Yersiniosis can be complicated by nonsuppurative, extraintestinal, inflammatory sequelae—e.g., reactive arthritis and erythema nodosum (Chap. 8). Other nonplague *Yersinia* species, including *Y. intermedia, Y. frederiksenii*, and *Y. kristensenii*, have been associated with enteritis or enterocolitis in humans (particularly immunocompromised adults), but little is known about their pathogenicity, public health importance, or clinical management.

ETIOLOGIC AGENTS

Y. enterocolitica and *Y. pseudotuberculosis* are pleomorphic gram-negative bacilli in the family Enterobacteriaceae. These organisms can multiply within a wide temperature range (–1°C to 45°C). Pathogenic *Y. enterocolitica* isolates are most commonly identified by biotyping based on biochemical profiles and serotyping according to somatic O and H antigens. Six biotypes and >60 serotypes of *Y. enterocolitica* are recognized. A separate serotyping system for *Y. pseudotuberculosis* (also based on somatic antigens) has distinguished six major serotypes (I–VI) and their subtypes.

EPIDEMIOLOGY

Yersinia Enterocolitica

Y. enterocolitica is distributed worldwide and has been isolated from soil, fresh water, contaminated foodstuffs (e.g., meat, milk, and vegetables), and a wide variety of wild and domestic animals. Many serotypes isolated from environmental sources, however, evidently are not human pathogens. Most human infections have been caused by *Y. enterocolitica* serotypes O:3; O:5,27; O:8; and O:9. These serotypes are primarily associated with wild and domestic mammals. The recognized incidence of these infections and their sequelae is highest in Scandinavia and some other northern European countries, but reliable population-based estimates of incidence are unavailable.

All age groups are susceptible to *Y. enterocolitica* infections, but the majority of cases of enterocolitis are in children 1–4 years old. These infections show a modest predilection for males. Mesenteric adenitis and terminal ileitis are most common among older children and young adults. Risk factors for *Y. enterocolitica* septicemia and metastatic focal infections include chronic liver disease, malignancy, diabetes mellitus, immunosuppressive therapy, HIV disease, alcoholism, malnutrition, advanced age, iron overload (see "Pathogenesis and Pathology," below), and hemolytic anemias (including the thalassemias). The nonsuppurative sequelae of yersiniosis are most common among adults. HLA-B27 is expressed in 70–80% of patients who develop reactive arthritis associated with yersiniosis. HLA-B27 is not a risk factor for *Yersinia*-induced erythema nodosum; females with this condition outnumber males by 2 to 1.

Among *Y. enterocolitica* strains isolated from patients in recent decades, serotypes O:3 and O:9 have predominated in Europe, whereas serotype O:3 has predominated in Canada, Japan, and the United States. The apparent incidence of *Yersinia*-induced nonsuppurative sequelae reportedly is 10–30% in Scandinavia and much lower in most other countries, including the United States.

Common-source outbreaks of *Y. enterocolitica* enteritis have been traced to such vehicles as raw milk, contaminated pasteurized milk, and foods prepared with contaminated fresh water. Because *Y. enterocolitica* commonly colonizes the gastrointestinal tracts of swine, sporadic human cases and outbreaks of yersiniosis have also been associated with the preparation or ingestion of raw pork products (e.g., chitterlings). In some cases of yersiniosis, circumstantial evidence suggests transmission via contact with dogs and cats or their feces. Several nosocomial outbreaks of *Y. enterocolitica* infection have been described; fecal-oral transmission from person to person was suspected. Fecal-oral transmission among family members may also explain occasional secondary cases in households. In a prospective study of 50 children with *Y. enterocolitica* enteritis, fecal excretion of the organism persisted for an average of 27 days (range, 4–79 days) after the cessation of symptoms. A chronic carrier state, however, has not been demonstrated. *Y. enterocolitica* is a rare but often lethal cause of transfusion-associated septicemia. The explanation is that blood donors occasionally have transient, occult *Y. enterocolitica* bacteremia and that this organism can slowly multiply to high concentrations in blood refrigerated for at least 10 days.

Yersinia Pseudotuberculosis

The ecology of *Y. pseudotuberculosis* seems to parallel that of *Y. enterocolitica* closely. *Y. pseudotuberculosis* is also widespread in wild and domestic animals and is isolated from many environmental sources. Swine appear to be an important reservoir for pathogenic strains. Although human infections appear to be relatively rare, large common-source epidemics can occur.

PATHOGENESIS AND PATHOLOGY

With rare exceptions (e.g., transmission via contaminated blood products or direct cutaneous inoculation), the enteropathogenic yersiniae are thought to enter the host via the oral route. The incubation period averages 5 days (range, 1–11 days). Studies of animals have shown that the organisms initially invade the ileal epithelium, then are translocated via M cells into the lamina propria, and finally enter Peyer's patches, where they replicate. They subsequently drain into the mesenteric lymph nodes, which undergo hyperplasia and from which the bacteria can be disseminated. The mesenteric lymph nodes can become intensely swollen and matted and are occasionally detected on physical examination as a tender right-lower-quadrant mass. Intestinal inflammation (most commonly of the distal ileum and less commonly of the ascending colon) develops and may be accompanied by mucosal ulcerations and by the shedding of PMNs and red blood cells into the intestinal lumen. In relatively severe cases, thrombosis of mesenteric blood vessels, intestinal hemorrhage, and necrosis can occur. In patients with enteropathogenic yersinial infections who undergo exploratory laparotomy, the appendix usually is histologically normal or shows only lymphoid hyperplasia, but frank suppuration is sometimes evident.

A plasmid of ~70 kb is essential for virulence of the enteropathogenic yersiniae because it encodes at least six *Yersinia* outer-membrane proteins, which confer a variety of pathogenic properties—e.g., cytotoxicity; resistance to phagocytosis by PMNs; and the ability to cause monocyte apoptosis (programmed cell death), to suppress the host's expression of tumor necrosis factor α, and to interfere with platelet aggregation and host complement activation. A chromosomal gene (*inv*) encodes for the surface protein invasin, which is necessary for yersinial invasion of nonphagocytic host cells (e.g., epithelial cells) in vitro and which facilitates the translocation of bacteria across the intestinal epithelium. Both *Y. enterocolitica* and *Y. pseudotuberculosis* can express at least one protein superantigen that selectively stimulates the proliferation of T cells. Many strains of *Y. enterocolitica* produce a heat-stable enterotoxin that is similar to *Escherichia coli* enterotoxin. The cell walls of *Y. enterocolitica* and *Y. pseudotuberculosis* contain a lipopolysaccharide (endotoxin). Some *Yersinia* strains are unable to synthesize bacterial iron chelators called *siderophores*. However, they can exploit host-chelated iron stores and the drug deferoxamine (a siderophore produced by *Streptomyces pilosus*). Therefore, iron overload (e.g., caused by hemodialysis or multiple transfusions) and deferoxamine therapy appear to be independent risk factors for *Y. enterocolitica* bacteremia, especially that involving serotypes O:3 and O:9, and to a lesser degree for *Y. pseudotuberculosis* bacteremia.

Immunogenetic factors and cell-mediated immune responses are clearly involved in the pathogenesis of reactive arthritis after infection with the enteropathogenic yersiniae. As noted above, most patients with *Yersinia*-induced reactive arthritis express HLA-B27. In addition, *Y. pseudotuberculosis* shares at least one cross-reactive epitope with HLA-B27, and *Y. enterocolitica* infection alters the expression of serologic HLA-B27 epitopes on lymphocytes and monocytes. In patients with reactive arthritis after *Y. enterocolitica* infection, yersinial antigens are commonly detectable in synovial fluid cells in the apparent absence of whole organisms. Thus it is unknown whether the arthritis results from occult bacterial persistence through self-tolerance of HLA-B27 with a failure of cross-reactive immune responses to yersiniae, from an immune response to common antigenic determinants shared by the bacteria and host HLA-B27 (i.e., molecular mimicry), or from other mechanisms. The pathogenesis of *Yersinia*-induced erythema nodosum is obscure.

In some assays, patients with Graves' disease have an increased prevalence of serum antibodies to *Y. enterocolitica*, and the immunoglobulins of patients recovering from *Y. enterocolitica* infections react with the human thyroid-stimulating hormone receptor. However, a link between *Y. enterocolitica* infection and the subsequent development of autoimmune thyroiditis has not been convincingly demonstrated. Similarly, the hypothesis that the nonplague yersinioses can trigger ulcerative colitis or Crohn's disease remains intriguing but unproven.

CLINICAL MANIFESTATIONS

Yersinia Enterocolitica

The principal clinical manifestations of *Y. enterocolitica* infection are enteritis, enterocolitis, mesenteric adenitis, and terminal ileitis. Less common manifestations include exudative pharyngitis, septicemia, metastatic focal infections, reactive polyarthritis, and erythema nodosum. When age groups are combined, the most common presentation of *Y. enterocolitica* infection is acute diarrhea from enteritis or enterocolitis. Low-grade fever and cramping abdominal pain occur in most cases, nausea and vomiting in 15–40%, hematochezia in up to 30%, and a generalized maculopapular skin rash in a few cases. Diarrhea persists for an average of 2 weeks (range, 1 day to many months), during which the frequency of bowel movements diminishes. Uncommonly, enteritis or enterocolitis can be complicated by severe abdominal pain and high fever. Rare (and sometimes fatal) complications include diffuse inflammation, ulceration, hemorrhage, and necrosis of the small bowel and colon; intestinal perforation; peritonitis; ascending cholangitis; mesenteric vein thrombosis; diverticulitis; toxic megacolon; and ileocecal intussusception.

The syndrome of mesenteric adenitis and terminal ileitis without diarrhea is easily confused with appendicitis. Low-grade fever and right-lower-quadrant pain, tenderness, guarding, and rebound tenderness are common. During six recognized common-source outbreaks in the United States, 10% of 444 patients with symptomatic undiagnosed *Y. enterocolitica* infections underwent laparotomy for suspected appendicitis; surgical incisions became infected with *Y. enterocolitica* in a few of these cases.

Acute pharyngitis and pharyngotonsillitis, with or without cervical adenitis or intestinal illness, are less common but potentially lethal manifestations of *Y. enterocolitica* infection, particularly in adults. *Y. enterocolitica* septicemia generally presents as a severe illness with fever and leukocytosis, often with abdominal pain and jaundice and without localized signs of infection. Metastatic focal *Y. enterocolitica* infections can occur with or without clinically apparent bacteremia and can affect almost any organ system. Examples include abscess formation (e.g., in liver, spleen, kidney, lung, skeletal muscle, lymph node, or cutaneous tissue), osteomyelitis, meningitis, peritonitis, urinary tract infection, pneumonia, empyema, endocarditis, pericarditis, mycotic aneurysm, septic arthritis, suppurative conjunctivitis, panophthalmitis, Parinaud's oculoglandular syndrome, and cutaneous pustules or bullae.

In Scandinavia, the incidence of reactive arthritis after *Y. enterocolitica* infection among adults is estimated to be at least 10%. About 80% of these patients have prior symptoms such as fever, diarrhea, or abdominal pain. Typically, these symptoms precede the arthritis by 1 week and are of short duration. The most commonly affected joints are the knees and ankles, but other joints can be involved. Typically, multiple (two to eight) joints become involved sequentially and asymmetrically over a period of a few days to 2 weeks, after which no additional joints are affected. Monarticular arthritis occurs less commonly. In two-thirds of cases, the acute arthritis remits spontaneously within 1–3 months. Chronic joint disease is documented in a minority of cases. A few HLA-B27-positive patients with *Y. enterocolitica*–induced arthritis have subsequent ankylosing spondylitis, but this development is best explained by the fact that HLA-B27 is a major risk factor for each of these diseases. Mild, self-limited myocarditis accompanies ~10% of cases of *Yersinia*-induced arthritis and can occur independently. Typical manifestations include cardiac murmurs and transient electrocardiographic abnormalities, such as prolongation of the PR interval and nonspecific ST-segment and T-wave changes. The syndrome of *Yersinia*-induced arthritis and carditis can be confused with acute rheumatic fever. In Scandinavia, erythema nodosum occurs in 15–20% of patients with yersiniosis, usually within a few days to 3 weeks after the onset of intestinal illness. Lesions typically are located on the lower extremities and resolve within 1 month. Less commonly reported nonsuppurative sequelae of *Y. enterocolitica* infections include reactive uveitis, iritis, conjunctivitis, urethritis, and glomerulonephritis. The complete triad of Reiter's syndrome (arthritis, conjunctivitis, and urethritis) is seen in 5–10% of patients with *Yersinia*-induced arthritis.

Yersinia Pseudotuberculosis

The most common clinical presentation of *Y. pseudotuberculosis* infection is fever and abdominal pain caused by mesenteric adenitis; diarrheal illness is less common than in *Y. enterocolitica* infection. Systemic manifestations, including septicemia, focal infections, reactive arthritis, and erythema nodosum, are generally similar to those associated with *Y. enterocolitica* infection. In addition, *Y. pseudotuberculosis* has been associated with a scarlet fever–like syndrome, acute interstitial nephritis, and hemolytic-uremic syndrome.

LABORATORY FINDINGS AND DIAGNOSIS

Results of routine laboratory tests in most patients with yersiniosis are nonspecific. Leukocyte counts are usually normal or slightly elevated, often with a modest left shift. Standard microbiologic methods are sufficient to isolate *Y. enterocolitica* and *Y. pseudotuberculosis* from otherwise-sterile sites, such as blood, CSF, lymph node tissue, and peritoneal fluid, and from abscesses. Isolation of these organisms from feces is impeded by their slow growth and the overgrowth of normal fecal flora on culture media routinely used to select for enteric bacteria. The yield from feces and other grossly contaminated specimens can be increased by the use of *Yersinia*-selective [e.g., cefsulodin-Irgasan-novobiocin (CIN)] agar and by cold enrichment. Because bacteriologic procedures designed to isolate yersiniae from feces are not considered cost-effective, many laboratories undertake them by special request only.

The results of serologic tests can be used to support a diagnosis of yersiniosis. Agglutination tests or ELISAs are used most commonly; immunoblotting has also been used. The existence of multiple serotypes makes routine serologic tests laborious; thus these tests are generally conducted only in research laboratories or large commercial laboratories. Since these tests are experimental and are neither standardized nor well validated, and since some strains of *Yersinia* cross-react with other bacteria (e.g., *Brucella*, *Salmonella*, *Vibrio*, and *Borrelia*) and with serum from some patients with thyroiditis, results should be interpreted with caution. In typical uncomplicated cases of yersiniosis, agglutinin titers begin to rise within the first week of illness, peak in the second week, and then gradually diminish and return to normal within 3–6 months, although agglutinating antibody may remain detectable for several years in some cases. Because an initial serum specimen is often collected ≥1 week after the onset of illness, when agglutinin titers are already high, it is usually impossible to document a fourfold or greater rise in titer between paired specimens (although a fourfold or greater fall in titer may be found). Immunohistochemical techniques and PCR tests to detect yersinial antigens and DNA, respectively, in clinical specimens are experimental at this time.

In patients with *Yersinia*-induced reactive arthritis, synovial fluid is sterile and the leukocyte count ranges from a few hundred to 60,000/μL, with a majority of PMNs. The erythrocyte sedimentation rate is often >100 mm/h. Rheumatoid factor and antinuclear antibodies are usually absent. The diagnosis of *Yersinia*-induced reactive arthritis or other nonsuppurative inflammatory sequelae can be difficult, especially when triggering infections are asymptomatic or clinically mild or occur several weeks before the diagnosis is attempted. Because the isolation of a pathogenic *Yersinia* strain from feces is the most specific diagnostic test in such cases, it should be attempted. Since culture is of limited sensitivity in this clinical setting, a high index of suspicion and positive results of serologic tests for *Y. enterocolitica* or *Y. pseudotuberculosis* are usually required for diagnosis.

℞ Treatment: OTHER *YERSINIA* INFECTIONS

The effectiveness of antimicrobial agents in the treatment of yersinial enteritis, enterocolitis, mesenteric adenitis, or terminal ileitis has not been established. These conditions are usually self-limited, and their treatment is symptom-based and supportive. In uncomplicated cases, diarrhea should be treated with fluid and electrolyte replacement, with the route of delivery dependent on clinical severity. Enteric precautions are advisable for patients hospitalized with yersinial diarrhea. In general, antimicrobial treatment should be reserved for patients with septicemia, metastatic focal infections, or immunosuppression and enterocolitis. Controlled clinical comparisons of antimicrobial agents in the treatment of severe cases of yersiniosis have not yet been conducted. In such cases, drug selection should ultimately be guided by clinical response and bacterial sensitivity patterns. Clinical isolates of *Y. enterocolitica* and *Y. pseudotuberculosis* are usually susceptible in vitro to aminoglycosides, third-generation cephalosporins, chloramphenicol, quinolones, tetracyclines, and TMP-SMX. In laboratory animals infected with enteropathogenic yersiniae, the fluoroquinolones have exerted the strongest bactericidal effects in vivo; clinical experience with these drugs against these pathogens in humans is promising but limited. Because they produce β-lactamases, isolates typically are resistant to penicillin, ampicillin, carbenicillin, and first-generation and most second-generation cephalosporins. Optimal dosages and durations of therapy have not been established. Mortality rates from *Y. enterocolitica* septicemia are ~10% despite treatment. Focal extraintestinal infections may require at least 3 weeks of therapy. No role for antimicrobial agents in the management of the nonsuppurative inflammatory manifestations of yersiniosis has been established. Patients with reactive arthritis may benefit from treatment with nonsteroidal anti-inflammatory drugs, intraarticular steroid injections, and physical therapy.

PREVENTION AND CONTROL

The importance of safe food-handling and food-preparation practices in the prevention of yersiniosis cannot be overemphasized. Caution is particularly warranted in the case of pork and other animal products. The consumption of raw or undercooked meats, especially pork, should be avoided. Increased efforts to prevent the spread of enteric pathogens in household, pet-care, day-care, and hospital settings and in the food industry would be likely to decrease the incidence of yersiniosis. Current regulations of the U.S. Food and Drug Administration require visual inspection of packed red cell units before transfusion, with the discarding of units in which bacterial contamination is suspected on the basis of darkening (reflecting decreased oxygen saturation and hemolysis). Since the risk is minimal, more specific measures to further decrease the likelihood of transfusion of *Y. enterocolitica*–contaminated blood products (e.g., limiting the period for which red cells can be stored before transfusion) have not been widely implemented.

Yersiniosis is not routinely reportable to public health authorities in most jurisdictions. However, clinicians who suspect a common-source outbreak (e.g., because they have documented a familial case cluster) or some other public health threat (e.g., because they have found *Y. enterocolitica* bacteremia in a recent blood donor) should consult promptly with local public health officials.

FURTHER READINGS

ABDEL-HAQ NM et al: Antibiotic susceptibilities of *Yersinia enterocolitica* recovered from children over a 12-year period. Int J Antimicrob Agents 27:449, 2006

DAS R et al: Study of proinflammatory responses induced by *Yersinia pestis* in human monocytes using cDNA arrays. Genes Immun 8:308, 2007

EISEN RJ et al: Human plague in the southwestern United States, 1957–2004: Spatial models of elevated risk of human exposure to *Yersinia pestis*. J Med Entomol 44:530, 2007

GRAHEK-OGDEN D: Outbreak of *Yersinia enterocolitica* serogroup O:9 infection and processed pork, Norway. Emerg Infect Dis 13:754, 2007

PERDIKOGIANNI C et al: *Yersinia enterocolitica* infection mimicking surgical conditions. Pediatr Surg Int 22:589, 2006

PRENTICE MB, RAHALISON L: Plague. Lancet 369:1196, 2007

CHAPTER 61

BARTONELLA INFECTIONS, INCLUDING CAT-SCRATCH DISEASE

David H. Spach ■ Emily Darby

Bartonella species are gram-negative bacteria that can cause an array of infectious diseases, including cat-scratch disease (CSD), bacillary angiomatosis, bacteremia, culture-negative endocarditis, trench fever, and bartonellosis (Table 61-1). Three *Bartonella* species play a major role in causing human disease: *B. bacilliformis*, *B. quintana*, and *B. henselae*. Recent advances in molecular diagnostics have expanded the list of diseases known to be caused by *Bartonella* species.

CAT-SCRATCH DISEASE

DEFINITION AND ETIOLOGY

CSD is typically a self-limited illness characterized by regional lymphadenopathy lasting weeks to months. *B. henselae* is the primary causative agent. Infrequently, patients with CSD develop disseminated *B. henselae* infection.

EPIDEMIOLOGY

CSD has a global distribution. In the United States, the annual incidence is ~4–9 cases per 100,000 persons, with ~40% of cases involving adults. Cats are the primary host for *B. henselae* and transmit the infection to humans via a scratch, bite, or lick. In cats (particularly kittens), the incidence of asymptomatic *B. henselae* bacteremia is high. The cat flea (*Ctenocephalides felis*) serves as the vector for transmission between animals. Rarely, CSD occurs after exposure to dogs.

CLINICAL PRESENTATION

The initial clinical manifestation—the primary inoculation lesion—consists of a 0.5- to 1-cm papule, vesicle, or nodule that appears at the site where *B. henselae* is introduced and persists for ~1–3 weeks. Adenopathy typically develops 2–3 weeks after the initial scratch or bite (range, 3–50 days). Unilateral solitary or regional lymphadenopathy (Fig. 61-1) occurs in more than 90% of patients; its location corresponds with the route of lymphatic drainage. Lymph nodes are tender, firm, and mobile, and ~10% suppurate; overlying erythema is occasionally present. Nonspecific systemic symptoms, such as fever, anorexia, headache, myalgias, malaise, and abdominal pain, are variably present at this stage. Lymphadenopathy usually resolves within 3 months.

Atypical presentations of CSD are described in up to one-quarter of cases. Parinaud's oculoglandular syndrome is a frequently reported atypical presentation that follows inoculation of bacteria onto the conjunctiva or eyelid. Patients develop unilateral manifestations that may include conjunctivitis, granulomatous lesions, and preauricular lymphadenopathy. Systemic spread of *B. henselae* may occur independent of lymphadenopathy or may follow the more typical manifestations of the disease. Disseminated disease most often involves the nervous system, visceral organs, or bone. Patients with neuroretinitis generally present with sudden, painless loss of vision. Most ocular abnormalities caused by CSD usually resolve within several months without residual damage; however, some patients have long-lasting visual deficits. Other rare complications include encephalitis, peripheral nerve abnormalities, myelitis, facial palsy, and granulomatous hepatitis or splenitis.

TABLE 61-1

MAJOR DISEASES CAUSED BY *BARTONELLA* SPECIES

DISEASE	ORGANISM	RISK FACTOR
Cat-scratch disease	*B. henselae*	Cat scratch or bite
Bacillary angiomatosis	*B. quintana, B. henselae*	Cat scratch or bite
Bacillary peliosis	*B. henselae*	Cat scratch or bite
Trench fever	*B. quintana*	Homelessness, body louse infestation, alcoholism
Endocarditis	*B. quintana, B. henselae, B. elizabethae*	As for cat-scratch disease and trench fever
Bartonellosis	*B. bacilliformis*	Sandfly bite

PATHOLOGY

Early in the course of CSD, histologic examination of lymph nodes reveals follicular hyperplasia and arteriolar proliferation. Cortical granulomas, with occasional multinucleated giant cells, neutrophilic infiltrates, and coalescing microabscesses (stellate microabscesses), appear within weeks; the granulomas are surrounded by histiocytes and peripheral lymphocytes. Warthin-Starry stain may reveal typical clusters of pleomorphic gram-negative organisms within areas of necrosis, blood vessel walls, or erythrocytes.

DIAGNOSIS

A suspected diagnosis of CSD is usually based on a typical clinical presentation in conjunction with a history of recent cat exposure. Results of routine laboratory studies are generally normal. The differential diagnosis most often includes lymphoma, mycobacterial infection, and soft tissue infection caused by methicillin-resistant *Staphylococcus aureus*. Not only can CSD overlap clinically with lymphoma and mycobacterial infection; it can also occur in

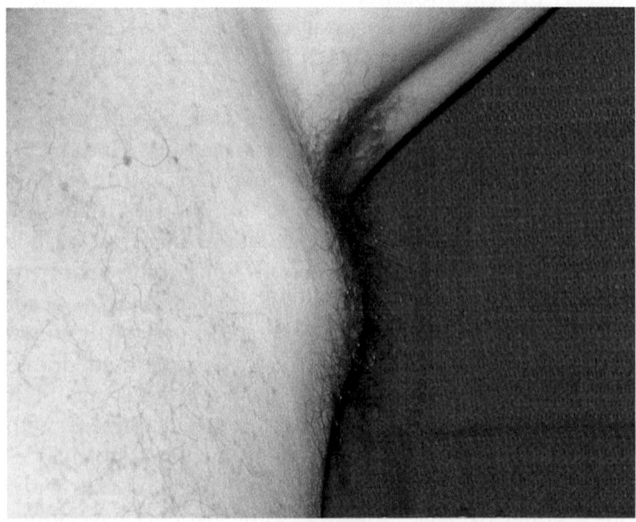

FIGURE 61-1

Characteristic regional (axillary) lymphadenopathy in a patient with cat-scratch disease.

TABLE 61-2

TREATMENT OF ADULTS WITH DISEASE CAUSED BY *BARTONELLA* SPECIES[a]

DISEASE	TREATMENT
Cat-scratch disease	
Lymphadenopathy	Consider azithromycin (500 mg PO on day 1, then 250 mg PO qd for 4 days)
Retinitis	Doxycycline (100 mg PO bid for 4–6 weeks) *plus* Rifampin (300 mg PO bid for 4–6 weeks)
Bacillary angiomatosis	Erythromycin (500 mg PO qid for 3 months) *or* Doxycycline (100 mg PO bid for 3 months)
Bacillary peliosis	Erythromycin (500 mg PO qid for 4 months) *or* Doxycycline (100 mg PO bid for 4 months)
Bartonella endocarditis	
Suspected	Gentamicin (3 mg/kg qd IV for 14 days) *plus* ceftriaxone (2 g IV qd for 6 weeks) *with or without* Doxycycline (100 mg PO bid for 6 weeks)
Confirmed	Gentamicin (3 mg/kg qd IV for 14 days) *plus* Doxycycline (100 mg PO bid for 6 weeks)
Trench fever	Doxycycline (200 mg PO qd for 4 weeks) *plus* Gentamicin (3 mg/kg qd IV for 14 days)
Bartonellosis	
Oroya fever	Chloramphenicol (500 mg PO or IV qid for 14 days) *plus* a β-lactam agent *or* Ciprofloxacin (500 mg bid for 10 days)
Verruga peruana	Rifampin (10 mg/kg qd PO for 14 days) *or* Streptomycin (15–20 mg/kg qd IM for 10 days)

[a]Based on recommendations from Rolain et al, 2004.

conjunction with these diseases. Serologic tests for antibody to *B. henselae* can support the clinical diagnosis but do not have optimal sensitivity and specificity. Accordingly, in most instances, lymph node biopsy or aspiration is required to rule out other diseases and establish the diagnosis. In this situation, polymerase chain reaction (PCR) analysis of the tissue sample is generally preferred. Cultures of lymph node tissue are rarely positive.

℞ Treatment: CAT-SCRATCH DISEASE

(Table 61-2) In most cases of typical CSD, illness eventually resolves without therapy. Studies of antimicrobial treatment for CSD in immunocompetent patients have demonstrated only modest benefit. Some experts advocate reassurance and supportive care for management of lymphadenopathy in immunocompetent patients, whereas others recommend treatment with azithromycin to expedite resolution of lymphadenopathy. Antimicrobial therapy is uniformly recommended for immunosuppressed patients with CSD. Most clinicians treat atypical manifestations of CSD, but there are few data to guide the management of atypical disease.

BARTONELLA INFECTIONS IN HIV-INFECTED PERSONS

B. henselae and *B. quintana* can cause a broad spectrum of disease in HIV-infected individuals, including bacillary angiomatosis, peliosis hepatis, osteomyelitis, unexplained fever, bacteremia, and endocarditis. Bacillary angiomatosis is the most common of these manifestations (Chap. 90). Regardless of the manifestations, serologic tests may help support the diagnosis. (See below for a full discussion of all these specific conditions.)

℞ Treatment: *BARTONELLA* INFECTIONS IN HIV-INFECTED PERSONS

As detailed in the next section, antibiotic therapy (Table 61-2) is strongly recommended for all HIV-infected patients with *Bartonella* infections. Indeed, visceral disease may be progressive and fatal without appropriate antibiotic therapy. Relapses of *Bartonella* infections in HIV-infected persons are common, particularly after relatively short antibiotic courses.

BACILLARY ANGIOMATOSIS AND PELIOSIS HEPATIS

ETIOLOGY AND EPIDEMIOLOGY

Bacillary angiomatosis and peliosis hepatis occur primarily in HIV-infected persons whose CD4+ T-cell counts are <100/μL. Earlier studies suggested that ~1 in 1000 HIV-infected persons developed bacillary angiomatosis; however, this incidence has declined in recent years, probably as a result of effective antiretroviral therapy and the consequent decrease in the number of patients with advanced immunodeficiency. Cutaneous bacillary angiomatosis is caused by *B. henselae* or *B. quintana*, subcutaneous nodules and lytic bone predominantly by *B. quintana*, and bacillary peliosis by *B. henselae*. Risk factors for *B. henselae* infection consist of contact with cats or fleas, whereas *B. quintana* infections are associated with low income, homelessness, and louse infestation.

CLINICAL PRESENTATION

Patients with bacillary angiomatosis most often present with painless cutaneous lesions, but other manifestations include subcutaneous masses or nodules (Fig. 61-2), superficial ulcerated plaques, and verrucous growths. The cutaneous lesions may be single or multiple and may vary in color from tan to red to deep purple. The differential diagnosis of cutaneous bacillary angiomatosis includes Kaposi's sarcoma, pyogenic granuloma, and subcutaneous tumors. Painful osseous lesions may develop beneath the cutaneous lesions. Bacillary angiomatosis may rarely involve the oropharynx, lungs, heart, intestines, lymph nodes, muscle, or brain. Patients with bacillary peliosis usually present with nonspecific systemic symptoms, with or without cutaneous involvement. Radiographic studies of osseous bacillary angiomatosis typically demonstrate lytic bone lesions on plain films and focal uptake of technetium on bone scans. Imaging of patients with peliosis hepatis generally reveals hypodense regions in the liver. In patients with advanced immunodeficiency, *B. henselae* and *B. quintana* can cause unexplained fever. In addition, *B. henselae* or *B. quintana* is occasionally identified as the cause of endocarditis in HIV-infected persons.

PATHOLOGY

Histologic examination of bacillary angiomatosis lesions demonstrates lobular proliferation of blood vessels lined by enlarged endothelial cells with a mixed infiltrate of

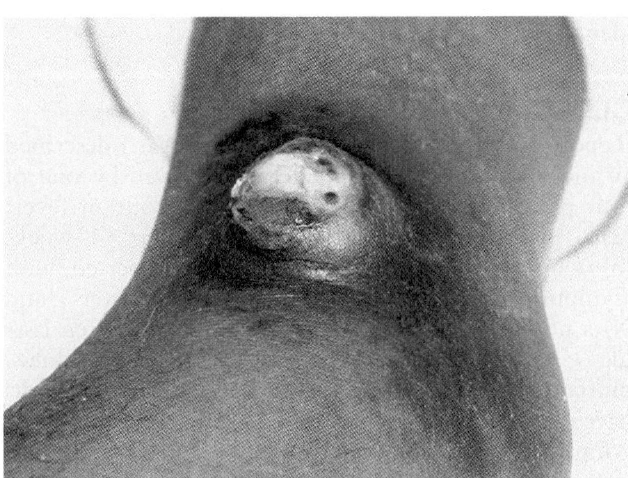

FIGURE 61-2
Nodular lesion of bacillary angiomatosis with superficial ulceration in an AIDS patient with advanced immunodeficiency.

neutrophils and lymphocytes. Examination of bacillary peliosis tissue reveals small blood-filled cystic lesions partially lined by endothelial cells and generally surrounded by a fibromyxoid stroma containing a mixture of inflammatory cells, dilated capillaries, and clumps of granular material. Warthin-Starry stain may reveal bacilli.

DIAGNOSIS

The diagnosis of bacillary angiomatosis is ideally based on histologic findings (see "Pathology" earlier in the chapter).

Rx Treatment: BACILLARY ANGIOMATOSIS AND PELIOSIS HEPATIS

(Table 61-2) As stated above, prolonged therapy with oral erythromycin or doxycycline is recommended for both bacillary angiomatosis and peliosis hepatis.

TRENCH FEVER

DEFINITION AND ETIOLOGY

Trench fever, a febrile illness caused by *B. quintana*, was initially described in World War I, during which the disease developed in an estimated 1 million soldiers on the western and eastern European fronts. In modern times, *B. quintana* infection has resurfaced as "urban trench fever."

EPIDEMIOLOGY

Available data suggest that *B. quintana* has a global distribution, and cases of trench fever have now been reported sporadically throughout the world. Risk factors associated with urban trench fever include poverty, homelessness, and alcoholism. Multiple studies have established the body louse as the principal vector for transmitting *B. quintana* to humans. No animal reservoirs have been identified.

CLINICAL PRESENTATION

Reports of classic trench fever in World War I described an incubation period of 5–20 days followed by one of four patterns of illness: (1) a solitary episode of fever; (2) a brief febrile period typically lasting <1 week; (3) febrile episodes lasting ~5 days interspersed with asymptomatic intervals of ~5 days ("quintan fever"); and (4) a persistent and debilitating febrile illness, often lasting >1 month. Despite the seriousness of the illness, mortality rates are low. In modern-day cases, patients have presented with nonspecific and inconsistent clinical symptoms that have included fever, headache, weight loss, and leg pain. Many patients in contemporary case series have been diagnosed with chronic bacteremia (often asymptomatic), and occasional patients have been diagnosed with culture-negative endocarditis (see below).

DIAGNOSIS

The diagnosis of urban trench fever is most often made on the basis of serologic studies or by isolating *B. quintana* from blood cultures. In patients with endocarditis who require valve replacement surgery, PCR testing of valve tissue can establish the diagnosis.

Rx Treatment: TRENCH FEVER

(Table 61-2) Relatively few data exist regarding optimal therapy for urban trench fever. Mild cases can be treated with doxycycline. However, patients with bacteremia should receive both doxycycline and gentamicin, mainly to prevent the development of endocarditis. Patients with documented endocarditis also should receive doxycycline plus gentamicin.

ENDOCARDITIS

DEFINITION AND ETIOLOGY

Bartonella species have now been established as an important cause of "culture-negative" endocarditis. Although reports have identified five *Bartonella* species as causes of infective endocarditis in humans, >95% of cases have involved either *B. quintana* or *B. henselae*.

EPIDEMIOLOGY

Sporadic cases of *Bartonella*-associated endocarditis have been reported in multiple regions of the world. Most cases have involved adults, and most have affected native heart valves. Identified risk factors for *B. quintana* endocarditis consist of homelessness and infestation with body lice, whereas exposure to cats and previous valvular heart disease are associated with *B. henselae* endocarditis.

CLINICAL PRESENTATION

Clinical findings in *Bartonella* endocarditis resemble the typical findings in subacute bacterial endocarditis. Because blood cultures usually have no evident growth in the first 7–10 days, *Bartonella* endocarditis often is initially diagnosed as culture-negative endocarditis.

DIAGNOSIS

The diagnosis of endocarditis is based on clinical, laboratory, and echocardiographic findings. The identification of *Bartonella* as the specific pathogen causing endocarditis can prove challenging, especially since only ~25% of patients with *Bartonella* endocarditis have *Bartonella* isolated from blood cultures. The yield of blood cultures is enhanced by extended incubation (for 4–6 weeks). In patients from whose blood cultures *Bartonella* is not isolated, the diagnosis is usually based on either a strongly positive serologic test or evidence (most often obtained with a PCR-based method) of *Bartonella* in cardiac valve tissue.

℞ Treatment: ENDOCARDITIS

(Table 61-2) For "culture-negative" endocarditis in which *Bartonella* is the suspected cause, empirical treatment consists of ceftriaxone plus gentamicin, with or without doxycycline. For confirmed *Bartonella* endocarditis, treatment consists of doxycycline plus gentamicin. If gentamicin cannot be used, rifampin should be considered as a substitute.

BARTONELLOSIS (CARRIÓN'S DISEASE)

DEFINITION AND ETIOLOGY

Bartonellosis, or Carrión's disease, is caused by *B. bacilliformis*. The disease is characterized by two distinct phases: (1) an acute febrile hematic phase, known as Oroya fever; and (2) an eruptive phase manifested by cutaneous lesions, known as verruga peruana. In 1885, Daniel Carrión, a Peruvian medical student, established the common source of the two phases of this illness by inoculating himself with material from a verruga peruana lesion and subsequently developing fatal Oroya fever.

EPIDEMIOLOGY

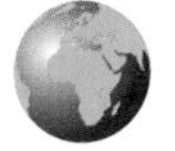

Bartonellosis occurs endemically in certain regions of South America. It has been reported predominantly in river valleys of the Andes Mountains in Peru as well as in some localized regions of Colombia and Ecuador. The sandfly *Lutzomyia verrucarum* serves as the vector for *B. bacilliformis* and transmits the organism to humans via a bite on the skin. Most patients with acute bartonellosis are immunologically naïve, and most cases involve tourists and transient workers. In contrast, the eruptive phase of bartonellosis most often occurs among the native population in the Andes.

CLINICAL PRESENTATION

The clinical manifestations of acute bartonellosis typically begin ~3 weeks after inoculation of *B. bacilliformis* and include fever, malaise, changes in mental status, hepatomegaly, lymphadenopathy, and profound macrocytic anemia. Patients are typically bacteremic with *B. bacilliformis* at this phase. Without antimicrobial therapy, the mortality rate exceeds 40%; infections with other pathogens and noninfectious complications contribute to this high mortality rate. Treatment with chloramphenicol during the acute phase decreases, but does not eliminate, the risk of developing eruptive bartonellosis. Only ~5% of persons with eruptive cutaneous verrugas recall having experienced an acute febrile illness in the preceding 3 months. The cutaneous verrugas typically manifest as reddish-purple pruritic papules or nodules and may resemble the cutaneous lesions of bacillary angiomatosis. Untreated, the lesions can persist for years.

DIAGNOSIS

The diagnosis of acute bartonellosis can reliably be made by detection of intraerythrocytic organisms in a Wright-Giemsa-stained thin blood smear. In addition, most patients have positive blood cultures, but 2–3 weeks are typically required for the organism's isolation. For patients with cutaneous verrugas in the eruptive phase, biopsy should be performed. Histopathologic examination characteristically shows intense proliferation of newly formed capillaries and marked endothelial hyperplasia. The yield of blood smear and blood culture is markedly lower among patients in the eruptive phase. The utility of serologic tests is high for patients in both phases.

℞ Treatment: BARTONELLOSIS

(Table 61-2) Use of chloramphenicol plus a second antimicrobial agent (generally a β-lactam) is generally recommended to provide effective treatment of *B. bacilliformis* and to cover any likely concomitant secondary bacterial infection. Treatment with ciprofloxacin, streptomycin, tetracycline, and erythromycin is also effective. Rifampin or streptomycin should be used to treat chronic bartonellosis.

FURTHER READINGS

Eremeeva ME et al: Bacteremia, fever, and splenomegaly caused by a newly recognized *Bartonella* species. N Engl J Med 356:2381, 2007

Florin TA et al: Beyond cat scratch disease: Widening spectrum of *Bartonella henselae* infection. Pediatrics 121:e1413, 2008

Foucault C et al: *Bartonella quintana* characteristics and clinical management. Emerg Infect Dis 12:217, 2006

Hansmann Y et al: Diagnosis of cat scratch disease with detection of *Bartonella henselae* by PCR: A study of patients with lymph node enlargement. J Clin Microbiol 43:3800, 2005

Houpikian P, Raoult D: Blood culture–negative endocarditis in a reference center: Etiologic diagnosis of 348 cases. Medicine (Baltimore) 84:162, 2005

Maguina C et al: Bartonellosis (Carrión's disease) in the modern era. Clin Infect Dis 33:772, 2001

Mohle-Boetani JC et al: Bacillary angiomatosis and bacillary peliosis in patients infected with human immunodeficiency virus: Clinical characteristics in a case-control study. Clin Infect Dis 22:794, 1996

Ohl ME, Spach DH: *Bartonella quintana* and urban trench fever. Clin Infect Dis 31:131, 2000

Rolain JM et al: Lymph node biopsy specimens and diagnosis of cat scratch disease. Emerg Infect Dis 12:1338, 2006

Rolain JM et al: Recommendations for treatment of human infections caused by *Bartonella* species. Antimicrob Agents Chemother 48:1921, 2004

Spach DH, Koehler JE: *Bartonella*-associated infections. Infect Dis Clin North Am 12:137, 1998

CHAPTER 62

DONOVANOSIS

Gavin Hart

Donovanosis is a chronic, progressively destructive bacterial infection of the genital region that is generally regarded as sexually transmitted (see "Epidemiology," below). The disease has been known by many other names, the most common of which are *granuloma inguinale* and *granuloma venereum*.

ETIOLOGY

Donovanosis is caused by *Klebsiella granulomatis* (formerly known as *Calymmatobacterium granulomatis*), an intracellular, gram-negative, pleomorphic, encapsulated (when mature) bacterium measuring 1.5 by 0.7 μm. *K. granulomatis* shares many morphologic and serologic characteristics and >99% homology at the nucleotide level with *Klebsiella* species that are pathogenic to humans. Polymerase chain reaction (PCR) amplification of the *phoE* gene shows it to be closely related to that in *Klebsiella pneumoniae, K. rhinoscleromatis*, and *K. ozaenae*. Electron microscopy shows typical gram-negative morphology and a large capsule but no flagella. Filiform or vesicular protrusions occur on a corrugated cell wall.

EPIDEMIOLOGY

Donovanosis is endemic among Aborigines in central Australia as well as in Papua New Guinea, southeastern India, southern Africa, Vietnam, the Caribbean, Brazil, and Argentina. In the first half of the twentieth century, the disease was endemic in parts of the United States (with an estimated 5000–10,000 cases in 1947); small epidemics still occur in this country and in other developed countries. The decline in the United States to fewer than 20 reported cases annually in the past decade has probably resulted from lower transmission rates due to earlier presentation for increasingly effective antibiotic therapy. More than 70% of cases involve persons 20–40 years of age.

The infection is predominantly sexually transmitted, but extragenital skin lesions can follow transmission from concurrent genital lesions via the fingers or through other nonsexual contact, and autoinoculation may produce new lesions from contact with adjacent skin ("kissing" lesions). Infants born to infected mothers have acquired infection at birth.

CLINICAL MANIFESTATIONS

The incubation period is usually 1–4 weeks but may extend to 1 year. Skin lesions have been detected in infants 6 weeks to 6 months after birth. The disease begins as one or more subcutaneous nodules that erode through the skin to produce clean, granulomatous, sharply defined, usually painless lesions (Fig. 62-1). These lesions, which bleed readily on contact, slowly enlarge. The genitalia are involved in 90% of cases, the inguinal region in 10%, and the anal region in 5–10%. Genital swelling, particularly of the labia, is a common feature and occasionally progresses to pseudoelephantiasis. Phimosis and paraphimosis are common local complications, and progressive erosion of affected tissues may completely destroy the penis or other organs. Less common clinical variants include a hypertrophic form (cauliflower- or wartlike lesions), a necrotic form (destructive lesions with foul-smelling exudate, often resembling amebiasis), and a sclerotic or cicatricial form, which has a dry base with extensive scar tissue. Tissue destruction may be greater in patients co-infected with HIV than in those without HIV infection.

Extragenital lesions occur in at least 6% of cases. Oral donovanosis, the most common extragenital manifestation, presents as pain or bleeding in the mouth, lesions on the lips, or extensive swelling of the gums and palate. Donovanosis may affect most bones, and sometimes many bones are affected at the same time; the tibia is involved in >50% of such cases. Bony lesions are associated with constitutional symptoms (weight loss, fever, night sweats, and malaise) and are usually found in women. More than 50% of women with donovanosis have primary lesions on the cervix. Prompt pelvic examinations and early diagnosis are likely to substantially decrease the morbidity and mortality (likely outcomes in misdiagnosed spinal lesions) associated with extragenital donovanosis in women.

DIAGNOSIS

Laboratory Diagnosis

The preferred diagnostic method involves demonstration of typical intracellular Donovan bodies within large mononuclear cells visualized in smears prepared from lesions (Fig. 62-2) or biopsy specimens. With typical beefy lesions, a small piece of tissue is removed with

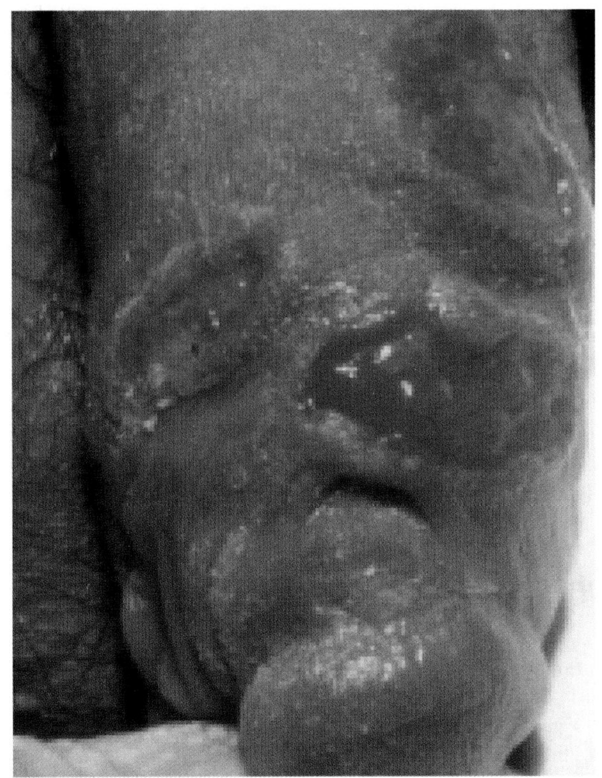

FIGURE 62-1
Multiple granulomatous lesions of the penis in a patient with donovanosis.

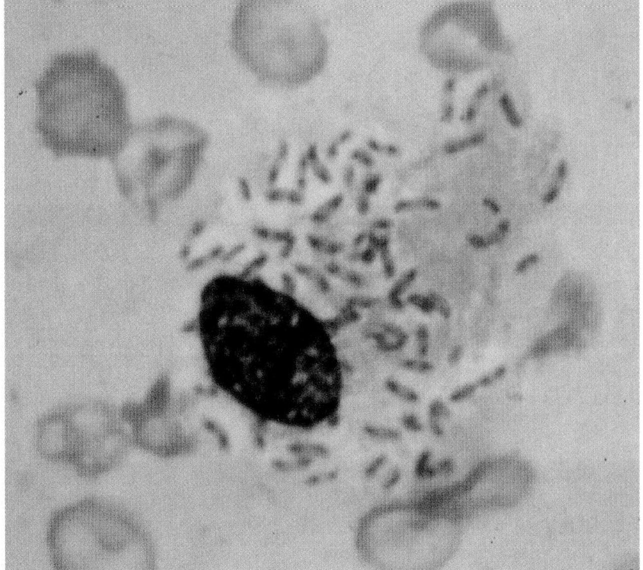

FIGURE 62-2
The typical appearance of Donovan bodies is seen in a large mononuclear cell (20–90 μm in diameter; Giemsa stain; original magnification, ×1000). The host cell nucleus is usually oval, eccentric, and vesicular or pyknotic. The causative organisms appear as bipolar-staining (closed safety-pin) forms that measure 1–1.5 μm in length and 0.5–0.7 μm in diameter and are contained in cytoplasmic vacuoles.

forceps and scalpel, and a crush impression of the deep surface is made on a glass slide. The smear is air-dried, heat-fixed, and stained with Giemsa, Leishman's, or Wright's stain. For dry, flat, or necrotic lesions, a punch-biopsy specimen should be obtained from the advancing edge. This specimen can be used to prepare a smear or embedded for histologic examination (with a silver stain). Histologic examination shows epithelial proliferation, often simulating neoplasia, with a heavy inflammatory infiltrate of plasma cells, some neutrophils, and few if any lymphocytes. *K. granulomatis* has never been grown on artificial solid media but has been cultured in chicken embryonic yolk sacs, on human monocytes, and on human epithelial (HEp-2) cells. A diagnostic PCR test has been developed and incorporated into a colorimetric detection system for *K. granulomatis*. A serologic test, based on indirect immunofluorescence, is more useful in confirming the diagnosis in cases with long-standing lesions than in early disease.

Differential Diagnosis

The differential diagnosis of donovanosis is summarized in Table 62-1. Syphilis and donovanosis frequently coexist because syphilis is usually highly prevalent in areas where donovanosis is endemic; thus positive syphilis serology does not exclude a diagnosis of donovanosis. Genital ulcers are a risk factor for HIV acquisition in developing countries, and patients with donovanosis should be tested for HIV infection.

TABLE 62-1

DIFFERENTIAL DIAGNOSIS OF DONOVANOSIS

DISEASE (CHAPTER)	DISTINGUISHING FEATURES
Secondary syphilis: condylomata lata (70)	White or pale moist plaques in anogenital region (as opposed to bright red donovanosis lesions); lesions subside within 1 week of treatment with benzathine penicillin, 2.4 mU (whereas donovanosis lesions remain unchanged)
Squamous cell carcinoma	Histologic appearance
Penile amebiasis (115)	Microscopic identification of *Entamoeba histolytica*
Chancroid: pseudogranuloma inguinale (47)	Culture of *Haemophilus ducreyi*
Tuberculosis (66)	Histologic features of bony lesions
Actinomycosis (64)	Microscopic identification of sulfur granules
Rhinoscleroma (16)	Histologic features
Leishmaniasis (119)	Histologic features
Histoplasmosis (103)	Histologic features

TABLE 62-2

THE MOST EFFECTIVE ANTIBIOTIC REGIMENS FOR TREATMENT OF DONOVANOSIS[a]

ANTIBIOTIC	ORAL DOSAGE
Azithromycin	1 g weekly or 500 mg/d
Erythromycin	500 mg qid
Tetracycline	500 mg qid
Doxycycline	100 mg bid
Trimethoprim-sulfamethoxazole	1 double-strength tablet[b] bid
Chloramphenicol	500 mg tid

[a]Patients should be examined weekly, and therapy should be continued until lesions have healed (3–5 weeks, except in severe cases).
[b]160 mg/800 mg.

℞ Treatment: DONOVANOSIS

Table 62-2 shows the most effective regimens for treating donovanosis. Doxycycline offers the advantage of convenient administration and has been widely used in developed countries, but azithromycin is increasingly being used as first-choice therapy. Extensive lesions have been cured with oral azithromycin at a dosage of 500 mg/d, but the more convenient dose of 1 g weekly is also effective. Although chloramphenicol is the drug of choice in some developing countries, it is unlikely to be acceptable in developed countries because of bone marrow toxicity. Penicillin is not effective for treating donovanosis. Patients should be examined weekly, and therapy should be continued until lesions have healed (3–5 weeks, except in severe cases). If antibiotic therapy is stopped earlier, lesions often continue to heal, but the relapse rate is higher. If the lesions are unchanged after 2 weeks of treatment, an alternative antibiotic regimen should be used.

The treatment regimens listed in Table 62-2—perhaps with increased duration—are usually adequate in HIV-infected patients without immunosuppression, but an increasing failure rate has been reported in immunosuppressed patients, for whom daily administration of azithromycin is recommended if other regimens fail to elicit a response.

FURTHER READINGS

See www.stdservices.on.net/std/donovanosis/Default.htm for an illustrated lecture and a comprehensive bibliography on donovanosis.

Hart G: Donovanosis (granuloma inguinale), in *Atlas of Infectious Diseases*, vol V: *Sexually Transmitted Diseases*, MF Rein (ed). Philadelphia, Churchill Livingstone, 1996, pp 17.1–17.10

———: Donovanosis. Clin Infect Dis 25:24, 1997

O'Farrell N: Donovanosis. Sex Transm Infect 78:452, 2002

Sardana K, Sehgal V: Genital ulcer disease and human immunodeficiency virus: A focus. Int J Dermatol 44:391, 2005

Wu JJ et al: Selected sexually transmitted diseases and their relationship to HIV. Clin Dermatol 22:499, 2004

PART 4 MISCELLANEOUS BACTERIAL INFECTIONS

CHAPTER 63 NOCARDIOSIS

Gregory A. Filice

Nocardiosis refers to disease caused by bacteria of the genus *Nocardia*. Pneumonia and disseminated disease are most common. Other forms include cellulitis, lymphocutaneous syndrome, actinomycetoma, and keratitis.

MICROBIOLOGY

Nocardiae are saprophytic aerobic actinomycetes and are common worldwide in soil, where they contribute to decay of organic matter. Nocardial taxonomy is complex and incompletely understood. As taxonomy continues to evolve, any nocardiae isolated from a human should be considered potential pathogens.

Nocardia asteroides, which is most commonly isolated from clinical material and associated with invasive disease, is actually a species complex. Six other *Nocardia* species [*N. brasiliensis*, *N. otitidiscaviarum* (formerly *N. caviae*), *N. farcinica*, *N. nova*, *N. transvalensis*, and *N. pseudobrasiliensis*] have been firmly established as human pathogens, and at least 11 additional species have been associated with human disease.

N. farcinica is a less common human pathogen than *N. asteroides* but is more virulent and prone to dissemination. *N. pseudobrasiliensis* is most often associated with invasive disease, and *N. brasiliensis* is usually associated with disease limited to the skin. *N. transvalensis* is generally associated with pulmonary or systemic disease in immunosuppressed patients or with actinomycetoma, an indolent, slowly progressive disease of skin and underlying tissues with nodular swellings and draining sinuses.

EPIDEMIOLOGY

Approximately 1100 cases of nocardial infection are diagnosed annually in the United States, 85% of them pulmonary and/or systemic. The annual incidence is ~0.375 cases per 100,000 persons. The disease is more common among adults than among children and among males than among females. Nearly all cases are sporadic, but outbreaks have been associated with contamination of the hospital environment, solutions, or drug injection equipment. Person-to-person spread is not well documented. There is no known seasonality.

The risk of pulmonary or disseminated disease is greater than usual among persons with deficient cell-mediated immunity, especially that associated with lymphoma, transplantation, glucocorticoid therapy, or AIDS. The incidence is ~140-fold greater among patients with AIDS and ~340-fold greater among bone marrow transplant recipients than in general populations. In AIDS, nocardiosis usually affects persons with <250 CD4+ T lymphocytes/μL. Nocardiosis has also been associated with pulmonary alveolar proteinosis, tuberculosis and other mycobacterial diseases, chronic granulomatous disease, interleukin 12 deficiency, and treatment with monoclonal antibodies to tumor necrosis factor. Any child with nocardiosis and no known cause of immunosuppression should undergo tests to determine the adequacy of the phagocytic respiratory burst.

Actinomycetoma associated with *N. brasiliensis*, *N. asteroides*, *N. otitidiscaviarum*, and *N. transvalensis* occurs mainly in tropical and subtropical regions, especially those of Mexico, Central and South America, Africa, and India. The most important risk factor is frequent contact with soil or vegetable matter.

PATHOLOGY AND PATHOGENESIS

Pneumonia and disseminated disease are both thought to follow inhalation of fragmented bacterial mycelia. The characteristic histologic feature of nocardiosis is an abscess with extensive neutrophil infiltration and prominent necrosis. Granulation tissue usually surrounds the lesions, but extensive fibrosis or encapsulation is uncommon. Actinomycetoma is characterized by suppurative inflammation with sinus tract formation. Granules—microcolonies composed of dense masses of bacterial filaments extending radially from a central core—are occasionally observed in histologic preparations. They are frequently found in discharges from lesions of actinomycetoma but almost never from lesions in other forms of nocardiosis. Infrequently, nocardiae and other indolent pathogens, including fungi or mycobacteria, are isolated from the same patient.

Nocardiae have evolved a number of properties that enable them to survive within phagocytes, including neutralization of oxidants, prevention of phagosome-lysosome fusion, and prevention of phagosome acidification. Neutrophils phagocytose the organisms and limit their growth but do not kill them efficiently. Cell-mediated immunity is important for definitive control and elimination of nocardiae.

CLINICAL MANIFESTATIONS

Respiratory Tract Disease

Pneumonia, the most common form of nocardial disease in the respiratory tract, is typically subacute; symptoms have usually been present for days or weeks at presentation. The onset is occasionally more acute in immunosuppressed patients. Cough is prominent and produces small amounts of thick, purulent sputum that is not malodorous. Fever, anorexia, weight loss, and malaise are common; dyspnea, pleuritic pain, and hemoptysis are less common. Remissions and exacerbations over several weeks are frequent. Roentgenographic patterns vary, but some are highly suggestive of nocardial pneumonia. Infiltrates vary in size and are typically of at least moderate density. Single or multiple nodules are common (Fig. 63-1 and 63-2), sometimes suggesting tumor metastases. Infiltrates and nodules tend to cavitate (Fig. 63-2). Empyema is present in one-third of cases.

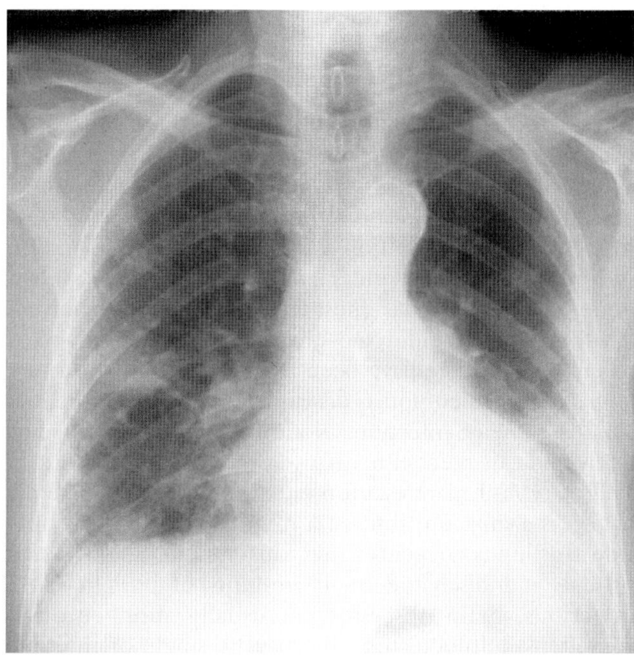

FIGURE 63-1

Nocardial pneumonia. Discrete nodular infiltrates are present in midlung fields on both sides.

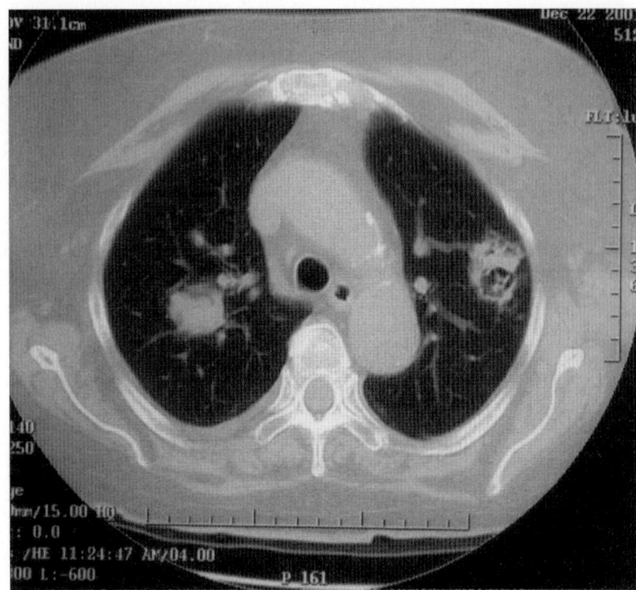

FIGURE 63-2
Nocardial pneumonia. A CT scan shows bilateral nodules, with cavitation in the nodule in the left lung.

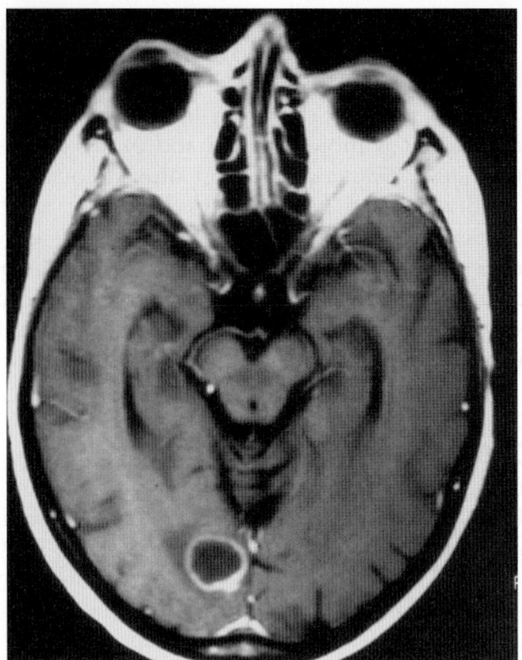

FIGURE 63-3
Nocardial abscesses in the right occipital lobe.

Nocardiosis may spread directly from the lungs to adjacent tissues. Pericarditis, mediastinitis, and the superior vena cava syndrome have all been reported. Nocardial laryngitis, tracheitis, and bronchitis are much less common than pneumonia. In the major airways, disease often presents as a nodular or granulomatous mass. A few cases of sinusitis have been reported.

Nocardiae are sometimes isolated from respiratory secretions of patients without apparent nocardial disease. These patients usually have chronic pulmonary disease with airway or parenchymal abnormalities and do not necessarily require treatment for nocardiosis (see "Diagnosis" later in the chapter).

Extrapulmonary Disease

In half of all cases of pulmonary nocardiosis, disease appears outside the lungs. In one-fifth of cases of disseminated disease, lung disease is not apparent. The most common site of dissemination is the brain. Other common sites include the skin and supporting structures, kidneys, bone, and muscle, but almost any organ can be involved. Peritonitis and epididymo-orchitis have been reported recently. Nocardiae have been recovered from blood in a few cases of pneumonia, disseminated disease, or central venous catheter infection. Nocardial endocarditis occurs rarely and can affect either native or prosthetic valves.

The typical manifestation of extrapulmonary dissemination is a subacute abscess. A minority of abscesses outside the lungs or central nervous system (CNS) form fistulae and discharge small amounts of pus. In CNS infections, brain abscesses are usually supratentorial, are often multiloculated, and may be single or multiple (Fig. 63-3). Brain abscesses tend to burrow into the ventricles or extend out into the subarachnoid space. The symptoms and signs are somewhat more indolent than those of other types of bacterial brain abscess. Meningitis is uncommon and is usually due to spread from a nearby brain abscess. Nocardiae are not easily recovered from cerebrospinal fluid (CSF).

Disease After Transcutaneous Inoculation

Disease that follows transcutaneous nocardial inoculation usually takes one of three forms: cellulitis, lymphocutaneous syndrome, or actinomycetoma.

Cellulitis generally begins 1–3 weeks after a recognized breach of the skin, often with soil contamination. Subacute cellulitis, with pain, swelling, erythema, and warmth, develops over days to weeks. The lesions are usually firm and not fluctuant. Disease may progress to involve underlying muscles, tendons, bones, or joints. Dissemination is rare. *N. brasiliensis* is the most common isolate, but *N. asteroides* is often isolated from people living in cooler climates.

Lymphocutaneous disease usually begins as a pyodermatous lesion at the site of inoculation, with central ulceration and purulent or honey-colored drainage. Subcutaneous nodules often appear along lymphatics that drain the primary lesion. The lymphangitic form closely resembles lymphocutaneous sporotrichosis (Chap. 110). Most cases of the lymphocutaneous syndrome are associated with *N. brasiliensis*.

Actinomycetoma (Fig. 63-4) usually begins with a nodular swelling, sometimes at a site of local trauma. Lesions typically develop on the feet or hands but may involve the posterior part of the neck, the upper back, the head, and other sites. The nodule eventually breaks down, and a fistula appears. This fistula is typically followed by others. The fistulae tend to come and go, with new ones forming

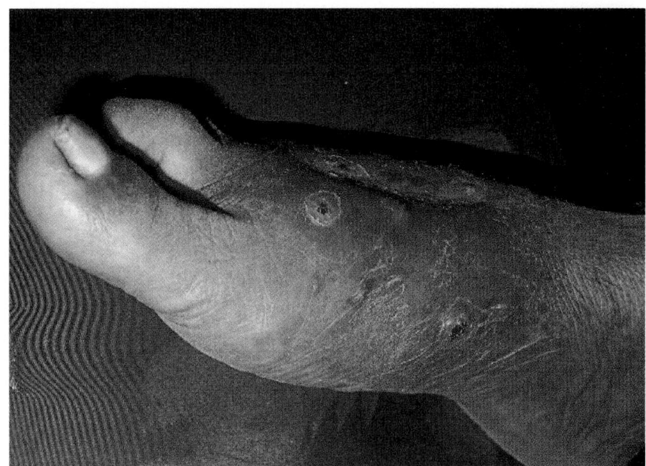

FIGURE 63-4
Nocardial actinomycetoma illustrating common features including swelling, multiple sinus tracts, and involvement of the foot. (*Image provided by Amor Khachemoune and Ronald O. Perelman, New York University School of Medicine.*)

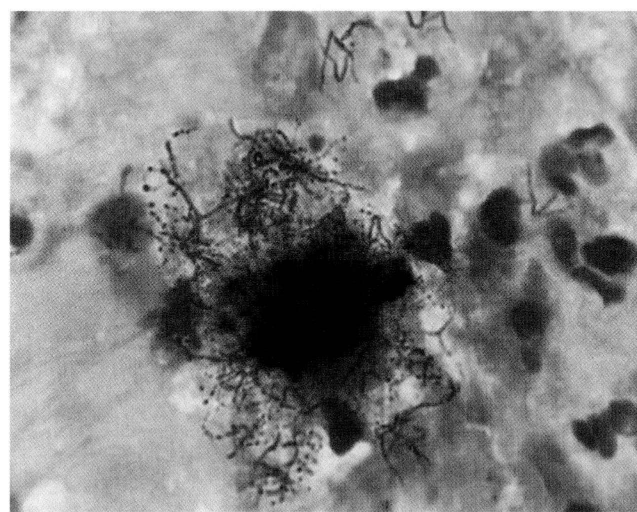

FIGURE 63-5
Gram-stained sputum from a patient with nocardial pneumonia. (*Image provided by Charles Cartwright and Susan Nelson, Hennepin County Medical Center, Minneapolis, MN.*)

as old ones disappear. The discharge is serous or purulent, may be bloody, and often contains 0.1- to 2-mm white granules consisting of masses of mycelia. The lesions spread slowly along fascial planes to involve adjacent areas of skin, subcutaneous tissue, and bone. Over months or years, there may be extensive deformation of the affected part. Lesions involving soft tissues are only mildly painful; those affecting bones or joints are more so. Systemic symptoms are absent or minimal. Infection rarely disseminates from actinomycetoma, and lesions on the hands and feet usually cause only local disability. Lesions on the head, neck, and trunk can invade locally to involve deep organs, with consequent severe disability or death.

Eye Infections

Nocardia species (particularly *N. asteroides*) are uncommon causes of subacute keratitis, usually after eye trauma. Nocardial endophthalmitis can develop after eye surgery. In one series, nocardiae accounted for more than half of culture-proved cases of endophthalmitis after cataract surgery. Endophthalmitis can also occur during disseminated disease. Nocardial infection of lachrymal glands has been reported.

DIAGNOSIS

The first step in diagnosis is examination of sputum or pus for crooked, branching, beaded, gram-positive filaments 1 μm wide and up to 50 μm long (Fig. 63-5). Most nocardiae are acid-fast in direct smears if a weak acid is used for decolorization (e.g., in the modified Kinyoun, Ziehl-Neelsen, and Fite-Faraco methods). The organisms often take up silver stains. Nocardiae grow relatively slowly; colonies may take up to 2 weeks to appear and may not develop their characteristic appearance for up to 4 weeks. Several blood culture systems support nocardial growth. Yield in manual systems is enhanced when blood cultures are incubated aerobically for up to 4 weeks and when blind subcultures are performed. Nocardial growth is so different from that of more common pathogens that the laboratory should be alerted when nocardiosis is suspected in order to maximize the likelihood of isolation. Since nocardiae are among the few aerobic microorganisms that use paraffin as a carbon source, paraffin baiting can be used to isolate the organisms from mixed cultures.

In nocardial pneumonia, sputum smears are often negative. Unless the diagnosis can be made in smear-negative cases by sampling lesions in more accessible sites, bronchoscopy or lung aspiration is usually necessary. Transtracheal aspiration should be avoided, as it frequently leads to nocardial cellulitis in tissues around the puncture wound.

To evaluate the possibility of dissemination in patients with nocardial pneumonia, a careful history should be obtained and a thorough physical examination performed. Suggestive symptoms or signs should be pursued with further diagnostic tests. CT or MRI of the head, with and without contrast material, should be undertaken if signs or symptoms suggest brain involvement. Some authorities recommend brain imaging in all cases of pulmonary or disseminated disease.

When clinically indicated, CSF or urine should be concentrated and then cultured. In actinomycetoma, granules should be sought in the discharge. Suspect particles should be washed in saline, examined microscopically, and cultured.

Isolation of nocardiae from sputum or blood occasionally represents colonization, transient infection, or contamination. In typical cases of respiratory tract colonization, Gram-stained specimens are negative and cultures are only intermittently positive. A positive sputum culture in an immunosuppressed patient usually reflects disease.

When nocardiae are isolated from an immunocompetent patient without apparent nocardial disease, the patient should be observed carefully without treatment. A patient with a host-defense defect that increases the risk of nocardiosis should usually receive antimicrobial treatment.

Nocardia species are difficult to differentiate from one another with standard biochemical tests. The Clinical and Laboratory Standards Institute has published a broth microdilution method for nocardiae, but experience with nocardiae and quality-control testing are required for reliable results. Isolates from patients with systemic or severe disease should be sent to a reference laboratory for definitive identification and susceptibility testing.

Several presumptive diagnostic tests for nocardial infection have been studied, including tests for antibodies, nocardial metabolites, and nocardial DNA. None is ready for clinical use at this time.

℞ Treatment: NOCARDIOSIS

Sulfonamides are the drugs of choice for nocardiosis (Table 63-1). The combination of sulfamethoxazole (SMX) and trimethoprim (TMP) is probably equivalent to sulfonamides; some authorities believe that the combination may in fact be more effective, but it also poses a modestly greater risk of hematologic toxicity. At the outset, 10–20 mg of TMP per kg and 50–100 mg of SMX per kg should be given each day in two divided doses. Later, the daily doses can be decreased to as little as 5 mg/kg and 25 mg/kg, respectively. In difficult cases, sulfonamide levels should be measured and dosages adjusted to keep serum concentrations between 100 and 150 μg/mL. In persons with sulfonamide allergies, desensitization usually allows continuation of therapy with these effective and inexpensive drugs.

Minocycline is the best-established alternative oral drug and should be given in doses of 100–200 mg twice a day. Other tetracyclines are usually ineffective. Linezolid appears to be active in vitro and has been effective in a few clinical cases. *N. nova* infections can be treated with erythromycin (500–750 mg four times a day) and/or ampicillin (1 g four times a day), but other *Nocardia* species are often resistant to both drugs. Amoxicillin (500 mg) combined with clavulanic acid (125 mg), given three times a day, has been effective in a few cases but should be avoided in cases due to *N. nova*, in which clavulanate induces β-lactamase production. Ofloxacin (400 mg twice a day) and clarithromycin (500 mg twice a day) have each been successful in a few cases.

Amikacin, the best-established parenteral drug, is given in doses of 5–7.5 mg/kg every 12 h. Serum levels should be monitored during prolonged therapy in patients with diminished renal function and in the elderly. Newer β-lactam antibiotics, including cefotaxime, ceftizoxime, ceftriaxone, and imipenem, are usually effective. These agents may be less effective in some cases caused by *N. farcinica*.

In vitro, *N. farcinica* differs from most nocardiae in that it is resistant to cephalosporins in most cases and to imipenem in one-fifth of cases. *N. pseudobrasiliensis* often exhibits resistance to minocycline or amoxicillin/clavulanic acid and susceptibility to ciprofloxacin or clarithromycin. *N. transvalensis* displays increased resistance to many antimicrobial agents, including amikacin, tobramycin, cefotaxime, ceftriaxone, and amoxicillin/clavulanic acid.

TABLE 63-1

TREATMENT FOR NOCARDIOSIS

DISEASE	DURATION	DRUGS (DAILY DOSE)[a]
Pulmonary or systemic		Systemic therapy
Intact host defenses	6–12 mo	Oral
Deficient host defenses	12 mo[b]	1. Trimethoprim (10–20 mg/kg) and sulfamethoxazole (50–100 mg/kg)
CNS disease	12 mo[c]	2. Minocycline (200–400 mg)
Cellulitis, lymphocutaneous syndrome	2 mo	3. Linezolid (1200 mg)
Osteomyelitis, arthritis, laryngitis, sinusitis	4 mo	Parenteral
		1. Amikacin (10–15 mg/kg)
Actinomycetoma	6–12 mo after clinical cure	2. Cefotaxime (6 g), ceftizoxime (6 g), ceftriaxone (1–2 g), imipenem (2 g)
Keratitis	Topical: Until apparent cure	1. Sulfonamide drops 2. Amikacin drops
	Systemic: Until 2–4 mo after apparent cure	Drugs for systemic therapy as listed above

[a]For each category, choices are numbered in order of preference.

[b]In some patients with AIDS or chronic granulomatous disease, therapy for pulmonary or systemic disease must be continued indefinitely.

[c]If all apparent CNS disease has been excised, the duration of therapy may be reduced to 6 months.

N. nova isolates appear to be susceptible to ampicillin and erythromycin in vitro but also produce β-lactamase constitutively or in the presence of a β-lactam drug.

Use of SMX and TMP in high-risk populations to prevent *Pneumocystis* disease or urinary tract infections appears to reduce the risk of nocardiosis as well. However, the incidence of nocardiosis is low enough that prophylaxis of this disease is not recommended.

In patients with nocardiosis who need immunosuppressive therapy for an underlying disease or prevention of transplant rejection, such therapy should be continued. In many cases, two or more antimicrobial agents have been used to treat nocardiosis, often in combinations including drugs that are usually effective by themselves, like a sulfonamide or minocycline. Whether such combination therapy is better than monotherapy is not known, and it certainly increases the risk of toxicity. In treating patients with severe disease, some experts begin with a combination including TMP-SMX, amikacin, and ceftriaxone or imipenem. If combination therapy is used initially, a single drug should be used after clinical improvement, which usually occurs within the first week or two of treatment.

Surgical management of nocardial disease is similar to that of other bacterial diseases. Brain abscesses should be aspirated, drained, or excised if the diagnosis is unclear, if an abscess is large and accessible, or if an abscess fails to respond to chemotherapy. Small or inaccessible brain abscesses should be treated medically; clinical improvement should be noticeable within 1–2 weeks. Brain imaging should be repeated to document the resolution of lesions, although abatement on images often lags behind clinical improvement.

Antimicrobial therapy usually suffices for nocardial actinomycetoma. In deep or extensive cases, drainage or excision of heavily involved tissue may facilitate healing, but structure and function should be preserved whenever possible.

Nocardial infections tend to relapse (particularly in patients with chronic granulomatous disease), and long courses of antimicrobial therapy are necessary. If disease is unusually extensive, if the patient is immunosuppressed, or if the response to therapy is slow, the recommendations in Table 63-1 should be exceeded.

The mortality rate for pulmonary or disseminated nocardiosis outside the CNS should be <5%. CNS disease carries a higher mortality rate. Patients should be followed carefully for at least 6 months after therapy has ended.

FURTHER READINGS

Brown-Elliott BA et al: Clinical and laboratory features of the *Nocardia* spp. based on current molecular taxonomy. Clin Microbiol Rev 19:259, 2006

Chouciño C et al: Nocardial infections in bone marrow transplant recipients. Clin Infect Dis 23:1012, 1996

Fabre S et al: Primary cutaneous *Nocardia otitidiscaviarum* infection in a patient with rheumatoid arthritis treated with infliximab. J Rheumatol 32:2432, 2005

Filice GA: Nocardiosis in persons with human immunodeficiency virus infection, transplant recipients, and large, geographically defined populations. J Lab Clin Med 145:156, 2005

Lalitha P et al: Postcataract endophthalmitis in South India incidence and outcome. Ophthalmology 112:1884, 2005

Palmer DL et al: Diagnostic and therapeutic considerations in *Nocardia asteroides* infection. Medicine 53:391, 1974

Peleg AY et al: Risk factors, clinical characteristics, and outcome of *Nocardia* infection in organ transplant recipients: A matched case-control study. Clin Infect Dis 44:1307, 2007

Poonwan N et al: Characterization of clinical isolates of pathogenic *Nocardia* strains and related actinomycetes in Thailand from 1996 to 2003. Mycopathologia 159:361, 2005

Routh JC et al: Epididymo-orchitis and testicular abscess due to *Nocardia asteroides* complex. Urology 65:591, 2005

Rupprecht TA, Pfister HW: Clinical experience with linezolid for the treatment of central nervous system infections. Eur J Neurol 12:536, 2005

Safdar N et al: Clinical problem-solving. Into the woods. N Engl J Med 356:943, 2007

Uttamchandani RB et al: Nocardiosis in 30 patients with advanced human immunodeficiency virus infection: Clinical features and outcome. Clin Infect Dis 18:348, 1994

CHAPTER 64

ACTINOMYCOSIS

Thomas A. Russo

Actinomycosis is an indolent, slowly progressive infection caused by anaerobic or microaerophilic bacteria, primarily of the genus *Actinomyces*, that colonize the mouth, colon, and vagina. Mucosal disruption may lead to infection at virtually any site in the body. In vivo growth of actinomycetes usually results in the formation of characteristic clumps called *grains* or *sulfur granules*. The clinical presentations of actinomycosis are myriad. Common in the preantibiotic era, actinomycosis has diminished in incidence, as has its timely recognition. Actinomycosis has been called the most misdiagnosed disease, and it has been said that no disease is so often missed by experienced clinicians. Thus this entity remains a diagnostic challenge.

Three clinical presentations that should prompt consideration of this unique infection are (1) the combination of chronicity, progression across tissue boundaries, and mass-like features (mimicking malignancy, with which it is often confused); (2) the development of a sinus tract, which may spontaneously resolve and recur; and (3) a refractory or relapsing infection after a short course of therapy, since cure of established actinomycosis requires prolonged treatment. An awareness of the full spectrum of the disease will expedite its diagnosis and treatment and will minimize the unnecessary surgical interventions, morbidity, and mortality that are reported all too often.

ETIOLOGIC AGENTS

Actinomycosis is most commonly caused by *A. israelii*. *A. naeslundii*, *A. odontolyticus*, *A. viscosus*, *A. meyeri*, *A. gerencseriae*, and *Propionibacterium propionicum* are established but less common causes. Most if not all actinomycotic infections are polymicrobial. *Actinobacillus actinomycetemcomitans*, *Eikenella corrodens*, Enterobacteriaceae, and species of *Fusobacterium*, *Bacteroides*, *Capnocytophaga*, *Staphylococcus*, and *Streptococcus* are commonly isolated with actinomycetes in various combinations, depending on the site of infection. The contribution of these other species to the pathogenesis of actinomycosis is uncertain.

Comparative 16S rRNA gene sequencing has led to the identification of an ever-expanding list of *Actinomyces* spp., presently numbered at 92. Increasing data support *A. europaeus*, *A. neuii*, *A. radingae*, *A. graevenitzii*, *A. turicensis*, *A. cardiffensis*, *A. houstonensis*, *A. hongkongensis*, and *A. funkei* as additional causes of human actinomycosis.

EPIDEMIOLOGY

Actinomycosis has no geographic boundaries and occurs throughout life, with a peak incidence in the middle decades. Males have a threefold higher incidence than females, possibly because of poorer dental hygiene and/or more frequent trauma. Factors that have probably contributed to the decrease in actinomycosis incidence since the advent of antibiotics include improved dental hygiene and the initiation of antimicrobial treatment before the disease develops fully. Individuals who do not seek or have access to health care are undoubtedly at higher risk.

PATHOGENESIS AND PATHOLOGY

The etiologic agents of actinomycosis are members of the normal oral flora and are often cultured from the bronchi, the gastrointestinal tract, and the female genital tract. The critical step in the development of actinomycosis is disruption of the mucosal barrier. Local infection may ensue. Once established, actinomycosis spreads contiguously in a slow progressive manner, ignoring tissue planes. Although acute inflammation may initially develop at the infection site, the hallmark of actinomycosis is the characteristic chronic, indolent phase manifested by lesions that usually appear as single or multiple indurations. Central necrosis consisting of neutrophils and sulfur granules develops and is virtually diagnostic. The fibrotic walls of the mass are typically described as "wooden." The responsible bacterial and/or host factors have not been identified. Over time, sinus tracts to the skin, adjacent organs, or bone may develop. In rare instances, distant hematogenous seeding may occur. As mentioned above, these unique features of actinomycosis mimic malignancy, with which it is often confused.

Foreign bodies appear to facilitate infection. This association most frequently involves intrauterine contraceptive devices (IUCDs). An increasing number of reports have described an association of actinomycosis with HIV infection, transplantation, and radio- or chemotherapy. Ulcerative mucosal infections (e.g., by herpes simplex virus or cytomegalovirus) and abnormalities in host defenses may facilitate the development of actinomycosis in the latter settings.

CLINICAL MANIFESTATIONS

Oral-Cervicofacial Disease

Actinomycosis occurs most frequently at an oral, cervical, or facial site, usually as a soft tissue swelling, abscess, or mass lesion that is often mistaken for a neoplasm. The angle of the jaw is generally involved, but a diagnosis of actinomycosis should be considered with any mass lesion or relapsing infection in the head and neck (Chap. 16). Otitis, sinusitis, and canaliculitis also can develop. Pain, fever, and leukocytosis are variably reported. Contiguous extension to the cranium, cervical spine, or thorax is a potential sequela.

Thoracic Disease

Thoracic actinomycosis usually follows an indolent progressive course, with involvement of the pulmonary parenchyma and/or the pleural space. Chest pain, fever, and weight loss are common. A cough, when present, is variably productive. The usual radiographic finding is either a mass lesion or pneumonia. On computed tomography (CT), central areas of low attenuation and ringlike rim enhancement may be seen. Cavitary disease or hilar adenopathy may develop. More than 50% of cases include pleural thickening, effusion, or empyema (Fig. 64-1). Rarely, pulmonary nodules or endobronchial lesions occur. Pulmonary lesions suggestive of actinomycosis may cross fissures or pleura; may involve the mediastinum, contiguous bone, or chest wall; or may be associated with a sinus tract. In the absence of these findings, thoracic actinomycosis is usually mistaken for a neoplasm or for pneumonia due to more usual causes.

Mediastinal infection is uncommon, usually arising from thoracic extension but rarely resulting from perforation of the esophagus, from trauma, or from head and neck or abdominal disease. The structures within the

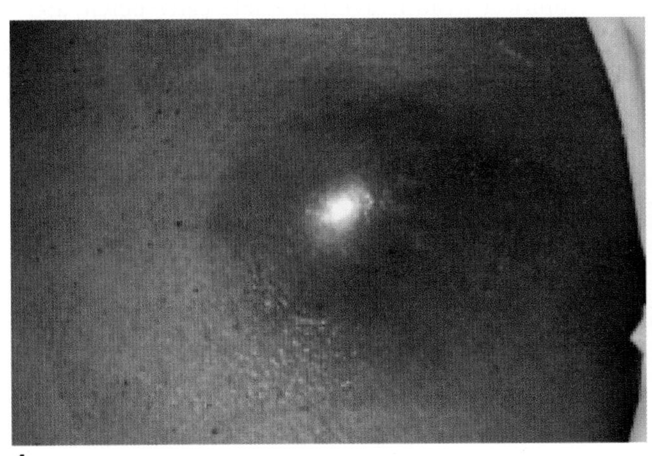

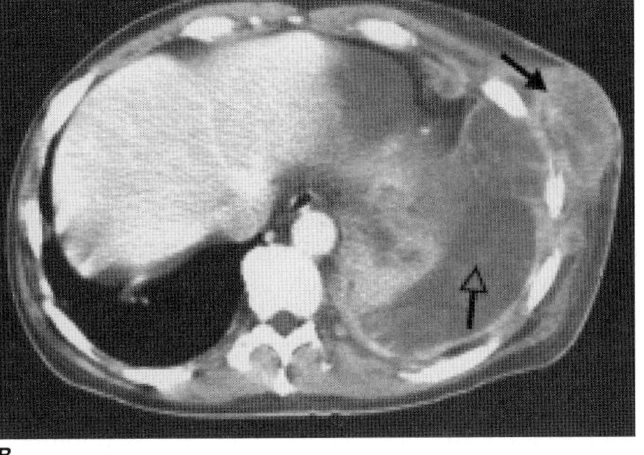

A B

FIGURE 64-1

Thoracic actinomycosis. *A.* A chest wall mass from extension of pulmonary infection. ***B.*** Pulmonary infection is complicated by empyema (*open arrow*) and extension to the chest wall (*closed arrow*). (*Courtesy of Dr. C.B. Hsiao, Division of Infectious Diseases, Department of Medicine, State University of New York at Buffalo; with permission.*)

mediastinum and the heart can be involved in various combinations; consequently, the possible presentations are diverse. Primary endocarditis and isolated disease of the breast have been described.

Abdominal Disease

Abdominal actinomycosis poses a great diagnostic challenge. Months or years usually pass from the inciting event (e.g., appendicitis, diverticulitis, peptic ulcer disease, foreign-body perforation, bowel surgery, or ascension from IUCD-associated pelvic disease) to clinical recognition. Because of the flow of peritoneal fluid and/or the direct extension of primary disease, virtually any abdominal organ, region, or space can be involved. The disease usually presents as an abscess, a mass, or a mixed lesion that is often fixed to underlying tissue and mistaken for a tumor. On CT, enhancement is most often heterogeneous and adjacent bowel is thickened. Sinus tracts to the abdominal wall, to the perianal region, or between the bowel and other organs may develop and mimic inflammatory bowel disease. Recurrent disease or a wound or fistula that fails to heal suggests actinomycosis.

Hepatic infection usually presents as one or more abscesses or masses (Fig. 64-2). Isolated disease presumably develops via hematogenous seeding from cryptic foci. Imaging and percutaneous techniques have resulted in improved diagnosis and treatment.

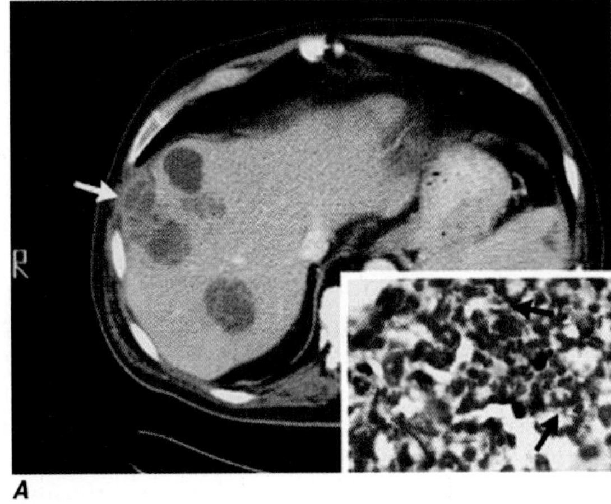

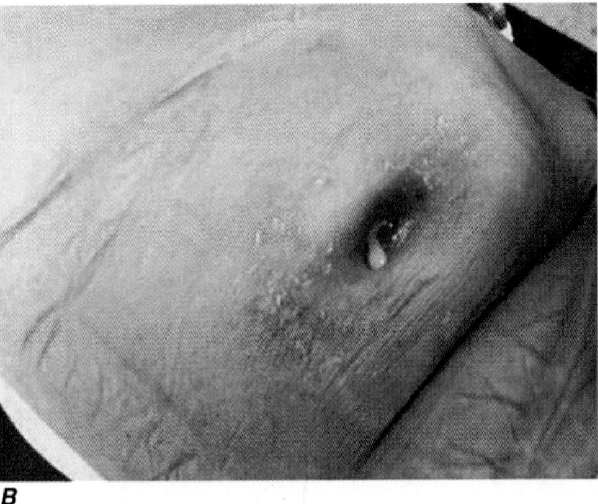

A B

FIGURE 64-2

Hepatic-splenic actinomycosis. *A.* Computed tomogram showing multiple hepatic abscesses and a small splenic lesion due to *A. israelii*. Arrow indicates extension outside the liver. ***Inset:*** Gram's stain of abscess fluid demonstrating beaded filamentous gram-positive rods. ***B.*** Subsequent formation of a sinus tract. (*Reprinted with permission from Saad M: Actinomyces hepatic abscess with cutaneous fistula. N Engl J Med 353:e16, 2005. © 2005 Massachusetts Medical Society. All rights reserved.*)

All levels of the urogenital tract can be infected. Renal disease usually presents as pyelonephritis and/or renal and perinephric abscess. Bladder involvement, usually due to extension of pelvic disease, may result in ureteral obstruction or fistulas to bowel, skin, or uterus. *Actinomyces* can be detected in urine with appropriate stains and cultures.

Pelvic Disease

Actinomycotic involvement of the pelvis occurs most commonly in association with an IUCD. When an IUCD is in place or has recently been removed, pelvic symptoms should prompt consideration of actinomycosis. The risk, although not quantified, appears small. The disease rarely develops when the IUCD has been in place for <1 year, but the risk increases with time. Actinomycosis can also present months after IUCD removal. Symptoms are typically indolent; fever, weight loss, abdominal pain, and abnormal vaginal bleeding or discharge are the most common. The earliest stage of disease—often endometritis—commonly progresses to pelvic masses or a tuboovarian abscess (Fig. 64-3). Unfortunately, because the diagnosis is often delayed, a "frozen pelvis" mimicking malignancy or endometriosis can develop by the time of recognition.

An unresolved issue is whether screening of cervical or endometrial specimens for *Actinomyces*-like organisms (ALOs) can predict or prevent IUCD-associated disease. Although the risk appears small, the consequences of infection are significant. Therefore, until more quantitative data become available, it seems prudent to remove the IUCD in the presence of symptoms that cannot be accounted for, regardless of whether ALOs or immunofluorescence-positive organisms are detected, and—if advanced disease is excluded—to initiate a 14-day course of empirical treatment for possible early pelvic actinomycosis. The detection of ALOs or immunofluorescence-positive organisms in the absence of symptoms warrants education of the patient and close follow-up but not removal of the IUCD unless a suitable contraceptive alternative is agreed on.

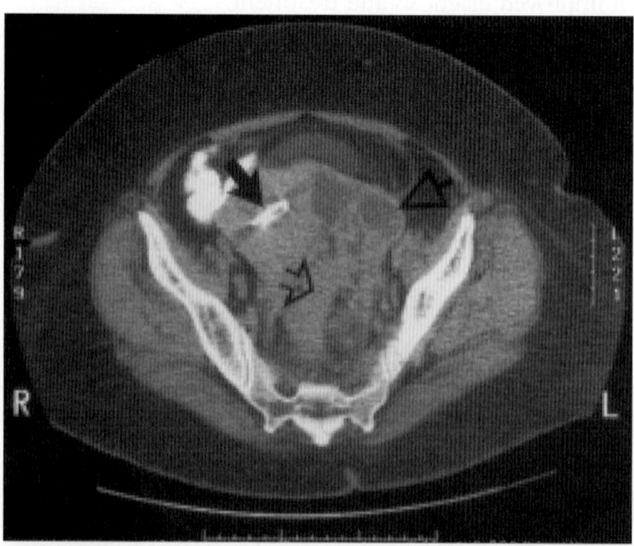

FIGURE 64-3

Computed tomogram showing pelvic actinomycosis associated with an intrauterine contraceptive device. The device is encased by endometrial fibrosis (*solid arrow*); also visible are paraendometrial fibrosis (*open triangular arrowhead*) and an area of suppuration (*open arrow*).

Central Nervous System Disease

Actinomycosis of the central nervous system (CNS) is rare. Single or multiple brain abscesses are most common. An abscess usually appears on CT as a ring-enhancing lesion with a thick wall that may be irregular or nodular. Meningitis, epidural or subdural space infection, and cavernous sinus syndrome also have been described.

Musculoskeletal and Soft Tissue Infection

Actinomycotic infection of bone is usually due to adjacent soft-tissue infection but may be associated with trauma (e.g., fracture of the mandible) or hematogenous spread. Because of slow disease progression, new bone formation and bone destruction are seen concomitantly. Infection of an extremity is uncommon and is usually a result of trauma. Skin, subcutaneous tissue, muscle, and bone (with periostitis or acute or chronic osteomyelitis) are involved alone or in various combinations. Cutaneous sinus tracts frequently develop.

Disseminated Disease

Hematogenous dissemination of disease from any location rarely results in multiple-organ involvement. The lungs and liver are most commonly affected, with the presentation of multiple nodules mimicking disseminated malignancy. The clinical presentation may be surprisingly indolent given the extent of disease.

DIAGNOSIS

The diagnosis of actinomycosis is rarely considered. All too often, the first mention of actinomycosis is by the pathologist after extensive surgery. Since medical therapy alone is often sufficient for cure, the challenge for the clinician is to consider the possibility of actinomycosis, to diagnose it in the least invasive fashion, and to avoid unnecessary surgery. The clinical and radiographic presentations that suggest actinomycosis are discussed above. Aspirations and biopsies (with or without CT or ultrasound guidance) are being used successfully to obtain clinical material for diagnosis, although surgery may be required. The diagnosis is most commonly made by microscopic identification of sulfur granules (an in vivo matrix of bacteria, calcium phosphate, and host material) in pus or tissues. Occasionally, these granules are identified grossly from draining sinus tracts or pus. Although sulfur granules are a defining characteristic of actinomycosis, granules are also found in mycetoma (Chaps. 63 and 110) and botryomycosis (a chronic suppurative bacterial infection of soft tissue or, in rare cases, visceral tissue that produces clumps of bacteria resembling granules). These entities can easily be differentiated from actinomycosis with appropriate histopathologic and microbiologic studies.

Microbiologic identification of actinomycetes is often precluded by prior antimicrobial therapy or failure to perform appropriate microbiologic cultures. For optimal yield, the avoidance of even a single dose of antibiotics is mandatory. Primary isolation usually requires 5–7 days but may take as long as 2–4 weeks. Although not routinely used, 16S rRNA gene amplification and sequencing have been successfully applied to increase diagnostic sensitivity. Because actinomycetes are components of the normal oral and genital-tract flora, their identification in the absence of sulfur granules in sputum, bronchial washings, and cervicovaginal secretions is of little significance.

℞ Treatment: ACTINOMYCOSIS

Decisions about treatment are based on the collective clinical experience of the past 50 years. Actinomycosis requires prolonged treatment with high doses of antimicrobial agents. The need for intensive treatment is presumably due to the drugs' poor penetration of the thick-walled masses common in this infection and/or the sulfur granules themselves. Although therapy must be individualized, the intravenous administration of 18–24 million units of penicillin daily for 2–6 weeks, followed by oral therapy with penicillin or amoxicillin (total duration, 6–12 months), is a reasonable guideline for serious infections and bulky disease. Less extensive disease, particularly that involving the oral-cervicofacial region, may be cured with a shorter course. If therapy is extended beyond the resolution of measurable disease, the risk of relapse—a clinical hallmark of this infection—will be minimized; CT and magnetic resonance imaging (MRI) are generally the most sensitive and objective techniques by which to accomplish this goal. A similar approach is reasonable for immunocompromised patients, although refractory disease has been described in HIV-infected individuals. Suitable alternative antimicrobial agents and those deemed unreliable are listed in Table 64-1. Although the role played by "companion" microbes in actinomycosis is unclear, many isolates are pathogens in their own right, and a regimen covering these organisms during the initial treatment course is reasonable.

Combined medical-surgical therapy is still advocated by some authorities. However, an increasing body of literature now supports an initial attempt at cure with medical therapy alone, even in extensive disease. CT and MRI should be used to monitor the response to therapy. In most cases, either surgery can be avoided or a less extensive procedure can be used. This approach is particularly valuable in sparing critical organs, such as the bladder or the reproductive organs in women of child-bearing age. For a well-defined abscess, percutaneous drainage in combination with medical therapy is a reasonable approach. When a critical location is involved (e.g., the epidural space, the CNS) or when suitable medical therapy fails, surgical intervention may be appropriate.

TABLE 64-1

APPROPRIATE AND INAPPROPRIATE ANTIBIOTIC THERAPY FOR ACTINOMYCOSIS[a]

CATEGORY	AGENT
Extensive successful clinical experience[b]	Penicillin: 18–24 mU/d IV q4h, 1–2 g/d PO q6h Erythromycin: 2–4 g/d IV q6h, 1–2 g/d PO q6h Tetracycline: 1–2 g/d PO q6h Doxycycline: 200 mg/d IV or PO q12–24h Minocycline: 200 mg/d IV or PO q12h Clindamycin: 2.7 g/d IV q8h, 1.2–1.8 g/d PO q6–8h
Anecdotal successful clinical experience	Ceftriaxone Ceftizoxime Imipenem Piperacillin-tazobactam
Agents that should be avoided	Metronidazole Aminoglycosides Oxacillin Dicloxacillin Cephalexin
Agents predicted to be efficacious on the basis of in vitro activity	Moxifloxacin Vancomycin Linezolid Quinupristin-dalfopristin

[a]Additional coverage for concomitant "companion" bacteria may be required.

[b]Controlled evaluations have not been performed. Dose and duration require individualization depending on the host, site, and extent of infection. As a general rule, a maximal parenteral antimicrobial dose for 2–6 weeks followed by oral therapy, for a total duration of 6–12 months, is required for serious infections and bulky disease, whereas a shorter course may suffice for less extensive disease, particularly in the oral-cervicofacial region.

FURTHER READINGS

Clarridge JE III, Zhang Q: Genotypic diversity of clinical *Actinomyces* species: Phenotype, source, and disease correlation among genospecies. J Clin Microbiol 40:3442, 2002

Colmegna I et al: Disseminated *Actinomyces meyeri* infection resembling lung cancer with brain metastases. Am J Med Sci 326:152, 2003

Kayikcioglu F et al: *Actinomyces* infection in the female genital tract. Eur J Obstet Gynecol Reprod Biol 118:77, 2005

Lecouvet F et al: The etiologic diagnosis of infectious discitis is improved by amplification-based DNA analysis. Arthritis Rheum 50:2985, 2004

Pulverer G et al: Human cervicofacial actinomycoses: Microbiologic data for 1997 cases. Clin Infect Dis 37:490, 2003

Russo TA: Actinomycosis, in *Principles and Practice of Infectious Diseases*, 6th ed, GL Mandell et al (eds). New York, Churchill Livingstone, 2005, pp 2924–2934

CHAPTER 65

INFECTIONS DUE TO MIXED ANAEROBIC ORGANISMS

Dennis L. Kasper ■ Ronit Cohen-Poradosu

DEFINITIONS

Anaerobic bacteria are organisms that require reduced oxygen tension for growth, failing to grow on the surface of solid media in 10% CO_2 in air. (In contrast, *microaerophilic bacteria* can grow in an atmosphere of 10% CO_2 in air or under anaerobic or aerobic conditions, although they grow best in the presence of only a small amount of atmospheric oxygen, and *facultative bacteria* can grow in the presence or absence of air.) This chapter describes infections caused by nonsporulating anaerobic bacteria. In general, anaerobes associated with human infections are relatively aerotolerant. They can survive for as long as 72 h in the presence of oxygen, although generally they do not multiply in this environment. A far smaller number of pathogenic anaerobic bacteria (which are also part of the normal flora) die after brief contact with oxygen, even in low concentrations.

The nonsporulating anaerobic bacteria exist as components of the normal flora on the mucosal surfaces of humans and animals. The major reservoirs of these bacteria are the mouth, lower gastrointestinal (GI) tract, skin, and female genital tract (Table 65-1). Among the constituents of the oral flora, anaerobes are the predominant commensal organisms, ranging in concentration from 10^9/mL in saliva to 10^{12}/mL in gingival scrapings. In the oral cavity, the ratio of anaerobic to aerobic bacteria ranges from 1:1 on the surface of a tooth to 1000:1 in the gingival crevices. Anaerobic bacteria are not found in appreciable numbers in the normal upper intestine until the distal ileum. In the colon, the proportion of anaerobes increases significantly, as does the overall bacterial count. In the colon, for example, there are 10^{11}–10^{12} organisms per gram of stool, and >99% of these organisms are anaerobic, with an anaerobe-to-aerobe ratio of ~1000:1. In the female genital tract, there are ~10^9 organisms per milliliter of secretions, with an anaerobe-to-aerobe ratio of ~10:1.

Anaerobes play a key role in maintaining the balance between the host and its colonizing organisms. Hundreds of species of anaerobic bacteria have been identified as part of the normal flora of humans. Identification of as many as 500 anaerobic species in fecal specimens reflects the diversity of the anaerobic flora. Despite the complex array of bacteria in the normal flora, relatively few species are isolated commonly from human infection. Anaerobic infections occur when the harmonious relationship between the host and the bacteria is disrupted. Any site in the body is susceptible to infection with these indigenous organisms when a mucosal barrier or the skin is compromised by surgery, trauma, tumor, ischemia, or necrosis, all of which can reduce local tissue redox potentials. Because the sites that are colonized by anaerobes contain many species of bacteria, disruption of anatomic barriers allows the penetration of many organisms, resulting in mixed infections involving multiple species of anaerobes combined with facultative or microaerophilic organisms. Such mixed infections are seen in the head and neck (chronic sinusitis, chronic otitis media, Ludwig's angina, and periodontal abscesses). Brain abscesses and subdural empyema are the most common anaerobic infections of the central nervous system (CNS). Anaerobes are responsible for pleuropulmonary diseases such as aspiration pneumonia, necrotizing pneumonia, lung abscess, and empyema. These organisms also play an important role in various intraabdominal infections, such as peritonitis and intraabdominal and hepatic abscesses (Chap. 24). They are isolated frequently in female genital tract infections, such as salpingitis, pelvic peritonitis, tuboovarian abscess, vulvovaginal abscess, septic abortion, and endometritis (Chap. 28). Anaerobic bacteria are also found often in infections of the skin, soft tissues, and bones and in bacteremia.

ETIOLOGY

The taxonomic classification of anaerobes is rapidly evolving, with frequent changes in nomenclature based on newly discovered relationships among bacterial species. The major anaerobic gram-positive cocci that produce disease are *Peptostreptococcus* spp. The major species of this genus that are involved in infections are *Peptostreptococcus micros*, *P. magnus*, *P. asaccharolyticus*, *P. anaerobius*, and *P. prevotii*. Clostridia (Chap. 42) are gram-positive rods that are isolated from wounds, abscesses, sites of abdominal infection, and blood. The principal anaerobic gram-negative bacilli found in human infections are the *Bacteroides fragilis* group as well as *Fusobacterium*, *Prevotella*, and *Porphyromonas* spp. Other members of the Bacteroidaceae family include *Bilophila wadsworthia*, an organism that has been isolated from infected sites and has been reported to cause serious infections. Gram-positive anaerobic non–spore-forming bacilli are uncommon as

TABLE 65-1

ANAEROBIC HUMAN FLORA: AN OVERVIEW

ANATOMIC SITE	TOTAL BACTERIA[a]	AEROBIC/ ANAEROBIC RATIO	POTENTIAL PATHOGENS
Oral cavity			
Saliva	10^8–10^9	1:1	*Fusobacterium nucleatum*, *Prevotella melaninogenica*, *Prevotella oralis* group, *Bacteroides ureolyticus* group, *Peptostreptococcus* spp.
Tooth surface	10^{10}–10^{11}	1:1	
Gingival crevices	10^{11}–10^{12}	10^3:1	
Gastrointestinal tract			
Stomach	0–10^5	1:1	
Jejunum/ileum	10^4–10^7	1:1	
Terminal ileum and colon	10^{11}–10^{12}	10^3:1	*Bacteroides* spp. (principally members of the *B. fragilis* group), *Prevotella* spp., *Clostridium* spp., *Peptostreptococcus* spp.
Female genital tract	10^7–10^9	10:1	*Peptostreptococcus* spp., *Bacteroides* spp., *Prevotella bivia*

[a]Per gram or milliliter.

etiologic agents of human infection. *Propionibacterium acnes*, a rare cause of foreign-body infections, is one of the few nonclostridial gram-positive rods associated with infections.

The *B. fragilis* group contains the anaerobic pathogens most frequently isolated from clinical infections. Members of this group are part of the normal bowel flora; they include several distinct species, such as *B. fragilis*, *B. thetaiotaomicron*, *B. vulgatus*, *B. uniformis*, *B. ovatus*, and *Parabacteroides distasonis*. *B. fragilis* is the most important clinical isolate. However, in cultures of commensal fecal flora, *B. fragilis* is isolated in lower numbers than some of the other *Bacteroides* spp.

A second major group of phenotypically similar organisms is part of the indigenous oral flora. Thus these organisms are found at infected sites that can be seeded with oral microflora. Many of these species are pigment-producing bacteria belonging to two distinct genera, *Prevotella* and *Porphyromonas*; these genera comprise several pathogenic species, including *Porphyromonas gingivalis*, *Porphyromonas asaccharolytica*, and *Prevotella oralis*. *Porphyromonas* and *Prevotella* spp. cause localized infections that can spread contiguously.

In female genital tract infections, organisms normally colonizing the vagina (e.g., *Prevotella bivia* and *Prevotella disiens*) are the most frequent isolates, although *B. fragilis* is not uncommon. The *Fusobacterium* species *F. necrophorum*, *F. nucleatum*, and *F. varium*, which reside primarily in the oral cavity and the GI tract, are also isolated from clinical infections, including necrotizing pneumonia and abscesses. The skin flora contains anaerobic bacteria as well: *Propionibacterium* (mainly *P. acnes*) and peptostreptococci.

Infections caused by anaerobic bacteria most frequently are due to more than one organism. These polymicrobial infections may be caused by one or several anaerobic species or by a combination of anaerobic organisms and microaerophilic or facultative bacteria acting synergistically.

Approach to the Patient:
INFECTIONS DUE TO MIXED ANAEROBIC ORGANISMS

The physician must consider several points when approaching the patient with presumptive infection due to anaerobic bacteria.

1. Most of the organisms colonizing mucosal sites are harmless commensals; very few cause disease. When these organisms do cause disease, it often occurs in proximity to the mucosal site they colonize.
2. For anaerobes to cause tissue infection, they must spread beyond the normal mucosal barriers.
3. Conditions favoring the propagation of these bacteria, particularly a lowered oxidation-reduction potential, are necessary. These conditions exist at sites of trauma, tissue destruction, compromised vascular supply, and complications of preexisting infection, which produce necrosis.
4. There is a complex array of infecting flora. For example, as many as 12 types of organisms can be isolated from a suppurative site.
5. Anaerobic organisms tend to be found in abscess cavities or in necrotic tissue. The failure of an abscess to yield organisms on routine culture is a clue that the abscess is likely to contain anaerobic bacteria. Often smears of this "sterile pus" are found to be teeming with bacteria when Gram's stain is applied. Malodorous pus suggests anaerobic infection. Although some facultative organisms (e.g., *Staphylococcus aureus*) are also capable of causing abscesses, abscesses in organs or deeper body tissues should call to mind anaerobic infection.
6. Gas is found in many anaerobic infections of deep tissues but is not diagnostic because it can be produced by aerobic bacteria as well.

7. Although a putrid-smelling infection site or discharge is considered diagnostic for anaerobic infection, this manifestation usually develops late in the course and is present in only 30–50% of cases.
8. Some species (the best example being the *B. fragilis* group) require specific therapy. However, many synergistic infections can be cured with antibiotics directed at some but not all of the organisms involved. Antibiotic therapy, combined with debridement and drainage, disrupts the interdependent relationship among the bacteria, and some species that are resistant to the antibiotic do not survive without the co-infecting organisms.
9. Manifestations of severe sepsis and disseminated intravascular coagulation (DIC) are unusual in patients with purely anaerobic infection.

EPIDEMIOLOGY

Difficulties in the performance of appropriate cultures, contamination of cultures by aerobic bacteria or components of the normal flora, and the lack of readily available, reliable culture techniques have made it impossible to obtain accurate data on incidence or prevalence. However, anaerobic infections are encountered frequently in hospitals with active surgical, trauma, and obstetric and gynecologic services. Depending on the institution, anaerobic bacteria account for 0.5–12% of all cases of bacteremia.

PATHOGENESIS

Anaerobic bacterial infections usually occur when an anatomic barrier becomes disrupted and constituents of the local flora enter a site that was previously sterile. Because of the specific growth requirements of anaerobic organisms and their presence as commensals on mucosal surfaces, conditions must arise that allow these organisms to penetrate mucosal barriers and enter tissue with a lowered oxidation-reduction potential. Therefore, tissue ischemia, trauma, surgery, perforated viscus, shock, and aspiration provide environments conducive to the proliferation of anaerobes. In the case of a perforated viscus, hundreds of species of anaerobic bacteria are spilled into the peritoneal cavity, but many of these organisms are unable to survive because the highly vascularized tissue provides a sufficiently high redox potential. The entry of oxygen into the environment results in the selection of the more aerotolerant anaerobic organisms.

The ability of an organism to adhere to host tissues is important to the establishment of infection. Some oral species adhere to crevicular epithelium in the oral cavity. *Prevotella melaninogenica* actually attaches to other microorganisms; *P. gingivalis* is a common isolate in periodontal disease. These organisms have fimbriae that facilitate attachment. Some *Bacteroides* strains appear to be piliated, a characteristic that may account for their ability to adhere.

The most extensively studied virulence factor of the nonsporulating anaerobes is the capsular polysaccharide complex of *B. fragilis*. This organism is unique among anaerobes in its potential for virulence during growth at normally sterile sites. Although it constitutes only 0.5–1% of the normal colonic flora, *B. fragilis* is the anaerobe most commonly isolated from intraabdominal infections and bacteremia. One polysaccharide of *B. fragilis* possesses distinct biologic properties, such as the ability (owing to a unique zwitterionic motif of charged sugars) to promote abscess formation. Intraabdominal abscess induction is related to the capacity of the polysaccharide to stimulate the release of cytokines and chemokines—in particular, interleukin (IL) 8, IL-17, and tumor necrosis factor (TNF) α—from resident peritoneal cells. The release of cytokines and chemokines results in the chemotaxis of polymorphonuclear neutrophils (PMNs) into the peritoneum, where they adhere to mesothelial cells induced by TNF-α to upregulate their expression of intercellular adhesion molecule 1 (ICAM-1). PMNs adherent to ICAM-1–expressing cells probably represent the nidus for an abscess. Prophylactic or therapeutic administration of the polysaccharide to experimental animals confers protection against abscess induction after challenge with intestinal microorganisms capable of inducing abscesses. This protection is mediated by T cells controlling cytokine release; IL-10 appears to be the cytokine primarily responsible for downregulating the tissue response of abscess formation. Although abscesses constitute a host response that localizes and contains infecting bacteria, abscess formation in patients with sepsis often results in severe and chronic illness that requires surgical drainage in combination with antimicrobial therapy.

Anaerobic bacteria produce a number of exoproteins that are capable of enhancing the organisms' virulence. The collagenase produced by *P. gingivalis* may enhance tissue destruction. An enterotoxin has been identified in *B. fragilis* strains associated with diarrheal disease in animals and young children. Anaerobic gram-negative bacteria such as *B. fragilis* possess lipopolysaccharides (LPSs, endotoxins) that are 100–1000 times less biologically potent than endotoxins associated with aerobic gram-negative bacteria. This relative biologic inactivity may account for the lower frequency of DIC and purpura in *Bacteroides* bacteremia than in facultative and aerobic gram-negative bacillary bacteremia. An exception is the LPS from *Fusobacterium*, which may account for the severity of Lemierre's syndrome.

CLINICAL MANIFESTATIONS

Anaerobic Infections of the Mouth, Head, and Neck

(See also Chap. 16) Anaerobic bacteria are commonly involved in infections of the mouth, head, and neck. The predominant isolates are components of the normal flora of the upper airways—mainly the *Bacteroides oralis* group, pigmented *Prevotella* spp., *P. asaccharolytica*, *Fusobacterium* spp., peptostreptococci, and microaerophilic streptococci.

Soft tissue infections of the oral-facial area may or may not be odontogenic. Odontogenic infections—primarily dental caries and periodontal disease—are common and have both local consequences (especially tooth loss) and the potential for life-threatening spread to the deep fascial spaces of the head and neck. Infections of the mouth can arise from either the supragingival or the subgingival dental plaque composed of bacteria colonizing the tooth surface. Supragingival plaque formation begins with the adherence of gram-positive bacteria to the tooth surface. This form of plaque is influenced by salivary and dietary components, oral hygiene, and local host factors. Supragingival plaque can lead to dental caries and, with further invasion, to pulpitis (endodontic infection) that can further perforate the alveolar bone, causing periapical abscess. Subgingival plaque is associated with periodontal infections (e.g., gingivitis, periodontitis, and periodontal abscess) that can further disseminate to adjacent structures such as the mandible, causing osteomyelitis of the maxillary sinuses. Periodontitis may also result in spreading infection that can involve adjacent bone or soft tissues.

Necrotizing Ulcerative Gingivitis

Gingivitis may become a necrotizing infection (trench mouth, Vincent's stomatitis). The onset of disease is usually sudden and is associated with tender bleeding gums, foul breath, and a bad taste. The gingival mucosa, especially the papillae between the teeth, becomes ulcerated and may be covered by a gray exudate, which is removable with gentle pressure. Patients may become systemically ill, developing fever, cervical lymphadenopathy, and leukocytosis. Occasionally, ulcerative gingivitis can spread to the buccal mucosa, the teeth, and the mandible or maxilla, resulting in widespread destruction of bone and soft tissue. This infection is termed *acute necrotizing ulcerative mucositis* (cancrum oris, noma). It destroys tissue rapidly, causing the teeth to fall out and large areas of bone—or even the whole mandible—to be sloughed. A strong putrid odor is frequently detected, although the lesions are not painful. The gangrenous lesions eventually heal, leaving large disfiguring defects. This infection most commonly follows a debilitating illness or affects severely malnourished children. It has been known to complicate leukemia or to develop in individuals with a genetic deficiency of catalase.

Acute Necrotizing Infections of the Pharynx

These infections usually occur in association with ulcerative gingivitis. Symptoms include an extremely sore throat, foul breath, and a bad taste accompanied by fever and a sensation of choking. Examination of the pharynx demonstrates that the tonsillar pillars are swollen, red, ulcerated, and covered with a grayish membrane that peels easily. Lymphadenopathy and leukocytosis are common. The disease may last for only a few days or, if not treated, may persist for weeks. Lesions begin unilaterally but may spread to the other side of the pharynx or the larynx. Aspiration of the infected material by the patient can result in lung abscesses.

Peripharyngeal Space Infections

These infections arise from the spread of organisms from the upper airways to potential spaces formed by the fascial planes of the head and neck. The etiology is typically polymicrobial and represents the normal flora of the mucosa of the originating site.

Peritonsillar abscess (*quinsy*) is a complication of acute tonsillitis caused mainly by a mixed flora containing anaerobes and group A *Streptococcus*. In submandibular space infection (*Ludwig's angina*), 80% of cases are caused by infection of the tissues surrounding the second and third molar teeth. This infection results in marked local swelling of tissues, with pain, trismus, and superior and posterior displacement of the tongue. Submandibular swelling of the neck can impair swallowing and cause respiratory obstruction. In some cases, tracheotomy may be life-saving. *Cervicofacial actinomycosis* (Chap. 64) is caused by a branching, gram-positive, non–spore-forming, strict/facultative anaerobe that is a part of the normal oral flora. This chronic disease is characterized by abscesses, draining sinus tracts, fistula, bone destruction, and fibrosis. It can easily be mistaken for malignancy or granulomatous disease. Actinomycosis less frequently involves the thorax, abdomen, pelvis, and CNS.

Sinusitis and Otitis

Anaerobic bacteria have been implicated in chronic sinusitis but play little role in acute sinusitis. In chronic sinusitis, anaerobic bacteria are found in 0–52% of cases, depending on the method used to collect specimens. In one study, cultures of samples from patients with chronic sinusitis and patients with an acute exacerbation of chronic sinusitis yielded aerobes only in 25% and 27% of cases, respectively; anaerobes only in 34% and 37%; and mixed organisms in 41% and 37%. The predominant aerobic bacteria were Enterobacteriaceae and *S. aureus* in both groups; in addition, *Streptococcus pneumoniae* was commonly isolated from the acute-exacerbation group. The predominant anaerobic bacteria in both groups were *Peptostreptococcus* spp., *Fusobacterium* spp., anaerobic gram-negative bacilli, and *P. acnes*.

Anaerobic bacteria are much more easily implicated in chronic suppurative otitis media than in acute otitis media. Purulent exudate from chronically draining ears has been found to contain anaerobes, particularly *Bacteroides* spp., in up to 50% of cases. *B. fragilis* has been isolated from up to 28% of patients with chronic otitis media.

Complications of Anaerobic Head and Neck Infections

Contiguous craniad spread of these infections may result in osteomyelitis of the skull or mandible or in intracranial infections such as brain abscess and subdural empyema. Caudal spread can produce mediastinitis or pleuropulmonary infection. Hematogenous complications may also result from anaerobic infections of the head and neck. Bacteremia, which occasionally is polymicrobial, can lead to endocarditis or other distant infections. Lemierre's syndrome, which has been uncommon in the antimicrobial era, is an acute oropharyngeal infection with secondary septic thrombophlebitis of the internal jugular vein and frequent metastasis, most commonly to the lung. *F. necrophorum* is the usual cause. This infection typically begins with pharyngitis, which is followed by local invasion in the lateral pharyngeal space with resultant internal jugular vein thrombophlebitis. A typical clinical triad seen in recent series is pharyngitis, a tender/swollen neck, and noncavitating pulmonary infiltrates.

CNS Infections

CNS infections associated with anaerobic bacteria are brain abscess (Chap. 29), epidural abscess, and subdural empyema. Anaerobic meningitis is rare and is usually related to parameningeal collection or shunt infection. If optimal bacteriologic techniques are employed, as many as 85% of brain abscesses yield anaerobic bacteria, which usually originate from otolaryngeal infection. Commonly isolated are peptostreptococci, *Fusobacterium* spp., *Bacteroides* spp., and *Prevotella* spp. Facultative or microaerophilic streptococci and coliforms are often part of a mixed infecting flora in brain abscesses.

Pleuropulmonary Infections

Anaerobic pleuropulmonary infections result from the aspiration of oropharyngeal contents, often in the context of an altered state of consciousness or an absent gag reflex. Four clinical syndromes are associated with anaerobic pleuropulmonary infection produced by aspiration: simple aspiration pneumonia, necrotizing pneumonia, lung abscess, and empyema.

Aspiration Pneumonitis

Bacterial aspiration pneumonitis must be distinguished from two other clinical syndromes associated with aspiration that are not of bacterial etiology. One syndrome results from aspiration of solids, usually food. Obstruction of major airways typically results in atelectasis and moderate nonspecific inflammation. Therapy consists of removal of the foreign body.

The second aspiration syndrome is more easily confused with bacterial aspiration. *Mendelson's syndrome,* a chemical pneumonitis, results from regurgitation of stomach contents and aspiration of chemical material, usually acidic gastric juices. Pulmonary inflammation—including the destruction of the alveolar lining, with transudation of fluid into the alveolar space—occurs with remarkable rapidity. Typically this syndrome develops within hours, often after anesthesia when the gag reflex is depressed. The patient becomes tachypneic, hypoxic, and febrile. The leukocyte count may rise, and the chest x-ray may evolve suddenly from normal to a complete bilateral "whiteout" within 8–24 h. Sputum production is minimal. The pulmonary signs and symptoms can resolve quickly with symptom-based therapy or can culminate in respiratory failure, with the subsequent development of bacterial superinfection over a period of days. Antibiotic therapy is not indicated unless bacterial infection supervenes.

In contrast to these syndromes, bacterial aspiration pneumonia develops over a period of several days or weeks rather than hours. It is seen in patients who are hospitalized and have a depressed gag reflex, impaired swallowing, or a tracheal or nasogastric tube; elderly patients; and patients with transiently impaired consciousness in the wake of seizures, cerebrovascular accidents, or alcoholic blackouts. Patients who enter the hospital with this syndrome typically have been ill for several days and generally report low-grade fever, malaise, and sputum production. In some patients, weight loss and anemia reflect a more chronic process. Usually the history reveals factors predisposing to aspiration, such as alcohol overdose or residence in a nursing home. Examination sometimes yields evidence of periodontal disease. Sputum characteristically is not malodorous unless the process has been underway for at least a week. A mixed bacterial flora with many PMNs is evident on Gram's staining of sputum. Expectorated sputum is unreliable for anaerobic cultures because of inevitable contamination by normal oral flora. Reliable specimens for culture can be obtained by transtracheal or transthoracic aspiration—techniques that are rarely used at present. Culture of protected-brush specimens or bronchoalveolar lavage fluid obtained by bronchoscopy is controversial.

Chest x-rays show consolidation in dependent pulmonary segments: in the basilar segments of the lower lobes if the patient has aspirated while upright and in either the posterior segment of the upper lobe (usually on the right side) or the superior segment of the lower lobe if the patient has aspirated while supine. The organisms isolated from the lungs reflect the pharyngeal flora; pigmented and nonpigmented *Prevotella* spp., *Peptostreptococcus* spp., *Bacteroides* spp., *Fusobacterium* spp., and anaerobic cocci are the most common isolates. The patient who aspirates in the hospital may also have a mixed infection involving enteric gram-negative rods. In a study on the microbiology of severe aspiration pneumonia in institutionalized elderly patients, gram-negative bacilli were cultured in 49% of cases (with an anaerobe also recovered in 14% of this group), anaerobes in 16%, and *S. aureus* in 12%.

Necrotizing Pneumonitis

This form of anaerobic pneumonitis is characterized by numerous small abscesses that spread to involve several pulmonary segments. The process can be indolent or fulminating. This syndrome is less common than either aspiration pneumonia or lung abscess and includes features of both types of infection.

Anaerobic Lung Abscesses

These abscesses result from subacute anaerobic pulmonary infection. The clinical syndrome typically involves a history of constitutional signs and symptoms (including malaise, weight loss, fever, night sweats, and foul-smelling sputum), perhaps over a period of weeks (Chap. 17). Patients who develop lung abscesses characteristically have dental infection and periodontitis, but lung abscesses in edentulous patients have been reported. Abscess cavities may be single or multiple and generally occur in dependent pulmonary segments (Fig. 65-1). Anaerobic abscesses must be distinguished from lesions associated with tuberculosis, neoplasia, and other conditions. Oral anaerobes predominate and are found in 60–80% of cases. There is also an important role for microaerophilic streptococci such as *S. milleri. S. aureus* and enteric gram-negative bacilli may be found as well. Septic pulmonary emboli may originate from intraabdominal or female genital tract infections and can produce anaerobic pneumonia.

Empyema

Empyema is a manifestation of long-standing anaerobic pulmonary infection. The clinical presentation, which

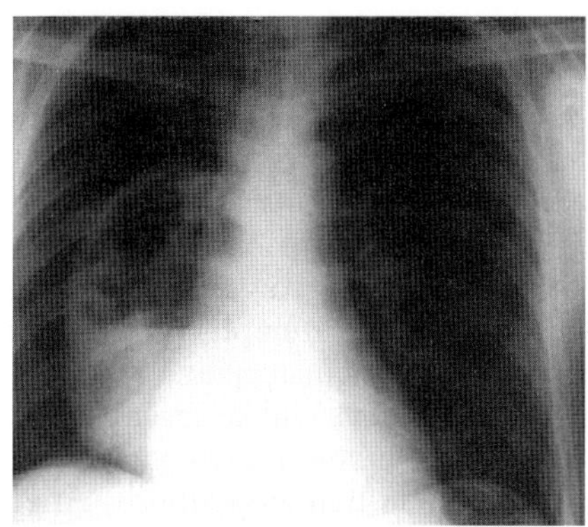

FIGURE 65-1

Chest radiograph of right-lower-lobe lung abscess in a 60-year-old alcoholic patient. [*From GL Mandell (ed): Atlas of Infectious Diseases, Vol VI. Philadelphia, Current Medicine Inc, Churchill Livingstone, 1996; with permission.*]

includes foul-smelling sputum, resembles that of other anaerobic pulmonary infections. Patients may report pleuritic chest pain and marked chest-wall tenderness.

Empyema may be masked by overlying pneumonitis and should be considered especially in cases of persistent fever despite antibiotic therapy. Diligent physical examination and the use of ultrasound to localize a loculated empyema are important diagnostic tools. The collection of a foul-smelling exudate by thoracentesis is typical. Cultures of infected pleural fluid yield an average of 3.5 anaerobes and 0.6 facultative or aerobic bacterial species. Drainage is required. Defervescence, a return to a feeling of well-being, and resolution of the process may require several months.

Extension from a subdiaphragmatic infection may also result in anaerobic empyema.

Intraabdominal Infections

Intraabdominal infections—mainly peritonitis and abscesses—are usually polymicrobial and represent the normal intestinal (especially colonic) flora. These infections usually follow a breach in the mucosal barrier occurring as a result of appendicitis, diverticulitis, neoplasm, inflammatory bowel disease, surgery, or trauma. On average, four to six species are isolated per specimen submitted to the microbiology laboratory, with a predominance of coliforms, anaerobes, and enterococci. The most common isolates are *Escherichia coli* and *B. fragilis.* Disease originating from proximal-bowel perforation reflects the flora of this site, with a predominance of aerobic and anaerobic gram-positive bacteria and *Candida.*

Enterotoxigenic *B. fragilis* has been associated with watery diarrhea in a few young children and adults. In case-control studies of children with undiagnosed diarrheal disease, enterotoxigenic *B. fragilis* was isolated from significantly more children with diarrhea than children in the control group. Neutropenic enterocolitis (typhlitis) has been associated with anaerobic infection of the cecum but—in the setting of neutropenia (Chap. 11)—may involve the entire bowel. Patients usually present with fever; abdominal pain, tenderness, and distention; and watery diarrhea. The bowel wall is edematous with hemorrhage and necrosis. The primary pathogen is thought by some authorities to be *Clostridium septicum*, but other clostridia and mixed anaerobic infections have also been implicated. More than 50% of patients developing early clinical signs can benefit from antibiotic therapy and bowel rest. Surgery is sometimes required to remove gangrenous bowel.

See Chap. 24 for a complete discussion of intraabdominal infections.

Pelvic Infections

The vagina of a healthy woman is one of the major reservoirs of anaerobic and aerobic bacteria. In the normal flora of the female genital tract, anaerobes outnumber aerobes by a ratio of ~10:1 and include anaerobic gram-positive cocci and *Bacteroides* spp. Anaerobes are isolated from most women with genital tract infections that are not caused by a sexually transmitted pathogen. The major anaerobic pathogens are *B. fragilis*, *P. bivia*, *P. disiens*, *P. melaninogenica*, anaerobic cocci, and *Clostridium* spp. Anaerobes are frequently encountered in tuboovarian abscess, septic abortion, pelvic abscess, endometritis, and postoperative wound infection, particularly after hysterectomy. Although these infections are often of mixed etiology, involving both anaerobes and coliforms, pure anaerobic infections without coliform or other facultative bacterial species occur more often in pelvic than in intraabdominal sites and are characterized by drainage of foul-smelling pus or blood from the uterus, generalized uterine or local pelvic tenderness, and continued fever and chills. Suppurative thrombophlebitis of the pelvic veins may complicate the infections and lead to repeated episodes of septic pulmonary emboli.

Anaerobic bacteria have been thought to be contributing factors in the etiology of bacterial vaginosis. This syndrome of unknown etiology is characterized by a profuse malodorous discharge and a change in the bacterial ecology that results in replacement of the *Lactobacillus*-dominated normal flora with an overgrowth of bacterial species including *Gardnerella vaginalis*, *Prevotella* spp., *Mobiluncus* spp., peptostreptococci, and genital mycoplasmas. A study based on 16S rRNA identification found other anaerobes that were predominant in cases but not in controls: *Atopobium, Leptotrichia, Megasphaera*, and *Eggerthella*. Anaerobic bacteria are thought to play a role in the etiology of pelvic inflammatory disease (Chap. 28), and several investigations have shown an association between bacterial vaginosis and the development of pelvic inflammatory disease.

Pelvic infections due to *Actinomyces* spp. have been associated with the use of intrauterine devices (Chap. 64).

Skin and Soft Tissue Infections

Injury to skin, bone, or soft tissue by trauma, ischemia, or surgery creates a suitable environment for anaerobic infections. These infections are most frequently found in sites prone to contamination with feces or with upper airway secretions—e.g., wounds associated with intestinal surgery, decubitus ulcers, or human bites. Deep soft-tissue infections associated with anaerobic bacteria are crepitant cellulitis, synergistic cellulitis, gangrene, and necrotizing fasciitis (Chaps. 21 and 42). Moreover, these organisms have been isolated from cutaneous abscesses, rectal abscesses, and axillary sweat gland infections (hidradenitis suppurativa). Anaerobes are frequently cultured from foot ulcers of diabetic patients.

These soft tissue or skin infections are usually polymicrobial. A mean of 4.8 bacterial species are isolated, with an anaerobe-to-aerobe ratio of ~3:2. The most frequently isolated organisms include *Bacteroides* spp., peptostreptococci, enterococci, clostridia, and *Proteus* spp. The involvement of anaerobes in these types of infections is associated with a higher frequency of fever, foul-smelling lesions, gas in the tissues, and visible foot ulcer.

Anaerobic bacterial synergistic gangrene (*Meleney's gangrene*), a rare infection of the superficial fascia, is characterized by exquisite pain, redness, and swelling followed by induration. Erythema surrounds a central zone of necrosis. A granulating ulcer forms at the original center as necrosis and erythema extend outward. Symptoms are limited to pain; fever is not typical. These infections usually involve a combination of *Peptostreptococcus* spp. and *S. aureus*; the usual site of infection is an abdominal surgical wound or the area surrounding an ulcer on an extremity. Treatment includes surgical removal of necrotic tissue and antimicrobial administration.

Necrotizing fasciitis, a rapidly spreading destructive disease of the fascia, is usually attributed to group A streptococci (Chap. 36), but can also be a mixed infection involving anaerobes and aerobes, usually after surgeries and in patients with diabetes or peripheral vascular disease. The most frequently isolated anaerobes in these infections are *Peptostreptococcus* and *Bacteroides* spp. Gas may be found in the tissues. Similarly, myonecrosis can be associated with mixed anaerobic infection. *Fournier's gangrene* consists of cellulitis involving the scrotum, perineum, and anterior abdominal wall, with mixed anaerobic organisms spreading along deep external fascial planes and causing extensive loss of skin.

Bone and Joint Infections

Although actinomycosis (Chap. 64) accounts on a worldwide basis for most anaerobic infections in bone, organisms including peptostreptococci or microaerophilic cocci, *Bacteroides* spp., *Fusobacterium* spp., and *Clostridium* spp. can also be involved. These infections frequently arise adjacent to soft tissue infections. Hematogenous seeding of bone is uncommon. *Prevotella* and *Porphyromonas* spp. are detected in infections involving the maxilla and mandible, whereas *Clostridium* spp. have been reported as anaerobic pathogens in cases of osteomyelitis of the long bones after fracture or trauma. Fusobacteria have been isolated in pure culture from sites of osteomyelitis adjacent to the perinasal sinuses. Peptostreptococci and microaerophilic cocci have been reported as significant pathogens in infections involving the skull, mastoid, and prosthetic implants placed in bone. In patients with osteomyelitis (Chap. 22), the most reliable culture specimen is a bone biopsy sample free of normal uninfected skin and subcutaneous tissue. In patients with anaerobic osteomyelitis, a mixed flora is frequently isolated from a bone biopsy specimen.

In cases of anaerobic septic arthritis, the most common isolates are *Fusobacterium* spp. Most of the patients involved have uncontrolled peritonsillar infections progressing to septic cervical venous thrombophlebitis (Lemierre's syndrome) and resulting in hematogenous dissemination with a predilection for the joints. Unlike anaerobic osteomyelitis, anaerobic pyoarthritis in most cases is not polymicrobial and may be acquired hematogenously. Anaerobes are important pathogens in infections involving prosthetic joints; in these infections, the causative organisms (such as *Peptostreptococcus* spp. and *P. acnes*) are part of the normal skin flora.

Bacteremia

Transient bacteremia is a well-known event in healthy people whose anatomic mucosal barriers have been injured (e.g., during dental extractions or dental scaling). These bacteremic episodes, which are often due to anaerobes, have no pathologic consequences. However, anaerobic bacteria are found in cultures of blood from clinically ill patients when proper culture techniques are used. Anaerobes have accounted for 0.5–12% of all bacteremias, depending on the institution. *B. fragilis* is the single most common anaerobic isolate from the bloodstream, accounting for 60–80% of anaerobic bacteremias.

In recent years, the rate of isolation of anaerobic bacteria from blood cultures has been decreasing. Studies from the 1970s and early 1980s found that 10–15% of positive blood cultures yielded anaerobes, whereas more recent surveys have found rates as low as 4%. This change may be related to the administration of antibiotic prophylaxis before intestinal surgery, the earlier recognition of localized infections, and the empirical use of broad-spectrum antibiotics for presumed infection. However, anaerobic bacteremia may be reemerging. Comparing two periods (1993–1996 and 2001–2004), investigators at the Mayo Clinics found a 74% increase in the incidence of anaerobic bacteremias per 100,000 patient-days; this finding contrasts with a 45% decrease in incidence from 1977 to 1988 at the same institution.

Once the organism in the blood has been identified, both the portal of bloodstream entry and the underlying problem that probably led to seeding of the bloodstream can often be deduced from an understanding of the organism's normal site of residence. For example, mixed anaerobic bacteremia including *B. fragilis* usually implies colonic pathology with mucosal disruption from neoplasia, diverticulitis, or some other inflammatory lesion. The initial manifestations are determined by the portal of entry and reflect the localized condition. When bloodstream invasion occurs, patients can become extremely ill, with rigors and hectic fevers. The clinical picture may be quite similar to that seen in sepsis involving aerobic gram-negative bacilli. Although complications of anaerobic bacteremia (e.g., septic thrombophlebitis and septic shock) have been reported, their incidence in association with anaerobic bacteremia is low. Anaerobic bacteremia is potentially fatal and requires rapid diagnosis and appropriate therapy. The mortality rate appears to increase with the age of the patient (with reported rates of >66% among patients >60 years old), with the isolation of multiple species from the bloodstream, and with the failure to surgically remove a focus of infection.

Endocarditis and Pericarditis

(See also Chap. 19) Endocarditis due to anaerobes is uncommon. However, anaerobic streptococci, which are often classified incorrectly, are responsible for this disease more frequently than is generally appreciated. Gram-negative anaerobes are unusual causes of endocarditis. Signs and symptoms of anaerobic endocarditis are similar to those of endocarditis due to facultative organisms. Mortality rates of 21–43% have been reported for anaerobic endocarditis.

Anaerobes, particularly *B. fragilis* and *Peptostreptococcus* spp., are uncommonly found in infected pericardial fluids. Anaerobic pericarditis is associated with a mortality rate of >50%.

DIAGNOSIS

There are three critical steps in the diagnosis of anaerobic infection: (1) proper specimen collection; (2) rapid transport of the specimens to the microbiology laboratory, preferably in anaerobic transport media; and (3) proper handling of the specimens by the laboratory. Specimens must be collected by meticulous sampling of infected sites, with avoidance of contamination by the normal flora. When such contamination is likely, the specimen is unacceptable. Examples of specimens unacceptable for anaerobic culture include sputum collected by expectoration or nasal tracheal suction, bronchoscopy specimens, samples collected directly through the vaginal vault, urine collected by voiding, and feces. Specimens appropriate for anaerobic culture include sterile body fluids such as blood, pleural fluid, peritoneal fluid, cerebrospinal fluid, and aspirates or biopsies from normally sterile sites.

Because even brief exposure to oxygen may kill some anaerobic organisms and result in failure to isolate them in the laboratory, air must be expelled from the syringe used to aspirate the abscess cavity, and the needle must be capped with a sterile rubber stopper. It is also important to remember that prior antibiotic therapy reduces cultivability of these bacteria. Specimens can be injected into transport bottles containing a reduced medium or taken immediately in syringes to the laboratory for direct culture on anaerobic media. In general, swabs should not be used. If a swab must be used, it should be placed in a reduced semisolid carrying medium before transport to the laboratory. Delays in transport may lead to a failure to isolate anaerobes due to exposure to oxygen or overgrowth of facultative organisms, which may eliminate or obscure any anaerobes that are present. All clinical specimens from suspected anaerobic infections should be Gram-stained and examined for organisms with characteristic morphology. It is not unusual for organisms to be observed on Gram's staining but not isolated in culture. If purulent materials are found to be sterile or organisms are seen on Gram's staining but do not grow in the culture, the involvement of anaerobes should be suspected.

Because of the time and difficulty involved in the isolation of anaerobic bacteria, diagnosis of anaerobic infections must frequently be based on presumptive evidence. Certain sites with lowered oxidation-reduction potential (e.g., avascular necrotic tissues) favor the diagnosis of an anaerobic infection. When infections occur in proximity to mucosal surfaces normally harboring an anaerobic flora, such as the GI tract, female genital tract, or oropharynx, anaerobes should be considered as potential etiologic agents. A foul odor is often indicative of anaerobes, which produce certain organic acids as they proliferate in necrotic tissue. Although these odors are nearly pathognomonic for anaerobic infection, the absence of odor does not exclude an anaerobic etiology. Because anaerobes often coexist with other bacteria to cause mixed or synergistic infection, Gram's staining of exudate frequently reveals numerous pleomorphic cocci and bacilli suggestive of anaerobes. Sometimes these organisms have morphologic characteristics associated with specific species.

The presence of gas in tissues is highly suggestive, but not diagnostic, of anaerobic infection. When cultures of obviously infected sites yield no growth, streptococci only, or a single aerobic species (such as *E. coli*) and Gram's staining reveals a mixed flora, the implication is that the anaerobic microorganisms failed to grow because of inadequate transport and/or culture techniques. Failure of an infection to respond to antibiotics that are not active against anaerobes (e.g., aminoglycosides and—in some circumstances—penicillin, cephalosporins, or tetracyclines) suggests an anaerobic etiology.

℞ Treatment: ANAEROBIC INFECTIONS

Successful therapy for anaerobic infections requires the administration of a combination of appropriate antibiotics, surgical resection, debridement of devitalized tissues, and drainage either by surgery or percutaneously (guided by an imaging technique such as CT, MRI, or ultrasound). Perforations must be closed promptly, closed spaces drained, tissue compartments decompressed, and an adequate blood supply established. Abscess cavities should be drained as soon as fluctuation or localization occurs.

ANTIBIOTIC THERAPY AND RESISTANCE

Decisions about the treatment of anaerobic infections with antibiotics are usually based on known resistance patterns in certain species, on the likelihood of encountering a given species in the case at hand, and on Gram's stain findings. Antibiotics active against clinically relevant anaerobes can be grouped into four categories on the basis of their predicted activity (Table 65-2). (Nearly all the drugs listed have toxic side effects, which are described in detail in Chap. 33.) In many infections, anaerobes are mixed with coliforms and other facultative

TABLE 65-2

ANTIMICROBIAL THERAPY FOR INFECTIONS INVOLVING COMMONLY ENCOUNTERED ANAEROBIC GRAM-NEGATIVE RODS

CATEGORY 1 (<2% RESISTANCE)	CATEGORY 2 (<15% RESISTANCE)	CATEGORY 3 (VARIABLE RESISTANCE)	CATEGORY 4 (RESISTANCE)
Carbapenems (imipenem, meropenem) Metronidazole[a] β-Lactam/β-lactamase inhibitor combination (ampicillin/sulbactam, ticarcillin/clavulanic acid, piperacillin/tazobactam) Chloramphenicol[b]	Cephamycins Clindamycin High-dose antipseudomonal penicillins	Penicillin Cephalosporins Tetracycline Vancomycin Erythromycin Tigecycline Newer quinolones (moxifloxacin)	Aminoglycosides Monobactams Trimethoprim-sulfamethoxazole

[a]Usually needs to be given in combination with aerobic bacterial coverage. For infections originating below the diaphragm, aerobic gram-negative coverage is essential. For infections from an oral source, aerobic gram-positive coverage is added. Metronidazole also is not active against *Actinomyces*, *Propionibacterium*, or other gram-positive non–spore-forming bacilli (e.g., *Eubacterium*, *Bifidobacterium*) and is unreliable against peptostreptococci.

[b]Chloramphenicol is probably not as effective as other category 1 antimicrobials in treating anaerobic infections.

organisms. The best therapeutic regimens, therefore, are usually those active against both aerobic and anaerobic bacteria. The choice of empirical antibiotics for the anaerobes in mixed infections can nearly always be made reliably, since patterns of antimicrobial susceptibility are usually predictable (Chap. 33 and Table 65-2).

Antibiotic susceptibility testing of anaerobic bacteria has been difficult and controversial. Owing to the slow growth rate of many anaerobes, the lack of standardized testing methods and of clinically relevant standards for resistance, and the generally good results obtained with empirical therapy, there has been limited interest in testing these organisms for antibiotic susceptibility. However, a recent study of antibiotic-treated patients with *Bacteroides* isolates from blood found mortality rates of 45% among those whose isolates were deemed resistant to the agent used and 16% among those whose isolates were deemed sensitive. These figures suggest that in vitro susceptibility testing should be performed for *Bacteroides* isolates from hospitalized patients with bacteremia and that the results of this testing should guide treatment. In general, cure rates of >80% can be attained among *Bacteroides*-infected patients with appropriate antimicrobial therapy and drainage. Of the drugs active against most clinically relevant anaerobes, metronidazole, β-lactam/β-lactamase inhibitor combinations, and carbapenems are preferred.

Antibiotic resistance in anaerobic bacteria is an increasing problem. Nearly all organisms in the *B. fragilis* group (>97%) are resistant to penicillin G. The cephamycins (cefoxitin and cefotetan) are more active against this group, but resistance rates between 8% and 14% were observed between 1987 and 2000. Rates of resistance to β-lactam agents among anaerobes other than *Bacteroides* are lower but highly variable. β-Lactam/β-lactamase inhibitor combinations such as ampicillin/sulbactam, ticarcillin/clavulanic acid, and piperacillin/tazobactam are usually a good option. Metronidazole is active against gram-negative anaerobes, including the *B. fragilis* group; resistance is rare but has been reported. Resistance to metronidazole is more common among gram-positive anaerobes, including *P. acnes*, *Actinomyces* spp., lactobacilli, and anaerobic streptococci. In the United States, rates of clindamycin resistance among isolates of the *B. fragilis* group increased from 3% in 1982 to 16% in 1996 and 26% in 2000, with figures as high as 44% in some series. Rates of resistance to clindamycin among non-*Bacteroides* anaerobes are much lower (<10%).

If a patient fails to respond to one of the category 1 or category 2 drugs (Table 65-2), consideration should be given to alternative therapy and to determination of the resistance patterns among *Bacteroides* isolates. Although in vitro resistance of *Bacteroides* spp. to chloramphenicol has not been reported, this drug may not be as effective as other category 1 drugs. Newer available options include tigecycline, the first glycylcycline to be approved by the U.S. Food and Drug Administration. Tigecycline is active against some anaerobic bacteria, including *Peptostreptococcus* spp., *Propionibacterium* spp., *Prevotella* spp., *Fusobacterium* spp., and most *Bacteroides* spp. Its efficacy for treatment of intraabdominal infections was comparable to that of imipenem in two phase 2 clinical trials. Data from in vitro susceptibility studies and clinical trials suggest that the newer fluoroquinolones (e.g., moxifloxacin and gemifloxacin) will be useful in the treatment of mixed aerobic-anaerobic infections. However, these drugs exhibit relatively weak in vitro activity against many *Bacteroides* spp. other than *B. fragilis*, including *B. thetaiotaomicron, B. vulgatus, and B. uniformis.*

TREATMENT OF INFECTIONS AT SPECIFIC SITES In clinical situations, specific regimens must be tailored to the initial site of infection. The duration of therapy also depends on the infection site; the reader is referred to specific chapters on sites of infection for recommendations.

β-Lactamase production has been reported in anaerobic strains that are usually isolated from infections originating above the diaphragm. Up to 60% of clinical isolates classified as *Prevotella* or *Porphyromonas* spp., non–*B. fragilis* species of *Bacteroides*, or *Fusobacterium* spp. reportedly produce β-lactamase. The clinical significance of resistance in these organisms has been suggested by studies showing clindamycin to be superior to penicillin (which for many years was considered the therapeutic "gold standard") for the treatment of lung abscesses. Presumably, the success of clindamycin is attributable to a broader spectrum of activity against oral anaerobes; thus a combination of penicillin and metronidazole or another antibiotic combination that is active against both oral anaerobes and aerobes is likely to be as effective as clindamycin. Bronchoscopy in lung abscess is indicated only to rule out airway obstruction and does not enhance drainage; in any event, it should be delayed until the antimicrobial regimen has begun to affect the disease process so that the procedure does not spread the infection. Surgery is almost never indicated because of the danger of spilling the abscess contents into the lungs.

Although many oral anaerobic infections and most cases of anaerobic pneumonia still respond to penicillin therapy, some infections due to oral organisms fail to respond to this drug, and in these cases the use of a drug that is effective against penicillin-resistant anaerobes is recommended (Table 65-2). Life-threatening infections involving the anaerobic flora of the mouth, such as space infections of the head and neck, should be treated empirically as if penicillin-resistant anaerobes are involved. Less serious infections involving the oral microflora can be treated with penicillin alone; metronidazole can be added (or clindamycin can be substituted) if the patient responds poorly to penicillin therapy. Combinations of antibiotics used to treat mixed infections of oral origin must include drugs active against the gram-positive aerobic flora of the mouth.

Chloramphenicol has been used successfully against anaerobic CNS infections at doses of 30–60 mg/kg per day, with the exact dose depending on the severity of illness. However, penicillin G and metronidazole also cross the blood-brain barrier and are bactericidal for many anaerobic organisms (Chap. 29).

Anaerobic infections arising below the diaphragm (e.g., colonic and intraabdominal infections) must be treated specifically with agents active against *Bacteroides* spp. (Table 65-2). In intraabdominal sepsis (Chap. 24), the use of antibiotics effective against penicillin-resistant anaerobes has clearly reduced the incidence of postoperative infections and serious infectious complications. Specifically, a drug from category 1 (Table 65-2) must be included for broad-spectrum coverage. Recommended doses for commonly used category 1 drugs are given in Table 65-3. Therapy for intraabdominal sepsis must also include drugs active against the gram-negative aerobic flora of the bowel. If the involvement of gram-positive bacteria such as enterococci is suspected, either ampicillin or vancomycin should be added. A meta-analysis of 40 randomized or quasi-randomized controlled trials of 16 antibiotic regimens for secondary peritonitis showed equivalent clinical success for all regimens.

TABLE 65-3

DOSES AND SCHEDULES FOR TREATMENT OF SERIOUS INFECTIONS DUE TO COMMONLY ENCOUNTERED ANAEROBIC GRAM-NEGATIVE RODS

FIRST-LINE THERAPY	DOSE	SCHEDULE[a]
Metronidazole[b]	500 mg	q6h
Ticarcillin/clavulanic acid	3.1 g	q4h
Piperacillin/tazobactam	3.375 g	q6h
Imipenem	0.5 g	q6h
Meropenem	1.0 g	q8h

[a]See disease-specific chapters for recommendations on duration of therapy.

[b]Should generally be used in conjunction with drugs active against aerobic or facultative organisms.

Note: All drugs are given by the IV route.

Cases of anaerobic osteomyelitis in which a mixed flora is isolated from a bone biopsy specimen should be treated with a regimen that covers all the isolates. When an anaerobic organism is recognized as a major or sole pathogen infecting a joint, the duration of treatment should be similar to that used for arthritis caused by aerobic bacteria (Chap. 23). Therapy includes the management of underlying disease states, the administration of appropriate antimicrobial agents, temporary joint immobilization, percutaneous drainage of effusions, and (usually) the removal of infected prostheses or internal fixation devices. Surgical drainage and debridement procedures such as sequestrectomy are essential for the removal of necrotic tissue that can sustain anaerobic infections.

The outcome of anaerobic bacteremia is significantly better in patients either initially given or switched to appropriate therapy based on known antibiotic susceptibilities.

FAILURE OF THERAPY Anaerobic infections that fail to respond to treatment or that relapse should be reassessed. Consideration should be given to additional surgical drainage or debridement. Superinfections with resistant gram-negative facultative or aerobic bacteria should be ruled out. The possibility of drug resistance must be entertained; if resistance is involved, repeated cultures may yield the pathogenic organism.

SUPPORTIVE MEASURES Other supportive measures in the management of anaerobic infections include careful attention to fluid and electrolyte balance (since extensive local edema may lead to hypoalbuminemia), hemodynamic support for septic shock, immobilization of infected extremities, maintenance of adequate nutrition during chronic infections by parenteral hyperalimentation, relief of pain, and anticoagulation with heparin for thrombophlebitis. For patients with severe anaerobic infections of soft tissues, hyperbaric oxygen therapy is advocated by some experts, but its value has not been proven in controlled trials.

FURTHER READINGS

ALDRIDGE KE et al: Bacteremia due to *Bacteroides fragilis* group: Distribution of species, beta-lactamase production and antimicrobial susceptibility patterns. Antimicrob Agents Chemother 47:148, 2003

KURIYAMA T et al: Antimicrobial susceptibility of 800 anaerobic isolates from patients with dentoalveolar infection to 13 oral antibiotics. Oral Microbiol Immunol 22:285, 2007

LASSMAN B et al: Reemergence of anaerobic bacteremia. Clin Infect Dis 44:895, 2007

LIU CY et al: Increasing trends in antimicrobial resistance among clinically important anaerobes and *Bacteroides fragilis* causing nosocomial infections: Emerging resistance to carbapenems. Antimicrob Agents Chemother 52:3161, 2008

MAZMANIAN SK et al: The love-hate relationship between bacterial polysaccharides and the immune system. Nat Rev Immunol 6:849, 2006

SALONEN JH et al: Clinical significance and outcome of anaerobic bacteremia. Clin Infect Dis 26:1413, 1998

SNYDMAN DR et al: National survey on the susceptibility of *Bacteroides fragilis* group: Report and analysis of trends in the United States from 1997 to 2004. Antimicrob Agents Chemother 51:1649, 2007

SOLOMKIN JS et al: Guidelines for the selection of anti-infective agents for complicated intra-abdominal infections. Clin Infect Dis 37:997, 2003

TZIANABOS AO et al: Anaerobic infections: General concepts, in *Principles and Practice of Infectious Diseases*, 6th ed, GL Mandell et al (eds). Philadelphia, Elsevier Churchill Livingstone, 2005, pp 2810–2816

PART 5 MYCOBACTERIAL DISEASES

CHAPTER 66

TUBERCULOSIS

Mario C. Raviglione ■ Richard J. O'Brien

Tuberculosis, one of the oldest diseases known to affect humans, is a major cause of death worldwide. This disease, which is caused by bacteria of the *Mycobacterium tuberculosis* complex, usually affects the lungs, although other organs are involved in up to one-third of cases. If properly treated, tuberculosis caused by drug-susceptible strains is curable in virtually all cases. If untreated, the disease may be fatal within 5 years in 50–65% of cases. Transmission usually takes place through the airborne spread of droplet nuclei produced by patients with infectious pulmonary tuberculosis.

ETIOLOGIC AGENT

Mycobacteria belong to the family Mycobacteriaceae and the order Actinomycetales. Of the pathogenic species belonging to the *M. tuberculosis* complex, the most common and important agent of human disease is *M. tuberculosis*. The complex includes *M. bovis* (the bovine tubercle bacillus—characteristically resistant to pyrazinamide, once an important cause of tuberculosis transmitted by unpasteurized milk, and currently the cause of a small percentage of cases worldwide), *M. caprae* (related to *M. bovis*), *M. africanum* (isolated from cases in West, Central, and East Africa), *M. microti* (the "vole" bacillus, a less virulent and rarely encountered organism), *M. pinnipedii* (a bacillus infecting seals and sea lions in the southern hemisphere and recently isolated from humans), and *M. canettii* (a rare isolate from East African cases that produces unusual smooth colonies on solid media and is considered closely related to a supposed progenitor type).

M. tuberculosis is a rod-shaped, non–spore-forming, thin aerobic bacterium measuring 0.5 μm by 3 μm. Mycobacteria, including *M. tuberculosis*, are often neutral on Gram's staining. However, once stained, the bacilli cannot be decolorized by acid alcohol; this characteristic justifies their classification as acid-fast bacilli (AFB; Fig. 66-1). Acid fastness is due mainly to the organisms' high content of mycolic acids, long-chain cross-linked fatty acids, and other cell-wall lipids. Microorganisms other than mycobacteria that display some acid fastness include

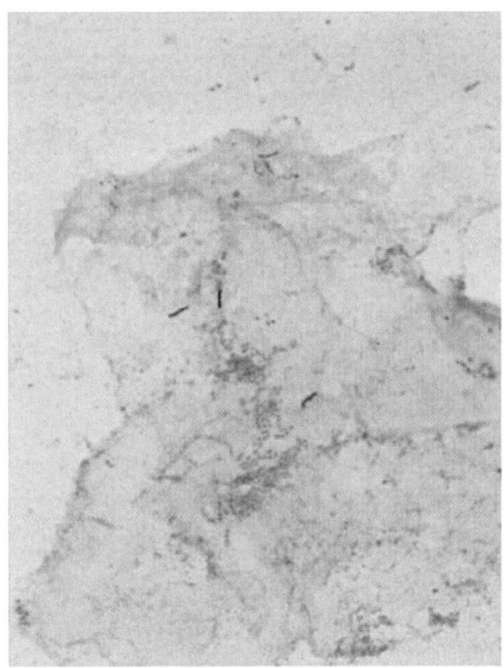

FIGURE 66-1
Acid-fast bacillus smear showing *M. tuberculosis* bacilli. (*Courtesy of the CDC, Atlanta.*)

species of *Nocardia* and *Rhodococcus*, *Legionella micdadei*, and the protozoa *Isospora* and *Cryptosporidium*. In the mycobacterial cell wall, lipids (e.g., mycolic acids) are linked to underlying arabinogalactan and peptidoglycan. This structure confers very low permeability of the cell wall, thus reducing the effectiveness of most antibiotics. Another molecule in the mycobacterial cell wall, lipoarabinomannan, is involved in the pathogen-host interaction and facilitates the survival of *M. tuberculosis* within macrophages. The complete genome sequence of *M. tuberculosis* comprises 4043 genes encoding 3993 proteins and 50 genes encoding RNAs; its high guanine-plus-cytosine content (65.6%) is indicative of an aerobic lifestyle. A large proportion of genes are devoted to the production of enzymes involved in cell wall metabolism.

EPIDEMIOLOGY

More than 5 million new cases of tuberculosis (all forms, both pulmonary and extrapulmonary) were reported to the World Health Organization (WHO) in 2005; >90% of cases were reported from developing countries. However, because of insufficient case detection and incomplete notification, reported cases represent only ~60% of total estimated cases. The WHO estimated that 8.8 million new cases of tuberculosis occurred worldwide in 2005, 95% of them in developing countries of Asia (4.9 million), Africa (2.6 million), the Middle East (0.6 million), and Latin America (0.4 million). It is further estimated that 1.6 million deaths from tuberculosis occurred in 2005, 95% of them in developing countries. Estimates of tuberculosis incidence rates (per 100,000 population) and numbers of tuberculosis-related deaths in 2005 are depicted in Fig. 66-2 and Fig. 66-3, respectively.

During the late 1980s and early 1990s, numbers of reported cases of tuberculosis increased in industrialized

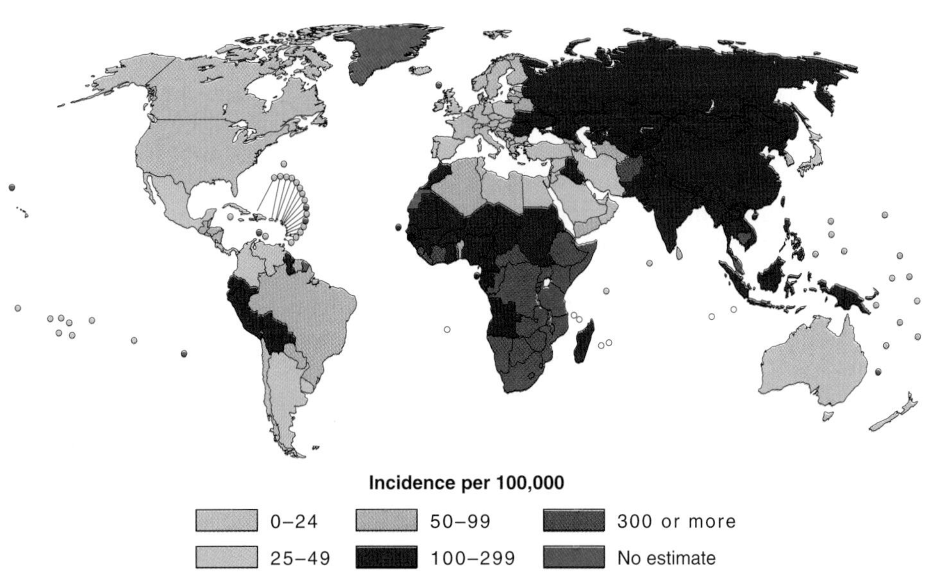

FIGURE 66-2
Estimated tuberculosis incidence rates (per 100,000 population) in 2005. The designations employed and the presentation of material on this map do not imply the expression of any opinion whatsoever on the part of the WHO concerning the legal status of any country, territory, city, or area or of its authorities or concerning the delimitation of its frontiers or boundaries. White lines on maps represent approximate border lines for which there may not yet be full agreement. (*Courtesy of the Stop TB Department, WHO; with permission.*)

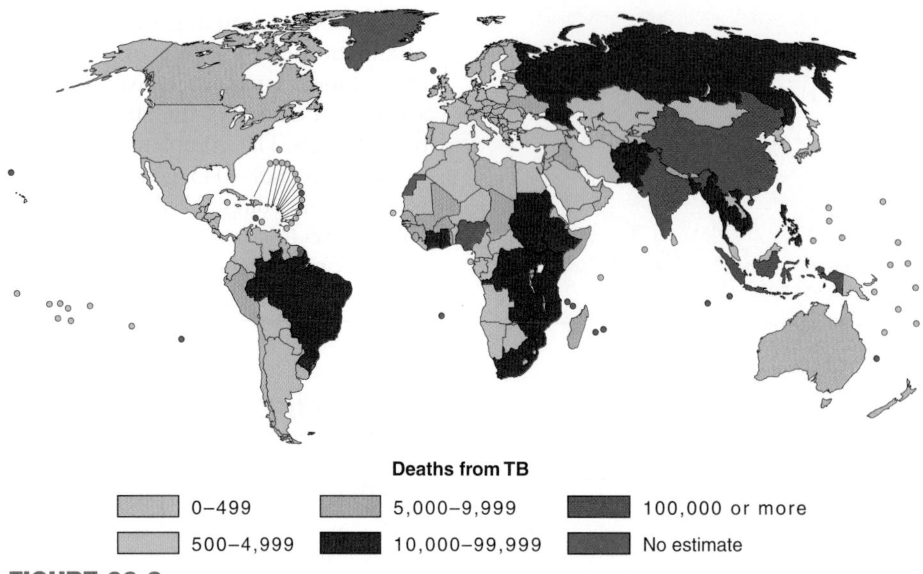

FIGURE 66-3

Estimated numbers of tuberculosis-related deaths in 2005. *(See also disclaimer in Fig. 66-2. Courtesy of the Stop TB Department, WHO; with permission.)*

countries. These increases were related largely to immigration from countries with a high prevalence of tuberculosis; infection with HIV; social problems, such as increased urban poverty, homelessness, and drug abuse; and dismantling of tuberculosis services. During the past few years, numbers of reported cases have begun to decline again or stabilized in industrialized nations. In the United States, with the implementation of stronger control programs, the decrease resumed in 1993. In 2005, 14,097 cases of tuberculosis (4.8 cases per 100,000 population) were reported to the Centers for Disease Control and Prevention (CDC).

In the United States, tuberculosis is uncommon among young adults of European descent, who have only rarely been exposed to *M. tuberculosis* infection during recent decades. In contrast, because of a high risk in the past, the prevalence of *M. tuberculosis* infection is relatively high among elderly Caucasians, who remain at increased risk of developing active tuberculosis. Tuberculosis in the United States is also a disease of young adult members of the HIV-infected, immigrant, and disadvantaged/marginalized populations. Similarly, in Europe, tuberculosis has reemerged as an important public health problem, mainly as a result of cases among immigrants from high-prevalence countries.

Recent data on trends indicate that in 2005, tuberculosis incidence was stable or falling in most regions; the result is a small decline globally from figures in previous years. This global reduction is due largely to an apparent peaking in Sub-Saharan Africa, where incidence had risen steeply since the 1980s as a result of the HIV epidemic and the paucity of health services. In eastern Europe, incidence increased during the 1990s because of deterioration in socioeconomic conditions and the health care infrastructure; however, after peaking in 2001, incidence has recently stabilized.

FROM EXPOSURE TO INFECTION

M. tuberculosis is most commonly transmitted from a person with infectious pulmonary tuberculosis to others by droplet nuclei, which are aerosolized by coughing, sneezing, or speaking. The tiny droplets dry rapidly; the smallest (<5–10 μm in diameter) may remain suspended in the air for several hours and may reach the terminal air passages when inhaled. There may be as many as 3000 infectious nuclei per cough. Other routes of transmission of tubercle bacilli (e.g., through the skin or the placenta) are uncommon and of no epidemiologic significance.

The probability of contact with a person who has an infectious form of tuberculosis, the intimacy and duration of that contact, the degree of infectiousness of the case, and the shared environment in which the contact takes place are all important determinants of the likelihood of transmission. Several studies of close-contact situations have clearly demonstrated that tuberculosis patients whose sputum contains AFB visible by microscopy are the most likely to transmit the infection. The most infectious patients have cavitary pulmonary disease or, much less commonly, laryngeal tuberculosis and produce sputum containing as many as 10^5–10^7 AFB/mL. Patients with sputum smear–negative/culture-positive tuberculosis are less infectious, and those with culture-negative pulmonary disease and extrapulmonary tuberculosis are essentially noninfectious. Because persons with both HIV infection and tuberculosis are less likely to have cavitations, they may be less infectious than persons without HIV co-infection. Crowding in poorly ventilated rooms is one of the most important factors in the transmission of tubercle bacilli, since it increases the intensity of contact with a case.

In short, the risk of acquiring *M. tuberculosis* infection is determined mainly by exogenous factors. Because of delays in seeking care and in making a diagnosis, it is estimated that, in high-prevalence settings, up to 20 contacts may be infected by each AFB-positive case before the index case is found to have tuberculosis.

FROM INFECTION TO DISEASE

Unlike the risk of acquiring infection with *M. tuberculosis*, the risk of developing disease after being infected depends largely on endogenous factors, such as the individual's innate immunologic and nonimmunologic defenses and level of function of cell-mediated immunity (CMI). Clinical illness directly after infection is classified as *primary tuberculosis* and is common among children up to 4 years of age and among immunocompromised persons. Although primary tuberculosis may be severe and disseminated, it is not generally associated with high-level transmissibility. When infection is acquired later in life, the chance is greater that the mature immune system will contain it at least temporarily. The majority of infected individuals who ultimately develop tuberculosis do so within the first year or two after infection. Dormant bacilli, however, may persist for years before reactivating to produce *secondary* (or *postprimary*) *tuberculosis*, which, because of frequent cavitation, is more often infectious than is primary disease. Overall, it is estimated that up to 10% of infected persons will eventually develop active tuberculosis in their lifetime. The risk is much higher among HIV-infected persons. Reinfection of a previously infected individual, which is common in areas with high rates of tuberculosis transmission, may also favor the development of disease. At the height of the tuberculosis resurgence in the United States in the early 1990s, molecular typing and comparison of strains of *M. tuberculosis* suggested that up to one-third of cases of active tuberculosis in some inner-city communities were due to recent transmission rather than to reactivation of latent infection.

Age is an important determinant of the risk of disease after infection. Among infected persons, the incidence of tuberculosis is highest during late adolescence and early adulthood; the reasons are unclear. The incidence among women peaks at 25–34 years of age. In this age group, rates among women may be higher than those among men, whereas at older ages, the opposite is true. The risk may increase in the elderly, possibly because of waning immunity and comorbidity.

A variety of diseases and conditions favor the development of active tuberculosis (Table 66-1). The most potent risk factor for tuberculosis among infected individuals is clearly HIV co-infection, which suppresses cellular immunity. The risk that latent *M. tuberculosis* infection will proceed to active disease is directly related to the patient's degree of immunosuppression. In a study of HIV-infected, tuberculin skin test (TST)–positive persons, this risk varied from 2.6 to 13.3 cases per 100 person-years and increased as the CD4+ T-cell count decreased.

TABLE 66-1

RISK FACTORS FOR ACTIVE TUBERCULOSIS AMONG PERSONS WHO HAVE BEEN INFECTED WITH TUBERCLE BACILLI

FACTOR	RELATIVE RISK/ODDS[a]
Recent infection (<1 year)	12.9
Fibrotic lesions (spontaneously healed)	2–20
Comorbidity	
HIV infection	100
Silicosis	30
Chronic renal failure/hemodialysis	10–25
Diabetes	2–4
Intravenous drug use	10–30
Immunosuppressive treatment	10
Gastrectomy	2–5
Jejunoileal bypass	30–60
Posttransplantation period (renal, cardiac)	20–70
Malnutrition and severe underweight	2

[a]Old infection = 1.

NATURAL HISTORY OF DISEASE

Studies conducted in various countries before the advent of chemotherapy showed that untreated tuberculosis is often fatal. About one-third of patients died within 1 year after diagnosis, and one-half died within 5 years. The 5-year mortality rate among sputum smear–positive cases was 65%. Of the survivors at 5 years, ~60% had undergone spontaneous remission, whereas the remainder were still excreting tubercle bacilli.

With effective, timely, and proper chemotherapy, patients have a very high chance of being cured. However, improper use of antituberculosis drugs, while reducing mortality rates, may also result in large numbers of chronic infectious cases, often with drug-resistant bacilli.

PATHOGENESIS AND IMMUNITY

INFECTION AND MACROPHAGE INVASION

The interaction of *M. tuberculosis* with the human host begins when droplet nuclei containing microorganisms from infectious patients are inhaled. Although the majority of inhaled bacilli are trapped in the upper airways and expelled by ciliated mucosal cells, a fraction (usually <10%) reach the alveoli. There, alveolar macrophages that have not yet been activated phagocytize the bacilli. Invasion of macrophages by mycobacteria results largely from binding of the bacterial cell wall with a variety of macrophage cell-surface molecules, including complement receptors, mannose receptor, immunoglobulin GFcγ receptor, and type A scavenger receptors. Phagocytosis is enhanced by complement activation leading to opsonization of bacilli with C3 activation products such as C3b. After a phagosome forms, the survival of *M. tuberculosis* within it seems to depend on reduced acidification due to lack of accumulation of vesicular proton-adenosine triphosphatase. A complex series of events is probably generated by the bacterial cell-wall glycolipid lipoarabinomannan (LAM). LAM inhibits the intracellular increase of Ca^{2+}. Thus the Ca^{2+}/calmodulin pathway (leading to phagosome-lysosome fusion) is impaired, and the bacilli may survive within the phagosomes. If the bacilli are successful in arresting phagosome maturation, then replication begins and the macrophage eventually ruptures and releases its bacillary contents.

VIRULENCE OF TUBERCLE BACILLI

Several genes thought to confer virulence to *M. tuberculosis* have been identified. The *katG* gene encodes for catalase/peroxidase enzymes that protect against oxidative stress; *rpoV* is the main sigma factor initiating transcription of several genes. Defects in these two genes result in loss of virulence. The *erp* gene, encoding a protein required for multiplication, also contributes to virulence. Strains of the Beijing/W genotype family have been identified in outbreak conditions in a variety of settings worldwide and have been associated with higher mortality rates and occasionally with multidrug resistance.

INNATE RESISTANCE TO INFECTION

Several observations suggest that genetic factors play a key role in innate nonimmune resistance to infection with *M. tuberculosis* and the development of disease. The existence of this resistance, which is polygenic in nature, is suggested by the differing degrees of susceptibility to tuberculosis in different populations. In mice, a gene called *Nramp1* (natural resistance–associated macrophage protein 1) plays a regulatory role in resistance/susceptibility to mycobacteria. The human homologue NRAMP1, which maps to chromosome 2q, may play a role in determining susceptibility to tuberculosis, as is suggested by a study among West Africans. Polymorphisms in multiple genes, such as those encoding for histocompatibility leukocyte antigen (HLA), interferon γ (IFN-γ), T-cell growth factor β (TGF-β), interleukin (IL) 10, mannose-binding protein, IFN-γ receptor, Toll-like receptor (TLR) 2, vitamin D receptor, and IL-1, have been associated with susceptibility to tuberculosis.

THE HOST RESPONSE

In the initial stage of host-bacterium interaction, either fusion between phagosomes and lysosomes occurs, preventing bacillary survival, or the bacilli begin to multiply, ultimately killing the macrophage. A variety of chemoattractants that are released after cell lysis (e.g., complement components, bacterial molecules, and cytokines) recruit additional immature monocyte-derived macrophages, including dendritic cells, which migrate to the draining lymph nodes and present mycobacterial antigens to T lymphocytes. At this point, the development of CMI and humoral immunity begins. These initial stages of infection are usually asymptomatic.

About 2–4 weeks after infection, two host responses to *M. tuberculosis* develop: a macrophage-activating CMI response and a tissue-damaging response. The *macrophage-activating response* is a T-cell–mediated phenomenon resulting in the activation of macrophages that are capable of killing and digesting tubercle bacilli. The *tissue-damaging response* is the result of a delayed-type hypersensitivity (DTH) reaction to various bacillary antigens; it destroys unactivated macrophages that contain multiplying bacilli but also causes caseous necrosis of the involved tissues (see below). Although both of these responses can inhibit mycobacterial growth, it is the balance between the two that determines the form of tuberculosis that will develop subsequently.

GRANULOMA FORMATION

With the development of specific immunity and the accumulation of large numbers of activated macrophages at the site of the primary lesion, granulomatous lesions (tubercles) are formed. These lesions consist of accumulations of lymphocytes and activated macrophages that evolve toward epithelioid and giant cell morphologies. Initially, the tissue-damaging response can limit mycobacterial growth within macrophages. As stated above, this response, mediated by various bacterial products, not only destroys macrophages but also produces early solid necrosis in the center of the tubercle. Although *M. tuberculosis* can survive, its growth is inhibited within this necrotic environment by low oxygen tension and low pH. At this point, some lesions may heal by fibrosis, with subsequent calcification, whereas inflammation and necrosis occur in other lesions.

THE MACROPHAGE-ACTIVATING RESPONSE

CMI is critical at this early stage. In the majority of infected individuals, local macrophages are activated when bacillary antigens processed by macrophages stimulate T lymphocytes to release a variety of lymphokines. These activated macrophages aggregate around the lesion's center and effectively neutralize tubercle bacilli without causing further tissue destruction. In the central part of the lesion, the necrotic material resembles soft cheese (*caseous necrosis*)—a phenomenon that may also be observed in other conditions, such as neoplasms. Even when healing takes place, viable bacilli may remain dormant within macrophages or in the necrotic material for many years. These "healed" lesions in the lung parenchyma and hilar lymph nodes may later undergo calcification.

THE DELAYED-TYPE HYPERSENSITIVITY REACTION

In a minority of cases, the macrophage-activating response is weak, and mycobacterial growth can be inhibited only by intensified DTH reactions, which lead to lung tissue destruction. The lesion tends to enlarge further, and the surrounding tissue is progressively damaged. At the center of the lesion, the caseous material liquefies. Bronchial walls as well as blood vessels are invaded and destroyed, and cavities are formed. The liquefied caseous material, containing large numbers of bacilli, is drained through bronchi. Within the cavity, tubercle bacilli multiply, spill into the airways, and are discharged into the environment through expiratory maneuvers such as coughing and talking.

In the early stages of infection, bacilli are usually transported by macrophages to regional lymph nodes, from which they gain access to the bloodstream and disseminate widely throughout the body. The resulting lesions may undergo the same evolution as those in the lungs, although most tend to heal. In young children with poor natural immunity, hematogenous dissemination may result in fatal miliary tuberculosis or tuberculous meningitis.

ROLE OF MACROPHAGES AND MONOCYTES

Although CMI confers partial protection against *M. tuberculosis*, humoral immunity plays a less well-defined role in protection (although evidence is accumulating on the existence of LAM antibodies, which may prevent dissemination of infection in children). In the case of CMI, two types of cells are essential: macrophages, which directly phagocytize tubercle bacilli, and T cells (mainly CD4+ T lymphocytes), which induce protection through the production of cytokines, especially IFN-γ.

After infection with *M. tuberculosis*, alveolar macrophages secrete various cytokines responsible for a number of events (e.g., the formation of granulomas) as well as systemic effects (e.g., fever and weight loss). Monocytes and macrophages attracted to the site are key components of the immune response. Their primary mechanism is probably related to production of nitric oxide, which has antimycobacterial activity and increases synthesis of cytokines such as tumor necrosis factor α (TNF-α) and IL-1, which in turn regulate release of reactive nitrogen intermediates. In addition, macrophages can undergo apoptosis—a defensive mechanism to prevent release of cytokines and bacilli via their sequestration in the apoptotic cell.

ROLE OF T LYMPHOCYTES

Alveolar macrophages, monocytes, and dendritic cells are also critical in processing and presenting antigens to T lymphocytes, primarily CD4+ and CD8+ T cells; the result is the activation and proliferation of CD4+ T lymphocytes, which are crucial to the host's defense against *M. tuberculosis*. Qualitative and quantitative defects of CD4+ T cells explain the inability of HIV-infected individuals to contain mycobacterial proliferation. Activated CD4+ T lymphocytes can differentiate into cytokine-producing T_H1 or T_H2 cells. T_H1 cells produce IFN-γ—an activator of macrophages and monocytes—and IL-2. T_H2 cells produce IL-4, IL-5, IL-10, and IL-13 and also may promote humoral immunity. The interplay of these various cytokines and their cross-regulation determine the host's response. The role of cytokines in promoting intracellular killing of mycobacteria, however, has not been entirely elucidated. IFN-γ may induce the generation of reactive nitrogen intermediates and regulate genes involved in bactericidal effects. TNF-α also seems to be important.

Observations made originally in transgenic knockout mice and more recently in humans suggest that other T-cell subsets, especially CD8+ T cells, may play an important role. CD8+ T cells have been associated with protective activities via cytotoxic responses and lysis of infected cells as well as with production of IFN-γ and TNF-α. Finally, natural killer cells act as co-regulators of CD8+ T-cell lytic activities, and γδ T cells are increasingly thought to be involved in protective responses in humans.

MYCOBACTERIAL LIPIDS AND PROTEINS

Lipids have been involved in mycobacterial recognition by the innate immune system, and lipoproteins (such as 19-kDa lipoprotein) have been proven to trigger potent signals through TLRs present in blood dendritic cells. *M. tuberculosis* possesses various protein antigens. Some are present in the cytoplasm and cell wall; others are secreted. That the latter are more important in eliciting a T-lymphocyte response is suggested by experiments documenting the appearance of protective immunity in animals after immunization with live, protein-secreting mycobacteria. Among the antigens that may play a protective role are the 30-kDa (or 85B) and ESAT-6 antigens. Protective immunity is probably the result of reactivity to many different mycobacterial antigens.

SKIN TEST REACTIVITY

Coincident with the appearance of immunity, DTH to *M. tuberculosis* develops. This reactivity is the basis of the TST, which is used primarily for the detection of *M. tuberculosis* infection in persons without symptoms. The cellular mechanisms responsible for TST reactivity are related mainly to previously sensitized CD4+ T lymphocytes, which are attracted to the skin-test site. There, they proliferate and produce cytokines.

Although DTH is associated with protective immunity (TST-positive persons being less susceptible to a new *M. tuberculosis* infection than TST-negative persons), it by no means guarantees protection against reactivation. In fact, cases of active tuberculosis are often accompanied by strongly positive skin-test reactions. There is also evidence of reinfection with a new strain of *M. tuberculosis* in patients previously treated for active disease. This evidence underscores the fact that previous latent or active tuberculosis may not confer fully protective immunity.

CLINICAL MANIFESTATIONS

Tuberculosis is classified as pulmonary, extrapulmonary, or both. Before the advent of HIV infection, ~80% of all new cases of tuberculosis were limited to the lungs. However, up to two-thirds of HIV-infected patients with tuberculosis may have both pulmonary and extrapulmonary disease or extrapulmonary disease alone.

PULMONARY TUBERCULOSIS

Pulmonary tuberculosis can be categorized as primary or postprimary (secondary).

Primary Disease

Primary pulmonary tuberculosis occurs soon after the initial infection with tubercle bacilli. In areas of high tuberculosis transmission, this form of disease is often seen in children. Because most inspired air is distributed to the middle and lower lung zones, these areas of the lungs are most commonly involved in primary tuberculosis. The lesion forming after infection is usually peripheral and accompanied in more than half of cases by hilar or paratracheal lymphadenopathy, which may not be detectable on chest radiography. In the majority of cases, the lesion heals spontaneously and may later be evident as a small calcified nodule (*Ghon lesion*).

In children and in persons with impaired immunity (e.g., those with malnutrition or HIV infection), primary pulmonary tuberculosis may progress rapidly to clinical illness. The initial lesion increases in size and can evolve in different ways. Pleural effusion, which is found in up to two-thirds of cases, results from the penetration of bacilli into the pleural space from an adjacent subpleural focus. In severe cases, the primary site rapidly enlarges, its central portion undergoes necrosis, and cavitation develops (*progressive primary tuberculosis*). Tuberculosis in young children is almost invariably accompanied by hilar or mediastinal lymphadenopathy due to the spread of bacilli from the lung parenchyma through lymphatic vessels. Enlarged lymph nodes may compress bronchi, causing obstruction and subsequent segmental or lobar collapse. Partial obstruction may cause obstructive emphysema, and bronchiectasis may also develop. Hematogenous dissemination, which is common and often asymptomatic, may result in the most severe manifestations of primary *M. tuberculosis* infection. Bacilli reach the bloodstream from the pulmonary lesion or the lymph nodes and disseminate into various organs, where they may produce granulomatous lesions. Although healing frequently takes place, immunocompromised persons (e.g., patients with HIV infection) may develop miliary tuberculosis and/or tuberculous meningitis.

Postprimary Disease

Also called *adult-type*, *reactivation*, or *secondary tuberculosis*, postprimary disease results from endogenous reactivation of latent infection and is usually localized to the apical and posterior segments of the upper lobes, where the substantially higher mean oxygen tension (compared with that in the lower zones) favors mycobacterial growth. In addition, the superior segments of the lower lobes are frequently involved. The extent of lung parenchymal involvement varies greatly, from small infiltrates to extensive cavitary disease. With cavity formation, liquefied necrotic contents are ultimately discharged into the airways, resulting in satellite lesions within the lungs that may in turn undergo cavitation (Figs. 66-4 and 66-5). Massive involvement of pulmonary segments or lobes, with coalescence of lesions, produces tuberculous pneumonia. Although up to one-third of untreated patients reportedly succumb to severe pulmonary tuberculosis within a few weeks or months after onset (the classical "galloping consumption" of the past), others undergo a process of spontaneous remission or proceed along a chronic, progressively debilitating course ("consumption"). Under these circumstances, some pulmonary lesions become fibrotic and may later calcify, but cavities persist in other parts of the lungs. Individuals with such chronic disease continue to discharge tubercle bacilli into the environment. Most patients respond to treatment, with defervescence, decreasing cough, weight gain, and a general improvement in well-being within several weeks.

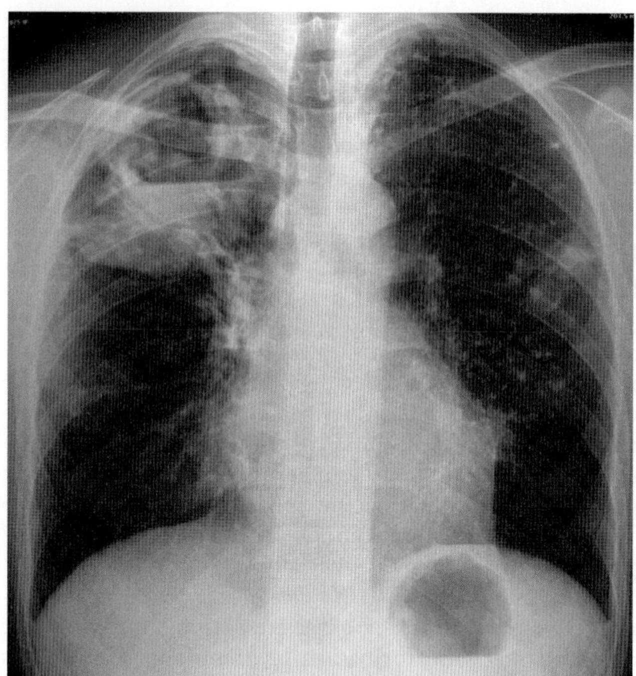

FIGURE 66-4
Chest radiograph showing a right upper-lobe infiltrate and a cavity with an air-fluid level in a patient with active tuberculosis. *(Courtesy of Dr. Andrea Gori, Department of Infectious Diseases, S. Paolo University Hospital, Milan, Italy; with permission.)*

Early in the course of disease, symptoms and signs are often nonspecific and insidious, consisting mainly of fever and night sweats, weight loss, anorexia, general

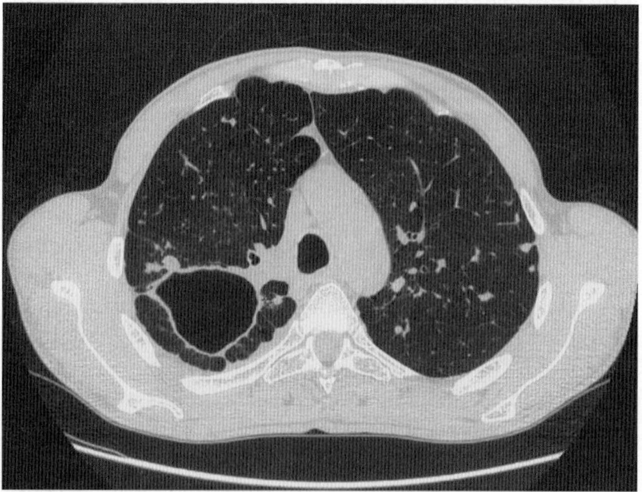

FIGURE 66-5
CT scan showing a large cavity in the right lung of a patient with active tuberculosis. *(Courtesy of Dr. Enrico Girardi, National Institute for Infectious Diseases, Spallanzani Hospital, Rome, Italy; with permission.)*

malaise, and weakness. However, in the majority of cases, cough eventually develops—often initially nonproductive and subsequently accompanied by the production of purulent sputum, sometimes with blood streaking. Massive hemoptysis may ensue as a consequence of the erosion of a blood vessel in the wall of a cavity. Hemoptysis, however, may also result from rupture of a dilated vessel in a cavity (*Rasmussen's aneurysm*) or from aspergilloma formation in an old cavity. Pleuritic chest pain sometimes develops in patients with subpleural parenchymal lesions. Extensive disease may produce dyspnea and, in rare instances, adult respiratory distress syndrome (ARDS).

Physical findings are of limited use in pulmonary tuberculosis. Many patients have no abnormalities detectable by chest examination, whereas others have detectable rales in the involved areas during inspiration, especially after coughing. Occasionally, rhonchi due to partial bronchial obstruction and classic amphoric breath sounds in areas with large cavities may be heard. Systemic features include fever (often low-grade and intermittent) in up to 80% of cases and wasting. Absence of fever, however, does not exclude tuberculosis. In some cases, pallor and finger clubbing develop. The most common hematologic findings are mild anemia and leukocytosis. Hyponatremia due to the syndrome of inappropriate secretion of antidiuretic hormone (SIADH) has also been reported.

EXTRAPULMONARY TUBERCULOSIS

In order of frequency, the extrapulmonary sites most commonly involved in tuberculosis are the lymph nodes, pleura, genitourinary tract, bones and joints, meninges, peritoneum, and pericardium. However, virtually all organ systems may be affected. As a result of hematogenous dissemination in HIV-infected individuals, extrapulmonary tuberculosis is seen more commonly today than in the past.

Lymph-Node Tuberculosis (Tuberculous Lymphadenitis)

The most common presentation of extrapulmonary tuberculosis (>40% of cases in the United States in recent series), lymph-node disease is particularly frequent among HIV-infected patients. In the United States, children and women (particularly non-Caucasians) also seem to be especially susceptible. Once caused mainly by *M. bovis*, tuberculous lymphadenitis is today due largely to *M. tuberculosis*. Lymph-node tuberculosis presents as painless swelling of the lymph nodes, most commonly at posterior cervical and supraclavicular sites (a condition historically referred to as *scrofula*). Lymph nodes are usually discrete and nontender in early disease but may be inflamed and have a fistulous tract draining caseous material. Associated pulmonary disease is seen in >40% of cases. Systemic symptoms are usually limited to HIV-infected patients. The diagnosis is established only by fine-needle aspiration or surgical biopsy. AFB are seen in up to 50% of cases, cultures are positive in 70–80%, and histologic examination shows granulomatous lesions. Among HIV-infected patients, granulomas usually are not seen. Differential diagnosis includes a variety of infectious conditions, neoplastic diseases such as lymphomas or metastatic carcinomas, and rare disorders like Kikuchi's disease (necrotizing histiocytic lymphadenitis), Kimura's disease, and Castleman's disease.

Pleural Tuberculosis

Involvement of the pleura, which accounts for ~20% of extrapulmonary cases in the United States, is common in primary tuberculosis and may result from either contiguous spread of parenchymal inflammation or, as in many cases of pleurisy accompanying postprimary disease, actual penetration by tubercle bacilli into the pleural space. Depending on the extent of reactivity, the effusion may be small, remain unnoticed, and resolve spontaneously or may be sufficiently large to cause symptoms such as fever, pleuritic chest pain, and dyspnea. Physical findings are those of pleural effusion: dullness to percussion and absence of breath sounds. A chest radiograph reveals the effusion and, in up to one-third of cases, also shows a parenchymal lesion. Thoracentesis is required to ascertain the nature of the effusion and to differentiate it from manifestations of other etiologies. The fluid is straw-colored and at times hemorrhagic; it is an exudate with a protein concentration >50% of that in serum (usually ~4–6 g/dL), a normal to low glucose concentration, a pH of ~7.3 (occasionally <7.2), and detectable white blood cells (usually 500–6000/μL). Neutrophils may predominate in the early stage, whereas mononuclear cells are the typical finding later. Mesothelial cells are generally rare or absent. AFB are seen on direct smear in only 10–25% of cases, but cultures may be positive for *M. tuberculosis* in 25–75% of cases; positive cultures are more common among postprimary cases. Determination of the pleural concentration of adenosine deaminase (ADA) is a useful screening test: tuberculosis is virtually excluded if the value is very low. Needle biopsy of the pleura is often required for diagnosis and reveals granulomas and/or yields a positive culture in up to 80% of cases. This form of pleural tuberculosis responds well to chemotherapy and may resolve spontaneously. The usefulness of glucocorticoid administration is doubtful.

Tuberculous empyema is a less common complication of pulmonary tuberculosis. It is usually the result of the rupture of a cavity, with spillage of a large number of organisms into the pleural space. This process may create a bronchopleural fistula with evident air in the pleural space. A chest radiograph shows hydropneumothorax with an air-fluid level. The pleural fluid is purulent and thick and contains large numbers of lymphocytes. Acid-fast smears and mycobacterial cultures are often positive. Surgical drainage is usually required as an adjunct to chemotherapy. Tuberculous empyema may result in severe pleural fibrosis and restrictive lung disease. Removal of the thickened visceral pleura (decortication) is occasionally necessary to improve lung function.

Tuberculosis of the Upper Airways

Nearly always a complication of advanced cavitary pulmonary tuberculosis, tuberculosis of the upper airways may involve the larynx, pharynx, and epiglottis. Symptoms include hoarseness, dysphonia, and dysphagia in addition to chronic productive cough. Findings depend on the site of involvement, and ulcerations may be seen on laryngoscopy. Acid-fast smear of the sputum is often positive, but biopsy may be necessary in some cases to establish the diagnosis. Carcinoma of the larynx may have similar features but is usually painless.

Genitourinary Tuberculosis

Genitourinary tuberculosis, which accounts for ~15% of all extrapulmonary cases in the United States, may involve any portion of the genitourinary tract. Local symptoms predominate, and up to one-third of patients may concomitantly have pulmonary disease. Urinary frequency, dysuria, nocturia, hematuria, and flank or abdominal pain are common presentations. However, patients may be asymptomatic and the disease discovered only after severe destructive lesions of the kidneys have developed. Urinalysis gives abnormal results in 90% of cases, revealing pyuria and hematuria. The documentation of culture-negative pyuria in acidic urine raises the suspicion of tuberculosis. Intravenous pyelography, abdominal CT, or MRI (Fig. 66-6) may show deformities and obstructions, and calcifications and ureteral strictures are suggestive findings. Culture of three morning urine specimens yields a definitive diagnosis in nearly 90% of cases. Severe ureteral strictures may lead to hydronephrosis and renal damage.

Genital tuberculosis is diagnosed more commonly in female than in male patients. In female patients, it affects the fallopian tubes and the endometrium and may cause infertility, pelvic pain, and menstrual abnormalities.

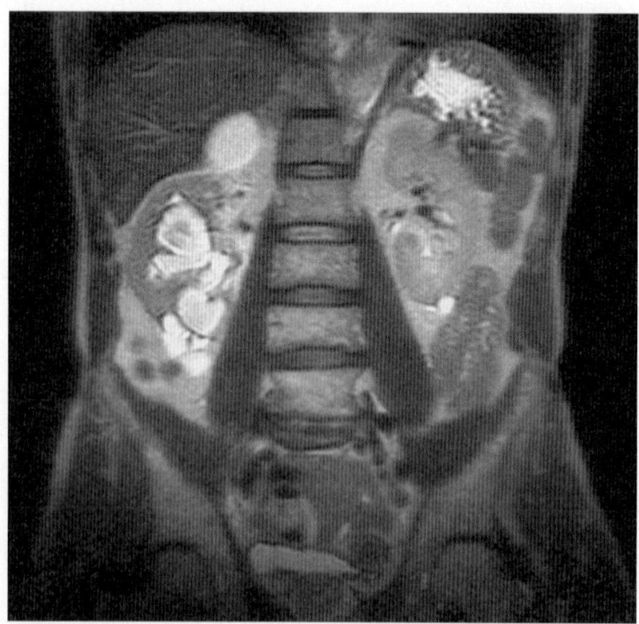

FIGURE 66-6
MRI of culture-confirmed renal tuberculosis. T2-weighted coronary plane: coronal sections showing several renal lesions in both the cortical and the medullary tissues of the right kidney. *(Courtesy of Dr. Alberto Matteelli, Department of Infectious Diseases, University of Brescia, Italy; with permission.)*

Diagnosis requires biopsy or culture of specimens obtained by dilatation and curettage. In male patients, tuberculosis preferentially affects the epididymis, producing a slightly tender mass that may drain externally through a fistulous tract; orchitis and prostatitis may also develop. In almost half of cases of genitourinary tuberculosis, urinary tract disease is also present. Genitourinary tuberculosis responds well to chemotherapy.

Skeletal Tuberculosis

In the United States, tuberculosis of the bones and joints is responsible for ~10% of extrapulmonary cases. In bone and joint disease, pathogenesis is related to reactivation of hematogenous foci or to spread from adjacent paravertebral lymph nodes. Weight-bearing joints (the spine in 40% of cases, the hips in 13%, and the knees in 10%) are most commonly affected. Spinal tuberculosis (Pott's disease or tuberculous spondylitis; Fig. 66-7) often involves two or more adjacent vertebral bodies. Although the upper thoracic spine is the most common site of spinal tuberculosis in children, the lower thoracic and upper lumbar vertebrae are usually affected in adults. From the anterior superior or inferior angle of the vertebral body, the lesion slowly reaches the adjacent body, later affecting the intervertebral disk. With advanced disease, collapse of vertebral bodies results in kyphosis (*gibbus*). A paravertebral "cold" abscess may also form. In the upper spine, this abscess may track to and penetrate the chest wall, presenting as a soft tissue mass; in the lower spine, it may reach the inguinal ligaments or present as a psoas abscess. CT or MRI reveals the characteristic lesion and suggests its etiology. The differential diagnosis includes tumors and other infections. Pyogenic bacterial osteomyelitis, in particular, involves the disk very early and produces rapid sclerosis. Aspiration of the abscess or bone biopsy confirms the tuberculous etiology, as cultures are usually positive and histologic findings highly typical. A catastrophic complication of Pott's disease is paraplegia, which is usually due to an abscess or a lesion compressing the spinal

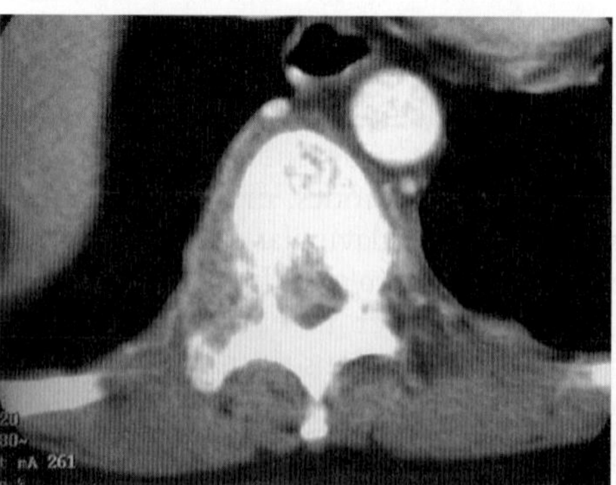

FIGURE 66-7
CT scan demonstrating destruction of the right pedicle of T10 due to Pott's disease. The patient, a 70-year-old Asian woman, presented with back pain and weight loss and had biopsy-proven tuberculosis. *(Courtesy of Charles L. Daley, M.D., University of California, San Francisco; with permission.)*

cord. Paraparesis due to a large abscess is a medical emergency and requires rapid drainage. Tuberculosis of the hip joints, usually involving the head of the femur, causes pain; tuberculosis of the knee produces pain and swelling. If the disease goes unrecognized, the joints may be destroyed. Diagnosis requires examination of the synovial fluid, which is thick in appearance, with a high protein concentration and a variable cell count. Although synovial fluid culture is positive in a high percentage of cases, synovial biopsy and tissue culture may be necessary to establish the diagnosis. Skeletal tuberculosis responds to chemotherapy, but severe cases may require surgery.

Tuberculous Meningitis and Tuberculoma

Tuberculosis of the central nervous system (CNS) accounts for ~5% of extrapulmonary cases in the United States. It is seen most often in young children but also develops in adults, especially those infected with HIV. Tuberculous meningitis results from the hematogenous spread of primary or postprimary pulmonary disease or from the rupture of a subependymal tubercle into the subarachnoid space. In more than half of cases, evidence of old pulmonary lesions or a miliary pattern is found on chest radiography. The disease often presents subtly as headache and slight mental changes after a prodrome of weeks of low-grade fever, malaise, anorexia, and irritability. If not recognized, tuberculous meningitis may evolve acutely with severe headache, confusion, lethargy, altered sensorium, and neck rigidity. Typically, the disease evolves over 1–2 weeks, a course longer than that of bacterial meningitis. Paresis of cranial nerves (ocular nerves in particular) is a frequent finding, and the involvement of cerebral arteries may produce focal ischemia. The ultimate evolution is toward coma, with hydrocephalus and intracranial hypertension.

Lumbar puncture is the cornerstone of diagnosis. In general, examination of the cerebrospinal fluid (CSF) reveals a high leukocyte count (up to 1000/μL), usually with a predominance of lymphocytes but sometimes with a predominance of neutrophils in the early stage; a protein content of 1–8 g/L (100–800 mg/dL); and a low glucose concentration. However, any of these three parameters can be within the normal range. AFB are seen on direct smear of CSF sediment in up to one-third of cases, but repeated lumbar punctures increase the yield. Culture of CSF is diagnostic in up to 80% of cases and remains the gold standard. Polymerase chain reaction (PCR) has a sensitivity of up to 80%, but rates of false-positivity reach 10%. The ADA concentration may be a sensitive test but has low specificity. Imaging studies (CT and MRI) may show hydrocephalus and abnormal enhancement of basal cisterns or ependyma.

If unrecognized, tuberculous meningitis is uniformly fatal. This disease responds to chemotherapy; however, neurologic sequelae are documented in 25% of treated cases, in most of which the diagnosis has been delayed. Clinical trials have demonstrated that patients given adjunctive glucocorticoids may experience faster resolution of CSF abnormalities and elevated CSF pressure. In a recent study, adjunctive dexamethasone (0.4 mg/kg per day given IV and tapering by 0.1 mg/kg per week until the fourth week, when 0.1 mg/kg per day was administered; followed by 4 mg/d given by mouth and tapering by 1 mg per week until the fourth week, when 1 mg/d was administered) significantly enhanced the chances of survival among persons >14 years of age but did not reduce the frequency of neurologic sequelae.

Tuberculoma, an uncommon manifestation of CNS tuberculosis, presents as one or more space-occupying lesions and usually causes seizures and focal signs. CT or MRI reveals contrast-enhanced ring lesions, but biopsy is necessary to establish the diagnosis.

Gastrointestinal Tuberculosis

Gastrointestinal tuberculosis is uncommon, making up 3.5% of extrapulmonary cases in the United States. Various pathogenetic mechanisms are involved: swallowing of sputum with direct seeding, hematogenous spread, or (largely in developing areas) ingestion of milk from cows affected by bovine tuberculosis. Although any portion of the gastrointestinal tract may be affected, the terminal ileum and the cecum are the sites most commonly involved. Abdominal pain (at times similar to that associated with appendicitis) and swelling, obstruction, hematochezia, and a palpable mass in the abdomen are common findings at presentation. Fever, weight loss, anorexia, and night sweats are also common. With intestinal-wall involvement, ulcerations and fistulae may simulate Crohn's disease; the differential diagnosis with this entity is always difficult. Anal fistulae should prompt an evaluation for rectal tuberculosis. As surgery is required in most cases, the diagnosis can be established by histologic examination and culture of specimens obtained intraoperatively.

Tuberculous peritonitis follows either the direct spread of tubercle bacilli from ruptured lymph nodes and intraabdominal organs (e.g., genital tuberculosis in women) or hematogenous seeding. Nonspecific abdominal pain, fever, and ascites should raise the suspicion of tuberculous peritonitis. The coexistence of cirrhosis in patients with tuberculous peritonitis complicates the diagnosis. In tuberculous peritonitis, paracentesis reveals an exudative fluid with a high protein content and leukocytosis that is usually lymphocytic (although neutrophils occasionally predominate). The yield of direct smear and culture is relatively low; culture of a large volume of ascitic fluid can increase the yield, but peritoneal biopsy (with a specimen best obtained by laparoscopy) is often needed to establish the diagnosis.

Pericardial Tuberculosis (Tuberculous Pericarditis)

Due to direct progression of a primary focus within the pericardium, to reactivation of a latent focus, or to rupture of an adjacent subcarinal lymph node, pericardial tuberculosis has often been a disease of the elderly in countries with low tuberculosis prevalence but also develops frequently in HIV-infected patients. Case-fatality rates are as high as 40% in some series. The onset may be subacute, although an acute presentation, with dyspnea, fever, dull retrosternal pain, and a pericardial friction rub, is possible. An effusion eventually develops in many cases; cardiovascular symptoms and signs of cardiac tamponade may ultimately appear (Chap. 20). In the presence of effusion, tuberculosis must be suspected if the patient belongs to a high-risk population (HIV-infected, originating in a high-prevalence country), if there is evidence of previous tuberculosis in other organs, or if echocardiography, CT, or MRI shows effusion and thickness across the pericardial space. A definitive diagnosis can be obtained by pericardiocentesis under echocardiographic guidance. The pericardial fluid must be submitted for biochemical, cytologic, and microbiologic study. The effusion is exudative in nature, with a high count of leukocytes (predominantly mononuclear cells). Hemorrhagic effusion is frequent. Direct smear examination is very rarely positive. Culture of pericardial fluid reveals *M. tuberculosis* in up to two-thirds of cases, whereas pericardial biopsy has a higher yield. High levels of ADA and IFN-γ may also suggest a tuberculous etiology.

Without treatment, pericardial tuberculosis is usually fatal. Even with treatment, complications may develop, including chronic constrictive pericarditis with thickening of the pericardium, fibrosis, and sometimes calcification, which may be visible on a chest radiograph. A course of glucocorticoid treatment (e.g., prednisone, 20–60 mg/d for up to 6 weeks) is useful in the management of acute disease, reducing effusion, facilitating hemodynamic recovery, and thus decreasing mortality rates. Progression to chronic constrictive pericarditis, however, seems unaffected by such therapy.

Miliary or Disseminated Tuberculosis

Miliary tuberculosis is due to hematogenous spread of tubercle bacilli. Although in children it is often the consequence of primary infection, in adults it may be due to either recent infection or reactivation of old disseminated foci. The lesions are usually yellowish granulomas 1–2 mm in diameter that resemble millet seeds (thus the term *miliary*, coined by nineteenth-century pathologists).

Clinical manifestations are nonspecific and protean, depending on the predominant site of involvement. Fever, night sweats, anorexia, weakness, and weight loss are presenting symptoms in the majority of cases. At times patients have a cough and other respiratory symptoms due to pulmonary involvement, as well as abdominal symptoms. Physical findings include hepatomegaly, splenomegaly, and lymphadenopathy. Eye examination may reveal choroidal tubercles, which are pathognomonic of miliary tuberculosis, in up to 30% of cases. Meningismus occurs in <10% of cases.

A high index of suspicion is required for the diagnosis of miliary tuberculosis. Frequently, chest radiography reveals a miliary reticulonodular pattern (more easily seen on underpenetrated film), although no radiographic abnormality may be evident early in the course and among HIV-infected patients. Other radiologic findings include large infiltrates, interstitial infiltrates (especially in HIV-infected patients), and pleural effusion. Sputum smear microscopy is negative in 80% of cases. Various hematologic abnormalities may be seen, including anemia with leukopenia, lymphopenia, neutrophilic leukocytosis and leukemoid reactions, and polycythemia. Disseminated intravascular coagulation has been reported. Elevation of alkaline phosphatase levels and other abnormal values in liver function tests are detected in patients with severe hepatic involvement. The TST may be negative in up to half of cases, but reactivity may be restored during chemotherapy. Bronchoalveolar lavage and transbronchial biopsy are more likely to provide bacteriologic confirmation, and granulomas are evident in liver or bone-marrow biopsy specimens from many patients. If it goes unrecognized, miliary tuberculosis is lethal; with proper early treatment, however, it is amenable to cure. Glucocorticoid therapy has not proved beneficial.

A rare presentation seen in the elderly is *cryptic miliary tuberculosis*, which has a chronic course characterized by mild intermittent fever, anemia, and—ultimately—meningeal involvement preceding death. An acute septicemic form, *nonreactive miliary tuberculosis*, occurs very rarely and is due to massive hematogenous dissemination of tubercle bacilli. Pancytopenia is common in this form of disease, which is rapidly fatal. At postmortem examination, multiple necrotic but nongranulomatous ("nonreactive") lesions are detected.

Less Common Extrapulmonary Forms

Tuberculosis may cause chorioretinitis, uveitis, panophthalmitis, and painful hypersensitivity-related phlyctenular conjunctivitis. Tuberculous otitis is rare and presents as hearing loss, otorrhea, and tympanic membrane perforation. In the nasopharynx, tuberculosis may simulate Wegener's granulomatosis. Cutaneous manifestations of tuberculosis include primary infection due to direct inoculation, abscesses and chronic ulcers, scrofuloderma, lupus vulgaris (a smoldering disease with nodules, plaques, and fissures), miliary lesions, and erythema nodosum. Adrenal tuberculosis is a manifestation of disseminated disease presenting rarely as adrenal insufficiency. Finally, congenital tuberculosis results from transplacental spread of tubercle bacilli to the fetus or from ingestion of contaminated amniotic fluid. This rare disease affects the liver, spleen, lymph nodes, and various other organs.

HIV-ASSOCIATED TUBERCULOSIS

(See also Chap. 90) Tuberculosis is one of the most common diseases among HIV-infected persons worldwide. In some African countries, the rate of HIV infection among tuberculosis patients reaches 70–80% in certain urban settings. A person with a positive TST who acquires HIV infection has a 3–13% annual risk of developing active tuberculosis. A new tuberculosis infection acquired by an HIV-infected individual may evolve to active disease in a matter of weeks rather than months or years.

Tuberculosis can appear at any stage of HIV infection, and its presentation varies with the stage. When CMI is only partially compromised, pulmonary tuberculosis presents in a typical manner (Figs. 66-4 and 66-5), with upper-lobe infiltrates and cavitation and without significant lymphadenopathy or pleural effusion. In late stages of HIV infection, a primary tuberculosis–like pattern, with diffuse interstitial or miliary infiltrates, little or no cavitation, and intrathoracic lymphadenopathy, is more common. Overall, sputum smears may be positive less frequently among tuberculosis patients with HIV infection than among those without; thus the diagnosis of tuberculosis may be unusually difficult, especially in view of the variety of HIV-related pulmonary conditions mimicking tuberculosis.

Extrapulmonary tuberculosis is common among HIV-infected patients. In various series, extrapulmonary tuberculosis—alone or in association with pulmonary disease—has been documented in 40–60% of all cases in HIV–co-infected individuals. The most common forms are lymphatic, disseminated, pleural, and pericardial. Mycobacteremia and meningitis are also frequent, particularly in advanced HIV disease.

The diagnosis of tuberculosis in HIV-infected patients may be difficult not only because of the increased frequency of sputum-smear negativity (up to 40% in culture-proven pulmonary cases), but also because of atypical radiographic findings, a lack of classic granuloma formation in the late stages, and a negative TST. Delays in treatment may prove fatal. Recommendations for the prevention and treatment of tuberculosis in HIV-infected individuals are provided below.

DIAGNOSIS OF TUBERCULOSIS

The key to the diagnosis of tuberculosis is a high index of suspicion. Diagnosis is not difficult with a high-risk patient—e.g., a homeless alcoholic who presents with typical symptoms and a classic chest radiograph showing upper-lobe infiltrates with cavities (Fig. 66-4). On the other hand, the diagnosis can easily be missed in an elderly nursing home resident or a teenager with a focal infiltrate.

Often, the diagnosis is first entertained when the chest radiograph of a patient being evaluated for respiratory symptoms is abnormal. If the patient has no complicating medical conditions that cause immunosuppression, the chest radiograph may show typical upper-lobe infiltrates with cavitation (Fig. 66-4). The longer the delay between the onset of symptoms and the diagnosis, the more likely is the finding of cavitary disease. In contrast, immunosuppressed patients, including those with HIV infection, may have "atypical" findings on chest radiography—e.g., lower-zone infiltrates without cavity formation.

AFB MICROSCOPY

A presumptive diagnosis is commonly based on the finding of AFB on microscopic examination of a diagnostic specimen, such as a smear of expectorated sputum or of tissue (e.g., a lymph node biopsy). Although rapid and inexpensive, AFB microscopy has relatively low sensitivity (40–60%) in confirmed cases of pulmonary tuberculosis. Most modern laboratories processing large numbers of diagnostic specimens use auramine-rhodamine staining and fluorescence microscopy. The more traditional method—light microscopy of specimens stained with Kinyoun or Ziehl-Neelsen basic fuchsin dyes—is satisfactory, although more time-consuming. For patients with suspected pulmonary tuberculosis, three sputum specimens, preferably collected early in the morning, should be submitted to the laboratory for AFB smear and mycobacterial culture. If tissue is obtained, it is critical that the portion of the specimen intended for culture not be put in formaldehyde. The use of AFB microscopy on urine or gastric lavage fluid is limited by the presence of commensal mycobacteria that can cause false-positive results.

MYCOBACTERIAL CULTURE

Definitive diagnosis depends on the isolation and identification of *M. tuberculosis* from a clinical specimen or the identification of specific sequences of DNA in a nucleic acid amplification test (see below). Specimens may be inoculated onto egg- or agar-based medium (e.g., Löwenstein-Jensen or Middlebrook 7H10) and incubated at 37°C (under 5% CO_2 for Middlebrook medium). Because most species of mycobacteria, including *M. tuberculosis*, grow slowly, 4–8 weeks may be required before growth is detected. Although *M. tuberculosis* may be presumptively identified on the basis of growth time and colony pigmentation and morphology, a variety of biochemical tests have traditionally been used to speciate mycobacterial isolates. In modern, well-equipped laboratories, the use of broth-based culture for isolation and speciation by molecular methods or high-pressure liquid chromatography of mycolic acids has replaced isolation on solid media and identification by biochemical tests. These new methods have decreased the time required for bacteriologic confirmation to 2–3 weeks.

NUCLEIC ACID AMPLIFICATION

Several test systems based on amplification of mycobacterial nucleic acid are available. These systems permit the diagnosis of tuberculosis in as little as several hours, with high specificity and sensitivity approaching that of culture. These tests are most useful for the rapid confirmation of tuberculosis in persons with AFB-positive specimens, but also have utility for the diagnosis of AFB-negative pulmonary and extrapulmonary tuberculosis.

DRUG SUSCEPTIBILITY TESTING

In general, the initial isolate of *M. tuberculosis* should be tested for susceptibility to isoniazid, rifampin, and ethambutol. In addition, expanded susceptibility testing is mandatory when resistance to one or more of these drugs is found or the patient either fails to respond to initial therapy or has a relapse after the completion of treatment (see "Treatment Failure and Relapse" later in the chapter). Susceptibility testing may be conducted directly (with the clinical specimen) or indirectly (with mycobacterial cultures) on solid or liquid medium. Results are obtained most rapidly by direct susceptibility testing on liquid medium, with an average reporting time of 3 weeks. With indirect testing on solid medium, results may be unavailable for ≥8 weeks. Molecular methods for the rapid identification of genetic mutations known to be associated with resistance to rifampin and isoniazid have been developed but are not marketed in the United States.

RADIOGRAPHIC PROCEDURES

As noted above, the initial suspicion of pulmonary tuberculosis is often based on abnormal chest radiographic findings in a patient with respiratory symptoms. Although the "classic" picture is that of upper-lobe disease with infiltrates and cavities (Fig. 66-4), virtually any radiographic pattern—from a normal film or a solitary pulmonary nodule to diffuse alveolar infiltrates in a patient with ARDS—may be seen. In the era of AIDS, no radiographic pattern can be considered pathognomonic. CT (Fig. 66-5) may be useful in interpreting questionable findings on plain chest radiography and may be helpful in diagnosing some forms of extrapulmonary tuberculosis [e.g., Pott's disease (Fig. 66-7)]. MRI is useful in the diagnosis of intracranial tuberculosis.

ADDITIONAL DIAGNOSTIC PROCEDURES

Other diagnostic tests may be used when pulmonary tuberculosis is suspected. Sputum induction by ultrasonic nebulization of hypertonic saline may be useful for patients who cannot produce a sputum specimen spontaneously. Frequently, patients with radiographic abnormalities that are consistent with other diagnoses (e.g., bronchogenic carcinoma) undergo fiberoptic bronchoscopy with bronchial brushings and endobronchial or transbronchial biopsy of the lesion. Bronchoalveolar lavage of a lung segment containing an abnormality may also be performed. In all cases, it is essential that specimens be submitted for AFB smear and mycobacterial culture. For the diagnosis of primary pulmonary tuberculosis in children, who often do not expectorate sputum, specimens from early-morning gastric lavage may yield positive cultures.

Invasive diagnostic procedures are indicated for patients with suspected extrapulmonary tuberculosis. In addition to testing of specimens from involved sites (e.g., CSF for tuberculous meningitis, pleural fluid and biopsy samples for pleural disease), biopsy and culture of bone marrow and liver tissue have a good diagnostic yield in disseminated (miliary) tuberculosis, particularly in HIV-infected patients, who also have a high frequency of positive blood cultures.

In some cases, cultures are negative but a clinical diagnosis of tuberculosis is supported by consistent epidemiologic evidence (e.g., a history of close contact with an infectious patient), a positive TST, and a compatible clinical and radiographic response to treatment. In the United States and other industrialized countries with low rates of tuberculosis, some patients with limited abnormalities on chest radiographs and sputum positive for AFB are infected with nontuberculous mycobacteria, most commonly organisms of the *M. avium* complex (MAC) or *M. kansasii* (Chap. 68). Factors favoring the diagnosis of nontuberculous mycobacterial disease over tuberculosis include an absence of risk factors for tuberculosis, a negative TST, and underlying chronic pulmonary disease.

Patients with HIV-associated tuberculosis pose several diagnostic problems (see "HIV-Associated Tuberculosis" earlier in the chapter). Moreover, HIV-infected patients with sputum culture–positive, AFB-positive tuberculosis may present with a normal chest radiograph. With the advent of highly active antiretroviral therapy, the occurrence of disseminated MAC disease that can be confused with tuberculosis has become much less common.

SEROLOGIC AND OTHER DIAGNOSTIC TESTS FOR ACTIVE TUBERCULOSIS

A number of serologic tests based on detection of antibodies to a variety of mycobacterial antigens are marketed in developing countries but not in the United States. Careful independent assessments of these tests suggest that they are not useful as diagnostic aids, especially in persons with a low probability of tuberculosis. Various methods aimed at detection of mycobacterial antigens in diagnostic specimens are being investigated but are limited at present by low sensitivity. Determination of ADA levels in pleural fluid may be useful in the diagnosis of pleural tuberculosis; the utility of this test in the diagnosis of other forms of extrapulmonary tuberculosis (e.g., pericardial, peritoneal, and meningeal) is less clear.

DIAGNOSIS OF LATENT *M. TUBERCULOSIS* INFECTION

Tuberculin Skin Testing

In 1891, Robert Koch discovered that components of *M. tuberculosis* in a concentrated liquid culture medium, subsequently named "old tuberculin" (OT), were capable of eliciting a skin reaction when injected subcutaneously into patients with tuberculosis. In 1932, Seibert and Munday purified this product by ammonium sulfate precipitation to produce an active protein fraction known as *tuberculin purified protein derivative (PPD)*. In 1941, PPD-S, developed by Seibert and Glenn, was chosen as the international standard. Later, the WHO and UNICEF sponsored large-scale production of a master batch of PPD (RT23) and made it available for general use. The greatest limitation of PPD is its lack of mycobacterial species specificity, a property due to the large number of proteins in this product that are highly conserved in the various species. In addition, subjectivity of the skin-reaction interpretation, deterioration of the product, and batch-to-batch variations limit the usefulness of PPD.

Skin testing with tuberculin-PPD (TST) is most widely used in screening for latent *M. tuberculosis* infection (LTBI). The test is of limited value in the diagnosis of active tuberculosis because of its relatively low sensitivity and specificity and its inability to discriminate between latent infection and active disease. False-negative reactions are common in immunosuppressed patients and in those with overwhelming tuberculosis. False positive reactions may be caused by infections with nontuberculous mycobacteria (Chap. 68) and by bacille Calmette-Guérin (BCG) vaccination.

IFN-γ Release Assays (IGRAs)

Recently, two in vitro assays that measure T-cell release of IFN-γ in response to stimulation with the highly tuberculosis-specific antigens ESAT-6 and CFP-10 have become commercially available. QuantiFERON-TB Gold® (Cellestis Ltd., Carnegie, Australia) is a whole-blood enzyme-linked immunosorbent assay (ELISA) for measurement of IFN-γ, and T-SPOT.TB® (Oxford Immunotec, Oxford, UK) is an enzyme-linked immunospot (ELISpot) assay.

IGRAs are more specific than the TST as a result of less cross-reactivity due to BCG vaccination and sensitization by nontuberculous mycobacteria. IGRAs also appear to be at least as sensitive as the TST for active tuberculosis (used as a surrogate for LTBI). Although diagnostic sensitivity for LTBI cannot be directly estimated because of the absence of a gold standard, these tests have shown better correlation than the TST with exposure to *M. tuberculosis* in contact investigations in low-incidence settings.

Other potential advantages of IGRAs include logistical convenience, the need for fewer patient visits to complete testing, the avoidance of unreliable and somewhat subjective measurements such as skin induration, and the ability to perform serial testing without inducing the boosting phenomenon (a spurious TST conversion due to boosting of reactivity on subsequent TSTs among BCG-vaccinated persons and those infected with other mycobacteria). Because of the high specificity and other potential advantages, IGRAs are likely to replace the TST for LTBI diagnosis in low-incidence, high-income settings where cross-reactivity due to BCG might adversely impact the interpretation and utility of the TST. Direct comparative studies in routine practice thus far suggest that the ELISpot has a lower rate of indeterminate results and probably a higher degree of diagnostic sensitivity than the whole-blood ELISA. Further studies are underway to assess the performance of these tests in contact investigations and in persons with suspected tuberculosis disease, health care workers, HIV-infected individuals, persons with iatrogenic immunosuppression, and children.

℞ Treatment: TUBERCULOSIS

The two aims of tuberculosis treatment are to interrupt tuberculosis transmission by rendering patients noninfectious and to prevent morbidity and death by curing patients with tuberculosis. Chemotherapy for tuberculosis became possible with the discovery of streptomycin in the mid-1940s. Randomized clinical trials clearly indicated that the administration of streptomycin to patients with chronic tuberculosis reduced mortality rates and led to cure in the majority of cases. However, monotherapy with streptomycin was frequently associated with the development of resistance to this drug and the attendant failure of treatment. With the discovery of para-aminosalicylic acid (PAS) and isoniazid, it became axiomatic that cure of tuberculosis required the concomitant administration of at least two agents to which the organism was susceptible. Furthermore, early clinical trials demonstrated that a long period of treatment—i.e., 12–24 months—was required to prevent recurrence.

The introduction of rifampin in the early 1970s heralded the era of effective short-course chemotherapy, with a treatment duration of <12 months. The discovery that pyrazinamide, which was first used in the 1950s, augmented the potency of isoniazid/rifampin regimens led to the use of a 6-month course of this triple-drug regimen as standard therapy.

DRUGS Four major drugs are considered the first-line agents for the treatment of tuberculosis: isoniazid, rifampin, pyrazinamide, and ethambutol (Table 66-2). These drugs are well absorbed after oral administration, with peak serum levels at 2–4 h and nearly complete elimination within 24 h. These agents are recommended on the basis of their bactericidal activity (i.e., their ability to rapidly reduce the number of viable organisms and render patients noninfectious), their sterilizing activity (i.e., their ability to kill all bacilli and thus sterilize the affected tissues, measured in terms of the ability to prevent relapses), and their low rate of induction of drug resistance. Rifapentine and rifabutin, two drugs related to rifampin, are also available in the United States and are useful for selected patients. For a detailed discussion of the drugs used for the treatment of tuberculosis, see Chap. 69.

TABLE 66-2

RECOMMENDED DOSAGE[a] FOR INITIAL TREATMENT OF TUBERCULOSIS IN ADULTS[b]

	DOSAGE	
DRUG	DAILY DOSE	THRICE-WEEKLY DOSE[c]
Isoniazid	5 mg/kg, max 300 mg	15 mg/kg, max 900 mg
Rifampin	10 mg/kg, max 600 mg	10 mg/kg, max 600 mg
Pyrazinamide	20–25 mg/kg, max 2 g	30–40 mg/kg, max 3 g
Ethambutol[d]	15–20 mg/kg	25–30 mg/kg

[a]The duration of treatment for individual drugs varies by regimen, as detailed in Table 66-3.

[b]Dosages for children are similar, except that some authorities recommend higher doses of isoniazid (10–15 mg/kg daily; 20–30 mg/kg intermittent) and rifampin (10–20 mg/kg).

[c]Dosages for twice-weekly administration are the same for isoniazid and rifampin but are higher for pyrazinamide (50 mg/kg, with a maximum of 4 g/d) and ethambutol (40–50 mg/d).

[d]In certain settings, streptomycin (15 mg/kg daily, with a maximum dose of 1 g; or 25–30 mg/kg thrice weekly, with a maximum dose of 1.5 g) can replace ethambutol in the initial phase of treatment. However, streptomycin is no longer considered a first-line drug by the ATS, the IDSA, or the CDC.

Source: Based on recommendations of the American Thoracic Society (ATS), the Infectious Diseases Society of America (IDSA), and the Centers for Disease Control and Prevention (CDC).

Because of a lower degree of efficacy and a higher degree of intolerability and toxicity, six classes of second-line drugs are generally used only for the treatment of patients with tuberculosis resistant to first-line drugs. Included in this group are the injectable aminoglycosides streptomycin (formerly a first-line agent), kanamycin, and amikacin; the injectable polypeptide capreomycin; the oral agents ethionamide, cycloserine, and PAS; and the fluoroquinolone antibiotics. Of the quinolones, third-generation agents are preferred: levofloxacin, gatifloxacin (no longer marketed in the United States), and moxifloxacin. Amithiozone (thiacetazone) is still used in some developing countries but is associated with severe and sometimes even fatal skin reactions among HIV-infected patients. Other drugs of unproven efficacy that have been used in the treatment of patients with resistance to most of the first- and second-line agents include clofazimine, amoxicillin/clavulanic acid, and linezolid.

REGIMENS Standard short-course regimens are divided into an initial, or bactericidal, phase and a continuation, or sterilizing, phase. During the initial phase, the majority of the tubercle bacilli are killed, symptoms resolve, and usually the patient becomes noninfectious. The continuation phase is required to eliminate persisting mycobacteria and prevent relapse.

The treatment regimen of choice for virtually all forms of tuberculosis in both adults and children consists of a 2-month initial phase of isoniazid, rifampin, pyrazinamide, and ethambutol followed by a 4-month continuation phase of isoniazid and rifampin (Table 66-3). Treatment may be given daily throughout the course or intermittently (either three times weekly throughout the course or twice weekly after an initial phase of daily therapy, although the twice-weekly option is not recommended by the WHO). A continuation phase of once-weekly rifapentine and isoniazid is equally effective for HIV-seronegative patients with noncavitary pulmonary tuberculosis who have negative sputum cultures at 2 months. Intermittent treatment is especially useful for patients whose therapy is being directly observed (see below). Patients with cavitary pulmonary tuberculosis

TABLE 66-3

RECOMMENDED ANTITUBERCULOSIS TREATMENT REGIMENS

	INITIAL PHASE		CONTINUATION PHASE	
INDICATION	**DURATION, MONTHS**	**DRUGS**	**DURATION, MONTHS**	**DRUGS**
New smear- or culture-positive cases	2	HRZE[a,b]	4	HR[a,c,d]
New culture-negative cases	2	HRZE[a]	2	HR[a]
Pregnancy	2	HRE[e]	7	HR
Failure and relapse[f]	—	—	—	—
Resistance (or intolerance) to H	Throughout (6)	RZE[g]		
Resistance to H + R	Throughout (12–18)	ZEQ + S (or another injectable agent[h])		
Resistance to all first-line drugs	Throughout (24)	1 injectable agent[h] + 3 of these 4: ethionamide, cycloserine, Q, PAS		
Standardized re-treatment (susceptibility testing unavailable)	3	HRZES[i]	5	HRE
Drug intolerance to R	Throughout (12)[j]	HZE		
Drug intolerance to Z	2	HRE	7	HR

[a]All drugs can be given daily or intermittently (three times weekly throughout or twice weekly after 2–8 weeks of daily therapy during the initial phase).
[b]Streptomycin can be used in place of ethambutol but is no longer considered to be a first-line drug by ATS/IDSA/CDC.
[c]The continuation phase should be extended to 7 months for patients with cavitary pulmonary tuberculosis who remain sputum culture–positive after the initial phase of treatment.
[d]HIV-negative patients with noncavitary pulmonary tuberculosis who have negative sputum AFB smears after the initial phase of treatment can be given once-weekly rifapentine/isoniazid in the continuation phase.
[e]The 6-month regimen with pyrazinamide can probably be used safely during pregnancy and is recommended by the WHO and the International Union Against Tuberculosis and Lung Disease. If pyrazinamide is not included in the initial treatment regimen, the minimum duration of therapy is 9 months.
[f]Regimen is tailored according to the results of drug susceptibility tests.
[g]A fluoroquinolone may strengthen the regimen for patients with extensive disease.
[h]Amikacin, kanamycin, or capreomycin. All these agents should be discontinued after 2–6 months, depending upon tolerance and response.
[i]Streptomycin should be discontinued after 2 months. This regimen is less effective for patients in whom treatment has failed, who have an increased probability of rifampin-resistant disease. In such cases, the re-treatment regimen might include second-line drugs chosen in light of the likely pattern of drug resistance.
[j]Streptomycin for the initial 2 months or a fluoroquinolone might strengthen the regimen for patients with extensive disease.
Note: H, isoniazid; R, rifampin; Z, pyrazinamide; E, ethambutol; S, streptomycin; Q, a quinolone antibiotic; PAS, para-aminosalicylic acid.

and delayed sputum-culture conversion (i.e., those who remain culture-positive at 2 months) should have the continuation phase extended by 3 months, for a total course of 9 months. For patients with sputum culture–negative pulmonary tuberculosis, the duration of treatment may be reduced to a total of 4 months. To prevent isoniazid-related neuropathy, pyridoxine (10–25 mg/d) should be added to the regimen given to persons at high risk of vitamin B6 deficiency (e.g., alcoholics; malnourished persons; pregnant and lactating women; and patients with conditions such as chronic renal failure, diabetes, and HIV infection, which are also associated with neuropathy). A full course of therapy (completion of treatment) is defined more accurately by the total number of doses taken than by the duration of treatment. Specific recommendations on the required numbers of doses for each of the various treatment regimens have been published jointly by the American Thoracic Society, the Infectious Diseases Society of America, and the CDC. In some developing countries where the ability to ensure compliance with treatment is limited, a continuation-phase regimen of daily isoniazid and ethambutol for 6 months is acceptable. However, this regimen is associated with a higher rate of relapse and failure, especially among HIV-infected patients.

Lack of adherence to treatment is recognized worldwide as the most important impediment to cure. Moreover, the tubercle bacilli infecting patients who do not adhere to the prescribed regimen are likely to become drug resistant. Both patient- and provider-related factors may affect compliance. Patient-related factors include a lack of belief that the illness is significant and/or that treatment will have a beneficial effect, the existence of concomitant medical conditions (notably substance abuse), lack of social support, and poverty, with attendant joblessness and homelessness. Provider-related factors that may promote compliance include the education and encouragement of patients, the offering of convenient clinic hours, and the provision of incentives and enablers such as meals and travel vouchers.

In addition to specific measures addressing noncompliance, two other strategic approaches are used: direct observation of treatment and provision of fixed-drug-combination (FDC) products. Because it is difficult to predict which patients will adhere to the recommended treatment, all patients should have their therapy directly supervised, especially during the initial phase. In the United States, personnel to supervise therapy are usually available through tuberculosis control programs of local public health departments. Supervision increases the proportion of patients completing treatment and greatly lessens the chances of relapse and acquired drug resistance. FDC products (e.g., isoniazid/rifampin, isoniazid/rifampin/pyrazinamide, and isoniazid/rifampin/pyrazinamide/ethambutol) are available (except, in the United States, for the four-drug FDC) and are strongly recommended as a means of minimizing the likelihood of prescription error and of the development of drug resistance as the result of monotherapy. In some formulations of these combination products, the bioavailability of rifampin has been found to be substandard. In North America and Europe, regulatory authorities ensure that combination products are of good quality; however, this type of quality assurance cannot be assumed to take place in less affluent countries. Alternative regimens for patients who exhibit drug intolerance or adverse reactions are listed in Table 66-3. However, severe side effects prompting discontinuation of any of the first-line drugs and use of these alternative regimens are uncommon.

MONITORING TREATMENT RESPONSE AND DRUG TOXICITY Bacteriologic evaluation is the preferred method of monitoring the response to treatment for tuberculosis. Patients with pulmonary disease should have their sputum examined monthly until cultures become negative. With the recommended regimen, >80% of patients will have negative sputum cultures at the end of the second month of treatment. By the end of the third month, virtually all patients should be culture-negative. In some patients, especially those with extensive cavitary disease and large numbers of organisms, AFB smear conversion may lag behind culture conversion. This phenomenon is presumably due to the expectoration and microscopic visualization of dead bacilli. As noted above, patients with cavitary disease who do not achieve sputum culture conversion by 2 months require extended treatment. When a patient's sputum cultures remain positive at ≥3 months, treatment failure and drug resistance or poor adherence with the regimen should be suspected (see below). A sputum specimen should be collected by the end of treatment to document cure. If mycobacterial cultures are not practical, then monitoring by AFB smear examination should be undertaken at 2, 5, and 6 months. Smears that are positive after 5 months of treatment in a patient known to be adherent are indicative of treatment failure.

Bacteriologic monitoring of patients with extrapulmonary tuberculosis is more difficult and often not feasible. In these cases, the response to treatment must be assessed clinically and radiographically.

Monitoring of the response to treatment during chemotherapy by serial chest radiographs is not recommended, as radiographic changes may lag behind bacteriologic response and are not highly sensitive. After the completion of treatment, neither sputum examination nor chest radiography is recommended for routine follow-up purposes. However, a chest radiograph obtained at the end of treatment may be useful for comparative purposes should the patient develop symptoms of recurrent tuberculosis months or years later. Patients should be instructed to report promptly for medical assessment should they develop any such symptoms.

During treatment, patients should be monitored for drug toxicity (see Table 69-3). The most common adverse reaction of significance is hepatitis. Patients should be carefully educated about the signs and symptoms of drug-induced hepatitis (e.g., dark urine, loss of appetite) and should be instructed to discontinue treatment promptly and see their health care provider should these symptoms occur. Although biochemical monitoring is not routinely recommended, all adult patients should undergo baseline assessment of liver function (e.g., measurement of serum levels of hepatic aminotransferases and serum bilirubin). Older patients, those with concomitant diseases, those with a history of hepatic disease (especially hepatitis C), and those using alcohol daily should be monitored especially closely (i.e., monthly), with repeated measurements of aminotransferases, during the initial phase of treatment. Up to 20% of patients have small increases in aspartate aminotransferase (up to three times the upper limit of normal) that are not accompanied by symptoms and are of no consequence. For patients with symptomatic hepatitis and those with marked (five- to sixfold) elevations in serum levels of aspartate aminotransferase, treatment should be stopped and drugs reintroduced one at a time after liver function has returned to normal.

Hypersensitivity reactions usually require the discontinuation of all drugs and rechallenge to determine which agent is the culprit. Because of the variety of regimens available, it is usually not necessary—although it is possible—to desensitize patients. Hyperuricemia and arthralgia caused by pyrazinamide can usually be managed by the administration of acetylsalicylic acid; however, pyrazinamide treatment should be stopped if the patient develops gouty arthritis. Individuals who develop autoimmune thrombocytopenia secondary to rifampin therapy should not receive the drug thereafter. Similarly, the occurrence of optic neuritis with ethambutol is an indication for permanent discontinuation of this drug. Other common manifestations of drug intolerance, such as pruritus and gastrointestinal upset, can generally be managed without the interruption of therapy.

TREATMENT FAILURE AND RELAPSE As stated above, treatment failure should be suspected when a patient's sputum cultures remain positive after 3 months or when AFB smears remain positive after 5 months. In the management of such patients, it is imperative that the current isolate be tested for susceptibility to first- and second-line agents. When the results of susceptibility testing are expected to become available within a few weeks, changes in the regimen can be postponed until that time. However, if the patient's clinical condition is deteriorating, an earlier change in regimen may be indicated. A cardinal rule in the latter situation is always to add more than one drug at a time to a failing regimen: at least two and preferably three drugs that have never been used and to which the bacilli are likely to be susceptible should be added. The patient may continue to take isoniazid and rifampin along with these new agents pending the results of susceptibility tests.

The mycobacterial strains infecting patients who experience a relapse after apparently successful treatment are less likely to have acquired drug resistance (see below) than are strains from patients in whom treatment has failed. However, if the regimen administered initially does not contain rifampin, the probability of isoniazid resistance is high. Acquired resistance is uncommon among strains from patients who relapse after completing a standard short-course regimen. However, it is prudent to begin the treatment of all patients who have relapsed with all four first-line drugs plus streptomycin, pending the results of susceptibility testing. In less affluent countries and other settings where facilities for culture and drug susceptibility testing are not available, a standard regimen should be used in all instances of relapse and treatment failure (Table 66-3).

DRUG-RESISTANT TUBERCULOSIS Strains of *M. tuberculosis* resistant to individual drugs arise by spontaneous point mutations in the mycobacterial genome, which occur at low but predictable rates. Because there is no cross-resistance among the commonly used drugs, the probability that a strain will be resistant to two drugs is the product of the probabilities of resistance to each drug and thus is low. The development of drug-resistant tuberculosis is invariably the result of monotherapy—i.e., the failure of the health care provider to prescribe at least two drugs to which tubercle bacilli are susceptible or of the patient to take properly prescribed therapy.

Drug-resistant tuberculosis may be either primary or acquired. Primary drug resistance is that in a strain infecting a patient who has not previously been treated. Acquired resistance develops during treatment with an inappropriate regimen. In North America and Europe, rates of primary resistance are generally low, and isoniazid resistance is most common. In the United States, although primary isoniazid resistance was stable at ~7–8% between 1993 and 2002, the rate of primary multidrug-resistant (MDR) tuberculosis (defined as tuberculosis due to a strain resistant at least to isoniazid and rifampin) declined from 2.5% to 1%. Resistance rates are higher among foreign-born and HIV-infected patients. Worldwide, MDR tuberculosis is a serious problem in some regions, especially in the former Soviet Union and parts of Asia (Fig. 66-8). As noted above, drug-resistant tuberculosis can be prevented by adherence to the principles of sound therapy: the inclusion of at least two bactericidal drugs to which the organism is susceptible, the use of FDC products, and the verification that patients complete the prescribed course.

Although the 6-month regimen described in Table 66-3 is generally effective for patients with initial isoniazid-resistant disease, it is prudent to include ethambutol and pyrazinamide for the full 6 months. In such cases, isoniazid probably does not contribute to a successful outcome and should be omitted. MDR tuberculosis is more difficult to manage than is disease caused by a drug-susceptible organism, especially because resistance to other first-line drugs as well as to isoniazid and rifampin is common. For strains resistant to isoniazid and rifampin, combinations of a fluoroquinolone, ethambutol, pyrazinamide, and streptomycin (or, for strains resistant to streptomycin as well, another injectable agent such as amikacin or kanamycin), given for 18–24 months and for at least 9 months after sputum culture conversion, may be effective. For patients with bacilli resistant to all of the first-line agents, cure may be attained with a combination of four second-line drugs, including one injectable agent (Table 66-3). The optimal duration of treatment in this situation is not known; however, a duration of

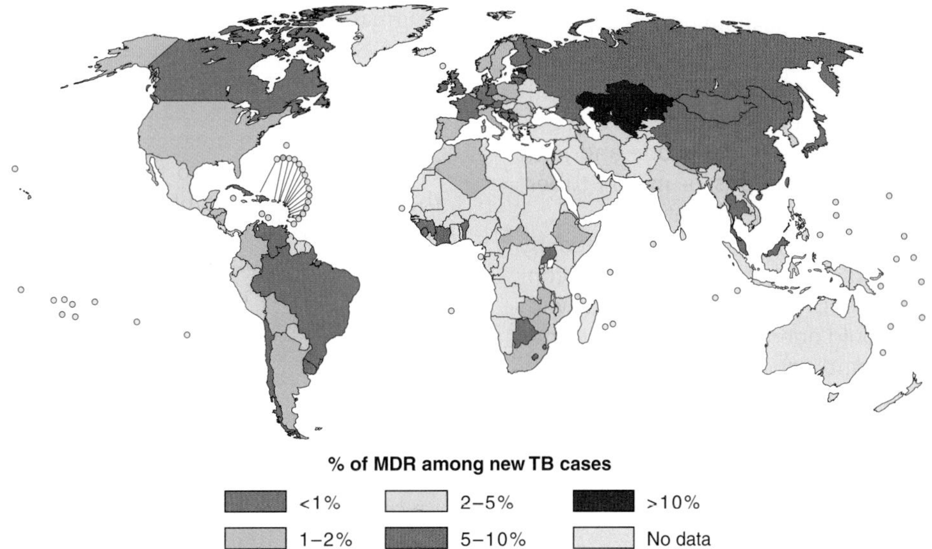

FIGURE 66-8

Percentage of new tuberculosis cases exhibiting multidrug resistance in all countries surveyed by the WHO/Union Global Drug Resistance Surveillance Project during 1994–2005. *(See also disclaimer in Fig. 66-2. Courtesy of the Stop TB Department, WHO; with permission.)*

24 months is recommended. MDR strains of *M. tuberculosis* that are also resistant to at least the fluoroquinolones and one or more of the injectable drugs amikacin, kanamycin, or capreomycin [extensive drug-resistant (XDR) strains] have fewer treatment options and a much poorer prognosis. For patients with localized disease and sufficient pulmonary reserve, lobectomy or pneumonectomy may be helpful. Because the management of patients with MDR and XDR tuberculosis is complicated by both social and medical factors, care of these patients should be restricted to those tuberculosis control programs with resources and capacity and to specialized centers.

HIV-ASSOCIATED TUBERCULOSIS In general, the standard treatment regimens are equally efficacious in HIV-negative and HIV-positive patients. However, adverse drug effects may be more pronounced in HIV-infected patients. Since these effects may include serious or even fatal skin reactions to amithiozone (thiacetazone), this drug, which has been used in place of ethambutol in developing countries, is no longer recommended by the WHO.

Three important considerations are relevant to tuberculosis treatment in HIV-infected patients: an increased frequency of paradoxical reactions, drug interactions between antiretroviral therapy and rifamycins, and development of rifampin monoresistance with widely spaced intermittent treatment. Exacerbations in symptoms, signs, and laboratory or radiographic manifestations of tuberculosis—termed the *immune reconstitution inflammatory syndrome* (IRIS)—have been associated with the administration of antiretroviral regimens. IRIS is more common among patients with advanced immunosuppression and extrapulmonary tuberculosis. The presumed pathogenesis of IRIS is an immune response that is elicited by antigens released as bacilli are killed during effective chemotherapy and that is temporally associated with improving immune function. The first priority in the management of a possible case of IRIS is to ensure that the clinical syndrome does not represent a failure of tuberculosis treatment or the development of another infection. Mild paradoxical reactions can be managed with symptom-based treatment. Glucocorticoids have been used for more severe reactions, although their use in this setting has not been formally evaluated in clinical trials.

Most HIV-infected tuberculosis patients are candidates for antiretroviral therapy, although the optimal timing of this treatment is not known. Rifampin, a potent inducer of enzymes of the cytochrome P450 system, lowers serum levels of many HIV protease inhibitors and some nonnucleoside reverse transcriptase inhibitors—essential drugs used in antiretroviral regimens. In such cases, rifabutin, which has much less enzyme-inducing activity, has been recommended in place of rifampin. However, dosage adjustment for rifabutin and/or the antiretroviral drugs may be necessary. Because recommendations are frequently updated, consultation of the CDC website is advised (*http://www.cdc.gov/tb*).

Several clinical trials of HIV-associated tuberculosis have found that patients with advanced immunosuppression (CD4+ T-cell counts of <100/μL) are prone to treatment failure and relapse with rifampin-resistant organisms when treated with "highly intermittent" (i.e., once- or twice-weekly) rifamycin-containing regimens. Consequently, it is recommended that these patients receive daily or thrice-weekly therapy for the entire course.

SPECIAL CLINICAL SITUATIONS Although comparative clinical trials of treatment for extrapulmonary tuberculosis are limited, the available evidence indicates that most forms of disease can be treated with the 6-month regimen recommended for patients with pulmonary disease. The American Academy of Pediatrics recommends that children with bone and joint tuberculosis, tuberculous meningitis, or miliary tuberculosis receive 9–12 months of treatment.

Treatment for tuberculosis may be complicated by underlying medical problems that require special consideration (see Table 69-1). As a rule, patients with chronic renal failure should not receive aminoglycosides and should receive ethambutol only if serum levels can be monitored. Isoniazid, rifampin, and pyrazinamide may be given in the usual doses in cases of mild to moderate renal failure, but the dosages of isoniazid and pyrazinamide should be reduced for all patients with severe renal failure except those undergoing hemodialysis. Patients with hepatic disease pose a special problem because of the hepatotoxicity of isoniazid, rifampin, and pyrazinamide. Patients with severe hepatic disease may be treated with ethambutol, streptomycin, and possibly another drug (e.g., a fluoroquinolone); if required, isoniazid and rifampin may be administered under close supervision. The use of pyrazinamide by patients with liver failure should be avoided. Silicotuberculosis necessitates the extension of therapy by at least 2 months.

The regimen of choice for pregnant women (Tables 69-1 and 66-3) is 9 months of treatment with isoniazid and rifampin supplemented by ethambutol for the first 2 months. Although the WHO has recommended routine use of pyrazinamide in pregnant women, this drug has not been recommended in the United States because of insufficient data documenting its safety in pregnancy. Streptomycin is contraindicated because it is known to cause eighth-cranial-nerve damage in the fetus. Treatment for tuberculosis is not a contraindication to breast-feeding; most of the drugs administered will be present in small quantities in breast milk, albeit at concentrations far too low to provide any therapeutic or prophylactic benefit to the child.

Medical consultation on difficult-to-manage cases is provided by the CDC Regional Training and Medical Consultation Centers (*http://www.cdc.gov/tb/education/rtmcc/default.htm*).

PREVENTION

By far the best way to prevent tuberculosis is to diagnose and isolate infectious cases rapidly and administer appropriate treatment until patients are rendered noninfectious and the disease is cured. Additional strategies include BCG vaccination and treatment of persons with latent tuberculosis infection who are at high risk of developing active disease.

BCG VACCINATION

BCG was derived from an attenuated strain of *M. bovis* and first administered to humans in 1921. Many BCG vaccines are available worldwide; all are derived from the original strain, but the vaccines vary in efficacy, ranging from 80% to nil in randomized, placebo-controlled trials. A similar range of efficacy was found in recent observational studies (case-control, historic cohort, and cross-sectional) in areas where infants are vaccinated at birth. These studies also found higher rates of efficacy in the protection of infants and young children from relatively serious forms of tuberculosis, such as tuberculous meningitis and miliary tuberculosis.

BCG vaccine is safe and rarely causes serious complications. The local tissue response begins 2–3 weeks after vaccination, with scar formation and healing within 3 months. Side effects—most commonly, ulceration at the vaccination site and regional lymphadenitis—occur in 1–10% of vaccinated persons. Some vaccine strains have caused osteomyelitis in ~1 case per million doses administered. Disseminated BCG infection and death have occurred in 1–10 cases per 10 million doses administered, although this problem is restricted almost exclusively to persons with impaired immunity, such as children with severe combined immunodeficiency syndrome or adults with HIV infection. BCG vaccination induces TST reactivity, which tends to wane with time. The presence or size of TST reactions after vaccination does not predict the degree of protection afforded.

BCG vaccine is recommended for routine use at birth in countries with high tuberculosis prevalence. However, because of the low risk of transmission of tuberculosis in the United States, the unreliable protection afforded by BCG, and its impact on the TST, the vaccine has never been recommended for general use in the United States. The CDC has recommended that HIV-infected adults and children not receive BCG vaccine, although the WHO has recommended that asymptomatic HIV-infected children residing in tuberculosis-endemic areas receive BCG.

℞ Treatment: LATENT TUBERCULOSIS INFECTION

Treatment of selected persons with LTBI aims at preventing active disease. This intervention (formerly called *preventive chemotherapy* or *chemoprophylaxis*) is based on the results of a large number of randomized, placebo-controlled clinical trials demonstrating that a 6- to 12-month course of isoniazid reduces the risk of active tuberculosis in infected people by up to 90%. Analysis of available data indicates that the optimal duration of treatment is 9–10 months. In the absence of reinfection, the protective effect is believed to be lifelong. Clinical trials have shown that isoniazid reduces rates of tuberculosis among TST-positive persons with HIV infection. Studies in HIV-infected patients have also demonstrated the effectiveness of shorter courses of rifampin-based treatment.

In most cases, candidates for treatment of LTBI (Table 66-4) are identified by the TST of persons in defined high-risk groups. For skin testing, 5 tuberculin units of polysorbate-stabilized PPD should be injected intradermally into the volar surface of the forearm (Mantoux method). Multipuncture tests are not recommended.

TABLE 66-4

TUBERCULIN REACTION SIZE AND TREATMENT OF LATENT TUBERCULOSIS INFECTION

RISK GROUP	TUBERCULIN REACTION SIZE, mm
HIV-infected persons or persons receiving immunosuppressive therapy	≥5
Close contacts of tuberculosis patients	≥5[a]
Persons with fibrotic lesions on chest radiography	≥5
Recently infected persons (≤2 years)	≥10
Persons with high-risk medical conditions[b]	≥10
Low-risk persons[c]	≥15

[a]Tuberculin-negative contacts, especially children, should receive prophylaxis for 2–3 months after contact ends and should then undergo repeat TST. Those whose results remain negative should discontinue prophylaxis. HIV-infected contacts should receive a full course of treatment regardless of TST results.

[b]Includes diabetes mellitus, some hematologic and reticuloendothelial diseases, injection drug use (with HIV seronegativity), end-stage renal disease, and clinical situations associated with rapid weight loss.

[c]Except for employment purposes where longitudinal TST screening is anticipated, TST is not indicated for these low-risk persons. A decision to treat should be based on individual risk/benefit considerations.

Reactions are read at 48–72 h as the transverse diameter (in millimeters) of induration; the diameter of erythema is not considered. In some persons, TST reactivity wanes with time but can be recalled by a second skin test administered ≥1 week after the first (i.e., two-step testing). For persons periodically undergoing the TST, such as health care workers and individuals admitted to long-term-care institutions, initial two-step testing may preclude subsequent misclassification of persons with boosted reactions as TST converters.

The cutoff for a positive TST (and thus for treatment) is related both to the probability that the reaction represents true infection and to the likelihood that the individual, if truly infected, will develop tuberculosis (Table 66-4). Thus positive reactions for close contacts of infectious cases, persons with HIV infection, persons receiving drugs that suppress the immune system, and previously untreated persons whose chest radiograph is consistent with healed tuberculosis are defined as an area of induration ≥5 mm in diameter. A 10-mm cutoff is used to define positive reactions in most other at-risk persons. For persons with a very low risk of developing tuberculosis if infected, a cutoff of 15 mm is used. (Except for employment purposes where longitudinal screening is anticipated, the TST is not indicated for these low-risk persons.) Treatment should be considered for persons from tuberculosis-endemic countries who have a history of BCG vaccination. A positive reaction in an IGRA is not based on the degree of response—i.e., the level of IFN-γ induced.

Some TST-negative individuals are also candidates for treatment. Infants and children who have come into contact with infectious cases should be treated and should have a repeat skin test 2 or 3 months after contact ends. Those whose test results remain negative should discontinue treatment. HIV-infected persons who have been exposed to an infectious tuberculosis patient should receive treatment regardless of the TST result.

Isoniazid is administered at a daily dose of 5 mg/kg (up to 300 mg/d) for 9 months (Table 66-5). On the basis of cost-benefit analyses, a 6-month period of treatment has been recommended in the past and may be considered for HIV-negative adults with normal chest radiographs when financial considerations are important. When supervised treatment is desirable and feasible, isoniazid may be given at a dose of 15 mg/kg (up to 900 mg) twice weekly. An alternative regimen for adults is 4 months of daily rifampin. A 3-month regimen of isoniazid and rifampin is recommended in the United Kingdom for both adults and children. A previously recommended regimen of 2 months of rifampin and pyrazinamide has been associated with serious and fatal hepatotoxicity and now is generally not recommended. The rifampin regimen should be considered for persons who are likely to have been infected with an isoniazid-resistant strain.

Isoniazid should not be given to persons with active liver disease. All persons at increased risk of hepatotoxicity (e.g., those abusing alcohol daily and those with a history of liver disease) should undergo baseline and then monthly assessment of liver function. All patients should be carefully educated about hepatitis and instructed to discontinue use of the drug immediately should any symptoms develop. Moreover, patients should be seen and questioned monthly during therapy about adverse reactions and should be given no more than 1 month's supply of drug at each visit.

It may be more difficult to ensure compliance when treating persons with latent infection than when treating those with active tuberculosis. If family members of active cases are being treated, compliance and monitoring may be easier. When feasible, twice-weekly supervised therapy may increase the likelihood of completion. As in active cases, the provision of incentives may also be helpful.

PRINCIPLES OF TUBERCULOSIS CONTROL

The highest priority in any tuberculosis control program is the prompt detection of cases and the provision of short-course chemotherapy to all tuberculosis patients under proper case-management conditions, including directly observed therapy. In addition, in low-prevalence countries with adequate resources, screening of high-risk groups (such as immigrants from high-prevalence countries, migratory workers, prisoners, the homeless, substance

TABLE 66-5

REVISED DRUG REGIMENS FOR TREATMENT OF LATENT TUBERCULOSIS INFECTION (LTBI) IN ADULTS

DRUG	INTERVAL AND DURATION	COMMENTS[a]	RATING[b] (EVIDENCE[c]) HIV-NEGATIVE	RATING[b] (EVIDENCE[c]) HIV-INFECTED
Isoniazid	Daily for 9 months[d,e]	In HIV-infected persons, isoniazid may be administered concurrently with nucleoside reverse transcriptase inhibitors, protease inhibitors, or nonnucleoside reverse transcriptase inhibitors (NNRTIs).	A (II)	A (II)
	Twice weekly for 9 months[d,e]	Directly observed therapy (DOT) must be used with twice-weekly dosing.	B (II)	B (II)
	Daily for 6 months[e]	Regimen is not indicated for HIV-infected persons, those with fibrotic lesions on chest radiographs, or children.	B (I)	C (I)
	Twice weekly for 6 months[e]	DOT must be used with twice-weekly dosing.	B (II)	C (I)
Rifampin[f]	Daily for 4 months	Regimen is used for contacts of patients with isoniazid-resistant, rifampin-susceptible tuberculosis. In HIV-infected persons, most protease inhibitors and delavirdine should not be administered concurrently with rifampin. Rifabutin, with appropriate dose adjustments, can be used with protease inhibitors (saquinavir should be augmented with ritonavir) and NNRTIs (except delavirdine). Clinicians should consult web-based updates for the latest specific recommendations.	B (II)	B (III)
Rifampin plus pyrazinamide (RZ)	Daily for 2 months	Regimen generally should not be offered for treatment of LTBI in either HIV-infected or HIV-negative persons.	D (II)	D (II)
	Twice weekly for 2–3 months		D (III)	D (III)

[a]Interactions with HIV-related drugs are updated frequently and are available at *http://aidsinfo.nih.gov*.

[b]Strength of the recommendation: A. Both strong evidence of efficacy and substantial clinical benefit support recommendation for use. Should always be offered. B. Moderate evidence for efficacy or strong evidence for efficacy but only limited clinical benefit supports recommendation for use. Should generally be offered. C. Evidence for efficacy is insufficient to support a recommendation for or against use, or evidence for efficacy might not outweigh adverse consequences (e.g., drug toxicity, drug interactions) or cost of the treatment or alternative approaches. Optional. D. Moderate evidence for lack of efficacy or for adverse outcome supports a recommendation against use. Should generally not be offered. E. Good evidence for lack of efficacy or for adverse outcome supports a recommendation against use. Should never be offered.

[c]Quality of evidence supporting the recommendation: I. Evidence from at least one properly randomized controlled trial. II. Evidence from at least one well-designed clinical trial without randomization, from cohort or case-controlled analytic studies (preferably from more than one center), from multiple time-series studies, or from dramatic results in uncontrolled experiments. III. Evidence from opinions of respected authorities based on clinical experience, descriptive studies, or reports of expert committees.

[d]Recommended regimen for persons aged <18 years.

[e]Recommended regimen for pregnant women.

[f]The substitution of rifapentine for rifampin is not recommended because rifapentine's safety and effectiveness have not been established for patients with LTBI.

Source: Adapted from CDC: Targeted tuberculin testing and treatment of latent tuberculosis infection. MMWR 49(RR-6), 2000.

abusers, and HIV-seropositive persons) is recommended. TST-positive high-risk persons should be treated for latent infection. Contact investigation is an important component of efficient tuberculosis control. In the United States, a great deal of attention has been given to the transmission of tuberculosis (particularly in association with HIV infection) in institutional settings such as hospitals, homeless shelters, and prisons. Measures to limit such transmission include respiratory isolation of persons with suspected tuberculosis until they are proven to be noninfectious (i.e., by sputum AFB smear negativity), proper ventilation in rooms of patients with infectious tuberculosis, use of ultraviolet irradiation in areas of increased risk of tuberculosis transmission, and periodic screening of personnel who may come into contact with known or unsuspected cases of tuberculosis. In the past, radiographic surveys, especially those conducted with portable equipment and miniature films, were advocated for case finding. Today, however, the prevalence of tuberculosis in industrialized countries is sufficiently low that "mass miniature radiography" is not cost-effective.

In high-prevalence countries, many tuberculosis control programs have made good progress in reducing morbidity and mortality during the past decade by adopting and implementing the DOTS strategy promoted by the WHO. This strategy consists of: (1) political commitment with increased and sustained financing; (2) case detection through quality-assured bacteriology (starting with microscopic examination of sputum from patients with cough of >2–3 weeks' duration); (3) administration of standardized treatment, with supervision and patient support; (4) an effective drug supply and management system; and (5) a monitoring and evaluation system, with impact measurement (including assessment of treatment outcomes—e.g., cure, completion of treatment without bacteriologic proof of cure, death, treatment failure, and default—in all cases registered and notified). In 2006, the WHO indicated that, although DOTS remains the essential component of any control strategy, additional steps must be undertaken to reach the 2015 tuberculosis control targets set within the United Nations Millennium Development Goals. Thus a new "Stop TB Strategy" with six components has been promoted: (1) Pursue high-quality DOTS expansion and enhancement. (2) Address HIV-associated tuberculosis, MDR tuberculosis, and other special challenges. (3) Contribute to health system strengthening. (4) Engage all care providers. (5) Empower people with tuberculosis and communities. (6) Enable and promote research. As part of the fourth component, new evidence-based International Standards for Tuberculosis Care, focused on diagnosis, treatment, and public health responsibilities, have recently been introduced for wide adoption by medical and professional societies, academic institutions, and all practitioners worldwide.

FURTHER READINGS

American Thoracic Society, Centers for Disease Control and Prevention: Targeted tuberculin testing and treatment of latent tuberculosis infection. Am J Respir Crit Care Med 161:S221, 2000

American Thoracic Society, Infectious Diseases Society of America, Centers for Disease Control and Prevention: Treatment of tuberculosis. Am J Respir Crit Care Med 167:603, 2003

Centers for Disease Control and Prevention: Control of tuberculosis in the United States: Recommendations from the American Thoracic Society, CDC, and the Infectious Diseases Society of America. MMWR 54:RR1, 2005

Hopewell PC et al: International standards for tuberculosis care. Lancet Infect Dis 6:710, 2006

Menzies D et al: Meta-analysis: New tests for the diagnosis of latent tuberculosis infection: Areas of uncertainty and recommendations for research. Ann Intern Med 146:340, 2007

Nahid P et al: Treatment outcomes of patients with HIV and tuberculosis. Am J Respir Crit Care Med 175:1199, 2007

Onyebujoh PC et al: Treatment options for HIV-associated tuberculosis. J Infect Dis 196(Suppl 1):S35, 2007

Pai M et al: New tools and emerging technologies for the diagnosis of tuberculosis. Part I: Latent tuberculosis. Part II: Active tuberculosis and drug resistance. Expert Rev Mol Diagn 6:413, 2006

Raviglione MC, Smith IM: XDR tuberculosis—Implications for global public health. N Engl J Med 356:656, 2007

———, Uplekar M: WHO's new Stop TB Strategy. Lancet 367:952, 2006

Reid A et al: Towards universal access to HIV prevention, treatment, care and support: The role of tuberculosis/HIV collaboration. Lancet Infect Dis 6:483, 2006

Volmink J, Garner P: Directly observed therapy for treating tuberculosis. Cochrane Database Syst Rev Oct 17(4):CD003343, 2007

World Health Organization: Guidelines for the programmatic management of drug-resistant tuberculosis. Geneva, WHO, 2006

Wright A et al: Global project on anti-tuberculosis drug resistance surveillance. Epidemiology of antituberculosis drug resistance 2002–07: An updated analysis of the Global Project on Anti-Tuberculosis Drug Resistance Surveillance. Lancet 373:186, 2009

CHAPTER 67

LEPROSY (HANSEN'S DISEASE)

Robert H. Gelber

Leprosy, first described in ancient Indian texts from the sixth century B.C., is a nonfatal, chronic infectious disease caused by *Mycobacterium leprae*, whose clinical manifestations are largely confined to the skin, peripheral nervous system, upper respiratory tract, eyes, and testes. The unique tropism of *M. leprae* for peripheral nerves (from large nerve trunks to microscopic dermal nerves) and certain immunologically mediated reactional states are the major causes of morbidity in leprosy. The propensity of the disease, when untreated, to result in characteristic deformities and the recognition in most cultures that the disease is communicable from person to person have resulted historically in a profound social stigma. Today, with early diagnosis and the institution of appropriate and effective antimicrobial therapy, patients can lead productive lives in the community, and deformities and other visible manifestations can largely be prevented.

ETIOLOGY

M. leprae is an obligate intracellular bacillus (0.3–1 μm wide and 1–8 μm long) that is confined to humans, armadillos in certain locales, and sphagnum moss. The organism is acid-fast, indistinguishable microscopically from other mycobacteria, and ideally detected in tissue sections by a modified Fite stain. Strain variability has been documented in this organism. *M. leprae* produces no known toxins and is well adapted to penetrate and reside within macrophages, yet it may survive outside the body for months. In untreated patients, only ~1% of *M. leprae* organisms are viable. The morphologic index (MI), a measure of the number of acid-fast bacilli (AFB) in skin scrapings that stain uniformly bright, correlates with viability. The bacteriologic index (BI), a logarithmic-scaled measure of the density of *M. leprae* in the dermis, may be as high as 4–6+ in untreated patients, falling by 1 unit per year during effective therapy; the rate of decrease is independent of the relative potency of effective antimicrobial therapy. A rising MI or BI suggests relapse and perhaps—if the patient is being treated—drug resistance. The latter possibility can be confirmed or excluded in the mouse model.

As a result of reductive evolution, almost half of the *M. leprae* genome contains nonfunctional genes; only 1605 genes encode for proteins, and 1439 genes are shared with *Mycobacterium tuberculosis*. In contrast, *M. tuberculosis* uses 91% of its genome to encode for 4000 proteins. Among the lost genes in *M. leprae* are those for catabolic and respiratory pathways; transport systems; purine, methionine, and glutamine synthesis; and nitrogen regulation. The genome of *M. leprae* provides a metabolic rationale for its obligate intracellular existence and reliance on host biochemical support, a template for targets of drug development, and ultimately a pathway to cultivation. The finding of strain variability among *M. leprae* isolates has provided a powerful tool with which to address anew the organism's epidemiology and pathobiology and to determine whether relapse represents reactivation or reinfection. The bacterium's complex cell wall contains large amounts of an *M. leprae*–specific phenolic glycolipid (PGL-1), which is detected in serologic tests. The unique trisaccharide of *M. leprae* binds to the basal lamina of Schwann cells; this interaction is probably relevant to the fact that *M. leprae* is the only bacterium to invade peripheral nerves.

Although it was the first bacterium to be etiologically associated with human disease, *M. leprae* remains one of the few bacterial species that still has not been cultivated on artificial medium or tissue culture. The multiplication of *M. leprae* in mouse footpads (albeit limited, with a doubling time of ~2 weeks) has provided a means to evaluate antimicrobial agents, monitor clinical trials, and screen vaccines. *M. leprae* grows best in cooler tissues (the skin, peripheral nerves, anterior chamber of the eye, upper respiratory tract, and testes), sparing warmer areas of the skin (the axilla, groin, scalp, and midline of the back).

EPIDEMIOLOGY

Demographics

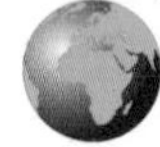

Leprosy is almost exclusively a disease of the developing world, affecting areas of Asia, Africa, Latin America, and the Pacific (Fig. 67-1). Although Africa has the highest disease prevalence, Asia has the most cases. More than 80% of the world's cases occur in a few countries: India, China, Myanmar, Indonesia, Brazil, Nigeria, Madagascar, and Nepal. Within endemic locales, the distribution of leprosy is quite uneven, with areas of high prevalence bordering on areas with little or no disease. In Brazil the majority of cases occur in the Amazon basin and two western states, whereas in Mexico leprosy is mostly confined to the Pacific coast. Except as imported cases, leprosy is largely absent from the United States, Canada, and northwestern Europe. In the United States, ~4000 persons have leprosy and 100–200 new cases are reported annually, most of them in California, Texas, New York, and Hawaii among immigrants from Mexico, Southeast Asia, the Philippines, and the Caribbean. The comparative genomics of single-nucleotide polymorphisms support the likelihood that four distinct strains exist, having originated in East Africa or Central Asia. A mutation spread to Europe and subsequently underwent two separate mutations that were then followed by spread to West Africa and the Americas.

The global prevalence of leprosy is difficult to assess, given that many of the locales with high prevalence lack a significant medical or public health infrastructure. Estimates range from 0.6 to 8 million affected individuals. The lower estimate includes only persons who have not completed chemotherapy, excluding those who may be physically or psychologically damaged from leprosy and who may yet relapse or develop immune-mediated reactions. The higher figure includes patients whose infections probably are already cured and many who have no leprosy-related deformity or disability. Although the figures on the worldwide prevalence of leprosy are debatable, it is not falling; there are an estimated 600,000 new cases annually, 60% of them in India.

Leprosy is associated with poverty and rural residence. It appears not to be associated with AIDS, perhaps because of leprosy's long incubation period. Most people appear to be naturally immune to leprosy and do not develop disease manifestations after exposure. The time of peak onset is in the second and third decades of life. The most severe lepromatous form of leprosy is twice as common among men as among women and is rarely encountered in children. The frequency of the polar forms of leprosy in different countries varies widely and may in part be genetically determined; certain HLA associations are known for both polar forms of leprosy (see below). In India and Africa, 90% of cases are tuberculoid; in Southeast Asia, 50% are tuberculoid

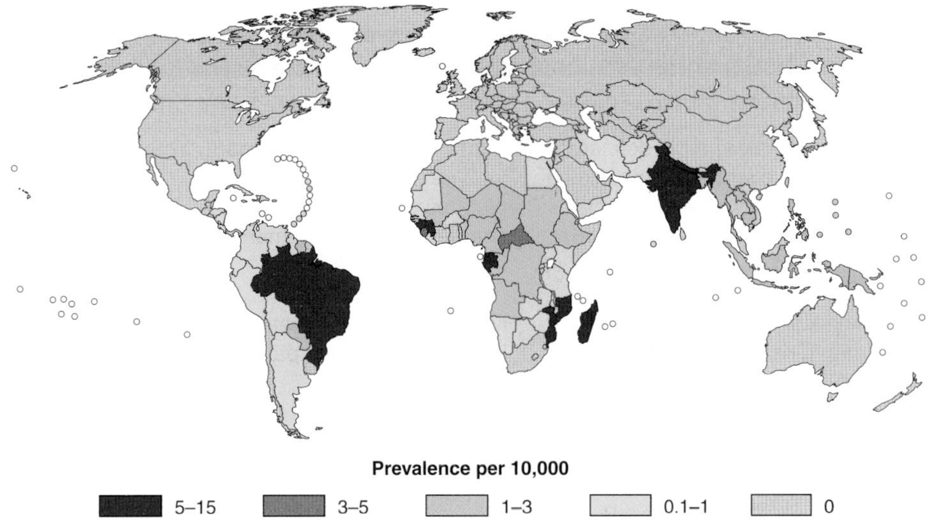

FIGURE 67-1

Estimated prevalence of leprosy at the turn of the millennium. Because data on leprosy prevalence in many endemic countries are unreliable, global prevalence is difficult to assess with any great degree of accuracy; however, it is not falling (see text). (*Courtesy of Patrick J. Brennan, Ph.D., with permission; www.cvmbs.colostate.edu/microbiology/leprosy/globalleprosy3.html.*)

and 50% lepromatous; and in Mexico, 90% are lepromatous. (For definitions of disease types, see Table 67-1 and "Clinical, Histologic, and Immunologic Spectrum.")

Transmission

The route of transmission of leprosy remains uncertain, and transmission routes may in fact be multiple. Nasal droplet infection, contact with infected soil, and even insect vectors have been considered the prime candidates.

Aerosolized *M. leprae* can cause infection in immunosuppressed mice, and a sneeze from an untreated lepromatous patient may contain $>10^{10}$ AFB. Furthermore, both IgA antibody to *M. leprae* and genes of *M. leprae*—demonstrable by polymerase chain reaction (PCR)—have been found in the nose of individuals without signs of leprosy from endemic areas and in 19% of occupational contacts of lepromatous patients.

Several lines of evidence implicate soil transmission. (1) In endemic countries such as India, leprosy is primarily a rural and not an urban disease. (2) *M. leprae* products reside in soil in endemic locales. (3) Direct dermal inoculation (e.g., during tattooing) may transmit *M. leprae*, and common sites of leprosy in children are the buttocks and thighs, suggesting that microinoculation of infected soil may transmit the disease.

Evidence for insect vectors of leprosy includes the demonstration that bedbugs and mosquitoes in the vicinity of leprosaria regularly harbor *M. leprae* and that experimentally infected mosquitoes can transmit infection to mice. Skin-to-skin contact is generally not considered an important route of transmission.

In endemic countries, ~50% of leprosy patients have a history of intimate contact with an infected person (often a household member), whereas, for unknown reasons, leprosy patients in nonendemic locales can identify such contact only 10% of the time. Moreover, household contact with an infected lepromatous case carries an eventual risk of disease acquisition of ~10% in endemic areas as opposed to only 1% in nonendemic locales. Contact with a tuberculoid case carries a very low risk. Physicians and nurses caring for leprosy patients and the co-workers of these patients are not at risk for leprosy.

M. leprae causes disease primarily in humans. However, in Texas and Louisiana, 15% of nine-banded armadillos are infected, and armadillo contact occasionally results in human disease. Armadillos develop disseminated infection after IV inoculation of live *M. leprae*.

CLINICAL, HISTOLOGIC, AND IMMUNOLOGIC SPECTRUM

The incubation period before manifestation of clinical disease can vary between 2 and 40 years, although it is generally 5–7 years in duration. Leprosy presents as a spectrum of clinical manifestations that have bacteriologic, pathologic, and immunologic counterparts. The spectrum from polar tuberculoid (TT) to borderline tuberculoid (BT) to mid-borderline (BB, which is rarely encountered) to borderline lepromatous (BL) to polar lepromatous (LL) disease is associated with an evolution from asymmetric localized macules and plaques to nodular and indurated symmetric generalized skin manifestations, an increasing bacterial load, and loss of *M. leprae*–specific cellular immunity (Table 67-1). Distinguishing dermatopatho logic characteristics include the number of lymphocytes, giant cells, and AFB as well as the nature of epithelioid cell differentiation. Where a patient presents on the clinical spectrum largely determines prognosis, complications, reactional states, and the intensity of antimicrobial therapy required.

TABLE 67-1

CLINICAL, BACTERIOLOGIC, PATHOLOGIC, AND IMMUNOLOGIC SPECTRUM OF LEPROSY

FEATURE	TUBERCULOID (TT, BT) LEPROSY	BORDERLINE (BB, BL) LEPROSY	LEPROMATOUS (LL) LEPROSY
Skin lesions	One or a few sharply defined annular asymmetric macules or plaques with a tendency toward central clearing, elevated borders	Intermediate between BT and LL type lesions; ill-defined plaques with an occasional sharp margin; few or many in number	Symmetric, poorly marginated, multiple infiltrated nodules and plaques or diffuse infiltration; xanthoma-like or dermatofibroma papules; leonine facies and eyebrow alopecia
Nerve lesions	Skin lesions anesthetic early; nerve near lesions sometimes enlarged; nerve abscesses most common in BT	Hypesthetic or anesthetic skin lesions; nerve trunk palsies, at times symmetric	Hypesthesia a late sign; nerve palsies variable; acral, distal, symmetric anesthesia common
Acid-fast bacilli (BI[a])	0–1+	3–5+	4–6+
Lymphocytes	2+	1+	0–1+
Macrophage differentiation	Epithelioid	Epithelioid in BB; usually undifferentiated, but may have foamy changes in BL	Foamy change the rule; may be undifferentiated in early lesions
Langhans' giant cells	1–3+	—	—
Lepromin skin test	+++	—	—
Lymphocyte transformation test	Generally positive	1–10%	1–2%
CD4+/CD8+ T-cell ratio in lesions	1.2	BB (NT); BL: 0.48	0.50
M. leprae PGL-1 antibodies	60%	85%	95%

[a]See text.

Note: BB, mid-borderline; BL, borderline lepromatous; BT, borderline tuberculoid; TT, polar tuberculoid; LL, polar lepromatous; BI, bacteriologic index; NT, not tested; PGL-1, phenolic glycolipid 1.

Tuberculoid Leprosy

At the less severe end of the spectrum is tuberculoid leprosy, which encompasses TT and BT disease. In general, these forms of leprosy result in symptoms confined to the skin and peripheral nerves. The skin lesions of tuberculoid leprosy consist of one or a few hypopigmented macules or plaques (Fig. 67-2) that are sharply demarcated and hypesthetic, often have erythematous or raised borders, and are devoid of the normal skin organs (sweat glands and hair follicles) and thus are dry, scaly, and anhidrotic. AFB are generally absent or few in number. Tuberculoid leprosy patients may have asymmetric enlargement of one or a few peripheral nerves. Indeed, leprosy and certain rare hereditary neuropathies are the only human diseases associated with peripheral-nerve enlargement. Although any peripheral nerve may be enlarged (including small digital and supraclavicular nerves), those most commonly affected are the ulnar, posterior auricular, peroneal, and posterior tibial nerves, with associated hypesthesia and myopathy. TT leprosy is the most common form of the disease encountered in India and Africa but is virtually absent in Southeast Asia, where BT leprosy is frequent.

In tuberculoid leprosy, T cells breach the perineurium, and destruction of Schwann cells and axons may be evident, resulting in fibrosis of the epineurium, replacement of the endoneurium with epithelial granulomas, and occasionally caseous necrosis. Such invasion and destruction of nerves in the dermis by T cells are pathognomonic for leprosy.

Circulating lymphocytes from patients with tuberculoid leprosy readily recognize *M. leprae* and its constituent

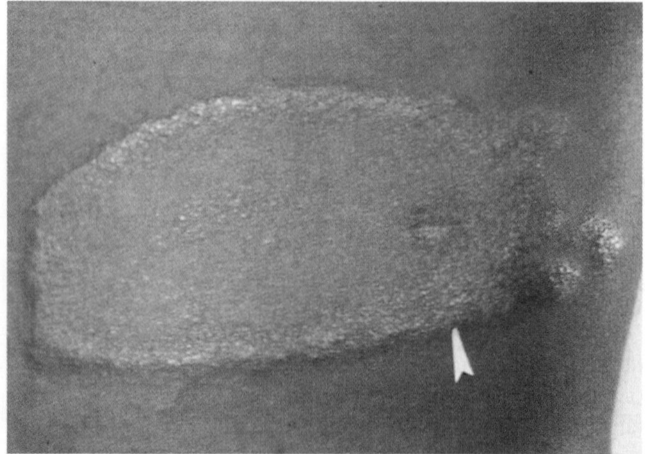

FIGURE 67-2

Tuberculoid (TT) leprosy: a well-defined, hypopigmented, anesthetic macule with anhidrosis and a raised granular margin *(arrowhead)*.

proteins, patients have positive lepromin skin tests (see "Diagnosis" later in the chapter), and—owing to a type 1 cytokine pattern in tuberculoid tissues—strong T-cell and macrophage activation results in a localized infection. In tuberculoid leprosy tissue, there is a 2:1 predominance of helper CD4+ over CD8+ T lymphocytes. Tuberculoid tissues are rich in the mRNAs of the proinflammatory T_H1 family of cytokines: interleukin (IL) 2, interferon γ (IFN-γ), and IL-12; in contrast, IL-4, IL-5, and IL-10 mRNAs are scarce.

Lepromatous Leprosy

Lepromatous leprosy patients present with symmetrically distributed skin nodules (Fig. 67-3), raised plaques, or diffuse dermal infiltration, which, when on the face, results in leonine facies. Late manifestations include loss of eyebrows (initially the lateral margins only) and eyelashes, pendulous earlobes, and dry scaling skin, particularly on the feet. In LL leprosy, bacilli are numerous in the skin (as many as 10^9/g), where they are often found in large clumps (*globi*), and in peripheral nerves, where they initially invade Schwann cells, resulting in foamy degenerative myelination and axonal degeneration and later in Wallerian degeneration. In addition, bacilli are plentiful in circulating blood and in all organ systems except the lungs and the central nervous system. Nevertheless, patients are afebrile, and there is no evidence of major organ system dysfunction. Found almost exclusively in western Mexico and the Caribbean is a form of lepromatous leprosy without visible skin lesions but with diffuse dermal infiltration and a demonstrably thickened dermis, termed *diffuse lepromatosis*. In lepromatous leprosy, nerve enlargement and damage tend to be symmetric, result from actual bacillary invasion, and are more insidious but ultimately more extensive than in tuberculoid leprosy. Patients with LL leprosy have acral, distal, symmetric peripheral neuropathy and a tendency toward symmetric nerve-trunk enlargement. They may also have signs and symptoms related to involvement of the upper respiratory tract, the anterior chamber of the eye, and the testes.

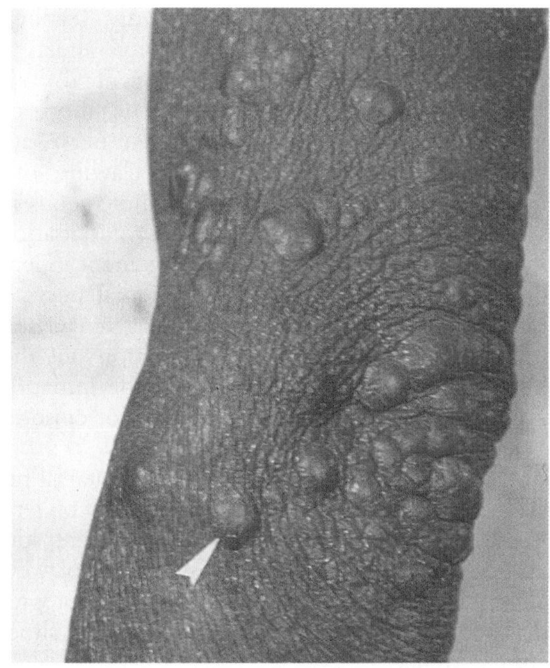

FIGURE 67-3
Lepromatous (LL) leprosy: advanced nodular lesions.

In untreated LL patients, lymphocytes regularly fail to recognize either *M. leprae* or its protein constituents, and lepromin skin tests are negative (see "Diagnosis," below). This loss of protective cellular immunity appears to be antigen-specific, as patients are not unusually susceptible to opportunistic infections, cancer, or AIDS and maintain delayed-type hypersensitivity to *Candida*, *Trichophyton*, mumps, tetanus toxoid, and even purified protein derivative of tuberculin. At times, *M. leprae*–specific anergy is reversible with effective chemotherapy. In LL tissues, there is a 2:1 ratio of CD8+ to CD4+ T lymphocytes. LL patients have a predominant T_H2 response and hyperglobulinemia, and LL tissues demonstrate a T_H2 cytokine profile, being rich in mRNAs for IL-4, IL-5, and IL-10 and poor in those for IL-2, IFN-γ, and IL-12. It appears that cytokines mediate a protective tissue response in leprosy, as injection of IFN-γ or IL-2 into lepromatous lesions causes a loss of AFB and histopathologic conversion toward a tuberculoid pattern. Macrophages of lepromatous leprosy patients appear to be functionally intact; circulating monocytes exhibit normal microbicidal function and responsiveness to IFN-γ.

Reactional States

Lepra reactions comprise several common immunologically mediated inflammatory states that cause considerable morbidity. Some of these reactions precede diagnosis and the institution of effective antimicrobial therapy; indeed, these reactions may precipitate presentation for medical attention and diagnosis. Other reactions occur after the initiation of appropriate chemotherapy and may cause patients to perceive that their leprosy is worsening and to lose confidence in conventional therapy. Only by warning patients of the potential for these reactions and describing their manifestations can physicians treating leprosy patients ensure continued credibility.

Type 1 Lepra Reactions (Downgrading and Reversal Reactions)

Type 1 lepra reactions occur in almost half of patients with borderline forms of leprosy but not in patients with pure lepromatous disease. Manifestations include classic signs of inflammation within previously involved macules, papules, and plaques and, on occasion, the appearance of new skin lesions, neuritis, and (less commonly) fever—generally low-grade. The nerve trunk most commonly involved in this process is the ulnar nerve at the elbow, which may be painful and exquisitely tender. If patients with affected nerves are not treated promptly with glucocorticoids (see below), irreversible nerve damage may result in as little as 24 h. The most dramatic manifestation is footdrop, which occurs when the peroneal nerve is involved.

When type 1 lepra reactions precede the initiation of appropriate antimicrobial therapy, they are termed *downgrading reactions*, and the case becomes histologically more lepromatous; when they occur after the initiation of therapy, they are termed *reversal reactions*, and the case becomes more tuberculoid. Reversal reactions often occur in the first months or years after the initiation of therapy, but may also develop several years thereafter.

Edema is the most characteristic microscopic feature of type 1 lepra lesions, whose diagnosis is primarily clinical. Reversal reactions are typified by a T_H1 cytokine profile, with an influx of CD4+ helper cells and increased levels of IFN-γ and IL-2. In addition, type 1 reactions are associated with large numbers of T cells bearing γ/δ receptors—a unique feature of leprosy.

Type 2 Lepra Reactions: Erythema Nodosum Leprosum

Erythema nodosum leprosum (ENL) (Fig. 67-4) occurs exclusively in patients near the lepromatous end of the leprosy spectrum (BL-LL), affecting nearly 50% of this group. Although ENL may precede leprosy diagnosis and initiation of therapy (sometimes, in fact, prompting the diagnosis), in 90% of cases it follows the institution of chemotherapy, generally within 2 years. The most common features of ENL are crops of painful erythematous papules that resolve spontaneously in a few days to a week but may recur, malaise, and fever that can be profound. However, patients may also experience symptoms of neuritis, lymphadenitis, uveitis, orchitis, and glomerulonephritis and may develop anemia, leukocytosis, and abnormal liver function tests (particularly increased aminotransferase levels). Individual patients may have either a single bout of ENL or chronic recurrent manifestations. Bouts may be either mild or severe and generalized; in rare instances, ENL results in death.

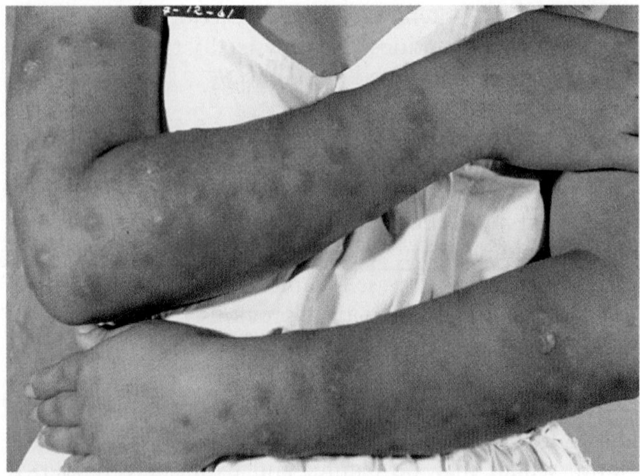

FIGURE 67-4
Moderately severe skin lesions of erythema nodosum leprosum (ENL), some with postulation and ulceration.

Skin biopsy of ENL papules reveals vasculitis or panniculitis, sometimes with many lymphocytes, but characteristically with polymorphonuclear leukocytes as well.

Elevated levels of circulating tumor necrosis factor (TNF) have been demonstrated in ENL; thus TNF may play a central role in the pathobiology of this syndrome. ENL is thought to be a consequence of immune complex deposition, given its T_H2 cytokine profile and its high levels of IL-6 and IL-8. However, in ENL tissue, the presence of HLA-DR framework antigen of epidermal cells—considered a marker for a delayed-type hypersensitivity response—and evidence of higher levels of IL-2 and IFN-γ than are usually seen in polar lepromatous disease suggest an alternative mechanism.

Lucio's Phenomenon

Lucio's phenomenon is an unusual reaction seen exclusively in patients from the Caribbean and Mexico who have the diffuse lepromatosis form of lepromatous leprosy, most often those who are untreated. Patients with this reaction develop recurrent crops of large, sharply marginated, ulcerative lesions—particularly on the lower extremities—that may be generalized and, when so, are frequently fatal as a result of secondary infection and consequent septic bacteremia. Histologically, the lesions are characterized by ischemic necrosis of the epidermis and superficial dermis, heavy parasitism of endothelial cells with AFB, and endothelial proliferation and thrombus formation in the larger vessels of the deeper dermis. Like ENL, Lucio's phenomenon is probably mediated by immune complexes.

Complications

The Extremities

Complications of the extremities in leprosy patients are primarily a consequence of neuropathy leading to insensitivity and myopathy. Insensitivity affects fine touch, pain, and heat receptors, but generally spares position and vibration appreciation. The most commonly affected nerve trunk is the ulnar nerve at the elbow, whose involvement results in clawing of the fourth and fifth fingers, loss of dorsal interosseous musculature in the affected hand, and loss of sensation in these distributions. Median nerve involvement in leprosy impairs thumb opposition and grasp; radial nerve dysfunction, although rare in leprosy, leads to wristdrop. Tendon transfers can restore hand function but should not be performed until 6 months after the initiation of antimicrobial therapy and the conclusion of episodes of acute neuritis.

Plantar ulceration, particularly at the metatarsal heads, is probably the most frequent complication of leprous neuropathy. Therapy requires careful debridement; administration of appropriate antibiotics; avoidance of weight-bearing until ulcerations are healed, with slowly progressive ambulation thereafter; and wearing of special shoes to prevent recurrence.

Footdrop as a result of peroneal nerve palsy should be treated with a simple nonmetallic brace within the shoe or with surgical correction attained by tendon transfers. Although uncommon, Charcot's joints, particularly of the foot and ankle, may result from leprosy.

The loss of distal digits in leprosy is a consequence of insensitivity, trauma, secondary infection, and—in lepromatous patients—a poorly understood and sometimes profound osteolytic process. Conscientious protection of the extremities during cooking and work and the early institution of therapy have substantially reduced the frequency and severity of distal digit loss in recent times.

The Nose

In lepromatous leprosy, bacillary invasion of the nasal mucosa can result in chronic nasal congestion and epistaxis. Saline nose drops may relieve these symptoms. Long-untreated LL leprosy may further result in destruction of the nasal cartilage, with consequent saddle-nose deformity or anosmia (more common in the preantibiotic era than at present). Nasal reconstructive procedures can ameliorate significant cosmetic defects.

The Eye

Owing to cranial nerve palsies, lagophthalmos and corneal insensitivity may complicate leprosy, resulting in trauma, secondary infection, and (without treatment) corneal ulcerations and opacities. For patients with these conditions, eyedrops during the day and ointments at night provide some protection from such consequences. Furthermore, in LL leprosy, the anterior chamber of the eye is invaded by bacilli, and ENL may result in uveitis, with consequent cataracts and glaucoma. Thus leprosy is a major cause of blindness in the developing world. Slit-lamp evaluation of LL patients often reveals "corneal beading," representing globi of *M. leprae*.

The Testes

M. leprae invades the testes, while ENL may cause orchitis. Thus males with lepromatous leprosy often manifest mild to severe testicular dysfunction, with an elevation of luteinizing and follicle-stimulating hormones, decreased testosterone, and aspermia or hypospermia in 85% of LL patients but in only 25% of BL patients. LL patients may become impotent and infertile. Impotence is sometimes responsive to testosterone replacement.

Amyloidosis

Secondary amyloidosis is a complication of LL leprosy and ENL that is encountered infrequently in the antibiotic era. This complication may result in abnormalities of hepatic and particularly renal function.

Nerve Abscesses

Patients with various forms of leprosy, but particularly those with the BT form, may develop abscesses of nerves (most commonly the ulnar) with an adjacent cellulitic appearance of the skin. In such conditions, the affected nerve is swollen and exquisitely tender. Although glucocorticoids may reduce signs of inflammation, rapid surgical decompression is necessary to prevent irreversible sequelae.

DIAGNOSIS

Leprosy most commonly presents with both characteristic skin lesions and skin histopathology. Thus the disease should be suspected when a patient from an endemic area has suggestive skin lesions or peripheral neuropathy. The diagnosis should be confirmed by histopathology. In tuberculoid leprosy, lesional areas—preferably the advancing edge—must be biopsied because normal-appearing skin does not have pathologic features. In lepromatous leprosy, nodules, plaques, and indurated areas are optimal biopsy sites, but biopsies of normal-appearing skin are also generally diagnostic. Lepromatous leprosy is associated with diffuse hyperglobulinemia, which may result in false-positive serologic tests (e.g., VDRL, RA, ANA) and therefore may cause diagnostic confusion. On occasion, tuberculoid lesions may not (1) appear typical, (2) be hypesthetic, and (3) contain granulomas but only nonspecific lymphocytic infiltrates. In such instances, two of these three characteristics are considered sufficient for a diagnosis. It is preferable to overdiagnose leprosy rather than to allow a patient to remain untreated.

IgM antibodies to PGL-1 are found in 95% of untreated lepromatous leprosy patients; the titer decreases with effective therapy. However, in tuberculoid leprosy—the form of disease most often associated with diagnostic uncertainty owing to the absence or paucity of AFB—patients have significant antibodies to PGL-1 only 60% of the time; moreover, in endemic locales, exposed individuals without clinical leprosy may harbor antibodies to PGL-1. Thus PGL-1 serology is of little diagnostic utility in tuberculoid leprosy. Heat-killed *M. leprae* (lepromin) has been used as a skin test reagent. It generally elicits a reaction in tuberculoid leprosy patients, may do so in individuals without leprosy, and gives negative results in lepromatous leprosy patients; consequently, it is likewise of little diagnostic value. Unfortunately, PCR of the skin for *M. leprae*, although positive in LL and BL leprosy, yields negative results in 50% of tuberculoid leprosy cases, again offering little diagnostic assistance.

Included in the differential diagnosis of lesions that resemble leprosy are sarcoidosis, leishmaniasis, lupus vulgaris, dermatofibroma, histiocytoma, lymphoma, syphilis, yaws, granuloma annulare, and various other disorders causing hypopigmentation (notably pityriasis alba, tinea, and vitiligo). Sarcoidosis may result in perineural inflammation, but actual granuloma formation within dermal nerves is pathognomonic for leprosy. In lepromatous leprosy, sputum specimens may be loaded with AFB—a finding that can be inappropriately interpreted as representing pulmonary tuberculosis.

℞ Treatment: LEPROSY

ANTIMICROBIAL THERAPY (SEE ALSO CHAP. 69)

Active Agents Established agents used to treat leprosy include dapsone (50–100 mg/d), clofazimine (50–100 mg/d, 100 mg three times weekly, or 300 mg monthly), and rifampin (600 mg daily or monthly). Of these drugs, only rifampin is bactericidal. The sulfones (folate antagonists), the foremost of which is dapsone, were the first antimicrobial agents found to be effective for the treatment of leprosy and are still the mainstay of therapy. With sulfone treatment, skin lesions resolve and numbers of viable bacilli in the skin are reduced. Although primarily bacteriostatic, dapsone monotherapy results in only a 2.5% resistance-related relapse rate; after ≥18 years of therapy and subsequent discontinuation, only another 10% of patients relapse, developing new, usually asymptomatic, shiny, "histoid" nodules. Dapsone is generally safe and inexpensive. Individuals with glucose-6-phosphate dehydrogenase deficiency who are treated with dapsone may develop severe hemolysis; those without this deficiency also have reduced red cell survival and a hemoglobin decrease averaging 1 g/dL. Dapsone's usefulness is limited occasionally by allergic dermatitis and rarely by the sulfone syndrome (including high fever, anemia, exfoliative dermatitis, and a mononucleosis-type blood picture). It must be remembered that rifampin induces microsomal enzymes, necessitating increased doses of medications such as glucocorticoids and oral birth control regimens. Clofazimine is often cosmetically unacceptable to light-skinned leprosy patients because it causes a red-black skin discoloration that accumulates, particularly in lesional areas, and makes the patient's diagnosis obvious to members of the community.

Other antimicrobial agents active against *M. leprae* in animal models and at the usual daily doses used in clinical trials include ethionamide/prothionamide; the aminoglycosides streptomycin, kanamycin, and amikacin (but not gentamicin or tobramycin); minocycline; clarithromycin; and several fluoroquinolones, particularly ofloxacin. Next to rifampin, minocycline, clarithromycin, and ofloxacin appear to be most bactericidal for *M. leprae*, but these drugs have not been used extensively in leprosy control programs. Most recently, rifapentine and moxifloxacin have been found to be especially potent against *M. leprae*. In preliminary clinical trials, moxifloxacin has been matched in potency only by rifampin.

Choice of Regimens Antimicrobial therapy for leprosy must be individualized, depending on the clinical/pathologic form of the disease encountered. Tuberculoid leprosy, which is associated with a low bacterial burden and a protective cellular immune response, is the easiest form to treat and can be reliably cured with a finite course of chemotherapy. In contrast, lepromatous leprosy may have a higher bacillary load than any other human bacterial disease, and the absence of a salutary T-cell repertoire requires prolonged or even lifelong chemotherapy. Hence careful classification of disease before therapy is important.

In developed countries, clinical experience with leprosy classification is limited; fortunately, however, the resources needed for skin biopsy are highly accessible and pathologic interpretation is readily available. In developing countries, clinical expertise is greater but is now waning substantially as the care of leprosy patients is integrated into general health services. In addition, access to dermatopathology services is often limited. In such instances, skin smears may prove useful, but in many locales, access to the resources needed for their preparation and interpretation may also be unavailable. Use of skin smears is no longer encouraged by the World Health Organization (WHO) and is often replaced by mere counting of lesions, which, together with the lack of histopathology, may negatively affect decisions about chemotherapy, increase the potential for reactions, and worsen the ultimate prognosis.

A reasoned approach to the treatment of leprosy is confounded by these and several other issues:

1. Even without therapy, TT leprosy may heal spontaneously, and prolonged dapsone monotherapy (even for LL leprosy) is generally curative in 80% of cases.
2. In tuberculoid disease, there are often no bacilli found in the skin before therapy, and thus there is no objective measure of therapeutic success. Furthermore, despite adequate treatment, TT and particularly BT lesions often resolve little or incompletely, whereas relapse and late type 1 lepra reactions can be difficult to distinguish.
3. LL leprosy patients commonly harbor viable persistent *M. leprae* organisms after prolonged intensive therapy; the propensity of these organisms to initiate clinical relapse is unclear. Because relapse in LL patients after discontinuation of rifampin-containing regimens usually begins only after 7–10 years, follow-up over the very long term is necessary to assess ultimate clinical outcomes.
4. Even though primary dapsone resistance is exceedingly rare and multidrug therapy is generally recommended (at least for lepromatous leprosy), there is a paucity of information from experimental animals and clinical trials on the optimal combination of antimicrobial agents, dosing schedule, or duration of therapy.

In 1982, the WHO made recommendations for "the chemotherapy of leprosy for control programs." These recommendations came on the heels of the demonstration of the relative success of long-term dapsone monotherapy and in the context of concerns about dapsone resistance. Other complicating considerations included the limited resources available for leprosy care in the very areas where it is most prevalent and the frustration and discouragement of patients and program managers with the previous requirement for lifelong therapy for many leprosy patients. The WHO delineated for the first time a finite duration of therapy for all forms of leprosy and—given the prohibitive cost of daily rifampin treatment in developing countries—encouraged the monthly administration of this agent as part of a multidrug regimen.

Over the ensuing years, these WHO recommendations have been broadly implemented, and the duration of therapy required, particularly for lepromatous leprosy, has been progressively shortened. For treatment purposes, the WHO classifies patients as *paucibacillary* or *multibacillary.* Previously, patients without demonstrable AFB in the dermis were classified as paucibacillary and those with AFB as multibacillary. Currently, owing to the perceived unreliability of skin smears in the field, patients are classified as multibacillary if they have six or more skin lesions and as paucibacillary if they have fewer. The WHO recommends that paucibacillary adults be treated with 100 mg of dapsone daily and 600 mg of rifampin monthly (supervised) for 6 months (Table 67-2). For patients with single-lesion paucibacillary leprosy, the WHO recommends as an alternative a single dose of rifampin (600 mg), ofloxacin (400 mg), and minocycline (100 mg). Multibacillary adults should be treated with 100 mg of dapsone plus 50 mg of clofazimine daily (unsupervised) and with 600 mg of rifampin plus 300 mg of clofazimine monthly (supervised). Originally, the WHO recommended that lepromatous patients be treated for 2 years or until smears became negative (generally in ~5 years); subsequently, the acceptable course was reduced to 1 year—a change that remains especially controversial in the absence of supporting clinical trials.

Several factors have caused many authorities to question the WHO recommendations and to favor a more intensive approach. Among these factors are—for multibacillary patients—a high (double-digit) relapse rate in three locales (reaching 20–40% in one locale, with the rate directly related to the initial bacterial burden) and—for paucibacillary patients—demonstrable lesional activity for years in fully half of patients after the completion of therapy. The more intensive approach (Table 67-2) calls for tuberculoid leprosy to be treated with dapsone (100 mg/d) for 5 years and for lepromatous leprosy to be treated with rifampin (600 mg/d) for 3 years and with dapsone (100 mg/d) throughout life.

On effective antimicrobial therapy, new skin lesions and signs and symptoms of peripheral neuropathy cease appearing. Nodules and plaques of lepromatous leprosy noticeably flatten in 1–2 months and resolve in 1 year or a few years, whereas tuberculoid skin lesions may disappear, improve, or remain relatively unchanged. Although the peripheral neuropathy of leprosy may improve somewhat in the first few months of therapy, rarely is it significantly ameliorated by treatment.

TABLE 67-2

ANTIMICROBIAL REGIMENS RECOMMENDED FOR THE TREATMENT OF LEPROSY IN ADULTS

FORM OF LEPROSY	MORE INTENSIVE REGIMEN	WHO RECOMMENDED REGIMEN (1982)
Tuberculoid (paucibacillary)	Dapsone (100 mg/d) for 5 years	Dapsone (100 mg/d, unsupervised) *plus* rifampin (600 mg/month, supervised) for 6 months
Lepromatous (multibacillary)	Rifampin (600 mg/d) for 3 years *plus* dapsone (100 mg/d) indefinitely	Dapsone (100 mg/d) *plus* clofazimine (50 mg/d), unsupervised; *and* rifampin (600 mg) *plus* clofazimine (300 mg) monthly (supervised) for 1–2 years

Note: See text for discussion and comparison of WHO recommendations and more intensive approach as well as alternative WHO regimen for single-lesion paucibacillary leprosy.

THERAPY FOR REACTIONS

Type 1 Type 1 lepra reactions are best treated with glucocorticoids (e.g., prednisone, initially at doses of 40–60 mg/d). As the inflammation subsides, the glucocorticoid dose can be tapered, but steroid therapy must be continued for at least 3 months lest recurrence supervene. Because of the myriad toxicities of prolonged glucocorticoid therapy, the indications for its initiation are strictly limited to lesions whose intense inflammation poses a threat of ulceration; lesions at cosmetically important sites, such as the face; and cases in which neuritis is present. Mild to moderate lepra reactions that do not meet these criteria should be tolerated and glucocorticoid treatment withheld. Thalidomide is ineffective against type 1 lepra reactions. Clofazimine (200–300 mg/d) is of questionable benefit, but in any event is far less efficacious than glucocorticoids.

Type 2 Treatment of ENL must be individualized. If ENL is mild (i.e., without fever or other organ involvement, with occasional crops of only a few skin papules), it may be treated with antipyretics alone. However, in cases with many skin lesions, fever, malaise, and other tissue involvement, brief courses (1–2 weeks) of glucocorticoids (initially 40–60 mg/d) are often effective. With or without therapy, individual inflamed papules last for >1 week. Successful therapy is defined by the cessation of skin lesion development and the disappearance of other systemic signs and symptoms. If, despite two courses of glucocorticoid therapy, ENL appears to be recurring and persisting, treatment with thalidomide (100–300 mg nightly) should be initiated, with the dose depending on the initial severity of the reaction. Because even a single dose of thalidomide administered early in pregnancy may result in severe birth defects, including phocomelia, the use of this drug in the United States for the treatment of fertile female patients is tightly regulated and requires informed consent, prior pregnancy testing, and maintenance of birth control measures. Although the mechanism of thalidomide's dramatic action against ENL is not entirely clear, the drug's efficacy is probably attributable to its reduction of TNF levels and IgM synthesis and its slowing of polymorphonuclear leukocyte migration. After the reaction is controlled, lower doses of thalidomide (50–200 mg nightly) are effective in preventing relapses of ENL.

Clofazimine in high doses (300 mg nightly) has some efficacy against ENL, but its use permits only a modest reduction of the glucocorticoid dose necessary for ENL control.

Lucio's Phenomenon Neither glucocorticoids nor thalidomide is effective against this syndrome. Optimal wound care and therapy for bacteremia are indicated. Ulcers tend to be chronic and heal poorly. In severe cases, exchange transfusion may prove useful.

PREVENTION AND CONTROL

Vaccination at birth with bacille Calmette-Guérin (BCG) has proved variably effective in preventing leprosy: the results have ranged from total inefficacy to 80% efficacy. The addition of heat-killed *M. leprae* to BCG does not increase vaccine efficacy. Because whole mycobacteria contain large amounts of lipids and carbohydrates that have proven in vitro to be immunosuppressive for lymphocytes and macrophages, *M. leprae* proteins may prove to be superior vaccines. Data from a mouse model support this possibility.

Chemoprophylaxis with dapsone may reduce the number of cases of tuberculoid leprosy but not of lepromatous leprosy and hence is not recommended, even for household contacts. Because leprosy transmission appears to require close prolonged household contact, hospitalized patients need not be isolated.

In 1992, the WHO—on the basis of that organization's treatment recommendations—launched a landmark campaign to eliminate leprosy as a public health problem by the year 2000 (goal, <1 case per 10,000 population). The campaign mobilized and energized nongovernmental organizations and national health services to treat leprosy with multiple drugs and to clean up outdated registries. In these respects, the effort has proven hugely successful, with >6 million patients completing therapy. However, the target of leprosy elimination has not yet been reached. In fact, the success of the WHO campaign in reducing the number of cases worldwide has been largely attributable to the redefinition of what constitutes a case of leprosy. Formerly calculated by disease prevalence, the case count is now limited to those not yet treated with multiple drugs. In each of the 23 countries with the largest number of leprosy cases, the annual incidence of leprosy is stable or actually rising. Furthermore, after the completion of therapy, when a patient is no longer considered to represent a "case," half of all patients continue to manifest disease activity for years; relapse rates (at least for multibacillary patients) are unacceptably high; disabilities and deformities go unchecked; and the social stigma of the disease persists.

During most of the twentieth century, nongovernmental organizations, particularly Christian missionaries, provided a medical infrastructure devoted to the care and treatment of leprosy patients—the envy of those with other medical priorities in the developing world. With the public perception that leprosy is near eradication, resources for patient care are rapidly being diverted, and the burden of patient care is being transferred to nonexistent or overloaded national health services and to health workers who lack the tools and skills needed for disease diagnosis, classification, and nuanced therapy (particularly in cases of reactional neuritis). Thus the prerequisites for a salutary outcome increasingly go unmet.

FURTHER READINGS

COLE ST et al: Massive gene decay in the leprosy bacillus. Nature 409:1007, 2001

GELBER RH: The chemotherapy of leprosy: Lessons learned, some forgotten, current status and future prospects. Malaysian J Dermatol 18:10, 2005

——— et al: The relapse rate in MB leprosy patients treated with 2-years of WHO-MDT is not low. Int J Lepr Other Mycobact Dis 72:493, 2004

LOCKWOOD D: Leprosy elimination—a virtual phenomenon or a reality? BMJ 324:1516, 2002

MODLIN RL, REA TH: Immunology of leprosy granulomas. Springer Semin Immunopathol 10:359, 1998

MONET M et al: On the origin of leprosy. Science 308:1040, 2005

RIDLEY DS: Histological classification and the immunological spectrum of leprosy. Bull World Health Organ 51:451, 1974

SHEPARD CC: The experimental disease that follows injection of human leprosy bacilli into foot pads of mice. J Exp Med 112:445, 1960

VAN VEEN NH et al: Corticosteroids for treating nerve damage in leprosy. Cochrane Database Syst Rev April 18(2):CD005491, 2007

WARWICK JB, LOCKWOOD D: Leprosy. Lancet 363:1209, 2004

WHO EXPERT COMMITTEE ON LEPROSY: Seventh Report. WHO Tech Rep Ser No. 874. Geneva, World Health Organization, 1998

CHAPTER 68

NONTUBERCULOUS MYCOBACTERIA

C. Fordham von Reyn

The designation *nontuberculous mycobacteria* (NTM) encompasses the mycobacterial species other than organisms of the *Mycobacterium tuberculosis* complex and *M. leprae*. The NTM are distributed widely in the environment, are typically acquired from environmental sources, and therefore are also referred to as *environmental mycobacteria*. Most species are less virulent for humans than *M. tuberculosis*. Thus symptomatic infections are often associated with local or generalized defects in host defenses. Because isolation of NTM from a clinical specimen may represent true infection, colonization, or environmental contamination, strict criteria are required to assess the clinical significance of a positive culture. Although the >90 species of NTM have been associated with a wide variety of infections, most infections are due to a relatively limited number of species that cause characteristic patterns of disease (Table 68-1).

MICROBIOLOGY

Like *M. tuberculosis*, NTM organisms are acid-fast bacilli (AFB), resisting decolorization after staining. NTM have conventionally been characterized by the time required for clinical specimens to yield visible growth on solid media. Rapidly growing NTM species, such as *M. abscessus*, *M. fortuitum*, and *M. chelonae*, appear within 7 days. These organisms grow on standard microbiologic media and thus may be reported even when the clinician has not explicitly requested cultures for mycobacteria. Slow-growing species, in contrast, often take 2–3 weeks to grow on solid media and require special mycobacterial media such as Lowenstein-Jensen or Middlebrook. Accordingly, slow-growing NTM species are usually isolated only when the clinician specifically requests cultures for mycobacteria. Representative slow-growing species include *M. avium*, *M. kansasii*, *M. ulcerans*, and *M. marinum*. The automated broth culture systems now used in many laboratories may permit isolation of slow-growing NTM organisms within 10–14 days.

Further classification based on colony pigmentation (Runyon's classification) has been replaced by the use of DNA probes for identification of common species such as *M. avium*, *M. intracellulare*, *M. gordonae* (which is rarely pathogenic), and *M. kansasii*. Less common species may be identified rapidly on the basis of fatty acid composition or DNA sequencing. Molecular strain typing ("fingerprinting") based on analysis of polymorphisms among large restriction fragments can be used to determine whether two or more isolates are genotypically and, by implication, epidemiologically related. This technique has been useful for identifying common-source outbreaks of infection or contamination.

Antibiotic susceptibility testing should be performed for rapidly growing NTM species. However, susceptibility testing of slow-growing species is of limited value: testing methods are not well standardized, and the relevance of the results to outcome is uncertain since patients are usually treated with multiple-drug regimens. As discussed later in this chapter, testing of *M. avium* or *M. kansasii* for susceptibility to specific drugs may be useful in certain situations.

DISTRIBUTION

NTM have a waxy, hydrophobic, triple-layered cell wall that renders them unusually resistant to varied physical conditions and chemical agents (including disinfectants such as chlorine at concentrations used in drinking water). These organisms can make use of a wide variety of carbon and nitrogen sources and can survive in nutrient-poor environments. Thus they are widely distributed in water, biofilms, and soil as well as in numerous animal species. Optimal growth temperatures vary and may influence distribution. For example, *M. avium* and *M. intracellulare* are often isolated from potable hot-water sources, whereas *M. marinum* is found in the cooler water of fish tanks. Most species of NTM are obligate aerobes and grow best at acid pH. Soil and natural water samples from most regions of the world contain numerous species of NTM, which are as common in northern regions (e.g., Finland) as they are in more temperate areas (e.g., the southern United States).

EPIDEMIOLOGY

Asymptomatic infections with NTM are common in humans and are probably acquired most often from childhood contact with soil, water, and possibly animals. Studies with skin-test agents derived from NTM indicate that 30–40% of adults in the northern and southern United States have had prior unrecognized or asymptomatic infection with NTM—most often with organisms of the *M. avium* complex (MAC). Since latent infection is not a recognized characteristic of NTM, most symptomatic infections are thought to represent recent exposure. Molecular methods have identified clusters of infections

TABLE 68-1

MAIN SPECIES OF NONTUBERCULOUS MYCOBACTERIA (NTM) AND PATTERNS OF DISEASE

SPECIES	GROWTH ON SOLID MEDIA	ENVIRONMENTAL RESERVOIR	PATTERNS OF DISEASE[a] CUTANEOUS	PULMONARY	DISSEMINATED	OTHER
M. avium	Slow	Hot water systems, natural water, soil	–	++	+++	Lymphadenitis
M. intracellulare	Slow	Hot water systems, natural water, soil	–	+++	+	Lymphadenitis
M. kansasii	Slow	Potable and natural water	–	+++	++	–
M. abscessus, *M. chelonae*, *M. fortuitum*	Rapid	Potable and natural water, soil	++	+	–	Sporotrichoid spread
M. marinum	Slow	Fish tanks, salt water	++	–	–	Sporotrichoid spread
M. ulcerans	Slow	Natural water	++	–	–	"Buruli ulcer," osteomyelitis

[a]Symbols indicate relative prevalence among NTM infections of the indicated species and pattern of disease: +++, most common; ++, common; +, reported but uncommon; –, rare or not reported.

and pseudoinfections associated with potable water as well as nosocomial infections related to clinical procedures such as endoscopy and surgery. Environmental exposures are assumed to cause most symptomatic infections; however, this point has been difficult to document by molecular methods, presumably because there are many potential exposures (some of which are sporadic) and because a specific NTM species may be present only transiently or in low numbers in any given source.

PATHOGENESIS

NTM may be acquired through cutaneous, respiratory, gastrointestinal, or (rarely) parenteral exposure. Organisms are ingested by host macrophages and may survive within these cells to replicate and cause symptomatic infection. Disease manifestations in immunocompetent hosts are due to host cellular immune responses and the formation of granulomas. Intracellular killing of mycobacteria, with ultimate control of infection, requires the action of cellular immune mechanisms including proliferation of CD4+ T lymphocytes and elaboration of interferon γ (IFN-γ) and interleukin 12. Deficiencies in CD4+ T-cell function due to HIV infection, anti–tumor necrosis factor (TNF) therapy, and inherited deficiencies in the production of or response to IFN-γ are associated with disseminated NTM infection (Chap. 90).

The cellular immune response to NTM may be evident in tuberculin skin testing or newer interferon-γ release assays (IGRAs). Tuberculin skin testing with *M. tuberculosis* purified protein derivative may elicit small reactions with some NTM and larger reactions (comparable to those in tuberculosis) among immunocompetent individuals infected with *M. marinum* or *M. kansasii*. IGRAs that employ *M. tuberculosis*–specific antigens (ESAT-6, CFP-10) are negative in most NTM infections but may be positive with *M. marinum* or *M. kansasii*.

There is no convincing evidence that NTM can establish latent infection with subsequent clinical reactivation—a pattern characteristic of *M. tuberculosis*. Asymptomatic infection with NTM in a healthy host may induce beneficial immunity; persons with skin-test reactivity to NTM antigens (e.g., *M. intracellulare*) are at decreased risk for the subsequent development of tuberculosis. Likewise, immunization with bacille Calmette-Guérin (BCG) from *M. bovis* provides protection against childhood cervical adenitis due to NTM.

CLINICAL SYNDROMES

Cutaneous Disease

NTM can cause a variety of cutaneous disease syndromes when inoculated directly from an environmental source into an area of open or diseased skin or into a surgical wound. These organisms are also associated with localized or disseminated cutaneous disease in immunosuppressed patients. *M. abscessus*, *M. fortuitum*, *M. chelonae*, *M. marinum*, and *M. ulcerans* are the most commonly involved species. Cutaneous disease may be nodular or ulcerating, sometimes with reddish-blue discoloration and typically with minimal drainage. Lesions may be single, or the infection may spread proximally up the lymphatics, producing additional nodules (sporotrichoid spread). In compromised hosts, disseminated lesions may appear as a result of bacteremic spread. Clinical suspicion of NTM infection is based on chronicity, the absence of bacterial growth on routine culture, and the failure to respond to standard antibacterial therapy. Biopsies often reveal granuloma formation, and acid-fast stains may be positive.

Pulmonary Disease

NTM species cause chronic progressive pulmonary infection both in normal hosts and in those with underlying pulmonary disease or immunosuppression. The clinical features may resemble slowly progressive pulmonary tuberculosis, which is often the initial diagnosis in patients with positive AFB smears. Among patients born in the United States, pulmonary disease due to AFB is more likely to be due to NTM than to *M. tuberculosis*.

The diagnosis of pulmonary infection with NTM is complicated by the variability in clinical and radiologic manifestations, the frequent presence of significant prior pulmonary disease, and the fact that isolation of NTM from the sputum may represent harmless colonization of the lower respiratory tract. The diagnosis should be based on specific, validated criteria that emphasize a compatible clinical syndrome, characteristic findings on chest x-ray or CT, and repeated isolation of NTM from the sputum or growth of NTM from a lung biopsy (Table 68-2).

In immunocompetent hosts, infection may result in the onset of chronic cough, dyspnea, and fatigue; fever is unusual. Pathologic and radiologic manifestations of pulmonary infection due to NTM include the formation of solitary or multiple nodules, chronic pneumonitis, bronchiectasis, cavity formation, or a combination of these features. In some patients with NTM pulmonary disease, CT shows a characteristic pattern of small cylindrical bronchiectasis and multiple small (<5-mm) nodules and fibrosis. Compared with patients who have tuberculosis, those who have lung disease caused by NTM are more likely to have bilateral and midzone infiltrates and less likely to have pleural effusions. Patients with characteristic radiologic findings and negative results of routine sputum cultures for mycobacteria should have bronchoscopy and transbronchial biopsy performed in an attempt to identify granulomas and AFB. In patients with chronic pulmonary disease, the superimposition of infection with NTM may not be associated with easily recognizable changes in symptoms or radiologic features.

TABLE 68-2

ATS/IDSA CRITERIA FOR THE DIAGNOSIS OF PULMONARY DISEASE DUE TO NONTUBERCULOUS MYCOBACTERIA[a]

CATEGORY	REQUIREMENT
Clinical	Pulmonary symptoms (e.g., chronic cough) and appropriate exclusion of other diagnoses
Radiologic	Chest x-ray: nodular or cavitary opacities *or* High-resolution CT: multifocal bronchiectasis with multiple small nodules
Bacteriologic	Sputum: ≥2 positive cultures *or* Bronchial wash or lavage: ≥1 positive culture *or* Lung biopsy: granulomatous inflammation or positive stain for acid-fast bacilli plus ≥1 positive culture (of biopsy, sputum, or bronchial wash sample)

[a]Diagnosis requires the fulfillment of clinical criteria plus one radiologic criterion and one bacteriologic criterion. ATS, American Thoracic Society; IDSA, Infectious Diseases Society of America.
Source: Griffith et al, 2007.

Together, MAC organisms (especially *M. intracellulare*) are the most common cause of pulmonary disease due to NTM in developed countries; next in frequency are *M. kansasii* (United States, Europe, South Africa), *M. abscessus* (United States), *M. xenopi* (Europe, Canada), and *M. malmoense* (United Kingdom, northern Europe). However, isolation of NTM from the sputum must be considered in the context of clinical manifestations. For example, NTM (most prominently, MAC organisms; less commonly, *M. abscessus*) can be cultured from 13% of cystic fibrosis patients in the United States; however, not all of these patients appear to have invasive NTM disease. Although invasive disease should be strongly suspected when the same NTM species is isolated on multiple occasions from a patient with lung disease, even persistent organisms may represent colonization or slowly progressive disease apparent only on long-term follow-up. Additional laboratory tests (e.g., immunologic assessments) are of no value in the diagnosis.

Although treatment should be considered in patients who meet the clinical, radiologic, and microbiologic criteria for NTM disease (Table 68-2), several other factors require consideration. For example, whereas species such as *M. kansasii* are usually pathogenic and a single isolate may be significant, species such as *M. gordonae* are rarely pathogenic, even when isolated repeatedly. In addition, in some patients with true invasive disease, infection may progress so slowly that it is unlikely to have much impact on longevity determined by age or comorbid illness. Since therapy for NTM requires prolonged administration of multiple drugs and is associated with significant side effects, the decision to institute treatment in patients with noncavitary disease who do not have clearly progressive pulmonary disease should be made with careful deliberation after a period of clinical and radiologic follow-up.

Disseminated Disease

Patients with impaired cellular immunity—most notably, patients with advanced HIV disease (Chap. 90), immunosuppressed recipients of solid-organ or hematopoietic stem-cell transplants (Chap. 12), and patients receiving anti-TNF therapy—are susceptible to disseminated disease due to NTM. Other predisposing conditions include treatment with glucocorticoids, lymphoma and leukemia (especially hairy cell leukemia), and heritable disorders of IFN-γ production and function. *M. avium* and *M. kansasii* are the species most commonly isolated in disseminated disease, but numerous other organisms (e.g., *M. genavense*, *M. haemophilum*) have also been recovered.

Patients with disseminated infection present with fever, weight loss, and fatigue and sometimes with hepatosplenomegaly or lymphadenopathy. Chest radiographs are typically normal in infection with *M. avium* (although they may show a miliary pattern) but are usually abnormal with *M. kansasii*. Laboratory studies may demonstrate anemia and an elevated level of alkaline phosphatase in serum. Disseminated disease is characterized by the widespread presence of foamy macrophages with AFB, which may be demonstrated in biopsy samples of bone marrow, intestine, or liver. Granulomas are typically absent in patients with impaired cellular immunity. In most cases, the diagnosis can be established by one or two sets of mycobacterial blood cultures, which will be positive for the etiologic mycobacteria in 2–3 weeks. Treatment requires long-term administration of a multiple-drug antimycobacterial regimen and attempts to ameliorate the defect in cellular immunity [e.g., institution of antiretroviral therapy (ART) and discontinuation of glucocorticoid administration].

Other Disease

NTM have been associated with disease at numerous other anatomic locations, including ocular infections, mastoiditis, sinusitis, mastitis, catheter site infections, endocarditis, meningitis, peritonitis, appendicitis, pericarditis, pyelonephritis, prostatitis, tenosynovitis, bursitis, septic arthritis, osteomyelitis, and lymphadenitis (especially in children). Accumulating data support an association between infection with *M. avium* subspecies *paratuberculosis* and Crohn's disease.

ORGANISMS

M. AVIUM COMPLEX

Pulmonary Disease

MAC organisms (*M. avium*, *M. intracellulare*, and genetically related unnamed species) are more common than *M. tuberculosis* as a cause of mycobacterial pulmonary disease among persons born in the United States. Epidemiologic data support a marked increase in the incidence of MAC infection over the past two to three decades. Two patterns of MAC disease are recognized: one form is typically the primary basis for a diagnosis of pulmonary disease and is often nodular/bronchiectatic, whereas the other form develops as a secondary complication of underlying pulmonary disease and is sometimes fibrocavitary (Table 68-3). The description of subtle defects in cellular immune responses and body morphotype in patients with primary disease raises the possibility of an as-yet-undefined immune defect predisposing to MAC infection. Patients with secondary disease include those with chronic obstructive pulmonary disease, prior tuberculosis, cystic fibrosis, or pulmonary alveolar proteinosis. The sources of infection have not been identified.

Clinical Features and Diagnosis

Symptoms and diagnostic studies are described above (see "Clinical Syndromes"). CT identifies characteristic cylindrical bronchiectasis with nodule formation, documents the extent of disease, and establishes a baseline for possible treatment. Standard diagnostic criteria should be applied (Table 68-2). Isolates from patients with prolonged prior macrolide exposure or prior treatment failure should be tested for susceptibility to clarithromycin.

℞ Treatment: MAC PULMONARY DISEASE

Treatment should be initiated in most patients with secondary MAC pulmonary disease. For patients with primary MAC pulmonary disease, decisions about treatment must be made on an individual basis. A period of observation before consideration of treatment may be useful when there is no evidence of a progressive pulmonary process and when the patient's age or underlying disease is likely to be the critical determinant of survival over the next few years.

Recommended treatment for MAC pulmonary disease includes two drugs: daily clarithromycin (or daily or thrice-weekly azithromycin) and ethambutol. Some authorities recommend a three-drug regimen including these two agents plus rifampin, although there are no comparative data for two- versus three-drug regimens, and concomitant administration of rifampin lowers serum levels of clarithromycin (Table 68-4). For seriously ill patients with advanced disease, a four-drug regimen

TABLE 68-3

TYPICAL FEATURES OF PRIMARY AND SECONDARY PULMONARY DISEASE DUE TO THE *M. AVIUM* COMPLEX

FEATURE	PRIMARY	SECONDARY
Age	>50 years	30–70 (mean, 60) years
Sex	F >M	M >F
Underlying disease	None definitively identified; subtle defect in cellular immunity postulated	Chronic obstructive pulmonary disease, cystic fibrosis, prior tuberculosis, alveolar proteinosis
Radiologic features	Typically nodular (<5 mm)/ bronchiectatic (cylindrical) with midzone involvement	Sometimes fibrocavitary; infiltrates or nodules in some cases

TABLE 68-4

REGIMENS FOR PREVENTION AND TREATMENT OF DISEASE DUE TO THE *M. AVIUM* COMPLEX

CATEGORY	REGIMEN	INDICATION AND DURATION
Pulmonary Disease		
Treatment	Clarithromycin (250–500 mg bid[a]) or azithromycin (250 mg/daily or thrice weekly[b]) ***plus*** Ethambutol (15 mg/kg qd)[c]	Treat when patient meets ATS/IDSA criteria (Table 68-2) and has secondary MAC disease or has primary MAC disease plus indication for treatment (see text). Treat for 18 months or until 12 months after conversion of sputum culture.
Disseminated Disease		
Treatment	Clarithromycin (500 mg PO bid) or azithromycin (500 mg daily[d]) ***plus*** Ethambutol (15 mg/kg qd[b])	Treat when MAC blood culture is positive or MAC is isolated from ordinarily sterile site. Continue with secondary prevention.
Prevention	Azithromycin (1200 mg PO weekly[b]) or clarithromycin (500 mg PO bid)	Treat when CD4+ T-cell count is <50/μL. Discontinue if CD4+ T-cell count exceeds 100/μL for >3 months during antiretroviral therapy.

[a]Give 250 mg of clarithromycin bid if the patient weighs <50 kg.
[b]Azithromycin is preferred to clarithromycin in pregnancy.
[c]An intermittent three-drug regimen with concomitant rifampin, rather than a daily two-drug regimen, is recommended in the current ATS/IDSA guidelines (Griffith et al, 2007) but not by this author; a four-drug regimen including streptomycin may be indicated in severe cases.
[d]Concomitant rifabutin (150–300 mg/d) may protect against the development of clarithromycin resistance and be associated with a modest clinical benefit but can cause interactions with antiretroviral therapy.

including the three drugs listed above as well as streptomycin or amikacin for the first 2 months should be considered. In many cases, treatment may serve only to halt the progression of radiologic findings; in some cases, symptoms and radiologic findings improve. The response to treatment is best in patients whose isolates have the lowest minimum inhibitory concentrations of clarithromycin. As many as 30% of patients treated with standard drugs at standard doses cannot tolerate therapy, generally because of gastrointestinal side effects. Rifabutin appears to have the highest rate of side effects. Stepwise introduction of drugs at 1-week intervals, starting with half the usual dose, may improve tolerance. In many cases, final doses need to be reduced or drugs eliminated or replaced with alternatives. Gatifloxacin and moxifloxacin exhibit in vitro activity against many strains but have not been studied for the treatment of pulmonary disease due to MAC.

For patients with positive sputum cultures who receive a macrolide-containing regimen, treatment should be continued for at least 12 months after cultures revert to negative; the typical duration is 18 months. The duration of therapy with other regimens may need to be extended to 24 months. Approximately 20% of patients experience treatment failure or relapse; some apparent treatment failures may actually represent reinfection. Surgical resection is an option for patients with localized disease who are intolerant of or unresponsive to multiple-drug therapy; however, this approach is associated with postoperative complications in as many as 20% of patients and should be undertaken only by surgeons who have considerable experience with this intervention.

Hot-Tub Lung

Hot-tub lung is a form of hypersensitivity pneumonitis due to NTM, most commonly MAC organisms. Affected individuals present with cough, fever, and dyspnea after repeated exposure to indoor hot tubs contaminated with MAC. Some patients are hypoxemic. The chest x-ray shows diffuse nodular infiltrates, and high-resolution CT may also demonstrate ground-glass infiltrates. MAC organisms can be isolated from expectorated sputum or lung tissue, and biopsy specimens display centrilobular and bronchocentric granuloma formation. Resolution typically follows avoidance of exposure and/or treatment with glucocorticoids. Most patients do not appear to require specific antimicrobial therapy.

Disseminated Disease

Disseminated MAC disease occurs principally among patients with immunosuppression (including those with advanced HIV disease) who live in developed countries but are not receiving ART. Almost all cases occur at CD4+ T-cell counts of <100/μL, and the risk is ~20% per year for untreated patients with CD4+ T-cell counts of <50/μL. The risk of disease is essentially eliminated for recipients of ART who have an increase in CD4+ T-cell count to >100/μL that is maintained for 3 months. Most cases are due to *M. avium*, and molecular studies indicate that as many as 25% of disseminated infections involve more than one strain. Strains causing bacteremia differ genetically from those typically isolated from respiratory sources or the environment. Molecular techniques have documented nosocomial acquisition from potable hot water and have demonstrated common genotypes among isolates from humans and those from peat used in potting soil. Epidemiologic studies have demonstrated an increased risk associated with consumption of untreated spring water and of raw or partially cooked fish or shellfish and a decreased risk associated with showering. Overall, sources of acquisition appear to be diverse and exposure is probably unavoidable; at this time, no specific behavioral changes can be recommended for at-risk patients.

Clinical Features and Diagnosis

Disseminated MAC infection in AIDS is associated with fever, weakness, and weight loss and usually presents as a wasting syndrome in patients who are not receiving ART or chemoprophylaxis for *M. avium* (Chap. 90). Untreated disease shortens the survival period of patients with advanced AIDS by 4–5 months. Laboratory findings may include anemia, hypoalbuminemia, and elevated serum levels of alkaline phosphatase and lactate dehydrogenase. HIV-infected patients with prior disseminated MAC infection or unrecognized or subclinical MAC infection may experience an immune reconstitution syndrome when they start to receive ART (Chap. 90). This syndrome presents 1–12 weeks after the institution of ART and often manifests as localized (or generalized) culture-positive lymphadenitis with blood cultures negative for *M. avium*.

℞ Treatment: DISSEMINATED MAC DISEASE

Disseminated MAC disease requires treatment with the combination of clarithromycin and ethambutol, with or without rifabutin (Table 68-4), along with ART for HIV. Antimycobacterial treatment should be continued for at least 12 months and until the CD4+ T-cell count has been >100/μL for at least 6 months. The immune reconstitution syndrome should be treated with initiation or continuation of the same antimycobacterial regimen.

Prevention

Chemoprophylaxis is highly effective for the prevention of disseminated MAC infection in AIDS (Table 68-4). Weekly azithromycin administration should be instituted when the CD4+ T-cell count is <50/μL or when a patient with HIV infection has had an AIDS-defining opportunistic infection (e.g., *Pneumocystis* infection). Chemoprophylaxis may be discontinued when the CD4+ T-cell count has been >100/μL for >3 months.

M. KANSASII

Pulmonary Disease

Pulmonary disease due to *M. kansasii* has been reported from many areas of the world, including North America, Europe, and South Africa. In the United States, *M. kansasii* is the second most common cause of lung disease due to NTM and is distributed largely in central and southern states and California. The average age of onset is 60 years, and most patients have predisposing factors, such as chronic obstructive pulmonary disease, carcinoma of the lung, silicosis, or prior tuberculosis. However, pulmonary infection sometimes occurs in persons without predisposing disease and has also been associated with poverty. Disease may sometimes wax and wane over many years; this pattern is assumed to represent chronic infection rather than reactivation. Localized pulmonary infection has been described in South African miners with early HIV infection and preserved CD4+ T-cell counts. The source of infection has not been identified, although *M. kansasii* has been isolated from both potable and natural water sources.

Clinical Features and Diagnosis

M. kansasii is the most pathogenic nontuberculous mycobacterial species affecting the lung, and the clinical features of *M. kansasii* disease resemble those of tuberculosis. Most cases include cough and sputum production; 30% include frank hemoptysis. Systemic signs and symptoms, including fever, night sweats, and weight loss, are reported by as many as 50% of patients. However, symptoms may be subtle or absent in patients with underlying malignancy. Chest radiographs show cavitation in 50% of patients, pleural scarring in 40%, and infiltrates in 30%; abnormalities are most prominent in the apices. Clinical and radiographic effects progress in the absence of treatment.

Sputum samples should be obtained for AFB staining and mycobacterial culture. The isolation of *M. kansasii* sometimes represents colonization; the diagnostic criteria in Table 68-2 are useful when multiple sputum samples can be obtained. However, the growth of *M. kansasii* from even a single sputum culture should be considered to have potential clinical significance, especially in HIV-positive patients. Testing of *M. kansasii* isolates for susceptibility to rifampin is recommended.

℞ Treatment: *M. KANSASII* PULMONARY DISEASE

For rifampin-susceptible strains of *M. kansasii*, the recommended regimen is daily rifampin (600 mg), isoniazid (300 mg), and ethambutol (15 mg/kg). Sputum cultures almost always become negative by 4 months; patients should be treated for at least 12 months after the last positive culture. Resistance to rifampin may develop, in which case clarithromycin or azithromycin may be substituted.

Disseminated Disease

Disseminated *M. kansasii* disease occurs principally among patients with advanced AIDS and CD4+ T-cell counts of <100/μL. It has also been reported in patients with leukemia, lymphoma, or solid-organ transplantation.

Clinical Features and Diagnosis

Symptoms are similar to those reported for disseminated MAC infection, although in disseminated *M. kansasii* infection, cough is more common, and chest radiographs more often demonstrate alveolar or interstitial infiltrates or cavities. An immune reconstitution syndrome may follow the institution of ART in HIV-infected patients, manifesting as cervical or mediastinal lymphadenitis (Chap. 90).

The diagnosis is established by the isolation of *M. kansasii* from a normally sterile parenchymal site or from blood. In one series of cases, concurrent disseminated infection with a second NTM species (most often *M. avium*) was found in one-third of patients. The isolation of *M. kansasii* from sputum from a patient with advanced HIV disease suggests disseminated infection and is an indication for mycobacterial blood culture.

℞ Treatment: *M. KANSASII* DISSEMINATED DISEASE

Treatment of disseminated *M. kansasii* disease is the same as that for pulmonary disease due to this organism. Patients with AIDS should receive an ART regimen that is compatible with a rifamycin (rifampin or rifabutin). Untreated disease is associated with shortened survival, and the response to treatment is good in patients who do not have rapidly progressive HIV infection. HIV-positive patients who experience clearing of systemic symptoms and have positive cultures with sustained recovery of the CD4+ T-cell count can probably have treatment discontinued (as described above for *M. avium* infection). There is no recommended prophylactic regimen, although the azithromycin regimen given to prevent disseminated *M. avium* infection may also be effective in preventing disseminated *M. kansasii* infection.

M. ABSCESSUS, M. CHELONAE, AND *M. FORTUITUM*

Three rapidly growing NTM species are prominent in reports of human infection and colonization: *M. abscessus*, *M. chelonae*, and *M. fortuitum*. These organisms are acquired from water, soil, or nosocomial sources. The most common clinical manifestation of infection is disseminated cutaneous disease in patients who have defects in cellular immunity or are receiving glucocorticoid therapy. Immunocompetent hosts can develop localized cutaneous infection in surgical or traumatic wounds, from contaminated injections, or after body piercing. Cutaneous lesions are cellulitic or nodular; are typically erythematous, indurated, and tender; and may progress to ulceration and purulent drainage. Proximal sporotrichoid spread has also been reported. Pulmonary infection (usually due to *M. abscessus*) is the next most common manifestation and occurs principally in patients with underlying lung disease, such as cystic fibrosis.

The rapidly growing NTM species may be isolated from clinical specimens submitted for routine microbiologic testing. However, reliable evaluation requires inoculation onto special mycobacterial media and an extended incubation period. Because rapidly growing NTM species are also common laboratory contaminants, numerous false alarms in the form of pseudoepidemics have been reported.

℞ Treatment: *M. ABSCESSUS, M. CHELONAE*, AND *M. FORTUITUM* INFECTIONS

Treatment varies with the patient group and with the species of rapidly growing NTM. Susceptibility tests should be performed and used to guide antibiotic selection. All three species are usually susceptible to clarithromycin and amikacin; *M. abscessus* and *M. fortuitum* are also susceptible to cefoxitin and imipenem. Other agents that may be active include doxycycline and fluoroquinolones. Patients with localized cutaneous disease may respond to a single active agent (e.g., clarithromycin at a dosage of 500 mg twice daily by mouth for ≥2 weeks). Up to 6 months of therapy may be optimal for bacteremic or disseminated cutaneous disease, and a second agent should be added on the basis of susceptibility tests. Pulmonary disease due to *M. fortuitum* or *M. chelonae* should be treated with two active agents (usually including clarithromycin) until sputum cultures have been negative for 12 months. Pulmonary disease due to *M. abscessus* is especially difficult to treat since prolonged therapy is necessary and the most active drugs require parenteral administration and carry a significant risk of toxicity with prolonged use. The most potent regimen is typically IV amikacin (10–15 mg/kg daily) and IV cefoxitin (3 g every 6 h) or imipenem (500 mg every 6–12 h) with oral clarithromycin (500 mg twice daily). Expert consultation should be sought for management of this chronic, often incurable pulmonary infection.

M. MARINUM

M. marinum is widely distributed in water and causes chronic cutaneous infection when an open cutaneous lesion is exposed to a colonized water source. Most infections are due to hand or upper-extremity exposure to fish tanks, and some are due to shellfish or marine exposures. Swimming pools are no longer a common source of infection because of current chlorination standards. *M. marinum* grows optimally at 30°C—a lower temperature than is optimal for most pathogenic mycobacteria. After a median incubation period of 21 days (≥30 days in 35% of cases), a granulomatous or ulcerating skin lesion develops at the site of entry, with subsequent sporotrichoid spread in many cases. In some patients, especially those with serious underlying disease and those receiving immunosuppressive therapy, infection may extend to deeper structures, producing tenosynovitis or osteomyelitis. The diagnosis is established by mycobacterial culture of a biopsied lesion or by demonstration of granulomas or AFB in a biopsy sample from a patient with a compatible exposure history.

℞ Treatment: *M. MARINUM* INFECTIONS

Treatment consists of the combination of clarithromycin and ethambutol; the regimen is given for 1–2 months after resolution of lesions—typically 3–4 months in total. Surgical debridement may be necessary in extensive or deep disease; however, routine incision and drainage are not helpful. Rifampin should be added in cases of osteomyelitis. Persons with occupational or avocational exposure to fish tanks or salt water should wear waterproof gloves to prevent infection of open cutaneous lesions.

M. ULCERANS

M. ulcerans causes cutaneous infection (Buruli ulcer) in endemic regions of Central and West Africa, Central and South America, Malaysia, Indonesia, Papua New Guinea, and Australia. The organism is closely related to *M. marinum*, has a similar temperature for optimal growth, and has been isolated from natural bodies of water. Most cases of human infection occur on the bare arms or legs of children or young adults living near rivers, lakes, or swamps. Transmission is thought to result from minor trauma or the bite of an aquatic insect. The initial lesion is a small painless nodule that progresses to a deep ulcer. The ulcer expands, resulting in sloughing of skin and subcutaneous tissue; osteomyelitis may also occur. Stellate scarring and deforming contractures may result from extensive necrosis.

Biopsy analyses demonstrate extracellular AFB in early lesions, with a limited inflammatory reaction. Tissue destruction extends beyond the area of demonstrable bacterial infection and has been attributed to a unique mycobacterial toxin, mycolactone.

℞ Treatment: *M. ULCERANS* INFECTIONS

Antimicrobial therapy has not yet been shown to be beneficial, although rifampin, dapsone, clarithromycin, streptomycin, and amikacin display in vitro activity against *M. ulcerans*. Surgical treatment is of primary importance, and skin grafting may be required. Immunization with BCG reduces the risk of disease by ~50%.

OTHER NTM SPECIES

Numerous other NTM species have been associated with human disease, although they may represent contaminants in clinical specimens. Species and sites of possible infection include *M. celatum* (lung, lymph nodes), *M. genavense* (disseminated), *M. gordonae* (skin, contaminant), *M. haemophilum* (skin, disseminated), *M. malmoense* (lung), *M. simiae* (lung, disseminated), *M. scrofulaceum* (lymphadenitis), *M. szulgai* (skin, lung), and *M. xenopi* (lung, disseminated).

FURTHER READINGS

Doucette K, Fishman JA: Nontuberculous mycobacterial infection in hematopoietic stem cell and solid organ transplant recipients. Clin Infect Dis 38:1428, 2004

Glassroth J: Pulmonary disease due to nontuberculous mycobacteria. Chest 133:243, 2008

Griffith DE et al: An official ATS/IDSA statement: Diagnosis, treatment and prevention of nontuberculous mycobacterial diseases. Am J Respir Crit Care Med 175:367, 2007

Hanak V et al: Hot tub lung: Presenting features and clinical course of 21 patients. Respir Med 100:610, 2006

Kobashi Y et al: Relationship between clinical efficacy of treatment of pulmonary *Mycobacterium avium* complex disease and drug-sensitivity testing of *M. avium* complex isolates. J Infect Chemother 12:195, 2006

Phillips M, von Reyn CF: Nosocomial infections due to nontuberculous mycobacteria. Clin Infect Dis 33:1363, 2001

Reed C et al: Environmental risk factors for infection with *Mycobacterium avium* complex. Am J Epidemiol 164:32, 2006

von Reyn CF et al: Skin test reactions to *Mycobacterium tuberculosis* purified protein derivative and *Mycobacterium avium* sensitin among health care workers and medical students in the United States. Int J Tuberc Lung Dis 5:1122, 2001

CHAPTER 69

ANTIMYCOBACTERIAL AGENTS

Richard J. Wallace, Jr. ■ David E. Griffith

The physician is greatly challenged to provide optimal therapy for mycobacterial illnesses because of the increase in both drug-susceptible and multidrug-resistant tuberculosis; the increasing number of pathogenic nontuberculous mycobacteria (NTM); drug-related toxicities and drug-drug interactions (especially in patients who have AIDS, with their complex antiretroviral drug regimens); and the plethora of new antibiotics with antimycobacterial potential. This chapter reviews the therapeutic agents used for treatment of tuberculosis, leprosy (Hansen's disease), and diseases caused by NTM, including the *Mycobacterium avium* complex (MAC), *M. kansasii*, the rapidly growing mycobacteria, and *M. marinum*. The use of first-line antimycobacterial agents in patients with renal or hepatic disease and in pregnant women is summarized in Table 69-1. The effects of antimycobacterial agents on the levels, activity, and toxicity of other commonly used drugs are summarized in Table 69-2. The reader is referred to the other chapters in this section for a more complete discussion of therapy for specific mycobacterial diseases.

TUBERCULOSIS

Drugs used to treat tuberculosis have been classified into first-line and second-line agents. *First-line essential* antituberculous agents are the most effective and are a necessary component of any short-course therapeutic regimen. The four drugs in this category are rifampin, isoniazid, ethambutol, and pyrazinamide. The *first-line supplemental* agents, which are highly effective with acceptable toxicity, include rifabutin, rifapentine, and streptomycin. *Second-line* antituberculous drugs are clinically much less effective than first-line agents and elicit severe reactions much more frequently. These drugs are rarely used in therapy and then only by caregivers experienced with their use. The older agents include para-aminosalicylic acid (PAS), ethionamide, cycloserine, amikacin, and capreomycin. Favorable experience in patients with tuberculosis resistant to or intolerant of first-line drugs suggests that the fluoroquinolones levofloxacin and moxifloxacin are important additions to multidrug antituberculous regimens;

TABLE 69-1

USE OF FIRST-LINE ANTIMYCOBACTERIAL AGENTS IN PATIENTS WITH RENAL OR HEPATIC DISEASE AND IN PREGNANT WOMEN

	USE IN INDICATED CIRCUMSTANCES			
		RENAL DISEASE: CREATININE CLEARANCE RATE		
AGENT	SEVERE HEPATIC DISEASE	<60 BUT >30 mL/min	≤30 mL/min	PREGNANCY[a]
Azithromycin	No change	No change	?Decrease dose	No evidence of risk (B)
Clarithromycin	No change	No change	Decrease dose	Risk cannot be ruled out (C)
Ethambutol	No change	No change	No change	Risk cannot be ruled out (C)
Isoniazid	Avoid use or monitor carefully	No change	No change	Risk cannot be ruled out (C)
Pyrazinamide	Avoid use or monitor carefully	No change	Decrease dose[b]	Risk cannot be ruled out (C)[c]
Rifabutin	No change	No change	No change	No evidence of risk (B)
Rifampin	Avoid use or monitor carefully	No change	No change	Risk cannot be ruled out (C)
Rifapentine	Avoid use or monitor carefully	No change	No change	Risk cannot be ruled out (C)
Streptomycin	No change	Decrease dose	Decrease dose and frequency	Definite evidence of risk (D)

[a]Based on Food and Drug Administration pregnancy categories of A–D, X.
[b]Prudent but not absolutely necessary.
[c]Use in pregnancy is recommended by international organizations outside the United States.

TABLE 69-2

EFFECTS OF MAJOR ANTIMYCOBACTERIAL AGENTS ON LEVELS/ACTIVITY/TOXICITY OF OTHER COMMONLY USED DRUGS[a]

Rifampin/rifabutin[b]	Isoniazid
Acetaminophen (↓)	Alcohol (↑ in risk of hepatitis)
Antiarrhythmics (↓)	Carbamazepine (↑)
Anticonvulsants (↓)	Diphenylhydantoin (↑)
Azole antifungals (↓)	Enflurane (↑ in risk of renal failure)
Barbiturates (↓)	Warfarin (↑)
β Blockers (↓)	**Clarithromycin**
Calcium channel blockers (↓)	Astemizole (↑)
Chloramphenicol (↓)	Carbamazepine (↑)
Clarithromycin (↓)	Digoxin (↑)
Cyclosporine (↓)	Rifabutin (↑)
Dapsone (↓)	Ritonavir (↓)
Delavirdine (↓)	Terfenadine (↑)
Diazepam (↓)	Zidovudine (↓)
Digoxin (↓)	
Doxycycline (↓)	
Fluoroquinolones (↓)	
Glucocorticoids (↓)	
Halothane (↓)	
Hormonal contraceptives (↓)	
Narcotics (↓)	
NNRTIs[c] (↓)	
Oral hypoglycemics (↓)	
Probenecid (↓)	
Protease inhibitors (↓)	
Quinidine (↓)	
Theophylline (↓)	
Tricyclic antidepressants (↓)	
Warfarin (↓)	
Zidovudine (↓)	

[a]The following antimycobacterial agents have no or minimal effects on other drugs: amikacin, azithromycin, capreomycin, ethambutol, streptomycin, pyrazinamide.
[b]Rifabutin, which induces the cytochrome P450 system, has the same effects (↓) as rifampin but to a lesser degree. All drugs whose half-life is decreased by rifampin induction of hepatic microsomal enzymes may be subject to the same effect when coadministered with rifabutin; however, this point has not yet been studied.
[c]NNRTIs, nonnucleoside reverse transcriptase inhibitors.

thus these agents have now been added to the list of second-line drugs.

FIRST-LINE ESSENTIAL ANTITUBERCULOUS DRUGS

Rifampin

Rifampin, a semisynthetic derivative of *Streptomyces mediterranei*, is considered the most important and potent antituberculous agent. It is also active against a wide spectrum of other organisms, including some gram-positive and gram-negative bacteria, *Legionella* spp., *M. kansasii*, and *M. marinum*.

Mechanism of Action

Rifampin has both intracellular and extracellular bactericidal activity. It blocks RNA synthesis by specifically binding and inhibiting DNA-dependent RNA polymerase. Susceptible strains of *M. tuberculosis* as well as *M. kansasii* and *M. marinum* are inhibited by ≤1 μg/mL.

Pharmacology

Rifampin is a fat-soluble complex macrocyclic antibiotic that is absorbed readily after either PO or IV administration. Serum levels of 10–20 μg/mL follow a standard adult oral dose of 600 mg. Rifampin distributes well throughout most body tissues, including inflamed meninges. The fact that rifampin turns body fluids (urine, saliva, sputum, tears) a red-orange color makes it simple and inexpensive to check on patients' compliance with therapy. Rifampin is excreted primarily through the bile and the enterohepatic circulation, whereas 30–40% of a dose is excreted via the kidneys. The drug is administered three times weekly, twice weekly, or daily at a dose of 600 mg for adults (10 mg/kg) and 10–20 mg/kg for children. As mentioned above, rifampin is also available for IV administration.

Adverse Effects

(Table 69-3) Rifampin is generally well tolerated; the most common adverse event is gastrointestinal upset. This drug rarely causes hepatocellular injury when given alone; however, hepatitis is more common when rifampin is given in combination with isoniazid or pyrazinamide. Other adverse effects of rifampin include rash (0.8%), hemolytic anemia (<1%), thrombocytopenia, and immunosuppression of unknown clinical importance. Rifampin is a potent inducer of the hepatic microsomal enzymes and thereby decreases the half-life of a number of drugs, including digoxin, warfarin, prednisone, cyclosporine, methadone, oral contraceptives, clarithromycin, the HIV protease inhibitors, the HIV nonnucleoside reverse transcriptase inhibitors, and quinidine (Table 69-2). The dose of rifampin generally does not require reduction in patients with renal failure, especially those receiving intermittent rifampin treatment (Table 69-1).

Resistance

Acquired resistance to rifampin results from spontaneous point mutations that alter the β subunit of the RNA polymerase (*rpoB*) gene. Studies have shown that 96% of rifampin-resistant strains have a missense mutation within a 91-bp central core region of the gene. Rifampin-resistant strains of *M. leprae* have similar mutations that alter a single serine residue (Ser-425) in the same core region of the *rpoB* gene. Intrinsic resistance to rifampin is relatively common among most species of rapidly growing and slowly growing NTM; the mechanisms underlying this resistance have yet to be determined.

Isoniazid

After rifampin, isoniazid is considered the best antituberculous drug available. Isoniazid should be included in all tuberculosis treatment regimens unless the organism is resistant. This agent is inexpensive, readily synthesized, available worldwide, highly selective for mycobacteria, and well tolerated, with only 5% of patients exhibiting adverse effects.

TABLE 69-3

MONITORING SIDE EFFECTS OF COMMON ANTITUBERCULOUS DRUGS

DRUG	SIDE EFFECT	MANAGEMENT
Rifampin	Rash	Observe patient/stop drug if significant
	Liver dysfunction	Monitor AST/limit alcohol consumption/monitor for hepatitis symptoms
	Flulike syndrome	Administer at least twice weekly/limit dose to 10 mg/kg (adults)
	Red-orange urine	Reassure patient
	Drug interactions	Consider monitoring levels of other drugs affected by rifampin, especially with contraceptives, anticoagulants, and digoxin/avoid use with protease inhibitors
	Fever, chills	Stop drug
Isoniazid	Hepatitis	Monitor AST/limit alcohol consumption/monitor for hepatitis symptoms/educate patient/stop drug at first symptoms of hepatitis (nausea, vomiting, anorexia, flulike syndrome)
	Peripheral neuritis	Administer vitamin B_6
	Optic neuritis	Administer vitamin B_6/stop drug
	Seizures	Administer vitamin B_6
Pyrazinamide	Hepatitis	Monitor AST/limit daily dosage to 15–30 mg/kg/discontinue with signs or symptoms of hepatitis
	Hyperuricemia	Monitor uric acid level only in cases of gout or renal failure
Ethambutol	Optic neuritis	Use 25 mg/kg daily only for first 2 months (except in drug-resistant tuberculosis), then use lower daily dose (15 mg/kg) when possible/monitor visual acuity (eye chart) and red-green color vision (Ishihara Color Book) at baseline and with any visual complaint/educate patient/stop drug at first change in vision, get ophthalmologic evaluation
Streptomycin, amikacin, capreomycin	Ototoxicity, renal toxicity	Limit dose and duration of therapy as much as possible/avoid daily therapy in patients >50 years old/monitor BUN and serum creatinine levels and possibly conduct audiometry before and as needed during therapy/question patient regularly about tinnitus, dizziness, vertigo, and decreased hearing/measure serum drug levels if possible/educate patient/stop drug at first development of adverse effect (usually tinnitus)

Note: AST, aspartate aminotransferase; BUN, blood urea nitrogen.

Mechanism of Action

Isoniazid is the hydrazide of isonicotinic acid, a small, water-soluble molecule that easily penetrates the cell. Its mechanism of action involves inhibition of mycolic acid cell-wall synthesis via oxygen-dependent pathways such as the catalase-peroxidase reaction. Isoniazid is bacteriostatic against resting bacilli and bactericidal against rapidly multiplying organisms, both extracellularly and intracellularly. The minimal inhibitory concentrations (MICs) of isoniazid for wild-type (untreated) strains of *M. tuberculosis* are <0.1 μg/mL, whereas those for *M. kansasii* are usually 0.5–2.0 μg/mL. The MICs of this drug for other NTM are often higher.

Pharmacology

Both oral and IM preparations of isoniazid are readily absorbed. The standard adult daily oral dose of 300 mg produces peak serum levels of 3–5 μg/mL. Isoniazid diffuses well throughout the body and reaches therapeutic concentrations in serum, cerebrospinal fluid (CSF), and infected tissue, including caseous granulomas. Isoniazid is metabolized in the liver via acetylation and hydrolysis; its metabolites are excreted into the urine. The rate of acetylation is genetically controlled. The recommended daily dose for the treatment of tuberculosis in the United States is 5 mg/kg for adults and 10–20 mg/kg for children, with a maximal daily dose of 300 mg for both groups. (Tuberculosis organizations outside the United States have recommended 5 mg/kg daily for both groups.) For intermittent therapy (usually directly observed), a maximal dose of 900 mg twice or thrice weekly is used. Isoniazid does not require dosage adjustment in patients with renal insufficiency or with end-stage renal disease requiring chronic hemodialysis. Although not approved by the U.S. Food and Drug Administration (FDA), IV isoniazid can be given in an urgent situation.

Adverse Effects

(Table 69-3) The two most important adverse effects of isoniazid therapy are hepatotoxicity and peripheral neuropathy. Other adverse reactions are either rare or less significant and include rash (2%), fever (1.2%), anemia, acne, arthritic symptoms, a systemic lupus erythematosus–like syndrome, optic atrophy, seizures, and psychiatric symptoms. Isoniazid-associated hepatotoxicity includes asymptomatic transient elevation in aminotransferase levels (20%), symptomatic hepatitis (<1%), and fulminant hepatitis with hepatic failure (<0.01%). Isoniazid-associated hepatitis is idiosyncratic and increases in incidence with age, daily alcohol consumption, concomitant rifampin administration, and active hepatitis B infection, as well as in women who are pregnant or in the immediate postpartum period (up to 3 months after delivery). Appropriate clinical monitoring of patients receiving isoniazid includes at least monthly questioning about hepatitis-related symptoms and filling of prescriptions for no more than 1 month's worth of medication. Clinical monitoring is essential for all patients since discontinuation of the drug at the onset of hepatitis symptoms reduces the risk of progression to fatal hepatitis. The Centers for Disease Control and Prevention (CDC) and the American Thoracic Society (ATS) recommend that serum concentrations of alanine aminotransferase (ALT) be determined at baseline in patients with liver disorders or HIV infection, in women who are pregnant or in the immediate postpartum period (3 months), in persons with a history of liver disease (e.g., hepatitis B or C, alcoholic hepatitis, or cirrhosis), in persons who use alcohol regularly, and in other individuals at risk for chronic liver disease who are receiving isoniazid for treatment of latent tuberculosis. Baseline testing is no longer routinely indicated in persons >35 years of age. Routine laboratory monitoring during isoniazid treatment is indicated for patients whose baseline liver function tests yield abnormal results and for persons at risk for hepatic disease, including the groups just mentioned. Measurement of the ALT level is mandatory whenever a patient notices the onset of symptoms suggestive of isoniazid-associated hepatitis (e.g., fever, anorexia, nausea, vomiting, and/or a flulike syndrome including fever and myalgias), and treatment should be discontinued until the relationship between therapy and symptoms is ascertained. The CDC and the ATS recommend that isoniazid should be discontinued whenever (1) an asymptomatic elevation of the ALT level exceeds five times the upper limit of normal or (2) the ALT is three times the upper limit of normal in conjunction with hepatitis symptoms or jaundice. Peripheral neuritis associated with isoniazid is uncommon and probably relates to interference with pyridoxine (vitamin B_6) metabolism. The risk of isoniazid-related neurotoxicity is greatest for patients with preexisting disorders that also pose a risk of neuropathy, such as diabetes, alcohol abuse, or malnutrition. In these patients, the prophylactic administration of 25–50 mg of pyridoxine daily should be considered.

Resistance

The molecular sites of isoniazid resistance have been detailed. Most isoniazid-resistant strains have amino acid changes in either the catalase-peroxidase gene (*katG*) or the promoter of a two-gene locus known as *inhA*. Missense mutations or deletion of *katG* is also associated with reduced catalase and peroxidase activity. Rates of primary isoniazid resistance in untreated patients are much higher in many foreign-born populations than in populations born in the United States.

Ethambutol

A derivative of ethylenediamine, ethambutol is a water-soluble compound that is active only against mycobacteria. Susceptible species include *M. tuberculosis*, *M. marinum*, *M. kansasii*, and MAC organisms. Among first-line drugs, ethambutol is the least potent against *M. tuberculosis*. It is used most often with rifampin for treatment of tuberculosis in patients who cannot tolerate isoniazid or who are thought or known to be infected with isoniazid-resistant organisms.

Mechanism of Action

Ethambutol at standard doses is bacteriostatic against *M. tuberculosis*. Its primary mechanism of action appears to be inhibition of an arabinosyltransferase that mediates the polymerization of arabinose into arabinogalactan within the cell wall.

Pharmacology

After oral administration, 75–80% of a dose of ethambutol is absorbed from the gastrointestinal tract. Peak serum levels of 2–4 μg/mL are achieved 2–4 h after the standard adult daily dose of 15 mg/kg. The drug's distribution throughout the body is adequate except in the CSF, where it reaches only low levels. However, ethambutol can reach CSF levels up to 50% as high as peak plasma levels when administered at a daily dosage of 25 mg/kg (which may be given in one daily dose) for the first 2 months, with subsequent reduction to 15 mg/kg. In cases of drug-resistant tuberculosis or where re-treatment is necessary, the higher dose may be given for the duration. For intermittent therapy, the dosage is 50 mg/kg twice weekly or 30 mg/kg thrice weekly. The dosage must be lowered for patients with renal insufficiency (a creatinine clearance rate of <50 mL/min) to prevent drug accumulation and toxicity.

Adverse Effects

(Table 69-3) Ethambutol is usually well tolerated. Retrobulbar optic neuritis is the most serious adverse effect; axial or central neuritis—the only form reported in patients taking doses of <30 mg/kg—involves the papillomacular bundle of fibers and results in reduced visual acuity, central scotoma, and loss of ability to see green. Symptoms of ocular toxicity typically develop several months after initiation of therapy, but rapid-onset optic neuritis has been reported. The risk of optic neuritis depends on the dose and duration of therapy: this reaction develops in 5% of patients receiving a daily dose of 25 mg/kg but in fewer than 1% of patients given a daily dose of 15 mg/kg. Patients taking the lower dose should be tested for visual acuity and red-green color discrimination at baseline and whenever there is a subjective change in vision. Patients taking the higher dose should be tested at baseline, monthly thereafter, and whenever there is a subjective change in vision. Intermittent (three times weekly) administration of ethambutol at 25 mg/kg per dose appears to be better tolerated than daily administration of 15 mg/kg, especially in elderly populations being treated for MAC infection. Optic neuritis with associated visual loss is usually reversible, but recovery may take >6 months.

Other adverse effects of ethambutol are infrequent. Hyperuricemia occurs but is usually asymptomatic. Peripheral sensory neuropathy occurs in rare instances. Optic neuritis is rare at the low dose in children; however, the use of ethambutol in very young children is problematic because visual complications are difficult to monitor.

Resistance

Ethambutol resistance in *M. tuberculosis* most commonly relates to missense mutations in the *embB* gene that encodes for arabinosyltransferase. Such mutations have been found in 70% of resistant strains and involve amino acid replacements at position 306 or 406 in ~90% of cases. Species of NTM that are intrinsically resistant to ethambutol have variant amino acids in this region of the gene, whereas susceptible species have the same amino acid sequences as *M. tuberculosis*.

Pyrazinamide

A derivative of nicotinic acid, pyrazinamide is an important bactericidal drug used in short-course therapy for tuberculosis.

Mechanism of Action

Pyrazinamide is similar to isoniazid in its narrow spectrum of antibacterial activity, which essentially includes only *M. tuberculosis*. The drug is bactericidal to slowly metabolizing organisms located within the acidic environment of the phagocyte or caseous granuloma; it is active only at a pH of <6.0. Pyrazinamide is considered a prodrug and is converted by the tubercle bacillus to the active form pyrazinoic acid. The target for this compound is thought to be a fatty acid synthase gene (*fasI*). Susceptible strains of *M. tuberculosis* are inhibited by 20 μg/mL.

Pharmacology

Pyrazinamide is well absorbed after oral administration, with a plasma concentration range of 20–60 μg/mL 1–2 h after oral ingestion of the currently recommended adult daily dose of 15–30 mg/kg (maximum, 2 g/d). The drug is well distributed throughout the body. Levels in CSF are excellent, reaching 50–100% of levels in serum. The serum half-life of the drug is 9–11 h. Pyrazinamide is metabolized by at least two major pathways and one minor pathway in the liver; its several metabolites include pyrazinoic acid, 5-hydroxypyrazinamide, and 5-hydroxypyrazinoic acid. Pyrazinamide is not available in a parenteral formulation.

Adverse Effects

(Table 69-3) At the high dosages used in the past, hepatotoxicity was a prominent complication of pyrazinamide therapy. However, at the currently recommended dosages, the frequency of hepatotoxicity is no higher than that for concomitant isoniazid and rifampin therapy. Although pyrazinamide is recommended by international tuberculosis organizations for routine use in pregnancy, it is not recommended in the United States because of inadequate teratogenicity data (Table 69-1). The combination of rifampin/pyrazinamide once recommended for treatment of latent tuberculosis has recently been shown to be associated with an unacceptably high rate of hepatitis. Hyperuricemia is a common adverse effect of pyrazinamide therapy; the incidence is probably reduced by concurrent rifampin therapy. Clinical gout is seen only rarely. Polyarthralgias are encountered fairly commonly but are not related to the hyperuricemia.

Resistance

Resistance to pyrazinamide is associated with loss of pyrazinamidase activity such that pyrazinamide is no longer converted to pyrazinoic acid. More than 90% of isolates with MICs of >100 μg/mL have mutations in the *pncA* gene, which encodes for pyrazinamidase. All strains of *M. bovis* are naturally resistant to pyrazinamide and have a point substitution within the *pncA* gene.

FIRST-LINE SUPPLEMENTAL DRUGS

Streptomycin

An aminoglycoside isolated from *Streptomyces griseus*, streptomycin is available for IM and IV administration only. In the United States, it is the least-used first-line supplemental drug for tuberculosis because of its toxicity, the difficulty in obtaining adequate CSF levels, and the inconvenience of parenteral administration. In developing countries, however, streptomycin is frequently used because of its low cost. The drug is active against untreated strains of *M. tuberculosis*, *M. kansasii*, and *M. marinum* and against some strains of MAC organisms at achievable serum levels.

Mechanism of Action

Streptomycin inhibits protein synthesis by disruption of ribosomal function.

Pharmacology

Serum levels of streptomycin peak at 25–40 μg/mL after a 1.0-g dose. Streptomycin is bactericidal for rapidly dividing extracellular mycobacteria but is ineffective in the acidic environment within the macrophage. It diffuses poorly into the meninges and, in patients with meningitis, reaches CSF levels that are only 20% of serum levels.

The usual adult dose of streptomycin for a 70-kg patient under age 50 is 0.5–1.0 g (10–15 mg/kg) given IM daily or five times per week; the pediatric dose is 20–40 mg/kg daily, with a maximum of 1 g/d. Because streptomycin is eliminated almost exclusively by the kidneys, the dosage must be lowered and the frequency of administration reduced (to only two or three times per week) in most patients >50 years of age and in any patient with renal impairment (Table 69-1) or reduced body weight. Streptomycin can be given IV, although this approach is not approved by the FDA.

Adverse Effects

(Table 69-3) Adverse reactions to streptomycin therapy occur in 10–20% of recipients. Ototoxicity and renal toxicity are the most common and the most serious.

Renal toxicity, usually manifested as nonoliguric renal failure, is less common with streptomycin than with other frequently used aminoglycosides, such as gentamicin. Ototoxicity involves both hearing loss and vestibular dysfunction. The latter is more common and includes loss of balance, vertigo, and tinnitus. Patients receiving streptomycin must be monitored carefully for these adverse effects. Less serious reactions include perioral paresthesia, eosinophilia, rash, and drug fever.

Resistance

In two-thirds of streptomycin-resistant strains of *M. tuberculosis*, mutations have been identified in one of two targets: a 16S rRNA gene (*rrs*) or the gene encoding ribosomal protein S12 (*rpsL*). Both targets are believed to be involved in streptomycin ribosomal binding. No mutational change has been identified in the other one-third of resistant isolates. Strains of *M. tuberculosis* resistant to streptomycin are not cross-resistant to capreomycin or amikacin.

Rifabutin

Rifabutin, a semisynthetic rifamycin spiropiperidyl derivative, shares many characteristics with rifampin, including activity against *M. tuberculosis*. Rifabutin is also active against some strains of rifampin-resistant *M. tuberculosis* and is more active than rifampin against the *M. avium* complex and other NTM. To date, rifabutin has been most useful in the prophylaxis of disseminated MAC infection and in the treatment of drug-resistant tuberculosis. Rifabutin is recommended in place of rifampin for the treatment of HIV-positive individuals who are also taking protease inhibitors because its effect on these agents is less pronounced (Table 69-2).

Mechanism of Action

In *Escherichia coli* and *Bacillus subtilis*, rifabutin inhibits DNA-dependent RNA polymerase in the same manner as rifampin. Its mode of action against mycobacteria is believed to be the same.

Pharmacology

The pharmacology of rifabutin is dramatically different from that of rifampin. Rifabutin is readily absorbed after a single oral dose of 300 mg and reaches peak serum levels (0.35 μg/mL) in 2–4 h. This lipophilic drug distributes best to tissues: tissue levels are 5–10 times higher than plasma levels. CSF concentrations are 30–70% of plasma levels in HIV-infected patients who have meningitis. The drug's slow clearance via hepatic metabolism and renal excretion results in a mean serum half-life of 45 h, which is much longer than the 3- to 5-h half-life of rifampin. Clarithromycin (but not azithromycin) and fluconazole appear to block the hepatic metabolism of rifabutin, with consequent increases in serum levels. Adjustment of dosage is usually unnecessary in elderly patients and in patients with reduced hepatic or renal function (Table 69-1).

Adverse Effects

The majority of rifabutin's adverse effects are dose related. These events occur most frequently in patients receiving >300 mg/d. The most common symptoms are gastrointestinal; other reactions include rash, headache, asthenia, chest pain, myalgia, and insomnia. Like those taking rifampin, most patients taking rifabutin have discolored (orange to tan) urine and other body fluids. Less common adverse reactions include fever, chills, a flulike syndrome, anterior uveitis, hepatitis, *Clostridium difficile*–associated diarrhea, a diffuse polymyalgia syndrome, and a yellow skin discoloration ("pseudojaundice"). Laboratory abnormalities include neutropenia, leukopenia, thrombocytopenia, and increased levels of liver enzymes. Rifabutin induces hepatic cytochrome P450 enzymes but does so much less strongly than rifampin.

Resistance

Resistance to rifabutin is attributable to the same mechanism as that to rifampin—i.e., mutations involving the *rpoB* gene. However, of the 14 mutant *rpoB* alleles that confer resistance to rifampin, only 9 confer high-level resistance to rifabutin; the remaining 5 result in only small changes in rifabutin MICs, which remain at ≤0.5 μg/mL. Thus rifabutin inhibits about one-quarter of rifampin-resistant strains of *M. tuberculosis*.

Rifapentine

A semisynthetic cyclopentyl rifamycin antibiotic, rifapentine received accelerated approval from the FDA for the treatment of tuberculosis. It is the first new drug approved for tuberculosis in the United States in 30 years. Although similar to rifampin, rifapentine is lipophilic and longer acting—characteristics that enhance patient compliance; the drug can be administered at a dose of 600 mg once or twice weekly. Rifapentine has not yet been approved for the treatment of patients with HIV disease because rifapentine/rifampin monoresistance frequently develops in HIV-positive patients receiving isoniazid plus once-weekly rifapentine.

Mechanism of Action

Rifapentine exerts its bactericidal effect by inhibiting DNA-dependent RNA polymerase in susceptible bacteria. The MICs of rifapentine for rifampin-susceptible strains of *M. tuberculosis* range from 0.03 to 0.12 μg/mL.

Pharmacology

After oral administration, rifapentine reaches peak serum concentrations in 5–6 h and achieves a steady state in 10 days. The half-life of rifapentine and its active metabolite 25-desacetyl rifapentine is ~13 h. The administered dose is excreted via the liver (70%).

Adverse Effects

Rifapentine's adverse-event pattern is similar to that of rifampin. Rifapentine induces the hepatic cytochrome P450 enzymes CYP3A4 and 2C8/9. Current induction studies suggest that its potential for drug-drug interaction may be lower than that of rifampin but greater than that of rifabutin. Drugs potentially affected by concomitant administration of rifapentine are listed under "Rifampin/rifabutin" in Table 69-2. Rifapentine is in category C for use in pregnancy (Table 69-1) because of its teratogenesis in rats and rabbits.

Resistance

Strains of *M. tuberculosis* resistant to rifapentine, rifampin, and rifabutin all involve spontaneous point mutations in the *rpoB* gene. All strains resistant to rifampin are also resistant to rifapentine.

SECOND-LINE ANTITUBERCULOUS DRUGS

Second-line and/or newer antituberculosis agents are used either when tuberculosis is drug resistant or when first-line supplemental drugs are not available. The more important second-line drugs are discussed below in their general (descending) order of usefulness.

Quinolones

The mode of action of the fluorinated quinolones presumably is the prevention of DNA synthesis through the inhibition of DNA gyrase. Ofloxacin, levofloxacin, ciprofloxacin, and moxifloxacin are active against many mycobacteria, including *M. tuberculosis*, *M. leprae*, *M. marinum*, *M. kansasii*, and *M. fortuitum*. Levofloxacin and moxifloxacin are the most active quinolones against *M. tuberculosis*. Recent studies suggest that use of moxifloxacin may reduce the duration of therapy for drug-susceptible tuberculosis. These drugs are well absorbed orally, reach high serum levels, and distribute well to body tissues and fluids. Although not approved for antituberculous therapy in the United States, ofloxacin—used in combination with isoniazid and rifampin for the treatment of pulmonary tuberculosis—has been as active and safe as ethambutol in initial trials. Adverse effects are relatively uncommon, occurring in 0.5–10% of cases and consisting mostly of benign reactions such as gastrointestinal intolerance, rashes, dizziness, and headache. The quinolones are rapidly becoming some of the most important and effective drugs for the treatment of patients who have resistant tuberculosis or are intolerant to first-line essential drugs. Some experts would classify the quinolones, especially moxifloxacin, as first-line supplemental agents. The quinolones can also be administered IV.

Mycobacterial resistance to the fluoroquinolones develops rapidly. Its molecular basis is complex; only some strains exhibit missense mutations in the A subunit (*gyrA* gene) of DNA gyrase. Fluoroquinolone-resistant tuberculosis is a source of growing concern. Because of their broad spectrum and the ease with which mutational resistance develops, antituberculous therapy with quinolones should be reserved (pending the results of ongoing studies) for patients with multidrug-resistant disease and for those who cannot tolerate first-line drugs.

Capreomycin

Capreomycin, a complex cyclic polypeptide antibiotic derived from *Streptomyces capreolus*, is similar to streptomycin in terms of dosing, mechanism of action, pharmacology, and toxicity. It is administered only by the IM route in doses of 10–15 mg/kg daily or five times per week (maximal daily dose, 1 g), with peak blood levels of 20–40 μg/mL. After 2–4 months, the dosage should be reduced to 1 g two or three times a week. Cross-resistance to kanamycin and amikacin—but not to streptomycin—is common. After streptomycin, capreomycin is the injectable drug of choice for tuberculosis.

Amikacin

This well-known aminoglycoside is bactericidal to extracellular organisms. Amikacin is active against *M. tuberculosis* and several of the nontuberculous species, including the rapidly growing mycobacteria, *M. kansasii*, *M. leprae*, and the *M. avium* complex. The usual adult dosage is 7–10 mg/kg IM or IV three to five times per week (generally no more than 500–750 mg/d). Resistance relates to a single A → G base-pair change at position 1408 in the 16S ribosomal RNA gene.

Ethionamide

Like isoniazid and pyrazinamide, ethionamide is a derivative of isonicotinic acid. This agent is bacteriostatic against metabolizing *M. tuberculosis* and some NTM. It is most useful in the treatment of multidrug-resistant tuberculosis. However, its use is severely limited by its toxicity and frequent side effects, which include intense gastrointestinal intolerance (anorexia, vomiting, and dysgeusia), serious neurologic reactions, reversible hepatitis (5% of cases), hypersensitivity reactions, and hypothyroidism.

Para-Aminosalicylic Acid

PAS as a calcium or sodium salt inhibits the growth of *M. tuberculosis* by impairing folate synthesis. It is rarely indicated for the treatment of tuberculosis because of its low level of antituberculous activity and its high level of gastrointestinal toxicity (manifesting as nausea, vomiting, and diarrhea). Enteric-coated PAS granules (4 g every 8 h) may be better tolerated than other formulations and produce higher therapeutic blood levels. The drug has a short half-life (1 h), and 80% of the dose is excreted in the urine.

Cycloserine

Cycloserine (D-4-amino-3-isoxazolidinone) is produced by *Streptomyces orchidaceus* and is active against a broad spectrum of bacteria, including *M. tuberculosis*. Cycloserine is well absorbed after oral administration and is widely distributed throughout body fluids, including the CSF. Serious side effects limit the use of this drug and include psychosis (with suicide in some cases), seizures, peripheral neuropathy, headaches, somnolence, and allergic reactions. Cycloserine should not be given to patients with epilepsy, active alcohol abuse, severe renal insufficiency, or a history of depression or psychosis.

NEWER ANTITUBERCULOUS DRUGS

A number of drugs are being evaluated for their antituberculous activity. This group includes newer rifamycins, fluoroquinolones, oxazolidinones (linezolid; see below), nitroimidazopyrans, and diarylquinolines. Although it is not clear how many of the new agents will prove to be clinically useful, there are currently more antituberculosis drugs in development than at any previous time.

Linezolid

Linezolid is one of a new class of gram-positive-active antimicrobial agents called oxazolidinones that inhibit protein synthesis by binding to the 70S ribosomal initiation complex. Linezolid has very low MICs against both drug-susceptible and drug-resistant *M. tuberculosis* in vitro and has been used successfully as a component of multidrug regimens in a small number of patients with drug-resistant tuberculosis. This agent is available in IV and oral forms. Linezolid is associated with frequent, severe adverse events, including bone marrow suppression (which appears to be dose dependent and reversible) and peripheral neuropathy (which appears to be neither dose dependent nor reversible).

LEPROSY (HANSEN'S DISEASE)

Therapy for leprosy remains difficult, especially in developing countries. Obstacles include the long courses of drug therapy required, the high cost and limited availability of most drugs, the frequency of adverse drug reactions, the difficulty of determining a treatment endpoint, and (given that *M. leprae* still cannot be grown in vitro) the difficulty of conducting susceptibility testing. Although many drugs are active against *M. leprae*, efficacy in the treatment of leprosy has been established only for dapsone, rifampin, clofazimine, and ethionamide; because of its potentially severe side effects, the WHO no longer recommends ethionamide for the treatment of leprosy. Initiation of multidrug treatment has reduced the problem of acquired drug resistance seen previously with dapsone monotherapy.

Rifampin

Rifampin is considered the most active agent for the treatment of leprosy. Its worldwide use is limited only by its cost. This drug is highly bactericidal against *M. leprae* and reduces the number of viable bacilli in patients' tissues faster than any other available agent. Rifampin must be combined with other antileprosy drugs to forestall resistance. For cost reasons, the drug dose of 600 mg is given once a month (supervised) outside the United States, but this dose is given daily in the United States. For details on pharmacology, adverse events, and resistance, see relevant sections under "Tuberculosis."

Dapsone

Dapsone (4,4′-diaminodiphenylsulfone) inhibits bacterial folic acid synthesis. It is now considered the second most active drug (after rifampin) in the treatment of leprosy because of its ready availability, low cost, and low toxicity and the susceptibility of untreated strains of *M. leprae* to low concentrations.

Pharmacology

Dapsone is well absorbed orally and distributes well throughout the body. The usual daily dosage is 100 mg for adults and 0.9–1.4 mg/kg for children. Plasma concentrations peak within 1–3 h. The median elimination half-life is 22 h. Dapsone is cleared by acetylation in the liver. The drug is 70% bound to plasma protein. Usual daily doses produce serum concentrations of 10–15 μg/mL, which far exceed the MIC for *M. leprae* (0.01–0.001 μg/mL).

Adverse Effects

Hemolysis and methemoglobinemia are common untoward reactions to dapsone. Patients should be screened for glucose-6-phosphate dehydrogenase deficiency to prevent serious drug-induced hemolysis. However, most patients tolerate dapsone therapy well with adequate clinical and laboratory supervision. Other side effects include gastrointestinal intolerance, headache, pruritus, peripheral neuropathies, nephrotic syndrome, fever, and rash.

Clofazimine

A phenazine iminoquinone dye, clofazimine is weakly bactericidal against *M. leprae*. It is useful in treating dapsone-resistant leprosy and may lessen the severity of erythema nodosum leprosum (ENL). Clofazimine's mode of action is not well understood. Its serum half-life is ~60–70 days; only a small proportion of the dose is excreted daily into the urine or bile. Bactericidal activity is very slow and is evident for ~50 days after administration. The usual adult dosage is 50–100 mg/d, 100 mg three times a week, or (for treatment of ENL) 300 mg/d. Untoward effects include skin discoloration and, less commonly, gastrointestinal intolerance.

Other Agents

A number of other drugs exhibit significant activity against *M. leprae*, but clinical experience with these agents is lacking. Thalidomide is now approved by the FDA for treatment of ENL. This drug is sedating and extremely teratogenic and should *never* be taken by anyone who is or may become pregnant. Physicians wishing to prescribe thalidomide must register with the System for Thalidomide Education and Prescribing Safety (S.T.E.P.S.) at 1-888-423-5436 (Celgene Corporation). The newer macrolide antibiotics (particularly clarithromycin), minocycline (a long-acting tetracycline), and a number of fluoroquinolones (including ofloxacin, sparfloxacin, and pefloxacin) have shown promising bactericidal activity against *M. leprae*. For the most minor form of leprosy, the WHO now suggests the use of single-dose rifampin/ofloxacin/minocycline (ROM).

NONTUBERCULOUS MYCOBACTERIA

Although less pathogenic than *M. tuberculosis*, NTM can cause pulmonary, skin, bone, joint, lymph node, and soft tissue infection as well as disseminated disease in immunocompromised hosts, including patients with AIDS. MAC organisms and *M. kansasii* are the two most common causes of NTM pulmonary infection. Up to 40% of AIDS patients with CD4+ T-cell counts of <50/μL develop disseminated disease due to *M. avium* unless they are receiving specific *M. avium* prophylaxis.

Clarithromycin

Clarithromycin (6-*0*-methylerythromycin) is a newer macrolide that is similar to erythromycin in its mechanism of action. It is well absorbed with or without meals but may elicit gastrointestinal intolerance. Clarithromycin distributes well into body tissues and fluids and is highly concentrated in macrophages. The drug is metabolized in the liver, with ~30% of a given dose excreted in the urine. The dosage should be reduced if the creatinine clearance rate is ≤30 mL/min. Like erythromycin, clarithromycin binds with plasma proteins (65–70%) and can raise the levels of drugs such as theophylline and carbamazepine. Serum levels of clarithromycin are reduced by rifampin and, to a lesser degree, by rifabutin; clarithromycin increases serum levels of rifabutin and some antihistamines (e.g., terfenadine), thus potentially increasing their toxicity. The drug is also highly active not only against MAC organisms but also against almost all other NTM, including *M. marinum*, *M. kansasii*, *M. haemophilum*, *M. genavense*, *M. xenopi*, *M. abscessus*, and *M. chelonae*. Recent studies have shown that most members of the *M. fortuitum* group are resistant to macrolides on the basis of chromosomal *erm* genes. Standard antimycobacterial doses have been 500 mg twice daily or, in the case of MAC pulmonary disease, three times weekly. The more common side effects of high doses include nausea, vomiting, and (occasionally) abnormal liver function tests. A bitter taste is common even with routine doses. Most gastrointestinal side effects can be minimized by reducing the dose or using slow-release formulations. Clarithromycin is teratogenic in laboratory animals and is in category C for use in pregnancy (Table 69-1). Resistance results from point mutations involving adenine at position 2058 or 2059 in the 23S ribosomal RNA gene macrolide binding site and is a major concern for all slowly growing species and the rapid growers *M. chelonae* and *M. abscessus*, which have only a single copy of the ribosomal genes.

Azithromycin

Azithromycin is a macrolide that belongs to the family of azalides. This drug reaches much lower serum levels than clarithromycin (usually ≤0.5 μg/mL), but its high tissue and macrophage concentrations and longer half-life suggest the feasibility of intermittent therapy. Azithromycin is involved in few drug interactions since it does not affect the cytochrome P450 system. The usual doses are 250–500 mg three times weekly (MAC therapy) or 1200 mg once a week (prophylaxis for disseminated *M. avium*). No alteration in dose is required in renal failure. The most common side effects are gastrointestinal symptoms and reversible hearing loss. Resistance to azithromycin develops by the same mechanism as that to clarithromycin, with cross-resistance between the two macrolides.

Therapy for Specific NTM Infections

MAC Organisms

The treatment of MAC lung disease involves the use of two or three drugs administered either daily or three times per week. Given the potential for drug-related toxicity and the remaining uncertainties about the optimal regimen and schedule, treatment frequently needs to be individualized.

Therapy for MAC lung disease in the adult patient with nodular disease and bronchiectasis usually involves the administration of clarithromycin (500 mg morning and night), ethambutol (25 mg/kg), and rifampin (600 mg) on a Monday–Wednesday–Friday schedule. For patients with upper-lobe cavitary disease, daily therapy is usually recommended. Therapy is generally continued until cultures have been negative for 12 months.

For disseminated disease in AIDS, daily administration of one of the newer macrolides (clarithromycin or azithromycin) and ethambutol (15 mg/kg) is considered an essential component of any treatment regimen, with rifabutin (300 mg) a commonly used third drug. Other alternative drugs include streptomycin and amikacin. Clofazimine appears to increase mortality risk and should be avoided. For prophylaxis of disseminated MAC disease, rifabutin (300 mg/d), clarithromycin (500 mg twice daily), and azithromycin (1200 mg once weekly) have all been effective in controlled or comparative clinical trials. Once-weekly azithromycin is the drug most often used.

M. Kansasii

M. kansasii is usually susceptible to most antituberculous drugs except for pyrazinamide. Current ATS recommendations for the treatment of *M. kansasii* pulmonary disease are daily isoniazid (300 mg), rifampin (600 mg), and ethambutol (15 mg/kg); this regimen is continued until 12 months after the last positive sputum culture. In patients taking protease inhibitors, rifabutin (150 mg/d) or clarithromycin (500 mg twice daily) should be substituted for rifampin. The potential advantages of the highly active rifabutin and the newer macrolides in immunocompetent patients have not been studied.

Rapidly Growing Mycobacteria

The *M. fortuitum* group, *M. abscessus*, and *M. chelonae* account for >80% of cases of clinical disease due to rapidly growing mycobacteria. These organisms are resistant to antituberculous agents other than amikacin but are variably susceptible to several traditional antibiotics. Clarithromycin has dramatically changed the approach to therapy for infections with rapidly growing mycobacteria, since it inhibits most species. Other drugs with good activity include amikacin, cefoxitin, doxycycline, imipenem, the fluorinated quinolones, sulfonamides, and linezolid.

M. Marinum

M. marinum, a cause of posttraumatic localized skin infection, is typically susceptible to minocycline, rifampin, ethambutol, clarithromycin, and trimethoprim-sulfamethoxazole and is resistant to isoniazid.

FURTHER READINGS

American Thoracic Society: Targeted tuberculin testing and treatment of latent tuberculosis infection. Am J Respir Crit Care Med 161:S221, 2000

———/Centers for Disease Control and Prevention/Infectious Diseases Society of America: Treatment of tuberculosis. Am J Respir Crit Care Med 167:603, 2003

Bock NN et al: A prospective, randomized, double-blind study of the tolerability of rifapentine 600, 900, and 1,200 mg plus isoniazid in the continuation phase of tuberculosis treatment. Am J Respir Crit Care Med 165:1526, 2002

Burman WJ et al: Moxifloxacin versus ethambutol in the first 2 months of treatment for pulmonary tuberculosis. Am J Respir Crit Care Med 174:331, 2006

Griffith DE et al: An official ATS/IDSA statement: Diagnosis, treatment, and prevention of nontuberculous mycobacterial diseases. Am J Respir Crit Care Med 175:367, 2007

Jasmer RM et al: Short-course rifampin and pyrazinamide compared with isoniazid for latent tuberculosis infection: A multicenter clinical trial. Ann Intern Med 137:640, 2002

Musser JM: Antimicrobial agent resistance in mycobacteria: Molecular genetic insights. Clin Microbiol Rev 8:496, 1995

Saukkonen JJ et al: An official ATS statement: Hepatotoxicity of antituberculosis therapy. Am J Respir Crit Care Med 174:935, 2006

WHO Expert Committee on Leprosy: Seventh Report. Geneva, World Health Organization, 1998, Technical Report Series, No. 874

PART 6 SPIROCHETAL DISEASES

CHAPTER 70

SYPHILIS

Sheila A. Lukehart

DEFINITION

Syphilis, a chronic systemic infection caused by *Treponema pallidum* subspecies *pallidum*, is usually sexually transmitted and is characterized by episodes of active disease interrupted by periods of latency. After an incubation period averaging 2–6 weeks, a primary lesion appears, often associated with regional lymphadenopathy. The secondary stage, associated with generalized mucocutaneous lesions and generalized lymphadenopathy, is followed by a latent period of subclinical infection lasting years or decades. In about one-third of untreated cases, the tertiary stage appears, characterized by progressive destructive mucocutaneous, musculoskeletal, or parenchymal lesions; aortitis; or symptomatic central nervous system (CNS) disease.

ETIOLOGY

The Spirochaetales include three genera that are pathogenic for humans and for a variety of other animals: *Leptospira*, which causes human leptospirosis (Chap. 72); *Borrelia*, which causes relapsing fever and Lyme disease (Chaps. 73 and 74); and *Treponema*, which causes the diseases known as treponematoses (see also Chap. 71). The genus *Treponema* includes *T. pallidum* subspecies *pallidum*, which causes venereal syphilis; *T. pallidum* subspecies *pertenue*, which causes yaws; *T. pallidum* subspecies *endemicum*, which causes endemic syphilis or bejel; and *T. carateum*, which causes pinta. Until recently, the subspecies were distinguished primarily by the clinical syndromes they produce. Researchers have now identified molecular signatures that can differentiate the three subspecies of *T. pallidum* by culture-independent, polymerase chain reaction (PCR)–based methods. Other *Treponema* species found in the human mouth, genital mucosa, and gastrointestinal tract have been associated with disease (e.g., periodontitis), but their role as primary etiologic agents is unclear.

T. pallidum subspecies *pallidum* (referred to hereafter simply as *T. pallidum*), a thin spiral organism, has a cell body surrounded by a trilaminar cytoplasmic membrane, a delicate peptidoglycan layer providing some structural rigidity, and a lipid-rich outer membrane containing relatively few integral membrane proteins. Endoflagella wind around the cell body in the periplasmic space and are responsible for motility.

T. pallidum cannot be cultured in vitro, and little was known about its metabolism until the genome was sequenced in 1998. This spirochete possesses severely limited metabolic capabilities, lacking the genes required for de novo synthesis of most amino acids, nucleotides, and lipids. In addition, *T. pallidum* lacks genes encoding the enzymes of the Krebs cycle and oxidative phosphorylation. To compensate, the organism contains numerous genes predicted to code for transporters of amino acids, carbohydrates, and cations. In addition, genome analyses and other studies have revealed the existence of a 12-member gene family (called *tpr*) that bears similarities to variable outer-membrane antigens of other spirochetes. One member, TprK, has discrete variable (V) regions that are targets of the humoral immune response. Data suggest that sequence variation occurs in TprK during infection and that this variation is a mechanism for immune invasion.

The only known natural host for *T. pallidum* is the human host. *T. pallidum* can infect many mammals, but only humans, higher apes, and a few laboratory animals regularly develop syphilitic lesions. Virulent strains of *T. pallidum* are grown in rabbits.

EPIDEMIOLOGY

Nearly all cases of syphilis are acquired by sexual contact with infectious lesions (i.e., the chancre, mucous patch, skin rash, or condylomata lata). Less common modes of transmission include nonsexual personal contact, infection in utero, blood transfusion, and organ transplantation.

SYPHILIS IN THE UNITED STATES

With the advent of penicillin therapy, the total number of cases of syphilis reported annually in the United States declined significantly to a low of 31,575 in 2000—a 95% decrease from 1943. In 2005, 33,278 cases were reported. Surveillance of the number of new cases of primary and secondary (infectious) syphilis, which is a better indicator of disease activity, has revealed multiple cycles of 7–10 years, each with a rapid rise and fall in incidence. The current increase in infectious syphilis (to 8724 cases in 2005) began in the western United States in 1997 and has particularly affected men who have sex with men (MSM), many of whom are co-infected with HIV. This outbreak has spread to large cities on the west coast of North America and to major cities elsewhere in the United States. It has been suggested that the regular fluctuation in syphilis rates is due to herd immunity in susceptible populations. Although there are no data to suggest that persons treated for syphilis possess significant resistance to reinfection, it has been recognized for many years that persons with untreated syphilis are refractory to symptomatic reinfection.

The populations at highest risk for acquiring syphilis have changed over time, with outbreaks among MSM in the late 1970s and early 1980s as well as at present. The epidemic that peaked in 1990 predominantly involved African-American heterosexual men and women and occurred largely in urban areas, where infectious syphilis was correlated significantly with the exchange of sex for crack cocaine. Since 1996, syphilis rates have declined among African Americans but remain higher than those for other racial/ethnic groups. Foci of syphilis still exist in a small number of counties in the southern United States.

The incidence of congenital syphilis roughly parallels that of infectious syphilis in females. The number of reported cases of congenital syphilis among infants ≤1 year of age fell to a low of 107 cases in 1978, when infectious syphilis was most prevalent among homosexual and bisexual men, and then rose dramatically from 1986 to 1991 during the epidemic in African-American women. In 2005, 329 cases were reported. It is important to note that the case definition for congenital syphilis was broadened in 1989 and now includes all live or stillborn infants delivered to women with untreated or inadequately treated syphilis.

One-third to one-half of individuals named as sexual contacts of persons with infectious syphilis become infected. Many sexual contacts will already have developed manifestations of syphilis when they are first seen, and ~30% of apparently uninfected contacts who are examined within 30 days of exposure actually have incubating infection and will later develop infectious syphilis if not treated. Thus identification and treatment of all recently exposed sexual contacts are important aspects of syphilis control. Also important is the identification of infected persons by serologic testing of pregnant women, persons admitted to hospitals, and military inductees. Routine premarital serologic testing for syphilis is controversial because of low yield.

GLOBAL SYPHILIS

Syphilis remains a significant health problem globally, with an estimated 12 million new infections per year. The regions that are most affected include Sub-Saharan Africa, South America, and Southeast Asia (Fig. 70-1). Some African studies have shown antenatal syphilis seropositivity rates as high as 30%, and congenital syphilis has been reported to account for up to 50% of stillbirths. Large increases in syphilis have occurred in the independent states of the former Soviet Union, and higher numbers of cases have recently been reported in European countries.

NATURAL COURSE AND PATHOGENESIS OF UNTREATED SYPHILIS

T. pallidum rapidly penetrates intact mucous membranes or microscopic abrasions in skin and within a few hours enters the lymphatics and blood to produce systemic infection and metastatic foci long before the appearance

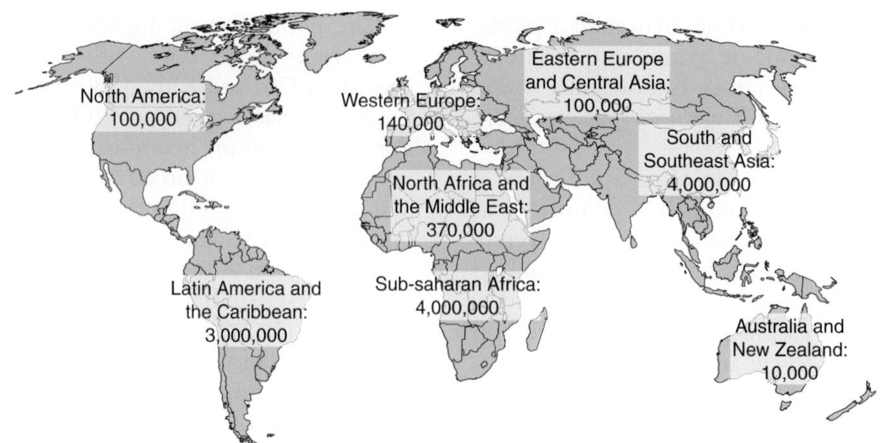

FIGURE 70-1

Estimated annual new cases of syphilis among adults, 1999. (*Courtesy of the World Health Organization.*)

of a primary lesion. Blood from a patient with incubating or early syphilis is infectious. The generation time of *T. pallidum* during early active disease in vivo is estimated to be ~30 h, and the incubation period of syphilis is inversely proportional to the number of organisms inoculated. The 50% infectious dose for intradermal inoculation in humans has been calculated to be 57 organisms, and the treponeme concentration generally reaches 10^7/g of tissue before a clinical lesion appears. The median incubation period in humans (~21 days) suggests an average inoculum of 500–1000 infectious organisms for naturally acquired disease; the incubation period rarely exceeds 6 weeks.

The primary lesion appears at the site of inoculation, usually persists for 4–6 weeks, and then heals spontaneously. Histopathologic examination shows perivascular infiltration, chiefly by CD4+ and CD8+ T lymphocytes, plasma cells, and macrophages, with capillary endothelial proliferation and subsequent obliteration of small blood vessels. The cellular infiltration displays a T_H1-type cytokine profile consistent with the activation of macrophages. Phagocytosis of opsonized organisms by activated macrophages ultimately causes their destruction, resulting in spontaneous resolution of the chancre.

The generalized parenchymal, constitutional, and mucocutaneous manifestations of secondary syphilis usually appear ~6–8 weeks after the chancre heals. Approximately 15% of patients with secondary syphilis still have persisting or healing chancres, and the stages may overlap more frequently in persons with concurrent HIV infection. In other patients, secondary lesions may appear several months after the chancre has healed, and some patients may enter the latent stage without ever recognizing secondary lesions. The histopathologic features of secondary maculopapular skin lesions are hyperkeratosis of the epidermis, capillary proliferation with endothelial swelling in the superficial corium, and dermal papillae with transmigration of polymorphonuclear leukocytes and, in the deeper corium, perivascular infiltration by CD8+ T lymphocytes, CD4+ T lymphocytes, macrophages, and plasma cells. Treponemes are found in many tissues, including the aqueous humor of the eye and the cerebrospinal fluid (CSF). Invasion of the CNS by *T. pallidum* occurs during the first weeks or months of infection, and CSF abnormalities are detected in as many as 40% of patients during the secondary stage. Clinical hepatitis and immune complex–induced membranous glomerulonephritis are relatively rare but recognized manifestations of secondary syphilis; liver function tests may yield abnormal results in up to one-quarter of patients with early syphilis. Generalized nontender lymphadenopathy is noted in 85% of patients with secondary syphilis. The paradoxical appearance of secondary manifestations despite high titers of antibody (including immobilizing antibody) to *T. pallidum* is unexplained but may result from antigenic variation or changes in expression of surface antigens. Secondary lesions subside within 2–6 weeks, and the infection enters the latent stage, which is detectable only by serologic testing. In the preantibiotic era, up to 25% of untreated patients experienced at least one generalized or localized mucocutaneous relapse, usually during the first year. Therefore, identification and examination of sexual contacts are most important for patients with syphilis of <1 year's duration. Recurrent generalized rash is now rare.

About one-third of patients with untreated latent syphilis developed clinically apparent tertiary disease in the preantibiotic era. In industrialized countries today, specific treatment for early and latent syphilis and coincidental therapy have nearly eliminated tertiary disease except for cases of neurosyphilis in HIV-infected persons. In the past, the most common types of tertiary disease were the gumma (a usually benign granulomatous lesion), cardiovascular syphilis (usually involving the vasa vasorum of the ascending aorta and resulting in aneurysm), and symptomatic neurosyphilis (tabes dorsalis and paresis). Asymptomatic CNS involvement, however, is still demonstrable in up to 25% of patients with late latent syphilis. The factors that contribute to the development and progression of tertiary disease are unknown.

The course of untreated syphilis was studied retrospectively in a group of nearly 2000 patients with primary or secondary disease diagnosed clinically (the Oslo Study, 1891–1951) and was assessed prospectively in 431 African-American men with seropositive latent syphilis of ≥3 years' duration (the notorious Tuskegee Study, 1932–1972). In the Oslo Study, 24% of patients developed relapsing secondary lesions within 4 years, and 28% eventually developed one or more manifestations of tertiary syphilis. Cardiovascular syphilis, including aortitis, was detected in 10% of patients, none of whom had been infected before age 15; 7% of patients developed symptomatic neurosyphilis, and 16% developed benign tertiary syphilis (gummas of the skin, mucous membranes, and skeleton). Syphilis was the primary cause of death in 15% of men and 8% of women. Cardiovascular syphilis was documented in 35% of men and 22% of women who eventually came to autopsy. In general, serious late complications were nearly twice as common among men as among women.

The Tuskegee Study showed that the death rate among untreated African-American men with syphilis (25–50 years old) was 17% higher than that among uninfected subjects and that 30% of all deaths were attributable to cardiovascular or CNS syphilis. By far the most important factor in increased mortality was cardiovascular syphilis. Anatomic evidence of aortitis was found in 40–60% of autopsied subjects with syphilis (vs 15% of control subjects), whereas CNS syphilis was found in only 4%. Rates of hypertension were also higher among the infected subjects. The ethical issues eventually raised by this study, begun in the preantibiotic era but continuing into the early 1970s, had a major influence on the development of current guidelines for human medical experimentation, and the history of the study may still contribute to a reluctance of some African Americans to participate as subjects in clinical research.

These two studies both showed that about one-third of patients with untreated syphilis develop clinical or pathologic evidence of tertiary syphilis, that about one-fourth die as a direct result of tertiary syphilis, and that there is additional excess mortality not directly attributable to tertiary syphilis.

CLINICAL MANIFESTATIONS

Primary Syphilis

The typical primary chancre usually begins as a single painless papule that rapidly becomes eroded and usually becomes indurated, with a characteristic cartilaginous consistency on palpation of the edge and base of the ulcer. In heterosexual men the chancre is usually located on the penis (Fig. 70-2), whereas in homosexual men it is often found in the anal canal or rectum, in the mouth, or on the external genitalia. In women, common primary sites are the cervix and labia. Consequently, primary syphilis goes unrecognized in women and homosexual men more often than in heterosexual men. Multiple primary lesions may be more common among men with concurrent HIV infection.

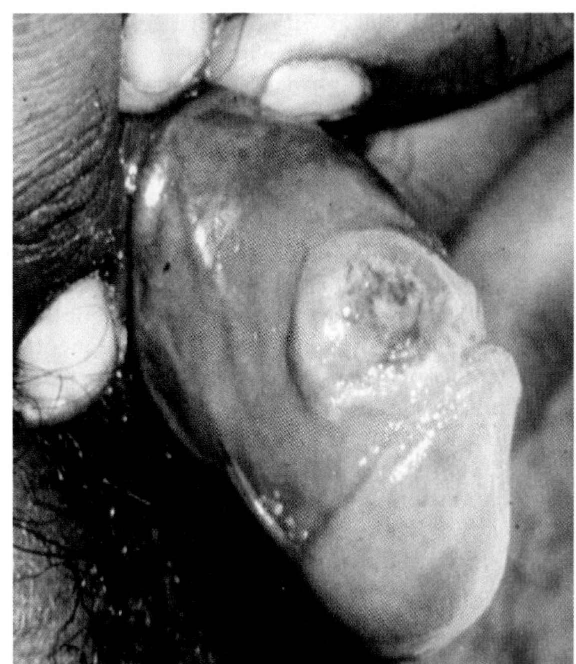

FIGURE 70-2
Primary syphilis with a firm, nontender chancre.

Atypical primary lesions are common. The clinical appearance depends on the number of treponemes inoculated and on the immunologic status of the patient. A large inoculum produces a dark-field-positive ulcerative lesion in nonimmune volunteers but may produce a small dark-field-negative papule, an asymptomatic but seropositive latent infection, or no response at all in some individuals with a history of syphilis. A small inoculum may produce only a papular lesion, even in nonimmune individuals. Therefore, syphilis should be considered even in the evaluation of trivial or atypical dark-field-negative genital lesions. The genital lesions that most commonly must be differentiated from those of primary syphilis include those caused by herpes simplex virus infection (Chap. 80), chancroid (Chap. 47), traumatic injury, and donovanosis (Chap. 62). *Primary genital herpes* may produce inguinal adenopathy, but the nodes are tender and the lesions consist of multiple painful vesicles, which later ulcerate and are often accompanied by systemic symptoms, including fever. *Recurrent genital herpes* typically begins with a unilateral cluster of painful vesicles, usually without associated adenopathy. *Chancroid* produces painful, superficial, exudative, nonindurated ulcers, more often multiple than in syphilis (see Fig. 47-2); adenopathy is common, can be either unilateral or bilateral, is tender, and may be suppurative. *Donovanosis*, which is rare in the United States and Europe, is usually seen as a granulomatous ulcer that, although painless, is friable.

Regional (usually inguinal) lymphadenopathy accompanies the primary syphilitic lesion, appearing within 1 week of lesion onset. The nodes are firm, nonsuppurative, and painless. Inguinal lymphadenopathy is bilateral and may occur with anal as well as with external genital chancres. The chancre generally heals within 4–6 weeks (range, 2–12 weeks), but lymphadenopathy may persist for months.

Secondary Syphilis

The protean manifestations of the secondary stage usually include localized or diffuse mucocutaneous lesions and generalized nontender lymphadenopathy. As stated above, the healing primary chancre is still present in 15% of cases, and the stages may overlap more frequently in persons with concurrent HIV infection than in those without this co-infection. The skin rash consists of macular, papular, papulosquamous, and occasionally pustular syphilides; often more than one form is present simultaneously. The eruption may be very subtle, and 25% of patients with a discernible rash may be unaware that they have dermatologic manifestations. Initial lesions are pale red or pink, nonpruritic, discrete macules distributed on the trunk and proximal extremities; these macules progress to papular lesions (Fig. 70-3) that are distributed widely and that frequently involve the palms and soles (Fig. 70-4*A*). Rarely, severe necrotic lesions (*lues maligna*) may appear. Involvement of the hair follicles may result in patchy alopecia of the scalp hair, eyebrows, or beard in up to 5% of cases.

In warm, moist, intertriginous areas (commonly the perianal region, vulva, and scrotum), papules can enlarge to produce broad, moist, pink or gray-white, highly infectious lesions (*condylomata lata*) in 10% of patients with secondary syphilis. Superficial mucosal erosions (*mucous patches*) occur in 10–15% of patients and commonly involve the oral or genital mucosa (Fig. 70-4*B*). The typical mucous patch is a painless silver-gray erosion surrounded by a red periphery.

Constitutional symptoms that may accompany or precede secondary syphilis include sore throat (15–30%), fever (5–8%), weight loss (2–20%), malaise (25%), anorexia (2–10%), headache (10%), and meningismus (5%).

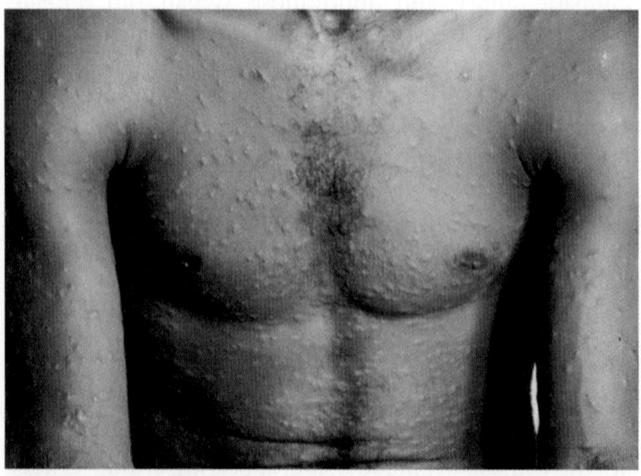

FIGURE 70-3
Secondary syphilis: the papulosquamous truncal eruption.

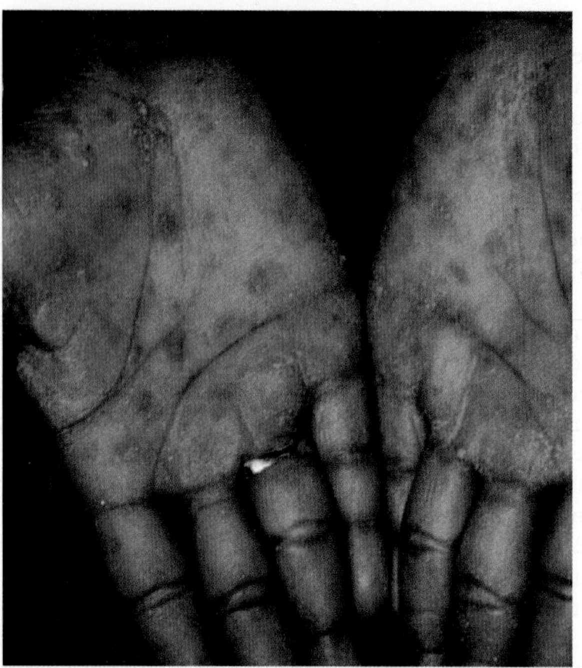

A

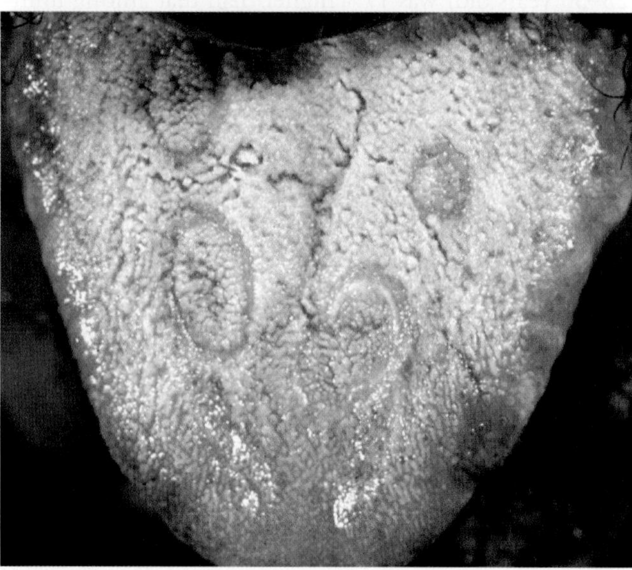

B

FIGURE 70-4
Secondary syphilis. *A.* Papules on the palms. ***B.*** Mucous patches on the tongue. (*Courtesy of Ron Roddy; with permission.*)

Acute meningitis occurs in only 1–2% of cases, but cell and protein concentrations in CSF are increased in ≥30% of cases. *T. pallidum* has been recovered from CSF during primary and secondary syphilis in 30% of cases; this finding is often but not always associated with other CSF abnormalities.

Less common complications of secondary syphilis include hepatitis, nephropathy, gastrointestinal involvement (hypertrophic gastritis, patchy proctitis, or a rectosigmoid mass), arthritis, and periostitis. Ocular findings that suggest secondary syphilis include pupillary abnormalities and optic neuritis as well as the classic iritis or uveitis. The diagnosis of secondary syphilis is often considered in the affected patients only after they fail to respond to steroid therapy. Anterior uveitis has been reported in 5–10% of patients with secondary syphilis, and *T. pallidum* has been demonstrated in the aqueous humor from such patients. Hepatic involvement is common in syphilis; although it is usually asymptomatic, up to 25% of patients may have abnormal liver function tests. Frank *syphilitic hepatitis* is distinguished by an unusually high serum level of alkaline phosphatase and by a nonspecific histologic appearance that is unlike that of viral hepatitis and includes moderate inflammation with polymorphonuclear leukocytes and lymphocytes, some hepatocellular damage, and no cholestasis. *Renal involvement* usually results from immune complex deposition and produces proteinuria associated with an acute nephrotic syndrome (or rarely with hemorrhagic glomerulonephritis). Like those of primary syphilis, the manifestations of the secondary stage resolve spontaneously, usually within 1–6 months.

Latent Syphilis

Positive serologic tests for syphilis, together with a normal CSF examination and the absence of clinical manifestations of syphilis, indicate a diagnosis of latent syphilis. The diagnosis is often suspected on the basis of a history of primary or secondary lesions, a history of exposure to syphilis, or the delivery of an infant with congenital syphilis. A previous negative serologic test or a history of lesions or exposure may help establish the duration of latent infection, which is an important factor in the selection of appropriate therapy. *Early latent* syphilis is limited to the first year after infection, whereas *late latent* syphilis is defined as that of ≥1 year's (or unknown) duration. *T. pallidum* may still seed the bloodstream intermittently during the latent stage, and pregnant women with latent syphilis may infect the fetus in utero. Moreover, syphilis has been transmitted through blood transfusion or organ donation from patients with latent syphilis. It was previously thought that untreated late latent syphilis had three possible outcomes: (1) persistent lifelong infection; (2) development of late syphilis; or (3) spontaneous cure, with reversion of serologic tests to negative. It is now apparent, however, that the more sensitive treponemal antibody tests rarely, if ever, become negative without treatment. Although progression to clinically evident late syphilis is very rare today, the occurrence of spontaneous cure is in doubt.

Involvement of the CNS

Traditionally, neurosyphilis has been considered a late manifestation of syphilis, but this view is inaccurate. CNS syphilis represents a continuum encompassing early invasion (usually within the first weeks or months of infection), months to years of asymptomatic involvement, and, in some cases, development of early or late neurologic manifestations.

Asymptomatic Neurosyphilis

The diagnosis of asymptomatic neurosyphilis is made in patients who lack neurologic symptoms and signs but who have CSF abnormalities including mononuclear pleocytosis, increased protein concentrations, or a reactive Venereal Disease Research Laboratory (VDRL) slide test. Such abnormalities are found in up to one-quarter of patients with untreated latent syphilis, and these patients are at risk for development of neurologic complications. In primary and secondary syphilis, such abnormalities may be found in up to 40% of untreated patients, and *T. pallidum* can be isolated from CSF of 30% of patients even in the absence of other CSF abnormalities. Although the therapeutic implications of these findings in early syphilis are uncertain, it seems appropriate to conclude that even patients with early syphilis who have such findings do indeed have asymptomatic neurosyphilis and should be treated for neurosyphilis. In patients with untreated asymptomatic neurosyphilis, the overall cumulative probability of progression to clinical neurosyphilis is ~20% in the first 10 years but increases with time; the likelihood is highest among patients with the greatest degree of pleocytosis or protein elevation. Patients with untreated latent syphilis and normal CSF probably run no risk of subsequent neurosyphilis. In one study, neurosyphilis was associated with a rapid plasma reagin (RPR) titer of ≥1:32, regardless of clinical stage or HIV infection status.

Symptomatic Neurosyphilis

Although mixed features are common, the major clinical categories of symptomatic neurosyphilis include meningeal, meningovascular, and parenchymatous syphilis. The last category includes general paresis and tabes dorsalis. The onset of symptoms usually comes <1 year after infection for meningeal syphilis, at 5–10 years for meningovascular syphilis, at 20 years for general paresis, and at 25–30 years for tabes dorsalis. However, symptomatic neurosyphilis, particularly in the antibiotic era, often presents not as a classic picture but rather as mixed and subtle or incomplete syndromes.

Meningeal syphilis may involve either the brain or the spinal cord, and patients may present with headache, nausea, vomiting, neck stiffness, cranial nerve involvement, seizures, and changes in mental status. This condition may be concurrent with or may follow the secondary stage. Patients presenting with uveitis or iritis frequently have meningeal syphilis.

Meningovascular syphilis reflects diffuse inflammation of the pia and arachnoid together with evidence of focal or widespread arterial involvement of small, medium, or large vessels. The most common presentation is a stroke syndrome involving the middle cerebral artery of a relatively young adult. However, unlike the usual thrombotic or embolic stroke syndrome of sudden onset, meningovascular syphilis often becomes manifest after a subacute encephalitic prodrome (with headaches, vertigo, insomnia, and psychological abnormalities), which is followed by a gradually progressive vascular syndrome.

The manifestations of *general paresis* reflect widespread late parenchymal damage and include abnormalities corresponding to the mnemonic *paresis: p*ersonality, *a*ffect, *r*eflexes (hyperactive), *e*ye (e.g., Argyll Robertson pupils), sensorium (illusions, delusions, hallucinations), intellect (a decrease in recent memory and in the capacity for orientation, calculations, judgment, and insight), and speech. *Tabes dorsalis* is a late manifestation of syphilis that presents as symptoms and signs of demyelination of the posterior columns, dorsal roots, and dorsal root ganglia. Symptoms include ataxic wide-based gait and footslap, paresthesia, bladder disturbances, impotence, areflexia, and loss of position, deep pain, and temperature sensations. Trophic joint degeneration (Charcot's joints) and perforating ulceration of the feet can result from loss of pain sensation. The small, irregular Argyll Robertson pupil, a feature of both tabes dorsalis and paresis, reacts to accommodation but not to light. *Optic atrophy* also occurs frequently in association with tabes.

Other Manifestations of Late Syphilis

The slowly progressive inflammatory disease leading to tertiary manifestations begins early during the pathogenesis of syphilis, although these manifestations may not become clinically apparent for years. Early syphilitic aortitis becomes evident soon after secondary lesions subside, and treponemes that trigger the development of gummas may have seeded the tissue years earlier.

Cardiovascular Syphilis

Cardiovascular manifestations, usually appearing 10–40 years after infection, are attributable to endarteritis obliterans of the vasa vasorum, which provide the blood supply to large vessels. This condition results in uncomplicated aortitis, aortic regurgitation, saccular aneurysm (usually of the ascending aorta), or coronary ostial stenosis. In the preantibiotic era, symptomatic cardiovascular complications developed in ~10% of persons with late untreated syphilis, although syphilitic aortitis was demonstrated at autopsy in about one-half of African-American men with untreated syphilis. Today, this form of late syphilis is rarely seen in the developed world.

Linear calcification of the ascending aorta on chest x-ray films suggests asymptomatic syphilitic aortitis, as arteriosclerosis seldom produces this sign. Syphilitic aneurysms—usually saccular, occasionally fusiform—do not lead to dissection. Only 1 in 10 aortic aneurysms of syphilitic origin involves the abdominal aorta.

Late Benign Syphilis (Gumma)

Gummas are usually solitary lesions ranging from microscopic to several centimeters in diameter. Histologic examination shows a granulomatous inflammation, with a central area of necrosis due to endarteritis obliterans. Although rarely demonstrated microscopically, *T. pallidum* has reportedly been recovered from these lesions, and penicillin treatment results in rapid resolution, confirming the treponemal stimulus for the inflammation. Common sites include the skin and skeletal system; however, any organ may be involved. Gummas of the skin produce indolent, painless, indurated nodular or ulcerative lesions that may resemble other chronic granulomatous conditions, including tuberculosis, sarcoidosis, leprosy, and deep fungal infections. Skeletal gummas most frequently involve the long bones, although any bone may be affected. Radiographic abnormalities with advanced gummas of bone include periostitis or destructive or sclerosing osteitis. Upper respiratory gummas can lead to perforation of the nasal septum or palate.

Congenital Syphilis

Transmission of *T. pallidum* from a syphilitic woman to her fetus across the placenta may occur at any stage of pregnancy, but fetal damage generally does not occur until after the fourth month of gestation, when fetal immunologic competence begins to develop. This timing suggests that the pathogenesis of congenital syphilis depends on the host immune response rather than on a direct toxic effect of *T. pallidum*. The risk of fetal infection during untreated early maternal syphilis is ~75–95%, decreasing to ~35% for maternal syphilis of >2 years' duration. Adequate treatment of the mother before the 16th week of pregnancy should prevent fetal damage, and treatment of the mother before the third trimester should adequately treat the infected fetus. Untreated maternal infection may result in a rate of fetal loss of up to 40% (with stillbirth more common than abortion because of the late onset of fetal pathology), prematurity, neonatal death, or nonfatal congenital syphilis. Among infants born alive, only fulminant congenital syphilis is clinically apparent at birth, and these babies have a very poor prognosis. The most common clinical problem is the healthy-appearing baby born to a mother with a positive serologic test. Routine serologic testing in early pregnancy is considered cost-effective in virtually all populations, even in areas with a low prenatal prevalence of syphilis. Where the prevalence of syphilis is high or when the patient is at high risk of reinfection, serologic testing should be repeated in the third trimester and at delivery. Neonatal congenital syphilis must be differentiated from other generalized congenital infections, including rubella, cytomegalovirus or herpes simplex virus infection, and toxoplasmosis, as well as from erythroblastosis fetalis.

The manifestations of congenital syphilis can be divided into three types according to their timing: (1) early manifestations, which appear within the first 2 years of life (often at 2–10 weeks of age), are infectious, and resemble the manifestations of severe secondary syphilis in the adult; (2) late manifestations, which appear after 2 years and are noninfectious; and (3) residual stigmata. The earliest sign of congenital syphilis (appearing 2–6 weeks after birth) is usually rhinitis, or "snuffles" (23%), which is soon followed by other mucocutaneous lesions (35–41%). These may include bullae (syphilitic pemphigus), vesicles, superficial desquamation, petechiae, and (later) papulosquamous lesions, mucous patches, and condylomata lata. The most common early manifestations are bone changes (61%), including osteochondritis, osteitis, and periostitis detectable by x-ray examination of long bones; hepatosplenomegaly (50%); lymphadenopathy (32%); anemia (34%); jaundice (30%); thrombocytopenia; and leukocytosis. CNS invasion by *T. pallidum* is detectable in 22% of infected neonates. Neonatal death is usually due to pulmonary hemorrhage, secondary bacterial infection, or severe hepatitis.

Late congenital syphilis (untreated after 2 years of age) is subclinical in 60% of cases; the clinical spectrum in the remainder of cases differs in certain respects from that of acquired late syphilis in the adult. For example, cardiovascular manifestations rarely develop in late congenital syphilis, whereas interstitial keratitis is much more common and occurs between the ages of 5 and 25. Other manifestations include eighth-nerve deafness and recurrent arthropathy. Bilateral knee effusions are known as *Clutton's joints*. Asymptomatic neurosyphilis is present in about one-third of untreated patients, and clinical neurosyphilis occurs in one-quarter of untreated individuals >6 years old. Gummatous periostitis occurs between the ages of 5 and 20 and, as in nonvenereal endemic syphilis, tends to cause destructive lesions of the palate and nasal septum.

Classic stigmata include *Hutchinson's teeth* (centrally notched, widely spaced, peg-shaped upper central incisors), "mulberry" molars (sixth-year molars with multiple, poorly developed cusps), saddle nose, and saber shins.

LABORATORY EXAMINATIONS

Demonstration of the Organism

T. pallidum cannot be detected by culture. Historically, dark-field microscopy and immunofluorescence antibody staining have been used to identify this spirochete in samples from moist lesions such as chancres or condylomata lata, but these tests are rarely available today outside of research laboratories. More sensitive PCR tests have been developed but are not commercially available.

T. pallidum can be found in tissue with appropriate silver stains, but these results should be interpreted with caution because artifacts resembling *T. pallidum* are often seen. Tissue treponemes can be demonstrated more reliably in research laboratories by PCR or by immunofluorescence or immunohistochemical methods using specific monoclonal or polyclonal antibodies to *T. pallidum*.

Serologic Tests for Syphilis

There are two types of serologic test for syphilis: nontreponemal and treponemal. Both are reactive in persons with any treponemal infection, including yaws, pinta, and endemic syphilis.

The most widely used nontreponemal antibody tests for syphilis are the RPR and VDRL tests, which measure IgG and IgM directed against a cardiolipin-lecithin-cholesterol antigen complex. The RPR test is easier to perform and uses unheated serum; it is the test of choice for rapid serologic diagnosis in a clinical setting and can be automated. The VDRL test remains the standard for examining CSF.

The RPR and VDRL tests are used for screening or for quantitation of serum antibody. The titer reflects disease activity, rising during the evolution of early syphilis and often exceeding 1:32 in secondary syphilis. A persistent fall by two dilutions (fourfold) or more after treatment of early syphilis is considered an adequate response to therapy. VDRL titers do not correspond directly to RPR titers, and sequential quantitative testing (as for response to therapy) must employ a single test.

The treponemal tests measure antibodies to native or recombinant *T. pallidum* antigens. These include the fluorescent treponemal antibody–absorbed (FTA-ABS) test and several agglutination assays. The microhemagglutination assay for *T. pallidum* (MHA-TP) has been replaced by the Serodia TP-PA test (Fujirebio, Tokyo), which is more sensitive for primary syphilis. The *T. pallidum* hemagglutination test (TPHA) is widely used in Europe but is not available in the United States. When used to confirm positive nontreponemal test results, treponemal tests have a very high positive predictive value for diagnosis of syphilis. In a screening setting, however, these tests give false-positive results at rates as high as 1–2%. New enzyme-linked immunosorbent assays have also been approved as confirmatory tests.

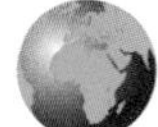

Considerable interest has recently been focused on point-of-care immunochromatographic strip tests that can be used in the field or in resource-poor settings.

The relative sensitivities of the standard tests for untreated syphilis are shown in Table 70-1. All tests may be nonreactive in early primary syphilis, although the treponemal tests have slightly higher sensitivity during this stage. All tests are reactive during secondary syphilis. (Fewer than 1% of patients with secondary syphilis have a VDRL test that is nonreactive or weakly reactive with undiluted serum but is positive at higher serum dilutions—the *prozone phenomenon*.) Whereas nontreponemal test titers will decline or the tests will become nonreactive after therapy for early syphilis, treponemal tests often remain reactive after therapy and are not helpful in determining infection status of persons with past syphilis.

For practical purposes, most clinicians need to be familiar with the three uses of serologic tests for syphilis: (1) screening or diagnostic purposes (RPR or VDRL), (2) quantitative measurement of antibody to assess clinical syphilis activity or to monitor response to therapy (RPR or VDRL), and (3) confirmation of a syphilis diagnosis in a patient with a reactive RPR or VDRL test (FTA-ABS or Serodia TP-PA).

IgM testing is not useful for adult syphilis. Moreover, no commercially available IgM test is recommended for evaluation of infants with suspected congenital syphilis.

False-Positive Serologic Tests for Syphilis

The lipid antigens of nontreponemal tests are found in human tissues, and the tests may be reactive (usually with titers ≤1:8) in persons without treponemal infection. Among patients selected on the basis of risk factors, clinical suspicion, or history of exposure, <1% of reactive tests are falsely positive. Modern VDRL and RPR tests are 97–99% specific, and false-positive reactions are largely limited to persons with autoimmune conditions

TABLE 70-1

SENSITIVITY OF SERODIAGNOSTIC TESTS IN UNTREATED SYPHILIS

	MEAN PERCENTAGE POSITIVE (RANGE) AT INDICATED STAGE OF DISEASE[b]			
TEST[a]	PRIMARY	SECONDARY	LATENT	TERTIARY
VDRL, RPR	78 (74–87)	100	95 (88–100)	71 (37–94)
FTA-ABS	84 (70–100)	100	100	96
TP-PA[c]	89	100	100	NA

[a]The specificity for each of these tests is 94–99%.
[b]In CDC studies.
[c]Limited numbers of sera have been evaluated by TP-PA.
Source: Modified from SA Larsen et al: Clin Microbiol Rev 8:1, 1995; and V Pope et al: J Clin Microbiol 38:2543, 2000.

or injection drug use. The prevalence of false-positive results increases with advancing age, approaching 10% among persons >70 years old. In a patient with a false-positive nontreponemal test, syphilis is excluded by a nonreactive treponemal test.

Evaluation for Neurosyphilis

Involvement of the CNS is detected by examination of CSF for pleocytosis (>5 white blood cells/mm^3), increased protein concentration (>45 mg/dL), or VDRL reactivity. CSF abnormalities can be demonstrated in up to 40% of cases of primary or secondary syphilis and in 25% of cases of latent syphilis. In older asymptomatic seropositive individuals, the yield of lumbar puncture is relatively low. *T. pallidum* has been recovered by CSF inoculation into rabbits from up to 30% of patients with primary or secondary syphilis but rarely from those with latent syphilis. The presence of *T. pallidum* in CSF is often associated with other CSF abnormalities; however, organisms can be recovered from patients with otherwise-normal CSF. Before the advent of penicillin, the risk of developing clinical neurosyphilis was roughly proportional to the intensity of CSF changes. CSF examination is recommended by the Centers for Disease Control and Prevention (CDC) in the evaluation of any seropositive patient with neurologic or ophthalmic signs and symptoms, patients with other late syphilis, cases of suspected treatment failure, and HIV-infected patients with untreated late latent syphilis or syphilis of unknown duration. The possibility of asymptomatic neurosyphilis in some patients with early disease is not addressed by these recommendations. Because standard therapy with penicillin G benzathine fails to result in treponemicidal drug levels in the CSF, some experts also advise lumbar puncture in early syphilis, particularly in patients with HIV infection or with nontreponemal test titers of ≥1:32.

The CSF VDRL test is highly specific but is insensitive and may be nonreactive even in cases of symptomatic neurosyphilis. The degree of sensitivity is highest in meningovascular syphilis and paresis and is lower in asymptomatic neurosyphilis and tabes dorsalis. The unabsorbed FTA test on CSF is reactive far more often than the CSF VDRL test in all stages of syphilis, but FTA reactivity may reflect passive transfer of serum antibody into the CSF. A nonreactive CSF FTA test, however, may be used to rule out neurosyphilis.

Evaluation for Syphilis in HIV-Infected Patients

Because persons at highest risk for syphilis are also at increased risk for HIV infection, these two infections frequently coexist. There is evidence that syphilis and other genital-ulcer diseases may be important risk factors for the acquisition and transmission of HIV infection.

The manifestations of syphilis may be altered in patients with concurrent HIV infection, and multiple cases of neurologic relapse after standard therapy have been reported in HIV-infected patients. *T. pallidum* has been isolated from the CSF of several patients after penicillin G benzathine therapy for early syphilis. A multicenter U.S. study of early syphilis found similar clinical responses to therapy in persons with and without concurrent HIV infection, although the study lacked sufficient statistical power to exclude an effect of HIV and 41% of subjects were lost to follow-up. Serologically defined treatment failure was more common among HIV-infected patients than among those without this co-infection. This investigation confirmed the high rate of CNS invasion in early syphilis and the persistence of *T. pallidum* after standard therapy: 11 of 43 HIV-infected patients and 21 of 88 HIV-uninfected patients had *T. pallidum* detectable in CSF before therapy; 7 of the 35 patients who underwent lumbar puncture after therapy (some HIV-infected and others uninfected) still had *T. pallidum* detectable in CSF.

There is no clear evidence that the sensitivity of serologic tests for syphilis differs in HIV-infected versus HIV-uninfected patients. Rates of decline of serologic titers appear to be slower in HIV-infected individuals. The clinical significance of this observation is unclear.

Persons with newly diagnosed HIV infection should be tested for syphilis; conversely, all patients with newly diagnosed syphilis should be tested for HIV infection. Some authorities, persuaded by reports of persistent *T. pallidum* in CSF of HIV-infected persons after standard therapy for early syphilis, recommend CSF examination for evidence of neurosyphilis for all co-infected patients, regardless of the stage of syphilis, with treatment for neurosyphilis if CSF abnormalities are found. Others believe that standard therapy is sufficient for all cases of early syphilis, without CSF examination. Serologic testing after treatment is important for all patients with syphilis, particularly for those also infected with HIV.

℞ Treatment: SYPHILIS

TREATMENT OF ACQUIRED SYPHILIS The CDC's 2006 guidelines for the treatment of syphilis are summarized in Table 70-2 and are discussed below. Penicillin G is the drug of choice for all stages of syphilis. *T. pallidum* is killed by very low concentrations of penicillin G, although a long period of exposure to penicillin is required because of the unusually slow rate of multiplication of the organism. The efficacy of penicillin against syphilis remains undiminished after 60 years of use. Other antibiotics effective in syphilis include the tetracyclines, erythromycin, and the cephalosporins. Aminoglycosides and spectinomycin inhibit *T. pallidum* only in very large doses, and the sulfonamides and the quinolones are inactive. Azithromycin has shown significant promise as an effective oral agent against *T. pallidum*; however, recent studies have documented clinical failures associated with a mutation in the 23S rRNA gene known to confer macrolide resistance. Strains harboring this mutation are present in >50% of recent isolates from Seattle and San Francisco. In contrast, an ongoing trial of single-dose azithromycin for early syphilis in Madagascar and several eastern U.S. sites has not documented clinical failures. Thus the prevalence of resistant strains varies by geographic location. In all cases, careful follow-up should be assured for any patient treated for syphilis with azithromycin.

EARLY SYPHILIS PATIENTS AND THEIR CONTACTS Penicillin G benzathine is the most widely used agent for the treatment of early syphilis; a single dose of 2.4 million units is recommended. Preventive treatment is also recommended for individuals who have been exposed to infectious syphilis within the previous 3 months. *The regimens recommended for prevention are the same as those recommended for early syphilis.*

Penicillin G benzathine cures >95% of cases of early syphilis. Clinical relapse can follow treatment with penicillin G benzathine in patients with both HIV infection and early syphilis. Because the risk of neurologic relapse may be higher in HIV-infected patients, some experts recommend examination of CSF from HIV-seropositive individuals with syphilis at any stage, particularly if the RPR or VDRL titer is ≥1:32. Therapy appropriate for

TABLE 70-2

RECOMMENDATIONS FOR THE TREATMENT OF SYPHILIS[a]

STAGE OF SYPHILIS	PATIENTS WITHOUT PENICILLIN ALLERGY	PATIENTS WITH CONFIRMED PENICILLIN ALLERGY
Primary, secondary, or early latent	Penicillin G benzathine (single dose of 2.4 mU IM)	Tetracycline hydrochloride (500 mg PO qid) or doxycycline (100 mg PO bid) for 2 weeks
Late latent (or latent of uncertain duration), cardiovascular, or benign tertiary	Lumbar puncture CSF normal: Penicillin G benzathine (2.4 mU IM weekly for 3 weeks) CSF abnormal: Treat as neurosyphilis	Lumbar puncture CSF normal and patient not infected with HIV: Tetracycline hydrochloride (500 mg PO qid) or doxycycline (100 mg PO bid) for 4 weeks CSF normal and patient infected with HIV: Desensitization and treatment with penicillin if compliance cannot be ensured CSF abnormal: Treat as neurosyphilis
Neurosyphilis (asymptomatic or symptomatic)	Aqueous penicillin G (18–24 mU/d IV, given as 3–4 mU q4h or continuous infusion) for 10–14 days *or* Aqueous penicillin G procaine (2.4 mU/d IM) plus oral probenecid (500 mg qid), both for 10–14 days	Desensitization and treatment with penicillin
Syphilis in pregnancy	According to stage	Desensitization and treatment with penicillin

[a]See text for full discussion of indications for lumbar puncture and syphilis therapy in HIV-infected individuals.
Note: mU, million units; CSF, cerebrospinal fluid.
Source: These recommendations are based on those issued by the Centers for Disease Control and Prevention in 2006.

neurosyphilis should be given if there is any evidence of CNS syphilis.

LATE LATENT AND LATE SYPHILIS If CSF abnormalities are found, the patient should be treated for neurosyphilis. If CSF is normal, the recommended treatment is penicillin G benzathine (7.2 million units total; Table 70-2). The clinical response to treatment for benign tertiary syphilis is usually impressive. However, responses to therapy for cardiovascular syphilis are not dramatic because aortic aneurysm and aortic regurgitation cannot be reversed by antibiotic treatment.

PENICILLIN-ALLERGIC PATIENTS For penicillin-allergic patients with syphilis, a 2-week (early syphilis) or 4-week (late or late latent syphilis) course of therapy with doxycycline or tetracycline is recommended. These regimens appear to be effective in early syphilis but have not been tested for late or late latent syphilis, and compliance may be problematic. Limited studies suggest that ceftriaxone (1 g/d, given IM or IV, for 8–10 days) is effective for early syphilis. These nonpenicillin regimens have not been carefully evaluated in HIV-infected individuals and should be used with caution. If compliance and follow-up cannot be ensured, penicillin-allergic HIV-infected persons with late latent or late syphilis should be desensitized and treated with penicillin.

NEUROSYPHILIS Penicillin G benzathine, given in total doses of up to 7.2 million units, does not produce detectable concentrations of penicillin G in CSF and should not be used for treatment of neurosyphilis. Asymptomatic neurosyphilis may relapse after treatment with benzathine penicillin, and the risk of relapse may be higher in HIV-infected patients. Administration of IV aqueous crystalline penicillin G in recommended doses is thought to ensure treponemicidal concentrations of penicillin G in CSF. The clinical response to penicillin therapy for meningeal syphilis is dramatic, but treatment of neurosyphilis with existing parenchymal damage may only arrest disease progression.

Some recent publications have reported neurologic relapse even after high-dose IV penicillin therapy for neurosyphilis in HIV-infected patients. No alternative therapies have been explored, but careful follow-up is essential, and re-treatment is warranted in such patients.

No data support the use of antibiotics other than penicillin G for the treatment of neurosyphilis. In patients with penicillin allergy demonstrated by skin testing, desensitization and treatment with penicillin is the recommended course.

MANAGEMENT OF SYPHILIS IN PREGNANCY Every pregnant woman should undergo a nontreponemal test at her first prenatal visit and, if at high risk of exposure, again in the third trimester and at delivery. In the untreated pregnant patient with presumed syphilis, expeditious treatment appropriate to the stage of the disease is essential. Patients should be warned of the risk of a Jarisch-Herxheimer reaction, which may be associated with mild premature contractions but rarely results in premature delivery.

Penicillin is the only recommended agent for the treatment of syphilis in pregnancy. If the patient has a documented penicillin allergy, desensitization and penicillin therapy should be undertaken according to the CDC's 2006 treatment guidelines. After treatment, a quantitative nontreponemal test should be repeated monthly throughout pregnancy to assess therapeutic efficacy. Treated women whose antibody titers rise by fourfold or who do not show a fourfold decrease in titer over a 3-month period should be re-treated.

EVALUATION AND MANAGEMENT OF CONGENITAL SYPHILIS Whether or not they are infected, newborn infants of mothers with reactive serologic tests may themselves have reactive tests because of transplacental transfer of maternal IgG antibody. For asymptomatic infants born to women treated adequately with penicillin during the first or second trimester of pregnancy, monthly quantitative nontreponemal tests may be performed to monitor for appropriate reduction in antibody titers. Rising or persistent titers indicate infection, and the infant should be treated. Detection of neonatal IgM antibody may be useful, but no commercially available test is currently recommended.

An infant should be treated at birth if the treatment status of the seropositive mother is unknown; if the mother has received inadequate or nonpenicillin therapy or has received penicillin therapy in the third trimester; or if the infant may be difficult to follow. The CSF should be examined to obtain baseline values before treatment. Penicillin is the only recommended drug for the treatment of syphilis in infants. Specific recommendations for the treatment of infants and older children are included in the CDC's 2006 guidelines.

JARISCH-HERXHEIMER REACTION A dramatic though usually mild reaction consisting of fever, chills, myalgias, headache, tachycardia, increased respiratory rate, increased circulating neutrophil count, and vasodilation with mild hypotension may follow the initiation of treatment for syphilis. This reaction is thought to be a response to lipoproteins released by dying *T. pallidum* organisms. The Jarisch-Herxheimer reaction occurs in ~50% of patients with primary syphilis, 90% of those with secondary syphilis, and a lower proportion of persons with later-stage disease. Defervescence takes place within 12–24 h. In patients with secondary syphilis, erythema and edema of the mucocutaneous lesions may increase. Patients should be warned to expect such symptoms, which can be managed with symptom-based treatment. Steroid and other anti-inflammatory therapy is not required for this mild transient reaction.

FOLLOW-UP EVALUATION OF RESPONSES TO THERAPY Efficacy of treatment should be assessed by monitoring of the quantitative VDRL or RPR titer (Table 70-3). More frequent serologic examination is

TABLE 70-3

RECOMMENDED FOLLOW-UP EVALUATION AFTER THERAPY FOR SYPHILIS

STAGE OF SYPHILIS	TESTS TO PERFORM	WHEN TO PERFORM	RE-TREATMENT[a] CONSIDERED IF:
Primary or secondary	Quantitative RPR or VDRL[b]	HIV-uninfected: 6 and 12 months HIV-infected: 3, 6, 9, 12, and 24 months	1. Titer increases by fourfold *or* 2. Titer fails to decline by fourfold or test fails to become nonreactive by 6 months *or* 3. Clinical signs persist or recur
Latent or late	Quantitative RPR or VDRL[b]	HIV-uninfected: 6, 12, and 24 months HIV-infected: 6, 12, 18, and 24 months	1. Titer increases by fourfold *or* 2. Initial titer of ≥1:32 fails to decline by fourfold by 6 months *or* 3. New clinical signs develop
Neurosyphilis (asymptomatic or symptomatic)	1. If CSF pleocytosis was documented initially, repeat CSF exam.	1. Every 6 months until CSF cell count is normal	1. CSF cell count has not decreased at 6 months *or*
	2. Monitor decline in CSF protein and CSF-VDRL. (Note: Rate of decline may be slow.)	2. Until normal	2. CSF is not normal after 2 years
	3. Quantitative serum RPR or VDRL.[b]	3. 6, 12, 18, and 24 months	

[a]Try to distinguish between reinfection and treatment failure. If no clear evidence of reinfection exists, perform CSF examination. If CSF is normal, treat as for late latent syphilis (Table 70-2). If CSF is abnormal, treat as for neurosyphilis (Table 70-2) .
[b]VDRL and RPR titers cannot be compared; use the same test for each follow-up sample.
Note: RPR, rapid plasma reagin; VDRL, Venereal Disease Research Laboratory; CSF, cerebrospinal fluid.

recommended for patients concurrently infected with HIV. Because the FTA-ABS and agglutination tests remain positive in most patients treated for seropositive syphilis, these tests are not useful in following the response to therapy. After successful treatment of seropositive first-episode primary or secondary syphilis, the VDRL or RPR titer progressively declines, becoming negative by 12 months in 40–75% of seropositive primary cases and in 20–40% of secondary cases. Patients with a history of syphilis have less rapid declines in titer and are less likely to become VDRL- or RPR-negative. Re-treatment should be considered if serologic responses are not adequate or if clinical signs persist or recur. Because it is difficult to differentiate treatment failure from reinfection, the CSF should be examined, with treatment for neurosyphilis if CSF is abnormal and treatment for late latent syphilis if CSF is normal.

Patients treated for late latent syphilis frequently have low initial VDRL or RPR titers and may not have a fourfold decline after therapy with penicillin. Re-treatment is not warranted unless the titer rises or signs and symptoms of syphilis appear. Because treponemal tests may remain positive despite treatment for seropositive syphilis, these tests are not useful in following the response to therapy.

The activity of neurosyphilis correlates best with CSF pleocytosis, and this measure provides the most sensitive index of response to treatment. An elevated CSF cell count falls to normal in 3–12 months in adequately treated HIV-uninfected patients. The persistence of mild pleocytosis in HIV-infected patients may be due to the presence of HIV in CSF; this scenario may be difficult to distinguish from treatment failure. Elevated levels of CSF protein fall more slowly, and the CSF VDRL titer declines gradually over a period of several years.

IMMUNITY TO SYPHILIS

The rate of development of acquired resistance to *T. pallidum* after natural or experimental infection is related to the size of the antigenic stimulus, which depends on both the size of the infecting inoculum and the duration of infection before treatment. The role of serum antibody in conferring immunity to syphilis remains undefined, although antibodies have been implicated in strain-specific immunity. Cellular immunity is considered to be of major importance in immunity and in the healing of early lesions. The cellular infiltration, predominantly T lymphocytes and macrophages, produces a T_H1 cytokine milieu consistent with the clearance of organisms by activated macrophages. Specific antibody enhances phagocytosis and is required for macrophage-mediated killing of *T. pallidum*. Recent studies indicate that sequence variation of TprK occurs during *T. pallidum* infection. This observation suggests a role for antigenic variation in the persistence of infection and in susceptibility to reinfection with another strain. No likely vaccine candidate antigens have been identified to date.

FURTHER READINGS

Centers for Disease Control and Prevention: 2006 Sexually transmitted diseases treatment guidelines. MMWR 55:22, 2006

Centurion-Lara A et al: Gene conversion: A mechanism for generation of heterogeneity in the *tprK* gene of *Treponema pallidum* during infection. Mol Microbiol 52:1579, 2004

Grassly NC et al: Host immunity and synchronized epidemics of syphilis across the United States. Nature 433:417, 2005

Lukehart SA et al: Macrolide resistance in *Treponema pallidum* in the United States and Ireland. N Engl J Med 351:154, 2004

Marra CM et al: Cerebrospinal fluid abnormalities in patients with syphilis: Association with clinical and laboratory features. J Infect Dis 189:369, 2004

——— et al: Normalization of cerebrospinal fluid abnormalities after neurosyphilis therapy: Does HIV status matter? Clin Infect Dis 38:1001, 2004

Michelow IC et al: Central nervous system infection in congenital syphilis. N Engl J Med 346:1792, 2002

Peeling R et al: Avoiding HIV and dying of syphilis. Lancet 364:1561, 2004

Rolfs RT et al: A randomized trial of enhanced therapy for early syphilis in patients with and without human immunodeficiency virus infection. N Engl J Med 337:307, 1997

Tobian AA et al: Male circumcision for the prevention of HSV-2 and HPV infections and syphilis. N Engl J Med 360:1298, 2009

Wolff T et al: Screening for syphilis infection in pregnant women: Evidence for the U.S. Preventive Services Task Force reaffirmation recommendation statement. Ann Intern Med 150:710, 2009

CHAPTER 71

ENDEMIC TREPONEMATOSES

Sheila A. Lukehart

The endemic, or nonvenereal, treponematoses are bacterial infections caused by close relatives of *Treponema pallidum* subspecies *pallidum*, the etiologic agent of venereal syphilis (Chap. 70). Yaws, pinta, and endemic syphilis are distinguished from venereal syphilis by mode of transmission, age of acquisition, geographic distribution, and clinical features. These infections are limited to rural areas of developing nations and are seen in developed countries only in recent immigrants from endemic regions. Our "knowledge" about the endemic treponematoses is based on observations of health care workers who have visited endemic areas; virtually no well-designed studies of the natural history, diagnosis, or treatment of these infections have been conducted. The treponemal infections are compared and contrasted in Table 71-1.

EPIDEMIOLOGY

The endemic treponematoses are chronic diseases transmitted by direct contact during childhood and, like syphilis, can cause severe late manifestations years after initial infection. In a World Health Organization (WHO)–sponsored mass eradication campaign from 1952 to 1969, more than 160 million people in Africa, Asia, and South America were examined for treponemal infections, and more than 50 million cases, contacts, and latent infections were treated. This campaign reduced the prevalence of active yaws from >20% to <1% in many areas. In recent decades, lack of focused surveillance and diversion of resources have resulted in a resurgence of these infections in some regions. The estimated geographic distribution of the endemic treponematoses in the 1990s is shown in Fig. 71-1. The most recent WHO estimate (1997) suggested that there are 460,000 new cases per year and a prevalence of 3 million infected persons. Areas of resurgent yaws morbidity include West Africa (Ivory Coast, Ghana, Togo, Benin), the Central African Republic, Nigeria, and rural Democratic Republic of Congo (formerly Zaire). The prevalence of endemic syphilis is estimated to be >10% in some regions of Mali, Niger, Burkina Faso, and Senegal. In Asia and the Pacific Islands, recent reports suggest active outbreaks of yaws in Papua New Guinea, East Timor, Vanuatu, Laos, Kampuchea, and Indonesia. India renewed its focus on yaws eradication in 1996 and reported no cases in 2004. In the Americas, foci of yaws persist in Haiti and other Caribbean islands, Peru, Colombia, Ecuador, Brazil, Guyana, and Surinam. Pinta is limited to Central America and northern South America, where it is found rarely and only in remote villages.

MICROBIOLOGY

The etiologic agents of the endemic treponematoses are *T. pallidum* subspecies *pertenue* (yaws), *T. pallidum* subspecies *endemicum* (endemic syphilis), and *T. carateum* (pinta). These little-studied organisms are morphologically identical to *T. pallidum* subspecies *pallidum*, and no antigenic differences among them have been identified to date. A controversy has existed about whether the pathogenic

TABLE 71-1

COMPARISON OF THE TREPONEMES AND ASSOCIATED DISEASES

FEATURE	VENEREAL SYPHILIS	YAWS	ENDEMIC SYPHILIS	PINTA
Organism	*T. pallidum* subsp. *pallidum*	*T. pallidum* subsp. *pertenue*	*T. pallidum* subsp. *endemicum*	*T. carateum*
Mode of transmission	Sexual, transplacental	Skin-to-skin	Household contacts: mouth-to-mouth or via shared drinking/eating utensils	Skin-to-skin
Usual age of acquisition	Adulthood	Early childhood	Early childhood	Late childhood
Primary lesion	Cutaneous ulcer (chancre)	Papilloma, often ulcerative	Rarely seen	Nonulcerating papule with satellites, pruritic
Location	Genital, oral, anal	Extremities	Oral	Extremities, face
Secondary lesions	Mucocutaneous lesions; condylomata lata	Cutaneous papulosquamous lesions; osteoperiostitis	Florid mucocutaneous lesions (mucous patch, split papule, condyloma latum); osteoperiostitis	Pintides, pigmented, pruritic
Infectious relapses	~25%	Common	Unknown	None
Late complications	Gummas, cardiovascular and CNS involvement[a]	Destructive gummas of skin, bone, cartilage	Destructive gummas of skin, bone, cartilage	Nondestructive, dyschromic, achromic macules

[a]CNS involvement in the endemic treponematoses has been postulated by some investigators (see text).

treponemes are truly different organisms. Three of the four organisms are classified as subspecies of *T. pallidum*; the fourth (*T. carateum*) remains a separate species simply because no organisms have been available for genetic studies. Molecular signatures that can differentiate the causative agents of venereal syphilis, yaws, and bejel have been identified by polymerase chain reaction amplification of *tpr* genes and restriction digestion. Whether these genetic differences are related to the distinct clinical courses of these diseases has not been determined.

CLINICAL FEATURES

All of the treponemal infections are chronic and are characterized by defined disease stages, with a localized primary lesion, disseminated secondary lesions, periods of latency, and possible late lesions. Primary and secondary stages are more frequently overlapping in yaws and endemic syphilis, and the late manifestations of pinta are very mild relative to the destructive lesions of the other treponematoses. The current preference is to divide the clinical course of the endemic treponematoses into "early" and "late" stages.

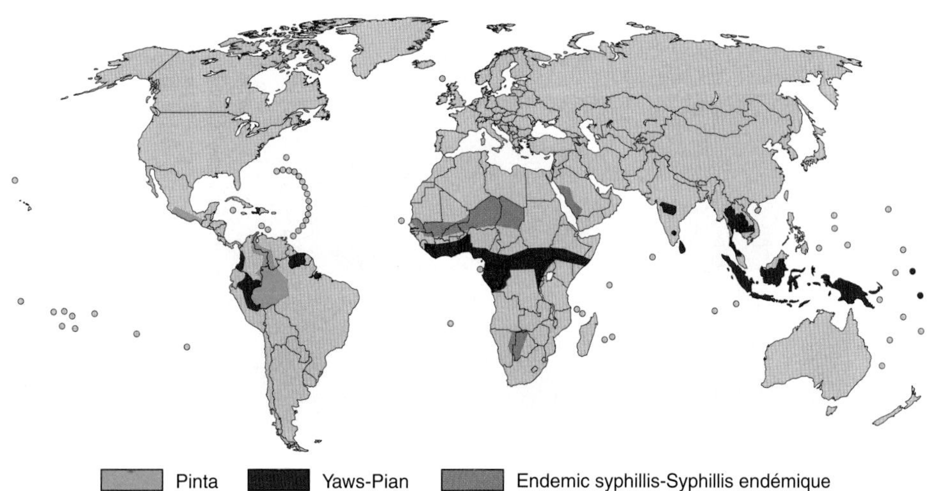

FIGURE 71-1

Geographic distribution of endemic treponematoses in the 1990s. (*Courtesy of the World Health Organization.*)

The major clinical features differing between venereal syphilis and the nonvenereal infections are the apparent lack of congenital transmission and of central nervous system (CNS) involvement in the nonvenereal infections. It is not known whether these distinctions are entirely accurate. Because of the high degree of genetic relatedness among the organisms, there is little biologic reason to think that *T. pallidum* subspecies *endemicum* and *T. pallidum* subspecies *pertenue* would be unable to cross the blood-brain barrier or to invade the placenta. These organisms are like *T. pallidum* subspecies *pallidum* in that they can disseminate from the site of primary infection and can persist for decades. The lack of recognized congenital infection may be due to the fact that childhood infections are in the latent stage (low bacterial load) before girls reach sexual maturity. Neurologic involvement may go unrecognized because of the lack of trained medical personnel in endemic regions, the delay of many years between infection and possible CNS manifestations, or a low rate of symptomatic CNS disease. Some published evidence supports congenital transmission as well as cardiovascular, ophthalmologic, and CNS involvement in yaws. Although the reported studies have been small, have failed to control for other causes of CNS abnormalities, have not included specific treponemal serologic tests, and have not analyzed the response to therapy, it may be erroneous to accept unquestioningly the frequently repeated belief that these organisms fail to cause such manifestations.

Yaws

Also known as *pian*, *framboesia*, or *bouba*, yaws is caused by *T. pallidum* subspecies *pertenue* and is characterized by the development of one or several primary lesions ("mother yaw"), which is followed by the appearance of multiple disseminated skin lesions. All early skin lesions are infectious and may persist for many months; cutaneous relapses are common during the first 5 years. Late manifestations, affecting 10% of untreated persons, are destructive and can involve skin, bone, and joints.

The infection is transmitted by direct contact with infectious lesions, often during play or group sleeping, and may be enhanced by disruption of the skin by insect bites or abrasions. After an average of 3–4 weeks, the first lesion begins as a papule—usually on an extremity—and then enlarges (particularly during moist warm weather) to become papillomatous or "raspberry-like" (thus the name "framboesia") (Fig. 71-2*A*). Regional lymphadenopathy develops, and the lesion usually heals within 6 months; dissemination is thought to occur during the early weeks of infection. A generalized secondary eruption, accompanied by generalized lymphadenopathy, appears either concurrent with or after the primary lesion, may take several forms (macular, papular, or papillomatous), and may become secondarily infected with other bacteria. Painful papillomatous lesions on the soles of the feet result in a painful crablike gait ("crab yaws"), and periostitis may result in nocturnal bone pain and polydactylitis. Late yaws is manifested by gummas of the skin and long bone, hyperkeratoses of the palms and soles, osteitis and periostitis, and hydrarthrosis. The late gummatous lesions are characteristically extensive. Destruction of the nose, maxilla, palate, and pharynx is termed *gangosa* and is similar to the destructive lesions seen in leprosy and leishmaniasis.

Endemic Syphilis

Endemic syphilis, also called *bejel*, *siti*, *dichuchwa*, *njovera*, or *skerljevo*, is caused by *T. pallidum* subspecies *endemicum*. The early lesions are localized primarily to the mucocutaneous and mucosal surfaces, and the infection may be transmitted by direct contact, by kissing, or by sharing drinking and eating utensils. A role for insects in transmission has been suggested but is

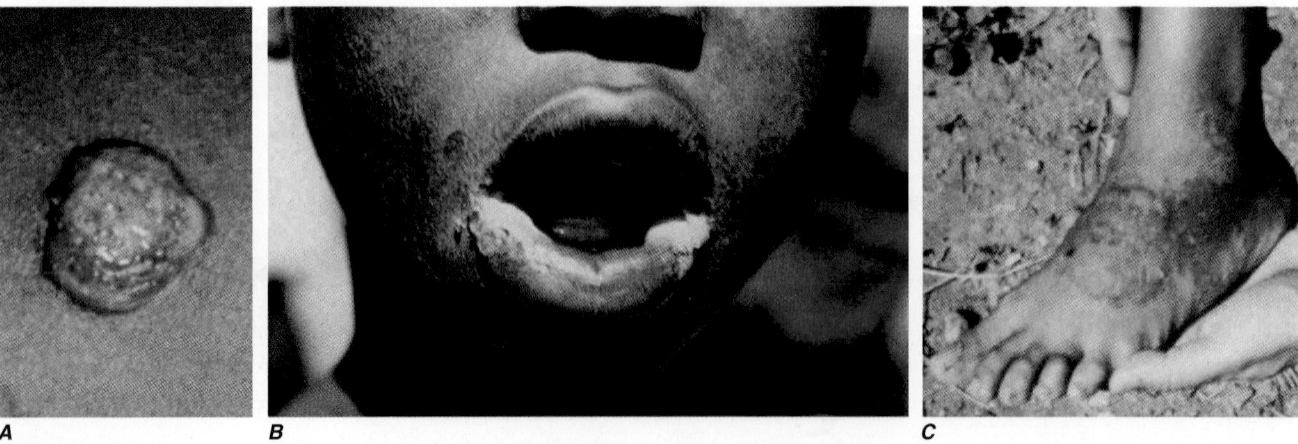

FIGURE 71-2

Clinical manifestations of endemic treponematoses. ***A.*** Papillomatous primary lesion of yaws. ***B.*** Split papules of early endemic syphilis. ***C.*** Pigmented macules of pinta. *(From PL Perine et al. Handbook of Endemic Treponematoses, Geneva, World Health Organization, 1984.)*

unproven. The initial lesion, usually an intraoral papule (Fig. 71-2*B*), often goes unrecognized and is followed by mucous patches on the oral mucosa and mucocutaneous lesions resembling the condylomata lata of secondary syphilis. This eruption may last for months or even years, and treponemes can readily be demonstrated in early lesions. Periostitis and regional lymphadenopathy are common. After a variable period of latency, late manifestations may appear, including osseous and cutaneous gummas. Destructive gummas, osteitis, and gangosa are more common in endemic syphilis than in late yaws.

Pinta

Pinta (also called *mal del pinto*, *carate*, *azul*, or *purupuru*) is the most benign of the treponemal infections and is caused by *T. carateum*. This disease has three stages that are characterized by marked changes in skin color (Fig. 71-2*C*), but it does not appear to cause destructive lesions or to involve other tissues. The initial papule is most often located on the extremities or face and is pruritic. After one to many months of infection, numerous disseminated secondary lesions (*pintides*) appear. These lesions are initially red but become deeply pigmented, ultimately turning a dark slate blue. The secondary lesions are infectious and highly pruritic and may persist for years. Late pigmented lesions are called *dyschromic macules* and contain treponemes. Over time, most pigmented lesions show varying degrees of depigmentation, becoming brown and eventually white and giving the skin a mottled appearance. White achromic lesions are characteristic of the late stage.

DIAGNOSIS

Diagnosis of the endemic treponematoses is based on clinical manifestations and, when available, dark-field microscopy and serologic testing. The same tests that are used for venereal syphilis (Chap. 70) become reactive during all treponemal infections, and there is no serologic test that can discriminate among the different infections. The nonvenereal treponemal infections should be considered in the evaluation of a reactive syphilis serology in any person who has emigrated from an endemic area.

Rx Treatment: ENDEMIC TREPONEMATOSES

The recommended therapy for patients and their contacts is benzathine penicillin (1.2 million units IM for adults; 600,000 units for children <10 years old). This dose is half of that recommended for early venereal syphilis, and no controlled efficacy studies have been conducted. Definitive evidence of resistance to penicillin is lacking, although relapsing lesions have been reported after penicillin treatment in Papua New Guinea. Limited data suggest the efficacy of tetracycline for treatment of yaws, but no data exist for other endemic treponematoses. Solely on the basis of experience with venereal syphilis, it is thought that doxycycline, tetracycline, and erythromycin (at doses appropriate for syphilis; Chap. 70) are alternatives for patients allergic to penicillin. A Jarisch-Herxheimer reaction (Chap. 70) may follow treatment of endemic treponematoses. Nontreponemal serologic titers [in the Venereal Disease Research Laboratory (VDRL) slide test or the rapid plasma reagin (RPR) test] usually decline after effective therapy, but patients may not become seronegative.

CONTROL

Lack of ongoing surveillance for the endemic treponematoses means that these potentially destructive diseases are not recognized by public health decision-makers and that control efforts are rarely undertaken, even though penicillin therapy is inexpensive and effective. There is concern that, as HIV spreads throughout developing countries, it may markedly affect the manifestations and transmission of the endemic treponematoses.

FURTHER READINGS

ANTAL GM et al: The endemic treponematoses. Microbes Infect 4:83, 2002

BORA D et al: Yaws and its eradication in India—a brief review. J Commun Dis 37:1, 2005

CENTURION-LARA A et al: Molecular differentiation of *Treponema pallidum* subspecies. J Clin Microbiol 44:3377, 2006

ENGELKENS HJH et al: Nonvenereal treponematoses in tropical countries. Clin Dermatol 17:143, 1999

WALKER SL et al: Yaws—a review of the last 50 years. Int J Dermatol 39:258, 2000

CHAPTER 72

LEPTOSPIROSIS

Peter Speelman ■ Rudy Hartskeerl

Leptospirosis is an emerging infectious disease of global importance, as illustrated by recent large outbreaks in Asia, Central and South America, and the United States. The disease is caused by pathogenic leptospires and is characterized by a broad spectrum of clinical manifestations, varying from inapparent infection to fulminant, fatal disease. In its mild form, leptospirosis may present as an influenza-like illness with headache and myalgias. Severe leptospirosis, characterized by jaundice, renal dysfunction, and hemorrhagic diathesis, is referred to as *Weil's syndrome*.

ETIOLOGIC AGENTS

Leptospires are spirochetes belonging to the order Spirochaetales and the family Leptospiraceae. Traditionally, the genus *Leptospira* comprised two species: the pathogenic *L. interrogans* and the free-living *L. biflexa*; the current designations are *L. interrogans sensu lato* and *L. biflexa sensu lato*, respectively. Seventeen genomospecies of pathogenic leptospires are now recognized on the basis of their DNA relatedness. The genome sequences of two strains have been published, and reporting of the genomes of other strains is in progress. This information will undoubtedly lead to a better understanding of the pathogenesis of leptospirosis. However, for clinical and epidemiologic reasons, it is still more practical to use a classification system based on serologic differences. The pathogenic leptospires are divided into serovars according to their antigenic composition. More than 250 serovars make up the 26 serogroups.

Leptospires are coiled, thin, highly motile organisms with hooked ends and two periplasmic flagella that permit burrowing into tissue (Fig. 72-1). These organisms are 6–20 μm long and ~0.1 μm wide. They stain poorly but can be seen microscopically by dark-field examination and after silver impregnation staining. Leptospires require special media and conditions for growth; it may take weeks for cultures to become positive.

EPIDEMIOLOGY

Leptospirosis is an important zoonosis with a worldwide distribution, affecting at least 160 mammalian species. Rodents, especially rats, are the most important reservoir, although other wild mammals as well as domestic and farm animals may also harbor leptospires. These microorganisms establish a symbiotic relationship with their host and can persist in the renal tubules for years. Some serovars are generally associated with particular animals (e.g., Icterohaemorrhagiae and Copenhageni with rats, Grippotyphosa with voles, Hardjo with cattle, Canicola with dogs, and Pomona with pigs) but may occur in other animals as well.

In most countries, leptospirosis in humans is an underestimated problem. This infection occurs most commonly in the tropics because the climate as well as the sometimes-poor hygienic conditions favor the pathogen's survival and distribution. Most cases occur in men, with a peak incidence during the summer and fall in Western countries and during the rainy season in the tropics. Transmission of leptospires to humans may follow direct contact with urine, blood, or tissue from an infected animal or exposure to a contaminated environment; human-to-human transmission is rare. Since leptospires are excreted in the urine and can survive in water for many months, water is an important vehicle in their transmission. Epidemics of leptospirosis may result from exposure to flood waters contaminated by urine from infected animals, as has been reported from Nicaragua.

Reliable data on morbidity and mortality from leptospirosis have gradually started to appear. In 1999, more than 500,000 cases were reported from China, with case-fatality rates ranging from 0.9 to 7.9%. In Brazil, more than 28,000 cases were reported in the same year. Although humans are commonly infected with leptospires, only a minority become symptomatic or develop severe leptospirosis. In an ongoing cohort study in Brazil, 5% of the persons studied have been infected, whereas the incidence of severe leptospirosis is 9.5 per 100,000 cases.

In the United States, the 40–120 cases reported annually to the Centers for Disease Control and Prevention (CDC) surely represent a significant underestimation of the total number. Certain occupational groups are at especially high risk; included are veterinarians, agricultural workers, sewage workers, slaughterhouse employees, and workers in the fishing industry. Such individuals may acquire leptospirosis through direct exposure to or contact with contaminated water and soil. Leptospirosis has also been recognized in deteriorating inner cities and suburbs where rat populations are expanding. One report described leptospirosis in urban residents of Baltimore who were sporadically exposed to rat urine.

Recreational exposure and domestic-animal contact are also prominent sources of leptospirosis. Recreational

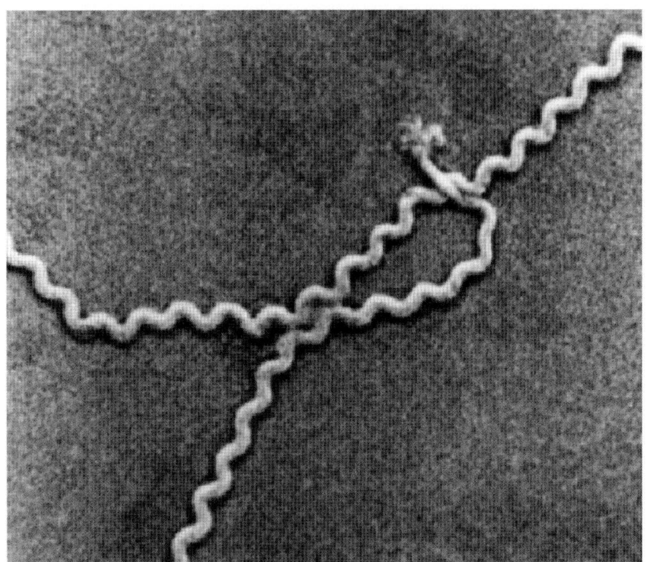

FIGURE 72-1
Scanning electron micrograph of leptospires.

water activities, such as canoeing, windsurfing, swimming, and waterskiing, place persons at risk. Several outbreaks have followed sporting events. For example, a large outbreak occurred in 1998 among athletes after a triathlon in Illinois. Ingestion of one or more swallows of lake water was a prominent risk factor for illness. Heavy rains that preceded the triathlon, with consequent agricultural runoff, are likely to have increased the level of leptospiral contamination in the lake water. In 2000, 80 participants contracted leptospirosis during an Eco-Challenge multisport endurance race in Malaysian Borneo. Swimming in the Segama River was an independent risk factor for infection.

In a study in the Netherlands, 14% of patients with confirmed leptospirosis had acquired the infection while traveling in tropical countries, most often in Southeast Asia. Transmission via laboratory accidents has been reported but is rare. Leptospirosis develops occasionally after unanticipated immersion in contaminated water (e.g., in an automobile accident) and rarely after an animal bite.

PATHOGENESIS

The pathogenesis of leptospirosis is incompletely understood. Leptospires enter the host through abrasions in the skin or through intact mucous membranes, especially the conjunctiva and the lining of the oro- and nasopharynx. Drinking of contaminated water may introduce leptospires through the mouth, throat, or esophagus. After entry of the organisms, leptospiremia develops, with subsequent spread to all organs. Multiplication takes place in blood and in tissues, and leptospires can be isolated from blood and cerebrospinal fluid (CSF) during the first 4–10 days of illness. CSF examination during this period documents pleocytosis in the majority of instances, but only a minority of patients develop symptoms and signs of meningitis at this point. All forms of leptospires can damage the wall of small blood vessels; this damage leads to vasculitis with leakage and extravasation of cells, including hemorrhages. The most important known pathogenic properties of leptospires are adhesion to cell surfaces and cellular toxicity.

Vasculitis is responsible for the most important manifestations of the disease. Although leptospires mainly infect the kidneys and liver, any organ may be affected. In the kidney, leptospires migrate to the interstitium, renal tubules, and tubular lumen, causing interstitial nephritis and tubular necrosis. Hypovolemia due to dehydration or altered capillary permeability may contribute to the development of renal failure. In the liver, centrilobular necrosis with proliferation of Kupffer's cells may be found. However, severe hepatocellular necrosis is not a feature of leptospirosis. Pulmonary involvement is the result of hemorrhage and not of inflammation. Invasion of skeletal muscle by leptospires results in swelling, vacuolation of the myofibrils, and focal necrosis. In severe leptospirosis, vasculitis may ultimately impair the microcirculation and increase capillary permeability, resulting in fluid leakage and hypovolemia.

When antibodies are formed, leptospires are eliminated from all sites in the host except the eye, the proximal renal tubules, and perhaps the brain, where they may persist for weeks or months. The persistence of leptospires in the aqueous humor occasionally causes chronic or recurrent uveitis. The systemic immune response is effective in eliminating the organism but may also produce symptomatic inflammatory reactions. A rise in antibody titer coincides with the development of meningitis; this association suggests that an immunologic mechanism is responsible.

After the start of antimicrobial treatment for leptospirosis, a Jarisch-Herxheimer reaction similar to that seen in other spirochetal diseases may develop. Although frequently described in older publications, this reaction seems to be a rare event in leptospirosis and is certainly less frequent in this infection than in other spirochetal diseases.

CLINICAL MANIFESTATIONS

(Fig. 72-2) Many *Leptospira*-infected persons remain asymptomatic. Serologic evidence of past inapparent infection is frequently found in persons who have been exposed to leptospires but have not become ill. In symptomatic cases of leptospirosis, clinical manifestations vary from mild to serious or even fatal. More than 90% of symptomatic persons have the relatively mild and usually anicteric form of leptospirosis, with or without meningitis. Severe leptospirosis with profound jaundice (Weil's syndrome) develops in 5–10% of infected individuals. The idea that distinct clinical syndromes are associated with specific serogroups has been refuted, although some serovars tend to cause more severe disease than others.

The incubation period is usually 1–2 weeks but ranges from 2 to 20 days (Fig. 72-2). Typically, an acute leptospiremic phase is followed by an immune leptospiruric phase. The distinction between the first and second phases is not always clear, and milder cases do not always include the second phase.

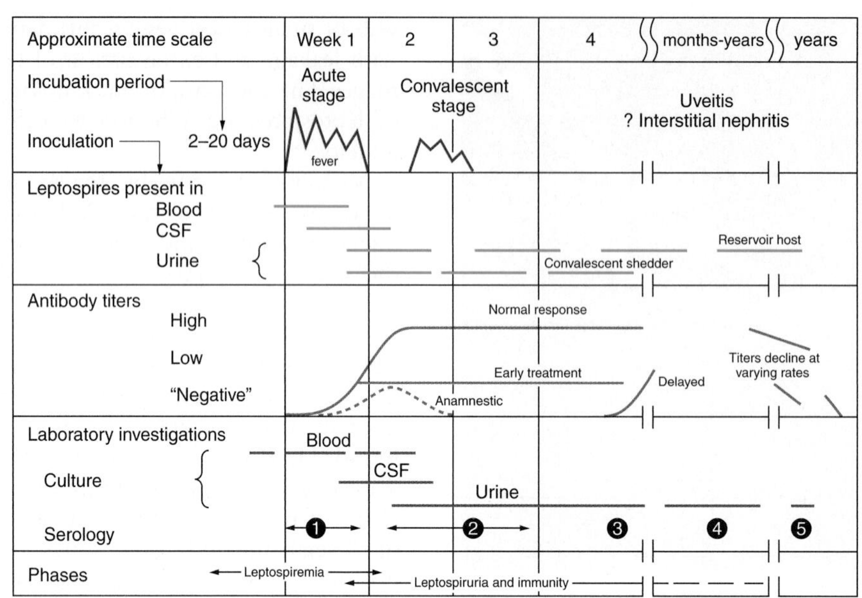

FIGURE 72-2

Biphasic nature of leptospirosis and relevant investigations at different stages of disease. Specimens 1 and 2 for serology are acute-phase serum samples, specimen 3 is a convalescent-phase serum sample that may facilitate detection of a delayed immune response, and specimens 4 and 5 are follow-up serum samples that can provide epidemiologic information, such as the presumptive infecting serogroup. [*Reprinted as adapted by Levett (from Turner LH: Leptospirosis. BMJ 1:231, 1969) with permission from the American Society for Microbiology and the BMJ Publishing Group.*]

Anicteric Leptospirosis

Leptospirosis may present as an acute influenza-like illness, with fever, chills, severe headache, nausea, vomiting, and myalgias. Muscle pain, which especially affects the calves, back, and abdomen, is an important feature of leptospiral infection. Less common features include sore throat and rash. The patient usually has an intense headache (frontal or retroorbital) and sometimes develops photophobia. Mental confusion may be evident. Pulmonary involvement, manifested in most cases by cough and chest pain and in a few cases by hemoptysis, is not uncommon.

The most common finding on physical examination is fever with conjunctival suffusion. Less common findings include muscle tenderness, lymphadenopathy, pharyngeal injection, rash, hepatomegaly, and splenomegaly. The rash may be macular, maculopapular, erythematous, urticarial, or hemorrhagic. Mild jaundice may be present.

Most patients become asymptomatic within 1 week. After an interval of 1–3 days, the illness recurs in a number of cases. The start of this second (immune) phase coincides with the development of antibodies. Symptoms are more variable than during the first (leptospiremic) phase. Usually the symptoms last for only a few days, but occasionally they persist for weeks. Often the fever is less pronounced and the myalgias are less severe than in the leptospiremic phase. An important event during the immune phase is the development of aseptic meningitis. Although no more than 15% of all patients have symptoms and signs of meningitis, many patients have CSF pleocytosis. Meningeal symptoms usually disappear within a few days but may persist for weeks. Similarly, pleocytosis generally disappears within 2 weeks but occasionally persists for months. Aseptic meningitis is more common among children than among adults. Iritis, iridocyclitis, and chorioretinitis—late complications that may persist for years—can become apparent as early as the third week but often present several months after the initial illness. One epidemic of uveitis among patients with leptospirosis has been reported. Mortality rates in anicteric leptospirosis are low, although death as a result of pulmonary hemorrhage occurred in 2.4% of cases in a Chinese outbreak.

Severe Leptospirosis (Weil's Syndrome)

Weil's syndrome, the most severe form of leptospirosis, is characterized by jaundice, renal dysfunction, and hemorrhagic diathesis; by pulmonary involvement in many cases; and by mortality rates of 5–15%. In Europe, this syndrome is frequently but not exclusively associated with infection due to serovar Icterohaemorrhagiae/Copenhageni. The onset of illness is no different from that of less severe leptospirosis; however, after 4–9 days, jaundice as well as renal and vascular dysfunction generally develop. Although some degree of defervescence may be noted after the first week of illness, a biphasic disease pattern like that seen in anicteric leptospirosis is lacking. The jaundice of Weil's syndrome, which can be profound and give an orange cast to the skin, is usually not associated with severe hepatic necrosis. Death is rarely due to liver failure. Hepatomegaly and tenderness in the right upper quadrant are usually detected. Splenomegaly is found in 20% of cases.

Renal failure may develop, often during the second week of illness. Hypovolemia and decreased renal perfusion contribute to the development of acute tubular necrosis with oliguria or anuria. Dialysis is sometimes required, although a fair number of cases can be managed without dialysis. Renal function may be completely regained.

Pulmonary involvement occurs frequently; in some clusters of cases, it is a major manifestation, resulting in cough, dyspnea, chest pain, and blood-stained sputum and sometimes in hemoptysis or even respiratory failure. Hemorrhagic manifestations are seen in Weil's syndrome: epistaxis, petechiae, purpura, and ecchymoses are found commonly, whereas severe gastrointestinal bleeding and adrenal or subarachnoid hemorrhage are detected rarely.

Rhabdomyolysis, hemolysis, myocarditis, pericarditis, congestive heart failure, cardiogenic shock, adult respiratory distress syndrome, necrotizing pancreatitis, and multiorgan failure have all been described during severe leptospirosis.

LABORATORY AND RADIOLOGIC FINDINGS

(Fig. 72-2) The kidneys are invariably involved in leptospirosis. Related findings range from urinary sediment changes (leukocytes, erythrocytes, and hyaline or granular casts) and mild proteinuria in anicteric leptospirosis to renal failure and azotemia in severe disease.

The erythrocyte sedimentation rate is usually elevated. In anicteric leptospirosis, peripheral leukocyte counts range from 3000 to 26,000/μL, with a left shift; in Weil's syndrome, leukocytosis is often marked. Mild thrombocytopenia occurs in up to 50% of patients and is associated with renal failure.

In contrast to patients with acute viral hepatitis, those with leptospirosis typically have elevated serum levels of bilirubin and alkaline phosphatase as well as mild increases (up to 200 U/L) in serum levels of aminotransferases. In Weil's syndrome, the prothrombin time may be prolonged but can be corrected with vitamin K. Levels of creatine phosphokinase, which are elevated in up to 50% of patients with leptospirosis during the first week of illness, may help to differentiate this infection from viral hepatitis.

When a meningeal reaction develops, polymorphonuclear leukocytes predominate initially and the number of mononuclear cells increases later. The protein concentration in the CSF may be elevated; CSF glucose levels are normal.

In severe leptospirosis, pulmonary radiographic abnormalities are more common than would be expected on the basis of physical examination. These abnormalities most frequently develop 3–9 days after the onset of illness. The most common radiographic finding is a patchy alveolar pattern that corresponds to scattered alveolar hemorrhage. Radiographic abnormalities most often affect the lower lobes in the periphery of the lung fields.

DIAGNOSIS

(Fig. 72-2) A definite diagnosis of leptospirosis is based either on isolation of the organism from the patient or on seroconversion or a rise in antibody titer in the microscopic agglutination test (MAT). In the United States, the MAT is performed only at the CDC. In cases with strong clinical evidence of infection, a single antibody titer of 1:200–1:800 (depending on whether the case occurs in a low- or high-endemic area) in the MAT is required. Preferably, a fourfold or greater rise in titer is detected between acute- and convalescent-phase serum specimens. Antibodies generally do not reach detectable levels until the second week of illness. The antibody response can be affected by early treatment.

The MAT, which uses a battery of live leptospiral strains, and the enzyme-linked immunosorbent assay (ELISA), which uses a broadly reacting antigen, are the standard serologic procedures. These tests usually are available only in specialized laboratories and are used for determination of the antibody titer and for tentative identification of the serogroup—and in some cases the serovar—involved (thus the importance of using antigens representative of the serovars prevalent in the particular geographic area). Since cross-reactions occur frequently, however, it is often impossible to identify the infecting serogroup or serovar. Serologic testing cannot be used as the basis for a decision about whether to start treatment.

In addition to the MAT and the ELISA, various rapid tests with diagnostic value (some of them commercially available) have been developed. These rapid tests, which mainly apply lateral flow, (latex) agglutination, or ELISA methodology, have reasonable sensitivity and specificity; variation in reported data probably reflects differences in test interpretation, (re)exposure risks, and serovar distribution and the use of biased serum panels. These methods do not require culture or MAT facilities. However, in endemic areas, pooled serum samples from the local population are required as positive and negative controls. Polymerase chain reaction techniques have been developed but so far have not found widespread use outside research and reference laboratories.

Leptospires can be isolated from blood and/or CSF during the first 10 days of illness and from urine for several weeks beginning at ~1 week. Cultures most often become positive after 2–4 weeks, with a range of 1 week to 6 months. Sometimes urine cultures remain positive for months or years after the start of illness. For isolation of leptospires from body fluids or tissues, Ellinghausen-McCullough-Johnson-Harris (EMJH) medium is useful; other possibilities are Fletcher's medium and Korthof's medium. Specimens can be mailed to a reference laboratory for culture, since leptospires remain viable in anticoagulated blood (heparin, EDTA, or citrate) for up to 11 days at room temperature. Isolation of leptospires is important since it is the only way the infecting serovar can be correctly identified. Dark-field examination of blood or urine frequently results in misdiagnosis and should not be used.

DIFFERENTIAL DIAGNOSIS

Leptospirosis should be differentiated from other febrile illnesses associated with headache and muscle pain, such as dengue, malaria, enteric fever, viral hepatitis, *Hantavirus* infections, and rickettsial diseases. In light of the strong similarity in epidemiology and clinical presentation between leptospirosis and *Hantavirus* infections and given the reported occurrence of dual infections, it is advisable to conduct serologic testing for *Hantavirus* in cases of suspected leptospirosis. When patients have a flulike disease with disproportionately severe myalgia or aseptic meningitis, a diagnosis of leptospirosis should be considered.

℞ Treatment: LEPTOSPIROSIS

Although a review of antibiotics for the treatment of leptospirosis concluded that there is insufficient evidence to provide clear guidelines for practice, the outcomes of the randomized clinical trials included in this review suggest that penicillin and doxycycline may be useful agents. Accordingly, these are the most commonly used antibiotics. Treatment should be initiated as early as possible; nevertheless, contrary to previous reports, treatment started after the first 4 days of illness is still effective. In milder cases, oral treatment with tetracycline, doxycycline, ampicillin, or amoxicillin should be considered. For severe cases of leptospirosis, intravenous administration of penicillin G, amoxicillin, ampicillin, or erythromycin is recommended (Table 72-1). One comparative trial of the efficacy of ceftriaxone and penicillin for the treatment of severe leptospirosis found no significant differences between the two drugs in terms of complications or mortality rates. Another open-label randomized study compared parenteral cefotaxime, penicillin G, and doxycycline for the treatment of suspected severe leptospirosis. Among 264 patients with leptospirosis confirmed by serologic testing or culture, the mortality rate was 5%. There were no significant differences between antibiotics with regard to associated mortality, defervescence, or time to resolution of abnormal laboratory findings. Thus doxycycline, cefotaxime, or ceftriaxone is a satisfactory alternative to penicillin G for the treatment of severe leptospirosis.

In rare cases, a Jarisch-Herxheimer reaction develops within hours after the start of antimicrobial therapy (see "Pathogenesis" earlier in the chapter). Although so far the only effective mode of management is supportive, the role of antibodies to tumor necrosis factor in the treatment of this reaction deserves further study. A beneficial effect of the use of such antibodies for the modulation of the reaction has been demonstrated in patients with louse-borne relapsing fever. Patients with severe leptospirosis and renal failure may require dialysis. Those with Weil's syndrome may need transfusions of whole blood and/or platelets. Intensive care may be necessary.

TABLE 72-1

TREATMENT AND CHEMOPROPHYLAXIS OF LEPTOSPIROSIS

PURPOSE OF DRUG ADMINISTRATION	REGIMEN
Treatment	
Mild leptospirosis	Doxycycline, 100 mg orally bid *or* Ampicillin, 500–750 mg orally qid *or* Amoxicillin, 500 mg orally qid
Moderate/severe leptospirosis	Penicillin G, 1.5 million units IV qid *or* Ampicillin, 1 g IV qid *or* Amoxicillin, 1 g IV qid *or* Ceftriaxone, 1 g IV once daily *or* Cefotaxime, 1 g IV qid *or* Erythromycin, 500 mg IV qid
Chemoprophylaxis	Doxycycline, 200 mg orally once a week

Note: All regimens used for treatment are administered for 7 days.

PROGNOSIS

Most patients with leptospirosis recover. Mortality rates are highest among patients who are elderly and those who have Weil's syndrome. Leptospirosis during pregnancy is associated with high rates of fetal mortality. Long-term follow-up of patients with renal failure and hepatic dysfunction has documented good recovery of renal and hepatic function.

PREVENTION

Individuals who may be exposed to leptospires through their occupations or their involvement in recreational water activities should be informed about the risks. Measures for controlling leptospirosis include avoidance of exposure to urine and tissues from infected animals, vaccination of animals, and rodent control. The animal vaccine used in a given area should contain the serovars known to be present in that area. Unfortunately, some vaccinated animals still excrete leptospires in their urine. Vaccination of humans against a specific serovar prevalent in an area has been undertaken in some European and Asian countries and has proved effective. Although a large-scale trial of vaccine in humans has been reported from Cuba, no conclusions can be drawn about efficacy and adverse reactions because of insufficient details on study design. Chemoprophylaxis with doxycycline (200 mg once a week) has appeared to be efficacious to some extent but is indicated only in rare instances of sustained short-term exposure (Table 72-1).

FURTHER READINGS

Bharti AR et al: Leptospirosis: A zoonotic disease of global importance. Lancet Infect Dis 3:757, 2003

Guidugli F et al: Antibiotics for leptospirosis. Cochrane Database Syst Rev 2:CD001306, 2000

Levett PN: Leptospirosis. Clin Microbiol Rev 14:296, 2001

MORGAN J et al: Outbreak of leptospirosis among triathlon participants and community residents in Springfield, Illinois, 1998. Clin Infect Dis 34:1593, 2002

PANAPHUT T et al: Ceftriaxone compared with sodium penicillin G for treatment of severe leptospirosis. Clin Infect Dis 36:1507, 2003

SEHGAL SC et al: Randomized controlled trial of doxycycline prophylaxis against leptospirosis in an endemic area. Int J Antimicrob Agents 13:249, 2000

SEJVAR J et al: Leptospirosis in "Eco-Challenge" athletes, Malaysian Borneo, 2000. Emerg Infect Dis 9:702, 2003

SUPPUTAMONGKOL Y et al: An open, randomized, controlled trial of penicillin, doxycycline, and cefotaxime for patients with severe leptospirosis. Clin Infect Dis 39:1417, 2004

VINETZ JM: Leptospirosis. Curr Opin Infect Dis 14:527, 2001

WORLD HEALTH ORGANIZATION/INTERNATIONAL LEPTOSPIROSIS SOCIETY: *Human Leptospirosis: Guidance for Diagnosis, Surveillance and Control.* Geneva, World Health Organization, 2003, 109 pp

CHAPTER 73

RELAPSING FEVER

David T. Dennis

DEFINITION

The term *relapsing fever* describes two distinct diseases. *Tick-borne (endemic)* relapsing fever (TBRF) is a zoonosis that is transmitted principally from rodents to humans by the bite of various soft ticks. *Louse-borne (epidemic)* relapsing fever (LBRF) is a disease of humans that is transmitted from one person to another by the body louse. Both diseases are characterized by recurrent acute episodes of spirochetemia and fever alternating with variable periods of remission.

ETIOLOGY

Relapsing fever is caused by infection with spirochetal gram-negative bacteria of the genus *Borrelia* (family Spirochaetaceae). The borreliae are helical in shape and average 0.2–0.5 μm in width and 5–20 μm in length. They comprise an outer membrane, an intermediate peptidoglycan layer, and an inner cytoplasmic membrane, which encloses the protoplasmic cylinder. A variable number of periplasmic flagella are situated beneath the outer membrane. Relapsing-fever borreliae are slow-growing and microaerophilic; they grow best at 30°–35°C in Barbour-Stoenner-Kelly (BSK II) medium.

B. recurrentis is the only species that causes LBRF. Most of the various species of *Borrelia* that cause TBRF are named after the species of *Ornithodoros* tick responsible for their transmission. In North America, TBRF is caused mostly by *B. hermsii* and only occasionally by *B. turicatae*; *B. duttoni* is the most common cause of TBRF in Sub-Saharan Africa, an area of high endemicity. Borreliae are unique among bacteria in having a genome composed of a linear chromosome and a series of linear and circular plasmids. The sequences of both the flagellin and the 16S ribosomal RNA genes are homogeneous among LBRF strains; in contrast, there is considerable heterogeneity of these genes between Old World and New World TBRF strains. A unique process of DNA rearrangement within *vmp* genes located on linear plasmids results in extensive variation in the expression of the surface antigens in relapsing fever borreliae. These *vmp* genes encode variable major proteins (VMPs) found on the spirochete's outer-membrane surface. The antigenic variation generated by sequential expression of previously silent *vmp* genes allows the borreliae to intermittently escape the immune response of the host and results in the febrile spirochetemic relapses that are characteristic of infection with these organisms.

EPIDEMIOLOGY

Louse-Borne Relapsing Fever

Body lice (*Pediculus humanus* var. *corporis*) become infected with *B. recurrentis* by feeding on spirochetemic humans, the only reservoirs of infection. In lice, *B. recurrentis* spirochetes are found almost exclusively in the hemolymph; humans acquire infection when body lice are crushed and their infective fluids enter breaks in the skin, typically abrasions caused by scratching of pruritic louse bites. Spirochetes are *not* transmitted directly by the bite of a louse (anterior station transmission) but may possibly be transmitted in a manner similar to epidemic typhus by percutaneous inoculation of louse feces (posterior station transmission). Lice have a life span of only a few weeks, feed at frequent intervals, and survive only a few days off the human host. Typically, body lice reside in seams of clothing and bedclothes, where they deposit their eggs (nits). Head lice have not been shown to be vectors of LBRF.

LBRF has severely affected military and civilian populations disrupted by war and other disasters. Historically, the disease has been most common among slum dwellers, prisoners, and others living in impoverished, overcrowded, and unhygienic conditions. In the first half of the twentieth century, during periods of war and famine, both LBRF and louse-borne typhus were epidemic in Eastern Europe, the Balkans, and the former Soviet Union. The global distribution and incidence of LBRF have been substantially reduced by improvements in standards of living, sanitation, and hygiene; LBRF is now an important disease only in northeastern Africa, especially the highlands of Ethiopia, where an estimated 10,000 cases occur annually. LBRF has repeatedly spilled out of Ethiopia into populations of displaced persons in neighboring Somalia and Sudan.

Short-term visitors to endemic areas are at almost no risk of LBRF. Persons who have close contact with LBRF-affected populations (such as relief workers) can acquire the disease from lice or by direct contact with contaminated blood.

Tick-Borne Relapsing Fever

Argasid ticks of the genus *Ornithodoros* transmit TBRF through their saliva and excreta when they take blood meals. Ticks typically become infected with TBRF borreliae as part of a zoonotic cycle when they feed on spirochetemic rodents and lagomorphs; the exception is *O. moubata*, a tick species that is thought to acquire *B. duttoni* only by feeding on infected humans. Ticks transmit TBRF borreliae vertically from one stage to the next; in some species, infection is transmitted transovarially over several generations. Soft ticks are hardy and can survive for as long as 10 years with only an occasional blood meal. These ticks feed painlessly, relatively quickly (for 20–45 min), and usually at night while hosts are sleeping. Thus patients with TBRF are often unaware of tick exposures.

TBRF borreliae are widely distributed throughout the world. Human infection with these organisms is generally underrecognized and underreported. TBRF is most highly endemic in Sub-Saharan Africa, but is also found in countries of the Mediterranean littoral, Middle Eastern states, southern Russia, the Indian subcontinent, Central Asia, and China and rarely in North, Central, and South America. The disease typically occurs sporadically or in small—often familial—clusters. Infected soft ticks may cause repeated infections among persons living or sleeping in the same dwelling. In Sub-Saharan Africa, *O. moubata*, the vector of *B. duttoni*, infests native huts and rest houses, hiding in crevices of floors and walls during the day and emerging at night to feed on sleeping inhabitants.

In the United States, TBRF occurs west of the Mississippi River, especially in forested mountainous areas of far western states, where *B. hermsii* is the causative agent. Less commonly, persons become infected with *B. turicatae* after exposures in tick-infested caves in semidesert areas of the Southwest. On average, ~35 cases of TBRF are reported annually in the United States. *B. hermsii* infections most often occur during spring and summer months among persons sleeping in rustic mountain cabins and vacation homes and occasionally in permanent residences and in outdoor settings. The vertebrate reservoirs of infection are chipmunks and other rodents that nest in foundations, wall spaces, and attics of these dwellings. Outbreaks caused by *B. hermsii* have taken place among persons staying in cabins along the north rim of the Grand Canyon and in the mountains of California, Idaho, and Colorado. In North America, most recent cases have been reported from Washington, California, Colorado, Idaho, Oregon, and British Columbia.

PATHOGENESIS AND PATHOLOGY

In humans, relapsing-fever borreliae pass through the skin or mucous membranes, multiply in the blood, and circulate in great numbers during febrile periods. The organisms have also been found in the liver, spleen, bone marrow, and central nervous system (CNS) and may be sequestered at these sites during periods of remission. The severity of disease is positively correlated with spirochete density in the blood. Even though the pathophysiologic manifestations of the disease resemble responses to endotoxin, and although plasma from some patients with relapsing fever coagulates *Limulus* amebocyte lysates, borreliae and other spirochetes have not been shown to express a true lipopolysaccharide (endotoxin) molecule. Infection with *B. recurrentis* has been shown, however, to activate protein mediators of inflammation, such as Hageman factor (factor XII), prekallikrein, and proteins of the complement system; furthermore, a spirochetal heat-stable pyrogenic factor stimulates mononuclear phagocytes to express increased amounts of leukocyte pyrogen and thromboplastin.

The treatment of relapsing fever with antibiotics may provoke a Jarisch-Herxheimer reaction (see "Treatment: Relapsing Fever" later in the chapter). In patients with LBRF, this reaction has been associated with a release of various cytokines into the plasma, including interleukin 6, interleukin 8, C-reactive protein, and large amounts of tumor necrosis factor α (TNF-α). Pretreatment of LBRF patients with antibody to TNF-α suppresses Jarisch-Herxheimer reactions and reduces plasma concentrations of certain cytokines.

Death due to TBRF is rare. In contrast, fatality rates of 20% have been recorded during outbreaks of LBRF in malnourished and stressed populations. Relapsing fever in pregnancy can result in abortion, stillbirth, and fatal neonatal infections. Autopsies of patients with relapsing fever most often reveal hepatosplenomegaly and variable edema and swelling of other organs, including brain, lungs, and kidneys. On microscopic examination, the spleen is congested and contains multiple microabscesses composed of mononuclear cells that replace the white pulp, the myocardium displays diffuse histiocytic inflammation and interstitial edema, and the liver has areas of midzonal necrosis. Petechial hemorrhages are commonly evident over the surfaces of the meninges, pleura, heart, spleen, liver, kidneys, and mesentery. Subcapsular and parenchymal hemorrhagic infarcts of the spleen, heart, liver, and brain are sometimes grossly visible.

CLINICAL MANIFESTATIONS

The clinical manifestations of LBRF and TBRF are similar. The common signs and symptoms of TBRF, as documented in North America, are listed in Table 73-1. The mean incubation period is 7 days (range, 2–18 days), and the onset of illness is sudden, with fever, headache, shaking chills, sweats, myalgias, and arthralgias. The arthralgia of relapsing fever can be severe, involving small and large joints, but there is no evidence of arthritis. Dizziness, nausea, and vomiting are common. Sleep may be difficult and is sometimes accompanied by disturbing dreams. The patient is coherent but withdrawn, thirsty, and uninterested in food and other outside stimuli. The fever is high from the first, with the temperature usually reaching ≥40°C (≥104°F) and then becoming irregular in pattern. High fever is sometimes accompanied by delirium. Patients are usually tachycardic and mildly tachypneic and become prostrate as the disease progresses. Some patients have meningismus. The conjunctivae are often injected, and photophobia is common. The sclerae may become icteric, particularly in the later stages of illness. The mucous membranes may be dry, and patients are often dehydrated. Scattered petechiae develop on the trunk, extremities, and mucous membranes in one-third or more of patients with LBRF but in a smaller proportion of patients with TBRF. A nonproductive cough is common, but chest sounds are usually normal; pleuritic pain and an accompanying pleuritic rub are sometimes noted. Cardiac findings are compatible with a high-output state; tachycardia and summation gallop are common. Tender enlargement of the spleen and liver frequently occurs in the acute phase of illness.

Epistaxis and blood-tinged sputum are common complications, and gastrointestinal and CNS hemorrhage can occur. Because of bleeding, outbreaks of LBRF have been initially confused with viral hemorrhagic fever. Other complications of variable incidence include iridocyclitis, optic neuritis, lymphocytic meningitis, coma, isolated cranial-nerve palsy, pneumonitis, myocarditis, and splenic rupture. Acute respiratory distress syndrome is becoming increasingly recognized as a complication of TBRF in the United States. However, life-threatening complications are unusual in otherwise healthy persons given supportive care, especially if the illness is diagnosed and treated early. Children generally have a milder course of illness than adults.

Without treatment, symptoms intensify over 2–7 days (average, 5 days in LBRF and 3 days in TBRF), ending in a spontaneous crisis that coincides with the disappearance of spirochetes from the circulation. The crisis comprises two phases over several hours: a *chill phase*, characterized by rigors, rising temperature, and hypermetabolism, and a *flush phase* of falling temperature, diaphoresis, and a decreased effective circulating blood volume. The pathophysiologic events associated with this crisis are magnified when precipitated by antibiotic treatment and are indistinguishable from the Jarisch-Herxheimer reaction of treated syphilis (see "Treatment: Relapsing Fever" later in the chapter). The crisis is followed by a period of exhaustion, sleep, and an uneventful recovery. Orthostatic hypotension is typical in the early recovery phase. Not uncommonly, in the first week of convalescence, the patient experiences 1 or 2 days of mild fever unassociated with detectable spirochetemia. In untreated patients, spirochetemia and symptoms may recur after a period of several days or weeks (average interval to first relapse, 9 days in LBRF and 7 days in TBRF). Only one or two relapses characteristically occur in untreated patients with LBRF, whereas as many as 10 (average, three) can occur in untreated patients with TBRF. In most cases, the illness becomes shorter and milder and the afebrile intervals longer with each relapse. Because of the great antigenic variation among *Borrelia* strains, infection confers only partial immunity, and repeated infections of the same individual have been recorded.

TABLE 73-1

MANIFESTATIONS OF TICK-BORNE RELAPSING FEVER ACQUIRED IN THE NORTHWESTERN UNITED STATES AND SOUTHWESTERN BRITISH COLUMBIA

SIGN OR SYMPTOM	%	SIGN OR SYMPTOM	%
Headache	94	Photophobia	25
Myalgia	92	Neck pain	24
Chills	88	Rash	18
Nausea	76	Dysuria	13
Arthralgia	73	Jaundice	10
Vomiting	71	Hepatomegaly	10
Abdominal pain	44	Splenomegaly	6
Confusion	38	Conjunctival injection	5
Dry cough	27	Eschar	2
Eye pain	26	Meningitis	2
Diarrhea	25	Nuchal rigidity	2
Dizziness	25		

Source: From a review of 182 cases reported in the period 1980–1995 (Dworkin et al. 2002).

DIFFERENTIAL DIAGNOSIS AND LABORATORY FINDINGS

Diseases that should be considered in the differential diagnosis of relapsing fever or that may complicate relapsing fever include typhus fever, typhoid fever, nontyphoidal salmonellosis, malaria, dengue and other arboviral illnesses, tuberculosis, leptospirosis, and viral hemorrhagic fevers. In the United States, the geographic distribution of Colorado tick fever (Chap. 99) overlaps that of TBRF, and the two diseases have similar manifestations early in their courses.

The diagnosis of relapsing fever is confirmed most easily by the detection of spirochetes in blood, bone marrow aspirates, or cerebrospinal fluid. Motile spirochetes can be seen when specimens are examined by dark-field microscopy. Fixed organisms are clearly visible in Wright-, Giemsa-, or acridine orange–stained preparations of thin or dehemoglobinized thick smears of peripheral blood or buffy-coat preparations (Fig. 73-1). Organisms are most numerous in specimens taken during

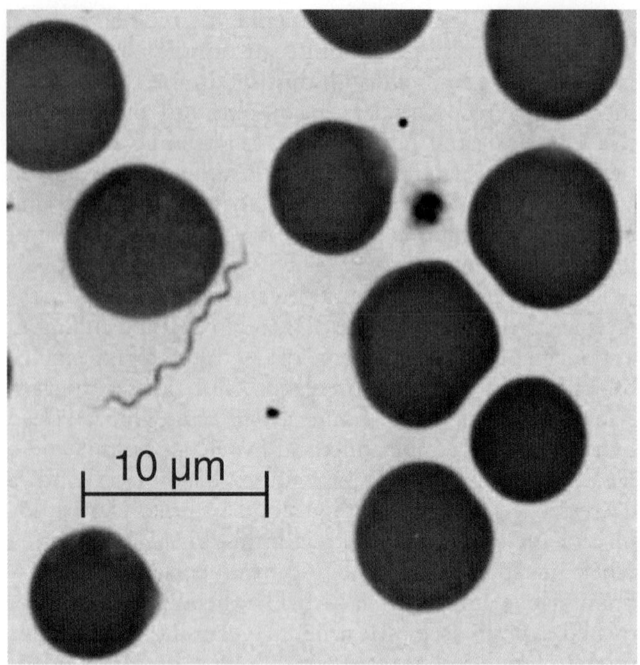

FIGURE 73-1

Photomicrograph of tick-borne relapsing fever spirochete (*B. hermsii*) in a Wright-Giemsa–stained peripheral blood film.

periods of high temperature preceding the crisis; smears of peripheral blood are positive in ≥70% of patients with LBRF and in a lower percentage of patients with TBRF. In reference laboratories, relapsing-fever spirochetes are cultured from blood by the inoculation of BSK II medium or by the intraperitoneal inoculation of immature laboratory mice. Serum antibodies to *Borrelia* can be detected by enzyme immunoassays, indirect fluorescent antibody (IFA) assay, and Western immunoblotting using whole-cell sonicates as antigen; however, these tests are unstandardized and are subject to insensitivity and cross-reactivity with other spirochetal agents, including *B. burgdorferi* (the agent of Lyme disease) and *Treponema pallidum*. The Western immunoblot test employing species-specific recombinant glycerophosphodiester phosphodiesterase (GlpQ) as antigen is more sensitive and specific than the whole-cell sonicate IFA test or the enzyme-linked immunosorbent assay.

Other laboratory findings in relapsing fever are nonspecific. The leukocyte count is normal or moderately elevated, with an unremarkable cell differential. Serum bilirubin levels are generally only slightly elevated. Thrombocytopenia commonly occurs in relapsing-fever patients during the acute phase of the illness; platelet counts rebound during early convalescence. Prothrombin and partial thromboplastin times are often moderately prolonged during acute illness, as are standardized bleeding times. Fibrinogen concentrations in the blood are normal, and fibrinolysis is mild or absent. Results of the Rumpel-Leede tourniquet test for capillary fragility are negative, despite the presence of petechiae.

℞ Treatment: RELAPSING FEVER

Relapsing-fever borreliae are exquisitely sensitive to antibiotics. Treatment with doxycycline (or another tetracycline), erythromycin, or chloramphenicol produces rapid clearance of spirochetes and a remission of symptoms (Table 73-2). The response to a single dose of penicillin may be delayed and incomplete. Although a single dose of doxycycline (or another tetracycline), erythromycin, or chloramphenicol is highly effective in the treatment of LBRF, less is known about the efficacy of single-dose treatment of TBRF. Empirical treatment of TBRF for 7 days is therefore recommended to reduce the risk of persisting or relapsing borreliosis. For children <8 years of age and for pregnant women, erythromycin or penicillin may be preferred, given the potential adverse effects of tetracyclines.

Treatment of LBRF with a rapidly acting antibiotic regularly precipitates a Jarisch-Herxheimer-like reaction within 1–4 h of the first dose. This reaction, which occurs in >50% of treated TBRF patients in North America, tends to be more severe when the patient has LBRF rather than TBRF and when high numbers of spirochetes are circulating in the bloodstream. In the chill phase of the reaction, rigors and rising fever are accompanied by an increasing metabolic rate, alveolar hyperventilation, high cardiac output, increasing peripheral vascular resistance, and decreased pulmonary arterial pressure. The body temperature commonly rises to ≥41°C (≥105.8°F). This high fever is accompanied often by agitation and confusion and sometimes by delirium. Fever can be partially controlled by the use of a cooling blanket and ice packs and by sponging of the patient with tepid water and alcohol. The chill phase terminates after 10–30 min, giving way to a flush phase characterized by a fall in body temperature, drenching

TABLE 73-2

ANTIBIOTIC TREATMENT OF LOUSE-BORNE AND TICK-BORNE RELAPSING FEVER IN ADULTS

MEDICATION	LOUSE-BORNE RELAPSING FEVER (SINGLE DOSE)	TICK-BORNE RELAPSING FEVER (7-DAY SCHEDULE)
Oral		
Erythromycin	500 mg	500 mg q6h
Tetracycline	500 mg	500 mg q6h
Doxycycline	100 mg	100 mg q12h
Chloramphenicol	500 mg	500 mg q6h
Parenteral[a]		
Erythromycin	500 mg	500 mg q6h
Tetracycline	250 mg	250 mg q6h
Doxycycline	100 mg	100 mg q12h
Chloramphenicol	500 mg	500 mg q6h
Penicillin G (procaine)	600,000 IU	600,000 IU daily

[a]For tick-borne relapsing fever, parenteral therapy is used only until oral treatment is tolerated.

sweats, and sometimes (more commonly in LBRF) a potentially dangerous fall in systemic arterial pressure and rise in pulmonary arterial pressure. Although cardiac output is maintained at high levels, the effective circulating blood volume decreases as peripheral vascular resistance falls. Vital signs must be monitored carefully during this period of the reaction, which usually lasts ≤8 h. Clinical and electrocardiographic evidence of myocarditis and myocardial dysfunction includes a prolonged QT_c interval, a third heart sound (S_3), elevated central venous pressure, arterial hypotension, and rare pulmonary congestion. The use of delayed-release IM penicillin may prolong or delay the clearance of spirochetes and thereby attenuate the accompanying Jarisch-Herxheimer reaction, but this response is not predictable; furthermore, single-dose penicillin treatment sometimes results in relapse of spirochetemia and symptoms. Glucocorticoids and nonsteroidal anti-inflammatory agents do not prevent or significantly modify the cardiopulmonary disturbances of the Jarisch-Herxheimer reaction, although hydrocortisone and acetaminophen given at the same time as antibiotics reduce peak body temperature. Although pretreatment with antibody to TNF-α may moderate the Jarisch-Herxheimer reaction in treated patients with LBRF, its use in LBRF is impractical and its use in TBRF (whose treatment is typically associated with a relatively mild Jarisch-Herxheimer reaction) is not warranted. Close monitoring of fluid balance, arterial and venous pressures, and myocardial function is advised in supportive management of the Jarisch-Herxheimer reaction in patients with LBRF.

The management of patients with relapsing fever–induced myocardial dysfunction requires caution in the administration of IV fluids and, in some cases, use of short-term inotropic therapy. The inability of heparin to control bleeding in LBRF suggests that disseminated intravascular coagulation is not important in its causation. Vitamin K and other soluble vitamins are sometimes given to counter dietary deficiencies in patients with LBRF. Because postural hypotension is often pronounced during the acute phase of relapsing fever and in the early stage of recovery, patients should be assisted when arising from bed.

Untreated LBRF has a high case-fatality rate, especially among persons in otherwise poor health, such as those in famine-affected populations. The fatality rate among treated persons is usually <5%. In general, TBRF is a milder disease than LBRF: the spontaneous crisis and the Jarisch-Herxheimer reactions are less pronounced and the case-fatality rates are lower for TBRF than for LBRF.

PREVENTION AND CONTROL

LBRF is best prevented by addressing socioeconomic circumstances that promote louse infestation (crowding, poverty, homelessness), by applying hygienic practices that reduce numbers of body lice (washing clothes, drying clothes in direct sunlight, changing clothes at frequent intervals), and by delousing. In infested situations like those in refugee camps, individuals, their clothes, and their bedding should be deloused with appropriate acaricides, such as 0.5% permethrin dust. Impregnation of clothing with liquid permethrin, a residual acaricide, can provide long-term protection against infestation. Spread of infection can be controlled by early case detection and treatment of infected persons and close contacts. In outbreaks of fever that involve louse-infested populations, empirical single-dose treatment with doxycycline will be effective against typhus as well as LBRF. *B. recurrentis* has a fragile life cycle and is eradicable.

In TBRF-endemic areas, risk of exposure can be reduced by avoiding rodent- and tick-infested dwellings and infested natural sites and by applying control measures. Access of rodents to foundation spaces, attics, and other harborages in dwellings, outbuildings, and their surroundings should be eliminated. Rodents and rodent nests should be removed from infested buildings. Tick harborages can be chemically treated by pest-control specialists using various acaricides, such as carbaryl, diazinon, chlorpyrifos, pyrethrins, and malathion. Persons who enter tick-infested sites can protect themselves by wearing clothing that denies ticks access to the skin, by applying repellents to exposed skin and to clothing, and by applying an acaricide containing permethrin to clothing. Reporting of suspected cases of relapsing fever to public health authorities is important so that an epidemiologic investigation and control measures can be initiated promptly. Prompt diagnosis and treatment of relapsing fever in pregnant women is important in avoiding the potentially severe consequences of fetal or neonatal infection.

FURTHER READINGS

Centers for Disease Control and Prevention: Acute respiratory distress syndrome in persons with tickborne relapsing fever—three states, 2004-2005. MMWR Morb Mortal Wkly Rep 56: 1073, 2007

Cutler SJ et al: *Borrelia recurrentis* characterization and comparison with relapsing fever, Lyme-associated, and other *Borrelia* spp. Int J Syst Bacteriol 47:958, 1997

Dai Q et al: Antigenic variation by *Borrelia hermsii* occurs through recombination between extragenic repetitive elements on linear plasmids. Mol Microbiol 60:1329, 2006

Dworkin MS et al: Tick-borne relapsing fever. Infect Dis Clin North Am 22:449, 2008

——— et al: Tick-borne relapsing fever in North America. Med Clin North Am 86:417, 2002

Goodman JL et al (eds): *Tick-Borne Diseases of Humans.* Washington, DC, ASM Press, 2005

Londono D et al: Cardiac apoptosis in severe relapsing fever borreliosis. Infect Immun 73:7669, 2005

Parola P, Raoult D: Ticks and tickborne bacterial diseases in humans: An emerging infectious threat. Clin Infect Dis 32:897, 2001

Paul WS et al: Outbreak of tick-borne relapsing fever at the north rim of the Grand Canyon: Evidence for effectiveness of preventive measures. Am J Trop Med Hyg 66:71, 2002

Porcella SF et al: Serodiagnosis of louse-borne relapsing fever with glycerophosphodiester phosphodiesterase (GlpQ) from *Borrelia recurrentis*. J Clin Microbiol 38:3561, 2000

Tal H et al: Postexposure treatment with doxycycline for the prevention of tick-borne relapsing fever. N Engl J Med 355:148, 2006

Vial L et al: Incidence of tick-borne relapsing fever in west Africa: Longitudinal study. Lancet 368:37, 2006

CHAPTER 74

LYME BORRELIOSIS

Allen C. Steere

DEFINITION

Lyme borreliosis is caused by a spirochete, *Borrelia burgdorferi sensu lato*, that is transmitted by ticks of the *Ixodes ricinus* complex. The infection usually begins with a characteristic expanding skin lesion, erythema migrans (EM; stage 1, localized infection). After several days or weeks, the spirochete may spread to many different sites (stage 2, disseminated infection). Possible manifestations of disseminated infection include secondary annular skin lesions, meningitis, cranial neuritis, radiculoneuritis, peripheral neuritis, carditis, atrioventricular nodal block, or migratory musculoskeletal pain. Months or years later (usually after periods of latent infection), intermittent or chronic arthritis, chronic encephalopathy or polyneuropathy, or acrodermatitis may develop (stage 3, persistent infection). Most patients experience early symptoms of the illness during the summer, but the infection may not become symptomatic until it progresses to stage 2 or 3.

Lyme disease was recognized as a separate entity in 1976 because of geographic clustering of children in Lyme, Connecticut, who were thought to have juvenile rheumatoid arthritis. It became apparent that Lyme disease was a multisystem illness that affected primarily the skin, nervous system, heart, and joints. Epidemiologic studies of patients with EM implicated certain *Ixodes* ticks as vectors of the disease. Early in the twentieth century, EM had been described in Europe and attributed to *I. ricinus* tick bites. In 1982, a previously unrecognized spirochete, now called *Borrelia burgdorferi*, was recovered from *Ixodes scapularis* ticks and then from patients with Lyme disease. The entity is now called Lyme disease or Lyme borreliosis.

ETIOLOGIC AGENT

B. burgdorferi, the causative agent of Lyme disease, is a fastidious, microaerophilic bacterium. The spirochete's genome is quite small (~1.5 Mb) and consists of a highly unusual linear chromosome of 950 kb as well as 9 circular and 12 linear plasmids. The most remarkable aspect of the *B. burgdorferi* genome is that there are sequences for more than 100 known or predicted lipoproteins—a larger number than in any other organism. The spirochete has few proteins with biosynthetic activity and depends on its host for most of its nutritional requirements. It has no sequences for recognizable toxins.

Currently, 13 closely related borrelial species are collectively referred to as *Borrelia burgdorferi sensu lato* (*B. burgdorferi* in the general sense). The human infection Lyme borreliosis is caused primarily by three pathogenic genospecies: *B. burgdorferi sensu stricto* (*B. burgdorferi* in the strict sense, hereafter referred to as *B. burgdorferi*), *Borrelia garinii*, and *Borrelia afzelii*. *B. burgdorferi* is the sole cause of the infection in the United States; all three genospecies are found in Europe, and the latter two species occur in Asia.

EPIDEMIOLOGY

The 13 known genospecies of *B. burgdorferi sensu lato* live in nature in enzootic cycles involving 14 different species of ticks that are part of the *I. ricinus* complex. *I. scapularis* is the principal vector in the northeastern United States from Maine to Virginia and in the midwestern states of Wisconsin and Minnesota. *I. pacificus* is the vector in the western states of California and Oregon. The disease is acquired throughout Europe (from Great Britain to Scandinavia to European Russia), where *I. ricinus* is the vector, and in Asian Russia, China, and Japan, where *I. persulcatus* is the vector. These ticks may transmit other diseases as well. In the United States, *I. scapularis* also transmits babesiosis and human anaplasmosis; in Europe and Asia, *I. ricinus* and *I. persulcatus* also transmit tick-borne encephalitis.

Ticks of the *I. ricinus* complex have larval, nymphal, and adult stages. They require a blood meal at each stage. The risk of infection in a given area depends largely on the density of these ticks as well as their feeding habits and animal hosts, which have evolved differently in different locations. For *I. scapularis* in the northeastern United States, the white-footed mouse and certain other rodents are the preferred hosts of the immature larvae and nymphs. It is critical that both of the tick's immature stages feed on the same host, because the life cycle of the spirochete depends on horizontal transmission: in early summer from infected nymphs to mice and in late summer from infected mice to larvae, which then molt to become the infected nymphs that will begin the cycle again the following year. It is the tiny nymphal tick that is primarily responsible for transmission of the disease to humans during the early summer months. White-tailed deer, which are not involved in the life cycle of the spirochete, are the preferred host for the adult stage of *I. scapularis* and seem to be critical to the tick's survival.

Lyme disease is now the most common vector-borne infection in the United States and Europe. Since surveillance was begun by the Centers for Disease Control and Prevention (CDC) in 1982, the number of cases in the United States has increased dramatically. More than 20,000 new cases are now reported each summer. In Europe, the highest reported frequencies of the disease are in the middle of the continent and in Scandinavia.

PATHOGENESIS AND IMMUNITY

To maintain its complex enzootic cycle, *B. burgdorferi* must adapt to two markedly different environments: the tick and the mammalian host. The spirochete expresses outer-surface protein A (OspA) in the midgut of the tick, whereas OspC is upregulated as the organism travels to the tick's salivary gland. There, OspC binds a tick salivary-gland protein (Salp15), which is required for infection of the mammalian host. The tick must usually be attached for at least 24 h for transmission of *B. burgdorferi.*

After injection into the human skin, *B. burgdorferi* may migrate outward, producing EM, and may spread hematogenously or in the lymph to other organs. The only known virulence factors of *B. burgdorferi* are surface proteins that allow the spirochete to attach to mammalian proteins, integrins, glycosaminoglycans, or glycoproteins. For example, spread through the skin and other tissue matrices may be facilitated by the binding of human plasminogen and its activators to the surface of the spirochete. Some *Borrelia* strains bind complement regulator–acquiring surface proteins (FHL-1/reconectin, or factor H), which help to protect spirochetes from complement-mediated lysis. Dissemination of the organism in the blood is facilitated by binding to the fibrinogen receptor on activated platelets ($\alpha_{IIb}\beta_3$) and the vitronectin receptor ($\alpha_v\beta_3$) on endothelial cells. Spirochetal decorin-binding proteins A and B bind decorin, a glycosaminoglycan on collagen fibrils; this binding may explain why the organism is commonly aligned with collagen fibrils in the extracellular matrix in the heart, nervous system, or joints.

To control and eradicate *B. burgdorferi*, the host mounts both innate and adaptive immune responses, resulting in macrophage- and antibody-mediated killing of the spirochete. As part of the innate immune response, complement may lyse the spirochete in the skin. Chemokines released by constituent cells in the skin lead to the recruitment of neutrophils and macrophages; the latter release potent proinflammatory cytokines. The purpose of the adaptive immune response appears to be the production of specific antibodies, which opsonize the organism—a step necessary for optimal spirochetal killing. Histologic examination of all affected tissues reveals an infiltration of lymphocytes, macrophages, and plasma cells with some degree of vascular damage (including mild vasculitis or hypervascular occlusion). These findings suggest that the spirochete may have been present in or around blood vessels.

Despite the innate and adaptive immune responses, *B. burgdorferi* may sometimes survive in certain sites, such as collagen bundles in synovial tissue. The ability of the spirochete to downregulate the expression of surface-exposed protein antigens and, in the case of the VlsE lipoprotein, the ability to change amino acid sequences in the protein are important mechanisms of immune evasion. However, in the battle between *B. burgdorferi* survival factors and host immune responses, spirochetes do not seem to be able to survive indefinitely against the immune responses of normal human patients. Moreover, the organisms do not have mechanisms that help to protect them from antibiotic therapy. For example, *B. burgdorferi* has only been seen extracellularly in affected tissues; it has not been shown to "hide out" in intracellular locations, thereby evading antibiotic exposure.

CLINICAL MANIFESTATIONS

Early Infection: Stage 1 (Localized Infection)

Because of the small size of nymphal ixodid ticks, most patients do not remember the preceding tick bite. After an incubation period of 3–32 days, EM, which occurs at the site of the tick bite, usually begins as a red macule or papule that expands slowly to form a large annular lesion (Fig. 74-1). As the lesion increases in size, it often develops a bright red outer border and partial central clearing. The center of the lesion sometimes becomes intensely erythematous and indurated, vesicular, or necrotic. In other instances, the expanding lesion remains an even, intense red; several red rings are found within an outside ring; or the central area turns blue before the lesion clears. Although EM can be located anywhere, the thigh, groin, and axilla are particularly common sites. The lesion is warm but not often painful. Approximately 20% of patients do not exhibit this characteristic skin manifestation.

Early Infection: Stage 2 (Disseminated Infection)

In cases in the United States, *B. burgdorferi* often spreads hematogenously to many sites within days or weeks after the onset of EM. In these cases, patients may develop

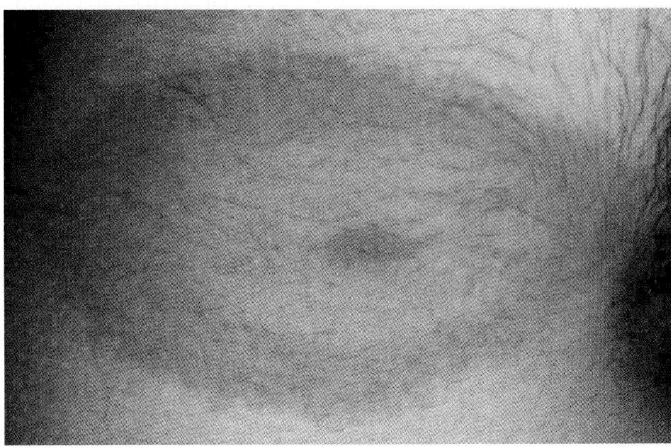

FIGURE 74-1

A classic erythema migrans lesion (9 cm in diameter) is shown near the right axilla. The lesion has partial central clearing, a bright red outer border, and a target center. *(Courtesy of Vijay K. Sikand, MD; with permission.)*

secondary annular skin lesions similar in appearance to the initial lesion. Skin involvement is commonly accompanied by severe headache, mild stiffness of the neck, fever, chills, migratory musculoskeletal pain, arthralgias, and profound malaise and fatigue. Less common manifestations include generalized lymphadenopathy or splenomegaly, hepatitis, sore throat, nonproductive cough, conjunctivitis, iritis, or testicular swelling. Except for fatigue and lethargy, which are often constant, the early signs and symptoms of Lyme disease are typically intermittent and changing. Even in untreated patients, the early symptoms usually become less severe or disappear within several weeks. In ~15% of patients, the infection presents with these nonspecific systemic symptoms.

Symptoms suggestive of meningeal irritation may develop early in Lyme disease when EM is present but usually are not associated with cerebrospinal fluid (CSF) pleocytosis or an objective neurologic deficit. After several weeks or months, ~15% of untreated patients develop frank neurologic abnormalities, including meningitis, subtle encephalitic signs, cranial neuritis (including bilateral facial palsy), motor or sensory radiculoneuropathy, peripheral neuropathy, mononeuritis multiplex, cerebellar ataxia, or myelitis—alone or in various combinations. In the United States, the usual pattern consists of fluctuating symptoms of meningitis accompanied by facial palsy and peripheral radiculoneuropathy. Lymphocytic pleocytosis (~100 cells/μL) is found in CSF, often along with elevated protein levels and normal or slightly low glucose concentrations. In Europe and Asia, the first neurologic sign is characteristically radicular pain, which is followed by the development of CSF pleocytosis (called meningopolyneuritis, or *Bannwarth's syndrome*); meningeal or encephalitic signs are frequently absent. In children, the optic nerve may be affected because of inflammation or increased intracranial pressure, which may lead to blindness. These early neurologic abnormalities usually resolve completely within months, but in rare cases, chronic neurologic disease may occur later.

Within several weeks after the onset of illness, ~8% of patients develop cardiac involvement. The most common abnormality is a fluctuating degree of atrioventricular block (first-degree, Wenckebach, or complete heart block). Some patients have more diffuse cardiac involvement, including electrocardiographic changes indicative of acute myopericarditis, left ventricular dysfunction evident on radionuclide scans, or (in rare cases) cardiomegaly or pancarditis. Cardiac involvement usually lasts for only a few weeks but may recur. Chronic cardiomyopathy caused by *B. burgdorferi* has been reported in Europe.

During this stage, musculoskeletal pain is common. The typical pattern consists of migratory pain in joints, tendons, bursae, muscles, or bones (usually without joint swelling) lasting for hours or days and affecting one or two locations at a time.

Late Infection: Stage 3 (Persistent Infection)

Months after the onset of infection, ~60% of patients in the United States who have received no antibiotic treatment develop frank arthritis. The typical pattern comprises intermittent attacks of oligoarticular arthritis in large joints (especially the knees), lasting for weeks or months in a given joint. A few small joints or periarticular sites may also be affected, primarily during early attacks. The number of patients who continue to have recurrent attacks decreases each year. However, in a small percentage of cases, involvement of large joints—usually one or both knees—becomes chronic and may lead to erosion of cartilage and bone.

White cell counts in joint fluid range from 500–110,000/μL (average, 25,000/μL); most of these cells are polymorphonuclear leukocytes. Tests for rheumatoid factor or antinuclear antibodies usually give negative results. Examination of synovial biopsy samples reveals fibrin deposits, villous hypertrophy, vascular proliferation, microangiopathic lesions, and a heavy infiltration of lymphocytes and plasma cells.

Although most patients with Lyme arthritis respond well to antibiotic therapy, a small percentage have persistent arthritis for months or even for several years after the apparent eradication of spirochetes from the joints by antibiotic therapy. Compared with antibiotic-responsive patients, those with antibiotic-refractory arthritis have a higher frequency of certain class II major histocompatibility complex molecules (particularly HLA-DRB1*0401 or -*0101 molecules) that bind an epitope of OspA ($OspA_{163-175}$), and they often exhibit T-cell recognition of this epitope. In addition, these patients have significantly higher levels of proinflammatory chemokines and cytokines in joint fluid (especially CXCL9 and interferon γ) than do antibiotic-responsive patients; these higher levels persist during the postantibiotic period, when polymerase chain reaction (PCR) results for *B. burgdorferi* DNA are uniformly negative. It has been postulated that, in these genetically susceptible individuals, *B. burgdorferi* may trigger autoimmunity within the proinflammatory milieu of the joints.

Although less common, chronic neurologic involvement may also become apparent months to several years after the onset of infection, sometimes after long periods of latent infection. The most common form of chronic central nervous system involvement is subtle encephalopathy affecting memory, mood, or sleep, and the most common form of peripheral neuropathy is an axonal polyneuropathy manifested as either distal paresthesia or spinal radicular pain. Patients with encephalopathy frequently have evidence of memory impairment in neuropsychological tests and abnormal results in CSF analyses. In cases of polyneuropathy, electromyography generally shows extensive abnormalities of proximal and distal nerve segments. Encephalomyelitis or leukoencephalitis, a rare manifestation of Lyme borreliosis associated primarily with *B. garinii* infection in Europe, is a severe neurologic disorder that may include spastic paraparesis, upper motor-neuron bladder dysfunction, and, rarely, lesions in the periventricular white matter.

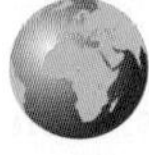

Acrodermatitis chronica atrophicans, the late skin manifestation of the disorder, has been associated primarily with *B. afzelii* infection in Europe and

Asia. It has been observed especially often in elderly women. The skin lesions, which are usually found on the acral surface of an arm or leg, begin insidiously with reddish-violaceous discoloration; they become sclerotic or atrophic over a period of years.

The basic patterns of Lyme borreliosis are similar worldwide, but there are regional variations, primarily between the illness found in America, which is caused exclusively by *B. burgdorferi*, and that found in Europe, which is caused primarily by *B. afzelii* and *B. garinii*. With each of the *Borrelia* spp., the infection usually begins with EM. However, *B. burgdorferi* often disseminates widely; it is particularly arthritogenic, and it may cause antibiotic-refractory arthritis. *B. garinii* typically disseminates less widely, but it is especially neurotropic and may cause borrelial encephalomyelitis. *B. afzelii* often infects only the skin but may persist in that site, where it may cause several different dermatoborrelioses, including acrodermatitis chronica atrophicans.

DIAGNOSIS

The culture of *B. burgdorferi* in Barbour-Stoenner-Kelly (BSK) medium permits definitive diagnosis, but this method has been used primarily in research studies. Moreover, with a few exceptions, positive cultures have been obtained only early in the illness—particularly from biopsy samples of EM skin lesions, less often from plasma samples, and occasionally from CSF samples. Later in the infection, PCR is greatly superior to culture for the detection of *B. burgdorferi* DNA in joint fluid—the major use for PCR testing in Lyme disease. However, the sensitivity of PCR determinations in CSF from patients with neuroborreliosis has been much lower. There seems to be little if any role for PCR in the detection of *B. burgdorferi* DNA in blood or urine samples. Moreover, this procedure, which must be carefully controlled to prevent contamination, is not routinely available.

Because of the problems associated with direct detection of *B. burgdorferi*, Lyme disease is usually diagnosed by the recognition of a characteristic clinical picture with serologic confirmation. Although serologic testing may yield negative results during the first several weeks of infection, most patients have a positive antibody response to *B. burgdorferi* after that time. The limitation of serologic tests is that they do not clearly distinguish between active and inactive infection. Patients with previous Lyme disease—particularly in cases progressing to late stages—often remain seropositive for years, even after adequate antibiotic treatment. In addition, ~10% of patients are seropositive because of asymptomatic infection. If these individuals subsequently develop another illness, the positive serologic test for Lyme disease may cause diagnostic confusion. According to an algorithm published by the American College of Physicians (Table 74-1), serologic testing for Lyme disease is recommended only for patients with at least an intermediate pretest probability of Lyme disease, such as those with oligoarticular arthritis. It should not be used as a screening procedure in patients with pain or fatigue syndromes. In such patients, the probability of a false-positive serologic result is higher than that of a true-positive result.

TABLE 74-1

ALGORITHM FOR TESTING FOR AND TREATING LYME DISEASE

PRETEST PROBABILITY	EXAMPLE	RECOMMENDATION
High	Patients with erythema migrans	Empirical antibiotic treatment without serologic testing
Intermediate	Patients with oligoarticular arthritis	Serologic testing and antibiotic treatment if test results are positive
Low	Patients with nonspecific symptoms (myalgias, arthralgias, fatigue)	Neither serologic testing nor antibiotic treatment

Source: Adapted from the recommendations of the American College of Physicians (G Nichol et al: Ann Intern Med 128:37, 1998, with permission).

For serologic analysis of Lyme disease in the United States, the CDC recommends a two-step approach in which samples are first tested by enzyme-linked immunosorbent assay (ELISA) and equivocal or positive results are then tested by Western blotting. During the first month of infection, both IgM and IgG responses to the spirochete should be determined, preferably in both acute- and convalescent-phase serum samples. Approximately 20–30% of patients have a positive response detectable in acute-phase samples, whereas ~70–80% have a positive response during convalescence (2–4 weeks later). After 1 month of infection (by which time most patients with active Lyme disease have disseminated infection), the sensitivity and specificity of the IgG response to the spirochete are both very high—in the range of 95–99%—as determined by the two-test approach of ELISA and Western blot. At this point and thereafter, a single test (that for IgG) is usually sufficient. In persons with illness of >1 month's duration, a positive IgM test result alone is likely to be false-positive and therefore should not be used to support the diagnosis.

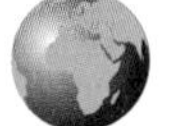

According to current criteria adopted by the CDC, an IgM Western blot is considered positive if two of the following three bands are present: 23, 39, and 41 kDa. However, the combination of the 23- and 41-kDa bands may still represent a false-positive result. An IgG blot is considered positive if 5 of the following 10 bands are present: 18, 23, 28, 30, 39, 41, 45, 58, 66, and 93 kDa. In European cases, there is less expansion of the antibody response, and no single set of criteria for the interpretation of immunoblots results in high levels of sensitivity and specificity in all countries.

Several second-generation tests that use recombinant spirochetal proteins or synthetic peptides have shown promising results. For example, an IgG ELISA employing a 26-mer peptide from invariant region 6 (IR_6) of the VlsE lipoprotein has a sensitivity and a specificity similar to those achieved with the IgM and IgG two-test approach using sonicated whole spirochetes. However, the IR_6 ELISA has a limitation similar to that affecting standard serology, in that a positive test result does not distinguish clearly between active and past infection. The IR_6 ELISA may be of value with regard to European as well as American strains of the spirochete.

DIFFERENTIAL DIAGNOSIS

Classic EM is a slowly expanding erythema, often with partial central clearing. If the lesion expands little, it may represent the red papule of an uninfected tick bite. If the lesion expands rapidly, it may represent cellulitis (e.g., streptococcal cellulitis) or an allergic reaction, perhaps to tick saliva. Patients with secondary annular lesions may be thought to have erythema multiforme, but neither the development of blistering mucosal lesions nor the involvement of the palms or soles is a feature of *B. burgdorferi* infection. In the southeastern United States, an EM-like skin lesion, sometimes with mild systemic symptoms, may be associated with *Amblyomma americanum* tick bites, but the cause of this illness has not yet been identified.

In the United States, *I. scapularis* ticks may transmit not only *B. burgdorferi* but also *Babesia microti*, a red blood cell parasite (Chap. 117), or *Anaplasma phagocytophilum*, the agent of human granulocytotropic anaplasmosis (formerly human granulocytotropic ehrlichiosis; Chap. 75). Although babesiosis and anaplasmosis are most often asymptomatic, infection with any of these three agents may cause nonspecific systemic symptoms, and co-infected patients may have more severe or persistent symptoms than patients infected with a single agent. Standard blood counts may yield clues regarding the presence of co-infection. Anaplasmosis may cause leukopenia or thrombocytopenia, and babesiosis may cause thrombocytopenia or (in severe cases) hemolytic anemia. IgM serologic responses may confuse the diagnosis. For example, *A. phagocytophilum* may elicit a positive IgM response to *B. burgdorferi*. The frequency of co-infection in different studies has been variable. In one prospective study, 4% of patients with EM had evidence of co-infection.

Facial palsy caused by *B. burgdorferi*, which occurs in the early disseminated phase of the infection (often in July, August, or September), is usually recognized by its association with EM. However, in rare cases, facial palsy without EM may be the presenting manifestation of Lyme disease. In such cases, both the IgM and the IgG responses to the spirochete are usually positive. The most common infectious agents that cause facial palsy are herpes simplex virus type 1 (Bell's palsy; Chap. 80) and varicella-zoster virus (Ramsay Hunt syndrome; Chap. 81).

Later in the infection, oligoarticular Lyme arthritis most resembles reactive arthritis in an adult or the pauciarticular form of juvenile rheumatoid arthritis in a child. Patients with Lyme arthritis usually have the highest IgG antibody responses seen in the infection, with reactivity to many spirochetal proteins.

The most common problem in diagnosis is to mistake Lyme disease for chronic fatigue syndrome (Chap. 31) or fibromyalgia. This difficulty is compounded by the fact that a small percentage of patients do in fact develop these chronic pain or fatigue syndromes in association with or soon after Lyme disease. Compared with Lyme disease, chronic fatigue syndrome or fibromyalgia tends to produce more generalized and disabling symptoms, including marked fatigue, severe headache, diffuse musculoskeletal pain, multiple symmetric tender points in characteristic locations, pain and stiffness in many joints, diffuse dysesthesia, difficulty with concentration, and sleep disturbances. Patients with chronic fatigue syndrome or fibromyalgia lack evidence of joint inflammation; they have normal results in neurologic tests; and they usually have a greater degree of anxiety and depression than patients with chronic neuroborreliosis.

℞ Treatment: LYME BORRELIOSIS

As outlined in the algorithm in Fig. 74-2, the various manifestations of Lyme disease can usually be treated

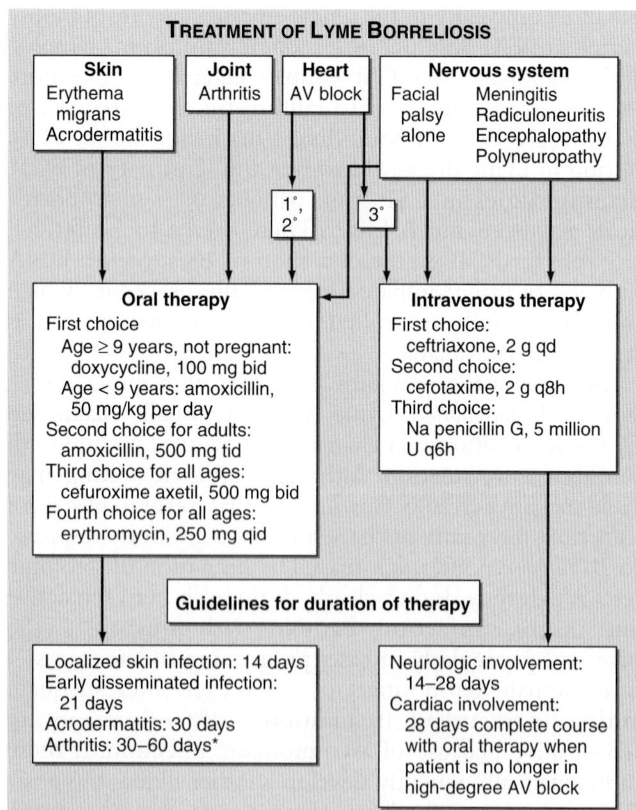

FIGURE 74-2

Algorithm for the treatment of the various acute or chronic manifestations of Lyme borreliosis. AV, atrioventricular. *For Lyme arthritis, IV ceftriaxone (2 g given once a day for 14–28 days) is also effective and is necessary for a small percentage of patients; however, compared with oral treatment, this regimen is less convenient to administer, has more side effects, and is more expensive.

successfully with orally administered antibiotics; the exceptions are objective neurologic abnormalities and third-degree atrioventricular heart block, which are generally treated with IV antibiotics. For early Lyme disease, doxycycline is effective in men and in nonpregnant women. An advantage of this regimen is that it is also effective against *A. phagocytophilum*, which is transmitted by the same tick that transmits the Lyme disease agent. Amoxicillin, cefuroxime axetil, and erythromycin or its congeners are second-, third-, and fourth-choice alternatives, respectively. In children, amoxicillin is effective (not more than 2 g/d); in cases of penicillin allergy, cefuroxime axetil or erythromycin may be used. In contrast to second- or third-generation cephalosporin antibiotics, first-generation cephalosporins, such as cephalexin, are not effective. For patients with infection localized to the skin, a 14-day course of therapy is generally sufficient; in contrast, for patients with disseminated infection, a 21-day course is recommended. Approximately 15% of patients experience a Jarisch-Herxheimer-like reaction during the first 24 h of therapy. In multicenter studies, >90% of patients whose early Lyme disease was treated with these regimens had satisfactory outcomes. Although some patients reported symptoms after treatment, objective evidence of persistent infection or relapse was rare, and re-treatment was usually unnecessary.

Oral administration of doxycycline or amoxicillin for 30 days is recommended for the initial treatment of Lyme arthritis in patients who do not have concomitant neurologic involvement. Among patients with arthritis who do not respond to oral antibiotics, re-treatment with IV ceftriaxone for 28 days is appropriate. In patients with arthritis in whom joint inflammation persists for months or even several years after both oral and IV antibiotics, despite a negative PCR result for *B. burgdorferi* DNA in joint fluid, treatment with anti-inflammatory agents or synovectomy may be successful.

For objective neurologic abnormalities (with the possible exception of facial palsy alone), parenteral antibiotic therapy is indicated. IV ceftriaxone, given for 14–28 days, is most commonly used for this purpose, but IV cefotaxime or IV penicillin G for the same duration may also be effective. In patients with high-degree atrioventricular block or a PR interval >0.3 s, IV therapy for at least part of the course and cardiac monitoring are recommended, but the insertion of a permanent pacemaker is not necessary.

It is unclear how and whether asymptomatic infection should be treated, but patients with such infection are often given a course of oral antibiotics. Because maternal-fetal transmission of *B. burgdorferi* seems to occur rarely (if at all), standard therapy for the manifestations of the illness is recommended for pregnant women. Long-term persistence of *B. burgdorferi* has not been documented in any large series of patients after treatment with currently recommended regimens. Therefore, there is no indication for multiple, repeated antibiotic courses in the treatment of Lyme disease.

After appropriately treated Lyme disease, a small percentage of patients continue to have subjective symptoms, primarily musculoskeletal pain, neurocognitive difficulties, or fatigue. This *chronic Lyme disease* or *post–Lyme syndrome* is a disabling condition that is similar to chronic fatigue syndrome or fibromyalgia. In a large study, one group of patients with post–Lyme syndrome received IV ceftriaxone for 30 days followed by oral doxycycline for 60 days, whereas another group received IV and oral placebo preparations for the same durations. No significant differences were found between groups in the numbers of patients reporting that their symptoms had improved, become worse, or stayed the same. Such patients are best treated for the relief of symptoms rather than with prolonged courses of antibiotics.

The risk of infection with *B. burgdorferi* after a recognized tick bite is so low that antibiotic prophylaxis is not routinely indicated. However, if an attached, engorged *I. scapularis* nymph is found or if follow-up is anticipated to be difficult, a single 200-mg dose of doxycycline, which usually prevents Lyme disease when given within 72 h after the tick bite, may be administered.

PROGNOSIS

The response to treatment is best early in the disease. Later treatment of Lyme borreliosis is still effective, but the period of convalescence may be longer. Eventually, most patients recover with minimal or no residual deficits.

REINFECTION

Reinfection may occur after EM when patients are treated with antimicrobial agents. In such cases, the immune response is not adequate to provide protection from subsequent infection. However, patients who develop an expanded immune response to the spirochete over a period of months (such as those with Lyme arthritis) have protective immunity for a period of years and do not acquire the infection again.

PREVENTION

Protective measures for the prevention of Lyme disease may include the avoidance of tick-infested areas, the use of repellents and acaricides, tick checks, and modification of landscapes in or near residential areas. Although a vaccine for Lyme disease used to be available, the manufacturer has discontinued its production. Therefore, no vaccine is now commercially available for the prevention of this infection.

FURTHER READINGS

BACON RM et al: Serodiagnosis of Lyme disease by kinetic immunosorbent assay using recombinant VlsE1 or peptide antigens of *Borrelia burgdorferi* compared with 2-tiered testing using whole-cell lysates. J Infect Dis 187:1187, 2003

FEDER HM et al: A critical appraisal of "chronic Lyme disease." N Engl J Med 357:1422, 2007

HALPERIN JJ et al: Practice Parameter: Treatment of nervous system Lyme disease (an evidence-based review). Report of the Quality Standards Subcommittee of the American Academy of Neurology. Neurology 69:91, 2007

KLEMPNER MS et al: Two controlled trials of antibiotic treatment in patients with persistent symptoms and a history of Lyme disease. N Engl J Med 345:85, 2001

NADELMAN RB et al: Prophylaxis with single-dose doxycycline for the prevention of Lyme disease after *Ixodes scapularis* tick bite. N Engl J Med 345:79, 2001

STEERE AC: Lyme disease. N Engl J Med 345:115, 2001

_____, ANGELIS SM: Therapy for Lyme arthritis: Strategies for the treatment of antibiotic-refractory arthritis. Arthritis Rheum 54:3079, 2006

_____ et al: Antibiotic-refractory Lyme arthritis is associated with HLA-DR molecules that bind a *Borrelia burgdorferi* peptide. J Exp Med 203:961, 2006

_____ et al: The emergence of Lyme disease. J Clin Invest 113:1093, 2004

TIBBLES CD, EDLOW JA: Does this patient have erythema migrans? JAMA 297:2617, 2007

WORMSER GP et al: The clinical assessment, treatment and prevention of Lyme disease, anaplasmosis, and babesiosis: Clinical practice guidelines of the Infectious Diseases Society of America. Clin Infect Dis 43:1089, 2006

PART 7 DISEASES CAUSED BY RICKETTSIAE, MYCOPLASMAS, AND CHLAMYDIAE

CHAPTER 75

RICKETTSIAL DISEASES

David H. Walker ■ J. Stephen Dumler ■ Thomas Marrie

The rickettsiae are a heterogeneous group of small, obligately intracellular, gram-negative coccobacilli and short bacilli, most of which are transmitted by a tick, mite, flea, or louse vector. Except for louse-borne typhus, humans are incidental hosts. Among rickettsiae, *Coxiella burnetii, Rickettsia prowazekii,* and *R. typhi* have the well-documented ability to survive for an extended period outside the reservoir or vector and to be extremely infectious: inhalation of a single *Coxiella* microorganism can cause pneumonia. High infectivity and severe illness after inhalation make *R. prowazekii, R. rickettsii, R. typhi, R. conorii,* and *C. burnetii* bioterrorism threats.

Clinical infections with rickettsiae can be classified according to (1) the taxonomy and diverse microbial characteristics of the agents, which belong to six genera (*Rickettsia, Orientia, Ehrlichia, Anaplasma, Neorickettsia,* and *Coxiella*); (2) epidemiology; or (3) clinical manifestations. The clinical manifestations of all the acute presentations are similar during the first 5 days: fever, headache, and myalgias with or without nausea, vomiting, and cough. As the course progresses, clinical manifestations—including occurrence of a macular, maculopapular, or vesicular rash; eschar; pneumonitis; and meningoencephalitis—vary from one disease to another. Given the 12 etiologic agents with varied mechanisms of transmission, geographic distributions, and associated disease manifestations, the consideration of rickettsial diseases as a single entity poses complex challenges (Table 75-1).

Establishing the etiologic diagnosis of rickettsioses is very difficult during the acute stage of illness, and definitive diagnosis usually requires the examination of paired serum samples after convalescence. Heightened clinical suspicion is based on epidemiologic data, history of exposure to vectors or reservoir animals, travel to endemic locations, clinical manifestations (sometimes including rash or eschar), and characteristic laboratory findings [including thrombocytopenia, normal or low white blood cell (WBC) counts, elevated hepatic enzyme levels, and hyponatremia]. Such suspicion should prompt empirical treatment. Doxycycline is the drug of choice for most of these infections. Only one agent, *C. burnetii*, has been documented to cause chronic illness. One other, *R. prowazekii*, causes recrudescent illness (Brill-Zinsser disease) when latent infection is reactivated years after resolution of the acute illness.

Rickettsial infections dominated by fever may resolve without further clinical evolution. However, after nonspecific early manifestations, the illnesses can also evolve along one or more of several principal clinical lines: (1) development of a macular or maculopapular rash; (2) development of an eschar at the site of tick or mite feeding; (3) development of a vesicular rash (often in rickettsialpox and African tick-bite fever); (4) development of

TABLE 75-1

FEATURES OF SELECTED RICKETTSIAL INFECTIONS

DISEASE	ORGANISM	TRANSMISSION	GEOGRAPHIC RANGE	INCUBATION PERIOD (DAYS)	DURATION (DAYS)	RASH (%)	ESCHAR (%)	LYMPHADENOPATHY[a]
Rocky Mountain spotted fever	*Rickettsia rickettsii*	Tick bite: *Dermacentor andersoni*	United States	2–14	10–20	90	<1	+
		D. variabilis	United States					
		Amblyomma cajennense, A. aureolatum	Central/South America					
		Rhipicephalus sanguineus	Mexico, United States					
Mediterranean spotted fever[b]	*R. conorii*	Tick bite: *R. sanguineus, R. pumilio*	Southern Europe, Africa, Middle East, Central Asia	5–7	7–14	97	50	+
African tick-bite fever	*R. africae*	Tick bite: *A. hebraeum, A. variegatum*	Sub-Saharan Africa, West Indies	4–10	?	50	90	++++
Rickettsialpox	*R. akari*	Mite bite: *Liponyssoides sanguineus*	United States, Ukraine, Croatia	10–17	3–11	100	90	+++
Flea-borne spotted fever	*R. felis*	Flea (mechanism undetermined): *Ctenocephalides felis*	North and South America, Europe	8–16	8–16	80	15	—
Epidemic typhus	*R. prowazekii*	Louse feces: *Pediculus humanus corporis,* fleas and lice of flying squirrels, or recrudescence	Worldwide	7–14	10–18	80	None	—
Tick-borne lymphadenopathy	*R. slovaca*	Tick bite: *Dermacentor marginatus, D. reticularis*	Europe	7–9	17–180	5	100	++++
Murine typhus	*R. typhi*	Flea feces: *Xenopsylla cheopis, C. felis*, others	Worldwide	8–16	8–16	80	None	—
Human monocytotropic ehrlichiosis	*Ehrlichia chaffeensis*	Tick bite: *Amblyomma americanum, D. variabilis*	United States	1–21	3–21	36	None	++
Human granulocytotropic anaplasmosis	*Anaplasma phagocytophilum*	Tick bite: *Ixodes scapularis, I. ricinus, I. pacificus*	United States, Europe, Asia	1–21	3–14	Rare	None	—
Scrub typhus	*Orientia tsutsugamushi*	Mite bite: *Leptotrombidium deliense,* others	Asia, Australia, New Guinea, Pacific Islands	9–18	6–21	50	35	+++
Q fever	*Coxiella burnetii*	Inhalation of aerosols of infected parturition material (sheep, dogs, others), ingestion of infected milk or milk products	Worldwide	3–30	5–57	<1	None	—

[a]++++, severe; +++, marked; ++, moderate; +, present in a small portion of cases; —, not a noted feature.
[b]Eschar is usually present at the bite site.

pneumonitis with chest radiographic opacities and/or rales [Q fever and severe cases of Rocky Mountain spotted fever (RMSF), Mediterranean spotted fever (MSF), louse-borne typhus, human monocytotropic ehrlichiosis (HME), human granulocytotropic anaplasmosis (HGA), scrub typhus, and murine typhus]; (5) development of meningoencephalitis [louse-borne typhus and severe cases of RMSF, scrub typhus, HME, murine typhus, MSF, and (rarely) Q fever]; and (6) progressive hypotension and multiorgan failure as seen with sepsis or toxic shock syndrome (RMSF, MSF, louse-borne typhus, murine typhus, scrub typhus, HME, and HGA).

Epidemiologic clues to the transmission of a particular pathogen include (1) environmental exposure to ticks, fleas, or mites during the season of activity of the vector species for the disease in the appropriate geographic region (spotted fever and typhus group rickettsioses, scrub typhus, ehrlichioses, anaplasmosis); (2) travel to or residence in an endemic geographic region during the incubation period (Table 75-1); (3) exposure to parturient ruminants, cats, and dogs (Q fever); (4) exposure to flying squirrels (*R. prowazekii* infection); and (5) history of previous louse-borne typhus (recrudescent typhus).

Clinical laboratory findings, such as thrombocytopenia (particularly in spotted fever and typhus rickettsioses, ehrlichioses, anaplasmosis, and scrub typhus), normal or low WBC counts, mild to moderate serum elevations of hepatic aminotransferases, and hyponatremia suggest some common pathophysiologic mechanisms.

Application of these clinical, epidemiologic, and laboratory principles requires a consideration of the possibility of a rickettsial diagnosis and a knowledge of the individual diseases.

TICK-, MITE-, LOUSE-, AND FLEA-BORNE RICKETTSIOSES

These diseases, caused by organisms of the genera *Rickettsia* and *Orientia* in the family Rickettsiaceae, result from endothelial infection and increased vascular permeability. Pathogenic rickettsial species are very closely related, have small genomes (as a result of reductive evolution, which eliminated genes for biosynthesis of intracellularly available molecules), and are traditionally separated into typhus and spotted fever groups on the basis of lipopolysaccharide antigens. Some diseases and their agents (e.g., *R. africae, R. parkeri*, and *R. sibirica*) are too similar to require separate descriptions. Indeed, the similarities among MSF (*R. conorii*, all strains), North Asian tick typhus (*R. sibirica*), Japanese spotted fever (*R. japonica*), and Flinders Island spotted fever (*R. honei*) far outweigh the minor variations. The Rickettsiaceae that cause life-threatening infections are, in order of decreasing case-fatality rate, *R. rickettsii* (RMSF); *R. prowazekii* (louse-borne typhus); *Orientia tsutsugamushi* (scrub typhus); *R. conorii* (MSF); *R. typhi* (murine typhus); and, in rare cases, other spotted fever group organisms. Some agents (e.g., *R. africae, R. akari, R. slovaca, R. honei, R. felis, R. aeschlimannii*, and *R. parkeri*) have never been documented to cause a fatal illness.

ROCKY MOUNTAIN SPOTTED FEVER

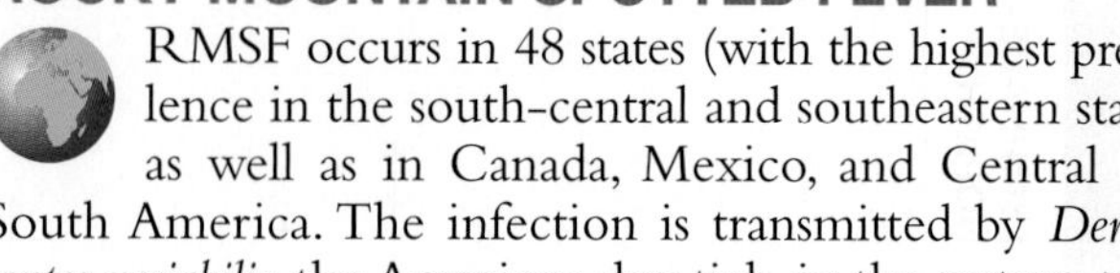

RMSF occurs in 48 states (with the highest prevalence in the south-central and southeastern states) as well as in Canada, Mexico, and Central and South America. The infection is transmitted by *Dermacentor variabilis*, the American dog tick, in the eastern two-thirds of the United States and California; by *D. andersoni*, the Rocky Mountain wood tick, in the western United States; by *Rhipicephalus sanguineus* in Mexico and Arizona; and by *Amblyomma cajennense* in Central and South America. Maintained principally by transovarian transmission from one generation of ticks to the next, *R. rickettsii* can be acquired by uninfected ticks through the ingestion of a blood meal from rickettsemic small mammals.

Humans become infected during tick season (in the Northern Hemisphere, from May to September), although some cases occur in winter. The mortality rate was 20–25% in the preantibiotic era and remains at ~3–5% principally because of delayed diagnosis and treatment. The case-fatality ratio increases with each decade of life above age 20.

Pathogenesis

R. rickettsii organisms are inoculated into the dermis along with secretions of the tick's salivary glands after ≥6 h of feeding. The rickettsiae spread lymphohematogenously throughout the body and infect numerous foci of contiguous endothelial cells. The dose-dependent incubation period is ~1 week (range, 2–14 days). Occlusive thrombosis and ischemic necrosis are not the fundamental pathologic basis for tissue and organ injury. Instead, increased vascular permeability, with resulting edema, hypovolemia, and ischemia, is responsible. Consumption of platelets results in thrombocytopenia in 32–52% of patients, but disseminated intravascular coagulation with hypofibrinogenemia is rare. Activation of platelets, generation of thrombin, and activation of the fibrinolytic system all appear to be homeostatic physiologic responses to endothelial injury.

Clinical Manifestations

Early in the illness, when medical attention usually is first sought, RMSF is difficult to distinguish from many self-limiting viral illnesses. Fever, headache, malaise, myalgia, nausea, vomiting, and anorexia are the most common symptoms during the first 3 days. The patient becomes progressively more ill as vascular infection and injury advance. In one large series, only one-third of patients were diagnosed with presumptive RMSF early in the clinical course and treated appropriately as outpatients. In the tertiary care setting, RMSF is all too often recognized only when late severe manifestations, developing at the end of the first week or during the second week of illness in patients without appropriate treatment, prompt return to a physician or hospital and admission to an intensive care unit.

The progressive nature of the infection is clearly manifested in the skin. Rash is evident in only 14% of

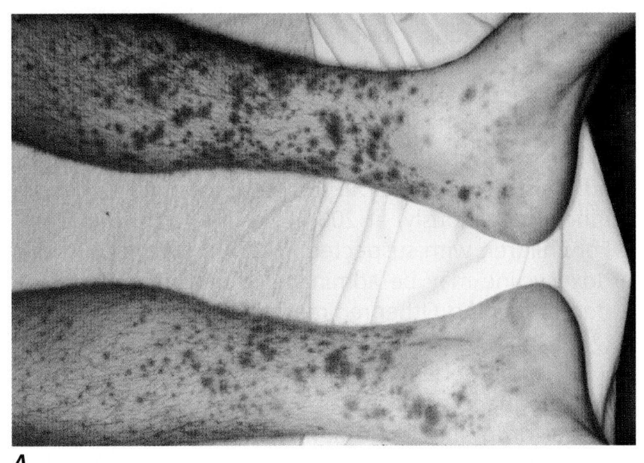

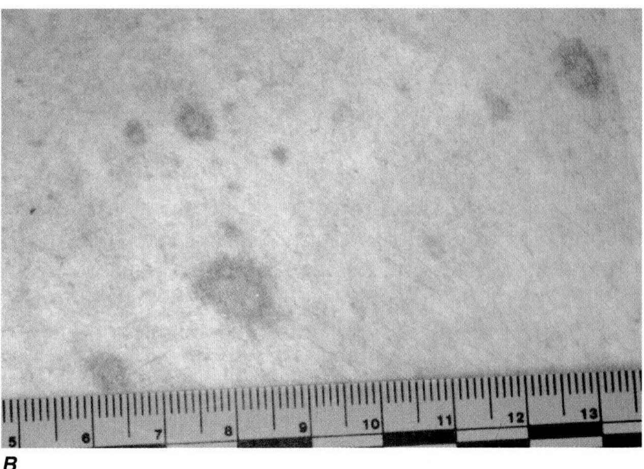

FIGURE 75-1

***A.* Petechial lesions of Rocky Mountain spotted fever** on the lower legs and soles of a young, previously healthy patient. ***B.* Close-up of lesions** from the same patient. (*Photos courtesy of Dr. Lindsey Baden; with permission.*)

patients on the first day of illness and in only 49% during the first 3 days. Macules (1–5 mm) appear first on the wrists and ankles and then on the remainder of the extremities and the trunk. Later, more severe vascular damage results in frank hemorrhage at the center of the maculopapule, producing a petechia that does not disappear upon compression (Fig. 75-1). This sequence of events is sometimes delayed or aborted by effective treatment. However, the rash is a variable manifestation, appearing on day 6 or later in 20% of cases and not appearing at all in 9–16% of cases. Petechiae occur in 41–59% of cases, appearing on or after day 6 in 74% of cases that include a rash. Involvement of the palms and soles, often considered diagnostically important, usually develops relatively late in the course (after day 5 in 43% of cases) and does not develop at all in 18–64% of cases.

Hypovolemia leads to prerenal azotemia and (in 17% of cases) hypotension. Infection of the pulmonary microcirculation leads to noncardiogenic pulmonary edema; 12% of patients have severe respiratory disease, and 8% require mechanical ventilation. Cardiac involvement manifests as dysrhythmia in 7–16% of cases.

Besides the preceding respiratory failure, central nervous system (CNS) involvement is the other important determinant of the outcome of RMSF. Encephalitis, presenting as confusion or lethargy, is apparent in 26–28% of cases. Progressively severe encephalitis manifests as stupor or delirium in 21–26% of cases, as ataxia in 18%, as coma in 10%, and as seizures in 8%. Numerous focal neurologic deficits have been reported. Meningoencephalitis results in cerebrospinal fluid (CSF) pleocytosis in 34–38% of cases; usually there are 10–100 cells/μL and a mononuclear predominance, but occasionally there are >100 cells/μL and a polymorphonuclear predominance. The CSF protein concentration is increased in 30–35% of cases, but the CSF glucose concentration is usually normal.

Renal failure, often reversible with rehydration, is caused by acute tubular necrosis in severe cases with shock. Hepatic injury with increased serum aminotransferase concentrations (38% of cases) is due to focal death of individual hepatocytes without hepatic failure. Jaundice is recognized in 9% of cases and an elevated serum bilirubin concentration in 18–30%.

Life-threatening bleeding is rare. Anemia develops in 30% of cases and is severe enough to require transfusions in 11%. Blood is detected in the stools or vomitus of 10% of patients, and death has followed massive upper gastrointestinal hemorrhage.

Other characteristic clinical laboratory findings include increased plasma levels of proteins of the acute-phase response (C-reactive protein, fibrinogen, ferritin, and others), hypoalbuminemia, and hyponatremia (in 56% of cases) due to the appropriate secretion of antidiuretic hormone in response to the hypovolemic state. Myositis occurs occasionally, with marked elevations in serum creatine kinase levels and multifocal rhabdomyonecrosis. Ocular involvement includes conjunctivitis in 30% of cases and retinal vein engorgement, flame hemorrhages, arterial occlusion, and papilledema with normal CSF pressure in some instances.

In untreated cases, the patient usually dies 8–15 days after onset. A rare presentation, fulminant RMSF, is fatal within 5 days after onset. This fulminant presentation is seen most often in black males with glucose-6-phosphate dehydrogenase (G6PD) deficiency and may be related to an undefined effect of hemolysis on the rickettsial infection. Although survivors of RMSF usually return to their previous state of health, permanent sequelae, including neurologic deficits and gangrene necessitating amputation of extremities, may follow severe illness.

Diagnosis

The diagnosis of RMSF during the acute stage is more difficult than is generally appreciated. The most important epidemiologic factor is a history of exposure to a potentially tick-infested environment within the 12 days preceding disease onset during a season of possible tick activity. However, only 60% of patients actually recall being bitten by a tick during the incubation period.

The differential diagnosis for early clinical manifestations of RMSF (fever, headache, and myalgia without a rash) includes influenza, enteroviral infection, infectious mononucleosis, viral hepatitis, leptospirosis, typhoid fever, gram-negative or gram-positive bacterial sepsis, HME, HGA, murine typhus, sylvatic flying-squirrel typhus, and rickettsialpox. Enterocolitis may be suggested by nausea, vomiting, and abdominal pain; prominence of abdominal tenderness has resulted in exploratory laparotomy. CNS involvement may masquerade as bacterial or viral meningoencephalitis. Cough, pulmonary signs, and chest radiographic opacities may lead to a diagnostic consideration of bronchitis or pneumonia.

At presentation during the first 3 days of illness, only 3% of patients exhibit the classic triad of fever, rash, and history of tick exposure. When a rash appears, a diagnosis of RMSF should certainly be considered. However, many illnesses considered in the differential diagnosis may also be associated with a rash, including rubeola, rubella, meningococcemia, disseminated gonococcal infection, secondary syphilis, toxic shock syndrome, drug hypersensitivity, idiopathic thrombocytopenic purpura, thrombotic thrombocytopenic purpura, Kawasaki syndrome, and immune complex vasculitis. Conversely, any person in an endemic area with a provisional diagnosis of one of the above illnesses may have RMSF. Thus, if a viral infection is suspected during RMSF season in an endemic area, it should always be kept in mind that RMSF can mimic viral infection early in the course; if the illness worsens over the next couple of days after initial presentation, the patient should return for reevaluation.

The most common serologic test for confirmation of the diagnosis is the indirect immunofluorescence assay. Not until 7–10 days after onset is a diagnostic titer of ≥1:64 usually detectable. The sensitivity and specificity of the indirect immunofluorescence assay are 94–100% and 100%, respectively. It is important to understand that serologic tests for RMSF are usually negative at the time of presentation for medical care and that treatment should not be delayed while a positive serologic result is awaited.

The only diagnostic test that is useful during the acute illness is immunohistologic examination of a cutaneous biopsy sample from a rash lesion for *R. rickettsii*. Examination of a 3-mm punch biopsy from such a lesion is 70% sensitive and 100% specific. Polymerase chain reaction (PCR) amplification and detection of *R. rickettsii* DNA in peripheral blood is a relatively insensitive approach except when the patient is already in the preterminal state. Rickettsiae are present in large quantities in heavily infected foci of endothelial cells but in relatively low quantities in the circulation. Cultivation of rickettsiae in cell culture is feasible but is seldom undertaken because of biohazard concerns.

℞ Treatment: ROCKY MOUNTAIN SPOTTED FEVER

The drug of choice for the treatment of both children and adults with RMSF is doxycycline, except when the patient is pregnant or allergic to this drug (see below). Because of the severity of RMSF, immediate empirical administration of doxycycline should be strongly considered for any patient with a consistent clinical presentation in the appropriate epidemiologic setting. Doxycycline is administered orally (or, in the presence of coma or vomiting, intravenously) at 200 mg/d in two divided doses. For children with suspected RMSF, up to five courses of doxycycline may be administered with minimal risk of dental staining. Other regimens include oral tetracycline (25–50 mg/kg per day) in four divided doses. Treatment with chloramphenicol is advised only for patients who are pregnant or allergic to doxycycline. The antirickettsial drug should be administered until the patient has been afebrile and improving clinically for 2–3 days. β-Lactam antibiotics, erythromycin, and aminoglycosides have no role in the treatment of RMSF, and sulfa-containing drugs are likely to exacerbate this infection. There is little clinical experience with fluoroquinolones, clarithromycin, and azithromycin, which are not recommended. The most seriously ill patients are managed in intensive care units, with careful administration of fluids to achieve optimal tissue perfusion without precipitating noncardiogenic pulmonary edema. In some severely ill patients, hypoxemia requires intubation and mechanical ventilation, oliguric or anuric acute renal failure requires hemodialysis, seizures necessitate the use of antiseizure medication, anemia or severe hemorrhage necessitates transfusions of packed red blood cells, or bleeding with severe thrombocytopenia requires platelet transfusions. Heparin is not a useful component of treatment, and there is no evidence that glucocorticoids affect outcome.

Prevention

Avoidance of tick bites is the only available preventive approach. Use of protective clothing and tick repellents, inspection of the body once or twice a day, and removal of ticks before they inoculate rickettsiae reduce the risk of infection.

MEDITERRANEAN SPOTTED FEVER (BOUTONNEUSE FEVER), AFRICAN TICK-BITE FEVER, AND OTHER TICK-BORNE SPOTTED FEVERS

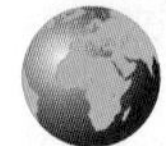

R. conorii is prevalent in southern Europe, Africa, and southwestern and south-central Asia. Regional names for the disease caused by this organism include Mediterranean spotted fever, Kenya tick typhus, Indian tick typhus, Israeli spotted fever, and Astrakhan spotted fever. The disease is characterized by high fever, rash, and—in most geographic locales—an inoculation eschar (*tâche noire*) at the site of the tick bite. A severe form of the disease (mortality rate, 50%) occurs in patients with diabetes, alcoholism, or heart failure.

African tick-bite fever, caused by *R. africae*, occurs in rural areas of Sub-Saharan Africa and in the Caribbean islands and is transmitted by *Amblyomma hebraeum* and *A. variegatum* ticks. The average incubation period is 7 days.

The mild illness consists of headache, fever, eschar, and regional lymphadenopathy. *Amblyomma* ticks often feed in groups, with the consequent development of multiple eschars. Rash may be vesicular, sparse, or absent altogether. Because of tourism in Sub-Saharan Africa, African tick-bite fever is the most frequently imported rickettsiosis in Europe and North America. A similar disease caused by the very closely related *R. parkeri* is transmitted by *A. maculatum* in the United States and *A. triste* in South America.

R. japonica causes *Japanese spotted fever,* which also occurs in Korea. A similar disease in northern Asia is caused by *R. sibirica. Queensland tick typhus* due to *R. australis* is transmitted by *Ixodes holocyclus. Flinders Island spotted fever,* found on the island for which it is named as well as in other parts of Tasmania, in mainland Australia, and in southeastern Asia, is caused by *R. honei.* In Europe, patients infected with *R. slovaca* after a wintertime *Dermacentor* tick bite manifest an afebrile illness with an eschar (usually on the scalp) and regional lymphadenopathy.

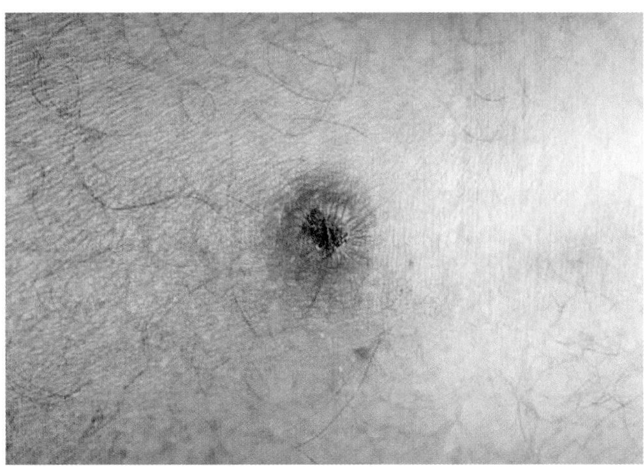

FIGURE 75-2
Eschar at the site of the mite bite in a patient with rickettsialpox. *(Reprinted from A Krusell et al: Emerg Infect Dis 8:727, 2002. Photo obtained by Dr. Kenneth Kaye.)*

Diagnosis

Diagnosis of these tick-borne spotted fevers is based on clinical and epidemiologic findings and is confirmed by serology, immunohistochemical demonstration of rickettsiae in skin biopsy specimens, cell-culture isolation of rickettsiae, or PCR of skin biopsy or blood samples. The serologic identification of the etiologic species requires knowledge of all the potential agents as well as expensive, laborious cross-adsorption of the patient's serum. In an endemic area, patients presenting with fever, rash, and/or a skin lesion consisting of a black necrotic area or a crust surrounded by erythema should be considered to have one of these rickettsial spotted fevers.

℞ Treatment: TICK-BORNE SPOTTED FEVERS

Successful therapeutic agents include doxycycline (100 mg bid orally for 1–5 days), ciprofloxacin (750 mg bid orally for 5 days), and chloramphenicol (500 mg qid orally for 7–10 days). Pregnant patients may be treated with josamycin (3 g/d orally for 5 days). Data on the efficacy of treatment of mildly ill children with clarithromycin or azithromycin should not be extrapolated to adults or to patients with moderate or severe illness.

RICKETTSIALPOX

R. akari infects mice and their mites (*Liponyssoides sanguineus*), which maintain the organisms by transovarian transmission.

Epidemiology

Rickettsialpox is recognized principally in New York City, but cases have also been reported in other urban and rural locations in the United States and in Ukraine, Croatia, and Turkey. Investigation of eschars suspected of representing bioterrorism-associated cutaneous anthrax has revealed that rickettsialpox occurs more frequently than previously realized.

Clinical Manifestations

A papule forms at the site of the mite's feeding, develops a central vesicle, and becomes a 1- to 2.5-cm painless black crusted eschar surrounded by an erythematous halo (Fig. 75-2). Enlargement of the regional lymph nodes draining the eschar suggests initial lymphogenous spread. After an incubation period of 10–17 days, during which the eschar and regional lymphadenopathy frequently go unnoticed, onset is marked by malaise, chills, fever, headache, and myalgia. A macular rash appears 2–6 days after onset and evolves sequentially into papules, vesicles, and crusts that heal without scarring (Fig. 75-3). The rash may remain macular or maculopapular. Some patients develop nausea, vomiting, abdominal pain, cough, conjunctivitis, or photophobia. If untreated, fever lasts 6–10 days.

Diagnosis and Treatment

Clinical, epidemiologic, and convalescent serologic data establish the diagnosis of a spotted fever group rickettsiosis that is seldom pursued further. Doxycycline is the drug of choice for treatment.

FLEA-BORNE SPOTTED FEVER

An emerging rickettsiosis caused by *R. felis* probably occurs worldwide. Maintained transovarially in the geographically widespread cat flea *Ctenocephalides felis*, the infection has been described as moderately severe, with fever, rash, headache, and CNS and gastrointestinal symptoms.

ENDEMIC MURINE TYPHUS

Epidemiology

R. typhi is maintained in mammalian host/flea cycles, with rats (*Rattus rattus* and *R. norvegicus*) and the Oriental

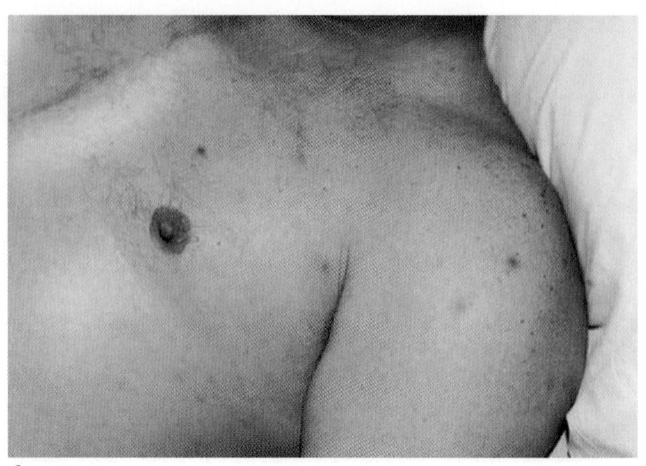

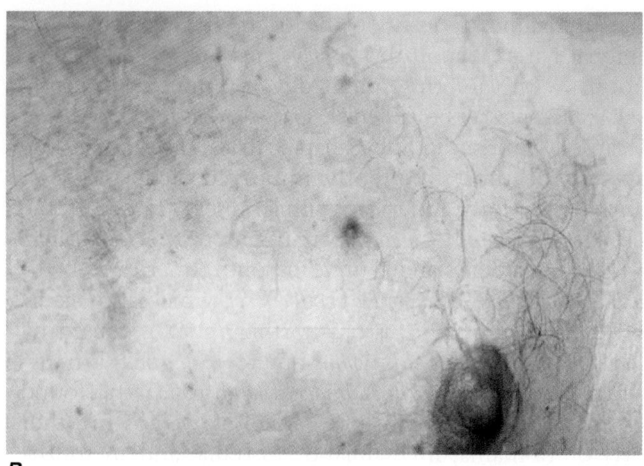

FIGURE 75-3

***A.* Papulovesicular lesions on the trunk of the patient with rickettsialpox** shown in Fig. 75-2. ***B.* Close-up of lesions** from the same patient. (*Reprinted from A Krusell et al: Emerg Infect Dis 8:727, 2002. Photos obtained by Dr. Kenneth Kaye.*)

rat flea (*Xenopsylla cheopis*) as the classic zoonotic niche. Fleas acquire *R. typhi* from rickettsemic rats and carry the organism throughout their life span. Nonimmune rats and humans are infected when rickettsia-laden flea feces contaminate pruritic bite lesions; less frequently, the flea bite transmits the organisms. Transmission also may occur via inhalation of aerosolized rickettsiae from flea feces. Infected rats appear healthy, although they are rickettsemic for ~2 weeks.

Murine typhus occurs mainly in southern Texas and southern California, where the classic rat/flea cycle is absent and an opossum/cat flea (*C. felis*) cycle is prominent. Globally, endemic typhus occurs year-round, mainly in warm (often coastal) areas throughout the tropics and subtropics, where it is highly prevalent though often unrecognized. The incidence peaks from April through June in southern Texas and during the warm months of summer and early fall in other geographic locations. Patients seldom recall exposure to fleas, although exposure to animals such as cats, opossums, and rats is reported in nearly 40% of cases.

Clinical Manifestations

The incubation period of experimental murine typhus averages 11 days (range, 8–16 days). Headache, myalgia, arthralgia, nausea, and malaise develop 1–3 days before onset of chills and fever. Nearly all patients experience nausea and vomiting early in the illness.

The duration of untreated illness averages 12 days (range, 9–18 days). Rash is present in only 13% of patients at presentation for medical care (usually ~4 days after onset of fever), appearing an average of 2 days later in half of the remaining patients and never appearing in the others. The initial macular rash is often detected by careful inspection of the axilla or the inner surface of the arm. Subsequently, the rash becomes maculopapular, involving the trunk more often than the extremities; it is seldom petechial and rarely involves the face, palms, or soles. A rash is detected in only 20% of patients with darkly pigmented skin.

Pulmonary involvement is frequently prominent; 35% of patients have a hacking, nonproductive cough, and 23% of patients who undergo chest radiography have pulmonary densities due to interstitial pneumonia, pulmonary edema, and pleural effusions. Bibasilar rales are the most common pulmonary sign. Less common clinical manifestations include abdominal pain, confusion, stupor, seizures, ataxia, coma, and jaundice. Clinical laboratory studies frequently reveal anemia and leukopenia early in the course, leukocytosis late in the course, thrombocytopenia, hyponatremia, hypoalbuminemia, mildly increased serum hepatic aminotransferases, and prerenal azotemia. Complications may include respiratory failure, hematemesis, cerebral hemorrhage, and hemolysis. Severe illness necessitates the admission of 10% of hospitalized patients to an intensive care unit. Greater severity is generally associated with old age, underlying disease, and treatment with a sulfonamide; the case-fatality rate is 1%. In a study of children with murine typhus, 50% suffered only nocturnal fevers, feeling well enough for active daytime play.

Diagnosis and Treatment

Cultivation, PCR, or cross-adsorption serologic studies of acute- and convalescent-phase sera can provide a specific diagnosis, and an immunohistochemical method for identification of typhus group-specific antigens has been developed. Nevertheless, most patients are treated empirically with doxycycline (100 mg bid orally for 7–15 days) on the basis of clinical suspicion. Serologic methods are usually used when laboratory confirmation of the diagnosis is sought.

EPIDEMIC (LOUSE-BORNE) TYPHUS

The human body louse (*Pediculus humanus corporis*) lives in clothing under poor hygienic conditions and usually in impoverished cold areas. Lice acquire *R. prowazekii* when they ingest blood from a rickettsemic patient. The rickettsiae multiply in the midgut epithelial cells of the louse and are shed in the louse's feces. The infected louse leaves a febrile person and deposits infected feces on its subsequent host during its blood meal; the patient autoinoculates the organisms by scratching. The louse is killed by the rickettsiae and does not pass *R. prowazekii* to its offspring.

Epidemic typhus haunts regions afflicted by wars and disasters. An outbreak involved 100,000 people in refugee camps in Burundi in 1997. A small focus occurred in Russia in 1998; sporadic cases have been reported from Algeria, and frequent outbreaks have occurred in Peru. Eastern flying-squirrels (*Glaucomys volans*) and their lice and fleas maintain *R. prowazekii* in a zoonotic cycle. The fleas transmit the infection sporadically to humans.

Brill-Zinsser disease is a recrudescent illness occurring years after acute epidemic typhus, probably as a result of waning immunity. Typhus infection remains latent for years; its reactivation results in sporadic cases of disease in louse-free populations or in epidemics in louse-infested populations.

Rickettsiae are potential agents of bioterrorism (Chap. 6). Infections with *R. prowazekii* and *R. rickettsii* have high case-fatality ratios. These organisms cause difficult-to-diagnose diseases, are highly infectious when inhaled as aerosols, and have been selected for resistance to tetracycline or chloramphenicol in the laboratory.

Clinical Manifestations

After an incubation period of ~1 week, the onset of illness is abrupt, with prostration, severe headache, and fever rising rapidly to 38.8°–40.0°C (102°–104°F). Cough is prominent, occurring in 70% of patients. Myalgias are usually severe. In the outbreak in Burundi, the disease was referred to as sutama ("crouching"), a designation reflecting the posture of patients attempting to alleviate the pain. A rash begins on the upper trunk, usually on the fifth day, and then becomes generalized, involving the entire body except the face, palms, and soles. Initially, this rash is macular; without treatment, it becomes maculopapular, petechial, and confluent. The rash often is not detected on black skin; 60% of African patients have spotless epidemic typhus. Photophobia, with considerable conjunctival injection and eye pain, is frequent. The tongue may be dry, brown, and furred. Confusion and coma are common. Skin necrosis and gangrene of the digits as well as interstitial pneumonia may occur in severe cases. Untreated disease is fatal in 7–40% of cases, with outcome depending primarily on the condition of the host. Patients with untreated infections develop renal insufficiency and multiorgan involvement in which neurologic manifestations are frequently prominent. Overall, 12% of patients with epidemic typhus have neurologic involvement. Infection associated with North American flying squirrels is a milder illness; whether this milder disease is due to host factors (e.g., better health status) or attenuated virulence is unknown.

Diagnosis and Treatment

Epidemic typhus is sometimes misdiagnosed as typhoid fever in tropical countries (Chap. 54). The means even for serologic studies are often unavailable in settings of louse-borne typhus. Epidemics may be recognized by the serologic or immunohistochemical diagnosis of a single case or by detection of *R. prowazekii* in a louse found on a patient. Cross-adsorption indirect fluorescent antibody (IFA) studies can distinguish *R. prowazekii* and *R. typhi* infections. Doxycycline (200 mg/d, given in two divided doses) is administered orally or—if the patient is comatose or vomiting—intravenously. Although under epidemic conditions a single 200-mg dose has proved effective, treatment is generally continued until 2–3 days after defervescence. Pregnant patients should be evaluated individually and treated with either chloramphenicol early in pregnancy or, if necessary, doxycycline late in pregnancy.

Prevention

Prevention of epidemic typhus involves control of body lice. Clothes should be changed regularly, and insecticides should be used every 6 weeks to control the louse population.

SCRUB TYPHUS

O. tsutsugamushi differs substantially from *Rickettsia* species both genetically and in terms of cell wall composition (i.e., it lacks lipopolysaccharide and peptidoglycan). *O. tsutsugamushi* is maintained by transovarian transmission in trombiculid mites. After hatching, infected larval mites (chiggers, the only stage that feeds on a host) inoculate organisms into the skin. Infected chiggers are found particularly in areas of heavy scrub vegetation during the wet season, when mites lay eggs.

Scrub typhus is endemic in eastern and southern Asia, northern Australia, and islands of the western Pacific and Indian Oceans. Infections are prevalent in these regions; in some areas, >3% of the population is infected or reinfected each month. Immunity wanes over 1–3 years, and the organism exhibits remarkable antigenic diversity.

Clinical Manifestations

Illness varies from mild and self-limiting to fatal. After an incubation period of 6–21 days, onset is characterized by fever, headache, myalgia, cough, and gastrointestinal symptoms. Some patients recover spontaneously after a few days. The classic case description includes an eschar where the chigger feeds, regional lymphadenopathy, and a maculopapular rash—signs that are seldom seen in indigenous patients. Fewer than 50% of Westerners develop an eschar, and fewer than 40% develop a rash (on day 4–6 of illness). Severe cases typically include encephalitis and interstitial pneumonia due to vascular injury. The case-fatality rate for untreated classic cases is 7% but would probably be lower if all mild cases were diagnosed.

Diagnosis and Treatment

Serologic assays (IFA, indirect immunoperoxidase, and enzyme immunoassays) are the mainstays of laboratory diagnosis. Patients are treated with doxycycline (100 mg bid orally for 7–15 days) or chloramphenicol (500 mg qid orally for 7–15 days).

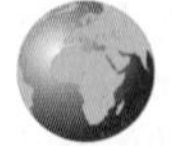

Some cases of scrub typhus in Thailand are caused by doxycycline- or chloramphenicol-resistant strains that are susceptible to rifampin. Azithromycin and clarithromycin have been used successfully in a few patients.

EHRLICHIOSES AND ANAPLASMOSIS

Ehrlichioses are acute febrile infections caused by members of the family Anaplasmataceae, which is made up of obligately intracellular organisms transmitted by ticks and contains four genera: *Ehrlichia*, *Anaplasma*, *Wolbachia*, and *Neorickettsia*. The bacteria reside in vertebrate reservoirs and target vacuoles of hematopoietic cells (Fig. 75-4). Two *Ehrlichia* species and one *Anaplasma* species cause human infections that can be severe and frequent. *E. chaffeensis*, the agent of HME, infects predominantly mononuclear phagocytic cells. *E. ewingii* and *A. phagocytophilum* infect neutrophils.

Ehrlichia and *Anaplasma* are maintained by horizontal tick-mammal-tick transmission, and humans are only inadvertently infected. Wolbachiae are associated with human diseases caused by filariae, since they are important for filarial viability and pathogenicity; antibiotic treatment targeting wolbachiae is a strategy for the control of filariasis. Neorickettsiae parasitize flukes that in turn parasitize aquatic snails, fish, and insects. Only a single human neorickettsiosis has been described: sennetsu fever, an infectious mononucleosis–like illness that was first identified in 1953. Transmission is probably due to the ingestion of raw fish containing *N. sennetsu*–infected flukes.

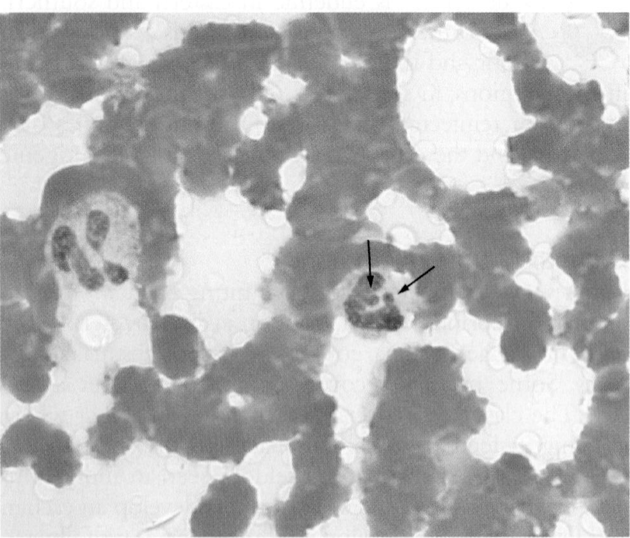

FIGURE 75-4
Peripheral blood smear from a patient with human granulocytotropic anaplasmosis. A neutrophil contains two morulae (vacuoles filled with *A. phagocytophilum*). (*Photo courtesy of Dr. J. Stephen Dumler.*)

HUMAN MONOCYTOTROPIC EHRLICHIOSIS

Epidemiology

More than 2657 cases of *E. chaffeensis* infection had been reported to the Centers for Disease Control and Prevention (CDC) as of September 2006. However, active prospective surveillance has demonstrated an incidence as high as 414 cases per 100,000 population in some regions of the United States. Most *E. chaffeensis* infections are identified in the south-central, southeastern, and mid-Atlantic states, but cases have also been recognized in California. All life stages of the Lone Star tick *(A. americanum)* vector feed on white-tailed deer—a major reservoir host. Subclinically infected dogs and coyotes also serve as reservoirs. Tick bites and exposures are reported by patients, frequently in rural areas and especially in May through July. The median age of HME patients is 53 years; however, severe and fatal infections in children are also well recognized. Of patients with HME, 61% are male.

Clinical Manifestations

E. chaffeensis disseminates hematogenously from the dermal blood pool created by the feeding tick. After a median incubation period of 8 days, illness develops. Clinical manifestations are undifferentiated and include fever (97% of cases), headache (80%), myalgia (57%), and malaise (82%). Less frequently observed are nausea, vomiting, and diarrhea (23–64%); cough (26%); rash (31% overall, 6% at presentation); and confusion (19%). HME can be severe: 62% of patients with documented cases are hospitalized, and ~3% die. Severe complications include toxic shock–like or septic shock–like syndromes, adult respiratory distress syndrome, cardiac failure, hepatitis, meningoencephalitis, hemorrhage, and—in immunocompromised patients—overwhelming infection. Laboratory findings are valuable in the differential diagnosis of HME; 62% of patients have leukopenia (initially lymphopenia, later neutropenia), 71% have thrombocytopenia, and 83% have elevated serum levels of hepatic aminotransferases. Despite low blood cell counts, the bone marrow is hypercellular, and noncaseating granulomas may be present. Vasculitis is not a component of HME.

Diagnosis

Because HME can be fatal, empirical antibiotic therapy based on clinical diagnosis is required. This diagnosis is suggested by fever with a known tick exposure during the preceding 3 weeks, thrombocytopenia and/or leukopenia, and increased serum aminotransferase activities. Morulae are infrequently demonstrated on peripheral blood smears. Active HME can be confirmed by PCR amplification of *E. chaffeensis* nucleic acids in blood obtained before the start of doxycycline therapy. Retrospective serodiagnosis requires a consistent clinical picture and a fourfold increase in *E. chaffeensis* antibody titer (to ≥1:64 in paired sera obtained ~3 weeks apart). Separate specific diagnostic tests are necessary for HME and HGA.

EHRLICHIOSIS EWINGII

Ehrlichia ewingii, originally a neutrophil pathogen causing febrile lameness in dogs, resembles *E. chaffeensis* in its tick vector (*A. americanum*) and vertebrate reservoirs (white-tailed deer and dogs). *E. ewingii* illness is similar to but less severe than HME. The majority of cases have occurred in immunocompromised patients. No specific diagnostic test for ehrlichiosis ewingii is readily available.

℞ Treatment: EHRLICHIOSES

Doxycycline is effective for HME and ehrlichiosis ewingii. Therapy with doxycycline (100 mg given orally or intravenously twice daily) or tetracycline (250–500 mg given orally every 6 h) lowers hospitalization rates and shortens fever duration. *E. chaffeensis* is not susceptible to chloramphenicol in vitro, and the use of this drug is controversial. Although a few reports document *E. chaffeensis* persistence in humans, this finding is rare; most infections are cured by short courses of doxycycline (continuing for 3–5 days after defervescence). Although poorly studied, rifampin may be suitable when doxycycline is contraindicated.

Prevention

HME and ehrlichiosis ewingii are prevented by the avoidance of ticks in endemic areas. The use of protective clothing and tick repellents, careful postexposure tick searches, and prompt removal of attached ticks markedly diminish infection risk.

HUMAN GRANULOCYTOTROPIC ANAPLASMOSIS

Epidemiology

As of September 2006, 3257 cases of HGA had been reported to the CDC, most in the upper midwestern and northeastern United States; the case distribution is similar to that for Lyme disease because of the shared *I. scapularis* tick vector. White-footed mice and white-tailed deer in the United States and red deer in Europe are natural reservoirs for *A. phagocytophilum*. HGA incidence peaks in May through July, but the disease can occur throughout the year with exposure to *Ixodes* ticks. HGA often affects males (57%) and older persons (median age, 51 years).

Clinical Manifestations

Seroprevalence rates are high in endemic regions; thus it seems likely that most individuals develop subclinical infections. The incubation period for HGA is 4–8 days, after which the disease manifests as fever (93% of cases), myalgia (77%), headache (76%), and malaise (94%). A minority of patients develop nausea, vomiting, or diarrhea (16–38%); cough (19%); or confusion (17%). Rash (6%) is almost invariably concurrent erythema migrans attributable to Lyme disease. Most patients develop thrombocytopenia (71%) and/or leukopenia (49%) with increased serum hepatic aminotransferase activities (71%).

Severe complications occur most often in the elderly and include adult respiratory distress syndrome, a toxic shock–like syndrome, and life-threatening opportunistic infections. Meningoencephalitis has not been conclusively documented with HGA, but brachial plexopathy and demyelinating polyneuropathy are reported. For HGA, 7% of patients require intensive care, and the case-fatality rate is 0.5%. Neither vasculitis nor granulomas are components of HGA. Although co-infections with *Borrelia burgdorferi* and *Babesia microti* [transmitted by the same tick vector(s)] occur, there is little evidence of comorbidity or persistence.

Diagnosis

HGA should be included in the differential diagnosis of influenza-like illnesses during seasons with *Ixodes* tick activity (May through December), especially with tick bite or exposure. Concurrent thrombocytopenia, leukopenia, or elevation in serum alanine or aspartate aminotransferase further increases the likelihood of HGA. Many HGA patients develop Lyme disease antibodies in the absence of clinical findings consistent with that diagnosis. Thus HGA should be considered in the differential diagnosis of atypical severe Lyme disease presentations. Peripheral blood film examination for neutrophil morulae can yield a diagnosis in 20–75% of infections. PCR testing of blood from patients with active disease before doxycycline therapy is sensitive and specific. Serodiagnosis is retrospective, requiring a fourfold increase in *A. phagocytophilum* antibody titer (to ≥1:80) in paired serum samples obtained 1 month apart. In regions where seroprevalence is high, a single acute-phase titer may be misleading.

℞ Treatment: HUMAN GRANULOCYTOTROPIC ANAPLASMOSIS

No prospective studies of therapy for HGA have been conducted. However, doxycycline (100 mg by mouth twice daily) is effective. Rifampin therapy is associated with improvement of HGA in pregnant women and children. Most treated patients defervesce within 24–48 h.

Prevention

HGA prevention requires tick avoidance. Transmission can be documented as few as 4 h after a tick bite.

Q FEVER

Q fever results from infection with *C. burnetii*, which can exist as a highly infectious phase I form within humans or as an avirulent phase II form. This organism forms spores that allow its survival in harsh environments. *Coxiella* escapes intracellular killing in macrophages by inhibiting the final phagosome maturation step (cathepsin fusion) and adapts to the acidic phagolysosome.

Q fever encompasses two broad clinical syndromes: acute and chronic infection. The host's immune response (rather than the infecting strain) most likely determines whether chronic Q fever develops. *C. burnetii* survives in monocytes from patients with chronic Q fever but not in those from patients with acute Q fever or from uninfected persons. Impairment of the bactericidal activity of the *C. burnetii*–infected monocyte seems to be due to overproduction of interleukin 10. The CD4+/CD8+ ratio is decreased in Q fever endocarditis. Very few organisms and a strong cellular response are observed in patients with acute Q fever, whereas many organisms and a moderate cellular response are seen in chronic Q fever. Immunologic control of *C. burnetii* is T cell–dependent, but 80–90% of bone marrow aspirates obtained after recovery from Q fever contain *C. burnetii* DNA.

Epidemiology

Q fever is a zoonosis. The primary sources of human infection are infected cattle, sheep, and goats. However, cats, rabbits, pigeons, and dogs have also transmitted *C. burnetii* to humans. The wildlife reservoir includes ticks. In the infected female mammal, *C. burnetii* localizes to the uterus and the mammary glands. Infection is reactivated during pregnancy. High concentrations of *C. burnetii* are found in the placenta. At the time of parturition, *C. burnetii* organisms are released into the air, and infection follows inhalation of aerosolized organisms by a susceptible host. Soil is contaminated during parturition, and *C. burnetii* aerosols can be generated months later during windstorms. Individuals up to 18 km from the source have been infected. *C. burnetii* is a potential agent of bioterrorism.

Persons at risk for Q fever include abattoir workers, veterinarians, and other individuals who have contact with infected animals, particularly newborn animals or products of conception. The organism is shed in milk for weeks to months after parturition. The ingestion of contaminated milk in some geographic areas probably represents a major route of transmission to humans, although the experimental evidence on this point is contradictory. In rare instances, human-to-human transmission has followed labor and childbirth in an infected woman, autopsy of an infected individual, or blood transfusion. Some evidence suggests that *C. burnetii* can be sexually transmitted among humans. Nevertheless, the vast majority of Q fever cases result from inhalation of contaminated aerosols.

Infections due to *C. burnetii* occur in most geographic locations except New Zealand and Antarctica. The primary manifestations of acute Q fever vary with the area. For example, the primary manifestation is pneumonia in Nova Scotia (Canada) but is granulomatous hepatitis in Marseille (France). These differences may reflect the route of infection—i.e., the ingestion of contaminated milk for hepatitis and inhalation of contaminated aerosols for pneumonia.

Young age seems to be protective against infection with *C. burnetii*. In a large outbreak in Switzerland, symptomatic infection occurred five times more often among persons >15 years of age than among those <15 years old. In many outbreaks, men are affected more commonly than women. In France, despite similar occupational exposure of the sexes, the male-to-female ratio is 2.45:1; this difference reflects the fact that female sex hormones are partially protective against infection.

Clinical Manifestations

Acute Q Fever

The incubation period for acute Q fever is 3–30 days. The symptoms are nonspecific; common among them are fever, extreme fatigue, and severe headache. Other symptoms include chills, sweats, nausea, vomiting, and diarrhea, which occur in 5–20% of patients. Cough develops in about half of patients with Q fever pneumonia. Neurologic manifestations of acute Q fever are uncommon; however, in one outbreak in the United Kingdom, 23% of 102 patients had neurologic signs and symptoms as the major manifestation. A nonspecific rash may be evident in 4–18% of patients. The WBC count is usually normal. Thrombocytopenia occurs in ~25% of patients, and reactive thrombocytosis (with platelet counts sometimes exceeding $10^6/\mu L$) frequently develops during recovery. Chest radiography may show an opacity that is indistinguishable from that seen in pneumonia of other etiologies. Multiple rounded opacities are common. In one study of 1070 patients with acute Q fever in southern France, 40% of patients presented with hepatitis, 17% with pneumonia, 20% with both pneumonia and hepatitis, 14% with isolated fever, 2% with CNS disease, and 1% with pericarditis and myocarditis.

Acute Q fever occasionally complicates pregnancy. In one series, Q fever in pregnancy resulted in premature birth in 35% of cases, and 43% of pregnancies ended in abortion or neonatal death. In Halifax, Nova Scotia, a current or previous neonatal death was three times more likely among women seropositive for *C. burnetii* than among seronegative women. Up to 70% of cases of Q fever in children are asymptomatic. Only a few cases of Q fever endocarditis have been reported in children.

In Australia and the United Kingdom, a fatigue state lasting 5–10 years has followed Q fever in 8–15% of cases. Low levels of *C. burnetii* DNA have been detected in the affected patients 0.75–5 years after infection. Patients who develop Q fever fatigue syndrome have a higher frequency of carriage of HLA-DRB1*11 and of the 2/2 genotype of the interferon γ intron 1 microsatellite.

Patients with acute Q fever and lesions of native heart valves, prosthetic heart valves, or prosthetic intravascular material should undergo serologic monitoring every 4 months for 2 years. If the phase I IgG titer is >1:800, further investigation is warranted. Some authorities recommend that patients with valvulopathy and acute Q fever receive doxycycline and hydroxychloroquine for 12 months to prevent chronic Q fever.

Chronic Q Fever

Chronic Q fever, which almost always implies endocarditis, usually occurs in patients with previous valvular heart disease, immunosuppression, or chronic renal insufficiency. Fever is usually absent or low grade. Patients may have nonspecific symptoms for up to 1 year before diagnosis. Valvular vegetations are detected in only 12% of patients by transthoracic echocardiography, but the rate of detection may be higher with transesophageal echocardiography. The vegetations in chronic Q fever endocarditis differ from those in bacterial endocarditis, manifesting as endothelialized nodules on the valves. A high index of suspicion is necessary for a correct diagnosis. The disease should be suspected in all patients with culture-negative endocarditis. In addition, all patients with valvular heart disease and an unexplained purpuric eruption, renal insufficiency, stroke, and/or progressive heart failure should be tested for *C. burnetii* infection. Patients with chronic Q fever have hepatomegaly and/or splenomegaly, which, in combination with rheumatoid factor, elevated erythrocyte sedimentation rate, high C-reactive protein level, and/or increased γ-globulin concentrations (up to 60–70 g/L), suggests this diagnosis. Other manifestations of chronic Q fever include infection of vascular prostheses, aneurysms, and bone, as well as chronic sternal wound infection. Unusual manifestations include chronic thrombocytopenia, mixed cryoglobulinemia, and livedo reticularis.

Diagnosis

Isolation of *C. burnetii* from buffy-coat blood samples or tissue specimens by a shell-vial technique is seldom attempted because of biohazard concerns. PCR detects *C. burnetii* DNA in tissues, including paraffin-embedded tissues. Serology is the most commonly used diagnostic tool. Indirect immunofluorescence is sensitive and specific and is the method of choice. Rheumatoid factor should be adsorbed from the specimen before testing. An IgG titer of ≥1:800 to phase I antigen is suggestive of chronic Q fever. In chronic infection, the antibody titer to phase I antigen is usually much higher than that to phase II antigen; the reverse is true in acute infection, in which a fourfold rise in titer may be demonstrated between acute- and convalescent-phase serum samples.

℞ Treatment: Q FEVER

Treatment of acute Q fever with doxycycline (100 mg twice daily for 14 days) is usually successful. Quinolones are also effective. When Q fever is diagnosed in a pregnant woman, treatment with trimethoprim-sulfamethoxazole is recommended for the duration of the pregnancy.

The treatment of chronic Q fever is difficult and requires careful follow-up. Addition of hydroxychloroquine (to alkalinize the phagolysosome) renders doxycycline bactericidal against *C. burnetii,* and this combination is currently the favored regimen. Treatment with doxycycline (100 mg bid) and hydroxychloroquine (200 mg tid; plasma concentration maintained at 0.8–1.2 μg/mL) for 18 months is superior to a regimen of doxycycline and ofloxacin. Optimal management of Q fever endocarditis entails determination of the minimal inhibitory concentration (MIC) of doxycycline for the patient's isolate and measurement of serum doxycycline levels. A serum level–to–doxycycline MIC ratio of ≥1 is associated with a rapid decline in phase I antibodies. Patients treated with this regimen must be advised about photosensitivity and retinal toxicity risks. The doxycycline-hydroxychloroquine regimen was successful in one patient with HIV infection and Q fever endocarditis. The Jarisch-Herxheimer reaction occasionally complicates the treatment of chronic Q fever.

Treatment of *C. burnetii*–infected aortic aneurysms is the same as that for Q fever endocarditis. Surgical intervention is often required.

If doxycycline-hydroxychloroquine cannot be used, the regimen should include at least two antibiotics active against *C. burnetii.* Rifampin (300 mg once daily) combined with doxycycline (100 mg twice daily) or ciprofloxacin (750 mg twice daily) has been used successfully. The optimal duration of antibiotic therapy for chronic Q fever remains undetermined. The authors recommend at least 3 years of treatment, with discontinuation only if the phase I IgA antibody titer is ≤1:50 and the IgG phase I titer is ≤1:200.

THERAPY WITH BIOLOGIC MODIFYING AGENTS Interferon γ was successful in the treatment of a 3-year-old boy with prolonged fever, abdominal pain, and thrombocytopenia due to *C. burnetii* that was not eradicated with conventional antibiotic therapy. Many patients with granulomatous hepatitis due to Q fever have a prolonged febrile illness that is unresponsive to antibiotics. For these individuals, treatment with prednisone (0.5 mg/kg) has resulted in defervescence within 2–15 days. After defervescence, the glucocorticoid dose is tapered over the next month.

Prevention

A whole-cell vaccine (Q-Vax) licensed in Australia effectively prevents Q fever in abattoir workers. Before administration of the vaccine, skin testing with intradermal diluted *C. burnetii* vaccine is performed, serologic testing is undertaken, and a history of possible Q fever is sought. Vaccine is given only to patients with no history of Q fever and negative results in serologic and skin tests.

Good animal-husbandry practices are important in preventing widespread contamination of the environment by *C. burnetii*. These practices include isolating aborting animals for up to 14 days, raising feed bunks to prevent contamination of feed by excreta, destroying aborted materials (i.e., burning and burying fetal membranes and stillborn animals), and wearing masks and gloves when handling aborted materials. Only seronegative pregnant animals should be used in research settings, and only seronegative animals should be permitted in petting zoos.

ACKNOWLEDGMENT

The contributions of Didier Raoult, MD, to this chapter in previous editions of Harrison's Principles of Internal Medicine are gratefully acknowledged.

FURTHER READINGS

BLANCO JR et al (eds): *Century of Rickettsiology: Emerging, Reemerging Rickettsioses, Molecular Diagnostics, and Emerging Veterinary Rickettsioses.* Malden, MA, Blackwell Scientific, 2006

CHAPMAN AS et al: Diagnosis and management of tickborne rickettsial diseases: Rocky Mountain spotted fever, ehrlichioses, and anaplasmosis—United States. MMWR 55:1, 2006

DUMLER JS: *Anaplasma* and *Ehrlichia* infection. Ann NY Acad Sci 1063:361, 2005

MCQUISTON JH et al: National surveillance and the epidemiology of Q fever in the United States, 1978–2004. Am J Trop Med Hyg 75:36, 2006

RAOULT D et al: Q fever 1985–1998. Clinical and epidemiologic features of 1,383 infections. Medicine (Baltimore) 79:109, 2000

WALKER DH et al: Emerging and re-emerging tick-transmitted rickettsial and ehrlichial infections. Med Clin North Am 92:1345, 2008

WALKER DH: Rickettsiae and rickettsial infections: The current state of knowledge. Clin Infect Dis 45(Suppl1):539, 2007

CHAPTER 76

INFECTIONS DUE TO MYCOPLASMAS

William M. McCormack

Mycoplasmas, the smallest free-living organisms known, are prokaryotes that are bounded only by a plasma membrane. Their lack of a cell wall is associated with cellular pleomorphism and resistance to cell wall–active antimicrobial agents, such as penicillins and cephalosporins. The organisms' small genome limits biosynthesis and explains the difficulties encountered with in vitro cultivation. Mycoplasmas typically colonize mucosal surfaces of the respiratory and urogenital tracts of many animal species. Of the 17 species of mycoplasmas recovered from humans, most are commensals. *Mycoplasma pneumoniae* causes upper and lower respiratory tract infections. *M. genitalium* and ureaplasmas are established causes of urethritis and have been implicated in other genital conditions. *M. hominis* and ureaplasmas are part of the complex microbial flora of bacterial vaginosis (Chap. 28). The two biovars of *Ureaplasma*, previously classified together as *U. urealyticum*, have recently been separated into two species: *U. parvum* and *U. urealyticum*.

MECHANISMS OF PATHOGENICITY

Adherence of mycoplasmas to the surface of the host cell is necessary for colonization and infection. Some pathogenic mycoplasmas are flask-shaped, with specialized tips that enhance adherence. *M. pneumoniae* adheres via a network of interactive adhesins and accessory proteins and produces hydrogen peroxide, which may cause injury to host cells. *M. hominis* metabolizes arginine, with the production of potentially cytotoxic amounts of ammonia. Ureaplasmas have been placed in a separate genus because of their unique urease activity; the metabolism of urea also produces ammonia. *M. pneumoniae* may evoke IgM autoantibodies that agglutinate human erythrocytes at 4°C. These cold agglutinins can cause anemia and other complications.

MYCOPLASMA PNEUMONIAE

Epidemiology

M. pneumoniae causes upper and lower respiratory tract symptoms in all age groups, with the highest attack rates in 5- to 20-year-olds. Infection with *M. pneumoniae* is acquired by inhalation of aerosols. The incubation period is 2–3 weeks, considerably longer than that of most other respiratory infections. Although epidemics have taken place in closed populations, such as those at schools and military installations, most cases occur sporadically or in families. Cases in families typically occur serially and are separated by 2- to 3-week intervals. Infections in adults are often the result of contact with children.

Infection with *M. pneumoniae* occurs worldwide and year round, with epidemics every few years. Some studies have noted an increase in the number of cases during the autumn months in temperate climates. Although pneumonia is the classic presentation, nonpneumonic infection is considerably more common. In very young children, most infections result only in upper respiratory symptoms, whereas children >5 years of age and adults may have bronchitis and pneumonia.

Clinical Presentation

After the prolonged incubation period, fever and constitutional symptoms develop along with headache and cough, both of which can be prominent and distressing.

Symptoms typically progress less rapidly than those of viral respiratory tract infections. In the minority (perhaps 5–10%) of infected individuals who develop tracheobronchitis or pneumonia, cough becomes more prominent. Sputum, if produced at all, is usually white and may be tinged with blood. The temperature seldom rises above 38.9°–39.4°C (102°–103°F). Shaking chills, myalgias, and gastrointestinal symptoms (e.g., nausea, vomiting, and diarrhea) are unusual. Chest muscle soreness may result from frequent and prolonged coughing, but true pleuritic pain is uncommon.

Pharyngeal injection is often noted. Cervical lymph node enlargement is unusual. Ear pain due to bullous myringitis (blisters on the tympanic membrane) is a unique but uncommon manifestation. As in other "atypical" pneumonias, findings on auscultation of the lung may be normal or nearly normal despite striking radiographic abnormalities. Pleural effusions develop in <20% of patients.

M. pneumoniae infection may be particularly severe in patients who have sickle cell disease and other hemoglobin S–related hemoglobinopathies. The functional asplenia seen in sickle cell disease may contribute to severe disease as it does in pneumococcal infection. Severe respiratory distress and large pleural effusions may occur.

Extrapulmonary Manifestations

A broad array of extrapulmonary abnormalities have been associated with *M. pneumoniae* infection (Table 76-1). Although these events are unusual, they complicate other respiratory diseases even more rarely and often provide the only clue that an otherwise-unremarkable respiratory infection may be mycoplasmal. Erythema multiforme (Stevens-Johnson syndrome) typically occurs in young male patients with *M. pneumoniae* infection. Digital necrosis has been seen in patients with sickle cell disease who develop very high titers of cold agglutinins. Arthralgias are not unusual in patients who have mycoplasmal pneumonia; mycoplasmal arthritis is rare except in patients who have hypogammaglobulinemia.

The pathogenesis of the extrapulmonary manifestations of *M. pneumoniae* infection is controversial. Occasional reports have described the identification of *M. pneumoniae* or its nucleic acids in involved tissues. The fact that most attempts at detection have yielded negative results, however, suggests that these extrapulmonary complications have an immunologic basis.

TABLE 76-1

EXTRAPULMONARY MANIFESTATIONS OF *MYCOPLASMA PNEUMONIAE* INFECTION

SYSTEM	MANIFESTATIONS
Dermatologic	Erythema multiforme Maculopapular exanthems Vesicular exanthems Erythema nodosum Urticaria
Cardiovascular	Myocarditis Pericarditis
Neurologic	Encephalitis Aseptic meningitis Cerebellar ataxia Guillain-Barré syndrome Transverse myelitis Polyradiculopathy
Rheumatologic	Arthralgias Arthritis Juvenile-onset spondyloarthropathy
Hematologic	Hemolytic anemia Coagulopathies

Diagnosis

Most infections with *M. pneumoniae* are not diagnosed, as they are indistinguishable from upper and lower respiratory tract infections caused by myriad other viral and bacterial pathogens. When the diagnosis is suspected, it is usually because illness is prolonged or extrapulmonary manifestations develop. The white blood cell count is generally somewhat elevated, with few immature cells. Gram's staining of sputum shows leukocytes without a predominance of any bacterial morphologic type. Since *M. pneumoniae* lacks a cell wall, it cannot be detected on Gram's stain. In patients who have pneumonia, the chest radiograph may show reticulonodular or interstitial infiltration, primarily in the lower lobes. As in other "atypical" pneumonias, radiographic abnormalities may be more prominent than would be predicted by auscultation of the chest.

M. pneumoniae can be grown on artificial media, but the process is exacting, requires special media, and takes upwards of 2 weeks. Thus mycoplasmal cultures do not provide timely information to aid in patient management. The same, unfortunately, is true of serologic diagnosis. Specific antibodies can be detected by enzyme-linked immunoassays, indirect immunofluorescence, or complement fixation, but do not develop early enough to guide decisions regarding treatment. As with most serologic tests, examination of paired acute- and convalescent-phase serum specimens is required for good sensitivity and specificity.

Cold agglutinins are nonspecific but develop within the first 7–10 days in more than half of patients with *M. pneumoniae* pneumonia and may be detectable when the patient presents to a health care provider. In a patient with a compatible clinical picture, a cold agglutinin titer of ≥1:32 supports the diagnosis of mycoplasmal pneumonia. Cold agglutinin determinations are readily available from diagnostic laboratories. The test can also be performed at the bedside by the addition of 1 mL of the patient's blood to a tube containing anticoagulant (e.g., a tube used to collect blood for determination of prothrombin activity). Before cooling, the nonaggregated red blood cells coat the sides of the inverted tube. The blood is cooled to 4°C when the tube is placed in an ice bath for 3–5 min or in a standard refrigerator. In a positive test, clumps of red blood cells can be observed when the tube is inverted. Rewarming of the sample to 37°C in an incubator or by exposure to body heat should reverse the agglutination. A positive "bedside" cold agglutinin test is equivalent to a laboratory titer of ≥1:64.

The lack of sensitive, specific, and timely diagnostic tests has prompted the development of a variety of antigen detection tests (e.g., nucleic acid amplification) that do not involve serology or the cultivation of live organisms. Since many viral and bacterial infections result in clinical presentations similar to that caused by *M. pneumoniae*, examination of specimens for single antigens is unlikely to be useful. Multiplex nucleic acid amplification tests that examine a single throat swab or sputum sample for the most likely causative microorganisms have been developed. Such tests may provide more precise etiologic diagnosis of upper and lower respiratory tract infections.

℞ Treatment: PNEUMONIA CAUSED BY *M. PNEUMONIAE*

Pneumonia due to *M. pneumoniae* is usually self-limited and is seldom life-threatening. Effective antimicrobial agents do shorten the duration of illness and, by reducing coughing, may conceivably render the patient less infectious. Although symptoms are alleviated by antimicrobial treatment, the organism usually is not eradicated. Cultures positive for *M. pneumoniae* may persist for months despite clinically effective antimicrobial therapy. The beneficial effects, if any, of such treatment on extrapulmonary manifestations of *M. pneumoniae* infection are unknown.

Because most mycoplasmal infections are not specifically diagnosed, management is directed at one of two syndromes: upper respiratory tract infection or community-acquired pneumonia. Upper respiratory infections, whether caused by viruses or by *M. pneumoniae*, do not require antimicrobial treatment. Community-acquired pneumonia (Chap. 17) may be caused by bacteria such as *Streptococcus pneumoniae* and *Haemophilus influenzae* or by "atypical" agents such as *Chlamydophila pneumoniae*, *Legionella pneumophila*, and *M. pneumoniae*. Recommended treatment regimens are detailed in Tables 76-2 and 76-3. Treatment of documented *M. pneumoniae* pneumonia is usually continued for 14–21 days.

TABLE 76-2

ORAL ANTIMICROBIAL AGENTS FOR THE TREATMENT OF AMBULATORY PATIENTS WITH COMMUNITY-ACQUIRED PNEUMONIA

AGENT	DOSE AND SCHEDULE
Doxycycline	100 mg bid
Erythromycin	500 mg qid
Clarithromycin	500 mg bid
Azithromycin	500 mg qd
Levofloxacin	750 mg qd
Moxifloxacin	400 mg qd
Gemifloxacin	320 mg qd

Note: Treatment of documented *M. pneumoniae* pneumonia is usually continued for 14–21 days.

TABLE 76-3

ANTIMICROBIAL AGENTS FOR THE TREATMENT OF HOSPITALIZED PATIENTS WITH COMMUNITY-ACQUIRED PNEUMONIA

1. Intravenous ceftriaxone (1.0 g/d) *or*
   Intravenous cefotaxime (1.0 g q8h) *or*
   Intravenous ampicillin/sulbactam (1.5–3.0 g q6h)
   plus
   Intravenous or oral erythromycin (500 mg qid) *or*
   Intravenous or oral azithromycin (500 mg qd) *or*
   Oral clarithromycin (500 mg bid)
2. Intravenous or oral levofloxacin (750 mg qd)
3. Intravenous or oral moxifloxacin (400 mg qd)

Note: Treatment of documented *M. pneumoniae* pneumonia is usually continued for 14–21 days.

GENITAL MYCOPLASMAS

(See also Chap. 28)

Epidemiology

M. hominis, *U. urealyticum*, and *U. parvum* are the most prevalent genital mycoplasmas. Infants may become colonized with these organisms during passage through a colonized birth canal. Neonatal colonization tends not to persist. Only ~10% of prepubertal girls and even fewer prepubertal boys are colonized with ureaplasmas. After puberty, colonization occurs mainly as a result of sexual activity. Among adults, disadvantaged populations have higher colonization rates. Ureaplasmas can be cultured from the vaginas of ~80% of women cared for in public clinics and about half of women cared for by private obstetricians and gynecologists. Similarly, vaginal *M. hominis* is found in ~50% of women attending public clinics and in ~20% of private patients. Men have somewhat lower rates of genital colonization than women. In short, *U. urealyticum*, *U. parvum*, and *M. hominis* are frequently detected in genital specimens from healthy, sexually experienced adults. Evaluation of the role of these organisms in human disease must take into account their high prevalence among healthy people.

M. fermentans colonizes both the respiratory and genital tracts in >20% of adults. There is no convincing evidence that *M. fermentans* causes human disease. *M. genitalium* is a fastidious organism that is difficult to cultivate. Polymerase chain reaction (PCR) studies have identified the organism more successfully.

Association with Human Disease

Nongonococcal Urethritis (NGU)

Although *Chlamydia trachomatis* is the organism most firmly implicated in the etiology of NGU, there is no doubt that sexually transmitted ureaplasmas and *M. genitalium* also cause some cases. The ubiquity of ureaplasmas among men who do not have urethritis and the difficulty of identifying *M. genitalium* do not allow precise estimation of the proportion of cases of NGU caused by each of these mycoplasmas.

Epididymitis and Prostatitis

Ureaplasmas may be an occasional cause of epididymitis. *M. hominis* has not been implicated in this disease. Neither organism has been convincingly associated with prostatitis.

Pelvic Inflammatory Disease (PID)

M. hominis and ureaplasmas are prominent components of the complex microbial flora of bacterial vaginosis. Since bacterial vaginosis is associated with PID, it is difficult to determine whether these organisms play an independent role in this condition. Although *M. genitalium* is not associated with bacterial vaginosis, preliminary studies have linked it to cervicitis, PID, and tubal factor infertility in women who are not infected with either *Neisseria gonorrhoeae* or *C. trachomatis*.

Disorders of Reproduction

Ureaplasmas have been considered as causes of involuntary infertility in both men and women, but there is no convincing evidence for such an association. These organisms have been associated with chorioamnionitis and preterm birth. Given the close association of ureaplasmas with bacterial vaginosis, a condition that is strongly associated with chorioamnionitis and preterm birth, it is difficult to define an independent role for ureaplasmas in these conditions. In infants of very low birth weight, ureaplasmas have been shown to cause pneumonia and long-term respiratory dysfunction. *M. hominis* can cause postpartum fever, which has been associated with isolation of this organism from blood and its occasional dissemination to joints, resulting in septic arthritis.

Extragenital Infections

Sexually acquired reactive arthritis and Reiter's syndrome may be triggered by ureaplasmas, although *C. trachomatis* is the usual triggering agent. Patients who have hypogammaglobulinemia may develop chronic arthritis due to ureaplasmas and some other mycoplasmal species. *M. hominis* has been identified in patients with postthoracotomy sternal wound infection and in rare instances of prosthetic heart valve and prosthetic joint infection.

Diagnosis

There is seldom any reason to examine specimens from the lower genital tract (vagina, male urethra) for mycoplasmas. The ubiquity of the organisms among healthy individuals makes a positive result uninterpretable. The organisms should be sought only in specimens from normally sterile areas, such as joint fluid with evidence of inflammation and cultures negative for conventional microorganisms.

M. hominis can replicate in many routine blood culture media without changing the appearance of the media. Although the organism forms nonhemolytic pinpoint colonies on blood agar, it cannot be visualized in gram-stained smears of these colonies. Neither ureaplasmas nor *M. genitalium* will grow in ordinary microbiologic media.

Microbiologic diagnosis of genital mycoplasmal infection requires specially prepared media and is beyond the capability of all but reference and research laboratories. Nucleic acid amplification tests such as PCR have been developed.

℞ Treatment: GENITAL MYCOPLASMAS

Ureaplasmas, *M. genitalium*, and *M. hominis* are usually susceptible to tetracyclines (e.g., doxycycline). Infections caused by tetracycline-resistant ureaplasmas can be treated with erythromycin, whereas those due to tetracycline-resistant strains of *M. hominis* respond to treatment with clindamycin. As noted above, a specific microbiologic diagnosis of mycoplasmal infection is seldom made. Appropriate treatment provides antimicrobial coverage for the organisms that cause the particular syndrome. Accordingly, NGU is treated with doxycycline (100 mg orally twice a day for 7 days) or azithromycin (1.0 g as a single oral dose) to provide activity against *C. trachomatis, U. urealyticum, U. parvum,* and *M. genitalium.* Recommended regimens for the treatment of PID provide antimicrobial activity against gonococci, chlamydiae, and anaerobes as well as genital mycoplasmas.

FURTHER READINGS

Alexander ER et al: Pneumonia due to *Mycoplasma pneumoniae*. N Engl J Med 275:131, 1966

Mandell LA et al: Update of practice guidelines for the management of community-acquired pneumonia in immunocompetent adults. Clin Infect Dis 37:1405, 2003

Morozumi M et al: Simultaneous detection of pathogens in clinical samples from patients with community-acquired pneumonia by real-time PCR with pathogen-specific molecular beacon probes. J Clin Microbiol 44:1440, 2006

Murray HW et al: The protean manifestations of *Mycoplasma pneumoniae* in adults. Am J Med 58:229, 1975

Taylor SN: *Mycoplasma genitalium*. Curr Infect Dis Rep 7:453, 2005

Waites KB et al: Mycoplasmas and ureaplasmas as neonatal pathogens. Clin Microbiol Rev 18:757, 2005

Walter ND et al: Community outbreak of *Mycoplasma pneumoniae* infection: school-based cluster of neurologic disease associated with household transmission of respiratory illness. J Infect Dis 198:1365, 2008

CHAPTER 77

CHLAMYDIAL INFECTIONS

Walter E. Stamm

Three chlamydial species cause human infections: *Chlamydia trachomatis, Chlamydophila psittaci*, and *Chlamydophila pneumoniae*. *C. psittaci* is widely distributed in nature, producing genital, conjunctival, intestinal, or respiratory infections in many mammalian and avian species. Genital infections with *C. psittaci* have been well characterized in several species and cause abortion and infertility. Although mammalian strains of *C. psittaci* are not known to infect humans, avian strains occasionally do so, causing pneumonia and the systemic illness known as *psittacosis*. *C. pneumoniae* is a fastidious chlamydial species that appears to be a common cause of upper respiratory tract infection and pneumonia, primarily in children and young adults, and is a cause of recurrent respiratory infections in older adults. Studies have also linked *C. pneumoniae* infection to atherosclerotic cardiovascular disease and perhaps to asthma. No animal reservoir has been identified for *C. pneumoniae*; it appears to be an exclusively human pathogen spread via the respiratory route through close personal contact. *C. trachomatis* is also an exclusively human pathogen and was identified as the cause of trachoma in the 1940s. Since then, *C. trachomatis* has been recognized as a major cause of sexually transmitted and perinatal infection.

Chlamydiae are obligate intracellular bacteria that are classified in their own order, Chlamydiales (Fig. 77-1). They possess both DNA and RNA, have a cell wall and ribosomes similar to those of gram-negative bacteria, and are inhibited by antibiotics such as tetracycline. A unique feature of all chlamydiae is their complex reproductive cycle (Fig. 77-2). Two forms of the microorganism—the extracellular elementary body (EB) and the intracellular reticulate body (RB)—participate in this cycle. The EB is adapted for extracellular survival and is the infective form transmitted from one person to another. EBs attach to susceptible target cells (usually columnar or transitional epithelial cells) and enter the cells inside a phagosome. Within 8 h of cell entry, the EBs reorganize into RBs, which are adapted to intracellular survival and multiplication. They undergo binary fission, eventually producing numerous replicates contained within the intracellular membrane-bound "inclusion body," which occupies much of the infected host cell. Chlamydial inclusions resist lysosomal fusion until late in the developmental cycle. After 24 h, the RBs condense and form EBs still contained within the inclusion. The inclusion then lyses, releasing EBs from the cell to initiate infection of adjacent cells or transmission to another person. Under some conditions [e.g., exposure to interferon γ (IFN-γ) or antibiotics], an altered life cycle is induced in which large, metabolically inactive RBs persist but do not replicate. Removal of the IFN-γ or antibiotics is followed by restoration of the normal life cycle.

Studies with monoclonal antibodies and nucleotide sequencing of the major outer-membrane protein have delineated at least 20 serotypes of *C. trachomatis*. According to the classification of Wang and Grayston, strains associated with trachoma are generally of the A, B, Ba, and C serovars, whereas serovars D through K are largely associated with sexually transmitted and perinatally acquired infections. Serovars L_1, L_2, and L_3 produce lymphogranuloma venereum (LGV) and hemorrhagic proctocolitis. The LGV strains exhibit unique biologic behavior in that they are more invasive than the other serovars, produce disease in lymphatic tissue, grow readily in cell culture systems and macrophages, and are lethal when inoculated intracerebrally into mice and monkeys. Non-LGV strains of *C. trachomatis* characteristically produce infections involving the superficial columnar epithelium of the eye, genitalia, and respiratory tract.

C. trachomatis is an infrequent cause of endocarditis, peritonitis, pleuritis, and possibly periappendicitis and occasionally causes respiratory infections in older children and adults. Some immunosuppressed patients with pneumonia have had either serologic or cultural evidence of *C. trachomatis* infection, but more data are necessary to define a pathogenic role for this organism in these patients.

C. TRACHOMATIS INFECTIONS

GENITAL INFECTIONS

Genital infections caused by *C. trachomatis* represent the most common bacterial sexually transmitted infections (STIs) in the United States (Chap. 28). An estimated 4 million cases occur each year. In adults, the clinical spectrum of sexually transmitted *C. trachomatis* infections parallels that of gonococcal infections. Both infections have been associated with urethritis, proctitis, and conjunctivitis in both sexes; with epididymitis in men; and with mucopurulent cervicitis (MPC), acute salpingitis, bartholinitis, and the Fitz-Hugh Curtis syndrome (perihepatitis) in women. Moreover, both infections can be associated with septic arthritis. In general, however,

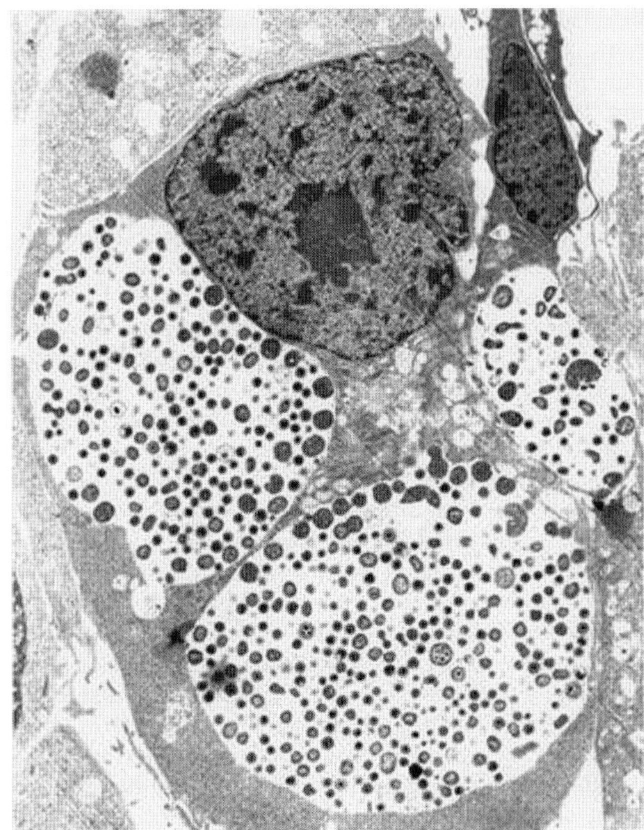

FIGURE 77-1
Chlamydial intracellular inclusions filled with smaller dense elementary bodies and larger reticulate bodies.

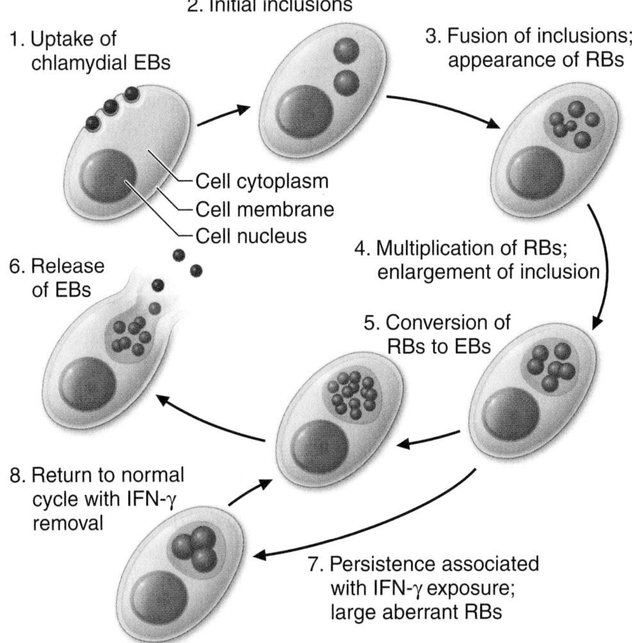

FIGURE 77-2
Chlamydial life cycle. EBs, elementary bodies; RBs, reticulate bodies; IFN-γ, interferon γ.

chlamydial infections produce fewer symptoms and signs than gonococcal infections at the same anatomic site; in fact, chlamydial infections are often totally asymptomatic. Increasing evidence suggests that many chlamydial infections of the genital tract, especially in women, persist for months without producing symptoms. Simultaneous infection with *C. trachomatis* often occurs in women with cervical gonococcal infection and in heterosexual men with gonococcal urethritis.

Epidemiology

Infections due to *C. trachomatis* have been reportable in the United States since 1985, and national incidence data show steadily rising numbers of reported infections, probably reflecting both increased testing and increased reporting more than increasing incidence. Most testing to date has focused on women, and thus the reported incidence is severalfold greater among women than among men; this difference likely represents a surveillance artifact.

The age of peak incidence of genital *C. trachomatis* infections, as of other STIs, is the late teens and early twenties. The prevalence of chlamydial urethral infection among young men is at least 3–5% for those seen in general medical settings or in urban high schools and is >10% for asymptomatic soldiers undergoing routine physical examination; 15–20% of heterosexual men seen in sexually transmitted disease (STD) clinics may be positive for *C. trachomatis*. In areas where chlamydial control programs have been implemented, the overall prevalence may be markedly reduced. In short, the prevalence among men varies widely with the population group studied and with the geographic locale. With the newer, more sensitive nucleic acid amplification tests (NAATs), such as polymerase chain reaction (PCR) and transcription-mediated amplification (TMA), prevalences in most populations have been 10–30% higher than those measured with older, less sensitive tests.

The prevalence of cervical infection among women is ~5% for asymptomatic college students and prenatal patients in the United States, >10% for women seen in family planning clinics, and >20% for women seen in STD clinics. As in men, the prevalence of genital *C. trachomatis* infections varies substantially by geographic locale, with the highest rates in the southeastern United States. However, substantial prevalences (~8%) of asymptomatic chlamydial infection have been demonstrated among young female military recruits from all parts of the United States. In this country, the prevalence of *C. trachomatis* in the cervix of pregnant women is 5–10 times higher than that of *Neisseria gonorrhoeae*. The prevalence of genital infection with either agent is highest among individuals who are between the ages of 18 and 24, single, and non-Caucasian (e.g., African-American or Latino). Recurrent chlamydial infections occur frequently in these same risk groups and are often acquired from untreated sexual partners. Use of oral contraceptive pills and the presence of cervical ectopy also confer an increased risk of chlamydial infection. The proportion of infections that are asymptomatic appears to be higher for *C. trachomatis* than for *N. gonorrhoeae*, and symptomatic *C. trachomatis* infections are clinically less severe. Mild or asymptomatic chlamydial infections of the fallopian tubes nonetheless cause ongoing tubal damage and infertility. Furthermore, because the total number of *C. trachomatis* infections exceeds the total number of *N. gonorrhoeae* infections in industrialized countries, the total morbidity caused by *C. trachomatis* genital infections in these countries exceeds that caused by *N. gonorrhoeae*. The prevalence of *C. trachomatis* is higher than that of *N. gonorrhoeae* in industrialized countries, in part because measures such as treatment of sex partners and routine cultures for case detection in asymptomatic individuals have been applied much longer and more effectively to the control of gonorrhea than to the control of *C. trachomatis* infection.

Pathogenesis

C. trachomatis preferentially infects the columnar epithelium of the eye and the respiratory and genital tracts. The infection induces an immune response but often persists for months or years in the absence of antimicrobial therapy. Serious sequelae often occur in association with repeated or persistent infections. The precise mechanism through which repeated or persistent infection elicits an inflammatory response that leads to tubal scarring and damage in the female upper genital tract is not yet clear. One antigen, the chlamydial 60-kDa heat-shock protein, may be involved in inducing a pathologic immune response or may elicit antibodies that cross-react with human heat-shock proteins. Several complete chlamydial genomes have been sequenced, and genetic studies may soon offer further insights into the pathogenic mechanisms of *C. trachomatis*.

Clinical Manifestations

Nongonococcal and Postgonococcal Urethritis

Nongonococcal urethritis (NGU) is a diagnosis of exclusion that is applied to men with symptoms and/or signs of urethritis who do not have gonorrhea. Postgonococcal urethritis (PGU) refers to NGU developing in men 2–3 weeks after treatment of gonococcal urethritis with single doses of agents such as penicillins or cephalosporins that lack antimicrobial activity against chlamydiae. Since current treatment regimens for gonorrhea include tetracycline, doxycycline, or azithromycin for possible concomitant chlamydial infection, both the incidence of PGU and the causative role of chlamydiae in this syndrome have declined. *C. trachomatis* causes 20–40% of cases of NGU in heterosexual men but is less commonly isolated from homosexual men with this syndrome. The cause of most of the remaining cases of NGU is uncertain; considerable evidence suggests that *Ureaplasma urealyticum* and *Mycoplasma genitalium* cause many cases of NGU, whereas *Trichomonas vaginalis* and herpes simplex virus (HSV) cause some cases.

NGU is diagnosed by documentation of a leukocytic urethral exudate and by exclusion of gonorrhea by Gram's staining or culture. *C. trachomatis* urethritis is generally less severe than gonococcal urethritis, although in an individual patient, these two forms of urethritis cannot be reliably differentiated solely on clinical grounds. Symptoms include urethral discharge (often whitish and mucoid rather than frankly purulent), dysuria, and urethral itching. Physical examination may reveal meatal erythema and tenderness and a urethral exudate that is often demonstrable only by stripping of the urethra.

At least one-third of males with *C. trachomatis* urethral infection have no demonstrable signs or symptoms of urethritis. Use of NAATs on first-void urine specimens to diagnose chlamydial infections in men has facilitated broader-based testing for asymptomatic infection in males. As a result, asymptomatic chlamydial urethritis has been demonstrated in 5–10% of sexually active adolescent males screened in school-based clinics or community centers. Such patients generally have first-glass pyuria (≥15 leukocytes per 400× microscopic field in the sediment of first-void urine), a positive leukocyte esterase test, or an increased number of leukocytes on a Gram-stained smear prepared from a urogenital swab inserted 1–2 cm into the anterior urethra. For the enumeration of leukocytes, the smear is first scanned at low power to identify areas of the slide containing the highest concentration of leukocytes. These areas are then examined under oil immersion (1000×). An average of four or more leukocytes in at least three of five 1000× oil-immersion fields is indicative of urethritis and correlates with the recovery of *C. trachomatis*. To differentiate between true urethritis and functional symptoms among symptomatic patients or to make a presumptive diagnosis of *C. trachomatis* infection in "high-risk" but asymptomatic men (e.g., male patients in STD clinics, sex partners of women with nongonococcal salpingitis or MPC, fathers of children with inclusion conjunctivitis), the examination of an endourethral specimen for increased leukocytes is useful if specific diagnostic tests for chlamydiae are not available. Alternatively, urethritis can be assayed noninvasively by examination of a first-void urine sample for pyuria, either by microscopy or by the leukocyte esterase test. Urine (or a urethral swab) can also be directly tested for chlamydiae or gonococci by DNA amplification methods, as described below.

Epididymitis

C. trachomatis is the foremost cause of epididymitis in sexually active heterosexual men <35 years of age, accounting for ~70% of cases. *N. gonorrhoeae* causes most of the remaining cases, and some men have simultaneous infections with both pathogens, usually accompanied by asymptomatic urethritis as defined above. In homosexual men, sexually transmitted coliform infection acquired via insertive rectal intercourse may cause epididymitis. Coliform bacteria and *Pseudomonas aeruginosa*, usually detected in association with preceding urologic instrumentation or surgery, are the most common causes of epididymitis in men over 35. Men with chlamydial epididymitis typically present with unilateral scrotal pain, fever, and epididymal tenderness or swelling on examination. The illness may be mild enough to treat with oral antibiotics on an outpatient basis or severe enough to require hospitalization and parenteral therapy. Testicular torsion should be excluded promptly by radionuclide scan, Doppler flow study, or surgical exploration in a teenager or young adult who presents with acute unilateral testicular pain without urethritis. The possibility of testicular tumor or chronic infection (e.g., tuberculosis) should be excluded when a patient with unilateral intrascrotal pain and swelling does not respond to appropriate antimicrobial therapy.

Reiter's Syndrome

Reiter's syndrome consists of conjunctivitis, urethritis (or, in female patients, cervicitis), arthritis, and characteristic mucocutaneous lesions. *C. trachomatis* has been recovered from the urethra of up to 70% of men with untreated nondiarrheal Reiter's syndrome and associated urethritis. In the absence of overt urethritis, it is important to exclude subclinical urethritis in the men in whom this diagnosis is suspected.

The pathogenesis of Reiter's syndrome remains obscure. However, since more than 80% of affected patients have the HLA-B27 phenotype and since other mucosal infections (with *Salmonella*, *Shigella*, or *Campylobacter*, for example) produce an identical syndrome, chlamydial infection is thought to initiate an aberrant and hyperactive immune response that produces inflammation at the involved target organs in these genetically predisposed individuals. Evidence of exaggerated cell-mediated and humoral immune responses to chlamydial antigens in Reiter's syndrome supports this hypothesis. The presumptive demonstration of chlamydial EBs and chlamydial DNA in the joint fluid and synovial tissue of patients with Reiter's syndrome suggests that chlamydiae may actually spread from genital to joint tissues in these patients, perhaps in macrophages.

Proctitis

C. trachomatis strains of either the genital immunotypes D through K or the LGV immunotypes cause proctitis in homosexual men who practice receptive anorectal intercourse. In the United States, the vast majority of cases are due to immunotypes D through K and present either as asymptomatic infection or as mild proctitis not unlike gonococcal proctitis. These infections may develop in heterosexual women as well. Patients present with mild rectal pain, mucous discharge, tenesmus, and (occasionally) bleeding. Nearly all have neutrophils in Gram-stained rectal samples. Anoscopy in these non-LGV cases of chlamydial proctitis reveals mild, patchy mucosal friability and mucopurulent discharge, and the disease process is limited to the distal rectum. LGV strains produce more severe ulcerative proctitis or proctocolitis that can be confused clinically with HSV proctitis (severe rectal pain, rectal bleeding, discharge, and tenesmus) and that histologically resembles Crohn's disease in that giant cell formation and granulomas can be seen. In the United States, these cases of LGV proctitis occur almost exclusively in homosexual men, many of whom are positive for HIV.

Mucopurulent Cervicitis

Although many women with *C. trachomatis* infection of the cervix have no symptoms or signs, a careful speculum examination reveals evidence of MPC in 30–50% of cases. As is discussed more fully in Chap. 28, MPC is associated with yellow mucopurulent endocervical discharge and with ≥20 neutrophils per 1000× microscopic field within strands of cervical mucus on a thinly smeared, Gram-stained preparation of endocervical exudate. Other characteristic findings include edema of the zone of cervical ectopy and a propensity of the mucosa to bleed on minor trauma—e.g., when specimens are collected with a swab. A Pap smear shows increased numbers of neutrophils as well as a characteristic pattern of mononuclear inflammatory cells, including plasma cells, transformed lymphocytes, and histiocytes. Cervical biopsy shows a predominantly mononuclear cell infiltrate of the subepithelial stroma, often with follicular cervicitis.

Pelvic Inflammatory Disease

(See also Chap. 28) In the United States, *C. trachomatis* has been identified in the fallopian tubes or endometrium of up to 50% of women with pelvic inflammatory disease (PID), and its role as an important etiologic agent in this syndrome is well accepted. PID occurs via ascending intraluminal spread of *C. trachomatis* from the lower genital tract. MPC is thus followed by endometritis, endosalpingitis, and finally pelvic peritonitis. Evidence of MPC is usually found in women with laparoscopically verified salpingitis. Similarly, endometritis, demonstrated by endometrial biopsy showing plasma cell infiltration of the endometrial epithelium, is documented in most women with laparoscopically verified chlamydial (or gonococcal) salpingitis. Chlamydial endometritis can also occur in the absence of clinical evidence of salpingitis: ~40–50% of women with MPC have plasma cell endometritis. Histologic evidence of endometritis has been correlated with an "endometritis syndrome" consisting of vaginal bleeding, lower abdominal pain, and uterine tenderness in the absence of adnexal tenderness. Chlamydial salpingitis produces milder symptoms than does gonococcal salpingitis and may be associated with less marked adnexal tenderness. Thus mild adnexal or uterine tenderness in sexually active women with cervicitis suggests PID.

Infertility associated with fallopian-tube scarring has been strongly linked to antecedent *C. trachomatis* infection in serologic studies. Since many infertile women with tubal scarring and antichlamydial antibody have no history of PID, it appears that subclinical tubal infection ("silent salpingitis") may produce scarring. Studies in animals and humans with salpingitis and tubal scarring suggest the continuing presence of persistent, slowly replicating chlamydial infection in tubal tissue. Although the pathogenesis of *C. trachomatis*–induced tubal scarring remains poorly understood, antibodies to the chlamydial 60-kDa heat-shock protein have been correlated with tubal infertility, ectopic pregnancy, and Fitz-Hugh–Curtis syndrome (see below). Thus this antigen may initiate an immune-mediated process that ultimately damages the fallopian tube. Host genetic susceptibility, as defined by HLA type, may also play an important role.

Perihepatitis, or the Fitz-Hugh–Curtis syndrome, was originally described as a complication of gonococcal PID.

The syndrome should be suspected whenever a young, sexually active woman presents with an illness resembling cholecystitis (fever and right-upper-quadrant pain of subacute or acute onset). Symptoms and signs of salpingitis may be minimal. Cultural and/or serologic evidence of *C. trachomatis* infection is found in three-quarters of women with this syndrome.

Urethral Syndrome in Women

In the absence of infection with uropathogens such as coliforms or *Staphylococcus saprophyticus*, *C. trachomatis* is the pathogen most commonly isolated from college women with dysuria, frequency, and pyuria (Chap. 27). This organism can also be isolated from the urethra of women without symptoms of urethritis, and up to 25% of female STD clinic patients with chlamydial urogenital infection have cultures positive for *C. trachomatis* from the urethra only.

Infection in Pregnancy and the Neonatal Period

Studies in the United States have demonstrated that 5–25% of pregnant women have *C. trachomatis* infections of the cervix. In these studies, approximately one-half to two-thirds of children exposed during birth have acquired *C. trachomatis* infection. Roughly half of the infected infants (25% of the group exposed) have developed clinical evidence of inclusion conjunctivitis. In addition to infecting the eye, *C. trachomatis* has been isolated frequently and persistently from the nasopharynx, rectum, and vagina of such infants, occasionally for >1 year in the absence of treatment. Pneumonia develops in 10% of children infected perinatally, and otitis media may in some cases result from perinatally acquired chlamydial infection.

Neonatal chlamydial conjunctivitis has an acute onset 5–14 days after birth and often produces a profuse mucopurulent discharge. However, it is impossible to differentiate chlamydial conjunctivitis from other forms of neonatal conjunctivitis (such as that due to *N. gonorrhoeae*, *Haemophilus influenzae*, *Streptococcus pneumoniae*, or HSV) on clinical grounds; thus laboratory diagnosis is required. Inclusions within epithelial cells are often detected in Giemsa-stained conjunctival smears, but these smears are considerably less sensitive than cultures, antigen detection tests, or NAATs for chlamydiae. Gram-stained smears may show gonococci or occasional small gram-negative coccobacilli in *Haemophilus* conjunctivitis, but smears should be accompanied by cultures for these agents.

C. trachomatis causes a distinctive pneumonia syndrome in infants. Epidemiologic studies have linked chlamydial pulmonary infection in infants with increased occurrence of subacute lung disease (bronchitis, asthma, wheezing) in later childhood.

Lymphogranuloma Venereum

Definition

LGV is an STI caused by *C. trachomatis* strains of the L_1, L_2, and L_3 serovars. In the United States, most cases are caused by L_2 organisms. Classically, acute LGV is characterized by a transient primary genital lesion followed by multilocular suppurative regional lymphadenopathy. However, patients exposed via insertive rectal intercourse usually develop hemorrhagic proctitis with regional lymphadenitis. Acute LGV is almost always associated with systemic symptoms such as fever and leukocytosis but is rarely associated with systemic complications such as meningoencephalitis. Without treatment, late complications that develop after a period of years include genital elephantiasis due to lymphatic involvement, strictures, and fistulas of the penis, urethra, and rectum.

Epidemiology

LGV is usually sexually transmitted, but occasional transmission by nonsexual personal contact, fomites, or laboratory accidents has been documented. Laboratory work involving the creation of aerosols of LGV organisms (e.g., sonication, homogenization) must be conducted only with appropriate measures for biologic containment.

The peak incidence of LGV corresponds to the age of greatest sexual activity: the second and third decades of life. The worldwide incidence of LGV is falling, but the disease is still endemic and a major cause of morbidity in Asia, Africa, South America, and parts of the Caribbean. In the Bahamas, an apparent outbreak of LGV was described in association with a concurrent increase in heterosexual infection with HIV. For more than a decade, however, the reported incidence of LGV in the United States has been only 0.1 case per 100,000 persons. Recently, clusters of LGV cases have been described in the United States and in Western Europe, largely among men having sex with men. These cases have usually presented as hemorrhagic proctocolitis in HIV-positive men. More widespread use of NAATs for identification of rectal infections may have enhanced case recognition.

The frequency of infection after exposure is believed to be much lower for LGV than for gonorrhea and syphilis. Early manifestations are recognized more often in men than in women, who usually present with late complications. In the United States, where the reported male-to-female ratio of cases is 3.4:1, most cases involve homosexually active men and persons returning from abroad (travelers, sailors, and military personnel). The main reservoir of infection, although it has not been directly demonstrated, is presumed to be asymptomatically infected individuals.

Clinical Manifestations

A *primary genital lesion* develops 3 days to 3 weeks after exposure. It is a small, painless vesicle or nonindurated ulcer or papule located on the penis in men and on the labia, posterior vagina, or fourchette in women. The primary lesion is noticed by fewer than one-third of men with LGV and only rarely by women. It heals in a few days without scarring and, even when noticed, is usually recognized as LGV only in retrospect. LGV strains of *C. trachomatis* have occasionally been recovered from genital ulcers and from the urethra of men and the endocervix of women who present with inguinal adenopathy; these areas may be the primary site of infection in some cases.

Primary anal or *rectal infection* develops after receptive anorectal intercourse. In women, rectal infection with LGV (or non-LGV) strains of *C. trachomatis* presumably can also arise by the contiguous spread of infected secretions along the perineum (as in rectal gonococcal infections in women) or perhaps by spread to the rectum via the pelvic lymphatics.

From the site of the primary urethral, genital, anal, or rectal infection, the organism spreads via the regional lymphatics. Penile, vulvar, or anal infection can lead to inguinal and femoral lymphadenitis. Rectal infection produces hypogastric and deep iliac lymphadenitis. Upper vaginal or cervical infection results in enlargement of the obturator and iliac nodes.

The most common presenting picture in heterosexual men is the *inguinal syndrome*, which is characterized by painful inguinal lymphadenopathy beginning 2–6 weeks after presumed exposure; in rare instances, the onset comes after a few months. The inguinal adenopathy is unilateral in two-thirds of cases, and palpable enlargement of the iliac and femoral nodes is often evident on the same side as the enlarged inguinal nodes. The nodes are initially discrete, but progressive periadenitis results in a matted mass of nodes that becomes fluctuant and suppurative. The overlying skin becomes fixed, inflamed, and thin and finally develops multiple draining fistulas. Extensive enlargement of chains of inguinal nodes above and below the inguinal ligament ("the sign of the groove") is not specific and, although not uncommon, is documented in only a minority of cases. On histologic examination, infected nodes are initially found to have characteristic small stellate abscesses surrounded by histiocytes. These abscesses coalesce to form large, necrotic, suppurative foci. Spontaneous healing usually takes place after several months; inguinal scars or granulomatous masses of various sizes persist for life. Massive pelvic lymphadenopathy may lead to exploratory laparotomy.

As NAATs for *C. trachomatis* are being used more often, increasing numbers of cases of LGV proctitis are being recognized in homosexual men. Such patients present with anorectal pain and mucopurulent, bloody rectal discharge. Although these patients may report diarrhea, they are often referring not to diarrhea but rather to frequent, painful, unsuccessful attempts at defecation (tenesmus). Sigmoidoscopy reveals ulcerative proctitis or proctocolitis, with purulent exudate and mucosal bleeding. The histopathologic findings in the rectal mucosa include granulomas with giant cells, crypt abscesses, and extensive inflammation. These clinical, sigmoidoscopic, and histopathologic findings may closely resemble those of Crohn's disease of the rectum.

Constitutional symptoms are common during the stage of regional lymphadenopathy and, in cases of proctitis, may include fever, chills, headache, meningismus, anorexia, myalgias, and arthralgias. These findings in the presence of lymphadenopathy are sometimes mistakenly interpreted as malignant lymphoma. Other systemic complications are infrequent but include arthritis with sterile effusion, aseptic meningitis, meningoencephalitis, conjunctivitis, hepatitis, and erythema nodosum. Chlamydiae have been recovered from the cerebrospinal fluid and in one case were isolated from the blood of a patient with severe constitutional symptoms—a result indicating the dissemination of infection. Laboratory-acquired infections suspected of being due to the inhalation of aerosols have been associated with mediastinal lymphadenitis, pneumonitis, and pleural effusion.

Complications of untreated anorectal infection include perirectal abscess, fistula in ano, and rectovaginal, rectovesical, and ischiorectal fistulas. Secondary bacterial infection probably contributes to these complications. Rectal stricture is a late complication of anorectal infection and usually develops 2–6 cm from the anal orifice—i.e., at a site within reach on digital rectal examination. Proximal extension of the stricture for several centimeters may lead to a mistaken clinical and radiographic diagnosis of carcinoma.

A small percentage of cases of LGV in men present as chronic progressive infiltrative, ulcerative, or fistular lesions of the penis, urethra, or scrotum. Associated lymphatic obstruction may produce elephantiasis. When urethral stricture occurs, it usually involves the posterior urethra and causes incontinence or difficulty with urination.

Approach to the Diagnosis and Treatment of C. Trachomatis *Genital Infections*

Four types of laboratory procedure are available to confirm *C. trachomatis* infection: direct microscopic examination of tissue scrapings for typical intracytoplasmic inclusions or EBs; isolation of the organism in cell culture; demonstration of chlamydial antigens by immunologic detection or demonstration of chlamydial genes in NAATs; and detection of antibody in serum or in local secretions.

Except in conjunctivitis, direct microscopic examination of Giemsa-stained cell scrapings for typical inclusions has an unacceptably low degree of sensitivity, and false-positive interpretations by inexperienced observers are also common. Even for conjunctivitis, this approach has been replaced by direct fluorescent antibody staining of conjunctival smears to identify chlamydial EBs with specific monoclonal antibodies (see below) or, where available, NAATs.

Cell culture techniques for isolation of *C. trachomatis* are available only in large medical centers. In addition to limited availability, other disadvantages of cell culture include its low and variable level of sensitivity (40–80%), its requirement for rigorous transport conditions, and its high cost and technically demanding nature. Therefore, nonculture alternatives involving antigen detection or nucleic acid amplification have been developed. In the direct immunofluorescent antibody (DFA) slide test, potentially infected genital or ocular secretions are smeared onto a slide, fixed, and stained with fluorescein-conjugated monoclonal antibody specific for chlamydial antigens. The observation of fluorescing EBs confirms the diagnosis. Enzyme-linked immunosorbent assay (ELISA) techniques for the detection of chlamydial antigens provide another alternative to culture. The reported sensitivity and specificity of these tests for genital infections (as compared with culture) have been 60–80% and

97–99%, respectively, in high-risk populations. More recently, NAATs have been developed for chlamydial diagnosis using PCR, ligase chain reaction (LCR), TMA, and other techniques. These tests are quite clearly the most sensitive and specific chlamydial diagnostic methods available; they are also the most expensive. Because of their very high analytic sensitivity, NAATs allow the use of novel specimens: these tests can detect chlamydial genes in first-void urine samples or patient-collected vaginal swabs with a high degree of sensitivity and specificity. The use of urine specimens and patient-collected vaginal swabs rather than conventional urethral and cervical swabs is particularly appealing for public-health chlamydial screening programs because of the ease of sample collection and transport, even in community-based settings. These tests have also facilitated population-based studies of chlamydial infections.

Serologic tests are of limited usefulness in the diagnosis of most chlamydial oculogenital infections. The complement fixation test with heat-stable, genus-specific antigen has been used with some success to diagnose LGV but is insensitive in infections due to non-LGV strains of *C. trachomatis*. The microimmunofluorescence (micro-IF) test with *C. trachomatis* antigens is more sensitive but is generally available only in research laboratories. The test measures antibodies by serovar specificity and by immunoglobulin class (IgM, IgG, IgA, secretory IgA) in both serum and local secretions. Cross-reacting antibodies to *C. pneumoniae* may sometimes be problematic. Serologic diagnosis by the micro-IF test may be useful in infant pneumonia (in which high-titer IgM antibody and/or fourfold rises in titer are often demonstrated), in chlamydial salpingitis (especially Fitz-Hugh–Curtis syndrome), and in LGV. In all of these more invasive syndromes, high antibody levels are present.

Table 77-1 summarizes the diagnostic tests of choice for patients with suspected *C. trachomatis* infection. It is clear that, in most settings and for most purposes, sensitivity and specificity will be greatest with NAATs. For patients to whom medicolegal considerations may apply (victims of sexual or child abuse), cultures or NAATs should always be used. In men with suspected urethritis, application of NAATs to a first-void urine specimen offers a sensitive and noninvasive diagnostic method other than the use of urethral swabs. For the diagnosis of urogenital (cervical or urethral) infections in women, testing of a first-void urine specimen by nucleic acid amplification methods is about as sensitive as testing of a cervical swab. Patient-collected vaginal swabs analyzed by NAAT have also been used successfully and with equal sensitivity and specificity. Since chlamydial diagnostic testing has become more widely available and is now more sensitive and specific than in the past, its use for specific diagnosis in patients with suspected chlamydial syndromes (e.g., MPC, NGU, and PID) and their partners should be promoted. High priority should also be given to the screening of asymptomatic high-risk women who would not otherwise receive treatment for presumptive chlamydial infection, especially those seen in high-risk settings (e.g., STD clinics or abortion clinics) and those with a high-risk profile (e.g., sexually active and ≤ 21 years of age, new sex partner within the preceding 2 months, or more than one current sex partner). Similar screening programs should be used to detect and treat asymptomatic urethritis in high-risk adolescent males. Where implemented, screening programs of this type have generally been associated with reductions in the prevalence of chlamydial infection and of its complications, such as PID, ectopic pregnancy, and infertility.

Rx Treatment: C. TRACHOMATIS GENITAL AND PERINATAL INFECTIONS

Until the introduction of azithromycin, chlamydial infections could not be eradicated by single-dose or short-term antimicrobial regimens, and most uncomplicated genital infections in adults were treated with a 7-day course of doxycycline or tetracycline. A 2-week course is recommended for complicated chlamydial infections (e.g., PID, epididymitis) and at least a 3-week course of doxycycline (100 mg orally bid) or erythromycin base (500 mg orally qid) for LGV. Failure of treatment with a tetracycline in genital infections usually indicates poor compliance or reinfection rather than the involvement of a drug-resistant strain. To date, clinically significant drug resistance has not been observed in *C. trachomatis* infection.

Therapy for *C. trachomatis* urethritis is more efficacious than therapy for nonchlamydial NGU. *C. trachomatis* is eradicated from the urethra in nearly all cases by treatment with tetracycline hydrochloride (500 mg qid for 7 days) or doxycycline (100 mg by mouth bid for 7 days).

Eradication of *C. trachomatis* from the cervix by tetracycline and doxycycline, with doses and durations similar to those specified above for urethritis, has been demonstrated. Azithromycin (a single oral 1-g dose) is the regimen of choice for pregnant women with *C. trachomatis* infection. However, amoxicillin (500 mg tid for 7 days) can also be given to pregnant women. Tetracycline hydrochloride (500 mg qid) or doxycycline (100 mg bid) for 14 days produces clinical and microbiologic cure of epididymitis and PID associated with *C. trachomatis* infection, but in this situation a tetracycline should always be used together with a drug that is highly effective against gonorrhea.

Azithromycin is highly active against *C. trachomatis*, exhibits prolonged bioavailability, is concentrated intracellularly, and has, for the first time, made it possible to use single-dose therapy for chlamydial infection. In comparative trials, a 1-g single dose of azithromycin has been as effective as 7 days of doxycycline therapy for uncomplicated chlamydial infection. Azithromycin causes fewer adverse gastrointestinal reactions than do older macrolides such as erythromycin. The single-dose regimen of azithromycin has great appeal for the treatment of patients with uncomplicated chlamydial infection (especially those without symptoms and those with a likelihood of poor compliance) and of sexual partners of

TABLE 77-1

DIAGNOSTIC TESTS FOR SEXUALLY TRANSMITTED AND PERINATAL *CHLAMYDIA TRACHOMATIS* INFECTION

INFECTION	SUGGESTIVE SIGNS/SYMPTOMS	PRESUMPTIVE DIAGNOSIS[a]	CONFIRMATORY TEST OF CHOICE
Men			
NGU, PGU	Discharge, dysuria	Gram's stain with >4 neutrophils per oil-immersion field; no gonococci	Urine or urethral NAAT for *C. trachomatis*
Epididymitis	Unilateral intrascrotal swelling, pain, tenderness; fever; NGU	Gram's stain with >4 neutrophils per oil-immersion field; no gonococci; urinalysis with pyuria	Urine or urethral NAAT for *C. trachomatis*
Women			
Cervicitis	Mucopurulent cervical discharge, bleeding and edema of the zone of cervical ectopy	Cervical Gram's stain with ≥20 neutrophils per oil-immersion field in cervical mucus	Urine, cervical, or vaginal NAAT for *C. trachomatis*
Salpingitis	Lower abdominal pain, cervical motion tenderness, adnexal tenderness or masses	*C. trachomatis* always potentially present in salpingitis	Urine, cervical, or vaginal NAAT for *C. trachomatis*
Urethritis	Dysuria and frequency without hematuria	MPC; sterile pyuria; negative routine urine culture	Urine or urethral NAAT for *C. trachomatis*
Adults of Either Sex			
Proctitis	Rectal pain, discharge, tenesmus, bleeding; history of receptive anorectal intercourse	Negative gonococcal culture and Gram's stain; at least 1 neutrophil per oil-immersion field in rectal Gram's stain	Rectal NAAT for *C. trachomatis* or culture
Reiter's syndrome	NGU, arthritis, conjunctivitis, typical skin lesions	Gram's stain with >4 neutrophils per oil-immersion field; lack of gonococci indicative of NGU	Urine or urethral NAAT for *C. trachomatis*
LGV	Regional adenopathy, primary lesion, proctitis, systemic symptoms	None	Culture of LGV strain from node or rectum, occasionally from urethra or cervix; NAAT for *C. trachomatis* from these sites; LGV CF titer, ≥1:64; micro-IF titer, ≥1:512
Neonates			
Conjunctivitis	Purulent conjunctival discharge 6–18 days after delivery	Negative culture and Gram's stain for gonococci, *Haemophilus* spp., pneumococci, staphylococci	Conjunctival NAAT for *C. trachomatis*; FA-stained scraping of conjunctival material
Infant pneumonia	Afebrile, staccato cough, diffuse rales, bilateral hyperinflation, interstitial infiltrates	None	Chlamydial culture or NAAT of sputum, pharynx, eye, rectum; micro-IF antibody to *C. trachomatis*—fourfold change in IgG or IgM antibody titer

[a]A presumptive diagnosis of chlamydial infection is often made in the syndromes listed when gonococci are not found. A positive test for *Neisseria gonorrhoeae* does not exclude the involvement of *C. trachomatis*, which often is present in patients with gonorrhea.

Note: CF, complement-fixing; FA, fluorescent antibody; LGV, lymphogranuloma venereum; micro-IF, microimmunofluorescence; MPC, mucopurulent cervicitis; NAAT, nucleic acid amplification test; NGU, nongonococcal urethritis; PGU, postgonococcal urethritis.

infected patients. These advantages must be weighed against the considerably greater cost of azithromycin. Whenever possible, the single 1-g dose should be given as directly observed therapy. Although not approved by the U.S. Food and Drug Administration for the treatment of pregnant women, the 1-g single-dose regimen of azithromycin appears to be safe and effective for this purpose.

Of the fluoroquinolones, ofloxacin (300 mg by mouth bid for 7 days) and levofloxacin (500 mg/d by mouth for 7 days) are as effective as doxycycline for the treatment of chlamydial infection and appear to be safe and well tolerated. These drugs cannot be used in pregnancy.

TREATMENT OF SEX PARTNERS The continued high prevalence of chlamydial infections in most parts of the United States is due primarily to the failure to diagnose—and therefore treat—patients with symptomatic or asymptomatic infection and their sex partners. *C. trachomatis* urethral or cervical infection has been well documented in a high proportion of the sex partners of patients with NGU, epididymitis, Reiter's syndrome, salpingitis, or endocervicitis. If possible, confirmatory laboratory tests for *Chlamydia* should be undertaken in these individuals, but even those without positive tests or evidence of clinical disease who have recently been exposed to proven or possible chlamydial infection (e.g., NGU) should be offered therapy. A novel approach is the use of partner-delivered therapy, in which the infected patient receives treatment and is also provided with single-dose azithromycin to give to his or her sex partner(s).

TREATMENT OF NEONATES AND INFANTS In neonates with conjunctivitis or infants with pneumonia, erythromycin ethylsuccinate or estolate can be given orally at a dosage of 50 mg/kg per day, preferably in four divided doses, for 2 weeks. Careful attention must be given to compliance with therapy—a frequent problem. Relapses of eye infection are common after treatment with topical erythromycin or tetracycline ophthalmic ointment and may also follow oral erythromycin therapy. Thus follow-up cultures should be performed after treatment. Both parents should be examined for *C. trachomatis* infection and, if diagnostic testing is not readily available, should be treated with doxycycline or azithromycin.

Prevention

Efforts to develop a vaccine for chlamydial infection have not yet been successful. Early diagnosis and treatment shorten the duration of the infectious period and therefore constitute primary prevention of chlamydial infection. By the early 1990s, one of the 10 regions of the United States (Region X, the Pacific Northwest) had formally undertaken a chlamydial control program involving widespread screening of women attending family planning clinics. In women meeting the criteria for high risk, ~500,000 tests per year were conducted at 150 such clinics throughout the region. Within 5 years, the prevalence of chlamydial infection had been reduced by >30% in this population. However, the chlamydial prevalence in Region X has since leveled off and even begun to increase once again. Thus further study of chlamydial screening programs and their impact on *Chlamydia*-associated reproductive sequelae is needed. Although most regions of the United States have now initiated screening programs, some family planning and STD clinics still do not offer chlamydial testing. The availability of highly sensitive and specific diagnostic tests that can be done with urine specimens and of single-dose therapy makes it feasible to mount an effective chlamydial control program nationwide, with screening of high-risk persons both in traditional health care settings and in novel community- and school-based settings.

TRACHOMA AND ADULT INCLUSION CONJUNCTIVITIS

Definition

Trachoma is a chronic conjunctivitis associated with infection by *C. trachomatis* serovar A, B, Ba, or C. It has been responsible for an estimated 20 million cases of blindness throughout the world and remains an important cause of preventable blindness. *Inclusion conjunctivitis* is an acute ocular infection caused by sexually transmitted *C. trachomatis* strains (usually serovars D through K) in adults exposed to infected genital secretions and in their newborn offspring.

Epidemiology

In trachoma-endemic areas where the classic eye disease is seen, *C. trachomatis* is transmitted from eye to eye via hands, flies, towels, and other fomites; serovar A, B, Ba, or C is usually involved. The worldwide incidence and severity of trachoma have decreased dramatically during the past 35 years, mainly as a result of improving hygienic and economic conditions. However, endemic trachoma is still the major cause of preventable blindness in northern Africa, Sub-Saharan Africa, the Middle East, and parts of Asia. Transmission occurs primarily through close personal contact, particularly among young children in rural communities with limited water supplies. In endemic areas, trachoma is associated with repeated exposure and reinfection, but the infection can also become chronic and persistent. Acute relapse of old trachoma occasionally follows treatment with cortisone eye ointment or develops in very old persons who were exposed in their youth.

Clinical Manifestations

Both endemic trachoma and adult inclusion conjunctivitis present initially as a conjunctivitis characterized by small lymphoid follicles in the conjunctiva. In regions with hyperendemic classic blinding trachoma, the disease usually starts insidiously before the age of 2 years. Reinfection is common and probably contributes to the pathogenesis of trachoma. Studies using PCR techniques indicate that chlamydial DNA is often present in the ocular secretions of patients with trachoma, even in the absence of positive cultures. Thus persistent infection may be more common than was previously thought.

The cornea becomes involved, with inflammatory leukocytic infiltrations and superficial vascularization (pannus formation). As the inflammation continues, conjunctival scarring eventually distorts the eyelids, causing them to turn inward so that the inturned lashes constantly abrade the eyeball (trichiasis and entropion); eventually the corneal epithelium is abraded and may ulcerate, with subsequent corneal scarring and blindness. Destruction of the conjunctival goblet cells, lacrimal ducts, and lacrimal gland may produce a "dry-eye" syndrome, with resultant corneal opacity due to drying (xerosis) or secondary bacterial corneal ulcers.

Communities with blinding trachoma often experience seasonal epidemics of conjunctivitis due to *H. influenzae* that contribute to the intensity of the inflammatory process. In such areas, the active infectious process usually resolves spontaneously in affected persons at 10–15 years of age, but the conjunctival scars continue to shrink, producing trichiasis and entropion and subsequent corneal scarring in adults. In areas with milder and less prevalent disease, the process may be much slower, with active disease continuing into adulthood; blindness is rare in these cases.

Eye infection with genital *C. trachomatis* strains in sexually active young adults presents as the acute onset of unilateral follicular conjunctivitis and preauricular lymphadenopathy similar to that seen in acute adenovirus or herpesvirus conjunctivitis. If untreated, the disease may persist for 6 weeks to 2 years. It is frequently associated with corneal inflammation in the form of discrete opacities ("infiltrates"), punctate epithelial erosions, and minor degrees of superficial corneal vascularization. Very rarely, conjunctival scarring and eyelid distortion occur, particularly in patients treated for many months with topical glucocorticoids. Recurrent eye infections develop most often in patients whose sexual consorts are not treated with antimicrobial agents.

Diagnosis

The clinical diagnosis of classic trachoma can be made if two of the following signs are present: (1) lymphoid follicles on the upper tarsal conjunctiva; (2) typical conjunctival scarring; (3) vascular pannus; or (4) limbal follicles or their sequelae, Herbert's pits. The clinical diagnosis of endemic trachoma should be confirmed by laboratory tests in children with more marked degrees of inflammation. Intracytoplasmic chlamydial inclusions are found in 10–60% of Giemsa-stained conjunctival smears in such populations, but chlamydial NAATs are more sensitive and are often positive when smears or cultures are negative. Follicular conjunctivitis in adult Europeans or Americans living in trachomatous regions is rarely due to trachoma.

℞ Treatment: ADULT INCLUSION CONJUNCTIVITIS

Adult inclusion conjunctivitis responds well to treatment with the same regimens used for treatment of uncomplicated genital infections—namely, azithromycin (a 1-g single oral dose) or doxycycline (100 mg bid for 7 days). Simultaneous treatment of all sexual consorts of the patient is also necessary to prevent ocular reinfection and to avoid chlamydial genital disease. Topical antibiotic treatment is not required for patients who receive systemic antibiotics.

Prevention

Efforts to develop a trachoma vaccine have not yet been successful. General hygienic measures associated with improved living standards are effective in the elimination of endemic trachoma. An adequate water supply for personal cleanliness may be a critical factor. In some areas the reduction of numbers of flies in the household is important. The key elements of the World Health Organization's Global Campaign to Eliminate Trachoma are encompassed in the S-A-F-E strategy: *s*urgery for deformed eyelids; periodic mass treatment with *a*zithromycin; *f*ace washing; and *e*nvironmental improvements. Mass treatment of entire villages with single-dose azithromycin has been associated with marked declines in chlamydial infection and eye disease.

C. PSITTACI INFECTIONS

Definition

Psittacosis is primarily an infectious disease of birds and mammals that is caused by *C. psittaci*. Transmission of infection from birds to humans results in a febrile illness characterized by pneumonitis and systemic manifestations. Inapparent infections or mild influenza-like illnesses may also occur. The term *ornithosis* is sometimes applied to infections contracted from birds other than parrots or parakeets, but *psittacosis* is the preferred generic term for all forms of the disease.

Epidemiology

Almost any avian species can harbor *C. psittaci*. Psittacine birds (parrots, parakeets, budgerigars) are most commonly infected, but human cases have been traced to contact with pigeons, ducks, turkeys, chickens, and many other birds. Psittacosis may be considered an occupational disease of pet-shop owners, poultry workers, pigeon fanciers, taxidermists, veterinarians, and zoo attendants. Incidence has increased during the past 25 years, with cases and outbreaks occurring primarily among employees of poultry-processing plants. It is suspected that many cases go undiagnosed and unreported.

C. psittaci is present in nasal secretions, excreta, tissues, and feathers of infected birds. Although the disease can be fatal, infected birds frequently show only minor evidence of illness, such as ruffled feathers, lethargy, and anorexia. Asymptomatic avian carriers are common, and complete recovery may be followed by continued shedding of the organism for many months.

Psittacosis is almost always transmitted to humans by the respiratory route. On rare occasions the disease may be acquired from the bite of a pet bird. Prolonged contact is not essential for transmission of the disease; spending a few minutes in an environment previously occupied by an infected bird has resulted in human infection. In one outbreak, gardening rather than direct exposure to birds was associated with infection. A psittacosis-like agent has been transmitted among hospital personnel, with severe and sometimes fatal infections. There is evidence that these "human" strains are more virulent than avian organisms. There is no record of infection acquired by the ingestion of poultry products.

Pathogenesis

The psittacosis agent gains entrance to the body through the upper respiratory tract, spreads via the bloodstream, and eventually localizes in the pulmonary alveoli and in the reticuloendothelial cells of the spleen and liver. Invasion of the lung probably takes place by way of the bloodstream rather than by direct extension from the upper air passages. A lymphocytic inflammatory response occurs on both the interstitial and the respiratory surfaces of the alveoli as well as in the perivascular spaces. The alveolar walls and interstitial tissues of the lung are thickened, edematous, necrotic, and occasionally hemorrhagic. Histologic examination of the affected areas reveals alveolar spaces filled with fluid, erythrocytes, and lymphocytes. The picture is not pathognomonic for psittacosis unless macrophages containing characteristic cytoplasmic inclusion bodies (Levinthal-Coles-Lillie bodies) are identified. The respiratory epithelium of the bronchi and bronchioles usually remains intact.

Clinical Manifestations

The clinical manifestations and course of psittacosis are extremely variable. After an incubation period of 7–14 days or longer, the disease may start abruptly with shaking chills and fever, with temperatures ranging as high as 40.5°C (105°F); however, the onset is often gradual, with fever increasing over 3–4 days. Headache is almost always prominent, is usually diffuse and excruciating, and is often the chief complaint.

Many patients present with a dry hacking cough that is usually nonproductive, but small amounts of mucoid or bloody sputum may be raised as the disease progresses. Cough may begin early in the course of the disease or as late as 5 days after the onset of fever. Chest pain, pleurisy with effusion, or a friction rub may all occur but are rare. Pericarditis and myocarditis have been reported. Most patients have a normal or slightly increased respiratory rate; marked dyspnea with cyanosis occurs only in severe psittacosis with extensive pulmonary involvement. In psittacosis, as in mycoplasmal pneumonias, the physical signs of pneumonitis tend to be less prominent than symptoms and x-ray findings would suggest. The initial examination may reveal fine sibilant rales, or clinical evidence of pneumonia may be completely lacking. Rales usually become audible and more numerous as the illness progresses. Signs of frank pulmonary consolidation are usually absent. Symptoms of upper respiratory tract infection are not prominent, although mild sore throat, pharyngitis, and cervical adenopathy are often documented; on occasion, the last may be the only manifestation of illness. Epistaxis is encountered early in the course of nearly one-fourth of cases. Photophobia is also common.

Patients often report generalized myalgia, and spasm and stiffness of the muscles of the back and neck may lead to an erroneous diagnosis of meningitis. Lethargy, mental depression, agitation, insomnia, and disorientation have been prominent features of the illness in some epidemics but not in others; delirium and stupor develop near the end of the first week in severe cases. Occasional patients are comatose when first seen; the diagnosis of psittacosis may be elusive in these cases. Gastrointestinal manifestations such as abdominal pain, nausea, vomiting, or diarrhea are noted in some cases; constipation and abdominal distention sometimes occur as late complications. Icterus, the result of severe hepatic involvement, is a rare and ominous finding. A faint macular rash (Horder's spots) resembling the rose spots of typhoid fever has been described.

Patients without cough or other clinical evidence of respiratory involvement present with fever of unknown origin (Chap. 9). The pulse rate is slow in relation to the fever. When splenomegaly is noted in a patient with acute pneumonitis, psittacosis should be considered; the reported incidence of splenomegaly in this disease ranges from 10 to 70%. Nontender hepatic enlargement also occurs, but jaundice is rare. Thrombophlebitis is not unusual during convalescence; indeed, pulmonary infarction is sometimes a late complication and may be fatal.

In untreated cases of psittacosis, sustained or mildly remittent fever persists for 10 days to 3 weeks or occasionally for as long as 3 months. Over this period, the respiratory manifestations gradually abate. Psittacosis contracted from parrots or parakeets is more likely to be a severe, prolonged illness than infection acquired from pigeons or barnyard fowl. Relapses occur but are rare. Occasional patients develop endocarditis, and *C. psittaci* infection should be considered in cases of culture-negative endocarditis. Secondary bacterial infections are uncommon. Immunity to reinfection is probably permanent.

Laboratory Findings

The chest x-ray in psittacosis is nonspecific and may show pneumonic lesions that are usually patchy in appearance but can be hazy, diffuse, homogeneous, lobar, atelectatic, wedge-shaped, nodular, or miliary. The white blood cell count is normal or moderately decreased in the acute phase of the disease but may rise in convalescence. The erythrocyte sedimentation rate frequently is not elevated. Transient proteinuria is common. The cerebrospinal fluid sometimes contains a few mononuclear cells but is otherwise normal. Despite hepatomegaly, the results of liver function tests are generally normal or only mildly elevated.

The diagnosis can be confirmed only by isolation of the causative microorganism or by serologic studies. The agent is present in the blood during the acute phase of the disease and in the bronchial secretions for weeks or sometimes years after infection, but it is difficult to isolate. Further, the organism is hazardous to work within the laboratory, and most clinical laboratories do not offer culture for *C. psittaci*. Thus psittacosis is most readily diagnosed by the demonstration of a rising titer of complement fixation antibody in the serum of a patient with a compatible clinical syndrome. Both an acute-phase and a convalescent-phase specimen should always be tested. *C. trachomatis*, *C. psittaci*, and *C. pneumoniae* all share a genus-specific "group" antigen, which is the basis of the complement fixation test. Thus acute infections with *C. trachomatis* or *C. pneumoniae* can also produce titer rises in this test. However, these three species have different major outer-membrane proteins that are the principal antigens in the micro-IF test. If there is doubt as to the interpretation of the complement fixation test, the micro-IF test can be used to differentiate among these antigens. The prompt initiation of treatment with tetracycline has been shown to delay an antibody rise in convalescence for several weeks or months.

Differential Diagnosis

A history of exposure to birds may be the only clinical basis for differentiating psittacosis from a variety of infectious and noninfectious febrile disorders. The list of pulmonary diseases that may be confused with psittacosis includes *Mycoplasma* pneumonia, *C. pneumoniae* pneumonia, legionellosis, viral pneumonia, Q fever, coccidioidomycosis, tuberculosis, enterovirus infection, carcinoma of the lung with bronchial obstruction, and common bacterial pneumonias. In the early stages, before pneumonitis appears, psittacosis may be mistaken for influenza, typhoid fever, miliary tuberculosis, or infectious mononucleosis.

℞ Treatment: *C. PSITTACI* INFECTIONS

The tetracyclines are consistently effective in the treatment of psittacosis. Defervescence and alleviation of symptoms usually take place within 24–48 h after the institution of therapy with 2 g daily in four divided doses. To avoid relapse, treatment should probably be continued for at least 7–14 days after defervescence. Doxycycline (100 mg by mouth bid) can also be used. In severe cases, hospitalization and pulmonary intensive care may be indicated. Sulfonamides are not active against *C. psittaci*. Erythromycin can be used in patients allergic to or intolerant of tetracyclines. Limited data from studies in vitro and in animal models suggest that azithromycin and some fluoroquinolones are active against *C. psittaci*.

C. PNEUMONIAE INFECTIONS

Definition

C. pneumoniae can be distinguished from the other two chlamydial species causing human infections on the basis of DNA hybridization and EB morphology. Although *C. pneumoniae* can be grown in a variety of cell cultures, it is considerably more difficult to culture than other chlamydiae, especially from clinical specimens. HL cells appear to be the most effective cell line for isolation of *C. pneumoniae*.

Epidemiology

Knowledge of the epidemiology of *C. pneumoniae* infections comes primarily from serologic studies. Infections begin to occur in late childhood, achieve peak incidence in early adulthood, and continue throughout adult life. Seroprevalence in the many adult populations that have been tested throughout the world exceeds 40%—a figure suggesting that *C. pneumoniae* infections are ubiquitous. Secondary episodes (reinfections) appear to occur commonly in older adults throughout life. *C. pneumoniae* also produces epidemics of pneumonia and respiratory illness, especially in close residential quarters such as military barracks. The incidence of infections outside of epidemics remains poorly defined. The organism appears to be transmitted from person to person, probably primarily in schools and family units.

Pathogenesis

Little is known about the pathogenesis of *C. pneumoniae* infection. The infection begins in the upper respiratory tract and in many persons is a long-lived asymptomatic condition of the upper respiratory mucosal surfaces. However, evidence of replication within vascular endothelium and synovial membranes of joints shows that, in at least some individuals, the organism is transported to distant sites, perhaps within macrophages. A *C. pneumoniae* outer-membrane protein may induce host immune responses whose cross-reaction with human proteins results in an autoimmune reaction.

Clinical Manifestations

The clinical spectrum of *C. pneumoniae* infection includes acute pharyngitis, sinusitis, bronchitis, and pneumonitis, primarily in young adults. The clinical manifestations of primary infection appear to be more severe and prolonged than those of reinfection. The pneumonitis resembles that of *Mycoplasma* pneumonia in that leukocytosis is frequently lacking and patients often have prominent antecedent upper respiratory tract symptoms, fever, nonproductive cough, mild to moderate illness, minimal findings on chest auscultation, and small segmental infiltrates on chest x-ray. In elderly patients, pneumonia due to *C. pneumoniae* can be especially severe and may necessitate hospitalization and respiratory support.

Epidemiologic studies have demonstrated an association between serologic evidence of *C. pneumoniae* infection and atherosclerotic disease of the coronary and other arteries. In addition, *C. pneumoniae* has been identified in atherosclerotic plaques by electron microscopy, DNA hybridization, and immunocytochemistry. The organism has also been recovered in culture from atheromatous plaque—a result indicating the presence of viable replicating bacteria in vessels. Evidence from animal models supports the hypothesis that *C. pneumoniae* infection of the upper respiratory tract is followed by recovery of the organism from atheromatous lesions in the aorta and that the infection accelerates the process of atherosclerosis, especially in hypercholesterolemic animals. Antimicrobial treatment of the infected animals reverses the increased risk of atherosclerosis. In humans, two small trials in patients with unstable angina or recent myocardial infarction suggested that antibiotics reduce subsequent untoward cardiac events. However, larger trials have not demonstrated that various antibiotic regimens affect the risk of these events.

Diagnosis

Diagnosis of *C. pneumoniae* infection is difficult because cell culture techniques are not available for routine clinical use and nonculture tests using antigen detection methods or DNA probes have not been developed for commercial use. Acute- and convalescent-phase sera can be tested for chlamydial complement fixation antibody to make a retrospective diagnosis. However, this test does not distinguish *C. pneumoniae* infection from infection due to *C. trachomatis* or *C. psittaci*.

Treatment: *C. PNEUMONIAE* INFECTIONS

Although few controlled trials of treatment have been reported, *C. pneumoniae* is inhibited in vitro by erythromycin, tetracycline, azithromycin, clarithromycin, gatifloxacin, and gemifloxacin. Recommended therapy consists of 2 g/d of either tetracycline or erythromycin for 10–14 days. Other macrolides (e.g., azithromycin) and some fluoroquinolones (e.g., levofloxacin and gatifloxacin) also appear to be effective.

FURTHER READINGS

Adimora AA: Treatment of uncomplicated genital *Chlamydia trachomatis* infections in adults. Clin Infect Dis 35(Suppl 2):S183, 2002

Cassell JA et al: Trends in sexually transmitted infections in general practice 1990–2000: Population based study using data from the UK general practice research database. BMJ 332:332, 2006

Chidambaran JD et al: Effect of a single mass antibiotic distribution on the prevalence of infectious trachoma. JAMA 295:1142, 2006

Datta SD et al: Gonorrhea and chlamydia in the United States among persons 14 to 39 years of age, 1999 to 2002. Ann Intern Med 147:89, 2007

Golden MR et al: Effect of expedited treatment of sex partners on recurrent or persistent gonorrhea or chlamydial infection. N Engl J Med 352:676, 2005

Grayston JT et al: Azithromycin for the secondary prevention of coronary events. N Engl J Med 352:1637, 2005

———: Infections caused by *Chlamydia pneumoniae*, strain TWAR. Clin Infect Dis 15:757, 1992

Holmes KK, Stamm WE: Lower genital tract infections in women: Cystitis, urethritis, vulvovaginitis, and cervicitis, in *Sexually Transmitted Diseases*, 4th ed, KK Holmes et al (eds). New York, McGraw-Hill, 2008

Meyers DS et al: Screening for chlamydial infection: an evidence update for the U.S. Preventive Services Task Force. Ann Intern Med 147:135, 2007

Solomon AW et al: Mass treatment with single-dose azithromycin for trachoma. N Engl J Med 351:1962, 2004

Stamm WE: *Chlamydia trachomatis* infections in adults, in *Sexually Transmitted Diseases*, 4th ed, KK Holmes et al (eds). New York, McGraw-Hill, 2008

———: *Chlamydia* screening: Expanding the scope. Ann Intern Med 141:570, 2004

———: *Chlamydia trachomatis*: The persistent pathogen. Sex Transm Dis 13:684, 2001

SECTION V

VIRAL INFECTIONS

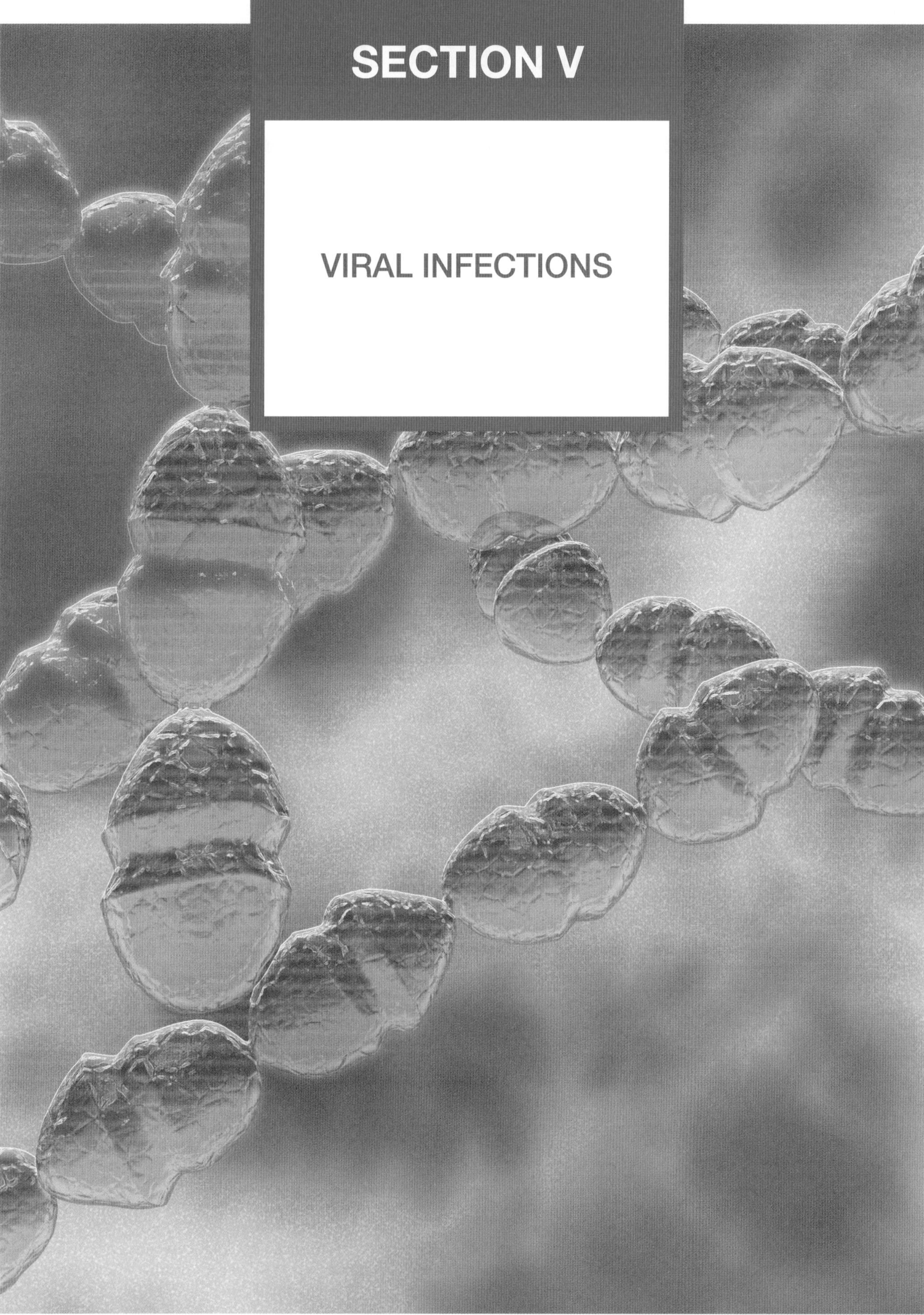

PART 1 VIRAL DISEASES: GENERAL CONSIDERATIONS

CHAPTER 78

MEDICAL VIROLOGY

Fred Wang ■ Elliott Kieff

DEFINING A VIRUS

Viruses consist of a nucleic acid surrounded by one or more proteins. Some viruses also have an outer-membrane envelope. Viruses are obligate intracellular parasites: they can replicate only within cells since their nucleic acids do not encode the many enzymes necessary for protein, carbohydrate, or lipid metabolism and for the generation of high-energy phosphates. Typically, viral nucleic acids encode proteins necessary for replicating and packaging their nucleic acids within the biochemical milieu of host cells.

Viruses differ from viroids, prions, and virusoids. *Virusoids* are nucleic acids that depend on helper viruses to package their nucleic acids into virus-like particles. *Viroids* are naked, cyclical, mostly double-stranded, small RNAs. Viroids appear to be restricted to plants, spread from cell to cell, and are replicated by cellular RNA polymerase II. *Prions* (Chap. 101) are abnormal protein molecules that can spread. These molecules reproduce by changing the structure of their normal cellular protein counterparts. Prions have been implicated in neurodegenerative conditions such as Creutzfeldt-Jakob disease, Gerstmann-Straüssler disease, kuru, and human bovine spongiform encephalopathy ("mad cow disease").

VIRAL STRUCTURE

Viruses have from a few to several hundred genes. These genes may be in a single-strand or double-strand DNA genome or in a single-strand sense, a single-strand or segmented antisense, or a double-strand segmented RNA genome. Sense-strand RNA genomes can be translated directly into protein. Sense and antisense genomes are also referred to as *positive-strand* and *negative-strand genomes*, respectively. The viral nucleic acid is usually associated with one or more virus-encoded nucleoproteins in the core of the viral particle. The viral nucleic acid and nucleoproteins are almost always enclosed in a protein shell called a *capsid*. Because of the limited genetic complexity of viruses, their capsids are usually composed of multimers of identical capsomeres. Capsomeres are in turn composed of one or a few proteins. Capsids have icosahedral or helical symmetry. Icosahedral structures approximate spheres but have two-, three-, and fivefold axes of symmetry, whereas helical structures have only a twofold axis of symmetry. The entire structural unit of nucleic acid, nucleoprotein(s), and capsid is called a *nucleocapsid*.

Many human viruses are simply composed of a core and a capsid. For these viruses, the outer surface of the capsid mediates contact with uninfected cells. Other viruses are more complex and have an outer lipid-containing envelope derived from virus-modified membranes of the infected cell. The piece of infected-cell membrane that becomes the viral envelope has usually been modified during infection by the insertion of virus-encoded glycoproteins, which usually mediate contact of enveloped viruses with uninfected cells. Matrix or tegument proteins fill the space between the nucleocapsid and the envelope in many enveloped viruses. In general, enveloped viruses are sensitive to lipid solvents and nonionic detergents that can dissolve the envelope, whereas viruses that consist only of nucleocapsids are somewhat resistant. A schematic diagram for large and complex herpesviruses is shown in Fig. 78-1. Prototypical pathogenic human viruses are listed in Table 78-1. The relative sizes and structures of typical pathogenic human viruses are shown in Fig. 78-2.

TAXONOMY OF PATHOGENIC HUMAN VIRUSES

As is apparent from Table 78-1 and Fig. 78-2, the classification of viruses into orders and families is based on nucleic acid composition, nucleocapsid size and symmetry, and presence or absence of an envelope. Viruses of a single family have similar types of genomes and are often morphologically indistinguishable in electron micrographs. Further subclassification into genera depends on similarities in epidemiology and biologic effects and on the degree of colinear nucleic acid sequence homology.

Most human viruses have a common name related to their pathologic effects or the circumstances of their

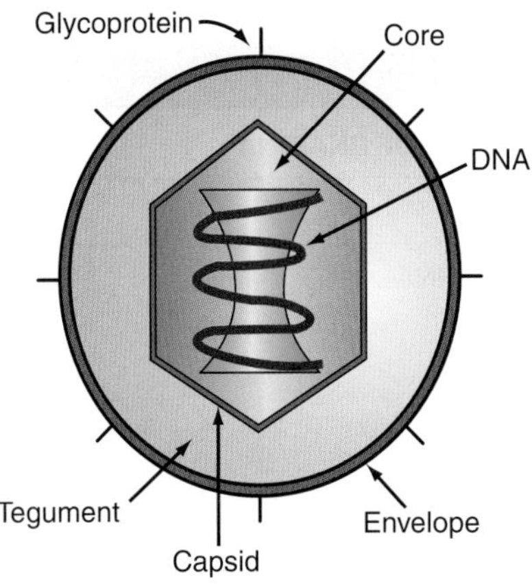

FIGURE 78-1
Schematic diagram of an enveloped herpesvirus with an icosahedral nucleocapsid. The approximate respective dimensions of the nucleocapsid and the enveloped particles are 110 and 180 nm. The capsid is composed of 162 capsomeres: 150 with sixfold and 12 with fivefold axes of symmetry.

discovery. Formal species names have been assigned by the International Committee on Taxonomy of Viruses. The formal designation consists of the name of the host followed by the family or genus of the virus and a number. This dual terminology has created a confusing situation in which viruses are referred to and referenced by either name—e.g., varicella-zoster virus (VZV) or human herpesvirus (HHV) 3.

VIRAL INFECTION IN VITRO

STAGES OF VIRAL INFECTION AT THE CELLULAR LEVEL

Viral Interactions with the Cell Surface and Cell Entry

Viral infection is initiated by adsorption of the virus to the cell surface. Adsorption results from the molecular interaction of viral surface proteins with receptors on the cell's plasma membrane (see Table 2-1). For example, a

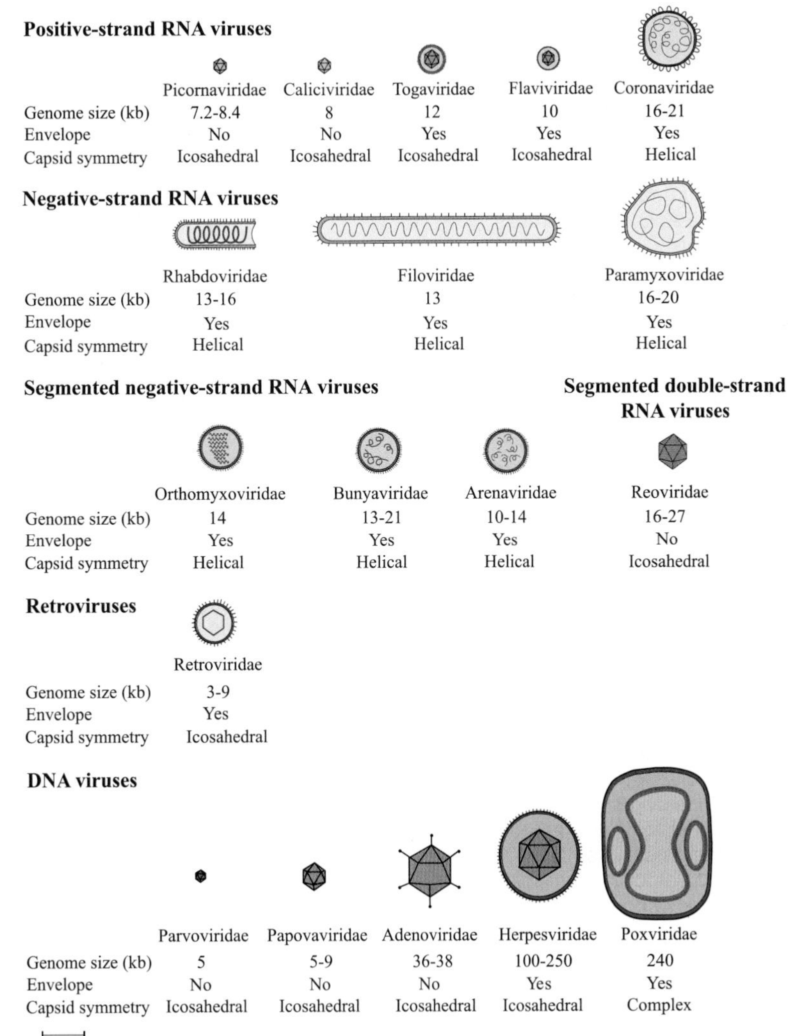

Positive-strand RNA viruses
Picornaviridae Caliciviridae Togaviridae Flaviviridae Coronaviridae
Genome size (kb) 7.2-8.4 8 12 10 16-21
Envelope No No Yes Yes Yes
Capsid symmetry Icosahedral Icosahedral Icosahedral Icosahedral Helical
Negative-strand RNA viruses
Rhabdoviridae Filoviridae Paramyxoviridae
Genome size (kb) 13-16 13 16-20
Envelope Yes Yes Yes
Capsid symmetry Helical Helical Helical
Segmented negative-strand RNA viruses
Segmented double-strand RNA viruses
Orthomyxoviridae Bunyaviridae Arenaviridae Reoviridae
Genome size (kb) 14 13-21 10-14 16-27
Envelope Yes Yes Yes No
Capsid symmetry Helical Helical Helical Icosahedral
Retroviruses
Retroviridae
Genome size (kb) 3-9
Envelope Yes
Capsid symmetry Icosahedral
DNA viruses
Parvoviridae Papovaviridae Adenoviridae Herpesviridae Poxviridae
Genome size (kb) 5 5-9 36-38 100-250 240
Envelope No No No Yes Yes
Capsid symmetry Icosahedral Icosahedral Icosahedral Icosahedral Complex
100 nm

FIGURE 78-2
Schematic diagrams of the major virus families including species that infect humans. The viruses are grouped by genome type and are drawn approximately to scale. Prototype viruses of each family that cause human disease are listed in Table 78-1.

TABLE 78-1

VIRUS FAMILIES PATHOGENIC FOR HUMANS

FAMILY	REPRESENTATIVE VIRUSES	TYPE OF RNA/DNA	LIPID ENVELOPE
RNA Viruses			
Picornaviridae	Poliovirus Coxsackievirus Echovirus Enterovirus Rhinovirus Hepatitis A virus	(+) RNA	No
Caliciviridae	Norwalk agent Hepatitis E virus	(+) RNA	No
Togaviridae	Rubella virus Eastern equine encephalitis virus Western equine encephalitis virus	(+) RNA	Yes
Flaviviridae	Yellow fever virus Dengue virus St. Louis encephalitis virus West Nile virus Hepatitis C virus Hepatitis G virus	(+) RNA	Yes
Coronaviridae	Coronaviruses[a]	(+) RNA	Yes
Rhabdoviridae	Rabies virus Vesicular stomatitis virus	(–) RNA	Yes
Filoviridae	Marburg virus Ebola virus	(–) RNA	Yes
Paramyxoviridae	Parainfluenza virus Respiratory syncytial virus Newcastle disease virus Mumps virus Rubeola (measles) virus	(–) RNA	Yes
Orthomyxoviridae	Influenza A, B, and C viruses	(–) RNA, 8 segments	Yes
Bunyaviridae	Hantavirus California encephalitis virus Sandfly fever virus	(–) RNA, 3 circular segments	Yes
Arenaviridae	Lymphocytic choriomeningitis virus Lassa fever virus South American hemorrhagic fever virus	(–) RNA, 2 circular segments	Yes
Reoviridae	Rotavirus Reovirus Colorado tick fever virus	ds RNA, 10–12 segments	No
Retroviridae	Human T-lymphotropic virus types I and II Human immunodeficiency virus types 1 and 2	(+) RNA, 2 identical segments	Yes
DNA Viruses			
Hepadnaviridae	Hepatitis B virus	ds DNA with ss portions	Yes
Parvoviridae	Parvovirus B19	ss DNA	No
Papovaviridae	Human papillomaviruses JC virus BK virus	ds DNA	No
Adenoviridae	Human adenoviruses	ds DNA	No
Herpesviridae	Herpes simplex virus types 1 and 2[b] Varicella-zoster virus[c] Epstein-Barr virus[d] Cytomegalovirus[e] Human herpesvirus 6 Human herpesvirus 7 Kaposi's sarcoma–associated herpesvirus[f]	ds DNA	Yes
Poxviridae	Variola (smallpox) virus Orf virus Molluscum contagiosum virus	ds DNA	Yes

[a]Including the coronavirus causing severe acute respiratory syndrome (SARS).
[b]Also called human herpesvirus (HHV) 1 and 2, respectively.
[c]Also called HHV-3.
[d]Also called HHV-4.
[e]Also called HHV-5.
[f]Also called HHV-8.
Note: ds, double-strand; ss, single-strand.

poliovirus capsid protein binds to a cell plasma-membrane protein of the immunoglobulin superfamily type. A rhinovirus capsid protein binds to intercellular adhesion molecule 1. An echovirus capsid protein binds to an integrin. The influenza A virus envelope hemagglutinin protein binds to sialic acid. The HIV envelope glycoprotein binds to CD4 and then engages one of several chemokine receptors that function as co-receptors for the virus. Herpes simplex virus (HSV) envelope glycoproteins bind to heparan sulfate on cell surfaces and then engage one of several immunoglobulin superfamily or tumor necrosis factor (TNF) receptors. Epstein-Barr virus (EBV) glycoprotein gp350 binds to the B lymphocyte complement receptor CD21 and then engages major histocompatibility complex (MHC) class II molecules as a co-receptor. Adsorption characteristically proceeds almost as well at 4°C as at 37°C. Adsorbed virus can still be neutralized by antibody. Adsorption frequently initiates changes in virion surface proteins that destabilize the viral surface proteins and prepare the way for the next stage of entry into the cell.

After adsorption, viruses penetrate the cell membrane by fusing with it. The fusion reaction results in the virus's partial decomposition. The virus becomes insensitive to neutralizing antibody as it penetrates, becomes uncoated, and enters the cytoplasm. Penetration and uncoating result in viral nucleocapsid or nucleoprotein entry into the cytoplasm. Penetration and uncoating as well as subsequent steps in viral replication depend on the cell's energy metabolism and on biochemical changes in the cell's plasma membrane and cytoskeleton. Therefore, penetration proceeds slowly at temperatures <37°C. Interaction of viral surface proteins with cell receptors can induce receptor aggregation at the site of adsorption. Receptor aggregation can trigger signaling events within the cytoplasm and changes in the plasma membrane. The cell frequently misperceives that the receptor has encountered its "normal ligand." Aggregated receptor may be internalized with the attached virus in an endocytic process. Viral endocytosis may proceed through clathrin-coated pits. Endocytosis is important in the entry of viruses as diverse as picornaviruses, influenza viruses, HIV, adenoviruses, and herpesviruses. In many cases, entry of the virus into the cytoplasm depends on acidification of the viral endosome.

Influenza virus provides a well-studied example of the effect of low pH on viral penetration. Influenza hemagglutinin mediates adsorption, receptor aggregation, and endocytosis. In low-pH endosomes, changes in the conformation of the hemagglutinin expose amphipathic domains that interact chemically with the cell membrane and initiate fusion of the viral and cellular membranes. (The HIV envelope glycoprotein undergoes similar conformational changes after interaction with CD4 and chemokine receptors.) For influenza virus, the M2 membrane protein also plays a key role in the uncoating of the viral envelope by providing an ion channel in the envelope. The fusion of viral proteins with cell membranes is a crucial step in viral infection, resulting in the mixture of viral envelope lipids and proteins with cell membrane lipids and proteins and (in this case) in the penetration of the influenza nucleocapsid into the cytoplasm. Viral glycoproteins other than the protein that mediates initial adsorption may be critical in mediating envelope fusion with cell membranes, which involves hydrophobic interactions. The hydrophobic interactions required for fusion can be susceptible to chemical inhibition or blockade.

Viral Gene Expression and Replication

After uncoating and release of viral nucleoprotein into the cytoplasm, the viral genome is transported to a site for expression and replication. In order to produce infectious progeny, viruses must (1) produce proteins necessary to replicate their nucleic acid, (2) produce structural proteins, and (3) assemble the nucleic acid and proteins into progeny virions. Different viruses use different strategies and gene repertoires to accomplish these goals. DNA viruses, except for poxviruses, replicate their nucleic acid and assemble into nucleocapsid complexes in the cell nucleus. RNA viruses, except for influenza viruses, transcribe and replicate their nucleic acid and assemble entirely in the cytoplasm. Thus the replication strategies of DNA and RNA viruses are presented separately below. Positive-strand and negative-strand RNA viruses are discussed separately. Medically important viruses of each group are used for illustrative purposes.

Positive-Strand RNA Viruses

Medically important positive-strand RNA viruses include picornaviruses, flaviviruses, togaviruses, caliciviruses, and coronaviruses. Genomic RNA from positive-strand RNA viruses is released into the cytoplasm without associated enzymes. Cell ribosomes recognize and associate with an internal ribosome entry sequence in the viral genomic RNA and translate a polyprotein that is a fusion of many or all of the viral proteins. The viral RNA polymerase and other viral proteins are cleaved from the polyprotein by protease components of the polyprotein. Antigenomic RNA is then transcribed from the genomic RNA template. Positive-strand genomes and mRNAs are next transcribed from the antigenomic RNA by the viral RNA polymerase. Positive-strand genomic RNA is encapsidated in the cytoplasm.

Negative-Strand RNA Viruses

Medically important negative-strand RNA viruses include rhabdoviruses, filoviruses, paramyxoviruses, myxoviruses, and bunyaviruses. Negative-strand RNA virus genomes are released into the cytoplasm with an associated RNA polymerase and one or more accessory proteins. Some of these genomes are segmented. Except for influenza viruses, negative-strand RNA viruses replicate entirely in the cytoplasm. The viral RNA polymerase transcribes messenger RNAs (mRNAs) as well as full-length antigenomic RNA, which is the template for replication of genomic RNA. These mRNAs encode for the viral RNA polymerase and accessory factors as well as for viral structural proteins. Influenza virus is an unusual negative-strand RNA virus that transcribes its mRNAs and antigenomic RNAs in the cell's nucleus. All negative-strand RNA viruses, including influenza viruses, assemble in the cytoplasm.

Double-Strand Segmented RNA Viruses

These viruses, which are taxonomically grouped in the reovirus family, have 10–12 RNA segments that make up their genome. The medically important viruses in this group are rotaviruses and Colorado tick fever virus. Reovirus virions include an RNA polymerase complex. Reoviruses replicate and assemble in the cytoplasm.

DNA Viruses

Medically important DNA viruses include parvoviruses, papovaviruses [e.g., human papillomaviruses (HPVs) and polyomaviruses], adenoviruses, herpesviruses, and poxviruses. Other than poxviruses, most DNA virus genomes must get to the cell's nucleus for transcription by cellular RNA polymerase II. For example, after receptor binding and fusion, herpesvirus nucleocapsids are released into the cytoplasm along with tegument proteins. The complex is then transported along microtubules to nuclear pores, and the DNA is released into the nucleus.

Transcriptional regulation and mRNA processing for nuclear DNA viruses depend on both viral and cellular proteins. For HSVs, a virus tegument protein activates transcription of viral immediate-early genes, a class of genes expressed immediately after infection. Transcription of immediate-early genes requires the viral tegument protein and preexisting cellular transcription factors. One of the key preexisting cellular factors for HSV-1 immediate-early gene transcription is docked in the cytoplasm in neurons. Nuclear absence of this cell factor important for viral gene transcription may explain why HSV-1 goes into a latent state in neurons and how lytic infection is activated by signaling in a latently infected cell.

DNA virus gene transcription is usually regulated and proceeds in an organized cascade. Transcription and expression of adenovirus and herpesvirus immediate-early genes turn on the promoters for early genes, whereas poxvirus virions carry all the factors necessary for early-gene transcription. Smaller DNA viruses are not as dependent on transactivators encoded from the viral genome for early-gene transcription. Most early genes encode proteins that are necessary for viral DNA synthesis and for the turn-on of late-gene transcription. Late genes encode mostly viral structural proteins or viral proteins necessary for the assembly and egress of the virus from the infected cell. Late-gene transcription is continuously dependent on DNA replication. Therefore, inhibitors of DNA replication also stop late-gene transcription.

Each DNA virus family uses unique mechanisms for replicating its DNA. Herpesvirus DNAs are linear in the virion but circularize in the infected cell. In lytic virus infection, circular herpesvirus genomes are replicated into linear concatemers through a "rolling-circle" mechanism. Herpesviruses encode a DNA polymerase and at least six other viral proteins necessary for viral DNA replication; these viruses also encode several enzymes that increase the pool of precursor deoxynucleotide triphosphates. Adenovirus genomes are linear in the virion and are replicated into complementary linear copies by a virus-encoded DNA polymerase and an initiator protein complex. The double-strand circular papovavirus genomes are replicated into progeny circular DNA molecules by cellular DNA replication enzymes. Two viral early proteins contribute to viral DNA replication and to the persistence of papovavirus DNA in latently infected cells. Early papovavirus proteins stimulate cells to remain in cycle, thus facilitating viral DNA replication.

Parvoviruses are the smallest DNA viruses: their genomes are half the size of the papovavirus genomes and include only two genes. Parvoviruses have negative single-strand DNA genomes. The replication of autonomous parvoviruses, such as B19, depends on cellular DNA replication and requires the virus-encoded Rep protein. Other parvoviruses, such as adeno-associated virus (AAV), are not autonomous and require helper viruses of the adenovirus or herpesvirus family for their replication. AAV has been touted as a potentially safe human gene therapy vector because its Rep protein causes its integration at a single chromosomal site.

Poxviruses are the largest DNA viruses and are unique among DNA viruses in replicating and assembling in the cytoplasm. Poxviruses encode transcription factors and an RNA polymerase as well as enzymes for RNA capping and polyadenylation and for DNA synthesis. Poxvirus DNA also has a unique structure. The two strands of the double-strand linear DNA are covalently linked at the ends so that the genome is also a covalently closed single-strand circle. In addition, there are inverted repeats at the ends of the DNA. During DNA replication, the genome is cleaved within the terminal inverted repeat, and the inverted repeats self-prime complementary-strand synthesis by the virus-encoded DNA polymerase. Like herpesviruses, poxviruses encode several enzymes that increase deoxynucleotide triphosphate precursor levels and thus facilitate viral DNA synthesis.

Viruses with Both RNA and DNA Genomes

Retroviruses and hepatitis B virus (HBV) are not purely RNA or DNA viruses. Retroviruses are enveloped RNA viruses with two identical sense-strand genomes and associated reverse transcriptase and integrase enzymes. Retroviruses differ from all other viruses in that they reverse-transcribe themselves into partially duplicated double-strand DNA copies and then routinely integrate into the host genome as part of their replication strategy. Cellular RNA polymerase II and transcription factors regulate transcription from the integrated provirus genome. Some retroviruses also encode for regulators of transcription and RNA processing, such as Tax and Rex in human T-lymphotropic virus (HTLV) types I and II and Tat and Rev in HIV-1 and HIV-2. HIV genomes also encode for the additional accessory proteins Vpr, Vpu, and Vif, which are important for efficient infection and immune escape. Full-length proviral transcripts are made from a promoter in the viral terminal repeat and serve as both genomic RNAs that will be packaged in the nucleocapsids and mRNAs that encode for the viral Gag protein, polymerase/integrase protein, and envelope glycoprotein. The Gag protein includes a protease that cleaves it into several components, including a viral matrix protein that coats the viral RNA. Viral RNA polymerase/integrase, matrix protein, and cellular tRNA are key components of the viral nucleocapsid. The HIV Gag protease has been an important target for inhibition of HIV replication. Remnants and even complete copies of simple retroviral DNA in the human genome indicate that there may be replication-competent simple human retroviruses. However, replication has not been documented or associated with any disease. Integrated retroviral DNAs are also present in other animal species, such as pigs. These porcine retroviruses are a potential cause for concern in xenotransplantation because retroviral replication could cause disease in humans. Since the retroviral DNA is integrated into the porcine genome, special pathogen-free breeding practices cannot cleanse the donor herd of retroviral infection.

HBV is unique because virion DNA expression in infected cells results in the packaging of reverse transcriptase and genomic RNA in the virion. The genomic RNA is then copied into an incomplete double-strand circular DNA genome before the virion matures and is released from the infected cell. On entry of HBV into the cytoplasm of an infected cell, the virion reverse transcriptase/DNA polymerase completes DNA synthesis, and the covalently closed circular genome resides in the nucleus. Viral mRNAs are transcribed from the closed circular viral episome by cellular RNA polymerase II. A capped and polyadenylated, full-genome-length, terminally redundant transcript is packaged into virus core particles in the cytoplasm of infected cells. This RNA associates with the viral reverse transcriptase. The reverse transcriptase converts the full-length, terminally redundant, core-particle, encapsidated RNA genome into partially double-strand DNA. HBV is believed to mature by budding through the cell's plasma membrane, which has been modified by the insertion of viral surface antigen protein.

Viral Assembly and Egress

For most viruses, nucleic acid and structural protein synthesis is accompanied by the assembly of protein and nucleic acid complexes. The assembly and egress of mature infectious virus mark the end of the eclipse phase of infection, during which infectious virus cannot be recovered from the infected cell. Nucleic acids from RNA viruses and poxviruses assemble into nucleocapsids in the cytoplasm. For all DNA viruses except poxviruses, viral DNA assembles into nucleocapsids in the nucleus. In general, the capsid proteins of viruses with icosahedral nucleocapsids can self-assemble into densely packed and highly ordered capsid structures. Herpesviruses require an assemblin protein as a scaffold for capsid assembly. Viral nucleic acid then spools into the assembled capsid. For herpesviruses, a full unit of the viral DNA genome is packaged into the capsid, and a capsid-associated nuclease cleaves the viral DNA at both ends. In the case of viruses with helical nucleocapsids, the protein component appears to assemble around the nucleic acid, which contributes to capsid organization.

Viruses must egress from the infected cell and not bind back to their receptor(s) on the outer surface of the plasma membrane. In many cases, enveloped viruses simply egress and acquire their envelope by budding through the cell's plasma membrane. Excess viral membrane glycoproteins are synthesized to saturate cell receptors and facilitate virus separation from the infected cell. Some viruses encode membrane proteins with enzymatic activity for receptor destruction. Influenza virus, for example, encodes a glycoprotein with neuraminidase activity, which destroys sialic acid on the infected cell's plasma membrane. Herpesvirus nucleocapsids acquire their initial envelope by assembling in the nucleus and then budding through the nuclear membrane into the endoplasmic reticular space. The enveloped herpesvirus is then released from the cell either by maturation in cytoplasmic vesicles, which fuse with the plasma membrane and release the virus by exocytosis, or by "de-envelopment" into the cytoplasm and "re-envelopment" at the Golgi or plasma membrane. In most instances, nonenveloped viruses appear to depend on the death and dissolution of the infected cell for their release.

FIDELITY OF VIRAL REPLICATION

Hundreds or thousands of progeny may be produced from a single virus-infected cell. Many particles partially assemble and never mature into virions. Many mature-appearing virions are imperfect and have only incomplete or nonfunctional genomes. Despite the inefficiency of assembly, a typical virus-infected cell releases 10–1000 infectious progeny. Some of these progeny may contain genomes that differ from those of the virus that infected the cell. Smaller, "defective" virus genomes have been noted with the replication of many RNA and DNA viruses. Virions with defective genomes can be produced in large numbers through packaging of incompletely synthesized nucleic acid. Adenovirus packaging is notoriously inefficient, and a high ratio of particle to infectious virus may limit the amount of recombinant adenovirus that can be administered for gene therapy. Mutant viral genomes are also produced and can be of medical significance. In general, viral nucleic acid replication is more error-prone than cellular nucleic acid replication. RNA polymerases and reverse transcriptases are significantly more error-prone than DNA polymerases. Mutant viruses can be virulent and may preferentially cause disease through evasion of the host immune response or through resistance to antiviral drugs. Persistent hepatitis C virus (HCV) infection is due in part to genome mutation and persistent immune escape. Viral nucleic acids can also mutate by recombination or reassortment between two related viruses in a single infected cell. Although this occurrence is unusual under most circumstances of natural infection, the changes can be substantial and can significantly alter virulence or epidemiology. Reassortment of an avian or mammalian influenza A hemagglutinin gene into a human influenza background is believed to play a role in the emergence of new epidemic influenza A strains.

VIRAL GENES NOT REQUIRED FOR VIRAL REPLICATION

Viruses frequently have genes encoding proteins that are not directly involved in replication or packaging of the viral nucleic acid, in virion assembly, or in regulation of the transcription of viral genes involved in those processes. Most of these proteins fall into five classes: (1) proteins that directly or indirectly alter cell growth; (2) proteins that inhibit cellular RNA or protein synthesis so that viral mRNA can be efficiently transcribed or translated; (3) proteins that promote cell survival or inhibit apoptosis so that progeny virus can mature and escape from the infected cell; (4) proteins that inhibit the host interferon response; and (5) proteins that downregulate host inflammatory or immune responses so that virus infection can proceed in an infected person to the extent consistent with the survival of the virus and its efficient transmission to a new host. More complex viruses of the poxvirus or herpesvirus family encode many proteins that serve these functions. Some of these viral proteins have motifs similar to those of cell proteins, whereas others are quite novel. Virology has increasingly focused on these more sophisticated strategies evolved by viruses to permit the establishment of long-term infection in humans and other animals. These strategies often provide unique insights into the control of cell growth, cell survival, macromolecular synthesis, proteolytic processing, immune or inflammatory suppression, immune resistance, cytokine mimicry, or cytokine blockade.

HOST RANGE

The concept of host range was originally based on the cell types in which a virus replicated in tissue culture. For the most part, the host range is limited by specific cell-surface proteins required for viral adsorption or penetration—i.e., to the cell types that express receptors or co-receptors for a specific virus. Another common basis for host-range limitation is the degree of transcriptional activity from viral promoters in different cell types. Most DNA viruses depend not only on cellular RNA polymerase II and the basal components of the cellular transcription complex, but also on activated components and transcriptional accessory factors, both of which differ among differentiated tissues, among cells at various phases of the cell cycle, and between resting and cycling cells.

The importance of host range factors is illustrated by the identification of determinants that prevent certain animal viruses from infecting humans. The SARS coronavirus and the influenza virus strain from the 1918 pandemic are believed to have originated from animal viruses in which minor genetic mutations resulted in more efficient human infection or enhanced transmission among humans.

VIRAL CYTOPATHIC EFFECTS AND INHIBITORS OF APOPTOSIS

The replication of almost all viruses has adverse effects on the infected cell, inhibiting cellular synthesis of DNA, RNA, or proteins. This inhibitory effect probably stems from the viruses' need to prevent or limit nonspecific, innate host resistance factors, including interferon (IFN). Most commonly, viruses specifically inhibit host protein synthesis by attacking a component of the translational initiation complex—frequently, a component that is not required for efficient translation of viral RNAs. Poliovirus protease 2A, for example, cleaves a cellular component of the complex that ordinarily facilitates translation of cell mRNAs by interacting with their cap structure. Poliovirus RNA is efficiently translated without a cap since it has an internal ribosome entry sequence. Influenza virus inhibits the processing of mRNA by snatching cap structures from nascent cell RNAs and using them as primers in the synthesis of viral mRNA. HSV has a virion tegument protein that inhibits cellular mRNA translation.

Apoptosis is the expected consequence of virus-induced inhibition of cellular macromolecular synthesis and viral nucleic acid replication. Although the induction of apoptosis may be important for the release of some viruses (particularly nonenveloped viruses), many viruses have acquired genes or parts of genes that enable them to forestall infected-cell apoptosis. This delay may be advantageous in allowing the completion of viral replication. Adenoviruses and herpesviruses encode analogues of the cellular Bc12 protein, which blocks mitochondrial enhancement of proapoptotic stimuli. Poxviruses and some herpesviruses encode caspase inhibitors. Many viruses, including HPVs and adenoviruses, encode proteins that inhibit p53 or its downstream proapoptotic effects.

VIRAL INFECTION IN VIVO

TRANSMISSION

The capsid and envelope of a virus protect its genome and permit its efficient transmission from cell to cell and to prospective hosts. Most common viral infections are spread by direct contact, by ingestion of contaminated water or food, or by inhalation of aerosolized particles. In all these situations, infection begins on an epithelial or mucosal surface and spreads along it or from it to deeper tissues. Infection may then spread through the body via the bloodstream, lymphatics, or neural circuits. Parenteral inoculation can also transmit some viral infections among humans or from animals (including insects) to humans.

Some viruses are transmitted only between humans. The dependence of smallpox and poliovirus infections on interhuman transmission makes it feasible to eliminate these viruses from human circulation by mass vaccination. In contrast, herpesviruses survive over time by establishing persistent infection in humans for decades, with eventual reactivation and infection of new and naïve generations.

Animals are important reservoirs and vectors for transmission of viruses causing human disease. Herpes B, monkeypox, and viral hemorrhagic fevers are examples of zoonotic infections caused by direct contact with animals or transmission from animals through other vectors. These infections may not be sustainable among humans alone because of the lack of efficient interhuman transmission. SARS resulted when an animal coronavirus apparently gained access to the human population concomitant with a mutation that enhanced its pathogenicity and spread in humans. Avian influenza viruses have drawn increased public attention because of their potential to undergo genetic changes and contribute to human disease.

PRIMARY INFECTION

The first (primary) episode of viral infection usually lasts from several days to several weeks. During this period, the concentration of virus at sites of infection rises and then falls, usually to unmeasurable levels. The rate at which the intensity of viral infection rises and falls at a given site depends on the accessibility of that organ or tissue to both the virus and systemic immune effectors, the intrinsic ability of the virus to replicate at that site, and endogenous nonspecific and specific resistance. Typically, infections with enterovirus, mumps virus, measles virus, rubella virus, rotavirus, influenza virus, AAV, adenovirus, HSV, and VZV are cleared from almost all sites within 3–4 weeks. Some of these viruses are especially proficient in altering or evading the innate and acquired immune responses; thus primary infection with AAV, EBV, or cytomegalovirus (CMV) can last for several months. Characteristically, primary infections due to HBV, HCV, hepatitis D virus (HDV), HIV, HPV, and molluscum contagiosum virus extend beyond several weeks. For some of these viruses (e.g., HPV, HBV, HCV, HDV, and molluscum contagiosum virus), the primary phase of infection is almost indistinguishable from the persistent phase.

Disease manifestations usually arise as a consequence of viral replication and the resultant inflammatory response at a specific site, but do not necessarily correlate with levels of replication at that site. For example, the clinical manifestations of limited infection with poliovirus, enterovirus, rabies virus, measles virus, mumps virus, or HSV in neural cells are severe relative to the level of viral replication at mucosal surfaces. Similarly, significant morbidity may accompany in utero fetal infection with rubella virus or CMV.

Primary infections are cleared by nonspecific innate and specific adaptive immune responses. Thereafter, an immunocompetent host is usually immune to the disease manifestations of reinfection by the same virus. Immunity frequently does not prevent transient surface colonization on reexposure, persistent colonization, or even limited deep infection.

PERSISTENT AND LATENT INFECTIONS

Relatively few viruses cause persistent or latent infections. HBV, HCV, rabies virus, measles virus, HIV, HTLV, HPV, HHV, and some poxviruses are notable exceptions. The mechanisms for persistent infection vary widely. HCV RNA polymerase and HIV reverse transcriptase have high mutation rates, and the generation of variant genomes that evade the host immune response facilitates persistent infection. HIV is also directly immunosuppressive, depleting CD4+ T lymphocytes and compromising CD8+ cytotoxic T-cell immune responsiveness. Moreover, HIV encodes a Nef protein that downmodulates MHC class I expression, rendering HIV-infected cells partially resistant to immune CD8+ cytolysis.

In contrast, DNA viruses have much lower mutation rates. Their persistence in human populations can be due to their ability to establish latent infection and to reactivate from latency. In this instance, *latency* is defined as a state of infection in which the virus is not replicating. Viral genes associated with lytic infection are not expressed, and infectious virus is not made. The complete viral genome is present and may be replicated by cellular DNA polymerase in conjunction with the cell genome replication. HPVs establish latent infection in basal epithelial cells, which replicate. Some of the progeny cells provide a stable supply of latently infected basal cells, whereas others go on to squamous differentiation and, in the process, become permissive for lytic viral infection. For herpesviruses, latent infection is established in nonreplicating neural cells (HSV and VZV) or in replicating cells of hematopoietic lineages [EBV and probably CMV, HHV-6, HHV-7, and Kaposi's sarcoma–associated herpesvirus (KSHV, also known as HHV-8)]. In their latent stage, HPV and herpesvirus genomes are largely hidden from the normal immune response. It is still not fully understood how partially latent and reactivated HPV and herpesvirus infections escape immediate and effective immune responses in highly immune hosts. HPV, HSV, and VZV may be somewhat protected because they replicate in middle and upper layers of the squamous epithelium—sites not routinely visited by immune and inflammatory cells. HSV and CMV are also known to encode proteins that downregulate MHC class I expression and antigenic peptide presentation on infected cells, thereby enabling these cells to escape CD8+ T-lymphocyte cytotoxicity.

Like other poxviruses, molluscum contagiosum virus cannot establish latent infection but rather causes persistent infection in hypertrophic lesions that last for months or years. This virus encodes a chemokine homologue that probably blocks inflammatory responses and an MHC class I analogue that may block cytotoxic T-lymphocyte attack.

PERSISTENT VIRAL INFECTIONS AND CANCER

Persistent viral infection is estimated to be the root cause of as many as 20% of human malignancies. For the most part, cancer is an accidental and highly unusual or long-term effect of infection with oncogenic human viruses. In these malignancies, viral infection is a critical and ultimately determinative early step, forcing infected cells to enter the cell cycle and enhancing their survival. An unusual virus-infected cell undergoes the subsequent genetic changes that permit the enhanced autonomous growth and survival characteristic of a malignant cell.

Most hepatocellular carcinoma is now believed to be caused by chronic inflammatory, immune, and regenerative responses to HBV or HCV infection. Epidemiologic data firmly link HBV and HCV infections to hepatocellular carcinoma. These infections elicit repetitive cycles of virus-induced liver injury followed by tissue repair and regeneration. Over decades, chronic virus infection, repetitive tissue regeneration, and acquired chromosomal changes can result in enhanced cell proliferation and survival and eventually in hepatocellular carcinoma. In rare instances, HBV DNA integrates into cellular DNA—an event that probably contributes to the development of some tumors.

Almost all cervical carcinoma is caused by persistent infection with "high-risk" genital HPV strains. Whereas HBV and HCV infections stimulate cell growth indirectly in response to virus-induced injury, proteins E6 and E7 of HPV type 16 or 18 can directly affect cell growth by causing the loss of p53 and RB, two cell proteins with tumor-suppressive function. These viral proteins can also increase genomic instability. However, like HBV and HCV infections, HPV infection alone is not sufficient for carcinogenesis. Cervical carcinoma is inevitably associated with persistent HPV infection and integration of the HPV genome into chromosomal DNA. Integrations that result in overexpression of E6 and E7 from HPV type 16 or 18 can cause profound changes in cell growth and survival, and subsequent chromosomal changes accumulating over ensuing cycles of cell growth can lead to malignant conversion and cervical carcinoma.

EBV infection and expression of the latent-infection viral proteins can immortalize B lymphocyte growth in tissue culture. In most humans, the immune response to the strongly antigenic EBV latent-infection proteins prevents uncontrolled B-cell lymphoproliferation. However, when humans are immunosuppressed by posttransplantation medications, HIV infection, or genetic immunodeficiencies, EBV-induced B-cell malignancies can emerge.

EBV infection also plays a role in the long-term development of certain B lymphocyte and epithelial cell malignancies. Persistent EBV infection and expression of the EBV oncogene LMP1 in latently infected epithelial cells appear to be critical early steps in the evolution of anaplastic nasopharyngeal carcinoma, a common malignancy in Chinese and North African populations. As in other virus-associated malignancies, genomic instability and chromosomal abnormalities contribute to the development of EBV-associated nasopharyngeal carcinomas. High-level LMP1 expression in Reed-Sternberg cells is also a hallmark of many cases of Hodgkin's disease. LMP1-induced nuclear factor κB (NF-κB) activity may rescue and prolong the survival of defective B cells that are normally eliminated by apoptosis, thereby allowing the acquisition of other genetic changes leading to malignant Reed-Sternberg cells.

The HTLV-I Tax and Rex proteins appear to be critical to the initiation of cutaneous adult T-cell lymphoma/leukemias that may occur long after primary HTLV I infection. Tax-induced NF-κB activation may contribute to cytokine production, infected cell survival, and eventual outgrowth of malignant cells.

Molecular data confirm the presence of KSHV DNA in all Kaposi's tumors, including those associated with HIV infection, transplantation, and familial transmission. KSHV infection is also etiologically implicated in pleural-effusion lymphomas and multicentric Castleman's disease, which are more common among HIV-infected than among HIV-uninfected people. Several KSHV proteins that can be expressed in latently infected cells, such as v-cyclin, v-interferon regulatory factor (v-IRF), and latency-associated nuclear antigen (LANA), are implicated in increased cell proliferation and survival.

Evidence supporting a causal role of viral infection in these malignancies includes (1) epidemiologic data, (2) the presence of viral DNA in all tumor cells, (3) the ability of the viruses to transform human cells in culture, (4) the results of in vitro assays for transforming effects of specific viral genes on cell growth or survival, and (5) pathologic data indicating the expression of transforming viral genes in premalignant or malignant cells in vivo. Virus-related malignancies provide an opportunity to expand our understanding of the biologic mechanisms important in the development of cancer; they also offer unique opportunities for the development of vaccines and therapeutics that could prevent or specifically treat cancers associated with virus infection. Widespread immunization against hepatitis B has resulted in a decreased prevalence of HBV-associated hepatitis and will likely prevent most HBV-related liver cancers. Studies of an HPV vaccine have shown reduced rates of colonization with high-risk HPV strains and a decreased risk of cervical cancer. The successful use of in vitro–expanded EBV-specific T-cell populations to treat or prevent EBV-associated post-transplantation lymphoproliferative disease demonstrates the potential of immunotherapy against virus-associated cancers.

RESISTANCE TO VIRAL INFECTIONS

Resistance to viral infections is initially provided by factors that are not virus-specific. Physical protection is afforded by the cornified layers of the skin and by mucous secretions that continuously sweep over mucosal surfaces. Once the first cell is infected, IFNs are induced and confer resistance to virus replication. Viral infection may also trigger the release of other cytokines from infected cells; these cytokines may be chemotactic to inflammatory and immune cells. Viral protein epitopes expressed on the cell surface in the context of MHC class I and II proteins stimulate the expansion of T-cell populations with T-cell receptors that can recognize the virus-encoded peptides. Cytokines, inflammatory agents, and antigens released by virus-induced cell death further attract inflammatory cells, dendritic cells, granulocytes, natural killer (NK) cells, and B lymphocytes to the sites of initial infection and to draining lymph nodes. IFNs and NK cells are particularly important in containing viral infection for the first several days. Granulocytes and macrophages are also important in the phagocytosis and degradation of viruses, especially after an initial antibody response.

By 7–10 days after infection, virus-specific antibody responses, virus-specific HLA class II–restricted CD4+

helper T-lymphocyte responses, and virus-specific HLA class I–restricted CD8+ cytotoxic T-lymphocyte responses have developed. These responses, whose magnitude typically increases over the second and third weeks of infection, are important in rapid recovery. Also between the second and third weeks, the antibody type usually changes from IgM to IgG; IgG or IgA antibody can then be detected at infected mucosal surfaces. Antibody may directly neutralize virus by binding to its surface and preventing its adsorption or penetration. Complement usually enhances antibody-mediated virus neutralization. Antibody and complement can also lyse virus-infected cells that express viral proteins on their surface. A cell infected with a replicating enveloped virus usually expresses the virus-envelope glycoproteins on the cell plasma membrane. Specific antibodies can bind to the glycoproteins, fix complement, and lyse the infected cell.

Antibody and CD4+/CD8+ T-lymphocyte responses tend to persist for several months after primary infection. Antibody-producing lymphocytes persist in small numbers as memory cells and begin to proliferate rapidly in response to a second infection, providing an early barrier to reinfection with the same virus. Immunologic memory for T-cell responses appears to be shorter-lived. Redevelopment of T-cell immunity may take longer than secondary antibody responses, particularly when many years have elapsed between primary infection and reexposure. However, persistent infections or frequent reactivations from latency can result in sustained high-level T-cell responses. For example, EBV and CMV typically induce high-level CD4+ and CD8+ T-cell responses that are sustained for decades after primary infection.

Some viruses have genes that alter innate and acquired host defenses. Adenoviruses encode small RNAs that inhibit IFN-induced, PKR-mediated shutoff of infected-cell protein synthesis. Furthermore, adenovirus E1A can directly inhibit IFN-mediated changes in cell gene transcription. Moreover, adenovirus E3 proteins prevent TNF-induced cytolysis and block HLA class I antigen synthesis by the infected cell. HSV ICP47 and CMV US11 block class I antigen presentation. EBV encodes an interleukin (IL) 10 homologue that inhibits NK and T-cell responses. Vaccinia virus encodes a soluble receptor for IFN-α and binding proteins for IFN-γ, IL-1, IL-18, and TNF, which inhibit host innate and adaptive immune responses. Vaccinia virus also encodes a caspase inhibitor that inhibits the ability of CD8+ cytotoxic cells to kill virus-infected cells. Some poxviruses and herpesviruses also encode chemokine-binding proteins that inhibit cellular inflammatory responses. The adoption of these strategies by viruses highlights the importance of the corresponding host resistance factors in containing viral infection and the importance of redundancy in host resistance.

The host inflammatory and immune response to viral infection does not come without a price. This response contributes to the symptoms, signs, and other pathophysiologic manifestations of viral infection. Inflammation at sites of viral infection can subvert an effective immune response and induce tissue death and dysfunction. Moreover, immune responses to viral infection could, in principle, result in immune attack upon cross-reactive epitopes on normal cells, with consequent autoimmunity. Although such effects have been demonstrated in experimental models, their role in the autoimmune manifestations of primary or recurrent human viral infections is uncertain.

INTERFERONS

All human cells can synthesize IFN-α or -β in response to viral infection. These IFN responses are usually induced by the presence of double-strand viral RNA, which can be made by both RNA and DNA viruses and sensed by double-strand RNA binding proteins in the cell cytoplasm, such as PKR and RIG-I. IFN-γ is not highly related to IFN-α or -β and is produced mainly by NK cells and by immune T lymphocytes responding to IL-12. IFN-α and -β bind to the IFN-α receptor, whereas IFN-γ binds to a different but related receptor. Both receptors signal through receptor-associated JAK kinases and other cytoplasmic proteins, including "STAT" proteins. STAT proteins are tyrosine-phosphorylated by JAK kinases, translocate to the nucleus, and activate promoters for specific cell genes. Three types of antiviral effects are induced by IFN at the transcriptional level. The first effect is attributable to the induction of 2′-5′ oligo(A) synthetases, which require double-strand RNA for their activation. Activated synthetase polymerizes oligo(A) and thereby activates RNAse L, which in turn degrades single-strand RNA. The second effect takes place through the induction of PKR, a serine and threonine kinase that is also activated by double-strand RNA. PKR phosphorylates and negatively regulates the translational initiation factor eIF2-α, shutting down protein synthesis in the infected cell. A third effect is initiated through the induction of Mx proteins, a family of GTPases that is particularly important in inhibiting the replication of influenza virus and vesicular stomatitis virus (VSV). These IFN effects are mostly directed against the infected cell, causing both viral and cellular dysfunction and thereby limiting viral replication.

DIAGNOSTIC VIROLOGY

A wide variety of methods are now used to diagnose viral infection. Serology and viral isolation in tissue culture remain important standards. Acute- and convalescent-phase sera with rising titers of antibody to virus-specific antigens and a shift from IgM to IgG antibodies are generally accepted as diagnostic of acute viral infection. Serologic diagnosis is based on a more than fourfold rise in IgG antibody concentration when acute- and convalescent-phase serum samples are analyzed at the same time.

Immunofluorescence, hemadsorption, and hemagglutination assays for antiviral antibodies are labor-intensive and are being replaced by enzyme-linked immunosorbent assays (ELISAs). ELISAs generally use specific viral proteins that are most frequently targeted by the antibody response. The proteins are purified from virus-infected cells or produced by recombinant DNA technology and are attached to a solid phase, where they can be incubated with serum, washed to eliminate nonspecific antibodies, and allowed to react with an enzyme-linked reagent to detect human IgG or IgM antibody specifically adhering to the viral antigen. The amount of antibody can then be quantitated by the intensity of a color reaction mediated by the linked enzyme. ELISAs can be sensitive and automated. Western blots can confirm the presence of antibody to multiple specific viral proteins simultaneously. The proteins are separated by size and transferred to an inert membrane, where they are incubated with serum antibodies. Western blots have an internal specificity control, since the level of reactivity for viral proteins can be compared with that for cellular proteins in the same sample. Western blots require individual evaluation and are inherently difficult to quantitate or automate.

Virus isolation in tissue culture depends on infection of susceptible cells and amplification by replication in infected cells. Virus growth in cell cultures can frequently be identified by its effects on cell morphology under light microscopy. For example, HSV produces a typical cytopathic effect in rabbit kidney cells within 3 days. Other viral cytopathic effects may not be as diagnostically useful. Identification usually requires confirmation by staining with virus-specific monoclonal antibodies. The efficiency and speed of virus identification can be enhanced by combining short-term culture with immune detection. In assays with "shell vials" of tissue culture cells growing on a coverslip, viral infection can be detected by staining of the culture with a monoclonal antibody to a specific viral protein expressed early in viral replication. Thus virus-infected cells can be detected within hours or days of inoculation; several rounds of infection would be required to produce a visible cytopathic effect.

Virus isolation in tissue culture also depends on the collection of specimens from the appropriate site and the rapid transport of these specimens in the appropriate medium to the virology laboratory. Rapid transport maintains viral viability and limits bacterial and fungal overgrowth. Enveloped viruses are generally much more sensitive to freezing and thawing than nonenveloped viruses. The most appropriate site for culture depends on the pathogenesis of the virus in question. Nasopharyngeal, tracheal, or endobronchial aspirates are most appropriate for the identification of respiratory viruses. Sputum cultures generally are less appropriate because bacterial contamination and viscosity threaten tissue-culture cell viability. Aspirates of vesicular fluid are useful for isolation of HSV and VZV. Nasopharyngeal aspirates and stool specimens may be useful when the patient has fever and a rash and an enteroviral infection is suspected. Adenoviruses can be cultured from the urine of patients with hemorrhagic cystitis. CMV can frequently be isolated from cultures of urine or buffy coat. Biopsy material can be effectively cultured when viruses infect major organs, as in HSV encephalitis or adenovirus pneumonia.

Virus isolation does not necessarily establish disease causality. Viruses can persistently or intermittently colonize normal human mucosal surfaces. Saliva can be positive for herpesviruses, and normal urine samples can be positive for CMV. Isolations from blood, cerebrospinal fluid (CSF), or tissue are more often diagnostic of significant viral infection.

Another method aimed at increasing the speed of viral diagnosis is direct testing for antigen or cytopathic effects. Virus-infected cells from the patient may be detected by staining with virus-specific monoclonal antibodies; e.g., epithelial cells obtained by nasopharyngeal aspiration can be stained with a variety of monoclonal antibodies to respiratory viruses.

Nucleic acid amplification techniques bring speed, sensitivity, and specificity to diagnostic virology. The ability to directly amplify minute amounts of viral nucleic acids present in specimens means that detection no longer depends on viable virus and its replication. For example, amplification and detection of HSV nucleic acids in the CSF of patients with HSV encephalitis is a more sensitive detection method than culture of virus from CSF. The extreme sensitivity of these tests can be a problem, since subclinical infection or contamination can lead to false-positive results. Detection of viral nucleic acids does not necessarily indicate virus-induced disease.

Measurement of the amount of viral RNA or DNA in peripheral blood is an important means of determining which patients are at increased risk for virus-induced disease and of evaluating clinical responses to antiviral chemotherapy. Nucleic acid technologies for RNA quantification are routinely used in AIDS patients to evaluate responses to antiviral agents and to detect virus resistance or noncompliance with therapy. Viral-load measurements are also useful for evaluating the treatment of patients with HBV and HCV infections. Nucleic acid testing or direct staining with CMV-specific monoclonal antibodies to quantitate virus-infected cells in the peripheral blood (CMV antigenemia) is useful for identifying immunosuppressed patients who may be at risk for CMV-induced disease.

DRUG TREATMENT FOR VIRAL INFECTIONS

Multiple steps in the viral life cycle can be effectively targeted by antiviral drugs. Nucleoside and nonnucleoside reverse transcriptase inhibitors prevent synthesis of the HIV provirus, whereas protease inhibitors block maturation of the HIV polyprotein after infection of the cell. Enfuvirtide is a small peptide derived from HIV gp41 that acts before infection by preventing a conformational change required for virus fusion. Integrase inhibitors are now in clinical testing. Amantadine and rimantadine inhibit the influenza M2 protein, preventing release of viral RNA early during infection, whereas zanamivir and oseltamivir inhibit the influenza neuraminidase, which is necessary for the efficient release of mature virions from infected cells.

Virus genomes can evolve resistance to drugs by mutation and selection, by recombination with a drug-resistant virus, or (in the case of influenza virus and other multicomponent RNA virus genomes) by reassortment. The emergence of drug-resistant strains can limit therapeutic efficacy. As with antibacterial therapy, excessive and inappropriate use of antiviral therapy can select for the emergence of drug-resistant strains. HIV genotyping is a rapid method for identifying drug-resistant viruses. Resistance to reverse transcriptase or protease inhibitors has been associated with specific mutations in the reverse transcriptase or protease genes. Identification of these mutations by polymerase chain reaction amplification and nucleic acid sequencing can be clinically useful for determining which antiviral agents may still be effective. Drug resistance in herpesviruses is a more unusual problem.

IMMUNIZATION FOR THE PREVENTION OF VIRAL INFECTIONS

Viral vaccines are among the outstanding accomplishments of medical science. Smallpox has been eradicated except as a potential weapon of biological warfare or bioterrorism (Chap. 6). Poliovirus eradication may soon follow. Measles can be contained or eliminated. Excess mortality due to influenza virus epidemics can be prevented, and the threat of influenza pandemics can be decreased by contemporary killed or live attenuated influenza vaccines. Mumps, rubella, and chickenpox are well controlled by childhood vaccination in the developed world. Reimmunization of mature adults can be used to control herpes zoster. New rotavirus vaccines are entering the market. Widespread HBV vaccination has dramatically lowered the frequency of acute and chronic hepatitis and is expected to lead to a dramatic decrease in the incidence of hepatocellular carcinoma. Use of purified proteins, genetically engineered live-virus vaccines, and recombinant DNA–based strategies will make it possible to immunize against severe infections with other viruses. The development of effective vaccines against HIV and HCV is complicated by the high mutation rate of RNA polymerase and reverse transcriptase, the evolutionary and individual divergence of HIV and HCV genomes, and repeated high-level exposure in some populations. Concerns about the use of smallpox and other viruses as weapons necessitate maintenance of immunity to agents that are not naturally encountered.

VIRUSES AS NOVEL THERAPEUTIC TOOLS OR AGENTS

Viruses are being experimentally developed for the delivery of biotherapeutics or novel vaccines. Foreign genes can be inserted into viral nucleic acids, and the recombinant virus vectors can be used to infect the patient or the patient's cells ex vivo. Retroviruses integrate into the cell genome and have been used to functionally replace the abnormal gene in T cells of patients with severe combined immunodeficiency, thereby restoring immune function. Recombinant adenovirus, AAV, and retroviruses are being explored for use in diseases due to single-gene defects, such as cystic fibrosis and hemophilia. Recombinant poxviruses and adenoviruses are also being used experimentally as vaccine vectors. Viral vectors are being tested experimentally for expressing cytokines that can enhance immunity against tumor cells or for expressing proteins that can increase the sensitivity of tumor cells to chemotherapy. Live HSV is now being used experimentally to kill glioblastoma cells after injections into tumors.

For improved safety, nonreplicating viruses are frequently employed in clinical trial settings. Potential adverse events associated with virus-mediated gene transfer include the induction of inflammatory and antiviral immune responses. Integration is useful for permanent gene therapy, but integrations can induce disease by enhancing or interrupting the expression of important cellular genes.

FURTHER READINGS

FINLAY BB, MCFADDEN G: Anti-immunology: Evasion of the host immune system by bacterial and viral pathogens. Cell 124:767, 2006

HILLEMAN MR: Strategies and mechanisms for host and pathogen survival in acute and persistent viral infections. Proc Natl Acad Sci USA 101(Suppl 2):14560, 2004

KNIPE DM et al (eds): *Fields Virology,* 6th ed. New York, Lippincott Williams & Wilkins, 2006

MUNGER K et al: Viral carcinogenesis and genomic instability. EXS 96:179, 2006

CHAPTER 79

ANTIVIRAL CHEMOTHERAPY, EXCLUDING ANTIRETROVIRAL DRUGS

Lindsey R. Baden ■ Raphael Dolin

The field of antiviral therapy—both the number of antiviral drugs and our understanding of their optimal use—continues to lag behind the field of antibacterial drug treatment, in which >70 years of experience have now been accumulated, but significant progress has been made in recent years on new drugs for several viral infections.

The development of antiviral drugs poses several challenges. Viruses replicate intracellularly and often employ host cell enzymes, macromolecules, and organelles for synthesis of viral particles. Therefore, useful antiviral compounds must discriminate between host and viral functions with a high degree of specificity; agents without such selectivity are likely to be too toxic for clinical use.

The development of laboratory assays to assist clinicians in the appropriate use of antiviral drugs is also in its early stages. Phenotypic and genotypic assays for resistance to antiviral drugs are becoming more widely available, and correlations of laboratory results with clinical outcomes in various settings are beginning to be defined. Of particular note has been the development of highly sensitive and specific methods that measure the concentration of virus in blood (*virus load*) and permit direct assessment of the antiviral effect of a given drug regimen in that compartment in the host. Virus load measurements have been useful in recognizing the risk of disease progression in patients with certain viral infections and in identifying patients to whom antiviral chemotherapy might be of greatest benefit. Like any in vitro laboratory test, these tests yield results that are highly dependent on (and likely to vary with) the laboratory techniques employed.

Information regarding the pharmacokinetics of some antiviral drugs, particularly in diverse clinical settings, is limited. Assays to measure the concentrations of these drugs, especially of their active moieties within cells, are primarily research procedures and are not widely available to clinicians. Thus there are relatively few guidelines for adjusting dosages of antiviral agents to maximize antiviral activity and minimize toxicity. Consequently, clinical use of antiviral drugs must be accompanied by particular vigilance with regard to unanticipated adverse effects.

Like that of other infections, the course of viral infections is profoundly affected by an interplay of the pathogen with a complex set of host defenses. The presence or absence of preexisting immunity, the ability to mount humoral and/or cell-mediated immune responses, and the stimulation of innate immunity are important determinants of the outcome of viral infections. The state of the host's defenses needs to be considered when antiviral agents are used or evaluated.

As with any therapy, the optimal use of antiviral compounds requires a specific and timely diagnosis. For some viral infections, such as herpes zoster, the clinical manifestations are so characteristic that a diagnosis can be made on clinical grounds alone. For other viral infections, such as influenza A, epidemiologic information (e.g., the documentation of a community-wide outbreak) can be used to make a presumptive diagnosis with a high degree of accuracy. However, for most other viral infections, including herpes simplex encephalitis, cytomegaloviral infections other than retinitis, and enteroviral infections, diagnosis on clinical grounds alone cannot be accomplished with certainty. For such infections, rapid viral diagnostic techniques are of great importance. Considerable progress has been made in recent years in the development of such tests, which are now widely available for a number of viral infections.

Despite these complexities, the efficacy of a number of antiviral compounds has been clearly established in rigorously conducted and controlled studies. As summarized in Table 79-1, this chapter reviews the antiviral drugs that are currently approved or are likely to be considered for approval in the near future for use against viral infections other than those caused by HIV. Antiretroviral drugs are reviewed in Chap. 90.

ANTIVIRAL DRUGS ACTIVE AGAINST RESPIRATORY INFECTIONS

ZANAMIVIR AND OSELTAMIVIR

Zanamivir and oseltamivir are inhibitors of the influenza viral neuraminidase enzyme, which is essential for release of the virus from infected cells and for its subsequent spread throughout the respiratory tract of the infected host. The enzyme cleaves terminal sialic acid residues and thus destroys the cellular receptors to which the viral hemagglutinin attaches. Zanamivir and oseltamivir are sialic acid transition-state analogues and are highly active and specific inhibitors of the neuraminidases of both influenza A and B viruses. The antineuraminidase activity of the two drugs is similar, although zanamivir has somewhat greater in vitro activity against influenza B. Both zanamivir and oseltamivir act through competitive and reversible inhibition of the active site of influenza A and B viral neuraminidases and have relatively little effect on mammalian cell enzymes.

Oseltamivir phosphate is an ethyl ester prodrug that is converted to oseltamivir carboxylate by esterases in the liver. Orally administered oseltamivir has a bioavailability of >60% and a plasma half-life of 7–9 h. The drug is excreted unmetabolized, primarily by the kidneys. Zanamivir has low oral bioavailability and is administered orally via a hand-held inhaler. By this route, ~15% of the dose is deposited in the lower respiratory tract, and low plasma levels of the drug are detected.

Orally inhaled zanamivir is generally well tolerated, although exacerbations of asthma may occur. The toxicities most frequently encountered with orally administered oseltamivir are nausea, gastrointestinal discomfort, and (less commonly) vomiting. Gastrointestinal discomfort is usually transient and is less likely if the drug is administered with food. Recently, neuropsychiatric events (delirium, self-injury) have been reported in children who have been taking oseltamivir, primarily in Japan.

Inhaled zanamivir and orally administered oseltamivir have been effective in the treatment of naturally occurring influenza A or B in otherwise-healthy adults. In placebo-controlled studies, illness has been shortened by 1.0–1.5 days of therapy with either of these drugs when treatment is administered within 2 days of onset. A recent meta-analysis of clinical studies of oseltamivir suggests that treatment may reduce the likelihood of certain respiratory tract complications of influenza. Once-daily inhaled zanamivir or once-daily orally administered oseltamivir provides effective prophylaxis against laboratory-documented influenza A– and influenza B–associated illness.

The emergence of viruses resistant to zanamivir or oseltamivir occurs but appears to be less frequent than the emergence of resistance to the adamantanes in clinical studies carried out thus far. In one pediatric study, 5.5% of patients treated with oseltamivir developed

TABLE 79-1

ANTIVIRAL CHEMOTHERAPY AND CHEMOPROPHYLAXIS

INFECTION	DRUG	ROUTE	DOSAGE	COMMENT
Influenza A and B				
Prophylaxis	Oseltamivir	Oral	Adults: 75 mg/d Children ≥1 yr: 30–75 mg/d, depending on weight	Prophylaxis must continue for the duration of the outbreak and can be administered simultaneously with inactivated vaccine. Unless the sensitivity of isolates is known, neither amantadine nor rimantadine is currently recommended for prophylaxis or therapy because of the high rate of resistance in influenza A/H3N2 viruses since the 2005–2006 season.
	Zanamivir	Inhaled orally	Adults and children ≥5 yrs: 10 mg/d	
	Amantadine[a] or rimantadine[a]	Oral	Adults: 200 mg/d Children 1–9 yrs: 5 mg/kg per day (maximum, 150 mg/d)	
Treatment	Oseltamivir	Oral	Adults: 75 mg bid for 5 days Children 1–12 yrs: 30–75 mg bid for 5 days	When started within 2 days of onset, zanamivir and oseltamivir reduce symptoms by 1.0–1.5 and 1.3 days, respectively, in uncomplicated disease. Zanamivir may exacerbate bronchospasm in patients with asthma. Oseltamivir's side effects of nausea and vomiting can be reduced in frequency by drug administration with food. Amantadine and rimantadine are similarly effective in uncomplicated influenza caused by sensitive viruses. None of the listed drugs has been thoroughly studied in complicated cases (e.g., pneumonia).
	Zanamivir	Inhaled orally	Adults and children ≥7 yrs: 10 mg bid for 5 days	
	Amantadine[a]	Oral	Adults: 100 qd or bid Children 1–9 yrs: 5 mg/kg per day (maximum, 150 mg/d) for 5–7 days	
	Rimantadine[a]	Oral	100 qd or bid for 5–7 days in adults	
RSV infection	Ribavirin	Small-particle aerosol	Administered continuously from reservoir containing 20 mg/mL for 3–6 days	Ribavirin is used for treatment of infants and young children hospitalized with RSV pneumonia and bronchiolitis.
CMV retinitis in immunocompromised host (AIDS)	Ganciclovir	IV	5 mg/kg bid for 14–21 days; then 5 mg/kg per day as maintenance dose	Ganciclovir, valganciclovir, foscarnet, and cidofovir are approved for treatment of CMV retinitis in patients with AIDS. They are also used for colitis, pneumonia, or "wasting" syndrome associated with CMV and for prevention of CMV disease in transplant recipients.
		Oral	1 g tid as maintenance dose	
	Valganciclovir	Oral	900 mg bid for 21 days; then 900 mg/d as maintenance dose	Valganciclovir has largely supplanted oral ganciclovir and is frequently used in place of IV ganciclovir.
	Foscarnet	IV	60 mg/kg q8h for 14–21 days; then 90–120 mg/kg per day as maintenance dose	Foscarnet is not myelosuppressive and is active against acyclovir- and ganciclovir-resistant herpesviruses.
	Cidofovir	IV	5 mg/kg once weekly for 2 weeks, then once every other week; given with probenecid and hydration	
	Fomivirsen	Intravitreal	330 mg on day 1 and day 15, followed by 330 mg monthly as maintenance	Fomivirsen has reduced the rate of progression of CMV retinitis in patients in whom other regimens have failed or have not been well tolerated. The major form of toxicity is ocular inflammation.

(*Continued*)

TABLE 79-1 (*CONTINUED*)

ANTIVIRAL CHEMOTHERAPY AND CHEMOPROPHYLAXIS

INFECTION	DRUG	ROUTE	DOSAGE	COMMENT
Varicella				
Immunocompetent host	Acyclovir	Oral	20 mg/kg (maximum, 800 mg) 4 or 5 times daily for 5 days	Treatment confers modest clinical benefit when administered within 24 h of rash onset.
Immunocompromised host	Acyclovir	IV	10 mg/kg q8h for 7 days	A change to oral valacyclovir can be considered once fever has subsided if there is no evidence of visceral involvement.
Herpes simplex encephalitis	Acyclovir	IV	10 mg/kg q8h for 14–21 days	Results are optimal when therapy is initiated early. Some authorities recommend treatment for 21 days to prevent relapses.
Neonatal herpes simplex	Acyclovir	IV	10 mg/kg q8h for 14–21 days	Serious morbidity is common despite therapy. Prolonged oral administration of acyclovir after initial IV therapy has been suggested because of long-term sequelae associated with cutaneous recurrences of HSV infection.
Genital herpes simplex				
Primary (treatment)	Acyclovir	IV	5 mg/kg q8h for 5–10 days	The IV route is preferred for infections severe enough to warrant hospitalization or with neurologic complications.
		Oral	200 mg 5 times daily for 10 days	The oral route is preferred for patients whose condition does not warrant hospitalization. Adequate hydration must be maintained.
	Acyclovir	Topical	5% ointment; 4–6 applications daily for 7–10 days	Topical use—largely supplemented by oral therapy—may obviate systemic administration to pregnant women. Systemic symptoms and untreated areas are not affected.
	Valacyclovir	Oral	1 g bid for 10 days	Valacyclovir appears to be as effective as acyclovir but can be administered less frequently.
	Famciclovir	Oral	250 mg tid for 5–10 days[b]	Famciclovir appears to be similar in effectiveness to acyclovir.
Recurrent (treatment)	Acyclovir	Oral	200 mg 5 times daily for 5 days	Clinical effect is modest and is enhanced if therapy is initiated early. Treatment does not affect recurrence rates.
	Famciclovir	Oral	1000 mg bid for 1 day	
	Valacyclovir	Oral	500 mg bid for 3 days	
Recurrent (suppression)	Acyclovir	Oral	400 mg bid for ≥12 months	Suppressive therapy is recommended only for patients with at least 6–10 recurrences per year. "Breakthrough" occasionally takes place, and asymptomatic shedding of virus occurs. The need for suppressive therapy should be reevaluated after 1 year. Suppression with valacyclovir reduces transmission of genital HSV among discordant couples.
	Valacyclovir	Oral	500–1000 mg/d	
	Famciclovir	Oral	125–250 mg bid	

(*Continued*)

TABLE 79-1 (*CONTINUED*)

ANTIVIRAL CHEMOTHERAPY AND CHEMOPROPHYLAXIS

INFECTION	DRUG	ROUTE	DOSAGE	COMMENT
Mucocutaneous herpes simplex in immunocompromised host				
Treatment	Acyclovir	IV	5 mg/kg q8h for 7 days	The choice of the IV or oral route depends on the severity of infection and the patient's ability to take oral medication. Oral or IV treatment has supplanted topical therapy except for small, easily accessible lesions. Foscarnet is used for acyclovir-resistant viruses.
		Oral	400 mg 5 times daily for 10 days	
		Topical	5% ointment; 4–6 applications daily for 7 days or until healed	
	Valacyclovir	Oral	1 g tid for 7 days[b]	
	Famciclovir	Oral	500 mg bid for 4 days[c]	
Prevention of recurrence during intense immunosuppression	Acyclovir	Oral	200 mg bid	Treatment is administered during periods when intense immunosuppression is expected—e.g., during antitumor chemotherapy or after transplantation—and is usually continued for 2–3 months.
		IV	5 mg/kg q12h	
	Valacyclovir	Oral	1 g tid[b]	
	Famciclovir	Oral	500 mg bid[b]	
Herpes simplex orolabialis (recurrent)	Penciclovir	Topical	1.0% cream applied q2h during waking hours for 4 days	Treatment shortens healing time and symptoms by 0.5–1.0 day (compared with placebo).
	Valacyclovir	Oral	2 g q12h for 1 day	Therapy begun at the earliest symptom reduces disease duration by 1 day.
	Famciclovir[b]	Oral	500 mg tid for 5 days	Therapy begun 48 h after UV light exposure decreases time to healing by 2 days.
	Docosonal[d]	Topical	10% cream 5 times daily until healed	Application at initial symptoms reduces healing time by 1 day.
Herpes simplex keratitis	Trifluridine	Topical	1 drop of 1% ophthalmic solution q2h while awake (maximum, 9 drops daily)	Therapy should be undertaken in consultation with an ophthalmologist.
	Vidarabine	Topical	0.5-in. ribbon of 3% ophthalmic ointment 5 times daily	
Herpes zoster				
Immunocompetent host	Valacyclovir	Oral	1 g tid for 7 days	Valacyclovir may be more effective than acyclovir for pain relief; otherwise, it has a similar effect on cutaneous lesions and should be given within 72 h of rash onset.
	Famciclovir	Oral	500 mg q8h for 7 days	The duration of postherpetic neuralgia is shorter than with placebo. Famciclovir showed overall efficacy similar to that of acyclovir in a comparative trial. It should be given ≤72 h after rash onset.
	Acyclovir	Oral	800 mg 5 times daily for 7–10 days	Acyclovir causes faster resolution of skin lesions than placebo and provides some relief of acute symptoms if given within 72 h of rash onset. Combined with tapering doses of prednisone, acyclovir improves quality-of-life outcomes.
Immunocompromised host	Acyclovir	IV	10 mg/kg q8h for 7 days	Effectiveness in localized zoster is most marked when treatment is given early. Foscarnet may be used for VZV infections that are resistant to acyclovir.
		Oral	800 mg 5 times daily for 7 days	
	Famciclovir	Oral	500 mg tid for 10 days[b]	

(*Continued*)

TABLE 79-1 (CONTINUED)

ANTIVIRAL CHEMOTHERAPY AND CHEMOPROPHYLAXIS

INFECTION	DRUG	ROUTE	DOSAGE	COMMENT
Herpes zoster ophthalmicus	Acyclovir	Oral	600 mg 5 times daily for 10 days	Treatment reduces ocular complications, including ocular keratitis and uveitis.
Condyloma acuminatum	IFN-α2b	Intralesional	1 million units per wart (maximum of 5) thrice weekly for 3 weeks	Intralesional treatment frequently results in regression of warts, but lesions often recur. Parenteral administration may be useful if lesions are numerous.
	IFN-αn3	Intralesional	250,000 units per wart (maximum of 10) twice weekly for up to 8 weeks	
Chronic hepatitis B	IFN-α2b	SC	5 million units daily or 10 million units thrice weekly for 16–24 weeks	HBeAg and DNA are eliminated in 33–37% of cases. Histopathologic improvement is also seen.
	Pegylated IFN-α2a	SC	180 μg weekly for 48 weeks	HBeAg and DNA are eliminated in 32–43% of recipients.
	Lamivudine	Oral	100 mg/d for 12–18 months; 150 mg bid as part of therapy for HIV infection	The efficacy of lamivudine is similar to that of IFN, but lamivudine is better tolerated. Resistance develops in 24% of recipients when lamivudine is used as monotherapy for 1 year.
	Adefovir dipivoxil	Oral	10 mg/d for 48 months	A return of ALT levels to normal is documented in 48–72% of recipients and improved liver histopathology in 53–64%. Adefovir is effective in lamivudine-resistant hepatitis B. Renal function should be monitored.
	Entecavir	Oral	0.5 mg/d for 48 weeks (1 mg/d if HBV is resistant to lamivudine)	Normalization of ALT is seen in 68–78% of recipients and loss of HBeAg in 21%. Entecavir is active against lamivudine-resistant HBV.
	Telbivudine	Oral	600 mg/d for 52 weeks	Reduction of HBV DNA by >5 $\log_{10}$ copies/mL along with either normalization of ALT or loss of serum HBeAg is seen in 75% of recipients. Myopathy may occur.
Chronic hepatitis C	IFN-α2a or IFN-α2b	SC	3 million units thrice weekly for 12–18 months	A return of ALT levels to normal is documented in 54% of recipients but is sustained in only 28%. Improvement in liver histopathology is seen.
	IFN-α2b/ ribavirin	SC (IFN)/oral (ribavirin)	3 million units thrice weekly (IFN)/1000–1200 mg daily (ribavirin) for 6–12 months	Combination therapy results in sustained responses in up to 40–50% of all recipients.
	Pegylated IFN-α2b	SC	1 μg/kg weekly for 12–24 months	The slower clearance of pegylated IFNs than of standard IFNs permits once-weekly administration. The pegylated formulations appear to be superior to standard IFNs in tolerability and efficacy, both as monotherapy and in combination with ribavirin. Sustained virologic responses were seen in 42–46% of genotype 1 patients and in 76–82% of those infected with genotype 2 or 3.
	Pegylated IFN-α2a	SC	180 μg weekly for 12–24 months	
	Pegylated IFN-α2b/ ribavirin	SC (IFN)/oral (ribavirin)	1.5 μg/kg weekly (IFN)/ 800–1200 mg daily (ribavirin)[d] for 24–48 weeks	
	Pegylated IFN-α2a/ ribavirin	SC (IFN)/oral (ribavirin)	180 μg weekly (IFN)/ 800–1200 mg daily (ribavirin) for 24–48 weeks	

(Continued)

TABLE 79-1 (CONTINUED)

ANTIVIRAL CHEMOTHERAPY AND CHEMOPROPHYLAXIS

INFECTION	DRUG	ROUTE	DOSAGE	COMMENT
Chronic hepatitis C (*continued*)	IFN-alfacon	SC	9–15 μg thrice weekly for 6–12 months	Doses of 9 and 15 μg are equivalent to IFN-α2a and IFN-α2b doses of 3 million and 5 million units, respectively.
Chronic hepatitis D	IFN-α2a or IFN-α2b	SC	9 million units thrice weekly for 12 months	The overall efficacy and the optimal regimen and duration of therapy have not been established. Responses usually are not sustained when therapy is stopped.

[a]Influenza A only. Unless isolate sensitivity is known, not recommended for prophylaxis or therapy since 2005–2006 because of high rates of resistance in influenza A/H3N2 viruses.
[b]Not approved for this indication by the U.S. Food and Drug Administration (FDA).
[c]Approved by the FDA for treatment of HIV-infected individuals.
[d]Active ingredient: benzyl alcohol. Available without prescription.
Note: ALT, alanine aminotransferase; CMV, cytomegalovirus; HBeAg, hepatitis B e antigen; HBV, hepatitis B virus; HSV, herpes simplex virus; IFN, interferon; RSV, respiratory syncytial virus; UV, ultraviolet; VZV, varicella-zoster virus.

resistant isolates. A somewhat higher rate of resistance was noted in a recent pediatric study of oseltamivir from Japan. Resistance to the neuraminidase inhibitors may develop by changes in the viral neuraminidase enzyme, by changes in the hemagglutinin that make it more resistant to the actions of the neuraminidase, or by both mechanisms. Some isolates that are resistant to oseltamivir may remain sensitive to zanamivir. Since the mechanisms of action of the neuraminidase inhibitors differ from those of the adamantanes (see below), zanamivir and oseltamivir are active against strains of influenza A virus that are resistant to amantadine and rimantadine.

Zanamivir and oseltamivir have been approved by the U.S. Food and Drug Administration (FDA) for treatment of influenza in adults and in children (those ≥7 years old for zanamivir and those ≥1 year old for oseltamivir) who have been symptomatic for ≤2 days. Oseltamivir is approved for prophylaxis of influenza in individuals ≥1 year of age and zanamivir for those ≥5 years of age (Table 79-1).

AMANTADINE AND RIMANTADINE

Amantadine and the closely related compound rimantadine are primary symmetric amines that display antiviral activity limited to influenza A viruses. Amantadine and rimantadine have been shown to be efficacious in the prophylaxis and treatment of influenza A infections in humans for >40 years. High frequencies of resistance to these drugs were noted among influenza A/H3N2 viruses in the 2005–2006 influenza season and continue to be seen up to the present (2006–2007). Therefore, these agents are no longer recommended unless the sensitivity of the individual influenza A isolate is known, in which case their use may be considered. Amantadine and rimantadine act through inhibition of the ion channel function of the influenza A M2 matrix protein, on which appropriate uncoating of the virus depends. A substitution of a single amino acid at critical sites in the M2 protein can result in a virus that is resistant to amantadine and rimantadine.

Amantadine and rimantadine have been shown to be effective in the prophylaxis of influenza A in large-scale studies of young adults and in less extensive studies of children and elderly persons. In such studies, efficacy rates of 55–80% in the prevention of influenza-like illness were noted, and even higher rates were reported when virus-specific attack rates were calculated. Amantadine and rimantadine have also been found to be effective in the treatment of influenza A infection in studies involving predominantly young adults and, to a lesser extent, children. Administration of these compounds within 24–72 h after the onset of illness has resulted in a reduction of the duration of signs and symptoms by ~50% from that in placebo recipients. The effect on signs and symptoms of illness is superior to that of commonly used antipyretic-analgesic agents. Only anecdotal reports are available concerning the efficacy of amantadine or rimantadine in the prevention or treatment of complications of influenza (e.g., pneumonia).

Amantadine and rimantadine are available only in oral formulations and are ordinarily administered to adults once or twice daily, with a dosage of 100–200 mg/d. Despite their structural similarities, the two compounds have different pharmacokinetics. Amantadine is not metabolized and is excreted almost entirely by the kidney, with a half-life of 12–17 h and peak plasma concentrations of 0.4 μg/mL. In contrast, rimantadine is extensively metabolized to hydroxylated derivatives and has a half-life of 30 h. Only 30–40% of an orally administered dose of rimantadine is recovered in the urine. The peak plasma levels of rimantadine are approximately half those of amantadine, but rimantadine is concentrated in respiratory secretions to a greater extent than amantadine. For prophylaxis, the compounds must be administered daily for the period at risk (i.e., the peak duration of the outbreak). For therapy, amantadine or rimantadine is generally administered for 5–7 days.

Although these compounds are generally well tolerated, 5–10% of amantadine recipients experience mild central nervous system side effects consisting primarily of dizziness, anxiety, insomnia, and difficulty in concentrating. These effects are rapidly reversible upon cessation of the drug's administration. At a dose of 200 mg/d, rimantadine is better tolerated than amantadine; in a large-scale study of young adults, adverse effects were no more frequent among rimantadine recipients than among placebo recipients. Seizures and worsening of congestive heart failure have also been reported in patients treated with amantadine, although a causal relationship has not been established. The dosage of amantadine should be reduced to 100 mg/d in patients with renal insufficiency [i.e., a creatinine clearance rate (Cr_{Cl}) of <50 mL/min] and in the elderly. A rimantadine dose of 100 mg/d should be used for patients with a Cr_{Cl} of <10 mL/min and in the elderly.

RIBAVIRIN

Ribavirin is a synthetic nucleoside analogue that inhibits a wide range of RNA and DNA viruses. The mechanism of action of ribavirin is not completely defined and may be different for different groups of viruses. Ribavirin-5′-monophosphate blocks the conversion of inosine-5′-monophosphate to xanthosine-5′-monophosphate and interferes with the synthesis of guanine nucleotides as well as that of both RNA and DNA. Ribavirin-5′-monophosphate also inhibits capping of virus-specific messenger RNA in certain viral systems. In studies demonstrating the effectiveness of ribavirin in the treatment of respiratory syncytial virus (RSV) infection in infants, the compound was administered as a small-particle aerosol. In infants with RSV infection who were given ribavirin by continuous aerosol for 3–6 days, illness and lower respiratory tract signs resolved more rapidly and arterial oxygen desaturation was less pronounced than in placebo-treated groups. In addition, ribavirin has had a beneficial clinical effect in infants with RSV infection who require mechanical ventilation. Aerosolized ribavirin has also been administered to older children and adults with severe RSV and parainfluenza virus infections (including immunosuppressed patients) and to older children and adults with influenza A or B infection, but the benefit of this treatment, if any, is unclear. In RSV infections in immunosuppressed patients, ribavirin is often given in combination with immunoglobulins.

Orally administered ribavirin has not been effective in the treatment of influenza A virus infections. IV or oral ribavirin has reduced mortality rates among patients with Lassa fever; it has been particularly effective in this regard when given within the first 6 days of illness. IV ribavirin has been reported to be of clinical benefit in the treatment of hemorrhagic fever with renal syndrome caused by Hantaan virus and as therapy for Argentinian hemorrhagic fever. Moreover, oral ribavirin has been recommended for the treatment and prophylaxis of Congo-Crimean hemorrhagic fever. An open-label trial suggested that oral ribavirin may be beneficial in the treatment of Nipah virus encephalitis. Use of IV ribavirin in patients with hantavirus pulmonary syndrome in the United States has not been associated with clear-cut benefits. Oral administration of ribavirin reduces serum aminotransferase levels in patients with chronic hepatitis C virus (HCV) infection; since it appears not to reduce serum HCV RNA levels, the mechanism of this effect is unclear. The drug provides added benefit when given by mouth in doses of 800–1200 mg/d in combination with interferon (IFN) α2b or α2a (see below), and the ribavirin/IFN combination has been approved for the treatment of patients with chronic HCV infection.

Large doses of ribavirin (800–1000 mg/d PO) have been associated with reversible hematopoietic toxicity. This effect has not been observed with aerosolized ribavirin, apparently because little drug is absorbed systemically. Aerosolized administration of ribavirin is generally well tolerated but occasionally is associated with bronchospasm, rash, or conjunctival irritation. Aerosolized ribavirin has been approved for treatment of RSV infection in infants and should be administered under close supervision—particularly in the setting of mechanical ventilation, where precipitation of the drug is possible. Health care workers exposed to the drug have experienced minor toxicity, including eye and respiratory tract irritation. Because ribavirin is mutagenic, teratogenic, and embryotoxic, its use is generally contraindicated in pregnancy. Its administration as an aerosol poses a risk to pregnant health care workers.

ANTIVIRAL DRUGS ACTIVE AGAINST HERPESVIRUS INFECTIONS

ACYCLOVIR AND VALACYCLOVIR

Acyclovir is a highly potent and selective inhibitor of the replication of certain herpesviruses, including herpes simplex virus (HSV) types 1 and 2, varicella-zoster virus (VZV), and Epstein-Barr virus (EBV). It is relatively ineffective in the treatment of human cytomegalovirus (CMV) infections; however, some studies have indicated its effectiveness in the prevention of CMV-associated disease in immunosuppressed patients. Valacyclovir, the L-valyl ester of acyclovir, is converted almost entirely to acyclovir by intestinal and hepatic hydrolysis after oral administration. Valacyclovir has pharmacokinetic advantages over orally administered acyclovir: it exhibits significantly greater oral bioavailability, results in higher blood levels, and can be given less frequently than acyclovir (two or three rather than five times daily).

The high degree of selectivity of acyclovir is related to its mechanism of action, which requires that the compound first be phosphorylated to acyclovir monophosphate. This phosphorylation occurs efficiently in herpesvirus-infected cells by means of a virus-coded thymidine kinase. In uninfected mammalian cells, little phosphorylation of acyclovir occurs, and the drug is therefore concentrated in herpesvirus-infected cells. Acyclovir monophosphate is subsequently converted by host cell kinases to a triphosphate that is a potent inhibitor of virus-induced DNA polymerase but has relatively little effect on host-cell DNA polymerase. Acyclovir triphosphate can also be incorporated into viral DNA, with early chain termination.

Acyclovir is available in IV, oral, and topical forms, whereas valacyclovir is available in an oral formulation. IV acyclovir is markedly effective in the treatment of mucocutaneous HSV infections in immunocompromised hosts, in whom it reduces time to healing, duration of pain, and virus shedding. When administered prophylactically during periods of intense immunosuppression (e.g., related to chemotherapy for leukemia or transplantation) and before the development of lesions, IV acyclovir reduces the frequency of HSV-associated disease. After prophylaxis is discontinued, HSV lesions recur. IV acyclovir is also effective in the treatment of HSV encephalitis; two comparative trials have indicated that acyclovir is more effective than vidarabine for this indication (see below).

Because VZV is generally less sensitive to acyclovir than is HSV, higher doses of acyclovir must be used to treat VZV infections. In immunocompromised patients with herpes zoster, IV acyclovir reduces the frequency of cutaneous dissemination and visceral complications and—in one comparative trial—was more effective than vidarabine. Acyclovir, administered at doses of 800 mg PO five times a day, had a modest beneficial effect on localized herpes zoster lesions in both immunocompromised and immunocompetent patients. Combination of acyclovir with a tapering regimen of prednisone appeared to be more effective than acyclovir alone in terms of quality-of-life outcomes in immunocompetent patients over age 50 with herpes zoster. A comparative study of acyclovir (800 mg PO five times daily) and valacyclovir (1 g PO tid) in immunocompetent patients with herpes zoster indicated that the latter drug may be more effective in eliciting the resolution of zoster-associated pain. Orally administered acyclovir (600 mg five times a day) reduced complications of herpes zoster ophthalmicus in a placebo-controlled trial.

In chickenpox, a modest overall clinical benefit is attained when oral acyclovir therapy is begun within 24 h of the onset of rash in otherwise-healthy children (20 mg/kg, up to a maximum of 800 mg, four times a day) or adults (800 mg five times a day). IV acyclovir has also been reported to be effective in the treatment of immunocompromised children with chickenpox.

The most widespread use of acyclovir is in the treatment of genital HSV infections. IV or oral acyclovir or oral valacyclovir has shortened the duration of symptoms, reduced virus shedding, and accelerated healing when employed for the treatment of primary genital HSV infections. Oral acyclovir and valacyclovir have also had a modest effect in treatment of recurrent genital HSV infections. However, the failure of treatment of either primary or recurrent disease to reduce the frequency of subsequent recurrences has indicated that acyclovir is ineffective in eliminating latent infection. Chronic oral administration of acyclovir for ≥1–6 years or of valacyclovir for ≥1 year has reduced the frequency of recurrences markedly during therapy; once the drug is discontinued, lesions recur. In one study, suppressive therapy with valacyclovir (500 mg once daily for 8 months) reduced transmission of HSV-2 genital infections among discordant couples by 50%. A modest effect on herpes labialis (i.e., a reduction of disease duration by 1 day) was seen when valacyclovir was administered upon detection of the first symptom of a lesion at a dose of 2 g every 12 h for 1 day. In AIDS patients, chronic or intermittent administration of acyclovir has been associated with the development of HSV and VZV strains resistant to the action of the drug and with clinical failures. The most common mechanism of resistance is a deficiency of the virus-induced thymidine kinase. Patients with HSV or VZV infections resistant to acyclovir have frequently responded to foscarnet.

With the availability of the oral and IV forms, there are few indications for topical acyclovir, although treatment with this formulation has been modestly beneficial in primary genital HSV infections and in mucocutaneous HSV infections in immunocompromised hosts.

Overall, acyclovir is remarkably well tolerated and is generally free of toxicity. The most frequently encountered form of toxicity is renal dysfunction because of drug crystallization, particularly after rapid IV administration or with inadequate hydration. Central nervous system changes, including lethargy and tremors, are occasionally reported, primarily in immunosuppressed patients. However, whether these changes are related to acyclovir, to concurrent administration of other therapy, or to underlying infection remains unclear. Acyclovir is excreted primarily unmetabolized by the kidney via both glomerular filtration and tubular secretion. Approximately 15% of a dose of acyclovir is metabolized to 9-[(carboxymethoxy) methyl]guanine or other minor metabolites. Reduction in dosage is indicated in patients with a Cr_{Cl} of <50 mL/min. The half-life of acyclovir is ~3 h in normal adults, and the peak plasma concentration after a 1-h infusion of a dose of 5 mg/kg is 9.8 μg/mL. Approximately 22% of an orally administered acyclovir dose is absorbed, and peak plasma concentrations of 0.3–0.9 μg/mL are attained after administration of a 200-mg dose. Acyclovir penetrates relatively well into the cerebrospinal fluid (CSF), with concentrations approaching half of those found in plasma.

Acyclovir causes chromosomal breakage at high doses, but its administration to pregnant women has not been associated with fetal abnormalities. Nonetheless, the potential risks and benefits of acyclovir should be carefully assessed before the drug is used in pregnancy.

Valacyclovir exhibits three to five times greater bioavailability than acyclovir. The concentration-time curve for valacyclovir, given as 1 g PO three times daily, is similar to that for acyclovir, given as 5 mg/kg IV every 8 h. The safety profiles of valacyclovir and acyclovir are similar, although thrombotic thrombocytopenic purpura/hemolytic-uremic syndrome has been reported in immunocompromised patients who have received high doses of valacyclovir (8 g/d). Valacyclovir is approved for the treatment of herpes zoster, of initial and recurrent episodes of genital HSV infections in immunocompetent adults, and of herpes labialis, as well as for suppressive treatment of genital herpes. Although it has not been extensively studied in other clinical settings involving HSV or VZV infections, many consultants use valacyclovir rather than oral acyclovir in settings where the latter has been approved because of valacyclovir's superior pharmacokinetics and more convenient dosing schedule.

CIDOFOVIR

Cidofovir is a phosphonate nucleotide analogue of cytosine. Its major use is in CMV infections, particularly retinitis, but it is active against a broad range of herpesviruses, including HSV, human herpesvirus (HHV) type 6, HHV-8, and certain other DNA viruses such as polyomaviruses, papillomaviruses, adenoviruses, and poxviruses, including variola (smallpox) and vaccinia. Cidofovir does not require initial phosphorylation by virus-induced kinases; the drug is phosphorylated by host cell enzymes to cidofovir diphosphate, which is a competitive inhibitor of viral DNA polymerases and, to a lesser extent, of host cell DNA polymerases. Incorporation of cidofovir diphosphate slows or terminates nascent DNA chain elongation. Cidofovir is active against HSV isolates that are resistant to acyclovir because of absent or altered thymidine kinase and against CMV isolates that are resistant to ganciclovir because of UL97 phosphotransferase mutations. Cidofovir is usually active against foscarnet-resistant CMV, although cross-resistance to foscarnet as well as to ganciclovir has been described.

Cidofovir has poor oral availability and is administered IV. It is excreted primarily by the kidney and has a plasma half-life of 2.6 h. Cidofovir diphosphate's intracellular half-life of >48 h is the basis for the recommended dosing regimen of 5 mg/kg once a week for the initial 2 weeks and then 5 mg/kg every other week. The major toxic effect of cidofovir is proximal renal tubular injury, as manifested by elevated serum creatinine levels and proteinuria. The risk of nephrotoxicity can be reduced by vigorous saline hydration and by concomitant oral administration of probenecid. Neutropenia, rashes, and gastrointestinal tolerance may also occur.

IV cidofovir has been approved for the treatment of CMV retinitis in AIDS patients who are intolerant of ganciclovir or foscarnet or in whom those drugs have failed. In a controlled study, a maintenance dosage of 5 mg/kg per week administered to AIDS patients reduced the progression of CMV retinitis from that seen at 3 mg/kg. IV cidofovir has been reported anecdotally to be effective for treatment of acyclovir-resistant mucocutaneous HSV infections. Likewise, topically administered cidofovir is reportedly beneficial against these infections in HIV-infected patients; it is also being studied for the treatment of anogenital warts. Anecdotal use of IV cidofovir has been described in disseminated adenoviral infections in immunosuppressed patients, but its efficacy, if any, is not known. An ophthalmic formulation is being studied as treatment for adenoviral keratoconjunctivitis. Intravitreal cidofovir has been used to treat CMV retinitis but has been associated with significant toxicity.

FOMIVIRSEN

Fomivirsen is the first antisense oligonucleotide approved by the FDA for therapy in humans. This phosphorothioate oligonucleotide, 21 nucleotides in length, inhibits CMV replication through interaction with CMV messenger RNA. Fomivirsen is complementary to messenger transcripts of the major immediate early region 2 (IE2) of CMV, which codes for proteins regulating viral gene expression. In addition to its antisense mechanism of action, fomivirsen may exert activity against CMV through inhibition of viral adsorption to cells as well as direct inhibition of viral replication. Because of its different mechanism of action, fomivirsen is active against CMV isolates that are resistant to nucleoside or nucleotide analogues, such as ganciclovir, foscarnet, or cidofovir.

Fomivirsen has been approved for intravitreal administration in the treatment of CMV retinitis in AIDS patients who have failed to respond to other treatments or cannot tolerate them. Injections of 330 mg for two doses 2 weeks apart, followed by maintenance doses of 330 mg monthly, significantly reduce the rate of progression of CMV retinitis. The major toxicity is ocular inflammation, including vitritis and iritis, which usually responds to topically administered glucocorticoids.

GANCICLOVIR AND VALGANCICLOVIR

An analogue of acyclovir, ganciclovir is active against HSV and VZV and is markedly more active than acyclovir against CMV. Ganciclovir triphosphate inhibits CMV DNA polymerase and can be incorporated into CMV DNA, whose elongation it eventually terminates. In HSV- and VZV-infected cells, ganciclovir is phosphorylated by virus-encoded thymidine kinases; in CMV-infected cells, it is phosphorylated by a viral kinase encoded by the UL97 gene. Ganciclovir triphosphate is present in tenfold higher concentrations in CMV-infected cells than in uninfected cells. Ganciclovir is approved for the treatment of CMV retinitis in immunosuppressed patients and for the prevention of CMV disease in transplant recipients. It is widely used for the treatment of other CMV-associated syndromes, including pneumonia, esophagogastrointestinal infections, hepatitis, and "wasting" illness.

Ganciclovir is available for IV or oral administration. Because its oral bioavailability is low (5–9%), relatively large doses (1 g three times daily) must be administered by this route. Oral ganciclovir has largely been supplanted by valganciclovir, which is the L-valyl ester of ganciclovir. Valganciclovir is well absorbed orally, with a bioavailability of 60%, and is rapidly hydrolyzed to ganciclovir in the intestine and liver. The area under the curve for a 900-mg dose of valganciclovir is equivalent to that for 5 mg/kg of ganciclovir given IV, although peak serum concentrations are ~40% lower for valganciclovir. The serum half-life is 3.5 h after IV administration of ganciclovir and 4.0 h after PO administration of valganciclovir. Ganciclovir is excreted primarily by the kidneys in an unmetabolized form, and its dosage should be reduced in cases of renal failure. The most commonly employed dosage for initial IV therapy is 5 mg/kg every 12 h for 14–21 days; this regimen is followed by an IV maintenance dose of 5 mg/kg per day or five times per week. For oral therapy with valganciclovir, the dose is 900 mg twice daily for 21 days followed by 900 mg once a day for maintenance, with dose adjustment in patients with renal dysfunction. Intraocular ganciclovir, given by either intravitreal injection or intraocular implantation, has also been used to treat CMV retinitis.

Ganciclovir is effective as prophylaxis against CMV-associated disease in organ and bone marrow transplant recipients. Oral ganciclovir administered prophylactically to AIDS patients with CD4+ T-cell counts of <100/μL has provided protection against the development of CMV retinitis. However, the long-term benefits of this approach to prophylaxis in AIDS patients have not been established, and most experts do not recommend the use of oral ganciclovir for this purpose. As already mentioned, valganciclovir has supplanted oral ganciclovir in settings where oral prophylaxis or therapy is considered.

The administration of ganciclovir has been associated with profound bone marrow suppression, particularly neutropenia, which significantly limits the drug's use in many patients. Bone marrow toxicity is potentiated in the setting of renal dysfunction and when other bone marrow suppressants, such as zidovudine, are used concomitantly.

Resistance has been noted in CMV isolates obtained after therapy with ganciclovir, especially in patients with AIDS. Such resistance may develop through a mutation in either the viral UL97 gene or the viral DNA polymerase. Ganciclovir-resistant isolates are usually sensitive to foscarnet (see below) or cidofovir (see above).

FAMCICLOVIR AND PENCICLOVIR

Famciclovir is the diacetyl 6-deoxyester of the guanosine analogue penciclovir. Famciclovir is well absorbed orally, has a bioavailability of 77%, and is rapidly converted to penciclovir by deacetylation and oxidation in the intestine and liver. Penciclovir's spectrum of activity and mechanism of action are similar to those of acyclovir. Thus penciclovir is usually not active against acyclovir-resistant viruses. However, some acyclovir-resistant viruses with altered thymidine kinase or DNA polymerase substrate specificity may be sensitive to penciclovir. This drug is phosphorylated initially by a virus-encoded thymidine kinase and subsequently by cellular kinases to penciclovir triphosphate, which inhibits HSV-1, HSV-2, VZV, and EBV as well as hepatitis B virus (HBV). The serum half-life of penciclovir is 2 h, but the intracellular half-life of penciclovir triphosphate is 7–20 h—markedly longer than that of acyclovir triphosphate. The latter is the basis for the less frequent (twice-daily) dosing schedule for famciclovir than for acyclovir. Penciclovir is eliminated primarily in the urine by both glomerular filtration and tubular secretion. The usually recommended dosage interval should be adjusted for renal insufficiency.

Clinical trials involving immunocompetent adults with herpes zoster showed that famciclovir was superior to placebo in eliciting the resolution of skin lesions and virus shedding and in shortening the duration of postherpetic neuralgia; moreover, administered at 500 mg every 8 h, famciclovir was at least as effective as acyclovir administered at a dose of 800 mg PO five times daily. Famciclovir was also effective in the treatment of herpes zoster in immunosuppressed patients. Clinical trials have demonstrated its effectiveness in the suppression of genital HSV infections for up to 1 year and in the treatment of initial and recurrent episodes of genital herpes. Famciclovir is effective as therapy for mucocutaneous HSV infections in HIV-infected patients. Application of a 1% penciclovir cream reduces the duration of signs and symptoms of herpes labialis in immunocompetent patients (by 0.5–1.0 day) and has been approved for that purpose by the FDA. Famciclovir is generally well tolerated, with occasional headache, nausea, and diarrhea reported in frequencies similar to those among placebo recipients. The administration of high doses of famciclovir for 2 years was associated with an increased incidence of mammary adenocarcinomas in female rats, but the clinical significance of this effect is unknown.

FOSCARNET

Foscarnet (phosphonoformic acid) is a pyrophosphate-containing compound that potently inhibits herpesviruses, including CMV. This drug inhibits DNA polymerases at the pyrophosphate binding site at concentrations that have relatively little effect on cellular polymerases. Foscarnet does not require phosphorylation to exert its antiviral activity and is therefore active against HSV and VZV isolates that are resistant to acyclovir because of deficiencies in thymidine kinase as well as against most ganciclovir-resistant strains of CMV. Foscarnet also inhibits the reverse transcriptase of HIV and is active against HIV in vivo.

Foscarnet is poorly soluble and must be administered IV via an infusion pump in a dilute solution over 1–2 h. The plasma half-life of foscarnet is 3–5 h and increases with decreasing renal function, since the drug is eliminated primarily by the kidneys. It has been estimated that 10–28% of a dose may be deposited in bone, where it can persist for months. The most common initial dosage of foscarnet—60 mg/kg every 8 h for 14–21 days—is followed by a maintenance dose of 90–120 mg/kg once a day.

Foscarnet is approved for the treatment of CMV retinitis in patients with AIDS and of acyclovir-resistant mucocutaneous HSV infections. In a comparative clinical trial, the drug appeared to be about as efficacious as ganciclovir against CMV retinitis but was associated with a longer survival period, possibly because of its activity against HIV. Intraocular foscarnet has been used to treat CMV retinitis. Foscarnet has also been employed to treat acyclovir-resistant HSV and VZV infections as well as ganciclovir-resistant CMV infections, although resistance to foscarnet has been reported in CMV isolates obtained during therapy. Foscarnet has also been used to treat HHV-6 infections in immunosuppressed patients.

The major form of toxicity associated with foscarnet is renal impairment. Thus renal function should be monitored closely, particularly during the initial phase of therapy. Since foscarnet binds divalent metal ions, hypocalcemia, hypomagnesemia, hypokalemia, and hypo- or hyperphosphatemia can develop. Saline hydration and slow infusion appear to protect the patient against nephrotoxicity and electrolyte disturbances. Although hematologic abnormalities have been documented (most commonly anemia), foscarnet is not generally myelosuppressive and may be administered concomitantly with myelosuppressive medications such as zidovudine.

TRIFLURIDINE

Trifluridine is a pyrimidine nucleoside active against HSV-1, HSV-2, and CMV. Trifluridine monophosphate irreversibly inhibits thymidylate synthetase, and trifluridine triphosphate inhibits viral and, to a lesser extent, cellular DNA polymerases. Because of systemic toxicity, its use is limited to topical therapy. Trifluridine is approved for treatment of HSV keratitis, for which trials have shown that it is more effective than topical idoxuridine but similar in efficacy to topical vidarabine. The drug has benefited some patients with HSV keratitis who have failed to respond to idoxuridine or vidarabine. Topical application of trifluridine to sites of acyclovir-resistant HSV mucocutaneous infections has also been beneficial in some cases.

VIDARABINE

Vidarabine is a purine nucleoside analogue with activity against HSV-1, HSV-2, VZV, and EBV. Vidarabine inhibits viral DNA synthesis through its 5′-triphosphorylated metabolite, although its precise molecular mechanisms of action are not completely understood. IV-administered vidarabine has been shown to be effective in the treatment of herpes simplex encephalitis, mucocutaneous HSV infections, herpes zoster in immunocompromised patients, and neonatal HSV infections. Its use has been supplanted by that of IV acyclovir, which is more effective and easier to administer. Production of the IV preparation has been discontinued by the manufacturer, but vidarabine is available as an ophthalmic ointment, which is effective in the treatment of HSV keratitis.

ANTIVIRAL DRUGS ACTIVE AGAINST HEPATITIS VIRUSES

LAMIVUDINE

Lamivudine is a pyrimidine nucleoside analogue that is used primarily in combination therapy against HIV infection (Chap. 90). It is also active against HBV through inhibition of the viral DNA polymerase and has been approved for the treatment of chronic HBV infection. At doses of 100 mg/d for 1 year, lamivudine is well tolerated and results in suppression of HBV DNA levels, normalization of serum aminotransferase levels in 50–70% of patients, and reduction of hepatic inflammation and fibrosis in 50–60% of patients. Loss of hepatitis B e antigen (HBeAg) occurs in 30% of patients. Resistance to lamivudine develops in 24% of patients treated for 1 year and is associated with changes in the YMDD motif of HBV DNA polymerase. This is an important limitation of monotherapy with the drug. Lamivudine is being evaluated as a component of combination regimens (with IFNs and other nucleoside or nucleotide analogues listed below) for the treatment of hepatitis B. Lamivudine appears to be useful in the prevention or suppression of HBV infection associated with liver transplantation.

ADEFOVIR

Adefovir dipivoxil is an acyclic nucleotide analogue of adenosine monophosphate that has activity against HBV, HIV, HSV, and CMV. It is phosphorylated by cellular kinases to the active triphosphate moiety, which is a competitive inhibitor of HBV DNA polymerase and results in chain termination after incorporation into nascent viral DNA. Adefovir is administered orally and is eliminated primarily by the kidneys, with a plasma half-life of 7.5 h. In clinical studies, therapy with adefovir at a dose of 10 mg/d for 48 weeks resulted in normalization of alanine aminotransferase (ALT) levels in 48–72% of patients and improved liver histology in 53–64%; it also resulted in a 3.6-$\log_{10}$ reduction in the number of HBV DNA copies per milliliter of plasma. Adefovir was effective in treatment-naive patients as well as in those infected with lamivudine-resistant HBV. Resistance to adefovir appears to develop less readily than that to lamivudine, but adefovir resistance rates of 15–18% have been reported after 192 weeks of treatment. This agent is generally well tolerated. Significant nephrotoxicity attributable to adefovir is uncommon at the dose employed in the treatment of HBV infections (10 mg/d) but is a treatment-limiting adverse effect at the higher doses used in therapy for HIV infections (30–120 mg/d). In any case, renal function should be monitored in patients taking adefovir, even at the lower dose. Adefovir is approved only for treatment of chronic HBV infection.

TENOFOVIR

Tenofovir disoproxil fumarate is a nucleotide analogue of adenosine monophosphate with activity against both retroviruses and hepadnaviruses. In patients co-infected with HIV and HBV, tenofovir reduces HBV loads by 3–4 $\log_{10}$ copies/mL at 24 weeks and is effective against lamivudine-resistant HBV. The drug is approved only for treatment of HIV infection, but its use should be considered in patients co-infected with HIV and HBV.

For a more detailed discussion of tenofovir, see Chap. 90.

ENTECAVIR

Entecavir is a cyclopentyl guanosine analogue that inhibits HBV through inhibition of HBV DNA polymerase by entecavir triphosphate and is also active against HIV. In vitro, entecavir is more potent than lamivudine or adefovir against HBV and is also effective against lamivudine-resistant HBV. Administration of entecavir at a dose of 0.5 mg/d PO for 48 weeks results in a reduction of HBV DNA by 5.0–6.9 $\log_{10}$ copies/mL, normalization of ALT values in 68–78% of recipients, and loss of HBeAg in 21%. Entecavir is highly bioavailable but should be taken on an empty stomach since food interferes with its absorption. The drug is eliminated primarily in unchanged form by the kidneys, and its dosage should be adjusted for patients with Cr_{Cl} values of <50 mg/min. Overall, entecavir is well tolerated. Resistance to entecavir has not been observed during the treatment of naïve patients; however, resistance was noted in 7–10% of lamivudine-refractory patients at 48 weeks of treatment with entecavir. Entecavir-resistant strains appear to be sensitive to adefovir. As with other anti-HBV treatments, exacerbation of hepatitis may occur when entecavir therapy is stopped. Entecavir is approved for treatment of chronic hepatitis B in adults.

TELBIVUDINE

Telbivudine is the β-L enantiomer of thymidine and is a potent inhibitor of HBV. Its active form is telbivudine triphosphate, which inhibits HBV DNA polymerase but has little or no activity against human DNA polymerase. Administration of telbivudine at a dose of 600 mg/d PO for 52 weeks to patients with chronic hepatitis B resulted in reduction of HBV DNA by >5 $\log_{10}$ copies/mL along with either loss of serum HBeAg or normalization of ALT in 75% of recipients. After 2 years of therapy, resistance to telbivudine was noted in isolates from 8.6–21.6% of patients. Telbivudine-resistant HBV is usually resistant to lamivudine as well but is generally susceptible to adefovir.

Telbivudine is eliminated primarily by the kidneys, and the dosage should be reduced in patients with a Cl_{Cr} value of <50 mL/min. Telbivudine is generally well tolerated, but increases in serum creatinine kinases and clinically evident myopathy have been observed. As with other anti-HBV drugs, hepatitis may be exacerbated in patients who have discontinued telbivudine therapy. Telbivudine has been approved for treatment of adults with chronic hepatitis B who have evidence of viral replication and either persistent elevation in serum aminotransferases or histologically active disease.

INTERFERONS

IFNs are cytokines that exhibit a broad spectrum of antiviral activities as well as immunomodulating and antiproliferative properties. IFNs are not available for oral administration but must be given IM, SC, or IV. Early studies with human leukocyte IFN demonstrated an effect in the prophylaxis of experimentally induced rhinovirus infections in humans and in the treatment of VZV infections in immunosuppressed patients. DNA recombinant technology has made available highly purified α, β, and γ IFNs that have been evaluated in a variety of viral infections. Results of such trials have confirmed the effectiveness of intranasally administered IFN in the prophylaxis of rhinovirus infections, although its use has been associated with nasal mucosal irritation. Studies have also demonstrated a beneficial effect of intralesionally or systemically administered IFNs on genital warts. The effect of systemic administration consists primarily of a reduction in the size of the warts, and this mode of therapy may be useful in persons who have numerous warts that cannot easily be treated by individual intralesional injections. However, lesions frequently recur after either intralesional or systemic IFN therapy is discontinued.

IFNs have undergone extensive study in the treatment of chronic HBV infection. The administration of IFN-α2b (5 million units daily or 10 million units three times a week for 16–24 weeks) to patients with stable chronic HBV infection resulted in loss of markers of HBV replication, such as HBeAg and HBV DNA, in 33–37% of cases; 8% of patients also became negative for hepatitis B surface antigen. In >80% of patients who lose HBeAg and HBV DNA markers, serum aminotransferases return to normal levels, and both short- and long-term improvements in liver histopathology have been described. Predictors of a favorable response to therapy include low pretherapy levels of HBV DNA, high pretherapy serum levels of ALT, a short duration of chronic HBV infection, and active inflammation in liver histopathology. Poor responses are seen in immunosuppressed patients, including those with HIV infection. A longer duration of therapy (12–24 months) is recommended for HBeAg-negative chronic hepatitis B. Adverse effects of the above doses of IFN are common and include fever, chills, myalgia, fatigue, neurotoxicity (primarily manifested as somnolence, depression, anxiety, and confusion), and leukopenia. Approximately 25% of patients receiving a daily dose of 5 million units require dose reduction, but <5% require discontinuation of therapy. Pegylated IFNs, which are covalently linked with monomethoxy polyethylene glycol, have a markedly reduced clearance rate. Therefore, they can be administered less frequently, are better tolerated, and may be more effective in some settings than standard IFNs (see discussion of hepatitis C below). Pegylated IFN-α2a is approved for the treatment of patients with chronic hepatitis B who are either positive or negative for HBeAg (Table 79-1).

Several IFN preparations, including IFN-α2a, IFN-α2b, IFN-alfacon-1, and IFN-αm1 (lymphoblastoid), have been studied as therapy for chronic HCV infections. A variety of monotherapy regimens have been employed, of which the most common is IFN-α2b or -α2a at 3 million units three times per week for 12–18 months. The addition of oral ribavirin to IFN-α2b—either as initial therapy or after failure of IFN therapy alone—results in significantly higher rates of sustained virologic and/or serum ALT responses (40–50%) than are obtained with monotherapy. Comparative studies indicate that pegylated IFN-α2b or -α2a therapy is more effective than standard IFN treatment against chronic HCV infection. The combination of SC pegylated IFN and oral ribavirin is more convenient and appears to be the most effective regimen for treatment of chronic hepatitis C. With this combination regimen, sustained virologic responses were seen in 42–46% of patients with genotype 1 infection and in 76–82% of patients with genotype 2 or 3 infection. Ribavirin appears to have a small antiviral effect in HCV infection, but may also be working through an immunomodulatory effect in combination with IFN. Optimal results with ribavirin appear to be associated with weight-based dosing. Prognostic factors for a favorable response include an age of <45 years, a short duration of infection, low levels of HCV RNA, and infection with HCV genotypes other than 1. IFN-alfacon, a synthetic "consensus" α interferon, appears to produce response rates similar to those elicited by IFN-α2a or -α2b alone and is also approved in the United States for the treatment of chronic hepatitis C.

The efficacy of IFN-α treatment for chronic hepatitis D remains unestablished. Anecdotal reports suggested that doses ranging from 5 million units daily to 9 million units three times per week for 12 months elicit biochemical and virologic responses. Results from small controlled trials have been inconsistent, and observed responses have not generally been sustained. Limited experience has been published with the use of pegylated IFN-α2b for treatment of hepatitis D, but some consultants prefer this agent for this indication because of its pharmacologic advantages over standard IFN.

FURTHER READINGS

BEUTNER KR et al: Valacyclovir compared with acyclovir for improved therapy for herpes zoster in immunocompetent adults. Antimicrob Agents Chemother 39:1546, 1995

COUCH RB: Drug therapy: Prevention and treatment of influenza. N Engl J Med 343:1778, 2000

CRUMPACKER CS: Ganciclovir. N Engl J Med 335:721, 1996

DOLIN R et al: A controlled trial of amantadine and rimantadine in the prophylaxis of influenza A infection. N Engl J Med 307:580, 1982

FIELD JJ, HOOFNAGLE JH: Mechanism of action of interferon and ribavirin in treatment of hepatitis C. Nature 436:967, 2005

GISH RG et al: Safety and antiviral activity of emtricitabine (FTC) for the treatment of chronic hepatitis B infection: A two-year study. J Hepatol 43:60, 2005

HALL CB et al: Aerosolized ribavirin treatment of infants with respiratory syncytial viral infection: A randomized double-blind study. N Engl J Med 308:1443, 1983

HAYDEN FG: Antiviral drugs (other than antiretrovirals), in *Principles and Practice of Infectious Diseases*, 6th ed, JE Bennett et al (eds). Philadelphia, Elsevier Churchill Livingstone, 2005, pp 514–551

LAI CL et al: Entecavir versus lamivudine for patients with HBeAg-negative chronic hepatitis B. N Engl J Med 354:186, 2006

LALEZARI JP et al: Randomized controlled study of the safety and efficacy of IV cidofovir for the treatment of relapsing cytomegalovirus retinitis in patients with AIDS. J AIDS 17:339, 1998

LOK AS et al: Management of hepatitis B: 2000—summary of a workshop. Gastroenterology 120:1828, 2001

MARTIN DF et al: A controlled trial of valganciclovir as induction therapy for cytomegalovirus retinitis. N Engl J Med 346:1119, 2002

NATIONAL INSTITUTES OF HEALTH CONSENSUS DEVELOPMENT CONFERENCE STATEMENT: Management of hepatitis C. September 12, 2002 (available at *www.niaid.nih.gov*)

TREANOR JJ et al: Efficacy and safety in treating acute influenza: A randomized controlled trial. U.S. Oral Neuraminidase Study Group. JAMA 283:1016, 2000

PART 2 INFECTIONS DUE TO DNA VIRUSES

CHAPTER 80

HERPES SIMPLEX VIRUSES

Lawrence Corey

DEFINITION

Herpes simplex viruses (HSV-1, HSV-2; *Herpesvirus hominis*) produce a variety of infections involving mucocutaneous surfaces, the central nervous system (CNS), and—on occasion—visceral organs. Prompt recognition and treatment reduce the morbidity and mortality associated with HSV infections.

ETIOLOGIC AGENT

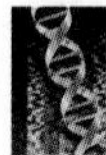

The genome of HSV is a linear, double-strand DNA molecule (molecular weight, ~100 × 10^6 units) that encodes >90 transcription units with 84 identified proteins. The genomic structures of the two HSV subtypes are similar. The overall genomic sequence homology between HSV-1 and HSV-2 is ~50%, whereas the proteome homology is >80%. The homologous sequences are distributed over the entire genome map, and most of the polypeptides specified by one viral type are antigenically related to polypeptides of the other viral type. Many type-specific regions unique to HSV-1 and HSV-2 proteins do exist, however, and a number of them appear to be important in host immunity. These type-specific regions have been used to develop serologic assays that distinguish between the two viral subtypes. Either restriction endonuclease analysis of viral DNA or DNA sequencing can be used to distinguish between the two subtypes and among strains of each subtype. The variability of nucleotide sequences from clinical strains of HSV-1 and HSV-2 is such that HSV isolates obtained from two individuals can be differentiated by restriction enzyme patterns or genomic sequences. Moreover, epidemiologically related sources, such as sexual partners, mother-infant pairs, or persons involved in a common-source outbreak, can be inferred from such patterns.

The viral genome is packaged in a regular icosahedral protein shell (capsid) composed of 162 capsomeres (see Fig. 78-1). The outer covering of the virus is a lipid-containing membrane (envelope) acquired as the DNA-containing capsid buds through the inner nuclear membrane of the host cell. Between the capsid and lipid bilayer of the envelope is the tegument. Viral replication has both nuclear and cytoplasmic phases. Attachment and fusion of the viral envelope and the cell membrane involve several ubiquitous heparin-like surface receptors. Replication is highly regulated. After fusion and entry, the nucleocapsid enters the cytoplasm and several viral proteins are released from the virion. Some of these viral proteins shut off host protein synthesis (by increasing cellular RNA degradation), whereas others "turn on" the transcription of early genes of HSV replication. These early gene products, designated α *genes*, are required for synthesis of the subsequent polypeptide group, the β polypeptides, many of which are regulatory proteins and enzymes required for DNA replication. Most current antiviral drugs interfere with β proteins, such as the viral DNA polymerase enzyme. The third (γ) class of HSV genes requires viral DNA replication for expression and constitutes most of the structural proteins specified by the virus.

After replication of the viral genome and synthesis of structural proteins, nucleocapsids are assembled in the nucleus of the cell. Envelopment occurs as the nucleocapsids bud through the inner nuclear membrane into the perinuclear space. In some cells, viral replication in the nucleus forms two types of inclusion bodies: type A basophilic Feulgen-positive bodies that contain viral DNA and eosinophilic inclusion bodies that are devoid of viral nucleic acid or protein and represent a "scar" of viral infection. Enveloped virions are then transported via the endoplasmic reticulum and the Golgi apparatus to the cell surface.

HSV infection of some neuronal cells does not result in cell death. Instead, viral genomes are maintained by the cell in a repressed state compatible with survival and normal activities of the cell, a condition called *latency*. Latency is associated with transcription of only a limited number of virus-encoded proteins. Subsequently, the viral genome may become activated; its activation results in the normal pattern of regulated viral gene expression, viral replication, and viral release. The release of HSV from the neuron and its subsequent entry into epithelial cells result in viral replication in these cells, destruction of the cells, and the subsequent reappearance of virus on mucosal surfaces. This process is termed *reactivation*. Whereas infectious virus is rarely recovered from sensory or autonomic nervous system ganglia dissected from cadavers, maintenance and growth of the neural cells (as "explants") in tissue culture result in production of infectious virions and in subsequent permissive infection of susceptible cells (*cocultivation*). The mechanisms by which latency is established, maintained, or broken are incompletely understood. Two RNA "latency-associated" transcripts that overlap the immediate early (α) gene products, called *ICP-O*, are found in abundance in the nuclei of latently infected neurons. Deletion mutants of this region that can become latent have been made. However, the efficiency of their later reactivation is reduced; thus these latency-associated transcripts may play a role in maintaining rather than in establishing latency. Recent studies suggest that HSV-specific micro-RNAs in these and other regions of the viral genome may play an important role in virus maintenance in and release from neurons. CD8+ T cells have been found in ganglia of experimental animals and humans and appear to influence the process of reactivation, possibly by inducing antiviral factors such as interferon (IFN) γ. At present, strategies to interrupt latency or to maintain molecular latency in neurons are not available. In experimental animals, ultraviolet light, systemic and local immunosuppression, and trauma to the skin or ganglia are associated with reactivation.

PATHOGENESIS

Exposure to HSV at mucosal surfaces or abraded skin sites permits entry of the virus and initiation of its replication in cells of the epidermis and dermis. HSV infections are usually acquired subclinically. Whether clinical or subclinical, HSV acquisition is associated with sufficient viral replication to permit infection of either sensory or autonomic nerve endings. On entry into the neuronal cell, the virus—or, more likely, the nucleocapsid—is transported intra-axonally to the nerve cell bodies in ganglia. In humans, the transit interval from inoculation of virus in peripheral tissue to spread to the ganglia is unknown. During the initial phase of infection, viral replication occurs in ganglia and contiguous neural tissue. Virus then spreads to other mucocutaneous surfaces through centrifugal migration of infectious virions via peripheral sensory nerves. This mode of spread helps explain the large surface area involved, the high frequency of new lesions distant from the initial crop of vesicles that is characteristic in patients with primary genital or oral-labial HSV infection, and the ability to recover virus from neural tissue distant from neurons innervating the inoculation site. Contiguous spread of locally inoculated virus also may take place and allow further mucosal extension of disease. Recent studies have demonstrated HSV viremia—another mechanism for extension of infection throughout the body—in ~30–40% of persons with primary HSV-2 infection. Latent infection with both viral subtypes in both sensory and autonomic ganglia has been demonstrated.

Analysis of the DNA from sequential isolates of HSV or from isolates from multiple infected ganglia in any one individual has revealed similar, if not identical, restriction endonuclease or DNA sequence patterns in most persons. Occasionally (most frequently in immunocompromised persons), multiple strains of the same viral subtype are detected in one individual. As exposure to mucosal shedding is relatively common during a person's lifetime, these data suggest that exogenous infection with different strains of the same subtype is possible.

IMMUNITY

Host responses influence the acquisition of HSV disease, the severity of infection, resistance to the development of latency, the maintenance of latency, and the frequency of recurrences. Both antibody-mediated and cell-mediated reactions are clinically important. Immunocompromised patients with defects in cell-mediated immunity experience more severe and more extensive HSV infections than those with deficits in humoral immunity, such as agammaglobulinemia. Experimental ablation of lymphocytes indicates that T cells play a major role in preventing lethal disseminated disease, although antibodies help reduce virus titers in neural tissue. Some of the clinical manifestations of HSV appear to be related to the host immune response (e.g., stromal opacities associated with recurrent herpetic keratitis). The surface viral glycoproteins have been shown to be targets of antibodies that mediate neutralization and immune-mediated cytolysis (antibody-dependent cell-mediated cytotoxicity). Monoclonal antibodies specific for each of the known viral glycoproteins have, in experimental infections, conferred protection against subsequent neurologic disease or ganglionic latency. In humans, however, subunit glycoprotein vaccines have been only partially successful in reducing acquisition of infection. Multiple cell populations, including natural killer cells, macrophages, and a variety of T lymphocytes, play a role in host defenses against HSV infections, as do lymphokines generated by T lymphocytes. In animals, passive transfer of primed lymphocytes confers protection from subsequent challenge. Maximal protection usually requires the activation of multiple T-cell subpopulations, including cytotoxic T cells and T cells responsible for delayed hypersensitivity. The latter cells may confer protection by the antigen-stimulated release of lymphokines (e.g., IFNs), which in turn have a direct antiviral effect and both activate and enhance a variety of specific and nonspecific effector cells. Increasing evidence suggests that HSV-specific CD8+ T-cell responses are critical for clearance of virus from lesions. In addition, immunosuppressed patients with frequent and prolonged HSV lesions have fewer functional CD8+ T cells directed at HSV. The HSV virion contains a variety of genes that are directed at the inhibition of host responses. These include gene no. 12 (*US-12*), which can bind to the cellular transporter-activating protein TAP-1 and reduce the ability of this protein to bind HSV peptides to human leukocyte antigen (HLA) class I, thereby reducing recognition of viral proteins by cytotoxic T cells of the host. This effect can be overcome by the addition of IFN-γ, but this reversal requires 24–48 h; thus the virus has time to replicate and invade other host cells. To date, the immunodominant T-cell responses appear to be type-specific. Entry of infectious HSV-1 and HSV-2 inhibits several signaling pathways of both CD4+ and CD8+ T cells, leading to their functional impairment in killing and influencing the spectrum of their cytokine secretion.

EPIDEMIOLOGY

Seroepidemiologic studies have documented HSV infections worldwide. Serologic assays with whole-virus antigen preparations, such as complement fixation, neutralization, indirect immunofluorescence, passive hemagglutination, radioimmunoassay, and enzyme-linked immunosorbent assay, are useful for differentiating uninfected (seronegative) persons from those with past HSV-1 or HSV-2 infection, but they do not reliably distinguish between the two viral subtypes. Serologic assays that identify antibodies to type-specific surface proteins (epitopes) of the two viral subtypes have been developed and can distinguish reliably between the human antibody responses to HSV-1 and HSV-2. The most commonly used assays are those that measure antibodies to glycoprotein G of HSV-1 (gG1) and HSV-2 (gG2). A Western blot assay that can detect several HSV type-specific proteins can also be used.

Infection with HSV-1 is acquired more frequently and earlier than infection with HSV-2. More than 90% of adults have antibodies to HSV-1 by the fifth decade of life. In populations of low socioeconomic status, most persons acquire HSV-1 infection before the third decade of life.

Antibodies to HSV-2 are not detected routinely until puberty. Antibody prevalence rates correlate with past sexual activity and vary greatly among different population groups. There is some evidence that the prevalence of HSV-2 has decreased slightly over the past 5 years in the United States. Serosurveys indicate that 15–20% of the U.S. population has antibodies to HSV-2. In most routine obstetric and family planning clinics, 25% of women have HSV-2 antibodies, although only 10% of those who are seropositive for HSV-2 report a history of genital lesions. As many as 50% of heterosexual adults attending sexually transmitted disease clinics have antibodies to HSV-2.

A wide variety of serologic surveys have indicated a similar or even higher seroprevalence of HSV-2 in most parts of Central America, South America, and Africa. There is an epidemiologic synergy between HSV-2 and HIV-1. HSV-2 infection is associated with a two- to fourfold increase in HIV-1 acquisition. In addition, HSV-2 is reactivated and transmitted more frequently in persons co-infected with HIV-1 and HSV-2 than in persons not infected with HIV-1. Thus most areas of the world with a high HIV-1 prevalence also have a high HSV-2 prevalence. In Africa, HSV-2 seroprevalence has ranged from 40 to 70% in obstetric and other sexually experienced populations. Antibody prevalence rates average ~5–10% higher among women than among men.

Several studies suggest that many cases of "asymptomatic" genital HSV-2 infection are, in fact, simply unrecognized: when "asymptomatic" seropositive persons are shown pictures of genital lesions, >60% subsequently identify episodes of symptomatic reactivation. Most important, these asymptomatic seropositive persons with reactivation shed virus on mucosal surfaces almost as frequently as those with symptomatic disease. The large reservoir of unidentified carriers of HSV-2 and the frequent asymptomatic reactivation of the virus from the genital tract have fostered the continued spread of genital herpes throughout the world. HSV-2 infection is an independent risk factor for the acquisition and transmission of infection with HIV-1. Among co-infected persons, HIV-1 virions can be shed from herpetic lesions of the genital region. This shedding may facilitate the spread of HIV through sexual contact.

HSV infections occur throughout the year. Transmission can result from contact with persons who have active ulcerative lesions or with persons who have no clinical manifestations of infection but who are shedding HSV from mucocutaneous surfaces. Studies using the polymerase chain reaction (PCR) have shown that HSV reactivation on genital skin and mucosal surfaces is much more common than previously recognized. Among immunocompetent adults, HSV-2 can be cultured from the genital tract on 2–10% of days tested, and HSV DNA can be detected on 20–30% of days by PCR. Corresponding figures for HSV-1 in oral secretions are similar. Rates of shedding are highest during the initial years after acquisition, with viral shedding occurring on as many as 30–50% of days during this period. Immunosuppressed patients shed HSV from mucosal sites at an even higher frequency (20–80% of days). Reactivation rates vary widely among individuals. Among HIV-positive patients, a low CD4+ T-cell count and a heavy viral load are associated with increased rates of HSV reactivation. (Daily antiviral chemotherapy for HSV-2 can markedly reduce shedding rates, as measured by PCR.) These high rates of mucocutaneous reactivation suggest that exposure to HSV from sexual or other close contact (kissing, sharing of glasses or silverware) is common and help explain the continuing spread and high seroprevalence of HSV infections worldwide.

CLINICAL SPECTRUM

HSV has been isolated from nearly all visceral and mucocutaneous sites. The clinical manifestations and course of HSV infection depend on the anatomic site involved, the age and immune status of the host, and the antigenic type of the virus. Primary HSV infections (i.e., first infections with either HSV-1 or HSV-2 in which the host lacks HSV antibodies in acute-phase serum) are frequently accompanied by systemic signs and symptoms. Compared with recurrent episodes, primary infections, which involve both mucosal and extramucosal sites, are characterized by a longer duration of symptoms and virus isolation from lesions. The incubation period ranges from 1 to 26 days (median, 6–8 days). Both viral subtypes can cause genital and oral-facial infections, and the infections caused by the two subtypes are clinically indistinguishable. However, the frequency of reactivation of infection is influenced by anatomic site and virus type. Genital HSV-2 infection is twice as likely to reactivate and recurs 8–10 times more frequently than genital HSV-1 infection. Conversely, oral-labial HSV-1 infection recurs more frequently than oral-labial HSV-2 infection. Asymptomatic shedding rates follow the same pattern.

Oral-Facial Infections

Gingivostomatitis and pharyngitis are the most common clinical manifestations of first-episode HSV-1 infection, whereas recurrent herpes labialis is the most common clinical manifestation of reactivation HSV-1 infection. HSV pharyngitis and gingivostomatitis usually result from primary infection and are most commonly seen among children and young adults. Clinical symptoms and signs, which include fever, malaise, myalgias, inability to eat, irritability, and cervical adenopathy, may last 3–14 days. Lesions may involve the hard and soft palate, gingiva, tongue, lip, and facial area. HSV-1 or HSV-2 infection of the pharynx usually results in exudative or ulcerative lesions of the posterior pharynx and/or tonsillar pillars. Lesions of the tongue, buccal mucosa, or gingiva may occur later in the course in one-third of cases. Fever lasting 2–7 days and cervical adenopathy are common. It can be difficult to differentiate HSV pharyngitis clinically from bacterial pharyngitis, *Mycoplasma pneumoniae* infections, and pharyngeal ulcerations of noninfectious etiologies (e.g., Stevens-Johnson syndrome). No substantial evidence suggests that reactivation of oral-labial HSV infection is associated with symptomatic recurrent pharyngitis.

Reactivation of HSV from the trigeminal ganglia may be associated with asymptomatic virus excretion in the saliva, development of intraoral mucosal ulcerations, or herpetic ulcerations on the vermilion border of the lip or external facial skin. About 50–70% of seropositive patients undergoing trigeminal nerve-root decompression and 10–15% of those undergoing dental extraction develop oral-labial HSV infection a median of 3 days after these procedures. Clinical differentiation of intraoral mucosal ulcerations due to HSV from aphthous, traumatic, or drug-induced ulcerations is difficult.

In immunosuppressed patients, HSV infection may extend into mucosal and deep cutaneous layers. Friability, necrosis, bleeding, severe pain, and inability to eat or drink may result. The lesions of HSV mucositis are clinically similar to mucosal lesions caused by cytotoxic drug therapy, trauma, or fungal or bacterial infections. Persistent ulcerative HSV infections are among the most common infections in patients with AIDS. HSV and *Candida* infections often occur concurrently. Systemic antiviral therapy speeds the rate of healing and relieves the pain of mucosal HSV infections in immunosuppressed patients. The frequency of HSV reactivation during the early phases of transplantation or induction chemotherapy is high (50–90%), and prophylactic systemic antiviral agents such as IV acyclovir, penciclovir, or the oral congeners of these drugs are used to reduce reactivation rates. Patients with atopic eczema may also develop severe oral-facial HSV infections (*eczema herpeticum*), which may rapidly involve extensive areas of skin and occasionally disseminate to visceral organs. Extensive eczema herpeticum has resolved promptly with the administration of IV acyclovir. Erythema multiforme may also be associated with HSV infections; some evidence suggests that HSV infection is the precipitating event in ~75% of cases of cutaneous erythema multiforme. HSV antigen has been demonstrated both in circulatory immune complexes and in skin lesion biopsy samples from these cases.

Patients with severe HSV-associated erythema multiforme are candidates for chronic suppressive oral antiviral therapy.

HSV-1 and varicella-zoster virus (VZV) have been implicated in the etiology of Bell's palsy (flaccid paralysis of the mandibular portion of the facial nerve). Although uniform recommendations for treatment of this entity are not available, recent evidence suggests that antiviral chemotherapy in conjunction with a short course of glucocorticoids may result in improved outcomes.

Genital Infections

First-episode primary genital herpes is characterized by fever, headache, malaise, and myalgias. Pain, itching, dysuria, vaginal and urethral discharge, and tender inguinal lymphadenopathy are the predominant local symptoms. Widely spaced bilateral lesions of the external genitalia are characteristic (Fig. 80-1). Lesions may be present in varying stages, including vesicles, pustules, or painful erythematous ulcers. The cervix and urethra are involved in >80% of women with first-episode infections. First episodes of genital herpes in patients who have had prior HSV-1 infection are associated with systemic symptoms in a few patients and with faster healing than primary genital herpes. The clinical courses of acute first-episode genital herpes are similar for HSV-1 and HSV-2 infection. However, the recurrence rates of genital disease differ with the viral subtype: the 12-month recurrence rates among patients with first-episode HSV-2 and HSV-1 infections are ~90% and ~55%, respectively (median number of recurrences, 4 and <1, respectively). Recurrence rates for genital HSV-2 infections vary greatly among individuals and over time within the same individual. HSV has been isolated from the urethra and urine of men and women without external genital lesions. A clear mucoid discharge and dysuria are characteristics of symptomatic HSV urethritis. HSV has been isolated from the urethra of 5% of women with the dysuria-frequency syndrome. Occasionally, HSV genital tract disease is manifested by endometritis and salpingitis in women and by prostatitis in men. About 15% of cases of HSV-2 acquisition are associated with nonlesional clinical syndromes, such as aseptic meningitis, cervicitis, or urethritis. A more complete discussion of the differential diagnosis of genital herpes is presented in Chap. 28.

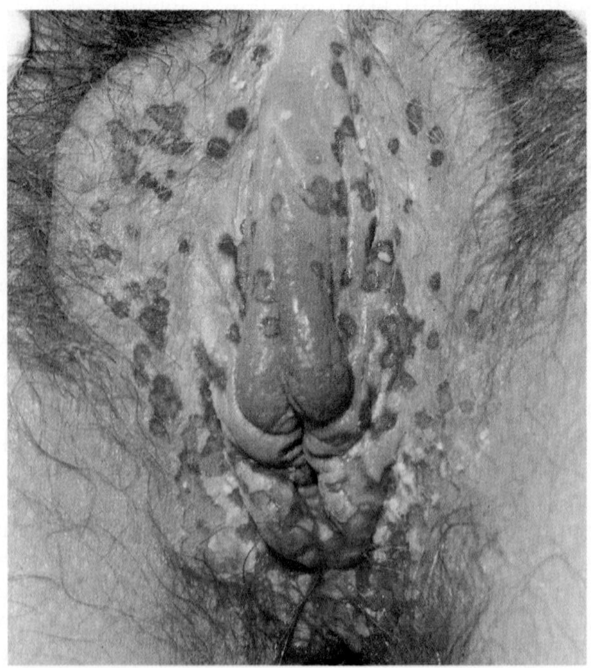

FIGURE 80-1
Genital herpes: primary vulvar infection. Multiple, extremely painful, punched-out, confluent, shallow ulcers on the edematous vulva and perineum. Micturition is often very painful. Associated inguinal lymphadenopathy is common. *(Reprinted with permission from K Wolff, RA Johnson, D Summond: Fitzpatrick's Color Atlas and Synopsis of Clinical Dermatology, 5th ed.)*

Both HSV-1 and HSV-2 can cause symptomatic or asymptomatic rectal and perianal infections. HSV proctitis is usually associated with rectal intercourse. However, subclinical perianal shedding of HSV is detected in women and men who report no rectal intercourse. This phenomenon is due to the establishment of latency in the sacral dermatome from prior genital tract infection, with subsequent reactivation in epithelial cells in the perianal region. Such reactivations are often subclinical. Symptoms of HSV proctitis include anorectal pain, anorectal discharge, tenesmus, and constipation. Sigmoidoscopy reveals ulcerative lesions of the distal 10 cm of the rectal mucosa. Rectal biopsies show mucosal ulceration, necrosis, polymorphonuclear and lymphocytic infiltration of the lamina propria, and (in occasional cases) multinucleated intranuclear inclusion–bearing cells. Perianal herpetic lesions are also found in immunosuppressed patients receiving cytotoxic therapy. Extensive perianal herpetic lesions and/or HSV proctitis is common among patients with HIV infection.

Herpetic Whitlow

Herpetic whitlow—HSV infection of the finger—may occur as a complication of primary oral or genital herpes by inoculation of virus through a break in the epidermal surface or by direct introduction of virus into the hand through occupational or some other type of exposure. Clinical signs and symptoms include abrupt-onset edema, erythema, and localized tenderness of the infected finger. Vesicular or pustular lesions of the fingertip that are indistinguishable from lesions of pyogenic bacterial infection are seen. Fever, lymphadenitis, and epitrochlear and axillary lymphadenopathy are common. The infection may recur. Prompt diagnosis (to avoid unnecessary and potentially exacerbating surgical therapy and/or transmission) is essential. Antiviral chemotherapy is usually recommended (see below).

Herpes Gladiatorum

HSV may infect almost any area of skin. Mucocutaneous HSV infections of the thorax, ears, face, and hands have been described among wrestlers. Transmission of these infections is facilitated by trauma to the skin sustained during wrestling. Several recent outbreaks have illustrated the importance of prompt diagnosis and therapy to contain the spread of this infection.

Eye Infections

HSV infection of the eye is the most common cause of corneal blindness in the United States. HSV keratitis presents as an acute onset of pain, blurred vision, chemosis, conjunctivitis, and characteristic dendritic lesions of the cornea. Use of topical glucocorticoids may exacerbate symptoms and lead to involvement of deep structures of the eye. Debridement, topical antiviral treatment, and/or IFN therapy hastens healing. However, recurrences are common, and the deeper structures of the eye may sustain immunopathologic injury. Stromal keratitis due to HSV appears to be related to T-cell–dependent destruction of deep corneal tissue. An HSV-1 epitope that is autoreactive with T-cell–targeting corneal antigens has been postulated to be a factor in this infection. Chorioretinitis, usually a manifestation of disseminated HSV infection, may occur in neonates or in patients with HIV infection. HSV and VZV can cause acute necrotizing retinitis as an uncommon but severe manifestation.

Central and Peripheral Nervous System Infections

HSV accounts for 10–20% of all cases of sporadic viral encephalitis in the United States. The estimated incidence is ~2.3 cases per 1 million persons per year. Cases are distributed throughout the year, and the age distribution appears to be biphasic, with peaks at 5–30 and >50 years of age. HSV-1 causes >95% of cases.

The pathogenesis of HSV encephalitis varies. In children and young adults, primary HSV infection may result in encephalitis; presumably, exogenously acquired virus enters the CNS by neurotropic spread from the periphery via the olfactory bulb. However, most adults with HSV encephalitis have clinical or serologic evidence of mucocutaneous HSV-1 infection before the onset of CNS symptoms. In ~25% of the cases examined, the HSV-1 strains from the oropharynx and brain tissue of the same patient differ; thus some cases may result from reinfection with another strain of HSV-1 that reaches the CNS. Two theories have been proposed to explain the development of actively replicating HSV in localized areas of the CNS in persons whose ganglionic and CNS isolates are similar. Reactivation of latent HSV-1 infection in trigeminal or autonomic nerve roots may be associated with extension of virus into the CNS via nerves innervating the middle cranial fossa. HSV DNA has been demonstrated by DNA hybridization in brain tissue obtained at autopsy—even from healthy adults. Thus reactivation of long-standing latent CNS infection may be another mechanism for the development of HSV encephalitis.

Recent studies have identified genetic polymorphisms in two separate genes among children with HSV encephalitis. Peripheral-blood mononuclear cells from these children appear to secrete reduced levels of IFN in response to HSV; if confirmed, this observation suggests that sporadic HSV encephalitis may be related to a variety of host genetic determinants.

The clinical hallmark of HSV encephalitis has been the acute onset of fever and focal neurologic symptoms and signs, especially in the temporal lobe (Fig. 80-2). Clinical differentiation of HSV encephalitis from other viral encephalitides, focal infections, or noninfectious processes is difficult. Elevated cerebrospinal fluid (CSF) protein levels, leukocytosis (predominantly lymphocytes), and red blood cell counts due to hemorrhagic necrosis are common. Although brain biopsy has been the gold standard for defining HSV encephalitis, the high sensitivity

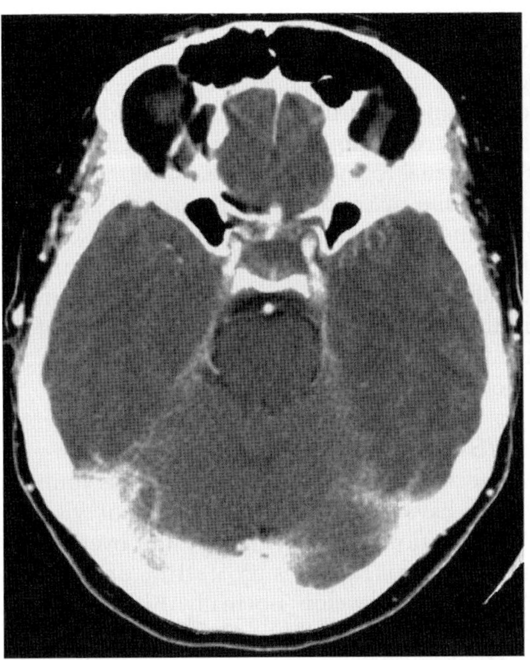

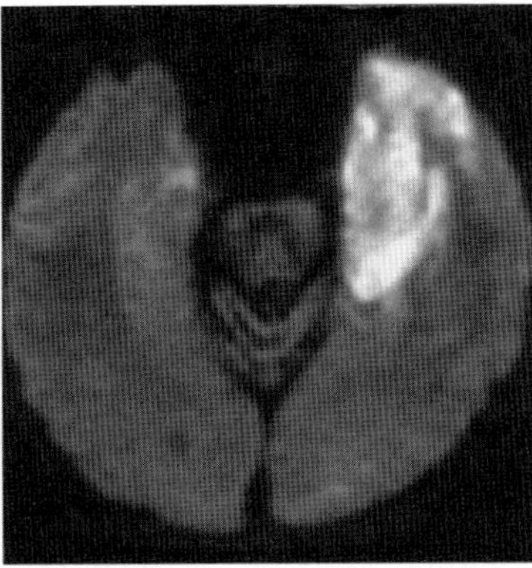

FIGURE 80-2
CT and diffusion-weighted MRI scans of the brain of a patient with left-temporal-lobe HSV encephalitis.

and specificity of HSV DNA detection by PCR in CSF has largely replaced biopsy for defining HSV CNS infection. Although titers of antibody to HSV in CSF and serum increase in most cases of HSV encephalitis, they rarely do so earlier than 10 days into the illness and therefore, although useful retrospectively, are generally not helpful in establishing an early clinical diagnosis. Demonstration of HSV antigen, HSV DNA, or HSV replication in brain tissue obtained by biopsy is highly sensitive and has a low complication rate; examination of such tissue also provides the best opportunity to identify alternative, potentially treatable causes of encephalitis. Antiviral chemotherapy with acyclovir reduces the rate of death from HSV encephalitis. Even with therapy, however, neurologic sequelae are common, especially in persons >50 years of age. Most authorities recommend the administration of IV acyclovir to patients with presumed HSV encephalitis until the diagnosis is confirmed or an alternative diagnosis is made. Among proven cases of HSV encephalitis, IV therapy is usually recommended until HSV DNA levels in CSF are substantially reduced or nearly undetectable.

HSV DNA has been detected in CSF from 3–15% of persons presenting to the hospital with aseptic meningitis. HSV meningitis, which is usually seen in association with primary genital HSV infection, is an acute, self-limited disease manifested by headache, fever, and mild photophobia and lasting 2–7 days. Lymphocytic pleocytosis in the CSF is characteristic. Neurologic sequelae of HSV meningitis are rare. HSV is the most commonly identified cause of recurrent lymphocytic meningitis (Mollaret's meningitis). Demonstration of HSV antibodies in CSF or persistence of HSV DNA in CSF can establish the diagnosis. For persons with frequent recurrences of HSV meningitis, antiviral therapy has reduced the occurrence of such episodes.

Autonomic nervous system dysfunction, especially of the sacral region, has been reported in association with both HSV and VZV infections. Numbness, tingling of the buttocks or perineal areas, urinary retention, constipation, CSF pleocytosis, and (in males) impotence may occur. Symptoms appear to resolve slowly over days or weeks. Occasionally, hypoesthesia and/or weakness of the lower extremities persists for many months. Rarely, transverse myelitis, manifested by a rapidly progressive symmetric paralysis of the lower extremities or Guillain-Barré syndrome, follows HSV infection. Similarly, peripheral nervous system involvement (Bell's palsy) or cranial polyneuritis may be related to reactivation of HSV-1 infection. Transitory hypoesthesia of the area of skin innervated by the trigeminal nerve and vestibular system dysfunction as measured by electronystagmography are the predominant signs of disease. Whether antiviral chemotherapy can abort these signs or reduce their frequency and severity is not yet known.

Visceral Infections

HSV infection of visceral organs usually results from viremia, and multiple-organ involvement is common. Occasionally, however, the clinical manifestations of HSV infection involve only the esophagus, lung, or liver. HSV esophagitis may result from direct extension of oral-pharyngeal HSV infection into the esophagus or may occur de novo by reactivation and spread of HSV to the esophageal mucosa via the vagus nerve. The predominant symptoms of HSV esophagitis are odynophagia, dysphagia, substernal pain, and weight loss. Multiple oval ulcerations appear on an erythematous base with or without a patchy white pseudomembrane. The distal esophagus is most commonly involved. With extensive disease, diffuse friability may spread to the entire esophagus. Neither endoscopic nor barium examination can reliably differentiate HSV esophagitis from *Candida* esophagitis or from esophageal ulcerations due to thermal injury, radiation, or corrosives. Endoscopically obtained secretions for cytologic examination and culture or DNA detection by PCR provide the most useful material for diagnosis. Systemic antiviral chemotherapy usually reduces symptoms and heals esophageal ulcerations.

HSV pneumonitis is uncommon except in severely immunosuppressed patients and may result from extension of herpetic tracheobronchitis into lung parenchyma. Focal necrotizing pneumonitis usually ensues. Hematogenous dissemination of virus from sites of oral or genital mucocutaneous disease may also occur, producing bilateral interstitial pneumonitis. Bacterial, fungal, and parasitic pathogens are commonly present in HSV pneumonitis. The mortality rate from untreated HSV pneumonia in immunosuppressed patients is high (>80%). HSV has also been isolated from the lower respiratory tract of persons with adult respiratory distress syndrome and prolonged intubation. The role of lower respiratory tract HSV infection in overall rates of morbidity and mortality associated with these conditions is unclear.

HSV is an uncommon cause of hepatitis in immunocompetent patients. HSV infection of the liver is associated with fever, abrupt elevations of bilirubin and serum aminotransferase levels, and leukopenia (<4000 white blood cells/μL). Disseminated intravascular coagulation may also develop.

Other reported complications of HSV infection include monarticular arthritis, adrenal necrosis, idiopathic thrombocytopenia, and glomerulonephritis. Disseminated HSV infection in immunocompetent patients is rare. In immunocompromised, burned, or malnourished patients, HSV occasionally disseminates to other visceral organs, such as the adrenal glands, pancreas, small and large intestines, and bone marrow. Rarely, primary HSV infection in pregnancy disseminates and may be associated with the death of both mother and fetus. This uncommon event is usually related to the acquisition of primary infection in the third trimester. Disseminated HSV infection is best detected by the presence of HSV DNA in plasma or blood.

Neonatal HSV Infections

Of all HSV-infected populations, neonates (infants younger than 6 weeks) have the highest frequency of visceral and/or CNS infection. Without therapy, the overall rate of death from neonatal herpes is 65%; <10% of neonates with CNS infection develop normally. Although skin lesions are the most commonly recognized features of disease, many infants do not develop lesions at all or do so only well into the course of disease. Neonatal infection is usually acquired perinatally from contact with infected genital secretions at delivery. Congenitally infected infants have been reported. In most series, 30% of neonatal HSV infections are due to HSV-1 and 70% to HSV-2. The risk of developing neonatal HSV infection is 10 times higher for an infant born to a mother who has recently acquired HSV than for other infants. Neonatal HSV-1 infections may also be acquired through postnatal contact with immediate family members who have symptomatic or asymptomatic oral-labial HSV-1 infection or through nosocomial transmission within the hospital. All neonates with presumed neonatal herpes should be treated with IV acyclovir. Antiviral chemotherapy with high-dose IV acyclovir (60 mg/kg per day) has reduced the mortality rate from neonatal herpes to ~15%. However, morbidity, especially among infants with HSV-2 infection involving the CNS, is still very high.

DIAGNOSIS

Both clinical and laboratory criteria are useful for diagnosing HSV infections. A clinical diagnosis can be made accurately when characteristic multiple vesicular lesions on an erythematous base are present. However, herpetic ulcerations may resemble skin ulcerations of other etiologies. Mucosal HSV infections may also present as urethritis or pharyngitis without cutaneous lesions. Thus laboratory studies to confirm the diagnosis and to guide therapy are recommended. Although staining of scrapings from the base of the lesions with Wright's, Giemsa's (Tzanck preparation), or Papanicolaou's stain to detect giant cells or intranuclear inclusions of *Herpesvirus* infection is a well-described procedure, few clinicians are skilled in these techniques, the sensitivity of staining is low (<30% for mucosal swabs), and these cytologic methods do not differentiate between HSV and VZV infections.

HSV infection is best confirmed in the laboratory by detection of virus, viral antigen, or viral DNA in scrapings from lesions. HSV DNA detection by PCR, when available, is the most sensitive laboratory technique. HSV causes a discernible cytopathic effect in a variety of cell culture systems, and this effect can be identified within 48–96 h after inoculation. Spin-amplified culture with subsequent staining for HSV antigen has shortened the time needed to identify HSV to <24 h. The sensitivity of all detection methods depends on the stage of the lesions (with higher sensitivity in vesicular than in ulcerative lesions), on whether the patient has a first or a recurrent episode of the disease (with higher sensitivity in first than in recurrent episodes), and on whether the sample is from an immunosuppressed or an immunocompetent patient (with more antigen or DNA in immunosuppressed patients). Laboratory confirmation permits subtyping of the virus; information on subtype may be useful epidemiologically and may help to predict the frequency of reactivation after first-episode oral-labial or genital HSV infection.

Acute- and convalescent-phase serum can be useful in demonstrating seroconversion during primary HSV-1 or HSV-2 infection. However, few available tests report titers, and increases in index values do not reflect first episodes in all patients. Serologic assays based on type-specific proteins should be used to identify asymptomatic carriers of HSV-1 or HSV-2 infection. No reliable IgM method for defining acute HSV infection is available.

Several studies have shown that persons with previously unrecognized HSV-2 infection can be taught to identify symptomatic reactivations. Individuals seropositive for HSV-2 should be told about the high frequency of subclinical reactivation in mucosal surfaces that are not visible to the eye (e.g., cervix, urethra, perianal skin) or in microscopic ulcerations that may not be clinically symptomatic. Transmission of infection during such episodes is well established. HSV-2–seropositive persons should be educated about the high likelihood of subclinical shedding and the role condoms (male or female) may play in reducing transmission. Antiviral therapy with valacyclovir (500 mg once daily) has been shown to reduce the transmission of HSV-2 between sexual partners.

℞ Treatment: HERPES SIMPLEX VIRUS INFECTIONS

Many aspects of mucocutaneous and visceral HSV infections are amenable to antiviral chemotherapy. For mucocutaneous infections, acyclovir and its congeners famciclovir and valacyclovir have been the mainstays of therapy. Several antiviral agents are available for topical use in HSV eye infections: idoxuridine, trifluorothymidine, topical vidarabine, and cidofovir. For HSV encephalitis and neonatal herpes, IV acyclovir is the treatment of choice.

All licensed antiviral agents for use against HSV inhibit the viral DNA polymerase. One class of drugs, typified by the drug acyclovir, is made up of substrates for the HSV enzyme thymidine kinase (TK). Acyclovir, ganciclovir, famciclovir, and valacyclovir are all selectively phosphorylated to the monophosphate form in virus-infected cells. Cellular enzymes convert the monophosphate form of the drug to the triphosphate, which is then incorporated into the viral DNA chain.

Acyclovir is the agent most frequently used for the treatment of HSV infections and is available in IV, oral, and topical formulations. Valacyclovir, the valyl ester of acyclovir, offers greater bioavailability than acyclovir and thus can be administered less frequently. Famciclovir, the oral formulation of penciclovir, is clinically effective in the treatment of a variety of HSV-1 and HSV-2 infections. Ganciclovir is active against both HSV-1 and HSV-2; however, it is more toxic than acyclovir, valacyclovir, and famciclovir and generally is not recommended for the treatment of HSV infections. Anecdotal case reports suggest that ganciclovir may also be less effective than acyclovir for treatment of HSV infections.

All three recommended compounds—acyclovir, valacyclovir, and famciclovir—have proved effective in shortening the duration of symptoms and lesions of mucocutaneous HSV infections in both immunocompromised and immunocompetent patients (Table 80-1). IV and oral formulations prevent reactivation of HSV in seropositive immunocompromised patients during induction chemotherapy or in the period immediately after

TABLE 80-1

ANTIVIRAL CHEMOTHERAPY FOR HSV INFECTION

I. Mucocutaneous HSV infections

A. *Infections in immunosuppressed patients*

1. *Acute symptomatic first or recurrent episodes:* IV acyclovir (5 mg/kg q8h) or oral acyclovir (400 mg qid), famciclovir (500 mg bid or tid), or valacyclovir (500 mg bid) is effective. Treatment duration may vary from 7 to 14 days.
2. *Suppression of reactivation disease (genital or oral-labial):* IV acyclovir (5 mg/kg q8h) or oral valacyclovir (500 mg bid) or acyclovir (400–800 mg 3–5 times per day) prevents recurrences during the 30-day period immediately after transplantation. Longer-term HSV suppression is often used for persons with continued immunosuppression. In bone marrow and renal transplant recipients, oral valacyclovir (2 g/d) is also effective in reducing cytomegalovirus infection. Oral valacyclovir at a dose of 4 g/d has been associated with thrombotic thrombocytopenic purpura after extended use in HIV-positive persons. In HIV-infected persons, oral acyclovir (400–800 mg bid), valacyclovir (500 mg bid), or famciclovir (500 mg bid) is effective in reducing clinical and subclinical reactivations of HSV-1 and HSV-2.

B. *Infections in immunocompetent patients*

1. *Genital herpes*
   a. *First episodes:* Oral acyclovir (200 mg 5 times per day or 400 mg tid), valacyclovir (1 g bid), or famciclovir (250 mg bid) for 7–14 days is effective. IV acyclovir (5 mg/kg q8h for 5 days) is given for severe disease or neurologic complications such as aseptic meningitis.
   b. *Symptomatic recurrent genital herpes:* Short-course (1- to 3-day) regimens are preferred because of low cost and convenience. Oral acyclovir (800 mg tid for 2 days), valacyclovir (500 mg bid for 3 days), or famciclovir (750 or 1000 mg bid for 1 day, a 1500-mg single dose, or 500 mg stat followed by 250 mg q12h for 3 days) effectively shortens lesion duration. Other options include oral acyclovir (200 mg 5 times per day), valacyclovir (500 mg bid), and famciclovir (125 mg bid for 5 days).
   c. *Suppression of recurrent genital herpes:* Oral acyclovir (200-mg capsules tid or qid, 400 mg bid, or 800 mg qd), famciclovir (250 mg bid), or valacyclovir (500 mg daily) is effective. Patients with >9 episodes per year should take oral valacyclovir at a dosage of 1 g daily or 500 mg bid.
2. *Oral-labial HSV infections*
   a. *First episode:* Oral acyclovir (200 mg) is given 4 or 5 times per day; an oral acyclovir suspension can be used (600 mg/m^2 qid). Oral famciclovir (250 mg bid) or valacyclovir (1 g bid) has been used clinically.
   b. *Recurrent episodes:* If initiated at the onset of the prodrome, single-dose or 1-day therapy effectively reduces pain and speeds healing. Regimens include oral famciclovir (a 1500-mg single dose or 750 mg bid for 1 day) or valacyclovir (a 2-g single dose or 2 g bid for 1 day). Self-initiated therapy with 6-times-daily topical penciclovir cream effectively speeds healing of oral-labial HSV. Topical acyclovir cream has also been shown to speed healing.
   c. *Suppression of reactivation of oral-labial HSV:* If started before exposure and continued for the duration of exposure (usually 5–10 days), oral acyclovir (400 mg bid) prevents reactivation of recurrent oral-labial HSV infection associated with severe sun exposure.
3. *Surgical prophylaxis of oral or genital HSV infection:* Several surgical procedures, such as laser skin resurfacing, trigeminal nerve-root decompression, and lumbar disk surgery, have been associated with HSV reactivation. IV acyclovir (5 mg/kg q8h) or oral acyclovir (800 mg bid), valacyclovir (500 mg bid), or famciclovir (250 mg bid) effectively reduces reactivation. Therapy should be initiated 48 h before surgery and continued for 3–7 days.
4. *Herpetic whitlow:* Oral acyclovir (200 mg) is given 5 times daily for 7–10 days.
5. *HSV proctitis:* Oral acyclovir (400 mg 5 times per day) is useful in shortening the course of infection. In immunosuppressed patients or in patients with severe infection, IV acyclovir (5 mg/kg q8h) may be useful.
6. *Herpetic eye infections:* In acute keratitis, topical trifluorothymidine, vidarabine, idoxuridine, acyclovir, penciclovir, and interferon are all beneficial. Debridement may be required. Topical steroids may worsen disease.

II. CNS HSV infections

A. *HSV encephalitis:* IV acyclovir (10 mg/kg q8h; 30 mg/kg per day) is given for 10 days or until HSV DNA is no longer detected in CSF.

B. *HSV aseptic meningitis:* No studies of systemic antiviral chemotherapy exist. If therapy is to be given, IV acyclovir (15–30 mg/kg per day) should be used.

C. *Autonomic radiculopathy:* No studies are available. Most authorities recommend a trial of IV acyclovir.

III. Neonatal HSV infections: Oral acyclovir (60 mg/kg per day, divided into 3 doses) is given. The recommended duration of treatment is 21 days. Monitoring for relapse should be undertaken, and some authorities recommend continued suppression with oral acyclovir suspension for 3–4 months.

IV. Visceral HSV infections

A. *HSV esophagitis:* IV acyclovir (15 mg/kg per day). In some patients with milder forms of immunosuppression, oral therapy with valacyclovir or famciclovir is effective.

B. *HSV pneumonitis:* No controlled studies exist. IV acyclovir (15 mg/kg per day) should be considered.

V. Disseminated HSV infections: No controlled studies exist. IV acyclovir (5 mg/kg q8h) should be tried. Adjustments for renal insufficiency may be needed. No definite evidence indicates that therapy will decrease the risk of death.

(*Continued*)

TABLE 80-1 (*CONTINUED*)

ANTIVIRAL CHEMOTHERAPY FOR HSV INFECTION

VI. Erythema multiforme associated with HSV: Anecdotal observations suggest that oral acyclovir (400 mg bid or tid) or valacyclovir (500 mg bid) will suppress erythema multiforme.

VII. Infections due to acyclovir-resistant HSV: IV foscarnet (40 mg/kg IV q8h) should be given until lesions heal. The optimal duration of therapy and the usefulness of its continuation to suppress lesions are unclear. Some patients may benefit from cutaneous application of trifluorothymidine or 5% cidofovir gel.

bone marrow or solid organ transplantation. Chronic daily suppressive therapy reduces the frequency of reactivation disease among patients with frequent genital or oral-labial herpes. Only valacyclovir has been subjected to clinical trials that demonstrated reduced transmission of HSV-2 infection between sexual partners.

IV acyclovir (30 mg/kg per day, given as a 10-mg/kg infusion over 1 h at 8-h intervals) is effective in reducing rates of death and morbidity from HSV encephalitis. Early initiation of therapy is a critical factor in outcome. The major side effect associated with IV acyclovir is transient renal insufficiency, usually due to crystallization of the compound in the renal parenchyma. This adverse reaction can be avoided if the medication is given slowly over 1 h and the patient is well hydrated. Because CSF levels of acyclovir average only 30–50% of plasma levels, the dosage of acyclovir used for treatment of CNS infection (30 mg/kg per day) is double that used for treatment of mucocutaneous or visceral disease (15 mg/kg per day). Even higher doses of IV acyclovir are used for neonatal HSV infection (60 mg/kg per day in three divided doses).

Among immunocompetent patients, recent studies have shown the effectiveness of short-course, high-dose oral therapy to reduce the signs and symptoms of oral and genital HSV infection. These regimens include valacyclovir (for 1–3 days) for oral-labial HSV and acyclovir (2 days), valacyclovir (3 days), or famciclovir (1 or 2 days) for recurrent-episode genital herpes (Table 80-1). These short-course regimens are less expensive and more convenient but should be reserved for immunocompetent hosts.

SUPPRESSION OF MUCOCUTANEOUS HERPES Recognition of the high frequency of subclinical reactivation provides a well-accepted rationale for the use of daily antiviral therapy to suppress reactivations of HSV, especially in persons with frequent clinical reactivations (e.g., those with recently acquired genital HSV infection). Immunosuppressed persons, including those with HIV infection, may also benefit from daily antiviral therapy. Recent studies have shown the efficacy of daily acyclovir and valacyclovir in reducing the frequency of HSV reactivations among HIV-positive persons. Regimens used include acyclovir (400 mg three times daily), famciclovir (500 mg twice daily), and valacyclovir (1 g twice daily); valacyclovir at a dose of 4 g daily was associated with thrombotic thrombocytopenic purpura in one study of HIV-infected persons.

In addition, daily treatment of HSV-2 reduces the titer of HIV RNA in plasma (0.5-log reduction) and in genital mucosa (0.33-log reduction).

REDUCED HSV TRANSMISSION TO SEXUAL PARTNERS Once-daily valacyclovir (500 mg) has been shown to reduce transmission of HSV-2 between sexual partners. Transmission rates are higher from males to females and among persons with frequent HSV-2 reactivation. Serologic screening can be used to identify at-risk couples. Daily valacyclovir appears more effective at reducing subclinical shedding than daily famciclovir.

ACYCLOVIR RESISTANCE Acyclovir-resistant strains of HSV have been identified. Most of these strains have an altered substrate specificity for phosphorylating acyclovir. Thus cross-resistance to famciclovir and valacyclovir is usually found. Occasionally, an isolate with altered TK specificity arises and is sensitive to famciclovir, but not to acyclovir. In some patients infected with TK-deficient virus, higher doses of acyclovir are associated with clearing of lesions. In others, clinical disease progresses despite high-dose therapy. Almost all clinically significant acyclovir resistance has been seen in immunocompromised patients, and HSV-2 isolates are more often resistant than HSV-1 strains. A study by the Centers for Disease Control and Prevention indicated that ~5% of HSV-2 isolates from HIV-positive persons exhibit some degree of in vitro resistance to acyclovir. Of HSV-2 isolates from immunocompetent patients attending sexually transmitted disease clinics, <0.5% show reduced in vitro sensitivity to acyclovir. The lack of appreciable change in the frequency of detection of such isolates in the past 20 years probably reflects the reduced transmission of TK-deficient mutants. Isolation of HSV from lesions persisting despite adequate dosages and blood levels of acyclovir should raise the suspicion of acyclovir resistance. Therapy with the antiviral drug foscarnet is useful in acyclovir-resistant cases (Chap. 79). Because of its toxicity and cost, this drug is usually reserved for patients with extensive mucocutaneous infections. Cidofovir is a nucleotide analogue and exists as a phosphonate or monophosphate form. Most TK-deficient strains of HSV are sensitive to cidofovir. Cidofovir ointment speeds healing of acyclovir-resistant lesions. No well-controlled trials of systemic cidofovir have been reported. True TK-negative variants of HSV appear to have a reduced capacity to spread because of altered neurovirulence—a feature important in the relatively infrequent presence of such strains in immunocompetent populations, even with increasing use of antiviral drugs.

PREVENTION

The success of efforts to control HSV disease on a population basis through suppressive antiviral chemotherapy and/or educational programs will be limited.

Barrier forms of contraception (especially condoms) decrease the likelihood of transmission of HSV infection, particularly during periods of asymptomatic viral excretion. When lesions are present, HSV infection may be transmitted by skin-to-skin contact despite the use of a condom. Nevertheless, the available data suggest that consistent condom use is an effective means of reducing the risk of genital HSV-2 transmission. Chronic daily antiviral therapy with valacyclovir can also be partially effective in reducing acquisition of HSV-2, especially among susceptible women. There are no comparative efficacy studies of valacyclovir versus condom use. Most authorities suggest both approaches. The need for a vaccine to prevent acquisition of HSV infection is great, especially in light of the role HSV-2 plays in enhancing the acquisition and transmission of HIV-1.

A substantial portion of neonatal HSV cases could be prevented by reducing the acquisition of HSV by women in the third trimester of pregnancy. Identification of women susceptible to HSV acquisition in pregnancy through serologic screening, with a focus on counseling against unprotected oral or genital sex, is receiving increasing attention. Neonatal HSV infection can result from either the acquisition of maternal infection near term or the reactivation of infection at delivery in the already-infected mother. Thus strategies for reducing neonatal HSV are complex. Some authorities have recommended that antiviral therapy with acyclovir or valacyclovir be given to HSV-2–infected women in late pregnancy as a means of reducing reactivation of HSV-2 at term. Data are not available to support the efficacy of this approach. Moreover, the high treatment-to-prevention ratio makes this a dubious public health approach, even though it can reduce the frequency of HSV-associated cesarean delivery.

FURTHER READINGS

Brown ZA et al: Effect of serologic status and cesarean delivery on transmission rates of herpes simplex virus from mother to infant. JAMA 289:203, 2003

Chilukuri S, Rosen T: Management of acyclovir-resistant herpes simplex virus. Dermatol Clin 21:311, 2003

Corey L et al: The effects of herpes simplex virus-2 on HIV-1 acquisition and transmission: A review of two overlapping epidemics. J AIDS 35:435, 2004

Gupta R et al: Genital herpes. Lancet 370:2127, 2007

Kimberlin DW et al: Safety and efficacy of high-dose intravenous acyclovir in the management of neonatal herpes simplex virus infections. Pediatrics 108:230, 2001

Nagot N et al: Reduction of HIV-1 RNA levels with therapy to suppress herpes simplex virus. N Engl J Med 356:790, 2007

Wald A et al: The relationship between condom use and herpes simplex virus acquisition. Ann Intern Med 143:707, 2005

Whitley RJ et al: Herpes simplex encephalitis: Adolescents and adults. Antiviral Res 71:141, 2006

CHAPTER 81

VARICELLA-ZOSTER VIRUS INFECTIONS

Richard J. Whitley

DEFINITION

Varicella-zoster virus (VZV) causes two distinct clinical entities: varicella (chickenpox) and herpes zoster (shingles). Chickenpox, a ubiquitous and extremely contagious infection, is usually a benign illness of childhood characterized by an exanthematous vesicular rash. With reactivation of latent VZV (which is most common after the sixth decade of life), herpes zoster presents as a dermatomal vesicular rash, usually associated with severe pain.

ETIOLOGY

A clinical association between varicella and herpes zoster has been recognized for nearly 100 years. Early in the twentieth century, similarities in the histopathologic features of skin lesions resulting from varicella and herpes zoster were demonstrated. Viral isolates from patients with chickenpox and herpes zoster produced similar alterations in tissue culture—specifically, the appearance of eosinophilic intranuclear inclusions and multinucleated giant cells. These results suggested that the viruses were biologically similar. Restriction endonuclease analyses of viral DNA from a patient with chickenpox who subsequently developed herpes zoster verified the molecular identity of the two viruses responsible for these different clinical presentations.

VZV is a member of the family Herpesviridae, sharing with other members such structural characteristics as a lipid envelope surrounding a nucleocapsid with icosahedral symmetry, a total diameter of ~180–200 nm, and centrally located double-stranded DNA that is ~125,000 bp in length.

PATHOGENESIS AND PATHOLOGY

Primary Infection

Transmission occurs readily by the respiratory route; the subsequent localized replication of the virus at an undefined site (presumably the nasopharynx) leads to seeding of the reticuloendothelial system and ultimately to the development of viremia. Viremia in patients with chickenpox is reflected in the diffuse and scattered nature of the skin lesions and can be verified in selected cases by the recovery of VZV from the blood or routinely by the detection of viral DNA in either blood or lesions by polymerase chain reaction (PCR). Vesicles involve the corium and dermis, with degenerative changes characterized by ballooning, the presence of multinucleated giant cells, and eosinophilic intranuclear inclusions. Infection may involve localized blood vessels of the skin, resulting in necrosis and epidermal hemorrhage. With the evolution of disease, the vesicular fluid becomes cloudy because of the recruitment of polymorphonuclear leukocytes and the presence of degenerated cells and fibrin. Ultimately, the vesicles either rupture and release their fluid (which includes infectious virus) or are gradually reabsorbed.

Recurrent Infection

The mechanism of reactivation of VZV that results in herpes zoster is unknown. Presumably, the virus infects dorsal root ganglia during chickenpox, where it remains latent until reactivated. Histopathologic examination of representative dorsal root ganglia during active herpes zoster demonstrates hemorrhage, edema, and lymphocytic infiltration.

Active replication of VZV in other organs, such as the lung or the brain, can occur during either chickenpox or herpes zoster but is uncommon in the immunocompetent host. Pulmonary involvement is characterized by interstitial pneumonitis, multinucleated giant cell formation, intranuclear inclusions, and pulmonary hemorrhage. Central nervous system (CNS) infection leads to histopathologic evidence of perivascular cuffing similar to that encountered in measles and other viral encephalitides. Focal hemorrhagic necrosis of the brain, characteristic of herpes simplex virus (HSV) encephalitis, is uncommon in VZV infection.

EPIDEMIOLOGY AND CLINICAL MANIFESTATIONS

Chickenpox

Humans are the only known reservoir for VZV. Chickenpox is highly contagious, with an attack rate of at least 90% among susceptible (seronegative) individuals. Persons of both sexes and all races are infected equally often. The virus is endemic in the population at large; however, it becomes epidemic among susceptible individuals during seasonal peaks—namely, late winter and early spring in the temperate zone. Historically, children 5–9 years old are most commonly affected and account for 50% of all cases. Most other cases involve children 1–4 and 10–14 years old. Approximately 10% of the population of the United States over the age of 15 is susceptible to infection. VZV vaccination during the second year of life is dramatically changing the epidemiology of infection. As a consequence, the annualized incidence of chickenpox is decreasing significantly.

The incubation period of chickenpox ranges from 10 to 21 days but is usually 14–17 days. Secondary attack rates in susceptible siblings within a household are 70–90%. Patients are infectious ~48 h before onset of the vesicular rash, during the period of vesicle formation (which generally lasts 4–5 days), and until all vesicles are crusted.

Clinically, chickenpox presents as a rash, low-grade fever, and malaise, although a few patients develop a prodrome 1–2 days before onset of the exanthem. In the immunocompetent patient, chickenpox is usually a benign illness associated with lassitude and with body temperatures of 37.8°–39.4°C (100°–103°F) of 3–5 days' duration. The skin lesions—the hallmark of the infection—include maculopapules, vesicles, and scabs in various stages of evolution (Fig. 81-1). These lesions, which evolve from maculopapules to vesicles over hours to days, appear on the trunk and face and rapidly spread to involve other areas of the body. Most are small and have an erythematous base with a diameter of 5–10 mm. Successive crops appear over a 2- to 4-day period. Lesions can also be found on the mucosa of the pharynx and/or the vagina. Their severity varies from one person to another. Some individuals have very few lesions, whereas others have as many as 2000. Younger children tend to have fewer vesicles than older individuals. Secondary and tertiary cases

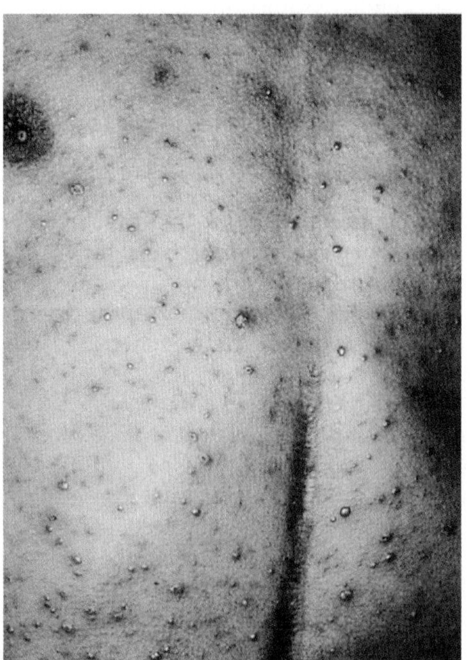

FIGURE 81-1

Numerous varicella lesions at various stages of evolution: vesicles on an erythematous base, umbilical vesicles, and crusts.

within families are associated with a relatively large number of vesicles. Immunocompromised patients—both children and adults, particularly those with leukemia—have lesions (often with a hemorrhagic base) that are more numerous and take longer to heal than those of immunocompetent patients. Immunocompromised individuals are also at greater risk for visceral complications, which occur in 30–50% of cases and are fatal 15% of the time in the absence of antiviral therapy.

The most common infectious complication of varicella is secondary bacterial superinfection of the skin, which is usually caused by *Streptococcus pyogenes* or *Staphylococcus aureus,* including strains that are methicillin resistant. Skin infection results from excoriation of lesions after scratching. Gram's staining of skin lesions should help clarify the etiology of unusually erythematous and pustulated lesions.

The most common extracutaneous site of involvement in children is the CNS. The syndrome of acute cerebellar ataxia and meningeal inflammation generally appears ~21 days after onset of the rash and rarely develops in the preeruptive phase. The cerebrospinal fluid (CSF) contains lymphocytes and elevated levels of protein. CNS involvement is a benign complication of VZV infection in children and generally does not require hospitalization. Aseptic meningitis, encephalitis, transverse myelitis, Guillain-Barré syndrome, and Reye's syndrome can also occur. Encephalitis is reported in 0.1–0.2% of children with chickenpox. Other than supportive care, no specific therapy is available for patients with CNS involvement.

Varicella pneumonia, the most serious complication following chickenpox, develops more commonly in adults (up to 20% of cases) than in children and is particularly severe in pregnant women. Pneumonia due to VZV usually has its onset 3–5 days into the illness and is associated with tachypnea, cough, dyspnea, and fever. Cyanosis, pleuritic chest pain, and hemoptysis are common. Roentgenographic evidence of disease consists of nodular infiltrates and interstitial pneumonitis. Resolution of pneumonitis parallels improvement of the skin rash; however, patients may have persistent fever and compromised pulmonary function for weeks.

Other complications of chickenpox include myocarditis, corneal lesions, nephritis, arthritis, bleeding diatheses, acute glomerulonephritis, and hepatitis. Hepatic involvement, distinct from Reye's syndrome and usually asymptomatic, is common in chickenpox and is generally characterized by elevated levels of liver enzymes, particularly aspartate and alanine aminotransferases.

Perinatal varicella is associated with a high mortality rate when maternal disease develops within 5 days before delivery or within 48 h thereafter. Because the newborn does not receive protective transplacental antibodies and has an immature immune system, the illness may be unusually severe. The reported mortality rate is as high as 30% in this group. *Congenital varicella*, with clinical manifestations of limb hypoplasia, cicatricial skin lesions, and microcephaly at birth, is extremely uncommon.

Herpes Zoster

Herpes zoster (also called shingles) is a sporadic disease that results from reactivation of latent VZV from dorsal root ganglia. Most patients have no history of recent exposure to other individuals with VZV infection. Herpes zoster occurs at all ages, but its incidence is highest (5–10 cases per 1000 persons) among individuals in the sixth decade of life and beyond. Recent data suggest that 1.2 million cases occur annually in the United States. Recurrent herpes zoster is exceedingly rare except in immunocompromised hosts, especially those with AIDS.

Herpes zoster is characterized by a unilateral vesicular eruption within a dermatome, often associated with severe pain. The dermatomes from T3 to L3 are most frequently involved. If the ophthalmic branch of the trigeminal nerve is involved, *zoster ophthalmicus* results. The factors responsible for the reactivation of VZV are not known. In children, reactivation is usually benign; in adults, it can be debilitating. The continuum of pain from onset to resolution is known as *zoster-associated pain*. The onset of disease is heralded by pain within the dermatome, which may precede lesions by 48–72 h; an erythematous maculopapular rash evolves rapidly into vesicular lesions (Fig. 81-2). In the normal host, these lesions may remain few in number and continue to form for only 3–5 days. The total duration of disease is generally 7–10 days; however, it may take as long as 2–4 weeks for the skin to return to normal. Patients with herpes zoster can transmit infection to seronegative individuals, with consequent chickenpox. In a few patients, characteristic localization of pain to a dermatome with serologic evidence of herpes zoster has been reported in the absence of skin lesions. When branches of the trigeminal nerve are involved, lesions may appear on the face, in the mouth, in the eye, or on the tongue. Zoster ophthalmicus is usually a debilitating condition that can result in blindness in the absence of antiviral therapy. In the *Ramsay Hunt syndrome*, pain and vesicles appear in the external auditory canal, and

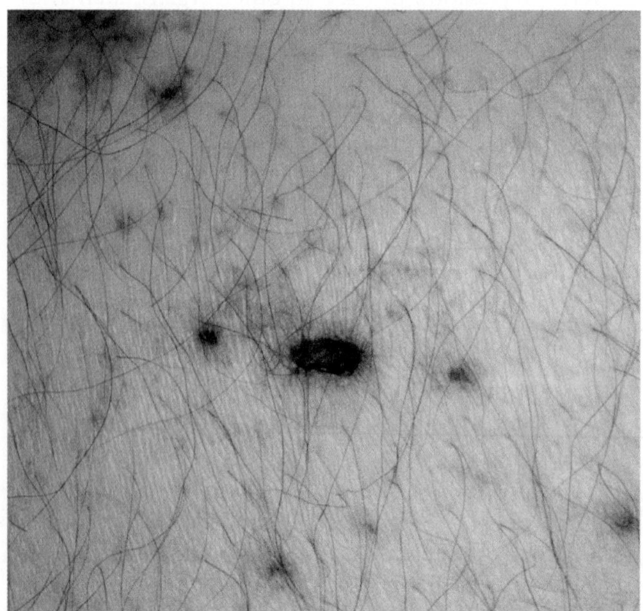

FIGURE 81-2
Close-up of lesions of disseminated zoster. Note lesions at different stages of evolution, including pustules and crusting. *(Photo courtesy of Lindsey Baden; with permission.)*

patients lose their sense of taste in the anterior two-thirds of the tongue while developing ipsilateral facial palsy. The geniculate ganglion of the sensory branch of the facial nerve is involved.

In both normal and immunocompromised hosts, the most debilitating complication of herpes zoster is pain associated with acute neuritis and postherpetic neuralgia. Postherpetic neuralgia is uncommon in young individuals; however, at least 50% of zoster patients over age 50 report some degree of pain in the involved dermatome months after the resolution of cutaneous disease. Changes in sensation in the dermatome, resulting in either hypo- or hyperesthesia, are common.

CNS involvement may follow localized herpes zoster. Many patients without signs of meningeal irritation have CSF pleocytosis and moderately elevated levels of CSF protein. Symptomatic meningoencephalitis is characterized by headache, fever, photophobia, meningitis, and vomiting. A rare manifestation of CNS involvement is granulomatous angiitis with contralateral hemiplegia, which can be diagnosed by cerebral arteriography. Other neurologic manifestations include transverse myelitis with or without motor paralysis.

Like chickenpox, herpes zoster is more severe in immunocompromised than immunocompetent individuals. Lesions continue to form for >1 week, and scabbing is not complete in most cases until 3 weeks into the illness. Patients with Hodgkin's disease and non-Hodgkin's lymphoma are at greatest risk for progressive herpes zoster. Cutaneous dissemination (Fig. 81-3) develops in ~40% of these patients. Among patients with cutaneous dissemination, the risk of pneumonitis, meningoencephalitis, hepatitis, and other serious complications is increased by 5–10%. However, even in immunocompromised patients, disseminated zoster is rarely fatal.

Recipients of hematopoietic stem-cell transplants are at particularly high risk of VZV infection. Of all cases of posttransplantation VZV infection, 30% occur within 1 year (50% of these within 9 months); 45% of the patients involved have cutaneous or visceral dissemination. The mortality rate in this situation is 10%. Postherpetic neuralgia, scarring, and bacterial superinfection are especially common in VZV infections occurring within 9 months of transplantation. Among infected patients, concomitant graft-versus-host disease increases the chance of dissemination and/or death.

DIFFERENTIAL DIAGNOSIS

The diagnosis of chickenpox is not difficult. The characteristic rash and a history of recent exposure should lead to a prompt diagnosis. Other viral infections that can mimic chickenpox include disseminated HSV infection in patients with atopic dermatitis and the disseminated vesiculopapular lesions sometimes associated with coxsackievirus infection, echovirus infection, or atypical measles. However, these rashes are more commonly morbilliform with a hemorrhagic component rather than vesicular or vesiculopustular. Rickettsialpox (Chap. 75) can be confused with chickenpox; however, rickettsialpox can be distinguished easily by detection of the "herald spot" at the site of the mite bite and the development of a more pronounced headache. Serologic testing is also useful in differentiating rickettsialpox from varicella and can confirm susceptibility in adults unsure of their chickenpox history. Concern about smallpox has recently increased because of the threat of bioterrorism (Chap. 6). The lesions of smallpox are larger than those of chickenpox and are all at the same stage of evolution at any given time.

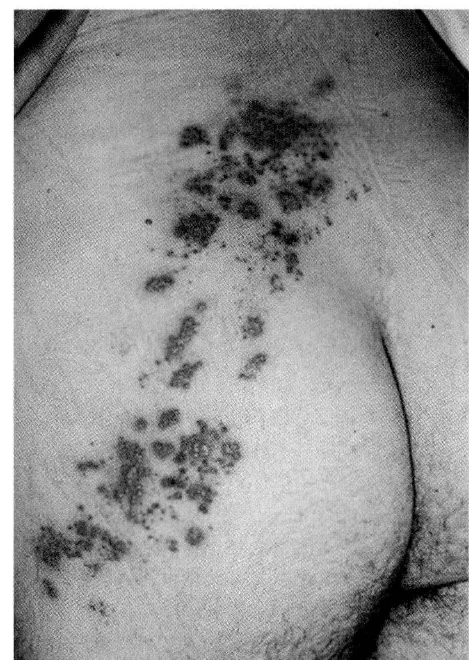

FIGURE 81-3

Herpes zoster is seen in this HIV-infected patient as hemorrhagic vesicles and pustules on an erythematous base grouped in a dermatomal distribution.

Unilateral vesicular lesions in a dermatomal pattern should lead rapidly to the diagnosis of herpes zoster, although the occurrence of shingles without a rash has been reported. Both HSV infections and coxsackievirus infections can cause dermatomal vesicular lesions. Supportive diagnostic virology and fluorescent staining of skin scrapings with monoclonal antibodies are helpful in ensuring the proper diagnosis. In the prodromal stage of herpes zoster, the diagnosis can be exceedingly difficult and may be made only after lesions have appeared or by retrospective serologic assessment.

LABORATORY FINDINGS

Unequivocal confirmation of the diagnosis is possible only through the isolation of VZV in susceptible tissue-culture cell lines, the demonstration of either seroconversion or a fourfold or greater rise in antibody titer between convalescent- and acute-phase serum specimens, or the detection of VZV DNA by PCR. A rapid impression can be obtained by a Tzanck smear, with scraping of the base of the lesions in an attempt to demonstrate multinucleated giant cells, although the sensitivity of this method is low (~60%). PCR technology for the detection of viral DNA in vesicular fluid is available in a limited number of diagnostic laboratories. Direct immunofluorescent staining of cells from the lesion base or detection of viral antigens by other assays (such as the immunoperoxidase assay) is also useful, although these tests are not commercially available. The most frequently employed serologic tools for assessing host response are the immunofluorescent detection of antibodies to VZV membrane antigens, the fluorescent antibody to membrane antigen (FAMA) test, immune adherence hemagglutination, and enzyme-linked immunosorbent assay (ELISA). The FAMA test and the ELISA appear to be most sensitive.

℞ Treatment: VARICELLA-ZOSTER VIRUS INFECTION

Medical management of chickenpox in the immunologically normal host is directed toward the prevention of avoidable complications. Obviously, good hygiene includes daily bathing and soaks. Secondary bacterial infection of the skin can be avoided by meticulous skin care, particularly with close cropping of fingernails. Pruritus can be decreased with topical dressings or the administration of antipruritic drugs. Tepid water baths and wet compresses are better than drying lotions for the relief of itching. Administration of aspirin to children with chickenpox should be avoided because of the association of aspirin derivatives with the development of Reye's syndrome. Acyclovir therapy (800 mg by mouth five times daily for 5–7 days) is recommended for adolescents and adults with chickenpox of ≤24 h duration. Likewise, acyclovir therapy may be of benefit to children <12 years of age if initiated early in the disease (<24 h) at a dose of 20 mg/kg every 6 h. The second-generation antiherpetic drugs valacyclovir and famciclovir are probably as efficacious or more so; however, no controlled clinical trials comparing these drugs have been reported. The advantages (i.e., pharmacokinetics) of the second-generation agents are described in Chap. 79.

Aluminum acetate soaks for the management of herpes zoster can be both soothing and cleansing. Patients with herpes zoster benefit from oral antiviral therapy, as evidenced by accelerated healing of lesions and resolution of zoster-associated pain with acyclovir, valacyclovir, or famciclovir. Acyclovir, now off patent, is administered at a dosage of 800 mg five times daily for 7–10 days. Famciclovir, the prodrug of penciclovir, is at least as effective as acyclovir and perhaps more so. One study showed twofold faster resolution of postherpetic neuralgia in famciclovir-treated patients with zoster than in recipients of placebo. The dose is 500 mg by mouth three times daily for 7 days. Valacyclovir, the prodrug of acyclovir, accelerates healing and resolution of zoster-associated pain more promptly than acyclovir. The dose is 1 g by mouth three times daily for 5–7 days. Compared with acyclovir, both famciclovir and valacyclovir offer the advantage of less frequent administration.

In severely immunocompromised hosts (e.g., transplant recipients, patients with lymphoproliferative malignancies), both chickenpox and herpes zoster (including disseminated disease) should be treated, at least at the outset, with intravenous acyclovir, which reduces the occurrence of visceral complications but has no effect on healing of skin lesions or pain. The dose is 10–12.5 mg/kg every 8 h for 7 days. For low-risk immunocompromised hosts, oral therapy with valacyclovir or famciclovir appears beneficial. Concomitant with the administration of intravenous acyclovir, it is desirable to wean these patients from immunosuppressive treatment.

Patients with varicella pneumonia may require removal of bronchial secretions and ventilatory support. Persons with zoster ophthalmicus should be referred immediately to an ophthalmologist. Therapy for this condition consists of the administration of analgesics for severe pain and the use of atropine. Acyclovir, valacyclovir, and famciclovir all accelerate healing.

The management of acute neuritis and/or postherpetic neuralgia can be particularly difficult. In addition to the judicious use of analgesics, ranging from nonnarcotics to narcotic derivatives, drugs such as gabapentin, pregabalin, amitriptyline hydrochloride, lidocaine patches, and fluphenazine hydrochloride are reportedly beneficial for pain relief. In one study, glucocorticoid therapy administered early in the course of localized herpes zoster significantly accelerated such quality-of-life improvements as a return to usual activity and termination of analgesia. The dose of prednisone administered orally was 60 mg/d on days 1–7, 30 mg/d on days 8–14, and 15 mg/d on days 15–21. This regimen is appropriate only for relatively healthy elderly persons with moderate or severe pain at presentation. Patients with osteoporosis, diabetes mellitus, glycosuria, or hypertension may not be appropriate candidates. Glucocorticoids should not be used without concomitant antiviral therapy.

PREVENTION

Three methods are used for the prevention of VZV infections. First, a live attenuated varicella vaccine (Oka) is recommended for all children >1 year of age (up to 12 years of age) who have not had chickenpox and for adults known to be seronegative for VZV. Two doses are recommended for all children: the first at 12–15 months of age and the second at ~4–6 years of age. VZV-seronegative persons >13 years of age should receive two doses of vaccine at least 1 month apart. The vaccine is both safe and efficacious. Breakthrough cases are mild and may result in spread of the vaccine virus to susceptible contacts. The universal vaccination of children is resulting in a decreased incidence of chickenpox in sentinel communities. Furthermore, inactivation of the vaccine virus significantly decreases the occurrence of herpes zoster after hematopoietic stem-cell transplantation. After administration of a vaccine with 18 times the viral content of the Oka vaccine to individuals >60 years of age, the incidence of shingles was found to decrease by 51%, the burden of illness by 61%, and the incidence of postherpetic neuralgia by 66%. The Advisory Committee on Immunization Practices has therefore recommended that persons in this age group be offered this vaccine in order to reduce the frequency of shingles and the severity of postherpetic neuralgia.

TABLE 81-1

RECOMMENDATIONS FOR VZIG ADMINISTRATION

Exposure Criteria

1. Exposure to person with chickenpox or zoster
   a. Household: residence in the same household
   b. Playmate: face-to-face indoor play
   c. Hospital
      Varicella: same 2- to 4-bed room or adjacent beds in large ward, face-to-face contact with infectious staff member or patient, visit by a person deemed contagious
      Zoster: intimate contact (e.g., touching or hugging) with a person deemed contagious
   d. Newborn infant: onset of varicella in the mother ≤5 days before delivery or ≤48 h after delivery; VZIG not indicated if the mother has zoster
2. Patient should receive VZIG as soon as possible but not >96 h after exposure

Candidates (Provided They Have Significant Exposure) Include

1. Immunocompromised susceptible children without a history of varicella or varicella immunization
2. Susceptible pregnant women
3. Newborn infants whose mother had onset of chickenpox within 5 days before or within 48 h after delivery
4. Hospitalized premature infant (≥28 weeks of gestation) whose mother lacks a reliable history of chickenpox or serologic evidence of protection against varicella
5. Hospitalized premature infant (<28 weeks of gestation or ≤1000-g birth weight), regardless of maternal history of varicella or varicella-zoster virus serologic status

A second approach is to administer varicella-zoster immune globulin (VZIG) to individuals who are susceptible, are at high risk for developing complications of varicella, and have had a significant exposure. This product should be given within 96 h (preferably within 72 h) of the exposure. Indications for administration of VZIG appear in Table 81-1. Unfortunately, the availability of this product in the future will be limited at best.

Lastly, antiviral therapy can be given as prophylaxis to individuals at high risk who are ineligible for vaccine or who are beyond the 96-h window after direct contact. Although the initial studies have used acyclovir, similar benefit can be anticipated with either valacyclovir or famciclovir. Therapy is instituted 7 days after intense exposure. At this time, the host is midway into the incubation period. This approach significantly decreases disease severity, if not totally preventing disease.

FURTHER READINGS

Arvin A: Aging, immunity, and the varicella-zoster virus. N Engl J Med 352:2266, 2005

Gnann JW, Whitley RJ: Herpes zoster. N Engl J Med 347:340, 2002

Harpaz R et al: Prevention of herpes zoster: Recommendations of the Advisory Committee on Immunization Practices (ACIP). MMWR Recomm Rep 57:1, 2008

He L et al: Corticosteroids for preventing postherpetic neuralgia. Cochrane Database Syst Rev CD005582, 2008

Izurieta HS et al: Postlicensure effectiveness of varicella vaccine during an outbreak in a child care center. JAMA 278:1495, 1997

Kimberlin DW, Whitley RJ: Varicella-zoster vaccine for the prevention of herpes zoster. N Engl J Med 356:1338, 2007

Nguyen HQ et al: Decline in mortality due to varicella after implementation of varicella vaccination in the United States. N Engl J Med 352:450, 2005

Oxman MN et al: A vaccine to prevent herpes zoster and postherpetic neuralgia in older adults. N Engl J Med 352:2271, 2005

Rowbotham M et al: Gabapentin for the treatment of postherpetic neuralgia. A randomized controlled trial. JAMA 280:1837, 1998

Seward JF et al: Contagiousness of varicella in vaccinated cases: A household contact study. JAMA 292:704, 2004

——— et al: Varicella disease after introduction of varicella vaccine in the United States, 1995-2000. JAMA 28:606, 2002

Wareham DW, Breuer J: Herpes zoster. BMJ 334:1211, 2007

CHAPTER 82

EPSTEIN-BARR VIRUS INFECTIONS, INCLUDING INFECTIOUS MONONUCLEOSIS

Jeffrey I. Cohen

DEFINITION

Epstein-Barr virus (EBV) is the cause of heterophile-positive infectious mononucleosis (IM), which is characterized by fever, sore throat, lymphadenopathy, and atypical lymphocytosis. EBV is also associated with several human tumors, including nasopharyngeal carcinoma, Burkitt's lymphoma, Hodgkin's disease, and (in patients with immunodeficiencies) B-cell lymphoma. The virus, a member of the family Herpesviridae, consists of a linear DNA core surrounded by a nucleocapsid and an envelope that contains glycoproteins. The two types of EBV that are widely prevalent in nature are not distinguishable by conventional serologic tests.

EPIDEMIOLOGY

EBV infections occur worldwide. These infections are most common in early childhood, with a second peak during late adolescence. By adulthood, more than 90% of individuals have been infected and have antibodies to the virus. IM is usually a disease of young adults. In lower socioeconomic groups and in areas of the world with lower standards of hygiene (e.g., developing countries), EBV tends to infect children at an early age, and symptomatic IM is uncommon. In areas with higher standards of hygiene, infection with EBV is often delayed until adulthood, and IM is more prevalent.

EBV is spread by contact with oral secretions. The virus is frequently transmitted from asymptomatic adults to infants and among young adults by transfer of saliva during kissing. Transmission by less intimate contact is rare. EBV has been transmitted by blood transfusion and by bone marrow transplantation. More than 90% of asymptomatic seropositive individuals shed the virus in oropharyngeal secretions. Shedding is increased in immunocompromised patients and those with IM.

PATHOGENESIS

EBV is transmitted by salivary secretions. The virus infects the epithelium of the oropharynx and the salivary glands and is shed from these cells. Although B cells may become infected after contact with epithelial cells, studies suggest that lymphocytes in the tonsillar crypts can be infected directly. The virus then spreads through the bloodstream. The proliferation and expansion of EBV-infected B cells along with reactive T cells during IM result in enlargement of lymphoid tissue. Polyclonal activation of B cells leads to the production of antibodies to host-cell and viral proteins. During the acute phase of IM, up to 1 in every 100 B cells in the peripheral blood is infected by EBV; after recovery, 1–50 in every 1 million B cells is infected. During IM, there is an inverted CD4+/CD8+ T-cell ratio. The percentage of CD4+ T cells decreases, whereas there are large clonal expansions of CD8+ T cells; up to 40% of CD8+ T cells are directed against EBV antigens during acute infection. Data suggest that memory B cells, not epithelial cells, are the reservoir for EBV in the body. When patients are treated with acyclovir, shedding of EBV from the oropharynx stops, but the virus persists in B cells.

The EBV receptor (CD21) on the surface of B cells is also the receptor for the C3d component of complement. EBV infection of epithelial cells results in viral replication and production of virions. When B cells are infected by EBV in vitro, they become transformed and can proliferate indefinitely. During latent infection of B cells, only the EBV nuclear antigens (EBNAs), latent membrane proteins (LMPs), and small EBV RNAs are expressed in vitro. EBV-transformed B cells secrete immunoglobulin; only a small fraction of cells produce virus.

Cellular immunity is more important than humoral immunity in controlling EBV infection. In the initial phase of infection, suppressor T cells, natural killer cells, and nonspecific cytotoxic T cells are important in controlling the proliferation of EBV-infected B cells. Levels of markers of T-cell activation and serum interferon (IFN) γ are elevated. Later in infection, HLA-restricted cytotoxic T cells that recognize EBNAs and LMPs and destroy EBV-infected cells are generated. Studies have shown that one of the late genes expressed during EBV replication, *BCRF1*, is a homologue of interleukin 10 and can inhibit the production of IFN-γ by mononuclear cells in vitro.

If T-cell immunity is compromised, EBV-infected B cells may begin to proliferate. When EBV is associated with lymphoma, virus-induced proliferation is but one step in a multistep process of neoplastic transformation. In many EBV-containing tumors, LMP-1 mimics members of the tumor necrosis factor receptor family (e.g., CD40), transmitting growth-proliferating signals.

CLINICAL MANIFESTATIONS

Signs and Symptoms

Most EBV infections in infants and young children either are asymptomatic or present as mild pharyngitis with or without tonsillitis. In contrast, up to 75% of infections in adolescents present as IM. IM in the elderly presents relatively often as nonspecific symptoms, including prolonged fever, fatigue, myalgia, and malaise. In contrast, pharyngitis, lymphadenopathy, splenomegaly, and atypical lymphocytes are relatively rare in elderly patients.

The incubation period for IM in young adults is ~4–6 weeks. A prodrome of fatigue, malaise, and myalgia may last for 1–2 weeks before the onset of fever, sore throat, and lymphadenopathy. Fever is usually low-grade and is most common in the first 2 weeks of the illness; however, it may persist for >1 month. Common signs and symptoms are listed along with their frequencies in Table 82-1. Lymphadenopathy and pharyngitis are most prominent during the first 2 weeks of the illness, whereas splenomegaly is more prominent during the second and third weeks. Lymphadenopathy most often affects the posterior cervical nodes but may be generalized. Enlarged lymph nodes are frequently tender and symmetric but are not fixed in place. Pharyngitis, often the most prominent sign, can be accompanied by enlargement of the tonsils with an exudate resembling that of streptococcal pharyngitis. A morbilliform or papular rash, usually on the arms or trunk, develops in ~5% of cases (Fig. 82-1). Most patients treated with ampicillin develop a macular rash; this rash is not predictive of future adverse reactions to penicillins. Erythema nodosum and erythema multiforme have also been described. Most patients have symptoms for 2–4 weeks, but malaise and difficulty concentrating can persist for months.

Laboratory Findings

The white blood cell count is usually elevated and peaks at 10,000–20,000/μL during the second or third week of

TABLE 82-1

SIGNS AND SYMPTOMS OF INFECTIOUS MONONUCLEOSIS

MANIFESTATION	MEDIAN PERCENTAGE OF PATIENTS (RANGE)
Symptoms	
Sore throat	75 (50–87)
Malaise	47 (42–76)
Headache	38 (22–67)
Abdominal pain, nausea, or vomiting	17 (5–25)
Chills	10 (9–11)
Signs	
Lymphadenopathy	95 (83–100)
Fever	93 (60–100)
Pharyngitis or tonsillitis	82 (68–90)
Splenomegaly	51 (43–64)
Hepatomegaly	11 (6–15)
Rash	10 (0–25)
Periorbital edema	13 (2–34)
Palatal enanthem	7 (3–13)
Jaundice	5 (2–10)

illness. Lymphocytosis is usually demonstrable, with >10% atypical lymphocytes. The latter cells are enlarged lymphocytes that have abundant cytoplasm, vacuoles, and indentations of the cell membrane (Fig. 82-2). CD8+ cells predominate among the atypical lymphocytes. Low-grade neutropenia and thrombocytopenia are common during the first month of illness. Liver function is abnormal in >90% of cases. Serum levels of aminotransferases and alkaline phosphatase are usually mildly elevated. The serum concentration of bilirubin is elevated in ~40% of cases.

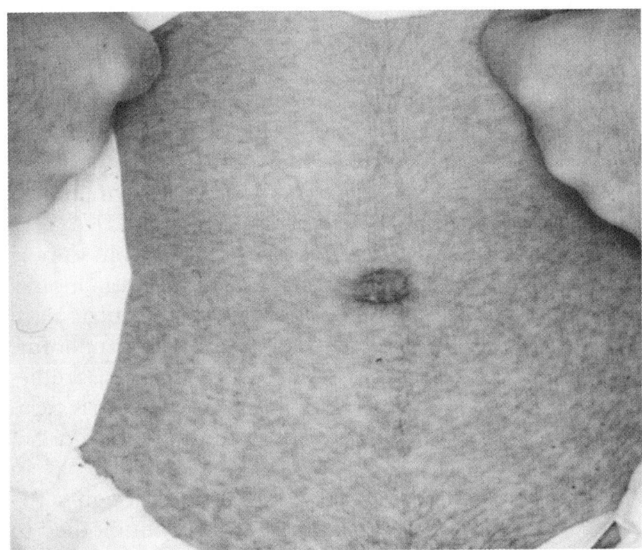

FIGURE 82-1
Rash in a patient with infectious mononucleosis due to Epstein-Barr virus. *(Courtesy of Maria Turner, MD; with permission.)*

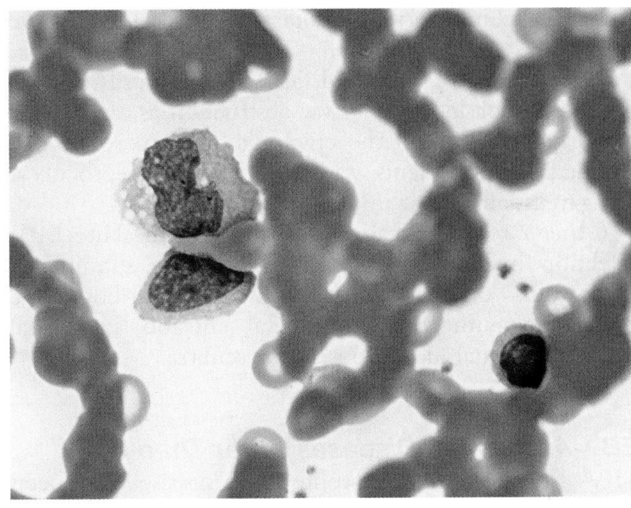

FIGURE 82-2
Atypical lymphocytes from a patient with infectious mononucleosis due to Epstein-Barr virus.

Complications

Most cases of IM are self-limited. Deaths are very rare and most often are due to central nervous system (CNS) complications, splenic rupture, upper airway obstruction, or bacterial superinfection.

When CNS complications develop, they usually do so during the first 2 weeks of EBV infection; in some patients, especially children, they are the only clinical manifestations of IM. Heterophile antibodies and atypical lymphocytes may be absent. Meningitis and encephalitis are the most common neurologic abnormalities, and patients may present with headache, meningismus, or cerebellar ataxia. Acute hemiplegia and psychosis have also been described. The cerebrospinal fluid (CSF) contains mainly lymphocytes, with occasional atypical lymphocytes. Most cases resolve without neurologic sequelae. Acute EBV infection has also been associated with cranial nerve palsies (especially those involving cranial nerve VII), Guillain-Barré syndrome, acute transverse myelitis, and peripheral neuritis.

Autoimmune hemolytic anemia occurs in ~2% of cases during the first 2 weeks. In most cases, the anemia is Coombs-positive, with cold agglutinins directed against the i red blood cell antigen. Most patients with hemolysis have mild anemia that lasts for 1–2 months, but some patients have severe disease with hemoglobinuria and jaundice. Nonspecific antibody responses may also include rheumatoid factor, antinuclear antibodies, anti–smooth muscle antibodies, antiplatelet antibodies, and cryoglobulins. IM has been associated with red-cell aplasia, severe granulocytopenia, thrombocytopenia, pancytopenia, and hemophagocytic syndrome. The spleen ruptures in <0.5% of cases. Splenic rupture is more common among male than female patients and may manifest as abdominal pain, referred shoulder pain, or hemodynamic compromise.

Hypertrophy of lymphoid tissue in the tonsils or adenoids can result in upper airway obstruction, as can inflammation and edema of the epiglottis, pharynx, or uvula. About 10% of patients with IM develop streptococcal pharyngitis after their initial sore throat resolves.

Other rare complications associated with acute EBV infection include hepatitis (which can be fulminant), myocarditis or pericarditis with electrocardiographic changes, pneumonia with pleural effusion, interstitial nephritis, genital ulcerations, and vasculitis.

EBV-Associated Diseases Other Than IM

EBV-associated lymphoproliferative disease has been described in patients with congenital or acquired immunodeficiency, including those with severe combined immunodeficiency, patients with AIDS, and recipients of bone marrow or organ transplants who are receiving immunosuppressive drugs (especially cyclosporine). Proliferating EBV-infected B cells infiltrate lymph nodes and multiple organs, and patients present with fever and lymphadenopathy or gastrointestinal symptoms. Pathologic studies show B-cell hyperplasia or poly- or monoclonal lymphoma. The X-linked lymphoproliferative syndrome (Duncan's disease) is a recessive disorder of young boys who have a normal response to childhood infections but develop fatal lymphoproliferative disorders after infection with EBV. The protein associated with this syndrome (SAP) binds to a protein that mediates interactions of B and T cells. Most patients with this syndrome die of acute IM. Others develop hypogammaglobulinemia, malignant B-cell lymphomas, aplastic anemia, or agranulocytosis. IM has also proved fatal to some patients with no obvious preexisting immune abnormality.

Oral hairy leukoplakia (Fig. 82-3) is an early manifestation of infection with HIV in adults (Chap. 90). Most patients present with raised, white corrugated lesions on the tongue (and occasionally on the buccal mucosa) that contain EBV DNA. Children infected with HIV can develop lymphoid interstitial pneumonitis; EBV DNA is often found in lung tissue from these patients.

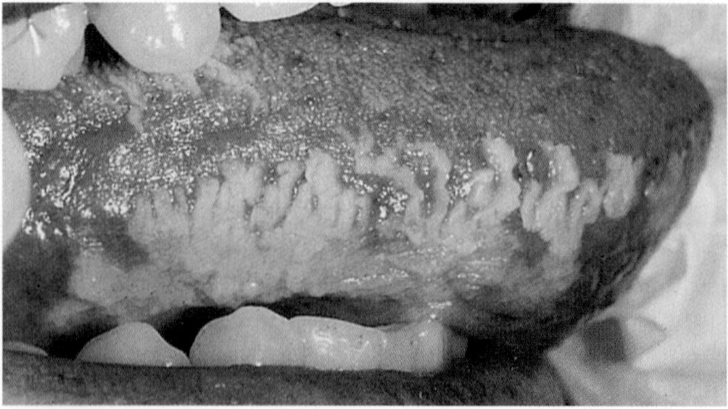

FIGURE 82-3

Oral hairy leukoplakia often presents as white plaques on the lateral surface of the tongue and is associated with Epstein-Barr virus infection.

Patients with chronic fatigue syndrome may have titers of antibody to EBV that are elevated but are not significantly different from those in healthy EBV-seropositive adults. Although some patients have malaise and fatigue that persist for weeks or months after IM, persistent EBV infection is not a cause of chronic fatigue syndrome. Chronic active EBV infection is very rare and is distinct from chronic fatigue syndrome. The affected patients have an illness lasting >6 months, with elevated levels of EBV DNA in the blood, very high titers of antibody to EBV, and evidence of organ involvement, including hepatosplenomegaly, lymphadenopathy, and pneumonitis, uveitis, or neurologic disease.

EBV is associated with several malignancies. About 15% of cases of Burkitt's lymphoma in the United States and ~90% of those in Africa are associated with EBV. African patients with Burkitt's lymphoma have high levels of antibody to EBV, and their tumor tissue usually contains viral DNA. Malaria infection in Africa may impair cellular immunity to EBV and induce polyclonal B cell activation with an expansion of EBV-infected B cells. These changes may enhance the proliferation of B cells, increasing the likelihood of a *c-myc* translocation—the hallmark of Burkitt's lymphoma. EBV-containing Burkitt's lymphoma also occurs in patients with AIDS.

Anaplastic nasopharyngeal carcinoma is uniformly associated with EBV; the affected tissues contain viral DNA and antigens. Patients with nasopharyngeal carcinoma often have elevated titers of antibody to EBV. High levels of EBV plasma DNA before treatment or detectable levels of EBV DNA after radiation therapy correlate with lower rates of overall survival and relapse-free survival among patients with nasopharyngeal carcinoma.

EBV has been associated with Hodgkin's disease, especially the mixed-cellularity type. Patients with Hodgkin's disease often have elevated titers of antibody to EBV. In about half of cases, viral DNA and antigens are found in Reed-Sternberg cells. The risk of EBV-positive Hodgkin's disease is significantly increased in young adults after EBV-seropositive IM. About 50% of non-Hodgkin's lymphomas in patients with AIDS are EBV-positive.

In some cases, EBV DNA has been detected in tumors from immunocompetent patients with tonsillar carcinoma, angioimmunoblastic lymphadenopathy, angiocentric nasal NK/T-cell immunoproliferative lesions, T-cell lymphoma, thymoma, gastric carcinoma, and CNS lymphoma. Studies have demonstrated viral DNA in leiomyosarcomas from AIDS patients and in smooth-muscle tumors from organ transplant recipients. Virtually all CNS lymphomas in AIDS patients are associated with EBV. Although serologic studies have found higher levels of antibodies to EBV before the onset of multiple sclerosis in persons ≥25 years old, other studies (including measurement of EBV antibody titers in the CSF) are needed to ascertain a possible causal relationship.

TABLE 82-2

SEROLOGIC FEATURES OF EBV-ASSOCIATED DISEASES

		RESULT IN INDICATED TEST[a]				
		ANTI-VCA		ANTI-EA		
CONDITION	HETEROPHILE	IgM	IgG	EA-D	EA-R	ANTI-EBNA
Acute infectious mononucleosis	+	+	++	+	−	−
Convalescence	±	−	+	−	±	+
Past infection	−	−	+	−	−	+
Reactivation with immunodeficiency	−	−	++	+	+	±
Burkitt's lymphoma	−	−	+++	±	++	+
Nasopharyngeal carcinoma	−	−	+++	++	±	+

[a]VCA, viral capsid antigen; EA, early antigen; EA-D antibody, antibody to early antigen in diffuse pattern in nucleus and cytoplasm of infected cells; EA-R antibody, antibody to early antigen restricted to the cytoplasm; and EBNA, Epstein-Barr nuclear antigen.
Source: Adapted from Okano, 1988.

DIAGNOSIS

Serologic Testing

The heterophile test is used for the diagnosis of IM in children and adults (Table 82-2). In the test for this antibody, human serum is absorbed with guinea pig kidney, and the heterophile titer is defined as the greatest serum dilution that agglutinates sheep, horse, or cow erythrocytes. Although heterophile antibody binds to certain animal erythrocytes, it does not interact with EBV proteins. A titer of ≥40-fold is diagnostic of acute EBV infection in a patient who has symptoms compatible with IM and atypical lymphocytes. Tests for heterophile antibodies are positive in 40% of patients with IM during the first week of illness and in 80–90% during the third week. Therefore, repeated testing may be necessary, especially if the initial test is performed early. Tests usually remain positive for 3 months after the onset of illness, but heterophile antibodies can persist for up to 1 year. These antibodies usually are not detectable in children <5 years of age, in the elderly, or in patients presenting with symptoms not typical of IM. The commercially available monospot test for heterophile antibodies is somewhat more sensitive than the classic heterophile test. The monospot test is ~75% sensitive and ~90% specific compared with EBV-specific serologies. False-positive monospot results are more common among persons with connective tissue disease, lymphoma, viral hepatitis, and malaria.

EBV-specific antibody testing is used for patients with suspected acute EBV infection who lack heterophile antibodies and for patients with atypical infections (Table 82-2). Titers of IgM and IgG antibodies to viral capsid antigen (VCA) are elevated in the serum of more than 90% of patients at the onset of disease. IgM antibody to VCA is most useful for the diagnosis of acute IM because it is present at elevated titers only during the first 2–3 months of the disease; in contrast, IgG antibody to VCA is usually not useful for diagnosis of IM but is often used to assess past exposure to EBV because it persists for life. Seroconversion to EBNA positivity is also useful for the diagnosis of acute infection with EBV. Antibodies to EBNA become detectable relatively late (3–6 weeks after the onset of symptoms) in nearly all cases of acute EBV infection and persist for the lifetime of the patient. These antibodies may be lacking in immunodeficient patients and in those with chronic active EBV infection.

Titers of other antibodies may also be elevated in IM; however, these elevations are less useful for diagnosis. Antibodies to early antigens (EAs) are found either in a diffuse pattern in the nucleus and cytoplasm of infected cells (EA-D antibody) or restricted to the cytoplasm (EA-R antibody). These antibodies are detectable 3–4 weeks after the onset of symptoms in patients with IM. About 70% of individuals with IM have EA-D antibodies during the illness; the presence of EA-D antibodies is especially likely in patients with relatively severe disease. These antibodies usually persist for only 3–6 months. Levels of EA-D antibodies are also elevated in patients with nasopharyngeal carcinoma or chronic active EBV infection. EA-R antibodies are only occasionally detected in patients with IM but are often found at elevated titers in patients with African Burkitt's lymphoma or chronic active EBV infection. IgA antibodies to EBV antigens have proved useful for the identification of patients with nasopharyngeal carcinoma and of persons at high risk for the disease.

Other Studies

Detection of EBV DNA, RNA, or proteins has been valuable in demonstrating the association of the virus with various malignancies. The polymerase chain reaction has been used to detect EBV DNA in the CSF of some AIDS patients with lymphomas and to monitor the amount of EBV DNA in the blood of patients with lymphoproliferative disease. Detection of high levels of EBV DNA in blood during the first few weeks of IM may be useful if serologic studies yield equivocal results. Culture of EBV from throat washings or blood is not helpful in the diagnosis of acute infection, since EBV commonly persists in the oropharynx and in B cells for the lifetime of the infected individual.

Differential Diagnosis

Whereas ~90% of cases of IM are due to EBV, 5–10% of cases are due to cytomegalovirus (CMV). CMV is the most common cause of heterophile-negative mononucleosis, usually presenting in older patients. IM caused by CMV is associated with a lower frequency of sore throat, splenomegaly, and lymphadenopathy than IM due to EBV. Less common causes of IM include acute infection with *Toxoplasma*, HIV, human herpesvirus 6, and hepatitis viruses as well as drug hypersensitivity reactions. Other diseases that share some of the features of IM include rubella, acute infectious lymphocytosis in children, and lymphoma or leukemia.

TABLE 82-3

TREATMENT OPTIONS FOR POSTTRANSPLANTATION EBV LYMPHOPROLIFERATIVE DISEASE
1. Reduction of immunosuppression, when possible
2. Excision of localized lesions
3. Interferon α
4. Monoclonal antibody to CD20 (rituximab)
5. Radiation therapy (especially for CNS lesions)
6. For stem-cell transplant recipients: donor lymphocyte infusions or donor EBV-specific cytotoxic T-cell infusions[a]
7. For solid organ transplant recipients: autologous or HLA-matched, EBV-specific, cytotoxic T-cell infusions[a]
8. Cytotoxic chemotherapy

[a] Infused T cells must be HLA-matched; lymphoproliferative lesions are usually of donor origin for stem-cell transplant recipients and of recipient origin for solid organ transplant recipients.

℞ Treatment: EBV-ASSOCIATED DISEASE

Therapy for IM consists of supportive measures, with rest and analgesia. Excessive physical activity during the first month should be avoided to reduce the possibility of splenic rupture, which necessitates splenectomy. Glucocorticoid therapy is not indicated for uncomplicated IM and in fact may predispose to bacterial superinfection. Prednisone (40–60 mg/d for 2–3 days, with subsequent tapering of the dose over 1–2 weeks) has been used for the prevention of airway obstruction in patients with severe tonsillar hypertrophy, for autoimmune hemolytic anemia, and for severe thrombocytopenia. Glucocorticoids have also been administered to a few selected patients with severe malaise and fever and to patients with severe CNS or cardiac disease.

Acyclovir has had no significant clinical impact on IM in controlled trials. In one study, the combination of acyclovir and prednisolone had no significant effect on the duration of symptoms of IM.

Acyclovir, at a dosage of 400–800 mg five times daily, has been effective for the treatment of oral hairy leukoplakia (despite common relapses). The posttransplantation EBV lymphoproliferative syndrome (Chap. 12) generally does not respond to antiviral therapy. When possible, therapy should be directed toward reduction of immunosuppression (Table 82-3). IFN-α or antibody to CD20 has been effective in some cases. Infusions of donor lymphocytes are often effective for stem-cell transplant recipients, although graft-versus-host disease can occur. Infusions of EBV-specific cytotoxic T cells have been used to prevent EBV lymphoproliferative disease in high-risk settings, as well as to treat the disease. Infusion of autologous EBV-specific cytotoxic T lymphocytes has shown promise in small studies of patients with nasopharyngeal carcinoma and Hodgkin's disease.

Treatment of two cases of X-linked lymphoproliferative syndrome with antibody to CD20 resulted in a successful outcome of what otherwise would probably have been fatal acute EBV infection.

PREVENTION

The isolation of patients with IM is unnecessary. Vaccines directed against the major EBV glycoprotein have been effective in animal studies and are undergoing clinical trials.

FURTHER READINGS

AUWAERTER PG: Infectious mononucleosis in middle age. JAMA 281:454, 1999

BOLLARD CM et al: Cytotoxic T lymphocyte therapy for Epstein-Barr virus positive Hodgkin's disease. J Exp Med 200:1623, 2004

CHOQUET S et al: Efficacy and safety of rituximab in B-cell post-transplant lymphoproliferative disorders: Results of a prospective multicenter phase 2 study. Blood 107:3053, 2006

COHEN JI: Epstein-Barr virus infection. N Engl J Med 343:481, 2000

FAFI-KREMER S et al: Long term shedding of infectious Epstein-Barr virus after infectious mononucleosis. J Infect Dis 191:985, 2005

HAQUE T et al: Allogeneic cytotoxic T-cell therapy for EBV-positive posttransplantation lymphoproliferative disease: results of a phase 2 multicenter clinical trial. Blood 110:1123, 2007

HIGGINS CD et al: A study of risk factors for acquisition of Epstein-Barr virus and its subtypes. J Infect Dis 195:474, 2007

MILNONE MC et al: Treatment of primary Epstein-Barr virus infection in patients with X-linked lymphoproliferative disease using B-cell-directed therapy. Blood 105:994, 2005

TORRE D, TAMBINI R: Acyclovir for treatment of infectious mononucleosis: A meta-analysis. Scand J Infect Dis 31:543, 1999

WILLIAMS H, CRAWFORD DH: Epstein-Barr virus: The impact of scientific advances on clinical practice. Blood 107:862, 2006

CHAPTER 83

CYTOMEGALOVIRUS AND HUMAN HERPESVIRUS TYPES 6, 7, AND 8

Martin S. Hirsch

CYTOMEGALOVIRUS

DEFINITION

Cytomegalovirus (CMV), which was initially isolated from patients with congenital cytomegalic inclusion disease, is now recognized as an important pathogen in all age groups. In addition to inducing severe birth defects, CMV causes a wide spectrum of disorders in older children and adults, ranging from an asymptomatic, subclinical infection to a mononucleosis syndrome in healthy individuals to disseminated disease in immunocompromised patients. Human CMV is one of several related species-specific viruses that cause similar diseases in various animals. All are associated with the production of characteristic enlarged cells—hence the name *cytomegalovirus*.

CMV, a β-herpesvirus, has double-strand DNA, four species of mRNA, a protein capsid, and a lipoprotein envelope. Like other herpesviruses, CMV demonstrates icosahedral symmetry, replicates in the cell nucleus, and can cause either a lytic and productive or a latent infection. CMV can be distinguished from other herpesviruses by certain biologic properties, such as host range and type of cytopathology. Viral replication is associated with production of large intranuclear inclusions and smaller cytoplasmic inclusions. CMV appears to replicate in a variety of cell types in vivo; in tissue culture it grows preferentially in fibroblasts. Although there is little evidence that CMV is oncogenic in vivo, it does transform fibroblasts in rare instances, and genomic transforming fragments have been identified.

EPIDEMIOLOGY

CMV has a worldwide distribution. Of newborns in the United States, ~1% are infected with CMV; the percentage is higher in many less-developed countries. Communal living and poor personal hygiene facilitate early spread. Perinatal and early childhood infections are common. CMV may be present in breast milk, saliva, feces, and urine. Transmission has occurred among young children in day-care centers and has been traced from infected toddler to pregnant mother to developing fetus. When an infected child introduces CMV into a household, 50% of susceptible family members seroconvert within 6 months.

CMV is not readily spread by casual contact but rather requires repeated or prolonged intimate exposure for transmission. In late adolescence and young adulthood, CMV is often transmitted sexually, and asymptomatic carriage in semen or cervical secretions is common. Antibody to CMV is present at detectable levels in a high proportion of sexually active men and women, who may harbor several strains simultaneously. Transfusion of whole blood or certain blood products containing viable leukocytes may transmit CMV, with a frequency of 0.14–10% per unit transfused.

Once infected, an individual generally carries CMV for life. The infection usually remains silent. However, CMV reactivation syndromes develop frequently when T-lymphocyte–mediated immunity is compromised—for example, after organ transplantation or in association with lymphoid neoplasms and certain acquired immunodeficiencies (in particular, HIV infection; Chap. 90). Most primary CMV infections in organ transplant recipients (Chap. 12) result from transmission in the graft itself. In CMV-seropositive transplant recipients, infection results from reactivation of latent virus or, less commonly, from reinfection by a new strain. CMV infection may be associated with coronary artery stenosis after heart transplantation or coronary angioplasty, but this association requires further validation.

PATHOGENESIS

Congenital CMV infection can result from either primary or reactivation infection of the mother. However, clinical disease in the fetus or newborn is almost exclusively related to primary maternal infection (Table 83-1). The factors determining the severity of congenital infection are unknown; a deficient capacity to produce precipitating antibodies and to mount T-cell responses to CMV is associated with relatively severe disease.

Primary infection in late childhood or adulthood is often associated with a vigorous T-lymphocyte response that may contribute to the development of a mononucleosis syndrome similar to that observed after Epstein-Barr virus (EBV) infection (Chap. 82). The hallmark of such infection is the appearance of atypical lymphocytes in the peripheral blood; these cells are predominantly activated CD8+ T lymphocytes. Polyclonal activation of B cells by

TABLE 83-1

CMV DISEASE IN THE IMMUNOCOMPROMISED HOST

POPULATION	RISK FACTORS	PRINCIPAL SYNDROMES	TREATMENT	PREVENTION
Fetus	Primary maternal infection/early pregnancy	Cytomegalic inclusion disease	None (?ganciclovir)	Avoidance of exposure or maternal treatment with CMV immunoglobulin during pregnancy
Organ transplant recipient	Serostatus of donor and recipient; immunosuppressive regimen; degree of rejection	Febrile leukopenia; pneumonia; gastrointestinal disease	Ganciclovir or valganciclovir	Donor matching; prophylaxis or preemptive therapy with ganciclovir or valganciclovir
Bone marrow transplant recipient	Graft-versus-host disease; older age; seropositive recipient; viremia	Pneumonia; gastrointestinal disease	Ganciclovir plus CMV immunoglobulin	Donor matching; prophylaxis or preemptive therapy with ganciclovir or valganciclovir
Person with AIDS	<100 CD4+ T cells per microliter; CMV seropositivity	Retinitis; gastrointestinal disease; neurologic disease	Ganciclovir, valganciclovir, foscarnet, or cidofovir	Oral valganciclovir

CMV contributes to the development of rheumatoid factors and other autoantibodies during mononucleosis.

Once acquired, CMV persists indefinitely in host tissues. The sites of persistent infection probably include multiple cell types and various organs. Transmission via blood transfusion or organ transplantation is due to silent infections in these tissues. Autopsy studies suggest that salivary glands and bowel may be sites of latent infection.

If the host's T-cell responses become compromised by disease or by iatrogenic immunosuppression, latent virus can be reactivated to cause a variety of syndromes. Chronic antigenic stimulation in the presence of immunosuppression (for example, after tissue transplantation) appears to be an ideal setting for CMV activation and CMV-induced disease. Certain particularly potent suppressants of T-cell immunity (e.g., antithymocyte globulin) are associated with a high rate of clinical CMV syndromes, which may follow either primary or reactivation infection. CMV may itself contribute to further T-lymphocyte hyporesponsiveness, which often precedes superinfection with other opportunistic pathogens, such as *Pneumocystis*. CMV and *Pneumocystis* are frequently found together in immunosuppressed patients with severe interstitial pneumonia.

PATHOLOGY

Cytomegalic cells in vivo (presumed to be infected epithelial cells) are two to four times larger than surrounding cells and often contain an 8- to 10-μm intranuclear inclusion that is eccentrically placed and is surrounded by a clear halo, producing an "owl's eye" appearance. Smaller granular cytoplasmic inclusions are demonstrated occasionally. Cytomegalic cells are found in a wide variety of organs, including the salivary gland, lung, liver, kidney, intestine, pancreas, adrenal gland, and central nervous system.

The cellular inflammatory response to infection consists of plasma cells, lymphocytes, and monocyte-macrophages. Granulomatous reactions occasionally develop, particularly in the liver. Immunopathologic reactions may contribute to CMV disease. Immune complexes have been detected in infected infants, sometimes in association with CMV-related glomerulopathies. Immune-complex glomerulopathy has also been observed in some CMV-infected patients after renal transplantation.

CLINICAL MANIFESTATIONS

Congenital CMV Infection

Fetal infections range from inapparent to severe and disseminated. Cytomegalic inclusion disease develops in ~5% of infected fetuses and is seen almost exclusively in infants born to mothers who develop primary infections during pregnancy. Petechiae, hepatosplenomegaly, and jaundice are the most common presenting features (60–80% of cases). Microcephaly with or without cerebral calcifications, intrauterine growth retardation, and prematurity are reported in 30–50% of cases. Inguinal hernias and chorioretinitis are less common. Laboratory abnormalities include elevated alanine aminotransferase levels, thrombocytopenia, conjugated hyperbilirubinemia, hemolysis, and elevated cerebrospinal fluid protein levels. The prognosis for severely infected infants is poor; the mortality rate is 20–30%, and few survivors escape intellectual or hearing difficulties later in childhood. The differential diagnosis of cytomegalic inclusion disease in infants includes syphilis, rubella, toxoplasmosis, infection with herpes simplex virus or enterovirus, and bacterial sepsis.

Most congenital CMV infections are clinically inapparent at birth. Of asymptomatically infected infants, 5–25% develop significant psychomotor, hearing, ocular, or dental abnormalities over the next several years.

Perinatal CMV Infection

The newborn may acquire CMV at delivery by passage through an infected birth canal or by postnatal contact with infected breast milk or other maternal secretions.

Of infants who are breast-fed for >1 month by seropositive mothers, 40–60% become infected. Iatrogenic transmission can result from neonatal blood transfusion; screening of blood products before transfusion into low-birth-weight seronegative infants or seronegative pregnant women decreases risk.

The great majority of infants infected at or after delivery remain asymptomatic. However, protracted interstitial pneumonitis has been associated with perinatally acquired CMV infection, particularly in premature infants, and occasionally has been accompanied by infection with *Chlamydia trachomatis*, *Pneumocystis*, or *Ureaplasma urealyticum*. Poor weight gain, adenopathy, rash, hepatitis, anemia, and atypical lymphocytosis may also be found, and CMV excretion often persists for months or years.

CMV Mononucleosis

The most common clinical manifestation of CMV infection in normal hosts beyond the neonatal period is a heterophile antibody–negative mononucleosis syndrome, which may develop spontaneously or follow transfusion of leukocyte-containing blood products. Although the syndrome occurs at all ages, it most often involves sexually active young adults. With incubation periods of 20–60 days, the illness generally lasts for 2–6 weeks. Prolonged high fevers, sometimes with chills, profound fatigue, and malaise, characterize this disorder. Myalgias, headache, and splenomegaly are common, but in CMV (as opposed to EBV) mononucleosis, exudative pharyngitis and cervical lymphadenopathy are rare. Occasional patients develop rubelliform rashes, often after exposure to ampicillin or certain other antibiotics. Less common are interstitial or segmental pneumonia, myocarditis, pleuritis, arthritis, and encephalitis. In rare cases, Guillain-Barré syndrome complicates CMV mononucleosis. The characteristic laboratory abnormality is relative lymphocytosis in peripheral blood, with >10% atypical lymphocytes. Total leukocyte counts may be low, normal, or markedly elevated. Although significant jaundice is uncommon, serum aminotransferase and alkaline phosphatase levels are often moderately elevated. Heterophile antibodies are absent; however, transient immunologic abnormalities are common and may include the presence of cryoglobulins, rheumatoid factors, cold agglutinins, and antinuclear antibodies. Hemolytic anemia, thrombocytopenia, and granulocytopenia complicate recovery in rare instances.

Most patients recover without sequelae, although postviral asthenia may persist for months. The excretion of CMV in urine, genital secretions, and/or saliva often continues for months or years. Rarely, CMV infection is fatal in immunocompetent hosts; survivors can have recurrent episodes of fever and malaise, sometimes associated with autonomic nervous system dysfunction (e.g., attacks of sweating or flushing).

CMV Infection in the Immunocompromised Host

(Table 83-1) CMV appears to be the most common and important viral pathogen complicating organ transplantation (Chap. 12). In recipients of kidney, heart, lung, and liver transplants, CMV induces a variety of syndromes, including fever and leukopenia, hepatitis, pneumonitis, esophagitis, gastritis, colitis, and retinitis. CMV disease may be an independent risk factor for both graft loss and death. The period of maximal risk is between 1 and 4 months after transplantation, although retinitis may be a later complication. Disease likelihood and viral replication levels generally are greater after primary infection than after reactivation. In addition, molecular studies indicate that seropositive transplant recipients are susceptible to reinfection with donor-derived, genotypically variant CMV, and such infection often results in disease. Reactivation infection, although common, is less likely than primary infection to be important clinically. The risk of clinical disease is related to various factors, such as the degree of immunosuppression; the use of antibodies to T-cell receptors; and co-infection with other pathogens. The transplanted organ is particularly vulnerable as a target for CMV infection; thus there is a tendency for CMV hepatitis to follow liver transplantation and for CMV pneumonitis to follow lung transplantation.

CMV pneumonia occurs in 15–20% of bone marrow transplant recipients; the case-fatality rate is 84–88%, although the risk of severe disease may be reduced by prophylaxis or preemptive therapy with antiviral drugs. The risk is greatest 5–13 weeks after transplantation, and identified risk factors include certain types of immunosuppressive therapy, acute graft-versus-host disease, older age, viremia, and pretransplantation seropositivity.

CMV is an important pathogen in patients with advanced HIV infection (Chap. 90), in whom it often causes retinitis or disseminated disease, particularly when peripheral-blood CD4+ T-cell counts fall below 50–100/μL. As treatment for underlying HIV infection has improved, the incidence of serious CMV infections (e.g., retinitis) has decreased. However, during the first few weeks after institution of highly active antiretroviral therapy, acute flare-ups of CMV retinitis may occur secondary to an immune reconstitution inflammatory syndrome.

Syndromes produced by CMV in immunocompromised hosts often begin with prolonged fever, malaise, anorexia, fatigue, night sweats, and arthralgias or myalgias. Liver function abnormalities, leukopenia, thrombocytopenia, and atypical lymphocytosis may be observed during these episodes. The development of tachypnea, hypoxia, and unproductive cough signals respiratory involvement. Radiologic examination of the lung often shows bilateral interstitial or reticulonodular infiltrates that begin in the periphery of the lower lobes and spread centrally and superiorly; localized segmental, nodular, or alveolar patterns are less common. The differential diagnosis includes *Pneumocystis* infection; other viral, bacterial, or fungal infections; pulmonary hemorrhage; and injury secondary to irradiation or to treatment with cytotoxic drugs.

Gastrointestinal CMV involvement may be localized or extensive and almost exclusively affects compromised hosts. Ulcers of the esophagus, stomach, small intestine, or colon may result in bleeding or perforation. CMV infection may lead to exacerbations of underlying ulcerative

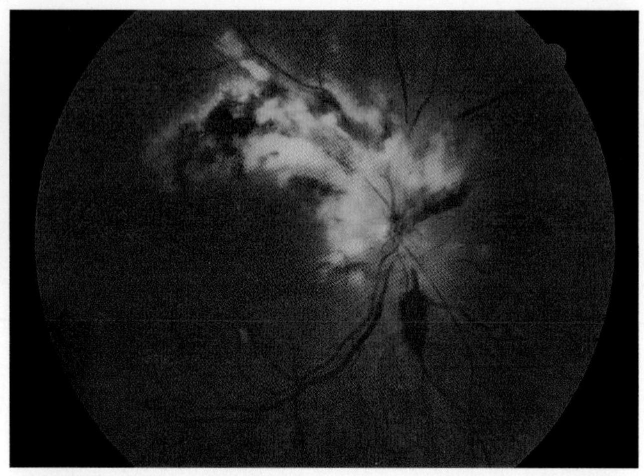

FIGURE 83-1
Cytomegalovirus infection in a patient with AIDS may appear as an arcuate zone of retinitis with hemorrhages and optic disk swelling. Often CMV is confined to the retinal periphery, beyond view of the direct ophthalmoscope.

colitis. Hepatitis occurs frequently, particularly after liver transplantation, and acalculous cholecystitis and adrenalitis have been described.

CMV rarely causes meningoencephalitis in otherwise-healthy individuals. Two forms of CMV encephalitis are seen in patients with AIDS. One resembles HIV encephalitis and presents as progressive dementia; the other is a ventriculoencephalitis characterized by cranial-nerve deficits, nystagmus, disorientation, lethargy, and ventriculomegaly. In immunocompromised patients, CMV can also cause subacute progressive polyradiculopathy, which is often reversible if recognized and treated promptly.

CMV retinitis is an important cause of blindness in immunocompromised patients, particularly patients with advanced AIDS (Chap. 90). Early lesions consist of small, opaque, white areas of granular retinal necrosis that spread in a centrifugal manner and are later accompanied by hemorrhages, vessel sheathing, and retinal edema (Fig. 83-1). CMV retinopathy must be distinguished from that due to other conditions, including toxoplasmosis, candidiasis, and herpes simplex virus infection.

Fatal CMV infections are often associated with persistent viremia and the involvement of multiple organ systems. Progressive pulmonary infiltrates, pancytopenia, hyperamylasemia, and hypotension are characteristic features that are frequently found in conjunction with a terminal bacterial, fungal, or protozoan superinfection. Extensive adrenal necrosis with CMV inclusions is often documented at autopsy, as is CMV involvement of many other organs.

DIAGNOSIS

The diagnosis of CMV infection usually cannot be made reliably on clinical grounds alone. Isolation of CMV or detection of its antigens or DNA in appropriate clinical specimens is the preferred approach. Virus excretion or viremia is readily detected by culture of appropriate specimens on human fibroblast monolayers. If CMV titers are high, as is common in congenital disseminated infection and in patients with AIDS, characteristic cytopathic effects may be detected within a few days. However, in some situations (e.g., CMV mononucleosis), viral titers are low, and cytopathic effects may take several weeks to appear. Many laboratories expedite diagnosis with an overnight tissue-culture method (shell vial assay) involving centrifugation and an immunocytochemical detection technique employing monoclonal antibodies to an immediate-early CMV antigen. Isolation of virus from urine or saliva does not, by itself, constitute proof of acute infection, since excretion from these sites may continue for months or years after illness. Detection of viremia is a better predictor of acute infection.

Detection of CMV antigens (pp65) in peripheral-blood leukocytes or of CMV DNA in blood or tissues may hasten diagnosis. Such assays may yield a positive result several days earlier than culture methods. The most sensitive way to detect CMV in blood or other fluids may be by amplifying CMV DNA by polymerase chain reaction (PCR). PCR detection of CMV DNA in blood may predict the risk for disease progression, and PCR detection of CMV DNA in cerebrospinal fluid is useful in the diagnosis of CMV encephalitis or polyradiculopathy.

A variety of serologic assays detect increases in titers of antibody to CMV antigens. An increased antibody level may not be detectable for up to 4 weeks after primary infection, and titers often remain high for years after infection. For this reason, single-sample antibody determinations are of no value in assessing the acuteness of infection. Detection of CMV-specific IgM is sometimes useful in the diagnosis of recent or active infection; circulating rheumatoid factors may result in occasional false-positive IgM tests.

℞ Treatment: CYTOMEGALOVIRUS INFECTION

Several measures are useful for the prevention of CMV infection in high-risk patients. The use of blood from seronegative donors or of blood that has been frozen, thawed, and deglycerolized greatly decreases the rate of transfusion-associated transmission. Matching of organ or bone marrow transplants by CMV serology, with exclusive use of organs from seronegative donors in seronegative recipients, reduces rates of primary infection after transplantation. Both live attenuated and CMV subunit vaccines have been evaluated, but neither is close to approval for general use.

CMV immune or hyperimmune globulin has been reported (1) to reduce rates of CMV-associated syndromes and of fungal or parasitic superinfections among seronegative renal transplant recipients and (2) to prevent congenital CMV infection in infants of women with primary infection during pregnancy. Studies in bone marrow transplant recipients have produced conflicting results. Prophylactic acyclovir or valacyclovir may reduce rates of CMV infection and disease in certain seronegative renal transplant recipients, although neither drug is effective in the treatment of active CMV disease.

Ganciclovir is a guanosine derivative that has considerably more activity against CMV than its congener acyclovir. After intracellular conversion by a viral phosphotransferase encoded by CMV gene region UL97, ganciclovir triphosphate is a selective inhibitor of CMV DNA polymerase. Several clinical studies have indicated response rates of 70–90% among patients with AIDS who are given ganciclovir for the treatment of CMV retinitis or colitis. In bone marrow transplant recipients with CMV pneumonia, ganciclovir is less effective when given alone, but it elicits a favorable clinical response 50–70% of the time when combined with CMV immune globulin. Prophylactic or suppressive ganciclovir may be useful in high-risk bone marrow or organ transplant recipients (e.g., those who are CMV-seropositive before transplantation or who are CMV culture–positive afterward). In many patients with AIDS, persistently low CD4+ T-cell counts, and CMV disease, clinical and virologic relapses occur promptly if treatment with ganciclovir is discontinued. Therefore, prolonged maintenance regimens are recommended for such patients. Resistance to ganciclovir is common among patients treated for >3 months and is usually related to mutations in the CMV UL97 gene.

Valganciclovir is an orally bioavailable prodrug that is rapidly metabolized to ganciclovir in intestinal tissues and the liver. Approximately 60% of an oral dose of valganciclovir is absorbed. An oral valganciclovir dose of 900 mg results in ganciclovir blood levels similar to those obtained with an IV ganciclovir dose of 5 mg/kg. Oral valganciclovir appears to be as effective as IV ganciclovir for both CMV retinitis induction and maintenance regimens. Furthermore, the adverse-event profiles and rates of resistance development for the two drugs are similar.

Ganciclovir or valganciclovir therapy for CMV retinitis consists of a 14- to 21-day induction course (5 mg/kg IV twice daily for ganciclovir or 900 mg twice daily for valganciclovir) followed by prolonged maintenance therapy. For parenteral maintenance, the ganciclovir dose is 5 mg/kg daily or 6 mg/kg 5 days per week; for oral maintenance, 900 mg of valganciclovir once daily is recommended. Peripheral-blood neutropenia develops in 16–29% of treated patients but may be ameliorated by granulocyte colony-stimulating factor or granulocyte-macrophage colony-stimulating factor. Discontinuation of maintenance therapy should be considered in patients with AIDS who, while receiving antiretroviral therapy, have a sustained (>6-month) increase in CD4+ T-cell counts to >100–150/μL.

Ganciclovir may also be administered via a slow-release pellet sutured into the eye. Although this intraocular device provides good local protection, contralateral eye disease and disseminated disease are not affected, and early retinal detachment is possible. A combination of intraocular and systemic therapy may be better than the intraocular implant alone.

Foscarnet (sodium phosphonoformate) inhibits CMV DNA polymerase. Because this agent does not require phosphorylation to be active, it is also effective against most ganciclovir-resistant isolates. Foscarnet is less well tolerated than ganciclovir and causes considerable toxicity, including renal dysfunction, hypomagnesemia, hypokalemia, hypocalcemia, genital ulcers, dysuria, nausea, and paresthesia. Moreover, foscarnet administration requires the use of an infusion pump and close clinical monitoring. With aggressive hydration and dose adjustments for renal dysfunction, the toxicity of foscarnet can be reduced. The use of foscarnet should be avoided when a saline load cannot be tolerated (e.g., in cardiomyopathy). The approved induction regimen is 60 mg/kg every 8 h for 2 weeks, although 90 mg/kg every 12 h is equally effective and no more toxic. Maintenance infusions should deliver 90–120 mg/kg once daily. No oral preparation is available. Foscarnet-resistant virus may emerge during extended therapy.

Cidofovir is a nucleotide analogue with a long intracellular half-life that allows intermittent IV administration. Induction regimens of 5 mg/kg weekly for 2 weeks are followed by maintenance regimens of 3–5 mg/kg every 2 weeks. Cidofovir can cause severe nephrotoxicity through dose-dependent proximal tubular cell injury; however, this adverse effect can be tempered somewhat by saline hydration and probenecid.

It is not clear whether universal prophylaxis or preemptive therapy is the preferable approach in CMV-seropositive immunocompromised hosts. Both ganciclovir and valganciclovir have been used successfully for prophylaxis and preemptive therapy in transplant recipients. For patients with advanced HIV infection (CD4+ T-cell counts of <50/μL), some authorities have advocated prophylaxis with oral ganciclovir or valganciclovir. However, side effects, lack of proven benefit, possible induction of viral resistance, and high cost have precluded the wide acceptance of this practice. Preemptive ganciclovir or valganciclovir therapy based on detection of CMV viremia by either antigenemia or PCR techniques is under study.

HUMAN HERPESVIRUS TYPES 6, 7, AND 8

Human herpesvirus (HHV) type 6 was first isolated in 1986 from peripheral-blood leukocytes of six persons with various lymphoproliferative disorders. The virus has a worldwide distribution, and two genetically distinct variants (HHV-6A and HHV-6B) are now recognized. HHV-6 appears to be transmitted by saliva and possibly by genital secretions.

Infection with HHV-6 frequently occurs during infancy as maternal antibody wanes. The peak age of acquisition is 9–21 months; by 24 months, seropositivity rates approach 80%. Older siblings appear to serve as a source of transmission. Congenital infection may also occur. Most infected children develop symptoms (fever, fussiness, and diarrhea). A minority develop exanthem subitum (roseola infantum), a common illness characterized by fever with subsequent rash. Approximately 10–20% of febrile seizures without rash during infancy are caused by HHV-6.

In older age groups, HHV-6 has been associated with mononucleosis syndromes, focal encephalitis, and (in immunocompromised hosts) pneumonitis and disseminated disease. In transplant recipients, HHV-6 infection may be associated with similar syndromes and with graft dysfunction. High plasma loads of HHV-6 DNA in stem-cell transplant recipients are associated with allelic-mismatched donors, use of steroids, delayed monocyte and platelet engraftment, development of limbic encephalitis, and increased all-cause mortality. Like many other viruses, HHV-6 has been implicated in the pathogenesis of multiple sclerosis, although further study is needed to distinguish between association and etiology.

HHV-7 was isolated in 1990 from T lymphocytes from the peripheral blood of a healthy 26-year-old man. The virus is frequently acquired during childhood, albeit at a later age than HHV-6. HHV-7 is commonly present in saliva, which is presumed to be the principal source of infection; breast milk can also carry the virus. Viremia can be associated with either primary or reactivation infection. The most common clinical manifestations of childhood HHV-7 infections are fever and seizures. Some children present with respiratory or gastrointestinal signs and symptoms. An association has been made between HHV-7 and pityriasis rosea, but evidence is insufficient to indicate a causal relationship.

HHV-6, HHV-7, and CMV infections may cluster in transplant recipients, making it difficult to sort out the roles of the various agents in individual clinical syndromes. HHV-6 and HHV-7 appear to be susceptible to ganciclovir and foscarnet, although definitive evidence of clinical responses is lacking.

Unique herpesvirus-like DNA sequences were reported during 1994 and 1995 in tissues derived from Kaposi's sarcoma (KS) and body cavity–based lymphoma occurring in patients with AIDS. The virus from which these sequences were derived is designated HHV-8 or Kaposi's sarcoma–associated herpesvirus (KSHV). HHV-8, which infects certain B lymphocytes and endothelium-derived spindle cells, appears to be causally related not only to KS but also to a subgroup of AIDS-related B-cell body cavity–based lymphomas (primary effusion lymphomas) and to multicentric Castleman's disease, a lymphoproliferative disorder of B cells. Initial suggestions that HHV-8 is associated with primary pulmonary hypertension have not been confirmed by subsequent studies.

Unlike other herpesvirus infections, HHV-8 infection is much more common in some geographic areas (e.g., central and southern Africa) than in others (North America, Asia, northern Europe). In high-prevalence areas, infection occurs in childhood, seropositivity is associated with having a seropositive mother or (to a lesser extent) older sibling, and HHV-8 may be transmitted in saliva. In low-prevalence areas, infections typically occur in adults, probably with sexual transmission. Concurrent epidemics of HIV-1 and HHV-8 infections among certain populations (e.g., homosexual and bisexual men) in the late 1970s and early 1980s appear to have resulted in the frequent association of AIDS and KS. Transmission of HHV-8 may also be associated with organ transplantation and injection drug use.

Primary HHV-8 infection in immunocompetent children may manifest as fever and maculopapular rash. Among individuals with intact immunity, chronic asymptomatic infection is the rule, and neoplastic disorders generally develop only after subsequent immunocompromise. Immunocompromised persons with primary infection may present with fever, splenomegaly, lymphoid hyperplasia, pancytopenia, or rapid-onset KS. Quantitative analysis of HHV-8 DNA suggests a predominance of latently infected cells in KS lesions and frequent lytic replication in multicentric Castleman's disease.

Effective antiretroviral therapy for HIV-infected individuals has led to a marked reduction in rates of KS among persons dually infected with HHV-8 and HIV in resource-rich areas. HHV-8 itself is susceptible in vitro to ganciclovir, foscarnet, and cidofovir, although clinical evidence for benefit of these agents is lacking.

FURTHER READINGS

Asahi-Ozaki Y et al: Quantitative analysis of Kaposi sarcoma–associated herpesvirus (KSHV) in KSHV-associated diseases. J Infect Dis 193:773, 2006

Cannon MJ et al: Blood-borne and sexual transmission of human herpesvirus 8 in women with or at risk for human immunodeficiency virus infection. N Engl J Med 344:637, 2001

Hall CB et al: Characteristics and acquisition of human herpesvirus (HHV)-7 infections in relation to infection with HHV-6. J Infect Dis 193:1063, 2006

Heineman TC et al: A phase 1 study of 4 live, recombinant human cytomegalovirus Towne/Toledo chimeric vaccines. J Infect Dis 193:1350, 2006

Kalil AC et al: Meta-analysis: The efficacy of strategies to prevent organ disease by cytomegalovirus in solid organ transplant recipients. Ann Intern Med 143:870, 2005

Martin DF et al: A controlled trial of valganciclovir as induction therapy for cytomegalovirus retinitis. N Engl J Med 346:1119, 2002

Mbulaiteye S et al: Molecular evidence for mother-to-child transmission of Kaposi sarcoma–associated herpesvirus in Uganda and K1 gene evolution within the host. J Infect Dis 193:1250, 2006

Nigro G et al: Passive immunization during pregnancy for congenital cytomegalovirus infection. N Engl J Med 353:1350, 2005

Ogata M et al: Human herpesvirus 6 DNA in plasma after allogeneic stem cell transplantation: Incidence and clinical significance. J Infect Dis 193:68, 2006

Pass RF et al: Vaccine prevention of maternal cytomegalovirus infection. N Engl J Med 360:1191, 2009

Seeley WW et al: Post-transplant acute limbic encephalitis: Clinical features and relationship to HHV6. Neurology 69:156, 2007

Zerr DM et al: A population-based study of primary human herpesvirus 6 infection. N Engl J Med 352:768, 2005

CHAPTER 84

MOLLUSCUM CONTAGIOSUM, MONKEYPOX, AND OTHER POXVIRUSES, EXCLUDING SMALLPOX VIRUS

Fred Wang

The poxvirus family includes a large number of related DNA viruses that infect various vertebrate hosts. The poxviruses responsible for infections in humans, along with the main manifestations of these infections, are listed in Table 84-1. Infections with orthopoxviruses—e.g., smallpox (variola major) virus (Chap. 6) or the zoonotic monkeypox virus—can result in systemic, potentially lethal human disease. Other poxvirus infections cause primarily localized skin disease in humans.

MOLLUSCUM CONTAGIOSUM

Molluscum contagiosum virus is an obligate human pathogen that causes distinctive proliferative skin lesions. These lesions measure 2–5 mm in diameter and are pearly, flesh-colored, and umbilicated, with a characteristic dimple at the center (Fig. 84-1). A relative lack of inflammation and necrosis distinguishes these proliferative lesions from other poxvirus lesions. Lesions may be found—singly or in clusters—anywhere on the body except on the palms and soles and may be associated with an eczematous rash.

Molluscum contagiosum is the most common human disease resulting from poxvirus infection and is transmitted by close contact, including sexual intercourse. Swimming pools are a common vector for transmission. Atopy and compromise of skin integrity increase the risk of infection. The incubation period ranges from 2 weeks to 6 months, with an average of 2–7 weeks. In most cases, the disease is self-limited and regresses spontaneously after 3–4 months in immunocompetent hosts. There are no systemic complications, but skin lesions may persist for 3–5 years. Molluscum contagiosum develops especially often in association with advanced HIV infection; the prevalence is 5–18% among HIV-infected patients (Chap. 90).

TABLE 84-1

POXVIRUSES AND HUMAN INFECTIONS

GENUS	SPECIES	HUMAN DISEASE
Orthopoxvirus	Variola[a]	Smallpox, systemic
	Monkeypox	Smallpox-like, systemic
	Vaccinia	Local pox lesion, occasionally systemic
	Cowpox	Local pox lesions
Molluscipoxvirus	Molluscum contagiosum	Molluscum contagiosum, multiple cutaneous lesions
Parapoxvirus	Orf	Contagious pustular dermatitis, local pox lesions
	Pseudocowpox	Milker's nodule, local pox lesions
Yatapoxvirus	Tanapox	Local pox lesions

[a]See Chap. 6.

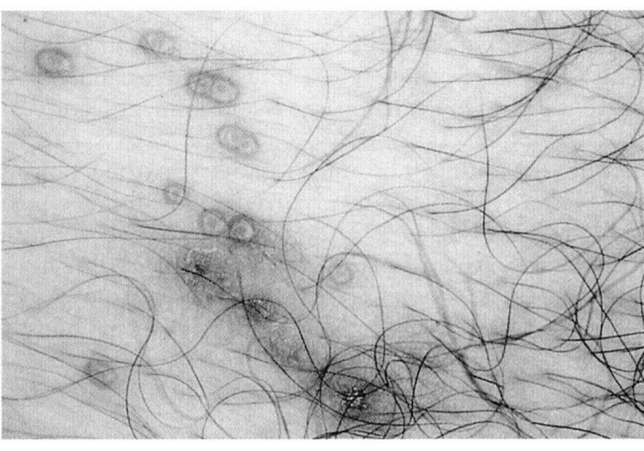

FIGURE 84-1

Molluscum contagiosum is a cutaneous poxvirus infection characterized by multiple umbilicated flesh-colored or hypopigmented papules.

The disease is often more generalized, severe, and persistent in AIDS patients than in other groups, frequently involving the face and upper body. Paradoxically, rates of molluscum contagiosum are reportedly elevated among patients receiving antiretroviral therapy. Moreover, the disease can be exacerbated in the immune reconstitution inflammatory syndrome (IRIS) associated with the initiation of antiretroviral therapy. Extensive molluscum contagiosum has also been reported in conjunction with other types of immunodeficiency.

The diagnosis of molluscum contagiosum is typically made by its clinical presentation and can be confirmed by histologic demonstration of the cytoplasmic eosinophilic inclusions, or *molluscum bodies*, that are characteristic of poxvirus replication. Molluscum contagiosum virus cannot be propagated in vitro, but electron microscopy and molecular studies can be used for its identification.

There is no specific systemic treatment for molluscum contagiosum, but a variety of techniques for physical ablation have been used. Cidofovir displays in vitro activity against many poxviruses, including smallpox virus and molluscum contagiosum virus, and case reports suggest that parenteral or topical cidofovir may have some efficacy in the treatment of recalcitrant molluscum contagiosum in immunosuppressed hosts.

MONKEYPOX

Although monkeypox virus was named after the animal from which it was originally isolated, rodents are the primary viral reservoir.

Human infections with monkeypox virus typically occur in Africa when humans come into direct contact with infected animals. Human disease is rare and is characterized by a systemic illness and a vesicular rash similar to those of variola. The clinical presentation of monkeypox can be confused with that of the more common varicella-zoster virus infection (Chap. 81). Compared with the lesions of this herpesvirus infection, monkeypox lesions tend to be more uniform (i.e., in the same stage of development), diffuse, and peripheral in distribution. Lymphadenopathy is a prominent feature of monkeypox infection.

The first outbreak of human monkeypox infection in the Western Hemisphere occurred in the midwestern United States during May and June 2003, when more than 70 cases were reported, of which 35 were laboratory confirmed. The outbreak was linked to contact with pet prairie dogs that had become infected while being housed with rodents imported from Ghana. Patients presented most frequently with fever, rash, and lymphadenopathy ~12 days after exposure. The median durations of fever and rash were 8 and 12 days, respectively. Of the nine patients who were hospitalized, five were judged to be severely ill, but there were no deaths. Smallpox vaccination can provide cross-reactive immunity to monkeypox infection; nevertheless, there were no significant clinical differences between vaccinated and unvaccinated individuals in this outbreak. Additional studies of people exposed in the outbreak detected subclinical infection in a few vaccinated individuals—an observation suggesting the possibility of long-term vaccine protection. The risk of human disease from animal orthopoxvirus infections may increase as smallpox immunity wanes in the general population and the popularity of exotic animals as household pets grows.

OTHER ZOONOTIC POXVIRUS INFECTIONS

Orf virus and *pseudocowpox* virus are parapoxviruses that naturally infect sheep and cattle. Direct contact with infected animals can result in human infections, typically on the hands, with the development of a nodular, highly vascular proliferative lesion that may ulcerate. Human orf virus infection is also called *ecthyma contagiosum*, and human pseudocowpox virus infection causes "milker's nodules."

Zoonotic infection with *cowpox* virus causes painful hemorrhagic lesions, mostly on the hands or face, with fever or flulike symptoms and lymphadenitis. Lesions generally resolve in 6–8 weeks. Human infection with *tanapox* virus occurs after contact with infected monkeys. In most cases, a febrile prodrome is followed by eruption of a single nodular lesion on the exposed area, but multiple lesions have also been reported. The lesions are relatively large, often break down to form an ulcer, and resolve in 5–6 weeks.

FURTHER READINGS

Centers For Disease Control And Prevention: Update: Multistate outbreak of monkeypox—Illinois, Indiana, Kansas, Missouri, Ohio, and Wisconsin, 2003. MMWR 52:642, 2003

Dhar AD et al: Tanapox infection in a college student. N Engl J Med 350:361, 2004

Hammarlund E et al: Multiple diagnostic techniques identify previously vaccinated individuals with protective immunity against monkeypox. Nat Med 11:1005, 2005

Huhn GD et al: Clinical characteristics of human monkeypox, and risk factors for severe disease. Clin Infect Dis 41:1742, 2005

Reed KD et al: The detection of monkeypox in humans in the Western Hemisphere. N Engl J Med 350:342, 2004

Taub DD et al: Immunity from smallpox vaccine persists for decades: A longitudinal study. Am J Med 121:1058, 2008

CHAPTER 85

PARVOVIRUS INFECTIONS

Kevin E. Brown

Parvoviruses, members of the family Parvoviridae, are small (diameter, ~22 nm), nonenveloped, icosahedral-shaped viruses with a linear single-stranded DNA genome of ~5000 nucleotides. These viruses are dependent on either rapidly dividing host cells or helper viruses for replication. At least four types of parvovirus infect humans: parvovirus B19, adeno-associated viruses (AAVs), the recently described PARV4/5 virus, and human bocavirus (HBoV). To date, only B19 has been shown definitively to be a human pathogen.

PARVOVIRUS B19

DEFINITION

B19 is the type member of the genus *Erythrovirus*. On the basis of viral sequence, B19 is divided into three genotypes (designated 1, 2, and 3), but only a single B19 antigenic type has been described. Genotypes 2 and 3 are detected relatively infrequently in Europe and the United States.

EPIDEMIOLOGY

B19 exclusively infects humans, and infection is endemic in virtually all parts of the world. Transmission occurs predominantly via the respiratory route and is followed by the onset of rash and arthralgia. By the age of 15 years, ~50% of children have detectable IgG; this figure rises to >90% among the elderly. In pregnant women, the estimated annual seroconversion rate is ~1%. Within households, secondary infection rates approach 50%.

Detection of high-titer B19 in blood is not unusual (see "Pathogenesis," below). Transmission can occur as a result of transfusion, most commonly of pooled components. To reduce the risk of transmission, plasma pools are screened by nucleic acid amplification technology, and high-titer pools are discarded. B19 is resistant to both heat and solvent-detergent inactivation.

PATHOGENESIS

B19 replicates primarily in erythroid progenitors. This specificity is due in part to the limited tissue distribution of the B19 receptor, blood group P antigen (globoside). Infection leads to high-titer viremia, with $>10^{12}$ virus particles/mL detectable in the blood at the apex (Fig. 85-1), and virus-induced cytotoxicity results in cessation of red cell production. In immunocompetent individuals, viremia and arrest of erythropoiesis are transient and resolve as the IgM and IgG antibody response is mounted. In individuals with normal erythropoiesis, there is only a minimal drop in hemoglobin levels; however, in those with increased erythropoiesis (especially with hemolytic anemia), this cessation of red cell production can induce a transient crisis with severe anemia (Fig. 85-1). Similarly, if an individual (or, after maternal infection, a fetus) does not mount a neutralizing antibody response and halt the lytic infection, erythroid production is compromised and chronic anemia develops (Fig. 85-1).

The immune-mediated phase of illness, which begins 2–3 weeks after infection as the IgM response peaks, manifests as the rash of fifth disease together with arthralgia and/or frank arthritis. Low-level B19 DNA can be detected by polymerase chain reaction (PCR) in blood and tissues for months to years after acute infection.

The B19 receptor is found in a variety of other cells and tissues, including megakaryocytes, endothelial cells, placenta, myocardium, and liver. Infection of these tissues by B19 may be responsible for some of the more unusual presentations of the infection. Rare individuals who lack P antigen are naturally resistant to B19 infection.

CLINICAL MANIFESTATIONS

Erythema Infectiosum

Most B19 infections are asymptomatic. The main manifestation of symptomatic B19 infection is erythema infectiosum, also known as *fifth disease* or *slapped-cheek disease* (Fig. 85-2). Infection begins with a minor febrile prodrome ~7–10 days after exposure, and the classic facial rash develops several days later. The rash may spread to the extremities in a lacy reticular pattern. However, its intensity and distribution vary, and the B19-induced rash is difficult to distinguish from other viral exanthems. Adults may not exhibit the "slapped-cheek" phenomenon.

Polyarthropathy Syndrome

Although uncommon among children, arthropathy occurs in ~50% of adults and is more common among women than among men. The distribution of the affected joints is often symmetrical, with arthralgia affecting the small joints of the hands and occasionally the ankles, knees, and wrists. Resolution usually occurs within a few weeks, but recurring symptoms can continue for months.

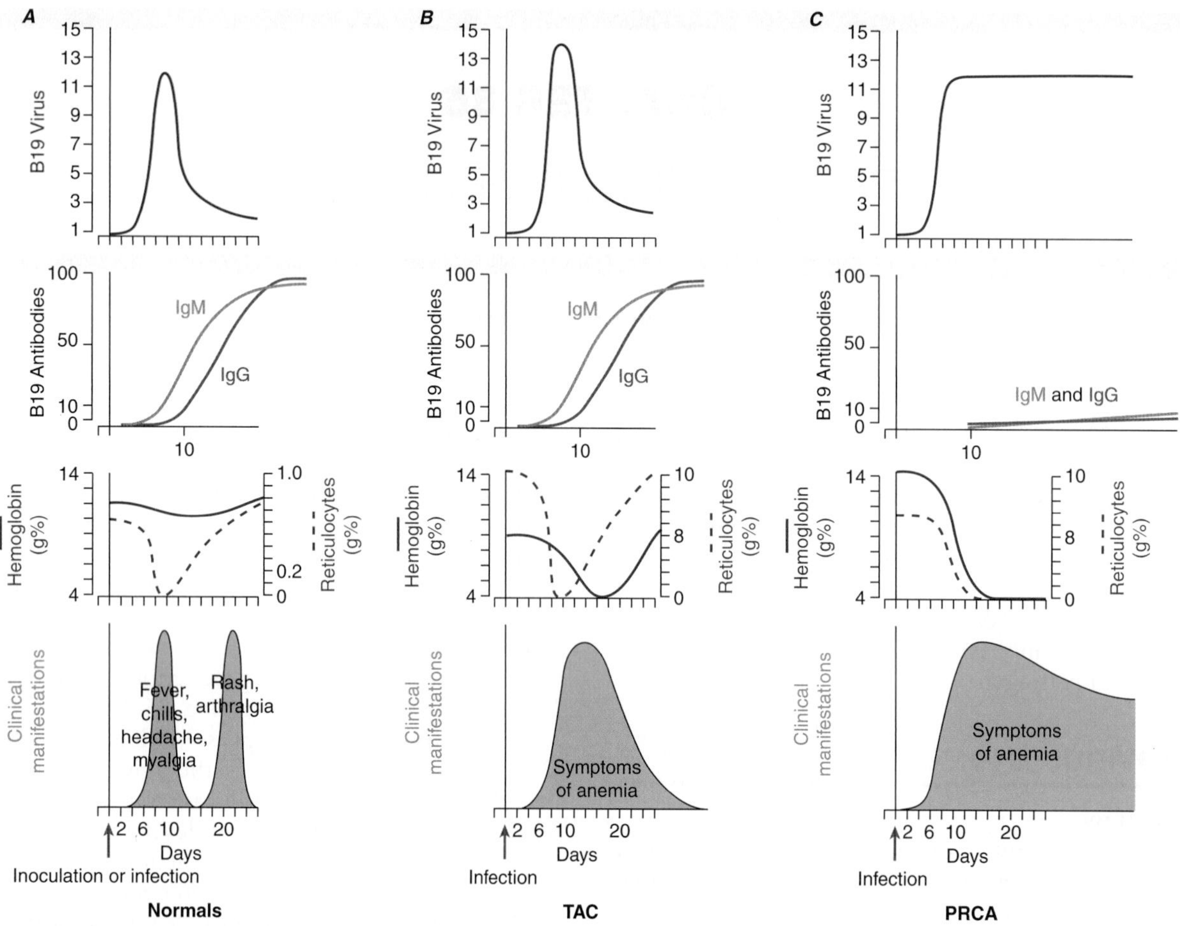

FIGURE 85-1

Schematic representation of the time course of B19 infection in (***A***) normals (erythema infectiosum), (***B***) transient aplastic crisis (TAC), and (***C***) chronic anemia/pure red-cell aplasia (PRCA). *(Reprinted with permission from Young and Brown, 2004. © 2004 Massachusetts Medical Society. All rights reserved.)*

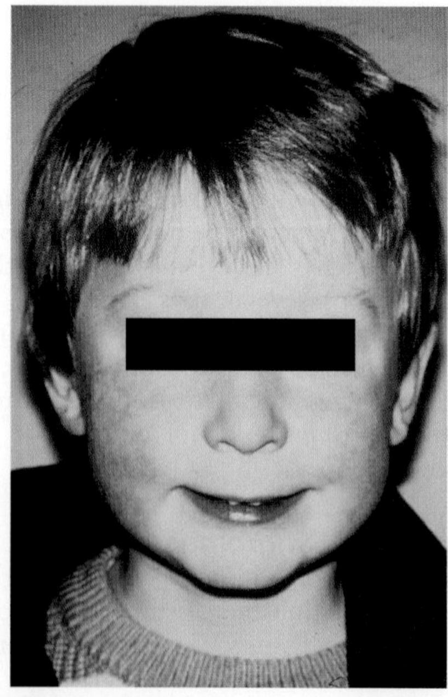

FIGURE 85-2

Child with erythema infectiosum, or fifth disease, showing typical "slapped-cheek" appearance. *(Courtesy of Bernard Cohen, Virus Reference Department, Health Protection Agency, London; with permission.)*

Transient Aplastic Crisis

Asymptomatic transient reticulocytopenia occurs in most individuals with B19 infection. However, in patients who depend on continual rapid production of red cells, infection can cause transient aplastic crisis (TAC). Affected individuals include those with hemolytic disorders, hemoglobinopathies, red cell enzymopathies, and autoimmune hemolytic anemias. Patients present with symptoms of severe anemia, and bone marrow examination reveals an absence of erythroid precursors and characteristic giant pronormoblasts.

Pure Red-Cell Aplasia/Chronic Anemia

Chronic B19 infection has been reported in a wide range of immunosuppressed patients, including those with congenital immunodeficiency, AIDS (Chap. 90), lymphoproliferative disorders (especially acute lymphocytic leukemia), and transplantation (Chap. 12). Patients have persistent anemia with reticulocytopenia, absent or low levels of B19 IgG, high levels of B19 DNA in serum, and—in many cases—scattered giant pronormoblasts in bone marrow. Rarely, nonerythroid hematologic lineages are also affected. Transient neutropenia, lymphopenia, and thrombocytopenia (including idiopathic thrombocytopenic purpura) have been observed. B19 occasionally causes a hemophagocytic syndrome.

A recent study in Papua New Guinea, where malaria is endemic, suggested that B19 infection plays a major role in the development of severe anemia. Further studies must determine whether B19 infection contributes to severe anemia in other malarial regions.

Hydrops Fetalis

B19 infection during pregnancy can lead to hydrops fetalis and/or fetal loss. The risk of transplacental fetal infection is ~30%, and the risk of fetal loss (predominantly early in the second trimester) is ~9%. The risk of congenital infection is <1%. Although B19 does not appear to be teratogenic, anecdotal cases of eye damage and CNS abnormalities have been reported. Cases of congenital anemia have also been described. B19 probably causes 10–20% of all cases of nonimmune hydrops.

Unusual Manifestations

Hepatitis, vasculitis, myocarditis, glomerulosclerosis, and central nervous system (CNS) disease have all been reported. However, B19 DNA can be detected by PCR for years in many tissues; this finding is of no known clinical significance, but its interpretation may cause confusion regarding B19 disease association.

DIAGNOSIS

Diagnosis of B19 infection in immunocompetent individuals is generally based on detection of B19 IgM antibodies (Table 85-1). IgM can be detected at the time of rash in erythema infectiosum and by the third day of TAC in patients with hematologic disorders; these antibodies remain detectable for ~3 months. B19 IgG is detectable by the seventh day of illness and persists throughout life. Detection of B19 DNA should be used for the diagnosis of early TAC or chronic anemia. Although B19 levels fall rapidly with the development of the immune response, DNA can be detectable by PCR for months or even years after infection, even in healthy individuals; therefore, quantitative PCR should be used. In acute infection at the height of viremia, >10^{12} B19 DNA genome equivalents (ge)/mL of serum can be detected; however, titers fall rapidly within 2 days. Patients with aplastic crisis or B19-induced chronic anemia generally have >10^5 B19 DNA ge/mL.

℞ Treatment: PARVOVIRUS INFECTION

No antiviral drug effective against B19 is available, and treatment of B19 infection often targets symptoms only. TAC precipitated by B19 infection frequently necessitates symptom-based treatment with blood transfusions. In patients receiving chemotherapy, temporary cessation of treatment may result in an immune response and resolution. If this approach is unsuccessful or not applicable, commercial immune globulin (IVIg; Gammagard, Sandoglobulin) from healthy blood donors can cure or ameliorate persistent B19 infection in immunosuppressed patients. Generally, the dose used is 400 mg/kg daily for 5–10 days. Like patients with TAC, immunosuppressed patients with persistent B19 infection should be considered infectious. Administration of IVIg is not beneficial for erythema infectiosum or B19-associated polyarthropathy. Intrauterine blood transfusion can prevent fetal loss in some cases of fetal hydrops.

PREVENTION

No vaccine has been approved for the prevention of B19 infection. A vaccine based on virus-like particles expressed in insect cells is under development; the results of phase 1 trials were promising.

TABLE 85-1

DISEASES ASSOCIATED WITH HUMAN PARVOVIRUS B19 INFECTION AND METHODS OF DIAGNOSIS

DISEASE	HOST(S)	IgM	IgG	PCR	QUANTITATIVE PCR
Fifth disease	Healthy children	Positive	Positive	Positive	
Polyarthropathy syndrome	Healthy adults (especially women)	Positive within 3 months of onset	Positive	Positive	
Transient aplastic crisis	Patients with increased erythropoiesis			Positive	Often >10^{12} ge/mL, but rapidly decreases
Persistent anemia/ pure red-cell aplasia	Immunodeficient or immunocompetent patients	Negative/weakly positive	Negative/ weakly positive	Positive	Often >10^{12} ge/mL, but should be >10^6 in the absence of treatment
Hydrops fetalis/ congenital anemia	Fetus (<20 weeks)			Positive amniotic fluid or tissue	

Note: ge, genome equivalents; PCR, polymerase chain reaction.

OTHER PARVOVIRUSES

ADENO-ASSOCIATED VIRUSES

Antibody studies indicate that AAV infections are common in childhood, but AAVs have not been associated with any disease and are considered nonpathogenic. Most of the interest in AAVs is related to their potential use as vectors for gene therapy.

PARV4/5

The PARV4 viral sequence was initially detected in a patient with an acute viral syndrome. Similar sequences, including the related PARV5 sequence, have been detected in pooled plasma collections. The DNA sequence of PARV4/5 is distinctly different from that of all other parvoviruses, and this virus cannot be classified within the current *Parvovirus* genus. Preliminary serologic studies indicate that PARV4/5 infection is common in childhood, but no association with disease has been shown.

HUMAN BOCAVIRUS

Animal bocaviruses are associated with mild respiratory symptoms and enteritis in young animals. HBoV was recently identified in the respiratory tract of young children with lower respiratory tract infections. However, its contribution to pathogenesis is unknown, and HBoV sequences are often found in the presence of other pathogens. The relation of HBoV and PARV4/5 viruses to the commonly observed fecal parvoviruses also remains to be established.

FURTHER READINGS

Allander T et al: Cloning of a human parvovirus by molecular screening of respiratory tract samples. Proc Natl Acad Sci USA 102:12891, 2005

Brown KE, Young NS: Parvovirus B19, in *Clinical Hematology*, NS Young et al (eds). Philadelphia, Mosby Elsevier, 2006, pp 981–991

——— et al: Resistance to parvovirus B19 infection due to lack of virus receptor (erythrocyte P antigen). N Engl J Med 330:1192, 1994

——— et al: Erythrocyte P antigen: Cellular receptor for B19 parvovirus. Science 262:114, 1993

Enders M et al: Improved diagnosis of gestational parvovirus B19 infection at the time of nonimmune fetal hydrops. J Infect Dis 197:58, 2008

Fryer JF et al: Novel parvovirus and related variant in human plasma. Emerg Infect Dis 12:151, 2006

Kerr JR et al: *Parvoviruses*. London, Hodder Arnold, 2006

Kurtzman GJ et al: Chronic bone marrow failure due to persistent B19 parvovirus infection. N Engl J Med 317:287, 1987

Wildig J et al: Parvovirus B19 infection contributes to severe anemia in young children in Papua New Guinea. J Infect Dis 194:146, 2006

Young NS, Brown KE: Parvovirus B19. N Engl J Med 350:586, 2004

CHAPTER 86

HUMAN PAPILLOMAVIRUS INFECTIONS

Richard C. Reichman

DEFINITION

Human papillomaviruses (HPVs) selectively infect the epithelium of skin and mucous membranes. These infections may be asymptomatic, produce warts, or be associated with a variety of both benign and malignant neoplasias.

ETIOLOGIC AGENT

Papillomaviruses are members of the family Papillomaviridae. They are nonenveloped, measure 50–55 nm in diameter, have icosahedral capsids composed of 72 capsomeres, and contain a double-strand circular DNA genome of ~7900 base pairs. The genomic organization of all papillomaviruses is similar and consists of an early (E) region, a late (L) region, and a noncoding upstream regulatory region (URR). Oncogenic HPV types can immortalize human keratinocytes, and this activity has been mapped to products of early genes E6 and E7. E6 protein facilitates the degradation of the p53 tumor-suppressor protein, and E7 protein binds the retinoblastoma gene product and related proteins. The E1 and E2 proteins modulate viral DNA replication and regulate gene expression. The L1 gene codes for the major capsid protein, which makes up 80% of the virion mass. L2 codes for a minor capsid protein. Type-specific conformational antigenic determinants are located on the virion surface. Papillomavirus types are distinguished from one another by the degree of nucleic acid sequence homology. Distinct types share <90% of their DNA sequences in L1. More than 100 HPV types are recognized, and individual types are associated with specific clinical manifestations. For example, HPV-1 causes plantar warts, HPV-6 causes anogenital warts, and HPV-16 infection can produce cervical dysplasia and invasive cervical cancer. HPVs are species-specific and have not been propagated in tissue culture or in common experimental animals. However, some HPV types have been produced in human tissues implanted in immunodeficient mice.

EPIDEMIOLOGY

There are few good studies of the incidence or prevalence of human warts in well-defined populations. Common warts (*verruca vulgaris*) are found in as many as 25% of some groups and are most prevalent among young children. Plantar warts (*verruca plantaris*) are also widely prevalent; they occur most often among adolescents and young adults. Anogenital warts (*condyloma acuminatum*) represent one of the most common sexually transmitted diseases in the United States. HPV infection of the uterine cervix produces the squamous cell abnormalities most frequently detected on Papanicolaou smears.

Most anogenital HPV infections are transmitted through direct contact with infectious lesions. However, lesion characteristics that are associated with transmission, including appearance, have not been defined, and individuals without obvious disease may transmit infection. Close personal contact is also assumed to play a role in the transmission of most cutaneous warts; the importance of fomites in this setting is not clear. Minor trauma at the site of inoculation may facilitate transmission. Recurrent respiratory papillomatosis in young children is an uncommon disease that is acquired from the infected maternal genital tract. In adults, orogenital sexual contact may transmit the disease.

According to a consensus panel gathered by the World Health Organization, a large body of epidemiologic and biologic data has established that some HPV infections cause cervical cancer. For example, >95% of cervical cancers contain HPV DNA of oncogenic (high-risk) types, such as 16, 18, 31, 33, and 45. HPV DNA is also present in the precursor lesions of cervical cancer (cervical intraepithelial neoplasias). Such lesions containing DNA of oncogenic types are more likely to progress than those associated with low-risk HPV types, such as 6 and 11. HPV DNA is transcribed in tumor tissues, and many epidemiologic studies have confirmed a strong relationship between HPV infection (with or without cofactors) and the development of cervical cancer. Definitive proof of the causative role of high-risk HPV types in the pathogenesis of high-grade cervical dysplasia has been provided by the results of recently conducted trials of HPV vaccines. However, it is important to realize that most cervical HPV infections, including those caused by high-risk types, are self-limited. Infection with high-risk HPV types has also been associated with squamous cell carcinomas and dysplasias of the penis, anus, vagina, and vulva. In patients with *epidermodysplasia verruciformis* (see "Clinical Manifestations" later in the chapter), squamous cell cancers develop frequently at sites infected with specific HPV types, including 5 and 8.

CLINICAL MANIFESTATIONS

The clinical manifestations of HPV infection depend on the location of lesions and the type of virus. Common warts usually occur on the hands as flesh-colored to brown, exophytic, and hyperkeratotic papules. Plantar warts may be quite painful; they can be differentiated from calluses by paring of the surface to reveal thrombosed capillaries. Flat warts (*verruca plana*) are most common among children and occur on the face, neck, chest, and flexor surfaces of the forearms and legs.

Anogenital warts develop on the skin and mucosal surfaces of external genitalia and perianal areas (Fig. 86-1). Among circumcised men, warts are most commonly found on the penile shaft. Lesions frequently occur at the urethral meatus and may extend proximally. Receptive anal intercourse predisposes both men and women to the development of perianal warts, but such lesions occasionally develop without such a history. In women, warts appear first at the posterior introitus and adjacent labia. They then spread to other parts of the vulva and commonly involve the vagina and cervix. In both sexes, external warts suggest the presence of internal lesions; however, internal lesions may be present without external warts, particularly in women. The differential diagnosis of anogenital warts includes condylomata lata of secondary syphilis, molluscum contagiosum, hirsutoid papillomatosis (pearly penile papules), fibroepitheliomas, and a variety of benign and malignant mucocutaneous neoplasms. Respiratory papillomatosis in young children, which may be life-threatening, presents as hoarseness, stridor, or respiratory distress. The disease in adults is usually milder.

Immunosuppressed patients, particularly those undergoing organ transplantation, often develop pityriasis

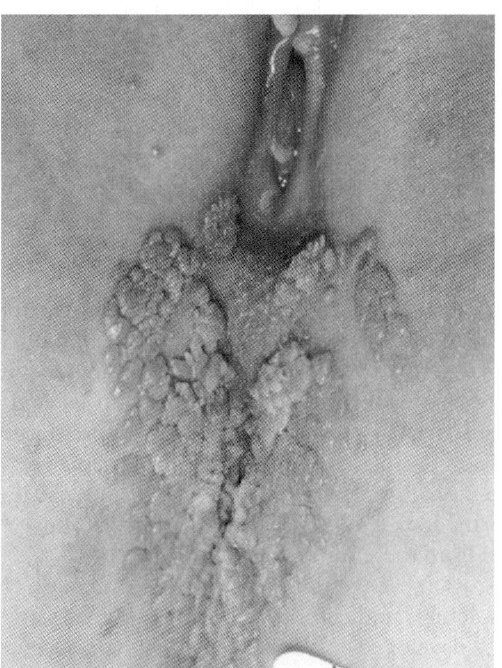

FIGURE 86-1

Anogenital warts are lesions produced by human papillomavirus and in this patient are seen as multiple verrucous papules coalescing into plaques.

versicolor–like lesions, from which DNA of several HPV types has been extracted. Occasionally, such lesions appear to undergo malignant transformation. Patients infected with HIV are often infected with uncommon HPV types, frequently have severe clinical manifestations of HPV infection, and are at high risk for cervical and anal dysplasia as well as for invasive cancer. HPV disease in patients with HIV infection may be associated with multiple HPV types, is difficult to treat, and often recurs (Chap. 90).

Epidermodysplasia verruciformis is a rare autosomal recessive disease characterized by an inability to control HPV infection. Patients are often infected with unique HPV types (i.e., types that affect only this group) and frequently develop cutaneous squamous cell malignancies, particularly in sun-exposed areas. The lesions resemble flat warts or macules similar to those of pityriasis versicolor.

The complications of warts include itching and occasionally bleeding. In rare cases, warts become secondarily infected with bacteria or fungi. Large masses of warts may cause mechanical problems, such as obstruction of the birth canal or the urinary tract. Dysplasias of the uterine cervix are generally asymptomatic until frank carcinoma develops. Patients with anogenital HPV disease may develop serious psychological symptoms due to anxiety and depression over this condition.

PATHOGENESIS

The incubation period of HPV disease is usually 3–4 months (range, 1 month to 2 years). All types of squamous epithelium can be infected by HPV, and the gross and histologic appearances of individual lesions vary with the site of infection and the type of virus. The replication of HPV begins with the infection of basal cells. As cellular differentiation proceeds, HPV DNA replicates and is transcribed. Ultimately, virions are assembled in the nucleus and released when keratinocytes are shed. This process is associated with proliferation of all epidermal layers except the basal layer and produces acanthosis, parakeratosis, and hyperkeratosis. Koilocytes—large round cells with pyknotic nuclei—appear in the granular layer. Histologically normal epithelium may contain HPV DNA, and residual DNA after treatment can be associated with recurrent disease.

Episomal HPV DNA is present in the nuclei of infected cells in benign lesions caused by HPV. However, in severe dysplasias and cancers, HPV DNA is generally integrated, with disruption of the E1/E2 open reading frames. This disruption leads to upregulation of E6 and E7 and subsequent interference with cellular tumor-suppressor proteins. Expression of E6 and E7 proteins of oncogenic HPV types is necessary for the development and maintenance of the transformed state in both cervical cancers and cell lines derived from these tumors.

Host defense responses to HPV infection remain incompletely understood. However, several studies of recently developed HPV vaccines have demonstrated that production of high titers of type-specific neutralizing antibodies by vaccinated individuals is associated with type-specific protection from HPV infection and disease. Because patients with defects in cell-mediated immune responses (including transplant recipients and patients with HIV infection) frequently develop severe HPV disease, such responses are probably important for the control of established virus replication and disease. Histologic studies demonstrating an epidermal lymphomonocytic infiltrate in resolving warts suggest that local immunity may be of particular importance in the resolution of disease. HPV infection also elicits a detectable serologic response in many patients. Using HPV virus-like particles (VLPs) as antigens, type-specific antibodies can be found in sera of about two-thirds of patients with anogenital infection. Antibodies to E-region proteins, most notably E7, have been detected among patients with cervical carcinoma.

DIAGNOSIS

Most warts that are visible to the naked eye can be diagnosed correctly by history and physical examination alone. The use of a colposcope is invaluable in assessing vaginal and cervical lesions and is helpful in the diagnosis of oral and cutaneous HPV disease as well. Application of 3–5% solutions of acetic acid may aid in the visualization of lesions, although the sensitivity and specificity of this procedure are unknown. Papanicolaou smears prepared from cervical or anal scrapings often show cytologic evidence of HPV infection. Persistent or atypical lesions should be biopsied and examined by routine histologic methods. The most sensitive and specific methods of virologic diagnosis use techniques such as the polymerase chain reaction or the hybrid capture assay to detect HPV nucleic acids and to identify specific virus types. Such tests may be useful in the diagnosis and management of cervical HPV disease, although their utility may vary according to the prevalence of disease and the availability of traditional cytologic and histologic testing. Serologic techniques to diagnose HPV infection are not helpful in individual cases and are not widely available.

℞ Treatment: HUMAN PAPILLOMAVIRUS INFECTIONS

(Table 86-1) Decisions regarding the initiation of therapy should be made with the recognition that currently available modes of treatment are not completely effective and some have significant side effects. In addition, treatment may be expensive, and many HPV lesions resolve spontaneously. Frequently used therapies include cryosurgery, application of caustic agents, electrodesiccation, surgical excision, and ablation with a laser. Topical antimetabolites such as 5-fluorouracil have also been used. Both failure and recurrence have been well documented with all of these methods of treatment. Cryosurgery is the initial treatment of choice for condyloma acuminatum. Topically applied podophyllum preparations as well as podofilox may also be used. Various interferon preparations have been employed with modest success in the treatment of respiratory papillomatosis and condyloma acuminatum. A topically applied interferon inducer, imiquimod, is also of benefit in the treatment of condyloma acuminatum. The diagnosis and management of anogenital dysplasias and of internal anogenital warts require special skills and resources, and patients with such lesions should be referred to a qualified specialist.

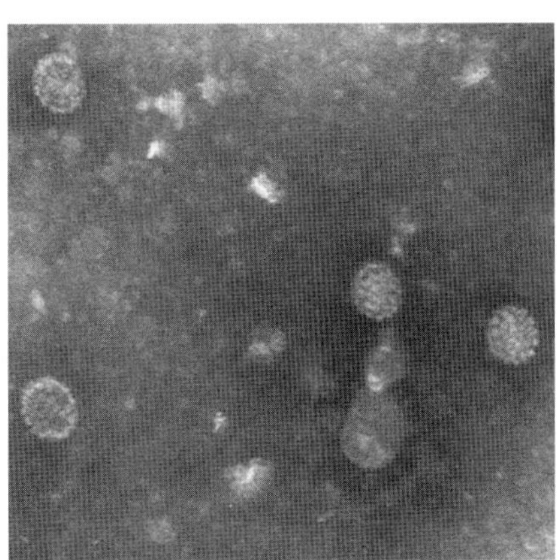

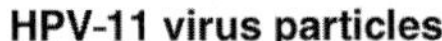

HPV-11 virus particles

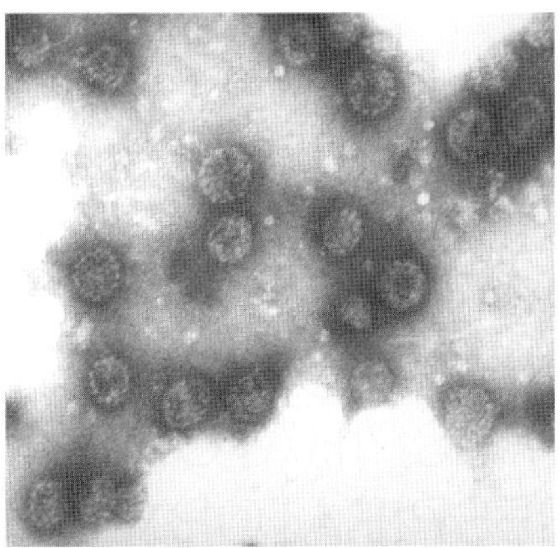

HPV-11 virus-like particles

FIGURE 86-2
HPV-11 virus-like particles produced in insect cells (***right***) are morphologically and antigenically indistinguishable from wild-type HPV-11 particles (***left***). *(Images courtesy of Drs. William Bonnez and Robert C. Rose; with permission.)*

PREVENTION

Recently developed HPV VLP vaccines dramatically reduce rates of infection and disease produced by the HPV types in the vaccines. These products are directed against virus types that cause anogenital tract disease and are derived from expression of the major capsid protein (L1) gene in tissue culture. When expressed using appropriate vectors and tissue culture systems, L1 self-assembles into a VLP that cannot be distinguished morphologically or antigenically from its wild-type counterpart (Fig. 86-2) but that contains no viral nucleic acid. Currently, one quadrivalent product (Gardasil, Merck) containing HPV types 6, 11, 16, and 18 has been licensed in the United States and recommended by the Centers for Disease Control and Prevention for administration to girls and young women 9–26 years of age. Another product (Cervarix, GlaxoSmithKline) contains HPV types 16 and 18 and is likely to be available in the near future. HPV types 6 and 11 cause 90% of anogenital warts, whereas types 16 and 18 are responsible for 70% of cervical cancers. Because 30% of cervical cancers are caused by HPV types not contained in the vaccines, no changes in cervical cancer screening programs are currently recommended. Barrier methods of contraception may also be helpful in preventing transmission of condyloma acuminatum and other anogenital HPV-associated diseases.

TABLE 86-1

TREATMENT OF EXTERNAL, EXOPHYTIC ANOGENITAL WARTS

I. Administered by provider
  A. Cryotherapy with liquid nitrogen or cryoprobe weekly
  B. Podophyllin resin, 10–25% weekly for up to 4 weeks
  C. Trichloroacetic acid or bichloroacetic acid, 80–90% weekly
  D. Surgical excision
  E. Other regimens
    1. Intralesionally administered interferon
    2. Laser surgery
II. Administered by patient
  A. Podofilox, 0.5% solution or gel twice daily for 3 days, followed by 4 days without therapy. This cycle may be repeated four times.
  B. Imiquimod, 5% cream 3 times per week for up to 16 weeks

Source: Modified from Centers for Disease Control and Prevention: MMWR 55(RR-11):1, 2006 *(www.cdc.gov/mmwr/preview/mmwrhtml/rr5511a1/htm).*

FURTHER READINGS

Bonnez W, Reichman RC: Papillomaviruses, in *Principles and Practice of Infectious Diseases*, 6th ed, GL Mandell et al (eds). Churchill Livingstone, New York, 2005, pp 1841–1856

Centers For Disease Control And Prevention: Sexually transmitted diseases treatment guidelines, 2006. MMWR 55(RR-11):1, 2006 (*www.cdc.gov/mmwr/preview/mmwrhtml/rr5511a1.htm*)

Datta SD et al: Human papillomavirus infection and cervical cytology in women screened for cervical cancer in the United States, 2003–2005. Ann Intern Med 148:493, 2008

D'Souza G et al: Case-control study of human papillomavirus and oropharyngeal cancer. N Engl J Med 356:1944, 2007

Dunne EF et al: Prevalence of HPV infection among females in the United States. JAMA 297:813, 2007

Garland SM et al: Quadrivalent vaccine against human papillomavirus to prevent anogenital diseases. N Engl J Med 356:1928, 2007

Harper DM et al: Sustained efficacy up to 4.5 years of a bivalent L1 virus-like particle vaccine against human papillomavirus types 16 and 18: Follow-up from a randomised control trial. Lancet 367:1247, 2006

Luque AE et al: Prevalence of human papillomavirus (HPV) genotypes and relation to cervical cytology among HIV-1 infected women in Rochester, New York. J Infect Dis 194:428, 2006

Markowitz LE et al: Quadrivalent Human Papillomavirus Vaccine: Recommendations of the Advisory Committee on Immunization Practices (ACIP). MMWR Recomm Rep 56:1, 2007

Van Seters M et al: Treatment of vulvar intraepithelial neoplasia with topical imiquimod. N Engl J Med 358:1465, 2008

Villa LL et al: High sustained efficacy of a prophylactic quadrivalent human papillomavirus types 6/11/16/18 L1 virus-like particle vaccine through 5 years of follow-up. Br J Cancer 11:1459, 2006

Winer RL et al: Risk of female human papillomavirus acquisition associated with first male sex partner. J Infect Dis 197:279, 2008

CHAPTER 87

COMMON VIRAL RESPIRATORY INFECTIONS AND SEVERE ACUTE RESPIRATORY SYNDROME (SARS)

Raphael Dolin

GENERAL CONSIDERATIONS

Acute viral respiratory illnesses are among the most common of human diseases, accounting for one-half or more of all acute illnesses. The incidence of acute respiratory disease in the United States is 3–5.6 cases per person per year. The rates are highest among children <1 year old (6.1–8.3 cases per year) and remain high until age 6, when a progressive decrease begins. Adults have 3–4 cases per person per year. Morbidity from acute respiratory illnesses accounts for 30–50% of time lost from work by adults and for 60–80% of time lost from school by children. The use of antibacterial agents to treat viral respiratory infections represents a major source of abuse of that category of drugs.

It has been estimated that two-thirds to three-fourths of cases of acute respiratory illnesses are caused by viruses. More than 200 antigenically distinct viruses from 10 genera have been reported to cause acute respiratory illness, and it is likely that additional agents will be described in the future. The vast majority of these viral infections involve the upper respiratory tract, but lower respiratory tract disease can also develop, particularly in younger age groups, in the elderly, and in certain epidemiologic settings.

The illnesses caused by respiratory viruses traditionally have been divided into multiple distinct syndromes, such as the "common cold," pharyngitis, croup (laryngotracheobronchitis), tracheitis, bronchiolitis, bronchitis, and pneumonia. Each of these general categories of illness has a certain epidemiologic and clinical profile; for example, croup occurs exclusively in very young children and has a characteristic clinical course. Some types of respiratory illness are more likely to be associated with certain viruses (e.g., the common cold with rhinoviruses), whereas others occupy characteristic epidemiologic niches (e.g., adenovirus infections in military recruits). The syndromes most commonly associated with infections with the major respiratory virus groups are summarized in Table 87-1. Most respiratory viruses clearly have the potential to cause more than one type of respiratory illness, and features of several types of illness may be found in the same patient. Moreover, the clinical illnesses induced by these viruses are rarely sufficiently distinctive to permit an etiologic diagnosis on clinical grounds alone, although the epidemiologic setting increases the likelihood that one group of viruses rather than another is involved. In general, laboratory methods must be relied on to establish a specific viral diagnosis.

This chapter reviews viral infections caused by six of the major groups of respiratory viruses: rhinoviruses, coronaviruses, respiratory syncytial viruses, metapneumoviruses, parainfluenza viruses, and adenoviruses. The extraordinary outbreaks of lower respiratory tract disease associated with coronaviruses (severe acute respiratory syndrome, or SARS) in 2002–2003 are also discussed. Influenza viruses, which are a major cause of death as well as morbidity, are reviewed in Chap. 88. Herpesviruses, which occasionally cause pharyngitis and which also cause lower respiratory tract disease in immunosuppressed patients, are reviewed in Chap. 80. Enteroviruses, which account for occasional respiratory illnesses during the summer months, are reviewed in Chap. 94.

RHINOVIRUS INFECTIONS

ETIOLOGIC AGENT

Rhinoviruses are members of the Picornaviridae family, small (15–30 nm) nonenveloped viruses that contain a single-stranded RNA genome. In contrast to other members of the picornavirus family, such as enteroviruses, rhinoviruses are acid-labile and are almost completely inactivated at pH ≤3. Rhinoviruses grow preferentially at 33°–34°C (the temperature of the human nasal passages) rather than at 37°C (the temperature of the lower respiratory tract). Of the 102 recognized serotypes of rhinovirus, 91 use intercellular adhesion molecule 1 (ICAM-1) as a cellular receptor and constitute the "major" receptor group, 10 use the low-density lipoprotein receptor and constitute the "minor" receptor group, and 1 uses decay-accelerating factor.

TABLE 87-1

ILLNESSES ASSOCIATED WITH RESPIRATORY VIRUSES

	FREQUENCY OF RESPIRATORY SYNDROMES		
VIRUS	**MOST FREQUENT**	**OCCASIONAL**	**INFREQUENT**
Rhinoviruses	Common cold	Exacerbation of chronic bronchitis and asthma	Pneumonia in children
Coronaviruses[a]	Common cold	Exacerbation of chronic bronchitis and asthma	Pneumonia and bronchiolitis
Human respiratory syncytial virus	Pneumonia and bronchiolitis in young children	Common cold in adults	Pneumonia in elderly and immunosuppressed patients
Parainfluenza viruses	Croup and lower respiratory tract disease in young children	Pharyngitis and common cold	Tracheobronchitis in adults; lower respiratory tract disease in immunosuppressed patients
Adenoviruses	Common cold and pharyngitis in children	Outbreaks of acute respiratory disease in military recruits[b]	Pneumonia in children; lower respiratory tract and disseminated disease in immunosuppressed patients
Influenza A viruses	Influenza[c]	Pneumonia and excess mortality in high-risk patients	Pneumonia in healthy individuals
Influenza B viruses	Influenza[c]	Rhinitis or pharyngitis alone	Pneumonia
Enteroviruses	Acute undifferentiated febrile illnesses[d]	Rhinitis or pharyngitis alone	Pneumonia
Herpes simplex viruses	Gingivostomatitis in children; pharyngotonsillitis in adults	Tracheitis and pneumonia in immunocompromised patients	Disseminated infection in immunocompromised patients
Human metapneumoviruses[e]	Lower respiratory tract disease in children	Upper respiratory tract illness in adults	Pneumonia in elderly and immunosuppressed patients

[a] SARS-associated coronavirus (SARS-CoV) caused epidemics of pneumonia from November 2002 to July 2003 (see text).
[b] Serotypes 4 and 7.
[c] Fever, cough, myalgia, malaise.
[d] May or may not have a respiratory component.
[e] Newly recognized human metapneumoviruses cause upper and lower respiratory tract illnesses; their relative frequency is under investigation.

EPIDEMIOLOGY

Rhinoviruses are a prominent cause of the common cold and have been detected in up to 50% of common cold–like illnesses by tissue culture and polymerase chain reaction (PCR) techniques. Overall rates of rhinovirus infection are higher among infants and young children and decrease with increasing age. Rhinovirus infections occur throughout the year, with seasonal peaks in early fall and spring in temperate climates. These infections are most often introduced into families by preschool or grade-school children <6 years old. Of initial illnesses in family settings, 25–70% are followed by secondary cases, with the highest attack rates among the youngest siblings at home. Attack rates also increase with family size.

Rhinoviruses appear to spread through direct contact with infected secretions, usually respiratory droplets. In some studies of volunteers, transmission was most efficient by hand-to-hand contact, with subsequent self-inoculation of the conjunctival or nasal mucosa. Other studies demonstrated transmission by large- or small-particle aerosol. Virus can be recovered from plastic surfaces inoculated 1–3 h previously; this observation suggests that environmental surfaces contribute to transmission. In studies of married couples in which neither partner had detectable serum antibody, transmission was associated with prolonged contact (≥122 h) during a 7-day period. Transmission was infrequent unless (1) virus was recoverable from the donor's hands and nasal mucosa, (2) at least 1000 $TCID_{50}$ of virus was present in nasal washes from the donor, and (3) the donor was at least moderately symptomatic with the "cold." Despite anecdotal observations, exposure to cold temperatures, fatigue, and sleep deprivation have not been associated with increased rates of rhinovirus-induced illness in volunteers, although some studies have suggested that psychologically defined "stress" may contribute to development of symptoms.

Infection with rhinoviruses is worldwide in distribution. By adulthood, nearly all individuals have neutralizing antibodies to multiple serotypes, although the prevalence of antibody to any one serotype varies widely. Multiple serotypes circulate simultaneously, and generally no single serotype or group of serotypes has been more prevalent than the others.

PATHOGENESIS

Rhinoviruses infect cells through attachment to specific cellular receptors; as mentioned above, most serotypes attach to ICAM-1, whereas a few use the low-density lipoprotein receptor. Relatively limited information is available on the histopathology and pathogenesis of acute rhinovirus infections in humans. Examination of biopsy specimens obtained during experimentally induced and naturally occurring illness indicates that the nasal mucosa is edematous, is often hyperemic, and—during acute illness—is covered by a mucoid discharge. There is a mild infiltrate with inflammatory cells, including neutrophils, lymphocytes, plasma cells, and eosinophils. Mucus-secreting glands in the submucosa appear hyperactive; the nasal turbinates are engorged, a condition that may lead to obstruction of nearby openings of sinus cavities. Several mediators—e.g., bradykinin; lysylbradykinin; prostaglandins; histamine; interleukins 1β, 6, and 8; and tumor necrosis factor α—have been linked to the development of signs and symptoms in rhinovirus-induced colds.

The incubation period for rhinovirus illness is short, generally 1–2 days. Virus shedding coincides with the onset of illness or may begin shortly before symptoms develop. The mechanisms of immunity to rhinovirus are not well worked out. In some studies, the presence of homotypic antibody has been associated with significantly reduced rates of subsequent infection and illness, but data conflict regarding the relative importance of serum and local antibody in protection from rhinovirus infection.

CLINICAL MANIFESTATIONS

The most common clinical manifestations of rhinovirus infections are those of the common cold. Illness usually begins with rhinorrhea and sneezing accompanied by nasal congestion. The throat is frequently sore, and in some cases sore throat is the initial complaint. Systemic signs and symptoms, such as malaise and headache, are mild or absent, and fever is unusual. Illness generally lasts for 4–9 days and resolves spontaneously without sequelae. In children, bronchitis, bronchiolitis, and bronchopneumonia have been reported; nevertheless, it appears that rhinoviruses are not major causes of lower respiratory tract disease in children. Rhinoviruses may cause exacerbations of asthma and chronic pulmonary disease in adults. The vast majority of rhinovirus infections resolve without sequelae, but complications related to obstruction of the eustachian tubes or sinus ostia, including otitis media or acute sinusitis, can develop. In immunosuppressed patients, particularly bone marrow transplant recipients, severe and even fatal pneumonias have been associated with rhinovirus infections.

DIAGNOSIS

Although rhinoviruses are the most frequently recognized cause of the common cold, similar illnesses are caused by a variety of other viruses, and a specific viral etiologic diagnosis cannot be made on clinical grounds alone. Rather, rhinovirus infection is diagnosed by isolation of the virus from nasal washes or nasal secretions in tissue culture. In practice, this procedure is rarely undertaken because of the benign, self-limited nature of the illness. In most settings, detection of rhinovirus RNA by PCR is more sensitive than that by tissue culture; however, PCR for rhinoviruses is largely a research procedure. Given the many serotypes of rhinovirus, diagnosis by serum antibody tests is currently impractical. Likewise, common laboratory tests, such as white blood cell count and erythrocyte sedimentation rate, are not helpful.

℞ Treatment: RHINOVIRUS INFECTIONS

Because rhinovirus infections are generally mild and self-limited, treatment is not usually necessary. Therapy in the form of first-generation antihistamines and nonsteroidal anti-inflammatory drugs may be beneficial in patients with particularly pronounced symptoms, and an oral decongestant may be added if nasal obstruction is particularly troublesome. Reduction of activity is prudent in instances of significant discomfort or fatigability. Antibacterial agents should be used only if bacterial complications such as otitis media or sinusitis develop. Specific antiviral therapy is not available.

PREVENTION

Intranasal application of interferon sprays has been effective in the prophylaxis of rhinovirus infections but is also associated with local irritation of the nasal mucosa. Studies of the prevention of rhinovirus infection by administration of antibodies to ICAM-1 or by the soluble purified receptors themselves have yielded disappointing results. Experimental vaccines to certain rhinovirus serotypes have been generated, but their usefulness is questionable because of the myriad serotypes and the uncertainty about mechanisms of immunity. Thorough hand washing, environmental decontamination, and protection against autoinoculation may help to reduce rates of transmission of infection.

CORONAVIRUS INFECTIONS, INCLUDING SARS

ETIOLOGIC AGENT

Coronaviruses are pleomorphic, single-stranded RNA viruses that measure 100–160 nm in diameter. The name derives from the crownlike appearance produced by the club-shaped projections that stud the viral envelope. Coronaviruses infect a wide variety of animal species and have been divided into three antigenic groups. Previously recognized coronaviruses that infect humans fell into two of these groups (serogroups I and II), which include human isolates HCoV-229E and HCoV-OC43, respectively. The coronavirus associated with SARS (SARS-CoV) was first believed to represent a novel group but now is considered to be a distantly related member of group II (Fig. 87-1). To date, the SARS-CoV strains that have been fully sequenced have shown only minimal variation.

In general, human coronaviruses have been difficult to cultivate in vitro, and some strains grow only in human tracheal organ cultures rather than in tissue culture. SARS-CoV is an exception whose ready growth in African green monkey kidney (Vero E6) cells greatly facilitates its study.

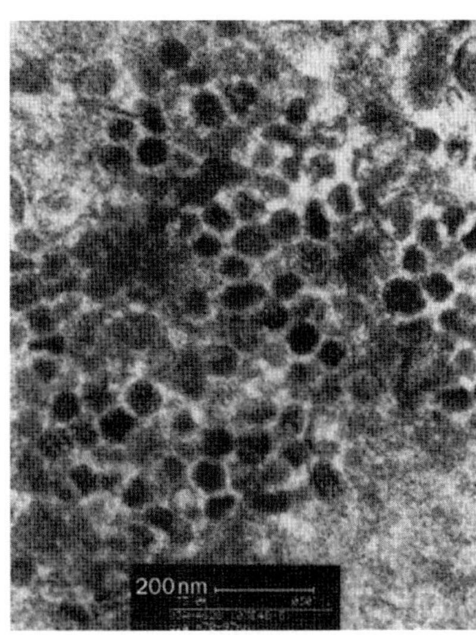

FIGURE 87-1
Electron micrograph of SARS-associated coronavirus (SARS-CoV) isolated in fetal rhesus kidney tissue culture from a lung biopsy sample from a patient with SARS. Viral particles are 55–90 mm in diameter. [*Reprinted with permission from Elsevier (JSM Peiris et al., Lancet 361:1319, 2003).*]

EPIDEMIOLOGY

Generally, human coronavirus infections are present throughout the world. Seroprevalence studies of strains HCoV-229E and HCoV-OC43 have demonstrated that serum antibodies are acquired early in life and increase in prevalence with advancing age, so that >80% of adult populations have antibodies as measured by enzyme-linked immunosorbent assay (ELISA). Overall, coronaviruses account for 10–35% of common colds, depending on the season. Coronavirus infections appear to be particularly prevalent in late fall, winter, and early spring—times when rhinovirus infections are less common.

An extraordinary outbreak of the coronavirus-associated illness known as SARS occurred in 2002–2003. The outbreak apparently began in southern China and eventually resulted in 8096 recognized cases in 28 countries in Asia, Europe, and North and South America; ~90% of cases occurred in China and Hong Kong. The natural reservoir of SARS-CoV appears to be the horseshoe bat, and the outbreak may have originated from human contact with infected semidomesticated animals such as the palm civet. In most cases, however, the infection was transmitted from human to human. Case-fatality rates varied among the outbreaks, with an overall figure of ~9.5%. The disease appeared to be somewhat milder in cases in the United States and was clearly less severe among children. The outbreak ceased in 2003; 17 cases were detected in 2004, mostly in laboratory-associated settings, and no cases were reported in 2005–2006.

The mechanisms of transmission of SARS are incompletely understood. Clusters of cases suggest that spread may occur by both large and small aerosols and perhaps by the fecal-oral route as well. The outbreak of illness in a large apartment complex in Hong Kong suggested that environmental sources, such as sewage or water, may also play a role in transmission. Some ill individuals ("superspreaders") appeared to be hyperinfectious and were capable of transmitting infection to 10–40 contacts, although most infections resulted in spread either to no one or to three or fewer individuals.

PATHOGENESIS

Coronaviruses that cause the common cold (e.g., strains HCoV-229E and HCoV-OC43) infect ciliated epithelial cells in the nasopharynx via the aminopeptidase N receptor (group I) or a sialic acid receptor (group II). Viral replication leads to damage of ciliated cells and induction of chemokines and interleukins, with consequent common-cold symptoms similar to those induced by rhinoviruses.

SARS-CoV infects cells of the respiratory tract via the angiotensin-converting enzyme 2 receptor. The result is a systemic illness in which virus is also found in the bloodstream, in the urine, and (for up to 2 months) in the stool. Virus persists in the respiratory tract for 2–3 weeks, and titers peak ~10 days after the onset of systemic illness. Pulmonary pathology consists of hyaline membrane formation, desquamation of pneumocytes in alveolar spaces, and an interstitial infiltrate made up of lymphocytes and mononuclear cells. Giant cells are frequently seen, and coronavirus particles have been detected in type II pneumocytes. Elevated levels of proinflammatory cytokines and chemokines have been detected in sera from patients with SARS.

CLINICAL MANIFESTATIONS

After an incubation period that generally lasts 2–7 days (range, 1–14 days), SARS usually begins as a systemic illness marked by the onset of fever, which is often accompanied by malaise, headache, and myalgias and is followed in 1–2 days by a nonproductive cough and dyspnea. Approximately 25% of patients have diarrhea. Chest x-rays can show a variety of infiltrates, including patchy areas of consolidation—most frequently in peripheral and lower lung fields—or interstitial infiltrates, which can progress to diffuse involvement (Fig. 87-2).

In severe cases, respiratory function may worsen during the second week of illness and progress to frank adult respiratory distress syndrome (ARDS) accompanied by multiorgan dysfunction. Risk factors for severe disease include an age of >50 years and comorbidities such as cardiovascular disease, diabetes, or hepatitis. Illness in pregnant women may be particularly severe, but SARS-CoV infection appears to be milder in children than in adults.

The clinical features of common colds caused by human coronaviruses are similar to those of illness caused by rhinoviruses. In studies of volunteers, the mean incubation period of colds induced by coronaviruses (3 days) is somewhat longer than that of illness caused by rhinoviruses, and the duration of illness is somewhat shorter (mean, 6–7 days). In some studies, the amount of nasal discharge was greater in colds induced by coronaviruses than in

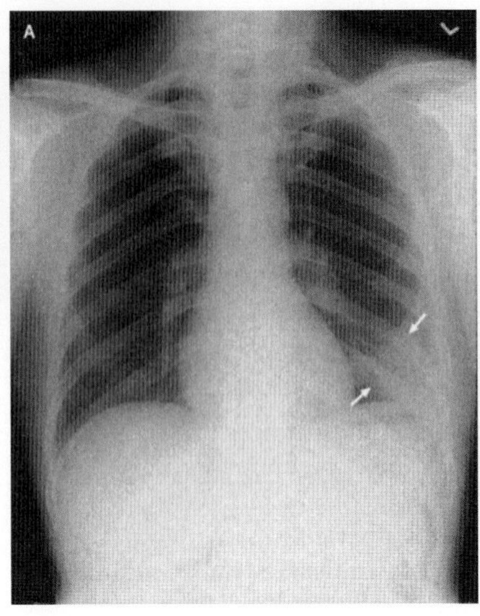

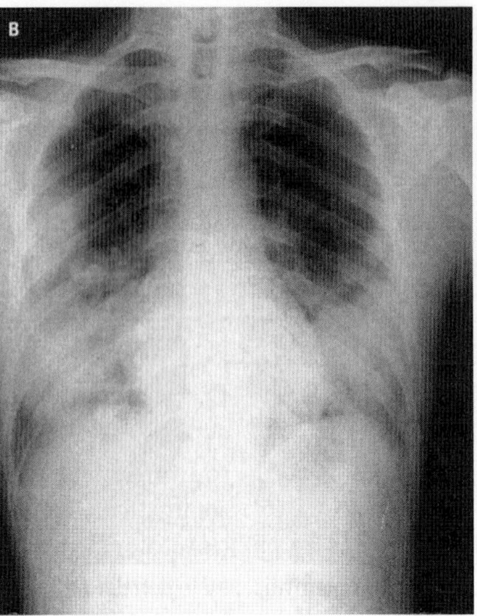

FIGURE 87-2
Chest x-rays of a 46-year-old man with SARS. The left lower lung infiltrate seen initially (***A***) progressed to multiple bilateral opacities (***B***). (*Reprinted with permission from N Lee et al. © 2003 Massachusetts Medical Society.*)

those induced by rhinoviruses. Coronaviruses other than SARS-CoV have been recovered occasionally from infants with pneumonia and from military recruits with lower respiratory tract disease and have been associated with worsening of chronic bronchitis. Two novel coronaviruses, HCoV-NL63 (group I) and HCoV-HKU1 (group II), have recently been isolated from patients hospitalized with acute respiratory illness. Their role as causes of human respiratory disease remains to be determined.

LABORATORY FINDINGS AND DIAGNOSIS

Laboratory abnormalities in SARS include lymphopenia, which is present in ~50% of cases and which mostly affects CD4+ T cells, but also involves CD8+ T cells and NK cells. Total white blood cell counts are normal or slightly low, and thrombocytopenia may develop as the illness progresses. Elevated serum levels of aminotransferases, creatine kinase, and lactate dehydrogenase have been reported.

A rapid diagnosis of SARS-CoV infection can be made by reverse-transcriptase PCR (RT-PCR) of respiratory tract samples and plasma early in illness and of urine and stool later on. SARS-CoV can also be grown from respiratory tract samples by inoculation into Vero E6 tissue culture cells, in which a cytopathic effect is seen within days. RT-PCR appears to be more sensitive than tissue culture, but only around one-third of cases are positive by PCR at initial presentation. Serum antibodies can be detected by ELISA or immunofluorescence, and nearly all patients develop detectable serum antibodies within 28 days after the onset of illness.

Laboratory diagnosis of coronavirus-induced colds is rarely required. Coronaviruses that cause those illnesses are frequently difficult to cultivate in vitro but can be detected in clinical samples by ELISA or immunofluorescence assays or by RT-PCR for viral RNA. These research procedures can be used to detect coronaviruses in unusual clinical settings.

℞ Treatment: CORONAVIRUS INFECTIONS

There is no specific therapy of established efficacy for SARS. Although ribavirin has frequently been used, it has little if any activity against SARS-CoV in vitro, and no beneficial effect on the course of illness has been demonstrated. Because of suggestions that immunopathology may contribute to the disease, glucocorticoids have also been widely used, but their benefit, if any, is likewise unestablished. Supportive care to maintain pulmonary and other organ system functions remains the mainstay of therapy.

The approach to the treatment of common colds caused by coronaviruses is similar to that discussed above for rhinovirus-induced illnesses.

PREVENTION

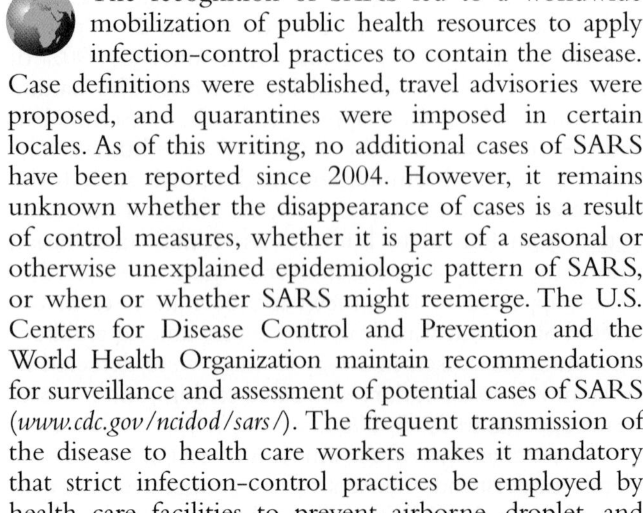

The recognition of SARS led to a worldwide mobilization of public health resources to apply infection-control practices to contain the disease. Case definitions were established, travel advisories were proposed, and quarantines were imposed in certain locales. As of this writing, no additional cases of SARS have been reported since 2004. However, it remains unknown whether the disappearance of cases is a result of control measures, whether it is part of a seasonal or otherwise unexplained epidemiologic pattern of SARS, or when or whether SARS might reemerge. The U.S. Centers for Disease Control and Prevention and the World Health Organization maintain recommendations for surveillance and assessment of potential cases of SARS (*www.cdc.gov/ncidod/sars/*). The frequent transmission of the disease to health care workers makes it mandatory that strict infection-control practices be employed by health care facilities to prevent airborne, droplet, and contact transmission from any suspected cases of SARS.

Health care workers who enter areas in which patients with SARS may be present should don gowns, gloves, and eye and respiratory protective equipment (e.g., an N95 filtering facepiece respirator certified by the National Institute for Occupational Safety and Health).

Vaccines have been developed against several animal coronaviruses but not against known human coronaviruses. The emergence of SARS-CoV has stimulated interest in the development of vaccines against such agents.

HUMAN RESPIRATORY SYNCYTIAL VIRUS INFECTIONS

ETIOLOGIC AGENT

Human respiratory syncytial virus, previously referred to as RSV and now designated HRSV, is a member of the Paramyxoviridae family (genus *Pneumovirus*). HRSV, an enveloped virus ~150–350 nm in diameter, is so named because its replication in vitro leads to the fusion of neighboring cells into large multinucleated syncytia. The single-stranded RNA genome codes for 11 virus-specific proteins. Viral RNA is contained in a helical nucleocapsid surrounded by a lipid envelope bearing two glycoproteins: the G protein, by which the virus attaches to cells, and the F (fusion) protein, which facilitates entry of the virus into the cell by fusing host and viral membranes. HRSV was once considered to be of a single antigenic type, but two distinct subgroups (A and B) and multiple subtypes within each subgroup have now been described. Antigenic diversity is reflected by differences in the G protein, whereas the F protein is highly conserved. Both antigenic groups can circulate simultaneously in outbreaks, although there are typically alternating patterns in which one subgroup predominates over 1- to 2-year periods. Infections with group B viruses may be somewhat milder than those with group A viruses.

EPIDEMIOLOGY

HRSV is a major respiratory pathogen of young children and the foremost cause of lower respiratory disease in infants. Infection with HRSV is seen throughout the world in annual epidemics that occur in late fall, winter, or spring and last up to 5 months. The virus is rarely encountered during the summer. Rates of illness are highest among infants 1–6 months of age, peaking at 2–3 months of age. The attack rates among susceptible infants and children are extraordinarily high, approaching 100% in settings such as day-care centers where large numbers of susceptible infants are present. By age 2, virtually all children will have been infected with HRSV. HRSV accounts for 20–25% of hospital admissions of young infants and children for pneumonia and for up to 75% of cases of bronchiolitis in this age group. It has been estimated that more than half of infants who are at risk will become infected during an HRSV epidemic.

In older children and adults, reinfection with HRSV is frequent but disease is milder than in infancy. A common cold–like syndrome is the illness most commonly associated with HRSV infection in adults. Severe lower respiratory tract disease with pneumonitis can occur in elderly (often institutionalized) adults and in patients with immunocompromising disorders or treatment, including recipients of stem-cell and solid-organ transplants. HRSV is also an important nosocomial pathogen; during an outbreak, it can infect pediatric patients and up to 25–50% of the staff on pediatric wards. The spread of HRSV among families is efficient: up to 40% of siblings may become infected when the virus is introduced into the family setting.

HRSV is transmitted primarily by close contact with contaminated fingers or fomites and by self-inoculation of the conjunctiva or anterior nares. Virus may also be spread by coarse aerosols produced by coughing or sneezing, but it is inefficiently spread by fine-particle aerosols. The incubation period is ~4–6 days, and virus shedding may last for ≥2 weeks in children and for shorter periods in adults. In immunosuppressed patients, shedding can continue for weeks.

PATHOGENESIS

Little is known about the histopathology of minor HRSV infection. Severe bronchiolitis or pneumonia is characterized by necrosis of the bronchiolar epithelium and a peribronchiolar infiltrate of lymphocytes and mononuclear cells. Interalveolar thickening and filling of alveolar spaces with fluid can also be found. The correlates of protective immunity to HRSV are incompletely understood. Because reinfection occurs frequently and is often associated with illness, the immunity that develops after single episodes of infection clearly is not complete or long-lasting. However, the cumulative effect of multiple reinfections is to temper subsequent disease and to provide some temporary measure of protection against infection. Studies of experimentally induced disease in healthy volunteers indicate that the presence of nasal IgA neutralizing antibody correlates more closely with protection than does the presence of serum antibody. Studies in infants, however, suggest that maternally acquired antibody provides some protection from lower respiratory tract disease, although illness can be severe even in infants who have moderate levels of maternally derived serum antibody. The relatively severe disease observed in immunosuppressed patients and experimental animal models indicates that cell-mediated immunity is an important mechanism of host defense against HRSV. Evidence suggests that class I MHC-restricted cytotoxic T cells may be particularly important in this regard.

CLINICAL MANIFESTATIONS

HRSV infection leads to a wide spectrum of respiratory illnesses. In infants, 25–40% of infections result in lower respiratory tract involvement, including pneumonia, bronchiolitis, and tracheobronchitis. In this age group, illness begins most frequently with rhinorrhea, low-grade fever, and mild systemic symptoms, often accompanied by cough and wheezing. Most patients recover gradually over 1–2 weeks. In more severe illness, tachypnea and dyspnea develop, and eventually frank hypoxia, cyanosis, and apnea can ensue. Physical examination may reveal diffuse wheezing, rhonchi, and rales. Chest radiography shows hyperexpansion, peribronchial thickening, and variable infiltrates ranging from diffuse interstitial infiltrates to segmental or lobar consolidation. Illness may be particularly severe in children born prematurely and in those with congenital cardiac disease, bronchopulmonary dysplasia, nephrotic syndrome, or immunosuppression. One study documented a 37% mortality rate among infants with HRSV pneumonia and congenital cardiac disease.

In adults, the most common symptoms of HRSV infection are those of the common cold, with rhinorrhea, sore throat, and cough. Illness is occasionally associated with moderate systemic symptoms such as malaise, headache, and fever. HRSV has also been reported to cause lower respiratory tract disease with fever in adults, including severe pneumonia in the elderly—particularly in nursing-home residents, among whom its impact can rival that of influenza. HRSV pneumonia can be a significant cause of morbidity and death among patients undergoing stem cell and solid-organ transplantation, where case-fatality rates of 20–80% have been reported. Sinusitis, otitis media, and worsening of chronic obstructive and reactive airway disease have also been associated with HRSV infection.

LABORATORY FINDINGS AND DIAGNOSIS

The diagnosis of HRSV infection can be suspected on the basis of a suggestive epidemiologic setting—that is, severe illness among infants during an outbreak of HRSV in the community. Infections in older children and adults cannot be differentiated with certainty from those caused by other respiratory viruses. The specific diagnosis is established by detection of HRSV in respiratory secretions, such as sputum, throat swabs, or nasopharyngeal washes. Virus can be isolated in tissue culture and is identified specifically by immunofluorescence, ELISA, or other immunologic techniques. Rapid viral diagnosis is available by immunofluorescence techniques or ELISA of nasopharyngeal washes, aspirates, and (less satisfactorily) nasopharyngeal swabs. With specimens from children, these techniques have sensitivities and specificities of 80–95%; they are somewhat less sensitive with specimens from adults. Serologic diagnosis may be made by comparison of acute- and convalescent-phase serum specimens by ELISA or by neutralization or complement-fixation tests. These tests may be useful in older children and adults but are less sensitive in children <4 months of age.

Treatment: ℞ HUMAN RESPIRATORY SYNCYTIAL VIRUS INFECTIONS

Treatment of upper respiratory tract HRSV infection is aimed primarily at the alleviation of symptoms and is similar to that for other viral infections of the upper respiratory tract. For lower respiratory tract infections, respiratory therapy, including hydration, suctioning of secretions, and administration of humidified oxygen and antibronchospastic agents, is given as needed. In severe hypoxia, intubation and ventilatory assistance may be required. Studies of infants with HRSV infection who were given aerosolized ribavirin, a nucleoside analogue active in vitro against HRSV, demonstrated a modest beneficial effect on the resolution of lower respiratory tract illness, including alleviation of blood-gas abnormalities. The American Academy of Pediatrics recommends that treatment with aerosolized ribavirin "may be considered" for infants who are severely ill or who are at high risk for complications of HRSV infection; included are premature infants and those with bronchopulmonary dysplasia, congenital heart disease, or immunosuppression. The efficacy of ribavirin against HRSV pneumonia in older children and adults, including those with immunosuppression, has not been established. Administration of standard immunoglobulin, immunoglobulin with high titers of antibody to HRSV (RSVIg), or chimeric mouse-human monoclonal IgG antibody to HRSV (palivizumab) has not been found to be beneficial in the treatment of HRSV pneumonia. Combined therapy with aerosolized ribavirin and palivizumab is being evaluated in immunosuppressed patients with HRSV pneumonia.

PREVENTION

Monthly administration of RSVIg or palivizumab has been approved as prophylaxis against HRSV for children <2 years of age who have bronchopulmonary dysplasia or cyanotic heart disease or who were born prematurely. Considerable interest exists in the development of vaccines against HRSV. Inactivated whole-virus vaccines have been ineffective; in one study, they actually potentiated disease in infants. Other approaches include immunization with purified F and G surface glycoproteins of HRSV or generation of stable, live attenuated virus vaccines. In settings such as pediatric wards where rates of transmission are high, barrier methods for the protection of hands and conjunctivae may be useful in reducing the spread of virus.

HUMAN METAPNEUMOVIRUS INFECTIONS

ETIOLOGIC AGENT

Human metapneumovirus (HMPV) is a recently described viral respiratory pathogen that has been assigned to the Paramyxoviridae family (genus *Metapneumovirus*). Its morphology and genomic organization are similar to those of avian metapneumoviruses, which are recognized respiratory pathogens of turkeys. HMPV particles may be spherical, filamentous, or pleomorphic in shape and measure 150–600 nm in diameter. Particles contain 15-nm projections from the surface that are similar in appearance to those of other Paramyxoviridae. The single-stranded RNA genome codes for nine proteins that, except for the absence of nonstructural proteins, generally correspond to those of HRSV. There is only one antigenic type; two closely related genetic subgroups (A and B) have been described.

EPIDEMIOLOGY

HMPV infections are worldwide in distribution, are most frequent during the winter, and occur early in life, so that serum antibodies to the virus are present in nearly all children by the age of 5. HMPV infections have been detected in older age groups, including elderly adults, and in both immunocompetent and immunosuppressed hosts. To date, studies indicate that HMPV infections account for 4% of respiratory tract illnesses requiring hospitalization of children, 12% of outpatient lower respiratory illnesses, and 2–4% of acute respiratory illnesses in ambulatory adults and elderly patients. HMPV has been detected in a few cases of SARS, but its role (if any) in these illnesses has not been established. Assessment of the overall significance of HMPV infections awaits the conduct of large-scale epidemiologic studies.

CLINICAL MANIFESTATIONS

The spectrum of clinical illnesses associated with HMPV is similar to that associated with HRSV and includes both upper and lower respiratory tract illnesses, such as bronchiolitis, croup, and pneumonia. Reinfection with HMPV is common in older children and adults and has manifestations ranging from subclinical infections to common cold syndromes and occasionally pneumonia, which is seen primarily in elderly patients and those with cardiopulmonary diseases. Serious HMPV infections occur in immunocompromised patients, including those with neoplasia and stem-cell transplants.

DIAGNOSIS

HMPV can be detected in nasal aspirates and respiratory secretions by PCR or by growth in rhesus monkey kidney (LLC-MK2) tissue cultures. Rapid immunodetection methods are under development. A serologic diagnosis can be made by ELISA, which uses HMPV-infected tissue culture lysates as sources of antigens.

Rx Treatment: HUMAN METAPNEUMOVIRUS INFECTIONS

Treatment for HMPV infections is primarily supportive and symptom-based. Ribavirin and RSVIg are both active against HMPV in vitro, but their efficacy in vivo is unknown.

PREVENTION

Vaccines against HMPV are in the early stages of development.

PARAINFLUENZA VIRUS INFECTIONS

ETIOLOGIC AGENT

Parainfluenza viruses belong to the Paramyxoviridae family (genera *Respirovirus* and *Rubulavirus*). They are 150–200 nm in diameter, are enveloped, and contain a single-stranded RNA genome. The envelope is studded with two glycoproteins: one possesses both hemagglutinin and neuraminidase activity, and the other contains fusion activity. The viral RNA genome is enclosed in a helical nucleocapsid and codes for six structural and several accessory proteins. There are four distinct serotypes of parainfluenza virus, all of which share certain antigens with other members of the Paramyxoviridae family, including mumps and Newcastle disease viruses.

EPIDEMIOLOGY

Parainfluenza viruses are distributed throughout the world; infection with type 4 (subtypes 4A and 4B) has been reported less widely, probably because type 4 is more difficult to grow in tissue culture. Infection is acquired in early childhood, so that by 5 years of age most children have antibodies to serotypes 1, 2, and 3. Types 1 and 2 cause epidemics during the fall, often occurring in an alternate-year pattern. Type 3 infection has been detected during all seasons of the year, but epidemics have occurred annually in the spring.

The contribution of parainfluenza infections to respiratory disease varies with both the location and the year. In studies conducted in the United States, parainfluenza virus infections have accounted for 4.3–22% of respiratory illnesses in children. In adults, parainfluenza infections are generally mild and account for <10% of respiratory illnesses. The major importance of parainfluenza viruses is as a cause of respiratory illness in young children, in whom they rank second only to HRSV as causes of lower respiratory tract illness. Parainfluenza virus type 1 is the most frequent cause of croup (laryngotracheobronchitis) in children, whereas serotype 2 causes similar, although generally less severe, disease. Type 3 is an important cause of bronchiolitis and pneumonia in infants, whereas illnesses associated with type 4 have generally been mild. Unlike types 1 and 2, type 3 frequently causes illness during the first month of life, when passively acquired maternal antibody is still present. Parainfluenza viruses are spread through infected respiratory secretions, primarily by person-to-person contact and/or by large droplets. The incubation period has varied from 3 to 6 days in experimental infections but may be somewhat shorter for naturally occurring disease in children.

PATHOGENESIS

Immunity to parainfluenza viruses is incompletely understood, but evidence suggests that immunity to infections with serotypes 1 and 2 is mediated by local IgA antibodies in the respiratory tract. Passively acquired serum neutralizing antibodies also confer some protection against infection with types 1, 2, and (to a lesser degree) 3. Studies in experimental animal models and in immunosuppressed patients suggest that T-cell–mediated immunity may also be important in parainfluenza virus infections.

CLINICAL MANIFESTATIONS

Parainfluenza virus infections occur most frequently among children, in whom initial infection with serotype 1, 2, or 3 is associated with an acute febrile illness 50–80%

of the time. Children may present with coryza, sore throat, hoarseness, and cough that may or may not be croupy. In severe croup, fever persists, with worsening coryza and sore throat. A brassy or barking cough may progress to frank stridor. Most children recover over the next 1 or 2 days, although progressive airway obstruction and hypoxia ensue occasionally. If bronchiolitis or pneumonia develops, progressive cough accompanied by wheezing, tachypnea, and intercostal retractions may occur. In this setting, sputum production increases modestly. Physical examination shows nasopharyngeal discharge and oropharyngeal injection, along with rhonchi, wheezes, or coarse breath sounds. Chest x-rays can show air trapping and occasionally interstitial infiltrates.

In older children and adults, parainfluenza infections tend to be milder, presenting most frequently as a common cold or as hoarseness, with or without cough. Lower respiratory tract involvement in older children and adults is uncommon, but tracheobronchitis in adults has been reported. Severe, prolonged, and even fatal parainfluenza infection has been reported in children and adults with severe immunosuppression, including stem-cell and solid-organ transplant recipients.

LABORATORY FINDINGS AND DIAGNOSIS

The clinical syndromes caused by parainfluenza viruses (with the possible exception of croup in young children) are not sufficiently distinctive to be diagnosed on clinical grounds alone. A specific diagnosis is established by detection of virus in respiratory tract secretions, throat swabs, or nasopharyngeal washings. Viral growth in tissue culture is detected either by hemagglutination or by a cytopathic effect. Rapid viral diagnosis may be made by identification of parainfluenza antigens in exfoliated cells from the respiratory tract with immunofluorescence or ELISA, although these techniques appear to be less sensitive than tissue culture. Highly specific and sensitive PCR assays have also been developed. Serologic diagnosis can be established by hemagglutination inhibition, complement-fixation, or neutralization tests of acute- and convalescent-phase specimens. However, since frequent heterotypic responses occur among the parainfluenza serotypes, the serotype causing illness often cannot be identified by serologic techniques alone.

Acute epiglottitis caused by *Haemophilus influenzae* type b must be differentiated from viral croup. Influenza A virus is also a common cause of croup during epidemic periods.

℞ Treatment: PARAINFLUENZA VIRUS INFECTIONS

For upper respiratory tract illness, symptoms can be treated as discussed for other viral respiratory tract illnesses. If complications such as sinusitis, otitis, or superimposed bacterial bronchitis develop, appropriate antibacterial antibiotics should be administered. Mild cases of croup should be treated with bed rest and moist air generated by vaporizers. More severe cases require hospitalization and close observation for the development of respiratory distress. If acute respiratory distress develops, humidified oxygen and intermittent racemic epinephrine are usually administered. Aerosolized or systemically administered glucocorticoids are beneficial; the latter have a more profound effect. No specific antiviral therapy is available, although ribavirin is active against parainfluenza viruses in vitro and anecdotal reports describe its use clinically, particularly in immunosuppressed patients.

PREVENTION

Vaccines against parainfluenza viruses are under development.

ADENOVIRUS INFECTIONS

ETIOLOGIC AGENT

Adenoviruses are complex DNA viruses that measure 70–80 nm in diameter. Human adenoviruses belong to the genus *Mastadenovirus*, which includes 51 serotypes. Adenoviruses have a characteristic morphology consisting of an icosahedral shell composed of 20 equilateral triangular faces and 12 vertices. The protein coat (capsid) consists of hexon subunits with group-specific and type-specific antigenic determinants and penton subunits at each vertex primarily containing group-specific antigens. A fiber with a knob at the end projects from each penton; this fiber contains type-specific and some group-specific antigens. Human adenoviruses have been divided into six subgenera (A through F) on the basis of the homology of DNA genomes and other properties. The adenovirus genome is a linear double-stranded DNA that codes for structural and nonstructural polypeptides. The replicative cycle of adenovirus may result either in lytic infection of cells or in the establishment of a latent infection (primarily involving lymphoid cells). Some adenovirus types can induce oncogenic transformation, and tumor formation has been observed in rodents; however, despite intensive investigation, adenoviruses have not been associated with tumors in humans.

EPIDEMIOLOGY

Adenovirus infections most frequently affect infants and children. Infections occur throughout the year but are most common from fall to spring. Adenoviruses account for ~10% of acute respiratory infections in children but for <2% of respiratory illnesses in civilian adults. Nearly 100% of adults have serum antibody to multiple serotypes—a finding indicating that infection is common in childhood. Types 1, 2, 3, and 5 are the most frequent isolates from children. Certain adenovirus serotypes—particularly 4 and 7 but also 3, 14, and 21—are associated with outbreaks of acute respiratory disease in military recruits in winter and spring. Adenovirus infection can be transmitted by inhalation of aerosolized virus, by inoculation of virus into conjunctival sacs, and probably by the fecal-oral route as well. Type-specific antibody generally develops after infection and is associated with protection, albeit incomplete, against infection with the same serotype.

CLINICAL MANIFESTATIONS

In children, adenoviruses cause a variety of clinical syndromes. The most common is an acute upper respiratory tract infection, with prominent rhinitis. On occasion, lower respiratory tract disease, including bronchiolitis and pneumonia, also develops. Adenoviruses, particularly types 3 and 7, cause pharyngoconjunctival fever, a characteristic acute febrile illness of children that occurs in outbreaks, most often in summer camps. The syndrome is marked by bilateral conjunctivitis in which the bulbar and palpebral conjunctivae have a granular appearance. Low-grade fever is frequently present for the first 3 to 5 days, and rhinitis, sore throat, and cervical adenopathy develop. The illness generally lasts for 1–2 weeks and resolves spontaneously. Febrile pharyngitis without conjunctivitis has also been associated with adenovirus infection. Adenoviruses have been isolated from cases of whooping cough with or without *Bordetella pertussis*; the significance of adenovirus in that disease is unknown.

In adults, the most frequently reported illness has been acute respiratory disease caused by adenovirus types 4 and 7 in military recruits. This illness is marked by a prominent sore throat and the gradual onset of fever, which often reaches 39°C (102.2°F) on the second or third day of illness. Cough is almost always present, and coryza and regional lymphadenopathy are frequently seen. Physical examination may show pharyngeal edema, injection, and tonsillar enlargement with little or no exudate. If pneumonia has developed, auscultation and x-ray of the chest may indicate areas of patchy infiltration.

Adenoviruses have been associated with a number of non–respiratory tract diseases, including acute diarrheal illness caused by types 40 and 41 in young children and hemorrhagic cystitis caused by types 11 and 21. Epidemic keratoconjunctivitis, caused most frequently by types 8, 19, and 37, has been associated with contaminated common sources such as ophthalmic solutions and roller towels. Adenoviruses have also been implicated in disseminated disease and pneumonia in immunosuppressed patients, including recipients of solid-organ or stem-cell transplants. In stem-cell transplant recipients, adenovirus infections have manifested as pneumonia, hepatitis, nephritis, colitis, encephalitis, and hemorrhagic cystitis. In solid-organ transplant recipients, adenovirus infection may involve the organ transplanted (e.g., hepatitis in liver transplants, nephritis in renal transplants) but can disseminate to other organs as well. In patients with AIDS, high-numbered and intermediate adenovirus serotypes have been isolated, usually in the setting of low CD4+ T-cell counts, but their isolation often has not been clearly linked to disease manifestations. Adenovirus nucleic acids have been detected in myocardial cells from patients with "idiopathic" myocardiopathies, and adenoviruses have been suggested as causative agents in some cases.

LABORATORY FINDINGS AND DIAGNOSIS

Adenovirus infection should be suspected in the epidemiologic setting of acute respiratory disease in military recruits and in certain of the clinical syndromes (such as pharyngoconjunctival fever or epidemic keratoconjunctivitis) in which outbreaks of characteristic illnesses occur. In most cases, however, illnesses caused by adenovirus infection cannot be differentiated from those caused by a number of other viral respiratory agents and *Mycoplasma pneumoniae*. A definitive diagnosis of adenovirus infection is established by detection of the virus in tissue culture (as evidenced by cytopathic changes) and by specific identification with immunofluorescence or other immunologic techniques. Rapid viral diagnosis can be established by immunofluorescence or ELISA of nasopharyngeal aspirates, conjunctival or respiratory secretions, urine, or stool. Highly sensitive and specific PCR assays and nucleic acid hybridization are also available. Adenovirus types 40 and 41, which have been associated with diarrheal disease in children, require special tissue-culture cells for isolation, and these serotypes are most commonly detected by direct ELISA of stool. Serum antibody rises can be demonstrated by complement-fixation or neutralization tests, ELISA, radioimmunoassay, or (for those adenoviruses that hemagglutinate red cells) hemagglutination inhibition tests.

℞ Treatment: ADENOVIRUS INFECTIONS

Only symptom-based treatment and supportive therapy are available for adenovirus infections, and clinically useful antiviral therapy has not been established. Ribavirin and cidofovir have activity in vitro against certain adenoviruses. Retrospective studies and anecdotes describe the use of these agents in disseminated adenovirus infections, but definitive efficacy data from controlled studies are not available.

PREVENTION

Live vaccines have been developed against adenovirus types 4 and 7 and have been used to control illness among military recruits. These vaccines consist of live, unattenuated virus administered in enteric-coated capsules. Infection of the gastrointestinal tract with types 4 and 7 does not cause disease but stimulates local and systemic antibodies that are protective against subsequent acute respiratory disease due to those serotypes. This vaccine has not been produced since 1999, and outbreaks of acute respiratory illness caused by adenovirus types 4 and 7 have emerged again among military recruits. Therefore, a program to redevelop type 4 and 7 vaccines is underway. Adenoviruses are also being studied as live-virus vectors for the delivery of vaccine antigens and for gene therapy.

FURTHER READINGS

American Academy of Pediatrics: Diagnosis and management of bronchiolitis. Pediatrics 118:1774, 2006

Chanock RM et al: Serious respiratory tract disease caused by respiratory syncytial virus: Prospects for improved therapy and effective immunization. Pediatrics 90:137, 1992

Christian MD et al: Severe acute respiratory syndrome. Clin Infect Dis 38:1420, 2004

Graham BS et al: Respiratory syncytial virus immunobiology and pathogenesis. Virology 297:1, 2002

GWALTNEY JM: Rhinoviruses, in *Principles and Practice of Infectious Diseases*, 6th ed, GF Mandell et al (eds). Philadelphia, Elsevier, 2005, pp 2185–2193

JEFFERSON T et al: Physical interventions to interrupt or reduce the spread of respiratory viruses: Systematic review. BMJ 336:77, 2008

LEE N et al: A major outbreak of severe acute respiratory syndrome in Hong Kong. N Engl J Med 348:1986, 2003

PEIRIS JS et al: Severe acute respiratory syndrome. Nat Med 10:S88, 2004

PERET T et al: Characterization of human metapneumoviruses isolated from patients in North America. J Infect Dis 185:1660, 2002

STOCKTON J et al: Human metapneumovirus as a cause of community-acquired respiratory illness. Emerg Infect Dis 8:897, 2002

TANSEY CM et al: One-year outcomes and health care utilization in survivors of severe acute respiratory syndrome. Arch Intern Med 167:1312, 2007

WRIGHT PF: Parainfluenza viruses, in *Viral Infections of the Respiratory Tract*, R Dolin, PF Wright (eds). New York, Marcel Dekker, 1999

CHAPTER 88

INFLUENZA

Raphael Dolin

DEFINITION

Influenza is an acute respiratory illness caused by infection with influenza viruses. The illness affects the upper and/or lower respiratory tract and is often accompanied by systemic signs and symptoms such as fever, headache, myalgia, and weakness. Outbreaks of illness of variable extent and severity occur nearly every winter. Such outbreaks result in significant morbidity in the general population and in increased mortality rates among certain high-risk patients, mainly as a result of pulmonary complications.

ETIOLOGIC AGENT

Influenza viruses are members of the Orthomyxoviridae family, of which influenza A, B, and C viruses constitute three separate genera. The designation of influenza viruses as type A, B, or C is based on antigenic characteristics of the nucleoprotein (NP) and matrix (M) protein antigens. Influenza A viruses are further subdivided (subtyped) on the basis of the surface hemagglutinin (H) and neuraminidase (N) antigens (see below); individual strains are designated according to the site of origin, isolate number, year of isolation, and subtype—for example, influenza A/Hiroshima/52/2005 (H3N2). Influenza A has 16 distinct H subtypes and 9 distinct N subtypes, of which only H1, H2, H3, N1, and N2 have been associated with epidemics of disease in humans. Influenza B and C viruses are similarly designated, but H and N antigens from these viruses do not receive subtype designations, since intratypic variations in influenza B antigens are less extensive than those in influenza A viruses and may not occur with influenza C virus.

Influenza A and B viruses are major human pathogens and the most extensively studied of the Orthomyxoviridae. Type A and type B viruses are morphologically similar. The virions are irregularly shaped spherical particles, measure 80–120 nm in diameter, and have a lipid envelope from the surface of which the H and N glycoproteins project (Fig. 88-1). The hemagglutinin is the site by which the virus binds to sialic acid cell receptors, whereas the neuraminidase degrades the receptor and plays a role in the release of the virus from infected cells after replication has taken place. Influenza viruses enter cells by receptor-mediated endocytosis, forming a virus-containing endosome. The viral hemagglutinin mediates fusion of the endosomal membrane with the virus envelope, and viral nucleocapsids are subsequently released into the cytoplasm. Immune responses to the H antigen are the major determinants of protection against infection with influenza virus, whereas those to the N antigen limit viral spread and contribute to reduction of the infection. The lipid envelope of influenza A virus also contains the M proteins M1 and M2, which are involved in stabilization of the lipid envelope and in virus assembly. The virion also contains the NP antigen, which is associated with the

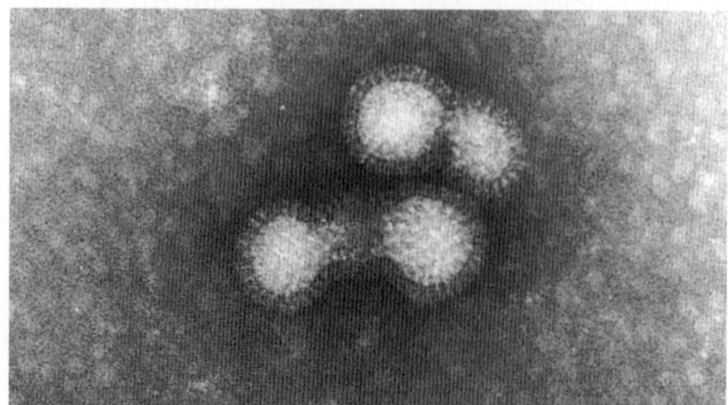

FIGURE 88-1
An electron micrograph of influenza A virus (×40,000).

TABLE 88-1

EMERGENCE OF ANTIGENIC SUBTYPES OF INFLUENZA A VIRUS ASSOCIATED WITH PANDEMIC OR EPIDEMIC DISEASE

YEARS	SUBTYPE	EXTENT OF OUTBREAK
1889–90	H2N8[a]	Severe pandemic
1900–03	H3N8[a]	?Moderate epidemic
1918–19	H1N1[b] (formerly HswN1)	Severe pandemic
1933–35	H1N1[b] (formerly H0N1)	Mild epidemic
1946–47	H1N1	Mild epidemic
1957–58	H2N2	Severe pandemic
1968–69	H3N2	Moderate pandemic
1977–78[c]	H1N1	Mild pandemic

[a]As determined by retrospective serologic survey of individuals alive during those years ("seroarcheology").
[b]Hemagglutinins formerly designated as Hsw and H0 are now classified as variants of H1.
[c]From this time until 2006–2007, viruses of the H1N1 and H3N2 subtypes circulated either in alternating years or concurrently. See text for a brief discussion of the ongoing pandemic of influenza A/H1N1 (swine influenza).

viral genome, as well as three polymerase (P) proteins that are essential for transcription and synthesis of viral RNA. Two nonstructural proteins function as an interferon antagonist and posttranscriptional regulator (NS1) and a nuclear export factor (NS2 or NEP).

The genomes of influenza A and B viruses consist of eight single-stranded RNA segments, which code for the structural and nonstructural proteins. Because the genome is segmented, the opportunity for gene reassortment during infection is high; reassortment often occurs during infection of cells with more than one influenza A virus.

EPIDEMIOLOGY

Influenza outbreaks are recorded virtually every year, although their extent and severity vary widely. Localized outbreaks take place at variable intervals, usually every 1–3 years. Global pandemics have occurred at variable intervals, but much less frequently than interpandemic outbreaks (Table 88-1). Apart from the recently declared pandemic of influenza A/H1N1 (swine influenza; see below), the most recent pandemic occurred in 1977—some 30 years ago as of this writing; because of this relatively long interval, concern exists that the next pandemic may be imminent.

Influenza A Virus

Antigenic Variation and Influenza Outbreaks

The most extensive and severe outbreaks are caused by influenza A viruses, in part because of the remarkable propensity of the H and N antigens of these viruses to undergo periodic antigenic variation. Major antigenic variations, called *antigenic shifts*, may be associated with pandemics and are restricted to influenza A viruses. Minor variations are called *antigenic drifts*. These types of antigenic variation may involve the hemagglutinin alone or both the hemagglutinin and the neuraminidase. An example of an antigenic shift involving both the hemagglutinin and the neuraminidase is that of 1957, when the predominant influenza A virus subtype shifted from H1N1 to H2N2; this shift resulted in a severe pandemic, with an estimated 70,000 excess deaths (i.e., deaths in excess of the number expected without an influenza epidemic) in the United States alone. In 1968, an antigenic shift involving only the hemagglutinin occurred (H2N2 to H3N2); the subsequent pandemic was less severe than that of 1957. In 1977, an H1N1 virus emerged and caused a pandemic that primarily affected younger individuals (i.e., those born after 1957). As can be seen in Table 88-1, H1N1 viruses circulated from 1918 to 1956; thus individuals born before 1957 would be expected to have some degree of immunity to H1N1 viruses. During most outbreaks of influenza A, a single subtype has circulated at a time. However, since 1977, H1N1 and H3N2 viruses have circulated simultaneously, resulting in outbreaks of varying severity. In some outbreaks, influenza B viruses have also circulated simultaneously with influenza A viruses.

Avian Influenza

In 1997, human cases of influenza caused by avian influenza viruses (A/H5N1) were detected in Hong Kong during an extensive outbreak of influenza in poultry. Between that time and January 2007, 261 cases of avian influenza in humans were reported in 10 countries in Asia and the Middle East. Nearly all of these cases were associated with contact with infected poultry. Efficient person-to-person transmission has not been observed to date. Mortality rates have been high (60%), and clinical manifestations have differed somewhat from those associated with "typical" outbreaks of influenza (see below). Transmission of avian influenza A/H7N7 viruses from infected poultry to humans has been observed in the Netherlands, resulting predominantly in cases of conjunctivitis and some respiratory illnesses. Infection with avian A/H9N2 viruses along with mild respiratory illness has been reported in children in Hong Kong. Because of the absence of widespread immunity to the H5, H7, and H9 viruses, concern has been raised that avian-to-human transmission may be the basis for the emergence of pandemic strains.

The origin of actual pandemic influenza A virus strains has now been partially elucidated with molecular virologic techniques. It appears that the pandemic strains of 1957 and 1968 resulted from a genetic reassortment between human viruses and avian viruses with novel surface glycoproteins (H2N2, H3). The influenza virus responsible for the most severe pandemic of modern times (1918–1919) appears to have represented an adaptation of an avian virus to efficient infection of humans. Close molecular surveillance of the avian viruses currently infecting humans is being conducted to provide early detection of possible pandemic strains.

Features of Pandemic and Interpandemic Influenza A

Pandemics provide the most dramatic evidence of the impact of influenza A. However, illnesses occurring between pandemics (interpandemic disease) account for extensive mortality and morbidity, albeit over a longer period. In the United States, influenza was associated with at least 19,000 excess deaths per season in 1976–1990 and with 36,000 excess deaths per season in 1990–1999. On average, there were 226,000 influenza-associated hospitalizations per year in this country in 1979–2001.

Influenza A viruses that circulate between pandemics demonstrate antigenic drifts in the H antigen. These antigenic drifts result from point mutations involving the RNA segment that codes for the hemagglutinin, which occur most frequently in five hypervariable regions. Epidemiologically significant strains—that is, those with the potential to cause widespread outbreaks—exhibit changes in amino acids in at least two of the major antigenic sites in the hemagglutinin molecule. Since two point mutations are unlikely to occur simultaneously, it is believed that antigenic drifts result from point mutations occurring sequentially during the spread of virus from person to person. Antigenic drifts have been reported nearly annually since 1977 for H1N1 viruses and since 1968 for H3N2 viruses.

Influenza A epidemics begin abruptly, peak over a 2- to 3-week period, generally last for 2–3 months, and often subside almost as rapidly as they began. The first indication of influenza activity in a community is an increase in the number of children with febrile respiratory illnesses who present for medical attention. This increase is followed by increases in rates of influenza-like illnesses among adults and eventually by an increase in hospital admissions for patients with pneumonia, worsening of congestive heart failure, and exacerbations of chronic pulmonary disease. Rates of absence from work and school also rise at this time. An increase in the number of deaths caused by pneumonia and influenza is generally a late observation in an outbreak. Attack rates have been highly variable from outbreak to outbreak but most commonly are in the range of 10–20% of the general population. During the pandemic of 1957, it was estimated that the attack rate of clinical influenza exceeded 50% in urban populations and that an additional 25% or more of individuals in these populations may have been subclinically infected with influenza A virus. Among institutionalized populations and in semiclosed settings with many susceptible individuals, even higher attack rates have been reported.

Epidemics of influenza A occur almost exclusively during the winter months in the temperate zones of the northern and southern hemispheres. In those locations, it is highly unusual to detect influenza A virus at other times, although rises in serum antibody titer or even outbreaks have been noted rarely during warm-weather months. In contrast, influenza virus infections occur throughout the year in the tropics. Where or how influenza A virus persists between outbreaks in temperate zones is unknown. It is possible that influenza A viruses are maintained in the human population on a worldwide basis by person-to-person transmission and that large population clusters support a low level of interepidemic transmission. Alternatively, human strains may persist in animal reservoirs. Convincing evidence to support either explanation is not available. In the modern era, rapid transportation may contribute to the transmission of viruses among widespread geographic locales.

The factors that result in the inception and termination of outbreaks of influenza A are incompletely understood. A major determinant of the extent and severity of an outbreak is the level of immunity in the population at risk. With the emergence of an antigenically novel influenza virus to which little or no immunity is present in a community, extensive outbreaks may occur. When the absence of immunity is worldwide, epidemic disease may spread around the globe, resulting in a pandemic. Such pandemic waves can continue for several years, until immunity in the population reaches a high level. In the years after pandemic influenza, antigenic drifts among influenza viruses result in outbreaks of variable severity in populations with high levels of immunity to the pandemic strain that circulated earlier. This situation persists until another antigenically novel pandemic strain emerges. On the other hand, outbreaks sometimes end despite the persistence of a large pool of susceptible individuals in the population. It has been suggested that certain influenza A viruses may be intrinsically less virulent and cause less severe disease than other variants, even in immunologically virgin subjects. If so, then other (undefined) factors besides the level of preexisting immunity must play a role in the epidemiology of influenza.

Pandemic Influenza A (H1N1)

In March 2009, an outbreak of influenza caused by a novel influenza A/H1N1 virus was detected in Mexico. Subsequently, cases were detected throughout the world, and in June 2009 the World Health Organization (WHO) declared that an influenza pandemic was underway. The 2009 influenza A/H1N1 virus that caused the pandemic was a reassortant between a virus previously circulating in North American swine and a Eurasian swine virus. This virus bore little antigenic relationship to the seasonal influenza A/H1N1 viruses that had circulated in recent years before 2009, but it did exhibit antigenic relatedness to A/H1N1 viruses that circulated before 1957.

Overall, the clinical illness induced by the pandemic influenza A/H1N1 virus appeared to be similar to that caused by seasonal influenza A virus. However, severe disease was prominent in pregnant women and young children, also occurring in young adults as well as in individuals with underlying medical illnesses (see "Influenza-Associated Morbidity and Mortality" later in the chapter).

Vaccines generated against seasonal influenza viruses, including A/H1N1 strains, do not provide protection against disease caused by the pandemic influenza A/H1N1 virus. A specific monovalent vaccine against the pandemic virus, A/California/07/2009 (H1N1), was manufactured and made available. As of November 2009, strains of the pandemic influenza A/H1N1 virus were sensitive to oseltamivir (with only a few exceptions) and to zanamivir. The virus is resistant to amantadine and rimantadine.

Updated information on the pandemic can be obtained from the Centers for Disease Control and

Prevention (*http://www.cdc.gov/h1n1flu/*) and WHO (*http://www.who.int/csr/disease/swineflu/en/index.html*).

Influenza B and C Viruses

Influenza B virus causes outbreaks that are generally less extensive and are associated with less severe disease than those caused by influenza A virus. The hemagglutinin and neuraminidase of influenza B virus undergo less frequent and less extensive variation than those of influenza A viruses; this characteristic may account, in part, for the lesser extent of disease. Influenza B outbreaks are seen most frequently in schools and military camps, although outbreaks in institutions in which elderly individuals reside have also been noted on occasion. The most serious complication of influenza B virus infection is Reye's syndrome.

In contrast to influenza A and B viruses, influenza C virus appears to be a relatively minor cause of disease in humans. It has been associated with common cold–like symptoms and occasionally with lower respiratory tract illness. Serum antibody to this virus is widely prevalent and indicates that asymptomatic infection may be common.

Influenza-Associated Morbidity and Mortality

The morbidity and mortality caused by influenza outbreaks continue to be substantial. Most individuals who die in this setting have underlying diseases that place them at high risk for complications of influenza. Excess hospitalizations for groups of adults and children with high-risk medical conditions ranged from 56 to 1900 per 100,000 during outbreaks of influenza in 1973–1993. The most prominent high-risk conditions are chronic cardiac and pulmonary diseases and old age. Mortality rates among individuals with chronic metabolic or renal disease or certain immunosuppressive diseases have also been elevated, albeit lower than those among patients with chronic cardiopulmonary diseases. The morbidity attributable to influenza in the general population is considerable. It is estimated that interpandemic outbreaks of influenza currently incur annual costs of more than $12 billion in the United States. If a pandemic were to occur, it is estimated that annual costs would range from $71 to $167 billion for attack rates of 15–35%.

PATHOGENESIS AND IMMUNITY

The initial event in influenza is infection of the respiratory epithelium with influenza virus acquired from respiratory secretions of acutely infected individuals. In all likelihood, the virus is transmitted via aerosols generated by coughs and sneezes, although hand-to-hand contact, other personal contact, and even fomite transmission may take place. Experimental evidence suggests that infection by a small-particle aerosol (particle diameter, <10 μm) is more efficient than that by larger droplets. Initially, viral infection involves the ciliated columnar epithelial cells, but it may also involve other respiratory tract cells, including alveolar cells, mucous gland cells, and macrophages. In infected cells, virus replicates within 4–6 h, after which infectious virus is released to infect adjacent or nearby cells. In this way, infection spreads from a few foci to a large number of respiratory cells over several hours. In experimentally induced infection, the incubation period of illness has ranged from 18 to 72 h, depending on the size of the viral inoculum. Histopathologic study reveals degenerative changes, including granulation, vacuolization, swelling, and pyknotic nuclei, in infected ciliated cells. The cells eventually become necrotic and desquamate; in some areas, previously columnar epithelium is replaced by flattened and metaplastic epithelial cells. The severity of illness is correlated with the quantity of virus shed in secretions; thus the degree of viral replication itself may be an important factor in pathogenesis. Despite the frequent development of systemic signs and symptoms such as fever, headache, and myalgias, influenza virus has only rarely been detected in extrapulmonary sites (including the bloodstream). Evidence suggests that the pathogenesis of systemic symptoms in influenza may be related to the induction of certain cytokines, particularly tumor necrosis factor α, interferon α, interleukin 6, and interleukin 8, in respiratory secretions and in the bloodstream.

The host response to influenza infections involves a complex interplay of humoral antibody, local antibody, cell-mediated immunity, interferon, and other host defenses. Serum antibody responses, which can be detected by the second week after primary infection, are measured by a variety of techniques: hemagglutination inhibition (HI), complement fixation (CF), neutralization, enzyme-linked immunosorbent assay (ELISA), and antineuraminidase antibody assay. Antibodies to the hemagglutinin appear to be the most important mediators of immunity; in several studies, HI titers of ≥40 have been associated with protection from infection. Secretory antibodies produced in the respiratory tract are predominantly of the IgA class and also play a major role in protection against infection. Secretory antibody neutralization titers of ≥4 have also been associated with protection. A variety of cell-mediated immune responses, both antigen-specific and antigen-nonspecific, can be detected early after infection and depend on the prior immune status of the host. These responses include T-cell proliferative, T-cell cytotoxic, and natural killer cell activity. In humans, CD8+ HLA class I–restricted cytotoxic T lymphocytes (CTLs) are directed at conserved regions of internal proteins (NP, M, and polymerases), as well as against the surface proteins (H and N). Interferons can be detected in respiratory secretions shortly after the shedding of virus has begun, and increases in interferon titers coincide with decreases in virus shedding.

The host defense factors responsible for cessation of virus shedding and resolution of illness have not been defined specifically. Virus shedding generally stops within 2–5 days after symptoms first appear, at a time when serum and local antibody responses often are not detectable by conventional techniques (although antibody increases may be detected earlier by use of highly sensitive techniques, particularly in individuals with previous immunity to the virus). It has been suggested that interferon, cell-mediated immune responses, and/or nonspecific inflammatory responses all contribute to the resolution of illness. CTL responses may be particularly important in this regard.

CLINICAL MANIFESTATIONS

Influenza has most frequently been described as an illness characterized by the abrupt onset of systemic symptoms, such as headache, feverishness, chills, myalgia, or malaise, and accompanying respiratory tract signs, particularly cough and sore throat. In many cases, the onset is so abrupt that patients can recall the precise time they became ill. However, the spectrum of clinical presentations is wide, ranging from a mild, afebrile respiratory illness similar to the common cold (with either a gradual or an abrupt onset) to severe prostration with relatively few respiratory signs and symptoms. In most of the cases that come to a physician's attention, the patient has a fever, with temperatures of 38°–41°C (100.4°–105.8°F). A rapid temperature rise within the first 24 h of illness is generally followed by gradual defervescence over 2–3 days, although, on occasion, fever may last as long as 1 week. Patients report a feverish feeling and chilliness, but true rigors are rare. Headache, either generalized or frontal, is often particularly troublesome. Myalgias may involve any part of the body but are most common in the legs and lumbosacral area. Arthralgias may also develop.

Respiratory symptoms often become more prominent as systemic symptoms subside. Many patients have a sore throat or persistent cough, which may last for ≥1 week and which is often accompanied by substernal discomfort. Ocular signs and symptoms include pain on motion of the eyes, photophobia, and burning of the eyes.

Physical findings are usually minimal in uncomplicated influenza. Early in the illness, the patient appears flushed, and the skin is hot and dry, although diaphoresis and mottled extremities are sometimes evident, particularly in older patients. Examination of the pharynx may yield surprisingly unremarkable results despite a severe sore throat, but injection of the mucous membranes and postnasal discharge are apparent in some cases. Mild cervical lymphadenopathy may be noted, especially in younger individuals. The results of chest examination are largely negative in uncomplicated influenza, although rhonchi, wheezes, and scattered rales have been reported with variable frequency in different outbreaks. Frank dyspnea, hyperpnea, cyanosis, diffuse rales, and signs of consolidation are indicative of pulmonary complications. Patients with apparently uncomplicated influenza have been reported to have a variety of mild ventilatory defects and increased alveolar-capillary diffusion gradients; thus subclinical pulmonary involvement may be more common than is appreciated.

In uncomplicated influenza, the acute illness generally resolves over 2–5 days, and most patients have largely recovered in 1 week, although cough may persist 1–2 weeks longer. In a significant minority (particularly the elderly), however, symptoms of weakness or lassitude (postinfluenzal asthenia) may persist for several weeks and may prove troublesome for persons who wish to resume their full level of activity promptly. The pathogenetic basis for this asthenia is unknown, although pulmonary function abnormalities may persist for several weeks after uncomplicated influenza.

COMPLICATIONS

Complications of influenza occur most frequently in patients >64 years old and in those with certain chronic disorders, including cardiac or pulmonary diseases, diabetes mellitus, hemoglobinopathies, renal dysfunction, and immunosuppression. Pregnancy in the second or third trimester also predisposes to complications with influenza. Children <2 years old (especially infants) are also at high risk for complications.

Pulmonary Complications

Pneumonia

The most significant complication of influenza is pneumonia: "primary" influenza viral pneumonia, secondary bacterial pneumonia, or mixed viral and bacterial pneumonia.

Primary Influenza Viral Pneumonia

Primary influenza viral pneumonia is the least common but most severe of the pneumonic complications. It presents as acute influenza that does not resolve but instead progresses relentlessly, with persistent fever, dyspnea, and eventual cyanosis. Sputum production is generally scanty, but the sputum can contain blood. Few physical signs may be evident early in the illness. In more advanced cases, diffuse rales may be noted, and chest x-ray findings consistent with diffuse interstitial infiltrates and/or acute respiratory distress syndrome may be present. In such cases, arterial blood-gas determinations show marked hypoxia. Viral cultures of respiratory secretions and lung parenchyma, especially if samples are taken early in illness, yield high titers of virus. In fatal cases of primary viral pneumonia, histopathologic examination reveals a marked inflammatory reaction in the alveolar septa, with edema and infiltration by lymphocytes, macrophages, occasional plasma cells, and variable numbers of neutrophils. Fibrin thrombi in alveolar capillaries, along with necrosis and hemorrhage, have also been noted. Eosinophilic hyaline membranes can be found lining alveoli and alveolar ducts.

Primary influenza viral pneumonia has a predilection for individuals with cardiac disease, particularly those with mitral stenosis, but has also been reported in otherwise-healthy young adults as well as in older individuals with chronic pulmonary disorders. In some epidemics of influenza (notably those of 1918 and 1957), pregnancy increased the risk of primary influenza pneumonia. Subsequent epidemics of influenza have been associated with increased rates of hospitalization among pregnant women.

Secondary Bacterial Pneumonia

Secondary bacterial pneumonia follows acute influenza. Improvement of the patient's condition over 2–3 days is followed by a reappearance of fever along with clinical signs and symptoms of bacterial pneumonia, including cough, production of purulent sputum, and physical and x-ray signs of consolidation. The most common bacterial pathogens in this setting are *Streptococcus pneumoniae*, *Staphylococcus aureus*, and *Haemophilus influenzae*—organisms that can colonize the nasopharynx and that cause infection in the wake of changes in bronchopulmonary defenses. The etiology can often be determined by Gram's staining and culture of an appropriately obtained sputum specimen. Secondary bacterial pneumonia occurs most frequently in high-risk individuals with chronic pulmonary and cardiac disease and in elderly individuals. Patients with secondary bacterial pneumonia often respond to antibiotic therapy when it is instituted promptly.

Mixed Viral and Bacterial Pneumonia

Perhaps the most common pneumonic complications during outbreaks of influenza have mixed features of viral and bacterial pneumonia. Patients may experience a gradual progression of their acute illness or may show transient improvement followed by clinical exacerbation, with eventual manifestation of the clinical features of bacterial pneumonia. Sputum cultures may contain both influenza A virus and one of the bacterial pathogens described above. Patchy infiltrates or areas of consolidation may be detected by physical examination and chest x-ray. Patients with mixed viral and bacterial pneumonia generally have less widespread involvement of the lung than those with primary viral pneumonia, and their bacterial infections may respond to appropriate antibacterial drugs. Mixed viral and bacterial pneumonia occurs primarily in patients with chronic cardiovascular and pulmonary diseases.

Other Pulmonary Complications

Other pulmonary complications associated with influenza include worsening of chronic obstructive pulmonary disease and exacerbation of chronic bronchitis and asthma. In children, influenza infection may present as croup. Sinusitis as well as otitis media (the latter occurring particularly often in children) may also be associated with influenza.

Extrapulmonary Complications

In addition to the pulmonary complications of influenza, a number of extrapulmonary complications may occur. These include *Reye's syndrome*, a serious complication in children that is associated with influenza B and to a lesser extent with influenza A virus infection as well as with varicella-zoster virus infection. An epidemiologic association between Reye's syndrome and aspirin therapy for the antecedent viral infection has been noted, and the syndrome's incidence has decreased markedly with widespread warnings regarding aspirin use by children with acute viral respiratory infections.

Myositis, rhabdomyolysis, and myoglobinuria are occasional complications of influenza infection. Although myalgias are exceedingly common in influenza, true myositis is rare. Patients with acute myositis have exquisite tenderness of the affected muscles, most commonly in the legs, and may not be able to tolerate even the slightest pressure, such as the touch of bedsheets. In the most severe cases, there is frank swelling and bogginess of muscles. Serum levels of creatine phosphokinase and aldolase are markedly elevated, and an occasional patient develops renal failure from myoglobinuria. The pathogenesis of influenza-associated myositis is also unclear, although the presence of influenza virus in affected muscles has been reported.

Myocarditis and pericarditis were reported in association with influenza virus infection during the 1918–1919 pandemic; these reports were based largely on histopathologic findings, and these complications have been reported only infrequently since that time. Electrocardiographic changes during acute influenza are common among patients who have cardiac disease but have been ascribed most often to exacerbations of the underlying cardiac disease rather than to direct involvement of the myocardium with influenza virus.

Central nervous system (CNS) diseases, including encephalitis, transverse myelitis, and Guillain-Barré syndrome, have been reported during influenza. The etiologic relationship of influenza virus to such CNS illnesses remains uncertain. Toxic shock syndrome associated with *S. aureus* or group A streptococcal infection after acute influenza infection has also been reported (Chaps. 35 and 36).

In addition to complications involving the specific organ systems described above, influenza outbreaks include a number of cases in which elderly and other high-risk individuals develop influenza and subsequently experience a gradual deterioration of underlying cardiovascular, pulmonary, or renal function—changes that occasionally are irreversible and lead to death. These deaths contribute to the overall excess mortality associated with influenza A outbreaks.

Complications of Avian Influenza

Cases of influenza caused by avian A/H5N1 virus are reportedly associated with high rates of pneumonia (>50%) and extrapulmonary manifestations such as diarrhea and CNS involvement. Deaths have been associated with multisystem dysfunction, including cardiac and renal failure.

LABORATORY FINDINGS AND DIAGNOSIS

During acute influenza, virus may be detected in throat swabs, nasopharyngeal washes, or sputum. The virus can be isolated by use of tissue culture—or, less commonly, chick embryos—within 48–72 h after inoculation. Most commonly, the laboratory diagnosis is established with rapid viral tests that detect viral nucleoprotein or neuraminidase by means of immunologic or enzymatic techniques that are highly sensitive and 60–90% as specific as tissue culture. Viral nucleic acids can also be detected in clinical samples by reverse transcriptase polymerase chain reaction. The type of the infecting influenza virus (A or B) may be determined by either immunofluorescence or HI techniques, and the hemagglutinin subtype of influenza A virus (H1, H2, or H3) may be identified by HI with use of subtype-specific antisera. Serologic methods for diagnosis require comparison of antibody titers in sera obtained during the acute illness with those in sera obtained 10–14 days after the onset of illness and are useful primarily in retrospect. Fourfold or greater titer rises as detected by HI or CF or significant rises as measured by ELISA are diagnostic of acute infection. CF tests are generally less sensitive than other serologic techniques, but, as they detect type-specific antigens, they may be particularly useful when subtype-specific reagents are not available.

Other laboratory tests generally are not helpful in the specific diagnosis of influenza virus infection. Leukocyte counts are variable, frequently being low early in illness and normal or slightly elevated later. Severe leukopenia has been described in overwhelming viral or bacterial infection, whereas leukocytosis with >15,000 cells/μL raises the suspicion of secondary bacterial infection.

DIFFERENTIAL DIAGNOSIS

During a community-wide outbreak, a clinical diagnosis of influenza can be made with a high degree of certainty in patients who present to a physician's office with the typical febrile respiratory illness described above. In the absence of an outbreak (i.e., in sporadic or isolated cases), influenza may be difficult to differentiate on clinical grounds alone from an acute respiratory illness caused by any of a variety of respiratory viruses or by *Mycoplasma pneumoniae*. Severe streptococcal pharyngitis or early bacterial pneumonia may mimic acute influenza, although bacterial pneumonias generally do not run a self-limited course. Purulent sputum in which a bacterial pathogen can be detected by Gram's staining is an important diagnostic feature in bacterial pneumonia.

℞ Treatment: INFLUENZA

In uncomplicated cases of influenza, symptom-based therapy with acetaminophen for the relief of headache, myalgia, and fever may be considered, but the use of salicylates should be avoided in children <18 years of age because of the possible association of salicylates with Reye's syndrome. Since cough is ordinarily self-limited, treatment with cough suppressants generally is not indicated, although codeine-containing compounds may be employed if the cough is particularly troublesome. Patients should be advised to rest and maintain hydration during acute illness and to return to full activity only gradually after illness has resolved, especially if it has been severe.

Specific antiviral therapy is available for influenza (**Table 88-2**): the neuraminidase inhibitors zanamivir and oseltamivir for both influenza A and influenza B and the adamantane agents amantadine and rimantadine for influenza A (Chap. 79). In 2005–2006, resistance to amantadine was reported in >90% of A/H3N2 viral isolates; thus amantadine and rimantadine are no longer recommended, but their use may be reconsidered if sensitivity becomes reestablished.

Oseltamivir (administered orally at a dose of 75 mg twice a day for 5 days) or zanamivir (which must be given by an oral inhalation device; 10 mg twice a day for 5 days) reduces the duration of signs and symptoms of influenza by 1–1.5 days if treatment is started within 2 days of the onset of illness. Zanamivir may exacerbate bronchospasm in asthmatic patients, and oseltamivir has been associated with nausea and vomiting, whose frequency can be reduced by administration of the drug with food. Oseltamivir has also been associated with neuropsychiatric side effects in children.

If begun within 48 h of the onset of illness due to sensitive influenza A virus strains, treatment with amantadine

TABLE 88-2

ANTIVIRAL MEDICATIONS FOR TREATMENT AND PROPHYLAXIS OF INFLUENZA

	AGE GROUP (YEARS)		
ANTIVIRAL DRUG	**CHILDREN (≤12)**	**13–64**	**≥65**
Oseltamivir			
Treatment, influenza A and B	Age 1–12, dose varies by weight[a]	75 mg PO bid	75 mg PO bid
Prophylaxis, influenza A and B	Age 1–12, dose varies by weight[b]	75 PO qd	75 mg PO qd
Zanamivir			
Treatment, influenza A and B	Age 7–12, 10 mg bid by inhalation	10 mg bid by inhalation	10 mg bid by inhalation
Prophylaxis, influenza A and B	Age 5–12, 10 mg qd by inhalation	10 mg qd by inhalation	10 mg qd by inhalation
Amantadine[c]			
Treatment, influenza A	Age 1–9, 5 mg/kg in 2 divided doses, up to 150 mg/d	Age ≥10, 100 mg PO bid	≤100 mg/d
Prophylaxis, influenza A	Age 1–9, 5 mg/kg in 2 divided doses, up to 150 mg/d	Age ≥10, 100 mg PO bid	≤100 mg/d
Rimantadine[c]			
Treatment, influenza A	Not approved	100 mg PO bid	100–200 mg/d
Prophylaxis, influenza A	Age 1–9, 5 mg/kg in 2 divided doses, up to 150 mg/d	Age ≥10, 100 mg PO bid	100–200 mg/d

[a]<15 kg: 30 mg bid; >15–23 kg: 45 mg bid; >23–40 kg: 60 mg bid; >40 kg: 75 mg bid.

[b]<15 kg: 30 mg qd; >15–23 kg: 45 mg qd; >23–40 kg: 60 mg qd; >40 kg: 75 mg qd.

[c]Amantadine and rimantadine were not recommended as of 2006–2007 because of widespread resistance in influenza A/H3N2 viruses. Their use may be reconsidered if viral susceptibility is reestablished.

or rimantadine reduces the duration of systemic and respiratory symptoms of influenza by ~50%. Of individuals who receive amantadine, 5–10% experience mild CNS side effects, primarily jitteriness, anxiety, insomnia, or difficulty concentrating. These side effects disappear promptly upon cessation of therapy. Rimantadine appears to be equally efficacious and is associated with less frequent CNS side effects than is amantadine. In adults, the usual dose of amantadine or rimantadine is 200 mg/d for 3–7 days. Since both drugs are excreted via the kidney, the dose should be reduced to ≤100 mg/d in elderly patients and in patients with renal insufficiency. Resistant viruses emerge frequently during treatment with amantadine or rimantadine and can be transmitted among family members. Development of resistance to zanamivir or oseltamivir appears to be less common but can occur. Ribavirin is a nucleoside analogue with activity against influenza A and B viruses in vitro. It has been reported to be variably effective against influenza when administered as an aerosol but ineffective when administered orally. Its efficacy in the treatment of influenza A or B is unestablished.

Studies demonstrating the therapeutic efficacy of antiviral compounds in influenza have primarily involved young adults with uncomplicated disease. A meta-analysis of studies with oseltamivir suggests that treatment may reduce the likelihood of some lower respiratory tract complications of influenza. However, it is not known whether antiviral agents are themselves effective in the treatment of influenza pneumonia or of other complications of influenza. Therapy for primary influenza pneumonia is directed at maintaining oxygenation and is most appropriately undertaken in an intensive care unit, with aggressive respiratory and hemodynamic support as needed. Bypass membrane oxygenators have been employed in this setting with variable results. When an acute respiratory distress syndrome develops, fluids must be administered cautiously, with close monitoring of blood gases and hemodynamic function.

Antibacterial drugs should be reserved for the treatment of bacterial complications of acute influenza, such as secondary bacterial pneumonia. The choice of antibiotics should be guided by Gram's staining and culture of appropriate specimens of respiratory secretions, such as sputum or transtracheal aspirates. If the etiology of a case of bacterial pneumonia is unclear from an examination of respiratory secretions, empirical antibiotics effective against the most common bacterial pathogens in this setting (*S. pneumoniae*, *S. aureus*, and *H. influenzae*) should be selected (Chaps. 34, 35, and 47).

PROPHYLAXIS

Inactivated and live attenuated vaccines against influenza are available, and their use represents the major public health measure for prevention of influenza. The vast majority of currently used vaccines are inactivated ("killed") preparations derived from influenza A and B viruses that circulated during the previous influenza season. If the vaccine virus and the currently circulating viruses are closely related, 50–80% protection against influenza would be expected from inactivated vaccines. The available inactivated vaccines have been highly purified and are associated with few reactions. Up to 5% of individuals experience low-grade fever and mild systemic symptoms 8–24 h after vaccination, and up to one-third develop mild redness or tenderness at the vaccination site. Since the vaccine is produced in eggs, individuals with true hypersensitivity to egg products either should be desensitized or should not be vaccinated. Although the 1976 swine influenza vaccine appears to have been associated with an increased frequency of Guillain-Barré syndrome, influenza vaccines administered since 1976 generally have not been. Possible exceptions were noted during the 1992–1993 and 1993–1994 influenza seasons, when there may have been an excess risk of Guillain-Barré syndrome of slightly more than 1 case per million vaccine recipients. However, the overall health risk following influenza outweighs the potential risk associated with vaccination.

The U.S. Public Health Service recommends the administration of inactivated influenza vaccine to individuals who, because of age or underlying disease, are at increased risk for complications of influenza and to the contacts of these individuals (Table 88-3). Inactivated vaccines may be administered safely to immunocompromised patients. Influenza vaccination is not associated with exacerbations of chronic nervous-system diseases such as multiple sclerosis. Vaccine should be administered early in the autumn before influenza outbreaks occur and should then be given annually to maintain immunity against the most current influenza virus strains.

A live attenuated influenza vaccine that is administered by intranasal spray is also available. The vaccine is generated by reassortment between currently circulating strains of influenza A and B virus and a cold-adapted, attenuated master strain. The cold-adapted vaccine is well tolerated and highly efficacious (92% protective) in young children; in one study, it provided protection against a circulating influenza virus that had drifted antigenically away from the vaccine strain. Live attenuated vaccine is approved for use in healthy persons 5–49 years of age.

Antiviral drugs may also be used as chemoprophylaxis against influenza (Table 88-2). Chemoprophylaxis with oseltamivir (75 mg/d by mouth) or zanamivir (10 mg/d inhaled) has been 84–89% efficacious against influenza A and B. Chemoprophylaxis with amantadine or rimantadine is no longer recommended because of reports of widespread resistance to these drugs. In earlier studies with sensitive viruses, prophylaxis with amantadine or rimantadine (100–200 mg/d) was 70–100% effective against illness associated with influenza A. Chemoprophylaxis is most likely to be used for high-risk individuals who have not received influenza vaccine or in a situation where the vaccines previously administered are relatively ineffective because of antigenic changes in the circulating virus. During an outbreak, antiviral chemoprophylaxis can be administered simultaneously with inactivated vaccine, since the drugs do not interfere with an immune response to the vaccine. In fact, there is evidence that

TABLE 88-3

PERSONS FOR WHOM ANNUAL INFLUENZA VACCINATION IS RECOMMENDED
Children 6–59 months old
Women who will be pregnant during the influenza season
Persons ≥50 years old
Children and adolescents (6 months to 18 years old) who are receiving long-term aspirin therapy and therefore may be at risk for developing Reye's syndrome after influenza
Adults and children who have chronic disorders of the pulmonary or cardiovascular systems, including asthma[a]
Adults and children who have required regular medical follow-up or hospitalization during the preceding year because of chronic metabolic diseases (including diabetes mellitus), renal dysfunction, hemoglobinopathies, or immunodeficiency (including immunodeficiency caused by medications or by HIV)
Adults and children who have any condition (e.g., cognitive dysfunction, spinal cord injuries, seizure disorders, or other neuromuscular disorders) that can compromise respiratory function or the handling of respiratory secretions or can increase the risk of aspiration
Residents of nursing homes and other chronic-care facilities that house persons of any age who have chronic medical conditions
Persons who live with or care for persons at high risk for influenza-related complications, including healthy household contacts of and caregivers for children from birth through 59 months of age
Health care workers

[a]Hypertension itself is not considered a chronic disorder for which influenza vaccination is recommended.

Source: Centers for Disease Control and Prevention: Prevention and control of influenza: Recommendations of the Advisory Committee on Immunization Practices (ACIP). MMWR 55(RR-11):1, 2006.

the protective effects of chemoprophylaxis and inactivated vaccine may be additive. However, concurrent administration of chemoprophylaxis and the live attenuated vaccine may interfere with the immune response to the latter. Antiviral drugs should not be administered until at least 2 weeks after administration of live vaccine, and vaccination with live vaccine should not begin until at least 48 h after antiviral drug administration has been stopped. Chemoprophylaxis may also be employed to control nosocomial outbreaks of influenza. For that purpose, prophylaxis should be instituted promptly when influenza activity is detected and must be continued daily for the duration of the outbreak.

FURTHER READINGS

Beigel JH et al: Avian influenza A (H5N1) infection in humans. N Engl J Med 353:1374, 2005

Belshe RB et al: The efficacy of live attenuated, cold adapted trivalent, intranasal influenza vaccine in children. N Engl J Med 38:1405, 1998

Centers For Disease Control And Prevention: Prevention and control of influenza. MMWR 55(RR–11):1, 2006

———: Severe methicillin-resistant *Staphylococcus aureus* community-acquired pneumonia associated with influenza—Louisiana and Georgia, December 2006–January 2007. MMWR 56:325, 2007

Cooper NJ et al: Effectiveness of neuraminidase inhibitors in treatment and prevention of influenza A and B: Systematic review and meta-analysis of randomized controlled trials. BMJ 326:1235, 2003

Dolin R: Interpandemic as well as pandemic disease. N Engl J Med 353:2535, 2005

Fiore AE et al: Prevention and control of influenza. Recommendations of the Advisory Committee on Immunization Practices (ACIP), 2007. MMWR Recomm Rep 56:1, 2007

Hatakeyama S et al: Emergence of influenza B viruses with reduced sensitivity to neuraminidase inhibitors. JAMA 297:1435, 2007

Hayden FG et al: Use of the selective oral neuraminidase inhibitor oseltamivir to prevent influenza. N Engl J Med 341:1336, 1999

Meltzer MI et al: The economic impact of pandemic influenza in the United States: Priorities for intervention. Emerg Infect Dis 5:659, 1999

MIST [Management of Influenza in the Southern Hemisphere Trialists] Study Group: Randomized trial of efficacy and safety of inhaled zanamivir in treatment of influenza A and B infections. Lancet 352:1871, 1998

Neuzil KM et al: Influenza-associated morbidity and mortality in young and middle-aged women. JAMA 281:901, 1999

Novel Swine-Origin Influenza A (H1N1) Virus Investigation Team et al: Emergence of a novel swine-origin influenza A (H1N1) virus in humans. N Engl J Med 360:2605, 2009

Rothberg MB et al: Complications of viral influenza. Am J Med 121:258, 2008

Shinde V et al. Triple-reassortant swine influenza A (H1) in humans in the United States, 2005-2009. N Engl J Med 360:2616, 2009

Simonsen L et al: Pandemic vs epidemic mortality: A pattern of changing age distribution. J Infect Dis 178:53, 1998

Treanor JJ: Influenza virus, in *Principles and Practice of Infectious Diseases*, 6th ed, GL Mandell et al (eds). Philadelphia, Elsevier, 2005, pp 2201–2203

Writing Committee of the Second World Health Organization Consultation on Clinical Aspects of Human Infection with Avian Influenza A (H5N1) Virus et al: Update on avian influenza A (H5N1) virus infection in humans. N Engl J Med 358:261, 2008

PART 4 INFECTIONS DUE TO HUMAN IMMUNODEFICIENCY VIRUS AND OTHER HUMAN RETROVIRUSES

CHAPTER 89

THE HUMAN RETROVIRUSES

Dan L. Longo ■ Anthony S. Fauci

The retroviruses, which make up a large family (Retroviridae), infect mainly vertebrates. These viruses have a unique replication cycle whereby their genetic information is encoded by RNA rather than DNA. Retroviruses contain an RNA-dependent DNA polymerase (a reverse transcriptase) that directs the synthesis of a DNA form of the viral genome after infection of a host cell. The designation *retrovirus* denotes that information in the form of RNA is transcribed into DNA in the host cell—a sequence that overturned a central dogma of molecular biology: that information passes unidirectionally from DNA to RNA to protein. The observation that RNA was the source of genetic information in the causative agents of certain animal tumors led to a number of paradigm-shifting biologic insights regarding not only the direction of genetic information passage but also the viral etiology of certain cancers and the concept of oncogenes as normal host genes scavenged and altered by a viral vector.

The family Retroviridae includes three subfamilies (Table 89-1): Oncovirinae, of which human T-cell lymphotropic virus (HTLV) type I is the most important in humans; Lentivirinae, of which HIV is the most important in humans; and Spumavirinae, the "foamy" viruses, named for the pathologic appearance of infected cells. A number of spumaviruses have been isolated from humans; however, they are not associated with any known disease and therefore are not discussed further in this chapter.

The wide variety of interactions of a retrovirus with its host range from completely benign events (e.g., silent carriage of endogenous retroviral sequences in the germline genome of many animal species) to rapidly fatal infections (e.g., exogenous infection with an oncogenic

TABLE 89-1

CLASSIFICATION OF RETROVIRUSES: THE FAMILY RETROVIRIDAE

SUBFAMILY, GROUP[a]	EXAMPLE(S)	FEATURE
Oncovirinae (oncogenic viruses)		
Avian leukosis	Rous sarcoma virus	Contains *src* oncogene
Mammalian C-type	Abelson leukemia virus	Contains *abl* oncogene
B-type	Murine mammary tumor virus	Can be endogenous or exogenous
D-type	Mason-Pfizer monkey virus	—
HTLV-BLV	HTLV-I	Causes T-cell lymphoma and neurologic disease
Lentivirinae (slow viruses)	HIV-1, HIV-2	Cause AIDS
	Visna virus	Causes lung and brain diseases in sheep
	Feline immunodeficiency virus	Causes immunodeficiency in cats
Spumavirinae (foamy viruses)	Simian foamy virus, human foamy virus	Cause no known disease

[a]The Oncovirinae were originally grouped into types A–D on the basis of morphologic features (size, core location, budding) under electron microscopy; however, this system has been replaced by groupings based on relationships of genome structure and sequence.

Note: HTLV, human T-cell lymphotropic virus; BLV, bovine leukemia virus.

virus such as Rous sarcoma virus in chickens). The ability of retroviruses to acquire and alter the structure and function of host cell sequences has revolutionized our understanding of molecular carcinogenesis. The viruses can insert into the germ-line genome of the host cell and behave as a transposable or movable genetic element. They can activate or inactivate genes near the site of integration into the genome. They can rapidly alter their own genome by recombination and mutation under selective environmental stimuli.

Most human viral diseases occur as a consequence of either tissue destruction by the virus itself or the host's response to the virus. Although these mechanisms are operative in retroviral infections, retroviruses have additional mechanisms of inducing disease, including the malignant transformation of an infected cell and the induction of an immunodeficiency state that leads to opportunistic diseases (infections and neoplasms; Chap. 90).

STRUCTURE AND LIFE CYCLE

Despite the wide range of biologic consequences of retroviral infection, all retroviruses are similar in structure, genome organization, and mode of replication. Retroviruses are 70–130 nm in diameter and have a lipid-containing envelope surrounding an icosahedral capsid with a dense inner core. The core contains two identical copies of the single-strand RNA genome. The RNA molecules are 8–10 kb long and are complexed with reverse transcriptase and tRNA. Other viral proteins, such as integrase, are also components of the virion particle. The RNA has features usually found in mRNA: a cap site at the 5' end of the molecule, which is important in the initiation of mRNA translation, and a polyadenylation site at the 3' end, which influences mRNA turnover (i.e., messages with shorter polyA tails turn over faster than messages with longer polyA tails). However, the retroviral RNA is not translated; instead it is transcribed into DNA. The DNA form of the retroviral genome is called a *provirus*.

The replication cycle of retroviruses proceeds in two phases (Fig. 89-1). In the first phase, the virus enters the cytoplasm after binding to a specific cell-surface receptor; the viral RNA and reverse transcriptase synthesize a double-strand DNA version of the RNA template; and the provirus moves into the nucleus and integrates into the host cell genome. This proviral integration is permanent. Although some animal retroviruses integrate into a single specific site of the host genome in every infected cell, the four known human retroviruses (HTLV-I, HTLV-II, HIV-1, and HIV-2) integrate randomly. This first phase of replication depends entirely on gene products in the virus. The second phase includes the synthesis and processing of viral genomes, mRNAs, and proteins using host cell machinery, often under the influence of viral gene products. Virions are assembled and released from the cell by budding from the membrane; host cell membrane proteins are frequently incorporated into the envelope of the virus. Proviral integration occurs during the S-phase of the cell cycle; thus, in general, nondividing cells are resistant to retroviral infection. Only the lentiviruses are able to infect nondividing cells. Once a host cell is infected, it is infected for the life of the cell.

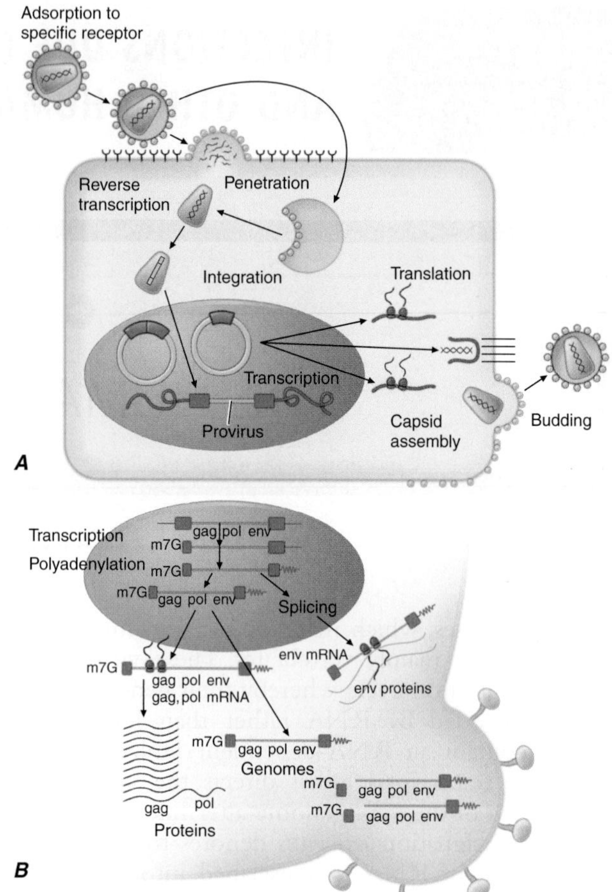

FIGURE 89-1

The life cycle of retroviruses. *A.* Overview of virus replication. The retrovirus enters a target cell by binding to a specific cell-surface receptor; once the virus is internalized, its RNA is released from the nucleocapsid and is reverse-transcribed into proviral DNA. The provirus is inserted into the genome and then transcribed into RNA; the RNA is translated; and virions assemble and are extruded from the cell membrane by budding. ***B.*** Overview of retroviral gene expression. The provirus is transcribed, capped, and polyadenylated. Viral RNA molecules then have one of three fates: they are exported to the cytoplasm, where they are packaged as the viral RNA in infectious viral particles; they are spliced to form the message for the envelope polyprotein; or they are translated into Gag and Pol proteins. Most of the messages for the Pol protein fail to initiate Pol translation because of a stop codon before its initiation; however, in a fraction of the messages, the stop codon is missed and the Pol proteins are translated. *[Modified from JM Coffin, in BN Fields, DM Knipe (eds): Fields Virology. New York, Raven, 1990; with permission.]*

Retroviral genomes include both coding and noncoding sequences (Fig. 89-2). In general, noncoding sequences are important recognition signals for DNA or RNA synthesis or processing events and are located in the 5' and 3' terminal regions of the genome. All retroviral genomes are terminally redundant, containing identical sequences called *long terminal repeats* (LTRs). The ends of the retroviral RNA genome differ slightly in sequence from the integrated retroviral DNA. In the latter, the

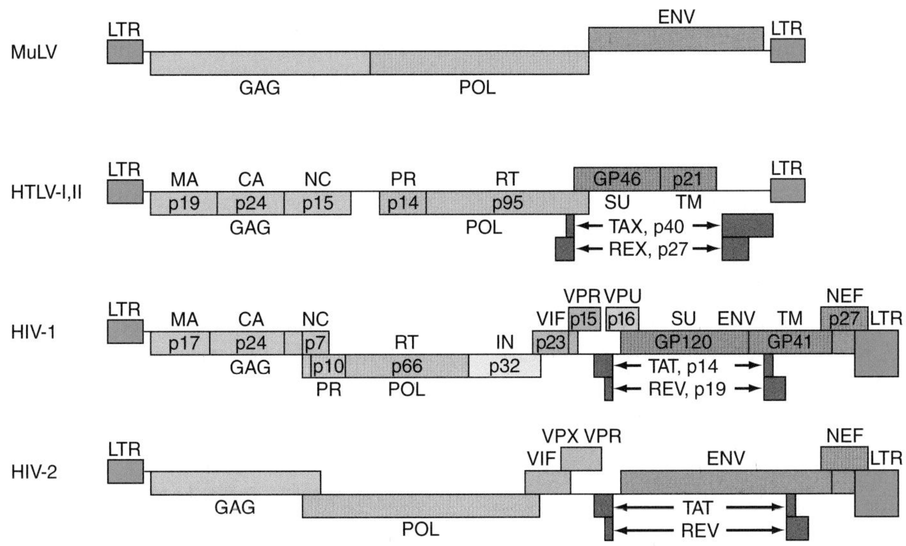

FIGURE 89-2

Genomic structure of retroviruses. The murine leukemia virus MuLV has the typical three structural genes: *gag*, *pol*, and *env*. The *gag* region gives rise to three proteins: matrix (MA), capsid (CA), and nucleic acid–binding (NC) proteins. The *pol* region encodes both a protease (PR) responsible for cleaving the viral polyproteins and a reverse transcriptase (RT). In addition, HIV *pol* encodes an integrase (IN). The *env* region encodes a surface protein (SU) and a small transmembrane protein (TM). The human retroviruses have additional gene products translated in each of the three possible reading frames. HTLV-I and HTLV-II have *tax* and *rex* genes with exons on either side of the *env* gene. HIV-1 and HIV-2 have six accessory gene products: *tat*, *rev*, *vif*, *nef*, *vpr*, and either *vpu* (in HIV-1) or *vpx* (in HIV-2). The genes for these proteins are located mainly between the *pol* and *env* genes. LTR, long terminal repeat.

LTR sequences are repeated in both the 5' and the 3' terminus of the virus. The LTRs contain sequences involved in initiating the expression of the viral proteins, the integration of the provirus, and the polyadenylation of viral RNAs. The primer binding site, which is critical for the initiation of reverse transcription, and the viral packaging sequences are located outside the LTR sequences. The coding regions include the *gag* (group-specific antigen, core protein), *pol* (RNA-dependent DNA polymerase), and *env* (envelope) genes. The *gag* gene encodes a precursor polyprotein that is cleaved to form three to five capsid proteins; a fraction of the Gag precursor proteins also contain a protease responsible for cleaving the Gag and Pol polyproteins. A Gag-Pol polyprotein gives rise to the protease that is responsible for cleaving the Gag-Pol polyprotein. The *pol* gene encodes three proteins: the reverse transcriptase, the integrase, and the protease. The reverse transcriptase functions to copy the viral RNA into the double-strand DNA provirus, which inserts itself into the host cell DNA via the action of integrase. The protease functions to cleave the Gag-Pol polyprotein into smaller protein products. The *env* gene encodes the envelope glycoproteins: one protein that binds to specific surface receptors and determines what cell types can be infected and a smaller transmembrane protein that anchors the complex to the envelope. Figure 89-3 shows how the retroviral gene products make up the virus structure.

HTLVs have a region between *env* and the 3' LTR that encodes at least two proteins in overlapping reading frames: Tax, a 40-kDa protein that does not bind to DNA but induces the expression of host cell transcription factors that alter host cell gene expression; and Rex, a 27-kDa protein that regulates the expression of viral mRNAs. These two proteins are produced from messages that are similar but that are spliced differently from overlapping but distinct exons.

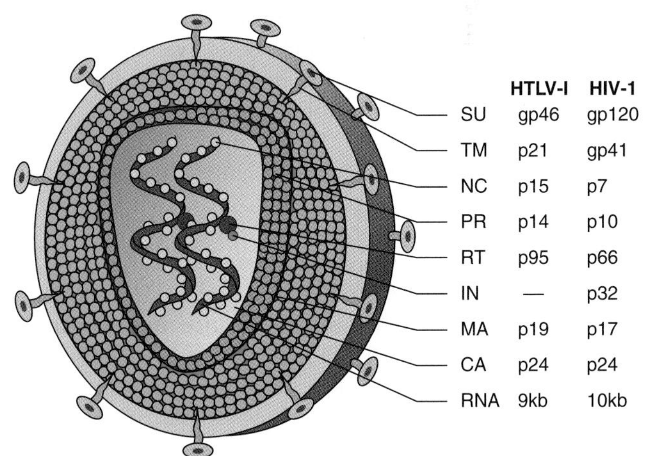

FIGURE 89-3

Schematic structure of human retroviruses. The surface glycoprotein (SU) is responsible for binding to receptors of host cells. The transmembrane protein (TM) anchors SU to the virus. NC is a nucleic acid–binding protein found in association with the viral RNA. A protease (PR) cleaves the polyproteins encoded by the *gag*, *pol*, and *env* genes into their functional components. RT is reverse transcriptase, and IN is an integrase present in some retroviruses (e.g., HIV-1) that facilitates insertion of the provirus into the host genome. The matrix protein (MA) is a Gag protein closely associated with the lipid of the envelope. The capsid protein (CA) forms the major internal structure of the virus, the core shell.

The lentiviruses in general, and HIV-1 and -2 in particular, contain a larger genome than other pathogenic retroviruses. They contain an untranslated region between *pol* and *env* that encodes portions of several proteins, varying with the reading frame into which the mRNA is spliced. Tat is a 14-kDa protein that augments the expression of virus from the LTR. The Rev protein of HIV-1, similar to the Rex protein of HTLV, regulates RNA splicing and/or RNA transport. The Nef protein downregulates CD4, the cellular receptor for HIV; alters host T-cell activation pathways; and enhances viral infectivity. The Vif protein is necessary for the proper assembly of the HIV nucleoprotein core in many types of cells; without Vif, proviral DNA is not efficiently produced in these infected cells. In addition, the Vif protein targets APOBEC (apolipoprotein B mRNA-editing enzyme catalytic polypeptide, a cytidine deaminase that mutates the viral sequence) for proteasomal degradation, thus blocking its virus-suppressing effect. Vpr, Vpu (HIV-1 only), and Vpx (HIV-2 only) are viral proteins encoded by translation of the same message in different reading frames. As noted above, oncogenic retroviruses depend on cell proliferation for their replication; lentiviruses can infect nondividing cells, largely through effects mediated by Vpr. Vpr facilitates transport of the provirus into the nucleus and can induce other cellular changes, such as G_2 growth arrest and differentiation of some target cells. Vpx is structurally related to Vpr, but its functions are not fully defined. Vpu promotes the degradation of CD4 in the endoplasmic reticulum and stimulates the release of virions from infected cells.

Retroviruses can be either exogenously acquired by infection with a virion capable of replication or transmitted in the germ line as endogenous virus. Endogenous retroviruses are often replication-defective. The human genome contains endogenous retroviral sequences, but there are no known replication-competent endogenous retroviruses in humans.

In general, viruses that contain only the *gag*, *pol*, and *env* genes either are not pathogenic or take a long time to induce disease; these observations indicate the importance of the other regulatory genes in viral disease pathogenesis. The pathogenesis of neoplastic transformation by retroviruses relies on the chance integration of the provirus at a spot in the genome that will result in the expression of a cellular gene (proto-oncogene) that becomes transforming by virtue of its unregulated expression. For example, avian leukosis virus causes B cell leukemia by inducing the expression of *myc*. Some retroviruses possess captured and altered cellular genes near their integration site, and these viral oncogenes are capable of transforming the infected host cell. Viruses that have oncogenes often have lost a portion of their genome that is required for replication. Such viruses need helper viruses to reproduce, a feature that may explain why these acute transforming retroviruses are rare in nature. All human retroviruses identified to date are exogenous and are not acutely transforming (i.e., they lack a transforming oncogene).

These remarkable properties of retroviruses have led to experimental efforts to use them as vectors to insert specific genes into particular cell types, a process known as *gene therapy* or *gene transfer*. The process could be used to repair a genetic defect or to introduce a new property that could be used therapeutically; for example, a gene (e.g., thymidine kinase) that would make a tumor cell susceptible to killing by a drug (e.g., ganciclovir) could be inserted. One source of concern about the use of retroviral vectors in humans is that replication-competent viruses might rescue endogenous retroviral replication, with unpredictable results. This concern is not merely hypothetical: the detection of proteins encoded by endogenous retroviral sequences on the surface of cancer cells implies that the genetic events leading to the cancer were able to activate the synthesis of these usually silent genes.

HUMAN T-CELL LYMPHOTROPIC VIRUS

HTLV-I was isolated in 1980 from a T-cell lymphoma cell line from a patient originally thought to have cutaneous T-cell lymphoma. Later it became clear that the patient had a distinct form of lymphoma (originally reported in Japan) called *adult T-cell leukemia/lymphoma* (ATL). Serologic data have determined that HTLV-I is the cause of at least two important diseases: ATL and tropical spastic paraparesis, also called *HTLV-I-associated myelopathy* (HAM). HTLV-I may also play a role in infective dermatitis and uveitis syndromes.

Two years after the isolation of HTLV-I, HTLV-II was isolated from a patient with an unusual form of hairy cell leukemia that affected T cells. Although early epidemiologic studies of HTLV-II failed to reveal a consistent disease association, more recent studies suggest an association of HTLV-II with human disease (see "Associated Diseases" under "Features of HTLV-II Infection" later in the chapter), particularly among injection drug users.

BIOLOGY AND MOLECULAR BIOLOGY

Because the biology of HTLV-I and that of HTLV-II are similar, the following discussion will focus on HTLV-I.

The human glucose transporter protein 1 (GLUT-1) functions as a receptor for HTLV-1, probably acting together with neuropilin-1 (NRP1). Generally, only T cells are productively infected, but infection of B cells and other cell types is occasionally detected. The most common outcome of HTLV-I infection is latent carriage of randomly integrated provirus in CD4+ T cells. HTLV-I does not contain an oncogene and does not insert into a unique site in the genome. Indeed, most infected cells express no viral gene products. The only viral gene product that is routinely expressed in tumor cells transformed by HTLV-I in vivo is *tax*, and even *tax* is not expressed in the tumor cells of many ATL patients. Cells transformed in vitro, by contrast, actively transcribe HTLV-I RNA and produce infectious virions. Most HTLV-I–transformed cell lines are the result of the infection of a normal host T cell in vitro. It is difficult to establish cell lines derived from authentic ATL cells.

Although *tax* does not itself bind to DNA, it does induce the expression of a wide range of host cell gene products, including transcription factors (especially c-rel/NF-κB, ets-1 and -2, and members of the fos/jun family), cytokines [e.g., interleukin (IL) 2, granulocyte-macrophage colony-stimulating factor, and tumor necrosis factor (TNF)], and membrane proteins and receptors [major histocompatibility (MHC) molecules and IL-2 receptor α]. The genes activated by *tax* are generally controlled by transcription factors of the c-rel/NF-κB and cyclic AMP response element binding (CREB) protein families. It is unclear how this induction of host gene expression leads to neoplastic transformation; *tax* can interfere with G_1 and mitotic cell-cycle checkpoints, block apoptosis, inhibit DNA repair, and promote antigen-independent T-cell proliferation. Induction of a cytokine-autocrine loop has been proposed; however, IL-2 is not the crucial cytokine. The involvement of IL-4, IL-7, and IL-15 has been proposed.

In light of the irregular expression of *tax* in ATL cells, it has been suggested that *tax* is important in the early phases of transformation but is not essential for the maintenance of the transformed state. As is clear from the epidemiology of HTLV-I infection, transformation of an infected cell is a rare event and may depend on heterogeneous second, third, or fourth genetic hits. No consistent chromosomal abnormalities have been described in ATL; however, individual cases with p53 mutations and translocations involving the T-cell receptor genes on chromosome 14 have been reported. *Tax* may repress certain DNA repair enzymes, permitting the accumulation of genetic damage that would normally be repaired. However, the molecular pathogenesis of HTLV-I–induced neoplasia is not fully understood.

FEATURES OF HTLV-I INFECTION

Epidemiology

HTLV-I infection is transmitted in at least three ways: from mother to child, especially via breast milk; through sexual activity, more commonly from men to women; and through the blood—via contaminated transfusions or contaminated needles. The virus is most commonly transmitted perinatally. Compared with HIV, which can be transmitted in cell-free form, HTLV-I is less infectious, and its transmission usually requires cell-to-cell contact.

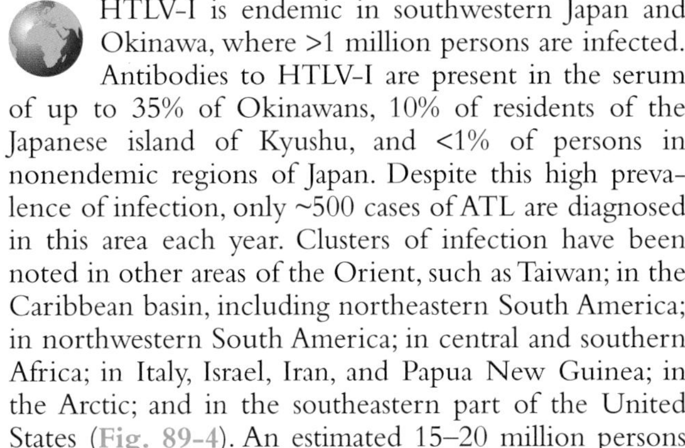

HTLV-I is endemic in southwestern Japan and Okinawa, where >1 million persons are infected. Antibodies to HTLV-I are present in the serum of up to 35% of Okinawans, 10% of residents of the Japanese island of Kyushu, and <1% of persons in nonendemic regions of Japan. Despite this high prevalence of infection, only ~500 cases of ATL are diagnosed in this area each year. Clusters of infection have been noted in other areas of the Orient, such as Taiwan; in the Caribbean basin, including northeastern South America; in northwestern South America; in central and southern Africa; in Italy, Israel, Iran, and Papua New Guinea; in the Arctic; and in the southeastern part of the United States (Fig. 89-4). An estimated 15–20 million persons have HTLV-I infection worldwide.

A progressive spastic or ataxic myelopathy developing in an individual who is HTLV-I positive (i.e., who has serum antibodies to HTLV-I) is likely to be due to direct infection of the nervous system with the virus; a similar disorder may result from infection with HIV or HTLV-II. In rare instances, patients with HAM are seronegative but have detectable antibody to HTLV-I in the cerebrospinal fluid (CSF).

The cumulative lifetime risk of developing ATL is 3% among HTLV-I–infected patients, with a threefold greater risk among men than among women; a similar cumulative risk is projected for HAM (4%), but with women more commonly affected than men. The distribution of the two diseases overlaps the distribution of HTLV-I, with >95% of affected patients showing serologic evidence of HTLV-I infection. The latency period between infection and the emergence of disease is 20–30 years for ATL. For HAM, the median latency period is ~3.3 years (range, 4 months to 30 years). The development of ATL is rare among

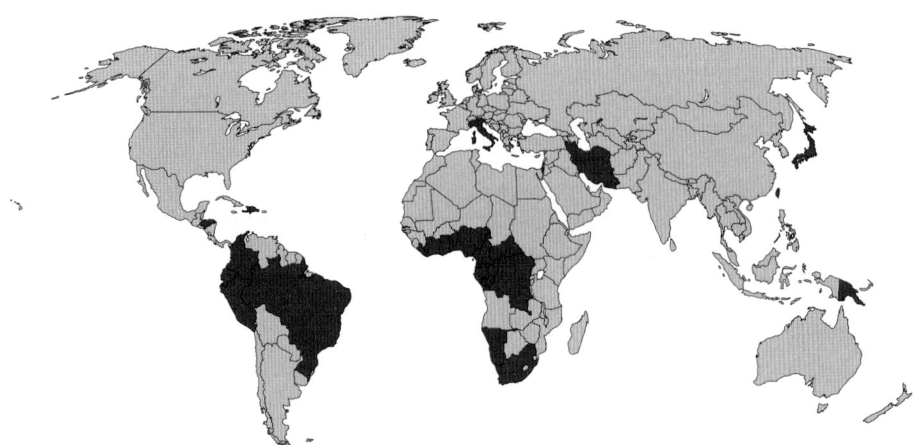

FIGURE 89-4

Global distribution of HTLV-I infection. Countries with a prevalence of HTLV-I infection of 1–5% are shaded darkly. Note that the distribution of infected patients is not uniform in endemic countries. For example, the people of southwestern Japan and northeastern Brazil are more commonly affected than those in other regions of those countries.

persons infected by blood products; however, ~20% of patients with HAM acquire HTLV-I from contaminated blood. ATL is more common among perinatally infected individuals, whereas HAM is more common among persons infected via sexual transmission.

Associated Diseases

ATL

Four clinical types of HTLV-I–induced neoplasia have been described: acute, lymphomatous, chronic, and smoldering. All of these tumors are monoclonal proliferations of CD4+ post-thymic T cells with clonal proviral integrations and clonal T-cell receptor gene rearrangements.

Acute ATL

About 60% of patients who develop malignancy have classic acute ATL, which is characterized by a short clinical prodrome (~2 weeks between the first symptoms and the diagnosis) and an aggressive natural history (median survival period, 6 months). The clinical picture is dominated by rapidly progressive skin lesions, pulmonary involvement, hypercalcemia, and lymphocytosis with cells containing lobulated or "flower-shaped" nuclei. The malignant cells have monoclonal proviral integrations and express CD4, CD3, and CD25 (low-affinity IL-2 receptors) on their surface. Serum levels of CD25 can be used as a tumor marker. Anemia and thrombocytopenia are rare. The skin lesions may be difficult to distinguish from those in mycosis fungoides. Lytic bone lesions, which are common, do not contain tumor cells, but rather are composed of osteolytic cells, usually without osteoblastic activity. Despite the leukemic picture, bone marrow involvement is patchy in most cases.

The hypercalcemia of ATL is multifactorial; the tumor cells produce osteoclast-activating factors (TNF-α, IL-1, lymphotoxin) and can also produce a parathyroid hormone–like molecule. Affected patients have an underlying immunodeficiency that makes them susceptible to opportunistic infections similar to those seen in patients with AIDS (Chap. 90). The pathogenesis of the immunodeficiency is unclear. Pulmonary infiltrates in ATL patients reflect leukemic infiltration half the time and opportunistic infections with organisms such as *Pneumocystis* and other fungi the other half. Gastrointestinal symptoms are nearly always related to opportunistic infection. *Strongyloides stercoralis* is a gastrointestinal parasite that has a pattern of endemic distribution similar to that of HTLV-I. HTLV-I–infected persons also infected with this parasite may develop ATL more often or more rapidly than those without *Strongyloides* infections. Serum concentrations of lactate dehydrogenase (LDH) and alkaline phosphatase are often elevated in ATL. About 10% of patients have leptomeningeal involvement leading to weakness, altered mental status, paresthesia, and/or headache. Unlike other forms of central nervous system (CNS) lymphoma, ATL may be accompanied by normal CSF protein levels. The diagnosis depends on finding ATL cells in the CSF.

Lymphomatous ATL

The lymphomatous type of ATL occurs in ~20% of patients and is similar to the acute form in its natural history and clinical course, except that circulating abnormal cells are rare and lymphadenopathy is evident. The histology of the lymphoma is variable but does not influence the natural history. In general, the diagnosis is suspected on the basis of the patient's birthplace (see "Epidemiology" earlier in the chapter) and the presence of skin lesions and hypercalcemia. The diagnosis is confirmed by the detection of antibodies to HTLV-I in serum.

Chronic ATL

Patients with the chronic form of ATL generally have normal serum levels of calcium and LDH and no involvement of the CNS, bone, or gastrointestinal tract. The median duration of survival for these patients is 2 years. In some cases, chronic ATL progresses to the acute form of the disease.

Smoldering ATL

Fewer than 5% of patients have the smoldering form of ATL. In this form, the malignant cells have monoclonal proviral integration; <5% of peripheral blood cells exhibit typical morphologic abnormalities; hypercalcemia, adenopathy, and hepatosplenomegaly do not develop; the CNS, the bones, and the gastrointestinal tract are not involved; and skin lesions and pulmonary lesions may be present. The median survival period of this small subset of patients appears to be ≥5 years.

HAM (Tropical Spastic Paraparesis)

In contrast to ATL, in which there is a slight predominance of male patients, HAM affects females disproportionately. HAM resembles multiple sclerosis in certain ways. The onset is insidious. Symptoms include weakness or stiffness in one or both legs, back pain, and urinary incontinence. Sensory changes are usually mild, but peripheral neuropathy may develop. The disease generally takes the form of slowly progressive and unremitting thoracic myelopathy; one-third of patients are bedridden within 10 years of diagnosis, and one-half are unable to walk unassisted by this point. Patients display spastic paraparesis or paraplegia with hyperreflexia, ankle clonus, and extensor plantar responses. Cognitive function is usually spared; cranial nerve abnormalities are unusual.

MRI reveals lesions in both the white matter and the paraventricular regions of the brain as well as in the spinal cord. Pathologic examination of the spinal cord shows symmetric degeneration of the lateral columns, including the corticospinal tracts; some cases involve the posterior columns as well. The spinal meninges and cord parenchyma contain an inflammatory infiltrate with myelin destruction.

HTLV-I is not usually found in cells of the CNS but may be detected in a small population of lymphocytes present in the CSF. In general, HTLV-I replication is greater in HAM than in ATL, and patients with HAM have a stronger immune response to the virus. Antibodies to HTLV-I are present in the serum and appear to be produced in the CSF of HAM patients, where titers are often higher than in the serum. The pathophysiology of HAM may involve the induction of autoimmune destruction of neural cells by T cells with specificity for viral components such as Tax or Env proteins. One theory is that susceptibility to HAM may be related to the presence of human leukocyte antigen (HLA) alleles capable of presenting viral antigens in a fashion that leads to autoimmunity. Insufficient data are available to confirm an HLA association. However, antibodies in the sera of HAM patients have been shown to bind a neuron-specific antigen [heteronuclear ribonuclear protein A1 (hnRNP A1)] and to interfere with neurotransmission in vitro.

It is unclear what factors influence whether HTLV-I infection will cause disease and, if it does, whether it will induce a neoplasm (ATL) or an autoimmune disorder (HAM). Differences in viral strains, the susceptibility of particular MHC haplotypes, the route of HTLV-I infection, the viral load, and the nature of the HTLV-I-related immune response are putative factors, but few definitive data are available.

Other Putative HTLV-I–Related Diseases

In areas where HTLV-I is endemic, diverse inflammatory and autoimmune diseases have been attributed to the virus, including uveitis, dermatitis, pneumonitis, rheumatoid arthritis, and polymyositis. However, a causal relationship between HTLV-I and these illnesses has not been established.

Prevention

Women in endemic areas should not breast-feed their children, and blood donors should be screened for serum antibodies to HTLV-I. As in the prevention of HIV infection, the practice of safe sex and the avoidance of needle sharing are important.

℞ Treatment: HTLV-I INFECTION

For the small number of patients who develop HTLV-I–related disease, therapies are not curative. In patients with the acute and lymphomatous types of ATL, the disease progresses rapidly. Hypercalcemia is generally controlled by glucocorticoid administration and cytotoxic therapy directed against the neoplasm. The tumor is highly responsive to combination chemotherapy that is employed against other forms of lymphoma; however, patients are susceptible to overwhelming bacterial and opportunistic infections, and ATL relapses within 4–10 months after remission in most cases. The combination of interferon α and zidovudine may extend survival. Because viral replication is not clearly associated with ATL progression, zidovudine is probably effective through its cytotoxic effects (as a chain-terminating thymidine analogue) rather than its antiviral effects. An experimental approach using an yttrium 90–labeled or toxin-conjugated antibody to the IL-2 receptor appears promising but is not widely available. Patients with the chronic or smoldering form of ATL may be managed with an expectant approach: treat any infections, and watch and wait for signs of progression to acute disease.

Patients with HAM may obtain some benefit from the use of glucocorticoids to reduce inflammation. Antiretroviral regimens have not been effective. In one study, danazol (200 mg three times daily) produced significant neurologic improvement in five of six treated patients, with resolution of urinary incontinence in two cases, decreased spasticity in three, and restoration of the ability to walk after confinement to a wheelchair in two. Physical therapy and rehabilitation are important components of management.

FEATURES OF HTLV-II INFECTION

Epidemiology

HTLV-II is endemic in certain Native American tribes and in Africa. It is generally considered to be a New World virus that was brought from Asia to the Americas 10,000–40,000 years ago during the migration of infected populations across the Bering land bridge. The mode of transmission of HTLV-II is probably the same as that of HTLV-I (see above). HTLV-II may be less readily transmitted sexually than HTLV-I.

Studies of large cohorts of injection drug users with serologic assays that reliably distinguish HTLV-I from HTLV-II indicated that the vast majority of HTLV-positive cohort members were infected with HTLV-II. The seroprevalence of HTLV in a cohort of 7841 injection drug users from drug treatment centers in Baltimore, Chicago, Los Angeles, New Jersey (Asbury Park and Trenton), New York City (Brooklyn and Harlem), Philadelphia, and San Antonio was 20.9%, with >97% of cases due to HTLV-II. The seroprevalence of HTLV-II was higher in the Southwest and the Midwest than in the Northeast. In contrast, the seroprevalence of HIV-1 was higher in the Northeast than in the Southwest or the Midwest. Approximately 3% of the cohort members were infected with both HTLV-II and HIV-1. The seroprevalence of HTLV-II increased linearly with age. Women were significantly more likely to be infected with HTLV-II than were men; the virus is thought to be more efficiently transmitted from male to female than from female to male.

Associated Diseases

Although HTLV-II was isolated from a patient with a T-cell variant of hairy cell leukemia, this virus has not been consistently associated with a particular disease and in fact has been thought of as "a virus searching for a disease." However, evidence is accumulating that HTLV-II may play a role in certain neurologic, hematologic, and dermatologic diseases. These data require confirmation, particularly in light of the previous confusion regarding the relative prevalences of HTLV-I and HTLV-II among injection drug users.

Prevention

Avoidance of needle sharing, adherence to safe-sex practices, screening of blood (by assays for HTLV-I, which also detect HTLV-II), and avoidance of breast-feeding by infected women are important principles in the prevention of spread of HTLV-II.

HUMAN IMMUNODEFICIENCY VIRUS

HIV-1 and HIV-2 are members of the lentivirus subfamily of Retroviridae and are the only lentiviruses known to infect humans. The lentiviruses are slow-acting by comparison with viruses that cause acute infection (e.g., influenza virus) but not by comparison with other retroviruses. The features of acute primary infection with HIV resemble those of more classic acute infections. The characteristic chronicity of HIV disease is consistent with the designation *lentivirus*. For a detailed discussion of HIV, see Chap. 90.

FURTHER READINGS

GHEZ D et al: Neuropilin-1 is involved in human T-cell lymphotropic virus type 1 entry. J Virol 80:6844, 2006

KASHANCHI F, BRADY JN: Transcriptional and post-transcriptional gene regulation of HTLV-1. Oncogene 24:5938, 2005

LEE SM et al: HTLV-1 induced molecular mimicry in neurological disease. Curr Top Microbiol Immunol 296:125, 2005

MANEL N et al: HTLV-I tropism and envelope receptor. Oncogene 24:6016, 2005

MATSUOKA M, JEANG KT: Human T-cell leukaemia virus type 1 (HTLV-1) infectivity and cellular transformation. Nat Rev Cancer 7:270, 2007

PELOPONESE JM et al: Modulation of nuclear factor-κB by human T cell leukemia virus type 1 Tax protein. Immunol Res 34:1, 2006

PROIETTI FA et al: Global epidemiology of HTLV-I infection and associated diseases. Oncogene 24:6058, 2005

TAYLOR GP, MATSUOKA M: Natural history of adult T-cell leukemia/lymphoma and approaches to therapy. Oncogene 24:6047, 2005

CHAPTER 90

HUMAN IMMUNODEFICIENCY VIRUS DISEASE: AIDS AND RELATED DISORDERS

Anthony S. Fauci ■ H. Clifford Lane

AIDS was first recognized in the United States in the summer of 1981, when the U.S. Centers for Disease Control and Prevention (CDC) reported the unexplained occurrence of *Pneumocystis jiroveci* (formerly *P. carinii*) pneumonia in five previously healthy homosexual men in Los Angeles and of Kaposi's sarcoma (KS) with or without *P. jiroveci* pneumonia in 26 previously healthy homosexual men in New York and Los Angeles. Within months, the disease became recognized in male and female injection drug users (IDUs) and soon thereafter in recipients of blood transfusions and in hemophiliacs. As the epidemiologic pattern of the disease unfolded, it became clear that an infectious agent transmissible by sexual (homosexual and heterosexual) contact and blood or blood products was the most likely etiologic cause of the epidemic.

In 1983, human immunodeficiency virus (HIV) was isolated from a patient with lymphadenopathy, and by 1984 it was demonstrated clearly to be the causative agent of AIDS. In 1985, a sensitive enzyme-linked immunosorbent assay (ELISA) was developed, which led to an appreciation of the scope and evolution of the HIV epidemic at first in the United States and other developed nations and ultimately among developing nations throughout the world (see below). The staggering worldwide evolution of the HIV pandemic has been matched by an explosion of information in the areas of HIV virology, pathogenesis (both immunologic and virologic), treatment of HIV disease, treatment and prophylaxis of the opportunistic diseases associated with HIV infection, prevention of infection, and vaccine development. The information flow related to HIV disease is enormous and continues to expand, and it has become almost impossible for the health care generalist to stay abreast of the literature. The purpose of this chapter is to present the most current information available on the scope of the epidemic; on its pathogenesis, treatment, and prevention; and on prospects for vaccine development. Above all, the aim is to provide a solid scientific basis and practical clinical guidelines for a state-of-the-art approach to the HIV-infected patient.

DEFINITION

The current CDC classification system for HIV-infected adolescents and adults categorizes persons on the basis of clinical conditions associated with HIV infection and CD4+ T-lymphocyte counts. The system is based on three ranges of CD4+ T-lymphocyte counts and three clinical categories and is represented by a matrix of nine mutually exclusive categories (Tables 90-1 and 90-2). Using this system, any HIV-infected individual with a CD4+ T-cell count of <200/μL has AIDS by definition, regardless of the presence of symptoms or opportunistic diseases (Table 90-1). Once individuals have had a clinical condition in category B, their disease classification cannot be reverted back to category A, even if the condition resolves; the same holds true for category C in relation to category B.

The definition of AIDS is indeed complex and comprehensive and was established not for the practical care of patients, but for surveillance purposes. Thus the clinician should not focus on whether or not the patient fulfills the strict definition of AIDS, but should view HIV disease as a spectrum ranging from primary infection, with or without the acute syndrome, to the asymptomatic stage, to advanced disease (see below).

ETIOLOGIC AGENT

The etiologic agent of AIDS is HIV, which belongs to the family of human retroviruses (Retroviridae) and the subfamily of lentiviruses (Chap. 89). Nononcogenic lentiviruses cause disease in other animal species, including sheep, horses, goats, cattle, cats, and monkeys. The four recognized human retroviruses belong to two distinct groups: the human T-lymphotropic viruses (HTLV)-I and HTLV-II, which are transforming retroviruses; and the human immunodeficiency viruses, HIV-1 and HIV-2, which cause cytopathic effects either directly or indirectly (see below and Chap. 89). The most common cause of HIV disease throughout the world, and certainly in the United States, is HIV-1, which comprises several subtypes with different geographic distributions (see below). HIV-2 was first identified in 1986 in

TABLE 90-1

1993 REVISED CLASSIFICATION SYSTEM FOR HIV INFECTION AND EXPANDED AIDS SURVEILLANCE CASE DEFINITION FOR ADOLESCENTS AND ADULTS[a]

	CLINICAL CATEGORIES		
CD4+ T-CELL CATEGORIES	A ASYMPTOMATIC, ACUTE (PRIMARY) HIV OR PGL[b]	B SYMPTOMATIC, NOT A OR C CONDITIONS	C AIDS-INDICATOR CONDITIONS
>500/μL	A1	B1	C1
200–499/μL	A2	B2	C2
<200/μL	A3	B3	C3

[a]The shaded areas indicate the expanded AIDS surveillance case definition.
[b]PGL, progressive generalized lymphadenopathy.
Source: MMWR 42(No. RR-17), December 18, 1992.

TABLE 90-2

CLINICAL CATEGORIES OF HIV INFECTION

Category A: Consists of one or more of the conditions listed below in an adolescent or adult (>13 years) with documented HIV infection. Conditions listed in categories B and C must not have occurred.
- Asymptomatic HIV infection
- Persistent generalized lymphadenopathy
- Acute (primary) HIV infection with accompanying illness or history of acute HIV infection

Category B: Consists of symptomatic conditions in an HIV-infected adolescent or adult that are not included among conditions listed in clinical category C and that meet at least one of the following criteria: (1) The conditions are attributed to HIV infection or are indicative of a defect in cell-mediated immunity; or (2) the conditions are considered by physicians to have a clinical course or to require management that is complicated by HIV infection. Examples include, but are not limited to, the following:
- Bacillary angiomatosis
- Candidiasis, oropharyngeal (thrush)
- Candidiasis, vulvovaginal; persistent, frequent, or poorly responsive to therapy
- Cervical dysplasia (moderate or severe)/cervical carcinoma in situ
- Constitutional symptoms, such as fever (38.5°C) or diarrhea lasting >1 month
- Hairy leukoplakia, oral
- Herpes zoster (shingles), involving at least two distinct episodes or more than one dermatome
- Idiopathic thrombocytopenic purpura
- Listeriosis
- Pelvic inflammatory disease, particularly if complicated by tuboovarian abscess
- Peripheral neuropathy

Category C: Conditions listed in the AIDS surveillance case definition.
- Candidiasis of bronchi, trachea, or lungs
- Candidiasis, esophageal
- Cervical cancer, invasive[a]
- Coccidioidomycosis, disseminated or extrapulmonary
- Cryptococcosis, extrapulmonary
- Cryptosporidiosis, chronic intestinal (>1 month's duration)
- Cytomegalovirus disease (other than liver, spleen, or nodes)
- Cytomegalovirus retinitis (with loss of vision)
- Encephalopathy, HIV-related
- Herpes simplex: chronic ulcer(s) (>1 month's duration); or bronchitis, pneumonia, or esophagitis
- Histoplasmosis, disseminated or extrapulmonary
- Isosporiasis, chronic intestinal (>1 month's duration)
- Kaposi's sarcoma
- Lymphoma, Burkitt's (or equivalent term)
- Lymphoma, primary, of brain
- Mycobacterium avium complex or *M. kansasii,* disseminated or extrapulmonary
- Mycobacterium tuberculosis, any site (pulmonary or extrapulmonary)
- Mycobacterium, other species or unidentified species, disseminated or extrapulmonary
- *Pneumocystis jiroveci* pneumonia
- Pneumonia, recurrent[a]
- Progressive multifocal leukoencephalopathy
- Salmonella septicemia, recurrent
- Toxoplasmosis of brain
- Wasting syndrome due to HIV

[a]Added in the 1993 expansion of the AIDS surveillance case definition.
Source: MMWR 42(No. RR-17), December 18, 1992.

West African patients and was originally confined to West Africa. However, a number of cases that can be traced to West Africa or to sexual contacts with West Africans have been identified throughout the world. Both HIV-1 and HIV-2 are zoonotic infections. The *Pan troglodytes troglodytes* species of chimpanzees has been established as the natural reservoir of HIV-1 and the most likely source of original human infection. HIV-2 is more closely related phylogenetically to the simian immunodeficiency virus (SIV) found in sooty mangabeys than it is to HIV-1. The taxonomic relationship among primate lentiviruses is shown in Fig. 90-1.

MORPHOLOGY OF HIV

Electron microscopy shows that the HIV virion is an icosahedral structure (Fig. 90-2*A*) containing numerous external spikes formed by the two major envelope proteins, the external gp120 and the transmembrane gp41. The virion buds from the surface of the infected cell and incorporates a variety of host proteins, including major histocompatibility complex (MHC) class I and II antigens, into its lipid bilayer. The structure of HIV-1 is schematically diagrammed in Fig. 90-2*B* (Chap. 89).

REPLICATION CYCLE OF HIV

HIV is an RNA virus whose hallmark is the reverse transcription of its genomic RNA to DNA by the enzyme *reverse transcriptase*. The replication cycle of HIV begins with the high-affinity binding of the gp120 protein via a portion of its V1 region near the N terminus to its receptor on the host cell surface, the CD4 molecule (Fig. 90-3). The CD4 molecule is a 55-kDa protein found predominantly on a subset of T lymphocytes that are responsible for helper function in the immune system. It is also expressed on the surface of monocytes/macrophages and dendritic/Langerhans cells. Once gp120 binds to CD4, the gp120 undergoes a conformational change that facilitates binding to one of a group of co-receptors. The two major co-receptors for HIV-1 are CCR5 and CXCR4. Both receptors belong to the family of seven-transmembrane-domain G protein–coupled cellular receptors, and the use of one or the other or both receptors by the virus for entry into the cell is an important determinant of the cellular tropism of the virus (see below for details). Certain dendritic cells express a diversity of C-type lectin receptors on their surface, one of which is called *DC-SIGN*, that also bind with high affinity to the HIV gp120 envelope protein, allowing the dendritic cell to facilitate the binding of virus to the CD4+ T cell upon engagement of dendritic cells with CD4+ T cells. After binding of the envelope protein to the CD4 molecule associated with the above-mentioned conformational change in the viral envelope gp120, fusion with the host cell membrane occurs via the newly exposed gp41 molecule penetrating the plasma membrane of the target cell and then coiling upon itself to bring the virion and target cell together. After fusion, the preintegration complex, composed of viral RNA and viral enzymes and surrounded by a capsid

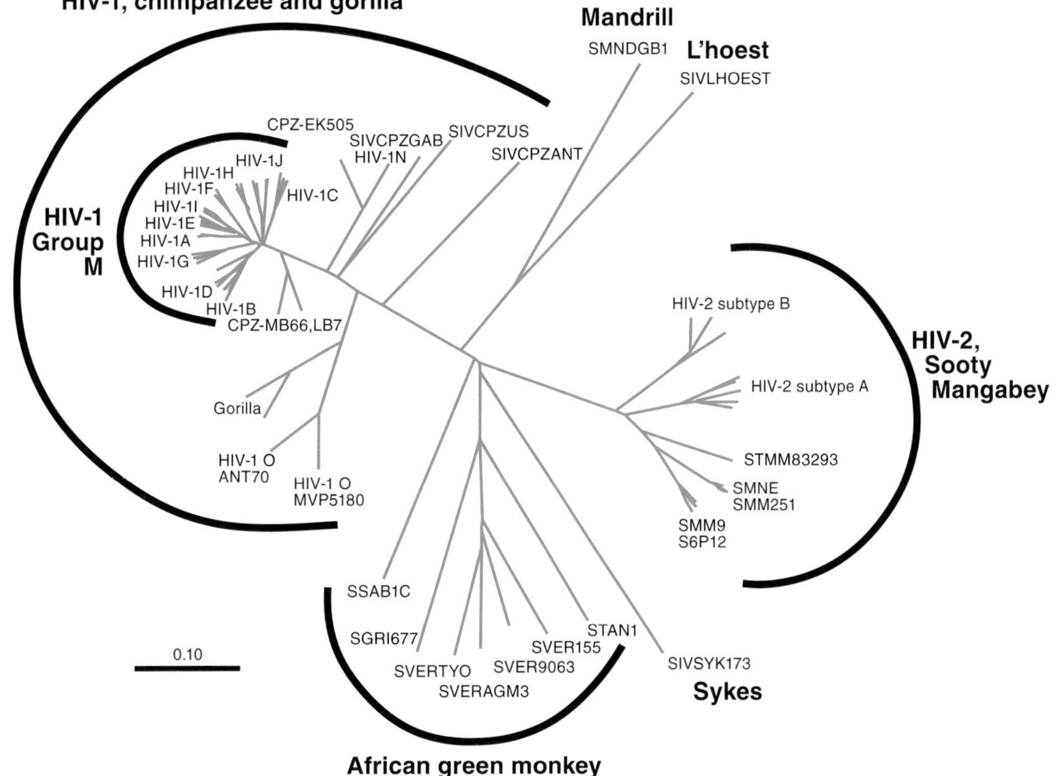

FIGURE 90-1

A phylogenetic tree, based on the complete genomes of primate immunodeficiency viruses. The scale at the bottom (0.10) indicates a 10% difference at the nucleotide level. *(Prepared by Brian Foley, PhD, of the HIV Sequence Database, Theoretical Biology and Biophysics Group, Los Alamos National Laboratory.)*

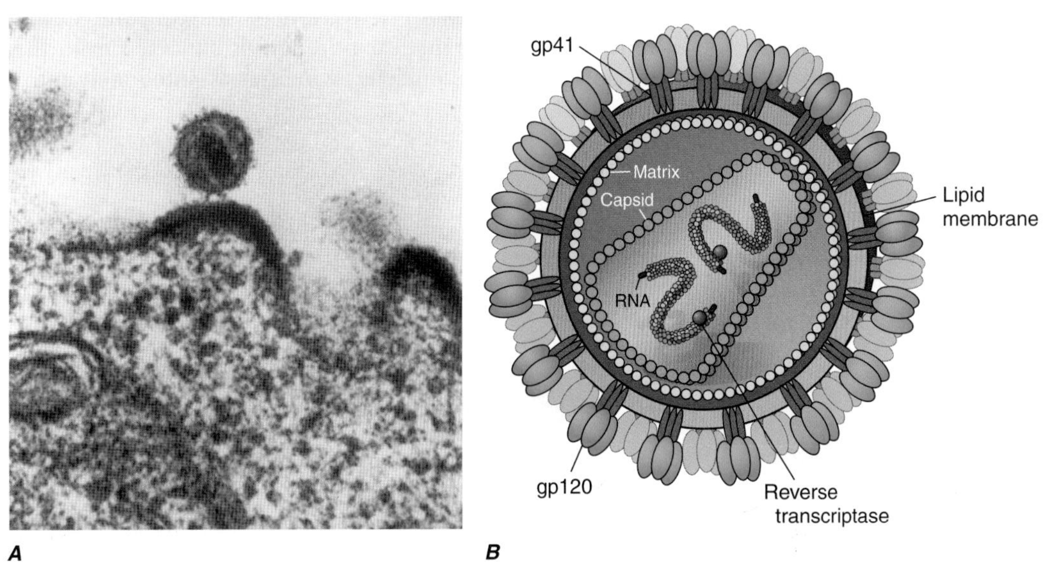

FIGURE 90-2

A.* Electron micrograph of HIV.** Figure illustrates a typical virion after budding from the surface of a CD4+ T lymphocyte, together with two additional incomplete virions in the process of budding from the cell membrane. ***B. Structure of HIV-1, including the gp120 outer membrane, gp41 transmembrane components of the envelope, genomic RNA, enzyme reverse transcriptase, p18(17) inner membrane (matrix), and p24 core protein (capsid) (copyright by George V. Kelvin). *(Adapted from RC Gallo: Sci Am 256:46, 1987.)*

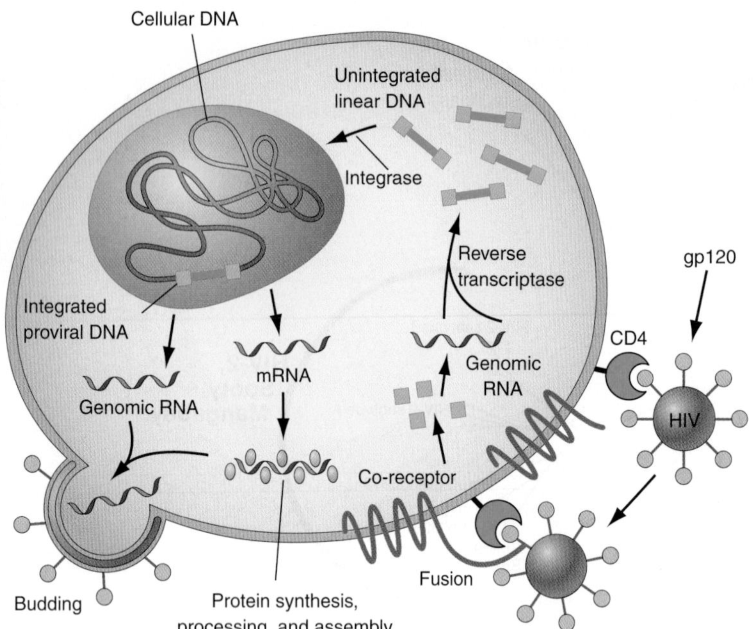

FIGURE 90-3
The replication cycle of HIV. See text for description. *(Adapted from Fauci, 1996.)*

protein coat, is released into the cytoplasm of the target cell (Fig. 90-4). As the preintegration complex traverses the cytoplasm to reach the nucleus (Fig. 90-3), the viral reverse transcriptase enzyme catalyzes the reverse transcription of the genomic RNA into DNA, and the protein coat opens to release the resulting double-stranded HIV-DNA. At this point in the replication cycle, the viral genome is vulnerable to cellular factors that can block the progression of infection. In particular, the cytoplasmic TRIM5-α protein in rhesus macaque cells blocks SIV replication at a point shortly after the virus fuses with the host cell. Although the exact mechanisms of action of TRIM5-α remain unclear, the human form is inhibited by cyclophilin A and is not effective in restricting HIV replication in human cells. The recently described APOBEC family of cellular proteins also inhibits progression of virus infection after virus has entered the cell. APOBEC proteins bind to nascent reverse transcripts and deaminate viral cytidine, causing hypermutation of HIV genomes. It is still not clear whether (1) viral replication is inhibited by the binding of APOBEC to the virus genome with subsequent accumulation of reverse transcripts, or (2) by the hypermutations caused by the enzymatic deaminase activity of APOBEC proteins. HIV has evolved a powerful strategy to protect itself from APOBEC. The viral protein Vif targets APOBEC for proteasomal degradation.

With activation of the cell, the viral DNA accesses the nuclear pore and is exported from the cytoplasm to the nucleus, where it is integrated into the host cell

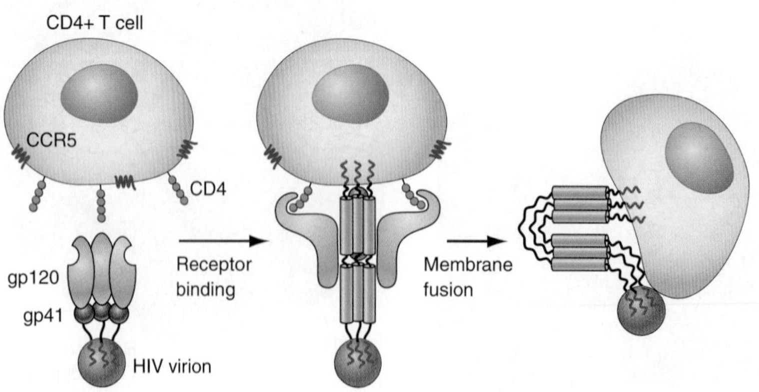

FIGURE 90-4
Binding and fusion of HIV-1 with its target cell. HIV-1 binds to its target cell via the CD4 molecule, leading to a conformational change in the gp120 molecule that allows it to bind to the co-receptor CCR5 (for R5-using viruses). The virus then firmly attaches to the host cell membrane in a coiled-spring fashion via the newly exposed gp41 molecule. Virus-cell fusion occurs as the transitional intermediate of gp41 undergoes further changes to form a hairpin structure that draws the two membranes into close proximity (see text for details). *(Adapted from D Montefiori, JP Moore: Science 283:336, 1999; with permission.)*

chromosomes through the action of another virally encoded enzyme, *integrase*. HIV provirus (DNA) selectively integrates into the nuclear DNA preferentially within introns of active genes and regional hotspots. This provirus may remain transcriptionally inactive (latent) or it may manifest varying levels of gene expression, up to active production of virus.

Cellular activation plays an important role in the replication cycle of HIV and is critical to the pathogenesis of HIV disease (see below). After initial binding and internalization of virions into the target cell, incompletely reverse-transcribed DNA intermediates are labile in quiescent cells and do not integrate efficiently into the host cell genome unless cellular activation occurs shortly after infection. Furthermore, some degree of activation of the host cell is required for the initiation of transcription of the integrated proviral DNA into either genomic RNA or mRNA. This latter process may not necessarily be associated with the detectable expression of the classic cell surface markers of activation. In this regard, activation of HIV expression from the latent state depends on the interaction of a number of cellular and viral factors. After transcription, HIV mRNA is translated into proteins that undergo modification through glycosylation, myristylation, phosphorylation, and cleavage. The viral particle is formed by the assembly of HIV proteins, enzymes, and genomic RNA at the plasma membrane of the cells. Budding of the progeny virion occurs through specialized regions in the lipid bilayer of the host cell membrane known as *lipid rafts*, where the core acquires its external envelope (Chap. 89). The virally encoded protease then catalyzes the cleavage of the gag-pol precursor (see below) to yield the mature virion. Progression through the virus replication cycle is profoundly influenced by a variety of viral regulatory gene products. Likewise, each point in the replication cycle of HIV is a real or potential target for therapeutic intervention (see below). Thus far, the reverse transcriptase, protease, and integrase enzymes as well as the process of virus–target cell binding and fusion have proven clinically to be susceptible to pharmacologic disruption (see below). Inhibitors of the maturation process of virions during the latter phase of the replication cycle are currently being evaluated in clinical trials.

HIV GENOME

Figure 90-5 illustrates schematically the arrangement of the HIV genome. Like other retroviruses, HIV-1 has genes that encode the structural proteins of the virus: *gag* encodes the proteins that form the core of the virion (including p24 antigen); *pol* encodes the enzymes responsible for protease processing of viral proteins, reverse transcription, and integration; and *env* encodes the envelope glycoproteins. However, HIV-1 is more complex than other retroviruses, particularly those of

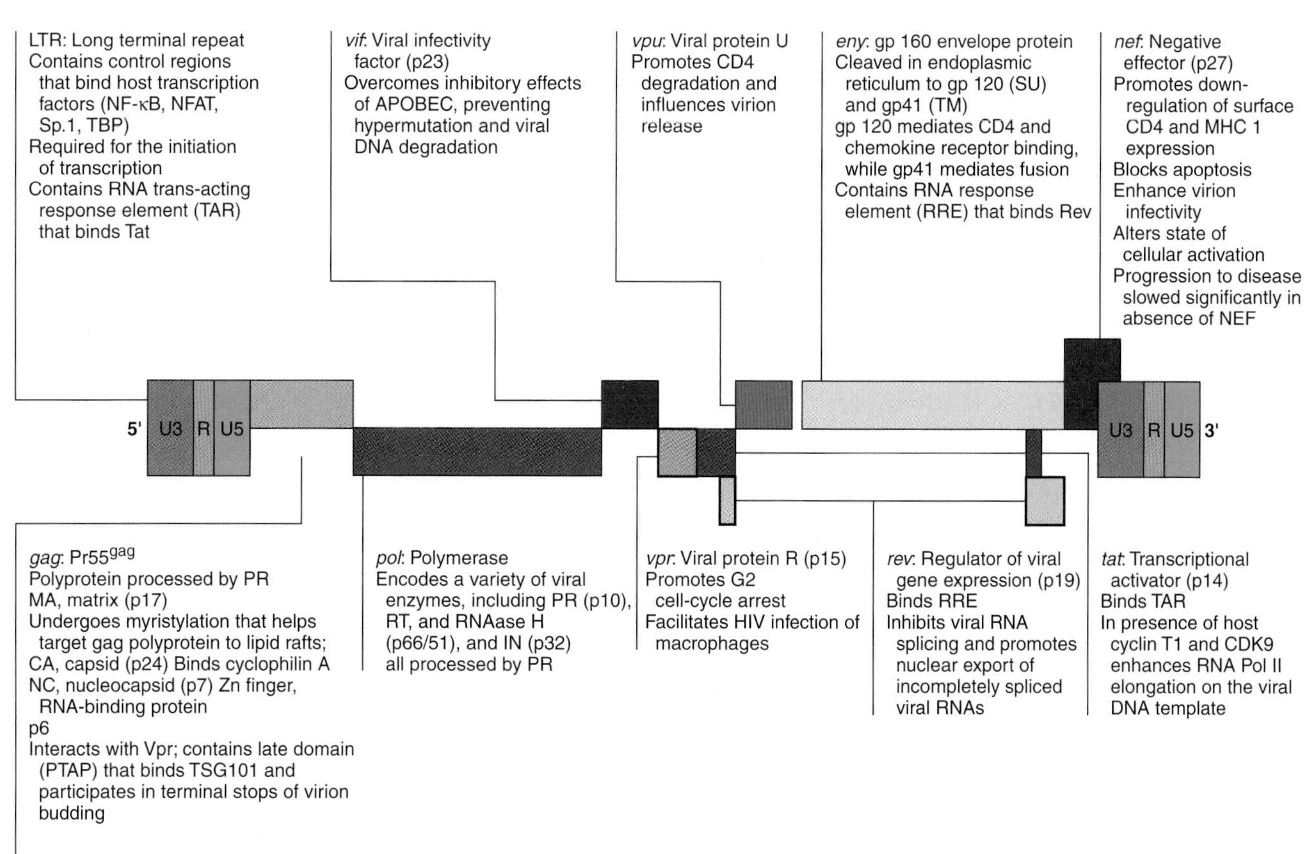

FIGURE 90-5

Organization of the genome of the HIV provirus together with a summary description of its nine genes encoding 15 proteins. *(Adapted from Greene and Peterlin.)*

the nonprimate group, in that it also contains at least six other genes (*tat, rev, nef, vif, vpr,* and *vpu*), which code for proteins involved in the modification of the host cell to enhance virus growth and the regulation of viral gene expression (Chap. 89). Several of these proteins are thought to play a role in the pathogenesis of HIV disease; their various functions are listed in Fig. 90-5. Flanking these genes are the long terminal repeats (LTRs), which contain regulatory elements involved in gene expression (Fig. 90-5). The major difference between the genomes of HIV-1 and HIV-2 is the fact that HIV-2 lacks the *vpu* gene and has a *vpx* gene not contained in HIV-1.

MOLECULAR HETEROGENEITY OF HIV-1

Molecular analyses of HIV isolates reveal varying levels of sequence diversity over all regions of the viral genome. For example, the degree of difference in the coding sequences of the viral envelope protein ranges from a few percent (very close, between isolates from the same infected individual) to 50% (extreme diversity, between isolates from the different groups of HIV-1, M, N, and O; see below). The changes tend to cluster in hypervariable regions. HIV can evolve by several means, including simple base substitution, insertions and deletions, recombination, and gain and loss of glycosylation sites. HIV sequence diversity arises directly from the limited fidelity of the reverse transcriptase. The balance of immune pressure and functional constraints on proteins influences the regional level of variation within proteins. For example, Envelope, which is exposed on the surface of the virion and is under immune selective pressure from both antibodies and cytolytic T lymphocytes, is extremely variable, with clusters of mutations in hypervariable domains. In contrast, Reverse Transcriptase, with important enzymatic functions, is relatively conserved, particularly around the active site. The extraordinary variability of HIV-1 is in marked contrast to the relative stability of HTLV-I and -II.

There are three groups of HIV-1: group M (major), which is responsible for most of the infections in the world; group O (outlier), a relatively rare viral form found originally in Cameroon, Gabon, and France; and group N, first identified in a Cameroonian woman with AIDS; only a few cases of the latter have been identified. Among primate lentiviruses, HIV-1 is most closely related to viruses isolated from chimpanzees and gorillas. The chimpanzee subspecies *Pan troglodytes troglodytes* has been established to be the natural reservoir of the HIV-1 M and N groups. The HIV-1 O group is most closely related to viruses found in Cameroonian gorillas. The M group comprises nine subtypes, or *clades*, designated A, B, C, D, F, G, H, J, and K, as well as a growing number of major and minor circulating recombinant forms (CRFs). CRFs are generated by infection of an individual with two subtypes that then recombine and create a virus with a selective advantage. These CRFs range from highly prevalent forms such as the AE virus, CRF01_AE, which is predominant in southeast Asia and often referred to simply as E, despite the fact that the

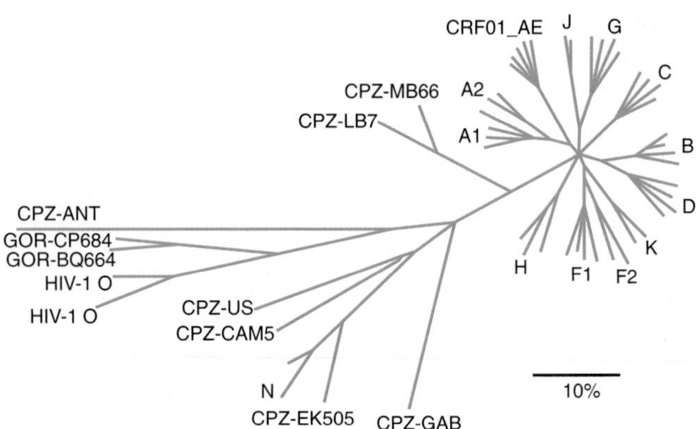

FIGURE 90-6

Phylogenetic tree constructed from representative viral envelope sequences of the subtypes and CRF01 in HIV-1 group M, some isolates from groups N and O (also HIV-1 human), CPZ (chimpanzee), and gorilla (GOR). The scale bar at the bottom indicates the genetic distances between the sequences. A1 and A2, F1 and F2 are subtypes; CRF01_AE is unique in the envelope gene but similar to subtype A in the rest of the genome. *(Courtesy of Brian Foley, PhD, Bette Korber, PhD, and Thomas Leitner, PhD, HIV Database, Los Alamos National Laboratory; with permission.)*

parental E virus has never been found, and CRF02_AG from west and central Africa, to a large number of CRFs that are relatively rare. The subtypes and CRFs create the major lineages of the M group of HIV-1. The picture has been complicated somewhat when it was found that some subtypes are not equidistant from one another, whereas others contained sequences so diverse that they could not properly be considered to be the same subtype. Thus the term *sub-subtype* was introduced, and subtypes A and F are now subdivided into A1 and A2, F1 and F2. It has also been argued that subtypes B and D are really too close to be separate subtypes and should be considered sub-subtypes; it was decided, however, not to increase the confusion by renaming the clades (Fig. 90-6).

The global patterns of HIV-1 variation likely result from accidents of viral trafficking. Subtype B viruses, which now differ by up to 17% in their *env* coding sequences, are the overwhelmingly predominant viruses seen in the United States, Canada, certain countries in South America, western Europe, and Australia. Other subtypes are also present in these countries to varying degrees. It is thought that, purely by chance, subtype B was seeded into the United States in the late 1970s, thereby establishing an overwhelming founder effect. Subtype C viruses (of the M group) are the most common form worldwide; many countries have co-circulating viral subtypes that are giving rise to new CRFs. Figure 90-7 schematically diagrams the worldwide distribution of HIV-1 subtypes by region. Seven strains account for the majority of HIV infections globally: HIV-1 subtypes A, B, C, D, G and two of the CRFs, CRF01_AE and CRF02_AG. The predominant subtype in Europe, Australia, and the Americas is subtype B. In Sub-Saharan Africa, home to

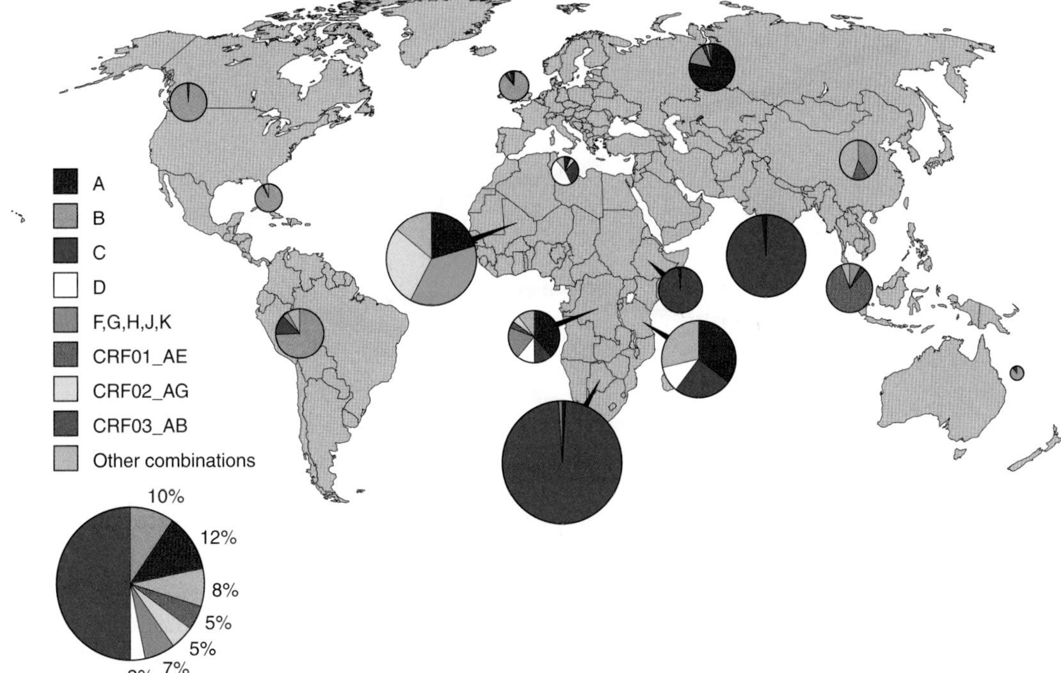

FIGURE 90-7

Geographic distribution of HIV-1 subtypes and recombinants. The prevalence of HIV-1 genetic subtypes varies by geographic region. The proportions of subtypes in different regions are indicated by pie charts. *(From J Hemelaar et al: AIDS 20:W13, 2006.)*

approximately two-thirds of all individuals living with HIV/AIDS, >50% of infections are caused by subtype C, with smaller proportions of infections caused by subtype A, subtype G, CRF02_AG, and other subtypes and recombinants. In Asia, HIV-1 isolates of the CRF01_AE lineage and subtypes C and B predominate. CRF01_AE accounts for most infections in south and southeast Asia, whereas subtype C is prevalent in India (see "HIV Infection and AIDS Worldwide" later in the chapter). Sequence analyses of HIV-1 isolates from infected individuals indicate that recombination among viruses of different clades likely occurs as a result of infection of an individual with viruses of more than one subtype, particularly in geographic areas where subtypes overlap.

TRANSMISSION

HIV is transmitted by both homosexual and heterosexual contact; by blood and blood products; and by infected mothers to infants either intrapartum, perinatally, or via breast milk. After >25 years of scrutiny, there is no evidence that HIV is transmitted by casual contact or that the virus can be spread by insects, such as by a mosquito bite.

SEXUAL TRANSMISSION

HIV infection is predominantly a sexually transmitted disease (STD) worldwide. In the United States, ~49% of the HIV/AIDS cases diagnosed in 2005 among adults and adolescents were attributed to male-to-male sexual contact. Heterosexual contact accounted for another 32%.

Worldwide, the most common mode of infection, particularly in developing countries, is clearly heterosexual transmission. Furthermore, the yearly incidence of new cases of AIDS attributed to heterosexual transmission of HIV is steadily increasing in the United States, mainly among minorities, particularly women in minority groups (Fig. 90-8).

HIV has been demonstrated in seminal fluid both within infected mononuclear cells and in cell-free material. The virus appears to concentrate in the seminal fluid, particularly in situations where there are increased numbers of lymphocytes and monocytes in the fluid, as in genital inflammatory states such as urethritis and epididymitis, conditions closely associated with other STDs (see below). The virus has also been demonstrated in cervical smears and vaginal fluid. There is a strong association of HIV transmission with receptive anal intercourse, probably because only a thin, fragile rectal mucosal membrane separates the deposited semen from potentially susceptible cells in and beneath the mucosa and trauma may be associated with anal intercourse. Anal douching and sexual practices that traumatize the rectal mucosa also increase the likelihood of infection. It is likely that anal intercourse provides at least two modalities of infection: (1) direct inoculation into blood in cases of traumatic tears in the mucosa; and (2) infection of susceptible target cells, such as Langerhans cells, in the mucosal layer in the absence of trauma (see below). Although the vaginal mucosa is several layers thicker than the rectal mucosa and less likely to be traumatized during intercourse, it is clear that the virus can be transmitted to either partner through vaginal intercourse.

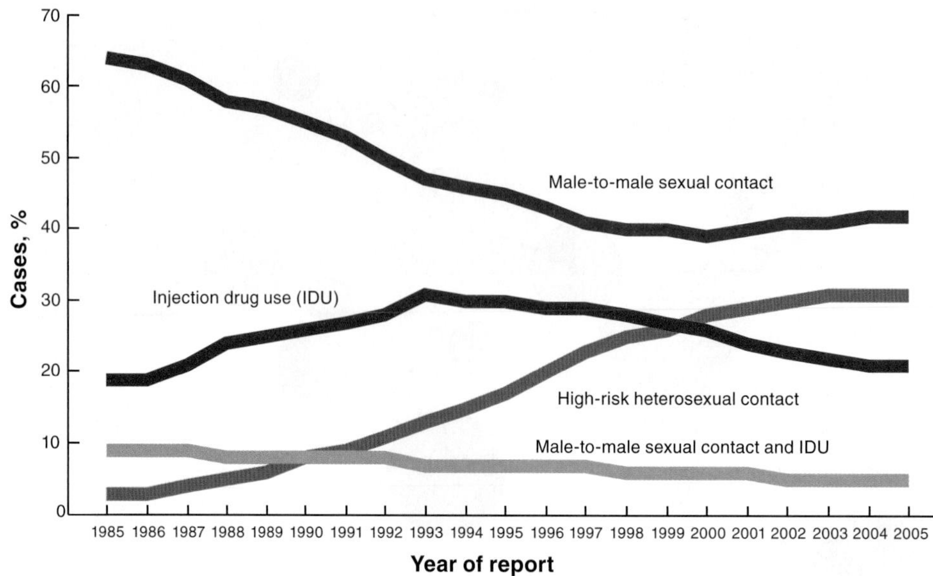

FIGURE 90-8

AIDS cases among U.S. adults and adolescents by exposure category and year of diagnosis. The proportion of AIDS cases attributed to heterosexual contact with a person known to have or at high risk for HIV infection (high-risk heterosexual) increased from 3% in 1985 to 31% in 2005. IDU, injection drug use. *[From The Centers for Disease Control and Prevention (CDC).]*

Studies in the United States and Europe have found that male-to-female HIV transmission is usually more efficient than female-to-male transmission, but small numbers of HIV-positive female index partners limit conclusive sex-specific estimates of transmission probabilities per sex act. The differences in reported transmission rates between men and women may be due in part to the prolonged exposure to infected seminal fluid of the vaginal and cervical mucosa, as well as the endometrium (when semen enters through the cervical os). By comparison, the penis and urethral orifice are exposed relatively briefly to infected vaginal fluid. Among various cofactors examined in studies of heterosexual HIV transmission, the presence of other sexually transmitted diseases (STDs; see below) has been strongly associated with HIV transmission. In this regard, there is a close association between genital ulcerations and transmission, from the standpoints of both susceptibility to infection and infectivity. Infections with microorganisms such as *Treponema pallidum* (Chap. 70), *Haemophilus ducreyi* (Chap. 47), and herpes simplex virus (HSV; Chap. 80) are important causes of genital ulcerations linked to transmission of HIV. In addition, pathogens responsible for nonulcerative inflammatory STDs such as those caused by *Chlamydia trachomatis* (Chap. 77), *Neisseria gonorrhoeae* (Chap. 45), and *Trichomonas vaginalis* (Chap. 122) are also associated with an increased risk of transmission of HIV infection. Bacterial vaginosis, an infection related to sexual behavior, but not strictly an STD, may also be linked to an increased risk of transmission of HIV infection. Several studies suggest that treating other STDs and genital tract syndromes may help prevent transmission of HIV. This effect is most prominent in populations in which the prevalence of HIV infection is relatively low. In studies conducted in Uganda, the chief predictor of heterosexual transmission of HIV was the level of plasma viremia. In a cohort of couples in which one partner was HIV-infected and one was initially uninfected, the mean serum HIV RNA level was significantly higher among HIV-infected subjects whose partners seroconverted than among those whose partners did not seroconvert. In fact transmission was rare when the infected partner had a plasma level of <1500 copies of HIV RNA per milliliter. The rate of HIV transmission per coital act was highest during the early stage of HIV infection when plasma HIV RNA levels are highest and in advanced disease as the viral set point increases (Fig. 90-9).

A number of studies have indicated that male *circumcision* is associated with a lower risk of HIV infection among men. This difference may be due to increased susceptibility of uncircumcised men to ulcerative STDs, as well as other factors such as microtrauma to the foreskin and glans penis. In addition, the highly vascularized inner foreskin tissue contains a high density of Langerhans cells as well as increased numbers of CD4+ T cells, macrophages, and other cellular targets for HIV. Finally, the moist environment under the foreskin may promote the presence or persistence of microbial flora that, via inflammatory changes, may lead to even higher concentrations of target cells for HIV in the foreskin. In some studies the use of oral contraceptives was associated with an increase in incidence of HIV infection over and above that which might be expected by not using a condom for birth control. This phenomenon may be due to drug-induced changes in the cervical mucosa, rendering it more vulnerable to penetration by the virus. Adolescent girls might also be more susceptible to

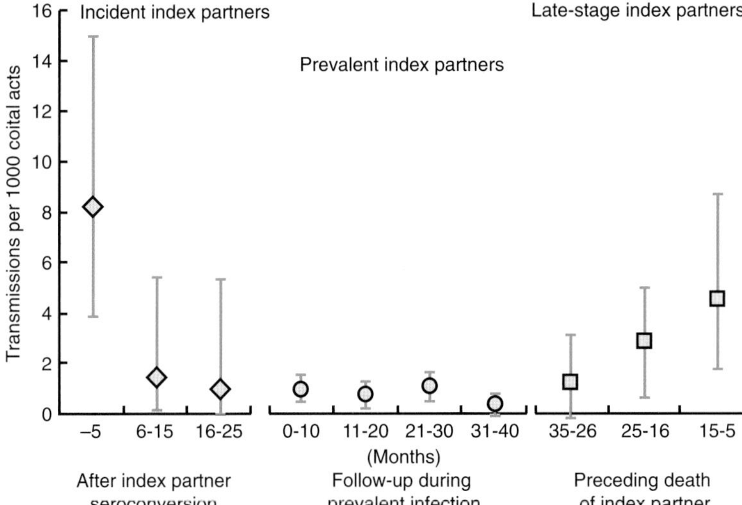

FIGURE 90-9
HIV transmission rate per coital act among 235 HIV serodiscordant couples in Uganda, and 95% confidence intervals, by follow-up interval. The risk of HIV transmission was highest during early-stage and late-stage infection. *(From Wawer et al.)*

infection upon exposure due to the properties of an immature genital tract with increased cervical ectopy or exposed columnar epithelium.

Oral sex is a much less efficient mode of transmission of HIV than is receptive anal intercourse. A number of studies have reported that the incidence of transmission of infection by oral sex among couples discordant for HIV was extremely low. However, there have been reports of documented HIV transmission resulting solely from receptive fellatio and insertive cunnilingus. Therefore, the assumption that receptive oral sex is completely safe is not warranted. The association of alcohol consumption and illicit drug use with unsafe sexual behavior, both homosexual and heterosexual, leads to an increased risk of sexual transmission of HIV. Methamphetamine ("crystal meth," "tina") and other so-called club drugs (e.g., ecstasy, ketamine, and gamma hydroxybutyrate), sometimes taken in conjunction with sildenafil (Viagra) or related drugs have been associated with risky sexual practices and increased risk of HIV infection, particularly among men who have sex with men.

TRANSMISSION BY BLOOD AND BLOOD PRODUCTS

HIV can be transmitted to individuals who receive HIV-tainted blood transfusions, blood products, or transplanted tissue as well as to IDUs who are exposed to HIV while sharing injection paraphernalia such as needles, syringes, the water in which drugs are mixed, or the cotton through which drugs are filtered. Parenteral transmission of HIV during injection drug use does not require IV puncture; SC ("skin popping") or IM ("muscling") injections can transmit HIV as well, even though these behaviors are sometimes erroneously perceived as low-risk. Among IDUs, the risk of HIV infection increases with the duration of injection drug use; the frequency of needle sharing; the number of partners with whom paraphernalia are shared, particularly in the setting of "shooting galleries" where drugs are sold and large numbers of IDUs may share a limited number of "works"; comorbid psychiatric conditions such as antisocial personality disorder; the use of cocaine in injectable form or smoked as "crack"; and the use of injection drugs in a geographic location with a high prevalence of HIV infection, such as certain inner-city areas in the United States.

The first transfusion-associated cases of AIDS were reported in 1982, and by the end of 2005, >9300 individuals in the United States who survived the illness for which they received HIV-contaminated blood transfusions, blood components, or transplanted tissue had developed AIDS. Virtually all these cases were due to HIV infection before the spring of 1985, when mandatory testing of donated blood for HIV-1 was initiated. It is estimated that 90–100% of individuals who were exposed to HIV-contaminated products became infected. Transfusions of whole blood, packed red blood cells, platelets, leukocytes, and plasma are all capable of transmitting HIV infection. In contrast, hyperimmune γ globulin, hepatitis B immune globulin, plasma-derived hepatitis B vaccine, and Rh_o immune globulin have not been associated with transmission of HIV infection. The procedures involved in processing these products either inactivate or remove the virus.

In addition to the above, an estimated 8000–10,000 individuals in the United States with hemophilia or other clotting disorders were infected with HIV by receipt of HIV-contaminated fresh-frozen plasma or concentrates of clotting factors; by the end of 2005, >5400 of these individuals had developed AIDS. Currently, in the United States and in most developed countries, the following measures have made the risk of transmission of HIV infection by transfused blood or blood products extremely small: (1) the screening of all blood for HIV nucleic acid, p24 antigen, and/or anti-HIV antibodies; (2) the self-deferral of donors on the basis of risk behavior; (3) the screening out of HIV-negative individuals with positive surrogate laboratory parameters of HIV infection, such as hepatitis B and C; and (4) serologic testing for syphilis. The chance of infection of a hemophiliac via clotting factor concentrates has essentially been eliminated because of the added layer of safety resulting from heat treatment of the concentrates.

It is currently estimated that the risk of infection with HIV in the United States via transfused screened blood is approximately 1 in 1.5 million donations. Therefore, among the ~15 million donations collected in the United States each year, about 10 infectious donations are available for transfusion. Thus, despite the best efforts of science, one cannot completely eliminate the risk of transfusion-related transmission of HIV since current technology cannot detect HIV RNA for the first 1–2 weeks after infection due to the low levels of viremia. There have been several reports of sporadic breakdowns in routinely available screening procedures in certain countries, where contaminated blood was allowed to be transfused, resulting in small clusters of patients becoming infected. In China, a disturbingly large number of persons have become infected by selling blood in situations where the collectors reused needles that were contaminated and, in some instances, mixed blood products from a number of individuals, separated the plasma, and reinfused red blood cells back into individual donors.

There have been no reported cases of transmission of HIV-2 in the United States via donated blood or tissues, and, currently, donated blood is screened for both HIV-1 and HIV-2 antibodies. Transmission of HIV (both HIV-1 and HIV-2) by blood or blood products is still an ongoing threat in certain developing countries, particularly in Sub-Saharan Africa, where routine screening of blood is not universally practiced.

Before the screening of donors, a small number of cases of transmission of HIV via semen used in artificial insemination and tissues used in organ transplantation were documented. At present, donors of such tissues are prescreened for HIV infection. However, laboratory errors can occur, and in 2007 an incorrect screening report led to the transplantation in Italy of two kidneys and a liver to three recipients from a deceased donor who was later discovered to have been HIV positive. With regard to HIV sero-discordant couples (male, HIV infected; female, HIV-uninfected) who wish to conceive a child, assisted reproductive techniques using sperm-washing to reduce the risk of HIV transmission have been successfully employed, with only one well-documented seroconversion in the uninfected female partner, reported in 1990.

OCCUPATIONAL TRANSMISSION OF HIV: HEALTH CARE WORKERS, LABORATORY WORKERS, AND THE HEALTH CARE SETTING

There is a small, but definite, occupational risk of HIV transmission to health care workers and laboratory personnel and potentially others who work with HIV-containing materials, particularly when sharp objects are used. An estimated 600,000–800,000 health care workers are stuck with needles or other sharp medical instruments in the United States each year.

Exposures that place a health care worker at potential risk of HIV infection are percutaneous injuries (e.g., a needle stick or cut with a sharp object) or contact of mucous membrane or nonintact skin (e.g., exposed skin that is chapped, abraded, or afflicted with dermatitis) with blood, tissue, or other potentially infectious body fluids. Large, multi-institutional studies have indicated that the risk of HIV transmission after skin puncture from a needle or a sharp object that was contaminated with blood from a person with documented HIV infection is ~0.3% and after a mucous membrane exposure it is 0.09% (see "HIV and the Health Care Worker" later in the chapter). HIV transmission after non-intact skin exposure has been documented, but the average risk for transmission by this route has not been precisely determined; however, it is estimated to be less than the risk for mucous membrane exposure. Transmission of HIV through intact skin has not been documented.

In addition to blood and visibly bloody body fluids, semen and vaginal secretions are also considered potentially infectious but have not been implicated in occupational transmission from patients to health care workers. The following fluids are also considered potentially infectious: cerebrospinal fluid, synovial fluid, pleural fluid, peritoneal fluid, pericardial fluid, and amniotic fluid. The risk for transmission after exposure to fluids or tissues other than HIV-infected blood also has not been quantified but is probably considerably lower than for blood exposures. Feces, nasal secretions, saliva, sputum, sweat, tears, urine, and vomitus are not considered potentially infectious unless they are visibly bloody. Rare cases of HIV transmission via human bites have been reported, but not after an occupational exposure.

An increased risk for HIV infection after percutaneous exposures to HIV-infected blood is associated with exposures involving a relatively large quantity of blood, as in the case of a device visibly contaminated with the patient's blood, a procedure that involves a needle placed directly in a vein or artery, or a deep injury. Factors that might be associated with mucocutaneous transmission of HIV include exposure to an unusually large volume of blood, prolonged contact, and a potential portal of entry. In addition, the risk increases for exposures to blood from patients with advanced-stage disease, owing to the higher titer of HIV in the blood as well as to other factors, such as the presence of more virulent strains of virus. The use of antiretroviral drugs as postexposure prophylaxis decreases the risk of infection compared with historic controls in occupationally exposed health care workers (see "HIV and the Health Care Worker" later in the chapter). The risk of hepatitis B virus (HBV) infection after a similar type of exposure is ~6–30% in nonimmune individuals; if a susceptible worker is exposed to HBV, postexposure prophylaxis with hepatitis B immune globulin and initiation of HBV vaccine is >90% effective in preventing HBV infection. The risk of hepatitis C virus (HCV) infection after percutaneous injury is ~1.8% (Chap. 92).

Since the beginning of the HIV epidemic, there have been at least three reported instances in which transmission of infection from a health care worker to patients seemed highly probable. One cluster of infections involved an HIV-infected dentist in Florida who apparently infected as many as six of his patients, most likely through contaminated instruments. Another case involved an HIV-infected orthopedic surgeon in France who apparently infected a patient during placement of a total hip prosthesis. A third case involved the apparent transmission of HIV from an HIV-infected nurse to a surgical patient in France. Breaches in infection control and the reuse of contaminated syringes have also resulted in the transmission of HIV from patient to patient in hospitals, nursing homes, and outpatient settings. For example, in the only report of HIV transmission from patient to patient during a surgical procedure, four patients in Australia were apparently infected by an HIV-negative general surgeon during routine outpatient surgery. Although the mechanism of transmission was not definitively identified, a failure on the part of the surgeon to sterilize instruments properly after prior surgery on an HIV-infected patient was considered a likely explanation for this outbreak. Three patients (two in hospitals in the United States and one in the Netherlands) undergoing nuclear medicine procedures were reported to have inadvertently received IV injections of blood or other material from patients infected with HIV. Hemodialysis centers have also been implicated in several reported HIV transmission incidents.

The most dramatic reports involved transmission of HIV to 8000–10,000 children in Romanian orphanages in the 1980s. Other large incidents occurred in hospitals in Russia and Libya in the late 1980s and late 1990s, respectively. Each of these incidents received considerable attention and likely was related to reuse of contaminated needles and/or administration of contaminated blood products. Despite the small number of documented cases, the risk of HIV transmission involving health care workers (infected or not) to patients is extremely low in developed countries; in fact, too low to be measured accurately. In this regard, several epidemiologic studies have been performed tracing thousands of patients of HIV-infected dentists, physicians, surgeons, obstetricians, and gynecologists, and no other cases of HIV infection that could be linked to the health care providers were identified. The very rare occurrence of transmission of HIV as well as HBV and HCV to and from health care workers in the workplace underscores the importance of the use of universal precautions when caring for all patients (see below and Chap. 13).

MATERNAL-FETAL/INFANT TRANSMISSION

HIV infection can be transmitted from an infected mother to her fetus during pregnancy, during delivery, or by breast-feeding. This is an extremely important form of transmission of HIV infection in certain developing countries, where the proportion of infected women to infected men is ~1:1. Virologic analysis of aborted fetuses indicate that HIV can be transmitted to the fetus as early as the first and second trimester of pregnancy. However, maternal transmission to the fetus occurs most commonly in the perinatal period. Two studies performed in Rwanda and the former Zaire indicated that the relative proportions of mother-to-child transmissions were 23–30% before birth, 50–65% during birth, and 12–20% via breast-feeding.

In the absence of prophylactic antiretroviral therapy to the mother during pregnancy, labor, and delivery, and to the fetus after birth (see below), the probability of transmission of HIV from mother to infant/fetus ranges from 15–25% in industrialized countries and from 25–35% in developing countries. These differences may relate to the adequacy of prenatal care as well as to the stage of HIV disease and the general health of the mother during pregnancy. Higher rates of transmission have been reported to be associated with many factors, the best documented of which is the presence of high maternal levels of plasma viremia. In one study of 552 singleton pregnancies in the United States, the rate of mother-to-baby transmission was 0% among women with <1000 copies of HIV RNA per milliliter of blood, 16.6% among women with 1000–10,000 copies/mL, 21.3% among women with 10,001–50,000 copies/mL, 30.9% among women with 50,001–100,000 copies/mL, and 40.6% among women with >100,000 copies/mL. However, there may not be a lower "threshold" below which transmission never occurs, since other studies have reported transmission by women with viral RNA levels <50 copies/mL. Low maternal CD4+ T-cell counts have also been associated with higher rates of transmission; however, since low CD4+ T-cell counts are often associated with high levels of plasma viremia, in one study using multivariate analysis including plasma viral load and CD4+ T-cell count, only the level of plasma HIV RNA was significant. Increased mother-to-child transmission is also correlated with closer HLA match between mother and child. A prolonged interval between membrane rupture and delivery is another well-documented risk factor for transmission. Other conditions that are potential risk factors, but which have not been consistently demonstrated, are the presence of chorioamnionitis at delivery; STDs during pregnancy; hard drug use during pregnancy; cigarette smoking; preterm delivery; and obstetrical procedures such as amniocentesis, amnioscopy, fetal scalp electrodes, and episiotomy. In a study conducted in the United States and France, zidovudine treatment of HIV-infected pregnant women from the beginning of the second trimester through delivery and of the infant for 6 weeks after birth dramatically decreased the rate of intrapartum and perinatal transmission of HIV infection from 22.6% in the untreated group to <5%. The rate of mother-to-child transmission is approaching 1% or less in pregnant women who are receiving combination antiretroviral therapy for their HIV infection. Such treatment, combined with cesarean section delivery, has rendered mother-to-child transmission of HIV an unusual event in the United States and other developed nations. In developed countries, current recommendations to reduce perinatal transmission of HIV include universal voluntary HIV testing and counseling of pregnant women, antiretroviral prophylaxis with one or more drugs in cases in which the mother does not require therapy for her HIV infection, combination therapy for women who do require therapy, obstetric management that attempts to minimize exposure of the infant to maternal blood and genital secretions, and avoidance of

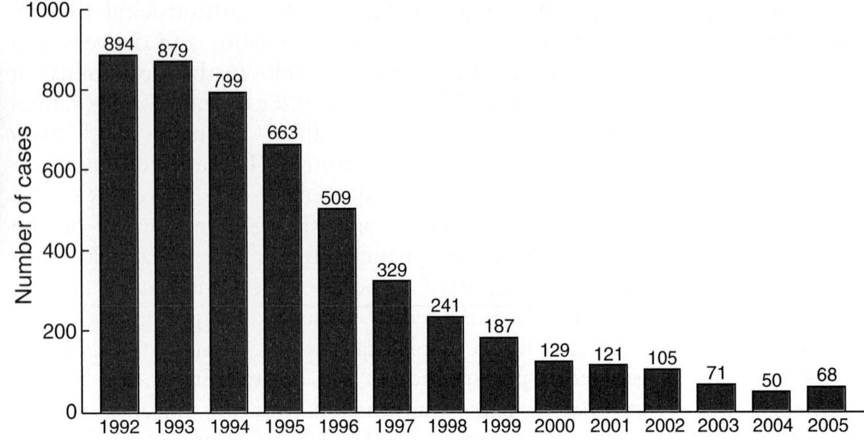

FIGURE 90-10
Estimated numbers of AIDS cases in children <13 years of age, by year of diagnosis, 1992–2005, 50 states and the District of Columbia. *(From CDC.)*

breast-feeding. It is recommended that the choice of antiretroviral therapy for pregnant women should be based on the same considerations used for women who are not pregnant, with discussion of the recognized and unknown risks and benefits of such therapy during pregnancy (see later in the chapter under "Treatment"). This approach has led to a remarkable decrease in the number of infants infected with HIV through mother-to-child transmission in the United States, from an estimated peak of 1750 HIV-infected infants born each year during the early to mid-1990s to 280–370 infants in 2000, and a dramatic decrease in reported AIDS cases among children (Fig. 90-10). Certain studies have demonstrated that truncated regimens of zidovudine alone or in combination with lamivudine given to the mother during the last few weeks of pregnancy or even only during labor and delivery, and to the infant for a week or less, significantly reduced transmission to the infant compared with placebo. Short-course prophylactic antiretroviral (ARV) regimens, such as a single dose of nevirapine given to the mother at the onset of labor and a single dose to the infant within 72 h of birth, are of particular relevance to low- to mid-income nations because of the low cost and the fact that in these regions perinatal care is often not available and pregnant women are often seen by a health care provider for the first time at or near the time of delivery. Indeed, short-course ARV regimens have now been used for several years in developing nations for the prevention of mother-to-child transmission. It is estimated that the successful implementation of such regimens has saved as many as 1000 babies per day from becoming infected with HIV, the vast majority of whom are in Sub-Saharan Africa. Given that combination ARV therapy is now increasingly available to individuals in developing countries due to the lower cost of drugs and programs that are making drugs available to these regions of the world, combinations of drugs are being used more frequently, where available, to treat HIV-infected pregnant women who require therapy notwithstanding their pregnancy. This has had the effect of benefitting the women, blocking HIV transmission to the fetus, and protecting against subsequent transmission by breast-feeding (see below).

Breast-feeding is an important modality of transmission of HIV infection in developing countries, particularly where mothers continue to breast-feed for prolonged periods. The risk factors for mother-to-child transmission of HIV via breast-feeding are not fully understood; factors that increase the likelihood of transmission include detectable levels of HIV in breast milk, the presence of mastitis, low maternal CD4+ T-cell counts, and maternal vitamin A deficiency. The risk of HIV infection via breast-feeding is highest in the early months of breast-feeding. In addition, exclusive breast-feeding has been reported to carry a lower risk of HIV transmission than mixed feeding. Certainly in developed countries, breast-feeding by an infected mother should be avoided. However, there is disagreement regarding recommendations for breast-feeding in certain developing countries, where breast milk is the only source of adequate nutrition as well as immunity against potentially serious infections for the infant. The optimal approach to prevent transmission by infected mothers who choose to breast-feed would be to provide continual treatment to the infected mother. This approach has become more feasible as ARV therapy becomes more widely available in developing countries. Despite progress in this regard, ARV therapy is currently available to only ~25% of persons in developing nations who require it. Therefore, alternative approaches to block transmission by breast-feeding are being tested. In this regard, studies are being conducted to determine whether intermittent administration of nevirapine, which has a relatively long half-life, to uninfected babies born of infected mothers decreases the incidence of infection via breast-feeding.

TRANSMISSION BY OTHER BODY FLUIDS

Although HIV can be isolated typically in low titers from saliva of a small proportion of infected individuals, there is no convincing evidence that saliva can transmit HIV infection, either through kissing or through other exposures, such as occupationally to health care workers. Saliva contains endogenous antiviral factors; among these factors, HIV-specific immunoglobulins of IgA, IgG, and IgM isotypes are detected readily in salivary secretions of infected individuals. It has been suggested that large glycoproteins such as mucins and thrombospondin-1 sequester HIV into aggregates for clearance by the host. In addition, a number of soluble salivary factors inhibit HIV to various degrees in vitro, probably by targeting host cell receptors rather than the virus itself. Perhaps the best-studied of these, secretory leukocyte protease inhibitor (SLPI), blocks HIV infection in several cell culture systems, and it is found in saliva at levels that approximate those required for inhibition of HIV in vitro. In this regard, higher salivary levels of SLPI in breast-fed infants were associated with a decreased risk of HIV transmission through breast milk. It has also been suggested that submandibular saliva reduces HIV infectivity by stripping gp120 from the surface of virions, and that saliva-mediated disruption and lysis of HIV-infected cells occurs because of the hypotonicity of oral secretions. There have been outlier cases of suspected transmission by saliva, but these have probably been blood-to-blood transmissions. Transmission of HIV by a human bite can occur but is a rare event; at least four cases of such transmission have been reported. In addition, a most unusual form of HIV transmission from infected children to mothers in the former Soviet Union has been identified. In those cases, the children (infected through transfusion) were said to have bleeding sores in the mouth, and the mothers were said to have lacerations and abrasions on and around the nipples of the breast resulting from trauma from the children's teeth. Breast-feeding had been continued until the children were older than is usual in other developed countries.

Although virus can be identified, if not isolated, from virtually any body fluid, there is no evidence that HIV transmission can occur as a result of exposure to tears, sweat, and urine. However, there have been isolated cases of transmission of HIV infection by body fluids that may or may not have been contaminated with blood. Most of these situations occurred in the setting of a close relative providing intensive nursing care for an HIV-infected person without observing universal precautions, underscoring the importance of observing such precautions in the handling of body fluids and wastes from HIV-infected individuals (see below).

EPIDEMIOLOGY

HIV INFECTION AND AIDS WORLDWIDE

HIV infection/AIDS is a global pandemic, with cases reported from virtually every country. At the end of 2007, 33.2 million individuals were living with HIV infection (range: 30.6–36.1 million) according to the Joint United Nations Programme on HIV/AIDS (UNAIDS). More than 95% of people living with HIV/AIDS reside in low- and middle-income countries; ~50% are female, and 2.5 million are children <15 years. The global distribution of these cases is illustrated in Fig. 90-11.

In 2007, there were an estimated 2.5 million new cases of HIV infection worldwide, including 420,000 in children <15 years. In 2007, global AIDS deaths totaled 2.1 million (including 330,000 children <15 years). UNAIDS estimates that global HIV prevalence has been level since 2001. HIV incidence likely peaked in the late 1990s at >3 million new infections per year (Fig. 90-12). Recent reductions in global HIV incidence likely reflect natural trends in the pandemic as well as the results of prevention programs resulting in behavior change.

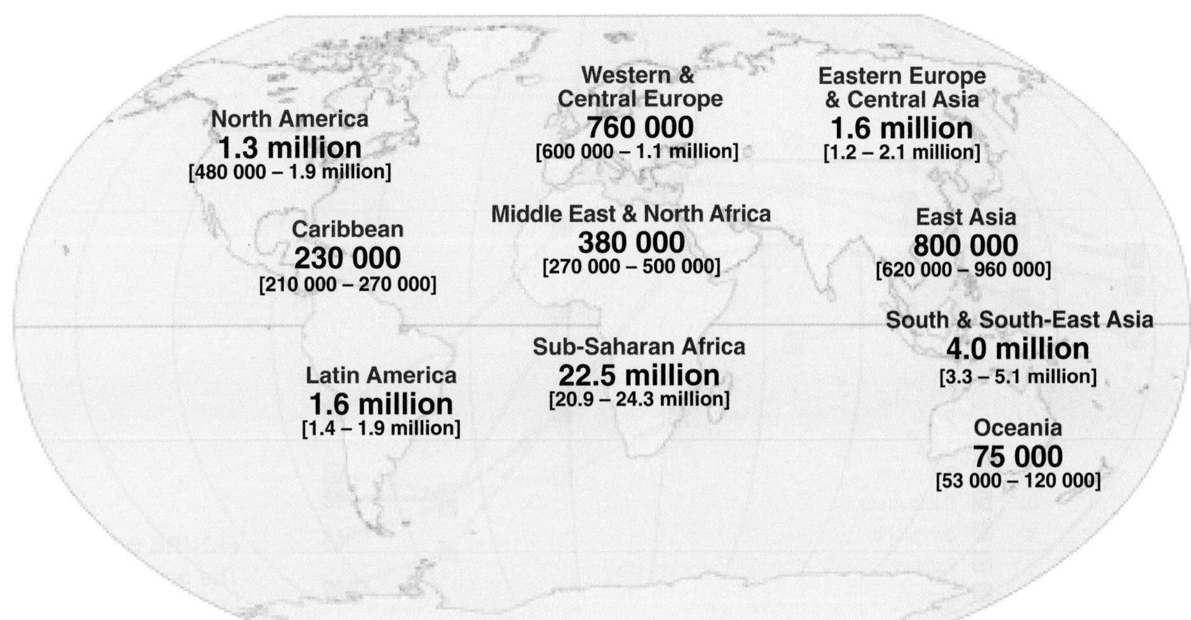

FIGURE 90-11

Estimated number of adults and children living with HIV infection as of December, 2007. Total: 33.2 (30.6–36.1) million. *[From United Nations AIDS Program (UNAIDS).]*

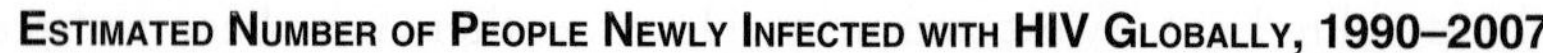

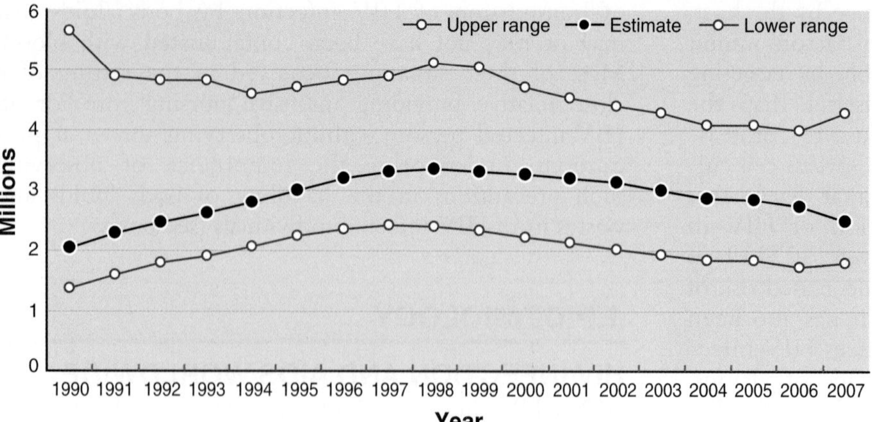

FIGURE 90-12
Estimated number of people newly infected with HIV globally, 1990–2007. *[From United Nations AIDS Program (UNAIDS).]*

The HIV epidemic has occurred in "waves" in different regions of the world, each wave having somewhat different characteristics depending on the demographics of the country and region in question and the timing of the introduction of HIV into the population. Although the AIDS epidemic was first recognized in the United States and shortly thereafter in Western Europe, it very likely began in Sub-Saharan Africa (see above), which has been particularly devastated by the epidemic. More than two-thirds of all people with HIV infection (~22.5 million) live in that region, even though Sub-Saharan Africa is home to just 10–11% of the world's population (Fig. 90-11). Within the region, southern Africa is worst-affected. In eight southern African countries, available seroprevalence data indicate that >15% of the adult population aged 15–49 is HIV-infected. In addition, among high-risk individuals (e.g., commercial sex workers, patients attending STD clinics) who live in urban areas of Sub-Saharan Africa, seroprevalence is now >50% in some countries. According to projections of the United Nations Population Division, life expectancies in several highly affected countries could drop to <40 years, well below what they would have been without HIV/AIDS and below levels reached in the pre-AIDS era (Fig. 90-13).

In Asia, an estimated 4.9 million people were living with HIV at the end of 2007. National HIV prevalence is highest in southeast Asia, with wide variation in trends between different countries. The epidemic in Asia lagged temporally behind that in Africa; however, the populations of many Asian nations are so large (especially India and China) that even low national HIV prevalence rates result in large numbers of people living with HIV. Encouragingly, HIV prevalence has declined in Myanmar, Cambodia, and Thailand; however, HIV prevalence continues to increase in other countries such as Indonesia and Vietnam.

The epidemic is expanding in Eastern Europe and Central Asia, where ~1.6 million people were living with

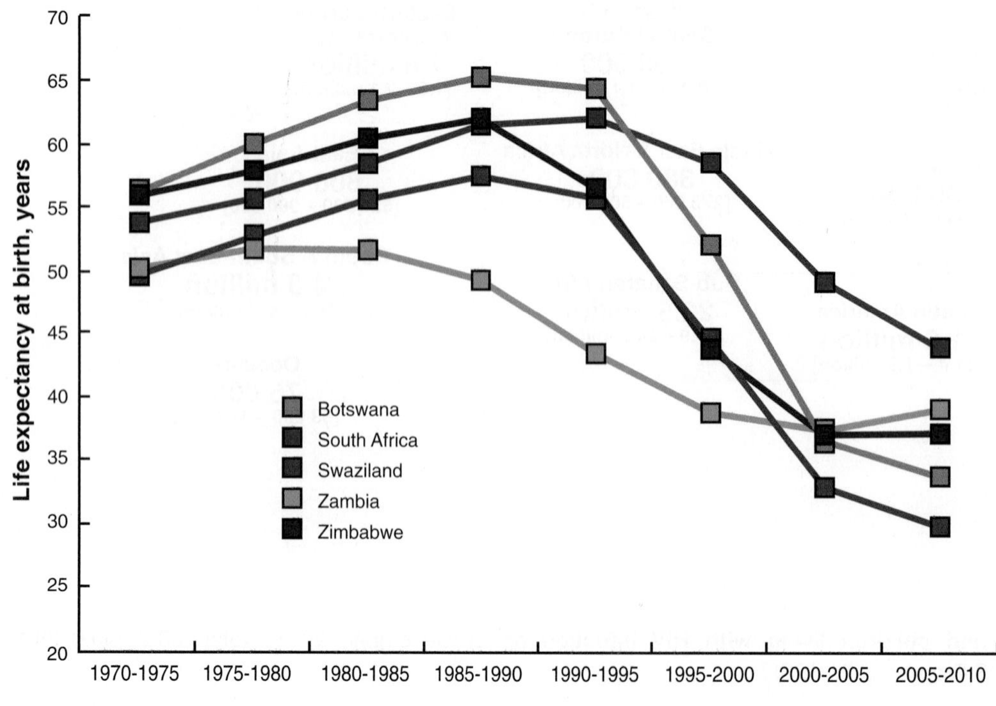

FIGURE 90-13
The impact of HIV/AIDS on life expectancy in five Sub-Saharan African countries, 1970–2010. *[From United Nations AIDS Program (UNAIDS).]*

HIV at the end of 2007. Ninety percent of new HIV infections reported in 2007 occurred in two countries, the Russian Federation and Ukraine. Driven initially by injection drug use and increasingly by heterosexual transmission, the number of new infections in this region has increased dramatically over the past decade.

Approximately 1.8 million people are living with HIV/AIDS in Latin America and the Caribbean. Brazil is home to the largest number of HIV-infected people in the region. However, the epidemic has been slowed in that country due to successful treatment and prevention efforts. The Caribbean region has the highest regional adult seroprevalence rate after Africa, due in large part to the huge case load in Haiti. Approximately 2.1 million people are living with HIV/AIDS in North America and in Western and Central Europe.

The major mode of HIV transmission worldwide is unquestionably heterosexual sex; this is particularly true, and has been so since the beginning of the epidemic, in developing countries, where the numbers of infected men and women are approximately equal. The epidemic in most developed countries was first introduced among men who have sex with men and, to a greater or lesser degree (depending on the individual country), among IDUs. In this regard, the total numbers of AIDS cases in those countries still reflect a high proportion of cases among these high-risk groups. However, in most developed countries, including the United States (see above and below), there has been a gradual shift toward heterosexual transmission (Fig. 90-8).

AIDS IN THE UNITED STATES

AIDS has had—and will continue to have—an extraordinary public health impact in the United States. As of January 1, 2006, an estimated 984,155 cases of AIDS had been diagnosed in the United States and dependent areas, and ~550,394 AIDS-related deaths had occurred. AIDS cases have been reported in all 50 states, the District of Columbia; and in U.S. dependencies, possessions, and associated nations. An estimated 1.1 million individuals in the United States are living with HIV infection, one-quarter of whom are unaware of their infection. The estimated HIV seroprevalence rate among adults aged 15–49 years in the United States is ~0.6%. Prevalence is highest among young adults in their late twenties and thirties and among minorities.

The number of AIDS cases and deaths rose steadily through the 1980s; AIDS cases peaked in 1993 and deaths in 1995 (Fig. 90-14). Since then, the annual numbers of AIDS-related deaths in the United States have fallen ~70%. This trend is due to several factors, including the improved prophylaxis and treatment of opportunistic infections, the growing experience among the health professions in caring for HIV-infected individuals, improved access to health care, and a decrease in new infections due to saturational effects and prevention efforts. However, the most influential factor clearly has been the increased use of potent ARV drugs, generally administered in a combination of three or four agents (see below).

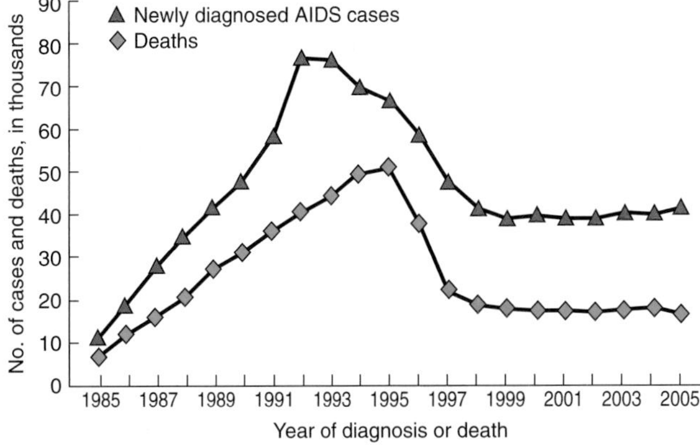

FIGURE 90-14

Estimated number of AIDS cases and AIDS deaths, United States, 1985–2005. *(From CDC.)*

Approximately 56,000 individuals are newly infected each year in the United States, a figure that has remained stable for at least 10 years. Among adults and adolescents newly diagnosed with HIV infection (regardless of AIDS status) in the United States in 2005, ~74% are men and ~26% are women (Fig. 90-15). Of new HIV/AIDS diagnoses among men, ~67% were due to male-to-male sexual contact, ~15% to heterosexual contact, ~13% to injection drug use, and ~5% to a combination of male-to-male sexual contact and injection drug use. Of new HIV/AIDS diagnoses among women, ~80% were due to heterosexual contact and ~20% to injection drug use.

HIV transmission patterns in the United States have shifted over time. When one looks at the totality of data collected from the beginning of the epidemic, ~46% of all AIDS cases are among men who have had sex with men. However, since the mid-1980s the proportion of newly reported cases of AIDS in this population has declined from ~64% of cases diagnosed in 1985 to ~42% of cases diagnosed in 2005 (Fig. 90-8). Meanwhile, the proportion of new AIDS cases attributed to heterosexual contact has increased dramatically, from 3% in 1985 to 31% in 2005. The share of AIDS diagnoses due to injection drug use was 19% in 1985, peaked at 31% in 1993, and was 21% in 2005. Women are increasingly affected: the proportion of AIDS cases among female adults and adolescents (age >13 years) increased from 7% in 1985 to 27% in 2005.

HIV infection and AIDS have disproportionately affected minority populations in the United States. Among those diagnosed with HIV (regardless of AIDS status) in 2005, 49% percent were African Americans, a group that comprises only 13% of the U.S. population (Fig. 90-16). An estimated 3% of black men and 1% of black women in their thirties are living with HIV infection. HIV/AIDS ranked ninth among all causes of mortality in the United States in 2004 among those aged 35–64 years, but among African Americans it ranked third.

As of January 1, 2006, an estimated 9112 cases of AIDS in children <13 years old had been diagnosed, and ~54% of these children have died. Approximately 93% of

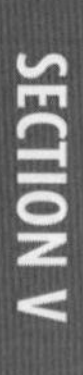
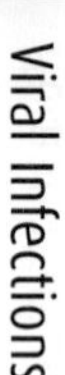
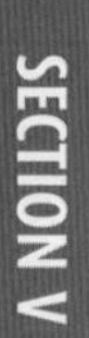
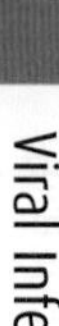
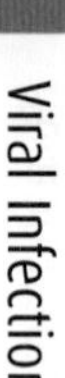
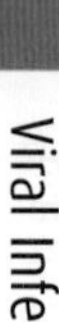
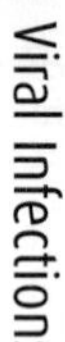
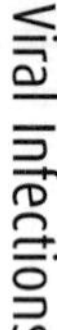
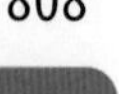
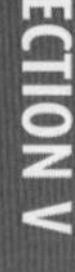
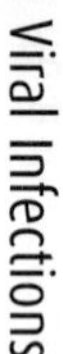

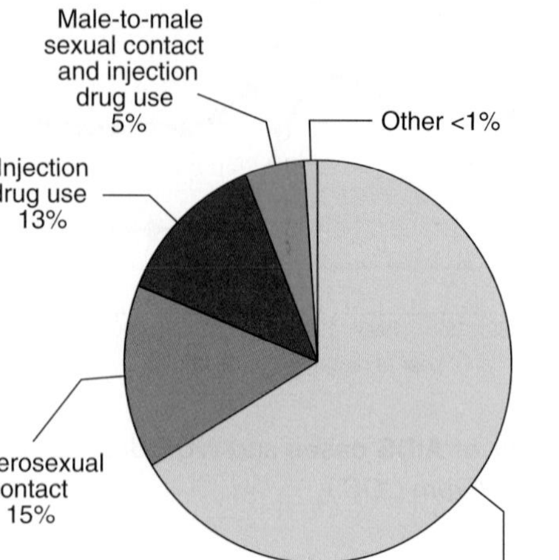

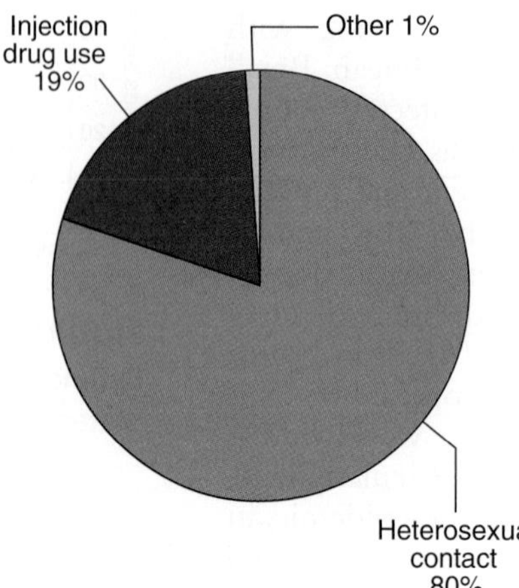

FIGURE 90-15

Transmission categories of adults and adolescents with HIV/AIDS diagnosed during 2005 in the United States. Estimates based on data from 33 states with long-term, confidential, name-based HIV infection reporting. Data include persons with a diagnosis of HIV infection regardless of AIDS status at diagnosis. *(From CDC.)*

these children were born to mothers who were HIV-infected or who were at risk for HIV infection and, in the majority of those cases, the mother was either an IDU or the heterosexual partner of an IDU. The estimated number of AIDS cases diagnosed among children perinatally exposed to HIV peaked in 1992 and has decreased in recent years (Fig. 90-10). The decline of these cases is likely associated with the implementation of guidelines for the universal counseling and voluntary HIV testing of pregnant women and the use of ARV therapy for pregnant women and newborn infants in order to prevent infection. Another contributing factor is the effective treatment of HIV infection in children who have become infected.

Although the HIV/AIDS epidemic on the whole is plateauing in the United States, it is spreading rapidly among certain populations, stabilizing in others, and decreasing in others. Similar to other STDs, HIV infection will not spread homogeneously throughout the population of the United States. However, it is clear that anyone who practices high-risk behavior is at risk for HIV infection. In addition, recent increases in infections and AIDS cases among young men who have sex with men and among heterosexuals (particularly sexual partners of IDUs, women, and adolescents) as well as the spread in pockets of poverty in both urban and rural regions (particularly among underserved minority populations in the southern United States with inadequate access to health care) testify to the fact that the epidemic of HIV infection in the United States remains a public health problem of major proportions.

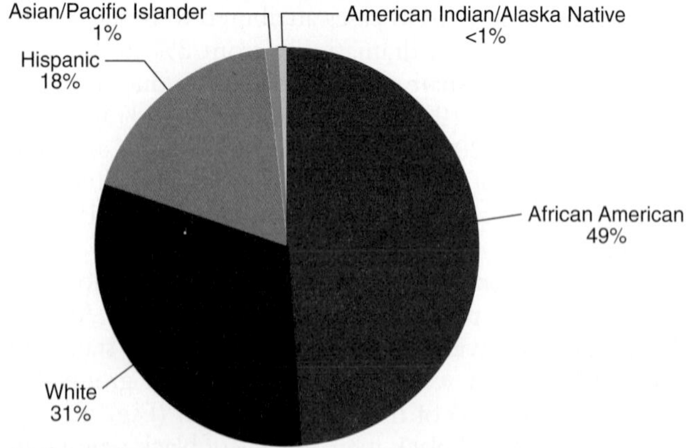

FIGURE 90-16

Race/ethnicity of persons (including children) with HIV/AIDS diagnosed during 2005 in the United States. Estimates based on data from 33 states with long-term, confidential, name-based HIV infection reporting. Data include persons with a diagnosis of HIV infection regardless of AIDS status at diagnosis. *(From CDC.)*

PATHOPHYSIOLOGY AND PATHOGENESIS

The hallmark of HIV disease is a profound immunodeficiency resulting primarily from a progressive quantitative and qualitative deficiency of the subset of T lymphocytes referred to as *helper T cells*. This subset of T cells is defined phenotypically by the presence on its surface of the CD4 molecule, which serves as the primary cellular receptor for HIV. A co-receptor must also be present together with CD4 for efficient fusion and entry of HIV-1 into its target cells (Figs. 90-3 and 90-4). HIV uses two major co-receptors for fusion and entry; these co-receptors are also the primary receptors for certain chemoattractive cytokines termed *chemokines* and belong to the seven-transmembrane-domain G protein–coupled family of receptors. CCR5 and CXCR4 are the major co-receptors used by HIV (see above and below). A number of mechanisms responsible for cellular depletion and/or immune dysfunction of CD4+ T cells have been demonstrated in vitro; these include direct infection and destruction of these cells by HIV and immune clearance of infected cells, as well as indirect effects such as immune exhaustion due to aberrant cellular activation and activation-induced cell death (see below). Patients with CD4+ T-cell levels below certain thresholds (see below) are at high risk of developing a variety of opportunistic diseases, particularly the infections and neoplasms that are AIDS-defining illnesses. Some features of AIDS, such as Kaposi's sarcoma and neurologic abnormalities (see below), cannot be explained completely by the immunodeficiency caused by HIV infection, since these complications may occur before the development of severe immunologic impairment.

The combination of viral pathogenic and immunopathogenic events that occurs during the course of HIV disease from the moment of initial (primary) infection through the development of advanced-stage disease is complex and varied. It is important to appreciate that the pathogenic mechanisms of HIV disease are multifactorial and multiphasic and are different at different stages of the disease. Therefore, it is essential to consider the typical clinical course of an untreated HIV-infected individual in order to more fully appreciate these pathogenic events (Fig. 90-17).

PRIMARY HIV INFECTION, INITIAL VIREMIA, AND DISSEMINATION OF VIRUS

The events associated with primary HIV infection are likely critical determinants of the subsequent course of HIV disease. In particular, the early dissemination of virus to lymphoid organs, particularly the gut-associated lymphoid tissue (GALT), is a major factor in the establishment of a chronic and persistent infection (see below). The initial infection of susceptible cells may vary somewhat with the route of infection. Virus that enters directly into the bloodstream via infected blood or blood products (i.e., transfusions, use of contaminated needles for injecting drugs, sharp-object injuries, maternal-to-fetal transmission either intrapartum or perinatally, or sexual intercourse where there is enough trauma to cause bleeding) is likely cleared from the circulation to the spleen and other lymphoid organs, where primary focal infections begin, followed by wider dissemination throughout other lymphoid tissues, particularly the GALT, leading to a burst of viremia. Dendritic cells play an important role in the initiation of HIV infection. These cells express a diversity of C-type lectin receptors on their surface, one of which is called *DC-SIGN* (see above). DC-SIGN binds with high affinity to the HIV envelope gp120 and can retain infectious particles for days in vitro. In this regard, dendritic cells can trap HIV and mediate the efficient transinfection of CD4+ T cells. In addition, DC-SIGN may also facilitate CD4-mediated infection of dendritic cells. These mechanisms likely operate in humans when HIV enters "locally" (as opposed to directly into the blood) and encounters mucosal dendritic cells via the vagina, rectum, or urethra during intercourse or via the upper gastrointestinal tract from swallowed infected breast milk or rarely semen or vaginal fluid. In primary HIV infection, virus replication in CD4+ T cells intensifies before the initiation of an HIV-specific immune response (see below, Fig. 90-17), with a

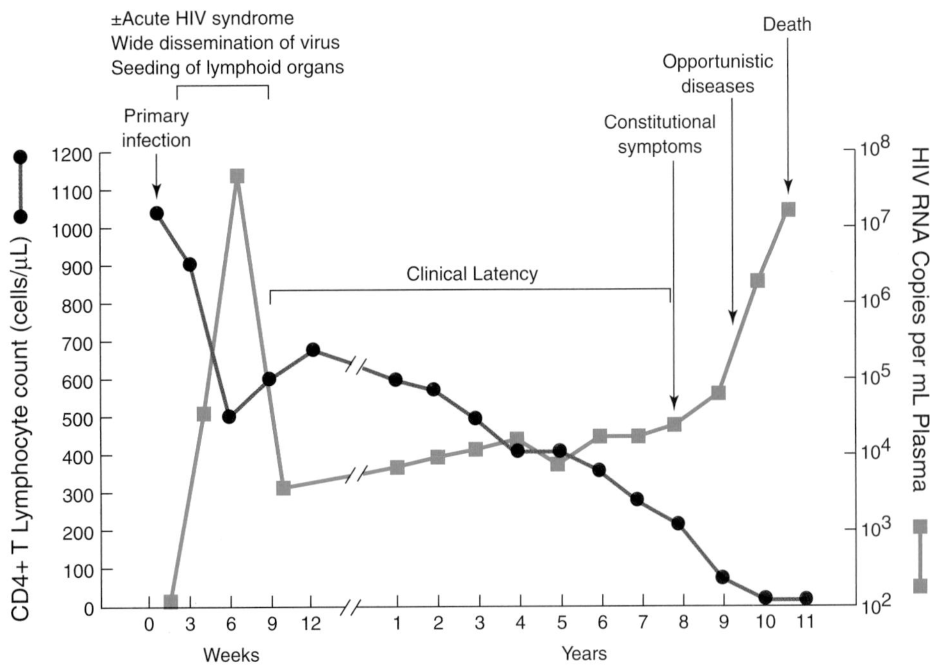

FIGURE 90-17

Typical course of an untreated HIV-infected individual. See text for detailed description. *[From G Pantaleo et al: N Engl J Med 328(5):327, 1993. Copyright 1993 Massachusetts Medical Society. All rights reserved.]*

burst of viremia resulting from the rapid replication of virus in susceptible cells in lymphoid organs (particularly the GALT), with subsequent dissemination of virus to the brain and other tissues. Of note, animal studies have demonstrated that a significant percentage of CD4+ T cells (particularly memory cells) in the GALT is depleted early after SIV infection, via either direct infection of cells or bystander cell killing. The repopulation of such cells may be extremely problematic, even after initiation of ARV therapy. Individuals who experience the "acute HIV syndrome," which occurs to varying degrees in ~50% of individuals with primary infection, have high levels of viremia measured in millions of copies of HIV RNA per milliliter that last for several weeks (see below). Acute mononucleosis-like symptoms are well correlated with the presence of viremia. Virtually all patients develop some degree of viremia during primary infection, which contributes to virus dissemination throughout the lymphoid tissue (see above), even though they may remain asymptomatic or not recall experiencing symptoms. It appears that the initial level of plasma viremia in primary HIV infection does not necessarily determine the rate of disease progression; however, the set point of the level of steady-state plasma viremia after ~1 year does seem to correlate with the slope of disease progression (see below).

ESTABLISHMENT OF CHRONIC AND PERSISTENT INFECTION

Persistent Virus Replication

HIV infection is unique among human viral infections. Despite the robust cellular and humoral immune responses that are mounted after primary infection (see below), once infection has been established, the virus succeeds in escaping immune-mediated clearance (see below), paradoxically seems to thrive on immune activation, and is never eliminated completely from the body. Rather, a chronic infection develops that persists with varying degrees of continual virus replication in the untreated patient for a median of ~10 years before the patient becomes clinically ill (see below). It is this establishment of a chronic, persistent infection that is the hallmark of HIV disease. Throughout the often protracted course of chronic infection, virus replication can invariably be detected in untreated patients, both by highly sensitive assays for plasma viremia as well as by demonstration of cell-associated HIV RNA in immunocompetent cells (predominantly CD4+ T cells and macrophages) in the circulation and in lymphoid tissue. Recent studies using highly sensitive molecular techniques have demonstrated that even in patients in whom plasma viremia is suppressed to below 50 copies of HIV RNA/mL by ARV therapy, there is a continual low level of virus replication (see below). In other human viral infections, with very few exceptions, if the host survives, the virus is completely cleared from the body and a state of immunity against subsequent infection develops. HIV infection very rarely kills the host during primary infection. Certain viruses, such as HSV (Chap. 80), are not completely cleared from the body after infection but instead enter a latent state; in these cases, clinical latency is accompanied by microbiologic latency. This is not the case with HIV infection as described above. Chronicity associated with persistent virus replication can also be seen in certain cases of HBV and HCV infections (Chap. 93); however, in these infections, the immune system is not a target of the virus.

Evasion of Immune System Control

Inherent to the establishment of chronicity of HIV infection is the ability of the virus to evade elimination and control by the immune system. There are a number of mechanisms whereby the virus accomplishes this evasion. Paramount among these is the establishment of a sustained level of replication associated with the generation of viral diversity via mutation and recombination, thus providing a means to evade control and elimination by the immune system. The selection of mutants that escape control by CD8+ cytolytic T lymphocytes (CTLs) is critical to the propagation and progression of HIV infection. The high rate of virus replication and the continual mutation of virus also contribute to the inability of neutralizing antibody to contain the virus quasispecies present in an individual at any given time. Molecular analysis of clonotypes has demonstrated that clones of CD8+ CTLs that expand greatly during primary HIV infection, and likely represent the high-affinity clones that would be expected to be most efficient in eliminating virus-infected cells, are no longer detectable after their initial burst of expansion. It is thought that the initially expanded clones may have been deleted or rendered dysfunctional owing to the overwhelming immune activation resulting from exposure to viral antigens during the initial burst of viremia, similar to the exhaustion of CD8+ CTLs that has been reported in the murine model of lymphocytic choriomeningitis virus (LCMV) infection. Recent studies have indicated that exhaustion of effector cells during prolonged immune activation is associated with expression of the programmed death (PD)-1 molecule (of the B7-CD28 family of molecules) on activated cells and its interaction with its ligands (L) PD-L1 and PD-L2 on antigen-presenting cells. This interaction results in a partially reversible signal for cell death and/or dysfunction. Another mechanism contributing to the evasion by HIV of immune system control is the downregulation of HLA class I molecules on the surface of HIV-infected cells by the Nef protein of HIV, resulting in the lack of ability of the CD8+ CTL to recognize and kill the infected target cell. Although this downregulation of HLA class I molecules would favor elimination of HIV-infected cells by natural killer (NK) cells, this latter mechanism does not seem to remove HIV-infected cells effectively (see below). The principal targets of neutralizing antibodies against HIV are the envelope proteins gp120 and gp41. HIV employs three mechanisms to evade neutralizing responses: hypervariability in the primary sequence of the envelope, extensive glycosylation of the envelope, and conformational masking of neutralizing epitopes.

CD4+ T-cell help is essential for the integrity of antigen-specific immune responses, both humoral and cell-mediated. HIV preferentially infects activated CD4+ T cells including HIV-specific CD4+ T cells, and so this loss of viral-specific helper T-cell responses has profound negative consequences for the immunologic control of HIV replication. Furthermore, this loss occurs early in the course of infection, and animal studies indicate that 40–70% of all memory CD4+ T cells in the GALT are eliminated during acute infection. Another means of escape of HIV-infected cells from elimination by CD8+ CTLs is the sequestration of infected cells in immunologically privileged sites such as the central nervous system (CNS).

Finally, the escape of HIV from elimination during primary infection allows the formation of a pool of latently infected cells that cannot be eliminated by virus-specific CTLs (see below). Thus, despite a potent immune response and the marked downregulation of virus replication after primary HIV infection, HIV succeeds in establishing a state of chronic infection with a variable degree of persistent virus replication. In most cases, during this period, patients make the clinical transition from acute primary infection to variable periods of clinical latency or smoldering disease activity (see below).

Reservoirs of HIV-Infected Cells: Obstacle to the Eradication of Virus

There exists in virtually all HIV-infected individuals a pool of latently infected, resting CD4+ T cells that serves as at least one component of the persistent reservoir of virus. Such cells manifest postintegration latency in that the HIV provirus integrates into the genome of the cell and can remain in this state until an activation signal drives the expression of HIV transcripts and ultimately replication-competent virus. This form of latency is to be distinguished from preintegration latency, in which HIV enters a resting CD4+ T cell and, in the absence of an activation signal, only a limited degree of reverse transcription of the HIV genome occurs. This period of preintegration latency may last hours to days, and if no activation signal is delivered to the cell, the proviral DNA loses its capacity to initiate a productive infection. If these cells do become activated, reverse transcription proceeds to completion and the virus continues along its replication cycle (see above and Fig. 90-18). The pool of cells that are in the postintegration state of latency is established early during the course of primary HIV infection. Despite the suppression of plasma viremia to <50 copies of HIV RNA per milliliter by potent combinations of several ARV drugs administered over several years, this pool of latently infected cells persists and can give rise to replication-competent virus. Modeling studies built on projections of decay curves (see below) have estimated that in such a setting of prolonged suppression, it would require from 7–70 years for the pool of latently infected cells to be completely eliminated. Furthermore, the reservoir of latently infected cells is replenished during minor detectable rebounds of virus replication that may occur intermittently, during the low levels of persistent virus replication that goes undetectable (see below) (Fig. 90-18), even in patients who for the most part are treated successfully, and certainly during major rebounds of viremia in patients whose therapy is interrupted for a period of weeks or longer. Over the past several years, attempts have been made to eliminate HIV in the latent viral reservoir using agents that stimulate resting CD4+ T cells during the course of antiretroviral therapy; however, such attempts have been unsuccessful. As more sophisticated techniques become available for measuring extremely low levels of virus replication, it is becoming clear that virus replication continually occurs at very low levels in a substantial proportion of individuals whose viral load is "undetectable" by the standard assays of plasma viremia (see above and below). Thus, although a small pool of truly resting, latently infected cells exists at any given point in time, this pool is continually being activated and replenished by ongoing low levels of virus replication. Reservoirs of HIV infected cells, latent or otherwise, can exist in a number of compartments including the lymphoid tissue, peripheral blood, and the CNS (likely in cells of the monocyte/macrophage lineage), as well as in other unidentified locations. Thus this persistent reservoir of infected cells at various stages of latency and/or low

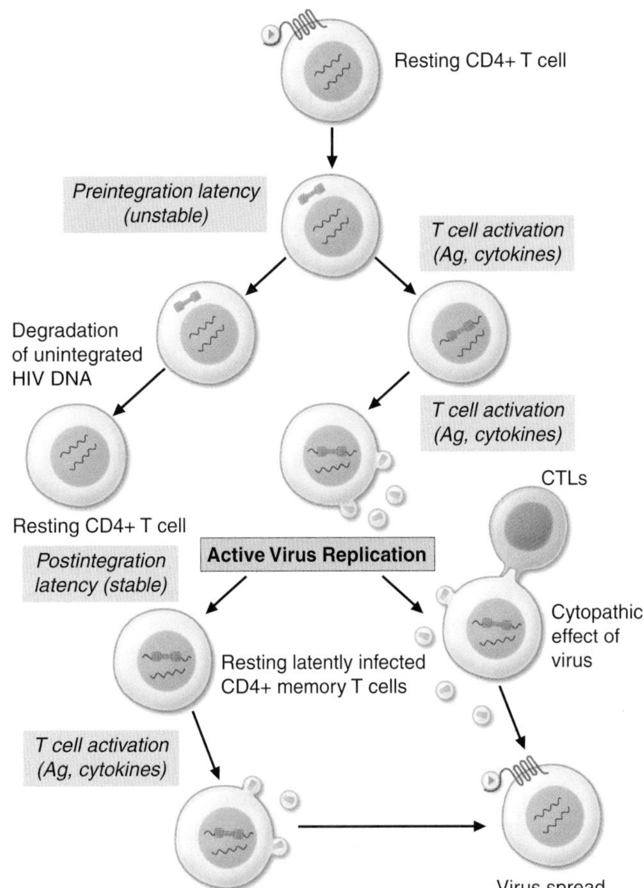

FIGURE 90-18
Generation of latently infected, resting CD4+ T cells in HIV-infected individuals. See text for details. Ag, antigen; CTLs, cytolytic T lymphocytes. *(Courtesy of TW Chun; with permission.)*

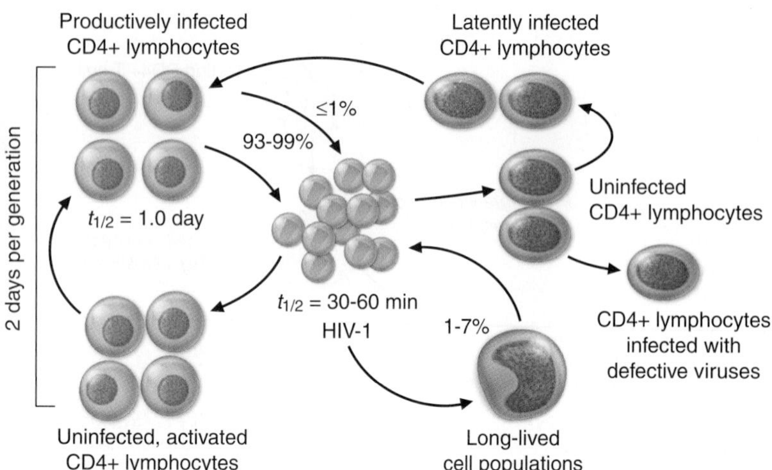

FIGURE 90-19

Dynamics of HIV infection in vivo. See text for detailed description. *(From AS Perelson et al: Science 271:1582, 1996.)*

levels of persistent virus replication are major obstacles to any goal of eradication of virus from infected individuals, despite the favorable clinical outcomes that have resulted from ARV therapy (see below).

Viral Dynamics

The dynamics of viral production and turnover have been quantified using mathematical modeling in the setting of the administration of reverse transcriptase and protease inhibitors to HIV-infected individuals in clinical studies. Treatment with these drugs resulted in a precipitous decline in the level of plasma viremia, which typically fell by well over 90% within 2 weeks. The number of CD4+ T cells in the blood increased concurrently, which suggested that the killing of CD4+ T cells was linked directly to the levels of replicating virus. However, a significant component of the early rise in CD4+ T cell numbers after the initiation of therapy may be due to the redistribution of cells into the peripheral blood from other body compartments as a consequence of therapy-related diminution in viremia-associated immune system activation. It was determined on the basis of modeling the kinetics of viral decline and the emergence of resistant mutants during therapy that 93–99% of the circulating virus originated from recently infected, rapidly turning over CD4+ T cells and that ~1–7% of circulating virus originated from longer-lived cells, likely monocytes/macrophages. A negligible amount of circulating virus originated from the pool of latently infected cells (see above) (Fig. 90-19). It was also determined that the half-life of a circulating virion was ~30–60 min and that of productively infected cells was 1 day. Given the relatively steady level of plasma viremia and of infected cells, it appears that extremely large amounts of virus (~10^{10}–10^{11} virions) are produced and cleared from the circulation each day. In addition, data suggest that the minimal duration of the HIV-1 replication cycle in vivo is ~2 days. Other studies have demonstrated that the decrease in plasma viremia that results from ARV therapy correlates closely with a decrease in virus replication in lymph nodes, further confirming that lymphoid tissue is the main site of HIV replication and the main source of plasma viremia.

The level of steady-state viremia, called the viral *set point*, at ~1 year has important prognostic implications for the progression of HIV disease. It has been demonstrated that as a group HIV-infected individuals who have a low set point at 6 months to 1 year progress to AIDS much more slowly than individuals whose set point is very high at that time (Fig. 90-20). Levels of viremia generally increase as disease progresses. Measurement of the level of viremia is critical in guiding therapeutic decisions in HIV-infected individuals (see below).

Clinical Latency Versus Microbiologic Latency

With the exception of long-term nonprogressors (see below), the level of CD4+ T cells in the blood decreases progressively in HIV-infected individuals. The decline in CD4+ T cells may be gradual or abrupt, the latter usually reflecting a significant spike in the level of plasma viremia. Most patients are relatively asymptomatic while this progressive decline is taking place (see below) and are often described as being in a state of *clinical latency*. However, this term is misleading; it does not mean disease latency, since progression, although slow in many cases, is generally relentless during this period. Furthermore, clinical latency should not be confused with microbiologic latency, since some level of virus replication invariably occurs during this period of clinical latency. Even in those rare patients who have <50 copies of HIV RNA per milliliter in the absence of therapy, there is virtually always some degree of ongoing virus replication.

ADVANCED HIV DISEASE

In untreated patients or in patients in whom therapy has not adequately controlled virus replication (see below), after a variable period, usually measured in years, the CD4+ T-cell count falls below a critical level (<200/μL) and the patient becomes highly susceptible to opportunistic disease (Fig. 90-17). For this reason, the CDC case definition of AIDS includes all HIV-infected individuals with CD4+ T-cell counts below this level (Table 90-1). Patients may experience constitutional signs and symptoms or may develop an opportunistic disease abruptly

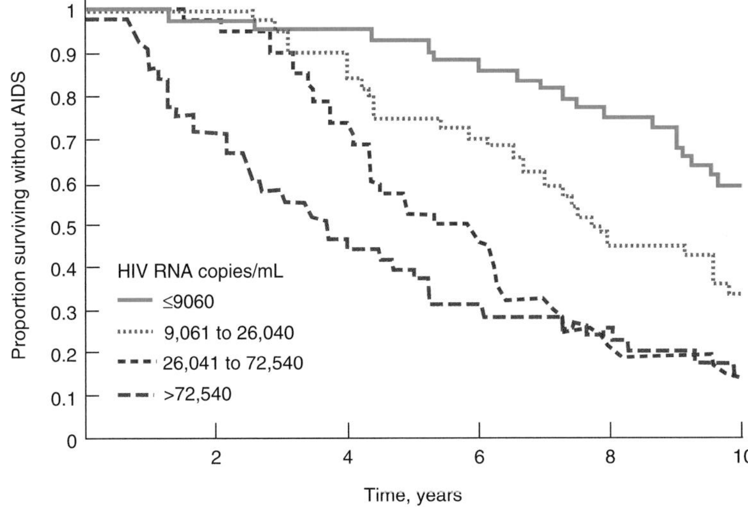

FIGURE 90-20

Relationship between levels of virus and rates of disease progression. Kaplan-Meier curves for AIDS-free survival stratified by baseline HIV-1 RNA categories (copies per milliliter). *(From Mellors et al.)*

without any prior symptoms, although the latter scenario is unusual. The depletion of CD4+ T cells continues to be progressive and unrelenting in this phase. It is not uncommon for CD4+ T-cell counts in the untreated patient to drop as low as 10/μL or even to zero. In countries where ARV therapy and prophylaxis and treatment for opportunistic infections are readily accessible to such patients, survival is increased dramatically even with this level of advanced disease. In contrast, untreated patients who progress to this severest form of immunodeficiency usually succumb to opportunistic infections or neoplasms (see below).

LONG-TERM SURVIVORS AND LONG-TERM NONPROGRESSORS

The prognosis for HIV-infected individuals who have access to health care and ARV therapy has improved greatly since the beginning of the epidemic. The median time from primary HIV infection to the development of AIDS in untreated individuals in the developed world is ~10 years. This period has been markedly extended by the wide availability of combinations of ARV drugs in the developed world, and increasingly in low- to mid-income countries; the full extent of this benefit is yet to be realized (see below). It is important to distinguish between the terms *long-term survivor* and *long-term nonprogressor.* Long-term nonprogressors are by definition long-term survivors; however, the reverse is not always true. The definitions of these categories are empirical and continue to change as more data are collected from prospective cohort studies. Predictions from one study that antedated the availability of effective ARV therapy estimated that ~13% of homosexual/bisexual men who were infected at an early age may remain free of clinical AIDS for >20 years. Originally, individuals were considered to be long-term survivors if they remained alive for 10–15 years after initial infection. Currently, individuals are considered to be long-term survivors if they remain alive for ≥20 years after initial infection. In most such individuals the disease has progressed, in that they have significant immunodeficiency, and many have experienced opportunistic diseases. Some of these individuals have CD4+ T-cell counts that have decreased to ≤200/μL but have remained stable at that level for years. The mechanisms of this stabilization are not entirely clear but may relate to the beneficial effects of ARV therapy and prophylaxis against opportunistic infections. In addition, a number of viral and/or host determinants likely contribute to the long-term survival of these individuals. Quantitative and qualitative aspects of the HIV-specific immune response, as well as recognized and unrecognized genetic factors (see below), may also contribute to the long-term survival of these individuals.

Definitions of long-term nonprogressors have varied considerably over the years, and so such individuals constitute a heterogeneous group. Originally, individuals considered to be long-term nonprogressors were those who had been infected with HIV for a long period (≥10 years), whose CD4+ T-cell counts were in the normal range and remained stable over years, and who had not received ARV therapy. Such patients had relatively low, but usually detectable, levels of plasma viremia, generally normal immune function according to commonly measured parameters (skin tests, in vitro lymphocyte responses to various mitogens and antigens), and normal-appearing lymphoid tissue architecture as determined on lymph node biopsy. In general, long-term nonprogressors manifested robust HIV-specific immune responses, both humoral (neutralizing antibodies) and cell-mediated (HIV-specific CTLs). However, this may also be true of some individuals early in the course of disease who ultimately progress to advanced disease. No qualitative abnormalities in the virus were detected in most of these patients. However, a small subset of patients did have defective virus; in particular, in one cohort of five long-term nonprogressors, the virus had a defect in the *nef* gene. In another report, a blood donor in Australia who was HIV-infected and a group of seven individuals who were infected by blood or blood products from that donor remained free of HIV-related disease and maintained normal and stable CD4+ T-cell counts for several years after infection. Sequence analysis of viruses isolated from the donor and recipients revealed similar deletions in the *nef* gene and the region of overlap of *nef* and the U3 region of the HIV LTR (Fig. 90-5). The vast majority of these originally reported long-term nonprogressors have now gone on to progressive disease. More recently, cohorts of rare long-term nonprogressors have been described who have been infected for 20 years with normal CD4+ T-cell counts and who typically maintain plasma viral RNA <50 copies per milliliter without ARV therapy. When these more stringent definitions based predominantly on levels of plasma viremia are applied, very strong associations with HLA B*5701 or HLA B*2705 alleles have been found. In addition, the HIV-specific CD8+ T-cell response in these patients is highly focused on B5701-restricted peptides, suggesting that the B5701 molecule plays a direct role in restriction of virus replication in these individuals, although the precise mechanisms of this effect remain unclear.

A number of other host genetic factors exert more modest effects on restriction of HIV replication, yet they also may be associated with slower progression of disease (see "Genetic Factors in HIV Pathogenesis" later in the chapter). The precise role of host factors in long-term nonprogression remains unclear. There is no single genetic determinant for nonprogression. However, several genetic variants and mutations have been demonstrated to result in a delay in the progression of HIV disease. These include heterozygosity for the *CCR5*-Δ32 deletion, heterozygosity for the *CCR2*-64I mutation, homozygosity for the *SDF1*-3'A mutation, and heterozygosity for the *RANTES*-28G mutation (see "Genetic Factors in HIV Pathogenesis" later in the chapter). Since CCR5 is the major co-receptor for R5 or macrophage-tropic strains of HIV and since individuals who are homozygous for the *CCR5*-Δ32 deletion are, with rare exceptions, protected against HIV infection, the potential mechanism for slow progression in heterozygotes is clear. In addition, certain single nucleotide polymorphisms in the *CCR5* promoter have been shown to be associated with slower progression of disease. The reason for the slowing of progression of HIV disease in individuals who are heterozygous for the *CCR2*-64I mutation is less clear; however, it has been demonstrated that CXCR4 can dimerize with the CCR2-64I mutant but not with wild-type CCR2. This dimerization may reduce the amount of CXCR4 on the cell surface and as a result inhibit infection with X4 viruses. Homozygosity for the *SDF1*-3' A mutation may upregulate the *SDF1* gene enabling SDF-1, which is the natural ligand for CXCR4, to compete more effectively with X4 virus for the CXCR4 co-receptor. The *RANTES*-28G mutation increases RANTES (CCL5) expression, which is the natural ligand for CCR5 and may thus inhibit infection with R5 viruses. The gene *CCL3L1* codes for MIP1αP and has an influence on both susceptibility to infection and disease progression based upon the gene copy number in the individual. Finally, maximal HLA heterozygosity of class I loci (A, B, and C) has been shown to be associated with delayed progression of HIV disease. Although most long-term nonprogressors have robust HIV-specific immune responses as well as competent CD8+ T-cell suppressors of HIV replication, it is unclear whether these factors are directly responsible for the state of nonprogression. A substantial proportion of HIV-infected individuals manifest comparable immune responses early in the course of their disease and still experience disease progression. As noted above, long-term nonprogressors likely represent a heterogeneous group. It has recently been reported in some cohorts that individuals co-infected with HIV and *GB virus C* (GBV-C) have lower mortality than HIV-infected individuals without GBV-C infection. The precise mechanisms of this apparent beneficial effect are unclear at present.

LYMPHOID ORGANS AND HIV PATHOGENESIS

Regardless of the portal of entry of HIV, lymphoid tissues are the major anatomic sites for the establishment and propagation of HIV infection (see above). Despite the use of measurements of plasma viremia to determine the level of disease activity, virus replication occurs mainly in lymphoid tissue and not in blood; indeed, the level of plasma viremia directly reflects virus production in lymphoid tissue.

Some patients experience progressive generalized lymphadenopathy (see below) early in the course of the infection; others experience varying degrees of transient lymphadenopathy. Lymphadenopathy reflects the cellular activation and immune response to the virus in the lymphoid tissue, which is generally characterized by follicular or germinal center hyperplasia. Lymphoid tissue involvement is a common denominator of virtually all patients with HIV infection, even those without easily detectable lymphadenopathy.

Simultaneous examinations of lymph tissue and peripheral blood in patients and monkeys during various stages of HIV and SIV infection, respectively, have led to substantial insight into the pathogenesis of HIV disease. In most of the original human studies, peripheral lymph nodes have been used predominantly as the source of lymphoid tissue. More recent studies in monkeys and humans have focused on the GALT, where the earliest burst of virus replication occurs associated with marked depletion of CD4+ T cells (see below). In detailed studies in peripheral lymph node tissue, using a combination of polymerase chain reaction (PCR) techniques for HIV DNA and HIV RNA in tissue and HIV RNA in plasma, in situ hybridization for HIV RNA, and light and electron microscopy, the following picture has emerged. During acute HIV infection, high levels of plasma viremia at first originating from virus replication in the GALT occurs with dissemination of virus to peripheral lymphoid tissue where extensive viral replication in individual cells is demonstrated. A profound degree of cellular activation occurs (see below) and is reflected in follicular or germinal center hyperplasia. At this time copious amounts of extracellular virions (both infectious and defective) are trapped on the processes of the follicular dendritic cells (FDCs) in the germinal centers of the lymph nodes. Virions that have bound complement components on their surfaces attach to the surface of FDCs via interactions with complement

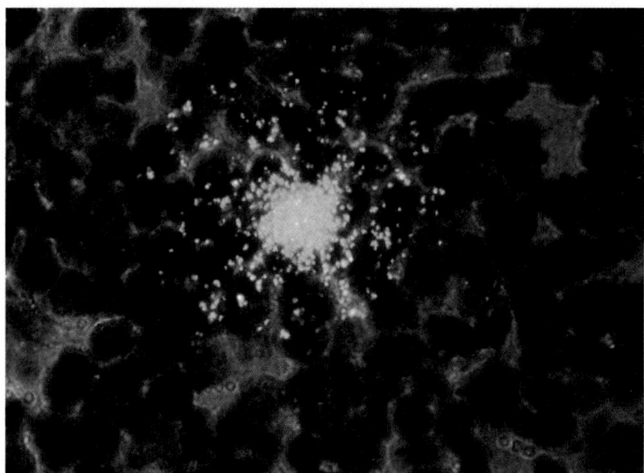

FIGURE 90-21
HIV in the lymph node of an HIV-infected individual. An individual cell infected with HIV shown expressing HIV RNA by in situ hybridization using a radiolabeled molecular probe. Original ×500. *(Adapted from G Pantaleo et al: Nature 362:355, 1993.)*

receptors and likely via Fc receptors that bind to antibodies that are attached to the virions. In situ hybridization reveals expression of virus in individual cells of the paracortical area and, to a lesser extent, the germinal center (Fig. 90-21). The persistence of trapped virus after the transition from acute to chronic infection likely reflects a steady state whereby trapped virus turns over and is replaced by fresh virions, which are continually produced to a greater or lesser degree in individual patients. The trapped virus, either as whole virion or shed envelope, serves as a continual activator of CD4+ T cells, thus driving further virus replication.

During early-stage HIV disease, the architecture of the germinal centers is generally preserved and may even be hyperplastic owing to in situ proliferation of cells (mostly B lymphocytes) and recruitment to the lymph nodes of a number of cell types (B cells, CD4+ and CD8+ T cells). Electron-microscopic studies have demonstrated a fine network of FDCs with many long, fingerlike processes that envelop virtually every lymphocyte in the germinal center. Extracellular virions can be seen attached to the processes, yet the FDCs appear to be relatively healthy. The trapping of antigen is a physiologically normal function for the FDCs, which present antigen to B cells and contribute to the generation of B-cell memory. However, in the case of HIV, the trapped virions serve as a persistent source of cellular activation, resulting in the secretion of proinflammatory cytokines such as interleukin (IL)-1β, tumor necrosis factor (TNF)-α, and IL-6, which can upregulate virus replication in infected cells (see below). Furthermore, although trapped virus is coated by neutralizing antibodies, it has been demonstrated that certain of these virions remain infectious for CD4+ T cells while attached to the processes of the FDCs. CD4+ T cells that migrate into the germinal center to provide help to B cells in the generation of an HIV-specific immune response are susceptible to infection by these trapped virions. Thus, in HIV infection, a normal physiologic function of the immune system, which contributes to the clearance of virus as well as to the generation of a specific immune response, can also have deleterious consequences.

As the disease progresses, the architecture of the germinal centers begins to show disruption, and the trapping efficiency of the lymphoid tissue diminishes. Electron microscopy reveals swollen organelles, and the FDCs begin to undergo cell death. The mechanisms of FDC death remain unclear; there is no indication by electron microscopy of copious virus replication or budding of virions off the cell in great quantities. This process of FDC death is accompanied by the deposition of collagen, leading to irreparable damage to the germinal centers. As the disease progresses to an advanced stage, there is complete disruption of the architecture of the germinal centers, accompanied by dissolution of the FDC network and massive dropout of FDCs. At this point, the lymph nodes are "burnt out." This destruction of lymphoid tissue compounds the immunodeficiency of HIV disease and contributes both to the inability to control HIV replication (leading usually to high levels of plasma viremia in the untreated or inadequately treated patient) and to the inability to mount adequate immune responses against opportunistic pathogens. The events from primary infection to the ultimate destruction of the immune system are illustrated in Fig. 90-22. Recently, nonhuman primate studies and some human studies have examined GALT at various stages of HIV disease. It is noteworthy that before infection approximately half of all CD4+ T cells in the jejunum express the HIV cellular co-receptor CCR5, rendering them highly susceptible to infection. Within the GALT, the basal level of activation combined with virus-mediated cellular activation results in the infection and elimination of an estimated 50–90% of CD4+ T cells in the gut. The extent of this early damage to GALT, which comprises a major component of lymphoid tissue in the body, plays a role in determining the potential for immunologic recovery of the memory cell subset.

CELLULAR ACTIVATION AND HIV PATHOGENESIS

Activation of the immune system is an essential component of an appropriate immune response to a foreign antigen. The immune system is normally in a state of homeostasis, awaiting perturbation by foreign antigenic stimuli. Once the immune response deals with and clears the antigen, the system returns to relative quiescence. In HIV infection, however, the immune system is chronically activated, providing the cell substrates necessary for persistent virus replication throughout the course of HIV disease, particularly in the untreated patient (see above) and to variable degrees even in certain patients receiving ARV therapy whose level of plasma viremia is suppressed to below the level of detection by standard assays (see below). Aberrant immune activation is the hallmark of HIV infection and is a critical component of the pathogenesis of HIV disease. This

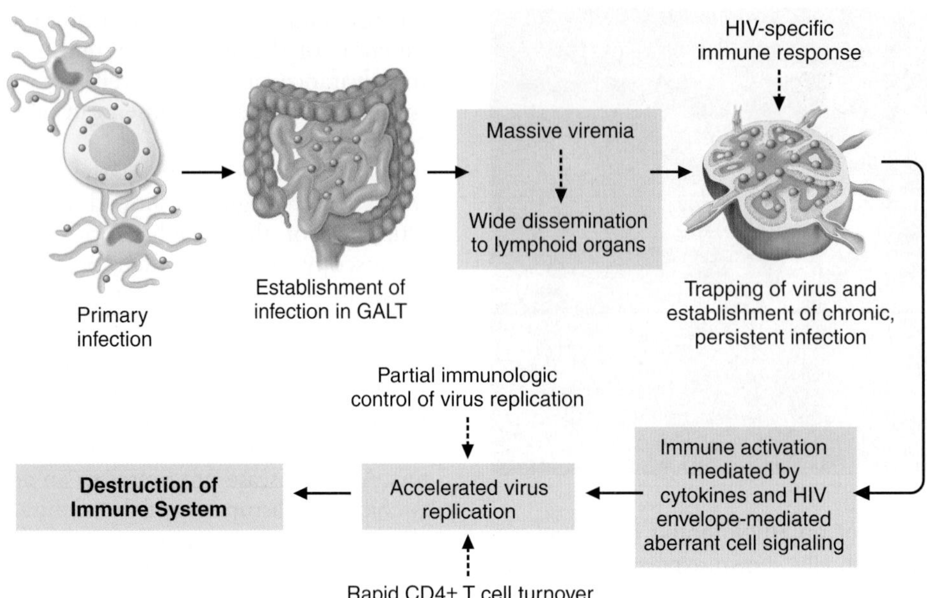

FIGURE 90-22

Events that transpire from primary HIV infection through the establishment of chronic persistent infection to the ultimate destruction of the immune system. See text for details. CTLs, cytolytic T lymphocytes; GALT, gut-associated lymphoid tissue.

activated state is reflected by hyperactivation of B cells leading to hypergammaglobulinemia; spontaneous lymphocyte proliferation; activation of monocytes; expression of activation markers on CD4+ and CD8+ T cells; increased activation-associated cellular apoptosis; lymph node hyperplasia, particularly early in the course of disease (see above); increased secretion of proinflammatory cytokines (see below); elevated levels of neopterin, β_2-microglobulin, acid-labile interferon, and soluble IL-2 receptors; and autoimmune phenomena (see below). Even in the absence of direct infection of a target cell, HIV envelope proteins can interact with cellular receptors (CD4 molecules and chemokine receptors) to deliver potent activation signals resulting in calcium flux, the phosphorylation of certain proteins involved in signal transduction, co-localization of cytoplasmic proteins including those involved in cell trafficking, immune dysfunction, and, under certain circumstances, apoptosis (see below). The secretion of certain proinflammatory and immunoregulatory cytokines is both a consequence of the aberrant immune activation associated with HIV infection and a mechanism of propagation of the process of aberrant cellular activation (see below).

In addition to endogenous factors such as cytokines, a number of exogenous factors such as other microbes that are associated with heightened cellular activation can enhance HIV replication and thus may have important effects on HIV pathogenesis. Co-infection in vivo or in vitro with a range of viruses, such as HSV types 1 and 2, cytomegalovirus (CMV), human herpesvirus (HHV) 6, Epstein-Barr virus (EBV), HBV, adenovirus, and HTLV-I have been shown to upregulate HIV expression. Other microbes, such as *Mycoplasma*, have been reported to contribute to the induction of HIV expression. In addition, infestation with nematodes has been shown to be associated with a heightened state of immune activation that facilitates HIV replication; in certain studies, deworming of the infected host has resulted in a decrease in plasma viremia. Two diseases of extraordinary global health significance, malaria and tuberculosis (TB), have been shown to increase HIV viral load in dually infected individuals. Globally, *Mycobacterium tuberculosis* is probably the most common opportunistic infection in HIV-infected individuals (see below and Chap. 66). In addition to the fact that HIV-infected individuals are more likely to develop active TB after exposure, it has been demonstrated that active TB can accelerate the course of HIV infection. It has also been shown that levels of plasma viremia are greatly elevated in HIV-infected individuals with active TB, compared with pre-TB levels and levels of viremia after successful treatment of the active TB. In vitro studies demonstrated that virus replication was markedly enhanced in lymphocytes of HIV-infected individuals who were skin test–positive for purified protein derivative (PPD) when PPD antigen was added to culture, resulting in cellular activation. Confirmatory evidence that antigen-induced activation was a major contributor to the accelerated viremia in HIV-infected individuals with active TB was provided by studies in which HIV-infected individuals were immunized with common recall antigens such as tetanus toxoid, influenza, or pneumococcal polysaccharide. Under these circumstances, a transient elevation of plasma viremia accompanied the cellular activation induced by the immunization. A greater degree of induction of virus was seen in those individuals with early-stage as opposed to advanced stage HIV disease (i.e., in those with more competent immune systems), and the degree of virus induction correlated with the level of immune system activation.

The situation is similar in the interaction between HIV and malaria parasites (Chap. 116). Acute infection of HIV-infected individuals with *Plasmodium falciparum* increases HIV viral load, and the increased viral load is reversed by effective malaria treatment.

Persistent immune activation may have several deleterious consequences. From a virologic standpoint, although quiescent CD4+ T cells can be infected with HIV, reverse transcription, integration, and virus spread are much more efficient in activated cells. Furthermore, cellular activation induces expression of virus in cells latently infected with HIV (see above). From an immunologic standpoint, chronic exposure of the immune system to a particular antigen over an extended period may ultimately lead to an inability to sustain an adequate immune response to the antigen in question. In many chronic viral infections, including HIV infection, persistent viremia is associated with "functional exhaustion" and apoptosis of virus-specific T cells. It has been demonstrated that this phenomenon may be mediated, at least in part, by the engagement of PD-1, which is highly expressed on the majority of HIV-specific T cells, with its ligands (PD-L1 and PD-L2) on antigen-presenting cells and epithelial cells, resulting in either T-cell death or anergy (see above). Furthermore, the ability of the immune system to respond to a broad spectrum of antigens may be compromised if immunocompetent cells are maintained in a state of chronic activation. In addition, activation of the immune system may favor the elimination of cells via programmed cell death (apoptosis) (see below) as well as the secretion of certain cytokines that can induce HIV expression (see below).

The deleterious effects of chronic immune activation on the progression of HIV disease are well established. As in most conditions of persistent antigen exposure, the host must maintain sufficient activation of antigen (HIV)-specific responses but must also prevent excessive activation and potential immune-mediated damage to tissues. Certain studies suggest that normal immunosuppressive mechanisms that act to keep hyperimmune activation in check, particularly CD4+, FoxP3+, CD25+ regulatory T cells (T-regs), may be dysfunctional or depleted in the context of advanced HIV disease.

Apoptosis

Apoptosis is a form of programmed cell death that is a normal mechanism for the elimination of effete cells in organogenesis as well as in the cellular proliferation that occurs during a normal immune response. Apoptosis is strictly dependent on cellular activation, and the aberrant cellular activation associated with HIV disease (see above) is correlated with a heightened state of apoptosis. It has been hypothesized that, in HIV infection, sequential activation signals delivered to CD4+ T cells induce apoptosis. Cross-linking of the CD4 molecule by gp120 or gp120/anti-gp120 complexes delivers the first of two signals required for apoptosis. The second signal supposedly leading to cell death is delivered via the T-cell receptor by antigen. According to this hypothesis, direct infection of CD4+ T cells is not required for apoptosis to occur, although it has been demonstrated that alterations in tyrosine kinase activity of HIV-infected cells may induce the cell to undergo apoptosis. HIV can trigger both Fas-dependent and Fas-independent pathways of apoptosis. Mechanisms involved in this process include upregulation of Fas and Fas ligand, upregulation of caspase-1 and caspase-6, downregulation of the anti-apoptotic Bcl-2 protein, and activation of cyclin-dependent kinases. Certain viral gene products have been associated with enhanced susceptibility to apoptosis including Env, Tat, and Vpr. In contrast, Nef has been shown to possess antiapoptotic properties. A number of studies, including those examining lymphoid tissue, have demonstrated that the rate of apoptosis is elevated in HIV infection and that apoptosis is seen in "bystander" cells such as CD8+ T cells and B cells as well as in CD4+ T cells. The intensity of apoptosis correlates with the general state of activation of the immune system and not with the stage of disease or with viral burden. It is likely that apoptosis of immunocompetent cells contributes to the immune abnormalities in HIV disease; however, this is probably a nonspecific mechanism that merely reflects the aberrant state of immune activation.

Autoimmune Phenomena

The autoimmune phenomena that are common in HIV-infected individuals reflect, at least in part, chronic immune system activation as well as molecular mimicry by viral components. Although these phenomena usually occur in the absence of autoimmune disease, a wide spectrum of clinical manifestations that may be associated with autoimmunity have been described (see below). Autoimmune phenomena include antibodies to lymphocytes and, less commonly, to platelets and neutrophils. Antiplatelet antibodies have some clinical relevance, in that they may contribute to the thrombocytopenia of HIV disease (see below). Antibodies to nuclear and cytoplasmic components of cells have been reported, as have antibodies to cardiolipin; CD4 molecules; CD43 molecules, C1q-A; variable regions of the T-cell receptor α, β, and γ chains; Fas; denatured collagen; and IL-2. In addition, autoantibodies to a range of serum proteins, including albumin, immunoglobulin, and thyroglobulin, have been reported. There is antigenic cross-reactivity between HIV viral proteins (gp120 and gp41) and MHC class II determinants, and anti-MHC class II antibodies have been reported in HIV infection. These antibodies could potentially lead to the elimination of MHC class II–bearing cells via antibody-dependent cellular cytotoxicity (ADCC), although this has not been clearly demonstrated to occur. In addition, regions of homology exist between HIV envelope glycoproteins and IL-2 as well as MHC class I molecules. With the widespread use of effective antiretroviral therapy, an *immune reconstitution inflammatory syndrome* (IRIS) has become increasingly more common. IRIS is an autoimmune-like phenomenon characterized by a paradoxical deterioration of clinical condition, which is usually compartmentalized to a particular organ system, in individuals in whom ARV therapy has recently been initiated. It is associated with a decrease in viral load and at least partial recovery of immune competence, usually associated with increases in CD4+ T-cell counts. The immunopathogenesis is felt to be related to an increase in immune response against the presence of residual antigens that are usually microbial and is commonly seen with underlying *Mycobacterium tuberculosis* and cryptococcosis. This syndrome is discussed in more detail below.

THE CYTOKINE NETWORK IN HIV PATHOGENESIS

The immune system is homeostatically regulated by a complex network of immunoregulatory cytokines, which are pleiotropic and redundant and operate in an autocrine and paracrine manner. They are expressed continuously, even during periods of apparent quiescence of the immune system. On perturbation of the immune system by antigenic challenge, the expression of cytokines increases to varying degrees. Cytokines that are important components of this immunoregulatory network have been demonstrated to play a major role in the regulation of HIV expression in vitro. Potent modulation of HIV expression has been demonstrated either by manipulating endogenous cytokines or by adding exogenous cytokines to culture. Cytokines that induce HIV expression in one or more of these systems include IL-1, IL-2, IL-3, IL-6, IL-12, TNF-α, TNF-β, macrophage colony-stimulating factor (M-CSF), and granulocyte-macrophage colony-stimulating factor (GM-CSF). Among these cytokines, the most consistent and potent inducers of HIV expression are the *proinflammatory cytokines* TNF-α, IL-1β, and IL-6. Interferon (IFN)-α and -β suppress HIV replication, whereas transforming growth factor (TGF) β, IL-4, IL-10, and IFN-γ can either induce or suppress HIV expression, depending on the system involved. The *CC-chemokines* RANTES (CCL5), macrophage inflammatory protein (MIP)-1α (CCL3), and MIP-1β (CCL4) inhibit infection by and spread of R5 HIV-1 strains, whereas *stromal cell–derived factor* (SDF) 1 inhibits infection by and spread of X4 strains (see below). The alpha defensin family of cytokines has been shown to inhibit both R5 and X4 viruses, and other soluble factors that have not yet been fully characterized have also been shown to suppress HIV replication.

The molecular mechanisms of HIV regulation are best understood for TNF-α, which activates NF-κB proteins that function as transcriptional activators of HIV expression. The HIV-inducing effect of IL-1β is thought to occur at the level of viral transcription in an NF-κB-independent manner. IL-6, GM-CSF, and IFN-γ regulate HIV expression mainly by posttranscriptional mechanisms. Elevated levels of TNF-α and IL-6 have been demonstrated in plasma and cerebrospinal fluid (CSF), and increased expression of TNF-α, IL-1β, IFN-γ, and IL-6 has been demonstrated in the lymph nodes of HIV-infected individuals. The mechanisms whereby the CC-chemokines RANTES (CCL5), MIP-1α (CCL3), and MIP-1β (CCL4) inhibit infection of R5 strains of HIV or SDF-1 blocks X4 strains of HIV involve blocking of the binding of the virus to its co-receptors, the CC-chemokine receptor CCR5 and the CXC-chemokine receptor CXCR4, respectively (see above and below). However, several CC-chemokines, including but not limited to CCL3, -4, and -5, induce intracellular signals that actually enhance infection by X4 strains of virus at both the entry and postentry levels. The mechanisms whereby other less well-characterized factors (see above) inhibit HIV replication are not completely understood.

Blocking of endogenous HIV-inducing cytokines or addition of inhibitors of HIV-suppressor cytokines in cultures of peripheral blood and lymph node mononuclear cells from HIV-infected individuals has demonstrated that HIV replication is controlled tightly by endogenous cytokines that act synergistically and in an autocrine and paracrine manner, similar to their physiologic function in the regulation of the immune system. Indeed, the net level of virus replication in an HIV-infected individual reflects at least in part a balance between inductive and suppressive host factors, mediated mainly by cytokines.

LYMPHOCYTE TURNOVER IN HIV INFECTION

The immune systems of patients with HIV infection are characterized by a profound increase in lymphocyte turnover that is immediately reduced with effective ARV therapy. Studies utilizing in vivo or in vitro labeling of lymphocytes in the S-phase of the cell cycle have demonstrated a tight correlation between the degree of lymphocyte turnover and plasma levels of HIV RNA. This increase in turnover is seen in CD4+ and CD8+ T lymphocytes as well as B lymphocytes and can be observed in peripheral blood and lymphoid tissue. Mathematical models derived from these data suggest that one can view the lymphoid pool as consisting of dynamically distinct subpopulations of cells that are differentially affected by HIV infection. A major consequence of HIV infection appears to be a shift in cells from a more quiescent pool to a pool with a higher turnover rate. It is likely that a consequence of a higher rate of turnover is a higher rate of cell death. The role of the thymus in adult human T-cell homeostasis and HIV pathogenesis is an area of controversy. Although some data point to an important role for the thymus in maintaining T-cell numbers and suggest that impairment of thymic function may be responsible for the declines in CD4+ T cells seen in the setting of HIV infection, other studies have concluded that the thymus plays a minor role in HIV pathogenesis. Among the data supporting an important role for the thymus are those that demonstrate an increase in the levels of T-cell receptor excision circles (TRECs) after initiation of ARV therapy. TRECs are a byproduct of T-cell development and represent episomal fragments of DNA that are excised during T-cell receptor gene rearrangement. Levels of TRECs will be the net result of changes in thymic output together with changes in T-cell turnover. An increase in thymic output and/or a decrease in T-cell turnover will lead to an increase in levels of TRECs. Although it is clear that levels of TRECs increase after initiation of

ARV therapy, it is not clear whether this is a consequence of increased thymic output or decreased T-cell turnover.

THE ROLE OF CO-RECEPTORS IN HIV PATHOGENESIS

As mentioned above, HIV-1 utilizes two major co-receptors along with CD4 to bind to, fuse with, and enter target cells; these co-receptors are CCR5 and CXCR4, which are also receptors for certain endogenous chemokines. Strains of HIV that utilize CCR5 as a co-receptor are referred to as *R5 viruses*. Strains of HIV that utilize CXCR4 are referred to as *X4 viruses*. Many virus strains are *dual tropic* in that they utilize both CCR5 and CXCR4; these are referred to as *R5X4 viruses*.

The natural chemokine ligands for the major HIV co-receptors can readily block entry of HIV. For example, the CC-chemokines RANTES (CCL5), MIP-1α (CCL3), and MIP-1β (CCL4), which are the natural ligands for CCR5, block entry of R5 viruses, whereas SDF-1, the natural ligand for CXCR4, blocks entry of X4 viruses. The mechanism of inhibition of viral entry is a steric inhibition of binding that is not dependent on signal transduction (Fig. 90-23).

The transmitting virus is almost invariably an R5 virus that predominates during the early stages of HIV disease. In ~40% of HIV-infected individuals, there is a transition to a predominantly X4 virus that is associated with a relatively rapid progression of disease. However, at least 60% of infected individuals progress in their disease while maintaining predominance of an R5 virus. It should be pointed out that clade C viruses, unlike other subgroups, almost never switch from CCR5 tropism to CXCR4 tropism; the reason for this difference is unclear. Other chemokine receptor family members may function as co-receptors for HIV and SIV entry, but to a much lesser extent than do CCR5 and CXCR4; these include CCR3, BOB/GPR15, CXCR6 (Bonzo/STRL33/TYMSTR), CCR2, CCR8, CX_3CR1(V28), and GPR1.

The basis for the tropism of different envelope glycoproteins for either CCR5 or CXCR4 relates to the ability of the HIV envelope, including the third variable region (V3 loop) of gp120, to interact with these co-receptors. In this regard, binding of gp120 to CD4 induces a conformational change in gp120 that increases its affinity for CCR5 (see above). Finally, R5 viruses are more efficient in infecting monocytes/macrophages and microglial cells of the brain (see "Neuropathogenesis" later in the chapter).

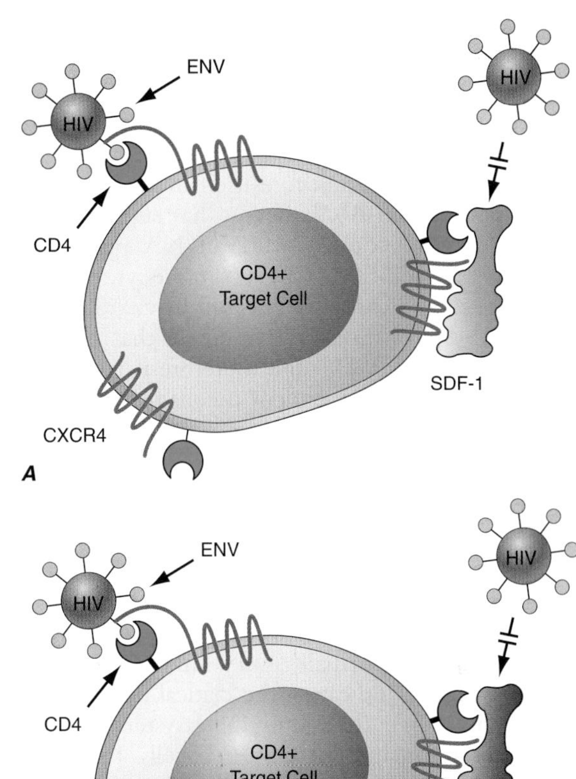

FIGURE 90-23

Model for the role of co-receptors CXCR4 and CCR5 in the efficient binding and entry of X4 (***A***) and R5 (***B***) strains of HIV-1, respectively, into CD4+ target cells. Blocking of this initial event in the virus life cycle can be accomplished by inhibition of binding to the co-receptor by the normal ligand for the receptor in question. The ligand for CXCR4 is stromal cell–derived factor (SDF-1); the ligands for CCR5 are RANTES, MIP-1α, and MIP-1β.

CELLULAR TARGETS OF HIV

Although the CD4+ T lymphocytes and CD4+ cells of monocyte lineage are the principal targets of HIV, virtually any cell that expresses the CD4 molecule together with co-receptor molecules (see above and below) can potentially be infected with HIV. Circulating dendritic cells have been reported to express low levels of CD4 and, depending on their stage of maturation, these cells can be infected with HIV (see below). Epidermal Langerhans cells express CD4 and have been infected by HIV in vivo. In vitro, HIV has been reported also to infect a wide range of cells and cell lines that express low levels of CD4, no detectable CD4, or only CD4 mRNA; among these are FDCs, megakaryocytes, eosinophils, astrocytes, oligodendrocytes, microglial cells, CD8+ T cells, B cells, and NK cells as well as a variety of organ-specific cells. Since the only cells that have been shown unequivocally to be infected with HIV and to support replication of the virus are CD4+ T lymphocytes and cells of monocyte/macrophage lineage, the relevance of the in vitro infection of these other cell types is questionable.

Of potentially important clinical relevance is the demonstration that thymic precursor cells, which were assumed to be negative for CD3, CD4, and CD8 molecules, actually do express low levels of CD4 and can be infected with HIV in vitro. In addition, human thymic epithelial cells transplanted into an immunodeficient mouse can be infected with HIV by direct inoculation of virus into the thymus. Since these cells may play a role in the normal regeneration of CD4+ T cells, it is possible that their infection and depletion contribute, at least in part, to the impaired ability of the CD4+ T-cell pool to completely reconstitute itself in certain infected individuals in whom ARV therapy has suppressed viral replication to <50 copies of HIV RNA per milliliter (see below). In addition, CD34+ monocyte precursor cells have been shown to be infected in vivo in patients with advanced HIV disease. It is likely that these cells express low levels of CD4, and therefore it is not essential to invoke CD4-independent mechanisms to explain the infection.

ABNORMALITIES OF MONONUCLEAR CELLS

CD4+ T Cells

The range of T-cell abnormalities in advanced HIV infection is broad. The defects are both quantitative and qualitative and affect virtually every limb of the immune system (see below), indicating the critical dependence of the integrity of the immune system on the inducer/helper function of CD4+ T cells. In advanced HIV disease, most of the observed immune defects can ultimately be explained by the quantitative depletion of CD4+ T cells. However, T-cell dysfunction (see below) can be demonstrated in patients early in the course of infection, even when the CD4+ T-cell count is in the low-normal range. The degree and spectrum of dysfunctions increase as the disease progresses. One of the first abnormalities to be detected is a defect in response to remote recall antigens, such as tetanus toxoid and influenza, at a time when mononuclear cells can still respond normally to mitogenic stimulation. Indeed, defects of central memory cells are a critical component of HIV immunopathogenesis. The progressive loss of antigen-specific CD4+ T cells has important implications for the control of HIV infection. In this regard, there is a correlation between the maintenance of HIV-specific CD4+ T-cell proliferative responses and improved control of infection. Essentially every T-cell function has been reported to be abnormal at some stage of HIV infection. These abnormalities include defective T-cell cloning and colony-forming efficiencies, impaired expression of IL-2 receptors, defective IL-2 production, reduced expression of the IL-7 receptor (CD127), and decreased IFN-γ production in response to antigens. The proportion of CD4+ T cells that express CD28, which is a major co-stimulatory molecule necessary for the normal activation of T cells, is reduced during HIV infection. Cells lacking expression of CD28 do not respond normally to activation signals and may express markers of terminal activation including HLA-DR, CD38, and CD45RO. CD4+ T cells from HIV-infected individuals express abnormally low levels of CD40 ligand, which may contribute to the dysregulation of B-cell function observed in HIV disease. As mentioned above (see "Cellular Activation and HIV Pathogenesis"), a subset of CD4+ T cells referred to as *T regulatory cells*, or T-regs, may be involved in dampening aberrant immune activation that propagates HIV replication. The presence of these T-reg cells correlates with lower viral loads and higher CD4+/CD8+ T-cell ratios. A loss of this T-reg capability with advanced disease may be detrimental to the control of virus replication.

TABLE 90-3

MECHANISMS OF CD4+ T-CELL DYSFUNCTION AND DEPLETION

DIRECT MECHANISMS	INDIRECT MECHANISMS
Loss of plasma membrane integrity due to viral budding	Aberrant intracellular signaling events
Accumulation of unintegrated viral DNA	Autoimmunity
Interference with cellular RNA processing	Innocent bystander killing of viral antigen–coated cells
Intracellular gp120-CD4 autofusion events	Apoptosis
Syncytia formation	Inhibition of lymphopoiesis
	Activation-induced cell death
	Elimination of HIV-infected cells by virus-specific immune responses

It is difficult to explain completely the profound immunodeficiency noted in HIV-infected individuals solely on the basis of direct infection and quantitative depletion of CD4+ T cells. This is particularly apparent during the early stages of HIV disease, when CD4+ T-cell numbers may be only marginally decreased.

In this regard, it is likely that CD4+ T-cell dysfunction results from a combination of depletion of cells due to direct infection of the cell and a number of virus-related but indirect effects on the cell (Table 90-3). Indeed, it has been demonstrated that patients with high levels of plasma viremia have a variety of subtle abnormalities of CD4+ T-cell function, particularly involving aberrancies in signal transduction pathways. These abnormalities could be due either to aberrant activation induced by the cascade of cytokines that are expressed in viremic patients or by the direct effect of virus on the cell. In this regard, certain of these abnormalities can be reproduced by exposing CD4+ T cells of normal individuals to oligomeric HIV envelope proteins in vitro (see below).

Single-cell killing and the formation of syncytia between infected and uninfected cells have been demonstrated clearly in vitro, although there is little evidence that this process occurs in vivo. Cytopathicity in an infected cell in vitro may result from a number of mechanisms, including copious budding of virions from the cell surface with resulting disruption of the integrity of the cell membrane; interference with cellular RNA processing or the accumulation of high levels of heterodisperse RNA molecules; disruption of cellular protein synthesis owing to high levels of viral RNA; accumulation of high levels of unintegrated viral DNA in the cell cytoplasm; induction of aberrant patterns of protein tyrosine phosphorylation; and the interaction between HIV gp120 and CD4 intracellularly. Strain differences in single-cell killing are determined largely by gp120 sequences, which supports the importance of the viral envelope in this process. Humoral and cellular immune responses to HIV may contribute to protective immunity by eliminating virus and virus-infected cells (see below). However, since the main targets of HIV infection are immunocompetent cells, these responses may contribute to immune cell depletion and immunologic dysfunction by eliminating both infected cells and "innocent bystander" cells. Soluble viral proteins, particularly gp120, can bind with high affinity to the CD4 molecules on uninfected T cells and monocytes; in addition, virus and/or viral proteins can bind to dendritic cells or FDCs. HIV-specific antibody can recognize these bound molecules and potentially collaborate in the elimination of the cells by ADCC.

Nonpolymorphic determinants of MHC class I products share a degree of homology with gp120 and gp41 proteins of HIV. Such similarities may lead to the generation of autoantibodies to self-MHC determinants. Anti-HLA-DR antibodies have been demonstrated in the sera of HIV-infected individuals (see "Autoimmune Phenomena" earlier in the chapter). These antibodies could contribute to the elimination of HLA-DR–expressing cells by ADCC; in addition, it has been suggested that these antibodies may inhibit certain T-cell functions that involve HLA-DR molecules.

HIV envelope glycoproteins gp120 and gp160 manifest high-affinity binding to CD4 as well as to various chemokine receptors (see above). Intracellular signals transduced by gp120 through both CD4 and CCR5/CXCR4 have been associated with a number of immunopathogenic processes including anergy, apoptosis, and abnormalities of cell trafficking. The molecular mechanisms responsible for these abnormalities include dysregulation of the T-cell receptor–phosphoinositide pathway, p56lck activation, phosphorylation of focal adhesion kinase, activation of the MAP kinase and ras signaling pathways, and downregulation of the co-stimulatory molecules CD40 ligand and CD80.

Finally, the inexorable decline in CD4+ T-cell counts that occurs in most HIV-infected individuals may result in part from the inability of the immune system to regenerate the rapidly turning over CD4+ T-cell pool efficiently enough to compensate for both HIV-mediated and naturally occurring attrition of cells. At least two major mechanisms may contribute to the failure of the CD4+ T-cell pool to reconstitute itself adequately over the course of HIV infection. The first is the destruction of lymphoid precursor cells, including thymic and bone marrow progenitor cells (see above); the other is the gradual disruption of the lymphoid tissue microenvironment, which is essential for efficient regeneration of immunocompetent cells (see above).

CD8+ T Cells

A relative CD8+ T lymphocytosis is generally associated with high levels of HIV plasma viremia and may in part reflect the expansion of clones of HIV-specific CD8+ CTLs. During the late stages of HIV infection, there may be a significant reduction in the numbers of CD8+ T cells despite the presence of high levels of viremia. HIV-specific CD8+ CTLs have been demonstrated in HIV-infected individuals early in the course of disease (see below). The emergence of HIV escape mutants may ultimately evade these HIV-specific CD8+ T cells. However, as the disease progresses, the functional capability of these cells may decrease and may be lost entirely. The cause of this loss of cytolytic activity is unclear. However, it has been demonstrated that, as disease progresses, CD8+ T cells assume an abnormal phenotype characterized by expression of activation markers such as HLA-DR and CD38 with an absence of expression of the IL-2 receptor (CD25), a loss of clonogenic potential, and a reduced expression of the IL-7 receptor (CD127). In this regard, it has been reported that nonprogressors can be distinguished from progressors by the maintenance in the former of a high proliferative capacity of their HIV-specific CD8+ T cells coupled to increases in perforin expression. It has been reported that the phenotype of CD8+ T cells in HIV-infected individuals may be of prognostic significance. Those individuals whose CD8+ T cells developed a phenotype of HLA-DR+/CD38– after seroconversion had stabilization of their CD4+ T-cell counts, whereas those whose CD8+ T cells developed a phenotype of HLA-DR+/CD38+ had a more aggressive course and a poorer prognosis. In addition to the defects in HIV-specific CTLs, functional defects in other MHC-restricted CTLs, such as those directed against influenza and CMV, have been demonstrated. CD8+ T cells secrete a variety of soluble factors that inhibit HIV replication including the CC-chemokines RANTES (CCL5), MIP-1α (CCL3), and MIP-1β (CCL4) as well as one or more as yet poorly identified factors (see above). The presence of high levels of HIV viremia in vivo as well as exposure of CD8+ T cells in vitro to HIV envelope, both of which are associated with aberrant immune activation, has been shown to be associated with a variety of cellular functional abnormalities. Furthermore, since the integrity of CD8+ T-cell function depends in part on adequate inductive signals from CD4+ T cells, the defect in CD8+ CTLs is likely compounded by the quantitative loss and qualitative dysfunction of CD4+ T cells. Finally, as mentioned above, certain cell surface negative regulatory molecules such as CTLA-4 and PD-1 are upregulated on activated T cells, and engagement of these molecules with their ligands may play a role in the exhaustion and death of CD8+, HIV-specific T cells.

B Cells

The predominant defect in B cells from HIV-infected individuals is one of aberrant cellular activation, which is reflected by spontaneous proliferation and immunoglobulin secretion and by increased spontaneous secretion of TNF-α and IL-6. In addition, B cells from HIV viremic patients manifest a decreased capacity to mount a proliferative response to ligation of the B-cell antigen receptor (surface IgM) at the same time as they are capable of robust differentiation in response to a variety of stimuli. B cells from

HIV-infected individuals manifest enhanced spontaneous in vitro transformation with EBV, a process that is likely due to defective T-cell immune surveillance. The in vivo counterpart of this phenomenon is an increase in the incidence of EBV-related B-cell lymphomas in HIV-infected individuals. Untransformed B cells cannot be infected with HIV. However, HIV or its products can activate B cells directly; portions of the HIV gp41 envelope protein have been reported to induce polyclonal B cell activation. In addition, it has been reported that products of the VH_3 genes on the surface of B cells can serve as a receptor for HIV. B cells from patients with high levels of viremia bind virions to their surface via the CD21 complement receptor. It is likely that in vivo activation of B cells by replication-competent or -defective virus as well as viral products during the viremic state account at least in part for the spontaneous activation of these cells noted ex vivo. B-cell subpopulations from HIV-infected individuals undergo a number of changes over the course of HIV disease, including the attrition of memory B cells; the appearance of mature, activated B cells defined by reduced expression of CD21, increased expression of activation markers, increased secretion of immunoglobulins, and increased susceptibility to Fas-mediated apoptosis; and the appearance of immature B cells associated with CD4+ T-cell lymphopenia. Cognate B cell–CD4+ T-cell interactions are abnormal in viremic HIV-infected individuals in that B cells respond poorly to CD4+ T-cell help and CD4+ T cells receive inadequate co-stimulatory signals from activated B cells. In vivo, the aberrant activated state of B cells manifests itself by hypergammaglobulinemia and by the presence of circulating immune complexes and autoantibodies (see above). HIV-infected individuals respond poorly to primary and secondary immunizations with protein and polysaccharide antigens. Using immunization with influenza vaccine, it has been demonstrated that there is a memory B-cell defect in HIV-infected individuals, particularly those with high levels of HIV viremia. Taken together, these B-cell defects are likely responsible in part for the increase in certain bacterial infections seen in advanced HIV disease in adults, as well as for the important role of bacterial infections in the morbidity and mortality of HIV-infected children, who cannot mount an adequate humoral response to common bacterial pathogens. The absolute number of circulating B cells may be depressed in HIV infection; this phenomenon likely reflects increased activation-induced apoptosis as well as a redistribution of cells out of the circulation and into the lymphoid tissue—phenomena that are associated with ongoing viral replication.

Monocytes/Macrophages

Circulating monocytes are generally normal in number in HIV-infected individuals. Monocytes express the CD4 molecule and several co-receptors for HIV on their surface, including CCR5, CXCR4, and CCR3, and thus are targets of HIV infection. The degree of cytopathicity of HIV for cells of the monocyte lineage is low, and HIV can replicate extensively in cells of the monocyte lineage with relatively little cytopathic effect. Hence monocyte-lineage cells may play a role in the dissemination of HIV in the body and can serve as reservoirs of HIV infection, thus representing an obstacle to the eradication of HIV by ARV drugs. In vivo infection of circulating monocytes is difficult to demonstrate; however, infection of tissue macrophages and macrophage-lineage cells in the brain (infiltrating macrophages or resident microglial cells) and lung (pulmonary alveolar macrophages) can be demonstrated easily. Tissue macrophages are an important source of HIV during the inflammatory response associated with opportunistic infections. Infection of monocyte precursors in the bone marrow may directly or indirectly be responsible for certain of the hematologic abnormalities in HIV-infected individuals. A number of abnormalities of circulating monocytes have been reported in HIV-infected individuals, including decreased secretion of IL-1 and IL-12; increased secretion of IL-10; defects in antigen presentation and induction of T-cell responses due to decreased MHC class II expression; and abnormalities of Fc receptor function, C3 receptor–mediated clearance, oxidative burst responses, and certain cytotoxic functions such as ADCC, possibly related to low levels of expression of Fc and complement receptors. Exposure of monocytes to viral proteins such as gp120 and Tat, as well as to certain cytokines, can cause abnormal activation, and this may play a role in cellular dysfunction (see above).

Dendritic and Langerhans Cells

Dendritic cells may play an important role in the initiation of HIV infection by virtue of the ability of HIV to bind to cell surface C-type lectin receptors, particularly DC-SIGN (see above). This allows efficient presentation of virus to CD4+ T-cell targets that become infected; complexes of infected CD4+ T cells and dendritic cells provide an optimal microenvironment for virus replication. There has been considerable disagreement regarding the HIV infectibility and hence the depletion as well as the dysfunction of dendritic cells themselves. Depending on their state of maturation, dendritic cells express varying levels of CD4 as well as several chemokine receptors. In this regard, it appears that the ability of a dendritic cell to become infected depends in part on its state of maturation. Mature dendritic cells have been demonstrated to be infectable by both R5 and X4 isolates of HIV-1. Immature tissue dendritic cells have been less well studied in their native state. Even in those dendritic cells in which infection occurs, the efficiency of infection and level of productivity of infection is quite low compared with CD4+ T cells.

Natural Killer Cells

The role of NK cells is to provide immunosurveillance against virus-infected cells, certain tumor cells, and allogeneic cells. Functional abnormalities in NK cells have been observed throughout the course of HIV disease, and the severity of these abnormalities increases as disease progresses. HIV infection of target cells downregulates HLA-A and -B, but not HLA-C and -D molecules;

this may explain in part the relative inability of NK cells to kill HIV-infected target cells. Most studies report that NK cells are normal in number; however, patients with high levels of virus replication manifest an abnormal representation of a functionally defective CD56–/CD16+ NK cell subset. This abnormal subset of NK cells manifests an increased expression of inhibitory NK cell receptors (iNKRs) and a substantial decrease in expression of natural cytotoxicity receptors (NCRs) and shows a markedly impaired lytic activity. The overrepresentation of this abnormal subset of NK cells may explain in part the observed defects in NK cell function in HIV-infected individuals. NK cells also serve as important sources of HIV-inhibitory CC-chemokines. NK cells isolated from HIV-infected individuals constitutively produce high levels of MIP-1α (CCL3), MIP-1β (CCL4), and RANTES (CCL5). In addition, high levels of these chemokines are seen when NK cells are stimulated with IL-2 or IL-15 or when CD16 is cross-linked or during the process of lytic killing of target cells. HIV-infected patients with high levels of plasma viremia manifest a decreased ability, compared with HIV-infected individuals who are aviremic, of their NK cells to block HIV replication in vitro in assays of both cell contact and supernatant-mediated suppression of virus. Finally, NK cell–dendritic cell interactions are important for normal immune function. NK cells and dendritic cells reciprocally modulate each other's activation and maturation. These interactions are markedly impaired in HIV-infected individuals with high levels of plasma viremia.

GENETIC FACTORS IN HIV PATHOGENESIS

MHC Genes

Several reports have described MHC alleles and other host factors that may influence the pathogenesis and course of HIV disease. These include associations with transmission and with the type of clinical course, such as slow or rapid rates of progression to AIDS (Table 90-4). For example, researchers recently employed a whole-genome association strategy to identify two independently acting groups of polymorphisms associated with HLA loci B and C, which explained 15% of the variation in viral load among individuals during the asymptomatic period of infection. A number of mechanisms have been proposed whereby MHC-encoded molecules might predispose an individual either to rapid progression or to nonprogression to AIDS. These proposed mechanisms include the ability to present certain immunodominant HIV T helper or CTL epitopes, leading to a relatively protective immune response against HIV and hence to a slower rate of disease progression. In contrast, certain MHC class I or class II alleles might predispose an individual to an immunopathogenic response against viral epitopes in certain tissues, such as the CNS or lungs, or against certain HIV-infected cell types, such as macrophages or dendritic cells/Langerhans cells. In addition, certain rare MHC class I and class II alleles might facilitate rapid recognition of HIV-infected cells from the infecting partner in primary HIV infection and promote rejection of these cells by alloreactive responses. Similarly, common MHC alleles could lead to less effective removal of HIV-infected allogeneic cells. In this regard, it has been demonstrated that allele sharing at HLA-B loci is associated with increased risk of transmission of HIV infection between heterosexual Zambian couples discordant for HIV. It has been clearly demonstrated that maximal *HLA* heterozygosity for class I loci (A, B, and C) is associated with a delayed onset of AIDS among HIV-infected individuals, whereas homozygosity for these loci was associated with a more rapid progression to AIDS and death. This observation is likely due to the fact that individuals who are heterozygous at *HLA* loci are able to present a greater variety of antigenic peptides to cytotoxic T lymphocytes than are homozygotes, resulting in a more effective immune response against a number of pathogens, including HIV. Of particular note is the fact that the HLA class I alleles B*35 and Cw*04 were consistently associated with rapid development of AIDS. Other data have indicated that transporter associated with antigen-processing (TAP) genes play a role in determining the outcome of HIV infection. HLA profiles that reflect certain combinations of MHC-encoded TAP and class I and class II genes are strongly associated with different rates of progression to AIDS. A recent finding of genetic association with HIV disease progression has highlighted the role for NK cells in HIV disease. A single nucleotide polymorphism (SNP) in the killer immunoglobulin-like receptor (KIR) gene was shown to be strongly associated with rapid progression to AIDS. However, when the KIR3 DS1 SNP was present with HLA-B Bw4-80I, the resultant phenotype was delayed progression to AIDS, even though this HLA-B allele alone has no effect on HIV disease progression. Furthermore, the KIR3 DS1/HLA-B Bw4-80I-carrying individuals had a significantly reduced viral load, beginning early in the course of infection, and protection against opportunistic infections during the later stages of the disease. This observation points to the potential role of NK cells in the maintenance of the viral set point, and strongly suggests that HLA-B Bw4-80I serves as the ligand activating the KIR, resulting in the death of the target cell. These gene-gene interactions between KIR and MHC genes are illustrated in Table 90-4.

Chemokine Receptors

The most dramatic example of a genetic factor influencing HIV infection and/or pathogenesis relates to the gene that codes for the HIV cellular co-receptor CCR5. Rare individuals have been reported who had repetitive sexual exposure to HIV in high-risk situations but remained uninfected. The peripheral blood mononuclear cells of two such individuals were found to be highly resistant to infection in vitro with R5 strains of HIV-1 but were readily infected with X4 strains. Genetic analysis revealed that these two individuals inherited a homozygous defect in the gene that codes for CCR5, the cellular co-receptor for R5 strains of HIV-1. The defective *CCR5* allele contained a 32-bp deletion corresponding to the second extracellular loop of the receptor (*Δ32* allele). The encoded protein was severely truncated and the receptor was nonfunctional, explaining the refractoriness to infection with R5 strains

TABLE 90-4

HOST GENETIC FACTORS THAT INFLUENCE RISK OF TRANSMISSION AND RATES OF DISEASE PROGRESSION TO AIDS

	MHC GENES	
	HLA CLASS I[a]	**HLA CLASS II[a]**
Disease Progression		
Rapid	**A23, A24,** *A26, A28, A29, A31, B7 supertype,* **B*08,** *B14, B21,* **B22,** *B25,* **B35,** *B37, B38,* **B53,** *B44, B49,* **C4, C7,** *C8, C16,* **homozygosity for class I alleles**	**DRB1*01, DRB1*03,** *DRB1*05, DRB1*11*
Slow	*A10, A19, A*30,* **A32,** *B14, B16, B17, B18,* **B27,** *B*39, B51,* **B57,** *B58, C8,* **heterozygosity for class I alleles**	*DRB1*03, DRB1*13*
Transmission		
Increased risk	*A2, B21, B35, Cw4,* ***allele sharing between HIV donor and recipient***	*DRB1*05, DRB1*06, DRB1*13*
Reduced risk	*A2/A6802 supertype, A11, B18, B52, B57, B58, C2*	

FACTOR	ASSOCIATION
Chemokine and Chemokine Receptor Genes	
CCR5	Homozygous defect involving a 32-bp deletion corresponding to the second extracellular loop of the receptor results in loss of surface expression and, consequently, resistance to infection; heterozygous defect appears to result in partial protection against transmission and disease progression. Several single nucleotide polymorphisms (SNPs) in the *CCR5* promoter have been identified that along with the CCR2-64I polymorphism define nine human haplogroups (HHA to HHE, HHF*1, HHF*2, HHG*1 and HHG*2). Homozygosity for the HHE haplotype is associated with an increased risk of transmission and an accelerated rate of disease progression.
CCR2	Heterozygosity for the CCR2-64I polymorphism is associated with a slower rate of disease progression, and in one study this effect was found to be more prominent in African Americans.
CX3CR1	Mutations 249I and 280M are associated with a rapid rate of disease progression to AIDS in a French-Caucasian cohort. Inconsistent effects were detected in other cohorts.
CCL3L1 (MIP-1αP)	The copy number of *CCL3L1* varies within and among populations (range 0–10 copies per diploid genome). A copy number lower than the average gene dose found in a population is associated with an increased risk of acquiring HIV and a more rapid rate of disease progression to AIDS.
CCL5 (RANTES)	SNPs in the promoter, intron, and 3'-untranslated region can influence transcription and protein production and, consequently, affect risk of acquiring HIV and rates of disease progression. For example, a haplotype defined by two promoter SNPs (-471A/-96C) is associated with a faster rate of disease progression in European Americans. However, the -471A/-96G haplotype is found mostly in populations from East Asia, and this haplotype was associated with a slow rate of disease progression in a Japanese cohort.
CCL2 (MCP-1)	The *MCP-1 -2578G* allele results in increased transcription, protein production, and monocyte recruitment. Homozygosity for the *MCP-1 -2578G* allele is associated with an enhanced risk of developing HIV-1–associated dementia and a rapid disease course.
CXCL12 (SDF-1)	The *SDF-1* 3'A SNP in the 3' untranslated region was initially reported to be associated with a slower disease rate of progression in a large U.S.-based cohort, but the results in other cohorts suggest an opposite effect.
Cytokine Genes	
IL-10	Individuals carrying the *IL-10* -592A promoter allele were at increased risk for HIV infection and, once infected, progressed more rapidly than did homozygotes for the alternative *IL-10-5'*-592 C/C genotype.
IL-4	The *IL-4*-589T results in higher levels of IL-4 production in vivo, resulting in downregulation of *CCR5*. However, the effects of this polymorphism on disease progression are inconsistent.
IL-6	A single report showed that possession of the IL-6 promoter polymorphism (-174G) is associated with an increased risk of developing Kaposi's sarcoma in HIV-1–positive individuals.
TNF-α	A single report showed that the SNP *TNF-α*-238A, but not the -308A allele, correlates with a higher frequency of lipodystrophy.
Other Genes	
APOBEC3G	The 186R allele is associated with a decline in CD4 T cells and an accelerated rate of progression to AIDS in African Americans.
VDR	Homozygosity for the vitamin D receptor gene polymorphism B (VDR-BB) correlates with a rapid progression to AIDS.
MBL2	Conflicting effects have been reported for MBL variants.

(*Continued*)

TABLE 90-4 (CONTINUED)

HOST GENETIC FACTORS THAT INFLUENCE RISK OF TRANSMISSION AND RATES OF DISEASE PROGRESSION TO AIDS

FACTOR	ASSOCIATION
Gene-Gene Interactions	
KIR gene with *HLA-B*	In the absence of *HLA-B* Bw4-80I, *KIR3DS1* is strongly associated with rapid progression to AIDS. This effect is reversed by the presence of *HLA-B* Bw4-80I. Individuals carrying both genes have a delayed progression to AIDS; in the absence of *KIR3DS1*, *HLA-B* Bw4-80I has no effect on disease progression.
CCL3L1 and *CCR5*	Based on possession of a low or high copy number of *CCL3L1* ($CCL3L1^{low}$ or $CCL3L1^{high}$) and a detrimental or nondetrimental ($CCR5^{det}$ or $CCR5^{nondet}$) *CCR5* genotype, variations in these two genes segregate into four genetic risk groups (GRGs). In HIV-infected adults followed in a U.S.-based cohort, an association for a low, moderate, and high risk of acquiring HIV or progressing rapidly to AIDS and death was detected in those possessing a $CCL3L1^{high}/CCR5^{nondet}$, $CCL3L1^{high}/CCR5^{det}$ or $CCL3L1^{low}/CCR5^{nondet}$, and $CCL3L1^{low}/CCR5^{det}$ GRG, respectively.

[a]For MHC genes, bold denotes alleles that in multiple reports have been shown to have consistent effects in different cohorts, whereas italic denotes alleles that have been show to have effects in a few cohorts. HH, human haplogroup.

Sources: Sunil K. Ahuja, MD, and adapted from HA Stephens: Trends Immunol 26(1):41, 2005; M Carrington, SJ O'Brien: Annu Rev Med 54:535 2003; Epub 2001 Dec 3; RA Kaslow et al: J Infect Dis. 191 [Suppl 1]:S68, 2005; A Telenti, G Bleiber: Future Virol 1:55, 2006.

of HIV-1. Population studies revealed that ~1% of the Caucasian population of western European ancestry possessed the homozygous defect. Up to 20% of individuals of European descent were found to be heterozygous for the *CCR5-Δ32* allele. Of note, cohort studies of hundreds of DNA samples originating from western and central Africa and Far East Asia indicate that the *CCR5-Δ32* allele is either absent or extremely rare in these populations. A number of studies found that the frequency of *CCR5-Δ32* allele was enriched in exposed, uninfected individuals. Furthermore, in a cohort of 1400 HIV-1–infected Caucasian individuals, no subject homozygous for the mutation was found, strongly supporting the concept that the homozygous defect confers protection against infection. This finding is particularly compelling in light of the fact that transmitting viruses are strongly biased toward R5 strains of HIV-1 (see above). Of note, several individuals have been identified who were homozygous for the *CCR5-Δ32* defect who in fact did become infected with HIV. These individuals were found to have an X4 strain of HIV that was associated in some cases with an accelerated course of disease. In some studies, HIV-infected individuals who are heterozygous for the *CCR5-Δ32* allele had a slower rate of disease progression. Slow progression of HIV disease is also seen in individuals who are heterozygous for the *CCR2-64I* polymorphism. This *CCR2-64I* allele–associated effect could be due to its linkage with SNPs in the *CCR5* promoter that are known to influence disease progression rates and/or due to dimerization of CXCR4 with the mutated *CCR2-64I* resulting in a decreased expression of CXCR4 on the cell surface.

A number of SNPs in the *CCR5* promoter have been associated with varied rates of disease progression. The promoter SNPs along the *CCR5-Δ32* and CCR2-V64I alleles define nine *CCR5* human haplogroups (HH) designated as HHA through HHE, and HHG*1, HHG*2, HHF*1 and HHF*2 (Table 90-4). Studies have shown that homozygosity for the HHE haplotype is associated with an increased risk of acquiring HIV and progressing rapidly to AIDS. Pairing of the HHC and the *CCR5-Δ32*-containing HHG*2 haplotype is associated with a slower rate of disease progression and reduced risk of acquiring HIV.

Chemokines

The varied distribution of the copy number of *CCL3L1* and *RANTES* polymorphisms provides some striking examples of the effect of chemokine genes on HIV pathogenesis. The *CCL3L1* gene encodes MIP-1αP, the most potent agonist of CCR5 and HIV-suppressive chemokine for R5 strains of HIV-1. This gene is present in a range of copy numbers in and among different racial groups. Individuals with fewer than average copy numbers for their racial group showed both an increased susceptibility to infection with HIV and a faster rate of progression to AIDS. When the interaction of this gene with the different *CCR5* alleles was examined, individuals with a low *CCL3L1* gene dose and certain *CCR5* alleles, which have a detrimental effect on disease progression, were shown to have a significantly greater risk of transmission and faster disease progression rates. SNPs have been identified in the gene that encodes for CCL5 (*RANTES*), another potent agonist of CCR5 and an R5 HIV-suppressive chemokine. Some of these SNPs correlate with either an increased or decreased *CCL5* gene transcription and this is thought to underlie the disease associations detected. For example, the *CCL5* -96G SNP upregulates *CCL5* gene transcription and is associated with delayed progression to AIDS in a Japanese cohort; the prevalence of this allele is very low in other populations. The opposite effects are observed for an intronic *CCL5* SNP designated as In1.1C. This SNP is associated with decreased *CCL5* gene transcription and correlates strongly with a rapid progression rate to AIDS. Other SNPs that decrease *CCL5* gene transcription are associated with a higher rate of HIV infection. The results of these genotype-phenotype studies with *CCL3L1* and *CCL5* genes reinforce the central role for R5 viruses in the establishment of HIV infection.

Additional associations for other chemokines have been noted. CCL2 is a one of the most potent chemokines that attracts and activates mononuclear phagocytes (MP). In a U.S. population-based study, homozygosity for the *CCL2* (*MCP-1*) -2578G allele was associated with a 50% reduction in the risk of acquiring HIV-1. However, once HIV-1 infection was established, this same *CCL2* genotype was associated with accelerated disease progression and a 4.5-fold increased risk of HIV-associated dementia. Possession of the *CCL2* -2578G allele is associated with increased CCL2 serum levels and recruitment of MPs to inflamed tissues. Since recruitment of MPs to the CNS and the activation status of MPs in the CNS is thought to be a key determinant of HIV-associated dementia, these association studies implicate a central role for CCL2 in the pathogenesis of HIV-related CNS disease.

Cytokines

In addition to the chemokine receptors and chemokines, polymorphisms in cytokine genes have also been found to influence intersubject differences in susceptibility to HIV/AIDS. Individuals who carry a certain allele (-592A) of the IL-10 promoter are at increased risk of infection and, once infected, progress more rapidly than homozygotes for the alternative genotype. The mechanism of this effect is felt to be a downregulation of the inhibitory cytokine IL-10 resulting in facilitation of HIV replication. The SNP, IL-4 -589T, increases IL-4 production. This allele associates with a slower progression to AIDS, presumably through the downregulation of CCR5 by higher and more sustained levels of IL-4. However, the effects of this IL-4 polymorphism on disease progression are inconsistent in different studies.

Other Genes

Additional genes such as those involved in innate immunity, lipid metabolism, and cell cycle have also been found to be associated with altered HIV/AIDS susceptibility. For example, a histidine-arginine change at position 186 in the gene that encodes APOBEC3G is found at a higher frequency in individuals of African descent and is associated with more rapid disease progression rates. Homozygosity for the vitamin D receptor form B correlates with rapid progression to AIDS. The mechanism is thought to relate to the known effects of vitamin D on immune modulation.

The effects of some genes [e.g., *CX3CR1*, *CXCL12 (SDF-1)*, *IL-4*, *IL-6*, *TNF-α*, and *MBL2*] on HIV pathogenesis are either from a single cohort or the findings are inconsistent in different cohorts. Nevertheless, there is growing appreciation that the evolutionary histories of human populations have had a significant impact on the distribution of variation of some genes that are thought to play a key role in HIV-1/AIDS pathogenesis, and that this might be responsible, in part, for the heterogeneous nature of the epidemiology of the HIV-1 pandemic.

NEUROPATHOGENESIS

Although there has been a remarkable decrease in the incidence of HIV encephalopathy among those with access to treatment in the era of effective ARV therapy, HIV-infected individuals can still experience a variety of neurologic abnormalities due either to opportunistic infections and neoplasms or to direct effects of HIV or its products (see below). With regard to the latter, HIV has been demonstrated in the brain and CSF of infected individuals with and without neuropsychiatric abnormalities. The main cell types that are infected in the brain in vivo are the perivascular macrophages and the microglial cells; monocytes that have already been infected in the blood can migrate into the brain, where they then reside as macrophages, or macrophages can be directly infected within the brain. The precise mechanisms whereby HIV enters the brain are unclear; however, they are thought to relate, at least in part, to the ability of virus-infected and immune-activated macrophages to induce adhesion molecules such as E-selectin and vascular cell adhesion molecule-1 (VCAM-1) on brain endothelium. Other studies have demonstrated that HIV gp120 enhances the expression of intercellular adhesion molecule-1 (ICAM-1) in glial cells; this effect may facilitate entry of HIV-infected cells into the CNS and may promote syncytia formation. Virus isolates from the brain are preferentially R5 strains as opposed to X4 strains (see above); in this regard, HIV-infected individuals who are heterozygous for *CCR5-Δ32* appear to be relatively protected against the development of HIV encephalopathy compared with wild-type individuals. Distinct HIV envelope sequences are associated with the clinical expression of the AIDS dementia complex (see below). There is no convincing evidence that brain cells other than those of monocyte/macrophage lineage can be productively infected in vivo. Astrocytes have been reported to be susceptible to HIV infection in vitro despite the fact that they do not express detectable levels of cell-surface CD4 or the main HIV co-receptors. Nonetheless, they do not support active virus replication. There is no convincing evidence that oligodendrocytes or neurons can be infected with HIV (see below).

HIV-infected individuals may manifest white matter lesions as well as neuronal loss. Given the absence of evidence of HIV infection of neurons either in vivo or in vitro, it is highly unlikely that direct infection of these cells accounts for their loss. Rather, the HIV-mediated effects on neurons and oligodendrocytes are thought to involve indirect pathways whereby viral proteins, particularly gp120 and Tat, trigger the release of endogenous neurotoxins from macrophages and to a lesser extent from astrocytes. In addition, it has been demonstrated that both HIV-1 Nef and Tat can induce chemotaxis of leukocytes, including monocytes, into the CNS. Neurotoxins can be released from monocytes as a consequence of infection and/or immune activation. Monocyte-derived neurotoxic factors have been reported to kill neurons via the *N*-methyl-D-aspartate (NMDA) receptor. In addition, HIV gp120 shed by virus-infected monocytes could cause neurotoxicity by antagonizing the function of vasoactive intestinal peptide (VIP), by elevating intracellular calcium levels, and by decreasing nerve growth factor levels in the cerebral cortex. A variety of monocyte-derived cytokines can contribute directly or indirectly to the neurotoxic effects in HIV infection; these include TNF-α, IL-1, IL-6, TGF-β, IFN-γ, platelet-activating factor, and endothelin. Furthermore, among the CC-chemokines, elevated levels of monocyte chemotactic protein (MCP)1 in the brain and CSF have been shown to correlate best with the presence and degree of HIV encephalopathy. In addition, infection and/or activation of monocyte-lineage cells can result in increased production of eicosanoids, nitric oxide, and quinolinic acid, which may contribute to neurotoxicity. Astrocytes may play diverse roles in HIV neuropathogenesis. Reactive gliosis or astrocytosis has been demonstrated in the brains of HIV-infected individuals, and TNF-α and IL-6 have been shown to induce astrocyte proliferation. In addition, astrocyte-derived IL-6 can induce HIV expression in infected cells in vitro. Furthermore, it has been suggested that astrocytes may downregulate macrophage-produced neurotoxins. It has been reported that HIV-infected individuals with the E4 allele for apolipoprotein E (apo E) are at increased risk for AIDS encephalopathy and peripheral neuropathy. The likelihood that HIV or its products are involved in neuropathogenesis is supported by the observation that neuropsychiatric abnormalities may undergo remarkable and rapid improvement upon the initiation of ARV therapy.

It has also been suggested that the CNS may serve as a relatively sequestered site for a reservoir of latently infected cells and for the slow, continual replication of HIV that might be a barrier for the eradication of virus by ARV therapy (see "Reservoirs of HIV-Infected Cells: Obstacle to the Eradication of Virus" earlier in the chapter).

PATHOGENESIS OF KAPOSI'S SARCOMA

There are at least four distinct epidemiologic forms of KS: (1) the classic form that occurs in older men of predominantly Mediterranean or eastern European Jewish backgrounds with no recognized contributing factors; (2) the equatorial African form that occurs in all ages, also without any recognized precipitating factors; (3) the form associated with organ transplantation and its attendant iatrogenic immunosuppressed state; and (4) the form associated with HIV-1 infection. In the latter two forms, KS is an opportunistic disease; in HIV-infected individuals, unlike typical opportunistic infections, its occurrence is not strictly related to the level of depression of CD4+ T-cell counts (see below). The pathogenesis of KS is complex; fundamentally, it is an angioproliferative disease that is not a true neoplastic sarcoma, at least not in its early stages. It is a manifestation of excessive proliferation of spindle cells that are believed to be of vascular origin and have features in common with endothelial and smooth-muscle cells. In HIV disease, the development of KS is dependent on the interplay of a variety of factors including HIV-1 itself, human herpes virus 8 (HHV-8), immune activation, and cytokine secretion. A number of epidemiologic and virologic studies have clearly linked HHV-8, which is also referred to as *Kaposi's sarcoma–associated herpesvirus* (KSHV), to KS not only in HIV-infected individuals, but also in individuals with the other forms of KS. HHV-8 is a γ-herpesvirus related to EBV and herpesvirus saimiri. It encodes a homologue to human IL-6 and in addition to KS has been implicated in the pathogenesis of body cavity lymphoma, multiple myeloma, and monoclonal gammopathy of undetermined significance. Sequences of HHV-8 are found universally in the lesions of KS, and patients with KS are virtually all seropositive for HHV-8. HHV-8 DNA sequences can be found in the B cells of 30–50% of patients with KS and 7% of patients with AIDS without clinically apparent KS.

Between 1 and 2% of eligible blood donors are positive for antibodies to HHV-8, whereas the prevalence of HHV-8 seropositivity in HIV-infected men is 30–35%. The prevalence in HIV-infected women is ~4%. This finding is reflective of the lower incidence of KS in women. It has been debated whether HHV-8 is actually the transforming agent in KS; the bulk of the cells in the tumor lesions of KS are not neoplastic cells. However, it has been demonstrated that endothelial cells can be transformed in vitro by HHV-8. In this regard, HHV-8 possesses a number of genes including homologues of the IL-8 receptor, Bcl-2, and cyclin D, which can potentially transform the host cell. Despite the complexity of the pathogenic events associated with the development of KS in HIV-infected individuals, HHV-8 is the etiologic agent of this disease. The initiation and/or propagation of KS requires an activated state and is mediated, at least in part, by cytokines. A number of factors, including TNF-α, IL-1β, IL-6, GM-CSF, basic fibroblast growth factor, and oncostatin M, function in an autocrine and paracrine manner to sustain the growth and chemotaxis of the KS spindle cells. In this regard, KSHV-derived IL-6 has been demonstrated to induce proliferation of lymphoma cells and to inhibit the cytostatic effects of INF-α on KSHV-infected lymphoma cells.

IMMUNE RESPONSE TO HIV

As detailed above and below, after the initial burst of viremia during primary infection, HIV-infected individuals mount robust immune responses that in most cases substantially curtail the levels of plasma viremia and likely contribute to delaying the ultimate development of clinically apparent disease for a median of 10 years in untreated individuals. This immune response contains elements of both humoral and cell-mediated immunity involving both innate and adaptive immune responses

TABLE 90-5

ELEMENTS OF THE IMMUNE RESPONSE TO HIV
Humoral immunity
Binding antibodies
Neutralizing antibodies
Type specific
Group specific
Antibodies participating in antibody-dependent cellular cytotoxicity (ADCC)
Protective
Pathogenic (bystander killing)
Enhancing antibodies
Complement
Cell-mediated immunity
Helper CD4+ T lymphocytes
Class I MHC–restricted cytotoxic CD8+ T lymphocytes
CD8+ T-cell–mediated inhibition (noncytolytic)
ADCC
Natural killer cells

(Table 90-5; Fig. 90-24). It is directed against multiple antigenic determinants of the HIV virion as well as against viral proteins expressed on the surface of infected cells. Ironically, those CD4+ T cells with T-cell receptors specific for HIV are theoretically those CD4+ T cells most likely to be activated and thus to serve as early targets for productive HIV infection and the cell death or dysfunction associated with infection. Thus an early consequence of HIV infection is interference with and decrease of the helper cell population needed to generate an effective immune response.

Although a great deal of investigation has been directed toward delineating and better understanding the components of this immune response, it remains unclear which immunologic effector mechanisms are most important in delaying progression of infection and which, if any, play a role in the pathogenesis of HIV disease. This lack of knowledge has also hampered the ability to develop an effective vaccine for HIV disease.

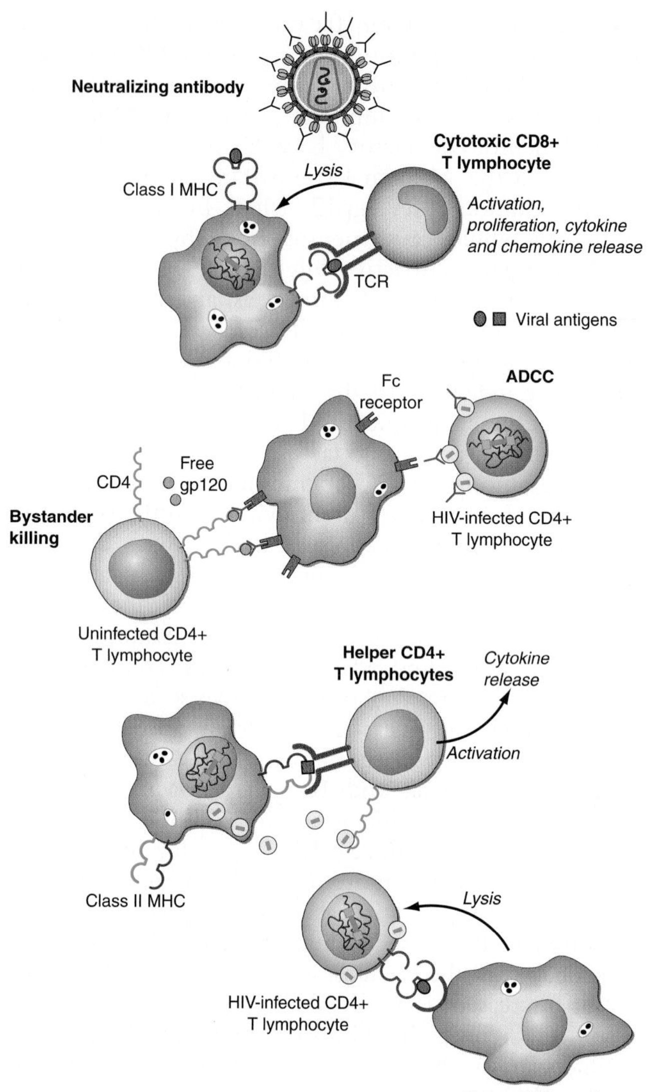

FIGURE 90-24

Schematic representation of the different immunologic effector mechanisms thought to be active in the setting of HIV infection. Detailed descriptions are given in the text. TCR, T-cell receptor; ADCC, antibody-dependent cellular cytotoxicity; MHC, major histocompatibility complex.

HUMORAL IMMUNE RESPONSE

Antibodies to HIV usually appear within 6 weeks and almost invariably within 12 weeks of primary infection (Fig. 90-25); rare exceptions are individuals who have defects in the ability to produce HIV-specific antibodies. Detection of these antibodies forms the basis of most diagnostic screening tests for HIV infection. The appearance of HIV-binding antibodies detected by ELISA and Western blot assays occurs before the appearance of neutralizing antibodies; the latter generally appear after the initial decreases in plasma viremia, which is more closely related to the appearance of HIV-specific CD8+ T lymphocytes. The first antibodies detected are those directed against the structural or gag proteins of HIV, p24 and p17, and the gag precursor p55. The development of antibodies to p24 is associated with a decrease in the serum levels of free p24 antigen. Antibodies to the gag proteins are followed by the appearance of antibodies to the envelope proteins (gp160, gp120, p88, and gp41) and to the products of the *pol* gene (p31, p51, and p66). In addition, one may see antibodies to the low-molecular-weight regulatory proteins encoded by the HIV genes *vpr*, *vpu*, *vif*, *rev*, *tat*, and *nef*. On rare occasion, levels of HIV-specific antibodies may decline during treatment of acute HIV infection.

Although antibodies to multiple antigens of HIV are produced, the precise functional significance of these different antibodies is unclear. The only viral proteins that elicit neutralizing antibodies are the envelope proteins gp120 and gp41. As noted above, the envelope of HIV consists of an outer envelope glycoprotein with a molecular mass of 120 kDa and a transmembrane glycoprotein with a molecular mass of 41 kDa. These are initially synthesized as a 160-kDa precursor that is cleaved by cellular proteases. Most of the antienvelope antibodies are directed either toward an epitope in the gp41 region

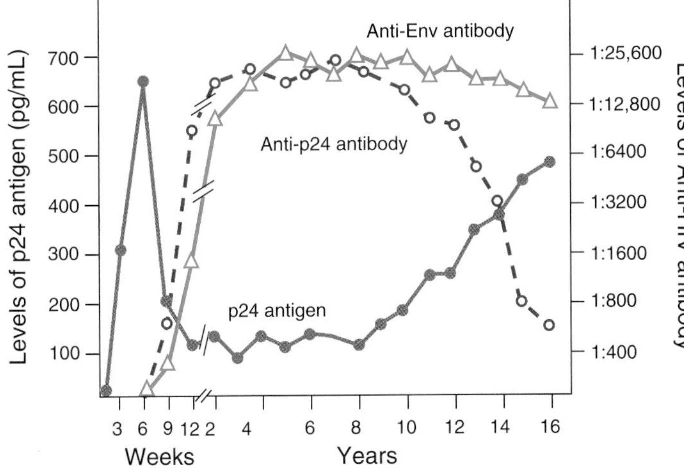

FIGURE 90-25

Relationship between antigenemia and the development of antibodies to HIV. Antibodies to HIV proteins are generally seen 6–12 weeks after infection and 3–6 weeks after the development of plasma viremia. Late in the course of illness, antibody levels to p24 decline, generally in association with a rising titer of p24 antigen.

comprising amino acids 579–613 or toward a hypervariable region in the gp120 molecule, known as the *V3 loop region*, comprising amino acids 303–338. This V3 region is a major site for the development of mutations that lead to variants of HIV that are not well recognized by the immune system.

Antibodies directed toward the envelope proteins of HIV have been characterized both as being protective and as possibly contributing to the pathogenesis of HIV disease. Among the protective antibodies are those that function to neutralize HIV directly and prevent the spread of infection to additional cells, as well as those that participate in ADCC. Within the first 6 months of infection neutralizing antibodies appear; however, the virus quickly escapes these neutralizing antibodies. One of the principal mechanisms of immune escape is the addition of N-linked glycosylation sites. The added carbohydrate moieties interfere with envelope recognition by these initial antibodies. The hyperglycosylation of the envelope protein has been termed the *glycan shield*. Neutralizing antibodies appear to be of two forms, type-specific and group-specific. *Type-specific neutralizing antibodies* are generally directed to the V3 loop region. These antibodies neutralize only viruses of a given strain and are present in low titer in most infected individuals. *Group-specific neutralizing antibodies* are capable of neutralizing a wide variety of HIV isolates. At least two forms of group-specific antibodies have been identified: those binding to amino acids 423–437 of gp120, which lie close to the CD4 binding site, and those binding to amino acids 728–745 of gp41, which lie proximal to the viral membrane. The other major class of protective antibodies are those that participate in ADCC, which is actually a form of cell-mediated immunity in which NK cells that bear Fc receptors are armed with specific anti-HIV antibodies that bind to the NK cells via their Fc portion. These armed NK cells then bind to and destroy cells expressing HIV antigens. Antibodies to both gp120 and gp41 have been shown to participate in ADCC-mediated killing of HIV-infected cells. The levels of antienvelope antibodies capable of mediating ADCC are highest in the earlier stages of HIV infection. In vitro, IL-2 can augment ADCC-mediated killing.

In addition to playing a role in host defense, HIV-specific antibodies have also been implicated in disease pathogenesis. Antibodies directed to gp41, when present in low titer, have been shown in vitro to be capable of facilitating infection of cells through an Fc receptor–mediated mechanism known as *antibody enhancement*. Thus the same regions of the envelope protein of HIV that give rise to antibodies capable of mediating ADCC also elicit the production of antibodies that can facilitate infection of cells in vitro. In addition, it has been postulated that anti-gp120 antibodies that participate in the ADCC killing of HIV-infected cells might also kill uninfected CD4+ T cells if the uninfected cells had bound free gp120, a phenomenon referred to as *bystander killing*. One of the most primitive components of the humoral immune system is the complement system. This element of innate immunity consists of ~30 proteins that are found circulating in blood or associated with cell membranes. Although HIV alone is capable of directly activating the complement cascade, the resulting lysis is weak due to the presence of host cell regulatory proteins captured in the virion envelope during budding. It is possible that complement-opsonized HIV virions have increased infectivity in a manner analogous to antibody-mediated enhancement.

CELLULAR IMMUNE RESPONSE

Given the fact that T-cell–mediated immunity is known to play a major role in host defense against most viral infections, it is generally thought to be an important component of the host immune response to HIV. T-cell immunity can be divided into two major categories, mediated respectively by the *helper/inducer CD4+ T cells* and the *cytotoxic/immunoregulatory CD8+ T cells*.

HIV-specific CD4+ T cells can be detected in the majority of HIV-infected patients through the use of flow cytometry to measure intracellular cytokine production in response to MHC class II tetramers pulsed with HIV peptides or through lymphocyte proliferation assays utilizing HIV antigens such as p24. HIV-specific CD4+ T cells may be preferential targets of HIV infection by HIV-infected antigen-presenting cells during the generation of an immune response to HIV (see above). However, they also are likely to undergo clonal expansions in response to HIV antigens and thus survive as a population of cells. No clear correlations exist between levels of HIV-specific CD4+ T lymphocytes and plasma HIV RNA levels; however, in the setting of high viral loads, CD4+ T-cell responses to HIV antigens appear to shift from one of proliferation and IL-2 production to one of IFN-γ production. Thus, although a reverse correlation exists between the level of p24-specific proliferation and levels of plasma HIV viremia, the nature of the causal relationship between these parameters is unclear.

MHC class I–restricted, HIV-specific CD8+ T cells have been identified in the peripheral blood of patients with HIV-1 infection. These cells include CTLs that produce perforins and T cells that can be induced by HIV antigens to express an array of cytokines such as IFN-γ. CTLs have been identified in the peripheral blood of patients within weeks of HIV infection. These CD8+ T lymphocytes, through their HIV-specific antigen receptors, bind to and cause the lytic destruction of target cells bearing autologous MHC class I molecules associated with HIV antigens. Two types of CTL activity can be demonstrated in the peripheral blood or lymph node mononuclear cells of HIV-infected individuals. The first type directly lyses appropriate target cells in culture without before vitro stimulation (*spontaneous CTL activity*). The other type of CTL activity reflects the *precursor frequency of CTLs* (CTLp); this type of CTL activity can be demonstrated by stimulation of CD8+ T cells in vitro with a mitogen such as phytohemagglutinin or anti-CD3 antibody.

In addition to CTLs, CD8+ T cells capable of being induced by HIV antigens to express cytokines such as IFN-γ also appear in the setting of HIV-1 infection. It is not clear whether these are the same or different effector pools compared with those cells mediating cytotoxicity; in addition, the relative roles of each in host defense against HIV are not fully understood. It does appear that these CD8+ T cells are driven to in vivo expansion by HIV antigen. There is a direct correlation between levels of CD8+ T cells capable of producing IFN-γ in response to HIV antigens and plasma levels of HIV-1 RNA. Thus, although these cells are clearly induced by HIV-1 infection, their overall ability to control infection remains unclear. Multiple HIV antigens, including Gag, Env, Pol, Tat, Rev, and Nef, can elicit CD8+ T-cell responses. Among patients who control viral replication in the absence of ARV drugs are a subset of patients whose peripheral blood contains a population of CD8+ T cells that undergo substantial proliferation and perforin expression in response to HIV antigens. It is possible that these cells play an important role in HIV-specific host defense.

At least three other forms of cell-mediated immunity to HIV have been described: CD8+ T-cell–mediated suppression of HIV replication, ADCC, and NK cell activity. *CD8+ T-cell–mediated suppression of HIV replication* refers to the ability of CD8+ T cells from an HIV-infected patient to inhibit the replication of HIV in tissue culture in a noncytolytic manner. There is no requirement for HLA compatibility between the CD8+ T cells and the HIV-infected cells. This effector mechanism is thus nonspecific and appears to be mediated by soluble factor(s) including the CC-chemokines RANTES (CCL5), MIP-1α (CCL3), and MIP-1β (CCL4) (see above). These CC-chemokines are potent suppressors of HIV replication and operate at least in part via blockade of the HIV co-receptor (*CCR5*) for R5 (macrophage-tropic) strains of HIV-1 (see above). *ADCC*, as described above in relation to humoral immunity, involves the killing of HIV-expressing cells by NK cells armed with specific antibodies directed against HIV antigens. Finally, *NK cells* alone have been shown to be capable of killing HIV-infected target cells in tissue culture. This primitive cytotoxic mechanism of host defense is directed toward nonspecific surveillance for neoplastic transformation and viral infection through recognition of altered class I MHC molecules.

DIAGNOSIS AND LABORATORY MONITORING OF HIV INFECTION

The establishment of HIV as the causative agent of AIDS and related syndromes early in 1984 was followed by the rapid development of sensitive screening tests for HIV infection. By March 1985, blood donors in the United States were routinely screened for antibodies to HIV. In June 1996, blood banks in the United States added the p24 antigen capture assay to the screening process to help identify the rare infected individuals who were donating blood in the time (up to 3 months) between infection and the development of antibodies. In 2002 the ability to detect early infection with HIV was further enhanced by the licensure of nucleic acid testing (NAT) as a routine part of blood donor screening. These refinements decreased the interval between infection and detection (window period) from 22 days for antibody testing to 16 days with p24 antigen testing and subsequently to 12 days with nucleic acid testing. The development of sensitive assays for monitoring levels of plasma viremia ushered in a new era of being able to monitor the progression of HIV disease more closely. Utilization of these tests, coupled with the measurement of levels of CD4+ T lymphocytes in peripheral blood, is essential in the management of patients with HIV infection.

DIAGNOSIS OF HIV INFECTION

The CDC has recommended that screening for HIV infection be performed as a matter of routine health care. The diagnosis of HIV infection depends upon the demonstration of antibodies to HIV and/or the direct detection of HIV or one of its components. As noted above, antibodies to HIV generally appear in the circulation 2–12 weeks after infection.

The standard blood screening test for HIV infection is the ELISA, also referred to as an *enzyme immunoassay* (EIA). This solid-phase assay is an extremely good screening test with a sensitivity of >99.5%. Most diagnostic laboratories use a commercial EIA kit that contains antigens from both HIV-1 and HIV-2 and thus are able to detect either. These kits use both natural and recombinant antigens and are continuously updated to increase their sensitivity to newly discovered species, such as group O viruses (Fig. 90-6). The fourth generation EIA tests combine detection of antibodies to HIV with detection of the p24 antigen of HIV. EIA tests are generally scored as positive (highly reactive), negative (nonreactive), or indeterminate (partially reactive). Although the EIA is an extremely sensitive test, it is not optimal with regard to specificity. This is particularly true in studies of low-risk individuals, such as volunteer blood donors. In this latter population, only 10% of EIA-positive individuals are subsequently confirmed to have HIV infection. Among the factors associated with false-positive EIA tests are antibodies to class II antigens, autoantibodies, hepatic disease, recent influenza vaccination, and acute viral infections. For these reasons, anyone suspected of having HIV infection based upon a positive or inconclusive EIA result must have the result confirmed with a more specific assay such as the Western blot. One can estimate whether or not an individual has a recent infection with HIV-1 by comparing the results on a standard assay that will score positive for all infected individuals to the results on an assay modified to be less sensitive ("detuned assay") that will score positive only for individuals with established HIV infection. In rare instances, an HIV-infected individual treated early in the course of infection may revert to a negative EIA. This does *not* indicate clearing of infection; rather, it signifies levels of ongoing exposure to virus insufficient to maintain a measurable antibody response. When these individuals have discontinued therapy, viruses and antibodies have reappeared.

The most commonly used confirmatory test is the Western blot (Fig. 90-26). This assay takes advantage of the fact that multiple HIV antigens of different, well-characterized molecular weights elicit the production of specific antibodies. These antigens can be separated on the basis of molecular weight, and antibodies to each component can be detected as discrete bands on the Western blot. A negative Western blot is one in which no bands are present at molecular weights corresponding to HIV gene products. In a patient with a positive or indeterminate EIA and a negative Western blot, one can conclude with certainty that the EIA reactivity was a false positive. On the other hand, a Western blot demonstrating antibodies to products of all three of the major genes of HIV (*gag*, *pol*, and *env*) is conclusive evidence of infection with HIV. Criteria established by the U.S. Food & Drug Administration (FDA) in 1993 for a positive Western blot state that a result is considered positive if antibodies exist to two of the three HIV proteins: p24, gp41, and gp120/160. Using these criteria, ~10% of all blood donors deemed positive for HIV-1 infection

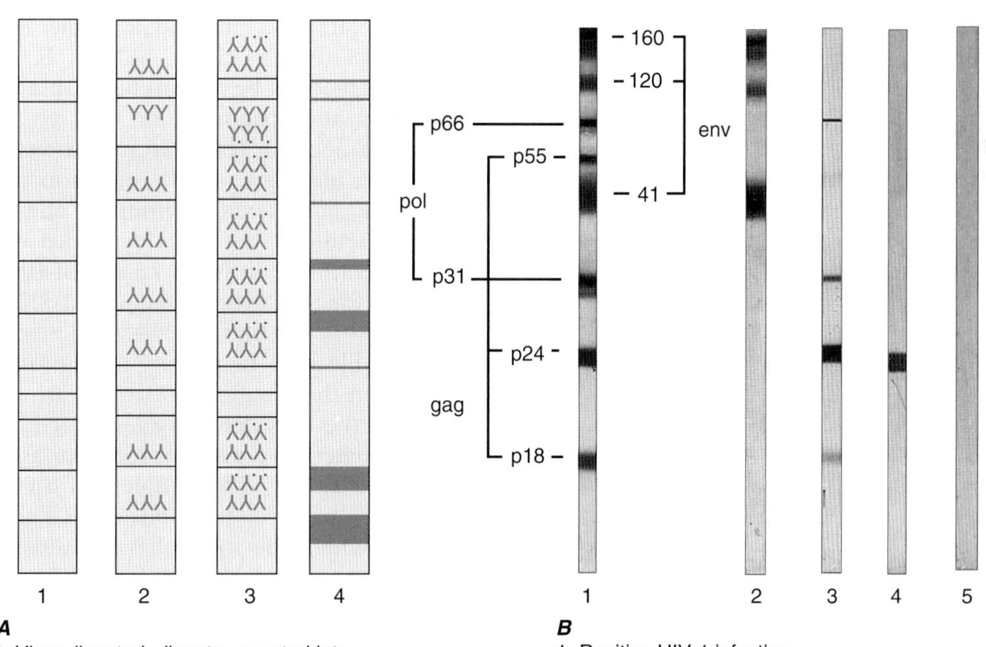

FIGURE 90-26

Western blot assay for detection of antibodies to HIV. ***A.*** Schematic representation of how a Western blot is performed. ***B.*** Examples of patterns of Western blot reactivity. In each instance, the Western blot strip contains antigens to HIV-1. The serum from the patient immunized to the HIV-1 envelope contains only antibodies to the HIV-1 envelope proteins. The serum from the patient with HIV-2 infection cross-reacts with both *reverse transcriptase* and *gag* gene products of HIV-1.

lacked an antibody band to the *pol* gene product p31. Some 50% of these blood donors were subsequently found to be false positives. Thus the absence of the p31 band should increase the suspicion that one may be dealing with a false-positive test result. In this setting it is prudent to obtain additional confirmation with an RNA-based test and/or a follow-up Western blot. By definition, Western blot patterns of reactivity that do not fall into the positive or negative categories are considered "indeterminate." There are two possible explanations for an indeterminate Western blot result. The most likely explanation in a low-risk individual is that the patient being tested has antibodies that cross-react with one of the proteins of HIV. The most common patterns of cross-reactivity are antibodies that react with p24 and/or p55. The least likely explanation in this setting is that the individual is infected with HIV and is in the process of mounting a classic antibody response. In either instance, the Western blot should be repeated in 1 month to determine whether or not the indeterminate pattern is a pattern in evolution. In addition, one may attempt to confirm a diagnosis of HIV infection with the p24 antigen capture assay or one of the tests for HIV RNA (discussed below). Although the Western blot is an excellent confirmatory test for HIV infection in patients with a positive or indeterminate EIA, it is a poor screening test. Among individuals with a negative EIA and PCR for HIV, 20–30% may show one or more bands on Western blot. Although these bands are usually faint and represent cross-reactivity, their presence creates a situation in which other diagnostic modalities (such as DNA PCR, RNA PCR, the bDNA assay, or p24 antigen capture) must be employed to ensure that the bands do not indicate early HIV infection.

A guideline for the use of these serologic tests in attempting to make a diagnosis of HIV infection is depicted in Fig. 90-27. In patients in whom HIV infection is suspected, the appropriate initial test is the EIA. If the result is negative, unless there is strong reason to suspect early HIV infection (as in a patient exposed within the previous 3 months), the diagnosis is ruled out and retesting should be performed only as clinically indicated. If the EIA is indeterminate or positive, the test should be repeated. If the repeat is negative on two occasions, one can assume that the initial positive reading was due to a technical error in the performance of the assay and that the patient is negative. If the repeat is indeterminate or positive, one should proceed to the HIV-1 Western blot. If the Western blot is positive, the diagnosis is HIV-1 infection. If the Western blot is negative, the EIA can be assumed to have been a false positive for HIV-1 and the diagnosis of HIV-1 infection is ruled out. It would be prudent at this point to perform specific serologic testing for HIV-2 following the same type of algorithm. If the Western blot for HIV-1 is indeterminate, it should be repeated in 4–6 weeks; in addition, one may proceed to a p24 antigen capture assay, HIV-1 RNA assay, or HIV-1 DNA PCR and specific serologic testing for HIV-2. If the p24 and HIV RNA assays are negative and there is no progression in the Western blot, a diagnosis of HIV-1 is ruled out. If either the p24 or HIV-1 RNA assay is positive and/or the HIV-1 Western blot shows progression, a tentative diagnosis of HIV-1 infection can be made and later confirmed with a follow-up Western blot demonstrating a positive pattern. In addition to these standard laboratory-based assays for detecting antibodies to HIV, a series of point-of-care tests are also available. Among the most popular of these is the OraQuick Rapid HIV-1 antibody test that can be run on blood, plasma, or saliva. The sensitivity and specificity of this test are each ~99%. Although negative results from this test are adequate to rule out a diagnosis of HIV infection, a positive finding should be considered preliminary and confirmed with standard serologic testing, as described above.

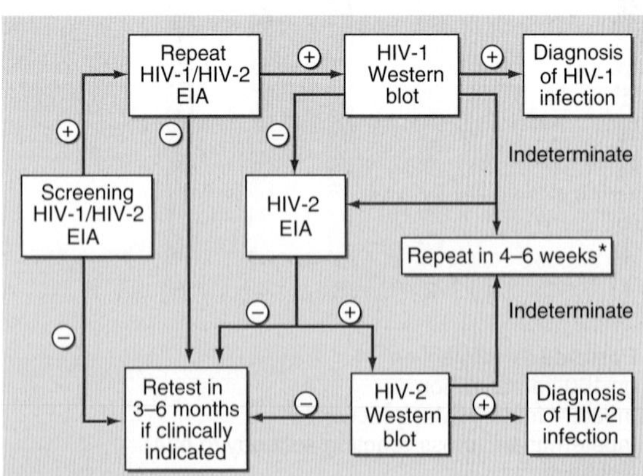

FIGURE 90-27

Algorithm for the use of serologic tests in the diagnosis of HIV-1 or HIV-2 infection. *Stable indeterminate Western blot 4–6 weeks later makes HIV infection unlikely. However, it should be repeated twice at 3-month intervals to rule out HIV infection. Alternatively, one may test for HIV-1 p24 antigen or HIV RNA. EIA, enzyme immunoassay.

As mentioned above, a variety of laboratory tests are available for the direct detection of HIV or its components (Table 90-6; Fig. 90-28). These tests may be of considerable help in making a diagnosis of HIV infection when the Western blot results are indeterminate. In addition, the tests detecting levels of HIV RNA can be used to determine prognosis and to assess the response to ARV therapies. The simplest of the direct detection tests is the *p24 antigen capture assay*. This is an EIA-type assay in which the solid phase consists of antibodies to the p24 antigen of HIV. It detects the viral protein p24 in the blood of HIV-infected individuals where it exists either as free antigen or complexed to anti-p24 antibodies. Overall, ~30% of individuals with untreated HIV infection have detectable levels of free p24 antigen. This increases to ~50% when samples are treated with a weak acid to dissociate antigen-antibody complexes. Throughout the course of HIV infection, an equilibrium exists between p24 antigen and anti-p24 antibodies. During the first few weeks of infection, before an immune response develops, there is a brisk rise in p24 antigen levels (Fig. 90-25). After the development of anti-p24 antibodies, these levels decline. Late in the course of infection, when circulating levels of virus are high, p24

TABLE 90-6

CHARACTERISTICS OF TESTS FOR DIRECT DETECTION OF HIV

TEST	TECHNIQUE	SENSITIVITY[a]	COST/TEST[b]
Immune complex–dissociated p24 antigen capture assay	Measurement of levels of HIV-1 core protein in an EIA-based format following dissociation of antigen-antibody complexes by weak acid treatment	Positive in 50% of patients; detects down to 15 pg/mL of p24 protein	$1–2
HIV RNA by PCR	PCR amplification of cDNA generated from viral RNA (target amplification)	Reliable to 40 copies/mL of HIV RNA	$75–150
HIV RNA by bDNA	Measurement of levels of particle-associated HIV RNA in a nucleic acid capture assay employing signal amplification	Reliable to 50 copies/mL of HIV RNA	$75–150
HIV RNA by NucliSens	Isothermic nucleic acid amplification with internal controls	Reliable to 80 copies/mL of HIV RNA	$75–150

[a]Sensitivity figures refer to those approved by the U.S. FDA.
[b]Prices may be lower in large volume settings.
Note: EIA, enzyme immunoassay; PCR, polymerase chain reaction.

antigen levels also increase, particularly when detected by techniques involving dissociation of antigen-antibody complexes. The p24 antigen capture assay has its greatest use as a screening test for HIV infection in patients suspected of having the acute HIV syndrome, as high levels of p24 antigen are present before the development of antibodies. Its use for routine blood donor screening for HIV infection has been replaced by use of nucleic acid testing. The ability to measure and monitor levels of HIV RNA in the plasma of patients with HIV infection has been of extraordinary value in furthering our understanding of the pathogenesis of HIV infection and in providing a diagnostic tool in settings where measurements of anti-HIV antibodies may be misleading, such as in acute infection and neonatal infection. Three assays are predominantly used for this purpose. They are reverse transcriptase PCR (*RT-PCR*; Amplicor); branched DNA (*bDNA*; VERSANT); and nucleic acid sequence–based amplification (*NASBA*; NucliSens). These tests are of value in making a diagnosis of HIV infection, in establishing initial prognosis, in determining the need for therapy, and for monitoring the effects of therapy. In addition to these three commercially available tests, the *DNA PCR* is also employed by research laboratories for making a diagnosis of HIV infection by amplifying HIV proviral DNA from peripheral blood mononuclear cells. The commercially available RNA detection tests have a sensitivity of 40–80 copies of HIV RNA per milliliter of plasma. Research laboratory–based RNA assays can detect as few as one HIV RNA copy per milliliter, although the DNA PCR tests can detect proviral DNA at a frequency of one copy per

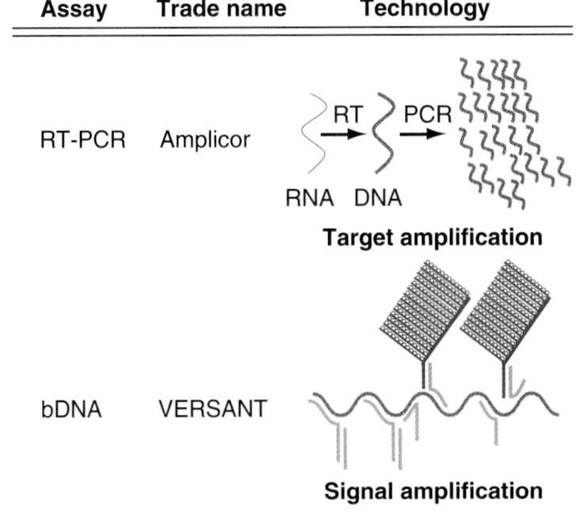

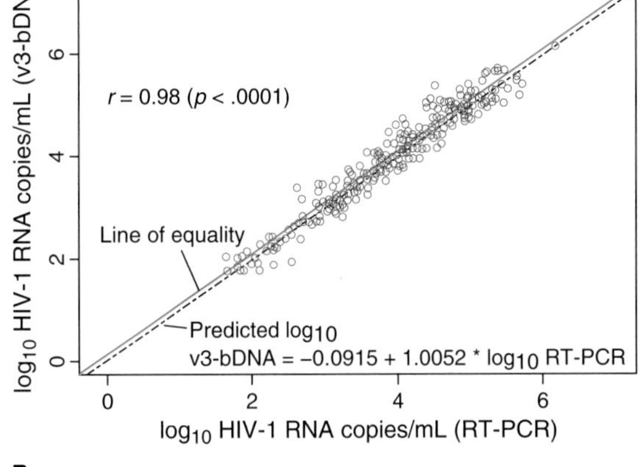

FIGURE 90-28

Comparison of RT-PCR and bDNA assays. *A.* Schematic representation of reverse transcriptase–polymerase chain reaction (RT-PCR) and bDNA assays. See text for detailed description. ***B.*** Scatter plot of $\log_{10}$ v3-bDNA versus $\log_{10}$ RT-PCR with the line of equity (solid) and the fitted regression line (hatched). The equation for the fitted regression line is given in the lower-right-hand corner. There is good agreement between the two assays. v3, version 3 of the bDNA assay. *(Adapted from HC Highbarger et al: J Clin Microbiol 37:3612, 1999.)*

10,000–100,000 cells. Thus these tests are extremely sensitive. One frequent consequence of a high degree of sensitivity is some loss of specificity, and false-positive results have been reported with each of these techniques. For this reason, a positive EIA with a confirmatory Western blot remains the "gold standard" for a diagnosis of HIV infection, and the interpretation of other test results must be done with this in mind.

In the RT-PCR technique, after DNase treatment, a cDNA copy is made of all RNA species present in plasma. Insofar as HIV is an RNA virus, this will result in the production of DNA copies of the HIV genome in amounts proportional to the amount of HIV RNA present in plasma. This cDNA is then amplified and characterized using standard PCR techniques, employing primer pairs that can distinguish genomic cDNA from messenger cDNA. The bDNA assay involves the use of a solid-phase nucleic acid capture system and signal amplification through successive nucleic acid hybridizations to detect small quantities of HIV RNA. Both tests can achieve a tenfold increase in sensitivity to 40–50 copies of HIV RNA per milliliter with a preconcentration step in which plasma undergoes ultracentrifugation to pellet the viral particles. The NASBA technique involves the isothermal amplification of a sequence within the gag region of HIV in the presence of internal standards and employs the production of multiple RNA copies through the action of T7-RNA polymerase. The resulting RNA species are quantitated through hybridization with a molecular beacon DNA probe that is quenched in the absence of hybridization. The lower limit of detection for the NucliSens assay is 80 copies/mL.

In addition to being a diagnostic and prognostic tool, RT-PCR is also useful for amplifying defined areas of the HIV genome for sequence analysis and has become an important technique for studies of sequence diversity and microbial resistance to ARV agents. In patients with a positive or indeterminate EIA test and an indeterminate Western blot, and in patients in whom serologic testing may be unreliable (such as patients with hypogammaglobulinemia or advanced HIV disease), these tests for quantitating HIV RNA in plasma provide valuable tools for making a diagnosis of HIV infection; however, they should be used for diagnosis only when standard serologic testing has failed to provide a definitive result.

LABORATORY MONITORING OF PATIENTS WITH HIV INFECTION

The epidemic of HIV infection and AIDS has provided the clinician with new challenges for integrating clinical and laboratory data to effect optimal patient management. The close relationship between clinical manifestations of HIV infection and CD4+ T-cell count has made measurement of the latter a routine part of the evaluation of HIV-infected individuals. Determinations of CD4+ T-cell counts and measurements of the levels of HIV RNA in serum or plasma provide a powerful set of tools for determining prognosis and monitoring response to therapy.

CD4+ T-Cell Counts

The CD4+ T-cell count is the laboratory test generally accepted as the best indicator of the immediate state of immunologic competence of the patient with HIV infection. This measurement, which can be made directly or calculated as the product of the percent of CD4+ T cells (determined by flow cytometry) and the total lymphocyte count [determined by the white blood cell count (WBC) and the differential percent], has been shown to correlate very well with the level of immunologic competence. Patients with CD4+ T-cell counts <200/μL are at high risk of disease from *P. jiroveci*, whereas patients with CD4+ T-cell counts <50/μL are at high risk of disease from CMV, mycobacteria of the *M. avium* complex (MAC), and/or *T. gondii* (Fig. 90-29). Patients with HIV infection should have CD4+ T-cell measurements performed at the time of diagnosis and every 3–6 months thereafter. More frequent measurements should be made if a declining trend is noted. According to most guidelines, a CD4 T-cell count <350/μL is an indication for consideration of initiating ARV therapy, and a decline in CD4+ T-cell count of >25% is an indication for considering a change in therapy. Once the CD4+ T-cell count is <200/μL, patients should be placed on a regimen for *P. jiroveci* prophylaxis, and once the count is <50/μL, primary prophylaxis for MAC infection is indicated. As with any laboratory measurement, one may wish to obtain two determinations before any significant changes in patient management based upon CD4+ T-cell count alone. In patients with hypersplenism or who have undergone splenectomy, the CD4+ T-cell percentage may be a more reliable indication of immune function than the CD4+ T-cell count. A CD4+ T-cell percent of 15 is comparable to a CD4+ T-cell count of 200/μL.

HIV RNA Determinations

Facilitated by highly sensitive techniques for the precise quantitation of small amounts of nucleic acids, the measurement of serum or plasma levels of HIV RNA has become an essential component in the monitoring of patients with HIV infection. As discussed under diagnosis of HIV infection, the two most commonly used techniques are the RT-PCR assay and the bDNA assay. Both assays generate data in the form of number of copies of HIV RNA per milliliter of serum or plasma. Standard assays can detect as few as 40–50 copies of HIV RNA per milliliter of plasma, whereas research-based assays can detect down to one copy per milliliter. Although earlier versions of the bDNA assay generated values that were ~50% of those of the RT-PCR assay, the more recent versions (version 3 or higher) provide numbers essentially identical to those of the RT-PCR test (Fig. 90-28). Although it is common practice to describe levels of HIV RNA below these cut-offs as "undetectable," this is a term that should be avoided, as it is imprecise and leaves the false impression that the level of virus is 0. By utilizing more sensitive, nested PCR techniques and by studying tissue levels of virus as well as plasma levels, HIV RNA can be detected in virtually every patient with HIV infection. Measurements of changes in

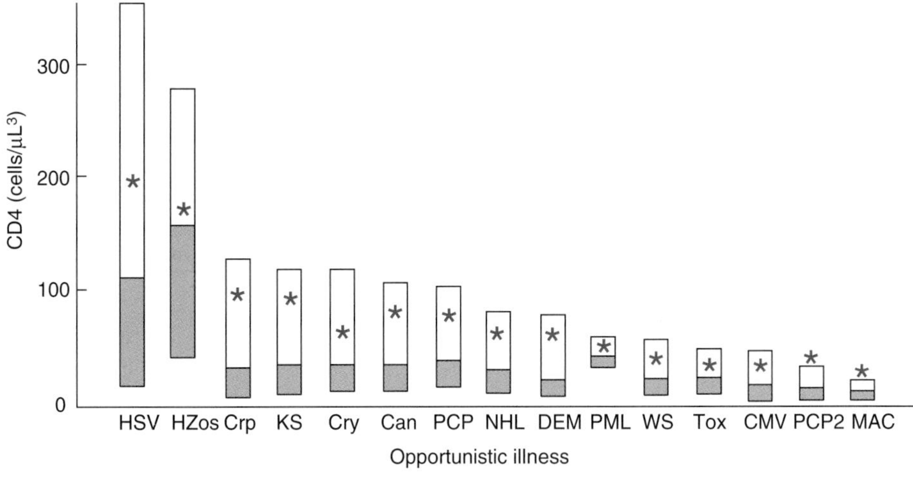

FIGURE 90-29

Relationship between CD4+ T-cell counts and the development of opportunistic diseases. Boxplot of the median (line inside the box), first quartile (bottom of the box), third quartile (top of the box), and mean (asterisk) CD4+ lymphocyte count at the time of the development of opportunistic disease. Can, candidal esophagitis; CMV, cytomegalovirus infection; Crp, cryptosporidiosis; Cry, cryptococcal meningitis; DEM, AIDS dementia complex; HSV, herpes simplex virus infection; HZos, herpes zoster; KS, Kaposi's sarcoma; MAC, *Mycobacterium avium* complex bacteremia; NHL, non-Hodgkin's lymphoma; PCP, primary *Pneumocystis jiroveci* pneumonia; PCP2, secondary *P. jiroveci* pneumonia; PML, progressive multifocal leukoencephalopathy; Tox, *Toxoplasma gondii* encephalitis; WS, wasting syndrome. *(From RD Moore, RE Chaisson: Ann Intern Med 124:633, 1996.)*

HIV RNA levels over time have been of great value in delineating the relationship between levels of virus and rates of disease progression (Fig. 90-20), the rates of viral turnover, the relationship between immune system activation and viral replication, and the time to development of drug resistance. HIV RNA measurements are greatly influenced by the state of activation of the immune system and may fluctuate greatly in the setting of secondary infections or immunization. For these reasons, decisions based upon HIV RNA levels should never be made on a single determination. Measurements of plasma HIV RNA levels should be made at the time of HIV diagnosis and every 3–6 months thereafter in the untreated patient. In general, most guidelines suggest that therapy be considered in patients with >100,000 copies of HIV RNA per milliliter (see below). After the initiation of therapy or any change in therapy, plasma HIV RNA levels should be monitored approximately every 4 weeks until the effectiveness of the therapeutic regimen is determined by the development of a new steady-state level of HIV RNA. In most instances of effective therapy this will be <50 copies per milliliter. This level of virus is generally achieved within 6 months of the initiation of effective treatment. During therapy, levels of HIV RNA should be monitored every 3–4 months to evaluate the continuing effectiveness of therapy.

HIV Resistance Testing

The availability of multiple ARV drugs as treatment options has generated a great deal of interest in the potential for measuring the sensitivity of an individual's HIV virus(es) to different ARV agents. HIV resistance testing can be done through either genotypic or phenotypic measurements. In the genotypic assays, sequence analyses of the HIV genomes obtained from patients are compared with sequences of viruses with known ARV resistance profiles. In the phenotypic assays, the in vivo growth of viral isolates obtained from the patient are compared with the growth of reference strains of the virus in the presence or absence of different ARV drugs. A modification of this phenotypic approach utilizes a comparison of the enzymatic activities of the reverse transcriptase or protease genes obtained by molecular cloning of patients' isolates to the enzymatic activities of genes obtained from reference strains of HIV in the presence or absence of different drugs targeted to these genes. These tests are quite good in identifying those ARV agents that have been utilized in the past and suggesting agents that may be of future value in a given patient. Drug resistance testing in the setting of virologic failure should be performed while the patient is still on the failing regimen because of the propensity for the pool of HIV quasispecies to rapidly revert to wild-type in the absence of the selective pressure of ARV therapy. In the hands of experts, resistance testing enhances the short-term ability to decrease viral load by ~0.5 log compared with changing drugs merely on the basis of drug history. In addition to the use of resistance testing to help in the selection of new drugs in patients with virologic failure, it may also be of value in selecting an initial regimen for treatment of therapy-naïve individuals. This is particularly true in geographic areas with a high level of background resistance.

Co-Receptor Tropism Assays

After the licensure of maraviroc as the first CCR5 antagonist for the treatment of HIV infection (see below), it became necessary to be able to determine whether or not a patient's virus was likely to respond to this treatment. Patients tend to have CCR5-tropic virus (see above) early in the course of infection, with a trend toward CXCR4 viruses later in disease. Maraviroc is only effective against CCR5-tropic viruses. Due to the fact that the genotypic determinants of cellular tropism are poorly defined, a phenotypic assay is necessary to determine this property of HIV. Two commercial assays; the Trofile assay (Monogram Biosciences) and the Phenoscript assay (VIRalliance), are available to make this determination. These assays clone the envelope regions of the patient's virus into an indicator virus that is then used to infect target cells expressing either CCR5 or CXCR4 as their co-receptor. These assays take weeks to perform and are expensive.

Other Tests

A variety of other laboratory tests have been studied as potential markers of HIV disease activity. Among these are quantitative culture of replication-competent HIV from plasma, peripheral blood mononuclear cells, or resting CD4+ T cells; circulating levels of β_2-microglobulin, soluble IL-2 receptor, IgA, acid-labile endogenous interferon, or TNF-α; and the presence or absence of activation markers such as CD38, HLA-DR, or PD-1 on CD8+ T cells. Although these measurements have value as markers of disease activity and help to increase our understanding of the pathogenesis of HIV disease, they do not currently play a major role in the monitoring of patients with HIV infection.

CLINICAL MANIFESTATIONS

The clinical consequences of HIV infection encompass a spectrum ranging from an acute syndrome associated with primary infection to a prolonged asymptomatic state to advanced disease. It is best to regard HIV disease as beginning at the time of primary infection and progressing through various stages. As mentioned above, active virus replication and progressive immunologic impairment occur throughout the course of HIV infection in most patients. With the exception of the rare true long-term nonprogressors (see above), HIV disease in untreated patients inexorably progresses even during the clinically latent stage. However, ARV therapy has had a major impact on blocking or slowing the progression of disease over extended periods of time in a substantial proportion of adequately treated patients (see below).

THE ACUTE HIV SYNDROME

It is estimated that 50–70% of individuals with HIV infection experience an acute clinical syndrome ~3–6 weeks after primary infection (Fig. 90-30). Varying degrees of clinical severity have been reported, and although it has been suggested that symptomatic seroconversion leading to the seeking of medical attention indicates an increased risk for an accelerated course of disease, there does not appear to be a correlation between the level of the initial burst of viremia in acute HIV infection and the subsequent course of disease. The typical clinical findings in the acute HIV syndrome are listed in Table 90-7; they occur along with a burst of plasma viremia. It has been reported that several symptoms of the acute HIV syndrome (fever, skin rash, pharyngitis, and myalgia) occur less frequently in those infected by injection drug use versus those infected by sexual contact. The syndrome is typical of an acute viral syndrome and has been likened to acute infectious mononucleosis. Symptoms usually persist for one to several weeks and gradually subside as an immune response to HIV develops and the levels of plasma viremia decrease. Opportunistic infections have been reported during this stage of infection, reflecting the immunodeficiency that results from reduced numbers of CD4+ T cells and likely also from the dysfunction of CD4+ T cells owing to viral protein and endogenous cytokine-induced perturbations of cells (see Table 90-3) associated with the extremely high levels of plasma viremia. A number of immunologic abnormalities accompany the acute HIV syndrome, including multiphasic perturbations of the numbers of circulating lymphocyte subsets. The number of total lymphocytes and T-cell

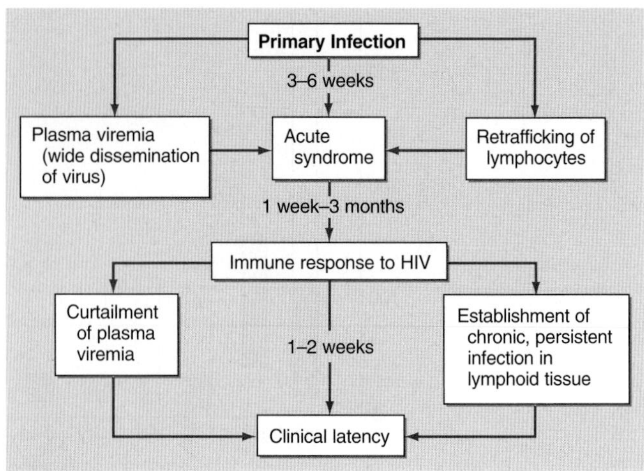

FIGURE 90-30

The acute HIV syndrome. See text for detailed description. *(Adapted from G Pantaleo et al: N Engl J Med 328:327, 1993. Copyright 1993 Massachusetts Medical Society. All rights reserved.)*

TABLE 90-7

CLINICAL FINDINGS IN THE ACUTE HIV SYNDROME

General	Neurologic
Fever	Meningitis
Pharyngitis	Encephalitis
Lymphadenopathy	Peripheral neuropathy
Headache/retroorbital pain	Myelopathy
Arthralgias/myalgias	Dermatologic
Lethargy/malaise	Erythematous maculopapular rash
Anorexia/weight loss	Mucocutaneous ulceration
Nausea/vomiting/diarrhea	

Source: From B Tindall, DA Cooper: AIDS 5:1, 1991.

subsets (CD4+ and CD8+) are initially reduced. An inversion of the CD4+/CD8+ T-cell ratio occurs later because of a rise in the number of CD8+ T cells. In fact, there may be a selective and transient expansion of CD8+ T-cell subsets, as determined by T-cell receptor analysis (see above). The total circulating CD8+ T-cell count may remain elevated or return to normal; however, CD4+ T-cell levels usually remain somewhat depressed, although there may be a slight rebound toward normal. Lymphadenopathy occurs in ~70% of individuals with primary HIV infection. Most patients recover spontaneously from this syndrome and many are left with only a mildly depressed CD4+ T-cell count that remains stable for a variable period before beginning its progressive decline (see below); in some individuals, the CD4+ T-cell count returns to the normal range. Approximately 10% of patients manifest a fulminant course of immunologic and clinical deterioration after primary infection, even after the disappearance of initial symptoms. In most patients, primary infection with or without the acute syndrome is followed by a prolonged period of clinical latency or smoldering low disease activity. A small percentage of HIV-infected individuals treated with ARV drugs during acute infection may revert to a negative EIA test during the time they remain on therapy. They rapidly re-seroconvert with the discontinuation of treatment.

THE ASYMPTOMATIC STAGE—CLINICAL LATENCY

Although the length of time from initial infection to the development of clinical disease varies greatly, the median time for untreated patients is ~10 years. As emphasized above, HIV disease with active virus replication is ongoing and progressive during this asymptomatic period. The rate of disease progression is directly correlated with HIV RNA levels. Patients with high levels of HIV RNA in plasma progress to symptomatic disease faster than do patients with low levels of HIV RNA (Fig. 90-20). Some patients referred to as *long-term nonprogressors* show little if any decline in CD4+ T-cell counts over extended periods of time. These patients generally have extremely low levels of HIV RNA, with a subset, referred to as *elite nonprogressors*, exhibiting HIV RNA levels <50 copies per milliliter. Certain other patients remain entirely asymptomatic despite the fact that their CD4+ T-cell counts show a steady progressive decline to extremely low levels. In these patients, the appearance of an opportunistic disease may be the first manifestation of HIV infection. During the asymptomatic period of HIV infection, the average rate of CD4+ T-cell decline is ~50/μL per year. When the CD4+ T-cell count falls to <200/μL, the resulting state of immunodeficiency is severe enough to place the patient at high risk for opportunistic infection and neoplasms and hence for clinically apparent disease.

SYMPTOMATIC DISEASE

Symptoms of HIV disease can appear at any time during the course of HIV infection. Generally speaking, the spectrum of illnesses that one observes changes as the CD4+ T-cell count declines. The more severe and life-threatening complications of HIV infection occur in patients with CD4+ T-cell counts <200/μL. A diagnosis of AIDS is made in anyone with HIV infection and a CD4+ T-cell count <200/μL and in anyone with HIV infection who develops one of the HIV-associated diseases considered to be indicative of a severe defect in cell-mediated immunity (category C, Table 90-2). Although the causative agents of the secondary infections are characteristically opportunistic organisms such as *P. jiroveci*, atypical mycobacteria, CMV, and other organisms that do not ordinarily cause disease in the absence of a compromised immune system, they also include common bacterial and mycobacterial pathogens. Fewer than 50% of deaths among AIDS patients are as a direct result of an AIDS-defining illness, and the average CD4+ T-cell count of an HIV-infected patient at the time of death is just over 300 cells/μL. Similarly, after the widespread use of combination ARV therapy and implementation of guidelines for the prevention of opportunistic infections (Table 90-8), the incidence of secondary infections has decreased dramatically (Fig. 90-31). Overall, the clinical

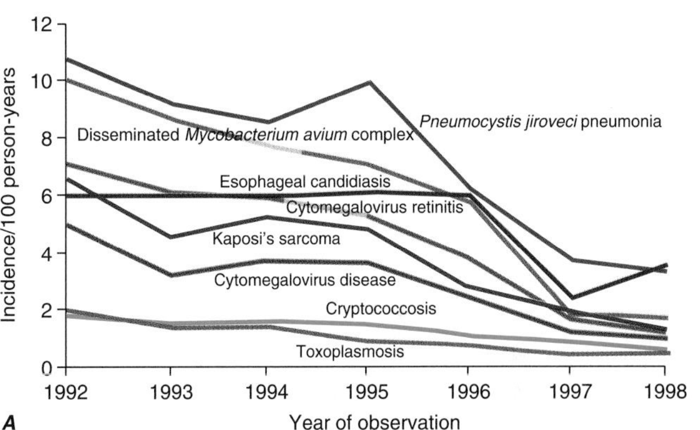

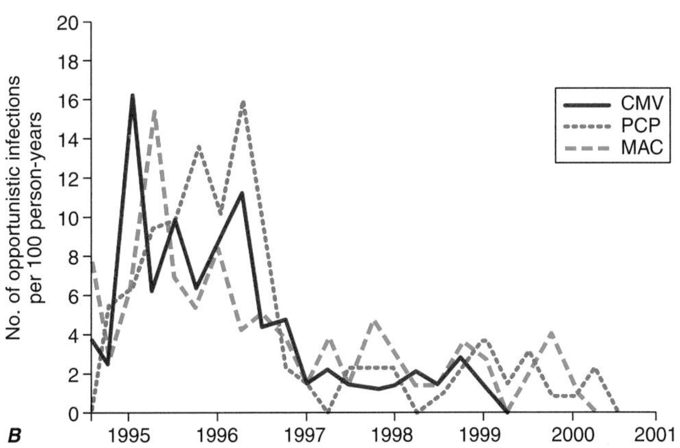

FIGURE 90-31

A. Decrease in the incidence of opportunistic infections and Kaposi's sarcoma in HIV-infected individuals with CD4+ *T-cell counts* <100/μL from 1992 through 1998. *[Adapted and updated from FJ Palella et al: N Engl J Med 338:853, 1998, and JE Kaplan et al: Clin Infect Dis 30(S1):S5, 2000, with permission.]* ***B.*** Quarterly incidence rates of cytomegalovirus (CMV), *Pneumocystis jiroveci* pneumonia (PCP), and *Mycobacterium avium* complex (MAC) from 1995–2001. *(From FJ Palella et al: AIDS 16:1617, 2002.)*

TABLE 90-8

NIH/CDC/IDSA 2008 GUIDELINES FOR THE PREVENTION OF OPPORTUNISTIC INFECTIONS IN PERSONS INFECTED WITH HIV

PATHOGEN	INDICATIONS	FIRST CHOICE(S)	ALTERNATIVES
Recommended as Standard of Care for Primary and Secondary Prophylaxis			
Pneumocystis jiroveci	CD4+ T-cell count <200/μL or Oropharyngeal candidiasis or Prior bout of PCP	Trimethoprim/sulfamethoxazole (TMP/SMZ), 1 DS tablet qd PO	Dapsone 50 mg bid PO or 100 mg/d PO Dapsone 50 mg/d PO + Pyrimethamine 50 mg/wk PO + Leucovorin 25 mg/wk PO
	May stop prophylaxis if CD4+ T-cell count >200/μL for ≥3 mo	TMP/SMZ, 1 SS tablet qd PO	Dapsone 200 mg PO + Pyrimethamine 75 mg PO + Leucovorin 25 mg PO weekly Aerosolized pentamidine, 300 mg qm via Respirgard II nebulizer Atovaquone 1500 mg/d PO TMP/SMZ 1 DS tablet PO 3×/wk
Mycobacterium tuberculosis			
Isoniazid sensitive	Skin test >5 mm or Prior positive test without treatment or Close contact with case of active pulmonary TB	Isoniazid 300 mg PO + Pyridoxine 50 mg PO qd ×9 mo Isoniazid 900 mg PO + Pyridoxine 100 mg PO 2 ×/wk ×9 mo	Isoniazid 900 mg PO + pyridoxine 50 mg PO 2×/wk × 9 mo Isoniazid 300 mg + rifampin 600 mg (or rifabutin 300 mg) + pyridoxine 50 mg/d ×4 mo
Isoniazid resistant	Same with high probability of exposure to isoniazid-resistant TB	Rifabutin 300 mg or Rifampin 600 mg PO qd ×4 mo	
Multidrug resistant	Same with high probability of exposure to multidrug resistant TB	Consult local public health authorities	
Mycobacterium-avium complex	CD4+ T-cell count <50/μL	Azithromycin 1200 mg weekly PO or Clarithromycin 500 mg bid PO	Rifabutin 300 mg/d PO Azithromycin 1200 mg weekly PO + Rifabutin 300 mg/d PO
	Prior documented disseminated disease	Clarithromycin 500 mg bid PO +	Azithromycin 500 mg/d PO +
	May stop prophylaxis if CD4+ T-cell count >100/μL for ≥3 mo	Ethambutol 15 (mg/kg)/d PO +/– Rifabutin 300 mg/d PO	Ethambutol 15 (mg/kg)/d PO +/– Rifabutin 300 mg/d PO
Toxoplasma gondii	TOXO IgG antibody and CD4+ T-cell count <100/μL	TMP/SMZ 1 DS tablet PO qd	TMP/SMZ 1 DS 3× weekly Dapsone 50 mg/d PO + Pyrimethamine 50 mg weekly PO + Leucovorin 25 mg weekly PO Dapsone 200 mg PO + Pyrimethamine 75 mg PO + Leucovorin 25 mg PO weekly Atovaquone 1500 mg PO +/– Pyrimethamine 25 mg PO + Leucovorin 10 mg PO daily
	Prior toxoplasmic encephalitis and CD4+ T-cell count <200	Sulfadiazine 500–1000 mg qid PO + pyrimethamine 25–50 mg/d PO + leucovorin 10–25 mg/d PO	Clindamycin 600 mg q8h PO + Pyrimethamine 25–50 mg/d PO + Leucovorin 10–25 mg/d PO
	May stop prophylaxis if CD4+ T-cell count >200/μL for ≥3 months		Atovaquone 750 mg PO q6–12 h +/– Pyrimethamine 25 mg/d + Leucovorin 10 mg/d PO
Varicella-zoster virus	Significant exposure to chickenpox or shingles in a patient with no history of immunization or prior exposure to either	Varicella zoster immune globulin 6.25 mL, IM, within 96 h of exposure	
Cryptococcus neoformans	Prior documented disease May stop prophylaxis if CD4+ T-cell count >200 for 6 mo and no evidence of active infection	Fluconazole 200 mg/d PO	Itraconazole 200 mg/d PO

(*Continued*)

TABLE 90-8 (*CONTINUED*)

NIH/CDC/IDSA 2008 GUIDELINES FOR THE PREVENTION OF OPPORTUNISTIC INFECTIONS IN PERSONS INFECTED WITH HIV

PATHOGEN	INDICATIONS	FIRST CHOICE(S)	ALTERNATIVES
Histoplasma capsulatum	Prior documented disease May stop prophylaxis after 1 year if CD4+ T-cell count >150 and patient on ARV therapy for ≥6 mo	Itraconazole 200 mg bid PO	Fluconazole 800 mg/d PO
Coccidioides immitis	Prior documented disease or Positive serology and CD4+ T-cell count <250 [for this indication, prophylaxis can be stopped if CD4+ T-cell count ≥250 for 6 mo]	Fluconazole 400 mg/d PO	Itraconazole 200 mg bid PO
Penicillium marneffei	Prior documented disease May stop secondary prophylaxis in patients on ARVs with CD4+ T-cell count >100 for ≥6 mo	Itraconazole 200 mg/d PO	
Salmonella species	Prior bacteremia	Ciprofloxacin 500 mg bid PO for 6 mo or more	
Bartonella	Prior infection May stop if CD4+ T-cell count >200 for >3 mo	Doxycycline 200 mg/d Azithromycin 1200 mg weekly PO Clarithromycin 500 mg bid PO	
Cytomegalovirus	Prior end-organ disease May stop prophylaxis if CD4+ T-cell count >100/μL for 6 mo and no evidence of active CMV disease Restart if prior retinitis and CD4+ T cells <100/μL	Ganciclovir, 5–6 mg/kg 5–7 d/wk IV Valganciclovir 900 mg bid PO Foscarnet 90–120 (mg/kg)/d IV Ganciclovir sustained-release implant q6–9 mo + Valganciclovir 900 mg bid PO	Cidofovir 5 mg/kg every other week IV + Probenecid Formivirsen 330 μg intravitreal q2–4 wk Valganciclovir 900 mg PO daily Formivirsen, 1 vial injected into the vitreous q2–4 wk
Immunizations Generally Recommended			
Hepatitis B virus	All susceptible (anti-HBc and anti-HBs negative) patients	Hepatitis B vaccine: 3 doses	
Hepatitis A virus	All susceptible (anti-HAV negative) patients	Hepatitis A vaccine: 2 doses	
Influenza virus	All patients annually	Inactivated trivalent influenza virus vaccine 1 dose yearly	Oseltamivir 75 mg PO qd Rimantadine or amantadine 100 mg PO bid (influenza A only)
Streptococcus pneumoniae	All patients, preferably before CD4+ T-cell count ≥200/μL	Pneumoccal vaccine 0.5 mL IM ×1 if CD4+ T-cell count >200/μL Reimmunize patients initially immunized at a CD4+ T-cell count <100/μL whose CD4+ T-cell count then increases to >200/μL	
Human papilloma-virus	Girls and women 9–26 years of age	HPV vaccine; 3 doses	
Recommended for Prevention of Severe or Frequent Recurrences			
Herpes simplex	Frequent/severe recurrences	Acyclovir 200 mg tid PO Acyclovir 400 mg bid PO Famciclovir 250 mg bid PO	Valacyclovir 500 mg PO bid
Candida	Frequent/severe recurrences	Fluconazole 100–200 mg/d PO	Itraconazole solution 200 mg/d PO

Note: DS, double strength; SS, single strength; PCP, *Pneumocystis carinii* pneumonia; TB, tuberculosis.

spectrum of HIV disease is constantly changing as patients live longer and new and better approaches to treatment and prophylaxis are developed. In addition to the classic AIDS-defining illnesses, patients with HIV infection also have an increase in serious non-AIDS illnesses, including cardiovascular, renal, and hepatic disease. The physician providing care to a patient with HIV infection must be well versed in general internal medicine as well as HIV-related infectious diseases and new clinical syndromes related to chronic illness and long-term ARV therapy. In general, it should be stressed that a key element of treatment of symptomatic complications of HIV disease, whether they are primary or secondary, is achieving good control of HIV replication through the use of combination ARV therapy and instituting primary and secondary prophylaxis for opportunistic infections as indicated.

Disease of the Respiratory System

Acute bronchitis and sinusitis are prevalent during all stages of HIV infection. The most severe cases tend to occur in patients with lower CD4+ T-cell counts. Sinusitis presents as fever, nasal congestion, and headache. The diagnosis is made by CT or MRI. The maxillary sinuses are most commonly involved; however, disease is also frequently seen in the ethmoid, sphenoid, and frontal sinuses. Although some patients may improve without antibiotic therapy, radiographic improvement is quicker and more pronounced in patients who have received antimicrobial therapy. It is postulated that this high incidence of sinusitis results from an increased frequency of infection with encapsulated organisms such as *H. influenzae* and *Streptococcus pneumoniae*. In patients with low CD4+ T-cell counts, one may see mucormycosis infections of the sinuses. In contrast to the course of this infection in other patient populations, mucormycosis of the sinuses in patients with HIV infection may progress more slowly. In this setting, aggressive, frequent local debridement in addition to local and systemic amphotericin B may be needed for effective treatment.

Pulmonary disease is one of the most frequent complications of HIV infection. The most common manifestation of pulmonary disease is pneumonia. The two most common causes of pneumonia are bacterial infections and the unicellular fungus *P. jiroveci* infection. Other major causes of pulmonary infiltrates include mycobacterial infections, other fungal infections, nonspecific interstitial pneumonitis, KS, and lymphoma.

Pneumonia is seen with an increased frequency in patients with HIV infection; they appear to be particularly prone to infections with encapsulated organisms. *S. pneumoniae* (Chap. 34) and *H. influenzae* (Chap. 47) are responsible for most cases of bacterial pneumonia in patients with AIDS. This may be a consequence of altered B-cell function and/or defects in neutrophil function that may be secondary to HIV disease (see above). *S. pneumoniae* (pneumococcal) infection may be the earliest serious infection to occur in patients with HIV disease. This can present as pneumonia, sinusitis, and/or bacteremia. Patients with untreated HIV infection have a sixfold increase in the incidence of pneumococcal pneumonia and a 100-fold increase in the incidence of pneumococcal bacteremia. Pneumococcal disease may be seen in patients with relatively intact immune systems. In one study, the baseline CD4+ T-cell count at the time of a first episode of pneumococcal pneumonia was ~300/μL. Of interest is the fact that the inflammatory response to pneumococcal infection appears proportional to the CD4+ T-cell count. Due to this high risk of pneumococcal disease, immunization with pneumococcal polysaccharide is one of the generally recommended prophylactic measures for patients with HIV infection. This is likely most effective if given while the CD4+ T-cell count is >200/μL. It is less clear whether this intervention is effective when given to patients with more advanced disease and high viral loads.

Pneumocystis pneumonia (PCP), once the hallmark of AIDS, has dramatically declined in incidence after the development of effective prophylactic regimens and the widespread use of combination ARV therapy. It is, however, the single most common cause of pneumonia in patients with HIV infection in the United States and can be identified as a likely etiologic agent in 25% of cases of pneumonia in patients with HIV infection. Approximately 25% of cases of HIV-associated PCP occur in patients who are unaware of their HIV status. The risk of PCP is greatest among those who have experienced a previous bout of PCP and those who have CD4+ T-cell counts of <200/μL. Overall, 79% of patients with PCP have CD4+ T-cell counts <100/μL and 95% of patients have CD4+ T-cell counts <200/μL. Recurrent fever, night sweats, thrush, and unexplained weight loss are also associated with an increased incidence of PCP. For these reasons, it is strongly recommended that all patients with CD4+ T-cell counts <200/μL (or a CD4 percentage <15) receive some form of PCP prophylaxis. The incidence of PCP is approaching zero in patients with known HIV infection receiving appropriate ARV therapy and prophylaxis. In the United States, primary PCP is now occurring at a median CD4+ T-cell count of 36/μL, whereas secondary PCP is occurring at a median CD4+ T-cell count of 10/μL. Patients with PCP generally present with fever and a cough that is usually nonproductive or productive of only scant amounts of white sputum. They may complain of a characteristic retrosternal chest pain that is worse on inspiration and is described as sharp or burning. HIV-associated PCP may have an indolent course characterized by weeks of vague symptoms and should be included in the differential diagnosis of fever, pulmonary complaints, or unexplained weight loss in any patient with HIV infection and <200 CD4+ T-cells/μL. The most common finding on chest x-ray is either a normal film, if the disease is suspected early, or a faint bilateral interstitial infiltrate. The classic finding of a dense perihilar infiltrate is unusual in patients with AIDS. In patients with PCP who have been receiving aerosolized pentamidine for prophylaxis, one may see an x-ray picture of upper lobe cavitary disease, reminiscent of TB. Other less common findings on chest x-ray include lobar infiltrates and pleural effusions. Routine laboratory evaluation is usually of little help in the differential diagnosis of PCP. A mild leukocytosis is common, although this may not be obvious in patients with prior neutropenia. Arterial blood gases may indicate hypoxemia with a decline in Pa_{O_2} and an increase in the arterial-alveolar (a − A) gradient. Arterial blood gas measurements not only aid in making the diagnosis of PCP, but also provide important information for staging the severity of the disease and directing treatment (see below). A definitive diagnosis of PCP requires demonstration of the organism in samples obtained from induced sputum, bronchoalveolar lavage, transbronchial biopsy, or open lung biopsy. PCR has been used to detect specific DNA sequences for *P. jiroveci* in clinical specimens where histologic examinations have failed to make a diagnosis.

In addition to pneumonia, a number of other clinical problems have been reported in HIV-infected patients as a result of infection with *P. jiroveci*. Otic involvement may be seen as a primary infection, presenting as a polypoid mass involving the external auditory canal. In patients receiving aerosolized pentamidine for prophylaxis against PCP, one may see a variety of extrapulmonary manifestations of *P. jiroveci*. These include ophthalmic lesions of the choroid, a necrotizing vasculitis that resembles Burger's disease, bone marrow hypoplasia, and intestinal obstruction. Other organs that have been involved include lymph nodes, spleen, liver, kidney, pancreas, pericardium, heart, thyroid, and adrenals. Organ infection may be associated with cystic lesions that may appear calcified on CT or ultrasound.

The standard treatment for PCP or disseminated pneumocystosis is trimethoprim/sulfamethoxazole (TMP/SMX). A high incidence of side effects, particularly skin rash and bone marrow suppression, is seen with TMP/SMX in patients with HIV infection. Alternative treatments for mild to moderate PCP include dapsone/trimethoprim and clindamycin/primaquine. Intravenous pentamidine is the treatment of choice for severe disease in the patient unable to tolerate TMP/SMX. For patients with a Pa_{O_2} < 70 mmHg or with an a − A gradient >35 mmHg, adjunct glucocorticoid therapy should be used in addition to specific antimicrobials. Overall, treatment should be for 21 days and followed by secondary prophylaxis. Prophylaxis for PCP is indicated for any HIV-infected individual who has experienced a prior bout of PCP, any patient with a CD4+ T-cell count of <200/μL or a CD4 percentage <15, any patient with unexplained fever for >2 weeks, and any patient with a history of oropharyngeal candidiasis. The preferred regimen for prophylaxis is TMP/SMX, one double-strength tablet daily. This regimen also provides protection against toxoplasmosis and some bacterial respiratory pathogens. For patients who cannot tolerate TMP/SMX, alternatives for prophylaxis include dapsone plus pyrimethamine plus leucovorin, aerosolized pentamidine administered by the Respirgard II nebulizer, and atovaquone. Primary or secondary prophylaxis for PCP can be discontinued in those patients treated with combination ARV therapy who maintain good suppression of HIV (<50 copies per milliliter) and CD4+ T-cell counts >200/μL for 3–6 months.

M. tuberculosis, once thought to be on its way to extinction in the United States, experienced a resurgence associated with the HIV epidemic (Chap. 66). Worldwide, approximately one-third of all AIDS-related deaths are associated with TB. In the United States ~5% of AIDS patients have active TB. HIV infection increases the risk of developing active TB by a factor of 100. For the patient with untreated HIV infection and a positive PPD skin test, the rate of reactivation TB is 7–10% per year. Untreated TB can accelerate the course of HIV infection. Levels of plasma HIV RNA increase in the setting of active TB and decline in the setting of successful TB treatment. Active TB is most common in patients 25–44 years of age, in African Americans and Hispanics, in patients in New York City and Miami, and in patients in developing countries. In these demographic groups, 20–70% of the new cases of active TB are in patients with HIV infection. The epidemic of TB embedded in the epidemic of HIV infection probably represents the greatest health risk to the general public and the health care profession associated with the HIV epidemic. In contrast to infection with atypical mycobacteria such as MAC, active TB often develops relatively early in the course of HIV infection and may be an early clinical sign of HIV disease. In one study, the median CD4+ T-cell count at presentation of TB was 326/μL. The clinical manifestations of TB in HIV-infected patients are quite varied and generally show different patterns as a function of the CD4+ T-cell count. In patients with relatively high CD4+ T-cell counts, the typical pattern of pulmonary reactivation occurs in which patients present with fever, cough, dyspnea on exertion, weight loss, night sweats, and a chest x-ray revealing cavitary apical disease of the upper lobes. In patients with lower CD4+ T-cell counts, disseminated disease is more common. In these patients, the chest x-ray may reveal diffuse or lower lobe bilateral reticulonodular infiltrates consistent with miliary spread, pleural effusions, and hilar and/or mediastinal adenopathy. Infection may be present in bone, brain, meninges, gastrointestinal tract, lymph nodes (particularly cervical lymph nodes), and viscera. Approximately 60–80% of patients have pulmonary disease, and 30–40% have extrapulmonary disease. Respiratory isolation and a negative-pressure room should be used for patients in whom a diagnosis of pulmonary TB is being considered. This approach is critical to limit nosocomial and community spread of infection. Culture of the organism from an involved site provides a definitive diagnosis. Blood cultures are positive in 15% of patients. This figure is higher in patients with lower CD4 +T-cell counts. In the setting of fulminant disease, one cannot rely upon the accuracy of a negative PPD skin test to rule out a diagnosis of TB. TB is one of the conditions associated with HIV infection for which cure is possible with appropriate therapy. Therapy for TB is generally the same in the HIV-infected patient as in the HIV-negative patient (Chap. 66). Due to the possibility of multidrug resistant or extensively drug-resistant TB, drug susceptibility testing should be performed to guide therapy. Due to pharmacokinetic interactions, adjusted doses of rifabutin should be substituted for rifampin in patients receiving the HIV protease inhibitors or nonnucleoside reverse transcriptase inhibitors. Treatment is most effective in programs that involve directly observed therapy. Initiation of ARV therapy and/or anti-TB therapy may be associated with clinical deterioration due to immune reconstitution inflammatory syndrome (IRIS) reactions. These are most common in patients initiating both treatments at the same time, occur several weeks after initiation of therapy, and are seen more frequently in patients with advanced HIV disease. Effective prevention of active TB can be a reality if the health care professional is aggressive in looking for evidence of latent TB by making sure that all patients with HIV infection receive a PPD skin test or evaluation with an interferon-γ release assay. Anergy testing is not of value in this setting. HIV-infected individuals with a skin test reaction of >5 mm, a positive interferon-γ release assay or those who are close household contacts of persons with active TB should receive treatment with 9 months of isoniazid.

Atypical mycobacterial infections are also seen with an increased frequency in patients with HIV infection. Infections with at least 12 different mycobacteria have been reported, including *M. bovis* and representatives of all four Runyon groups. The most common atypical mycobacterial infection is with *M. avium* or *M. intracellulare* species—MAC. Infections with MAC are seen mainly in patients in the United States and are rare in Africa. It has been suggested that prior infection with *M. tuberculosis* decreases the risk of MAC infection. MAC infections probably arise from organisms that are ubiquitous in the environment, including both soil and water. The presumed portals of entry are the respiratory and gastrointestinal tract. MAC infection is a late complication of HIV infection, predominantly occurring in patients with CD4+ T-cell counts of <50/μL. The average CD4+ T-cell count at the time of diagnosis is 10/μL. The most common presentation is disseminated disease with fever, weight loss, and night sweats. At least 85% of patients with MAC infection are mycobacteremic, and large numbers of organisms can often be demonstrated on bone marrow biopsy. The chest x-ray is abnormal in ~25% of patients, with the most common pattern being that of a bilateral, lower lobe infiltrate suggestive of miliary spread. Alveolar or nodular infiltrates and hilar and/or mediastinal adenopathy can also occur. Other clinical findings include endobronchial lesions, abdominal pain, diarrhea, and lymphadenopathy. The diagnosis is made by the culture of blood or involved tissue. The finding of two consecutive sputum samples positive for MAC is highly suggestive of pulmonary infection. Cultures may take 2 weeks to turn positive. Therapy consists of a macrolide, usually clarithromycin, with ethambutol. Some physicians elect to add a third drug from among rifabutin, ciprofloxacin, or amikacin in patients with extensive disease. Therapy is generally for life; however, with the use of highly active antiretroviral therapy (HAART), it is possible to discontinue therapy in patients with sustained suppression of HIV replication and CD4+ T-cell counts >100/μL for 3–6 months. Primary prophylaxis for MAC is indicated in patients with HIV infection and CD4+ T-cell counts <50/μL. This may be discontinued in patients in whom HAART induces a sustained suppression of viral replication and increases in CD4+ T-cell counts to >100/μL for 3–6 months.

Rhodococcus equi is a gram-positive pleomorphic acid-fast non–spore-forming bacillus that can cause pulmonary and/or disseminated infection in patients with HIV infection. Fever and cough are the most common presenting signs. Radiographically, one may see cavitary lesions and consolidation. Blood cultures are often positive. Treatment is based upon antimicrobial sensitivity testing.

Fungal infections of the lung, in addition to PCP, can be seen in patients with AIDS. Patients with pulmonary cryptococcal disease present with fever, cough, dyspnea, and in some cases, hemoptysis. A focal or diffuse interstitial infiltrate is seen on chest x-ray in >90% of patients. In addition, one may see lobar disease, cavitary disease, pleural effusions, and hilar or mediastinal adenopathy. Over half of patients are fungemic, and 90% of patients have concomitant CNS infection. *Coccidioides immitis* is a mold that is endemic in the southwest United States. It can cause a reactivation pulmonary syndrome in patients with HIV infection. Most patients with this condition will have CD4+ T-cell counts <250/μL. Patients present with fever, weight loss, cough, and extensive, diffuse reticulonodular infiltrates on chest x-ray. One may also see nodules, cavities, pleural effusions, and hilar adenopathy. Although serologic testing is of value in the immunocompetent host, serologies are negative in 25% of HIV-infected patients with coccidioidal infection. Invasive aspergillosis is not an AIDS-defining illness and is generally not seen in patients with AIDS in the absence of neutropenia or administration of glucocorticoids. *Aspergillus* infection may have an unusual presentation in the respiratory tract of patients with AIDS where it gives the appearance of a pseudomembranous tracheobronchitis. Primary pulmonary infection of the lung may be seen with *histoplasmosis*. The most common pulmonary manifestation of histoplasmosis, however, is in the setting of disseminated disease, presumably due to reactivation. In this setting, respiratory symptoms are usually minimal, with cough and dyspnea occurring in 10–30% of patients. The chest x-ray is abnormal in ~50% of patients, showing either a diffuse interstitial infiltrate or diffuse small nodules.

Two forms of *idiopathic interstitial pneumonia* have been identified in patients with HIV infection: lymphoid interstitial pneumonitis (LIP) and nonspecific interstitial pneumonitis (NIP). LIP, a common finding in children, is seen in about 1% of adult patients with untreated HIV infection. This disorder is characterized by a benign infiltrate of the lung and is thought to be part of the polyclonal activation of lymphocytes seen in the context of HIV and EBV infections. Transbronchial biopsy is diagnostic in 50% of the cases, with an open-lung biopsy required for diagnosis in the remainder of cases. This condition is generally self-limited and no specific treatment is necessary. Severe cases have been managed with brief courses of glucocorticoids. Although rarely a clinical problem since the use of HAART, evidence of NIP may be seen in up to half of all patients with untreated HIV infection. Histologically, interstitial infiltrates of lymphocytes and plasma cells in a perivascular and peribronchial distribution are present. When symptomatic, patients present with fever and nonproductive cough occasionally accompanied by mild chest discomfort. Chest x-ray is usually normal or may reveal a faint interstitial pattern. Similar to LIP, NIP is a self-limited process for which no therapy is indicated other than appropriate management of the underlying HIV infection. HIV-related pulmonary arterial hypertension (HIV-PAH) is seen in ~0.5% of HIV-infected individuals. Patients may present with an array of symptoms including shortness of breath, fatigue, syncope, chest pain, and signs of right-sided heart failure. Chest x-ray reveals dilated pulmonary vessels and right-sided cardiomegaly with right ventricular hypertrophy seen on electrocardiogram. ARV therapy does not appear to be of clear benefit, and the prognosis is quite poor, with a median survival in the range of 2 years.

Neoplastic diseases of the lung including KS and lymphoma are discussed below in the section on malignancies.

Diseases of the Cardiovascular System

Heart disease is a relatively common postmortem finding in HIV-infected patients (25–75% in autopsy series). Cardiovascular disease may be seen as a direct consequence of HIV infection or as a consequence of ARV therapy as part of the lipodystrophy syndrome. As a primary consequence of HIV infection, the most common clinically significant finding is a dilated cardiomyopathy associated with congestive heart failure (CHF), referred to as *HIV-associated cardiomyopathy*. This generally occurs as a late complication of HIV infection and, histologically, displays elements of myocarditis. For this reason, some have advocated treatment with intravenous immunoglobulin (IVIg). HIV can be directly demonstrated in cardiac tissue in this setting, and there is debate over whether or not it plays a direct role in this condition. Patients present with typical findings of CHF, namely edema and shortness of breath. Patients with HIV infection may also develop cardiomyopathy as side effects of IFN-α or nucleoside analogue therapy. These are reversible once therapy is stopped. KS, cryptococcosis, Chagas' disease, and toxoplasmosis can involve the myocardium, leading to cardiomyopathy. In one series, most patients with HIV infection and a treatable myocarditis were found to have myocarditis associated with toxoplasmosis. Most of these patients also had evidence of CNS toxoplasmosis. Thus MRI or double-dose contrast CT scan of the brain should be included in the workup of any patient with advanced HIV infection and cardiomyopathy.

A variety of other cardiovascular problems are found in patients with HIV infection. Pericardial effusions may be seen in the setting of advanced HIV infection. Predisposing factors include TB, CHF, mycobacterial infection, cryptococcal infection, pulmonary infection, lymphoma, and KS. Although pericarditis is quite rare, in one series, 5% of patients with HIV disease had pericardial effusions that were considered to be moderate or severe. Tamponade and death have occurred in association with pericardial KS, presumably owing to acute hemorrhage. Nonbacterial thrombotic endocarditis has been reported and should be considered in patients with unexplained embolic phenomena. Intravenous pentamidine, when given rapidly, can result in hypotension as a consequence of cardiovascular collapse. A high percentage of patients have hypertriglyceridemia and elevations in serum cholesterol, and coronary artery disease has been a relatively frequent finding at autopsy. This problem appears to be becoming even more prevalent as a side effect of HAART and in particular in patients with co-infection with HCV. Although the clinical significance of these findings has not been precisely defined, recent data suggest a linear relationship between time on HAART and development of ischemic heart disease. In one large series, the overall rate of myocardial infarction (MI) was 3.5/1000 years, 28% of these events were fatal, and MI was responsible for 7% of all deaths in the cohort. The risk of MI increased by 26% per year of HAART. This small increase in the risk of death from MI in the setting of HAART has to be balanced against the marked increase in overall survival brought about by HAART. Efforts to decrease the risk of cardiovascular diseases by minimizing the time on HAART were associated with a paradoxical increase in the rate of cardiovascular disease, suggesting that the pathogenesis of cardiovascular diseases in the setting of HIV infection is multifactorial, with HIV infection and the resulting immune activation and coagulopathy likely playing a significant role.

Diseases of the Oropharynx and Gastrointestinal System

Oropharyngeal and gastrointestinal diseases are common features of HIV infection. They are most frequently due to secondary infections. In addition, oral and gastrointestinal lesions may occur with KS and lymphoma.

Oral lesions, including *thrush*, *hairy leukoplakia*, and *aphthous ulcers* (Fig. 90-32), are particularly common in patients with untreated HIV infection. Thrush, due to *Candida* infection, and oral hairy leukoplakia, presumed due to EBV, are usually indicative of fairly advanced immunologic decline; they generally occur in patients with CD4+ T-cell counts of <300/μL. In one study, 59% of patients with oral candidiasis went on to develop AIDS in the next year. Thrush appears as a white, cheesy exudate, often on an erythematous mucosa in the posterior oropharynx. Although most commonly seen on the soft palate, early lesions are often found along the gingival border. The diagnosis is made by direct examination of a scraping for pseudohyphal elements. Culturing is of no diagnostic value, as most patients with HIV infection will have a positive throat culture for *Candida* even in the absence of thrush. Oral hairy leukoplakia presents as white, frondlike lesions, generally along the lateral borders of the tongue and sometimes on the adjacent buccal mucosa (Fig. 90-32). Despite its name, oral hairy

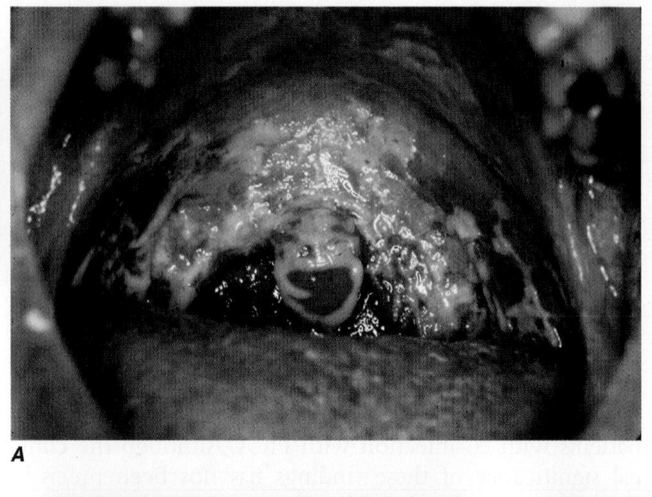

A

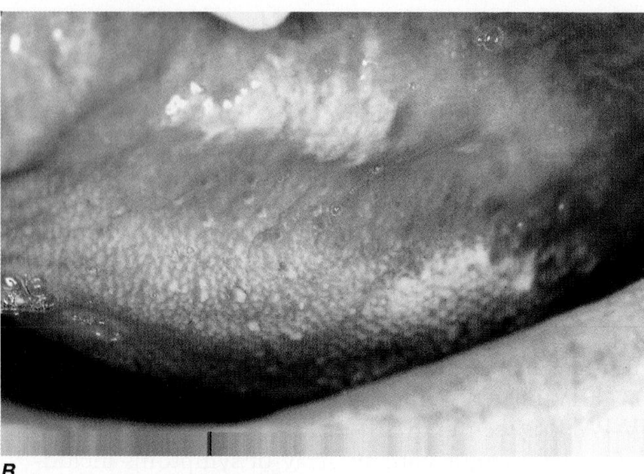

B

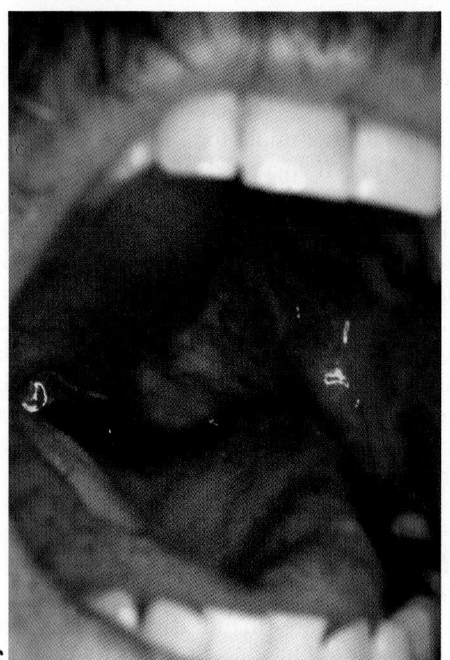

C

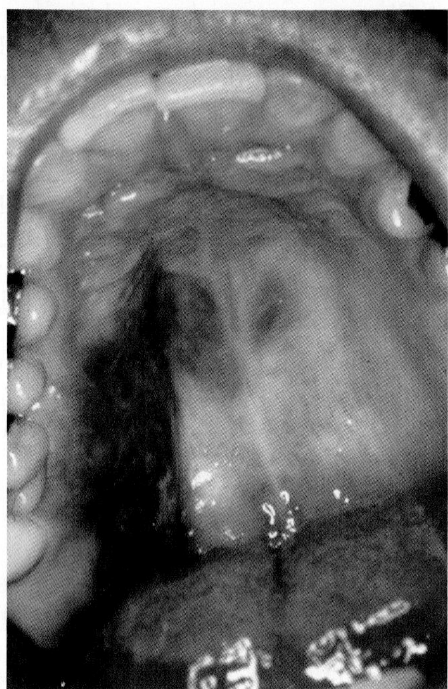

D

FIGURE 90-32

Various oral lesions in HIV-infected individuals. *A.* Thrush. ***B.*** Hairy leukoplakia. ***C.*** Aphthous ulcer. ***D.*** Kaposi's sarcoma.

leukoplakia is not considered a premalignant condition. Lesions are associated with florid replication of EBV. Although usually more disconcerting as a sign of HIV-associated immunodeficiency than a clinical problem in need of treatment, severe cases have been reported to respond to topical podophyllin or systemic therapy with anti-herpesvirus agents. Aphthous ulcers of the posterior oropharynx are also seen with regularity in patients with HIV infection (Fig. 90-32). These lesions are of unknown etiology and can be quite painful and interfere with swallowing. Topical anesthetics provide immediate symptomatic relief of short duration. The fact that thalidomide is an effective treatment for this condition suggests that the pathogenesis may involve the action of tissue-destructive cytokines. Palatal, glossal, or gingival ulcers may also result from cryptococcal disease or histoplasmosis.

Esophagitis (Fig. 90-33) may present with odynophagia and retrosternal pain. Upper endoscopy is generally required to make an accurate diagnosis. Esophagitis may be due to *Candida*, CMV, or HSV. Although CMV tends to be associated with a single large ulcer, HSV infection is more often associated with multiple small ulcers. The esophagus may also be the site of KS and lymphoma. Like the oral mucosa, the esophageal mucosa may have large, painful ulcers of unclear etiology that may respond to thalidomide. Although achlorhydria is a common problem in patients with HIV infection, other gastric problems are generally rare. Among the conditions involving the stomach are KS and lymphoma. Infections of the small and large intestine leading to diarrhea, abdominal pain, and occasionally fever are among the most significant gastrointestinal problems in HIV-infected patients. They include infections with bacteria, protozoa, and viruses.

Bacteria may be responsible for secondary infections of the gastrointestinal tract. Infections with enteric pathogens such as *Salmonella*, *Shigella*, and *Campylobacter* are more common in homosexual men and are often more severe and more apt to relapse in patients with HIV infection. Patients with untreated HIV have

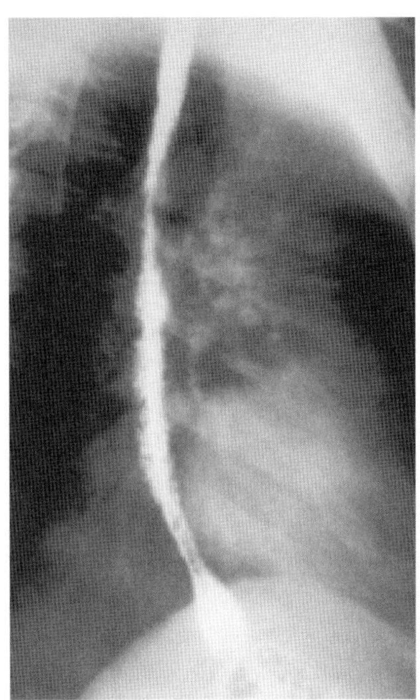

FIGURE 90-33

Barium swallow of a patient with *Candida* esophagitis. The flow of barium along the mucosal surface is grossly irregular.

approximately a 20-fold increased risk of infection with *S. typhimurium*. They may present with a variety of nonspecific symptoms including fever, anorexia, fatigue, and malaise of several weeks' duration. Diarrhea is common but may be absent. Diagnosis is made by culture of blood and stool. Long-term therapy with ciprofloxacin is the recommended treatment. HIV-infected patients also have an increased incidence of *S. typhi* infection in areas of the world where typhoid is a problem. *Shigella* spp., particularly *S. flexneri*, can cause severe intestinal disease in HIV-infected individuals. Up to 50% of patients will develop bacteremia. *Campylobacter* infections occur with an increased frequency in patients with HIV infection. Although *C. jejuni* is the strain most frequently isolated, infections with many other strains have been reported. Patients usually present with crampy abdominal pain, fever, and bloody diarrhea. Infection may present as proctitis. Stool examination reveals the presence of fecal leukocytes. Systemic infection can occur, with up to 10% of infected patients exhibiting bacteremia. Most strains are sensitive to erythromycin. Abdominal pain and diarrhea may be seen with MAC infection.

Fungal infections may also be a cause of diarrhea in patients with HIV infection. Histoplasmosis, coccidioidomycosis, and penicilliosis have all been identified as a cause of fever and diarrhea in patients with HIV infection. Peritonitis has been seen with *C. immitis*.

Cryptosporidia, microsporidia, and *Isospora belli* (Chap. 122) are the most common opportunistic protozoa that infect the gastrointestinal tract and cause diarrhea in HIV-infected patients. Cryptosporidial infection may present in a variety of ways, ranging from a self-limited or intermittent diarrheal illness in patients in the early stages of HIV infection to a severe, life-threatening diarrhea in severely immunodeficient individuals. In patients with untreated HIV infection and CD4+ T-cell counts of <300/μL, the incidence of cryptosporidiosis is ~1% per year. In 75% of cases, the diarrhea is accompanied by crampy abdominal pain, and 25% of patients have nausea and/or vomiting. Cryptosporidia may also cause biliary tract disease in the HIV-infected patient, leading to cholecystitis with or without accompanying cholangitis. The diagnosis of cryptosporidial diarrhea is made by stool examination. The diarrhea is noninflammatory, and the characteristic finding is the presence of oocysts that stain with acid-fast dyes. Therapy is predominantly supportive, and marked improvements have been reported in the setting of effective ARV therapy. Treatment with up to 2000 mg/d of nitazoxanide (NTZ) is associated with improvement in symptoms or a decrease in shedding of organisms in about half of patients. Its overall role in the management of this condition remains unclear. Patients can minimize their risk of developing cryptosporidiosis by avoiding contact with human and animal feces and by not drinking untreated water from lakes or rivers.

Microsporidia are small, unicellular, obligate intracellular parasites that reside in the cytoplasm of enteric cells (Chap. 122). The main species causing disease in humans is *Enterocytozoon bieneusi*. The clinical manifestations are similar to those described for cryptosporidia and include abdominal pain and diarrhea. The small size of the organism may make it difficult to detect; however, with the use of chromotrope-based stains, organisms can be identified in stool samples by light microscopy. Definitive diagnosis generally depends on electron-microscopic examination of a stool specimen, intestinal aspirate, or intestinal biopsy specimen. In contrast to cryptosporidia, microsporidia have been noted in a variety of extraintestinal locations, including the eye, muscle, and liver, and have been associated with conjunctivitis and hepatitis. Albendazole, 400 mg bid, has been reported to be of benefit in some patients.

I. belli is a coccidian parasite (Chap. 122) most commonly found as a cause of diarrhea in patients from the Caribbean and Africa. Its cysts appear in the stool as large, acid-fast structures that can be differentiated from those of cryptosporidia on the basis of size, shape, and number of sporocysts. The clinical syndromes of *Isospora* infection are identical to those caused by cryptosporidia. The important distinction is that infection with *Isospora* is generally relatively easy to treat with TMP/SMX. Although relapses are common, a thrice-weekly regimen of TMP/SMX appears adequate to prevent recurrence.

CMV colitis was once seen as a consequence of advanced immunodeficiency in 5–10% of patients with AIDS. It is much less common with the advent of HAART. CMV colitis presents as diarrhea, abdominal pain, weight loss, and anorexia. The diarrhea is usually nonbloody, and the diagnosis is achieved through endoscopy and biopsy. Multiple mucosal ulcerations are seen at endoscopy, and biopsies reveal characteristic intranuclear inclusion bodies. Secondary bacteremias may result as a consequence of thinning of the bowel wall.

Treatment is with either ganciclovir or foscarnet for 3–6 weeks. Relapses are common, and maintenance therapy is typically necessary in patients whose HIV infection is poorly controlled. Patients with CMV disease of the gastrointestinal tract should be carefully monitored for evidence of CMV retinitis.

In addition to disease caused by specific secondary infections, patients with HIV infection may also experience a chronic diarrheal syndrome for which no etiologic agent other than HIV can be identified. This entity is referred to as *AIDS enteropathy* or *HIV enteropathy*. It is most likely a direct result of HIV infection in the gastrointestinal tract. Histologic examination of the small bowel in these patients reveals low-grade mucosal atrophy with a decrease in mitotic figures, suggesting a hyporegenerative state. Patients often have decreased or absent small-bowel lactase and malabsorption with accompanying weight loss.

The initial evaluation of a patient with HIV infection and diarrhea should include a set of stool examinations, including culture, examination for ova and parasites, and examination for *Clostridium difficile* toxin. Approximately 50% of the time this workup will demonstrate infection with pathogenic bacteria, mycobacteria, or protozoa. If the initial stool examinations are negative, additional evaluation, including upper and/or lower endoscopy with biopsy, will yield a diagnosis of microsporidial or mycobacterial infection of the small intestine ~30% of the time. In patients for whom this diagnostic evaluation is nonrevealing, a presumptive diagnosis of HIV enteropathy can be made if the diarrhea has persisted for >1 month. An algorithm for the evaluation of diarrhea in patients with HIV infection is given in Fig. 90-34.

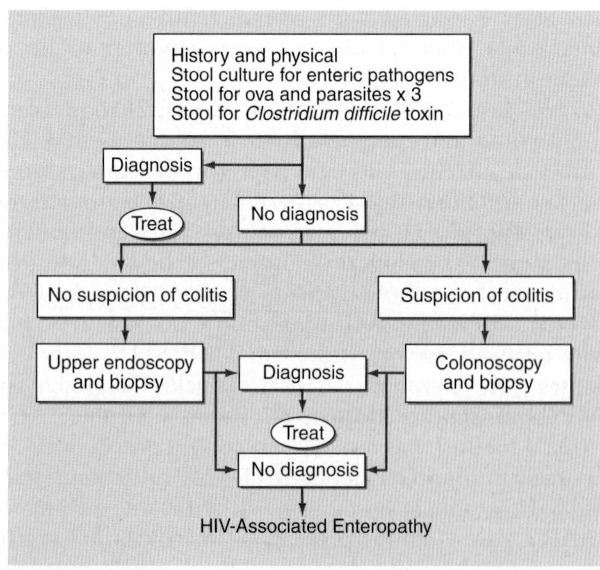

FIGURE 90-34

Algorithm for the evaluation of diarrhea in a patient with HIV infection. HIV-associated enteropathy is a diagnosis of exclusion and can be made only after other, generally treatable, forms of diarrheal illness have been ruled out.

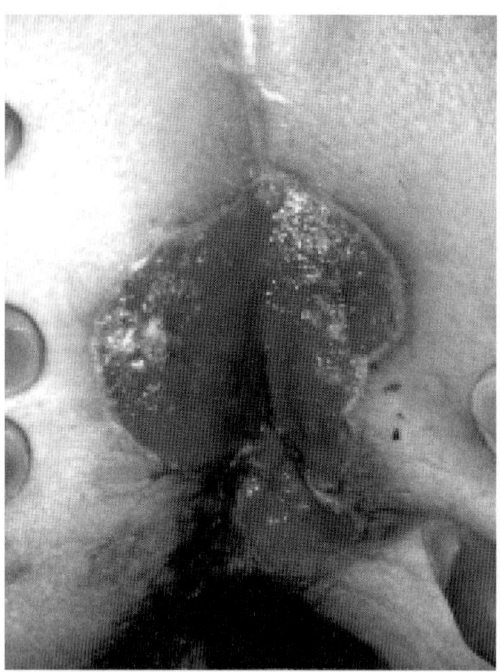

FIGURE 90-35

Severe, erosive perirectal herpes simplex in a patient with AIDS.

Rectal lesions are common in HIV-infected patients, particularly the perirectal ulcers and erosions due to the reactivation of HSV (Fig. 90-35). These may appear quite atypical, as denuded skin without vesicles, and they respond well to treatment with acyclovir, famciclovir, or foscarnet. Other rectal lesions encountered in patients with HIV infection include condylomata acuminata, KS, and intraepithelial neoplasia (see below).

Hepatobiliary Disease

Diseases of the hepatobiliary system are a major problem in patients with HIV infection. It has been estimated that approximately one-third of the deaths of patients with HIV infection are in some way related to liver disease. Although this is predominantly a reflection of the problems encountered in the setting of co-infection with hepatitis B or C, it is also a reflection of the hepatic injury, ranging from hepatic steatosis to hypersensitivity reactions to immune reconstitution, that can be seen in the context of ARV therapy.

The prevalence of co-infection with HIV and hepatitis viruses varies by geographic region. In the United States, ~90% of HIV-infected individuals have evidence of infection with HBV; 6–14% have chronic HBV infection; 5–50% of patients are co-infected with HCV; and co-infection with hepatitis D, E, and/or G viruses is common. Among IV drug users with HIV infection, rates of HCV infection range from 70–95%. HIV infection has a significant impact on the course of hepatitis virus infection. It is associated with approximately a threefold increase in the development of persistent hepatitis B surface antigenemia. Patients infected with both HBV and HIV have decreased evidence of inflammatory liver disease. The presumption that this is due to the immunosuppressive effects of HIV infection is supported by the observations that this situation can be reversed, and one may see the development of more severe hepatitis after the initiation of effective ARV therapy. In studies of the impact of HIV on HBV infection, four- to tenfold increases in liver-related mortality have been noted in patients with HIV and active HBV infection compared with rates in patients with either infection alone. There is a slight increase in overall mortality in HIV-infected individuals who are also hepatitis B surface antigen (HBsAg) positive. IFN-α is less successful as a treatment of HBV in patients with HIV co-infection, and lamivudine, emtricitabine, or adefovir/tenofovir and entecavir alone or in combination are useful in the treatment of hepatitis B in patients with HIV infection. It is important to remember that all the above-mentioned drugs also have activity against HIV and should not be used as single agents in patients with HIV infection, in order to avoid the rapid development of resistant quasispecies of HIV. HCV infection is more severe in the patient with HIV infection; it does not appear to affect overall mortality in HIV-infected individuals when other variables such as age, baseline CD4+ T-cell count, and use of HAART are taken into account. In the setting of HIV and HCV co-infection, levels of HCV are approximately tenfold higher than in the HIV-negative patient with HCV infection and there is a tenfold increased risk of death due to liver disease in co-infected patients. Treatment for HCV infection consists of pegylated IFN-α and ribavirin. If a 2-log drop in levels of HCV RNA is not seen within 12 weeks, it is unlikely that therapy will be of value. Hepatitis A virus infection is not seen with an increased frequency in patients with HIV infection. It is recommended that all patients with HIV infection who have not experienced natural infection be immunized with hepatitis A and/or hepatitis B vaccines. Infection with hepatitis G virus, also known as GB virus C, is seen in ~50% of patients with HIV infection. For reasons that are currently unclear, there are data to suggest that patients with HIV infection co-infected with this virus have a decreased rate of progression to AIDS.

A variety of other infections may also involve the liver. Granulomatous hepatitis may be seen as a consequence of mycobacterial or fungal infections, particularly MAC infection. Hepatic masses may be seen in the context of TB, peliosis hepatis, or fungal infection. Among the fungal opportunistic infections, *C. immitis* and *Histoplasma capsulatum* are those most likely to involve the liver. Biliary tract disease in the form of papillary stenosis or sclerosing cholangitis has been reported in the context of cryptosporidiosis, CMV infection, and KS.

Many of the drugs used to treat HIV infection are metabolized by the liver and can cause liver injury. Fatal hepatic reactions have been reported with a wide array of ARVs, including nucleoside analogues, nonnucleoside analogues, and protease inhibitors. Nucleoside analogues work by inhibiting DNA synthesis. This can result in toxicity to mitochondria, which can lead to disturbances in oxidative metabolism. This may manifest as hepatic steatosis and, in severe cases, lactic acidosis and fulminant liver failure. It is important to be aware of this condition and to watch for it in patients with HIV infection receiving nucleoside analogues. It is reversible if diagnosed early and the offending agent(s) discontinued. Nevirapine has been associated with at times fatal fulminant and cholestatic hepatitis, hepatic necrosis, and hepatic failure. Indinavir may cause mild to moderate elevations in serum bilirubin in 10–15% of patients in a syndrome similar to Gilbert's syndrome. A similar pattern of hepatic injury may be seen with atazanavir. In the patient receiving HAART with an unexplained increase in hepatic transaminases, strong consideration should be given to drug toxicity. *Pancreatic injury* is most commonly a consequence of drug toxicity, notably that secondary to pentamidine or dideoxynucleosides. Although up to half of patients in some series have biochemical evidence of pancreatic injury, <5% of patients show any clinical evidence of pancreatitis that is not linked to a drug toxicity.

Diseases of the Kidney and Genitourinary Tract

Diseases of the kidney or genitourinary tract may be a direct consequence of HIV infection, due to an opportunistic infection or neoplasm, or related to drug toxicity. *HIV-associated nephropathy* was first described in IDUs and was initially thought to be IDU nephropathy in patients with HIV infection; it is now recognized as a true direct complication of HIV infection. Although the majority of patients have CD4+ T-cell counts <200/μL, HIV-associated nephropathy can be an early manifestation of HIV infection and is also seen in children. Over 90% of reported cases have been in African-American or Hispanic individuals; the disease is not only more prevalent in these populations, but is also more severe and is the third leading cause of end-stage renal failure among African Americans aged 20–64 in the United States. Proteinuria is the hallmark of this disorder. Overall, microalbuminuria is seen in ~20% of untreated HIV-infected patients; significant proteinuria is seen in closer to 2%. Edema and hypertension are rare. Ultrasound examination reveals enlarged, hyperechogenic kidneys. A definitive diagnosis is obtained through renal biopsy. Histologically, focal segmental glomerulosclerosis is present in 80%, and mesangial proliferation in 10–15% of cases. Before effective antiretroviral therapy, this disease was characterized by relatively rapid progression to end-stage renal disease, and patients with HIV-associated nephropathy should be treated for their HIV infection regardless of CD4+ T-cell count. Treatment with angiotensin-converting enzyme (ACE) inhibitors and/or prednisone, 60 mg/d, has also been reported to be of benefit in some cases. The incidence of this disease in patients receiving adequate ARV therapy has not been well defined; however, the impression is that it has decreased in frequency and severity. It is the leading cause of end-stage renal disease in patients with HIV infection.

Among the drugs commonly associated with renal damage in patients with HIV disease are pentamidine, amphotericin, adefovir, cidofovir, tenofovir, and foscarnet.

TMP/SMX may compete for tubular secretion with creatinine and cause an increase in the serum creatinine level. Sulfadiazine may crystallize in the kidney and result in an easily reversible form of renal shutdown. One of the most common drug-induced renal complications is indinavir-associated renal calculi. This condition is seen in ~10% of patients receiving this HIV protease inhibitor. It may present with a variety of manifestations, ranging from asymptomatic hematuria to renal colic. Adequate hydration is the mainstay of treatment and prevention for this condition.

Genitourinary tract infections are seen with a high frequency in patients with HIV infection; they present with skin lesions, dysuria, hematuria, and/or pyuria and are managed in the same fashion as in patients without HIV infection. Infections with HSV are covered below under dermatologic disorders. Infections with *T. pallidum*, the etiologic agent of *syphilis*, play an important role in the HIV epidemic. In HIV-negative individuals, genital syphilitic ulcers as well as the ulcers of chancroid are major predisposing factors for heterosexual transmission of HIV infection. Although most HIV-infected individuals with syphilis have a typical presentation, a variety of formerly rare clinical problems may be encountered in the setting of dual infection. Among them are *lues maligna*, an ulcerating lesion of the skin due to a necrotizing vasculitis; unexplained fever; nephrotic syndrome; and neurosyphilis. The most common presentation of syphilis in the HIV-infected patient is that of *condylomata lata*, a form of secondary syphilis. Neurosyphilis may be asymptomatic or may present as acute meningitis, neuroretinitis, deafness, or stroke. The rate of neurosyphilis may be as high as 1% in patients with HIV infection. As a consequence of the immunologic abnormalities seen in the setting of HIV infection, diagnosis of syphilis through standard serologic testing may be challenging. On the one hand, a significant number of patients have false-positive Venereal Disease Research Laboratory (VDRL) tests due to polyclonal B cell activation. On the other hand, the development of a new positive VDRL may be delayed in patients with new infections, and the anti-fluorescent treponema antibody (anti-FTA) test may be negative due to immunodeficiency. Thus dark-field examination of appropriate specimens should be performed in any patient in whom syphilis is suspected, even if the patient has a negative VDRL. Similarly, any patient with a positive serum VDRL test, neurologic findings, and an abnormal spinal fluid examination should be considered to have neurosyphilis, regardless of the CSF VDRL result. In any setting, patients treated for syphilis need to be carefully monitored to ensure adequate therapy.

Vulvovaginal candidiasis is a common problem in women with HIV infection. Symptoms include pruritus, discomfort, dyspareunia, and dysuria. Vulvar infection may present as a morbilliform rash that may extend to the thighs. Vaginal infection is usually associated with a white discharge, and plaques may be seen along an erythematous vaginal wall. Diagnosis is made by microscopic examination of the discharge for pseudohyphal elements in a 10% potassium hydroxide solution. Mild disease can be treated with topical therapy. More serious disease can be treated with fluconazole. Other causes of vaginitis include *Trichomonas* and mixed bacteria.

Diseases of the Endocrine System and Metabolic Disorders

A variety of endocrine and metabolic disorders are seen in the context of HIV infection. Between 33 and 75% of patients with HIV infection receiving HAART develop a syndrome often referred to as *lipodystrophy*, consisting of elevations in plasma triglycerides, total cholesterol, and apolipoprotein B, as well as hyperinsulinemia and hyperglycemia. Many of the patients have been noted to have a characteristic set of body habitus changes associated with fat redistribution, consisting of truncal obesity coupled with peripheral wasting (Fig. 90-36). Truncal obesity is apparent as an increase in abdominal girth related to increases in mesenteric fat, a dorsocervical fat pad ("buffalo hump") reminiscent of patients with Cushing's syndrome, and enlargement of the breasts. The peripheral wasting or lipoatrophy is particularly noticeable in the face and buttocks and by the prominence of the veins in the legs. These changes may develop at any time ranging from ~6 weeks to several years after the initiation of HAART. Approximately 20% of the patients with HIV-associated lipodystrophy meet the criteria for the *metabolic syndrome* as defined by The International Diabetes Federation or The U.S. National Cholesterol Education Program Adult Treatment Panel III. The lipodystrophy syndrome has been reported in association with regimens containing a variety of different drugs, and although initially reported in the setting of protease inhibitor therapy, it appears similar changes can also be induced by potent protease-sparing regimens. It has been suggested that the lipoatrophy changes are particularly severe in patients receiving thymidine analogues. National Cholesterol Education Program (NCEP) guidelines should be followed in the management of these lipid abnormalities. Due to concerns regarding drug interactions, the most commonly utilized agents in this setting are gemfibrozil and atorvastatin. In addition to these abnormalities, patients with HIV infection treated with HAART have been found to have an increased incidence of osteonecrosis or avascular necrosis of the hip and shoulders. In a study of asymptomatic patients, 4.4% were found to have evidence of osteonecrosis on MRI. This complication has been associated with the use of lipid-lowering agents, systemic glucocorticoids, or testosterone; bodybuilding exercise; alcohol consumption; and the presence of anticardiolipin antibodies. Osteoporosis has been reported in 7% of women with HIV infection, with 41% of women demonstrating some degree of osteopenia. In addition, lactic acidosis is associated with ARV therapy. This is most commonly seen with nucleoside analogue reverse transcriptase inhibitors and can be fatal (see below).

Patients with advanced HIV disease may develop hyponatremia due to the syndrome of inappropriate antidiuretic hormone (vasopressin) secretion (SIADH) as a consequence of increased free water intake and

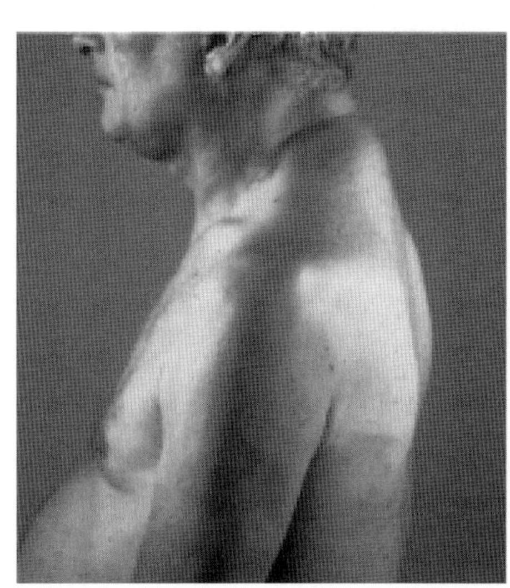
A

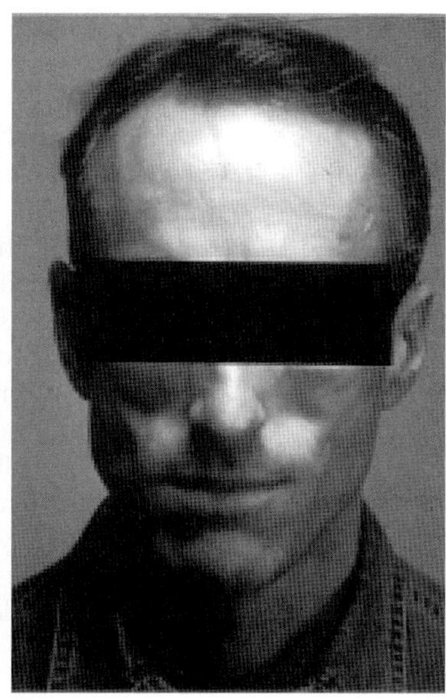
B

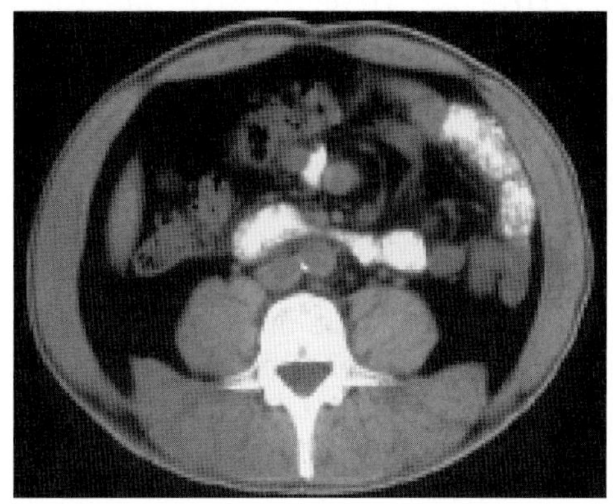
C

FIGURE 90-36
Characteristics of lipodystrophy. *A.* Truncal obesity and buffalo hump. ***B.*** Facial wasting. ***C.*** Accumulation of intraabdominal fat on CT scan.

decreased free water excretion. SIADH is usually seen in conjunction with pulmonary or CNS disease. Low serum sodium may also be due to adrenal insufficiency; concomitant high serum potassium should alert one to this possibility. Adrenal gland disease may be due to mycobacterial infections, CMV disease, cryptococcal disease, histoplasmosis, or ketoconazole toxicity.

Thyroid function may be altered in 10–15% of patients with HIV infection. Both hypo- and hyperthyroidism may be seen. The predominant abnormality is subclinical hypothyroidism. In the setting of HAART, up to 10% of patients have been noted to have elevated thyroid-stimulating hormone levels, suggesting that this may be a manifestation of immune reconstitution. Immune-reconstitution Graves' disease may occur as a late (9–48 months) complication of HAART. In advanced HIV disease, infection of the thyroid gland may occur with opportunistic pathogens, including *P. jiroveci*, CMV, mycobacteria, *Toxoplasma gondii*, and *Cryptococcus neoformans*. These infections are generally associated with a nontender, diffuse enlargement of the thyroid gland. Thyroid function is usually normal. Diagnosis is made by fine-needle aspirate or open biopsy.

Advanced HIV disease is associated with *hypogonadism* in ~50% of men. Although this is generally a complication of underlying illness, testicular dysfunction may also be a side effect of ganciclovir therapy. In some surveys, up to two-thirds of patients report decreased libido and one-third complain of impotence. Androgen-replacement therapy should be considered in patients with symptomatic hypogonadism. HIV infection does not seem to have a significant effect on the menstrual cycle outside the setting of advanced disease.

Rheumatologic Diseases

Immunologic and rheumatologic disorders are common in patients with HIV infection and range from excessive immediate-type hypersensitivity reactions to an increase in the incidence of reactive arthritis to conditions characterized by a diffuse infiltrative lymphocytosis. The occurrence of these phenomena is an apparent paradox in the setting of the profound immunodeficiency and immunosuppression that characterizes HIV infection.

Drug allergies are the most significant allergic reactions occurring in HIV-infected patients and appear to become more common as the disease progresses. They occur in up to 65% of patients who receive therapy with TMP/SMX for PCP. In general, these drug reactions are characterized by erythematous, morbilliform eruptions that are pruritic, tend to coalesce, and are often associated with fever. Nonetheless, ~33% of patients can be maintained on the offending therapy, and thus these reactions are not an immediate indication to stop the drug. Anaphylaxis is extremely rare in patients with HIV infection, and patients who have a cutaneous reaction during a single course of therapy can still be considered candidates for future treatment or prophylaxis with the same agent. The one exception to this is the nucleoside analogue abacavir, where fatal hypersensitivity reactions have been reported with rechallenge. This hypersensitivity is strongly associated with the HLA-B57 haplotype and a hypersensitivity reaction to abacavir is an absolute contraindication to future therapy. For other agents, including TMP/SMX, desensitization regimens are moderately successful. Although the mechanisms underlying these allergic-type reactions remain unknown, patients with HIV infection have been noted to have elevated IgE levels that increase as the CD4+ T-cell count declines. The numerous examples of patients with multiple drug reactions suggest that a common pathway is involved.

HIV infection shares many similarities with a variety of autoimmune diseases, including a substantial polyclonal B-cell activation that is associated with a high incidence of antiphospholipid antibodies, such as anticardiolipin antibodies, VDRL antibodies, and lupus-like anticoagulants. In addition, HIV-infected individuals have an increased incidence of antinuclear antibodies. Despite these serologic findings, there is no evidence that HIV-infected individuals have an increase in two of the more common autoimmune diseases, i.e., systemic lupus erythematosus and rheumatoid arthritis. In fact, it has been observed that these diseases may be somewhat ameliorated by the concomitant presence of HIV infection, suggesting that an intact CD4+ T-cell limb of the immune response plays an integral role in the pathogenesis of these conditions. Similarly, there are anecdotal reports of patients with common variable immunodeficiency, characterized by hypogammaglobulinemia, who have had a normalization of Ig levels after the development of HIV infection, suggesting a possible role for overactive CD4+ T-cell immunity in certain forms of that syndrome. The one autoimmune disease that may occur with an increased frequency in patients with HIV infection is a variant of primary Sjögren's syndrome. Patients with HIV infection may develop a syndrome consisting of parotid gland enlargement, dry eyes, and dry mouth that is associated with lymphocytic infiltrates of the salivary gland and lung. In contrast to Sjögren's syndrome, in which these infiltrates are composed predominantly of CD4+ T cells, in patients with HIV infection, the infiltrates are composed predominantly of CD8+ T cells. In addition, although patients with Sjögren's syndrome are mainly women who have autoantibodies to Ro and La and who frequently have HLA-DR3 or -B8 MHC haplotypes, HIV-infected individuals with this syndrome are usually African-American men who do not have anti-Ro or anti-La and who most often are HLA-DR5. This syndrome appears to be less common with the increased use of effective ARV therapy. The term *diffuse infiltrative lymphocytosis syndrome* (DILS) has been proposed to describe this entity and to distinguish it from Sjögren's syndrome.

Approximately one-third of HIV-infected individuals experience arthralgias; furthermore, 5–10% are diagnosed as having some form of reactive arthritis, such as Reiter's syndrome or psoriatic arthritis. These syndromes occur with increasing frequency as the competency of the immune system declines. This association may be related to an increase in the number of infections with organisms that may trigger a reactive arthritis with progressive immunodeficiency or to a loss of important regulatory T cells. Reactive arthritides in HIV-infected individuals generally respond well to standard treatment; however, therapy with methotrexate has been associated with an increase in the incidence of opportunistic infections and should be used with caution and only in severe cases.

HIV-infected individuals also experience a variety of joint problems without obvious cause that are referred to generically as *HIV-* or *AIDS-associated arthropathy*. This syndrome is characterized by subacute oligoarticular arthritis developing over a period of 1–6 weeks and lasting 6 weeks to 6 months. It generally involves the large joints, predominantly the knees and ankles, and is nonerosive with only a mild inflammatory response. X-rays of the joint are nonrevealing. Nonsteroidal anti-inflammatory drugs are only marginally helpful; however, relief has been noted with the use of intraarticular glucocorticoids. A second form of arthritis also thought to be secondary to HIV infection is called *painful articular syndrome*. This condition, reported as occurring in as many as 10% of AIDS patients, presents as an acute, severe, sharp pain in the affected joint. It affects primarily the knees, elbows, and shoulders; lasts 2–24 h; and may be severe enough to require narcotic analgesics. The cause of this arthropathy is unclear; however, it is thought to result from a direct effect of HIV on the joint. This condition is reminiscent of the fact that other lentiviruses, in particular the caprine arthritis-encephalitis virus, are capable of directly causing arthritis.

A variety of other immunologic or rheumatologic diseases have been reported in HIV-infected individuals, either de novo or in association with opportunistic infections or drugs. Using the criteria of widespread musculoskeletal pain of at least 3 months' duration and the presence of at least 11 of 18 possible tender points by digital palpation, 11% of an HIV-infected cohort containing 55% IDUs were diagnosed as having *fibromyalgia*. Although the incidence of frank arthritis was less in this population than in other studied populations that consisted predominantly of homosexual men, these data support the concept that there are musculoskeletal problems that occur as a direct result of HIV infection. In addition, there have been reports of leukocytoclastic vasculitis in the setting of zidovudine therapy. CNS angiitis and polymyositis have also been reported in HIV-infected individuals. Septic arthritis is surprisingly rare, especially given the increased incidence of staphylococcal bacteremias seen in this population. When septic arthritis has been reported, it has usually been due to *Staphylococcus aureus*, systemic fungal infections with *C. neoformans*, *Sporothrix schenckii*, or *H. capsulatum* or to systemic mycobacterial infection with *M. tuberculosis, M. haemophilum, M. avium*, or *M. kansasii*.

As noted above, 4.4% of patients with HIV infection were found to have some evidence of osteonecrosis by MRI during systematic screening of asymptomatic patients. The percentage of patients with symptomatic osteonecrosis has been estimated to be as high as 1%. Although this problem was first recognized in the setting of HAART, it has been difficult to establish a cause-and-effect relationship. Alcohol consumption and a history of glucocorticoid use have been particularly associated with this condition in patients with HIV infection.

Immune Reconstitution Inflammatory Syndrome

After the initiation of effective ARV therapy, a paradoxical worsening of preexisting, untreated, or partially treated opportunistic infections may be noted (Table 90-9). These IRISs are particularly common in patients with underlying untreated mycobacterial infections. They are seen in anywhere from 10–50% of patients, depending upon the clinical setting, and are most common in patients starting therapy with CD4+ T-cell counts <50 cells/μL who have a precipitous drop in HIV RNA levels after the initiation of HAART. Signs and symptoms may appear anywhere from 2 weeks to 2 years after the initiation of HAART and can include localized lymphadenitis, prolonged fever, pulmonary infiltrates, increased intracranial pressure, uveitis, and Graves' disease. The clinical course can be protracted and severe cases can be fatal. The underlying mechanism appears to be related to a phenomenon similar to type IV hypersensitivity reactions and reflects the immediate improvements in immune function that occur as levels of HIV RNA drop and the immunosuppressive effects of HIV infection are controlled. In severe cases, the use of immunosuppressive drugs such as glucocorticoids may be required to blunt the inflammatory component of these reactions while specific antimicrobial therapy takes effect.

Diseases of the Hematopoietic System

Disorders of the hematopoietic system including lymphadenopathy, anemia, leukopenia, and/or thrombocytopenia are common throughout the course of HIV

TABLE 90-9

CHARACTERISTICS OF IMMUNE RECONSTITUTION INFLAMMATORY SYNDROME (IRIS)

- Paradoxical worsening of clinical condition after the initiation of antiretroviral therapy
- Occurs weeks to months after the initiation of antiretroviral therapy
- Most common in patients starting therapy with a CD4+ T-cell count under 50/μL who experience a precipitous drop in viral load
- Frequently seen in the setting of tuberculosis
- Can be fatal

TABLE 90-10

CAUSES OF BONE MARROW SUPPRESSION IN PATIENTS WITH HIV INFECTION

HIV infection	Medications
Mycobacterial infections	Zidovudine
Fungal infections	Dapsone
B19 parvovirus infection	Trimethoprim/sulfamethoxazole
Lymphoma	Pyrimethamine
	5-Flucytosine
	Ganciclovir
	Interferon-α
	Trimetrexate
	Foscarnet

infection and may be the direct result of HIV, manifestations of secondary infections and neoplasms, or side effects of therapy (Table 90-10). Direct histologic examination and culture of lymph node or bone marrow tissue are often diagnostic. A significant percentage of bone marrow aspirates from patients with HIV infection have been reported to contain lymphoid aggregates, the precise significance of which is unknown. Initiation of HAART will lead to reversal of most hematologic complications that are the direct result of HIV infection.

Some patients, otherwise asymptomatic, may develop *persistent generalized lymphadenopathy* as an early clinical manifestation of HIV infection. This condition is defined as the presence of enlarged lymph nodes (>1 cm) in two or more extrainguinal sites for >3 months without an obvious cause. The lymphadenopathy is due to marked follicular hyperplasia in the node in response to HIV infection. The nodes are generally discrete and freely movable. This feature of HIV disease may be seen at any point in the spectrum of immune dysfunction and is not associated with an increased likelihood of developing AIDS. Paradoxically, a loss in lymphadenopathy or a decrease in lymph node size outside the setting of ARV therapy may be a prognostic marker of disease progression. In patients with CD4+ T-cell counts >200/μL, the differential diagnosis of lymphadenopathy includes KS, TB, Castleman's disease, and lymphoma. In patients with more advanced disease, lymphadenopathy may also be due to atypical mycobacterial infection, toxoplasmosis, systemic fungal infection, or bacillary angiomatosis. Although indicated in patients with CD4+ T-cell counts <200/μL, lymph node biopsy is not indicated in patients with early-stage disease unless there are signs and symptoms of systemic illness, such as fever and weight loss, or unless the nodes begin to enlarge, become fixed, or coalesce. Monoclonal gammopathy of unknown significance (MGUS), defined as the presence of a serum monoclonal IgG, IgA, or IgM in the absence of a clear cause, has been reported in 3% of patients with HIV infection. The overall clinical significance of this finding in patients with HIV infection is unclear, although it has been associated with other viral infections, non-Hodgkin's lymphoma, and plasma cell malignancy.

Anemia is the most common hematologic abnormality in HIV-infected patients and in the absence of a specific treatable cause is independently associated with a poor prognosis. Although generally mild, anemia can be quite severe and require chronic blood transfusions. Among the specific reversible causes of anemia in the setting of HIV infection are drug toxicity, systemic fungal and mycobacterial infections, nutritional deficiencies, and parvovirus B19 infections. Zidovudine may block erythroid maturation, before its effects on other marrow elements. A characteristic feature of zidovudine therapy is an elevated mean corpuscular volume (MCV). Another drug used in patients with HIV infection that has a selective effect on the erythroid series is dapsone. This drug can cause a serious hemolytic anemia in patients who are deficient in glucose-6-phosphate dehydrogenase and can create a functional anemia in others through induction of methemoglobinemia. Folate levels are usually normal in HIV-infected individuals; however, vitamin B_{12} levels may be depressed as a consequence of achlorhydria or malabsorption. True autoimmune hemolytic anemia is rare, although ~20% of patients with HIV infection may have a positive direct antiglobulin test as a consequence of polyclonal B-cell activation. Infection with parvovirus B19 may also cause anemia. It is important to recognize this possibility given the fact that it responds well to treatment with IVIg. Erythropoietin levels in patients with HIV infection and anemia are generally less than expected given the degree of anemia. Treatment with erythropoietin at doses of 100 μg/kg three times a week may result in an increase in hemoglobulin levels. An exception to this is a subset of patients with zidovudine-associated anemia in whom erythropoietin levels may be quite high.

During the course of HIV infection, neutropenia may be seen in approximately half of patients. In most instances it is mild; however, it can be severe and can put patients at risk of spontaneous bacterial infections. This is most frequently seen in patients with severely advanced HIV disease and in patients receiving any of a number of potentially myelosuppressive therapies. In the setting of neutropenia, diseases that are not commonly seen in HIV-infected patients, such as aspergillosis or mucormycosis, may occur. The potential role of colony-stimulating factors in the management of patients with HIV infection has undergone extensive evaluation. Both granulocyte colony-stimulating factor (G-CSF) and GM-CSF increase neutrophil counts in patients with HIV infection regardless of the cause of the neutropenia. Earlier concerns about the potential of these agents to also increase levels of HIV were not confirmed in controlled clinical trials.

Thrombocytopenia may be an early consequence of HIV infection. Approximately 3% of patients with untreated HIV infection and CD4+ T-cell counts ≥400/μL have platelet counts <150,000/μL. For untreated patients with CD4+ T-cell counts <400/μL, this incidence increases to 10%. Thrombocytopenia is rarely a serious clinical problem in patients with HIV infection and generally responds well to ARV therapy. Clinically, it resembles the thrombocytopenia seen in patients with idiopathic thrombocytopenic purpura. Immune complexes containing anti-gp120 antibodies and anti-anti-gp120 antibodies have been noted in the circulation and on the surface of platelets in patients with HIV infection. Patients with HIV infection have also been noted to have a platelet-specific antibody directed toward a 25-kDa component of the surface of the platelet. Other data suggest that the thrombocytopenia in patients with HIV infection may be due to a direct effect of HIV on megakaryocytes. Whatever the cause, it is very clear that the most effective medical approach to this problem has been the use of HAART. For patients with platelet counts <20,000/μL a more aggressive approach combining IVIg or anti-Rh Ig for an immediate response with ARV therapy for a more lasting response is appropriate. Rituximab has been used with some success in otherwise refractory cases. Splenectomy is a rarely needed option and is reserved for patients refractory to medical management. Because of the risk of serious infection with encapsulated organisms, all patients with HIV infection about to undergo splenectomy should be immunized with pneumococcal polysaccharide. It should be noted that, in addition to causing an increase in the platelet count, removal of the spleen will result in an increase in the peripheral blood lymphocyte count, making CD4+ T-cell counts unreliable. In this setting, the clinician should rely on the CD4+ T-cell percent for making diagnostic decisions with respect to the likelihood of opportunistic infections. A CD4+ T-cell percent of 15 is approximately equivalent to a CD4+ T-cell count of 200/μL. In patients with early HIV infection, thrombocytopenia has also been reported as a consequence of classic thrombotic thrombocytopenic purpura. This clinical syndrome, consisting of fever, thrombocytopenia, hemolytic anemia, and neurologic and renal dysfunction, is a rare complication of early HIV infection. As in other settings, the appropriate management is the use of salicylates and plasma exchange. Other causes of thrombocytopenia include lymphoma, mycobacterial infections, and fungal infections.

Approximately 4% of patients with HIV infection experience venous thrombotic events such as deep vein thrombosis or pulmonary embolism. Among the factors associated with clinical thrombosis are age over 45, history of an opportunistic infection, and estrogen use.

Abnormalities of the coagulation cascade including decreased protein S activity, increases in factor VIII, and the presence of anticardiolipin antibodies have been reported in patients with HIV infection.

Elevations in D-dimer appear predictive of a poor clinical outcome.

Dermatologic Diseases

Dermatologic problems occur in >90% of patients with HIV infection. From the macular, roseola-like rash seen with the acute seroconversion syndrome to extensive end-stage KS, cutaneous manifestations of HIV disease can be seen throughout the course of HIV infection. Among the more common nonneoplastic problems are seborrheic dermatitis, folliculitis, and opportunistic infections. Extrapulmonary pneumocystosis may cause a necrotizing vasculitis. Neoplastic conditions are covered below in the section on malignant diseases.

Seborrheic dermatitis occurs in 3% of the general population and in up to 50% of patients with HIV infection. Seborrheic dermatitis increases in prevalence and severity as the CD4+ T-cell count declines. In HIV-infected patients, seborrheic dermatitis may be aggravated by concomitant infection with *Pityrosporum*, a yeastlike fungus; use of topical antifungal agents has been recommended in cases refractory to standard topical treatment.

Folliculitis is among the most prevalent dermatologic disorders in patients with HIV infection and is seen in ~20% of patients. It is more common in patients with CD4+ T-cell counts <200 cells/μL. One form of folliculitis, *eosinophilic pustular folliculitis,* is a rare dermatologic condition that is seen with increased frequency in patients with HIV infection. It presents as multiple, urticarial perifollicular papules that may coalesce into plaquelike lesions. Skin biopsy reveals an eosinophilic infiltrate of the hair follicle, which in certain cases has been associated with the presence of a mite. Patients typically have an elevated serum IgE level and may respond to treatment with topical antihelminthics. Pruritus is a common symptom in patients with HIV infection and can lead to prurigo nodularis. Patients with HIV infection have also been reported to develop a severe form of *Norwegian scabies* with hyperkeratotic psoriasiform lesions.

Both *psoriasis* and *ichthyosis*, although they are not reported to be increased in frequency, may be particularly severe when they occur in patients with HIV infection. Preexisting psoriasis may become guttate in appearance and more refractory to treatment in the setting of HIV infection.

Reactivation herpes zoster (*shingles*) is seen in 10–20% of patients with HIV infection. This reactivation syndrome of varicella-zoster virus indicates a modest decline in immune function and may be the first indication of clinical immunodeficiency. In one series, patients who developed shingles did so an average of 5 years after HIV infection. In a cohort of patients with HIV infection and localized zoster, the subsequent rate of the development of AIDS was 1% per month. In that study, AIDS was more likely to develop if the outbreak of zoster was associated with severe pain, extensive skin involvement, or involvement of cranial or cervical dermatomes. The clinical manifestations of reactivation zoster in HIV-infected patients, although indicative of immunologic compromise, are not as severe as those seen in other immunodeficient conditions. Thus, although lesions may extend over several dermatomes and frank cutaneous dissemination may be seen, visceral involvement has not been reported. In contrast to patients without a known underlying immunodeficiency state, patients with HIV infection tend to have recurrences of zoster with a relapse rate of ~20%. Acyclovir or famciclovir is the treatment of choice. Foscarnet may be of value in patients with acyclovir-resistant virus.

Infection with *herpes simplex virus* in HIV-infected individuals is associated with recurrent orolabial, genital, and perianal lesions as part of recurrent reactivation syndromes (Chap. 80). As HIV disease progresses and the CD4+ T-cell count declines, these infections become more frequent and severe. Lesions often appear as beefy red, are exquisitely painful, and have a tendency to occur high in the gluteal cleft (Fig. 90-35). Perirectal HSV may be associated with proctitis and anal fissures. HSV should be high in the differential diagnosis of any HIV-infected patient with a poorly healing, painful perirectal lesion. In addition to recurrent mucosal ulcers, recurrent HSV infection in the form of *herpetic whitlow* can be a problem in patients with HIV infection, presenting with painful vesicles or extensive cutaneous erosion. Acyclovir or famciclovir is the treatment of choice in these settings. Of note is the fact that even subclinical reactivation of herpes simplex may be associated with increases in plasma HIV RNA levels. In a cohort of patients from Burkina Faso seropositive for HIV-1 and HSV-2 with CD4+ T-cell counts >200 cells/μL, chronic use of valacyclovir was associated with a 0.5-log decrease in HIV viral load. Thus consideration should be given to chronic suppressive therapy in patients with recurrent outbreaks of herpesvirus.

Diffuse skin eruptions due to *Molluscum contagiosum* may be seen in patients with advanced HIV infection. These flesh-colored, umbilicated lesions may be treated with local therapy. They tend to regress with effective ARV therapy. Similarly, *condyloma acuminatum* lesions may be more severe and more widely distributed in patients with low CD4+ T-cell counts. Atypical mycobacterial infections may present as erythematous cutaneous nodules, as may fungal infections, *Bartonella*, *Acanthamoeba*, and KS.

The skin of patients with HIV infection is often a target organ for drug reactions. Although most skin reactions are mild and not necessarily an indication to discontinue therapy, patients may have particularly severe cutaneous reactions, including erythroderma and *Stevens-Johnson syndrome*, as a reaction to drugs, particularly sulfa drugs, the nonnucleoside reverse transcriptase inhibitors, abacavir, amprenavir, darunavir, fosamprenavir, and tipranavir. Similarly, patients with HIV infection are often quite photosensitive and burn easily after exposure to sunlight or as a side effect of radiation therapy.

HIV infection and its treatment may be accompanied by cosmetic changes of the skin that are not of great clinical importance but may be troubling to patients. Yellowing of the nails and straightening of the hair, particularly in African-American patients, have been reported as a consequence of HIV infection. Zidovudine therapy has been associated with elongation of the eyelashes and the development of a bluish discoloration to the nails, again more common in African-American patients. Therapy with clofazimine may cause a yellow-orange discoloration of the skin and urine.

Neurologic Diseases

Clinical disease of the nervous system accounts for a significant degree of morbidity in a high percentage of patients with HIV infection (Table 90-11). The neurologic problems that occur in HIV-infected individuals may be either primary to the pathogenic processes of HIV infection or secondary to opportunistic infections or neoplasms (see above). Among the more frequent opportunistic diseases that involve the CNS are toxoplasmosis,

TABLE 90-11

NEUROLOGIC DISEASES IN PATIENTS WITH HIV INFECTION

Opportunistic infections	Myelopathy
Toxoplasmosis	Vacuolar myelopathy
Cryptococcosis	Pure sensory ataxia
Progressive multifocal leukoencephalopathy	Paresthesia/dysesthesia
Cytomegalovirus	Peripheral neuropathy
Syphilis	Acute inflammatory demyelinating polyneuropathy (Guillain-Barré syndrome)
Mycobacterium tuberculosis	Chronic inflammatory demyelinating polyneuropathy (CIDP)
HTLV-I infection	Mononeuritis multiplex
Neoplasms	Distal symmetric polyneuropathy
Primary CNS lymphoma	Myopathy
Kaposi's sarcoma	
Result of HIV-1 infection	
Aseptic meningitis	
HIV-associated neurocognitive impairment, including HIV encephalopathy/AIDS dementia complex	

cryptococcosis, progressive multifocal leukoencephalopathy, and primary CNS lymphoma. Other less common problems include mycobacterial infections; syphilis; and infection with CMV, HTLV-I, *T. cruzi*, or *Acanthamoeba*. Overall, secondary diseases of the CNS occur in approximately one-third of patients with AIDS. These data antedate the widespread use of combination ARV therapy, and this frequency is considerably less in patients receiving effective ARV drugs. Primary processes related to HIV infection of the nervous system are reminiscent of those seen with other lentiviruses, such as the Visna-Maedi virus of sheep.

Neurologic problems directly attributable to HIV occur throughout the course of infection and may be inflammatory, demyelinating, or degenerative in nature. The term *HIV-associated neurocognitive impairment* (HNCI) is used to describe a spectrum of disorders that range from asymptomatic to apparent only through extensive neuropsychiatric testing to clinically severe. The most severe form, the *AIDS dementia complex*, or *HIV encephalopathy*, is considered an AIDS-defining illness. Most HIV-infected patients have some neurologic problem during the course of their disease. As noted in the section on pathogenesis, damage to the CNS may be a direct result of viral infection of the CNS macrophages or glial cells or may be secondary to the release of neurotoxins and potentially toxic cytokines such as IL-1β, TNF-α, IL-6, and TGF-β. It has been reported that HIV-infected individuals with the E4 allele for apo E are at increased risk for AIDS encephalopathy and peripheral neuropathy. Virtually all patients with HIV infection have some degree of nervous system involvement with the virus. This is evidenced by the fact that CSF findings are abnormal in ~90% of patients, even during the asymptomatic phase of HIV infection. CSF abnormalities include pleocytosis (50–65% of patients), detection of viral RNA (~75%), elevated CSF protein (35%), and evidence of intrathecal synthesis of anti-HIV antibodies (90%). It is important to point out that evidence of infection of the CNS with HIV does not imply impairment of cognitive function. The neurologic function of an HIV-infected individual should be considered normal unless clinical signs and symptoms suggest otherwise.

Aseptic meningitis may be seen in any but the very late stages of HIV infection. In the setting of acute primary infection patients may experience a syndrome of headache, photophobia, and meningismus. Rarely, an acute encephalopathy due to encephalitis may occur. Cranial nerve involvement may be seen, predominantly cranial nerve VII but occasionally V and/or VIII. CSF findings include a lymphocytic pleocytosis, elevated protein level, and normal glucose level. This syndrome, which cannot be clinically differentiated from other viral meningitides (Chap. 30), usually resolves spontaneously within 2–4 weeks; however, in some patients, signs and symptoms may become chronic. Aseptic meningitis may occur any time in the course of HIV infection; however, it is rare after the development of AIDS. This fact suggests that clinical aseptic meningitis in the context of HIV infection is an immune-mediated disease.

C. neoformans is the leading infectious cause of meningitis in patients with AIDS (Chap. 106). It is the initial AIDS-defining illness in ~2% of patients and generally occurs in patients with CD4+ T-cell counts <100/μL. Cryptococcal meningitis is particularly common in patients with AIDS in Africa, occurring in ~20% of patients. Most patients present with a picture of subacute meningoencephalitis with fever, nausea, vomiting, altered mental status, headache, and meningeal signs. The incidence of seizures and focal neurologic deficits is low. The CSF profile may be normal or may show only modest elevations in WBC or protein levels and decreases in glucose. In addition to meningitis, patients may develop cryptococcomas and cranial nerve involvement. Approximately one-third of patients also have pulmonary disease. Uncommon manifestations of cryptococcal infection include skin lesions that resemble *molluscum contagiosum*, lymphadenopathy, palatal and glossal ulcers, arthritis, gastroenteritis, myocarditis, and prostatitis. The prostate gland may serve as a reservoir for smoldering cryptococcal infection. The diagnosis of cryptococcal meningitis is made by identification of organisms in spinal fluid with India ink examination or by the detection of cryptococcal antigen. A biopsy may be needed to make a diagnosis of CNS cryptococcoma. Treatment is with IV amphotericin B, at a dose of 0.7 mg/kg daily, with flucytosine, 25 mg/kg qid for 2 weeks, followed by fluconazole, 400 mg/d PO for 10 weeks, and then fluconazole, 200 mg/d until the CD4+ T-cell count has increased to >200 cells/μL for 6 months in response to HAART. Repeated lumbar puncture may be required to manage increased intracranial pressure. Symptoms may recur with initiation of HAART as an immune reconstitution syndrome (see above). Other fungi that may cause meningitis in patients with HIV infection are *C. immitis* and *H. capsulatum*. Meningoencephalitis has also been reported due to *Acanthamoeba* or *Naegleria*.

HIV encephalopathy, also called HIV-associated dementia or AIDS dementia complex, consists of a constellation of signs and symptoms of CNS disease. Although this is generally a late complication of HIV infection that progresses slowly over months, it can be seen in patients with CD4+ T-cell counts >350 cells/μL. A major feature of this entity is the development of dementia, defined as a decline in cognitive ability from a previous level. It may present as impaired ability to concentrate, increased forgetfulness, difficulty reading, or increased difficulty performing complex tasks. Initially these symptoms may be indistinguishable from findings of situational depression or fatigue. In contrast to "cortical" dementia (such as Alzheimer's disease), aphasia, apraxia, and agnosia are uncommon, leading some investigators to classify HIV encephalopathy as a "subcortical dementia" (see below). In addition to dementia, patients with HIV encephalopathy may also have motor and behavioral abnormalities. Among the motor problems are unsteady gait, poor balance, tremor, and difficulty with rapid alternating movements. Increased tone and deep tendon reflexes may be found in patients with spinal cord involvement. Late stages may be complicated by bowel and/or bladder incontinence. Behavioral problems include apathy and lack of initiative, with progression to a vegetative state in some instances. Some patients develop a state of agitation or mild mania. These changes usually occur without significant changes in level of alertness. This is in contrast to the finding of somnolence in patients with dementia due to toxic/metabolic encephalopathies.

HIV encephalopathy is the initial AIDS-defining illness in ~3% of patients with HIV infection and thus only rarely precedes clinical evidence of immunodeficiency. Clinically significant encephalopathy eventually develops in ~25% of patients with AIDS. As immunologic function declines, the risk and severity of HIV encephalopathy increase. Autopsy series suggest that 80–90% of patients with HIV infection have histologic evidence of CNS involvement. Several classification schemes have been developed for grading HIV encephalopathy; a commonly used clinical staging system is outlined in Table 90-12.

The precise cause of HIV encephalopathy remains unclear, although the condition is thought to be a result of a combination of direct effects of HIV on the CNS and associated immune activation. HIV has been found in the brains of patients with HIV encephalopathy by Southern blot, in situ hybridization, PCR, and electron microscopy. Multinucleated giant cells, macrophages, and microglial cells appear to be the main cell types harboring virus in the CNS. Histologically, the major changes are seen in the subcortical areas of the brain and include pallor and gliosis, multinucleated giant cell encephalitis, and vacuolar myelopathy. Less commonly, diffuse or focal spongiform changes occur in the white matter. Areas of the brain involved in motor, language, and judgment are most severely affected.

There are no specific criteria for a diagnosis of HIV encephalopathy, and this syndrome must be differentiated from a number of other diseases that affect the CNS of HIV-infected patients (Table 90-11). The diagnosis of dementia depends upon demonstrating a decline in cognitive function. This can be accomplished objectively with the use of a Mini-Mental Status Examination (MMSE) in patients for whom prior scores are available. For this reason, it is advisable for all patients with a diagnosis of HIV infection to have a baseline MMSE. However, changes in MMSE scores may be absent in patients with mild HIV encephalopathy. Imaging studies of the CNS, by either MRI or CT, often demonstrate evidence of cerebral atrophy (Fig. 90-37). MRI may also reveal small areas of increased density on T2-weighted images. Lumbar puncture is an important element of the evaluation of patients with HIV infection and neurologic

TABLE 90-12

CLINICAL STAGING OF HIV ENCEPHALOPATHY (AIDS DEMENTIA COMPLEX)

STAGE	DEFINITION
Stage 0 (normal)	Normal mental and motor function
Stage 0.5 (equivocal/subclinical)	Absent, minimal, or equivocal symptoms without impairment of work or capacity to perform activities of daily living. Mild signs (snout response, slowed ocular or extremity movements) may be present. Gait and strength are normal.
Stage 1 (mild)	Able to perform all but the more demanding aspects of work or activities of daily living but with unequivocal evidence (signs or symptoms that may include performance on neuropsychological testing) of functional, intellectual, or motor impairment. Can walk without assistance.
Stage 2 (moderate)	Able to perform basic activities of self-care but cannot work or maintain the more demanding aspects of daily life. Ambulatory, but may require a single prop.
Stage 3 (severe)	Major intellectual incapacity (cannot follow news or personal events, cannot sustain complex conversation, considerable slowing of all output) or motor disability (cannot walk unassisted, usually with slowing and clumsiness of arms as well).
Stage 4 (end-stage)	Nearly vegetative. Intellectual and social comprehension and output are at a rudimentary level. Nearly or absolutely mute. Paraparetic or paraplegic with urinary and fecal incontinence.

Source: Adapted from JJ Sidtis, RW Price, Neurology 40:197, 1990.

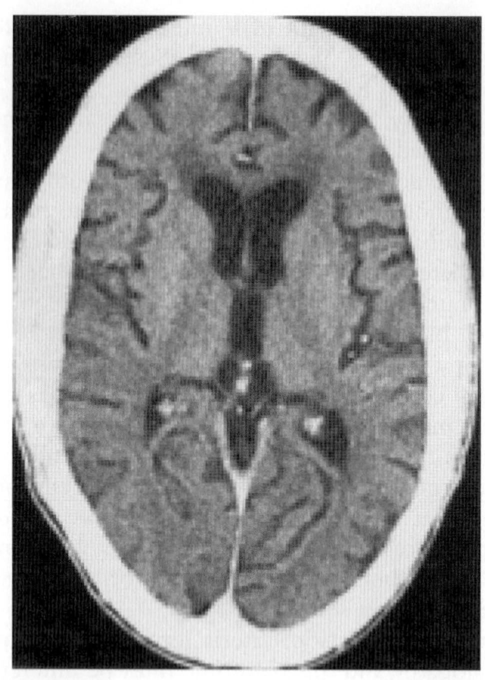

FIGURE 90-37
AIDS dementia complex. Postcontrast CT scan through the lateral ventricles of a 47-year-old man with AIDS, altered mental status, and dementia. The lateral and third ventricles and the cerebral sulci are abnormally prominent. Mild white matter hypodensity is also seen adjacent to the frontal horns of the lateral ventricles.

abnormalities. It is generally most helpful in ruling out or making a diagnosis of opportunistic infections. In HIV encephalopathy, patients may have the nonspecific findings of an increase in CSF cells and protein level. Although HIV RNA can often be detected in the spinal fluid and HIV can be cultured from the CSF, this finding is not specific for HIV encephalopathy. There appears to be no correlation between the presence of HIV in the CSF and the presence of HIV encephalopathy. Elevated levels of macrophage chemoattractant protein (MCP-1), β_2-microglobulin, neopterin, and quinolinic acid (a metabolite of tryptophan reported to cause CNS injury) have been noted in the CSF of patients with HIV encephalopathy. These findings suggest that these factors as well as inflammatory cytokines may be involved in the pathogenesis of this syndrome.

Combination ARV therapy is of benefit in patients with HIV encephalopathy. Improvement in neuropsychiatric test scores has been noted for both adult and pediatric patients treated with ARVs. The rapid improvement in cognitive function noted with the initiation of ARV therapy suggests that at least some component of this problem is quickly reversible, again supporting at least a partial role of soluble mediators in the pathogenesis. It should also be noted that these patients have an increased sensitivity to the side effects of neuroleptic drugs. The use of these drugs for symptomatic treatment is associated with an increased risk of extrapyramidal side effects; therefore, patients with HIV encephalopathy who receive these agents must be monitored carefully.

Seizures may be a consequence of opportunistic infections, neoplasms, or HIV encephalopathy (Table 90-13). The seizure threshold is often lower than normal in patients with advanced HIV infection due to the frequent presence of electrolyte abnormalities. Seizures are seen in 15–40% of patients with cerebral toxoplasmosis, 15–35% of patients with primary CNS lymphoma, 8% of patients with cryptococcal meningitis, and 7–50% of patients with HIV encephalopathy. Seizures may also be seen in patients with CNS tuberculosis, aseptic meningitis, and progressive multifocal leukoencephalopathy. Seizures may be the presenting clinical symptom of HIV disease. In one study of 100 patients with HIV infection presenting with a first seizure, cerebral mass lesions were the most common cause, responsible for 32 of the 100 new-onset seizures. Of these 32 cases, 28 were due to toxoplasmosis and 4 to lymphoma. HIV encephalopathy accounted for an additional 24 new-onset seizures. Cryptococcal meningitis was the third most common diagnosis, responsible for 13 of the 100 seizures. In 23 cases, no cause could be found, and it is possible that these cases represent a subcategory of HIV encephalopathy. Of these 23 cases, 16 (70%) had two or more seizures, suggesting that anticonvulsant therapy is indicated in all patients with HIV infection and seizures unless a rapidly correctable cause is found. Although phenytoin remains the initial treatment of choice, hypersensitivity reactions to this drug have been

TABLE 90-13

CAUSES OF SEIZURES IN PATIENTS WITH HIV INFECTION

DISEASE	OVERALL CONTRIBUTION TO FIRST SEIZURE, %	FRACTION OF PATIENTS WHO HAVE SEIZURES, %
HIV encephalopathy	24–47	7–50
Cerebral toxoplasmosis	28	15–40
Cryptococcal meningitis	13	8
Primary central nervous system lymphoma	4	15–30
Progressive multifocal leukoencephalopathy	1	

Source: From DM Holtzman et al: Am J Med 87:173, 1989.

reported in >10% of patients with AIDS, and therefore the use of phenobarbital or valproic acid must be considered as alternatives.

Patients with HIV infection may present with *focal neurologic deficits* from a variety of causes. The most common causes are toxoplasmosis, progressive multifocal leukoencephalopathy, and CNS lymphoma. Other causes include cryptococcal infections (discussed above; also Chap. 106), stroke, and reactivation Chagas' disease.

Toxoplasmosis has been one of the most common causes of secondary CNS infections in patients with AIDS, but its incidence is decreasing in the era of HAART. It is most common in patients from the Caribbean and from France. Toxoplasmosis is generally a late complication of HIV infection and usually occurs in patients with CD4+ T-cell counts <200/μL. Cerebral toxoplasmosis is thought to represent a reactivation syndrome. It is 10 times more common in patients with antibodies to the organism than in patients who are seronegative. Patients diagnosed with HIV infection should be screened for IgG antibodies to *T. gondii* during the time of their initial workup. Those who are seronegative should be counseled about ways to minimize the risk of primary infection including avoiding the consumption of undercooked meat and careful hand washing after contact with soil or changing the cat litter box. The most common clinical presentation of cerebral toxoplasmosis in patients with HIV infection is fever, headache, and focal neurologic deficits. Patients may present with seizure, hemiparesis, or aphasia as a manifestation of these focal deficits or with a picture more influenced by the accompanying cerebral edema and characterized by confusion, dementia, and lethargy, which can progress to coma. The diagnosis is usually suspected on the basis of MRI findings of multiple lesions in multiple locations, although in some cases only a single lesion is seen. Pathologically, these lesions generally exhibit inflammation and central necrosis and, as a result, demonstrate ring enhancement on contrast MRI (Fig. 90-38) or, if MRI is unavailable or contraindicated, on double-dose contrast CT. There is usually evidence of surrounding edema. In addition to toxoplasmosis, the differential diagnosis of single or multiple enhancing mass lesions in the HIV-infected patient includes primary CNS lymphoma (see below) and, less commonly, TB or fungal or bacterial abscesses. The definitive diagnostic procedure is brain biopsy. However, given the morbidity than can accompany this procedure, it is usually reserved for the patient who has failed 2–4 weeks of empirical therapy. If the patient is seronegative for *T. gondii*, the likelihood that a mass lesion is due to toxoplasmosis is <10%. In that setting, one may choose to be more aggressive and perform a brain biopsy sooner. Standard treatment is sulfadiazine and pyrimethamine with leucovorin as needed for a minimum of 4–6 weeks. Alternative therapeutic regimens include clindamycin in combination with pyrimethamine; atovaquone plus pyrimethamine; and azithromycin plus pyrimethamine plus rifabutin. Relapses are common, and it is recommended that patients with a history of prior toxoplasmic encephalitis receive maintenance therapy with sulfadiazine, pyrimethamine, and leucovorin as long as their CD4+ T-cell counts remain <200 cells/μL. Patients with CD4+ T-cell counts <100/μL and IgG antibody to *Toxoplasma* should

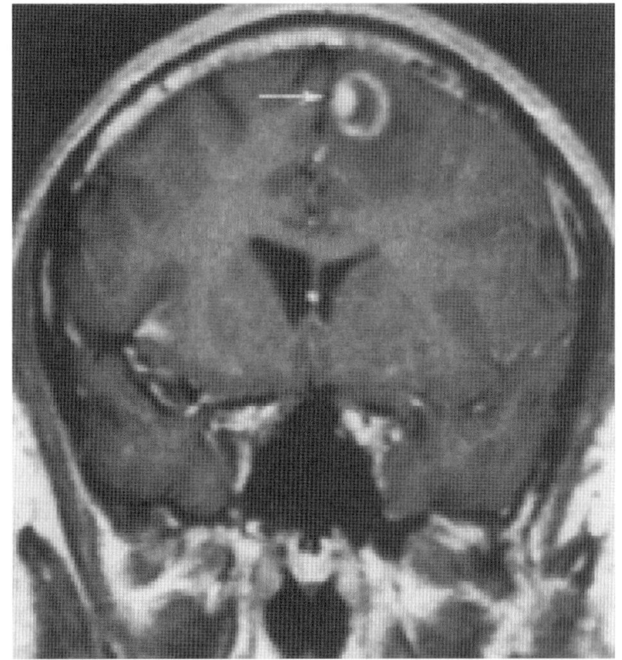

FIGURE 90-38

Central nervous system toxoplasmosis. A coronal post-contrast T1-weighted MR scan demonstrates a peripheral enhancing lesion in the left frontal lobe, associated with an eccentric nodular area of enhancement (*arrow*); this so-called eccentric target sign is typical of toxoplasmosis.

receive primary prophylaxis for toxoplasmosis. Fortunately, the same daily regimen of a single double-strength tablet of TMP/SMX used for *P. jiroveci* prophylaxis provides adequate primary protection against toxoplasmosis. Secondary prophylaxis/maintenance therapy for toxoplasmosis may be discontinued in the setting of effective ARV therapy and increases in CD4+ T-cell counts to >200/μL for 6 months.

JC virus, a human polyomavirus that is the etiologic agent of *progressive multifocal leukoencephalopathy* (PML), is an important opportunistic pathogen in patients with AIDS (Chap. 29). Although ~70% of the general adult population have antibodies to JC virus, indicative of prior infection, <10% of healthy adults show any evidence of ongoing viral replication. PML is the only known clinical manifestation of JC virus infection. It is a late manifestation of AIDS and is seen in ~4% of patients with AIDS. The lesions of PML begin as small foci of demyelination in subcortical white matter that eventually coalesce. The cerebral hemispheres, cerebellum, and brainstem may all be involved. Patients typically have a protracted course with multifocal neurologic deficits, with or without changes in mental status. Approximately 20% of patients experience seizures. Ataxia, hemiparesis, visual field defects, aphasia, and sensory defects may occur. MRI typically reveals multiple, nonenhancing white matter lesions that may coalesce and have a predilection for the occipital and parietal lobes. The lesions show signal hyperintensity on T2-weighted images and diminished signal on T1-weighted images. The measurement of JC virus DNA levels in CSF has a diagnostic sensitivity of 76% and a specificity of close to 100%. Before the availability of potent ARV combination therapy, the majority of patients with PML died within 3–6 months of the onset of symptoms. Paradoxical worsening of PML has been seen with initiation of HAART as an immune reconstitution syndrome. There is no specific treatment for PML; however, a minimal median survival of 18 months and survival of >7 years have been reported in patients with PML treated with HAART for their HIV disease. Unfortunately, only ~50% of patients with HIV infection and PML show neurologic improvement with HAART. Studies with other antiviral agents such as cidofovir have failed to show clear benefit. Factors influencing a favorable prognosis for PML in the setting of HIV infection include a CD4+ T-cell count >100/μL at baseline and the ability to maintain an HIV viral load of <500 copies per milliliter. Baseline HIV-1 viral load does not have independent predictive value of survival. PML is one of the few opportunistic infections that continues to occur with some frequency despite the widespread use of HAART.

Reactivation American trypanosomiasis may present as acute meningoencephalitis with focal neurologic signs, fever, headache, vomiting, and seizures. In South America, reactivation of *Chagas' disease* is considered to be an AIDS-defining condition and may be the initial AIDS-defining condition. Lesions appear radiographically as single or multiple hypodense areas, typically with ring enhancement and edema. They are found predominantly in the subcortical areas, a feature that differentiates them from the deeper lesions of toxoplasmosis. *Trypanosoma cruzi* amastigotes, or trypanosomes, can be identified from biopsy specimens or CSF. Other CSF findings include elevated protein and a mild (<100 cells/μL) lymphocytic pleocytosis. Organisms can also be identified by direct examination of the blood. Treatment consists of benzimidazole (2.5 mg/kg bid) or nifurtimox (2 mg/kg qid) for at least 60 days, followed by maintenance therapy for the duration of immunodeficiency with either drug at a dose of 5 mg/kg three times a week. As is the case with cerebral toxoplasmosis, successful therapy with ARVs may allow discontinuation of therapy for Chagas' disease.

Stroke may occur in patients with HIV infection. In contrast to the other causes of focal neurologic deficits in patients with HIV infection, the symptoms of a stroke are sudden in onset. Among the secondary infectious diseases in patients with HIV infection that may be associated with stroke are vasculitis due to cerebral varicella zoster or neurosyphilis and septic embolism in association with fungal infection. Other elements of the differential diagnosis of stroke in the patient with HIV infection include atherosclerotic cerebral vascular disease, thrombotic thrombocytopenic purpura, and cocaine or amphetamine use.

Primary CNS lymphoma is discussed below in the section on neoplastic diseases.

Spinal cord disease, or myelopathy, is present in ~20% of patients with AIDS, often as part of HIV encephalopathy. In fact, 90% of the patients with HIV-associated myelopathy have some evidence of dementia, suggesting that similar pathologic processes may be responsible for both conditions. Three main types of spinal cord disease are seen in patients with AIDS. The first of these is a vacuolar myelopathy, as discussed above under HIV encephalopathy. This condition is pathologically similar to subacute combined degeneration of the cord such as occurs with pernicious anemia. Although vitamin B_{12} deficiency can be seen in patients with AIDS as a primary complication of HIV infection, it does not appear to be responsible for the myelopathy seen in the majority of patients. Vacuolar myelopathy is characterized by a subacute onset and often presents with gait disturbances, predominantly ataxia and spasticity; it may progress to include bladder and bowel dysfunction. Physical findings include evidence of increased deep tendon reflexes and extensor plantar responses. The second form of spinal cord disease involves the dorsal columns and presents as a pure sensory ataxia. The third form is also sensory in nature and presents with paresthesias and dysesthesias of the lower extremities. In contrast to the cognitive problems seen in patients with HIV encephalopathy, these spinal cord syndromes do not respond well to ARV drugs, and therapy is mainly supportive.

One important disease of the spinal cord that also involves the peripheral nerves is a *myelopathy* and *polyradiculopathy* seen in association with CMV infection. This entity is generally seen late in the course of HIV infection and is fulminant in onset, with lower extremity and sacral paresthesias, difficulty in walking, areflexia, ascending sensory loss, and urinary retention. The clinical course is rapidly progressive over a period of weeks. CSF examination reveals a predominantly neutrophilic pleocytosis, and CMV DNA can be detected by CSF PCR. Therapy with ganciclovir or foscarnet can lead to rapid improvement, and prompt initiation of foscarnet or ganciclovir therapy is important in minimizing the degree of permanent neurologic damage. Combination therapy with both drugs should be considered in patients who have been previously treated for CMV disease. Other diseases involving the spinal cord in patients with HIV infection include HTLV-I–associated myelopathy (HAM) (Chap. 89), neurosyphilis (Chap. 70), infection with herpes simplex (Chap. 80) or varicella-zoster (Chap. 81), TB (Chap. 66), and lymphoma.

Peripheral neuropathies are common in patients with HIV infection. They occur at all stages of illness and take a variety of forms. Early in the course of HIV infection, an acute inflammatory demyelinating polyneuropathy resembling Guillain-Barré syndrome may occur. In other patients, a progressive or relapsing-remitting inflammatory neuropathy resembling chronic inflammatory demyelinating polyneuropathy (CIDP) has been noted. Patients commonly present with progressive weakness, areflexia, and minimal sensory changes. CSF examination often reveals a mononuclear pleocytosis, and peripheral nerve biopsy demonstrates a perivascular infiltrate suggesting an autoimmune etiology. Plasma exchange or IVIg has been tried with variable success. Because of the immunosuppressive effects of glucocorticoids, they should be reserved for severe cases of CIDP refractory to other measures. Another autoimmune peripheral neuropathy seen in patients with AIDS is mononeuritis multiplex due to a necrotizing arteritis of peripheral nerves. The most common peripheral neuropathy in patients with

HIV infection is a *distal sensory polyneuropathy* that may be a direct consequence of HIV infection or a side effect of dideoxynucleoside therapy. Two-thirds of patients with AIDS may be shown by electrophysiologic studies to have some evidence of peripheral nerve disease. Presenting symptoms are usually painful burning sensations in the feet and lower extremities. Findings on examination include a stocking-type sensory loss to pinprick, temperature, and touch sensation and a loss of ankle reflexes. Motor changes are mild and are usually limited to weakness of the intrinsic foot muscles. Response of this condition to ARVs has been variable, perhaps because ARVs are responsible for the problem in some instances. When due to dideoxynucleoside therapy, patients with lower extremity peripheral neuropathy may complain of a sensation that they are walking on ice. Other entities in the differential diagnosis of peripheral neuropathy include diabetes mellitus, vitamin B_{12} deficiency, and side effects from metronidazole or dapsone. For distal symmetric polyneuropathy that fails to resolve after the discontinuation of dideoxynucleosides, therapy is symptomatic; gabapentin, carbamazepine, tricyclics, or analgesics may be effective for dysesthesias. Treatment-naive patients may respond to combination ARV therapy.

Myopathy may complicate the course of HIV infection; causes include HIV infection itself, zidovudine, and the generalized wasting syndrome. HIV-associated myopathy may range in severity from an asymptomatic elevation in creatine kinase levels to a subacute syndrome characterized by proximal muscle weakness and myalgias. Quite pronounced elevations in creatine kinase may occur in asymptomatic patients, particularly after exercise. The clinical significance of this as an isolated laboratory finding is unclear. A variety of both inflammatory and noninflammatory pathologic processes have been noted in patients with more severe myopathy, including myofiber necrosis with inflammatory cells, nemaline rod bodies, cytoplasmic bodies, and mitochondrial abnormalities. Profound muscle wasting, often with muscle pain, may be seen after prolonged zidovudine therapy. This toxic side effect of the drug is dose-dependent and is related to its ability to interfere with the function of mitochondrial polymerases. It is reversible after discontinuation of the drug. Red ragged fibers are a histologic hallmark of zidovudine-induced myopathy.

Ophthalmologic Disease

Ophthalmologic problems occur in ~50% of patients with advanced HIV infection. The most common abnormal findings on funduscopic examination are cotton-wool spots. These are hard white spots that appear on the surface of the retina and often have an irregular edge. They represent areas of retinal ischemia secondary to microvascular disease. At times they are associated with small areas of hemorrhage and thus can be difficult to distinguish from CMV retinitis. In contrast to CMV retinitis, however, these lesions are not associated with visual loss and tend to remain stable or improve over time.

One of the most devastating consequences of HIV infection is CMV retinitis. Patients at high risk of CMV retinitis (CD4+ T-cell count <100/μL) should undergo an ophthalmologic examination every 3–6 months. The majority of cases of CMV retinitis occur in patients with a CD4+ T-cell count <50/μL. Before the availability of HAART, this CMV reactivation syndrome was seen in 25–30% of patients with AIDS. CMV retinitis usually presents as a painless, progressive loss of vision. Patients may also complain of blurred vision, "floaters," and scintillations. The disease is usually bilateral, although typically it affects one eye more than the other. The diagnosis is made on clinical grounds by an experienced ophthalmologist. The characteristic retinal appearance is that of perivascular hemorrhage and exudate. In situations where the diagnosis is in doubt due to an atypical presentation or an unexpected lack of response to therapy, vitreous or aqueous humor sampling with molecular diagnostic techniques may be of value. CMV infection of the retina results in a necrotic inflammatory process, and the visual loss that develops is irreversible. CMV retinitis may be complicated by rhegmatogenous retinal detachment as a consequence of retinal atrophy in areas of prior inflammation. Therapy for CMV retinitis consists of oral valganciclovir, IV ganciclovir, or IV foscarnet, with cidofovir as an alternative. Combination therapy with ganciclovir and foscarnet has been shown to be slightly more effective than either ganciclovir or foscarnet alone in the patient with relapsed CMV retinitis. A 3-week induction course is followed by maintenance therapy with oral valganciclovir. If CMV disease is limited to the eye, a ganciclovir-releasing intraocular implant, periodic injections of the antisense nucleic acid preparation fomivirsen, or intravitreal injections of ganciclovir or foscarnet may be considered; some choose to combine intraocular implants with oral valganciclovir. Intravitreal injections of cidofovir are generally avoided due to the increased risk of uveitis and hypotony. Maintenance therapy is continued until the CD4+ T-cell count remains >100–150/μL for >6 months. The majority of patients with HIV infection and CMV disease develop some degree of uveitis with the initiation of ARV therapy. The etiology of this is unknown; however, it has been suggested that this may be due to the generation of an enhanced immune response to CMV as an IRIS (see above). In some instances this has required the use of topical glucocorticoids.

Both HSV and varicella zoster virus can cause a rapidly progressing, bilateral necrotizing retinitis referred to as the *acute retinal necrosis syndrome*, or *progressive outer retinal necrosis* (PORN). This syndrome, in contrast to CMV retinitis, is associated with pain, keratitis, and iritis. It is often associated with orolabial HSV or trigeminal zoster. Ophthalmologic examination reveals widespread pale gray peripheral lesions. This condition is often complicated by retinal detachment. It is important to recognize and treat this condition with IV acyclovir as quickly as possible to minimize the loss of vision.

Several other secondary infections may cause ocular problems in HIV-infected patients. *P. jiroveci* can cause a lesion of the choroid that may be detected as an incidental finding on ophthalmologic examination. These lesions are typically bilateral, are from half to twice the disc diameter in size, and appear as slightly elevated yellow-white plaques. They are usually asymptomatic and may be confused with cotton-wool spots. Chorioretinitis due to toxoplasmosis can be seen alone or, more commonly, in association with CNS toxoplasmosis. KS may involve the eyelid or conjunctiva, whereas lymphoma may involve the retina.

Additional Disseminated Infections and Wasting Syndrome

Infections with species of the small, gram-negative rickettsia-like organism *Bartonella* (Chap. 61) are seen with increased frequency in patients with HIV infection. Although not considered an AIDS-defining illness by the CDC, many experts view infection with *Bartonella* as indicative of a severe defect in cell-mediated immunity. It is usually seen in patients with CD4+ T-cell counts <100/μL. Among the clinical manifestations of *Bartonella* infection are bacillary angiomatosis, cat-scratch disease, and trench fever. *Bacillary angiomatosis* is usually due to infection with *B. henselae*. It is characterized by a vascular proliferation that leads to a variety of skin lesions that have been confused with the skin lesions of KS. In contrast to the lesions of KS, the lesions of bacillary angiomatosis generally blanch, are painful, and typically occur in the setting of systemic symptoms. Infection can extend to the lymph nodes, liver (peliosis hepatis), spleen, bone, heart, CNS, respiratory tract, and gastrointestinal tract. *Cat-scratch disease* generally begins with a papule at the site of inoculation. This is followed several weeks later by the development of regional adenopathy and malaise. Infection with *B. quintana* is transmitted by lice and has been associated with case reports of trench fever, endocarditis, adenopathy, and bacillary angiomatosis. The organism is quite difficult to culture, and diagnosis often relies upon identifying the organism in biopsy specimens using the Warthin-Starry or similar stains. Treatment is with either erythromycin or doxycycline for at least 3 months.

Histoplasmosis is an opportunistic infection that is seen most frequently in patients in the Mississippi and Ohio River valleys, Puerto Rico, the Dominican Republic, and South America. These are all areas in which infection with *H. capsulatum* is endemic (Chap. 103). Because of this limited geographic distribution, the percentage of AIDS cases in the United States with histoplasmosis is only ~0.5. Histoplasmosis is generally a late manifestation of HIV infection; however, it may be the initial AIDS-defining condition. In one study, the median CD4+ T-cell count for patients with histoplasmosis and AIDS was 33/μL. Although disease due to *H. capsulatum* may present as a primary infection of the lung, disseminated disease, presumably due to reactivation, is the most common presentation in HIV-infected patients. Patients usually present with a 4- to 8-week history of fever and weight loss. Hepatosplenomegaly and lymphadenopathy are each seen in about 25% of patients. CNS disease, either meningitis or a mass lesion, is seen in 15% of patients. Bone marrow involvement is common, with thrombocytopenia, neutropenia, and anemia occurring in 33% of patients. Approximately 7% of patients have mucocutaneous lesions consisting of a maculopapular rash and skin or oral ulcers. Respiratory symptoms are usually mild, with chest x-ray showing a diffuse infiltrate or diffuse small nodules in ~50% of cases. Diagnosis is made by culturing the organisms from blood, bone marrow, or tissue. Treatment is typically with amphotericin B, 0.7–1.0 mg/kg daily to a total dose of 1 g followed by maintenance therapy with itraconazole. In the setting of mild infection, it may be appropriate to treat with itraconazole alone.

After the spread of HIV infection to southeast Asia, disseminated infection with the fungus *Penicillium marneffei* was recognized as a complication of HIV infection and is considered an AIDS-defining condition in those parts of the world where it occurs. *P. marneffei* is the third most common AIDS-defining illness in Thailand, following TB and cryptococcosis. It is more frequently diagnosed in the rainy than the dry season. Clinical features include fever, generalized lymphadenopathy, hepatosplenomegaly, anemia, thrombocytopenia, and papular skin lesions with central umbilication. Treatment is with amphotericin B followed by itraconazole.

Visceral leishmaniasis (Chap. 119) is recognized with increasing frequency in patients with HIV infection who live in or travel to areas endemic for this protozoal infection transmitted by sandflies. The clinical presentation is one of hepatosplenomegaly, fever, and hematologic abnormalities. Lymphadenopathy and other constitutional symptoms may be present. A chronic, relapsing course is seen in two-thirds of co-infected patients. Organisms can be isolated from cultures of bone marrow aspirates. Histologic stains may be negative, and antibody titers are of little help. Patients with HIV infection usually respond well initially to standard therapy with amphotericin B or pentavalent antimony compounds. Eradication of the organism is difficult, however, and relapses are common.

Patients with HIV infection are at increased risk of clinical malaria. This is particularly true for patients from nonendemic areas with presumed primary infection and in patients with lower CD4+ T-cell counts. HIV-positive individuals with CD4+ T-cell counts <300 cells/μL have a poorer response to malaria treatment than others. Co-infection with malaria is associated with a modest increase in HIV viral load. The risk of malaria may be decreased with TMP/SMX prophylaxis.

Generalized wasting is an AIDS-defining condition; it is defined as involuntary weight loss of >10% associated with intermittent or constant fever and chronic diarrhea or fatigue lasting >30 days in the absence of a defined cause other than HIV infection. It is the initial AIDS-defining condition in ~10% of patients with AIDS in the United States and is an indication for initiation of HAART. A constant feature of this syndrome is severe muscle wasting with scattered myofiber degeneration and occasional evidence of myositis. Glucocorticoids may be of some benefit; however, this approach must be carefully weighed against the risk of compounding the immunodeficiency of HIV infection. Androgenic steroids, growth hormone, and total parenteral nutrition have been used as therapeutic interventions with variable success.

Neoplastic Diseases

The neoplastic diseases clearly seen with an increased frequency in patients with HIV infection are KS and non-Hodgkin's lymphoma. In addition, there also appears to be an increased incidence of Hodgkin's disease; multiple myeloma; leukemia; melanoma; and cervical, brain, testicular, oral, lung, and anal cancers. Recent years have witnessed a marked reduction in the incidence of KS (Fig. 90-31) and improvements in the outcomes of HIV-infected patients with non-AIDS-defining malignancies. These changes are primarily due to the use of potent ARV therapy. Rates of non-Hodgkin's lymphoma have declined as well; however, this decline has not been as dramatic as the decline in rates of KS. In contrast, HAART has had little effect on human papilloma virus (HPV)–associated malignancies. As patients with HIV infection live longer, a wider array of cancers are being seen in this population of patients. Although some may only reflect known risk factors (i.e., smoking) that are increased in patients with HIV infection, some may be a direct consequence of HIV.

Kaposi's sarcoma is a multicentric neoplasm consisting of multiple vascular nodules appearing in the skin, mucous membranes, and viscera. The course ranges from indolent, with only minor skin or lymph node involvement, to fulminant, with extensive cutaneous and visceral involvement. In the initial period of the AIDS epidemic, KS was a prominent clinical feature of the first cases of AIDS, occurring in 79% of the patients diagnosed in 1981. By 1989 it was seen in only 25% of cases, by 1992 the number had decreased to 9%, and by 1997 the number was <1%. HHV-8 or KSHV has been strongly implicated as a viral cofactor in the pathogenesis of KS (see above).

Clinically, KS has varied presentations and may be seen at any stage of HIV infection, even in the presence of a normal CD4+ T-cell count. The initial lesion may be a small, raised reddish-purple nodule on the skin (Fig. 90-39), a discoloration on the oral mucosa (Fig. 90-32*D*), or a swollen lymph node. Lesions often appear in sun-exposed areas, particularly the tip of the nose, and have a propensity to occur in areas of trauma (Koebner phenomenon). Because of the vascular nature of the tumors and the presence of extravasated red blood cells in the lesions, their colors range from reddish to purple to brown and often take the appearance of a bruise, with yellowish discoloration and tattooing. Lesions range in size from a few millimeters to several centimeters in diameter and may be either discrete or confluent. KS lesions most commonly appear as raised macules; however, they can also be papular, particularly in patients with higher CD4+ T-cell counts. Confluent lesions may give rise to surrounding lymphedema and may be disfiguring when they involve the face and disabling when they involve the lower extremities or the surfaces of joints. Apart from skin, lymph nodes, gastrointestinal tract, and lung are the organ systems most commonly affected by KS. Lesions have been reported in virtually every organ, including the heart and the CNS. In contrast to most malignancies, in which lymph node involvement implies metastatic spread and a poor prognosis, lymph node involvement may be seen very early in KS and is of no special clinical significance. In fact, some patients may present with disease limited to the lymph nodes. These are generally patients with relatively intact immune function and thus the patients with the best prognosis. Pulmonary involvement with KS generally presents with shortness of breath. Some 80% of patients with pulmonary KS also have cutaneous lesions. The chest x-ray characteristically shows bilateral lower lobe infiltrates that obscure the margins of the mediastinum and diaphragm (Fig. 90-40). Pleural effusions are seen in 70% of cases of pulmonary KS, a fact that is often helpful in the differential diagnosis. Gastrointestinal

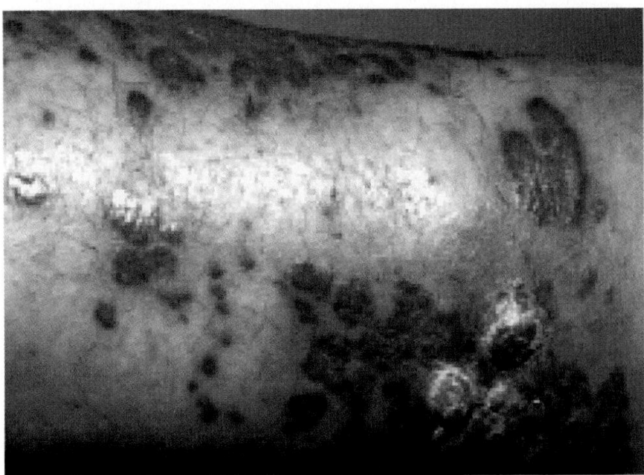

FIGURE 90-39
Kaposi's sarcoma in a patient with AIDS demonstrating patch, plaque, and tumor stages.

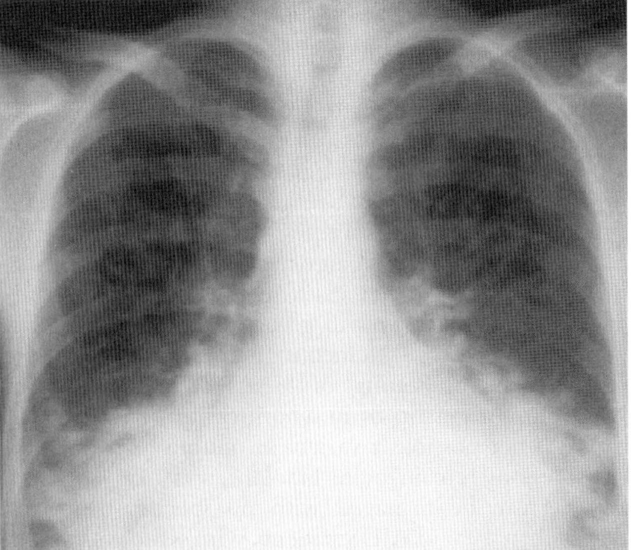

FIGURE 90-40
Chest x-ray of a patient with AIDS and pulmonary Kaposi's sarcoma. The characteristic findings include dense bilateral lower lobe infiltrates obscuring the heart borders and a pleural effusion.

TABLE 90-14

NATIONAL INSTITUTE OF ALLERGY AND INFECTIOUS DISEASES AIDS CLINICAL TRIALS GROUP TIS STAGING SYSTEM FOR KAPOSI'S SARCOMA

PARAMETER	GOOD RISK (STAGE 0): ALL OF THE FOLLOWING	POOR RISK (STAGE 1): ANY OF THE FOLLOWING
Tumor (T)	Confined to skin and/or lymph nodes and/or minimal oral disease	Tumor-associated edema or ulceration Extensive oral lesions Gastrointestinal lesions Nonnodal visceral lesions
Immune system (I)	CD4+ T-cell count ≥200/μL	CD4+ T-cell count <200/μL
Systemic illness (S)	No B symptoms[a] Karnofsky performance status ≥70 No history of opportunistic infection, neurologic disease, lymphoma, or thrush	B symptoms[a] present Karnofsky performance status <70 History of opportunistic infection, neurologic disease, lymphoma, or thrush

[a]Defined as unexplained fever, night sweats, >10% involuntary weight loss, or diarrhea persisting for more than 2 weeks.

involvement is seen in 50% of patients and usually takes one of two forms: (1) mucosal involvement, which may lead to bleeding that can be severe; these patients sometimes also develop symptoms of gastrointestinal obstruction if lesions become large; and (2) biliary tract involvement. KS lesions may infiltrate the gallbladder and biliary tree, leading to a clinical picture of obstructive jaundice similar to that seen with sclerosing cholangitis. Several staging systems have been proposed for KS. One in common use was developed by the National Institute of Allergy and Infectious Diseases AIDS Clinical Trials Group; it distinguishes patients on the basis of tumor extent, immunologic function, and presence or absence of systemic disease (Table 90-14).

A diagnosis of KS is based upon biopsy of a suspicious lesion. Histologically one sees a proliferation of spindle cells and endothelial cells, extravasation of red blood cells, hemosiderin-laden macrophages, and, in early cases, an inflammatory cell infiltrate. Included in the differential diagnosis are lymphoma (particularly for oral lesions), bacillary angiomatosis, and cutaneous mycobacterial infections.

Management of KS (Table 90-15) should be carried out in consultation with an expert since definitive treatment guidelines do not exist. In the majority of cases, effective ARV therapy will go a long way in achieving control. Indeed, spontaneous regressions have been reported in the setting of HAART. For patients in whom tumor persists or in whom control of HIV replication is not possible, a variety of options exist. In some cases, lesions remain quite indolent, and many of these patients can be managed with no specific treatment. Fewer than 10% of AIDS patients with KS die as a consequence of their malignancy, and death from secondary infections is considerably more common. Thus, whenever possible, one should avoid treatment regimens that may further suppress the immune system and increase susceptibility to opportunistic infections. Treatment is indicated under two main circumstances. The first is when a single lesion or a limited number of lesions are causing significant discomfort or cosmetic problems, such as with prominent facial lesions, lesions overlying a joint, or lesions in the oropharynx that interfere with swallowing or breathing. Under these circumstances, treatment with localized radiation, intralesional vinblastine, or cryotherapy may be helpful. It should be noted that patients with HIV infection are particularly sensitive to the side effects of radiation therapy. This is especially true with respect to the development of radiation-induced mucositis; doses of radiation directed at mucosal surfaces, particularly in the head and neck region, should be adjusted accordingly. The use of systemic therapy, either IFN-α or chemotherapy, should be considered in patients with a large number of lesions or in patients with visceral involvement. The single most important

TABLE 90-15

MANAGEMENT OF AIDS-ASSOCIATED KAPOSI'S SARCOMA

Observation and optimization of antiretroviral therapy
Single or limited number of lesions
- Radiation
- Intralesional vinblastine
- Cryotherapy

Extensive disease
- Initial therapy
  - Interferon-α (if CD4+ T cells >150/μL)
  - Liposomal daunorubicin
- Subsequent therapy
  - Liposomal doxorubicin
  - Paclitaxel
- Combination chemotherapy with low-dose doxorubicin, bleomycin, and vinblastine (ABV)
- Radiation treatment

determinant of response appears to be the CD4+ T-cell count. This relationship between response rate and baseline CD4+ T-cell count is particularly true for IFN-α. The response rate for patients with CD4+ T-cell counts >600/μL is ~80%, whereas the response rate for patients with counts <150/μL is <10%. In contrast to the other systemic therapies, IFN-α provides an added advantage of having ARV activity; thus it may be the appropriate first choice for single-agent systemic therapy for early patients with disseminated disease. A variety of chemotherapeutic agents have also been shown to have activity against KS. Three of them, liposomal daunorubicin, liposomal doxorubicin, and paclitaxel, have been approved by the FDA for this indication. Liposomal daunorubicin is approved as first-line therapy for patients with advanced KS. It has fewer side effects than conventional chemotherapy. In contrast, liposomal doxorubicin and paclitaxel are approved only for KS patients who have failed standard chemotherapy. Response rates vary from 23–88%, appear to be comparable to what had been achieved earlier with combination chemotherapy regimens, and are greatly influenced by CD4+ T-cell count.

Lymphomas occur with an increased frequency in patients with congenital or acquired T-cell immunodeficiencies. AIDS is no exception; at least 6% of all patients with AIDS develop lymphoma at some time during the course of their illness. This is a 120-fold increase in incidence compared with that of the general population. In contrast to the situation with KS, primary CNS lymphoma, and most opportunistic infections, the incidence of AIDS-associated systemic lymphomas has not experienced as dramatic a decrease as a consequence of the widespread use of effective ARV therapy. Lymphoma occurs in all risk groups, with the highest incidence in patients with hemophilia and the lowest incidence in patients from the Caribbean or Africa with heterosexually acquired infection. Lymphoma is a late manifestation of HIV infection, generally occurring in patients with CD4+ T-cell counts <200/μL. As HIV disease progresses, the risk of lymphoma increases. In contrast to KS, which occurs at a relatively constant rate throughout the course of HIV disease, the attack rate for lymphoma increases exponentially with increasing duration of HIV infection and decreasing level of immunologic function. At 3 years after a diagnosis of HIV infection, the risk of lymphoma is 0.8% per year; by 8 years after infection, it is 2.6% per year. As individuals with HIV infection live longer as a consequence of improved ARV therapy and better treatment and prophylaxis of opportunistic infections, it is anticipated that the incidence of lymphomas may increase.

Three main categories of lymphoma are seen in patients with HIV infection: grade III or IV immunoblastic lymphoma, Burkitt's lymphoma, and primary CNS lymphoma. Approximately 90% of these lymphomas are B cell in phenotype, and half contain EBV DNA. These tumors may be either monoclonal or oligoclonal in nature and are probably in some way related to the pronounced polyclonal B-cell activation seen in patients with AIDS.

Immunoblastic lymphomas account for ~60% of the cases of lymphoma in patients with AIDS. These are generally high grade and would have been classified as diffuse histiocytic lymphomas in earlier classification schemes. This tumor is more common in older patients, increasing in incidence from 0% in HIV-infected individuals <1 year old to >3% in those >50. One variant of immunoblastic lymphoma is body cavity lymphoma. This malignancy presents with lymphomatous pleural, pericardial, and/or peritoneal effusions in the absence of discrete nodal or extranodal masses. The tumor cells do not express surface markers for B cells or T cells. HHV-8 DNA sequences have been found in the genomes of the malignant cells from patients with body cavity lymphomas (see above).

Small noncleaved cell lymphoma (*Burkitt's lymphoma*) accounts for ~20% of the cases of lymphoma in patients with AIDS. It is most frequent in patients 10–19 years old and usually demonstrates characteristic c-*myc* translocations from chromosome 8 to chromosomes 14 or 22. Burkitt's lymphoma is not commonly seen in the setting of immunodeficiency other than HIV-associated immunodeficiency, and the incidence of this particular tumor is more than 1000-fold higher in the setting of HIV infection than in the general population. In contrast to African Burkitt's lymphoma, where 97% of the cases contain EBV genome, only 50% of HIV-associated Burkitt's lymphomas are EBV-positive.

Primary CNS lymphoma accounts for ~20% of the cases of lymphoma in patients with HIV infection. In contrast to HIV-associated Burkitt's lymphoma, primary CNS lymphomas are usually positive for EBV. In one study, the incidence of Epstein-Barr positivity was 100%. This malignancy does not have a predilection for any particular age group. The median CD4+ T-cell count at the time of diagnosis is ~50/μL. Thus CNS lymphoma generally presents at a later stage of HIV infection than systemic lymphoma. This fact may at least in part explain the poorer prognosis for this subset of patients.

The clinical presentation of lymphoma in patients with HIV infection is quite varied, ranging from focal seizures to rapidly growing mass lesions in the oral mucosa (Fig. 90-41) to persistent unexplained fever. At

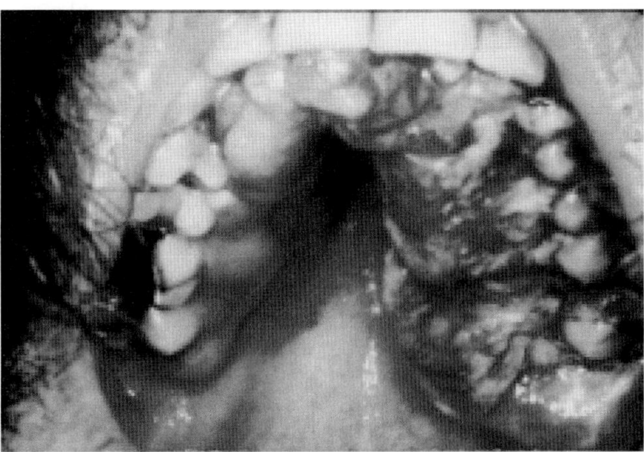

FIGURE 90-41
Diffuse histiocytic lymphoma involving the hard palate of a patient with AIDS.

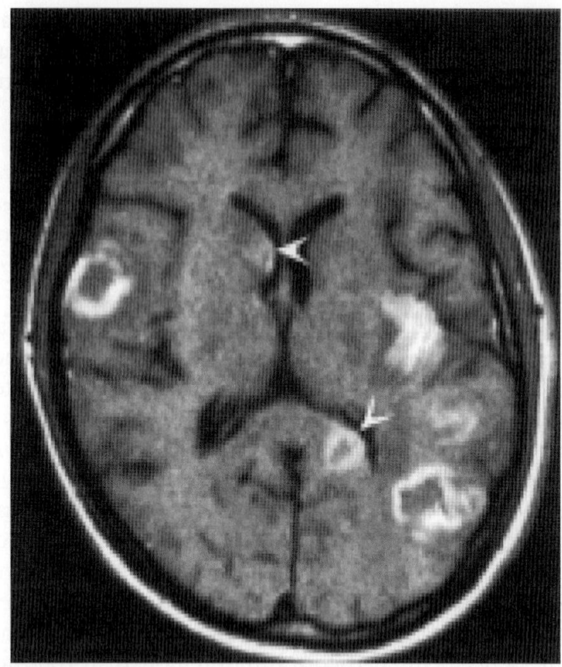

FIGURE 90-42

Central nervous system lymphoma. Postcontrast T1-weighted MR scan in a patient with AIDS, an altered mental status, and hemiparesis. Multiple enhancing lesions, some ring-enhancing, are present. The left Sylvian lesion shows gyral and subcortical enhancement, and the lesions in the caudate and splenium (*arrowheads*) show enhancement of adjacent ependymal surfaces.

least 80% of patients present with extranodal disease, and a similar percentage have B-type symptoms of fever, night sweats, or weight loss. Virtually any site in the body may be involved. The most common extranodal site is the CNS, which is involved in approximately one-third of all patients with lymphoma. Approximately 60% of these cases are primary CNS lymphoma. Primary CNS lymphoma generally presents with focal neurologic deficits, including cranial nerve findings, headaches, and/or seizures. MRI or CT generally reveals a limited number (one to three) of 3- to 5-cm lesions (Fig. 90-42). The lesions often show ring enhancement on contrast administration and may occur in any location. Locations that are most commonly involved with CNS lymphoma are deep in the white matter. Contrast enhancement is usually less pronounced than that seen with toxoplasmosis. The main diseases in the differential diagnosis are cerebral toxoplasmosis and cerebral Chagas' disease. In addition to the 20% of lymphomas in HIV-infected individuals that are primary CNS lymphomas, CNS disease is also seen in HIV-infected patients with systemic lymphoma. Approximately 20% of patients with systemic lymphoma have CNS disease in the form of leptomeningeal involvement. This fact underscores the importance of lumbar puncture in the staging evaluation of patients with systemic lymphoma.

Systemic lymphoma is seen at earlier stages of HIV infection than primary CNS lymphoma. In one series the mean CD4+ T-cell count was 189/μL. In addition to lymph node involvement, systemic lymphoma may commonly involve the gastrointestinal tract, bone marrow, liver, and lung. Gastrointestinal tract involvement is seen in ~25% of patients. Any site in the gastrointestinal tract may be involved, and patients may complain of difficulty swallowing or abdominal pain. The diagnosis is usually suspected on the basis of CT or MRI of the abdomen. Bone marrow involvement is seen in ~20% of patients and may lead to pancytopenia. Liver and lung involvement are each seen in ~10% of patients. Pulmonary disease may present as either a mass lesion, multiple nodules, or an interstitial infiltrate.

Both conventional and unconventional approaches have been employed in an attempt to treat HIV-related lymphomas. Systemic lymphoma is generally treated by the oncologist with combination chemotherapy. Earlier disappointing figures are being replaced with more optimistic results for the treatment of systemic lymphoma following the availability of more effective combination ARV therapy. As in most situations in patients with HIV disease, those with the higher CD4+ T-cell counts tend to do better. Response rates as high as 72% with a median survival of 33 months and disease-free intervals up to 9 years have been reported. Treatment of primary CNS lymphoma remains a significant challenge. Treatment is complicated by the fact that this illness usually occurs in patients with advanced HIV disease. Palliative measures such as radiation therapy provide some relief. The prognosis remains poor in this group, with a 2-year survival of 29%.

Multicentric Castleman's disease is an HHV-8 associated lymphoproliferative disorder that is seen with an increased frequency in patients with HIV infection. Although not a true malignancy, it shares many features with lymphoma, including generalized lymphadenopathy, hepatosplenomegaly, and systemic symptoms of fever, fatigue, and weight loss. Pulmonary symptoms may be seen in ~50% of patients. Kaposi's sarcoma is present in 75–82% of cases. Lymph node biopsies reveal a predominance of interfollicular plasma cells and/or germinal centers with vascularization and an "onion skin" appearance (hyaline vascular). Before the availability of HAART, HIV-infected patients with multicentric Castleman's disease had a 15-fold increased risk of developing non-Hodgkin's lymphoma compared with HIV-infected patients in general. Treatment typically involves chemotherapy. Anecdotal reports of success with rituximab suggest that more specific treatment may be successful, although in one series, treatment with rituximab was associated with worsening of coexisting KS. The median survival of patients with treated multicentric Castleman's disease pre-HAART was 14 months. This has increased to 4 years in the era of HAART.

Evidence of infection with *human papilloma virus* (HPV), associated with *intraepithelial dysplasia of the cervix* or *anus*, is approximately twice as common in HIV-infected individuals as in the general population and can lead to intraepithelial neoplasia and eventually invasive cancer. In separate studies, HIV-infected men were examined for evidence of anal dysplasia, and Papanicolaou (Pap) smears were found to be abnormal in 20–80%. These changes tend to persist and are generally not affected by HAART, raising the possibility of a subsequent transition to a more malignant condition. Although the incidence of an abnormal Pap smear of the cervix is ~5% in otherwise healthy women, the incidence of abnormal cervical smears in women with HIV infection is 30–60%, and *invasive cervical cancer* is included as an AIDS-defining condition. Thus far, however, only small increases in the incidence of cervical or anal cancer have been seen as a consequence of HIV infection. However, given this high rate of dysplasia, a comprehensive gynecologic and rectal examination, including Pap smear, is indicated at the initial evaluation and 6 months later for all patients with HIV infection. If these examinations are negative at both time points, the patient should be followed with yearly evaluations. If an initial or repeat Pap smear shows evidence of severe inflammation with reactive squamous changes, the next Pap smear should be performed at 3 months. If, at any time, a Pap smear shows evidence of squamous intraepithelial lesions, colposcopic examination with biopsies as indicated should be performed. The 2-year survival rate for HIV infected patients with invasive cervical cancer is 64% compared with 79% in non-HIV-infected patients. The most common HPV genotypes in the general population and the genotypes upon which current HPV vaccines are based are 16 and 18. This is not the case in the HIV-infected population, where other genotypes such as 56 and 53 predominate. This raises concerns as to the potential effectiveness of the current HPV vaccines for HIV-infected patients.

IDIOPATHIC CD4+ T LYMPHOCYTOPENIA

A syndrome was recognized in 1992 that was characterized by an absolute CD4+ T-cell count of <300/μL or <20% of total T cells on a minimum of two occasions at least 6 weeks apart; no evidence of HIV-1, HIV-2, HTLV-I, or HTLV-II on testing; and the absence of any defined immunodeficiency or therapy associated with decreased levels of CD4+ T cells. By mid-1993, ~100 patients had been described. After extensive multicenter investigations, a series of reports were published in early 1993, which together allowed a number of conclusions. Idiopathic CD4+ lymphocytopenia (ICL) is a very rare syndrome, as determined by studies of blood donors and cohorts of HIV-seronegative men who have sex with men. Cases were clearly identified as early as 1983, and cases remarkably similar to ICL had been identified decades ago. The definition of ICL based on CD4+ T-cell counts coincided with the ready availability of testing for CD4+ T cells in patients suspected of being immunosuppressed. Although, as a result of immune deficiency, certain patients with ICL develop some of the opportunistic diseases (particularly cryptococcosis) seen in HIV-infected patients, the syndrome is demographically, clinically, and immunologically unlike HIV infection and AIDS. Fewer than half of the reported ICL patients had risk factors for HIV infection, and there were wide geographic and age distributions. The fact that a significant proportion of patients did have risk factors probably reflects a selection bias, in that physicians who take care of HIV-infected patients are more likely to monitor CD4+ T cells. Approximately one-third of the patients are women, compared with 16% of women among HIV-infected individuals in the United States. Many patients with ICL remained clinically stable, and their condition did not deteriorate progressively as is common with seriously immunodeficient HIV-infected patients. Certain patients with ICL even experienced spontaneous reversal of the CD4+ T lymphocytopenia. Immunologic abnormalities in ICL are somewhat different from those of HIV infection. ICL patients often also have decreases in CD8+ T cells and in B cells. Furthermore, immunoglobulin levels were either normal or, more commonly, decreased in patients with ICL, compared with the usual hypergammaglobulinemia of HIV-infected individuals. Finally, virologic studies revealed no evidence of HIV-1, HIV-2, HTLV-I, or HTLV-II or of any other mononuclear cell–tropic virus. Furthermore, there was no epidemiologic evidence to suggest that a transmissible microbe was involved. The cases of ICL were widely dispersed, with no clustering. Close contacts and sexual partners who were studied were clinically well and were serologically, immunologically, and virologically negative for HIV. ICL is a heterogeneous syndrome, and it is highly likely that there is no common cause; however, there may be common causes among subgroups of patients that are currently unrecognized.

Patients who present with laboratory data consistent with ICL should be worked up for underlying diseases that could be responsible for the immune deficiency. If no underlying cause is detected, no specific therapy should be initiated. However, if opportunistic diseases occur, they should be treated appropriately (see above). Depending on the level of the CD4+ T-cell count, patients should receive prophylaxis for the commonly encountered opportunistic infections.

Rx Treatment: AIDS AND RELATED DISORDERS

GENERAL PRINCIPLES OF PATIENT MANAGEMENT The CDC guidelines call for the testing for HIV infection to be a part of routine medical care. It is recommended that the patient be informed of the intention to test as is the case with other routine laboratory determinations and be given the opportunity to "opt out." Such an approach is critical to the goal of identifying as many infected individuals as possible since ~25% of the >1 million individuals in the United States who are HIV-infected are not aware of their status. Under these circumstances of routine testing, although desirable, pretest counseling may not always be built into the testing process. However, no matter how well prepared a patient is for adversity, the discovery of a diagnosis of HIV infection is a devastating event. Thus physicians should be sensitive to this fact and, where possible, execute some degree of pretest counseling to at least partially prepare the patient should the results demonstrate the presence of HIV infection. After a diagnosis of HIV infection, the health care provider should be prepared to activate support systems immediately for the newly diagnosed patient. These should include an experienced social worker or nurse who can spend time talking to the person and ensuring that he or she is emotionally stable. Most communities have HIV support centers that can be of great help in these difficult situations.

The treatment of patients with HIV infection requires not only a comprehensive knowledge of the possible disease processes that may occur and up-to-date knowledge of and experience with ARV therapy, but also the ability to deal with the problems of a chronic, potentially life-threatening illness. A comprehensive knowledge of internal medicine is required to deal with the changing spectrum of illness associated with HIV infection. Great advances have been made in the treatment of patients with HIV infection. The appropriate use of potent combination ARV therapy and other treatment and prophylactic interventions is of critical importance in providing each patient with the best opportunity to live a long and healthy life despite the presence of HIV infection. In contrast to the earlier days of this epidemic, a diagnosis of HIV infection need no longer be equated with an inevitably fatal disease. In addition to medical interventions, the health care provider has a responsibility to provide each patient with appropriate counseling and education concerning their disease as part of a comprehensive care plan. Patients must be educated about the potential transmissibility of their infection and about the fact that although health care providers may refer to levels of the virus as "undetectable," this is more a reflection of the sensitivity of the assay being used to measure the virus than a comment on the presence or absence of the virus. It is important for patients to be aware that the virus is still present and capable of being transmitted at all stages of HIV disease. Thus there need to be frank discussions concerning sexual practices and the sharing of needles. The treating physician must not only be aware of the latest medications available for patients with HIV infection, but must also educate patients concerning the natural history of their illness and listen and be sensitive to their fears and concerns. As with other diseases, therapeutic decisions should be made in consultation with the patient, when possible, and with the patient's proxy if the patient is incapable of making decisions. In this regard, it is recommended that all patients with HIV infection, and in particular those with CD4+ T-cell counts <200/μL, designate a trusted individual with durable power of attorney to make medical decisions on their behalf, if necessary.

After a diagnosis of HIV infection, there are several examinations and laboratory studies that should be performed to help determine the extent of disease and provide baseline standards for future reference (Table 90-16). In addition to routine chemistry, fasting lipid profile, fasting glucose and hematology screening panels, Pap smear, and chest x-ray, one should also obtain a CD4+ T-cell count, two separate plasma HIV RNA levels, an HIV resistance test, an RPR or VDRL test, an anti-*Toxoplasma* antibody titer, and serologies for hepatitis A, B, and C. A PPD test should be done, and an MMSE performed and recorded. Patients should be immunized with pneumococcal polysaccharide and, if seronegative for these viruses, with hepatitis A and hepatitis B vaccines. The status of hepatitis C infection should be determined. In addition, patients should be counseled with regard to sexual practices and needle sharing, and counseling should be offered to those whom the patient knows or suspects may also be infected. Once these baseline activities are performed, short- and long-term medical management strategies should be developed based upon the most recent information available and modified as new information becomes available. The field of HIV medicine is changing rapidly, and it is difficult to remain fully up to date. Fortunately there are a series of excellent sites on the Internet that are frequently updated, and they provide the most recent information on a variety of topics, including consensus panel reports on treatment (Table 90-17).

TABLE 90-16

INITIAL EVALUATION OF THE PATIENT WITH HIV INFECTION
History and physical examination
Routine chemistry and hematology
Lipid profile and fasting glucose
CD4+ T-lymphocyte count
Two plasma HIV RNA levels
HIV resistance testing
RPR test
Anti-*Toxoplasma* antibody titer
PPD skin test
Mini-mental status examination
Serologies for hepatitis A, hepatitis B, and hepatitis C
Immunization with pneumococcal polysaccharide; influenza as indicated
Immunization with hepatitis A and hepatitis B if seronegative
Counseling regarding natural history and transmission
Help contacting others who might be infected

Note: VDRL, Venereal Disease Research Laboratory; PPD, purified protein derivative.

ANTIRETROVIRAL THERAPY Combination antiretroviral therapy (ART), or highly active antiretroviral therapy (HAART), is the cornerstone of management of patients with HIV infection. After the initiation of widespread use of HAART in the United States in 1995–1996, marked declines have been noted in the incidence of most AIDS-defining conditions (Fig. 90-31). Suppression of HIV replication is an important component in prolonging life as well as in improving the quality of life in patients with HIV infection. Adequate suppression requires strict adherence to prescribed regimens of ARV

TABLE 90-17

RESOURCES AVAILABLE ON THE WORLD WIDE WEB ON HIV DISEASE

http://www.aidsinfo.nih.gov	AIDS info, a service of the U.S. Department of Health and Human Services, posts federally approved treatment guidelines for HIV and AIDS; provides information on federally funded and privately funded clinical trials and CDC publications and data
http://www.cdcnpin.org	Updates on epidemiologic data from the CDC

Note: CDC, Centers for Disease Control and Prevention.

drugs. This has been facilitated by the coformulations of ARVs and the development of once-daily regimens. Unfortunately, many of the most important questions related to the treatment of HIV disease currently lack definitive answers. Among them are the questions of when should therapy be started, what is the best initial regimen, when should a given regimen be changed, and what should it be changed to when a change is made. Notwithstanding these uncertainties, the physician and patient must come to a mutually agreeable plan based upon the best available data. In an effort to facilitate this process, the U.S. Department of Health and Human Services has published a series of frequently updated guidelines including the "*Principles of Therapy of HIV Infection,*" "*Guidelines for the Use of Antiretroviral Agents in HIV-Infected Adults and Adolescents,*" and "*Guidelines for the Prevention of Opportunistic Infections in Persons Infected with Human Immunodeficiency Virus.*" At present, an extensive clinical trials network, involving both clinical investigators and patient advocates, is in place attempting to develop improved approaches to therapy. Consortia comprising representatives of academia, industry, independent foundations, and the federal government are involved in the process of drug development, including a wide-ranging series of clinical trials. As a result, new therapies and new therapeutic strategies are continually emerging. New drugs are often available through expanded access programs before official licensure. Given the complexity of this field, decisions regarding ARV therapy are best made in consultation with experts. Currently available drugs for the treatment of HIV infection fall into four categories: those that inhibit the viral reverse transcriptase enzyme, those that inhibit the viral protease enzyme, those that inhibit the viral integrase enzyme, and those that interfere with viral entry (**Table 90-18**, **Fig. 90-43**).

The FDA-approved reverse transcriptase inhibitors include the *nucleoside analogues* zidovudine, didanosine, zalcitabine, stavudine, lamivudine, abacavir, and

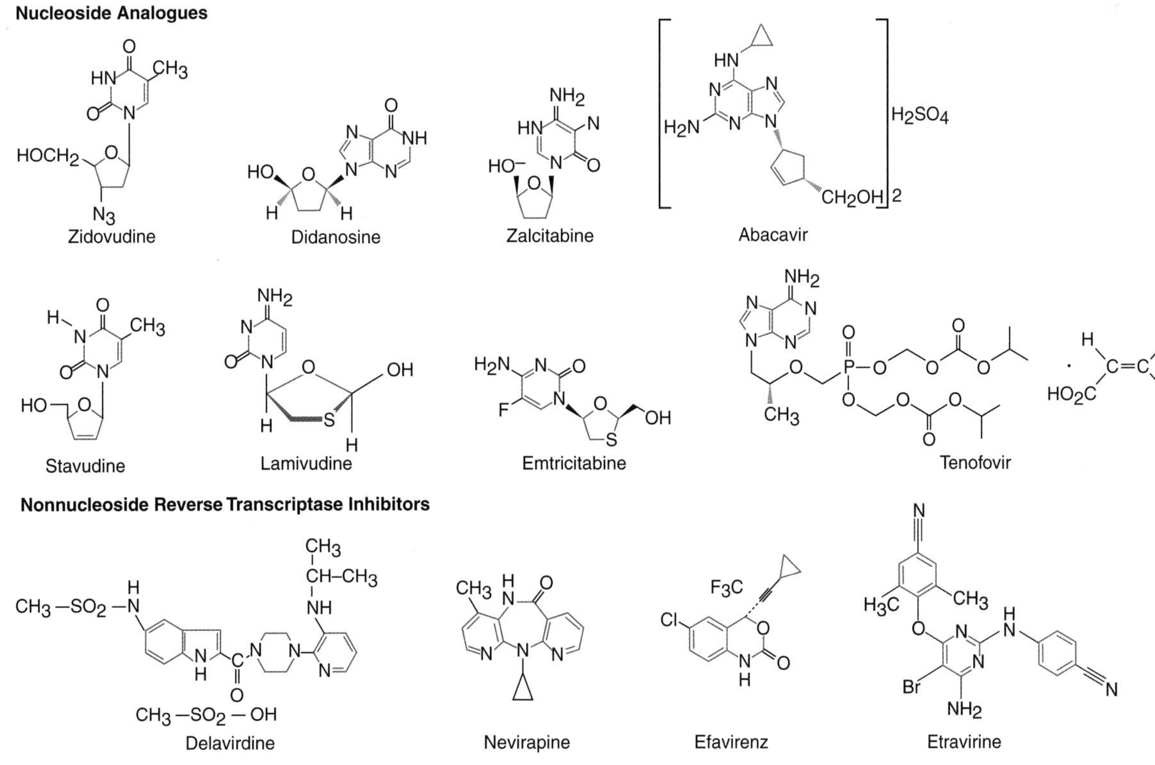

Nucleoside Analogues

Zidovudine Didanosine Zalcitabine Abacavir (H_2SO_4)

Stavudine Lamivudine Emtricitabine Tenofovir

Nonnucleoside Reverse Transcriptase Inhibitors

Delavirdine (CH_3-SO_2-OH) Nevirapine Efavirenz Etravirine

FIGURE 90-43
Molecular structures of antiretroviral agents. (*Continued on next page*)

 (Continued from preceding page)

Protease Inhibitors

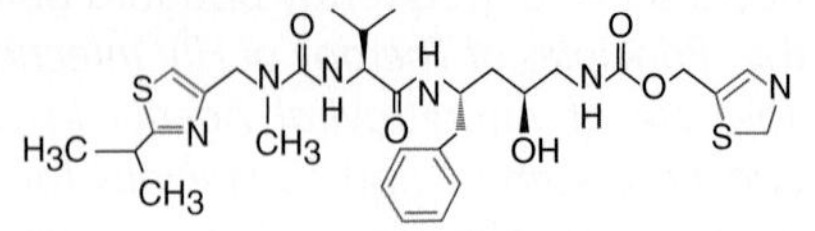

Ritonavir

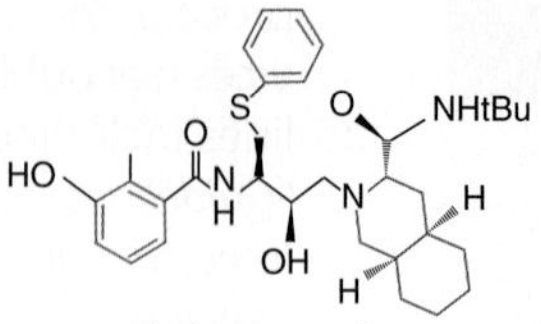

Nelfinavir mesylate

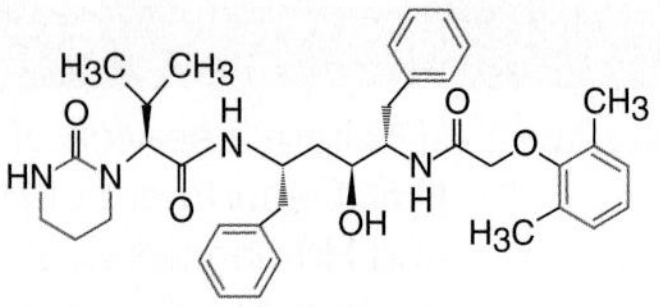

Lopinavir

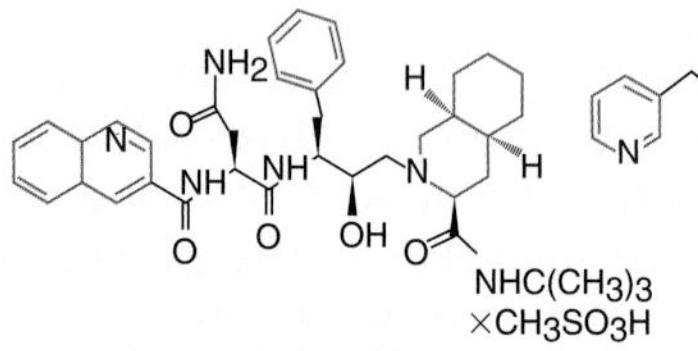

Saquinavir mesylate

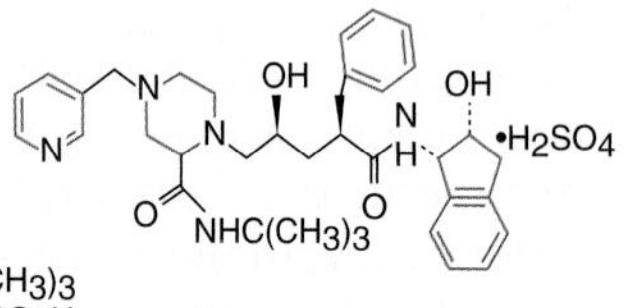

Indinavir sulfate

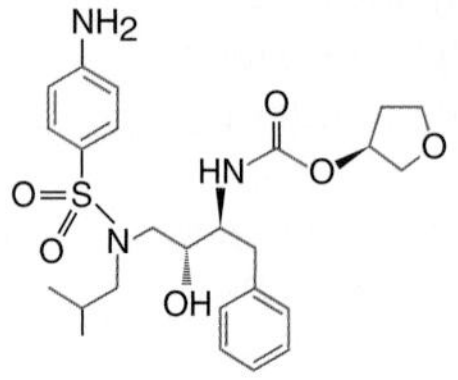

Amprenavir

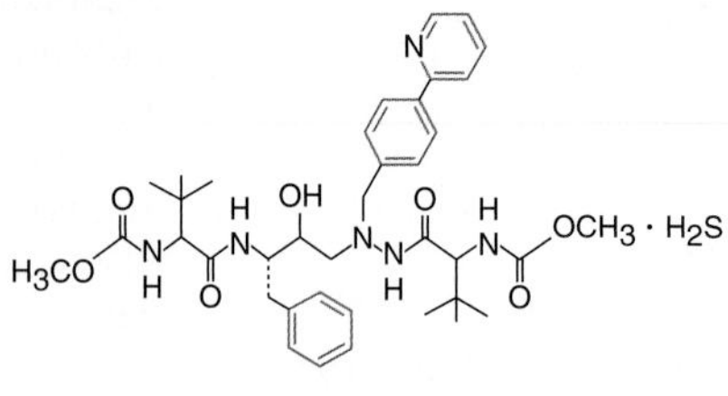

Atazanavir

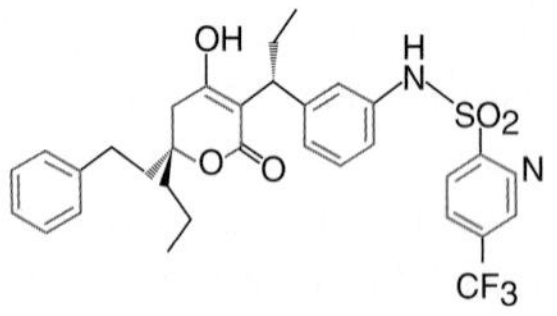

Tipranavir

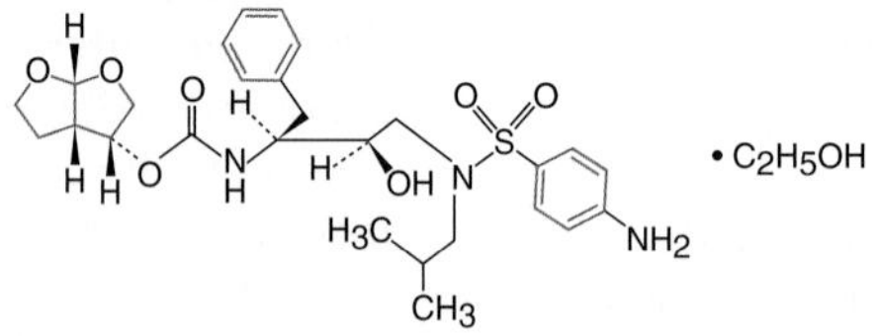

Darunavir

Entry Inhibitors

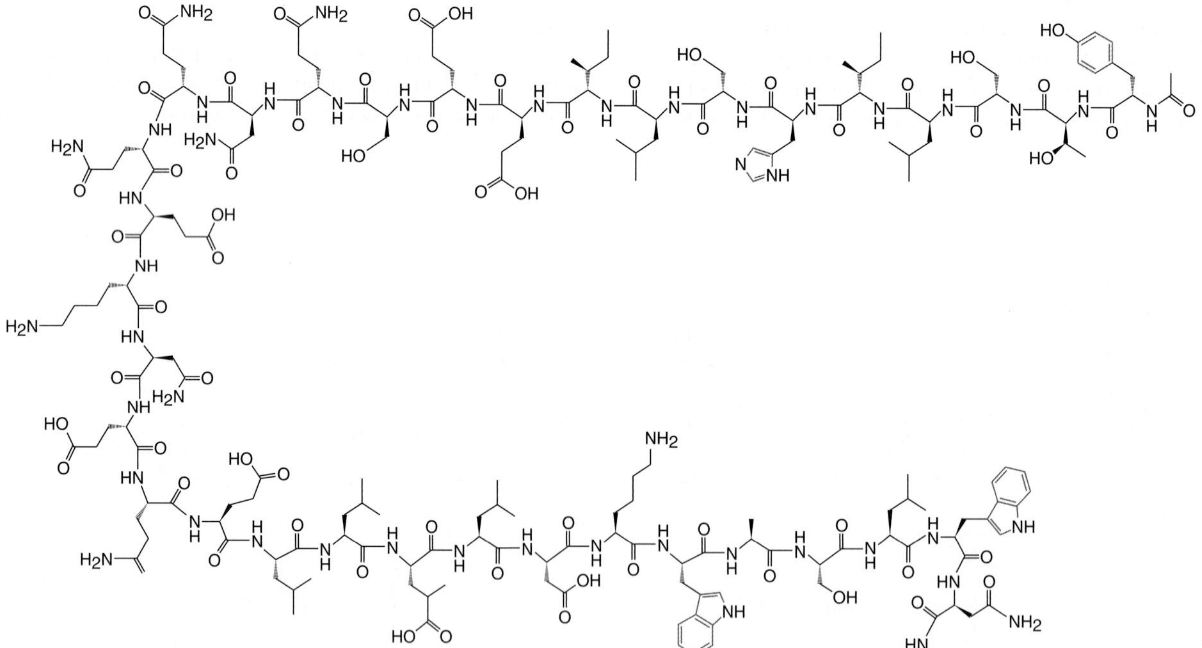

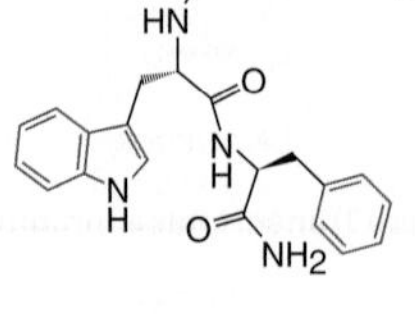

Enfuvirtide

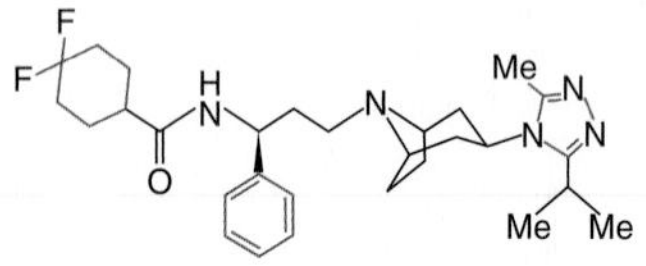

Maraviroc

Integrase Inhibitor

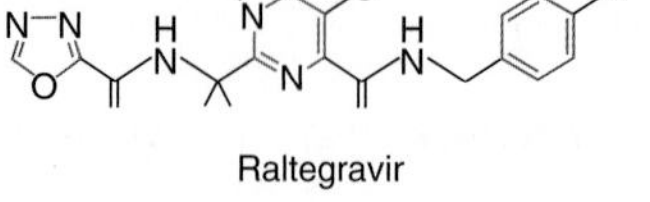

Raltegravir

FIGURE 90-43 (*Continued*)

TABLE 90-18

ANTIRETROVIRAL DRUGS USED IN THE TREATMENT OF HIV INFECTION

DRUG	STATUS	INDICATION	DOSE IN COMBINATION	SUPPORTING DATA	TOXICITY
Reverse Transcriptase Inhibitors					
Zidovudine (AZT, azidothymidine, Retrovir, 3'azido-3'-deoxythymidine)	Licensed	Treatment of HIV infection in combination with other antiretroviral agents Prevention of maternal-fetal HIV transmission	200 mg q8h or 300 mg bid	19 vs 1 death in original placebo-controlled trial in 281 patients with AIDS or ARC. Decreased progression to AIDS in patients with CD4+ T-cell counts <500/μL, $n = 2051$ In pregnant women with CD4+ T-cell count ≥200/μL, AZT PO beginning at weeks 14–34 of gestation plus IV drug during labor and delivery plus PO AZT to infant for 6 wk decreased transmission of HIV by 67.5% (from 25.5% to 8.3%), $n = 363$	Anemia, granulocytopenia, myopathy, lactic acidosis, hepatomegaly with steatosis, headache, nausea
Didanosine (Videx, Videx EC, ddI, dideoxyinosine, 2',3'-dideoxyinosine)	Licensed	For treatment of HIV infection in combination with other antiretroviral agents	Buffered: Requires 2 tablets to achieve adequate buffering of stomach acid; should be administered on an empty stomach ≥60 kg: 200 mg bid <60 kg: 125 mg bid Enteric coated: ≥60 kg: 400 mg qd < 60 kg: 250 mg qd	Clinically superior to AZT as monotherapy in 913 patients with prior AZT therapy. Clinically superior to AZT and comparable to AZT + ddI and AZT + ddC in 1067 AZT-naive patients with CD4+ T-cell counts of 200–500/μL	Pancreatitis, peripheral neuropathy, abnormalities on liver function tests, lactic acidosis, hepatomegaly with steatosis
Zalcitabine (ddC, HIVID, 2'3'-dideoxycytidine)	Licensed Discontinued in 2006	In combination with other antiretroviral agents for the treatment of HIV infection	0.75 mg tid	Clinically inferior to AZT monotherapy as initial treatment. Clinically as good as ddI in advanced patients intolerant to AZT. In combination with AZT, was clinically superior to AZT alone in patients with AIDS or CD4+ T-cell count <350/μL	Peripheral neuropathy, pancreatitis, lactic acidosis, hepatomegaly with steatosis, oral ulcers
Stavudine (d4T, Zerit, 2'3'-didehydro-3'-dideoxythymidine)	Licensed	Treatment of HIV-infected patients in combination with other antiretroviral agents	≥60 kg: 40 mg bid <60 kg: 30 mg bid	Superior to AZT with respect to changes in CD4+ T-cell counts in 359 patients who had received ≥24 wk of AZT. After 12 wk of randomization, the CD4+ T-cell count had decreased in AZT-treated controls by a mean of 22/μL, whereas in stavudine-treated patients, it had increased by a mean of 22/μL	Peripheral neuropathy, pancreatitis, lactic acidosis, hepatomegaly with steatosis, ascending neuromuscular weakness, lipodystrophy

(Continued)

TABLE 90-18 (*CONTINUED*)

ANTIRETROVIRAL DRUGS USED IN THE TREATMENT OF HIV INFECTION

DRUG	STATUS	INDICATION	DOSE IN COMBINATION	SUPPORTING DATA	TOXICITY
Lamivudine (Epivir, 2'3'-dideoxy-3'-thiacytidine, 3TC)	Licensed	In combination with other antiretroviral agents for the treatment of HIV infection	150 mg bid 300 mg qd	Superior to AZT alone with respect to changes in CD4 counts in 495 patients who were zidovudine-naive and 477 patients who were zidovudine-experienced. Overall CD4+ T-cell counts for the zidovudine group were at baseline by 24 wk, whereas in the group treated with zidovudine plus lamivudine, they were 10–50 cells/μL above baseline. 54% decrease in progression to AIDS/death compared with AZT alone	Hepatotoxicity
Emtricitabine (FTC, Emtriva)	Licensed	In combination with other antiretroviral agents for the treatment of HIV infection	200 mg qd	Comparable to d4T in combination with ddI and efavirenz in 571 treatment-naive patients. Similar to 3TC in combination with AZT or d4T + NNRT1 or PI in 440 patients doing well for at least 12 weeks on a 3TC regimen	Hepatotoxicity
Abacavir (Ziagen)	Licensed	For treatment of HIV infection in combination with other antiretroviral agents	300 mg bid	Abacavir + AZT + 3TC equivalent to indinavir + AZT + 3TC with regard to viral load suppression (~60% in each group with <400 HIV RNA copies/mL plasma) and CD4 cell increase (~100/μL in each group) at 24 weeks	Hypersensitivity reaction (can be fatal); fever, rash, nausea, vomiting, malaise or fatigue, and loss of appetite
Tenofovir (Viread)	Licensed	For use in combination with other antiretroviral agents when treatment is indicated	300 mg qd	Reduction of ~0.6 log in HIV-1 RNA levels when added to background regimen in treatment-experienced patients	Potential for renal toxicity
Delavirdine (Rescriptor)	Licensed	For use in combination with appropriate antiretrovirals when treatment is warranted	400 mg tid	Delavirdine + AZT superior to AZT alone with regard to viral load suppression at 52 weeks	Skin rash, abnormalities in liver function tests
Nevirapine (Viramune)	Licensed	In combination with other antiretroviral agents for treatment of progressive HIV infection	200 mg/d × 14 days then 200 mg bid	Increases in CD4+ T-cell count, decrease in HIV RNA when used in combination with nucleosides	Skin rash, hepatotoxicity

Efavirenz (Sustiva)	Licensed	For treatment of HIV infection in combination with other antiretroviral agents	600 mg qhs	Efavirenz + AZT + 3TC comparable to indinavir + AZT + 3TC with regard to viral load suppression (a higher percentage of the efavirenz group achieved viral load <50 copies/mL; however, the discontinuation rate in the indinavir group was unexpectedly high, accounting for most treatment "failures"); CD4 cell increase (~140/µL in each group) at 24 weeks	Rash, dysphoria, elevated liver function tests, drowsiness, abnormal dreams, depression
Etravirine	Expanded access 1-866-889-2074	Pending	Pending	Pending	Rash, headache, dizziness, nausea, diarrhea
Protease Inhibitors					
Saquinavir mesylate (Invirase—hard gel capsule)	Licensed	In combination with other antiretroviral agents when therapy is warranted	1000 mg + 100 mg ritonavir bid	Increases in CD4+ T-cell counts, reduction in HIV RNA most pronounced in combination therapy with ddC. 50% reduction in first AIDS-defining event or death in combination with ddC compared with either agent alone	Diarrhea, nausea, headaches, hyperglycemia, fat redistribution, lipid abnormalities
(Fortovase—soft gel capsule)	Licensed Discontinued 2006	For use in combination with other antiretroviral agents when treatment is warranted	1200 mg tid	Reduction in the mortality rate and AIDS-defining events for patients who received hard-gel formulation in combination with ddC	Diarrhea, nausea, abdominal pain, headaches, hyperglycemia, fat redistribution, lipid abnormalities
Ritonavir (Norvir)	Licensed	In combination with other antiretroviral agents for treatment of HIV infection when treatment is warranted	600 mg bid	Reduction in the cumulative incidence of clinical progression or death from 34 to 17% in patients with CD4+ T-cell count <100/µL treated for a median of 6 months	Nausea, abdominal pain, hyperglycemia, fat redistribution, lipid abnormalities, may alter levels of many other drugs, including saquinavir
Indinavir sulfate (Crixivan)	Licensed	For treatment of HIV infection in combination with other antiretroviral agents when antiretroviral treatment is warranted	800 mg q8h or 800 mg + 100 mg ritonavir bid or 1000 mg q8h when used with efavirenz or nevirapine	Increase in CD4+ T-cell count by 100/µL and 2-log decrease in HIV RNA levels when given in combination with zidovudine and lamivudine. Decrease of 50% in risk of progression to AIDS or death when given with zidovudine and lamivudine compared with zidovudine and lamivudine alone	Nephrolithiasis, indirect hyperbilirubinemia, hyperglycemia, fat redistribution, lipid abnormalities

(Continued)

TABLE 90-18 (*CONTINUED*)

ANTIRETROVIRAL DRUGS USED IN THE TREATMENT OF HIV INFECTION

DRUG	STATUS	INDICATION	DOSE IN COMBINATION	SUPPORTING DATA	TOXICITY
Nelfinavir mesylate (Viracept)	Licensed	For treatment of HIV infection in combination with other antiretroviral agents when antiretroviral therapy is warranted	750 mg tid or 1250 mg bid	2.0-log decline in HIV RNA when given in combination with stavudine	Diarrhea, loose stools, hyperglycemia, fat redistribution, lipid abnormalities May contain traces of the potential carcinogen/teratogen ethyl methane sulfonate
Amprenavir (Agenerase)	Licensed	In combination with other antiretroviral agents for treatment of HIV infection	1200 mg bid or 600 mg + 100 mg ritonavir bid or 1200 mg + 200 mg ritonavir qd	In treatment-naïve patients, amprenavir + AZT + 3TC superior to AZT + 3TC with regard to viral load suppression (53% vs 11% with <400 HIV RNA copies/mL plasma at 24 weeks). CD4+ T-cell responses similar between treatment groups. In treatment-experienced patients, amprenavir + NRTIs similar to indinavir + NRTIs with regard to viral load suppression (43% vs 53% with <400 HIV RNA copies/mL plasma at 24 weeks). CD4+ T-cell responses superior in the indinavir + NRTIs group	Nausea, vomiting, diarrhea, rash, oral paresthesias, elevated liver function tests, hyperglycemia, fat redistribution, lipid abnormalities
Fosamprenavir (Lexiva)	Licensed		1400 mg bid or 700 mg + 100 mg ritonavir bid		
Lopinavir/ritonavir (Kaletra)	Licensed	For treatment of HIV infection in combination with other antiretroviral agents	400 mg/100 mg bid	In treatment-naïve patients, lopinavir/ritonavir + d4T + 3TC superior to nelfinavir+ d4T + 3TC with regard to viral load suppression (79% vs 64% with <400 HIV RNA copies/mL at 40 weeks). CD4+ T-cell increases similar in both groups	Diarrhea, hyperglycemia, fat redistribution, lipid abnormalities
Atazanavir (Reyataz)	Licensed	For treatment of HIV infection in combination with other antiretroviral agents	400 mg qd or 300 mg qd + Ritonavir 100 mg qd when given with efavirenz	Comparable to efavirenz when given in combination with AZT + 3TC in a study of 810 treatment-naive patients. Comparable to nelfinavir when given in combination with d4T + 3TC in a study of 467 treatment-naive patients	Hyperbilirubinemia, PR prolongation, nausea, vomiting, hyperglycemia, fat maldistribution
Tipranavir (Aptivus)	Licensed	In combination with 200 mg ritonavir for combination therapy in treatment-experienced adults	500 mg + 200 mg ritonavir twice daily	At 24 weeks, patients with prior extensive exposure to ARVs showed a –0.8-log change in HIV RNA levels and a 34 cell increase in CD4+ T cells compound to –0.25 log and 4 cells in the control arm. Inferior to lopinavir/ritonavir in a randomized, controlled trial in naïve patients	Diarrhea, nausea, fatigue, headache, skin rash, hepatotoxicity, intracranial hemorrhage

Darunavir (Prezista)	Licensed	In combination with 100 mg ritonavir for combination therapy in treatment-experienced adults	600 mg + 100 mg ritonavir twice daily with food	At 24 weeks, patients with prior extensive exposure to antiretrovirals treated with a new combination including darunavir showed a –1.89-log change in HIV RNA levels and a 92 cell increase in CD4+ T cells compared with –0.48 log and 17 cells in the control arm	Diarrhea, nausea, headache
Entry Inhibitors					
Enfuvirtide (Fuzeon)	Licensed	In combination with other agents in treatment-experienced patients with evidence of HIV-1 replication despite ongoing antiretroviral therapy	90 mg SC bid	In treatment of experienced patients, superior to placebo when added to new optimized background (37% vs 16% with <400 HIV RNA copies/mL at 24 weeks; + 71 vs + 35 CD4+ T cells at 24 weeks)	Local injection reactions, hypersensitivity reactions, increased rate of bacterial pneumonia
Maraviroc (Selzentry)	Licensed	In combination with other antiretroviral agents in treatment experienced adults infected with only CCR5-tropic HIV-1 that is resistant to multiple antiretroviral agents	150–600 mg bid depending upon concomitant medications (see text)	At 24 weeks, among 635 patients with CCR5-tropic virus and HIV-1 RNA >5000 copies/mL despite at least 6 months of prior therapy with at least one agent from 3 of the 4 antiretroviral drug classes, 61% of patients randomized to maraviroc achieved HIV RNA levels <400 copies/mL compared to 28% of patients randomized to placebo	Hepatotoxicity, nasopharyngitis, fever, cough, rash, abdominal pain, dizziness, fever, musculoskeletal symptoms
Integrase Inhibitor					
Raltegravir (Isentress)	Licensed	In combination with other antiretroviral agents in treatment experienced patients with evidence of ongoing HIV-1 replication	400 mg bid	At 24 weeks, among 436 patients with three-class drug resistance, 76% of patients randomized to receive raltegravir achieved HIV RNA levels <400 copies/mL compared with 41% of patients randomized to receive placebo	Nausea, rash

Note: ARC, AIDS-related complex; NRTIs, nonnucleoside reverse transcriptase inhibitors.

emtricitabine; the *nucleotide analogue* tenofovir; and the *nonnucleoside reverse transcriptase inhibitors* nevirapine, delavirdine, and efavirenz (Fig. 90-43; Table 90-18). These were the first class of drugs that were licensed for the treatment of HIV infection. They are indicated for this use as part of combination regimens. It should be stressed that none of these drugs should be used as monotherapy for HIV infection due to the relative ease with which drug resistance may develop under such circumstances. Thus, when lamivudine or tenofovir are used to treat hepatitis B infection in the setting of HIV infection, one should ensure that the patient is also on additional ARV medication. The reverse transcriptase inhibitors block the HIV replication cycle at the point of RNA-dependent DNA synthesis, the reverse transcription step. Although the nonnucleoside reverse transcriptase inhibitors are quite selective for the HIV-1 reverse transcriptase, the nucleoside and nucleotide analogues inhibit a variety of DNA polymerization reactions in addition to those of the HIV-1 reverse transcriptase. For this reason, serious side effects are more varied with the nucleoside analogues and include mitochondrial damage that can lead to hepatic steatosis and lactic acidosis as well as peripheral neuropathy and pancreatitis. One of the more recently recognized problems that has been encountered with the widespread use of HAART therapy has been a syndrome of hyperlipidemia, glucose intolerance/insulin resistance, and fat redistribution often referred to as *lipodystrophy syndrome* (discussed above under metabolic abnormalities).

Zidovudine (AZT; 3'-azido-2',3'-dideoxythymidine) was the first drug approved for the treatment of HIV infection and is the prototype nucleoside analogue. These compounds, in which the hydroxyl group in the 3′ position of the ribose moiety is substituted with a hydrogen or other chemical group, act as DNA chain terminators owing to their inability to form a 3′-5′ phosphodiester linkage with another nucleoside. They bind much more avidly to the active site of the RNA-dependent DNA polymerase of HIV (reverse transcriptase) than to the active site of mammalian cell DNA polymerases; this explains their selective effect on HIV replication. Zidovudine also has a relatively high avidity for the DNA polymerase-γ of human mitochondria. This may contribute to the development of the fatty liver and the myopathy sometimes observed in patients taking zidovudine. As with all the nucleoside analogues, the active form of zidovudine is the triphosphate, and the rate of phosphorylation, a thymidine kinase–dependent pathway, may be different in different cells. This may explain why zidovudine is more effective at inhibiting HIV replication in some cells than others. The clinical benefit of zidovudine was clearly established in 1986 in a phase II, randomized, placebo-controlled trial in patients with advanced HIV disease. However, although treatment of patients with early stages of HIV infection with zidovudine monotherapy was associated with increases in CD4+ T-cell count, it was not associated with a better overall outcome than waiting until later to treat. Subsequent trials established the ability of this drug to dramatically decrease the incidence of perinatal transmission of HIV from infected mother to infant. Eventually a series of studies demonstrated the superiority of combination ARV regimens over zidovudine alone, and combination therapy (discussed below) remains the standard of treatment today. Among the side effects of zidovudine at the initiation of therapy are fatigue, malaise, nausea, and headache. These side effects often subside over time. Patients on zidovudine may develop a macrocytic anemia, neutropenia, myopathy, cardiomyopathy, and lactic acidosis associated with fatty infiltration of the liver. As with every ARV drug, HIV has the ability to develop resistance to zidovudine. Zidovudine resistance has been reported to occur ~6 months after the initiation of zidovudine monotherapy. More recently, zidovudine-resistant viruses have been noted in patients with acute infection before the initiation of therapy, implying that zidovudine-resistant viruses can be transmitted from person to person. Resistance emerges more rapidly in late-stage patients, presumably as a consequence of a greater degree of viral replication and thus a greater opportunity for mutation. A variety of amino acid changes including substitutions, insertions, and deletions have been reported to confer zidovudine resistance (Fig. 90-44). One combination preparation, Combivir, consists of zidovudine and lamivudine, whereas another, Trizivir, consists of zidovudine, lamivudine, and abacavir.

Didanosine (ddI; 2',3'-dideoxyinosine) was the second drug licensed for the treatment of HIV infection, followed shortly thereafter by zalcitabine. Didanosine is metabolized to dideoxyadenosine in vivo. It is best absorbed on an empty stomach at a high pH. The toxicity profile of didanosine is quite different from that of zidovudine. The most common toxicity is a painful sensory peripheral neuropathy that occurs in ~30% of patients receiving >400 mg/d. It generally resolves with discontinuation of the drug and may not recur if the drug is resumed at a reduced dose. At higher doses than are currently used, one may see pancreatitis in ~10% of patients. Pancreatitis associated with didanosine therapy can be fatal. Didanosine should be discontinued if a patient experiences abdominal pain consistent with pancreatitis or if an elevated serum amylase or lipase level is found in association with an edematous pancreas on ultrasound. Didanosine is contraindicated in patients with a prior history of pancreatitis, regardless of etiology. A higher incidence of didanosine-associated toxicities has been seen when it is used in combination with stavudine, hydroxyurea, ribavirin, or tenofovir.

Zalcitabine (ddC; 2',3'-dideoxycytidine) is rarely used today in the management of patients with HIV infection and was discontinued from the U.S. market in 2006. Among the nucleoside analogues licensed for the treatment of HIV infection, it is probably the weakest. The main toxicities of ddC are peripheral neuropathy and pancreatitis.

Stavudine (d4T; 2',3'-didehydro-3'-deoxythymidine) was the fourth drug licensed for the treatment of HIV

MUTATIONS IN THE REVERSE TRANSCRIPTASE GENE ASSOCIATED WITH RESISTANCE TO REVERSE TRANSCRIPTASE INHIBITORS

Nucleoside and Nucleotide Reverse Transcriptase Inhibitors (nRTIs)

Multi-nRTI Resistance: 69 Insertion Complex (affects all nRTIs currently approved by the US FDA)

Wild type	M	A	▼	K	L	T	K
Position	**41**	**62**	**69**	**70**	**210**	**215**	**219**
Substitution	L	V	Insert	R	W	Y F	Q E

Multi-nRTI Resistance: 151 Complex (affects all nRTIs currently approved by the US FDA except tenofovir)

Wild type	A	V	F	F	Q
Position	**62**	**75**	**77**	**116**	**151**
Substitution	V	I	L	Y	M

Multi-nRTI Resistance: Thymidine Analogue-Associated Mutations (TAMs; affects all nRTIs currently approved by the US FDA)

Wild type	M	D	K	L	T	K
Position	**41**	**67**	**70**	**210**	**215**	**219**
Substitution	L	N	R	W	Y F	Q E

Abacavir

Wild type	K	L	Y	M
Position	**65**	**74**	**115**	**184**
Substitution	R	V	F	V

Didanosine

Wild type	K	L
Position	**65**	**74**
Substitution	R	V

Emtricitabine

Wild type	K	M
Position	**65**	**184**
Substitution	R	V I

Lamivudine

Wild type	K	M
Position	**65**	**184**
Substitution	R	V I

Stavudine

Wild type	M	D	K	L	T	K
Position	**41**	**67**	**70**	**210**	**215**	**219**
Substitution	L	N	R	W	Y F	Q E

Tenofovir

Wild type	K	K
Position	**65**	**70**
Substitution	R	R

Zidovudine

Wild type	M	D	K	L	T	K
Position	**41**	**67**	**70**	**210**	**215**	**219**
Substitution	L	N	R	W	Y F	Q E

Nonnucleoside Reverse Transcriptase Inhibitors (NNRTIs)

Efavirenz

Wild type	L	K	V	V	Y	Y	G	P
Position	**100**	**103**	**106**	**108**	**181**	**188**	**190**	**225**
Substitution	I	N	M	I	C I	L	S A	H

Etravirine (expanded access)

Wild type	V	A	L	K	V	V	Y	G
Position	90	98	100	101	106	179	181	190
Substitution	I	G	I	E P	I	D F	C I V	S A

Nevirapine

Wild type	L	K	V	V	Y	Y	G
Position	**100**	**103**	**106**	**108**	**181**	**188**	**190**
Substitution	I	N	A M	I	C I	C L H	A

FIGURE 90-44 *(Continued on next page)*

Amino acid substitutions conferring resistance to antiretroviral drugs. For each amino acid residue, the letter above the bar indicates the amino acid associated with wild-type virus and the letter(s) below indicate the substitution(s) that confer viral resistance. The number shows the position of the mutation in the protein. Mutations selected by protease inhibitors in Gag cleavage sites are not listed. HR1 indicates first heptad repeat; NAMs indicates nRTI-associated mutations; nRTI indicates nucleoside reverse transcriptase inhibitor; NNRTI indicates nonnucleoside reverse transcriptase inhibitor; PI indicates protease inhibitor. Amino acid abbreviations: A, alanine; C, cysteine; D, aspartate; E, glutamine; F, phenylalanine; G, glycine; H, histidine; I, isoleucine; K, lysine; L, leucine; M, methionine; N, asparagine; P, proline; Q, glutamine; R, arginine;

 (Continued from preceding page)

MUTATIONS IN THE PROTEASE GENE ASSOCIATED WITH RESISTANCE TO PROTEASE INHIBITORS

Atazanavir +/– ritonavir

Wild-type	L	G	K	L	V	L	E	M	M	G	I	F	I	D	I	I	A	G	V	I	I	N	L	I
Position	10	16	20	24	32	33	34	36	46	48	**50**	53	54	60	62	64	71	73	82	**84**	85	**88**	90	93
Substitution	I F V C	E	R M I T V	I	I	I F V	Q	I L V	I L	V	L	L Y	L V M T A	E	V	L M V	V I T L	C S T A	A T F I	V	V	S	M	L M

Fosamprenavir/ ritonavir

Wild-type	L	V	M	I	I	I	G	L	V	I	L
Position	10	32	46	47	**50**	54	73	76	82	**84**	90
Substitution	F I R V	I	I L	V	V	L V M	S	V	A F S T	V	M

Darunavir/ ritonavir

Wild-type	V	V	L	I	I	I	G	L	I	L
Position	11	32	33	47	**50**	**54**	73	**76**	**84**	89
Substitution	I	I	F	V	V	M L	S	V	V	V

Indinavir/ ritonavir

Wild-type	L	K	L	V	M	M	I	A	G	L	V	V	I	L
Position	10	20	24	32	36	**46**	54	71	73	76	77	**82**	**84**	90
Substitution	I R V	M R	I	I	I	I L	V	V T	S A	V	I	A F T	V	M

Lopinavir/ ritonavir

Wild-type	L	K	L	V	L	M	I	I	F	I	L	A	G	L	V	I	L
Position	10	20	24	**32**	33	46	**47**	50	53	54	63	71	73	76	**82**	84	90
Substitution	F I R V	M R	I	I	F	I L	V A	V	L	V L A M T S	P	V T	S	V	A F T S	V	M

Nelfinavir

Wild-type	L	D	M	M	A	V	V	I	N	L
Position	10	**30**	36	46	71	77	82	84	88	**90**
Substitution	F I	N	I	I L	V T	I	A F T S	V	D S	M

Saquinavir/ ritonavir

Wild-type	L	L	G	I	I	A	G	V	V	I	L
Position	10	24	**48**	54	62	71	73	77	82	84	**90**
Substitution	I R V	I	V	V L	V	V T	S	I	A F T S	V	M

Tipranavir/ ritonavir

Wild-type	L	I	K	L	E	M	K	M	I	I	Q	H	T	V	N	I	L
Position	10	13	20	**33**	35	36	43	46	47	54	58	69	74	**82**	83	**84**	90
Substitution	V	V	M R	F	G	I	T	L	V	A M V	E	K	P	L T	D	V	M

MUTATIONS IN THE ENVELOPE GENE ASSOCIATED WITH RESISTANCE TO ENTRY INHIBITORS

Enfuvirtide

Wild-type	G	I	V	Q	Q	N	N
Position	36	37	38	39	40	42	43
Substitution	D S	V	A M E	R	H	T	D

Maraviroc: See User Note

MUTATIONS IN THE INTEGRASE GENE ASSOCIATED WITH RESISTANCE TO INTEGRASE INHIBITORS

Raltegravir (expanded access)

Wild-type	Q	N
Position	**148**	**155**
Substitution	H K R	H

MUTATIONS

Insertion

Amino acid, wild-type — L

Amino acid position

Major (boldface type; protease only) — **90** 54

Amino acid substitution conferring resistance — M

Minor (lightface type; protease only)

FIGURE 90-44 (*Continued*)

S, serine; T, threonine; V, valine; W, tryptophan; Y, tyrosine. *[Reprinted with permission from the International AIDS Society—USA. Johnson VA, Brun-Vézinet F, Clotet B, Günthard HF, Kuritzkes DR, Pillay D, Schapiro JM, and Richman DD. Update of the Drug Resistance Mutations in HIV-1: 2007. Topics in HIV Medicine. 2007; 15(4):119–125. Updated information (and thorough explanatory notes) is available at www.iasusa.org.]*

infection and was discontinued from the U.S. market in 2006. Like zidovudine, stavudine is a thymidine analogue. These two drugs are antagonistic in vitro and in vivo and should not be given together. Stavudine has been associated with a higher incidence of mitochondrial toxicity than the other licensed nucleoside analogues. Peripheral neuropathy, lipoatrophy, lactic acidosis, and hepatic steatosis are the main toxicities of stavudine.

Lamivudine (3TC; 2',3'-dideoxy-3'-thiacytidine) is the fifth of the nucleoside analogues to be licensed in the United States. In actual practice, lamivudine or the closely related drug emtricitabine is a frequent element of many different combination regimens currently in use. These two drugs and the nucleotide reverse transcriptase inhibitor tenofovir (see below) also have activity against hepatitis B virus. For this reason, flares of hepatitis may be seen in co-infected patients starting and or stopping these agents due to the confounding issues of direct effects of treatment and the potential for the IRIS (see above). To prevent the development of resistant strains of HIV, these drugs should never be used on their own for the treatment of hepatitis B in the patient with HIV infection. Lamivudine is available either alone or in coformulations including zidovudine and/or abacavir (Table 90-19). One reason behind the excellent synergy seen between lamivudine and the other nucleoside analogues may be that strains of HIV resistant to lamivudine (M184V substitution) appear to have enhanced sensitivity to other nucleosides, and thus development of dual resistance is more difficult. In addition, there is a suggestion that 3TC-resistant strains of HIV may be less virulent and are less able to generate new mutants than are strains of HIV that are 3TC-sensitive. Lamivudine is among the best tolerated and least toxic nucleoside analogues.

Emtricitabine (FTC; 5-fluoro-1-(2R,5S)-[2-(hydroxymethyl)-1,3-oxathiolan-5-y]cytosine) is the negative enantiomer of a thio analogue of cytidine with a fluorine in the 5 position. It is licensed for use in combination with other ARV agents for treatment of HIV-1 infection in adults. Compared with lamivudine, it is similar in activity and has a longer half-life. It is available either alone or coformulated with tenofovir or tenofovir and efavirenz (Table 90-19). Resistance to emtricitabine is associated with the M184V mutation in reverse transcriptase. Viruses showing the K65R mutation in reverse transcriptase may have reduced susceptibility to emtricitabine.

Abacavir {(1S,cis)-4-[2-amino-6-(cyclopropylamino)-9H-purin-9-yl]-2-cyclopentene-1-methanol sulfate (salt)(2:1)} is a synthetic carbocyclic analogue of the nucleoside guanosine. It is licensed to be used in combination with other ARV agents for the treatment of HIV-1 infection. Hypersensitivity reactions that may occur with initial therapy or rechallenge have been reported in ~4% of patients treated with this drug, and patients developing signs or symptoms of hypersensitivity such as fever, skin rash, fatigue, and gastrointestinal symptoms should discontinue the drug and not restart it. Fatal hypersensitivity reactions have been reported with rechallenge. Abacavir hypersensitivity appears to occur with a higher frequency in patients who are HLA-B57. It has been recommended that patients be screened for HLA-B57 before initiation of abacavir and that abacavir only be used as a last resort in patients who are HLA-B57 positive. Abacavir-resistant strains of HIV are typically also resistant to lamivudine, didanosine, and zalcitabine. Abacavir is formulated alone as well as in combination with lamivudine or zidovudine and lamivudine.

Tenofovir disoproxil fumarate (9-[(R)-2-[[bis[[(isopropoxycarbonyl)oxy]methoxy]phosphinyl]methoxy]propyl]adenine fumarate (1:1)) is an acyclic nucleoside phosphonate diester analogue of adenosine monophosphate. It undergoes diester hydrolysis to form the nucleoside monophosphate tenofovir and is the first nucleotide analogue to be licensed for treatment of HIV infection. It is indicated in combination with other ARV agents for the treatment of HIV-1 infection. HIV isolates with increased resistance typically express a K65R mutation in reverse transcriptase and a three- to fourfold reduction in sensitivity to tenofovir. Tenofovir is primarily eliminated by the kidneys, and renal impairment including a Fanconi-like syndrome with hypophosphatemia may occur. Tenofovir is contraindicated in patients with renal impairment. Coadministration with didanosine leads to a 60% increase in didanosine levels, and thus doses of didanosine need to be adjusted and patients monitored carefully if these two drugs are used in combination. In addition, CD4+ T-cell increases may be blunted in patients on this combination. Coadministration of tenofovir with atazanavir leads to a decrease in atazanavir levels, and thus low-dose ritonavir (see below) needs to be added when these drugs are used in combination. Tenofovir is available alone and coformulated with emtricitabine or emtricitabine and efavirenz.

Nevirapine, delavirdine, efavirenz, and *etravirine* are nonnucleoside inhibitors of the HIV-1 reverse transcriptase. They are licensed for use in combination with nucleoside analogues for the treatment of HIV-infected adults. Coformulations that include efavirenz or nevirapine are available (Table 90-19). These agents inhibit reverse transcriptase by binding to regions of the enzyme outside the active site and causing conformational changes in the enzyme that render it inactive.

TABLE 90-19

COMBINATION FORMULATIONS OF ANTIRETROVIRAL DRUGS

NAME	COMBINATION
Combivir	Zidovudine + lamivudine
Epzicom	Zidovudine + abacavir
Trizivir	Zidovudine + lamivudine + abacavir
Truvada	Tenofovir + emtricitabine
Atripla	Tenofovir + emtricitabine + efavirenz
Triomune[a]	Stavudine + lamivudine + nevirapine

[a]Not licensed in the United States.

Although these agents are active in the nanomolar range, they are also very selective for the reverse transcriptase of HIV-1, have no activity against HIV-2, and, when used as monotherapy, are associated with the rapid emergence of drug-resistant mutants (Table 90-18; Fig. 90-44). Efavirenz is administered once a day, nevirapine and etravirine twice a day, and delavirdine three times a day. All four drugs are associated with the development of a maculopapular rash, generally seen within the first few weeks of therapy. Although it is possible to treat through this rash, it is important to be sure that one is not dealing with a more severe eruption such as Stevens-Johnson syndrome by looking carefully for signs of mucosal involvement, significant fever, or painful lesions with desquamation. Severe, life-threatening, and in some cases fatal hepatotoxicity, including fulminant and cholestatic hepatitis, hepatic necrosis, and hepatic failure, have been reported in patients treated with nevirapine. There is a suggestion that this is more common in women with higher CD4+ T-cell counts. Many patients treated with efavirenz note a feeling of light-headedness, dizziness, or out of sorts after the initiation of therapy. Some complain of vivid dreams. These symptoms tend to disappear after several weeks of therapy. Aside from difficulties with dreams, taking efavirenz at bedtime may minimize the side effects. Efavirenz may cause fetal harm when administered during the first trimester to a pregnant woman. Women of childbearing potential should undergo pregnancy testing before initiation of efavirenz. Efavirenz is commonly used in combination with two nucleoside analogues as part of initial treatment regimens. Etravirine is a diarylpyrimidine derivative that is currently available on expanded access for treatment of HIV infection in combination with other agents. In contrast to the other nonnucleoside reverse transcriptase inhibitors, which all exhibit cross-resistance, etravirine may be active against strains of HIV that are resistant to other nonnucleoside reverse transcriptase inhibitors. Among its side effects are rash, headache, nausea, and diarrhea.

The HIV-1 protease inhibitors (saquinavir, indinavir, ritonavir, nelfinavir, amprenavir, fosamprenavir, lopinavir/ritonavir, atazanavir, tipranavir, and darunavir) are a major part of the therapeutic armamentarium of ARVs. When used as part of initial regimens in combination with reverse transcriptase inhibitors, these agents have been shown to be capable of suppressing levels of HIV replication to under 50 copies per milliliter in the majority of patients for a minimum of 5 years. As in the case of reverse transcriptase inhibitors, resistance to protease inhibitors can develop rapidly in the setting of monotherapy, and thus these agents should be used only as part of combination therapeutic regimens. A summary of known resistance mutations for protease inhibitors is shown in Fig. 90-44.

Saquinavir was the first of the HIV-1 protease inhibitors to be licensed. It is typically given with low doses of ritonavir to obtain therapeutic levels. Saquinavir is metabolized by the cytochrome P450 system in both the gastrointestinal tract and the liver. Low-dose ritonavir results in inhibition of cytochrome P450 action. Thus when both drugs are administered together, there is an increase in saquinavir levels. This use of low doses of ritonavir to provide pharmacodynamic boosting of other agents is a common strategy in HIV therapy. Saquinavir is among the best-tolerated protease inhibitors.

Ritonavir was the first protease inhibitor for which clinical efficacy was demonstrated. In a study of 1090 patients with CD4+ T-cell counts <100/μL who were randomized to receive either placebo or ritonavir in addition to any other licensed medications, patients receiving ritonavir had a reduction in the cumulative incidence of clinical progression or death from 34 to 17%. Mortality decreased from 10.1 to 5.8%. At full doses, ritonavir is poorly tolerated. Among the main side effects are nausea, diarrhea, abdominal pain, hyperlipidemia, and circumoral paresthesia. Ritonavir has a high affinity for several isoforms of cytochrome P450, and its use can result in large increases in the plasma concentrations of drugs metabolized by this pathway. Among the agents affected in this manner are most other protease inhibitors, macrolide antibiotics, R-warfarin, ondansetron, rifabutin, most calcium channel blockers, glucocorticoids, and some of the chemotherapeutic agents used to treat KS and/or lymphomas. In addition, ritonavir may increase the activity of glucuronyltransferases, thus decreasing the levels of drugs metabolized by this pathway. Overall, great care must be taken when prescribing additional drugs to patients taking protease inhibitors in general and ritonavir in particular. As mentioned above, the pharmacodynamic boosting property of ritonavir, seen with doses as low as 100–200 mg once or twice a day, is often used in the setting of combination ARV therapy for HIV infection to derive more convenient regimens. For example, when given with low-dose ritonavir, saquinavir and indinavir can both be given on twice-a-day schedules and taken with food.

Indinavir was the first protease inhibitor used in combination with dual nucleoside therapy. The combination of zidovudine, lamivudine, and indinavir was the first "triple combination" shown to have a profound effect on HIV replication. The main side effects of indinavir are nephrolithiasis (seen in 4% of patients) and asymptomatic indirect hyperbilirubinemia (seen in 10%). Indinavir is predominantly metabolized by the liver. The dose should be lowered in patients with cirrhosis. Levels of indinavir are decreased during concurrent therapy with rifabutin, efavirenz, or nevirapine and increased during concurrent therapy with ketoconazole, delavirdine, or ritonavir. Dosages should be modified appropriately in these circumstances (Table 90-18).

Nelfinavir was approved in 1997 and *amprenavir* was approved in 1999 for the treatment of adult or pediatric HIV infection when ARV therapy is warranted. As with most of the newer ARV agents, these approvals were based on randomized, controlled trials that demonstrated decreases in plasma HIV RNA levels and increases in CD4+ T-cell counts. The presence of the potential carcinogen and teratogen ethyl methanesulfonate in nelfinavir preparations makes it a drug to be avoided in pregnant women. Both nelfinavir and amprenavir have unique resistance profiles. Nelfinavir resistance is associated with a D30N substitution in the protease gene. Viruses harboring this single mutation retain sensitivity to other protease inhibitors. Although it has been suggested that for this reason nelfinavir is a good initial protease inhibitor, enthusiasm for its use has waned after the 48-week clinical trials data demonstrating the virologic inferiority of nelfinavir to lopinavir/ritonavir, to fosamprenavir, and to efavirenz. Protease inhibitor resistance typically involves multiple amino acid substitutions and reduced susceptibility across the class. Amprenavir resistance is associated with a unique substitution at amino acid 50 (I50V). Nelfinavir and amprenavir are both associated with gastrointestinal side effects. About 1% of patients receiving amprenavir have experienced severe and life-threatening skin reactions. An additional disadvantage of amprenavir is that the original formulation requires the patient to take 8 large capsules twice a day. Amprenavir has largely been replaced by fosamprenavir (see below).

Fosamprenavir was licensed in 2003 for the treatment of HIV infection in combination with other ARV agents in adults. It is a prodrug of amprenavir that is rapidly converted to amprenavir by cellular phosphatases. It is supplied as a 700-mg tablet. The recommended dosage is 1400 mg bid or 700 mg bid with ritonavir, 100 mg bid, or 1400 mg once a day with ritonavir, 200 mg once a day. As noted above, ritonavir-boosted fosamprenavir has been shown to be comparable to lopinavir/ritonavir and efavirenz in combination regimens.

Lopinavir/ritonavir (Kaletra) is a fixed-dose combination of the protease inhibitors lopinavir (200 mg) and ritonavir (50 mg). It was licensed in 2000 for treatment of HIV-1 infection in adults and children in combination with other agents. A main advantage of this pill is that it combines the pharmacologic enhancement of low-dose ritonavir with a second protease inhibitor in a single capsule. In a randomized, controlled trial, this combination capsule was found to be superior to nelfinavir. Its main complications are gastrointestinal upset and hyperlipidemia.

Atazanavir is an azapeptide inhibitor of the HIV-1 protease that was licensed in 2003. An advantage of atazanavir is that total cholesterol and triglyceride levels do not increase as much with atazanavir as with other protease inhibitors. This coupled with the fact that it can be given on a once-daily schedule has made atazanavir a popular component of initial treatment regimens. Atazanavir is associated with increases in serum bilirubin and prolongations of the ECG PR interval. Atazanavir-resistant isolates emerging in previously treatment-naïve individuals frequently harbor an I50L substitution. This mutation in some instances is associated with increased sensitivity to other protease inhibitors. Atazanavir requires an acidic gastric pH for absorption, and its use in combination with a proton pump inhibitor is contraindicated due to concerns about absorption. Atazanavir is an inhibitor of cytochrome P3A and its use may be associated with increased levels of calcium channel blockers, macrolide antibiotics, HMB-CoA reductase inhibitors, and sildenafil. Levels of atazanavir are lower in the presence of tenofovir or efavirenz. In these settings, levels of atazanavir should be boosted with the use of low-dose ritonavir.

Tipranavir is a non-peptidic HIV protease inhibitor licensed in 2005. It is licensed for use in combination with 200 mg ritonavir and is indicated for combination ARV therapy of HIV-1 infection in treatment-experienced adults or in adults with evidence of HIV-1 strains resistant to multiple protease inhibitors. Tipranavir was found to be inferior to lopinavir/ritonavir in a randomized controlled trial in naïve patients. In that study, at lower doses it was virologically inferior, whereas at higher doses it exhibited a greater degree of hepatotoxicity. The main side effects of tipranavir are gastrointestinal intolerance and skin rash; the latter is seen in ~10% of patients and may be related to the sulfonamide moiety in the molecule. Tipranavir coadministered with ritonavir has also been associated with reports of intracranial hemorrhage as well as reports of clinical hepatitis and hepatic decompensation, including some fatalities in both settings. The risk of hepatotoxicity is increased in patients with hepatitis B or C co-infection.

Darunavir is a non-peptidic HIV protease inhibitor licensed in 2006 to be coadministered with 100 mg of ritonavir and other ARV agents for the treatment of HIV infection in ARV treatment–experienced adults. This indication is based on the fact that the trials leading to licensure of darunavir were carried out in treatment-experienced patients. In these studies, 46% of patients achieved a reduction in HIV RNA viral loads to <50 copies per milliliter. Studies are underway in treatment-naïve patients. Skin rash, which may be severe, is seen in 7% of patients and may be related to the sulfonamide moiety contained in the molecule. Gastrointestinal intolerance and headache are the other most frequent side effects.

Entry inhibitors act by interfering with the binding of HIV to its receptor or co-receptor or by interfering with the process of fusion (see above). The first drug in this class to be licensed was the fusion inhibitor *enfuvirtide*, or T-20, followed by the CCR5 antagonist *maraviroc*. A variety of additional small molecules that bind to HIV-1 co-receptors are currently in clinical trials.

Enfuvirtide is a linear 36-amino-acid synthetic peptide with the *N*-terminus acetylated and the *C*-terminus a carboxamide. It is composed of naturally occurring L-amino acid residues and interferes with the fusion of the viral and cellular membranes by binding to the HR1 region in the gp41 subunit of the HIV-1 envelope. This binding interferes with the coil-coil interaction required to approximate the two membranes. Resistant isolates of HIV exhibit amino acid changes in positions 36–45 of gp41. In two independent studies, patients who had persistent viremia despite prior treatment with agents from all three available classes of drugs were randomized to receive an individualized regimen (based upon prior treatment history and resistance profile) with or without enfuvirtide. The change in plasma HIV-1 RNA from baseline was

~1 log greater (–1.53 vs –0.68) in patients randomized to receive enfuvirtide. Among the drawbacks of this agent are the requirement for twice-a-day injection, the occurrence of injection site reactions in close to 100% of patients, and an increase in bacterial pneumonia in the enfuvirtide-treated patients compared to the patients in the control arm (4.68 vs 0.61 events per 100 patient years) in the phase III studies.

Maraviroc is a CCR5 antagonist that interferes with HIV binding at the stage of co-receptor engagement. It was licensed in 2007 for treatment of HIV infection in combination with other agents in treatment-experienced patients infected with only CCR5-tropic virus resistant to multiple agents. A co-receptor tropism assay should be performed if one is considering the use of maraviroc to ensure that the potential patient is harboring R5 virus. In phase III trials of treatment-experienced patients randomized to receive optimal therapy plus maraviroc or placebo, 61% of patients randomized to maraviroc achieved HIV RNA levels <400 copies/mL compared with 28% of patients randomized to placebo. An allergic reaction-associated hepatotoxicity has been reported with maraviroc. Among the most common side effects of maraviroc are dizziness due to postural hypotension, cough, fever, colds, rash, muscle and joint pain, and stomach pain. Maraviroc is a substrate of CYP3A and Pgp, and the recommend dose varies depending upon concomitant medications. In combination with nucleoside analogues, tipranavir/ritonavir, enfuvirtide and/or nevirapine the dose is 300 mg twice daily. In the presence of CYP3A inhibitors such as most protease inhibitors the dose is 150 mg twice daily and in presence of CYP3A inducers such as efavirenz, the dose is 600 mg twice daily.

The newest class of ARV compounds are the *integrase inhibitors*. *Raltegravir* is an inhibitor of the viral enzyme integrase and the first of this class to be approved. It was approved in 2007 for treatment of HIV infection in combination with other agents in treatment experienced patients. Raltegravir exhibits a wide range of activity against HIV-1 and HIV-2, including viruses with multiple resistance mutations to other classes of drugs. As with several other compounds, resistance to raltegravir comes at the expense of replicative fitness. In two phase III studies in which 436 patients with 3-class ARV drug resistance were randomized to an optimized background regimen with raltegravir or placebo, 76% of patients receiving raltegravir achieved HIV RNA levels <400 copies/mL compared with 41% of patients randomized to the placebo arm. In contrast to many other antiretroviral drugs, the side effect profile of raltegravir is minimal, with similar side effect profiles noted for the raltegravir and placebo groups.

PRINCIPLES OF THERAPY The principles of therapy for HIV infection have been articulated by a panel sponsored by the U.S. Department of Health and Human Services as a working group of the NIH Office of AIDS Research Advisory Council These principles are summarized in Table 90-20. As noted in these guidelines, eradication of HIV infection has not yet been possible. Treatment decisions must take into account the fact that one is dealing with a chronic infection. Although early therapy is generally the rule in infectious diseases, immediate treatment of every HIV-infected individual upon diagnosis may not be prudent, and therapeutic decisions must take into account the balance between risks and benefits. Although it seems reasonable to assume that the complications associated with ARV therapy could be minimized by regimens designed to minimize exposure to the drugs in question, all efforts to do so have paradoxically been associated with an increase in serious adverse events in the patients randomized to intermittent therapy suggesting that some "non-AIDS" associated serious adverse events such as heart attack and stroke may be linked to HIV replication. Thus, unless contraindicated for reasons of toxicity, patients started on ARV therapy should remain on ARV therapy.

TABLE 90-20

PRINCIPLES OF THERAPY OF HIV INFECTION

1. Ongoing HIV replication leads to immune system damage and progression to AIDS.
2. Plasma HIV RNA levels indicate the magnitude of HIV replication and the rate of CD4+ T-cell destruction. CD4+ T-cell counts indicate the current level of competence of the immune system.
3. Rates of disease progression differ among individuals, and treatment decisions should be individualized based upon plasma HIV RNA levels and CD4+ T-cell counts.
4. Maximal suppression of viral replication is a goal of therapy; the greater the suppression, the less likely the appearance of drug-resistant quasispecies.
5. The most effective therapeutic strategies involve the simultaneous initiation of combinations of effective anti-HIV drugs with which the patient has not been previously treated and that are not cross-resistant with antiretroviral agents that the patient has already received.
6. The antiretroviral drugs used in combination regimens should be used according to optimum schedules and dosages.
7. The number of available drugs is limited. Any decisions on antiretroviral therapy have a long-term impact on future options for the patient.
8. Women should receive optimal antiretroviral therapy regardless of pregnancy status.
9. The same principles apply to children and adults. The treatment of HIV-infected children involves unique pharmacologic, virologic, and immunologic considerations.
10. Compliance is an important part of ensuring maximal effect from a given regimen. The simpler the regimen, the easier it is for the patient to be compliant.

Source: Modified from *Principles of Therapy of HIV Infection*, USPHS, and the Henry J. Kaiser Family Foundation.

TABLE 90-21

INDICATIONS FOR THE INITIATION OF ANTIRETROVIRAL THERAPY IN PATIENTS WITH HIV INFECTION

I. Acute infection syndrome
II. Chronic infection
   A. Symptomatic disease (including HIV-associated nephropathy)
   B. Asymptomatic diseases
      1. CD4+ T-cell count <350/μL[a]
      2. Pregnancy
III. Postexposure prophylaxis

[a]This is an area of controversy. Some experts would wait until the CD4 cell count declines to 200/μL, some would treat everyone with a viral load >100,000 copies/mL, whereas others would treat everyone regardless of CD4+ T-cell count.

Source: *Guidelines for the Use of Antiretroviral Agents in HIV-Infected Adults and Adolescents,* USPHS.

TABLE 90-22

INDICATIONS FOR CHANGING ANTIRETROVIRAL THERAPY IN PATIENTS WITH HIV INFECTION[a]

Less than a 1-log drop in plasma HIV RNA by 4 weeks after the initiation of therapy
A reproducible significant increase (defined as three-fold or greater) from the nadir of plasma HIV RNA level not attributable to intercurrent infection, vaccination, or test methodology
Persistently declining CD4+ T-cell numbers
Clinical deterioration
Side effects

[a]Generally speaking, a change should involve the initiation of at least two drugs felt to be effective in the given patient. The exception to this is when change is being made to manage toxicity, in which case a single substitution is reasonable.

Source: *Guidelines for the Use of Antiretroviral Agents in HIV-Infected Adults and Adolescents,* USPHS.

At present, a reasonable course of action is to initiate ARV therapy in anyone with the acute HIV syndrome; all pregnant women; patients with symptomatic disease; and patients with asymptomatic disease with CD4+ T-cell counts <350/μL (**Table 90-21**). In addition, one may wish to administer a 6-week course of therapy to uninfected individuals immediately after a high-risk exposure to HIV.

Once the decision has been made to initiate therapy, the health care provider must decide which drugs to use as the first regimen. The decision regarding choice of drugs not only will affect the immediate response to therapy but also will have implications regarding options for future therapeutic regimens. The initial regimen is usually the most effective insofar as the virus has yet to develop significant resistance. The two options for initial therapy most commonly in use today are two different three-drug regimens. The first regimen utilizes two nucleoside analogues (one of which is usually lamivudine or emtricitabine) and a nonnucleoside reverse transcriptase inhibitor. The second regimen utilizes two nucleoside analogues and a protease inhibitor. Unfortunately there are no clear data at present on which to base distinctions between these two approaches. After the initiation of therapy, one should expect a 1-log (tenfold) reduction in plasma HIV RNA levels within 1–2 months and eventually a decline in plasma HIV RNA levels to <50 copies per milliliter. During this same time there should be a rise in the CD4+ T-cell count of 100–150/μL that is particularly brisk during the first month of therapy. Many clinicians feel that failure to achieve this endpoint is an indication for a change in therapy. Other reasons for a change in therapy include a persistently declining CD4+ T-cell count, clinical deterioration, or drug toxicity (**Table 90-22**). As in the case of initiating therapy, changing therapy may have a lasting impact on future therapeutic options. When changing therapy because of treatment failure (clinical progression or worsening laboratory parameters), it is important to attempt to provide a regimen with at least two new active drugs. This decision can be guided by resistance testing (see below). In the patient in whom a change is made for reasons of drug toxicity, a simple replacement of one drug is reasonable. It should be stressed that in attempting to sort out a drug toxicity it may be advisable to hold all therapy for a period of time to distinguish between drug toxicity and disease progression. Drug toxicity will usually begin to show signs of reversal within 1–2 weeks. Before changing a treatment regimen because of drug failure, it is important to ensure that the patient has been adherent to the prescribed regimen. As in the case of initial therapy, the simpler the new therapeutic regimen, the easier it is for the patient to be compliant. Plasma HIV RNA levels and CD4+ T-lymphocyte counts should be monitored every 3–4 months during therapy and more frequently if one is contemplating a change in regimen or immediately after a change in regimen.

In an attempt to determine an optimal therapeutic regimen, one may attempt to measure ARV drug susceptibility through genotyping or phenotyping of HIV quasispecies and determine adequacy of dosing through measurement of drug levels. Genotyping may be done through dideoxynucleotide sequencing, DNA chip hybridization, or line probe assays. Phenotypic assays typically measure the enzymatic activity of viral enzymes in the presence or absence of different concentrations of different drugs and have also been used to determine coreceptor tropism. These assays will generally detect quasispecies present at a frequency of ≥10%. The precise role of resistance testing in the management of patients with HIV infection is not yet clear. It is generally recommended that resistance testing be used in selecting initial therapy in settings where the risk of transmission of resistant virus is high (such as the United States and Europe) and in determining new regimens for patients experiencing virologic failure while on therapy. Resistance testing may be of particular value in distinguishing drug-resistant virus from poor patient compliance. Due to the rapid rate at which drug-resistant viruses revert to wild-type, it is recommended that resistant testing performed in the setting of drug failure be carried out while the patient is still on the failing regimen. Measurement of plasma drug levels can also be used to tailor an individual treatment. The inhibitory quotient, defined as the trough blood level/IC50 of the patient's virus, is used by some to determine the adequacy of dosing of a given treatment regimen.

In addition to the licensed medications discussed above, a large number of experimental agents are being evaluated as possible therapies for HIV infection. Therapeutic strategies are being developed that interfere with virtually every step of the replication cycle of the virus (Fig. 90-3). In addition, as more is discovered about the role of the immune system in controlling viral replication, additional strategies, generically referred to as "immune-based therapies," are being developed as a complement to antiviral therapy. Among the antiviral agents in early clinical trials are additional nucleoside and nucleotide analogues, protease inhibitors, fusion inhibitors, receptor and co-receptor antagonists, and integrase inhibitors as well as new anti-viral strategies including antisense nucleic acids and maturation inhibitors. Among the immune-based therapies being evaluated are IFN-α, bone marrow transplantation, adoptive transfer of lymphocytes genetically modified to resist infection or enhance HIV-specific immunity, active immunotherapy with inactivated HIV or its components, IL-2, and IL-7.

HIV AND THE HEALTH CARE WORKER

Health care workers, especially those who deal with large numbers of HIV-infected patients, have a small but definite risk of becoming infected with HIV as a result of professional activities (see "Occupational Transmission of HIV: Health Care Workers, Laboratory Workers, and the Health Care Setting" earlier in the chapter). The first case of HIV transmission from a patient to health care worker was reported in 1984. By the end of 2002, 106 health care workers worldwide were documented as having seroconverted to HIV after occupational HIV exposure; another 238 possible occupational seroconversions had been reported. Only three of these cases were reported from Sub-Saharan Africa, where HIV is most prevalent. Hence it is likely that the global prevalence of occupationally acquired HIV infection is much higher than has been reported.

In the United States, 57 health care workers have become infected with HIV by occupational exposure; 26 have developed AIDS. The individuals who seroconverted include 19 laboratory workers (16 of whom were clinical laboratory workers), 24 nurses, 6 physicians, 2 surgical technicians, 1 dialysis technician, 1 respiratory therapist, 1 health aide, 1 embalmer/morgue technician, and 2 housekeeper/maintenance workers. The exposures included 48 percutaneous (puncture/cut injury), 5 mucocutaneous (mucous membrane and/or skin), 2 both percutaneous and mucocutaneous, and 2 unknown route of exposure. Forty-nine exposures were to HIV-infected blood, three to concentrated virus in a laboratory, one to visibly bloody fluid, and four to an unspecified fluid. As of January 1, 2003, there had been 139 other cases of HIV infection or AIDS among health care workers who have not reported other risk factors for HIV infection and who report a history of exposure to blood, body fluids, or HIV-infected laboratory material, but for whom seroconversion after exposure was not documented. The number of these workers who actually acquired their infection through occupational exposures is not known. Taken together, the data from several large studies suggest that the risk of HIV infection after a percutaneous exposure to HIV-contaminated blood is ~0.3%, and after a mucous membrane exposure, ~0.09%. Although episodes of HIV transmission after nonintact skin exposure have been documented, the average risk for transmission by this route has not been precisely quantified but is estimated to be less than the risk for mucous membrane exposures. The risk for transmission after exposure to fluids or tissues other than HIV-infected blood also has not been quantified but is probably considerably lower than for blood exposures. A seroprevalence survey of 3420 orthopedic surgeons, 75% of whom practiced in an area with a relatively high prevalence of HIV infection and 39% of whom reported percutaneous exposure to patient blood, usually through an accident involving a suture needle, failed to reveal any cases of possible occupational infection, suggesting that the risk of infection with a suture needle may be considerably less than that with a blood-drawing needle.

Most cases of health care worker seroconversion occur as a result of needle-stick injuries. When one considers the circumstances that result in needle-stick injuries, it is immediately obvious that adhering to the standard guidelines for dealing with sharp objects would result in a significant decrease in this type of accident. In one study, 27% of needle-stick injuries resulted from improper disposal of the needle (over half of these were due to recapping the needle), 23% occurred during attempts to start an IV line, 22% occurred during blood drawing, 16% were associated with an IM or SC injection, and 12% were associated with giving an IV infusion.

Clinicians should consider potential occupational exposures to HIV as urgent medical concerns to ensure timely postexposure management and possible administration of postexposure ARV prophylaxis (PEP). Recommendations regarding PEP must take into account that several circumstances determine the risk of transmission of HIV after occupational exposure. In this regard, several factors have been associated with an increased risk for occupational transmission of HIV infection, including deep injury, the presence of visible blood on the instrument causing the exposure, injury with a device that had been placed in the vein or artery of the source patient, terminal illness in the source patient, and lack of postexposure ARV therapy in the exposed health care worker. Other important considerations when considering PEP in the health care worker include known or suspected pregnancy or breastfeeding, the possibility of exposure to drug-resistant virus, and toxicities of PEP regimens. Regardless of the decision to use PEP, the wound should be cleansed immediately and antiseptic applied. If a decision is made to offer PEP, U.S. Public Health Service guidelines recommend (1) a combination of two nucleoside analogue reverse transcriptase inhibitors given for 4 weeks for less severe exposures, or (2) a combination of two nucleoside analogue reverse transcriptase inhibitors plus a third drug given for 4 weeks for more severe exposures. Most clinicians administer the latter regimen in all cases in which a decision is made to treat. Detailed guidelines are available from the *Updated U.S. Public Health Service Guidelines for the Management of Occupational Exposures to HIV and Recommendations for Postexposure Prophylaxis* (CDC, 2005). The report emphasizes the importance of adherence to PEP when it is indicated; follow-up of exposed workers to improve PEP adherences, monitoring for adverse events (including seroconversion), and expert consultation in the management of exposures.

For consultation on the treatment of occupational exposures to HIV and other bloodborne pathogens, the clinician managing the exposed patient can call the National Clinicians' Post-Exposure Prophylaxis Hotline (PEPline) at 888-HIV-4911 (888-448-4911). This service is available 24 h a day, at no charge (additional information on the Internet is available at *http://www.ucsf.edu/hivcntr*). PEPline support may be especially useful in challenging situations, such as when drug-resistant HIV strains are suspected or the health care worker is pregnant.

Health care workers can minimize their risk of occupational HIV infection by following the CDC guidelines of July 1991, which include adherence to universal precautions, refraining from direct patient care if one has exudative lesions or weeping dermatitis, and disinfecting and sterilizing reusable devices employed in invasive procedures. The premise of universal precautions is that every specimen should be handled as if it came from someone infected with a bloodborne pathogen. All samples should be double-bagged, gloves should be worn when drawing blood, and spills should be immediately disinfected with bleach.

In attempting to put this small but definite risk to the health care worker in perspective, it is important to point out that ~200 health care workers die each year as a result of occupationally acquired hepatitis B infection. The tragedy in this instance is that these infections and deaths due to HBV could be greatly decreased by more extended use of the HBV vaccine. The risk of HBV infection after a needle-stick injury from a hepatitis antigen–positive patient is much higher than the risk of HIV infection (see "Transmission" earlier in the chapter). There are multiple examples of needle-stick injuries where the patient was positive for both HBV and HIV and the health care worker became infected only with HBV. For these reasons, it is advisable, given the high prevalence of HBV infection in HIV-infected individuals, that all health care workers dealing with HIV-infected patients be immunized with the HBV vaccine.

TB is another infection common to HIV-infected patients that can be transmitted to the health care worker. For this reason, all health care workers should know their PPD status, have it checked yearly, and receive 6 months of isoniazid treatment if their skin test converts to positive. In addition, all patients in whom a diagnosis of TB is being entertained should be placed immediately in respiratory isolation, pending results of the diagnostic evaluation. The emergence of drug-resistant organisms, including the extensively drug resistant TB strains that have been identified in Africa, has made TB an increasing problem for health care workers. This is particularly true for the health care worker with preexisting HIV infection.

One of the most charged issues ever to come between health care workers and patients is that of transmission of infection from HIV-infected health care workers to their patients. This is discussed under "Occupational Transmission of HIV: Health Care Workers, Laboratory Workers, and the Health Care Setting" earlier in the chapter. Theoretically, the same universal precautions that are used to protect the health care worker from the HIV-infected patient will also protect the patient from the HIV-infected health care worker.

VACCINES

Given that human behavior, especially human sexual behavior, is extremely difficult to change, a critical modality for preventing the spread of HIV infection is the development of a safe and effective vaccine. Historically, vaccines have provided a safe, cost-effective, and efficient means of preventing illness, disability, and death from infectious diseases. Successful vaccines for the most part are predicated on the assumption that the body can mount an adequate immune response to the microbe or virus in question during natural infection, and that the vaccine will mimic the natural response to infection. Even with serious diseases such as smallpox, poliomyelitis, measles, and influenza among others, the body in the vast majority of cases clears the infectious agent and provides protection against future exposure. Unfortunately, this is not the case with HIV infection since the natural immune response to HIV infection is unable to clear the virus from the body and cases of superinfection have been reported. Some of the factors that contribute to the problematic nature of development of a preventive HIV vaccine are the high mutability of the virus, the fact that the infection can be transmitted by cell-free or cell-associated virus, the likely need for the development of effective mucosal immunity, and the fact that it has been difficult to establish the precise correlates of protective immunity to HIV infection. Some HIV-infected individuals are long-term nonprogressors (see above), and a number of individuals have been exposed to HIV multiple times but remain uninfected; these facts suggest that there are elements of an HIV-specific immune response that have the potential to be protective. Early attempts to develop a vaccine with the envelope protein gp120 aimed at inducing neutralizing antibodies in humans were performed based on the induction of neutralizing antibodies in non-human primates. The significance of the laboratory assays were unknown at the time, and the elicited antisera failed to neutralize primary isolates of HIV cultured and tested in fresh peripheral blood mononuclear cells. In this regard, two phase 3 trials were undertaken in the United States and Thailand using soluble gp120, and the vaccines failed to protect human volunteers from HIV infection. It should be pointed out that although the ideal goal of an HIV vaccine is to prevent infection, a vaccine given to an uninfected individual that significantly alters the course of disease or the infectivity of the individual, should that person become infected, could have an impact not only on the individual in question but also on the spread of infection in the community. In this regard, a number of studies in monkeys using vaccines that induce predominantly cellular (T-cell) immune responses have not protected the animals against infection but have lowered the initial burst of viremia after acute infection as well as decreased temporarily the viral set point. Since most sexually transmitted HIV infections occur when the transmitting partner is experiencing high levels of viremia such as during the acute phase of HIV infection or during the advanced stage of disease when the viral load is high, such a vaccine, which might limit the initial burst of viremia in primary infection and decrease the established viral set point, could have benefits for the individual as well as for their sexual partners. It is clear that it will take several years of clinical trials to establish the efficacy or lack thereof of a candidate vaccine for HIV.

PREVENTION

Education, counseling, and behavior modification are the cornerstones of an HIV prevention strategy. A major problem in the United States and elsewhere is that many infections are passed on by those who do not know that they are infected. Of the >1 million persons in the United States who are HIV-infected, it is estimated that ~25% do not know their HIV status and thus may be putting others at risk by their own behavior. In this regard, the CDC has recently recommended that HIV testing become part of routine medical care and that all individuals between the ages of 13 and 64 years be informed of the testing and be tested without the need for written informed consent. The individual could "opt out" of testing, but if not, testing would be routinely administered. In addition to identifying individuals who might benefit from ARV therapy, information gathered from such an approach should serve as the basis for behavior-modification programs, both for infected individuals who may be unaware of their HIV status and who could infect others and for uninfected individuals practicing high-risk behavior. The practice of "safer sex" is the most effective way for sexually active uninfected individuals to avoid contracting HIV infection and for infected individuals to avoid spreading infection. Abstinence from sexual relations is the only absolute way to prevent sexual transmission of HIV infection. However, for many individuals this may not be feasible, and there are a number of relatively safe practices that can markedly decrease the chances of transmission of HIV infection. Partners engaged in monogamous sexual relationships who wish to be assured of safety should both be tested for HIV antibody. If both are negative, it must be understood that any divergence from monogamy puts both partners at risk; open discussion of the importance of honesty in such relationships should be encouraged. When the HIV status of either partner is not known, or when one partner is positive, there are a number of options. Use of condoms can markedly decrease the chance of HIV transmission. It should be remembered that condoms are not 100% effective in preventing transmission of HIV infection, and there is an ~10% failure rate of condoms used for contraceptive purposes. Most condom failures result from breakage or improper usage, such as not wearing the condom for the entire period of intercourse. Latex condoms are preferable, since virus has been shown to leak through natural skin condoms. Petroleum-based gels should never be used for lubrication of the condom, since they increase the likelihood of condom rupture. Some men who have sex with men practice fellatio as a "minimal risk" activity compared with anal intercourse. It should be emphasized that receptive fellatio is definitely not safe sex, and although the incidence of transmission via fellatio is considerably less than that of rectal or vaginal intercourse, there has been documentation of transmission of HIV where receptive fellatio was the only sexual act performed (see "Transmission" earlier in the chapter). Topical microbicides for vaginal and anal use are being pursued actively as a means by which individuals could avoid infection when the insertive partner cannot be relied on to use a condom. Three clinical trials in South Africa, Uganda, and Kenya have shown that adult male circumcision results in an ~50% reduction in HIV acquisition in the circumcised subject. Clearly, this approach has considerable potential as a preventive strategy for HIV infection and is currently being pursued, particularly in developing nations, as a component of HIV prevention. Kissing is considered safe, although there is a theoretical possibility of transmission via virus in saliva. The low concentration of virus in saliva of infected individuals, as well as the presence in saliva of HIV-inhibitory proteins (see above), lessens any risk of transmission by kissing.

The most effective way to prevent transmission of HIV infection among IDUs is to stop the use of injectable drugs. Unfortunately, that is extremely difficult to accomplish unless the individual enters a treatment program. For those who will not or cannot participate in a drug treatment program and who will continue to inject drugs, the avoidance of sharing of needles and other paraphernalia ("works") is the next best way to avoid transmission of infection. However, the cultural and social factors that contribute to the sharing of paraphernalia are complex and difficult to overcome. In addition, needles and syringes may be in short supply. Under these circumstances, paraphernalia should be cleaned after each usage with a virucidal solution, such as undiluted sodium hypochlorite (household bleach). Data from a number of studies have indicated that programs that provide sterile needles to addicts in exchange for used needles have resulted in a decrease in HIV transmission without increasing the use of injection drugs. It is important for IDUs to be tested for HIV infection and counseled to avoid transmission to their sexual partners. Secondary and tertiary spread of HIV infection by the heterosexual route within settings of a high level of injection drug use has increased greatly in the United States, particularly among African Americans (see above). Studies are underway to determine the safety and efficacy of preexposure as well as postexposure administration of ARV drugs for the prevention of HIV infection.

Transmission of HIV via transfused blood or blood products has been decreased dramatically by a combination of screening of all blood donors for HIV infection by assays for both HIV antibody and nucleic acid and self-deferral of individuals at risk for HIV infection. In addition, clotting factor concentrates are heat-treated, essentially eliminating the risk to hemophiliacs who require these products. Autologous transfusions are preferable to transfusions from another individual. However, logistic constraints as well as the unpredictability of the need for most transfusions limit the feasibility of this approach. At present, the risk of becoming HIV-infected from a contaminated blood transfusion is approximately 1 in 1.5 million donations.

Treatment of an HIV-infected mother with ARV therapy during pregnancy and the infant during the first weeks after birth has proved very effective in dramatically decreasing mother-to-child transmission of HIV. In situations such as that seen in certain developing countries where pregnant women frequently present to a health care system during labor, administration of a short course (as little as a single dose of one drug) of ARV therapy to the mother during labor and to the infant within 48 h of birth has also been successful in decreasing the incidence of mother-to-child transmission of HIV.

HIV can be transmitted via breast milk and colostrum. The avoidance of breast-feeding may not be practical in developing countries, where nutritional concerns override the risk of HIV transmission. However, it is becoming appreciated that 5–15% of infants who were born of HIV-infected mothers and who were fortunate enough not to have been infected intrapartum or peripartum become infected via breast-feeding. Therefore, in developing countries, breast-feeding from an infected mother should be avoided if at all possible. Unfortunately, this is rarely the case, and given the disadvantages of withholding breast-feeding in developing countries (see above), health authorities in most developing countries continue to recommend breast-feeding despite the potential for HIV transmission. Treatment of the infected mother with ARV therapy, in addition to decreasing perinatal mother-to-child transmission, can also decrease transmission by breast-feeding. In developed countries such as the United States, where bottled formula and milk are readily accessible, breast-feeding is absolutely contraindicated when a mother is HIV positive.

FURTHER READINGS

Arthos J et al: HIV-1 envelope protein binds to and signals through integrin α4β7, the gut mucosal honing receptor for peripheral T cells. Nature Immunol 9:301, 2008

Bailey RC et al: Male circumcision for HIV prevention in young men in Casuum, Kenya: A randomised controlled trial. Lancet 369:643, 2007

Benson CA et al: Treating opportunistic infections among HIV-infected adults and adolescents. Recommendations from CDC, the National Institutes of Health, and the HIV Medicine Association/Infectious Diseases Society of America. MMWR 53(RR-15):1, 2004. Updates available at *http://www.aidsinfo.nih.gov*

Brenner BG et al: High rates of forward transmission events after acute/early HIV-1 infection. J Infect Dis 195:951, 2007

Centers for Disease Control and Prevention: Revised guidelines for HIV counseling, testing, and referral. MMWR Recomm Rep 50(RR-19):1, 2001

———: Updated U.S. Public Health Service guidelines for the management of occupational exposures to HIV and recommendations for postexposure prophylaxis. MMWR Recomm Rep 54(RR-9): 1, 2005

———: HIV/AIDS Surveillance Report, 2005;17 (Revised ed), 2007. Available at *http://www.cdc.gov/hiv/*

———: Revised recommendations for HIV testing of adults, adolescents, and pregnant women in health-care settings. MMWR Recomm Rep 55(RR-14):1, 2006

———: Essential Components of a Comprehensive Strategy to Prevent Domestic HIV, 2006. Available at *http://www.cdc.gov/Hiv/resources/reports/comp_hiv_prev/index.htm*

———; Health Resources and Services Administration; National Institutes of Health; HIV Medicine Association of the Infectious Diseases Society of America: Incorporating HIV prevention into the medical care of persons living with HIV. MMWR Recomm Rep 52(RR-12):1, 2003

Centlivre M et al: In HIV-1 pathogenesis the die is cast during primary infection. AIDS 21:1, 2007

Cohen MS, Pilcher CD: Amplified HIV transmission and new approaches to HIV prevention. J Infect Dis 191:1391, 2005

Collins LS et al: Multicentric Castleman's disease in HIV infection. Int J STD AIDS 17:19, 2006

Corey L: Synergistic copathogens—HIV-1 and HSV-2. N Engl J Med 356:854, 2007

Deeks SG, Walker BD: Human immunodeficiency virus controllers: Mechanisms of durable virus control in the absence of antiretroviral therapy. Immunity 27:406, 2007

Department of Health and Human Services Panel on Antiretroviral Guidelines for Adults and Adolescents: *Guidelines for the Use of Antiretroviral Agents in HIV-1-Infected Adults and Adolescents*, October 10, 2006. Updates available at *http://www.aidsinfo.nih.gov*

Dieffenbach CW, Fauci AS: Universal voluntary testing and treatment for prevention of HIV transmission. JAMA 301:2380, 2009

Dorak MT et al: Transmission of HIV-1 and HLA-B allele-sharing within serodiscordant heterosexual Zambian couples. Lancet 363:2137, 2004

Drumright L et al: Unprotected anal intercourse and substance use among men who have sex with men with recent HIV infection. J AIDS 43:344, 2006

Este JA, Telenti A: HIV entry inhibitors. Lancet 370:81, 2007

Fauci AS: Host factors and the pathogenesis of HIV-induced disease. Nature 384:529, 1996

———: The AIDS epidemic—considerations for the 21st century. N Engl J Med 341:1046, 1999

Fellay J et al: A whole-genome association study of major determinants for host control of HIV-1. Science 317:944, 2007

Freeman GJ et al: Reinvigorating exhausted HIV-specific T cells via PD-1–PD-1 ligand blockade. J Exp Med 203:2223, 2006

Freiberg M et al: The association between hepatitis C infection and prevalent cardiovascular disease among HIV-infected individuals. AIDS 21:193, 2007

GERETTI AM: Epidemiology of antiretroviral drug resistance in drug-naive persons. Curr Opin Infect Dis 20:22, 2007

GONZALEZ-SCARANO F, MARTIN-GARCIA J: The neuropathogenesis of AIDS. Nat Rev Immunol 5:69, 2005

GRAY RH et al: Male circumcision for HIV prevention in men in Rakai, Uganda: A randomised trial. Lancet 369:657, 2007

GREENE WC, PETERLIN BM: Charting HIV's remarkable voyage through the cell: Basic science as a passport to future therapy. Nat Med 8:673, 2002

GUTIERREZ F et al: Osteonecrosis in patients infected with HIV: Clinical epidemiology and natural history in a large case series from Spain. J AIDS 42(3):286, 2006

HAMMER SM et al: Treatment for adult HIV infection: 2006 recommendations of the International AIDS Society-USA panel. JAMA 296:827, 2006

HAN Y et al: Experimental approaches to the study of HIV-1 latency. Nat Rev Microbiol 5:95, 2007

HO DD et al: Rapid turnover of plasma virions and CD4 lymphocytes in HIV infection. Nature 373:123, 1995

HOFFMAN RM, CURRIER JS: Management of antiretroviral treatment-related complications. Infect Clin Dis North Am 21:103, 2007

HUANG L et al: Current concepts: Intensive care of patients with HIV Infection. N Engl J Med 355:173, 2006

IZZEDINE H, DERAY G: The nephrologist in the HAART era. AIDS 21:409, 2007

JOHNSTON MI, FAUCI AS: An HIV vaccine: Evolving concepts. N Engl J Med 356:2073, 2007

JOINT UNITED NATIONS PROGRAMME ON HIV/AIDS (UNAIDS): Report on the global AIDS epidemic, 2006

———: AIDS epidemic update, 2007

KAPLAN JE et al: Guidelines for preventing opportunistic infections among HIV-infected persons—2002. Recommendations of the U.S. Public Health Service and the Infectious Diseases Society of America. MMWR Recomm Rep 51(RR-8):1, 2002. Updates available at *http://www.aidsinfo.nih.gov*

KEELE BF et al: Chimpanzee reservoirs of pandemic and nonpandemic HIV-1. Science 313:523, 2006

KERULY JC, MOORE RD: Immune status at presentation to care did not improve among antiretroviral-naive persons from 1990 to 2006. Clin Infect Dis 45:1369, 2007

KITAHATA MM et al: Effect of early versus deferred antiretroviral therapy for HIV on survival. N Engl J Med 360:1815, 2009

KOZIEL MJ, PETERS MG: Current concepts: Viral hepatitis in HIV infection. N Engl J Med 356:1445, 2007

LIPMAN M, BREEN R: Immune reconstitution inflammatory syndrome in HIV. Curr Opin Infect Dis 19:20, 2006

LYLES CM et al: Best-evidence interventions: Findings from a systematic review of HIV behavioral interventions for US populations at high risk, 2000–2004. Am J Public Health 97:133, 2007

MANGILI A et al: Risk of cardiovascular disease in a cohort of HIV-infected adults: A study using carotid intima-media thickness and coronary artery calcium score. Clin Infect Dis 43:1482,2006

MASUR H, KAPLAN JE: New guidelines for the management of HIV-related opportunistic infections. JAMA 301:2378, 2009

MAY MT et al: HIV treatment response and prognosis in Europe and North America in the first decade of highly active antiretroviral therapy: A collaborative analysis. Lancet 368:451, 2006

MELLORS JW et al: Prognosis in HIV-1 infection predicted by the quantity of virus in plasma. Science 272:1167, 1996

MORSE CG, KOVACS JA: Metabolic and skeletal complications of HIV infection: The price of success. JAMA 296:844, 2006

PANTALEO G, FAUCI AS: HIV infection is active and progressive in lymphoid tissue during the clinically latent stage of disease. Nature 362:355, 1993

PALEFSKY JM et al: Anal intraepithelial neoplasia in the highly active antiretroviral therapy era among HIV-positive men who have sex with men. AIDS 19:1407, 2005

PALELLA FJ JR et al: Mortality in the highly active antiretroviral therapy era: Changing causes of death and disease in the HIV Outpatient Study. J AIDS 43(1):27, 2006

PERINATAL HIV GUIDELINES WORKING GROUP: U.S. Public Health Service Task Force recommendations for use of antiretroviral drugs in pregnant HIV-1-infected women for maternal health and interventions to reduce perinatal HIV-1 transmission in the United States, November 2, 2007. Updates available at *http://www.aidsinfo.nih.gov*

SHELBURNE SA et al: Incidence and risk factors for immune reconstitution inflammatory syndrome during highly active antiretroviral therapy. AIDS 19:399, 2005

SILVESTRI G et al: Understanding the benign nature of SIV infection in natural hosts. J Clin Invest 11:3148, 2007

SIMON V et al: HIV/AIDS epidemiology, pathogenesis, prevention, and treatment. Lancet 368:489, 2006

STEPHENS HA: HIV-1 diversity versus HLA class I polymorphism. Trends Immunol 26:41, 2005

THE STRATEGIES FOR MANAGEMENT OF ANTIRETROVIRAL THERAPY (SMART) STUDY GROUP: CD4+ count-guided interruption of antiretroviral treatment. N Engl J Med 355(22):2283, 2006

U.S. PUBLIC HEALTH SERVICE: Updated U.S. Public Health Service Guidelines for the Management of Occupational Exposures to HBV, HCV, and HIV and Recommendations for Postexposure Prophylaxis. MMWR Recomm Rep 50(RR-11):1, 2001. Updates available at *http://www.aidsinfo.nih.gov*

VOLMINK J et al: Antiretrovirals for reducing the risk of mother-to-child transmission of HIV infection. Cochrane Database Syst Rev 1:CD003510, 2007

WALENSKY RP et al: The survival benefits of AIDS treatment in the United States. J Infect Dis 194:11, 2006

Wawer MJ et al: Rates of HIV-1 transmission per coital act, by stage of HIV-1 infection, in Rakai, Uganda. J Infect Dis 191:1403, 2005

WEI X et al: Viral dynamics in human immunodeficiency virus type 1 infection. Nature 373:117, 1995

WELLS CD et al: HIV infection and multidrug-resistant tuberculosis: The perfect storm. J Infect Dis 196(Suppl 1):S86, 2007

WHEN TO START CONSORTIUM: Timing of initiation of antiretroviral therapy in AIDS-free HIV-1-infected patients: a collaborative analysis of 18 HIV cohort studies. Lancet 373:1352, 2009

ZANCANARO PCQ et al: Cutaneous manifestations of HIV in the era of highly active antiretroviral therapy: An institutional urban clinic experience. J Am Acad Dermatol 54(4):581, 2006

CHAPTER 91
VIRAL GASTROENTERITIS

Umesh D. Parashar ■ Roger I. Glass

Acute infectious gastroenteritis is a common illness that affects persons of all ages worldwide. It is a leading cause of mortality among children in developing countries, accounting for an estimated 2 million deaths each year, and is responsible for up to 10–12% of all hospitalizations among children in industrialized countries, including the United States. Elderly persons, especially those with debilitating health conditions, are also at risk of severe complications and death from acute gastroenteritis. Among healthy young adults, acute gastroenteritis is rarely fatal but incurs substantial medical and social costs, including those of time lost from work.

Several enteric viruses have been recognized as important etiologic agents of acute infectious gastroenteritis (Table 91-1, Fig. 91-1). Illness caused by these viruses is characterized by the acute onset of vomiting and/or diarrhea, which may be accompanied by fever, nausea, abdominal cramps, anorexia, and malaise. As shown in Table 91-2, several features can help distinguish gastroenteritis caused by viruses from that caused by bacterial agents. However, the distinction based on clinical and epidemiologic parameters alone is often difficult, and laboratory tests may be required to confirm the diagnosis.

HUMAN CALICIVIRUSES

Etiologic Agent

The Norwalk virus is the prototype strain of a group of nonenveloped, small (27–40 nm), round, icosahedral viruses with relatively amorphous surface features on visualization by electron microscopy. These viruses have been difficult to classify because they have not been adapted to cell culture, they often are shed in low titers for only a few days, and no animal models are available. Molecular cloning and characterization have demonstrated that these viruses have a single, positive-strand RNA genome ~7.5 kb in length and that they possess a single virion-associated protein—similar to that of typical caliciviruses—with a molecular mass of 60 kDa.

TABLE 91-1

VIRAL CAUSES OF GASTROENTERITIS AMONG HUMANS

VIRUS	FAMILY	GENOME	PRIMARY AGE GROUP AT RISK	CLINICAL SEVERITY	DETECTION ASSAYS[a]
Group A rotavirus	Reoviridae	Double-strand segmented RNA	Children <5 years	+++	EM, EIA (commercial), PAGE, RT-PCR
Norovirus	Caliciviridae	Positive-sense single-strand RNA	All ages	++	EM, EIA, RT-PCR
Sapovirus	Caliciviridae	Positive-sense single-strand RNA	Children <5 years	+	EM, EIA, RT-PCR
Astrovirus	Astroviridae	Positive-sense single-strand RNA	Children <5 years	+	EM, EIA, RT-PCR
Adenovirus (types 40 and 41)	Adenoviridae	Double-strand DNA	Children <5 years	+/++	EM, EIA (commercial), PCR

[a]EIA, enzyme immunoassay; EM, electron microscopy; PAGE, polyacrylamide gel electrophoresis; PCR, polymerase chain reaction; RT-PCR, reverse-transcriptase PCR.

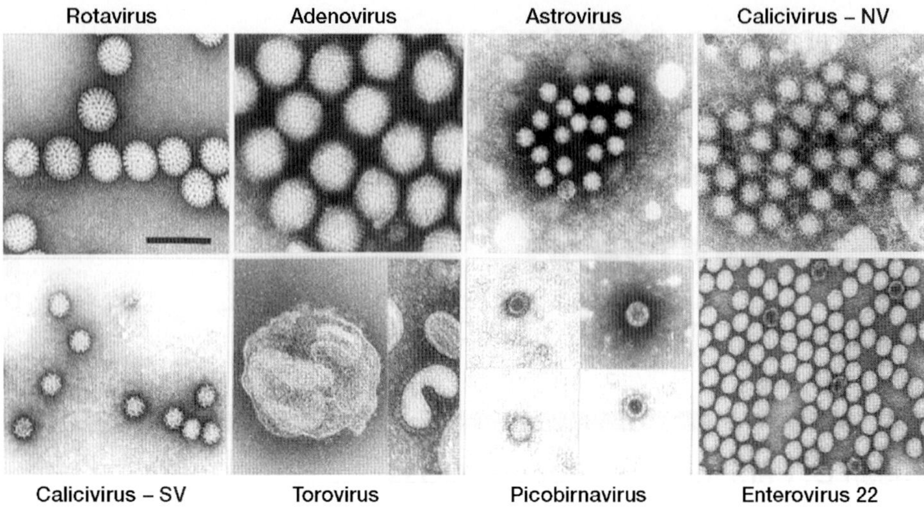

FIGURE 91-1
Viral agents of gastroenteritis. NV, Norwalk-like virus; SV, Sapporo-like virus.

TABLE 91-2

CHARACTERISTICS OF GASTROENTERITIS CAUSED BY VIRAL AND BACTERIAL AGENTS

FEATURE	VIRAL GASTROENTERITIS	BACTERIAL GASTROENTERITIS
Setting	Incidence similar in developing and developed countries	More common in settings with poor hygiene and sanitation
Infectious dose	Low (10–100 viral particles) for most agents	High (>10^5 bacteria) for *Escherichia coli*, *Salmonella*, *Vibrio*; medium (10^2–10^5 bacteria) for *Campylobacter jejuni*; low (10–100 bacteria) for *Shigella*
Seasonality	In temperate climates, winter seasonality for most agents; year-round occurrence in tropical areas	More common in summer or rainy months, particularly in developing countries with a high disease burden
Incubation period	1–3 days for most agents; can be shorter for norovirus	1–7 days for common agents (e.g., *Campylobacter*, *E. coli*, *Shigella*, *Salmonella*); a few hours for bacteria producing preformed toxins (e.g., *Staphylococcus aureus*, *Bacillus cereus*)
Reservoir	Primarily humans	Depending on species, human (e.g., *Shigella*, *Salmonella*), animal (e.g., *Campylobacter*, *Salmonella*, *E. coli*), and water (e.g., *Vibrio*) reservoirs exist.
Fever	Common with rotavirus and norovirus; uncommon with other agents	Common with agents causing inflammatory diarrhea (e.g., *Salmonella*, *Shigella*)
Vomiting	Prominent and can be the only presenting feature, especially in children	Common with bacteria producing preformed toxins; less prominent in diarrhea due to other agents
Diarrhea	Common; nonbloody in almost all cases	Prominent and frequently bloody with agents causing inflammatory diarrhea
Duration	1–3 days for norovirus and sapovirus; 2–8 days for other viruses	1–2 days for bacteria producing preformed toxins; 2–8 days for most other bacteria
Diagnosis	This is often a diagnosis of exclusion in clinical practice. Commercial enzyme immunoassays are available for detection of rotavirus and adenovirus, but identification of other agents is limited to research and public health laboratories.	Fecal examination for leukocytes and blood is helpful in differential diagnosis. Culture of stool specimens, sometimes on special media, can identify several pathogens. Molecular techniques are useful epidemiologic tools but are not routinely used in most laboratories.
Treatment	Supportive therapy to maintain adequate hydration and nutrition should be given. Antibiotics and antimotility agents are contraindicated.	Supportive hydration therapy is adequate for most patients. Antibiotics are recommended for patients with dysentery caused by *Shigella* or *Vibrio cholerae* and for some patients with *Clostridium difficile* colitis.

On the basis of these molecular characteristics, these viruses are presently classified in two genera belonging to the family Caliciviridae: the *noroviruses* and the *sapoviruses* (previously called Norwalk-like viruses and Sapporo-like viruses, respectively).

Epidemiology

Infections with the Norwalk and related human caliciviruses are common worldwide, and most adults have antibodies to these viruses. Antibody is acquired at an earlier age in developing countries—a pattern consistent with the presumed fecal-oral mode of transmission. Infections occur year-round, although, in temperate climates, a distinct increase has been noted in cold-weather months. Noroviruses may be the most common infectious agents of mild gastroenteritis in the community and affect all age groups, whereas sapoviruses primarily cause gastroenteritis in children. Noroviruses also cause traveler's diarrhea, and outbreaks have occurred among military personnel deployed to various parts of the world. The etiologic role of noroviruses in moderate and severe gastroenteritis requiring a visit to a physician or hospitalization is still being studied. However, the limited data available indicate that norovirus may be the second most common viral agent (after rotavirus) among young children and the most common agent among older children and adults. Noroviruses are also recognized as the major cause of epidemics of gastroenteritis worldwide. In the United States, >90% of outbreaks of nonbacterial gastroenteritis are caused by noroviruses. Epidemics occur throughout the year, in all age groups, and in a variety of settings.

Virus is transmitted predominantly by the fecal-oral route but is also present in vomitus. Because an inoculum with very few viruses can be infectious, transmission can occur by aerosolization, by contact with contaminated fomites, and by person-to-person contact. Viral shedding and infectivity are greatest during the acute illness, but challenge studies with Norwalk virus in volunteers indicate that viral antigen may be shed by asymptomatically infected persons and also by symptomatic persons before the onset of symptoms and for up to 2 weeks after the resolution of illness. In one study, 11 of 15 norovirus-infected children <2 years of age shed the virus for >2 weeks after onset; this group included 3 infants <6 months of age who shed virus for 42–47 days or even longer.

Pathogenesis

The exact sites and cellular receptors for attachment of viral particles have not been determined. Data suggest that carbohydrates that are similar to human histo-blood group antigens and are present on the gastroduodenal epithelium of individuals with the secretor phenotype may serve as ligands for the attachment of Norwalk virus. Additional studies must more fully elucidate norovirus-carbohydrate interactions, including potential strain-specific variations. After the infection of volunteers, reversible lesions are noted in the upper jejunum, with broadening and blunting of the villi, shortening of the microvilli, vacuolization of the lining epithelium, crypt hyperplasia, and infiltration of the lamina propria by polymorphonuclear neutrophils and lymphocytes. The lesions persist for at least 4 days after the resolution of symptoms and are associated with malabsorption of carbohydrates and fats and a decreased level of brush-border enzymes. Adenylate cyclase activity is not altered. No histopathologic changes are seen in the stomach or colon, but gastric motor function is delayed, and this alteration is believed to contribute to the nausea and vomiting that are typical of this illness.

Clinical Manifestations

Gastroenteritis caused by Norwalk and related human caliciviruses has a sudden onset, following an average incubation period of 24 h (range, 12–72 h). The illness generally lasts 12–60 h and is characterized by one or more of the following symptoms: nausea, vomiting, abdominal cramps, and diarrhea. Vomiting is more prevalent among children, whereas a greater proportion of adults develop diarrhea. Constitutional symptoms are common, including headache, fever, chills, and myalgias. Noroviruses appear to cause more severe illness than sapoviruses, although both illnesses are less severe than that due to rotavirus. The stools are characteristically loose and watery, without blood, mucus, or leukocytes. White cell counts are generally normal; rarely, leukocytosis with relative lymphopenia may be observed. Death is a rare outcome and usually results from severe dehydration in vulnerable persons (e.g., elderly patients with debilitating health conditions).

Immunity

Approximately 50% of persons challenged with Norwalk virus become ill and acquire short-term immunity against the infecting strain. Immunity to Norwalk virus appears to correlate inversely with level of antibody; i.e., persons with higher levels of preexisting antibody to Norwalk virus are more susceptible to illness. This observation suggests that some individuals have a genetic predisposition to illness. Recent data indicate that specific ABO, Lewis, and secretor blood group phenotypes may influence susceptibility to norovirus infection.

Diagnosis

Cloning and sequencing of the genomes of Norwalk and several other human caliciviruses have allowed the development of assays based on polymerase chain reaction (PCR) for detection of virus in stool and vomitus. Virus-like particles produced by expression of capsid proteins in a recombinant baculovirus vector have been used to develop enzyme immunoassays (EIAs) for detection of virus in stool or a serologic response to a specific viral antigen. These newer diagnostic techniques are considerably more sensitive than previous detection methods, such as electron microscopy, immune electron microscopy, and EIAs based on reagents derived from humans. However, no currently available single assay can detect all human caliciviruses because of their great genetic and antigenic diversity. In addition, the assays are still cumbersome and are available primarily in research laboratories, although they are increasingly being adopted by public health laboratories for routine screening of fecal specimens from patients affected by outbreaks of gastroenteritis. Commercial EIA kits have been developed but are still being evaluated to determine their optimal use for both outbreak-related and sporadic acute gastroenteritis cases.

Treatment: ℞ INFECTIONS WITH NORWALK AND RELATED HUMAN CALICIVIRUSES

The disease is self-limited, and oral rehydration therapy is generally adequate. If severe dehydration develops, IV fluid therapy is indicated. No specific antiviral therapy is available.

Prevention

Epidemic prevention relies on situation-specific measures, such as control of contamination of food and water, exclusion of ill food handlers, and reduction of person-to-person spread through good personal hygiene and disinfection of contaminated fomites. The role of immunoprophylaxis is not clear, given the lack of long-term immunity from natural disease and the paradoxical inverse association between the level of immune response and protection from disease.

ROTAVIRUS

Etiologic Agent

Rotaviruses are members of the family Reoviridae. The viral genome consists of 11 segments of double-strand RNA that are enclosed in a triple-layered, nonenveloped, icosahedral capsid 75 nm in diameter. Viral protein 6 (VP6), the major structural protein, is the target of commercial immunoassays and determines the group specificity of rotaviruses. There are seven major groups of rotavirus (A through G); human illness is caused primarily by group A and, to a much lesser extent, by groups B and C. Two outer-capsid proteins, VP7 (G-protein) and VP4 (P-protein), determine serotype specificity, induce neutralizing antibodies, and form the basis for binary classification of rotaviruses (G and P types). The segmented genome of rotavirus allows genetic reassortment (i.e., exchange of genome segments between viruses) during co-infection—a property that may play a role in viral evolution and has been utilized in the development of reassortant animal-human rotavirus–based vaccines.

Epidemiology

Worldwide, nearly all children are infected with rotavirus by 3–5 years of age. Neonatal infections are common but are often asymptomatic or mild, presumably because of protection from maternal antibody or breast-feeding. First infections after 3 months of age are likely to be symptomatic, and the incidence of disease peaks among children 4–23 months of age. Reinfections are common, but the severity of disease decreases with each repeat infection. Therefore, severe rotavirus infections are relatively uncommon among older children and adults. Nevertheless, rotavirus can cause illness in parents and caretakers of children with rotavirus diarrhea, immunocompromised persons, travelers, and elderly individuals and should be considered in the differential diagnosis of gastroenteritis among adults. In temperate climates, rotavirus disease occurs predominantly during the cooler fall and winter months. In the United States, the rotavirus season each year begins in the Southwest during the autumn (October through December) and migrates across the continent, peaking in the Northeast during the spring (March through May) (Fig. 91-2); the reasons for this characteristic pattern are not clear. In tropical settings, rotavirus disease occurs year-round, with less pronounced seasonal peaks.

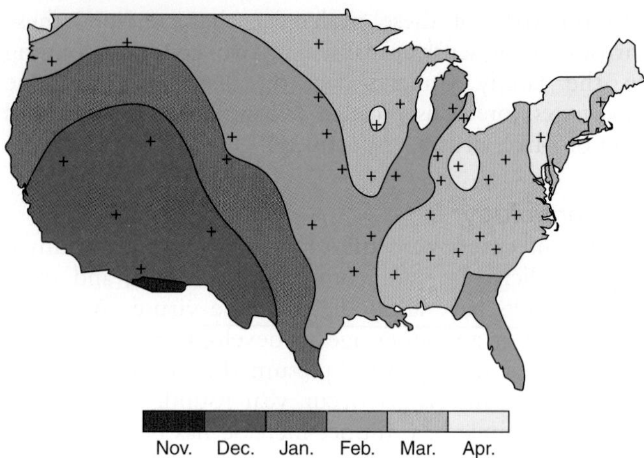

FIGURE 91-2

Time of peak rotavirus activity in the contiguous 48 states: United States, July 1991 to June 1997. Data are from ~90 U.S. laboratories. *(Adapted from TJ Torok et al: Visualizing geographic and temporal trends in rotavirus activity in the United States, 1991 to 1996. National Respiratory and Enteric Virus Surveillance System Collaborating Laboratories. Pediatr Infect Dis J 16:941, 1997.)*

Rotavirus gastroenteritis is more frequently associated with dehydration than is gastroenteritis caused by other pathogens. Therefore, the proportion of gastroenteritis cases that are attributable to rotavirus increases with increasing severity of illness, ranging from a median of 8% in the community to 18% among outpatients and 40% among hospitalized patients. Each year, rotavirus is estimated to cause ~500,000 childhood deaths worldwide.

During episodes of rotavirus-associated diarrhea, virus is shed in large quantities in stool (10^7–10^{12}/g). Viral shedding detectable by EIA usually subsides within 1 week but may persist for >30 days in immunocompromised individuals. Viral shedding may be detected for longer periods by sensitive molecular assays, such as PCR. The virus is transmitted predominantly through the fecal-oral route. Spread through respiratory secretions, person-to-person contact, or contaminated environmental surfaces has also been postulated to explain the rapid acquisition of antibody in the first 3 years of life, regardless of sanitary conditions.

At least 10 different G serotypes of group A rotavirus have been identified in humans, but only five types (G1 through G4 and G9) are common. While human rotavirus strains that possess a high degree of genetic homology with animal strains have been identified, animal-to-human transmission appears to be uncommon.

Group B rotaviruses have been associated with several large epidemics of severe gastroenteritis among adults in China since 1982 and have recently been identified in India but not in other parts of the world. Group C rotaviruses have been associated with a small proportion of pediatric gastroenteritis cases in several countries worldwide.

Pathogenesis

Rotaviruses infect and ultimately destroy mature enterocytes in the villous epithelium of the proximal small intestine. The loss of absorptive villous epithelium, coupled with the proliferation of secretory crypt cells, results in secretory diarrhea. Brush-border enzymes characteristic of differentiated cells are reduced, and this change leads to the accumulation of unmetabolized disaccharides and consequent osmotic diarrhea. Studies in mice indicate that a nonstructural rotavirus protein, NSP4, functions as an enterotoxin and contributes to secretory diarrhea by altering epithelial cell function and permeability. In addition, rotavirus may evoke fluid secretion through activation of the enteric nervous system in the intestinal wall. Recent data indicate that rotavirus antigenemia and viremia are common among children with acute rotavirus infection, although the antigen and RNA levels in serum are substantially lower than those in stool.

Clinical Manifestations

The clinical spectrum of rotavirus infection ranges from subclinical infection to severe gastroenteritis leading to life-threatening dehydration. After an incubation period of 1–3 days, the illness has an abrupt onset, with vomiting frequently preceding the onset of diarrhea. Up to one-third of patients may have a temperature of >39°C. The stools are characteristically loose and watery and only infrequently contain red or white cells. Gastrointestinal symptoms generally resolve in 3–7 days.

Respiratory and neurologic features in children with rotavirus infection have been reported, but causal associations have not been proven. Moreover, rotavirus infection has been associated with a variety of other clinical conditions (e.g., sudden infant death syndrome, necrotizing enterocolitis, intussusception, Kawasaki disease, and type 1 diabetes), but no causal relationship has been confirmed with any of these syndromes.

Rotavirus does not appear to be a major opportunistic pathogen in children with HIV infection. In severely immunodeficient children, rotavirus can cause protracted diarrhea with prolonged viral excretion and, in rare instances, can disseminate systemically. Persons who are immunosuppressed for bone marrow transplantation are also at risk for severe or even fatal rotavirus disease.

Immunity

Protection against rotavirus disease is correlated with the presence of virus-specific secretory IgA antibodies in the intestine and, to some extent, the serum. Because virus-specific IgA production at the intestinal surface is short-lived, complete protection against disease is only temporary. However, each infection and subsequent reinfection confers progressively greater immunity; thus severe disease is most common among young children with first or second infections. Immunologic memory is believed to be important in the attenuation of disease severity upon reinfection.

Diagnosis

Illness caused by rotavirus is difficult to distinguish clinically from that caused by other enteric viruses. Because large quantities of virus are shed in feces, the diagnosis can usually be confirmed by a wide variety of commercially available EIAs or by techniques for detecting viral RNA, such as gel electrophoresis, probe hybridization, or PCR.

℞ Treatment: ROTAVIRUS INFECTIONS

Rotavirus gastroenteritis can lead to severe dehydration. Thus appropriate treatment should be instituted early. Standard oral rehydration therapy is successful in most children who can take oral fluids, but IV fluid replacement may be required for patients who are severely dehydrated or are unable to tolerate oral therapy because of frequent vomiting. The therapeutic role of probiotics, bismuth subsalicylate, enkephalinase inhibitors, and nitazoxanide has been evaluated in clinical studies but is not clearly defined. Antibiotics and antimotility agents should be avoided. In immunocompromised children with chronic symptomatic rotavirus disease, orally administered immunoglobulins or colostrum may resolve symptoms, but the choice of agents and their doses have not been well studied and are often empirical.

Prevention

Efforts to develop rotavirus vaccines were pursued because it was apparent—given the similar rates in less developed and industrialized nations—that improvements in hygiene and sanitation were unlikely to reduce disease incidence. The first rotavirus vaccine licensed in the United States in 1998 was withdrawn from the market within 1 year because it was linked with intussusception, a severe bowel obstruction.

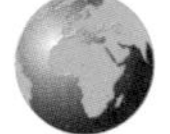

In 2006, promising safety and efficacy results for two new rotavirus vaccines were reported from large clinical trials conducted in North America, Europe, and Latin America. One of these vaccines, a multivalent bovine-human reassortant rotavirus-based preparation, was recommended for routine immunization of all U.S. infants in early 2006. The second vaccine, based on a single attenuated human rotavirus strain, is not licensed in the United States but has been introduced in immunization programs in several countries in Latin America and Europe.

Global Considerations

Rotavirus is ubiquitous and infects nearly all children worldwide by 5 years of age. However, compared with rotavirus disease in industrialized countries, that in developing countries occurs at a younger age, is less seasonal, is more often associated with severe outcomes (including death), and is more frequently caused by uncommon rotavirus strains. The different epidemiology of rotavirus disease and the greater prevalence of co-infection with other enteric pathogens, of comorbidities, and of malnutrition in developing countries may adversely affect the performance of rotavirus vaccines. Therefore, before global recommendations for vaccine use can be issued, it is vital to evaluate the efficacy of rotavirus vaccines in resource-poor settings of Africa and Asia. Trials in these areas are underway.

OTHER VIRAL AGENTS OF GASTROENTERITIS

Enteric *adenoviruses* of serotypes 40 and 41 belonging to subgroup F are 70- to 80-nm viruses with double-strand DNA that cause ~2–12% of all diarrhea episodes in young children. Unlike adenoviruses that cause respiratory illness, enteric adenoviruses are difficult to cultivate in cell lines, but they can be detected with commercially available EIAs.

Astroviruses, 28- to 30-nm viruses with a characteristic icosahedral structure, contain a positive-sense, single-strand RNA. At least seven serotypes have been identified, of which serotype 1 is most common. Astroviruses are primarily pediatric pathogens, causing ~2–10% of cases of mild to moderate gastroenteritis in children. The availability of simple immunoassays to detect virus in fecal specimens and of molecular methods to confirm and characterize strains will permit more comprehensive assessment of the etiologic role of these agents.

Toroviruses are 100- to 140-nm, enveloped, positive-strand RNA viruses that are recognized as causes of gastroenteritis in horses (Berne virus) and cattle (Breda virus). Their role as a cause of diarrhea in humans is still unclear, but studies from Canada have demonstrated associations between torovirus excretion and both nosocomial gastroenteritis and necrotizing enterocolitis in neonates. These associations require further evaluation.

Picobirnaviruses are small, bisegmented, double-strand RNA viruses that cause gastroenteritis in a variety of animals. Their role as primary causes of gastroenteritis in humans remains unclear, but several studies have found an association between picobirnaviruses and gastroenteritis in HIV-infected adults.

Several other viruses (e.g., enteroviruses, reoviruses, pestiviruses, and parvovirus B) have been identified in the feces of patients with diarrhea, but their etiologic role in gastroenteritis has not been proven. Diarrhea has also been noted as a manifestation of infection with two recently recognized viruses that primarily cause severe respiratory illness: the severe acute respiratory syndrome–associated coronavirus (SARS-CoV) and influenza A/H5N1 virus.

FURTHER READINGS

Dolin R: Noroviruses—challenges to control. N Engl J Med 357:1072, 2007

Greenberg HB, Estes MK: Rotaviruses: From pathogenesis to vaccination. Gastroenterology 136:1939, 2009

Huang P et al: Norovirus and histo-blood group antigens: Demonstration of a wide spectrum of strain specificities and classification of two major binding groups among multiple binding patterns. J Virol 79:6714, 2005

Ko G et al: Noroviruses as a cause of traveler's diarrhea among students from the United States visiting Mexico. J Clin Microbiol 43:6126, 2005

Leung WK et al: Enteric involvement of severe acute respiratory syndrome–associated coronavirus infection. Gastroenterology 125:1011, 2003

Lodha A et al: Human torovirus: A new virus associated with neonatal necrotizing enterocolitis. Acta Paediatr 94:1085, 2005

Murata T et al: Prolonged norovirus shedding in infants ≤6 months of age with gastroenteritis. Pediatr Infect Dis J 26:46, 2007

Parashar UD, Glass RI: Rotavirus vaccines—early success, remaining questions. N Engl J Med 360:1063, 2009

Ray P et al: Quantitative evaluation of rotaviral antigenemia in children with acute rotaviral diarrhea. J Infect Dis 194:588, 2006

Rossignol JF et al: Effect of nitazoxanide for treatment of severe rotavirus diarrhoea: Randomised double-blind placebo-controlled trial. Lancet 368:124, 2006

Ruiz-Palacios G et al: Safety and efficacy of an attenuated vaccine against severe rotavirus gastroenteritis. N Engl J Med 354:11, 2006

Tran TH et al: Avian influenza A (H5N1) in 10 patients in Vietnam. N Engl J Med 350:1179, 2004

Vesikari T et al: Safety and efficacy of a pentavalent human-bovine (WC3) reassortant rotavirus vaccine. N Engl J Med 354:23, 2006

CHAPTER 92

ACUTE VIRAL HEPATITIS

Jules L. Dienstag

Acute viral hepatitis is a systemic infection affecting the liver predominantly. Almost all cases of acute viral hepatitis are caused by one of five viral agents: hepatitis A virus (HAV), hepatitis B virus (HBV), hepatitis C virus (HCV), the HBV-associated delta agent or hepatitis D virus (HDV), and hepatitis E virus (HEV). Other transfusion-transmitted agents, e.g., "hepatitis G" virus and "TT" virus, have been identified but do not cause hepatitis. All these human hepatitis viruses are RNA viruses, except for hepatitis B, which is a DNA virus. Although these agents can be distinguished by their molecular and antigenic properties, all types of viral hepatitis produce clinically similar illnesses. These range from asymptomatic and inapparent to fulminant and fatal acute infections common to all types, on the one hand, and from subclinical persistent infections to rapidly progressive chronic liver disease with cirrhosis and even hepatocellular carcinoma, common to the bloodborne types (HBV, HCV, and HDV), on the other.

VIROLOGY AND ETIOLOGY

Hepatitis A

Hepatitis A virus is a nonenveloped 27-nm, heat-, acid-, and ether-resistant RNA virus in the hepatovirus genus of the picornavirus family (Fig. 92-1). Its virion contains four capsid polypeptides, designated VP1 to VP4, which are cleaved posttranslationally from the polyprotein product of a 7500-nucleotide genome. Inactivation of viral activity can be achieved by boiling for 1 min, by contact with formaldehyde and chlorine, or by ultraviolet irradiation. Despite nucleotide sequence variation of up to 20% among isolates of HAV, all strains of this virus are immunologically indistinguishable and belong to one serotype. Hepatitis A has an incubation period of ~4 weeks. Its replication is limited to the liver, but the virus is present in the liver, bile, stools, and blood during the late incubation period and acute preicteric phase of illness. Despite persistence of virus in the liver, viral shedding in feces, viremia, and infectivity diminish rapidly once jaundice becomes apparent. HAV can be cultivated reproducibly in vitro.

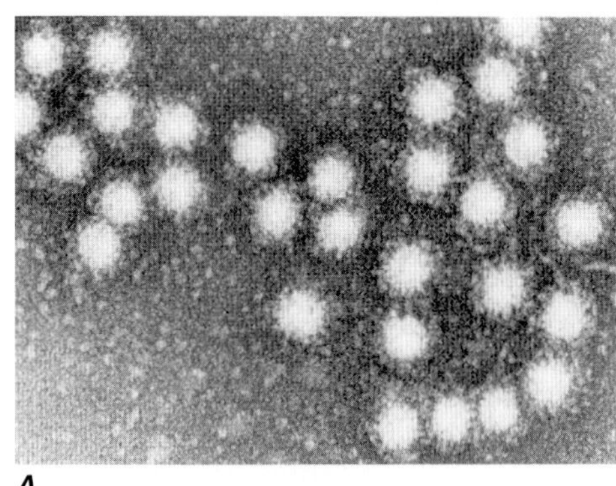

A

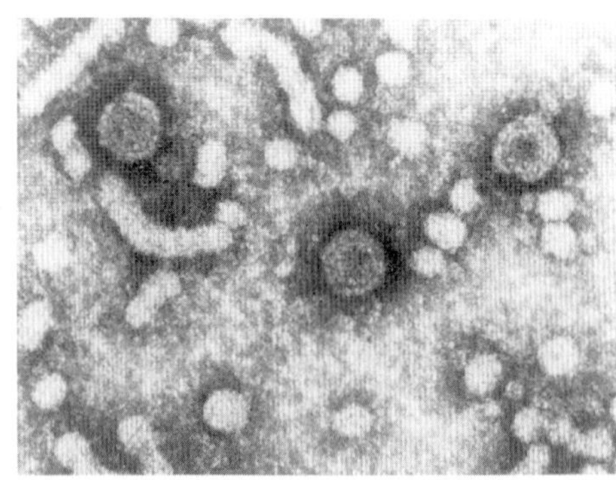

B

FIGURE 92-1

Electron micrographs of hepatitis A virus particles and serum from a patient with hepatitis B. *A.* 27-nm hepatitis A virus particles purified from stool of a patient with acute hepatitis A and aggregated by antibody to hepatitis A virus. ***B.*** Concentrated serum from a patient with hepatitis B, demonstrating the 42-nm virions, tubular forms, and spherical 22-nm particles of hepatitis B surface antigen. 132,000×. (Hepatitis D resembles 42-nm virions of hepatitis B but is smaller, 35–37 nm; hepatitis E resembles hepatitis A virus but is slightly larger, 32–34 nm; hepatitis C has been visualized as a 55-nm particle.)

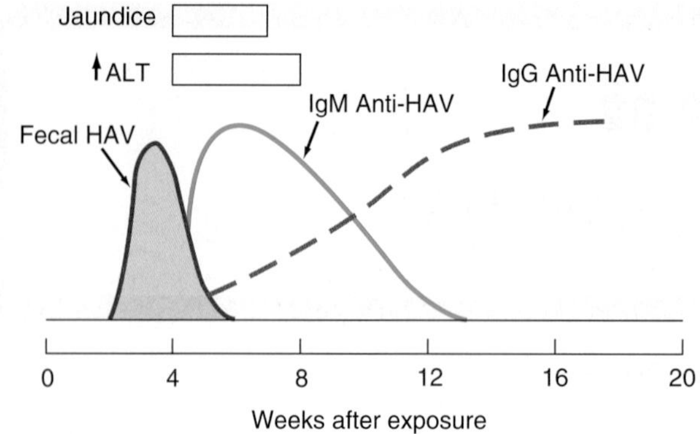

FIGURE 92-2

Scheme of typical clinical and laboratory features of hepatitis A.

Antibodies to HAV (anti-HAV) can be detected during acute illness when serum aminotransferase activity is elevated and fecal HAV shedding is still occurring. This early antibody response is predominantly of the IgM class and persists for several months, rarely for 6–12 months. During convalescence, however, anti-HAV of the IgG class becomes the predominant antibody (Fig. 92-2). Therefore, the diagnosis of hepatitis A is made during acute illness by demonstrating anti-HAV of the IgM class. After acute illness, anti-HAV of the IgG class remains detectable indefinitely, and patients with serum anti-HAV are immune to reinfection. Neutralizing antibody activity parallels the appearance of anti-HAV, and the IgG anti-HAV present in immune globulin accounts for the protection it affords against HAV infection.

Hepatitis B

Hepatitis B virus is a DNA virus with a remarkably compact genomic structure; despite its small, circular, 3200-bp size, HBV DNA codes for four sets of viral products with a complex, multiparticle structure. HBV achieves its genomic economy by relying on an efficient strategy of encoding proteins from four overlapping genes: S, C, P, and X (Fig. 92-3), as detailed below. Once thought to be unique among viruses, HBV is now recognized as one of a family of animal viruses, hepadnaviruses (hepatotropic DNA viruses), and is classified as hepadnavirus type 1. Similar viruses infect certain species of woodchucks, ground and tree squirrels, and Pekin ducks, to mention the most carefully characterized. Like HBV, all have the same distinctive three morphologic forms, have counterparts to the envelope and nucleocapsid virus antigens of HBV, replicate in the liver but exist in extrahepatic sites, contain their own endogenous DNA polymerase, have partially double-strand and partially single-strand genomes, are associated with acute and chronic hepatitis and hepatocellular carcinoma, and rely on a replicative strategy unique among DNA viruses but typical of retroviruses. Instead of DNA replication directly from a DNA template, hepadnaviruses rely on reverse transcription (effected by the DNA polymerase) of minus-strand DNA from a "pregenomic"

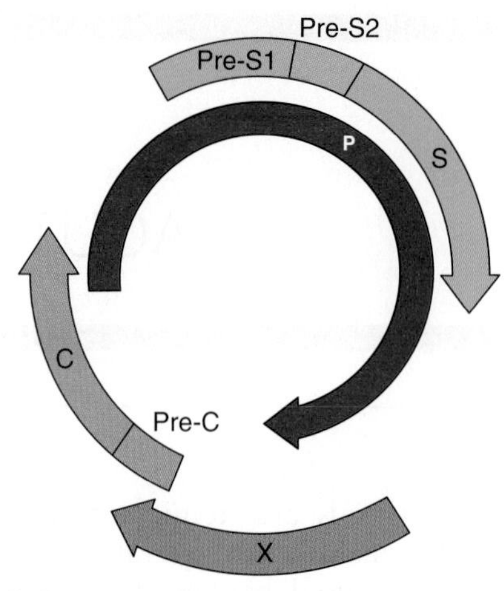

FIGURE 92-3

Compact genomic structure of HBV. This structure, with overlapping genes, permits HBV to code for multiple proteins. The S gene codes for the "major" envelope protein, HBsAg. Pre-S1 and pre-S2, upstream of S, combine with S to code for two larger proteins, "middle" protein, the product of pre-S2 + S, and "large" protein, the product of pre-S1 + pre-S2 + S. The largest gene, P, codes for DNA polymerase. The C gene codes for two nucleocapsid proteins, HBeAg, a soluble, secreted protein (initiation from the pre-C region of the gene) and HBcAg, the intracellular core protein (initiation after pre-C). The X gene codes for HBxAg, which can transactivate the transcription of cellular and viral genes; its clinical relevance is not known, but it may contribute to carcinogenesis by binding to p53.

RNA intermediate. Then plus-strand DNA is transcribed from the minus-strand DNA template by the DNA-dependent DNA polymerase and converted in the hepatocyte nucleus to a covalently closed circular DNA, which serves as a template for messenger RNA and pregenomic RNA. Viral proteins are translated by the messenger RNA, and the proteins and genome are packaged into virions and secreted from the hepatocyte. Although HBV is difficult to cultivate in vitro in the conventional sense from clinical material, several cell lines have been transfected with HBV DNA. Such transfected cells support in vitro replication of the intact virus and its component proteins.

Viral Proteins and Particles

Of the three particulate forms of HBV (Table 92-1), the most numerous are the 22-nm particles, which appear as spherical or long filamentous forms; these are antigenically indistinguishable from the outer surface or envelope protein of HBV and are thought to represent excess viral envelope protein. Outnumbered in serum by a factor of 100 or 1000 to 1 compared with the spheres and tubules are large, 42-nm, double-shelled spherical particles, which represent the intact hepatitis B virion (Fig. 92-1). The envelope protein expressed on the outer surface of the virion and on the smaller spherical and tubular structures is referred to as *hepatitis B surface antigen* (HBsAg). The concentration of HBsAg and virus particles in the blood may reach 500 μg/mL and 10 trillion

TABLE 92-1

NOMENCLATURE AND FEATURES OF HEPATITIS VIRUSES

HEPATITIS TYPE	VIRUS PARTICLE, nm	MORPHOLOGY	GENOME[a]	CLASSIFICATION	ANTIGEN(S)	ANTIBODIES	REMARKS
HAV	27	Icosahedral nonenveloped	7.5-kb RNA, linear, ss, +	Hepatovirus	HAV	Anti-HAV	Early fecal shedding Diagnosis: IgM anti-HAV Previous infection: IgG anti-HAV
HBV	42	Double-shelled virion (surface and core) spherical	3.2-kb DNA, circular, ss/ds	Hepadnavirus	HBsAg HBcAg HBeAg	Anti-HBs Anti-HBc Anti-HBe	Bloodborne virus; carrier state Acute diagnosis: HBsAg, IgM anti-HBc Chronic diagnosis: IgG anti-HBc, HBsAg Markers of replication: HBeAg, HBV DNA Liver, lymphocytes, other organs
	27	Nucleocapsid core			HBcAg HBeAg	Anti-HBc Anti-HBe	Nucleocapsid contains DNA and DNA polymerase; present in hepatocyte nucleus; HBcAg does not circulate; HBeAg (soluble, nonparticulate) and HBV DNA circulate—correlate with infectivity and complete virions
	22	Spherical and filamentous; represents excess virus coat material			HBsAg	Anti-HBs	HBsAg detectable in >95% of patients with acute hepatitis B; found in serum, body fluids, hepatocyte cytoplasm; anti-HBs appears following infection—protective antibody
HCV	Approx. 40–60	Enveloped	9.4-kb RNA, linear, ss, +	Hepacivirus	HCV C100-3 C33c C22-3 NS5	Anti-HCV	Bloodborne agent, formerly labeled non-A, non-B hepatitis Acute diagnosis: anti-HCV (C33c, C22-3, NS5), HCV RNA Chronic diagnosis: anti-HCV (C100-3, C33c, C22-3, NS5) and HCV RNA; cytoplasmic location in hepatocytes
HDV	35–37	Enveloped hybrid particle with HBsAg coat and HDV core	1.7-kb RNA, circular, ss, –	Resembles viroids and plant satellite viruses	HBsAg HDV antigen	Anti-HBs Anti-HDV	Defective RNA virus, requires helper function of HBV (hepadnaviruses); HDV antigen present in hepatocyte nucleus Diagnosis: anti-HDV, HDV RNA; HBV/HDV coinfection—IgM anti-HBc and anti-HDV; HDV superinfection—IgG anti-HBc and anti-HDV
HEV	32–34	Nonenveloped icosahedral	7.6-kb RNA, linear, ss, +	Hepevirus	HEV antigen	Anti-HEV	Agent of enterically transmitted hepatitis; rare in USA; occurs in Asia, Mediterranean countries, Central America Diagnosis: IgM/IgG anti-HEV (assays being developed); virus in stool, bile, hepatocyte cytoplasm

[a]ss, single-strand; ss/ds, partially single-strand, partially double-strand; –, minus-strand; +, plus-strand.

particles per milliliter, respectively. The envelope protein, HBsAg, is the product of the S gene of HBV.

A number of different HBsAg subdeterminants have been identified. There is a common group-reactive antigen, *a*, shared by all HBsAg isolates. In addition, HBsAg may contain one of several subtype-specific antigens, namely, *d* or *y*, *w* or *r*, as well as other more recently characterized specificities. Hepatitis B isolates fall into one of at least eight subtypes and eight genotypes (A–H). Geographic distribution of genotypes and subtypes varies; genotypes A (corresponding to subtype *adw*) and D (*ayw*) predominate in the United States and Europe, while genotypes B (*adw*) and C (*adr*) predominate in Asia. Clinical course and outcome are independent of subtype, but preliminary reports suggest that genotype B is associated with less rapidly progressive liver disease and a lower likelihood, or delayed appearance, of hepatocellular carcinoma than genotype C. Patients with genotype A appear to be more likely to clear circulating viremia and to achieve HBsAg seroconversion, both spontaneously and in response to antiviral therapy. In addition, "precore" mutations are favored by certain genotypes (see below).

Upstream of the S gene are the pre-S genes (Fig. 92-3), which code for pre-S gene products, including receptors on the HBV surface for polymerized human serum albumin and for hepatocyte membrane proteins. The pre-S region actually consists of both pre-S1 and pre-S2. Depending on where translation is initiated, three potential HBsAg gene products are synthesized. The protein product of the S gene is HBsAg (*major protein*), the product of the S region plus the adjacent pre-S2 region is the *middle protein*, and the product of the pre-S1 plus pre-S2 plus S regions is the *large protein*. Compared with the smaller spherical and tubular particles of HBV, complete 42-nm virions are enriched in the large protein. Both pre-S proteins and their respective antibodies can be detected during HBV infection, and the period of pre-S antigenemia appears to coincide with other markers of virus replication, as detailed below.

The intact 42-nm virion contains a 27-nm nucleocapsid core particle. Nucleocapsid proteins are coded for by the C gene. The antigen expressed on the surface of the nucleocapsid core is referred to as *hepatitis B core antigen* (HBcAg), and its corresponding antibody is anti-HBc. A third HBV antigen is *hepatitis B e antigen* (HBeAg), a soluble, nonparticulate, nucleocapsid protein that is immunologically distinct from intact HBcAg but is a product of the same C gene. The C gene has two initiation codons, a precore and a core region (Fig. 92-3). If translation is initiated at the precore region, the protein product is HBeAg, which has a signal peptide that binds it to the smooth endoplasmic reticulum and leads to its secretion into the circulation. If translation begins with the core region, HBcAg is the protein product; it has no signal peptide, it is not secreted, but it assembles into nucleocapsid particles, which bind to and incorporate RNA and which, ultimately, contain HBV DNA. Also packaged within the nucleocapsid core is a DNA polymerase, which directs replication and repair of HBV DNA. When packaging within viral proteins is complete, synthesis of the incomplete plus strand stops; this accounts for the single-strand gap and for differences in the size of the gap. HBcAg particles remain in the hepatocyte, where they are readily detectable by immunohistochemical staining, and are exported after encapsidation by an envelope of HBsAg. Therefore, naked core particles do not circulate in the serum. The secreted nucleocapsid protein, HBeAg, provides a convenient, readily detectable, qualitative marker of HBV replication and relative infectivity.

HBsAg-positive serum containing HBeAg is more likely to be highly infectious and to be associated with the presence of hepatitis B virions (and detectable HBV DNA, see below) than HBeAg-negative or anti-HBe-positive serum. For example, HBsAg carrier mothers who are HBeAg-positive almost invariably (>90%) transmit hepatitis B infection to their offspring, whereas HBsAg carrier mothers with anti-HBe rarely (10–15%) infect their offspring.

Early during the course of acute hepatitis B, HBeAg appears transiently; its disappearance may be a harbinger of clinical improvement and resolution of infection. Persistence of HBeAg in serum beyond the first 3 months of acute infection may be predictive of the development of chronic infection, and the presence of HBeAg during chronic hepatitis B is associated with ongoing viral replication, infectivity, and inflammatory liver injury.

The third of the HBV genes is the largest, the P gene (Fig. 92-3), which codes for the DNA polymerase; as noted above, this enzyme has both DNA-dependent DNA polymerase and RNA-dependent reverse transcriptase activities. The fourth gene, X, codes for a small, nonparticulate protein, *hepatitis B x antigen* (HBxAg), that is capable of transactivating the transcription of both viral and cellular genes (Fig. 92-3). In the cytoplasm, HBxAg effects calcium release (possibly from mitochondria), which activates signal-transduction pathways that lead to stimulation of HBV reverse transcription and HBV DNA replication. Such transactivation may enhance the replication of HBV, leading to the clinical association observed between the expression of HBxAg and antibodies to it in patients with severe chronic hepatitis and hepatocellular carcinoma. The transactivating activity can enhance the transcription and replication of other viruses besides HBV, such as HIV. Cellular processes transactivated by X include the human interferon γ gene and class I major histocompatibility genes; potentially, these effects could contribute to enhanced susceptibility of HBV-infected hepatocytes to cytolytic T cells. The expression of X can also induce programmed cell death (apoptosis).

Serologic and Virologic Markers

After a person is infected with HBV, the first virologic marker detectable in serum within 1–12 weeks, usually between 8–12 weeks, is HBsAg (Fig. 92-4). Circulating HBsAg precedes elevations of serum aminotransferase activity and clinical symptoms by 2–6 weeks and remains detectable during the entire icteric or symptomatic phase of acute hepatitis B and beyond. In typical cases, HBsAg becomes undetectable 1–2 months after the onset of jaundice and rarely persists beyond 6 months. After HBsAg disappears, antibody to HBsAg (anti-HBs) becomes detectable in serum and remains

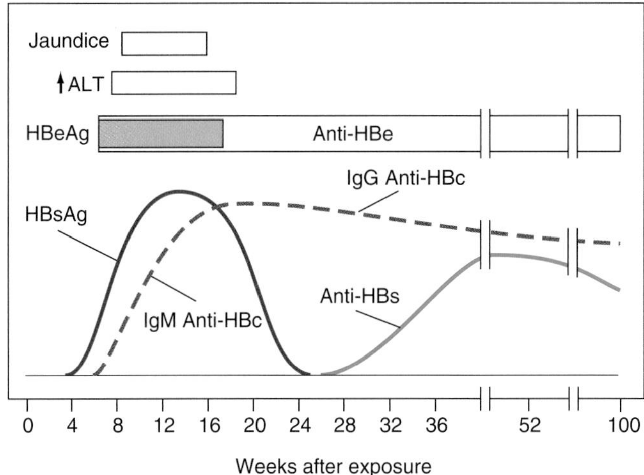

FIGURE 92-4

Scheme of typical clinical and laboratory features of acute hepatitis B.

detectable indefinitely thereafter. Because HBcAg is intracellular and, when in the serum, sequestered within an HBsAg coat, naked core particles do not circulate in serum and, therefore, HBcAg is not detectable routinely in the serum of patients with HBV infection. By contrast, anti-HBc is readily demonstrable in serum, beginning within the first 1–2 weeks after the appearance of HBsAg and preceding detectable levels of anti-HBs by weeks to months. Because variability exists in the time of appearance of anti-HBs after HBV infection, occasionally a gap of several weeks or longer may separate the disappearance of HBsAg and the appearance of anti-HBs. During this "gap" or "window" period, anti-HBc may represent the only serologic evidence of current or recent HBV infection, and blood containing anti-HBc in the absence of HBsAg and anti-HBs has been implicated in the development of transfusion-associated hepatitis B. In part because the sensitivity of immunoassays for HBsAg and anti-HBs has increased, however, this window period is rarely encountered. In some persons, years after HBV infection, anti-HBc may persist in the circulation longer than anti-HBs. Therefore, isolated anti-HBc does not necessarily indicate active virus replication; most instances of isolated anti-HBc represent hepatitis B infection in the remote past. Rarely, however, isolated anti-HBc represents low-level hepatitis B viremia, with HBsAg below the detection threshold; occasionally, isolated anti-HBc represents a cross-reacting or false-positive immunologic specificity. Recent and remote HBV infections can be distinguished by determination of the immunoglobulin class of anti-HBc. Anti-HBc of the IgM class (IgM anti-HBc) predominates during the first 6 months after acute infection, whereas IgG anti-HBc is the predominant class of anti-HBc beyond 6 months. Therefore, patients with current or recent acute hepatitis B, including those in the anti-HBc window, have IgM anti-HBc in their serum. In patients who have recovered from hepatitis B in the remote past as well as those with chronic HBV infection, anti-HBc is predominantly of the IgG class. Infrequently, in ≤1–5% of patients with acute HBV infection, levels of HBsAg are too low to be detected; in such cases, the presence of IgM anti-HBc establishes the diagnosis of acute hepatitis B. When isolated anti-HBc occurs in the rare patient with chronic hepatitis B whose HBsAg level is below the sensitivity threshold of contemporary immunoassays (a low-level carrier), the anti-HBc is of the IgG class. Generally, in persons who have recovered from hepatitis B, anti-HBs and anti-HBc persist indefinitely.

The temporal association between the appearance of anti-HBs and resolution of HBV infection as well as the observation that persons with anti-HBs in serum are protected against reinfection with HBV suggests that *anti-HBs are the protective antibody*. Therefore, strategies for prevention of HBV infection are based on providing susceptible persons with circulating anti-HBs (see below). Occasionally, in 10–20% of patients with chronic hepatitis B, low-level, low-affinity anti-HBs can be detected. This antibody is directed against a subtype determinant different from that represented by the patient's HBsAg; its presence is thought to reflect the stimulation of a related clone of antibody-forming cells, but it has no clinical relevance and does not signal imminent clearance of hepatitis B. These patients with HBsAg and such nonneutralizing anti-HBs should be categorized as having chronic HBV infection.

The other readily detectable serologic marker of HBV infection, HBeAg, appears concurrently with or shortly after HBsAg. Its appearance coincides temporally with high levels of virus replication and reflects the presence of circulating intact virions and detectable HBV DNA (with the notable exception of patients with precore mutations who cannot synthesize HBeAg—see the next section, "Molecular Variants"). Pre-S1 and pre-S2 proteins are also expressed during periods of peak replication, but assays for these gene products are not routinely available. In self-limited HBV infections, HBeAg becomes undetectable shortly after peak elevations in aminotransferase activity, before the disappearance of HBsAg, and anti-HBe then becomes detectable, coinciding with a period of relatively lower infectivity (Fig. 92-4). Because markers of HBV replication appear transiently during acute infection, testing for such markers is of little clinical utility in typical cases of acute HBV infection. In contrast, markers of HBV replication provide valuable information in patients with protracted infections.

Departing from the pattern typical of acute HBV infections, in chronic HBV infection, HBsAg remains detectable beyond 6 months, anti-HBc is primarily of the IgG class, and anti-HBs is either undetectable or detectable at low levels (see "Laboratory Features" later in the chapter) (Fig. 92-5). During early chronic HBV infection, HBV DNA can be detected both in serum and in hepatocyte nuclei, where it is present in free or episomal form. This *replicative stage* of HBV infection is the time of maximal infectivity and liver injury; HBeAg is a qualitative marker and HBV DNA a quantitative marker of this replicative phase, during which all three forms of HBV circulate, including intact virions. Over time, the replicative phase of chronic HBV infection gives way to a relatively *nonreplicative phase*. This occurs at

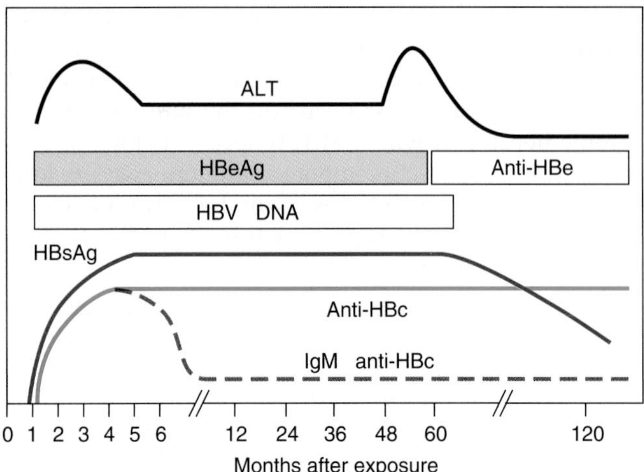

FIGURE 92-5

Scheme of typical laboratory features of wild-type chronic hepatitis B. HBeAg and HBV DNA can be detected in serum during the *replicative phase* of chronic infection, which is associated with infectivity and liver injury. Seroconversion from the replicative phase to the *nonreplicative phase* occurs at a rate of ~10% per year and is heralded by an acute hepatitis–like elevation of ALT activity; during the nonreplicative phase, infectivity and liver injury are limited. In HBeAg-negative chronic hepatitis B associated with mutations in the precore region of the HBV genome, replicative chronic hepatitis B occurs in the absence of HBeAg.

a rate of ~10% per year and is accompanied by seroconversion from HBeAg-positive to anti-HBe-positive. In most cases, this seroconversion coincides with a transient, acute hepatitis-like elevation in aminotransferase activity, believed to reflect cell-mediated immune clearance of virus-infected hepatocytes. In the nonreplicative phase of chronic infection, when HBV DNA is demonstrable in hepatocyte nuclei, it tends to be integrated into the host genome. In this phase, only spherical and tubular forms of HBV, *not intact virions*, circulate, and liver injury tends to subside. Most such patients would be characterized as *inactive HBV carriers*. In reality, the designations *replicative* and *nonreplicative* are only relative; even in the so-called nonreplicative phase, HBV replication can be detected at levels of ~$\leq 10^3$ virions with highly sensitive amplification probes such as the polymerase chain reaction (PCR); below this replication threshold, liver injury and infectivity of HBV are limited to negligible. Still, the distinctions are pathophysiologically and clinically meaningful. Occasionally, nonreplicative HBV infection converts back to replicative infection. Such spontaneous reactivations are accompanied by reexpression of HBeAg and HBV DNA, and sometimes of IgM anti-HBc, as well as by exacerbations of liver injury. Because high-titer IgM anti-HBc can reappear during acute exacerbations of chronic hepatitis B, relying on IgM anti-HBc versus IgG anti-HBc to distinguish between acute and chronic hepatitis B infection, respectively, may not always be reliable; in such cases, patient history is invaluable in helping to distinguish de novo acute hepatitis B infection from acute exacerbation of chronic hepatitis B infection.

Molecular Variants

Variation occurs throughout the HBV genome, and clinical isolates of HBV that do not express typical viral proteins have been attributed to mutations in individual or even multiple gene locations. For example, variants have been described that lack nucleocapsid proteins, envelope proteins, or both. Two categories of naturally occurring HBV variants have attracted the most attention. One of these was identified initially in Mediterranean countries among patients with an unusual serologic-clinical profile. They have severe chronic HBV infection and detectable HBV DNA but with anti-HBe instead of HBeAg. These patients were found to be infected with an HBV mutant that contained an alteration in the precore region rendering the virus incapable of encoding HBeAg. Although several potential mutation sites exist in the pre-C region, the region of the C gene necessary for the expression of HBeAg (see "Virology and Etiology" earlier in the chapter), the most commonly encountered in such patients is a single base substitution, from G to A, which occurs in the second to last codon of the pre-C gene at nucleotide 1896. This substitution results in the replacement of the TGG tryptophan codon by a stop codon (T*A*G), which prevents the translation of HBeAg. Another mutation, in the core-promoter region, prevents transcription of the coding region for HBeAg and yields an HBeAg-negative phenotype. Patients with such mutations in the precore region and who are unable to secrete HBeAg tend to have severe liver disease that progresses more rapidly to cirrhosis. Both "wild-type" HBV and precore-mutant HBV can coexist in the same patient, or mutant HBV may arise late during wild-type HBV infection. In addition, clusters of fulminant hepatitis B in Israel and Japan have been attributed to common-source infection with a precore mutant. Fulminant hepatitis B in North America and western Europe, however, occurs in patients infected with wild-type HBV, in the absence of precore mutants, and both precore mutants and other mutations throughout the HBV genome occur commonly even in patients with typical, self-limited, milder forms of HBV infection. HBeAg-negative chronic hepatitis with mutations in the precore region is now the most frequently encountered form of hepatitis B in Mediterranean countries and in Europe. In the United States, where HBV genotype A (less prone to G1896A mutation) is prevalent, precore-mutant HBV is much less common; however, as a result of immigration from Asia and Europe, the proportion of HBeAg-negative hepatitis B–infected individuals has increased in the United States, and they now represent approximately a third of patients with chronic hepatitis B. Characteristic of such HBeAg-negative chronic hepatitis B are lower levels of HBV DNA (usually $\leq 10^5$ copies/mL) and one of several patterns of aminotransferase activity—persistent elevations, periodic fluctuations above the normal range, and periodic fluctuations between the normal and elevated range.

The second important category of HBV mutants consists of *escape mutants*, in which a single amino acid substitution, from glycine to arginine, occurs at position 145 of the immunodominant *a* determinant common to all subtypes of HBsAg. This change in HBsAg leads to a critical conformational change that results in a loss of neutralizing activity by anti-HBs. This specific HBV/*a* mutant has been observed in two situations, active and passive immunization, in which humoral immunologic pressure may favor evolutionary change ("escape") in the virus—in a small number of hepatitis B vaccine recipients who acquired HBV infection despite the prior appearance of neutralizing anti-HBs and in liver transplant recipients who underwent the procedure for hepatitis B and who were treated with a high-potency human monoclonal anti-HBs preparation. Although such mutants have not been recognized frequently, their existence raises a concern that may complicate vaccination strategies and serologic diagnosis. Different types of mutations emerge during antiviral therapy of chronic hepatitis B with nucleoside analogues; such "YMDD" and similar mutations in the polymerase motif of HBV are described in Chap. 93.

Extrahepatic Sites

Hepatitis B antigens and HBV DNA have been identified in extrahepatic sites, including lymph nodes, bone marrow, circulating lymphocytes, spleen, and pancreas. Although the virus does not appear to be associated with tissue injury in any of these extrahepatic sites, its presence in these "remote" reservoirs has been invoked to explain the recurrence of HBV infection after orthotopic liver transplantation. A more complete understanding of the clinical relevance of extrahepatic HBV remains to be defined.

Hepatitis D

The delta hepatitis agent, or HDV, is a defective RNA virus that coinfects with and requires the helper function of HBV (or other hepadnaviruses) for its replication and expression. Slightly smaller than HBV, delta is a formalin-sensitive, 35- to 37-nm virus with a hybrid structure. Its nucleocapsid expresses delta antigen, which bears no antigenic homology with any of the HBV antigens, and contains the virus genome. The delta core is "encapsidated" by an outer envelope of HBsAg, indistinguishable from that of HBV except in its relative compositions of major, middle, and large HBsAg component proteins. The genome is a small, 1700-nucleotide, circular, single-strand RNA (minus strand) that is nonhomologous with HBV DNA (except for a small area of the polymerase gene) but that has features and the rolling circle model of replication common to genomes of plant satellite viruses or viroids. HDV RNA contains many areas of internal complementarity; therefore, it can fold on itself by internal base pairing to form an unusual, very stable, rodlike structure. HDV RNA requires host RNA polymerase II for its replication via RNA-directed RNA synthesis by transcription of genomic RNA to a complementary antigenomic (plus strand) RNA; the antigenomic RNA, in turn, serves as a template for subsequent genomic RNA synthesis. Between the genomic and antigenomic RNAs of HDV, there are coding regions for nine proteins. Delta antigen, which is a product of the antigenomic strand, exists in two forms, a small, 195-amino-acid species, which plays a role in facilitating HDV RNA replication, and a large, 214-amino-acid species, which appears to suppress replication but is required for assembly of the antigen into virions. Delta antigens have been shown to bind directly to RNA polymerase II, resulting in stimulation of transcription. Although complete hepatitis D virions and liver injury require the cooperative helper function of HBV, intracellular replication of HDV RNA can occur without HBV. Genomic heterogeneity among HDV isolates has been described; however, pathophysiologic and clinical consequences of this genetic diversity have not been recognized.

HDV can either infect a person simultaneously with HBV (*co-infection*) or superinfect a person already infected with HBV (*superinfection*); when HDV infection is transmitted from a donor with one HBsAg subtype to an HBsAg-positive recipient with a different subtype, the HDV agent assumes the HBsAg subtype of the recipient, rather than the donor. Because HDV relies absolutely on HBV, the duration of HDV infection is determined by the duration of (and cannot outlast) HBV infection. HDV antigen is expressed primarily in hepatocyte nuclei and is occasionally detectable in serum. During acute HDV infection, anti-HDV of the IgM class predominates, and 30–40 days may elapse after symptoms appear before anti-HDV can be detected. In self-limited infection, anti-HDV is low titer and transient, rarely remaining detectable beyond the clearance of HBsAg and HDV antigen. In chronic HDV infection, anti-HDV circulates in high titer, and both IgM and IgG anti-HDV can be detected. HDV antigen in the liver and HDV RNA in serum and liver can be detected during HDV replication.

Hepatitis C

Hepatitis C virus, which, before its identification was labeled "non-A, non-B hepatitis," is a linear, single-strand, positive-sense, 9600-nucleotide RNA virus, the genome of which is similar in organization to that of flaviviruses and pestiviruses; HCV is the only member of the genus *Hepacivirus* in the family Flaviviridae. The HCV genome contains a single large open reading frame (gene) that codes for a virus polyprotein of ~3000 amino acids, which is cleaved after translation to yield 10 viral proteins. The 5′ end of the genome consists of an untranslated region (containing an internal ribosomal entry site) adjacent to the genes for four structural proteins; the nucleocapsid core protein, C; two envelope glycoproteins, E1 and E2; and a membrane protein p7. The 5′ untranslated region and core gene are highly conserved among genotypes, but the envelope proteins are coded for by the hypervariable region, which varies from isolate to isolate and may allow the virus to evade host immunologic containment directed at accessible virus-envelope proteins. The 3′ end of the genome also includes an untranslated region and contains the genes for six nonstructural (NS) proteins NS2, NS3, NS4A, NS4B, NS5A, and NS5B. The NS2 cysteine protease cleaves NS3 from NS2, and the NS3-4A serine protease cleaves all the downstream proteins from the polyprotein. Important NS proteins

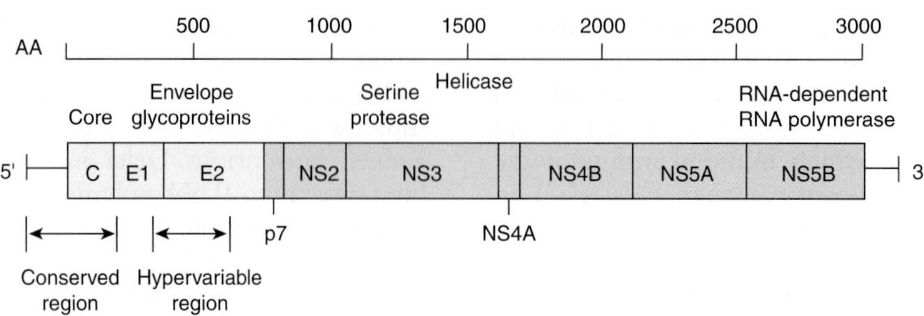

FIGURE 92-6

Organization of the hepatitis C virus genome and its associated, 3000-amino-acid (AA) proteins. The three structural genes at the 5′ end are the core region, C, which codes for the nucleocapsid, and the envelope regions, E1 and E2, which code for envelope glycoproteins. The 5′ untranslated region and the C region are highly conserved among isolates, while the envelope domain E2 contains the hypervariable region. Adjacent to the structural proteins is p7, a membrane protein that appears to function as an ion channel. At the 3′ end are six nonstructural (NS) regions, NS2, which codes for a cysteine protease; NS3, which codes for a serine protease and an RNA helicase; NS4 and NS4B; NS5A; and NS5B, which codes for an RNA-dependent RNA polymerase. After translation of the entire polyprotein, individual proteins are cleaved by both host and viral proteases.

involved in virus replication include the NS3 helicase, NS3-NS4A serine protease, and the NS5B RNA-dependent RNA polymerase (Fig. 92-6). Because HCV does not replicate via a DNA intermediate, it does not integrate into the host genome. Because HCV tends to circulate in relatively low titer, 10^3–10^7 virions/mL, visualization of virus particles, estimated to be 40–60 nm in diameter, remains difficult. Still, the replication rate of HCV is very high, 10^{12} virions per day; its half-life is 2.7 h. The chimpanzee is a helpful but cumbersome animal model. Although a robust, reproducible, small-animal model is lacking, HCV replication has been documented in an immunodeficient-mouse model containing explants of human liver and in transgenic mouse and rat models. Although in vitro replication has been difficult, hepatocellular carcinoma–derived cell lines have been described (replicon systems) that support replication of genetically manipulated, truncated or full-length HCV RNA (but not intact virions). Recently, complete replication of HCV and intact 55-nm virions has been described in cell culture systems. Preliminary data suggest that HCV gains entry into the hepatocyte via the CD81 receptor.

At least six distinct genotypes, as well as >50 subtypes within genotypes, of HCV have been identified by nucleotide sequencing. Genotypes differ one from another in sequence homology by ≥30%. Because divergence of HCV isolates within a genotype or subtype, and within the same host, may vary insufficiently to define a distinct genotype, these intragenotypic differences are referred to as *quasispecies* and differ in sequence homology by only a few percent. The genotypic and quasispecies diversity of HCV, resulting from its high mutation rate, interferes with effective humoral immunity. Neutralizing antibodies to HCV have been demonstrated, but they tend to be short-lived, and HCV infection does not induce lasting immunity against reinfection with different virus isolates or even the same virus isolate. Thus, neither *heterologous* nor *homologous* immunity appears to develop commonly after acute HCV infection. Some HCV genotypes are distributed worldwide, while others are more geographically confined (see "Epidemiology and Global Features" later in the chapter). In addition, differences exist among genotypes in responsiveness to antiviral therapy; however, early reports of differences in pathogenicity among genotypes have not been corroborated.

Currently available, third-generation immunoassays, which incorporate proteins from the core, NS3, and NS5 regions, detect anti-HCV antibodies during acute infection. The most sensitive indicator of HCV infection is the presence of HCV RNA, which requires molecular amplification by PCR or transcription-mediated amplification (TMA) (Fig. 92-7). To allow standardization of the quantification of HCV RNA among laboratories and commercial assays, HCV RNA is reported as international units (IU) per milliliter; quantitative assays are available that allow detection of HCV RNA with a sensitivity as low as 5 IU/mL. HCV RNA can be detected within a few days of exposure to HCV, well before the appearance of anti-HCV, and tends to persist for the duration of HCV infection; however, occasionally in patients with chronic HCV infection, HCV RNA may

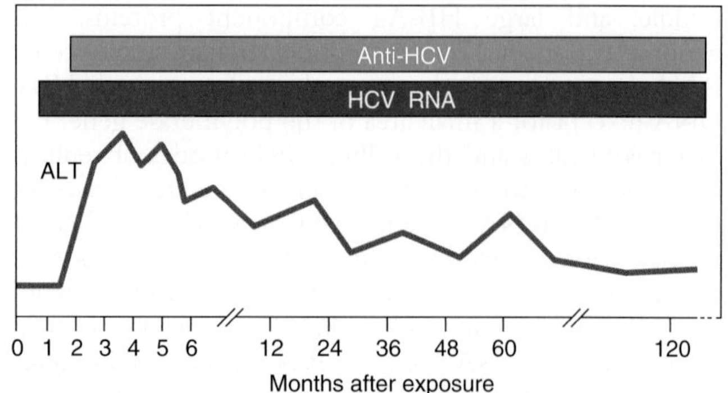

FIGURE 92-7

Scheme of typical laboratory features during acute hepatitis C progressing to chronicity. HCV RNA is the first detectable event, preceding ALT elevation and the appearance of anti-HCV.

be detectable only intermittently. Application of sensitive molecular probes for HCV RNA has revealed the presence of replicative HCV in peripheral blood lymphocytes of infected persons; however, as is the case for HBV in lymphocytes, the clinical relevance of HCV lymphocyte infection is not known.

Hepatitis E

Previously labeled *epidemic* or *enterically transmitted non-A, non-B hepatitis*, HEV is an enterically transmitted virus that occurs primarily in India, Asia, Africa, and Central America; in those geographic areas, HEV is the most common cause of acute hepatitis. This agent, with epidemiologic features resembling those of hepatitis A, is a 32- to 34-nm, nonenveloped, HAV-like virus with a 7600-nucleotide, single-strand, positive-sense RNA genome. HEV has three open reading frames (ORF) (genes), the largest of which, *ORF1*, encodes nonstructural proteins involved in virus replication. A middle-sized gene, *ORF2*, encodes the nucleocapsid protein, and the smallest, *ORF3*, encodes a structural protein whose function remains undetermined. All HEV isolates appear to belong to a single serotype, despite genomic heterogeneity of up to 25% and the existence of five genotypes, only four of which have been detected in humans; genotypes 1 and 2 appear to be more virulent, while genotypes 3 and 4 are more attenuated and account for subclinical infections. Contributing to the perpetuation of this virus are animal reservoirs, most notably in swine. There is no genomic or antigenic homology, however, between HEV and HAV or other picornaviruses; and HEV, although resembling caliciviruses, is sufficiently distinct from any known agent to merit a new classification of its own as a unique genus, *Hepevirus*, within the Hepeviridae family. The virus has been detected in stool, bile, and liver and is excreted in the stool during the late incubation period; immune responses to viral antigens occur very early during the course of acute infection. Both IgM anti-HEV and IgG anti-HEV can be detected, but both fall rapidly after acute infection, reaching low levels within 9–12 months. Currently, serologic testing for HEV infection is not available routinely.

PATHOGENESIS

Under ordinary circumstances, none of the hepatitis viruses is known to be directly cytopathic to hepatocytes. Evidence suggests that the clinical manifestations and outcomes after acute liver injury associated with viral hepatitis are determined by the immunologic responses of the host. Among the viral hepatitides, the immunopathogenesis of hepatitis B and C have been studied most extensively.

Hepatitis B

For HBV, the existence of inactive hepatitis B carriers with normal liver histology and function suggests that the virus is not directly cytopathic. The fact that patients with defects in cellular immune competence are more likely to remain chronically infected rather than to clear HBV is cited to support the role of cellular immune responses in the pathogenesis of hepatitis B–related liver injury. The model that has the most experimental support involves cytolytic T cells sensitized specifically to recognize host and hepatitis B viral antigens on the liver cell surface. Laboratory observations suggest that nucleocapsid proteins (HBcAg and possibly HBeAg), present on the cell membrane in minute quantities, are the viral target antigens that, with host antigens, invite cytolytic T cells to destroy HBV-infected hepatocytes. Differences in the robustness of CD8+ cytolytic T-cell responsiveness and in the elaboration of antiviral cytokines by T cells have been invoked to explain differences in outcomes between those who recover after acute hepatitis and those who progress to chronic hepatitis or between those with mild and those with severe (fulminant) acute HBV infection.

Although a robust cytolytic T-cell response occurs and eliminates virus-infected liver cells during acute hepatitis B, >90% of HBV DNA has been found in experimentally infected chimpanzees to disappear from the liver and blood before maximal T-cell infiltration of the liver and before most of the biochemical and histologic evidence of liver injury. This observation suggests that components of the innate immune system and inflammatory cytokines, independent of cytopathic antiviral mechanisms, participate in the early immune response to HBV infection; this effect has been shown to represent elimination of HBV replicative intermediates from the cytoplasm and covalently closed circular viral DNA from the nucleus of infected hepatocytes. Ultimately, HBV-HLA-specific cytolytic T-cell responses of the adaptive immune system are felt to be responsible for recovery from HBV infection.

Debate continues over the relative importance of viral and host factors in the pathogenesis of HBV-associated liver injury and its outcome. As noted above, precore genetic mutants of HBV have been associated with the more severe outcomes of HBV infection (severe chronic and fulminant hepatitis), suggesting that, under certain circumstances, relative pathogenicity is a property of the virus, not the host. The fact that concomitant HDV and HBV infections are associated with more severe liver injury than HBV infection alone and the fact that cells transfected in vitro with the gene for HDV (delta) antigen express HDV antigen and then become necrotic in the absence of any immunologic influences are also consistent with a viral effect on pathogenicity. Similarly, in patients who undergo liver transplantation for end-stage chronic hepatitis B, occasionally, rapidly progressive liver injury appears in the new liver. This clinical pattern is associated with an unusual histologic pattern in the new liver, *fibrosing cholestatic hepatitis*, which, ultrastructurally, appears to represent a choking of the cell with overwhelming quantities of HBsAg. This observation suggests that under the influence of the potent immunosuppressive agents required to prevent allograft rejection, HBV may have a direct cytopathic effect on liver cells, independent of the immune system.

Although the precise mechanism of liver injury in HBV infection remains elusive, studies of nucleocapsid proteins have shed light on the profound immunologic tolerance to HBV of babies born to mothers with highly replicative (HBeAg-positive), chronic HBV infection. In HBeAg-expressing transgenic mice, in utero exposure to HBeAg, which is sufficiently small to traverse the placenta, induces T cell tolerance to both nucleocapsid proteins. This, in turn, may explain why, when infection occurs so early in life, immunologic clearance does not occur, and protracted, lifelong infection ensues.

An important distinction should be drawn between HBV infection acquired at birth, common in endemic areas, such as the Far East, and infection acquired in adulthood, common in the west. Infection in the neonatal period is associated with the acquisition of immunologic tolerance to HBV, absence of an acute-hepatitis illness, but the almost invariable establishment of chronic, often lifelong infection. Neonatally acquired HBV infection can culminate decades later in cirrhosis and hepatocellular carcinoma (see "Complications and Sequelae" later in the chapter). In contrast, when HBV infection is acquired during adolescence or early adulthood, the host-immune response to HBV-infected hepatocytes tends to be robust, an acute hepatitis-like illness is the rule, and failure to recover is the exception. After adulthood-acquired infection, chronicity is uncommon, and the risk of hepatocellular carcinoma is very low. Based on these observations, some authorities categorize HBV infection into an "immunotolerant" phase, an "immunoreactive" phase, and an inactive phase. This somewhat simplistic formulation does not apply at all to the typical adult in the west with self-limited acute hepatitis B, in whom no period of immunologic tolerance occurs. Even among those with neonatally acquired HBV infection, in whom immunologic tolerance is established definitively, intermittent bursts of hepatic necroinflammatory activity punctuate the period during the early decades of life during which liver injury appears to be quiescent (labeled by some as the "immunotolerant" phase). In addition, even when clinically apparent liver injury and progressive fibrosis emerge during later decades (the so-called immunoreactive, or immunointolerant, phase), the level of immunologic tolerance to HBV remains substantial. More accurately, in patients with neonatally acquired HBV infection, a dynamic equilibrium exists between tolerance and intolerance, the outcome of which determines the clinical expression of chronic infection.

Hepatitis C

Cell-mediated immune responses and elaboration by T cells of antiviral cytokines contribute to the containment of infection and pathogenesis of liver injury associated with hepatitis C. Perhaps HCV infection of lymphoid cells plays a role in moderating immune responsiveness to the virus, as well. Intrahepatic HLA class I–restricted cytolytic T cells directed at nucleocapsid, envelope, and nonstructural viral protein antigens have been demonstrated in patients with chronic hepatitis C; however, such virus-specific cytolytic T cell responses do not correlate adequately with the degree of liver injury or with recovery. Yet, a consensus has emerged supporting a role in the pathogenesis of HCV-associated liver injury of virus-activated CD4 helper T cells that stimulate, via the cytokines they elaborate, HCV-specific CD8 cytotoxic T cells. These responses appear to be more robust (higher in number, more diverse in viral antigen specificity, more functionally effective, and more long-lasting) in those who recover from HCV than in those who have chronic infection. Several HLA alleles have been linked with self-limited hepatitis C, but such associations do not apply universally. Attention has been focused as well on adaptive immunity; the establishment of persistent infection correlates with failure of adaptive immune responses to HCV. Furthermore, HCV proteins have been shown to interfere with innate immunity by resulting in blocking of type 1 interferon responses and inhibition of interferon signaling and effector molecules in the interferon signaling cascade. Also shown to contribute to limiting HCV infection are natural killer cells of the innate immune system, which function when HLA class 1 molecules required for successful adaptive immunity are underexpressed. Of note, the emergence of substantial viral quasispecies diversity allows the virus to evade attempts by the host to contain HCV infection immunologically.

Finally, cross-reactivity between viral antigens (HCV NS3 and NS5A) and host autoantigens (cytochrome P450 2D6) has been invoked to explain the association between hepatitis C and a subset of patients with autoimmune hepatitis and antibodies to liver-kidney microsomal (LKM) antigen (anti-LKM) (Chap. 93).

EXTRAHEPATIC MANIFESTATIONS

Immune complex–mediated tissue damage appears to play a pathogenetic role in the extrahepatic manifestations of acute hepatitis B. The occasional prodromal serum sickness–like syndrome observed in acute hepatitis B appears to be related to the deposition in tissue blood vessel walls of HBsAg-anti-HBs circulating immune complexes, leading to activation of the complement system and depressed serum complement levels.

In patients with chronic hepatitis B, other types of immune-complex disease may be seen. Glomerulonephritis with the nephritic syndrome is occasionally observed; HBsAg, immunoglobulin, and C3 deposition has been found in the glomerular basement membrane. While polyarteritis nodosa develops in considerably fewer than 1% of patients with chronic HBV infection, 20–30% of patients with polyarteritis nodosa have HBsAg in serum. In these patients, the affected small and medium-size arterioles have been shown to contain HBsAg, immunoglobulins, and complement components. Another extrahepatic manifestation of viral hepatitis, essential mixed cryoglobulinemia (EMC), was reported initially to be associated with hepatitis B. The disorder is characterized clinically by arthritis, cutaneous vasculitis (palpable purpura), and occasionally with glomerulonephritis and serologically by the presence of circulating cryoprecipitable immune complexes of more than one immunoglobulin class. Many patients with this syndrome have chronic liver disease, but the association with HBV infection is limited; instead, a substantial proportion has chronic HCV infection, with circulating immune complexes containing HCV RNA. Immune-complex glomerulonephritis is another recognized extrahepatic manifestation of chronic hepatitis C.

PATHOLOGY

The typical morphologic lesions of all types of viral hepatitis are similar and consist of panlobular infiltration with mononuclear cells, hepatic cell necrosis, hyperplasia of Kupffer cells, and variable degrees of cholestasis. Hepatic cell regeneration is present, as evidenced by numerous mitotic figures, multinucleated cells, and "rosette" or "pseudoacinar" formation. The mononuclear infiltration consists primarily of small lymphocytes, although plasma cells and eosinophils occasionally are present. Liver cell damage consists of hepatic cell degeneration and necrosis, cell dropout, ballooning of cells, and acidophilic degeneration of hepatocytes (forming so-called Councilman or apoptotic bodies). Large hepatocytes with a ground-glass appearance of the cytoplasm may be seen in chronic but not in acute HBV infection; these cells contain HBsAg and can be identified histochemically with orcein or aldehyde fuchsin. In uncomplicated viral hepatitis, the reticulin framework is preserved.

In hepatitis C, the histologic lesion is often remarkable for a relative paucity of inflammation, a marked increase in activation of sinusoidal lining cells, lymphoid aggregates, the presence of fat (more frequent in genotype 3 and linked to increased fibrosis), and, occasionally, bile duct lesions in which biliary epithelial cells appear to be piled up without interruption of the basement membrane. Occasionally, microvesicular steatosis occurs in hepatitis D. In hepatitis E, a common histologic feature is marked cholestasis. A cholestatic variant of slowly resolving acute hepatitis A also has been described.

A more severe histologic lesion, *bridging hepatic necrosis*, also termed *subacute* or *confluent necrosis* or *interface hepatitis*, is occasionally observed in some patients with acute hepatitis. "Bridging" between lobules results from large areas of hepatic cell dropout, with collapse of the reticulin framework. Characteristically, the bridge consists of condensed reticulum, inflammatory debris, and degenerating liver cells that span adjacent portal areas, portal to central veins, or central vein to central vein. This lesion had been thought to have prognostic significance; in many of the originally described patients with this lesion, a subacute course terminated in death within several weeks to months, or severe chronic hepatitis and postnecrotic cirrhosis developed. Subsequent investigations have failed to uphold the association between bridging necrosis and such a poor prognosis in patients with acute hepatitis. Therefore, although demonstration of this lesion in patients with chronic hepatitis has prognostic significance (Chap. 93), its demonstration during acute hepatitis is less meaningful, and liver biopsies to identify this lesion are no longer undertaken routinely in patients with acute hepatitis. In *massive hepatic necrosis* (fulminant hepatitis, "acute yellow atrophy"), the striking feature at postmortem examination is the finding of a small, shrunken, soft liver. Histologic examination reveals massive necrosis and dropout of liver cells of most lobules with extensive collapse and condensation of the reticulin framework. When histologic documentation is required in the management of fulminant or very severe hepatitis, a biopsy can be done by the angiographically guided transjugular route, which permits the performance of this invasive procedure in the presence of severe coagulopathy.

Immunohistochemical and electron-microscopic studies have localized HBsAg to the cytoplasm and plasma membrane of infected liver cells. In contrast, HBcAg predominates in the nucleus, but occasionally, scant amounts are also seen in the cytoplasm and on the cell membrane. HDV antigen is localized to the hepatocyte nucleus, while HAV, HCV, and HEV antigens are localized to the cytoplasm.

EPIDEMIOLOGY AND GLOBAL FEATURES

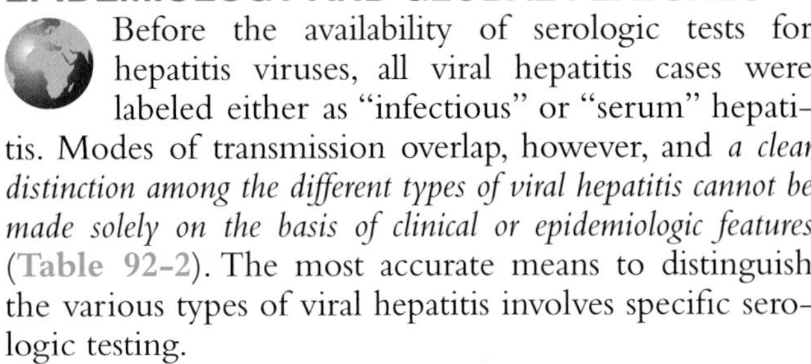

Before the availability of serologic tests for hepatitis viruses, all viral hepatitis cases were labeled either as "infectious" or "serum" hepatitis. Modes of transmission overlap, however, and *a clear distinction among the different types of viral hepatitis cannot be made solely on the basis of clinical or epidemiologic features* (Table 92-2). The most accurate means to distinguish the various types of viral hepatitis involves specific serologic testing.

Hepatitis A

This agent is transmitted almost exclusively by the fecal-oral route. Person-to-person spread of HAV is enhanced by poor personal hygiene and overcrowding; large outbreaks as well as sporadic cases have been traced to contaminated food, water, milk, frozen raspberries and strawberries, green onions imported from Mexico, and shellfish. Intrafamily and intrainstitutional spread are also common. Early epidemiologic observations supported a predilection for hepatitis A to occur in late fall and early winter. In temperate zones, epidemic waves have been recorded every 5–20 years as new segments of nonimmune population appeared; however, in developed countries, the incidence of hepatitis A has been declining, presumably as a function of improved sanitation, and these cyclic patterns are no longer observed. No HAV carrier state has been identified after acute hepatitis A; perpetuation of the virus in nature depends presumably on nonepidemic, inapparent subclinical infection and/or contamination linked to environmental reservoirs.

In the general population, anti-HAV, a marker for previous HAV infection, increases in prevalence as a function of increasing age and of decreasing socioeconomic status. In the 1970s, serologic evidence of prior hepatitis A infection occurred in ~40% of urban populations in the United States, most of whose members never recalled having had a symptomatic case of hepatitis. In subsequent decades, however, the prevalence of anti-HAV has been declining in the United States. In developing countries, exposure, infection, and subsequent immunity are almost universal in childhood. As the frequency of subclinical childhood infections declines in developed countries, a susceptible cohort of adults emerges. Hepatitis A tends to

TABLE 92-2

CLINICAL AND EPIDEMIOLOGIC FEATURES OF VIRAL HEPATITIS

FEATURE	HAV	HBV	HCV	HDV	HEV
Incubation (days)	15–45, mean 30	30–180, mean 60–90	15–160, mean 50	30–180, mean 60–90	14–60, mean 40
Onset	Acute	Insidious or acute	Insidious	Insidious or acute	Acute
Age preference	Children, young adults	Young adults (sexual and percutaneous), babies, toddlers	Any age, but more common in adults	Any age (similar to HBV)	Young adults (20–40 years)
Transmission					
Fecal-oral	+++	–	–	–	+++
Percutaneous	Unusual	+++	+++	+++	–
Perinatal	–	+++	±[a]	+	–
Sexual	±	++	±[a]	++	–
Clinical					
Severity	Mild	Occasionally severe	Moderate	Occasionally severe	Mild
Fulminant	0.1%	0.1–1%	0.1%	5–20%[b]	1–2%[e]
Progression to chronicity	None	Occasional (1–10%) (90% of neonates)	Common (85%)	Common[d]	None
Carrier	None	0.1–30%[c]	1.5–3.2%	Variable[f]	None
Cancer	None	+ (neonatal infection)	+	±	None
Prognosis	Excellent	Worse with age, debility	Moderate	Acute, good Chronic, poor	Good
Prophylaxis	IG Inactivated vaccine	HBIG Recombinant vaccine	None	HBV vaccine (none for HBV carriers)	Vaccine
Therapy	None	Interferon Lamivudine Adefovir Pegylated interferon Entecavir Telbivudine	Pegylated interferon plus ribavirin	Interferon ±	None

[a]Primarily with HIV co-infection and high-level viremia in index case; risk 5%.
[b]Up to 5% in acute HBV/HDV co-infection; up to 20% in HDV superinfection of chronic HBV infection.
[c]Varies considerably throughout the world and in subpopulations within countries; see text.
[d]In acute HBV/HDV co-infection, the frequency of chronicity is the same as that for HBV; in HDV superinfection, chronicity is invariable.
[e]10–20% in pregnant women.
[f]Common in Mediterranean countries, rare in North America and western Europe.

be more symptomatic in adults; therefore, paradoxically, as the frequency of HAV infection declines, the likelihood of clinically apparent, even severe, HAV illnesses increases in the susceptible adult population. Travel to endemic areas is a common source of infection for adults from nonendemic areas. More recently recognized epidemiologic foci of HAV infection include child-care centers, neonatal intensive care units, promiscuous men who have sex with men, and injection drug users. Although hepatitis A is rarely bloodborne, several outbreaks have been recognized in recipients of clotting factor concentrates. In the United States, the introduction of hepatitis A vaccination programs among children from high-incidence states has resulted in a >70% reduction in the annual incidence of new HAV infections and has shifted the burden of new infections from children to young adults.

Hepatitis B

Percutaneous inoculation has long been recognized as a major route of hepatitis B transmission, but the outmoded designation "serum hepatitis" is an inaccurate label for the epidemiologic spectrum of HBV infection recognized today. As detailed below, most of the hepatitis transmitted by blood transfusion is not caused by HBV; moreover, in approximately two-thirds of patients with acute type B hepatitis, no history of an identifiable percutaneous exposure can be elicited. We now recognize that many cases of hepatitis B result from less obvious modes of nonpercutaneous or covert percutaneous transmission. HBsAg has been identified in almost every body fluid from infected persons, and at least some of these body fluids—most notably semen and saliva—are infectious, albeit less so than serum, when administered percutaneously or nonpercutaneously to experimental animals. Among the nonpercutaneous modes of HBV transmission, oral ingestion has been documented as a potential but inefficient route of exposure. By contrast, the two nonpercutaneous routes considered to have the greatest impact are intimate (especially sexual) contact and perinatal transmission.

In Sub-Saharan Africa, intimate contact among toddlers is considered instrumental in contributing to the maintenance of the high frequency of hepatitis B in the population. Perinatal transmission occurs primarily in infants born to HBsAg carrier mothers or mothers with acute hepatitis B during the third trimester of pregnancy or during the early postpartum period. Perinatal transmission is uncommon in North America and western Europe but occurs with great frequency and is the most important mode of HBV perpetuation in the Far East and developing countries. Although the precise mode of perinatal transmission is unknown, and although ~10% of infections may be acquired in utero, epidemiologic evidence suggests that most infections occur approximately at the time of delivery and are not related to breast feeding. The likelihood of perinatal transmission of HBV correlates with the presence of HBeAg; 90% of HBeAg-positive mothers but only 10–15% of anti-HBe-positive mothers transmit HBV infection to their offspring. In most cases, acute infection in the neonate is clinically asymptomatic, but the child is very likely to become an HBsAg carrier.

The >350 million HBsAg carriers in the world constitute the main reservoir of hepatitis B in human beings. Serum HBsAg is infrequent (0.1–0.5%) in normal populations in the United States and western Europe. However, a prevalence of up to 5–20% has been found in the Far East and in some tropical countries; in persons with Down's syndrome, lepromatous leprosy, leukemia, Hodgkin's disease, polyarteritis nodosa; in patients with chronic renal disease on hemodialysis; and in injection drug users.

Other groups with high rates of HBV infection include spouses of acutely infected persons, sexually promiscuous persons (especially promiscuous men who have sex with men), health care workers exposed to blood, persons who require repeated transfusions especially with pooled blood product concentrates (e.g., hemophiliacs), residents and staff of custodial institutions for the developmentally handicapped, prisoners, and, to a lesser extent, family members of chronically infected patients. In volunteer blood donors, the prevalence of anti-HBs, a reflection of previous HBV infection, ranges from 5–10%, but the prevalence is higher in lower socioeconomic strata, older age groups, and persons—including those mentioned above—exposed to blood products. Because of highly sensitive virologic screening of donor blood, the risk of acquiring HBV infection from a blood transfusion is 1 in 230,000.

Prevalence of infection, modes of transmission, and human behavior conspire to mold geographically different epidemiologic patterns of HBV infection. In the Far East and Africa, hepatitis B, a disease of the newborn and young children, is perpetuated by a cycle of maternal-neonatal spread. In North America and western Europe, hepatitis B is primarily a disease of adolescence and early adulthood, the time of life when intimate sexual contact as well as recreational and occupational percutaneous exposures tend to occur. The introduction of hepatitis B vaccine in the early 1980s and adoption of universal childhood vaccination policies in many countries resulted in a dramatic, ~90%, decline in the incidence of new HBV infections in those countries as well as in the dire consequences of chronic infection.

Hepatitis D

Infection with HDV has a worldwide distribution, but two epidemiologic patterns exist. In Mediterranean countries (northern Africa, southern Europe, the Middle East), HDV infection is endemic among those with hepatitis B, and the disease is transmitted predominantly by nonpercutaneous means, especially close personal contact. In nonendemic areas, such as the United States and northern Europe, HDV infection is confined to persons exposed frequently to blood and blood products, primarily injection drug users and hemophiliacs. HDV infection can be introduced into a population through drug users or by migration of persons from endemic to nonendemic areas. Thus, patterns of population migration and human behavior facilitating percutaneous contact play important roles in the introduction and amplification of HDV infection. Occasionally, the migrating epidemiology of hepatitis D is expressed in explosive outbreaks of severe hepatitis, such as those that have occurred in remote South American villages as well as in urban centers in the United States. Ultimately, such outbreaks of hepatitis D—either of co-infections with acute hepatitis B or of superinfections in those already infected with HBV—may blur the distinctions between endemic and nonendemic areas. On a global scale, HDV infection is declining. Even in Italy, an HDV-endemic area, public health measures introduced to control HBV infection resulted during the 1990s in a 1.5%/year reduction in the prevalence of HDV infection.

Hepatitis C

Routine screening of blood donors for HBsAg and the elimination of commercial blood sources in the early 1970s reduced the frequency of, but did not eliminate, transfusion-associated hepatitis. During the 1970s, the likelihood of acquiring hepatitis after transfusion of voluntarily donated, HBsAg-screened blood was ~10% per patient (up to 0.9% per unit transfused); 90–95% of these cases were classified, based on serologic exclusion of hepatitis A and B, as "non-A, non-B" hepatitis. For patients requiring transfusion of pooled products, such as clotting factor concentrates, the risk was even higher, up to 20–30%.

During the 1980s, voluntary self-exclusion of blood donors with risk factors for AIDS and then the introduction of donor screening for anti-HIV reduced further the likelihood of transfusion-associated hepatitis to <5%. During the late 1980s and early 1990s, the introduction first of "surrogate" screening tests for non-A, non-B hepatitis [alanine aminotransferase (ALT) and anti-HBc, both shown to identify blood donors with a higher likelihood of transmitting non-A, non-B hepatitis to recipients] and, subsequently, after the discovery of HCV, first-generation immunoassays for anti-HCV reduced the frequency of transfusion-associated hepatitis even further. A prospective analysis of transfusion-associated hepatitis conducted between 1986 and 1990 showed that the incidence of transfusion-associated hepatitis at one urban university hospital fell from a baseline of 3.8% per patient (0.45% per unit transfused) to 1.5% per patient (0.19% per unit) after the introduction of surrogate testing and to 0.6% per patient (0.03% per unit) after the introduction of first-generation anti-HCV assays. The introduction of second-generation anti-HCV assays reduced the frequency of transfusion-associated hepatitis C to almost imperceptible levels, 1 in 100,000, and these gains were reinforced by the application of automated PCR testing of donated blood for HCV RNA, which has resulted in a reduction in the risk of transfusion-associated HCV infection to 1 in 2.3 million transfusions.

In addition to being transmitted by transfusion, hepatitis C can be transmitted by other percutaneous routes, such as injection drug use. In addition, this virus can be transmitted by occupational exposure to blood, and the likelihood of infection is increased in hemodialysis units. Although the frequency of transfusion-associated hepatitis C fell as a result of blood donor screening, the overall frequency of hepatitis C remained the same until the early 1990s, when the overall frequency fell by 80%, in parallel with a reduction in the number of new cases in injection drug users. After the exclusion of anti-HCV-positive plasma units from the donor pool, rare, sporadic instances have occurred of hepatitis C among recipients of immunoglobulin (IG) preparations for intravenous (but not intramuscular) use.

Serologic evidence for HCV infection occurs in 90% of patients with a history of transfusion-associated hepatitis (almost all occurring before 1992, when second-generation HCV-screening tests were introduced); hemophiliacs and others treated with clotting factors; injection drug users; 60–70% of patients with sporadic "non-A, non-B" hepatitis who lack identifiable risk factors; 0.5% of volunteer blood donors; and, in the most recent survey conducted in the United States between 1999 and 2000, 1.6% of the general population in the United States, which translates into 4.1 million persons (3.2 million with viremia). Comparable frequencies of HCV infection occur in most countries around the world, with 170 million persons infected worldwide, but extraordinarily high prevalences of HCV infection occur in certain countries, such as Egypt, where >20% of the population in some cities is infected. The high frequency in Egypt is attributable to contaminated equipment used for medical procedures and unsafe injection practices. In the United States, African Americans and Mexican Americans have higher frequencies of HCV infection than whites. Between 1988 and 1994, 30- to 40-year-old adult males had the highest prevalence of HCV infection; however, in a survey conducted between 1999 and 2000, the peak age decile had shifted to those age 40–49 years. Thus, despite an 80% reduction in new HCV infections during the 1990s, the prevalence of HCV infection in the population was sustained by an aging cohort that had acquired their infections two to three decades earlier, during the 1960s and 1970s, as a result predominantly of self inoculation with recreational drugs. Hepatitis C accounts for 40% of chronic liver disease, is the most frequent indication for liver transplantation, and is estimated to account for 8000–10,000 deaths per year in the United States.

The distribution of HCV genotypes varies in different parts of the world. Worldwide, genotype 1 is the most common. In the United States, genotype 1 accounts for 70% of HCV infections, while genotypes 2 and 3 account for the remaining 30%; among African Americans, the frequency of genotype 1 is even higher, i.e., 90%. Genotype 4 predominates in Egypt; genotype 5 is localized to South Africa and genotype 6 to Hong Kong.

Most asymptomatic blood donors found to have anti-HCV and ~20–30% of persons with reported cases of acute hepatitis C do not fall into a recognized risk group; however, many such blood donors do recall risk-associated behaviors when questioned carefully.

As a bloodborne infection, HCV potentially can be transmitted sexually and perinatally; however, both of these modes of transmission are inefficient for hepatitis C. Although 10–15% of patients with acute hepatitis C report having potential sexual sources of infection, most studies have failed to identify sexual transmission of this agent. The chances of sexual and perinatal transmission have been estimated to be ~5%, well below comparable rates for HIV and HBV infections. Moreover, sexual transmission appears to be confined to such subgroups as persons with multiple sexual partners and sexually transmitted diseases; transmission of HCV infection is rare between stable, monogamous sexual partners. Breast feeding does not increase the risk of HCV infection between an infected mother and her infant. Infection of health workers is not dramatically higher than among the general population; however, health workers are more likely to acquire HCV infection through accidental needle punctures, the efficiency of which is ~3%. Infection of household contacts is rare as well.

Other groups with an increased frequency of HCV infection include patients who require hemodialysis and organ transplantation and those who require transfusions in the setting of cancer chemotherapy. In immunosuppressed individuals, levels of anti-HCV may be undetectable, and a diagnosis may require testing for HCV RNA. Although new acute cases of hepatitis C are rare, newly diagnosed cases are common among otherwise healthy persons who experimented briefly with injection drugs, as noted above, two or three decades earlier. Such instances usually remain unrecognized for years, until unearthed by laboratory screening for routine medical examinations, insurance applications, and attempted blood donation.

Hepatitis E

This type of hepatitis, identified in India, Asia, Africa, the Middle East, and Central America, resembles hepatitis A in its primarily enteric mode of spread. The commonly recognized cases occur after contamination of water supplies such as after monsoon flooding, but sporadic, isolated cases occur. An epidemiologic feature that distinguishes HEV from other enteric agents is the rarity of secondary person-to-person spread from infected persons to their close contacts. Infections arise in populations that are immune to HAV and favor young adults. In endemic areas, the prevalence of antibodies to HEV is ≤40%. In nonendemic areas of the world, such as the United States, clinically apparent acute hepatitis E is extremely rare; however, the prevalence of antibodies to HEV can be as high as 20% in such areas. In nonendemic areas, HEV does not account for any of the sporadic "non-A, non-B" cases of hepatitis; however, cases imported from endemic areas have been found in the United States. Several reports suggest a zoonotic reservoir for HEV in swine.

CLINICAL AND LABORATORY FEATURES

Symptoms and Signs

Acute viral hepatitis occurs after an incubation period that varies according to the responsible agent. Generally, incubation periods for hepatitis A range from 15–45 days (mean, 4 weeks), for hepatitis B and D from 30–180 days (mean, 8–12 weeks), for hepatitis C from 15–160 days (mean, 7 weeks), and for hepatitis E from 14–60 days (mean, 5–6 weeks). The *prodromal symptoms* of acute viral hepatitis are systemic and quite variable. Constitutional symptoms of anorexia, nausea and vomiting, fatigue, malaise, arthralgias, myalgias, headache, photophobia, pharyngitis, cough, and coryza may precede the onset of jaundice by 1–2 weeks. The nausea, vomiting, and anorexia are frequently associated with alterations in olfaction and taste. A low-grade fever between 38° and 39°C (100°–102°F) is more often present in hepatitis A and E than in hepatitis B or C, except when hepatitis B is heralded by a serum sickness–like syndrome; rarely, a fever of 39.5°–40°C (103°–104°F) may accompany the constitutional symptoms. Dark urine and clay-colored stools may be noticed by the patient from 1–5 days before the onset of clinical jaundice.

With the onset of *clinical jaundice*, the constitutional prodromal symptoms usually diminish, but in some patients mild weight loss (2.5–5 kg) is common and may continue during the entire icteric phase. The liver becomes enlarged and tender and may be associated with right upper quadrant pain and discomfort. Infrequently, patients present with a cholestatic picture, suggesting extrahepatic biliary obstruction. Splenomegaly and cervical adenopathy are present in 10–20% of patients with acute hepatitis. Rarely, a few spider angiomas appear during the icteric phase and disappear during convalescence. During the *recovery phase*, constitutional symptoms disappear, but usually some liver enlargement and abnormalities in liver biochemical tests are still evident. The duration of the posticteric phase is variable, ranging 2–12 weeks, and is usually more prolonged in acute hepatitis B and C. Complete clinical and biochemical recovery is to be expected 1–2 months after all cases of hepatitis A and E and 3–4 months after the onset of jaundice in three-quarters of uncomplicated, self-limited cases of hepatitis B and C (among healthy adults, acute hepatitis B is self-limited in 95–99% while hepatitis C is self-limited in only ~15%). In the remainder, biochemical recovery may be delayed. A substantial proportion of patients with viral hepatitis never become icteric.

Infection with HDV can occur in the presence of acute or chronic HBV infection; the duration of HBV infection determines the duration of HDV infection. When acute HDV and HBV infection occur simultaneously, clinical and biochemical features may be indistinguishable from those of HBV infection alone, although occasionally they are more severe. As opposed to patients with *acute* HBV infection, patients with *chronic* HBV infection can support HDV replication indefinitely. This can happen when acute HDV infection occurs in the presence of a nonresolving acute HBV infection. More commonly, acute HDV infection becomes chronic when it is superimposed on an underlying chronic HBV infection. In such cases, the HDV superinfection appears as a clinical exacerbation or an episode resembling acute viral hepatitis in someone already chronically infected with HBV. Superinfection with HDV in a patient with chronic hepatitis B often leads to clinical deterioration (see below).

In addition to superinfections with other hepatitis agents, acute hepatitis–like clinical events in persons with chronic hepatitis B may accompany spontaneous HBeAg-to–anti-HBe seroconversion or spontaneous reactivation, i.e., reversion from nonreplicative to replicative infection. Such reactivations can occur as well in therapeutically immunosuppressed patients with chronic HBV infection when cytotoxic/immunosuppressive drugs are withdrawn; in these cases, restoration of immune competence is thought to allow resumption of previously checked cell-mediated immune cytolysis of HBV-infected hepatocytes. Occasionally, acute clinical exacerbations of chronic hepatitis B may represent the emergence of a precore mutant (see "Virology and Etiology" near the start of the chapter), and the subsequent course in such patients may be characterized by periodic exacerbations.

Laboratory Features

The serum aminotransferases aspartate aminotransferase (AST) and ALT (previously designated SGOT and SGPT) show a variable increase during the prodromal phase of acute viral hepatitis and precede the rise in bilirubin level (Figs. 92-2 and 92-4). The acute level of these enzymes, however, does not correlate well with the degree of liver cell damage. Peak levels vary from 400–4000 IU or more; these levels are usually reached at the time the patient is clinically icteric and diminish progressively during the recovery phase of acute hepatitis. The diagnosis of anicteric hepatitis is based on clinical features and on aminotransferase elevations.

Jaundice is usually visible in the sclera or skin when the serum bilirubin value is >43 μmol/L (2.5 mg/dL). When jaundice appears, the serum bilirubin typically rises to levels ranging from 85–340 μmol/L (5–20 mg/dL). The serum bilirubin may continue to rise despite falling serum aminotransferase levels. In most instances, the total bilirubin is equally divided between the conjugated and unconjugated fractions. Bilirubin levels >340 μmol/L (20 mg/dL) extending and persisting late into the course of viral hepatitis are more likely to be associated with severe disease. In certain patients with underlying hemolytic anemia, however, such as glucose-6-phosphate dehydrogenase deficiency and sickle cell anemia, a high serum bilirubin level is common, resulting from superimposed hemolysis. In such patients, bilirubin levels >513 μmol/L (30 mg/dL) have been observed and are not necessarily associated with a poor prognosis.

Neutropenia and lymphopenia are transient and are followed by a relative lymphocytosis. Atypical lymphocytes (varying between 2 and 20%) are common during the acute phase. Measurement of the prothrombin time (PT) is important in patients with acute viral hepatitis, for a prolonged value may reflect a severe hepatic synthetic defect, signify extensive hepatocellular necrosis, and indicate a worse prognosis. Occasionally, a prolonged PT may occur with only mild increases in the serum bilirubin and aminotransferase levels. Prolonged nausea and vomiting, inadequate carbohydrate intake, and poor hepatic glycogen reserves may contribute to hypoglycemia noted occasionally in patients with severe viral hepatitis. Serum alkaline phosphatase may be normal or only mildly elevated, while a fall in serum albumin is uncommon in uncomplicated acute viral hepatitis. In some patients, mild and transient steatorrhea has been noted as well as slight microscopic hematuria and minimal proteinuria.

A diffuse but mild elevation of the γ globulin fraction is common during acute viral hepatitis. Serum IgG and IgM levels are elevated in about one-third of patients during the acute phase of viral hepatitis, but the serum IgM level is elevated more characteristically during acute hepatitis A. During the acute phase of viral hepatitis, antibodies to smooth muscle and other cell constituents may be present, and low titers of rheumatoid factor, nuclear antibody, and heterophil antibody can also be found occasionally. In hepatitis C and D, antibodies to LKM may occur; however, the species of LKM antibodies in the two types of hepatitis are different from each other as well as from the LKM antibody species characteristic of autoimmune hepatitis type 2 (Chap. 93). The autoantibodies in viral hepatitis are nonspecific and can also be associated with other viral and systemic diseases. In contrast, virus-specific antibodies, which appear during and after hepatitis virus infection, are serologic markers of diagnostic importance.

As described above, serologic tests are available with which to establish a diagnosis of hepatitis A, B, D, and C. Tests for fecal or serum HAV are not routinely available. Therefore, a diagnosis of hepatitis A is based on detection of IgM anti-HAV during acute illness (Fig. 92-2). Rheumatoid factor can give rise to false-positive results in this test.

A diagnosis of HBV infection can usually be made by detection of HBsAg in serum. Infrequently, levels of HBsAg are too low to be detected during acute HBV infection, even with contemporary, highly sensitive immunoassays. In such cases, the diagnosis can be established by the presence of IgM anti-HBc.

The titer of HBsAg bears little relation to the severity of clinical disease. Indeed, an inverse correlation exists between the serum concentration of HBsAg and the degree of liver cell damage. For example, titers are highest in immunosuppressed patients, lower in patients with chronic liver disease (but higher in mild chronic than in severe chronic hepatitis), and very low in patients with acute fulminant hepatitis. These observations suggest that, in hepatitis B, the degree of liver cell damage and the clinical course are related to variations in the patient's immune response to HBV rather than to the amount of circulating HBsAg. In immunocompetent persons, however, there is a correlation between markers of HBV *replication* and liver injury (see below).

Another serologic marker that may be of value in patients with hepatitis B is HBeAg. Its principal clinical usefulness is as an indicator of relative infectivity. Because HBeAg is invariably present during early acute hepatitis B, HBeAg testing is indicated primarily during follow-up of chronic infection.

In patients with hepatitis B surface antigenemia of unknown duration, e.g., blood donors found to be HBsAg-positive and referred to a physician for evaluation, testing for IgM anti-HBc may be useful to distinguish between acute or recent infection (IgM anti-HBc-positive) and chronic HBV infection (IgM anti-HBc-negative, IgG anti-HBc-positive). A false-positive test for IgM anti-HBc may be encountered in patients with high-titer rheumatoid factor.

Anti-HBs is rarely detectable in the presence of HBsAg in patients with *acute* hepatitis B, but 10–20% of persons with *chronic* HBV infection may harbor low-level anti-HBs. This antibody is directed not against the common group determinant, *a*, but against the heterotypic subtype determinant (e.g., HBsAg of subtype *ad* with anti-HBs of subtype *y*). In most cases, this serologic pattern cannot be attributed to infection with two different HBV subtypes, and the presence of this antibody is not a harbinger of imminent HBsAg clearance. When such antibody is detected, its presence is of no recognized clinical significance (see "Virology and Etiology" earlier in the chapter).

After immunization with hepatitis B vaccine, which consists of HBsAg alone, anti-HBs is the only serologic marker to appear. The commonly encountered serologic patterns of hepatitis B and their interpretations are summarized in Table 92-3. Tests for the detection of HBV DNA in liver and serum are now available. Like HBeAg, serum HBV DNA is an indicator of HBV replication, but tests for HBV DNA are more sensitive and quantitative. First-generation hybridization assays for HBV DNA had a sensitivity of 10^5–10^6 virions/mL, a relative threshold below which infectivity and liver injury are limited and HBeAg is usually undetectable. Currently, testing for HBV DNA has shifted from insensitive hybridization assays to amplification assays, e.g., the PCR-based assay, which can detect as few as 10 or 100 virions/mL; among the commercially available PCR assays, the most useful are those with the highest sensitivity (5–10 IU/mL) and the largest dynamic range (10^0–10^9 IU/mL). With increased sensitivity, amplification assays remain reactive well below the threshold for infectivity and liver injury. These markers are useful in following the course of HBV replication in patients with chronic hepatitis B receiving antiviral chemotherapy, e.g., with interferon or nucleoside analogues (Chap. 93). In immunocompetent persons, a general correlation does appear to exist between the level of HBV replication, as reflected by the level of HBV DNA in serum, and the degree of liver injury. High serum HBV DNA levels, increased expression of viral antigens, and necroinflammatory activity in the liver go hand in hand unless immunosuppression interferes with cytolytic T cell responses to virus-infected cells; reduction of HBV replication with antiviral drugs tends to be

TABLE 92-3

COMMONLY ENCOUNTERED SEROLOGIC PATTERNS OF HEPATITIS B INFECTION

HBsAg	ANTI-HBs	ANTI-HBc	HBeAg	ANTI-HBe	INTERPRETATION
+	–	IgM	+	–	Acute hepatitis B, high infectivity
+	–	IgG	+	–	Chronic hepatitis B, high infectivity
+	–	IgG	–	+	1. Late acute or chronic hepatitis B, low infectivity 2. HBeAg-negative ("precore-mutant") hepatitis B (chronic or, rarely, acute)
+	+	+	+/–	+/–	1. HBsAg of one subtype and heterotypic anti-HBs (common) 2. Process of seroconversion from HBsAg to anti-HBs (rare)
–	–	IgM	+/–	+/–	1. Acute hepatitis B 2. Anti-HBc "window"
–	–	IgG	–	+/–	1. Low-level hepatitis B carrier 2. Hepatitis B in remote past
–	+	IgG	–	+/–	Recovery from hepatitis B
–	+	–	–	–	1. Immunization with HBsAg (after vaccination) 2. Hepatitis B in the remote past (?) 3. False-positive

accompanied by an improvement in liver histology. Among patients with chronic hepatitis B, high levels of HBV DNA increase the risk of cirrhosis, hepatic decompensation, and hepatocellular carcinoma (see "Complications and Sequelae" later in the chapter).

In patients with hepatitis C, an episodic pattern of aminotransferase elevation is common. A specific serologic diagnosis of hepatitis C can be made by demonstrating the presence in serum of anti-HCV. When contemporary immunoassays are used, anti-HCV can be detected in acute hepatitis C during the initial phase of elevated aminotransferase activity. This antibody may never become detectable in 5–10% of patients with acute hepatitis C, and levels of anti-HCV may become undetectable after recovery (albeit rare) from acute hepatitis C. In patients with chronic hepatitis C, anti-HCV is detectable in >95% of cases. Nonspecificity can confound immunoassays for anti-HCV, especially in persons with a low prior probability of infection, such as volunteer blood donors, or in persons with circulating rheumatoid factor, which can bind nonspecifically to assay reagents; testing for HCV RNA can be used in such settings to distinguish between true-positive and false-positive anti-HCV determinations. Assays for HCV RNA are the most sensitive tests for HCV infection and represent the "gold standard" in establishing a diagnosis of hepatitis C. HCV RNA can be detected even before acute elevation of aminotransferase activity and before the appearance of anti-HCV in patients with acute hepatitis C. In addition, HCV RNA remains detectable indefinitely, continuously in most but intermittently in some, in patients with chronic hepatitis C (detectable as well in some persons with normal liver tests, i.e., inactive carriers). In the small minority of patients with hepatitis C who lack anti-HCV, a diagnosis can be supported by detection of HCV RNA. If all these tests are negative and the patient has a well-characterized case of hepatitis after percutaneous exposure to blood or blood products, a diagnosis of hepatitis caused by another agent, as yet unidentified, can be entertained.

Amplification techniques are required to detect HCV RNA, and two types are available. One is a branched-chain complementary DNA (bDNA) assay, in which the detection signal (a colorimetrically detectable enzyme bound to a complementary DNA probe) is amplified. The other involves target amplification, i.e., synthesis of multiple copies of the viral genome. This can be done by PCR or TMA, in which the viral RNA is reverse transcribed to complementary DNA and then amplified by repeated cycles of DNA synthesis. Both can be used as quantitative assays and a measurement of relative "viral load"; PCR and TMA, with a sensitivity of $10–10^2$ IU/mL, are more sensitive than bDNA, with a sensitivity of 10^3 IU/mL; assays are available with a wide dynamic range ($10–10^7$ IU/mL). Determination of HCV RNA level is not a reliable marker of disease severity or prognosis but is helpful in predicting relative responsiveness to antiviral therapy. The same is true for determinations of HCV genotype (Chap. 93).

A proportion of patients with hepatitis C have isolated anti-HBc in their blood, a reflection of a common risk in certain populations of exposure to multiple bloodborne hepatitis agents. The anti-HBc in such cases is almost invariably of the IgG class and usually represents HBV infection in the remote past (HBV DNA undetectable), rarely current HBV infection with low-level virus carriage.

The presence of HDV infection can be identified by demonstrating intrahepatic HDV antigen or, more practically, an anti-HDV seroconversion (a rise in titer of anti-HDV or de novo appearance of anti-HDV). Circulating HDV antigen, also diagnostic of acute infection, is detectable only briefly, if at all. Because anti-HDV is often undetectable once HBsAg disappears, retrospective serodiagnosis of acute self-limited, simultaneous HBV and HDV infection is difficult. Early diagnosis of acute infection may be hampered by a delay of up to 30–40 days in the appearance of anti-HDV.

When a patient presents with acute hepatitis and has HBsAg and anti-HDV in serum, determination of the class of anti-HBc is helpful in establishing the relationship between infection with HBV and HDV. Although IgM anti-HBc does not distinguish *absolutely* between acute and chronic HBV infection, its presence is a reliable indicator of recent infection and its absence a reliable indicator of infection in the remote past. In simultaneous acute HBV and HDV infections, IgM anti-HBc will be detectable, while in acute HDV infection superimposed on chronic HBV infection, anti-HBc will be of the IgG class.

Tests for the presence of HDV RNA are useful for determining the presence of ongoing HDV replication and relative infectivity. Diagnostic tests for hepatitis E are commercially available in several countries outside the United States; in the United States, diagnostic assays can be performed at the Centers for Disease Control and Prevention.

Liver biopsy is rarely necessary or indicated in acute viral hepatitis, except when the diagnosis is questionable or when clinical evidence suggests a diagnosis of chronic hepatitis.

A diagnostic algorithm can be applied in the evaluation of cases of acute viral hepatitis. A patient with acute hepatitis should undergo four serologic tests: HBsAg, IgM anti-HAV, IgM anti-HBc, and anti-HCV (Table 92-4). The presence of HBsAg, with or without IgM anti-HBc, represents HBV infection. If IgM anti-HBc is present, the HBV infection is considered acute; if IgM anti-HBc is absent, the HBV infection is considered chronic. A diagnosis of acute hepatitis B can be made in the absence of HBsAg when IgM anti-HBc is detectable. A diagnosis of acute hepatitis A is based on the presence of IgM anti-HAV. If IgM anti-HAV coexists with HBsAg, a diagnosis of simultaneous HAV and HBV infections can be made; if IgM anti-HBc (with or without HBsAg) is detectable, the patient has simultaneous acute hepatitis A and B, and if IgM anti-HBc is undetectable, the patient has acute hepatitis A superimposed on chronic HBV infection. The presence of anti-HCV supports a diagnosis of acute hepatitis C. Occasionally, testing for HCV RNA or repeat anti-HCV testing later during the illness is necessary to establish the diagnosis. Absence of all serologic markers is consistent with a diagnosis of "non-A, non-B, non-C" hepatitis, if the epidemiologic setting is appropriate.

In patients with chronic hepatitis, initial testing should consist of HBsAg and anti-HCV. Anti-HCV supports and HCV RNA testing establishes the diagnosis of chronic hepatitis C. If a serologic diagnosis of chronic hepatitis B is made, testing for HBeAg and anti-HBe is indicated to evaluate relative infectivity. Testing for HBV DNA in such patients provides a more quantitative and sensitive measure of the level of virus replication and, therefore, is very helpful during antiviral therapy (Chap. 93). In patients with chronic hepatitis B and normal aminotransferase activity in the absence of HBeAg, serial testing over time is often required to distinguish between inactive carriage and HBeAg-negative chronic hepatitis B with fluctuating virologic and necroinflammatory activity. In patients with hepatitis B, testing for anti-HDV is useful under the following circumstances: patients with severe and fulminant disease, patients with severe chronic disease, patients with chronic hepatitis B who have acute hepatitis-like exacerbations, persons with frequent percutaneous exposures, and persons from areas where HDV infection is endemic.

TABLE 92-4

SIMPLIFIED DIAGNOSTIC APPROACH IN PATIENTS PRESENTING WITH ACUTE HEPATITIS

SEROLOGIC TESTS OF PATIENT'S SERUM				
HBsAg	IgM ANTI-HAV	IgM ANTI-HBc	ANTI-HCV	DIAGNOSTIC INTERPRETATION
+	–	+	–	Acute hepatitis B
+	–	–	–	Chronic hepatitis B
+	+	–	–	Acute hepatitis A superimposed on chronic hepatitis B
+	+	+	–	Acute hepatitis A and B
–	+	–	–	Acute hepatitis A
–	+	+	–	Acute hepatitis A and B (HBsAg below detection threshold)
–	–	+	–	Acute hepatitis B (HBsAg below detection threshold)
–	–	–	+	Acute hepatitis C

PROGNOSIS

Virtually all previously healthy patients with hepatitis A recover completely from their illness with no clinical sequelae. Similarly, in acute hepatitis B, 95–99% of previously healthy adults have a favorable course and recover completely. Certain clinical and laboratory features, however, suggest a more complicated and protracted course. Patients of advanced age and with serious underlying medical disorders may have a prolonged course and are more likely to experience severe hepatitis. Initial presenting features such as ascites, peripheral edema, and symptoms of hepatic encephalopathy suggest a poorer prognosis. In addition, a prolonged PT, low serum albumin level, hypoglycemia, and very high serum bilirubin values suggest severe hepatocellular disease. Patients with these clinical and laboratory features deserve prompt hospital admission. The case-fatality rate in hepatitis A and B is very low (~0.1%) but is increased by advanced age and underlying debilitating disorders. Among patients ill enough to be hospitalized for acute hepatitis B, the fatality rate is 1%. Hepatitis C is less severe during the acute phase than hepatitis B and is more likely to be anicteric; fatalities are rare, but the precise case-fatality rate is not known. In outbreaks of waterborne hepatitis E in India and Asia, the case-fatality rate is 1–2% and up to 10–20% in pregnant women. Patients with simultaneous acute hepatitis B and hepatitis D do not necessarily experience a higher mortality rate than do patients with acute hepatitis B alone; however, in several recent outbreaks of acute simultaneous HBV and HDV infection among injection drug users, the case-fatality rate has been ~5%. In the case of HDV superinfection of a person with chronic hepatitis B, the likelihood of fulminant hepatitis and death is increased substantially. Although the case-fatality rate for hepatitis D has not been defined adequately, in outbreaks of severe HDV superinfection in isolated populations with a high hepatitis B carrier rate, the mortality rate has been recorded in excess of 20%.

Complications and Sequelae

A small proportion of patients with hepatitis A experience *relapsing hepatitis* weeks to months after apparent recovery from acute hepatitis. Relapses are characterized by recurrence of symptoms, aminotransferase elevations, occasionally jaundice, and fecal excretion of HAV. Another unusual variant of acute hepatitis A is *cholestatic hepatitis*, characterized by protracted cholestatic jaundice and pruritus. Rarely, liver test abnormalities persist for many months, even up to a year. Even when these complications occur, hepatitis A remains self-limited and does not progress to chronic liver disease. During the prodromal phase of acute hepatitis B, a serum sickness–like syndrome characterized by arthralgia or arthritis, rash, angioedema, and rarely hematuria and proteinuria may develop in 5–10% of patients. This syndrome occurs before the onset of clinical jaundice, and these patients are often diagnosed erroneously as having rheumatologic diseases. The diagnosis can be established by measuring serum aminotransferase levels, which are almost invariably elevated, and serum HBsAg. As noted above, EMC is an immune-complex disease that can complicate chronic hepatitis C and is part of a spectrum of B cell lymphoproliferative disorders, which, in rare instances, can evolve to B cell lymphoma. Attention has been drawn as well to associations between hepatitis C and such cutaneous disorders as porphyria cutanea tarda and lichen planus. A mechanism for these associations is unknown.

The most feared complication of viral hepatitis is *fulminant hepatitis* (massive hepatic necrosis); fortunately, this is a rare event. Fulminant hepatitis is primarily seen in hepatitis B and D, as well as hepatitis E, but rare fulminant cases of hepatitis A occur primarily in older adults and in persons with underlying chronic liver disease, including, according to some reports, chronic hepatitis B and C. Hepatitis B accounts for >50% of fulminant cases of viral hepatitis, a sizable proportion of which are associated with HDV infection and another proportion with underlying chronic hepatitis C. Fulminant hepatitis is hardly ever seen in hepatitis C, but hepatitis E, as noted above, can be complicated by fatal fulminant hepatitis in 1–2% of all cases and in up to 20% of cases occurring in pregnant women. Patients usually present with signs and symptoms of encephalopathy that may evolve to deep coma. The liver is usually small and the PT excessively prolonged. The combination of rapidly shrinking liver size, rapidly rising bilirubin level, and marked prolongation of the PT, even as aminotransferase levels fall, together with clinical signs of confusion, disorientation, somnolence, ascites, and edema, indicates that the patient has hepatic failure with encephalopathy. Cerebral edema is common; brainstem compression, gastrointestinal bleeding, sepsis, respiratory failure, cardiovascular collapse, and renal failure are terminal events. The mortality rate is exceedingly high (>80% in patients with deep coma), but patients who survive may have a complete biochemical and histologic recovery. If a donor liver can be located in time, liver transplantation may be life-saving in patients with fulminant hepatitis.

Documenting the disappearance of HBsAg after apparent clinical recovery from acute hepatitis B is particularly important. Before laboratory methods were available to distinguish between acute hepatitis and acute hepatitis–like exacerbations (*spontaneous reactivations*) of chronic hepatitis B, observations suggested that ~10% of previously healthy patients remained HBsAg-positive for >6 months after the onset of clinically apparent acute hepatitis B. Half of these persons cleared the antigen from their circulations during the next several years, but the other 5% remained chronically HBsAg-positive. More recent observations suggest that the true rate of chronic infection after clinically apparent acute hepatitis B is as low as 1% in normal, immunocompetent, young adults. Earlier, higher estimates may have been confounded by inadvertent inclusion of acute exacerbations in chronically infected patients; these patients, chronically HBsAg-positive before exacerbation, were unlikely to seroconvert to HBsAg-negative thereafter. Whether the rate of chronicity is 10 or 1%, such patients have anti-HBc in serum; anti-HBs is either undetected or detected at low titer against the opposite subtype specificity of the antigen (see "Laboratory Features" earlier in the chapter). These patients may (1) be inactive carriers; (2) have low-grade, mild chronic hepatitis; or (3) have moderate to severe chronic hepatitis with or without cirrhosis. The likelihood of remaining chronically infected after acute HBV infection is especially high among neonates, persons with Down's syndrome, chronically hemodialyzed patients, and immunosuppressed patients, including persons with HIV infection.

Chronic hepatitis is an important late complication of acute hepatitis B occurring in a small proportion of patients with acute disease but more common in those who present with chronic infection without having experienced an acute illness, as occurs typically after neonatal infection or after infection in an immunosuppressed host (Chap. 93). Certain clinical and laboratory features suggest progression of acute hepatitis to chronic hepatitis: (1) lack of complete resolution of clinical symptoms of anorexia, weight loss, and fatigue and the persistence of hepatomegaly; (2) the presence of bridging/interface or multilobular hepatic necrosis on liver biopsy during protracted, severe acute viral hepatitis; (3) failure of the serum aminotransferase, bilirubin, and globulin levels to return to normal within 6–12 months after the acute illness; and (4) the persistence of HBeAg for >3 months or HBsAg for >6 months after acute hepatitis.

Although acute hepatitis D infection does not increase the likelihood of chronicity of simultaneous acute hepatitis B, hepatitis D has the potential for contributing to the severity of chronic hepatitis B. Hepatitis D superinfection can transform inactive or mild chronic hepatitis B into severe, progressive chronic hepatitis and cirrhosis; it also can accelerate the course of chronic hepatitis B. Some HDV superinfections in patients with chronic hepatitis B lead to fulminant hepatitis. Although HDV and HBV infections are associated with severe liver disease, mild hepatitis and even inactive carriage have been identified in some patients, and the disease may become indolent beyond the early years of infection. After acute HCV infection, the likelihood of remaining chronically *infected* approaches 85–90%. Although many patients with chronic hepatitis C have no symptoms, cirrhosis may develop in as many as 20% within 10–20 years of acute illness; in some series of cases reported by referral centers, cirrhosis has been reported in as many as 50% of patients with chronic hepatitis C. Although chronic hepatitis C accounts for at least 40% of cases of chronic liver disease and of patients undergoing liver transplantation for end-stage liver disease in the United States and Europe, in the majority of patients with chronic hepatitis C, morbidity and mortality are limited during the initial 20 years after the onset of infection. Progression of chronic hepatitis C may be influenced by age of acquisition, duration of infection, immunosuppression, coexisting excessive alcohol use, concomitant hepatic steatosis, other hepatitis virus infection, or HIV co-infection. In fact, instances of severe and rapidly progressive chronic hepatitis B and C are being recognized with increasing frequency in patients with HIV infection (Chap. 90). In contrast, neither HAV nor HEV causes chronic liver disease.

Rare complications of viral hepatitis include pancreatitis, myocarditis, atypical pneumonia, aplastic anemia, transverse myelitis, and peripheral neuropathy. Persons with chronic hepatitis B, particularly those infected in infancy or early childhood and especially those with HBeAg and/or high-level HBV DNA, have an enhanced risk of hepatocellular carcinoma. The risk of hepatocellular carcinoma is increased as well in patients with chronic hepatitis C, almost exclusively in patients with cirrhosis, and almost always after at least several decades, usually after three decades of disease. In children, hepatitis B may present rarely with anicteric hepatitis, a nonpruritic papular rash of the face, buttocks, and limbs, and lymphadenopathy (papular acrodermatitis of childhood, or Gianotti-Crosti syndrome).

Rarely, autoimmune hepatitis (Chap. 93) can be triggered by a bout of otherwise self-limited acute hepatitis, as reported after acute hepatitis A, B, and C.

DIFFERENTIAL DIAGNOSIS

Viral diseases such as infectious mononucleosis; those due to cytomegalovirus, herpes simplex, and coxsackieviruses; and toxoplasmosis may share certain clinical features with viral hepatitis and cause elevations in serum aminotransferase and less commonly in serum bilirubin levels. Tests such as the differential heterophile and serologic tests for these agents may be helpful in the differential diagnosis if HBsAg, anti-HBc, IgM anti-HAV, and anti-HCV determinations are negative. Aminotransferase elevations can accompany almost any systemic viral infection; other rare causes of liver injury confused with viral hepatitis are infections with *Leptospira*, *Candida*, *Brucella*, *Mycobacterium*, and *Pneumocystis*. A complete drug history is particularly important, for many drugs and certain anesthetic agents can produce a picture of either acute hepatitis or cholestasis. Equally important is a past history of unexplained "repeated episodes" of acute hepatitis. This history should alert the physician to the possibility that the underlying disorder is chronic hepatitis. Alcoholic hepatitis must also be considered, but usually the serum aminotransferase levels are not as markedly elevated and other stigmata of alcoholism may be present. The finding on liver biopsy of fatty infiltration, a neutrophilic inflammatory reaction, and "alcoholic hyaline" would be consistent with alcohol-induced rather than viral liver injury. Because acute hepatitis may present with right upper quadrant abdominal pain, nausea and vomiting, fever, and icterus, it is often confused with acute cholecystitis, common duct stone, or ascending cholangitis. Patients with acute viral hepatitis may tolerate surgery poorly; therefore, it is important to exclude this diagnosis, and in confusing cases, a percutaneous liver biopsy may be necessary before laparotomy. Viral hepatitis in the elderly is often misdiagnosed as obstructive jaundice resulting from a common duct stone or carcinoma of the pancreas. Because acute hepatitis in the elderly may be quite severe and the operative mortality high, a thorough evaluation including biochemical tests, radiographic studies of the biliary tree, and even liver biopsy may be necessary to exclude primary parenchymal liver disease. Another clinical constellation that may mimic acute hepatitis is right ventricular failure with passive hepatic congestion or hypoperfusion syndromes, such as those associated with shock, severe hypotension, and severe left ventricular failure. Also included in this general category is any disorder that interferes with venous return to the heart, such as right atrial myxoma, constrictive pericarditis, hepatic vein occlusion (Budd-Chiari syndrome), or venoocclusive disease. Clinical features are usually sufficient to distinguish between these vascular disorders and viral hepatitis. Acute fatty liver of pregnancy, cholestasis of pregnancy, eclampsia, and the HELLP syndrome (*h*emolysis, *e*levated *l*iver tests, and *l*ow *p*latelets) can be confused with viral hepatitis during pregnancy. Very rarely, malignancies metastatic to the liver can mimic acute or even fulminant viral hepatitis. Occasionally, genetic or metabolic liver disorders (e.g., Wilson's disease, α_1-antitrypsin deficiency) as well as nonalcoholic fatty liver disease are confused with viral hepatitis.

℞ Treatment: ACUTE VIRAL HEPATITIS

In hepatitis B, among previously healthy adults who present with clinically apparent acute hepatitis, recovery occurs in ~99%; therefore, antiviral therapy is not likely to improve the rate of recovery and is not required. In rare instances of severe acute hepatitis B, treatment with a nucleoside analogue, such as lamivudine, at the 100-mg/d oral dose used to treat chronic hepatitis B (Chap. 93), has been attempted successfully. Although clinical trials have not been done to establish the efficacy of this approach, although severe acute hepatitis B is not an approved indication for therapy, and although the duration of therapy has not been determined, nonetheless, most authorities would recommend institution of antiviral therapy for severe, but not mild-moderate, acute hepatitis B. In typical cases of acute hepatitis C, recovery is rare, progression to chronic hepatitis is the rule, and meta-analyses of small clinical trials suggest that antiviral therapy with interferon α monotherapy (3 million units SC three times a week) is beneficial, reducing the rate of chronicity considerably by inducing sustained responses in 30–70% of patients. In a German multicenter study of 44 patients with acute symptomatic hepatitis C, initiation of intensive interferon α therapy (5 million units SC daily for 4 weeks, then three times a week for another 20 weeks) within an average of 3 months after infection resulted in a sustained virologic response rate of 98%. Although treatment of acute hepatitis C is recommended, the optimum regimen, duration of therapy, and time to initiate therapy remain to be determined. Many authorities now opt for a 24-week course (beginning within 2–3 months after onset) of the best regimen identified for the treatment of chronic hepatitis C, long-acting pegylated interferon plus the nucleoside analogue ribavirin, the efficacy of which is superior to that of standard interferon monotherapy regimens (see Chap. 93 for doses). Because of the marked reduction over the past two decades in the frequency of acute hepatitis C, opportunities to identify and treat patients with acute hepatitis C are rare indeed, except in injection drug users. Hospital epidemiologists, however, will encounter health workers who sustain hepatitis C–contaminated needle sticks; when monitoring for ALT elevations and HCV RNA after these accidents identifies acute hepatitis C (risk only ~3%), therapy should be initiated.

Notwithstanding these specific therapeutic considerations, in most cases of typical acute viral hepatitis, specific treatment generally is not necessary. Although hospitalization may be required for clinically severe illness, most patients do not require hospital care. Forced and prolonged bed rest is not essential for full recovery, but many patients will feel better with restricted physical activity. A high-calorie diet is desirable, and because many patients may experience nausea late in the day, the major caloric intake is best tolerated in the morning. Intravenous feeding is necessary in the acute stage if the patient has persistent vomiting and cannot maintain oral intake. Drugs capable of producing adverse reactions such as cholestasis and drugs metabolized by the liver should be avoided. If severe pruritus is present, the use of the bile salt–sequestering resin cholestyramine is helpful. Glucocorticoid therapy has no value in acute viral hepatitis, even in severe cases associated with *bridging necrosis*, and may be deleterious, even increasing the risk of chronicity (e.g., of acute hepatitis B).

Physical isolation of patients with hepatitis to a single room and bathroom is rarely necessary except in the case of fecal incontinence for hepatitis A and E or uncontrolled, voluminous bleeding for hepatitis B (with or without concomitant hepatitis D) and hepatitis C. Because most patients hospitalized with hepatitis A excrete little if any HAV, the likelihood of HAV transmission from these patients during their hospitalization is low. Therefore, burdensome *enteric precautions are no longer recommended*. Although gloves should be worn when the bedpans or fecal material of patients with hepatitis A are handled, these precautions do not represent a departure from sensible procedure and contemporary universal precautions for all hospitalized patients. For patients with hepatitis B and hepatitis C, emphasis should be placed on blood precautions, i.e., avoiding direct, ungloved hand contact with blood and other body fluids. Enteric precautions are unnecessary. The importance of simple hygienic precautions, such as hand washing, cannot be overemphasized. Universal precautions that have been adopted for all patients apply to patients with viral hepatitis.

Hospitalized patients may be discharged following substantial symptomatic improvement, a significant downward trend in the serum aminotransferase and bilirubin values, and a return to normal of the PT. Mild aminotransferase elevations should not be considered contraindications to the gradual resumption of normal activity.

In *fulminant hepatitis*, the goal of therapy is to support the patient by maintenance of fluid balance, support of circulation and respiration, control of bleeding, correction of hypoglycemia, and treatment of other complications of the comatose state in anticipation of liver regeneration and repair. Protein intake should be restricted, and oral lactulose or neomycin administered. Glucocorticoid therapy has been shown in controlled trials to be ineffective. Likewise, exchange transfusion, plasmapheresis, human cross-circulation, porcine liver cross-perfusion, hemoperfusion, and extracorporeal liver-assist devices have not been proved to enhance survival. Meticulous intensive care that includes prophylactic antibiotic coverage is the one factor that does appear to improve survival. Orthotopic liver transplantation is resorted to with increasing frequency, with excellent results, in patients with fulminant hepatitis.

PROPHYLAXIS

Because application of therapy for acute viral hepatitis is limited, and because antiviral therapy for chronic viral hepatitis is cumbersome and costly but effective in only a proportion of patients (Chap. 93), emphasis is placed on prevention through immunization. The prophylactic approach differs for each of the types of viral hepatitis. In the past, immunoprophylaxis relied exclusively on passive immunization with antibody-containing globulin preparations purified by cold ethanol fractionation from the plasma of hundreds of normal donors. Currently, for hepatitis A and B, active immunization with vaccines is the preferable approach to prevention.

Hepatitis A

Both passive immunization with IG and active immunization with killed vaccines are available. All preparations of IG contain anti-HAV concentrations sufficient to be protective. When administered before exposure or during the early incubation period, IG is effective in preventing clinically apparent hepatitis A. For postexposure prophylaxis of intimate contacts (household, sexual, institutional) of persons with hepatitis A, the administration of 0.02 mL/kg is recommended as early after exposure as possible; it may be effective even when administered as late as 2 weeks after exposure. Prophylaxis is not necessary for those who have already received hepatitis A vaccine, casual contacts (office, factory, school, or hospital), for most elderly persons, who are very likely to be immune, or for those known to have anti-HAV in their serum. In day-care centers, recognition of hepatitis A in children or staff should provide a stimulus for immunoprophylaxis in the center and in the children's family members. By the time most common-source outbreaks of hepatitis A are recognized, it is usually too late in the incubation period for IG to be effective; however, prophylaxis may limit the frequency of secondary cases. For travelers to tropical countries, developing countries, and other areas outside standard tourist routes, IG prophylaxis had been recommended, before a vaccine became available. When such travel lasted <3 months, 0.02 mL/kg was given; for longer travel or residence in these areas, a dose of 0.06 mL/kg every 4–6 months was recommended. Administration of plasma-derived globulin is safe; all contemporary lots of IG are subjected to viral inactivation steps and must be free of HCV RNA as determined by PCR testing. Administration of IM lots of IG has not been associated with transmission of HBV, HCV, or HIV.

Formalin-inactivated vaccines made from strains of HAV attenuated in tissue culture have been shown to be safe, immunogenic, and effective in preventing hepatitis A. Hepatitis A vaccines are approved for use in persons who are at least 1 year old and appear to provide adequate protection beginning 4 weeks after a primary inoculation. If it can be given within 4 weeks of an expected exposure, such as by travel to an endemic area, hepatitis A vaccine is the preferred approach to *preexposure* immunoprophylaxis. If travel is more imminent, IG (0.02 mL/kg) should be administered at a different injection site, along with the first dose of vaccine. Because vaccination provides long-lasting protection (protective levels of anti-HAV should last 20 years after vaccination), persons whose risk will be sustained (e.g., frequent travelers or those remaining in endemic areas for prolonged periods) should be vaccinated, and vaccine should supplant the need for repeated IG injections. Shortly after its introduction, hepatitis A vaccine was recommended for children living in communities with a high incidence of HAV infection; in 1999, this recommendation was extended to include all children living in states, counties, and communities with high rates of HAV infection. As of 2006, the Advisory Committee on Immunization Practices of the U.S. Public Health Service recommended *routine hepatitis A vaccination of all children*. Other groups considered to be at increased risk for HAV infection and who are candidates for hepatitis A vaccination include military personnel, populations with cyclic outbreaks of hepatitis A (e.g., Alaskan natives), employees of day-care centers, primate handlers, laboratory workers exposed to hepatitis A or fecal specimens, and patients with chronic liver disease. Because of an increased risk of fulminant hepatitis A—observed in some experiences but not confirmed in others—among patients with chronic hepatitis C, patients with chronic hepatitis C have been singled out as candidates for hepatitis A vaccination. Other populations whose recognized risk of hepatitis A is increased should be vaccinated, including men who have sex with men, injection drug users, and persons with clotting disorders who require frequent administration of clotting-factor concentrates. Recommendations for dose and frequency differ for the two approved vaccine preparations (Table 92-5); all injections are IM. Hepatitis A vaccine has been reported to be effective in preventing secondary household cases of acute hepatitis A, but its role in other instances of postexposure prophylaxis remains to be demonstrated.

Hepatitis B

Until 1982, prevention of hepatitis B was based on *passive* immunoprophylaxis either with standard IG, containing

TABLE 92-5

HEPATITIS A VACCINATION SCHEDULES

AGE, YEARS	NO. OF DOSES	DOSE	SCHEDULE, MONTHS
HAVRIX (GlaxoSmithKline)[a]			
1–18	2	720 ELU[b] (0.5 mL)	0, 6–12
≥19	2	1440 ELU (1.0 mL)	0, 6–12
VAQTA (Merck)			
1–18	2	25 units (0.5 mL)	0, 6–18
≥19	2	50 units (1.0 mL)	0, 6–18

[a]A combination of this hepatitis A vaccine and hepatitis B vaccine, TWINRIX, is licensed for simultaneous protection against both of these viruses among adults (age ≥18 years). Each 1.0-mL dose contains 720 ELU of hepatitis A vaccine and 20 μg of hepatitis B vaccine. These doses are recommended at months 0, 1, and 6.
[b]Enzyme-linked immunoassay units.

modest levels of anti-HBs, or hepatitis B immune globulin (HBIG), containing high-titer anti-HBs. The efficacy of standard IG has never been established and remains questionable; even the efficacy of HBIG, demonstrated in several clinical trials, has been challenged, and its contribution appears to be in reducing the frequency of clinical *illness*, not in preventing *infection*. The first vaccine for *active* immunization, introduced in 1982, was prepared from purified, noninfectious 22-nm spherical forms of HBsAg derived from the plasma of healthy HBsAg carriers. In 1987, the plasma-derived vaccine was supplanted by a genetically engineered vaccine derived from recombinant yeast. The latter vaccine consists of HBsAg particles that are nonglycosylated but are otherwise indistinguishable from natural HBsAg; two recombinant vaccines are licensed for use in the United States. Current recommendations can be divided into those for preexposure and postexposure prophylaxis.

For *preexposure* prophylaxis against hepatitis B in settings of frequent exposure (health workers exposed to blood; hemodialysis patients and staff; residents and staff of custodial institutions for the developmentally handicapped; injection drug users; inmates of long-term correctional facilities; persons with multiple sexual partners; persons such as hemophiliacs who require long-term, high-volume therapy with blood derivatives; household and sexual contacts of HBsAg carriers; persons living in or traveling extensively in endemic areas; unvaccinated children under the age of 18; and unvaccinated children who are Alaskan natives, Pacific Islanders, or residents in households of first-generation immigrants from endemic countries), three IM (deltoid, not gluteal) injections of hepatitis B vaccine are recommended at 0, 1, and 6 months (other, optional schedules are summarized in Table 92-6). Pregnancy is *not* a contraindication to vaccination. In areas of low HBV endemicity such as the United States, despite the availability of safe and effective hepatitis B vaccines, a strategy of vaccinating persons in high-risk groups has not been effective. The incidence of new hepatitis B cases continued to increase in the United States after introduction of vaccines; <10% of all targeted persons in high-risk groups have actually been vaccinated, and ~30% of persons with sporadic acute hepatitis B do not fall into any high-risk-group category. Therefore, to have an impact on the frequency of HBV infection in an area of low endemicity such as the United States, universal hepatitis B vaccination in childhood has been recommended. For unvaccinated children born after the implementation of universal infant vaccination, vaccination during early adolescence, at age 11–12 years, was recommended, and this recommendation has been extended to include all unvaccinated children age 0–19 years. In HBV-hyperendemic areas, e.g., Asia, universal vaccination of children has resulted in a marked 10- to 15-year decline in hepatitis B and its complications.

The two available recombinant hepatitis B vaccines are comparable, one containing 10 μg of HBsAg (Recombivax-HB) and the other containing 20 μg of HBsAg (Engerix-B), and recommended doses for each injection vary for the two preparations (Table 92-6).

TABLE 92-6

PREEXPOSURE HEPATITIS B VACCINATION SCHEDULES

TARGET GROUP	NO. OF DOSES	DOSE	SCHEDULE, MONTHS
RECOMBIVAX-HB (Merck)[a]			
Infants, children (<1–10 years)	3	5 μg (0.5 mL)	0, 1–2, 4–6
Adolescents (11–19 years)	3 or 4	5 μg (0.5 mL)	0–2, 1–4, 4–6 *or* 0, 12, 24 *or* 0, 1, 2, 12
	or		
	2	10 μg (1.0 mL)	0, 4–6 (age 11–15)
Adults (≥20 years)	3	10 μg (1.0 mL)	0–2, 1–4, 4–6
Hemodialysis patients[b]			
<20 years	3	5 μg (0.5 mL)	0, 1, 6
≥20 years	3	40 μg (4.0 mL)	0, 1, 6
ENGERIX-B (GlaxoSmithKline)[c]			
Infants, children (<1–10 years)	3 or 4	10 μg (0.5 mL)	0, 1–2, 4–6 *or* 0, 1, 2,12
Adolescents (10–19 years)	3 or 4	10 μg (0.5 mL)	0, 1–2, 4–6 *or* 0, 12, 24 *or* 0, 1, 2, 12
Adults (≥20 years)	3 or 4	20 μg (1.0 mL)	0–2, 1–4, 4–6 *or* 0, 1, 2, 12
Hemodialysis patients[b]			
<20 years	4	10 μg (0.5 mL)	0, 1, 2, 6
≥20 years	4	40 μg (2.0 mL)	0, 1, 2, 6

[a]This manufacturer produces a licensed combination of hepatitis B vaccine and vaccines against *Haemophilus influenzae* type b and *Neisseria meningitidis*, Comvax, for use in infants and young children. Please consult product insert for dose and schedule.

[b]This group also includes other immunocompromised persons.

[c]This manufacturer produces two licensed combination hepatitis B vaccines: (1) Twinrix, recombinant hepatitis B vaccine plus inactivated hepatitis A vaccine, is licensed for simultaneous protection against both of these viruses among adults (age ≥ 18 years). Each 1.0-mL dose contains 720 enzyme-linked immunoassay units of hepatitis A vaccine and 20 μg of hepatitis B vaccine. These doses are recommended at months 0, 1, and 6. (2) Pediatrix, recombinant hepatitis B vaccine plus diphtheria and tetanus toxoid, pertussis, and inactivated poliovirus, is licensed for use in infants and young children. Please consult product insert for doses and schedules.

Combinations of hepatitis B vaccine with other childhood vaccines are available as well (Table 92-6).

For unvaccinated persons sustaining an exposure to HBV, *postexposure* prophylaxis with a combination of HBIG (for rapid achievement of high-titer circulating anti-HBs) and hepatitis B vaccine (for achievement of long-lasting immunity as well as its apparent efficacy in attenuating clinical illness after exposure) is recommended. For *perinatal* exposure of infants born to HBsAg-positive mothers, a single dose of HBIG, 0.5 mL, should be administered IM in the thigh *immediately after birth*, followed by a complete course of three injections of recombinant hepatitis B vaccine (see doses above) to be started within the first 12 h of life. For those experiencing a direct percutaneous inoculation or transmucosal exposure to HBsAg-positive blood or body fluids (e.g., accidental *needle stick*, other mucosal penetration, or ingestion), a single IM dose of HBIG, 0.06 mL/kg, administered as soon after exposure as possible, is followed by a complete course of hepatitis B vaccine to begin within the first week. For those exposed by *sexual* contact to a patient with acute hepatitis B, a single IM dose of HBIG, 0.06 mL/kg, should be given within 14 days of exposure, to be followed by a complete course of hepatitis B vaccine. When both HBIG and hepatitis B vaccine are recommended, they may be given at the same time but at separate sites.

The precise duration of protection afforded by hepatitis B vaccine is unknown; however, ~80–90% of immunocompetent vaccinees retain protective levels of anti-HBs for at least 5 years, and 60–80% for 10 years. Thereafter and even after anti-HBs becomes undetectable, protection persists against clinical hepatitis B, hepatitis B surface antigenemia, and chronic HBV infection. Currently, *booster* immunizations are not recommended routinely, except in immunosuppressed persons who have lost detectable anti-HBs or immunocompetent persons who sustain percutaneous HBsAg-positive inoculations after losing detectable antibody. Specifically, for hemodialysis patients, annual anti-HBs testing is recommended after vaccination; booster doses are recommended when anti-HBs levels fall to <10 mIU/mL. As noted above, for persons at risk of both hepatitis A and B, a combined vaccine is available containing 720 enzyme-linked immunoassay units of inactivated HAV and 20 μg of recombinant HBsAg (at 0, 1, and 6 months).

Hepatitis D

Infection with hepatitis D can be prevented by vaccinating susceptible persons with hepatitis B vaccine. No product is available for immunoprophylaxis to prevent HDV superinfection in HBsAg carriers; for them, avoidance of percutaneous exposures and limitation of intimate contact with persons who have HDV infection are recommended.

Hepatitis C

IG is ineffective in preventing hepatitis C and is no longer recommended for postexposure prophylaxis in cases of perinatal, needle stick, or sexual exposure. Although prototype vaccines that induce antibodies to HCV envelope proteins have been developed, currently, hepatitis C vaccination is not feasible practically. Genotype and quasispecies viral heterogeneity, as well as rapid evasion of neutralizing antibodies by this rapidly mutating virus, conspire to render HCV a difficult target for immunoprophylaxis with a vaccine. Prevention of transfusion-associated hepatitis C has been accomplished by the following successively introduced measures: Exclusion of commercial blood donors and reliance on a volunteer blood supply; screening donor blood with surrogate markers such as ALT (no longer recommended) and anti-HBc, markers that identify segments of the blood donor population with an increased risk of bloodborne infections; exclusion of blood donors in high-risk groups for AIDS and the introduction of anti-HIV screening tests; and progressively sensitive serologic and virologic screening tests for HCV infection.

In the absence of active or passive immunization, prevention of hepatitis C includes behavior changes and precautions to limit exposures to infected persons. Recommendations designed to identify patients with clinically inapparent hepatitis as candidates for medical management have as a secondary benefit the identification of persons whose contacts could be at risk of becoming infected. A so-called look-back program has been recommended to identify persons who were transfused before 1992 with blood from a donor found subsequently to have hepatitis C. In addition, anti-HCV testing is recommended for anyone who received a blood transfusion or a transplanted organ before the introduction of second-generation screening tests in 1992, those who ever used injection drugs, chronically hemodialyzed patients, persons with clotting disorders who received clotting factors made before 1987 from pooled blood products, persons with elevated aminotransferase levels, health workers exposed to HCV-positive blood or contaminated needles, and children born to HCV-positive mothers.

For stable, monogamous sexual partners, sexual transmission of hepatitis C is unlikely, and sexual barrier precautions are not recommended. For persons with multiple sexual partners or with sexually transmitted diseases, the risk of sexual transmission of hepatitis C is increased, and barrier precautions (latex condoms) are recommended. A person with hepatitis C should avoid sharing such items as razors, toothbrushes, and nail clippers with sexual partners and family members. No special precautions are recommended for babies born to mothers with hepatitis C, and breast feeding does not have to be restricted.

Hepatitis E

Whether IG prevents hepatitis E remains undetermined. A recombinant vaccine has been developed and is undergoing clinical testing.

FURTHER READINGS

Blum HE, Marcellin P: EASL Consensus Conference on Hepatitis B. J Hepatol 39(Suppl 1):1, 2003

Centers for Disease Control and Prevention: Updated U.S. Public Health Service guidelines for the management of occupational exposures to HBV, HCV, and HIV and recommendations for postexposure prophylaxis. MMWR 50(RR-11):1, 2001

———: General recommendations on immunization: Recommendations of the Advisory Committee on Immunization Practices and the American Academy of Family Physicians. MMWR 51(RR-2):1, 2002

CHEN CJ et al: Risk of hepatocellular carcinoma across a biological gradient of serum hepatitis B virus DNA level. JAMA 295:65, 2006

CHU C-J et al: Hepatitis B virus genotype B is associated with earlier HBeAg seroconversion compared with hepatitis B virus genotype C. Gastroenterology 122:1756, 2002

CONSENSUS STATEMENT: EASL International Consensus Conference on Hepatitis C. J Hepatol 30:956, 1999

DIENSTAG JL, MCHUTCHISON JG: American Gastroenterological Association technical review on the management of hepatitis C. Gastroenterology 130:231, 2006

FERRARI C et al: Immunopathogenesis of hepatitis B. J Hepatol 39(Suppl 1):S36, 2003

GISH RG, LOCARNINI SA: Chronic hepatitis B: Current testing strategies. Clin Gastroenterol Hepatol 4:666, 2006

HADZIYANNIS SJ, VASSILOPOULOS D: Hepatitis B e antigen-negative chronic hepatitis B. Hepatology 34:617, 2001

JAECKEL E et al: Treatment of acute hepatitis C with interferon alfa-2b. N Engl J Med 345:1452, 2001

LAUER GM, WALKER BD: Medical progress: Hepatitis C virus infection. N Engl J Med 345:41, 2001

LOK ASF, MCMAHON BJ: Chronic hepatitis B. Hepatology 34:1225, 2001

MAHESHWARI A et al: Acute hepatitis C. Lancet 372:321, 2008

MARGOLIS HS et al (eds): *Viral Hepatitis and Liver Disease*. Atlanta/London, International Medical Press, 2002

PATRA S et al: Maternal and fetal outcomes in pregnant women with acute hepatitis E virus infection. Ann Intern Med 147:28, 2007

PAWLOTSKY J-M: Molecular diagnosis of viral hepatitis. Gastroenterology 122:1554, 2002

REHERMANN B: Immune response in hepatitis B virus infection. Semin Liver Dis 23:21, 2003

SCHREIBER GB et al: The risk of transfusion-transmitted viral infection. N Engl J Med 334:1685, 1996

SEEFF LB: Natural history of chronic hepatitis C. Hepatology 36(Suppl 1):S35, 2002

STRADER DB et al: Diagnosis, management, and treatment of hepatitis C (AASLD practice guidelines). Hepatology 39:1147, 2004

THIMME R et al: Viral and immunological determinants of hepatitis C virus clearance, persistence, and disease. Proc Natl Acad Sci USA 99:15661, 2002

YANG H-I et al: Hepatitis B e antigen and the risk of hepatocellular carcinoma. N Engl J Med 347:168, 2002

CHAPTER 93
CHRONIC HEPATITIS

Jules L. Dienstag

Chronic hepatitis represents a series of liver disorders of varying causes and severity in which hepatic inflammation and necrosis continue for at least 6 months. Milder forms are nonprogressive or only slowly progressive, while more severe forms may be associated with scarring and architectural reorganization, which, when advanced, lead ultimately to cirrhosis. Several categories of chronic hepatitis have been recognized. These include chronic viral hepatitis, drug-induced chronic hepatitis, and autoimmune chronic hepatitis. In many cases, clinical and laboratory features are insufficient to allow assignment into one of these three categories; these "idiopathic" cases are also believed to represent autoimmune chronic hepatitis. Finally, clinical and laboratory features of chronic hepatitis are observed occasionally in patients with such hereditary/metabolic disorders as Wilson's disease (copper overload) and even occasionally in patients with alcoholic liver injury. Although all types of chronic hepatitis share certain clinical, laboratory, and histopathologic features, chronic viral and chronic autoimmune hepatitis are sufficiently distinct to merit separate discussions. For discussion of acute hepatitis, see Chap. 92.

CLASSIFICATION OF CHRONIC HEPATITIS

Common to all forms of chronic hepatitis are histopathologic distinctions based on localization and extent of liver injury. These vary from the milder forms, previously labeled *chronic persistent hepatitis* and *chronic lobular hepatitis*, to the more severe form, formerly called *chronic active hepatitis*. When first defined, these designations were felt to have prognostic implications, which have been challenged by more recent observations. Categorization of chronic hepatitis based primarily on histopathologic features has been replaced by a more informative classification based on a combination of clinical, serologic, and histologic variables. Classification of chronic hepatitis is based on (1) its *cause*; (2) its histologic activity, or *grade*; and (3) its degree of progression, or *stage*. Thus, neither clinical features alone nor histologic features—requiring liver biopsy—alone are sufficient to characterize and distinguish among the several categories of chronic hepatitis.

TABLE 93-1

CLINICAL AND LABORATORY FEATURES OF CHRONIC HEPATITIS

TYPE OF HEPATITIS	DIAGNOSTIC TEST(S)	AUTOANTIBODIES	THERAPY
Chronic hepatitis B	HBsAg, IgG anti-HBc, HBeAg, HBV DNA	Uncommon	IFN-α, PEG IFN-α, lamivudine, adefovir, entecavir
Chronic hepatitis C	Anti-HCV, HCV RNA	Anti-LKM1[a]	PEG IFN-α plus ribavirin
Chronic hepatitis D	Anti-HDV, HDV RNA, HBsAg, IgG anti-HBc	Anti-LKM3	IFN-α, PEG IFN-α[b]
Autoimmune hepatitis	ANA[c] (homogeneous), anti-LKM1(±), hyperglobulinemia	ANA, anti-LKM1, anti-SLA[d]	Prednisone, azathioprine
Drug-associated	—	Uncommon	Withdraw drug
Cryptogenic	All negative	None	Prednisone (?), azathioprine (?)

[a]Antibodies to liver-kidney microsomes type 1 (autoimmune hepatitis type II and some cases of hepatitis C).
[b]Clinical trials suggest benefit of IFN-α therapy or PEG IFN-α.
[c]Antinuclear antibody (autoimmune hepatitis type I).
[d]Antibodies to soluble liver antigen (autoimmune hepatitis type III).
Note: HBc, hepatitis B core; HBeAg, hepatitis B e antigen; HBsAg, hepatitis B surface antigen; HBV, hepatitis B virus; HCV, hepatitis C virus; HDV, hepatitis D virus; IFN-α, interferon α; IgG, immunoglobulin G; LKM, liver-kidney microsome; PEG-IFN-α, pegylated interferon α; SLA, soluble liver antigen.

CLASSIFICATION BY CAUSE

Clinical and serologic features allow the establishment of a diagnosis of *chronic viral hepatitis*, caused by hepatitis B, hepatitis B plus D, or hepatitis C; *autoimmune hepatitis*, including several subcategories, I and II (perhaps III), based on serologic distinctions; *drug-associated chronic hepatitis*; and a category of unknown cause, or *cryptogenic chronic hepatitis* (Table 93-1). These are addressed in more detail below.

CLASSIFICATION BY GRADE

Grade, a histologic assessment of necroinflammatory activity, is based on examination of the liver biopsy. An assessment of important histologic features includes the degree of *periportal necrosis* and the disruption of the limiting plate of periportal hepatocytes by inflammatory cells (so-called *piecemeal necrosis* or *interface hepatitis*); the degree of confluent necrosis that links or forms bridges between vascular structures—between portal tract and portal tract or even more important bridges between portal tract and central vein—referred to as *bridging necrosis*; the degree of hepatocyte degeneration and focal necrosis within the lobule; and the degree of *portal inflammation*. Several scoring systems that take these histologic features into account have been devised, and the most popular are the histologic activity index (HAI) and the METAVIR score (Table 93-2). Based on the presence and degree of these features of histologic activity, chronic hepatitis can be graded as mild, moderate, or severe.

CLASSIFICATION BY STAGE

The stage of chronic hepatitis, which reflects the level of progression of the disease, is based on the degree of hepatic fibrosis. When fibrosis is so extensive that fibrous septa surround parenchymal nodules and alter the normal architecture of the liver lobule, the histologic lesion is defined as *cirrhosis*. Staging is based on the degree of fibrosis as categorized on a numerical scale from 0–6 (HAI) or 0–4 (METAVIR) (Table 93-2).

CHRONIC VIRAL HEPATITIS

Both the enterically transmitted forms of viral hepatitis, hepatitis A and E, are self-limited and do not cause chronic hepatitis (rare reports notwithstanding in which acute hepatitis A serves as a trigger for the onset of autoimmune hepatitis in genetically susceptible patients). In contrast, the entire clinicopathologic spectrum of chronic hepatitis occurs in patients with chronic viral hepatitis B and C as well as in patients with chronic hepatitis D superimposed on chronic hepatitis B.

CHRONIC HEPATITIS B

The likelihood of chronicity after acute hepatitis B varies as a function of age. Infection at birth is associated with clinically silent acute infection but a 90% chance of chronic infection, while infection in young adulthood in immunocompetent persons is typically associated with clinically apparent acute hepatitis but a risk of chronicity of only approximately 1%. Most cases of chronic hepatitis B among adults, however, occur in patients who never had a recognized episode of clinically apparent acute viral hepatitis. The degree of liver injury (grade) in patients with chronic hepatitis B is variable, ranging from none in inactive carriers to mild to moderate to severe. Among adults with chronic hepatitis B, histologic features are of prognostic importance. In one long-term study of patients with chronic hepatitis B, investigators

TABLE 93-2

HISTOLOGIC GRADING AND STAGING IN CHRONIC HEPATITIS

	HISTOLOGIC ACTIVITY INDEX (HAI)[a]		METAVIR[b]	
HISTOLOGIC FEATURE	**SEVERITY**	**SCORE**	**SEVERITY**	**SCORE**
Necroinflammatory Activity (Grade)				
Perioportal necrosis,	None	0	None	0
including piecemeal	Mild	1	Mild	1
necrosis (PN) and/or	Mild/moderate	2	Moderate	2
bridging necrosis (BN)	Moderate	3	Severe	3
	Severe	4		
			Bridging necrosis	Yes
				No
Intralobular Confluent	—None	0	None or mild	0
necrosis	—Focal	1	Moderate	1
	—Zone 3 some	2	Severe	2
	—Zone 3 most	3		
	—Zone 3 + BN few	4		
	—Zone 3 + BN multiple	5		
	—Panacinar/multiacinar	6		
Focal	—None	0		
	—≤1 Focus/10× field	1		
	—2–4 Foci/10× field	2		
	—5–10 Foci/10× field	3		
	—>10 Foci/10× field	4		
Portal inflammation	None	0		
	Mild	1		
	Moderate	3		
	Moderate/marked	3		
	Marked	4		
	Total	0–18		
				A0–A3[c]
Fibrosis (Stage)				
None		0		F0
Portal fibrosis—some		1		F1
Portal fibrosis—most		2		F1
Bridging fibrosis—few		3		F2
Bridging fibrosis—many		4		F3
Incomplete cirrhosis		5		F4
Cirrhosis		6		F4
	Total	6		4

[a]J Hepatol 22:696, 1995.
[b]Hepatology 24:289, 1996.
[c]Necroinflammatory grade: A0 = none; A1 = mild; A2 = moderate; A3 = severe.

found a 5-year survival rate of 97% for patients with mild chronic hepatitis, 86% for patients with moderate to severe chronic hepatitis, and only 55% for patients with chronic hepatitis and postnecrotic cirrhosis. The 15-year survival in these cohorts was 77, 66, and 40%, respectively. On the other hand, more recent observations do not allow us to be so sanguine about the prognosis in patients with mild chronic hepatitis; among such patients followed for 1–13 years, progression to more severe chronic hepatitis and cirrhosis has been observed in more than a quarter of cases.

More important to consider than histology alone in patients with chronic hepatitis B is the degree of hepatitis B virus (HBV) replication. As reviewed in Chap. 92, chronic HBV infection can occur in the presence or absence of serum hepatitis B e antigen (HBeAg), and generally, for both HBeAg-reactive and HBeAg-negative chronic hepatitis B, the level of HBV DNA correlates with the level of liver injury and risk of progression. In *HBeAg-reactive chronic hepatitis B*, two phases have been recognized based on the relative level of HBV replication. The relatively *replicative phase* is characterized by the presence in the serum of HBeAg and HBV DNA levels well in excess of 10^5–10^6 virions/mL, by the presence in the liver of detectable intrahepatocyte nucleocapsid antigens [primarily hepatitis B core antigen (HBcAg)], by high infectivity, and by accompanying liver injury. In contrast, the relatively *nonreplicative phase* is characterized by the absence of the conventional serum marker of HBV replication (HBeAg), the appearance of anti-HBe, levels of HBV DNA below a threshold of ~10^3 virions/mL, the absence of intrahepatocytic HBcAg, limited infectivity, and minimal liver injury. Those patients in the replicative phase tend to have more severe chronic hepatitis, while those in the nonreplicative phase tend to have minimal or mild chronic hepatitis or to be inactive hepatitis B carriers; however, distinctions in HBV replication and in histologic category do not always coincide. The likelihood in a patient with HBeAg-reactive chronic hepatitis B of converting spontaneously from relatively replicative to nonreplicative infection is approximately 10–15% per year. In patients with HBeAg-reactive chronic HBV infection, especially when acquired at birth or in early childhood, as recognized commonly in Asian countries, a dichotomy is common between very high levels of HBV replication and negligible levels of liver injury. Yet despite the relatively immediate, apparently benign nature of liver disease for many decades in this population, patients with childhood-acquired HBV infection are the ones at ultimately increased risk later in life of cirrhosis and hepatocellular carcinoma (HCC). A discussion of the pathogenesis of liver injury in patients with chronic hepatitis B appears in Chap. 92.

HBeAg-negative chronic hepatitis B, i.e., chronic HBV infection with active virus replication, readily detectable HBV DNA but without HBeAg (anti-HBe-reactive), is more common than HBeAg-reactive chronic hepatitis B in Mediterranean and European countries and in Asia (and, correspondingly, in HBV genotypes other than A). Compared to patients with HBeAg-reactive chronic hepatitis B, patients with HBeAg-negative chronic hepatitis B have levels of HBV DNA that are several orders of magnitude lower (no more than 10^5–10^6 virions/mL) than those observed in the HBeAg-reactive subset. Most such cases represent precore or core-promoter mutations acquired late in the natural history of the disease (mostly early-life onset; age range 40–55 years, older than that for HBeAg-reactive chronic hepatitis B); these mutations prevent translation of HBeAg from the precore component of the HBV genome (precore mutants) or are characterized by down-regulated transcription of precore mRNA (core-promoter mutants; Chap. 92). Although their levels of HBV DNA tend to be lower than among patients with HBeAg-reactive chronic hepatitis B, patients with HBeAg-negative chronic hepatitis B can have progressive liver injury (complicated by cirrhosis and HCC) and experience episodic reactivation of liver disease reflected in fluctuating levels of aminotransferase activity ("flares"). The biochemical and histologic activity of HBeAg-negative disease tends to correlate closely with levels of HBV replication, unlike the case mentioned above of Asian patients with HBeAg-reactive chronic hepatitis B during the early decades of their HBV infection. An important point worth reiterating is the observation that the level of HBV replication is the most important risk factor for the ultimate development of cirrhosis and HCC in both HBeAg-reactive and HBeAg-negative patients. Although levels of HBV DNA are lower and more readily suppressed to undetectable levels in HBeAg-negative (compared to HBeAg-reactive) chronic hepatitis B, achieving sustained responses that permit discontinuation of antiviral therapy is less likely in HBeAg-negative patients (see below). Inactive carriers are patients with circulating hepatitis B surface antigen (HBsAg), normal serum aminotransferase levels, undetectable HBeAg, and levels of HBV DNA that are either undetectable or present at levels ≤10^3 virions/mL. This serologic profile can occur not only in inactive carriers but also in patients with HBeAg-negative chronic hepatitis B during periods of relative inactivity; distinguishing between the two requires sequential biochemical and virologic monitoring over many months.

The spectrum of *clinical features* of chronic hepatitis B is broad, ranging from asymptomatic infection to debilitating disease or even end-stage, fatal hepatic failure. As noted above, the onset of the disease tends to be insidious in most patients, with the exception of the very few in whom chronic disease follows failure of resolution of clinically apparent acute hepatitis B. The clinical and laboratory features associated with progression from acute to chronic hepatitis B are discussed in Chap. 92.

Fatigue is a common symptom, and persistent or intermittent *jaundice* is a common feature in severe or advanced cases. Intermittent deepening of jaundice and recurrence of malaise and anorexia, as well as worsening fatigue, are reminiscent of acute hepatitis; such exacerbations may occur spontaneously, often coinciding with evidence of virologic reactivation; may lead to progressive liver injury; and, when superimposed on well-established cirrhosis, may cause hepatic decompensation. Complications of cirrhosis occur in end-stage chronic hepatitis and include ascites, edema, bleeding gastroesophageal varices, hepatic encephalopathy, coagulopathy, or hypersplenism. Occasionally these complications bring the patient to initial clinical attention. Extrahepatic complications of chronic hepatitis B, similar to those seen during the prodromal phase of acute hepatitis B, are associated with deposition of circulating hepatitis B antigen–antibody immune complexes. These include arthralgias and arthritis, which are common, and the more rare purpuric cutaneous lesions (leukocytoclastic vasculitis), immune-complex glomerulonephritis, and generalized vasculitis (polyarteritis nodosa) (Chap. 92).

Laboratory features of chronic hepatitis B do not distinguish adequately between histologically mild and severe hepatitis. Aminotransferase elevations tend to be modest for chronic hepatitis B but may fluctuate in the range of 100–1000 units. As is true for acute viral hepatitis B, alanine aminotransferase (ALT) tends to be more elevated than aspartate aminotransferase (AST); however, once cirrhosis is established, AST tends to exceed ALT. Levels of alkaline phosphatase activity tend to be normal or only marginally elevated. In severe cases, moderate elevations in serum bilirubin [51.3–171 μmol/L (3–10 mg/dL)] occur. Hypoalbuminemia and prolongation of the prothrombin time occur in severe or end-stage cases. Hyperglobulinemia and detectable circulating autoantibodies are distinctly absent in chronic hepatitis B (in contrast to autoimmune hepatitis). Viral markers of chronic HBV infection are discussed in Chap. 92.

℞ Treatment: CHRONIC HEPATITIS B

Although progression to cirrhosis is more likely in severe than in mild or moderate chronic hepatitis B, all forms of chronic hepatitis B can be progressive, and progression occurs primarily in patients with active HBV replication. Moreover, in populations of patients with chronic hepatitis B who are at risk for HCC, the risk is highest for those with continued, high-level HBV replication. Therefore, management of chronic hepatitis B is directed at suppressing the level of virus replication. To date, five drugs have been approved for treatment of chronic hepatitis B: injectable interferon (IFN) α; pegylated interferon [long-acting IFN bound to polyethylene glycol (PEG), known as *PEG IFN*]; and the oral agents lamivudine, adefovir dipivoxil, and entecavir. Several other drugs, including emtricitabine, tenofovir, telbivudine, pradefovir, and clevudine, are in the process of efficacy testing in clinical trials.

Antiviral therapy for hepatitis B has evolved rapidly since the mid-1990s, as has the sensitivity of tests for HBV DNA. When IFN and lamivudine were evaluated in clinical trials, HBV DNA was measured by insensitive hybridization assays with detection thresholds of 10^5–10^6 virions/mL; when adefovir, entecavir, and PEG IFN were studied in clinical trials, HBV DNA was measured by sensitive amplification assays [polymerase chain reaction (PCR)] with detection thresholds of 10^2–10^3 virions/mL. Recognition of these distinctions is helpful when comparing results of clinical trials that established the efficacy of these therapies (reviewed below in chronological order of publication of these efficacy trials).

INTERFERON IFN-α was the first approved therapy for chronic hepatitis B. For immunocompetent adults with HBeAg-reactive chronic hepatitis B [who tend to have high-level HBV DNA (>10^5–10^6 virions/mL) and histologic evidence of chronic hepatitis on liver biopsy], a 16-week course of IFN given subcutaneously at a daily dose of 5 million units, or three times a week at a dose of 10 million units, results in a loss of HBeAg and hybridization-detectable HBV DNA (i.e., a reduction to levels below 10^5–10^6 virions/mL) in ~30% of patients, with a concomitant improvement in liver histology. Seroconversion from HBeAg to anti-HBe occurs in approximately 20%, and, in early trials, approximately 8% lost HBsAg. Successful INF therapy and seroconversion are often accompanied by an acute hepatitis-like elevation in aminotransferase activity, which has been postulated to result from enhanced cytolytic T cell clearance of HBV-infected hepatocytes. Relapse after successful therapy is rare (1 or 2%). The likelihood of responding to IFN is higher in patients with lower levels of HBV DNA and substantial elevations of ALT. Although children can respond as well as adults, IFN therapy has not been effective in very young children infected at birth. Similarly, IFN therapy has not been effective in immunosuppressed persons, Asian patients with minimal-to-mild ALT elevations, or patients with decompensated chronic hepatitis B (in whom such therapy can actually be detrimental, sometimes precipitating decompensation, often associated with severe adverse effects). Among patients with HBeAg loss during therapy, long-term follow-up has demonstrated that 80% experience eventual loss of HBsAg, i.e., all serologic markers of infection, and normalization of ALT over a 9-year posttreatment period. In addition, improved long-term and complication-free survival as well as a reduction in the frequency of HCC have been documented among interferon responders, supporting the conclusion that successful interferon therapy improves the natural history of chronic hepatitis B.

Retreatment of IFN nonresponders with another course of IFN may enhance response rates somewhat; currently, however, most would opt to address IFN nonresponders by offering them one of the newer, oral therapies.

Initial trials of brief-duration IFN therapy in patients with *HBeAg-negative chronic hepatitis B* were disappointing, suppressing HBV replication transiently during therapy but almost never resulting in sustained antiviral responses. In subsequent IFN trials among patients with HBeAg-negative chronic hepatitis B, however, more protracted courses, lasting up to a year and a half, have been reported to result in sustained remissions, with suppressed HBV DNA and aminotransferase activity, in ~20%.

Complications of IFN therapy include systemic "flu-like" symptoms; marrow suppression; emotional lability (irritability commonly, depression/anxiety less frequently); autoimmune reactions (especially autoimmune thyroiditis); and miscellaneous side effects such as alopecia, rashes, diarrhea, and numbness and tingling of the extremities. With the possible exception of autoimmune thyroiditis, all these side effects are reversible upon dose lowering or cessation of therapy.

Whether or not IFN remains competitive with the newer generation of antivirals, it did represent the first successful antiviral approach, and it set the standard against which subsequent drugs are measured—the achievement of durable virologic, serologic, biochemical, and histologic responses; consolidation of virologic and biochemical benefit in the ensuing years after therapy; and improvement in the natural history of chronic hepatitis B. For all practical purposes, standard IFN has been supplanted by long-acting PEG IFN (see below).

LAMIVUDINE The first of the nucleoside analogues to be approved, the dideoxynucleoside lamivudine, inhibits reverse transcriptase activity of both HIV and HBV and is a potent and effective agent for patients with chronic hepatitis B. In clinical trials among patients with HBeAg-reactive chronic hepatitis B, lamivudine therapy at daily doses of 100 mg for 48–52 weeks suppressed HBV DNA by a median of approximately 5.5 $\log_{10}$ copies/mL and to undetectable levels, as measured by PCR amplification assays, in approximately 40% of patients. Therapy was associated with HBeAg loss in 32–33%; HBeAg seroconversion (i.e., conversion from HBeAg-reactive to anti-HBe-reactive) in 16–21%; normalization of ALT in 40–75%; improvement in histology in 50–60%; retardation in fibrosis in 20–30%; and prevention of progression to cirrhosis. HBeAg responses can occur even in subgroups who are resistant to IFN (e.g., those with high-level HBV DNA) or who failed in the past to respond to it. As is true for IFN therapy of chronic hepatitis B, patients with near-normal ALT activity tend not to experience HBeAg responses (despite suppression of HBV DNA), and those with ALT levels exceeding five times the upper limit of normal can expect 1-year HBeAg seroconversion rates of 50–60%. Generally, HBeAg seroconversions are confined to patients who achieve suppression of HBV DNA to $<10^4$ genomes/mL. Among patients who undergo HBeAg responses during a year-long course of therapy and in whom the response is sustained for 4–6 months after cessation of therapy, the response is durable thereafter in the vast majority, >80%; therefore, the achievement of an HBeAg response represents a viable stopping point in therapy. Reduced durability has been reported in some Asian experiences; however, in most western and Asian patient study populations, long-term durability of HBeAg responses is the rule, which, at least in Western patients, is accompanied by a posttreatment HBsAg seroconversation rate comparable to that seen after IFN-induced HBeAg responses. If HBeAg is unaffected by lamivudine therapy, the current approach is to continue therapy until an HBeAg response occurs, but long-term therapy may be required to suppress HBV replication and, in turn, limit liver injury; HBeAg seroconversions can increase to a level of 50% after 5 years of therapy. Histologic improvement continues to accrue with therapy beyond the first year; after a cumulative course of 3 years of lamivudine therapy, necroinflammatory activity is reduced in the majority of patients, and even cirrhosis has been shown to regress to precirrhotic stages.

Losses of HBsAg have been few during the first year of lamivudine therapy, and this observation had been cited as an advantage of IFN over lamivudine; however, in head-to-head comparisons between standard IFN and lamivudine monotherapy, HBsAg losses were rare in both groups. Trials in which lamivudine and interferon were administered in combination failed to show a benefit of combination therapy over lamivudine monotherapy for either treatment-naïve patients or prior interferon nonresponders.

In patients with *HBeAg-negative chronic hepatitis B*, i.e., in those with precore and core-promoter HBV mutations, 1 year of lamivudine therapy results in HBV DNA suppression and normalization of ALT in three-quarters of patients and in histologic improvement in approximately two-thirds. Therapy has been shown to suppress HBV DNA by approximately 4.5 $\log_{10}$ copies/mL (baseline HBV DNA levels are lower than in patients with HBeAg-reactive hepatitis B) and to undetectable levels in 70%, as measured by sensitive PCR amplification assays. Lacking HBeAg at the outset, patients with HBeAg-negative chronic hepatitis B cannot achieve an HBeAg response—a stopping point in HBeAg-reactive patients; invariably, when therapy is discontinued, reactivation is the rule. Therefore, these patients require long-term therapy; with successive years, the proportion with suppressed HBV DNA and normal ALT increases.

Clinical and laboratory side effects of lamivudine are negligible, indistinguishable from those observed in placebo recipients. During lamivudine therapy, transient ALT elevations, resembling those seen during IFN therapy and during spontaneous HBeAg-to-anti-HBe seroconversions, occur in a quarter of patients. These ALT elevations may result from restored cytolytic T cell activation permitted by suppression of HBV replication. Similar ALT elevations, however, occur at an identical frequency in placebo recipients, but ALT elevations associated with HBeAg seroconversion are confined to lamivudine-treated patients. When therapy is stopped after a year of therapy, two- to threefold ALT elevations occur in 20–30% of lamivudine-treated patients, representing renewed liver-cell injury as HBV replication returns. Although these posttreatment flares are almost always transient and mild, rare severe exacerbations, especially in cirrhotic patients, have been observed, mandating close and careful clinical and virologic monitoring after discontinuation of treatment. Many authorities caution against discontinuing therapy in patients with cirrhosis, in whom posttreatment flares could precipitate decompensation.

Long-term monotherapy with lamivudine is associated with methionine-to-valine (M204V) or methionine-to-isoleucine (M204I) mutations, primarily at amino acid 204 in the tyrosine-methionine-aspartate-aspartate (YMDD) motif of HBV DNA polymerase, analogous to mutations that occur in HIV-infected patients treated with this drug. During a year of therapy, YMDD mutations occur in 15–30% of patients; the frequency increases with each year of therapy, reaching 70% at year 5. Although resistance to lamivudine may not lead to immediate loss of antiviral effect, patients with YMDD mutants ultimately experience degradation of clinical, biochemical, and histologic responses. Therefore, if treatment is begun with lamivudine monotherapy, the emergence of lamivudine resistance, reflected clinically by a breakthrough from suppressed levels of HBV DNA and ALT, is managed by adding another antiviral to which YMDD variants are sensitive (e.g., adefovir; see below).

Currently, although lamivudine is very safe and still used widely in other parts of the world, in the United States and Europe lamivudine has been eclipsed by more potent antivirals that have superior resistance profiles (see below). Still, as the first successful oral antiviral agent for use in hepatitis B, lamivudine has provided proof of the concept that polymerase inhibitors can achieve both virologic, serologic, biochemical, and histologic benefit. In addition, lamivudine has been shown to be effective in the treatment of patients with decompensated hepatitis B (for whom IFN is contraindicated), in some of whom decompensation can be reversed. Moreover, among patients with cirrhosis or advanced fibrosis, lamivudine has been shown to be effective in reducing the risk of progression to hepatic decompensation and, marginally, the risk of HCC.

Because lamivudine monotherapy can result universally in the rapid emergence of YMDD variants in persons with HIV infection, patients with chronic hepatitis B should be tested for anti-HIV prior to therapy; if HIV infection is identified, lamivudine monotherapy at the HBV daily dose of 100 mg is contraindicated. These patients should be treated with triple-drug antiretroviral therapy, including a lamivudine daily dose of 300 mg (Chap. 90). The safety of lamivudine during pregnancy has not been established; however, the drug is not teratogenic in rodents and has been used safely in pregnant women with HIV infection and with HBV infection. Limited data even suggest that administration of lamivudine during the last month of pregnancy to mothers with high-level hepatitis B viremia can reduce the likelihood of perinatal transmission of hepatitis B.

ADEFOVIR DIPIVOXIL The acyclic nucleotide analogue adefovir dipivoxil, the prodrug of adefovir, is a potent antiviral that, at an oral daily dose of 10 mg, reduces HBV DNA by approximately 3.5–4 $\log_{10}$ copies/mL and is equally effective in treatment-naïve patients and IFN nonresponders. In HBeAg-reactive chronic hepatitis B, a 48-week course of adefovir dipivoxil was shown to achieve histologic improvement (and reduce the progression of fibrosis) and normalization of ALT in half of patients, HBeAg seroconversion in 12%, HBeAg loss in 23%, and suppression to an undetectable level of HBV DNA in 20–30%, as measured by PCR. Similar to IFN and lamivudine, adefovir dipivoxil is more likely to achieve an HBeAg response in patients with high baseline ALT; for example, among adefovir-treated patients with ALT level >5 times the upper limit of normal, HBeAg seroconversions occurred in 25%. The durability of adefovir-induced HBeAg responses is high (91% in one study); therefore, HBeAg response can be relied upon as a stopping point for adefovir therapy. Although data on the impact of additional therapy beyond one year are limited, biochemical, serologic, and virologic outcomes improve progressively as therapy is continued.

In patients with *HBeAg-negative chronic hepatitis B*, a 48-week course of 10 mg/d of adefovir dipivoxil resulted in histologic improvement in two-thirds, normalization of ALT in three-quarters, and suppression of HBV DNA to PCR-undetectable levels in half. As was true for lamivudine, because HBeAg responses—a potential stopping point—cannot be achieved in this group, reactivation is the rule when adefovir therapy is discontinued, and indefinite, long-term therapy is required. Treatment beyond the first year consolidates the gain of the first year; after 5 years of therapy, improvement in hepatic inflammation and regression of fibrosis was observed in three-quarters of patients, ALT was normal in 70%, and HBV DNA was undetectable in almost 70%.

Adefovir contains a flexible acyclic linker instead of the L-nucleoside ring of lamivudine, avoiding steric hindrance by mutated amino acids. In addition, the molecular structure of phosphorylated adefovir is very similar to that of its natural substrate; therefore mutations to adefovir would also affect binding of the natural substrate, dATP. Hypothetically, these are among the reasons that resistance to adefovir dipivoxil is much less likely than resistance to lamivudine; no resistance was encountered in 1 year of clinical-trial therapy. In subsequent years, however, adefovir resistance begins to emerge [asparagine to threonine at amino acid 236 (N236T) and alanine to valine or threonine at amino acid 181 (A181V/T) primarily], occurring in 2.5% after 2 years, but in 29% after 5 years of therapy. Among patients coinfected with HBV and HIV and who have normal CD4+ T cell counts, adefovir dipivoxil is effective in suppressing HBV dramatically (by 5 $\log s_{10}$ in one study). Moreover, adefovir dipivoxil is effective in lamivudine-resistant, YMDD-mutant HBV and can be used when such lamivudine-induced variants emerge. When lamivudine resistance occurs, authorities have debated whether to add adefovir or switch to adefovir; however, adding adefovir, i.e., maintaining lamivudine to preempt the emergence of adefovir resistance, appears to be the favored approach. In this vein, almost invariably, patients with adefovir-mutant HBV respond to lamivudine. When, in the past, adefovir had been evaluated as therapy for HIV infection, doses of 60–120 mg were required to suppress HIV, and at these doses the drug was nephrotoxic. Even at 30 mg/d, creatinine elevations of 44 μmol/L (0.5 mg/dL) occur in 10% of patients; however, at the HBV-effective dose of 10 mg, such elevations of creatinine are rarely encountered. If any nephrotoxicity does occur, it rarely appears before 6–8 months of therapy. Although renal tubular injury is a rare potential side effect, and although creatinine monitoring is recommended during treatment, the therapeutic index of adefovir dipivoxil is high, and the nephrotoxicity observed in clinical trials at higher doses was reversible. For patients with underlying renal disease, adefovir dipivoxil dose reductions are recommended: administration reduced to every 48 h for creatinine clearances of 20–49 mL/min, to every 72 h for creatinine clearances of 10–19 mL/min, and once a week, following dialysis, for patients undergoing hemodialysis. Adefovir dipivoxil is very well tolerated, and ALT elevations during and after withdrawal of therapy are similar to those observed and described above in clinical trials of lamivudine. An advantage of adefovir is its relatively favorable resistance profile; however, it is not as potent as the other approved oral agents, it does not suppress HBV DNA as rapidly or as uniformly as the others, and a small proportion of patients have no demonstrable response to the drug ("primary nonresponders").

PEGYLATED INTERFERON After long-acting PEG IFN was shown to be effective in the treatment of hepatitis C (see below), this more convenient drug was evaluated in the treatment of chronic hepatitis B. Preliminary trials documented that once-a-week PEG IFN was more effective than the more frequently administered, standard IFN, following which several large-scale trials were conducted among patients with HBeAg-reactive and HBeAg-negative chronic hepatitis B.

In HBeAg-reactive chronic hepatitis B, two large-scale studies were done, one with PEG IFN-α2b (100 μg weekly for 32 weeks, then 50 μg weekly for another 20 weeks for a total of 52 weeks, with a comparison arm of combination PEG IFN with oral lamivudine) in 307 subjects; the other involved PEG IFN-α2a (180 μg weekly for 48 weeks) in 814 primarily Asian patients confined to those with ALT ≥2 × the upper limit of normal, with comparison arms of lamivudine monotherapy and combination PEG IFN plus lamivudine. At the end of therapy (48–52 weeks) in the PEG IFN monotherapy arms, HBeAg loss occurred in approximately 30%, HBeAg seroconversion in 22–27%, undetectable HBV DNA (<400 copies/mL by PCR) in 10–25%, normal ALT in 34–39%, and a mean reduction in HBV DNA of 2 $\log_{10}$ copies/mL (PEG IFN-α2b) to 4.5 $\log_{10}$ copies/mL (PEG IFN-α2a). Six months after completing PEG IFN monotherapy in these trials, HBeAg losses were present in approximately 35%, HBeAg seroconversion in approximately 30%, undetectable HBV DNA in 7–14%, normal ALT in 32–41%, and a mean reduction in HBV DNA of 2–2.4 $\log_{10}$ copies/mL. Although the combination of PEG IFN and lamivudine was superior at the end of therapy in one or more serologic, virologic, or biochemical outcomes, neither the combination arm (in both studies) nor the lamivudine monotherapy arm (in the PEG IFN-α2a trial) demonstrated any benefit compared to the PEG IFN monotherapy arms 6 months after therapy. Moreover, HBsAg seroconversion occurred in 3–7% of PEG IFN recipients (with or without lamivudine); some of these seroconversions were identified by the end of therapy, but many were identified during the posttreatment follow-up period. The likelihood of HBeAg loss in PEG IFN–treated HBeAg-reactive patients is associated with HBV genotype A > B > C > D.

Based on these results, some authorities concluded that PEG IFN monotherapy should be the first-line therapy of choice in HBeAg-reactive chronic hepatitis B; however, this conclusion has been challenged. Although a finite, 1-year course of PEG IFN results in a higher rate of sustained response (6 months after treatment) than is achieved with oral nucleoside/nucleotide analogue therapy, the comparison is confounded by the fact that oral agents are not discontinued at the end of a year. Instead, taken orally and free of side effects, therapy with oral agents is extended indefinitely or until after the occurrence of an HBeAg response. The rate of HBeAg responses after 2 years of oral-agent therapy is at least as high as, if not higher than, that achieved with PEG IFN after 1 year; favoring oral agents is the absence of injections and difficult-to-tolerate side effects as well as lower direct and indirect medical costs and inconvenience. The association of HBsAg responses with PEG IFN therapy occurs in such a small proportion of patients that subjecting everyone to PEG IFN for the marginal gain of HBsAg responses during or immediately after therapy in such a very small minority is questionable. Moreover, HBsAg responses occur in a comparable proportion of nucleoside/nucleotide-treated patients in the years after therapy. Of course, resistance is not an issue during PEG IFN therapy, but the risk of resistance is much lower with new agents (none recorded after 2 years in previously treatment-naïve entecavir-treated patients; see below). Finally, the level of HBV DNA inhibition that can be achieved with the newer agents, and even with lamivudine, exceeds that which can be achieved with PEG IFN, in some cases by several orders of magnitude.

In HBeAg-negative chronic hepatitis B, a trial of PEG IFN-α2a (180 μg weekly for 48 weeks versus comparison arms of lamivudine monotherapy and of combination therapy) in 564 patients showed that PEG IFN monotherapy resulted at the end of therapy in suppression of HBV DNA by a mean of 4.1 $\log_{10}$ copies/mL, undetectable HBV DNA (<400 copies/mL by PCR) in 63%, and normal ALT in 38%. Although lamivudine monotherapy and combination lamivudine–PEG IFN therapy were both superior to PEG IFN at the end of therapy, no advantage of lamivudine monotherapy or combination therapy was apparent over PEG IFN monotherapy 6 months after therapy—suppression of HBV DNA by a mean of 2.3 $\log_{10}$ copies/mL, undetectable HBV DNA in 19%, and normal ALT in 59%. As was the case for standard IFN therapy in HBeAg-negative patients, after longer periods of post-PEG IFN treatment observation, sustained response rates fell substantially, raising questions about the value of a finite period of PEG IFN in these patients.

ENTECAVIR Entecavir, an oral guanosine analogue polymerase inhibitor, appears to be the most potent of the HBV antivirals and is just as well tolerated as lamivudine. In a 709-subject clinical trial among HBeAg-reactive patients, oral entecavir, 0.5 mg daily, was compared to lamivudine, 100 mg daily. At 48 weeks, entecavir was superior to lamivudine in suppression of HBV DNA, mean 6.9 versus 5.5 $\log_{10}$ copies/mL and in percent with undetectable HBV DNA (<300 copies/mL by PCR), 67% versus 36%; histologic improvement (≥2-point improvement in necroinflammatory HAI score), 72% versus 62%; and normal ALT (68% versus 60%). The two treatments were indistinguishable in percent with HBeAg loss (22% versus 20%) and seroconversion (21% versus 18%). Among patients treated with entecavir for 96 weeks, HBV DNA was undetectable cumulatively in 80% (versus 39% for lamivudine), and HBeAg seroconversions had occurred in 31% (versus 26% for lamivudine). Similarly, in a 638-subject clinical trial among HBeAg-negative patients, at week 48, oral entecavir, 0.5 mg daily, was superior to lamivudine, 100 mg daily, in suppression of HBV DNA, mean 5.0 versus 4.5 $\log_{10}$ copies/mL and in percent with undetectable HBV DNA, 90% versus 72%; histologic improvement, 78% versus 71% and normal

ALT, 68% versus 60%. No resistance mutations were encountered in previously treatment-naïve entecavir-treated patients during 96 weeks of therapy.

Entecavir is also effective against lamivudine-resistant HBV infection. In a trial of 286 lamivudine-resistant patients, entecavir, at a higher daily dose of 1.0 mg, was superior to lamivudine, as measured at week 48, in achieving suppression of HBV DNA (mean 5.1 versus 0.48 $\log_{10}$ copies/mL); undetectable HBV DNA, in 72% versus 19%; normal ALT, in 61% versus 15%; HBeAg loss, in 10% versus 3%; and HBeAg seroconversion, in 8% versus 3%. In this population of lamivudine-experienced patients, however, entecavir resistance did emerge in 7% at 48 weeks and in 9% at 96 weeks. Therefore, entecavir is not as attractive a choice as adefovir (or off-label tenofovir) for patients with lamivudine-resistant hepatitis B.

At the end of 2 years of entecavir therapy in clinical trials among HBeAg-reactive patients, HBsAg seroconversion were observed in 5% (≤2% during the first year). In addition, on-treatment and posttreatment ALT flares are relatively uncommon and relatively mild in entecavir-treated patients.

A comparison of the four antiviral therapies in current use appears in Table 93-3.

COMBINATION THERAPY Although the combination of lamivudine and PEG IFN suppresses HBV DNA more profoundly during therapy than does monotherapy with either drug alone (and is much less likely to be associated with lamivudine resistance), this combination used for a year is no better than a year of PEG IFN in achieving sustained responses. To date, combinations of oral nucleoside/nucleotide agents have not achieved an enhancement in virologic, serologic, or biochemical efficacy over that achieved by the more potent of the combined drugs given individually. On the other hand, combining agents that are not cross-resistant (e.g., lamivudine and adefovir) has the potential to reduce the risk or perhaps even to preempt entirely the emergence of drug resistance. In the future, the treatment paradigm is likely to shift from the current approach of sequential monotherapy to preemptive combination therapy; clinical trials are warranted.

TREATMENT RECOMMENDATIONS Several learned societies and groups of expert physicians have issued treatment recommendations for patients with chronic hepatitis B. Although the recommendations differ slightly, a consensus has emerged on most of the important points (Table 93-4). No treatment is recommended or available for inactive "nonreplicative" hepatitis B carriers (undetectable HBeAg with normal ALT and HBV DNA $<10^4$ copies/mL documented serially over time). In patients with detectable HBeAg and HBV DNA levels $\geq 10^5$ copies/mL, treatment is recommended for those with elevated ALT levels (some authorities require the elevation to be at least twice the upper limit of normal). For those patients with normal ALT (or $\leq 2 \times$ the upper limit of normal), in whom sustained responses are not likely and who would require multiyear therapy, antiviral therapy is not recommended currently. For patients with HBeAg-negative chronic hepatitis B, elevated ALT ($\geq 2 \times$ the upper limit of normal according to some authorities), and HBV DNA $\geq 10^4$ (or 10^5 according to some authorities) copies/mL, antiviral therapy is recommended. If HBV DNA is $<10^4$–10^5 and ALT is normal (or near normal), treatment is not recommended; however, if HBV DNA is $\geq 10^4$ copies/mL but ALT is normal or near normal, some would recommend considering liver biopsy and basing a decision to treat on the presence of substantial liver injury.

For patients with compensated cirrhosis, because antiviral therapy has been shown to retard clinical progression, many authorities would choose to treat regardless of HBeAg status, HBV DNA level and ALT; however, some authorities favor monitoring without therapy for those with HBV DNA levels $<10^4$ copies/mL. For patients with decompensated cirrhosis, treatment is recommended by some authorities regardless of serologic, virologic, and biochemical status; however, other experts do not recommend therapy if HBV DNA is undetectable or low ($<10^5$ copies/mL). At the same time, patients with decompensated cirrhosis should be evaluated as candidates for liver transplantation.

Among the five available drugs for hepatitis B, PEG IFN has supplanted standard IFN. Because entecavir has been proved superior to lamivudine in clinical trials, entecavir has supplanted lamivudine in some countries. PEG IFN, lamivudine, adefovir, and entecavir can each be used as first-line therapy (Table 93-3). PEG IFN requires finite-duration therapy, achieves the highest rate of HBeAg responses after a year of therapy, and does not support viral mutations, but it requires subcutaneous injections and is associated with inconvenience and intolerability. Lamivudine, adefovir, and entecavir require long-term therapy in most patients, and when used alone, lamivudine fosters the emergence of viral mutations, adefovir much less so, and entecavir rarely at all, except in lamivudine-experienced patients. These oral agents do not require injections, are very well tolerated, lead to improved histology in 50–90% of patients, for the most part suppress HBV DNA more profoundly than does PEG IFN, and are effective even in patients who fail to respond to IFN-based therapy. Although these oral agents are less likely to result in HBeAg responses during the first year of therapy, as compared to PEG IFN, treatment with oral agents tends to be extended beyond the first year and, by the end of the second year, yields HBeAg responses (and even HBsAg responses) comparable in frequency to those achieved after 1 year of PEG IFN (and without the associated side effects). Although adefovir is safe, creatinine monitoring is recommended. Substantial experience with lamivudine during pregnancy (see above) has identified no teratogenicity. Standard IFN does not appear to cause congenital anomalies, and data on the safety of PEG IFN during pregnancy are not available. Adefovir during pregnancy has not been associated with birth defects; however, there may be an increased risk of spontaneous abortion.

TABLE 93-3

COMPARISON OF INTERFERON (PEG IFN), LAMIVUDINE, ADEFOVIR, AND ENTECAVIR THERAPY FOR CHRONIC HEPATITIS B[a]

FEATURE	PEG IFN[b]	LAMIVUDINE	ADEFOVIR	ENTECAVIR
Route of administration	Subcutaneous injection	Oral	Oral	Oral
Duration of therapy[c]	48–52 weeks	≥52 weeks	≥48 weeks	≥48 weeks
Tolerability	Poorly tolerated	Well tolerated	Well tolerated; creatinine monitoring recommended	Well tolerated
HBeAg loss 1 year	29–30%	20–33%	23%	22%
HBeAg seroconversion				
1 year Rx	18–20%	16–21%	12%	21%
>1 year Rx	NA	Up to 50% @ 5 years	43% @ 3 years[d]	31% @ 2 years
HBeAg seroconversion if ALT >5 × normal	Not reported	>50%	21%	Not reported
Log_{10} HBV DNA reduction (mean copies/mL)				
HBeAg-reactive	4.5	5.5	Median 3.5–5	6.9
HBeAg-negative	4.1	4.4–4.7	Median 3.5–3.9	5.0
HBV DNA PCR negative (<300–400 copies/mL; <1,000 copies/mL for adefovir) end of year 1				
HBeAg-reactive	10–25%	36–40%	12–21%	69% (80% @ 2 years)
HBeAg-negative	63%	39–73%	51% (79% @ 3 years)	90%
ALT normalization at end of year 1				
HBeAg-reactive	39%	41–75%	58% (81% @ 3 years)	78%
HBeAg-negative	34–38%	62–79%	48% (69% @ 3 years)	78%
HBsAg loss during year 1	0–7%	0–4%	0% (1–2% @ 2 years)	2% (5% @ 2 years)
HBsAg loss after therapy	3–7% after 6 months	23% after 2 years	Not reported	Not reported
Histologic improvement (≥2 point reduction in HAI) at year 1				
HBeAg-reactive	38% 6 months after	51–62%	53%	62%
HBeAg-negative	48% 6 months after	61–66%	64%	70%
Viral resistance	None	15–30% @ 1 year 70% @ 5 years	None @ 1 year 29% @ 5 years	None @ 2 years[e]
Durability of response 4–6 months after therapy[f]				
HBeAg-reactive	Limited data	70–80%	91%	82%
HBeAg-negative	36%	23–35%	Low	48%
Cost (U.S. $) for 1 year	~$18,000	~$2,500	~$6,500	~$8,700[g]

[a]Generally, these comparisons are based on data on each drug tested individually versus placebo in registration clinical trials. With rare exception, these comparisons are not based on head-to-head testing of these drugs, hence relative advantages and disadvantages should be interpreted cautiously.

[b]Although standard interferon α administered daily or three times a week is approved as therapy for chronic hepatitis B, it has been supplanted by pegylated interferon (PEG IFN), which is administered once a week and is more effective. Standard interferon has no advantages over PEG IFN.

[c]Duration of therapy in clinical efficacy trials; use in clinical practice may vary.

[d]Because of a computer-generated randomization error that resulted in misallocation of drug versus placebo during the second year of clinical-trial treatment, the frequency of HBeAg seroconversion beyond the first year is an estimate (Kaplan-Meier analysis) based on the small subset in whom adefovir was administered correctly.

[e]7% during a year of therapy (9% during 2 years) in lamivudine-resistant patients.

[f]In HBeAg-reactive patients, durability of HBeAg seroconversion; in HBeAg-negative patients, durability of virologic (HBV DNA undetectable by PCR) and biochemical (normal ALT) response.

[g]~17,400 for lamivudine-refractory patients.

Note: ALT, alanine aminotransferase; HAI, histologic activity index; HBeAg, hepatitis B e antigen; HBsAg, hepatitis B surface antigen; HBV, hepatitis B virus; NA, not applicable; Rx, therapy; PCR, polymerase chain reaction.

TABLE 93-4

RECOMMENDATIONS FOR TREATMENT OF CHRONIC HEPATITIS B

HBeAg STATUS	CLINICAL	HBV DNA (COPIES/ML)	ALT	RECOMMENDATION
HBeAg-reactive	[a]	$<10^5$	Normal ($\leq$2 × ULN)[b]	No treatment; monitor
	Chronic hepatitis	$\geq 10^5$	Normal ($\leq$2 × ULN)[b, c]	No treatment; current treatment of limited benefit (some suggest liver biopsy and treating if abnormal)
	Chronic hepatitis	$\geq 10^5$	Elevated (>2 × ULN)[b]	Treat[d]
	Cirrhosis compensated	+ or –[e]	Normal or elevated	Treat[e] with oral agents,[f] not PEG IFN
	Cirrhosis decompensated	+ or –[e]	Normal or elevated	Treat[e] with oral agents,[g] not PEG IFN; refer for liver transplantation
HBeAg-negative	[a]	$<10^4$ or 10^5[h]	Normal ($\leq$2 × ULN)[b]	Inactive carrier; treatment not necessary
	Chronic hepatitis	$\geq 10^4$ or 10^5[h]	Normal	Consider liver biopsy; treat if biopsy abnormal
	Chronic hepatitis	$\geq 10^4$ or 10^5[h]	Elevated (>2 × ULN)[b]	Treat[i]
	Cirrhosis compensated	+ or –	Elevated or normal	Treat with oral agents,[j] not PEG IFN (some authorities recommend either following or treating for HBV DNA $<10^4$ copies/mL)
	Cirrhosis decompensated	+ or –	Elevated or normal	Treat with oral agents,[j] not PEG IFN (some authorities would follow without therapy for undetectable HBV DNA; refer for liver transplantation)

[a]Liver disease tends to be mild or inactive clinically; most such patients do not undergo liver biopsy.

[b]In some guidelines, ALT categories are normal or elevated; in others, ALT categories are $\leq$ or > 2 times the upper limit of normal.

[c]Typical pattern in childhood-acquired infection, common in Asian populations.

[d]Any of the oral drugs (lamivudine, adefovir, entecavir) or PEG IFN can be used as first-line therapy (see text); although still used extensively in some parts of the world, lamivudine has been supplanted in some countries as first-line therapy because of its resistance profile. The oral agents, but not PEG IFN, should be used for interferon-refractory/intolerant and immunocompromised patients. PEG IFN is administered weekly by subcutaneous injection for a year; the oral agents are administered daily for at least a year and continued indefinitely or until at least 6 months after HBeAg seroconversion.

[e]Treating or monitoring without therapy are options for patients with HBV DNA $<10^4$ or $<10^5$ copies/mL.

[f]Some authorities would observe without treatment if HBV DNA is undetectable ($<10^4$ copies/mL), while others would treat regardless of the HBV DNA status. Lamivudine monotherapy is not an attractive choice because of its resistance profile.

[g]Some authorities recommend treating regardless of HBV DNA status, while others suggest referring for liver transplantation, without treatment, for those with undetectable HBV DNA ($<10^5$ copies/mL). Lamivudine is a less attractive choice because of its resistance profile. Because the emergence of resistance can lead to loss of antiviral benefit and further deterioration in decompensated cirrhosis, some authorities recommend combination therapy (e.g., lamivudine or entecavir plus adefovir) for patients with decompensated cirrhosis.

[h]Some authorities rely on a cutoff of 10^4 copies/mL, while others choose 10^5 copies/mL.

[i]Because HBeAg seroconversion is not an option, the goal of therapy is to suppress HBV DNA and maintain a normal ALT. Although any of the oral agents or PEG IFN can be used as first-line therapy, lamivudine is less favored because of its resistance profile and the need, in the vast majority of cases, for long-term therapy. PEG IFN is administered by subcutaneous injection weekly for a year (caution is warranted in relying on a 6-month posttreatment interval to define a sustained response; the majority of such responses are lost thereafter). Adefovir and entecavir are administered daily, usually indefinitely or, until, as occurs very rarely, virologic and biochemical responses are accompanied by an HBsAg seroconversion.

[j]Low-resistance regimen favored (i.e., adefovir or entecavir, not lamivudine) indefinitely.

Note: ALT, alanine aminotransferase; HBeAg, hepatitis B e antigen; HBsAg, hepatitis B surface antigen; HBV, hepatitis B virus; ULN, upper limits of normal; PEG IFN, pegylated interferon.

Data on the safety of entecavir during pregnancy have not been published. In general, except perhaps for lamivudine, and until additional data become available, the other antivirals for hepatitis B should be avoided or used with extreme caution during pregnancy.

As noted above, some physicians prefer to begin with PEG IFN, while other physicians and patients prefer oral agents as first-line therapy. For patients with decompensated cirrhosis, the emergence of resistance can result in further deterioration and loss of antiviral effectiveness. Therefore, in this patient subset, the threshold for relying on therapy with a very favorable resistance profile (e.g., entecavir) or on combination therapy (e.g., lamivudine or entecavir along with adefovir or the yet-to-be-approved tenofovir) is low. PEG IFN should not be used in patients with compensated or decompensated cirrhosis.

For patients with end-stage chronic hepatitis B who undergo liver transplantation, reinfection of the new liver is almost universal in the absence of antiviral therapy. The majority of patients become high-level viremic carriers with minimal liver injury. Before the availability of antiviral therapy, an unpredictable proportion experienced severe hepatitis B–related liver injury, sometimes a fulminant-like hepatitis, sometimes a rapid recapitulation of the original severe chronic hepatitis B. Currently, however, prevention of recurrent hepatitis B after liver transplantation has been achieved definitively by *combining* hepatitis B immune globulin with one of the oral nucleoside or nucleotide analogues (lamivudine, adefovir, or entecavir).

Patients with HBV-HIV co-infection can have progressive HBV-associated liver disease and, occasionally, a severe exacerbation of hepatitis B resulting from immunologic reconstitution following highly active antiretroviral therapy. Lamivudine should never be used as monotherapy in patients with HBV-HIV infection, because HIV resistance emerges rapidly to both viruses. Adefovir and entecavir have been used successfully to treat chronic hepatitis B in HBV-HIV co-infected patients. Tenofovir and the combination of tenofovir and emtricitabine in one pill are approved therapies for HIV and represent excellent choices for treating HBV infection in HBV-HIV co-infected patients.

Patients with chronic hepatitis B who undergo cytotoxic chemotherapy for treatment of malignancies experience enhanced HBV replication and viral expression on hepatocyte membranes during chemotherapy coupled with suppression of cellular immunity. When chemotherapy is withdrawn, such patients are at risk for reactivation of hepatitis B, often severe and occasionally fatal. Such rebound reactivation represents restoration of cytolytic T-cell function against a target organ enriched in HBV expression. Preemptive treatment with lamivudine prior to the initiation of chemotherapy has been shown to reduce the risk of such reactivation. In all likelihood, the newer, more potent oral antiviral agents will work as well and with a lower risk of antiviral drug resistance. The optimal duration of antiviral therapy after completion of chemotherapy is not known, but some authorities have suggested 3 months.

NOVEL ANTIVIRALS AND STRATEGIES In addition to the five approved antiviral drugs for hepatitis B, several others are being evaluated in clinical trials, as listed in Table 93-5. Telbivudine, a cytosine analogue, appears to be similar in efficacy to entecavir but slightly less potent in suppressing HBV DNA, and it is associated with low-level resistance (M204I, not M204V mutations). This drug was approved in October 2006. Resistance mutations after 2 years of treatment occur in ~20%. Tenofovir, a nucleotide analogue, is similar to adefovir but more potent in suppressing HBV DNA and inducing HBeAg responses; it is highly active against both wild-type and lamivudine-resistant HBV and active in patients with primary nonresponse to adefovir. Its safety and resistance profile are very favorable as well; in all likelihood, it will supplant adefovir once comparisons in clinical trials are complete. Emtricitabine is a fluorinated cytosine analogue very similar to lamivudine in structure, efficacy, and resistance profile. A combination of emtricitabine and tenofovir is approved for the treatment of HIV infection and is an appealing combination therapy for hepatitis B; however, neither emtricitabine nor the combination are approved yet for hepatitis B. Clevudine is a pyrimidine nucleoside analogue whose potency in the woodchuck model of hepatitis B is higher than that of any other antiviral agent; however, in human trials, maximal HBV DNA suppression has been 5 $\log_{10}$ copies/mL; after clevudine therapy, HBV DNA is much slower to rebound than after withdrawal of other agents. Because direct-acting antivirals have been so successful in the management of chronic hepatitis B, more unconventional approaches—e.g., immunologic or genetic manipulation—are not likely to be competitive. Finally, initial emphasis in the development of antiviral therapy for hepatitis B was placed on monotherapy; however, in the future, with or without additive or synergistic efficacy, combination therapy regimens that prevent resistance are likely to become the norm.

TABLE 93-5

NEW ANTIVIRAL DRUGS BEING DEVELOPED FOR THE TREATMENT OF CHRONIC HEPATITIS B

Telbivudine[a]	Emtricitabine (FTC)
Tenofovir[b]	Clevudine (L-MFAU)

[a]Approved in October 2006.
[b]Active against lamivudine-associated YMDD-mutant HBV. (YMDD, tyrosine-methionine-aspartate-aspartate.)

CHRONIC HEPATITIS D (DELTA HEPATITIS)

Chronic hepatitis D (HDV) may follow acute co-infection with HBV but at a rate no higher than the rate of chronicity of acute hepatitis B. That is, although HDV co-infection can increase the severity of acute hepatitis B, HDV does not increase the likelihood of progression to chronic hepatitis B. When, however, HDV superinfection occurs in a person who is already chronically infected with HBV, long-term HDV infection is the rule and a worsening of the liver disease the expected consequence. Except for severity, chronic hepatitis B plus D has similar clinical and laboratory features to those seen in chronic hepatitis B alone. Relatively severe chronic hepatitis, with or without cirrhosis, is the rule, and mild chronic hepatitis is the exception. Occasionally, mild hepatitis or even, rarely, inactive carriage occurs in patients with chronic hepatitis B plus D, and the disease may become indolent after several years of infection. A distinguishing serologic feature of chronic hepatitis D is the presence in the circulation of antibodies to liver-kidney microsomes (anti-LKM); however, the anti-LKM seen in hepatitis D, anti-LKM3, are directed against uridine diphosphate glucuronosyltransferase and are distinct from anti-LKM1 seen in patients with autoimmune hepatitis and in a subset of patients with chronic hepatitis C (see below). The clinical and laboratory features of chronic HDV infection are summarized in Chap. 92.

℞ Treatment: CHRONIC HEPATITIS D

Management is not well defined. Glucocorticoids are ineffective and are not used. Preliminary experimental trials of IFN-α suggested that conventional doses and durations of therapy lower levels of HDV RNA and aminotransferase activity only transiently during treatment but have no impact on the natural history of the disease. In contrast, high-dose IFN-α (9 million units three times a week) for 12 months may be associated with a sustained loss of HDV replication and clinical improvement in up to 50% of patients. Moreover, the beneficial impact of treatment has been observed to persist for 15 years and to be associated with a reduction in grade of hepatic necrosis and inflammation, reversion of advanced fibrosis (improved stage), and clearance of HDV RNA in some patients. A suggested approach to therapy has been high-dose, long-term IFN for at least a year and, in responders, extension of therapy until HDV RNA and HBsAg clearance. Although experience with PEG IFN in the treatment of chronic hepatitis D is limited, if future studies confirm its equivalence to, or superiority over, standard IFN, PEG IFN is likely to become a more convenient replacement for standard IFN. None of the new antiviral agents for hepatitis B—lamivudine, adefovir, entecavir—are effective in hepatitis D; however, preliminary indications in the woodchuck model of hepatitis B are that clevudine may be. In patients with end-stage liver disease secondary to chronic hepatitis D, liver transplantation has been effective. If hepatitis D recurs in the new liver without the expression of hepatitis B (an unusual serologic profile in immunocompetent persons but common in transplant patients), liver injury is limited. In fact, the outcome of transplantation for chronic hepatitis D is superior to that for chronic hepatitis B.

CHRONIC HEPATITIS C

Regardless of the epidemiologic mode of acquisition of hepatitis C virus (HCV) infection, chronic hepatitis follows acute hepatitis C in 50–70% of cases; chronic infection is common even in those with a return to normal in aminotransferase levels after acute hepatitis C, adding up to an 85% likelihood of chronic HCV infection after acute hepatitis C. Furthermore, in patients with chronic transfusion-associated hepatitis followed for 10–20 years, progression to cirrhosis occurs in about 20%. Such is the case even for patients with relatively clinically mild chronic hepatitis, including those without symptoms, with only modest elevations of aminotransferase activity and with mild chronic hepatitis on liver biopsy. Even in cohorts of well-compensated patients with chronic hepatitis C referred for clinical research trials (no complications of chronic liver disease and with normal hepatic synthetic function), the prevalence of cirrhosis may be as high as 50%. Most cases of hepatitis C are identified initially in asymptomatic patients who have no history of acute hepatitis C, e.g., those discovered while attempting to donate blood, while undergoing lab testing as part of an application for life insurance, or as a result of routine laboratory tests. The source of HCV infection in many of these cases is not defined, although a long-forgotten percutaneous exposure in the remote past can be elicited in a substantial proportion and probably accounts for most infections; most of these infections were acquired in the 1960s and 1970s, coming to clinical attention decades later.

Approximately a third of patients with chronic hepatitis C have normal or near-normal aminotransferase activity; although a third to a half of these patients have chronic hepatitis on liver biopsy, the grade of liver injury and stage of fibrosis tend to be mild in the vast majority. In some cases, more severe liver injury has been reported—even, rarely, cirrhosis, most likely the result of previous histologic activity. Among patients with persistent normal aminotransferase activity sustained over ≥5–10 years, histologic progression has been shown not to occur; however, approximately a quarter of patients with normal aminotransferase activity experience subsequent aminotransferase elevations, and histologic injury can be progressive once abnormal biochemical activity resumes. Therefore, continued clinical monitoring is indicated, even for patients with normal aminotransferase activity.

Despite this substantial rate of progression of chronic hepatitis C, and despite the fact that liver failure can result from end-stage chronic hepatitis C, the long-term prognosis for chronic hepatitis C in a majority of patients is relatively benign. Mortality over 10–20 years among patients with transfusion-associated chronic hepatitis C has been shown not to differ from mortality in a matched population of transfused patients in whom hepatitis C did not develop. Although death in the hepatitis group is more likely to result from liver failure, and although hepatic decompensation may occur in ~15% of such patients over the course of a decade, the majority (almost 60%) of patients remain asymptomatic and well compensated, with no clinical sequelae of chronic liver disease. Overall, then, chronic hepatitis C tends to be very slowly and insidiously progressive, if at all, in the vast majority of patients, while in approximately a quarter of cases, chronic hepatitis C will progress eventually to end-stage cirrhosis. In fact, because HCV infection is so prevalent, and because a proportion of patients progress inexorably to end-stage liver disease, hepatitis C is the most frequent indication for liver transplantation. Referral bias may account for the more severe outcomes described in cohorts of patients reported from tertiary care centers (20-year progression of 20%) versus the more benign outcomes in cohorts of patients monitored from initial blood-product-associated acute hepatitis or identified in community settings (20-year progression of only 4–7%). Still unexplained, however, are the wide ranges in reported progression to cirrhosis, from 2% over 17 years in a population of women with hepatitis C infection acquired from contaminated anti-D immune globulin to 30% over ≤11 years in recipients of contaminated intravenous immune globulin.

Progression of liver disease in patients with chronic hepatitis C has been reported to be more likely in patients with older age, longer duration of infection, advanced histologic stage and grade, genotype 1, more complex quasispecies diversity, increased hepatic iron, concomitant other liver disorders (alcoholic liver disease, chronic hepatitis B, hemochromatosis, α_1-antitrypsin deficiency, and steatohepatitis), HIV infection, and obesity. Among these variables, however, duration of infection appears to be the most important, and some of the others probably reflect disease duration to some extent (e.g., quasispecies diversity, hepatic iron accumulation). No other epidemiologic or clinical features of chronic hepatitis C (e.g., severity of acute hepatitis, level of aminotransferase activity, level of HCV RNA, presence or absence of jaundice during acute hepatitis) are predictive of eventual outcome. Despite the relatively benign nature of chronic hepatitis C over time in many patients, cirrhosis following chronic hepatitis C has been associated with the late development, after several decades, of HCC; the annual rate of HCC in cirrhotic patients with hepatitis C is 1–4%, occurring primarily in patients who have had HCV infection for 30 or more years.

Perhaps the best prognostic indicator in chronic hepatitis C is liver histology; the rate of hepatic fibrosis may be slow, moderate, or rapid. Patients with mild necrosis and inflammation as well as those with limited fibrosis have an excellent prognosis and limited progression to cirrhosis. In contrast, among patients with moderate to severe necroinflammatory activity or fibrosis, including septal or bridging fibrosis, progression to cirrhosis is highly likely over the course of 10–20 years. Among patients with compensated cirrhosis associated with hepatitis C, the 10-year survival is close to 80%; mortality occurs at a rate of 2–6% per year, decompensation at a rate of 4–5% per year, and, as noted above, HCC at a rate of 1–4% per year.

Clinical features of chronic hepatitis C are similar to those described above for chronic hepatitis B. Generally, *fatigue* is the most common symptom; jaundice is rare. Immune complex–mediated extrahepatic complications of chronic hepatitis C are less common than in chronic hepatitis B (despite the fact that assays for immune complexes are often positive in patients with chronic hepatitis C), with the exception of essential mixed cryoglobulinemia (Chap. 92). In addition, chronic hepatitis C has been associated with extrahepatic complications unrelated to immune-complex injury. These include Sjögren's syndrome, lichen planus, and porphyria cutanea tarda.

Laboratory features of chronic hepatitis C are similar to those in patients with chronic hepatitis B, but aminotransferase levels tend to fluctuate more (the characteristic episodic pattern of aminotransferase activity) and to be lower, especially in patients with long-standing disease. An interesting and occasionally confusing finding in patients with chronic hepatitis C is the presence of autoantibodies. Rarely, patients with autoimmune hepatitis (see below) and hyperglobulinemia have false-positive immunoassays for anti-HCV. On the other hand, some patients with serologically confirmable chronic hepatitis C have circulating anti-LKM. These antibodies are anti-LKM1, as seen in patients with autoimmune hepatitis type 2 (see below), and are directed against a 33-amino-acid sequence of cytochrome P450 IID6. The occurrence of anti-LKM1 in some patients with chronic hepatitis C may result from the partial sequence homology between the epitope recognized by anti-LKM1 and two segments of the HCV polyprotein. In addition, the presence of this autoantibody in some patients with chronic hepatitis C suggests that autoimmunity may be playing a role in the pathogenesis of chronic hepatitis C.

Histopathologic features of chronic hepatitis C, especially those that distinguish hepatitis C from hepatitis B, are described in Chap. 92.

℞ Treatment: CHRONIC HEPATITIS C

Therapy for chronic hepatitis C has evolved substantially in the decade and a half since IFN-α was introduced for this indication. When first approved, IFN-α was administered via subcutaneous injection three times a week for 6 months but achieved a sustained virologic response (a reduction of HCV RNA to undetectable levels by PCR when measured ≥6 months after completion of therapy) below 10%. Doubling the duration of therapy—but not increasing the dose or changing IFN preparations—increased the sustained virologic response rate to ~20%, and addition to the regimen of daily ribavirin, an oral guanosine nucleoside, increased sustained virologic responses to 40%. When used alone, ribavirin is ineffective and does not reduce HCV RNA levels, but ribavirin enhances the efficacy of IFN by reducing the likelihood of virologic relapse after the achievement of an end-treatment response (response measured during, and maintained to the end of, treatment). Proposed mechanisms to explain the role of ribavirin include subtle direct reduction of HCV replication, inhibition of host inosine monophosphate dehydrogenase activity (and associated depletion of guanosine pools), immune modulation, and induction of virologic mutational catastrophe.

Many important lessons about antiviral therapy for chronic hepatitis C were learned from the experience with IFN monotherapy and combination IFN-ribavirin therapy. Even in the absence of biochemical and virologic responses, histologic improvement occurs in approximately three-quarters of all treated patients. In chronic hepatitis C, unlike the case in hepatitis B, responses to therapy are not accompanied by transient, acute hepatitis-like aminotransferase elevations. Instead, ALT levels fall precipitously during therapy. Up to 90% of virologic responses are achieved within the first 12 weeks of therapy; responses thereafter are rare. Most relapses occur within the first 12 weeks after treatment. Sustained virologic responses are very durable; normal ALT, improved histology, and absence of HCV RNA in serum and liver have been documented 5–6 years after successful therapy, and "relapses" 2 years after sustained responses are almost unheard of. Thus, sustained virologic responses to antiviral therapy of chronic hepatitis C are tantamount to cures.

Patient variables that tend to correlate with sustained virologic responsiveness to IFN include favorable genotype (genotypes 2 and 3 as opposed to genotypes 1 and 4), low baseline HCV RNA level (<2 million copies/mL, which is equivalent to ~800,000 international units/mL, the current convention of quantitation), histologically mild hepatitis and minimal fibrosis, age <40, absence of obesity, and female gender. Patients with cirrhosis can respond, but they are less likely to do so. Studies of combination IFN-ribavirin therapy showed conclusively that in patients with genotype 1, therapy should last a full year, while in those with genotypes 2 and 3, a 6-month course of therapy suffices. The response rate in African Americans is disappointingly low for reasons that remain obscure. Finally, the likelihood of a sustained response is best if adherence to the treatment regimen is high, i.e., if patients receive ≥80% of the IFN and ribavirin doses and if they continue treatment for ≥80% of the anticipated duration of therapy. Other variables reported to correlate with increased responsiveness include brief duration of infection, low HCV quasispecies diversity, immunocompetence, and low liver iron levels. High levels of HCV RNA, more histologically advanced liver disease, and high quasispecies diversity all go hand in hand with advanced duration of infection, which may be the single most important variable determining IFN responsiveness. The ironic fact, then, is that patients whose disease is least likely to progress are the ones *most* likely to respond to interferon and vice versa. Finally, among patients with genotype 1b, responsiveness to IFN is enhanced in those with amino-acid-substitution mutations in the nonstructural protein 5A gene.

Side effects of IFN therapy are described above in the section on treatment of chronic hepatitis B. The most pronounced side effect of ribavirin therapy is hemolysis; a reduction in hemoglobin of up to 2–3 g or in hematocrit of 5–10% can be anticipated. A small, unpredictable proportion of patients experience profound, brisk hemolysis, resulting in symptomatic anemia; therefore, close monitoring of blood counts is crucial, and ribavirin should be avoided in patients with anemia or hemoglobinopathies and in patients with coronary artery disease or cerebrovascular disease, in whom anemia can precipitate an ischemic event. When symptomatic anemia occurs, ribavirin dose reductions or addition of erythropoietin to boost red blood cell levels may be required. In addition, ribavirin, which is renally excreted, should not be used in patients with renal insufficiency; the drug is teratogenic, precluding its use during pregnancy and mandating the scrupulous use of efficient contraception during therapy.

Ribavirin can also cause nasal and chest congestion, pruritus, and precipitation of gout. Combination IFN-ribavirin therapy is more difficult to tolerate than IFN monotherapy. In one large clinical trial of combination therapy versus monotherapy, among those in the 1-year treatment group, 21% of the combination group (but only 14% of the monotherapy group) had to discontinue treatment, while 26% of the combination group (but only 9% of the monotherapy group) required dose reductions.

Studies of viral kinetics have shown that despite a virion half-life in serum of only 2–3 h, the level of HCV is maintained by a high replication rate of 10^{12} hepatitis C virions per day. IFN-α blocks virion production or release with an efficacy that increases with increasing drug doses; moreover, the calculated death rate for infected cells during IFN therapy is inversely related to viral load; patients with the most rapid death rate of infected hepatocytes are more likely to achieve undetectable HCV RNA at 3 months; achieving this landmark is predictive of a subsequent sustained response. Therefore, to achieve rapid viral clearance from serum and the liver, *high-dose induction therapy* has been advocated. In practice, however, high-dose induction therapy has not yielded higher sustained response rates.

TREATMENT OF CHOICE For the treatment of chronic hepatitis C, standard IFNs have now been supplanted by PEG IFNs. These have elimination times up to sevenfold longer than standard IFNs, i.e., a substantially longer half-life, and achieve prolonged concentrations, permitting administration once (rather than three times) a week. Instead of the frequent drug peaks (linked to side effects) and troughs (when drug is absent) associated with frequent administration of short-acting IFNs, administration of PEG IFNs results in drug concentrations that are more stable and sustained over time. Once-a-week PEG IFN monotherapy is twice as effective as monotherapy with its standard IFN counterpart, approaches the efficacy of combination standard IFN plus ribavirin, and is as well tolerated as standard IFNs, without more difficult-to-manage thrombocytopenia and leukopenia than standard IFNs. The current standard of care, however, is a combination of PEG IFN plus ribavirin.

Two PEG IFNs are available: PEG IFN-α2b and α2a. In the registration trial for PEG IFN-α2b plus ribavirin, the best regimen was 48 weeks of 1.5 μg/kg of PEG IFN once a week plus 800 mg of ribavirin daily. A post hoc analysis suggested that weight-based dosing of ribavirin would have been more effective than the fixed 800-mg dose used in the study. In the first registration trial for PEG IFN-α2a plus ribavirin, the best regimen was 48 weeks of 180 μg of PEG IFN plus 1000 mg (for patients <75 kg) to 1200 mg (for patients ≥75 kg) of ribavirin. Sustained virologic responses of 54 and 56% were reported in these two studies, respectively. A subsequent study of PEG IFN-α2a plus ribavirin showed that, for patients with genotypes 2 and 3, a duration of 6 months and a ribavirin dose of 800 mg were sufficient. Among the three studies, for patients in the optimal treatment arm, sustained response rates for patients with genotype 1 were

42–51% and for patients with genotypes 2 and 3 rates were 76–82%. Subsequent studies have shown that, in patients with genotypes 2 and 3, if HCV RNA is undetectable at 4 weeks ("rapid virologic response"), the total duration of therapy required to achieve a sustained virologic response can be as short as 12–16 weeks, especially for patients with genotype 2 (less so for those with genotype 3). These clinical trials of abbreviated treatment, however, were conducted with full, weight-based ribavirin doses rather than the current convention of uniform, 800-mg flat dosing; studies of abbreviated-duration therapy with flat ribavirin dosing in patients with genotypes 2 and 3 are awaited. Between genotypes 2 and 3, genotype 3 is somewhat more refractory, and some authorities would extend therapy for a full 48 weeks in patients with genotype 3, especially if they have advanced hepatic fibrosis or cirrhosis and/or high-level HCV RNA.

In the initial registration trials for combination PEG IFN plus ribavirin, both combination PEG IFN regimens were compared to standard IFN-α2b plus ribavirin. Side effects of the combination PEG IFN-α2b regimen were comparable to those for the combination standard IFN regimen; however, when the combination PEG IFN-α2a regimen was compared to the combination standard IFN-α2b regimen, flulike symptoms and depression were less common in the combination PEG IFN group. Although the two combination PEG IFN regimens were not tested head-to-head, and although ascertainment of side effects differed between studies of the two drugs, when each was tested against standard IFN-α2b plus ribavirin, combination PEG IFN-α2a plus ribavirin appeared to be better tolerated. Recommended doses for the two PEG IFNs plus ribavirin and other comparisons between the two therapies are shown in Table 93-6.

Unless ribavirin is contraindicated (see above), combination PEG IFN plus ribavirin is the recommended course of therapy—24 weeks for genotypes 2 and 3 and 48 weeks for genotype 1. Measurement of quantitative HCV RNA levels at 12 weeks is helpful in guiding therapy; if a 2-$\log_{10}$ drop in HCV RNA has not been achieved by this time, chances for a sustained virologic response are negligible. If the 12-week HCV RNA has fallen by two $\log_{10}$ ("early virologic response"), the chances for a sustained virologic response at the end of therapy are approximately two-thirds; if the 12-week HCV RNA is undetectable, the chances for a sustained virologic response exceed 80%. If the goal of therapy is sustained virologic response, failure to achieve a 12-week 2-$\log_{10}$ drop in HCV RNA may be used as a signal to discontinue therapy, especially in those who do not tolerate the drugs well. Still, conceivably, some may achieve histologic benefit in the absence of a virologic response, and some clinicians choose to continue therapy even in the absence of a 2-$\log_{10}$ HCV RNA reduction at 12 weeks. Studies are underway to determine whether, even in the absence of a virologic response, maintenance therapy with PEG IFN can slow histologic and clinical progression of hepatitis C.

Studies have suggested that the frequency of sustained virologic responses to PEG IFN/ribavirin therapy can be increased by raising the dose of ribavirin

TABLE 93-6

PEGYLATED INTERFERON-α-2a AND α-2b FOR CHRONIC HEPATITIS C

	PEG IFN-α2b	PEG IFN-α2a
PEG size	12 kD linear	40 kD branched
Elimination half-life	54 h	65 h
Clearance	725 mL/h	60 mL/h
Best dose monotherapy[a]	1.0 μg/kg (weight-based)	180 μg
Best dose combination therapy	1.5 μg/kg (weight-based)	180 μg
Storage	Room temperature	Refrigerated
Ribavirin dose		
Genotype 1	800 mg[b]	1000–1200 mg[c]
Genotype 2/3	800 mg	800 mg
Duration of therapy		
Genotype 1	48 weeks	48 weeks
Genotype 2/3	48 weeks[d]	24 weeks
Efficacy of combination Rx[e]	54%	56%
Genotype 1	42%	46–51%
Genotype 2/3	82%	76–78%

[a]Reserved for patients in whom ribavirin is contraindicated or not tolerated.

[b]In the registration trial for PEG IFN-α2b plus ribavirin, the optimal regimen was 1.5 μg of PEG IFN plus 800 mg of ribavirin; however, a post hoc analysis of this study suggested that higher ribavirin doses are better. In addition, data from the study of PEG IFN-α2a supported weight-based dosing, 1000 mg (for patients weighing <75 kg) and 1200 mg (for patients weighing ≥75 kg) for genotype 1. Therefore, the higher ribavirin doses are recommended for both types of PEG IFN in patients with genotype 1.

[c]1000 mg for patients weighing <75 kg; 1200 mg for patients weighing ≥75 kg.

[d]In the registration trial for PEG IFN-α2b plus ribavirin, all patients were treated for 48 weeks; however, data from other trials of standard interferons and the other PEG IFN demonstrated that 24 weeks suffices for patients with genotypes 2 and 3. For patients with genotype 3 who have advanced fibrosis/cirrhosis and/or high-level HCV RNA, a full 48 weeks is preferable.

[e]To date, direct, head-to-head comparisons of the two PEG IFNs have not been reported. Attempts to compare the two PEG IFN preparations based on the results of registration clinical trials are confounded by differences between trials of the two agents in methodological details (different ribavirin doses, different methods for recording depression and other side effects) and study-population composition (different proportion with bridging fibrosis/cirrhosis, proportion from the United States versus international, mean weight, proportion with genotype 1, and proportion with high-level HCV RNA).

Note: HCV RNA, hepatitis C virus RNA; PEG, polyethylene glycol; PEG IFN, pegylated interferon.

(if tolerated or supplemented by erythropoietin) or by tailoring treatment based on viral response to prolong the duration of viral clearance before discontinuing therapy, i.e., extending therapy from 48 to 72 weeks for patients with genotype 1 and a slow virologic response, i.e., those whose HCV RNA has not fallen rapidly to undetectable levels within 4 weeks (absence of "rapid virologic

TABLE 93-7

INDICATIONS AND RECOMMENDATIONS FOR ANTIVIRAL THERAPY OF CHRONIC HEPATITIS C

Standard Indications for Therapy

Detectable HCV RNA (with or without elevated ALT)

Portal/bridging fibrosis or moderate to severe hepatitis on liver biopsy

Retreatment Recommended

Relapsers after a previous course of standard interferon monotherapy or combination standard interferon/ribavirin therapy

A course of PEG IFN plus ribavirin

Nonresponders to a previous course of standard IFN monotherapy or combination standard IFN/ribavirin therapy

A course of PEG IFN plus ribavirin—more likely to achieve a sustained virologic response in Caucasian patients without previous ribavirin therapy, with low baseline HCV RNA levels, with a 2-$\log_{10}$ reduction in HCV RNA during previous therapy, with genotypes 2 and 3, and without reduction in ribavirin dose

Antiviral Therapy Not Recommended Routinely but Management Decisions Made on an Individual Basis

Children (age <18 years)

Age >60

Mild hepatitis on liver biopsy

Long-Term Maintenance Therapy Recommended

Cutaneous vasculitis and glomerulonephritis associated with chronic hepatitis C

Long-Term Maintenance Therapy being Assessed in Clinical Trials

Relapsers

Nonresponders

Antiviral Therapy Not Recommended

Decompensated cirrhosis

Pregnancy (teratogenicity of ribavirin)

Therapeutic Regimens

First-line treatment: PEG IFN subcutaneously once a week plus daily ribavirin orally

HCV genotypes 1 and 4–48 weeks of therapy

PEG IFN-α2a 180 μg weekly plus ribavirin 1000 mg/d (weight <75 kg) to 1200 mg/d (weight ≥75 kg) or

PEG IFN-α2b 1.5 μg/kg weekly plus ribavirin 800 mg/d (the dose used in registration clinical trials, but the higher, weight-based ribavirin doses above are recommended for both types of PEG IFN)

HCV genotypes 2 and 3–24 weeks of therapy

PEG IFN-α2a 180 μg weekly plus ribavirin 800 mg/d or

PEG IFN-α2b 1.5 μg/kg weekly plus ribavirin 800 mg/d (for patients with genotype 3 who have advanced fibrosis and/or high-level HCV RNA, a full 48 weeks of therapy may be preferable)

Alternative regimen: PEG IFN (α2a 180 μg or α2b 1.0 μg/kg) subcutaneously once a week (primarily for patients in whom ribavirin is contraindicated or not tolerated) for 24 (genotypes 2 and 3) or 48 (genotypes 1 and 4) weeks

For HCV-HIV co-infected patients: 48 weeks, regardless of genotype, of weekly PEG IFN-α2a (180 μg) or PEG IFN-α2b (1.5 μg/kg) plus a daily ribavirin dose of at least 600–800 mg, up to full weight-based 1000–1200 mg dosing if tolerated

Features Associated with Reduced Responsiveness

Genotype 1

High-level HCV RNA (>2 million copies/mL or >800,000 IU/mL)

Advanced fibrosis (bridging fibrosis, cirrhosis)

Long-duration disease

Age >40

High HCV quasispecies diversity

Immunosuppression

African American

Obesity

Hepatic steatosis

Reduced adherence (lower drug doses and reduced duration of therapy)

Note: ALT, alanine aminotransferase; HCV, hepatitis C virus; IFN, interferon; PEG IFN, pegylated interferon; IU, international units (1 IU/mL is equivalent to ~2.5 copies/mL).

response"). Confirmatory studies are awaited. Tailoring therapy based on the kinetics of HCV RNA reduction has also been applied to abbreviating the duration of therapy in patients with genotype 1. The results of several clinical trials suggest that, in genotype 1 patients with a 4-week rapid virologic response, but only in the subset with a baseline low level of HCV RNA, 24 weeks of therapy with PEG IFN and weight-based ribavirin suffices, yielding sustained response rates comparable to those achieved with 48 weeks of therapy. Again, although regulatory agencies in Europe have adopted this treatment approach, broad adoption of this approach awaits confirmatory studies.

INDICATIONS FOR ANTIVIRAL THERAPY

Patients with chronic hepatitis C who have detectable HCV RNA in serum and chronic hepatitis of at least moderate grade and stage (portal or bridging fibrosis) are candidates for antiviral therapy with PEG IFN plus ribavirin. Most authorities recommend 800 mg of ribavirin for patients with genotypes 2 and 3 and weight-based 1000–1200 mg for patients with genotype 1 (and 4) for both types of PEG IFN, unless ribavirin is contraindicated (Table 93-7). Although patients with persistently normal ALT activity tend not to progress histologically, they respond to antiviral therapy just as well as do patients with elevated ALT levels; therefore, while observation without therapy is an option, such patients are potential candidates for antiviral therapy. Therapy with IFN has been shown to improve survival and complication-free survival and to slow progression of fibrosis.

Prior to therapy, HCV genotype should be determined, and the genotype dictates the duration of therapy: 1 year (48 weeks) for patients with genotype 1; 6 months (24 weeks) for those with genotypes 2 and 3;

and potentially only 12–16 weeks for patients with genotype 2 whose HCV RNA becomes undetectable within 4 weeks. As noted above, the absence of a 2-$\log_{10}$ drop in HCV RNA at week 12 (an *early virologic response*) weighs heavily against the likelihood of a sustained virologic response even if therapy is continued for the remainder of the planned full year. Therefore, measuring HCV RNA at baseline and at 12 weeks is recommended routinely, especially for patients with genotype 1. The consensus view is that therapy can be discontinued if an early virologic response is not achieved; however, histologic benefit may occur even in the absence of a virologic response. In addition, if current trials show that maintenance therapy can slow the progression of chronic hepatitis C, early virologic nonresponders may be identified as candidates for maintenance therapy; the results of these trials are awaited. Although response rates are lower in patients with certain pretreatment variables, selection for treatment should not be based on symptoms, genotype, HCV RNA level, mode of acquisition of hepatitis C, or advanced hepatic fibrosis. Patients with cirrhosis can respond and should not be excluded as candidates for therapy.

Patients who have relapsed after a course of IFN monotherapy are candidates for retreatment with PEG IFN plus ribavirin (i.e., a more effective treatment regimen is required). For nonresponders to a prior course of IFN monotherapy, retreatment with IFN monotherapy or combination IFN plus ribavirin therapy is unlikely to achieve a sustained virologic response; however, a trial of combination PEG IFN plus ribavirin may be worthwhile. End-treatment virologic responses as high as 40% can occur in this setting, but a sustained virologic response is the outcome in <15–20% of patients. Sustained virologic responses to retreatment of nonresponders are more frequent in those who had never received ribavirin in the past, those with genotypes 2 and 3, those with low pretreatment HCV RNA levels, and noncirrhotics, but less frequent in African Americans, those who failed to achieve a substantial reduction in HCV RNA during their previous course of therapy, and those who required ribavirin-dose reductions. Potential approaches to improving responsiveness to PEG IFN/ribavirin in prior nonresponders include longer duration of treatment; higher doses of either PEG IFN, ribavirin, or both; and switching to a different IFN preparation. However, none of these approaches is of proven efficacy.

Early treatment is indicated for persons with acute hepatitis C (Chap. 92). In patients with biochemically and histologically mild chronic hepatitis C, the rate of progression is slow, and monitoring without therapy is an option; however, such patients respond just as well to combination PEG IFN plus ribavirin therapy as those with elevated ALT and more histologically severe hepatitis. Therefore, therapy for these patients should be considered and the decision made based on such factors as patient motivation, genotype, stage of fibrosis, age, and comorbid conditions. A pretreatment liver biopsy to assess histologic grade and stage provides substantial information about progression of hepatitis C in the past and has prognostic value for future progression. As therapy has improved for patients with a broad range of histologic severity, and as noninvasive laboratory markers of fibrosis have gained popularity, some authorities have placed less value on pretreatment liver biopsies. On the other hand, serum markers of fibrosis are not considered sufficiently accurate, and histologic findings provide important prognostic information to physician and patient. Therefore, a pretreatment liver biopsy is still recommended in most cases.

Patients with compensated cirrhosis can respond to therapy, although their likelihood of a sustained response is lower than in noncirrhotics. Whether survival is improved after successful antiviral therapy in cirrhotics is controversial. Similarly, although several retrospective studies have suggested that antiviral therapy in cirrhotics with chronic hepatitis C reduces the frequency of HCC, less advanced disease in the treated cirrhotics, not treatment itself, may have accounted for the reduced frequency of HCC observed in the treated cohort; prospective studies to address this question are in progress. Patients with decompensated cirrhosis are not candidates for IFN-based antiviral therapy but should be referred for liver transplantation. Some liver transplantation centers have evaluated progressively escalated, low-dose antiviral therapy in an attempt to eradicate hepatitis C viremia prior to transplantation; however, data supporting this approach are limited. After liver transplantation, recurrent hepatitis C is the rule, and the pace of disease progression is more accelerated than in immunocompetent patients. Current therapy with PEG IFN and ribavirin is unsatisfactory in most patients, but attempts to minimize immunosuppression are beneficial. The cutaneous and renal vasculitis of HCV-associated essential mixed cryoglobulinemia (Chap. 92) may respond to antiviral therapy, but sustained responses are rare after discontinuation of therapy; therefore, prolonged, perhaps indefinite, therapy is recommended in this group. Anecdotal reports suggest that antiviral therapy may be effective in porphyria cutanea tarda or lichen planus associated with hepatitis C.

In patients with HCV/HIV co-infection, hepatitis C is more progressive and severe than in HCV-monoinfected patients. Although patients with HCV/HIV co-infection respond to antiviral therapy for hepatitis C, they do not respond as well as patients with HCV infection alone. Four large national and international trials of antiviral therapy among patients with HCV/HIV co-infection have shown that PEG IFN (both α2a and α2b) plus ribavirin (daily doses ranging from flat-dosed 600–800 mg to weight-based 1000/1200 mg) is superior to standard IFN regimens; however, sustained response rates were lower than in HCV-monoinfected patients, ranging from 14 to 38% for patients with genotypes 1 and 4 and from 44 to 73% for patients with genotypes 2 and 3. In the three largest trials, all patients, including those with genotypes 2 and 3, were treated for a full 48 weeks. In addition, tolerability of therapy was lower than in HCV-monoinfected patients; therapy was discontinued because of side effects in 12–39% of patients in these clinical trials. Based on these trials, weekly PEG IFN plus daily ribavirin at a daily dose of at least 600–800 mg, up to full weight-based doses if tolerated, is recommended for a full 48 weeks, regardless of genotype. An alternative recommendation for ribavirin doses was issued by a European Consensus Conference and consisted of standard, weight-based 1000–1200 mg for genotypes 1 and 4, but 800 mg for genotypes 2 and 3. In HCV/HIV-infected patients, ribavirin can potentiate the toxicity of—and should not be used together with—didanosine.

Persons with a history of injection-drug use and alcoholism can be treated successfully for chronic hepatitis C, preferably in conjunction with drug and alcohol treatment programs. Because ribavirin is excreted renally, patients with end-stage renal disease, including those undergoing dialysis (which does not clear ribavirin), are not candidates for ribavirin therapy. Rare reports suggest that reduced-dose ribavirin can be used, but the frequency of anemia is very high and data on efficacy are limited. In addition, the manufacturer of PEG IFN-α2a recommends a dose reduction from 180 to 135 μg daily in patients with renal failure. Neither the optimal regimen nor the efficacy of therapy is established in this population.

NOVEL ANTIVIRALS Among the new approaches to antiviral therapy are direct antivirals (so-called specifically targeted antiviral therapy), including orally administered polymerase and protease inhibitors. For example, in preliminary studies among small numbers of subjects, one of the protease inhibitors being investigated has been shown to suppress HCV RNA by 4 $\log_{10}$ in 14 days when used as monotherapy, to suppress HCV RNA by 5.5 $\log_{10}$ in 14 days when combined with PEG IFN injections, and to suppress HCV RNA to undetectable levels in 12 of 12 subjects treated for 28 days when combined with PEG IFN and ribavirin. Because resistance to these oral agents used alone has been both anticipated and observed, polymerase and protease inhibitors are being evaluated in combinations with PEG IFN (± ribavirin) to preempt the emergence of resistance. Potentially, in the future, combinations of specifically targeted antiviral agents will be used in drug cocktails that may replace IFN-based regimens entirely.

AUTOIMMUNE HEPATITIS

DEFINITION

Autoimmune hepatitis is a chronic disorder characterized by continuing hepatocellular necrosis and inflammation, usually with fibrosis, which can progress to cirrhosis and liver failure. When fulfilling criteria of severity, this type of chronic hepatitis, when untreated, may have a 6-month mortality of as high as 40%. Based on contemporary estimates of the natural history of treated autoimmune hepatitis, the 10-year survival is 80–90%. The prominence of extrahepatic features of autoimmunity as well as seroimmunologic abnormalities in this disorder supports an autoimmune process in its pathogenesis; this concept is reflected in the labels *lupoid*, *plasma cell*, or *autoimmune hepatitis*. Autoantibodies and other typical features of autoimmunity, however, do not occur in all cases; among the broader categories of "idiopathic" or cryptogenic chronic hepatitis, many, perhaps the majority, are probably autoimmune in origin. Cases in which hepatotropic viruses, metabolic/genetic derangements, and hepatotoxic drugs have been excluded represent a spectrum of heterogeneous liver disorders of unknown cause, a proportion of which are most likely autoimmune hepatitis.

IMMUNOPATHOGENESIS

The weight of evidence suggests that the progressive liver injury in patients with autoimmune hepatitis is the result of a cell-mediated immunologic attack directed against liver cells. In all likelihood, predisposition to autoimmunity is inherited, while the liver specificity of this injury is triggered by environmental (e.g., chemical or viral) factors. For example, patients have been described in whom apparently self-limited cases of acute hepatitis A, B, or C led to autoimmune hepatitis, presumably because of genetic susceptibility or predisposition. Evidence to support an autoimmune pathogenesis in this type of hepatitis includes the following: (1) In the liver, the histopathologic lesions are composed predominantly of cytotoxic T cells and plasma cells; (2) circulating autoantibodies (nuclear, smooth muscle, thyroid, etc.; see below), rheumatoid factor, and hyperglobulinemia are common; (3) other autoimmune disorders—such as thyroiditis, rheumatoid arthritis, autoimmune hemolytic anemia, ulcerative colitis, membranoproliferative glomerulonephritis, juvenile diabetes mellitus, celiac disease, and Sjögren's syndrome—occur with increased frequency in patients who have autoimmune hepatitis and in their relatives; (4) histocompatibility haplotypes associated with autoimmune diseases, such as HLA-B1, -B8, -DR3, and -DR4 as well as extended haplotype DRB1 alleles, are common in patients with autoimmune hepatitis; and (5) this type of chronic hepatitis is responsive to glucocorticoid/immunosuppressive therapy, effective in a variety of autoimmune disorders.

Cellular immune mechanisms appear to be important in the pathogenesis of autoimmune hepatitis. In vitro studies have suggested that in patients with this disorder, lymphocytes are capable of becoming sensitized to hepatocyte membrane proteins and of destroying liver cells. Abnormalities of immunoregulatory control over cytotoxic lymphocytes (impaired regulatory CD4+CD25+ T cell influences) may play a role as well. Studies of genetic predisposition to autoimmune hepatitis demonstrate that certain haplotypes are associated with the disorder, as enumerated above. The precise triggering factors, genetic influences, and cytotoxic and immunoregulatory mechanisms involved in this type of liver injury remain poorly defined.

Intriguing clues into the pathogenesis of autoimmune hepatitis come from the observation that circulating autoantibodies are prevalent in patients with this disorder. Among the autoantibodies described in these patients are antibodies to nuclei [so-called antinuclear antibodies (ANAs), primarily in a homogeneous pattern] and smooth muscle (so-called anti-smooth-muscle antibodies, directed at actin), anti-LKM (see below), antibodies to "soluble liver antigen/liver pancreas antigen" (directed against a uracil-guanine-adenine transfer RNA suppressor protein), as well as antibodies to the liver-specific asialoglycoprotein receptor (or "hepatic lectin") and other hepatocyte membrane proteins. Although some of these provide helpful diagnostic markers, their involvement in the pathogenesis of autoimmune hepatitis has not been established.

Humoral immune mechanisms have been shown to play a role in the extrahepatic manifestations of autoimmune and idiopathic hepatitis. Arthralgias, arthritis, cutaneous vasculitis, and glomerulonephritis occurring in patients with autoimmune hepatitis appear to be mediated by the deposition of circulating immune complexes in affected tissue vessels, followed by complement activation, inflammation, and tissue injury. While specific viral antigen-antibody complexes can be identified in acute and chronic viral hepatitis, the nature of the immune complexes in autoimmune hepatitis has not been defined.

Many of the *clinical features* of autoimmune hepatitis are similar to those described for chronic viral hepatitis. The onset of disease may be insidious or abrupt; the disease may present initially like, and be confused with, acute viral hepatitis; a history of recurrent bouts of what had been labeled *acute hepatitis* is not uncommon. A subset of patients with autoimmune hepatitis has distinct features. Such patients are predominantly young to middle-aged women with marked hyperglobulinemia and high-titer circulating ANAs. This is the group with positive lupus erythematosus (LE) preparations (initially labeled "lupoid" hepatitis) in whom other autoimmune features are common. Fatigue, malaise, anorexia, amenorrhea, acne, arthralgias, and jaundice are common. Occasionally arthritis, maculopapular eruptions (including cutaneous vasculitis), erythema nodosum, colitis, pleurisy, pericarditis, anemia, azotemia, and sicca syndrome (keratoconjunctivitis, xerostomia) occur. In some patients, complications of cirrhosis, such as ascites and edema (associated with hypoalbuminemia), encephalopathy, hypersplenism, coagulopathy, or variceal bleeding may bring the patient to initial medical attention.

The course of autoimmune hepatitis may be variable. In those with mild disease or limited histologic lesions (e.g., piecemeal necrosis without bridging), progression to cirrhosis is limited. In those with severe symptomatic autoimmune hepatitis (aminotransferase levels >10 times normal, marked hyperglobulinemia, "aggressive" histologic lesions—bridging necrosis or multilobular collapse, cirrhosis), the 6-month mortality without therapy may be as high as 40%. Such severe disease accounts for only 20% of cases; the natural history of milder disease is variable, often accentuated by spontaneous remissions and exacerbations. Especially poor prognostic signs include the presence histologically of multilobular collapse at the time of initial presentation and failure of the bilirubin to improve after 2 weeks of therapy. Death may result from hepatic failure, hepatic coma, other complications of cirrhosis (e.g., variceal hemorrhage), and intercurrent infection. In patients with established cirrhosis, HCC may be a late complication but occurs less frequently than in cirrhosis associated with viral hepatitis.

Laboratory features of autoimmune hepatitis are similar to those seen in chronic viral hepatitis. Liver biochemical tests are invariably abnormal but may not correlate with the clinical severity or histopathologic features in individual cases. Many patients with autoimmune hepatitis have normal serum bilirubin, alkaline phosphatase, and globulin levels with only minimal aminotransferase elevations. Serum AST and ALT levels are increased and fluctuate in the range of 100–1000 units. In severe cases, the serum bilirubin level is moderately elevated [51–171 μmol/L (3–10 mg/dL)]. Hypoalbuminemia occurs in patients with very active or advanced disease. Serum alkaline phosphatase levels may be moderately elevated or near normal. In a small proportion of patients, marked elevations of alkaline phosphatase activity occur; in such patients, clinical and laboratory features overlap with those of primary biliary cirrhosis. The prothrombin time is often prolonged, particularly late in the disease or during active phases.

Hypergammaglobulinemia (>2.5 g/dL) is common in autoimmune hepatitis. Rheumatoid factor is common as well. As noted above, circulating autoantibodies are also prevalent. The most characteristic are ANAs in a homogeneous staining pattern. Smooth-muscle antibodies are less specific, seen just as frequently in chronic viral hepatitis. Because of the high levels of globulins achieved in the circulation of some patients with autoimmune hepatitis, occasionally the globulins may bind nonspecifically in solid-phase binding immunoassays for viral antibodies. This has been recognized most commonly in tests for antibodies to hepatitis C virus, as noted above. In fact, studies of autoantibodies in autoimmune hepatitis have led to the recognition of new categories of autoimmune hepatitis. *Type I autoimmune hepatitis* is the classic syndrome occurring in young women, associated with marked hyperglobulinemia, lupoid features, circulating ANAs, and HLA-DR3 or HLA-DR4. Also associated with type I autoimmune hepatitis are autoantibodies against actin as well as atypical perinuclear antineutrophilic cytoplasmic antibodies (pANCA).

Type II autoimmune hepatitis, often seen in children, more common in Mediterranean populations, and linked to HLA-DRB1 and HLA-DQB1 haplotypes, is associated not with ANA but with anti-LKM. Actually, anti-LKM represent a heterogeneous group of antibodies. In type II autoimmune hepatitis, the antibody is anti-LKM1, directed against cytochrome P450 2D6. This is the same anti-LKM seen in some patients with chronic hepatitis C. Anti-LKM2 is seen in drug-induced hepatitis, and anti-LKM3 is seen in patients with chronic hepatitis D. Another autoantibody observed in type II autoimmune hepatitis is directed against liver cytosol formiminotransferase cyclodeaminase (anti-liver cytosol 1). Another type of autoimmune hepatitis has been recognized, *type III autoimmune hepatitis*. These patients lack ANA and anti-LKM1 but have circulating antibodies to soluble liver antigen/liver pancreas antigen. Most of these patients are women and have clinical features similar to, perhaps more severe than, those of patients with type I autoimmune hepatitis. Whether type III autoimmune hepatitis actually represents a distinct category or is part of the spectrum of type I autoimmune hepatitis remains controversial, and this subcategory has not been adopted by a consensus of international experts.

Liver biopsy abnormalities are similar to those described for chronic viral hepatitis. Expanding portal tracts and extending beyond the plate of periportal hepatocytes into the parenchyma (designated *interface hepatitis* or *piecemeal necrosis*) is a mononuclear cell infiltrate that, in autoimmune hepatitis, may include the presence of plasma cells. Necroinflammatory activity characterizes the lobular parenchyma, and evidence of hepatocellular regeneration is reflected by "rosette" formation, the occurrence of thickened liver cell plates, and regenerative "pseudolobules." Septal fibrosis, bridging fibrosis, and cirrhosis are frequent. Bile duct injury and granulomas are uncommon; however, a subgroup of patients with autoimmune hepatitis have histologic, biochemical, and serologic features overlapping those of primary biliary cirrhosis.

DIAGNOSTIC CRITERIA

An international group has suggested a set of criteria for establishing a diagnosis of autoimmune hepatitis. Exclusion of liver disease caused by genetic disorders, viral hepatitis, drug hepatotoxicity, and alcohol are linked with such inclusive diagnostic criteria as hyperglobulinemia, autoantibodies, and characteristic histologic features. This international group has also suggested a comprehensive diagnostic scoring system that, rarely required for typical cases, may be helpful when typical features are not present. Factors that weigh in favor of the diagnosis include female gender; predominant aminotransferase elevation; presence and level of globulin elevation; presence of nuclear, smooth muscle, LKM1, and other autoantibodies; concurrent other autoimmune diseases; characteristic histologic features (interface hepatitis, plasma cells, rosettes); HLA DR3 or DR4 markers; and response to treatment (see below). Weighing against the diagnosis are predominant alkaline phosphatase elevation, mitochondrial antibodies, markers of viral hepatitis, history of hepatotoxic drugs or excessive alcohol, histologic evidence of bile duct injury, or such atypical histologic features as fatty infiltration, iron overload, and viral inclusions.

DIFFERENTIAL DIAGNOSIS

Early during the course of chronic hepatitis, autoimmune hepatitis may resemble typical *acute viral hepatitis*. Without histologic assessment, severe chronic hepatitis cannot be readily distinguished based on clinical or biochemical criteria from mild chronic hepatitis. In adolescence, *Wilson's disease* may present with features of chronic hepatitis long before neurologic manifestations become apparent and before the formation of Kayser-Fleischer rings. In this age group, serum ceruloplasmin and serum and urinary copper determinations plus measurement of liver copper levels will establish the correct diagnosis. *Postnecrotic* or *cryptogenic cirrhosis* and *primary biliary cirrhosis* share clinical features with autoimmune hepatitis, and both alcoholic hepatitis and nonalcoholic steatohepatitis may present with many features common to autoimmune hepatitis; historic, biochemical, serologic, and histologic assessments are usually sufficient to allow these entities to be distinguished from autoimmune hepatitis. Of course, the distinction between autoimmune and chronic viral hepatitis is not always straightforward, especially when viral antibodies occur in patients with autoimmune disease or when autoantibodies occur in patients with viral disease. Furthermore, the presence of extrahepatic features such as arthritis, cutaneous vasculitis, or pleuritis—not to mention the presence of circulating autoantibodies—may cause confusion with *rheumatologic disorders* such as rheumatoid arthritis and systemic lupus erythematosus. The existence of clinical and biochemical features of progressive necroinflammatory liver disease distinguishes chronic hepatitis from these other disorders, which are not associated with severe liver disease.

Finally, occasionally, features of autoimmune hepatitis overlap with features of autoimmune biliary disorders such as primary biliary cirrhosis, primary sclerosing cholangitis, or, even more rarely, mitochondrial antibody-negative autoimmune cholangitis. Such overlap syndromes are difficult to categorize, and often response to therapy may be the distinguishing factor that establishes the diagnosis.

℞ Treatment: AUTOIMMUNE HEPATITIS

The mainstay of management in autoimmune hepatitis is glucocorticoid therapy. Several controlled clinical trials have documented that such therapy leads to symptomatic, clinical, biochemical, and histologic improvement as well as increased survival. A therapeutic response can be expected in up to 80% of patients. Unfortunately, therapy has not been shown to prevent ultimate progression to cirrhosis; however, instances of reversal of fibrosis and cirrhosis have been reported in patients responding to treatment. Although some advocate the use of prednisolone (the hepatic metabolite of prednisone), prednisone is just as effective and is favored by most authorities. Therapy may be initiated at 20 mg/d, but a popular regimen in the United States relies on an initiation dose of 60 mg/d. This high dose is tapered successively over the course of a month down to a maintenance level of 20 mg/d. An alternative but equally effective approach is to begin with half the prednisone dose (30 mg/d) along with azathioprine (50 mg/d). With azathioprine maintained at 50 mg/d, the prednisone dose is tapered over the course of a month down to a maintenance level of 10 mg/d. The advantage of the combination approach is a reduction, over the span of an 18-month course of therapy, in serious, life-threatening complications of steroid therapy from 66% down to under 20%. In combination regimens,

6-mercaptopurine may be substituted for its prodrug azathioprine, but this is rarely required. Azathioprine alone, however, is not effective in achieving remission, nor is alternate-day glucocorticoid therapy. Although therapy has been shown to be effective for severe autoimmune hepatitis (AST ≥10 times the upper limit of normal or ≥5 times the upper limit of normal in conjunction with serum globulin ≥ twice normal; bridging necrosis or multilobular necrosis on liver biopsy; presence of symptoms), therapy is not indicated for mild forms of chronic hepatitis, and the efficacy of therapy in mild or asymptomatic autoimmune hepatitis has not been established.

Improvement of fatigue, anorexia, malaise, and jaundice tends to occur within days to several weeks; biochemical improvement occurs over the course of several weeks to months, with a fall in serum bilirubin and globulin levels and an increase in serum albumin. Serum aminotransferase levels usually drop promptly, but improvements in AST and ALT alone do not appear to be a reliable marker of recovery in individual patients; histologic improvement, characterized by a decrease in mononuclear infiltration and in hepatocellular necrosis, may be delayed for 6–24 months. Still, if interpreted cautiously, aminotransferase levels are valuable indicators of relative disease activity, and many authorities do *not* advocate serial liver biopsies to assess therapeutic success or to guide decisions to alter or stop therapy. Therapy should continue for at least 12–18 months. After tapering and cessation of therapy, the likelihood of relapse is at least 50%, even if posttreatment histology has improved to show mild chronic hepatitis, and the majority of patients require therapy at maintenance doses indefinitely. Continuing azathioprine alone (2 mg/kg body weight daily) after cessation of prednisone therapy may reduce the frequency of relapse.

In medically refractory cases, an attempt should be made to intensify treatment with high-dose glucocorticoid monotherapy (60 mg daily) or combination glucocorticoid (30 mg daily) plus high-dose azathioprine (150 mg daily) therapy. After a month, doses of prednisone can be reduced by 10 mg a month, and doses of azathioprine can be reduced by 50 mg a month toward ultimate, conventional maintenance doses. Patients refractory to this regimen may be treated with cyclosporine, tacrolimus, or mycophenolate mofetil; however, to date only limited anecdotal reports support these approaches. If medical therapy fails, or when chronic hepatitis progresses to cirrhosis and is associated with life-threatening complications of liver decompensation, liver transplantation is the only recourse; failure of the bilirubin to improve after 2 weeks of therapy should prompt early consideration of the patient for liver transplantation. Recurrence of autoimmune hepatitis in the new liver occurs rarely in most experiences but in as many as 35–40% of cases in others.

ACKNOWLEDGMENT

Kurt J. Isselbacher, MD, contributed to this chapter in previous editions of Harrison's Principles of Internal Medicine.

FURTHER READINGS

BENHAMOU Y, SALMON D (guest ed): Proceedings of the 1st European consensus conference on the treatment of chronic hepatitis B and C in HIV co-infected patients. J Hepatol 44(Suppl 1):S1, 2006

CHANG T-T et al: A comparison of entecavir and lamivudine for HBeAg-positive chronic hepatitis B. N Engl J Med 354:1001, 2006

CZAJA AJ, FREESE DK: AASLD practice guidelines: Diagnosis and treatment of autoimmune hepatitis. Hepatology 36:479, 2002

DIENSTAG JL: American Gastroenterological Association medical position statement on the management of hepatitis C. Gastroenterology 130:225, 2006

———, MCHUTCHISON JG: American Gastroenterological Association technical review on the management of hepatitis C. Gastroenterology 130:231, 2006

EUROPEAN ASSOCIATION FOR THE STUDY OF THE LIVER: EASL Consensus Conference on Hepatitis B. J Hepatol 39(Suppl 1):S1, 2003

FUNG SK, LOK ASF: Treatment of chronic hepatitis B: Who to treat, what to use, and for how long? Clin Gastroenterol Hepatol 2:839, 2004

HÉZODE C et al: Telaprevir and peginterferon with or without ribavirin for chronic HCV infection. N Engl J Med 360:1839, 2009

JENSEN DM et al: Re-treatment of patients with chronic hepatitis C who do not respond to peginterferon-alpha2b: A randomized trial. Ann Intern Med 150:528, 2009

KRAWITT EL: Autoimmune hepatitis. N Engl J Med 354:54, 2006

LAI C-L et al: Entecavir versus lamivudine for patients with HBeAg-negative chronic hepatitis B. N Engl J Med 354:1011, 2006

LIAW Y-F et al: Asian-Pacific consensus statement on the management of chronic hepatitis B: A 2005 update. Liver International 25:472, 2005

———, CHU CM: Hepatitis B virus infection. Lancet 373:582, 2009

LOCARNINI SA (guest ed): The control of hepatitis B: The role for chemoprevention. Semin Liver Dis 26:1, 2006

MCHUTCHISON JG et al: Telaprevir with peginterferon and ribavirin for chronic HCV genotype 1 infection. N Engl J Med 360:1827, 2009

NATIONAL INSTITUTES OF HEALTH CONSENSUS DEVELOPMENT CONFERENCE: Management of hepatitis C. Hepatology 36(Suppl 1):1S, 2002

PAWLOTSKY J-M: Therapy of hepatitis C: From empiricism to eradication. Hepatology 43:S207, 2006

PEARLMAN BL: Chronic hepatitis C therapy: Changing the rules of duration. Clin Gastroenterol Hepatol 4:963, 2006

RODRIGUEZ-TORRES M et al: Latino Study Group. Peginterferon alfa-2a and ribavirin in Latino and non-Latino whites with hepatitis C. N Engl J Med 360:257, 2009

ROMEO R et al: A 28-year study of the course of hepatitis Delta infection: A risk factor for cirrhosis and hepatocellular carcinoma. Gastroenterology 136:1629, 2009

SHAMLIYAN TA et al: Antiviral therapy for adults with chronic hepatitis B: A systematic review for a National Institutes of Health Consensus Development Conference. Ann Intern Med 150:111, 2009

STRADER DB et al: AASLD practice guideline: Diagnosis, management, and treatment of hepatitis C. Hepatology 39:1147, 2004

CHAPTER 94

ENTEROVIRUSES AND REOVIRUSES

Jeffrey I. Cohen

ENTEROVIRUSES

CLASSIFICATION AND CHARACTERIZATION

Enteroviruses are so named because of their ability to multiply in the gastrointestinal tract. Despite their name, these viruses are not a prominent cause of gastroenteritis. Enteroviruses encompass 65 human serotypes: 3 serotypes of poliovirus, 23 serotypes of coxsackievirus A, 6 serotypes of coxsackievirus B, 29 serotypes of echovirus, and enteroviruses 68–71. Enteroviruses 73–102 have recently been identified in humans by molecular techniques, but their clinical features have not been described. Enterovirus surveillance conducted in the United States by the Centers for Disease Control and Prevention (CDC) in 2007–2008 showed that the most common serotype, coxsackievirus B1, was followed in frequency by echoviruses 18, 9, and 6, which together accounted for 52% of all isolates.

Human enteroviruses contain a single-stranded RNA genome surrounded by an icosahedral capsid comprising four viral proteins. These viruses have no lipid envelope and are stable in acidic environments, including the stomach. They are resistant to inactivation by standard disinfectants (e.g., alcohol, detergents) and can persist for days at room temperature.

PATHOGENESIS AND IMMUNITY

Much of what is known about the pathogenesis of enteroviruses has been derived from studies of poliovirus infection. After ingestion, poliovirus is thought to infect epithelial cells in the mucosa of the gastrointestinal tract and then to spread to and replicate in the submucosal lymphoid tissue of the tonsils and Peyer's patches. The virus next spreads to the regional lymph nodes, a viremic phase ensues, and the virus replicates in organs of the reticuloendothelial system. In some cases, a second viremia occurs and the virus replicates further in various tissues, sometimes causing symptomatic disease.

It is uncertain whether poliovirus reaches the central nervous system (CNS) during viremia or whether it also spreads via peripheral nerves. Since viremia precedes the onset of neurologic disease in humans and in experimentally infected chimpanzees, it has been assumed that the virus enters the CNS via the bloodstream. The poliovirus receptor is a member of the immunoglobulin superfamily. Poliovirus infection is limited to primates, largely because their cells express the viral receptor. Studies demonstrating the poliovirus receptor in the end-plate region of muscle at the neuromuscular junction suggest that, if the virus enters the muscle during viremia, it could travel across the neuromuscular junction up the axon to the anterior horn cells. Studies of monkeys and of transgenic mice expressing the poliovirus receptor show that, after IM injection, poliovirus does not reach the spinal cord if the sciatic nerve is cut. Taken together, these findings suggest that poliovirus can spread directly from muscle to the CNS by neural pathways. Intercellular adhesion molecule 1 (ICAM-1) is a receptor for coxsackieviruses A13, A18, and A21; CAR for coxsackievirus B; VLA-2 integrin for echovirus types 1 and 8; and CD55 for enterovirus 70 and some serotypes of coxsackievirus A and B and echovirus.

Poliovirus can usually be cultured from the blood 3–5 days after infection, before the development of neutralizing antibodies. While viral replication at secondary sites begins to slow 1 week after infection, it continues in the gastrointestinal tract. Poliovirus is shed from the oropharynx for up to 3 weeks after infection and from the gastrointestinal tract for as long as 12 weeks; immunodeficient patients can shed poliovirus for up to 20 years. During replication in the gastrointestinal tract, attenuated oral poliovirus can mutate, reverting to a more neurovirulent phenotype within a few days. The clinical significance of this increased neurovirulence is unknown.

Humoral and secretory immunity in the gastrointestinal tract is important for the control of enterovirus infections. Enteroviruses induce specific IgM, which usually persists for <6 months, and specific IgG, which persists for life. Capsid protein VP1 is the predominant target of neutralizing antibody, which generally confers lifelong protection against subsequent disease caused by the same serotype but does not prevent infection or virus shedding. Enteroviruses also induce cellular immunity, but the significance of this mechanism in limiting infection is uncertain. Patients with impaired cellular immunity are not known to develop unusually severe disease when infected with enteroviruses. In contrast, the severe infections in patients with agammaglobulinemia emphasize the importance of humoral immunity in controlling enterovirus infections. Disseminated enterovirus infections have occurred in stem cell transplant recipients. IgA antibodies are instrumental in reducing poliovirus replication in and shedding from the gastrointestinal tract. Breast milk contains IgA specific for enteroviruses and can protect humans from infection.

EPIDEMIOLOGY

Enteroviruses have a worldwide distribution. More than 50% of nonpoliovirus enterovirus infections and more than 90% of poliovirus infections are subclinical. When symptoms do develop, they are usually nonspecific and occur in conjunction with fever; only a minority of infections are associated with specific clinical syndromes. The incubation period for most enterovirus infections ranges from 2 to 14 days but usually is <1 week.

Enterovirus infection is more common in socioeconomically disadvantaged areas, especially in those where conditions are crowded and in tropical areas where hygiene is poor. Infection is most common among infants and young children; serious illness develops most often during the first few days of life and in older children and adults. In developing countries, where children are infected at an early age, poliovirus infection has less often been associated with paralysis; in countries with better hygiene, older children and adults are more likely to be seronegative, become infected, and develop paralysis. Passively acquired maternal antibody reduces the risk of symptomatic infection in neonates. Young children are the most frequent shedders of enteroviruses and are usually the index cases in family outbreaks. In temperate climates, enterovirus infections occur most often in the summer and fall; no seasonal pattern is apparent in the tropics.

Most enteroviruses are transmitted primarily by the fecal-oral route from fecally contaminated fingers or inanimate objects. Patients are most infectious shortly before and after the onset of symptomatic disease, when virus is present in the stool and throat. The ingestion of virus-contaminated food or water can also cause disease. Certain enteroviruses (such as enterovirus 70, which causes acute hemorrhagic conjunctivitis) can be transmitted by direct inoculation from the fingers to the eye. Airborne transmission is important for some viruses that cause respiratory tract disease, such as coxsackievirus A21. Enteroviruses can be transmitted across the placenta from mother to fetus, causing severe disease in the newborn. The transmission of enteroviruses through blood transfusions or insect bites has not been documented. Nosocomial spread of coxsackievirus and echovirus has taken place in hospital nurseries.

CLINICAL FEATURES

Poliovirus Infection

Most infections with poliovirus are asymptomatic. After an incubation period of 3–6 days, ~5% of patients present with a minor illness (abortive poliomyelitis) manifested by fever, malaise, sore throat, anorexia, myalgias, and headache. This condition usually resolves in 3 days. About 1% of patients present with aseptic meningitis (nonparalytic poliomyelitis). Examination of cerebrospinal fluid (CSF) reveals lymphocytic pleocytosis, a normal glucose level, and a normal or slightly elevated protein level; CSF polymorphonuclear leukocytes may be present early. In some patients, especially children, malaise and fever precede the onset of aseptic meningitis.

Paralytic Poliomyelitis

The least common presentation is that of paralytic disease. After one or several days, signs of aseptic meningitis are followed by severe back, neck, and muscle pain and by the rapid or gradual development of motor weakness. In some cases the disease appears to be biphasic, with aseptic meningitis followed first by apparent recovery but then (1–2 days later) by the return of fever and the development of paralysis; this form is more common among children than among adults. Weakness is generally asymmetric, is proximal more than distal, and may involve the legs (most commonly); the arms; or the abdominal, thoracic, or bulbar muscles. Paralysis develops during the febrile phase of the illness and usually does not progress after defervescence. Urinary retention may also occur. Examination reveals weakness, fasciculations, decreased muscle tone, and reduced or absent reflexes in affected areas. Transient hyperreflexia sometimes precedes the loss of reflexes. Patients frequently report sensory symptoms, but objective sensory testing usually yields normal results. Bulbar paralysis may lead to dysphagia, difficulty in handling secretions, or dysphonia. Respiratory insufficiency due to aspiration, involvement of the respiratory center in the medulla, or paralysis of the phrenic or intercostal nerves may develop, and severe medullary involvement may lead to circulatory collapse. Most patients with paralysis recover some function weeks to months after infection. About two-thirds of patients have residual neurologic sequelae.

Paralytic disease is more common among older individuals, pregnant women, and persons exercising strenuously or undergoing trauma at the time of CNS symptoms. Tonsillectomy predisposes to bulbar poliomyelitis, and IM injections increase the risk of paralysis in the involved limb(s).

Vaccine-Associated Poliomyelitis

Until recently, poliomyelitis due to live poliovirus vaccine occurred in the United States. The risk of developing poliomyelitis after oral vaccination is estimated at 1 case per 2.5 million doses. The risk is ~2000 times higher among immunodeficient persons, especially in persons with hypo- or agammaglobulinemia. Before 1997, an average of eight cases of vaccine-associated poliomyelitis occurred—in both vaccinees and their contacts—in the United States each year. With the change in recommendations first to a sequential regimen of inactivated poliovirus vaccine (IPV) and oral poliovirus vaccine (OPV) in 1997 and then to an all-IPV regimen in 2000, the number of cases of vaccine-associated polio declined. From 1997 to 1999, six such cases were reported in the United States; no cases have been reported since 1999.

Postpolio Syndrome

The *postpolio syndrome* presents as a new onset of weakness, fatigue, fasciculations, and pain with additional atrophy of the muscle group involved during the initial paralytic disease 20–40 years earlier. The syndrome is more common among women and with increasing time after acute disease. The onset is usually insidious, and weakness occasionally extends to muscles that were not involved during the initial illness. The prognosis is generally good; progression to further weakness is usually slow, with plateau periods of 1–10 years. The postpolio syndrome is thought to be due to progressive dysfunction and loss of motor neurons that compensated for the neurons lost during the original infection and not to persistent or reactivated poliovirus infection.

Other Enteroviruses

An estimated 5–10 million cases of symptomatic disease due to enteroviruses other than poliovirus occur in the United States each year. Among neonates, enteroviruses are the most common cause of aseptic meningitis and nonspecific febrile illnesses. Certain clinical syndromes are more likely to be caused by certain serotypes (Table 94-1), but there is much overlap. In 2002–2004, 85% of enterovirus infections were caused by only 9 human serotypes. Echoviruses 9 and 30 accounted for 60% of recognized enterovirus infections.

TABLE 94-1

MANIFESTATIONS COMMONLY ASSOCIATED WITH ENTEROVIRUS SEROTYPES

	SEROTYPE(S) OF INDICATED VIRUS	
MANIFESTATION	COXSACKIEVIRUS	ECHOVIRUS (E) AND ENTEROVIRUS (Ent)
Acute hemorrhagic conjunctivitis	A24	E70
Aseptic meningitis	A2, 4, 7, 9, 10; B1-5	E4, 6, 7, 9, 11, 13, 16, 18, 19, 30, 33; Ent70, 71
Encephalitis	A9; B1-5	E3, 4, 6, 9, 11, 25, 30; Ent71
Exanthem	A4, 5, 9, 10, 16; B1, 3-5	E4-7, 9, 11, 16-19, 25, 30; Ent71
Generalized disease of the newborn	B1-5	E4-6, 7, 9, 11, 14, 16, 18, 19
Hand-foot-and-mouth disease	A5, 7, 9, 10, 16; B1, 2, 5	Ent71
Herpangina	A1-10, 16, 22; B1-5	E6, 9, 11, 16, 17, 25; Ent71
Myocarditis, pericarditis	A4, 9, 16; B1-5	E6, 9, 11, 22
Paralysis	A4, 7, 9; B1-5	E2, 4, 6, 9, 11, 30; Ent70, 71
Pleurodynia	A1, 2, 4, 6, 9, 10, 16; B1-6	E1-3, 6, 7, 9, 11, 12, 14, 16, 19, 24, 25, 30
Pneumonia	A9, 16; B1-5	E6, 7, 9, 11, 12, 19, 20, 30; Ent68, 71

Nonspecific Febrile Illness (Summer Grippe)

The most common clinical manifestation of enterovirus infection is a nonspecific febrile illness. After an incubation period of 3–6 days, patients present with an acute onset of fever, malaise, and headache. Occasional cases are associated with upper respiratory symptoms, and some cases include nausea and vomiting. Symptoms often last for 3–4 days, and most cases resolve in a week. While infections with other respiratory viruses occur more often from late fall to early spring, enterovirus febrile illness frequently occurs in the summer and early fall.

Generalized Disease of the Newborn

Most serious enterovirus infections in infants develop during the first week of life, although severe disease can occur up to 3 months of age. Neonates often present with an illness resembling bacterial sepsis, with fever, irritability, and lethargy. Laboratory abnormalities include leukocytosis with a left shift, thrombocytopenia, elevated values in liver function tests, and CSF pleocytosis. The illness can be complicated by myocarditis and hypotension, fulminant hepatitis and disseminated intravascular coagulation, meningitis or meningoencephalitis, or pneumonia. It may be difficult to distinguish neonatal enterovirus infection from bacterial sepsis, although a history of a recent virus-like illness in the mother provides a clue.

Aseptic Meningitis and Encephalitis

Enteroviruses are the cause of up to 90% of cases of aseptic meningitis in children and young adults in which an etiologic agent can be identified. Patients with aseptic meningitis typically present with an acute onset of fever, chills, headache, photophobia, and pain on eye movement. Nausea and vomiting are also common. Examination reveals meningismus without localizing neurologic signs; drowsiness or irritability may also be apparent. In some cases, a febrile illness may be reported that remits but returns several days later in conjunction with signs of meningitis. Other systemic manifestations may provide clues to an enteroviral cause, including diarrhea, myalgias, rash, pleurodynia, myocarditis, and herpangina. Examination of the CSF invariably reveals pleocytosis; early in the course, polymorphonuclear leukocytes may be present or even predominant—a finding that raises the possibility of bacterial or other nonviral causes of meningitis. Partially treated bacterial meningitis may be particularly difficult to exclude in some instances. A useful rule is that the CSF cell count in enteroviral meningitis shows a shift to lymphocytic predominance within 24 h of presentation, and the total count generally does not exceed 1000 cells/μL. Additional CSF findings consist of a normal glucose content and a normal or only slightly elevated (by ≤100 mg/dL) level of protein. Enteroviruses and mumps virus may produce a similar picture of meningitis; a low CSF glucose level suggests mumps, whereas a normal CSF glucose level and transient CSF polymorphonuclear pleocytosis suggest enterovirus infection. Enteroviral meningitis is more frequent in summer and fall in temperate climates, while viral meningitis of other etiologies (e.g., mumps) is more common in winter and spring. Symptoms ordinarily resolve within a week, although CSF abnormalities can persist for several weeks. Enteroviral meningitis is often more severe in adults than in children. Neurologic sequelae are rare, and most patients have an excellent prognosis.

Enteroviral encephalitis is much less common than enteroviral aseptic meningitis. Occasional highly inflammatory cases of enteroviral meningitis may be complicated by a mild form of encephalitis that is recognized on the basis of progressive lethargy, disorientation, and sometimes seizures. Less commonly, severe primary encephalitis may develop. An estimated 10–20% of cases of viral encephalitis are due to enteroviruses. Immunocompetent patients generally have a good prognosis.

Patients with hypogammaglobulinemia or agammaglobulinemia or severe combined immunodeficiency may develop chronic meningitis or encephalitis; about half of these patients have a dermatomyositis-like syndrome, with peripheral edema, rash, and myositis. They may also have chronic hepatitis. Patients may develop neurologic disease while receiving gamma globulin replacement therapy. Echoviruses (especially echovirus 11) are the most common pathogens in this situation.

Paralytic disease due to enteroviruses other than poliovirus occurs sporadically and is usually less severe than poliomyelitis. Most cases are due to enterovirus 70 or 71 or to coxsackievirus A7 or A9. Guillain-Barré syndrome is also associated with enterovirus infection. While some studies have suggested a link between enteroviruses and the chronic fatigue syndrome, most recent studies have not demonstrated such an association.

Pleurodynia (Bornholm Disease)

Patients with pleurodynia present with an acute onset of fever and spasms of pleuritic chest or upper abdominal pain. Chest pain is more common in adults, and abdominal pain is more common in children. Paroxysms of severe, knifelike pain usually last 15–30 min and are associated with diaphoresis and tachypnea. Fever peaks within an hour after the onset of paroxysms and subsides when pain resolves. The involved muscles are tender to palpation, and a pleural rub may be detected. The white blood cell count and chest x-ray are usually normal. Most cases are due to coxsackievirus B and occur during epidemics. Symptoms resolve in a few days, and recurrences are rare. Treatment includes the administration of nonsteroidal anti-inflammatory agents or the application of heat to the affected muscles.

Myocarditis and Pericarditis

Enteroviruses are estimated to cause up to one-third of cases of acute myocarditis. Coxsackievirus B and its RNA have been detected in pericardial fluid and myocardial tissue in some cases of acute myocarditis and pericarditis. Most cases of enteroviral myocarditis or pericarditis occur in newborns, adolescents, or young adults. More than two-thirds of patients are male. Patients often present with an upper respiratory tract infection that is followed by fever, chest pain, dyspnea, arrhythmias, and occasionally heart failure. A pericardial friction rub is documented in half of cases, and the electrocardiogram shows ST-segment elevations or ST- and T-wave abnormalities. Serum levels of myocardial enzymes are often elevated. Neonates commonly have severe disease, while most older children and adults recover completely. Up to 10% of cases progress to chronic dilated cardiomyopathy. Chronic constrictive pericarditis may also be a sequela.

Exanthems

Enterovirus infection is the leading cause of exanthems in children in the summer and fall. While exanthems are associated with many enteroviruses, certain types have been linked to specific syndromes. Echoviruses 9 and 16 have frequently been associated with exanthem and fever. Rashes may be discrete (rubelliform) or confluent (morbilliform), beginning on the face and spreading to the trunk and extremities. Echovirus 9 is the most common cause of rubelliform rash. Unlike the rash of rubella, the enteroviral rash occurs in the summer and is not associated with lymphadenopathy. Roseola-like rashes develop after defervescence, with macules and papules on the face and trunk. The Boston exanthem, caused by echovirus 16, is a roseola-like rash that often affects multiple members of a family. A variety of other rashes have been associated with enteroviruses, including erythema multiforme and vesicular, urticarial, petechial, or purpuric lesions. Enanthems also occur, including lesions that resemble the Koplik's spots seen with measles.

Hand-Foot-and-Mouth Disease

After an incubation period of 4–6 days, patients with hand-foot-and-mouth disease present with fever, anorexia, and malaise; these manifestations are followed by the development of sore throat and vesicles (Fig. 94-1*A*) on the buccal mucosa and often on the tongue and then by the appearance of tender vesicular lesions on the dorsum of the hands, sometimes with involvement of the palms. The vesicles may form bullae and quickly ulcerate. About one-third of patients also have lesions on the palate, uvula, or tonsillar pillars, and one-third have a rash on the feet (including the soles) or on the buttocks. The disease is highly infectious, with attack rates of close to 100% among young children. The lesions usually resolve in 1 week. Most cases are due to coxsackievirus A16 or enterovirus 71.

An epidemic of enterovirus 71 infection in Taiwan in 1998 resulted in thousands of cases of hand-foot-and-mouth disease or herpangina. Severe complications included CNS disease, myocarditis, and pulmonary hemorrhage. About 90% of those who died were children ≤5 years old, and these deaths were associated with pulmonary edema or pulmonary hemorrhage. CNS disease included aseptic meningitis, flaccid paralysis (similar to poliomyelitis), or rhombencephalitis with myoclonus and tremor or ataxia. The mean age of patients with CNS complications was 2.5 years, and MRI in cases with encephalitis usually showed brain-stem lesions. Follow-up of children at 6 months showed persistent dysphagia,

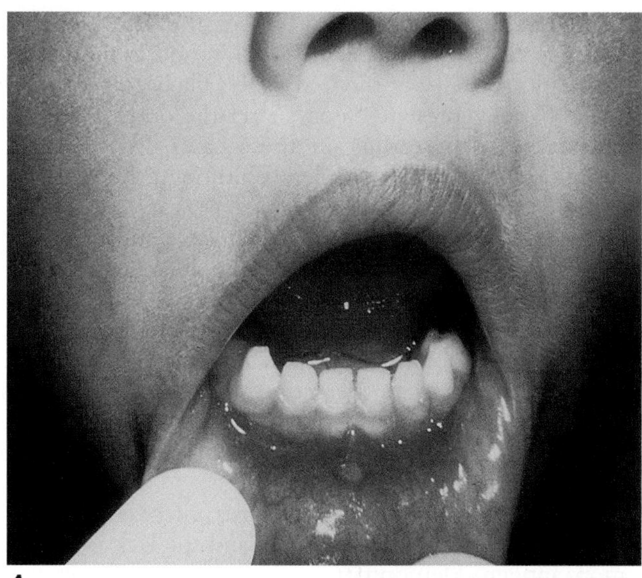
A

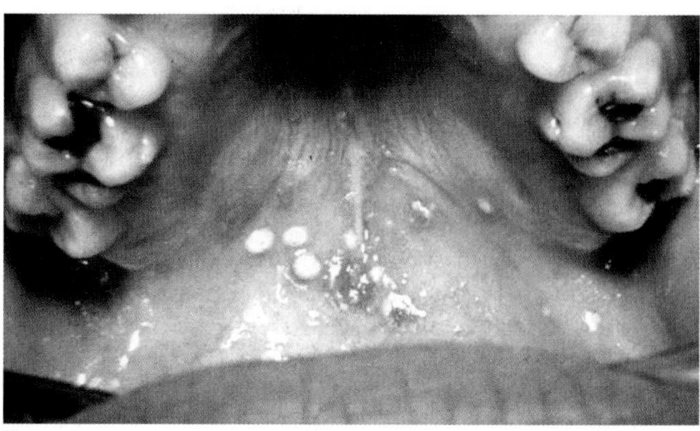
B

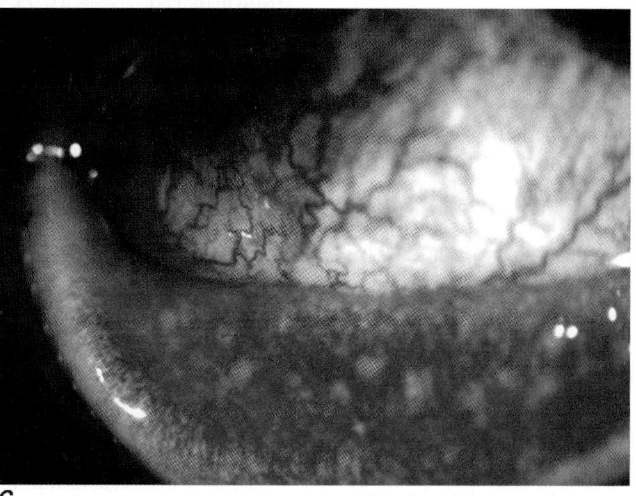
C

FIGURE 94-1
A. Tender vesicles and erosions in the mouth of a patient with hand-foot-and-mouth disease. ***B.*** Soft-palate lesions of herpangina due to coxsackievirus. ***C.*** Acute hemorrhagic conjunctivitis due to enterovirus 71. *(Images B and C are reprinted with permission from Redbook 2006: Committee on Infectious Diseases, 27th ed. Elk Grove Village, IL: American Academy of Pediatrics.)*

cranial nerve palsies, hypoventilation, limb weakness, and atrophy.

Herpangina

Herpangina is usually caused by coxsackievirus A and presents as acute-onset fever, sore throat, dysphagia, and grayish-white papulovesicular lesions on an erythematous base that ulcerate (Fig. 94-1*B*). The lesions can persist for weeks; are present on the soft palate, anterior pillars of the tonsils, and uvula; and are concentrated in the posterior portion of the mouth. In contrast to herpes stomatitis, enteroviral herpangina is not associated with gingivitis. Acute lymphonodular pharyngitis associated with coxsackievirus A10 presents as white or yellow nodules surrounded by erythema in the posterior oropharynx. The lesions do not ulcerate.

Acute Hemorrhagic Conjunctivitis

Patients with acute hemorrhagic conjunctivitis present with an acute onset of severe eye pain, blurred vision, photophobia, and watery discharge from the eye. Examination reveals edema, chemosis, and subconjunctival hemorrhage and often shows punctate keratitis and conjunctival follicles as well (Fig. 94-1*C*). Preauricular adenopathy is often found. Epidemics and nosocomial spread have been associated with enterovirus 70 and coxsackievirus A24. Systemic symptoms, including headache and fever, develop in 20% of cases, and recovery is usually complete in 10 days. The sudden onset and short duration of the illness help to distinguish acute hemorrhagic conjunctivitis from other ocular infections such as those due to adenovirus and *Chlamydia*. Paralysis has been associated with some cases of acute hemorrhagic conjunctivitis due to enterovirus 70 during epidemics.

Other Manifestations

Enteroviruses are an infrequent cause of childhood pneumonia and the common cold. Coxsackievirus B has been isolated at autopsy from the pancreas of a few children presenting with type 1 diabetes mellitus; however, most attempts to isolate the virus have been unsuccessful. Other diseases that have been associated with enterovirus infection include parotitis, bronchitis, bronchiolitis, croup, infectious lymphocytosis, polymyositis, acute arthritis, and acute nephritis.

DIAGNOSIS

Isolation of enterovirus in cell culture is the traditional diagnostic procedure. While cultures of stool, nasopharyngeal, or throat samples from patients with enterovirus diseases are often positive, isolation of the virus from these sites does not prove that it is directly associated with disease because these sites are frequently colonized for weeks in patients with subclinical infections. Isolation of virus from the throat is more likely to be associated with disease than isolation from the stool since virus is shed for shorter periods from the throat. Cultures of CSF, serum, fluid from body cavities, or tissues are positive less frequently, but a positive result is indicative of disease caused by enterovirus. In some cases, the virus is isolated only from the blood or only from the CSF; therefore, it is important to culture multiple sites. Cultures are more likely to be positive earlier than later in the course of infection. Most human enteroviruses can be detected within a week after inoculation of cell cultures. Cultures may be negative because of the presence of neutralizing antibody, lack of susceptibility of the cells used, or inappropriate handling of the specimen. Coxsackievirus A may require inoculation into special cell-culture lines or into suckling mice.

Identification of the enterovirus serotype is useful primarily for epidemiologic studies and, with a few exceptions, has little clinical utility. It is important to identify serious infections with enterovirus during epidemics and to distinguish the vaccine strain of poliovirus from the other enteroviruses in the throat or in the feces. Stool and throat samples for culture as well as acute- and convalescent-phase serum specimens should be obtained from all patients with suspected poliomyelitis. In the absence of a positive CSF culture, a positive culture of stool obtained within the first 2 weeks after the onset of symptoms is most often used to confirm the diagnosis of poliomyelitis. If poliovirus infection is suspected, two or more fecal and throat swab samples should be obtained at least 1 day apart and cultured for enterovirus as soon as possible. If poliovirus is isolated, it should be sent to the CDC for identification as either wild-type or vaccine virus.

The polymerase chain reaction (PCR) has been used to amplify viral nucleic acid from CSF, serum, urine, throat swabs, and tissues. A single pair of PCR primers can detect >92% of the serotypes that infect humans. With the proper controls, PCR of the CSF is highly sensitive (≥95%) and specific (>80%) and is more rapid than culture. PCR of the CSF is less likely to be positive when patients present ≥3 days after the onset of meningitis rather than earlier; in these cases, PCR of fecal specimens should be considered, although the test is less specific than PCR of CSF.

PCR of serum is also highly sensitive and specific in the diagnosis of disseminated disease. PCR may be particularly helpful for the diagnosis and follow-up of enterovirus disease in immunodeficient patients receiving immunoglobulin therapy, whose viral cultures may be negative. Antigen detection and hybridization of enterovirus sequences in human tissues with a specific probe are additional options, but these techniques are generally less sensitive than PCR.

Serologic diagnosis of enterovirus infection is limited by the large number of serotypes and the lack of a common antigen. Demonstration of seroconversion may be useful in rare cases for confirmation of culture results, but serologic testing is usually limited to epidemiologic studies. Serum should be collected and frozen soon after the onset of disease and again ~4 weeks later. Measurement of neutralizing titers is the most accurate method for antibody determination; measurement of complement-fixation titers is usually less sensitive. Titers of virus-specific IgM are elevated in both acute and chronic infection.

℞ Treatment: ENTEROVIRUS INFECTIONS

Most enterovirus infections are mild and resolve spontaneously; however, intensive supportive care may be needed for cardiac, hepatic, or CNS disease. IV, intrathecal, or intraventricular immunoglobulin has been used with apparent success for the treatment of chronic enterovirus meningoencephalitis and dermatomyositis in patients with hypogammaglobulinemia or agammaglobulinemia. The disease may stabilize or resolve during therapy; however, some patients decline inexorably despite therapy. IV administration of immunoglobulin with high titers of antibody to the infecting virus has been used in some cases of life-threatening infection in neonates, who may not have maternally acquired antibody. In one trial involving neonates with enterovirus infections, immunoglobulin containing very high titers of antibody to the infecting virus reduced rates of viremia; however, the study was too small to show a substantial clinical benefit. The level of enteroviral antibodies varies with the immunoglobulin preparation. For a time, pleconaril was given to patients with severe enterovirus infections on a compassionate-use basis, but this drug is no longer available for this use. Glucocorticoids are contraindicated.

Good hand-washing practices and the use of gowns and gloves are important in limiting nosocomial transmission of enteroviruses during epidemics. Enteric precautions are indicated for 7 days after the onset of enterovirus infections.

PREVENTION AND ERADICATION OF POLIOVIRUS

(See also Chap. 3) After a peak of 57,879 cases of poliomyelitis in the United States in 1952, the introduction of inactivated vaccine in 1955 and of oral vaccine in 1961 ultimately eradicated disease due to wild-type poliovirus in the Western Hemisphere. Such disease has not been documented in the United States since 1979, when cases occurred among religious groups who had declined immunization. In the Western Hemisphere, paralysis due to wild-type poliovirus was last documented in 1991.

In 1988, the World Health Organization adopted a resolution to eradicate poliomyelitis by the year 2000. From 1988 to 2001, the number of cases worldwide decreased by >99%, with fewer than 1000 confirmed cases reported in 2001. In 2002, however, there were ~1900 cases of polio, with ~1500 reported in India. Wild-type poliovirus type 2 has not been detected in the world since 1999. The Americas were certified free of indigenous wild-type poliovirus transmission in 1994, the Western Pacific Region in 2000, and the European Region in 2002. The total number of cases worldwide fell to a nadir of 498 in 2001. However, from 2002 to 2005, 21 countries previously free of polio reported cases imported from 6 polio-endemic countries. By 2006, polio transmission had been reduced in most of these 21 countries; in 2008, 1730 cases were reported, ~90% of them from Nigeria, India, Pakistan, and Afghanistan—the only countries where polio remains endemic (Table 94-2). Polio is a source of concern for unimmunized and partially immunized travelers to these regions. In 2008–2009, the importation of wild-type poliovirus into 15 countries in Africa resulted in 96 cases of polio, with persistent transmission of virus in 5 countries previously free of the virus. In 2008, ~8% of polio cases were imported from Nigeria and India. Outbreaks of polio in Europe and North America have been traced to cases imported from the Indian subcontinent. Clearly, global eradication of polio is necessary to eliminate the risk of importation of wild-type virus. Outbreaks are thought to have been facilitated by suboptimal rates of vaccination, isolated pockets of unvaccinated children, poor sanitation and crowding, improper vaccine-storage conditions, and a reduced level of response to one of the serotypes in the vaccine. While the global eradication campaign has markedly reduced the number of cases of polio, doubts have been raised as to whether eradication is a realistic goal given the large number of asymptomatic cases and the political instability in developing countries.

Outbreaks of poliomyelitis due to circulating vaccine-derived poliovirus have recently occurred. In Egypt, 30 cases of vaccine-derived polio occurred in 1988–1993; in the Dominican Republic and Haiti, 21 cases occurred in 2000–2001; and fewer than 5 cases each occurred in the Philippines (2001), Madagascar (2002), and China (2004). These OPV-derived viruses reverted to a more neurovirulent phenotype after undetected circulation (probably for >2 years). The epidemic in Hispaniola was rapidly terminated after intensive vaccination with OPV. In 2005, a case of vaccine-derived polio occurred in an unvaccinated U.S. woman returning from a visit to Central and South America. In the same year, an unvaccinated immunocompromised infant in Minnesota was found to be shedding vaccine-derived poliovirus; further investigation identified 3 other infants in the same community who were shedding the virus. All 4 infants were asymptomatic. These outbreaks emphasize the need for maintaining high levels of vaccine coverage and continued surveillance for circulating virus.

IPV is used in most industrialized countries and OPV in most developing countries, including those in which polio still is or recently was endemic. After several doses of OPV alone, the seropositivity rate for individual poliovirus serotypes may still be suboptimal for children in developing countries; one or more supplemental doses of IPV can increase the rate of seropositivity for these serotypes. While IM injections of other vaccines (live or attenuated) can be given concurrently with OPV, unnecessary IM injections should be avoided during the first month after vaccination because they increase the risk of vaccine-associated paralysis. Since 1988, an enhanced-potency inactivated poliovirus vaccine has been available in the United States.

OPV and IPV induce antibodies that persist for at least 5 years. Both vaccines induce IgG and IgA antibodies. Compared with recipients of IPV, recipients of OPV shed less virus and less frequently develop reinfection with wild-type virus after exposure to poliovirus. Although IPV is safe and efficacious, OPV offers the advantages of ease of administration, lower cost, and induction of intestinal immunity resulting in a reduction

TABLE 94-2

LABORATORY-CONFIRMED CASES OF POLIOMYELITIS IN 2008

COUNTRY	TYPE OF TRANSMISSION	NUMBER OF CASES
Nigeria	Endemic	860[a]
India	Endemic	559
Pakistan	Endemic	117
Chad	Imported	37
Afghanistan	Endemic	31
Angola	Imported	29
Sudan	Imported	26
Niger	Imported	12
Others[b]	Imported	42
Others[c]	Vaccine-derived	17
Total		1730

[a]Of these cases, 62 were vaccine-derived.

[b]Ghana, 8; Benin, 6; Burkina Faso, 6; Nepal, 6; Democratic Republic of the Congo, 5; Central African Republic, 3; Ethiopia, 3; Togo, 3; Cote d'Ivoire, 1; Mali, 1.

[c]Democratic Republic of the Congo, 14; Ethiopia, 3.

Source: World Health Organization.

TABLE 94-3

RECOMMENDATIONS FOR POLIOVIRUS VACCINATION OF ADULTS

1. Most adults in the United States have been vaccinated during childhood and have little risk of exposure to wild-type virus in the United States. Immunization is recommended for those with a higher risk of exposure than the general population, including:
   a. Travelers to areas where poliovirus is or may be epidemic or endemic;
   b. Members of communities or population groups with disease caused by wild-type polioviruses;
   c. Laboratory workers handling specimens that may contain wild-type polioviruses;
   d. Health care workers in close contact with patients who may be excreting wild-type polioviruses.
2. Three doses of IPV are recommended for adults who need to be immunized. The second dose should be given 1–2 months after the first dose; the third dose should be given 6–12 months after the second dose.
3. Adults who are at increased risk of exposure to wild-type poliovirus and who have previously completed primary immunization should receive a single dose of IPV. Adults who did not complete primary immunization should receive the remaining vaccinations with IPV.

Note: IPV, inactivated poliovirus vaccine.
Source: Modified from Pickering LK, ed. Redbook 2006: Committee on Infectious Diseases, 27th ed. Elk Grove Village, IL: American Academy of Pediatrics.

in the risk of community transmission of wild-type virus. Because of progress toward global eradication of polio (with a reduced risk of imported cases) and the continued occurrence of cases of vaccine-associated polio, an all-IPV regimen was recommended in 2000 for childhood poliovirus vaccination in the United States, with vaccine administration at 2, 4, and 6–18 months and 4–6 years of age. The risk of vaccine-associated polio should be discussed before OPV is administered. Recommendations for vaccination of adults are listed in Table 94-3.

There are concerns about discontinuing vaccination in the event that endemic spread of poliovirus is eliminated. Among the reasons for these concerns are that poliovirus is shed from some immunocompromised persons for several years, that vaccine-derived poliovirus can circulate and cause disease, and that wild-type poliovirus is present in a large number of laboratories. A national survey began in October 2002 to encourage laboratories to dispose of all unneeded wild-type poliovirus materials and to identify laboratories that have wild-type poliovirus or specimens that may contain virus.

REOVIRUSES

Reoviruses are double-stranded RNA viruses encompassing three serotypes. Serologic studies indicate that most humans are infected with reoviruses during childhood. Most infections either are asymptomatic or cause very mild disease. One outbreak of reovirus infection in children resulted in minor upper respiratory tract symptoms. Reovirus is considered a rare cause of mild gastroenteritis in infants and children. Speculation regarding an association of reovirus type 3 with idiopathic neonatal hepatitis and extrahepatic biliary atresia is based on an elevated prevalence of antibody to reovirus among some of these patients and the detection of viral RNA by PCR in hepatobiliary tissues in some studies.

FURTHER READINGS

Alexander LN et al: Vaccine policy changes and epidemiology of poliomyelitis in the United States. JAMA 292:1696, 2004

Arita I et al: Is polio eradication realistic? Science 312:852, 2006

Centers for Disease Control and Prevention: Enterovirus surveillance—United States, 2002–2004. MMWR 55:153, 2006

———: Resurgence of wild poliovirus type 1 transmission and consequences of importation—21 countries, 2002–2005. MMWR 55:145, 2006

Chang L-Y et al: Transmission and clinical features of enterovirus 71 infections in household contacts in Taiwan. JAMA 291:222, 2004

el Sayed N et al: Monovalent type 1 oral poliovirus vaccine in newborns. N Engl J Med 359:1655, 2008

Fowlkes AL et al: Enterovirus-associated encephalitis in the California encephalitis project, 1998-2005. J Infect Dis 198:1685, 2008

Jenkins HE et al: Effectiveness of immunization against paralytic poliomyelitis in Nigeria. N Engl J Med 359:1666, 2008

Jubelt B, Aagre JC: Characteristics and management of postpolio syndrome. JAMA 284:412, 2000

Kew O et al: Vaccine-derived polioviruses and the endgame strategy for global polio eradication. Annu Rev Microbiol 59:587, 2005

Kupilia L et al: Diagnosis of enteroviral meningitis by use of polymerase chain reaction of cerebrospinal fluid, stool, and serum specimens. Clin Infect Dis 40:982, 2005

MacLennan C et al: Failure to clear persistent vaccine-derived neurovirulent poliovirus infection in an immunocompromised man. Lancet 363:1509, 2004

Perez-Velez CM et al: Outbreak of neurologic enterovirus type 71 disease: A diagnostic challenge. Clin Infect Dis 45:950, 2007

Thompson KM, Tebbens RJ: Eradication versus control for poliomyelitis: An economic analysis. Lancet 369:1363, 2007

Yajima T, Knowlton KU: Viral myocarditis: from the perspective of the virus. Circulation 119:2615, 2009

CHAPTER 95

MEASLES (RUBEOLA)

Anne Gershon

DEFINITION

Measles (rubeola) is a highly contagious, acute, exanthematous respiratory disease with a characteristic clinical picture and a pathognomonic enanthem: Koplik's spots, an eruption on the buccal mucous membranes (Fig. 95-1). A successful live attenuated measles vaccine became available in 1963 in the United States and elsewhere, and measles is now an unusual disease in most developed countries where this vaccine is widely used. However, measles continues to occur sporadically in miniepidemics in the United States, and major epidemics in developing nations make this disease a persistent cause of childhood morbidity and mortality.

In 2000, measles was the fifth leading cause of childhood mortality worldwide, with an estimated 777,000 deaths. The global incidence of measles in 2004 is shown in Fig. 95-2.

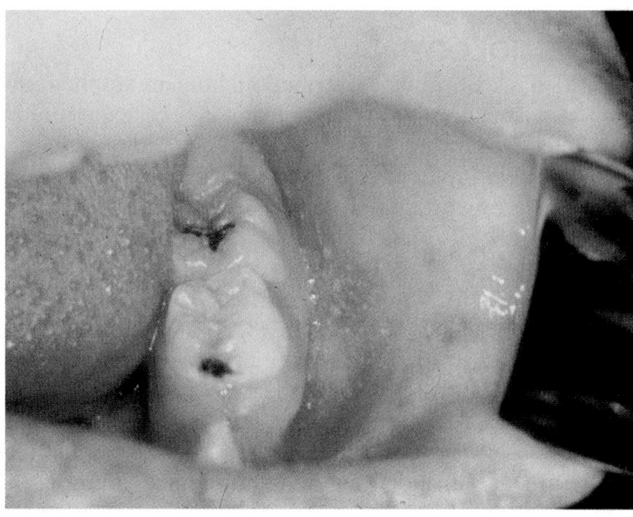

FIGURE 95-1
Koplik's spots, which manifest as white or bluish lesions with an erythematous halo on the buccal mucosa, usually occur in the first 2 days of measles symptoms and may briefly overlap the measles exanthem. The presence of the erythematous halo differentiates Koplik's spots from Fordyce's spots (ectopic sebaceous glands), which occur in the mouths of healthy individuals. *(Source: Centers for Disease Control and Prevention. Photo selected by Dr. Kenneth Kaye.)*

ETIOLOGIC AGENT

Measles virus is the only member of the genus *Morbillivirus* that infects humans. Part of the family Paramyxoviridae, it is related to viruses causing similar infections in other mammals: distemper, rinderpest, morbilli, and *peste des petits ruminants*. There is only one antigenic type. Virions—pleomorphic spheres with a diameter of

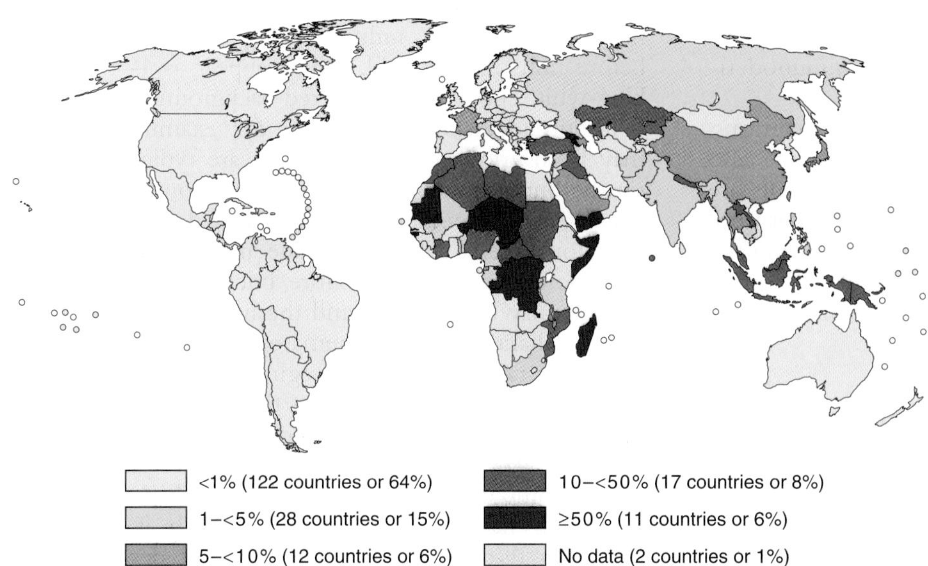

FIGURE 95-2
Worldwide reported measles incidence rate per 100,000 population, 2004. *(Source: WHO/IBV database, 2005. This map does not imply the expression of any opinion whatsoever on the part of the World Health Organization concerning the legal status of any country, territory, city, or area of its authorities or concerning the delimitation of its frontiers or boundaries.)*

100–250 nm—consist of six proteins. The inner capsid is composed of RNA and three proteins. The outer envelope consists of a matrix protein bearing short surface-glycoprotein projections or peplomers, one a hemagglutinin (H) and the other a fusion (F) protein. Sequencing of the single-stranded genome makes it possible to distinguish vaccine-type from wild-type virus. The genetic variability of wild-type virus (23 genotypes identified) permits identification of strains endemic within a given locale where measles cases have occurred. The cellular receptors for measles virus are the CD46 and CD150 molecules expressed on many human cells.

EPIDEMIOLOGY

Measles has a worldwide distribution; humans are the only natural hosts, although other primates can be experimentally infected. During the prevaccination era in the United States, measles epidemics took place every 2–5 years. In epidemic years, roughly half a million measles cases occurred; 99% of adults had serologic evidence of previous measles infection. After the live attenuated vaccine became available, the number of cases reported to the Centers for Disease Control and Prevention fell, with a nadir of 1497 cases in 1983. In 1990, after an upsurge to more than 27,000 cases (with 89 deaths), the disease was once more brought under control, mainly through the routine administration of two doses of vaccine. Reasons for the resurgence included failure to immunize young children, especially in inner-city areas; primary vaccine failure (rate, ~5%); and (rarely) waning immunity.

Between 1993 and 1996, fewer than 1000 cases per year were reported in the United States; 309 cases were reported in 1995, 116 in 2001, and only 37 in 2004. Molecular studies indicated interruption of transmission of indigenous measles in 1993. Most cases since have resulted from international importations of the virus by immigrants or U.S. citizens returning from travel abroad. Mortality rates are highest among children <2 years of age and among adults. Patients with impaired cell-mediated immunity are at especially high risk for severe or even fatal measles. The measles-associated mortality rate in the United States is ~0.3%; in developing countries, it frequently exceeds 1% and sometimes approaches 10% because of malnutrition and associated immunodeficiency and HIV infection.

Measles virus is transmitted by respiratory secretions, predominantly through exposure to aerosols but also through direct contact with larger droplets. Patients are contagious from 1 or 2 days before symptom onset until 4 days after the rash appears. Infectivity peaks during the prodromal phase. The mean intervals from infection to symptom onset and rash appearance are 10 and 14 days, respectively.

PATHOGENESIS, IMMUNITY, AND PATHOLOGY

Measles virus invades the respiratory epithelium and spreads via the bloodstream to the reticuloendothelial system, from which it infects white blood cells, thereby establishing infection of the skin, respiratory tract, and other organs. Both viremia and viruria develop. Multinucleated giant cells with inclusion bodies in the nucleus and cytoplasm (Warthin-Finkeldey cells) are found in respiratory and lymphoid tissues and are pathognomonic for measles. Direct invasion of T lymphocytes and increased levels of suppressive cytokines (e.g., interleukin 4) may play a role in the temporary depression of cellular immunity that accompanies and transiently follows measles. The major infected cell in the blood is the monocyte. Infection of the entire respiratory tract accounts for the characteristic cough and coryza of measles and for the less frequent manifestations of croup, bronchiolitis, and pneumonia. Generalized damage to the respiratory tract, with loss of cilia, predisposes to secondary bacterial infections such as pneumonia and otitis media.

Specific antibodies are not detectable before the onset of rash. Cellular immunity (consisting of cytotoxic T cells and possibly natural killer cells) plays a prominent role in host defense, and patients who are deficient in cellular immunity are at high risk for severe measles. Children with isolated agammaglobulinemia are not at increased risk. Immune reactions to the virus in the endothelial cells of dermal capillaries play a substantial role in the development of Koplik's spots (the pathognomonic enanthem) and rash; in immunodeficient hosts, measles may be severe despite the absence of these manifestations. Measles antigens have been demonstrated in involved skin during early stages of the illness.

Pathologic changes in measles encephalitis include focal hemorrhage, congestion, and perivascular demyelination. Measles virus is rarely isolated from cerebrospinal fluid (CSF) in cases of encephalitis, which are thought to be due to the interaction of virus-infected cells with local cellular immune factors.

CLINICAL MANIFESTATIONS

Measles begins with a 2- to 4-day respiratory prodrome of malaise, cough, coryza, conjunctivitis with lacrimation, nasal discharge, and increasing fever [with temperatures as high as 40.6°C (105°F), probably reflecting secondary viremia]. At this stage of the illness, in which the rash has not yet developed, influenza may be suspected. Just before rash onset, Koplik's spots appear as 1- to 2-mm blue-white spots on a bright red background (Fig. 95-1). Without adequate illumination for examination, they may be overlooked. Koplik's spots are typically located on the buccal mucosa, alongside the second molars, and may be extensive; they are not associated with any other infectious disease. The spots wane after the onset of rash and soon disappear. The entire buccal and inner labial mucosa may be inflamed, and the lips may be reddened.

The characteristic erythematous, nonpruritic, maculopapular rash of measles begins at the hairline and behind the ears, spreads down the trunk and limbs to include the palms and soles, and often becomes confluent (Fig. 95-3). At this time, the patient is at the most severe point of the illness. By the fourth day, the rash begins to fade in the order in which it appeared. Brownish discoloration of the skin and desquamation

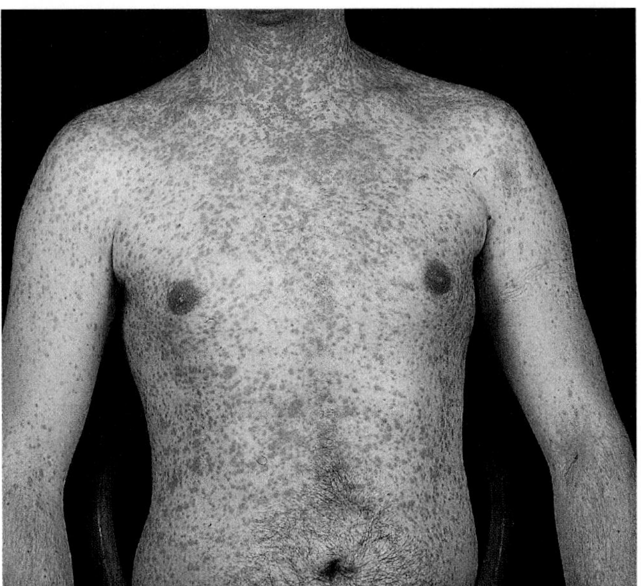

FIGURE 95-3

In measles, discrete erythematous lesions become confluent as the rash spreads downward. *(Reprinted with permission from Fitzpatrick TB et al: Color Atlas & Synopsis of Clinical Dermatology, 4th ed. New York, McGraw-Hill, 2001, p 775.)*

may occur later. Fever usually resolves by the fourth or fifth day after the onset of rash; prolonged fever suggests a complication of measles. Lymphadenopathy, diarrhea, vomiting, and splenomegaly are common features. The chest x-ray may be abnormal, even in uncomplicated measles, because of the propensity of measles virus to invade the respiratory tract. The entire illness, which usually lasts ~10 days, tends to be more severe in adults than in children, with higher fever, more prominent rash, and a higher incidence of complications.

Milder forms of the illness with less intense symptoms and a milder rash, termed *modified measles*, may occur in individuals with preexisting partial immunity induced by active or passive vaccination. These patients include infants <1 year of age who retain some proportion of passively acquired maternal antibodies. On occasion, individuals with a history of immunization may develop modified measles.

COMPLICATIONS

The complications of measles (Table 95-1) can be divided into three groups, according to the site involved: the respiratory tract, the central nervous system (CNS), and the gastrointestinal tract. Respiratory tract involvement, manifested as laryngitis, croup, or bronchitis, occurs in the majority of cases of uncomplicated measles. In young children, otitis media is the most common complication. Pneumonia is a frequent reason for hospitalization, especially of adults. The pneumonia is of viral origin in the majority of cases, but secondary bacterial infection (most commonly caused by streptococci, pneumococci, or staphylococci) also develops with some frequency. Primary giant-cell (Hecht's) pneumonia is most often documented in immunocompromised and/or malnourished patients.

TABLE 95-1

COMPLICATIONS OF MEASLES

COMPLICATION	COMMENTS
Otitis media	Very common in infants with measles
Pneumonia	May be primary viral pneumonia or bacterial superinfection; frequent reason for hospitalization of adults; measles rash sometimes lacking in immunocompromised patients with measles pneumonia
Croup	Occasionally severe, requiring intubation in infants
Gastroenteritis	Diarrhea can be life threatening in infants
Cervical adenitis	Due to lymphoid hyperplasia as host response to virus; common
Acute encephalitis	May be mild to severe/fatal; occurs in 1 in 1000 cases of measles; cerebral and cerebellar forms; immune-mediated pathogenesis
Subacute sclerosing panencephalitis (SSPE)	In 1 in 100,000 cases of measles, usually when measles occurs in infancy; seen 5–10 years later. In the United States, most children with SSPE were born in another country where measles vaccine is not routinely used.

Encephalographic abnormalities in the absence of symptoms of CNS disease are extremely common in measles. Symptomatic CNS disease may present with fever, headache, drowsiness, coma, and/or seizures. Symptoms usually begin within days after the onset of rash but occasionally appear for the first time several weeks later. About 10% of patients do not survive acute measles encephalitis; a significant percentage of survivors have permanent sequelae (e.g., mental retardation or epilepsy). Most cases appear to result from an immune-mediated response to myelin proteins (postinfectious encephalomyelitis) and not directly from viral infection of the CNS. Rarely, transverse myelitis follows measles. Immunocompromised patients are at risk for progressive fatal encephalitis 1–6 months after measles; in some cases, even though prior measles has not been recognized, the virus is identified at autopsy. Subacute sclerosing panencephalitis (SSPE)—a protracted, chronic, extremely rare form of measles encephalitis—sometimes follows measles and is particularly common among children who have measles before the age of 2 years (Chap. 29). As a result of widespread vaccination, SSPE has virtually disappeared in the United States. Typically, progressive dementia evolves over several months. SSPE is thought to be due to a complex interaction of the host with defective measles virus.

Gastrointestinal complications of measles include gastroenteritis, hepatitis, appendicitis, ileocolitis, and mesenteric adenitis. It is not uncommon to detect high levels of alanine and aspartate aminotransferases in the absence of gastrointestinal signs such as jaundice.

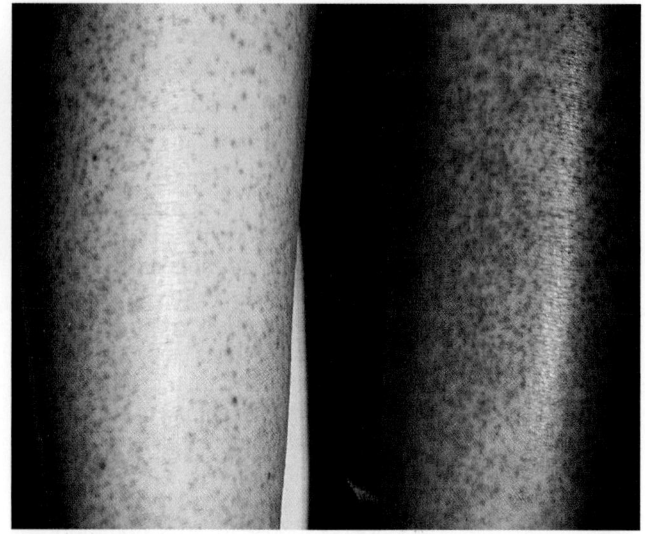

FIGURE 95-4
Petechial lesions in a patient with atypical measles. *(Photo courtesy of Stephen E. Gellis, MD; with permission.)*

Rare complications include myocarditis, glomerulonephritis, and postinfectious thrombocytopenic purpura. Measles can exacerbate preexisting tuberculosis, presumably through virus-induced depression of cellular immunity. Natural measles and immunization against measles can result in tuberculin skin-test anergy lasting for ~1 month.

ATYPICAL MEASLES

An atypical form of measles has been reported in individuals who received formalin-inactivated measles vaccine (used in the United States in 1963–1967 and in Canada until 1970) and subsequently were exposed to measles virus. After a several-day prodrome of fever, myalgia, and headache, the rash appears (Fig. 95-4); it begins peripherally and can be urticarial, maculopapular, hemorrhagic, and/or vesicular. Fever is high and accompanied by edema of the extremities, interstitial pulmonary infiltrates, hepatitis, and (on occasion) pleural effusion. The differential diagnosis includes Rocky Mountain spotted fever, Henoch-Schönlein purpura, meningococcemia, drug allergy, toxic shock syndrome, and varicella. Despite its severity, the illness is self-limited. Measles virus cannot be isolated from these patients. This disease is believed to be due to hypersensitivity to measles virus induced by the inactivated vaccine. To prevent it, adults who received formalin-inactivated measles vaccine should be immunized with live attenuated measles vaccine. Because inactivated measles vaccine has not been available for >35 years, atypical measles has virtually disappeared.

MEASLES IN THE IMMUNOCOMPROMISED HOST

Patients with defects in cell-mediated immunity are at risk for severe protracted and fatal measles. Included in this category are patients with congenital cellular immune defects or malignancy, recipients of immunosuppressive therapy, or persons infected with HIV. In these patients, measles may not be accompanied by a rash. Complications are primary measles (giant-cell) pneumonia, progressive encephalitis beginning weeks or months after initial infection, and (in HIV-infected patients) progression to AIDS.

MEASLES IN ADULTS

Measles is naturally a disease of childhood and, like many other viral infections, is more severe in adults than in children. About 3% of young adults with measles develop primary viral pneumonia and require hospitalization. Hepatitis and bronchospasm are more common among adults with measles than among children, and the rash is more severe and more confluent in adults. Bacterial superinfection is more common among adults, more than one-third of whom develop respiratory complications such as otitis media, sinusitis, and pneumonia. Adults may develop measles because they were never immunized or (more rarely) because their vaccine-induced immunity has waned. Very low titers of antibody to measles virus have been associated with lack of protection.

LABORATORY FINDINGS

Lymphopenia and neutropenia are common in measles and may be due to invasion of leukocytes by the virus, with subsequent cell death. Leukocytosis may herald a bacterial superinfection. Patients with measles encephalitis usually have an elevated protein concentration in CSF as well as lymphocytosis.

DIAGNOSIS

A specific diagnosis of measles can be made quickly by immunofluorescent staining of a smear of respiratory secretions for measles antigen; monoclonal antibodies conjugated to fluorescein are commercially available. Secretions can be examined microscopically for multinucleated giant cells. Measles virus can be demonstrated by culture or polymerase chain reaction in respiratory secretions or urine. A number of serologic tests are available. A serologic diagnosis by enzyme immunoassay (EIA) cannot necessarily be made rapidly if acute- and convalescent-phase serum specimens are examined. However, EIA measurement of specific IgM permits diagnosis on the basis of an acute-phase serum sample. Specific IgM antibodies are detectable within 1–2 days after rash onset, and the IgG titer rises significantly after 10 days. Atypical measles and SSPE are associated with extremely high levels of measles antibodies in blood and/or CSF.

DIFFERENTIAL DIAGNOSIS

Classic measles—with Koplik's spots, cough, coryza, conjunctivitis, and a rash beginning on the head—is easily diagnosed on clinical grounds. Modified measles is more difficult to diagnose because one or more characteristic signs or symptoms may be lacking. The differential diagnosis of measles includes Kawasaki disease, scarlet fever, infectious mononucleosis, toxoplasmosis, drug eruption, and

Mycoplasma pneumoniae infection. In the differential diagnosis of measles, attention should be paid to the current epidemiology of the disease in the community and to the patient's history of measles vaccination and foreign travel.

PREVENTION

The development of live attenuated measles vaccine by Enders and colleagues was a milestone in American medicine. This vaccine, used in the United States for the routine immunization of children since 1963, induces seroconversion in ~95% of recipients and probably confers lifelong protection. Waning immunity to measles after immunization is rare. For the past three decades, measles vaccine has been available as the combination vaccine measles-mumps-rubella (MMR); this vaccine should be administered to children at 12–15 months of age. (Vaccination at 12 months is preferred for infants whose mothers were immunized against measles in childhood.) A second dose of MMR vaccine is recommended for school-age children. This two-dose policy was developed in the late 1980s in response to measles outbreaks in the United States. MMR vaccine is likely to be supplanted by MMRV vaccine, which also covers varicella and was licensed by the U.S. Food and Drug Administration in 2005. MMRV vaccine is licensed only for children 1–13 years of age.

Older susceptible persons should be immunized. Individuals should be considered susceptible to measles unless they have documentation of physician-diagnosed measles or of the receipt of two doses of vaccine, have laboratory evidence of measles immunity, or were born before 1957. Rarely, individuals born before 1957 develop measles, and those who are at risk of exposure to measles (e.g., health care workers, teachers, and international travelers) should be tested for measles antibody and immunized if necessary. Approximately 10% of healthy vaccinees develop a fever, with temperatures up to 39.4°C (103°F), 5–7 days after vaccination; this fever lasts 1–5 days and is accompanied by a transient rash. Individuals previously immunized only with killed vaccine are considered susceptible and should receive at least one dose—preferably two doses—of MMR vaccine. Transient adverse reactions in these individuals include fever, malaise, and redness and swelling at the injection site.

Because of the severity of measles in this group and the lack of reported problems following vaccination, children with asymptomatic HIV infection should receive MMR vaccine; those with severe immunosuppression (<15% CD4+ T lymphocytes) should not. A case of fatal measles due to vaccine-type virus was reported in a college student with AIDS in 1998. Measles vaccine is contraindicated for persons with impaired cell-mediated immunity, for pregnant women, and for persons with a history of anaphylaxis due to egg protein or neomycin. Minor illnesses, with or without fever and a history of convulsions, are not contraindications to vaccination. Vaccination should be deferred for 6–11 months after the receipt of immune globulin or of blood products containing antibodies and for at least 3 months after the discontinuation of immunosuppressive treatment. Vaccine failures have been ascribed to faulty vaccine storage, the presence of maternally derived antibodies in infants, and simultaneous administration of measles vaccine and immune globulin.

The only temporally related causal complications of measles vaccination are febrile seizures, which rarely have long-term sequelae; self-limited thrombocytopenia; and rare anaphylaxis. An exhaustive analysis conducted in 2000 by a number of official committees, including those of the American Academy of Pediatrics and the Institute of Medicine, found no causal relationship between MMR vaccination and subsequent development of autism.

Children and adults who are susceptible to measles and are exposed to the disease should receive postexposure prophylaxis. Standard immune globulin, given intramuscularly within 6 days of exposure, can exert a protective or modifying effect. The dose is 0.25 mL/kg for healthy persons and 0.5 mL/kg for immunocompromised persons, with a maximum dose of 15 mL. Immune globulin is particularly strongly indicated for susceptible household contacts, especially those <1 year of age, and for immunocompromised persons. HIV-infected individuals, particularly those with severe immunosuppression, should be given immune globulin after exposure, regardless of their measles immune status and whether or not they are receiving intravenous immune globulin. Vaccination within 72 h of exposure may also provide protection against clinical measles but is contraindicated in immunocompromised patients. Vaccine and immune globulin should not be given concurrently.

℞ Treatment: MEASLES

Therapy for measles is largely supportive and symptom based. Patients with otitis media and pneumonia should be given standard antibiotics. Patients with encephalitis need supportive care, including observation for increased intracranial pressure. Controlled trials suggest clinical benefit from high doses of vitamin A in severe or potentially severe measles, especially in children <2 years old who are or may be malnourished. On the basis of limited data, a dose of 50,000 IU is used for infants 1–6 months old; 100,000 IU is recommended for infants 7–12 months old and 200,000 IU for children >1 year old. A single dose is administered on two consecutive days. In the United States, vitamin A treatment is recommended for young children hospitalized for measles and for pediatric measles patients with immunodeficiency, clinical evidence of vitamin A deficiency, impaired intestinal absorption, moderate to severe malnutrition, or recent immigration from an area where there is high mortality from measles. Transient vomiting and headache may be associated with the administration of vitamin A. Ribavirin is effective against measles virus in vitro and may be considered for use in immunocompromised individuals.

FURTHER READINGS

Centers for Disease Control and Prevention: Measles, mumps, and rubella—vaccine use and strategies for elimination of measles, rubella, and congenital rubella syndrome and control of mumps. MMWR Morb Mortal Wkly Rep 47:1, 1998

———: Measles—United States, 2004. MMWR Morb Mortal Wkly Rep 54:1229, 2005

———: Update: measles—United States, January–July 2008. MMWR Morb Mortal Wkly Rep 57:893, 2008

———: Progress toward measles elimination—European Region, 2005–2008. MMWR Morb Mortal Wkly Rep 58:142, 2009

D'Souza RM, D'Souza R: Vitamin A for preventing secondary infections in children with measles—a systematic review. J Trop Pediatr 48:72, 2002

Forni AL et al: Severe measles pneumonitis in adults: Evaluation of clinical characteristics and therapy with intravenous ribavirin. Clin Infect Dis 19:454, 1994

Gerber JS, Offit PA: Vaccines and autism: a tale of shifting hypotheses. Clin Infect Dis 48:456, 2009

Immunization Safety Review Committee, Institute of Medicine: *Immunization Safety Review: Measles-Mumps-Rubella Vaccine and Autism*, K Stratton et al (eds). Washington, DC, National Academy of Sciences, 2001 *(www.nap.edu/catalog/10101.html)*

Kaplan LJ et al: Severe measles in immunocompromised patients. JAMA 267:1237, 1992

Stalkup JR: A review of measles virus. Dermatol Clin 20:209, 2002

Yeung LF et al: A limited measles outbreak in a highly vaccinated US boarding school. Pediatrics 116:1287, 2005

CHAPTER 96
RUBELLA (GERMAN MEASLES)

Anne Gershon

DEFINITION

Rubella is an acute viral infection of children and adults that characteristically includes rash, fever, and lymphadenopathy and has a broad spectrum of other possible manifestations. However, a high percentage of rubella infections in both children and adults are subclinical. In addition, the illness can resemble a mild attack of measles (rubeola) and can cause arthritis, especially in adults. Rubella was formerly known as *German measles* because it was first distinguished clinically from rubeola in Germany, where it generated much medical interest in the mid-eighteenth and early nineteenth centuries. Rubella during pregnancy can lead to fetal infection, with the production of a significant constellation of malformations (*congenital rubella syndrome*) in a high proportion of infected fetuses. Rubella virus was first isolated in cell culture just before the last pandemic of the disease began in 1962. Since the licensing of rubella vaccine in the United States in 1969, there have been no further epidemics in this country.

ETIOLOGIC AGENT

Rubella virus, a togavirus, is the only member of the *Rubivirus* genus and is closely related to the alphaviruses. Unlike these agents, however, it does not require a vector for transmission. Moreover, there is no RNA sequence homology between rubella virus and the alphaviruses.

The rubella virion is composed of an inner icosahedral capsid of RNA and protein that is surrounded by a lipid-containing envelope with glycoprotein spikes and a diameter of ~60 nm. The structural proteins associated with rubella virus are E1 and E2 (transmembrane envelope glycoproteins) and C (the capsid protein that surrounds the viral RNA). Only one serotype has been identified.

EPIDEMIOLOGY

In the United States during the prevaccine era, rubella was most common in the spring and most often affected school-age children; only 80–90% of adults were immune; and major epidemics occurred every 6–9 years. The most recent epidemic in the United States occurred in 1964–1965, when more than 12 million cases of postnatal rubella and more than 20,000 cases of the congenital rubella syndrome were reported. Although there have been no epidemics since the introduction of live attenuated rubella vaccine in 1969, limited outbreaks have been reported in settings where susceptible individuals come into close contact with one another (e.g., schools and workplaces). Since 2001, the annual incidences of rubella have been the lowest ever recorded in the United States. In 2001–2004, an average of only 14 cases of postnatally acquired rubella were reported annually to the Centers for Disease Control and Prevention (CDC). During these 4 years, only 4 confirmed cases of congenital rubella syndrome were reported. Three of the affected infants were born to women who had immigrated to the United States. Currently, 91% of U.S. residents are estimated to be immune to rubella, and at least 95% of schoolchildren have been immunized. When rubella is reported in the United States, the genotype of the virus is consistent with an imported agent.

Although rubella is no longer considered endemic in the United States, global challenges remain. According to the World Health Organization, 57% of countries included rubella vaccine in their national programs in 2003, but rubella continues to be endemic in many areas of the world.

Whether symptomatic or subclinical, rubella is contagious, albeit less so than measles. Its incubation period is 18 days on average, with a range of 12–23 days. The virus, which is spread in droplets shed in respiratory secretions, infects the respiratory tract and then the bloodstream. In postnatally acquired infections, rubella virus is shed during the prodromal phase of the illness, and shedding from the pharynx can continue for ~1 week after onset. Despite high titers of specific neutralizing antibodies, infants with congenital rubella may excrete rubella virus from the respiratory tract and in the urine until the age of 2 years. This excretion raises important issues related to infection control in hospital and day-care settings. Persons recently immunized with live attenuated rubella vaccine do not transmit the vaccine virus to others, although low titers of rubella virus may be detected transiently in the pharynx.

After an attack of rubella, specific antibodies and cell-mediated immunity develop and probably play a significant role in protection against future disease. Asymptomatic reinfection at the level of the respiratory tract is common upon re-exposure to the virus but is rarely, if ever, associated with viremia.

Rubella virus has been cultured from respiratory secretions during reinfection. Fetal infection may occur during maternal reinfection but is acknowledged to be extremely rare because of the absence of maternal viremia under these circumstances. Viremia following reinfection of individuals immunized against rubella also is rare.

Although the current level of congenital rubella in the United States is exceedingly low, it has been observed that young immigrants to the United States from countries in Latin America and the Caribbean, where rubella vaccine is not routinely given to children, are at increased risk for rubella susceptibility. Because infants with the congenital rubella syndrome have been born to immigrant Hispanic women, increasing efforts have been made to identify and vaccinate such women before they become pregnant.

PATHOGENESIS AND PATHOLOGY

Little is known about the microscopic pathology of postnatally acquired rubella because the disease is invariably self-limited. Like that of measles, the rash of rubella is immunologically mediated; its onset coincides with the development of specific antibodies. Viremia can be demonstrated for ~1 week before and ends within a few days after the onset of rash.

The cause of the damage to cells and organs in congenital rubella is not well understood. Proposed mechanisms of fetal damage include mitotic arrest of cells, tissue necrosis without inflammation, and chromosomal damage. The growth of the fetus may be retarded. Other findings may include decreased numbers of megakaryocytes in the bone marrow, extramedullary hematopoiesis, and interstitial pneumonia.

CLINICAL MANIFESTATIONS

Postnatally Acquired Rubella

Infection acquired after birth usually results in an extremely mild or subclinical illness. A prodromal phase is uncommon in children; adults may have more severe disease, with a brief prodrome of malaise, fever, and anorexia. The foremost symptoms of postnatally acquired rubella include posterior auricular, cervical, and suboccipital lymphadenopathy; fever; and rash. The rash often begins on the face (Fig. 96-1) and spreads down the body. It is maculopapular but not confluent, is sometimes accompanied by mild coryza and conjunctivitis, and generally lasts for 3–5 days. A petechial enanthem on the soft palate, designated *Forschheimer spots*, may occur but is not specific for rubella. Fever may be absent entirely or may be present for only several days in the early phase of the illness.

Complications of postnatally acquired rubella are uncommon; bacterial superinfection is rare. One particularly troublesome complication is seen almost exclusively in women: arthritis, most frequently involving the fingers, wrists, and/or knees. Arthritis develops as the rash is appearing and may take several weeks to resolve. Chronic arthritis resulting from rubella is extremely rare. Rubella virus has been isolated from joint fluid during acute

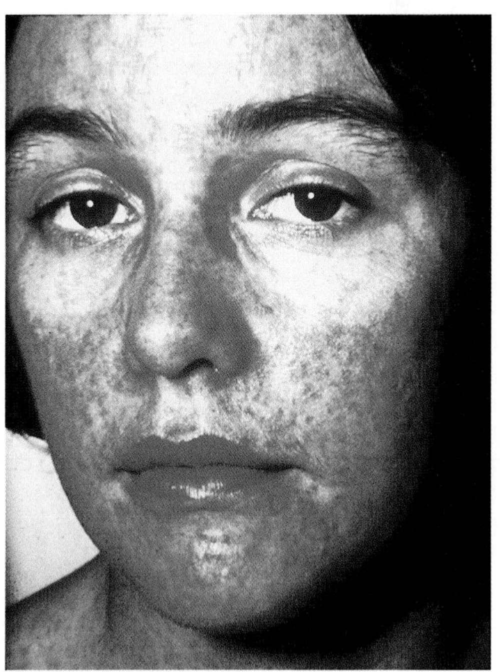

FIGURE 96-1

In rubella, an erythematous exanthem spreads from the hairline downward and clears as it spreads. *(Photo courtesy of Stephen E. Gellis, MD; with permission.)*

rubella arthritis and from peripheral blood in chronic rubella arthritis.

Another complication of postnatally acquired rubella is hemorrhage due to both thrombocytopenia and vascular damage; this complication occurs in 1 of every 3000 patients. Thrombocytopenia may last for weeks or months; it can have long-term consequences if there is bleeding into organs such as the eye or the brain.

Both children and adults may develop encephalitis after rubella; the incidence is about five times lower than that of encephalitis following measles. Adults are more likely than children to develop encephalitis; the mortality rate from this complication is 20–50%. Mild hepatitis is an unusual complication. Immunosuppressed patients are not at increased risk for rubella as they are for measles.

Congenital Rubella

Maternal infection in early pregnancy can lead to fetal infection, with resultant congenital rubella. The classic signs of congenital rubella are cataract, heart disease, deafness, and myriad other defects (Table 96-1). The most important factor in the pathogenicity of rubella virus for the fetus is gestational age at the time of infection. Maternal infection during the first trimester leads to fetal infection in ~50% of cases; maternal infection early in the second trimester leads to fetal infection in about one-third of cases. Fetal malformations not only are more common after maternal infection in the first trimester but also tend to be more severe and to involve more organ systems. Whereas a fetus infected in the fourth week of gestation may develop many problems, one infected later (e.g., in the twentieth week) may have isolated deafness as the only symptom.

TABLE 96-1

CLINICAL PROBLEMS ASSOCIATED WITH THE CONGENITAL RUBELLA SYNDROME

TRANSIENT SIGNS/ SYMPTOMS (AT BIRTH ONLY)	PERMANENT SIGNS/ SYMPTOMS (DEVELOPMENTAL)
Bony abnormalities	Autism
Cloudy cornea	Behavioral disorders
Hemolytic anemia	Congenital heart disease (patent ductus arteriosus, pulmonic stenosis)
Hepatitis	Cryptorchidism
Hepatosplenomegaly	Deafness
Jaundice	Degenerative brain disease
Low birth weight	Diabetes mellitus
Lymphadenopathy	Glaucoma
Meningoencephalitis	Inguinal hernia
Rubella viral pneumonia	Mental retardation
Thrombocytopenic purpura	Microcephaly
	Myopia
	Precocious puberty
	Retinopathy
	Seizures
	Spastic diplegia
	Thyroid disorders

DIAGNOSIS

Because postnatally acquired rubella is often a mild disease and because many cases are subclinical, diagnosis on clinical grounds can be difficult. Other diseases that may mimic rubella include toxoplasmosis, scarlet fever, modified measles, roseola, fifth disease (erythema infectiosum due to parvovirus B19), and enteroviral infection. Routine laboratory tests usually reveal leukopenia and atypical lymphocytes.

The isolation of rubella virus in cell cultures of throat samples, urine, or other secretions is difficult and expensive but is sometimes undertaken. Polymerase chain reaction (PCR) is also useful for diagnosis. These techniques are particularly useful when congenital rubella is suspected. A laboratory diagnosis may also be made serologically. The most commonly used test is an enzyme-linked immunosorbent assay (ELISA) for IgG and IgM antibodies. Acute rubella is diagnosed by the documentation of a fourfold or greater rise in the titer of IgG antibodies in paired acute- and convalescent-phase serum specimens or by the detection of rubella-specific IgM antibodies in one serum specimen. However, false-negative and false-positive IgM reactions are sometimes obtained. Moreover, true-positive IgM reactions can occur in both primary infection and reinfection. Congenital rubella is diagnosed by the isolation of rubella virus, a positive PCR assay, the detection of IgM antibodies in a single serum sample, and/or the documentation of either the persistence of rubella antibodies in serum beyond 1 year of age or a rising antibody titer anytime during infancy in an unvaccinated child. Biopsied tissues and/or blood and cerebrospinal fluid have also been used for the demonstration of rubella antigens with monoclonal antibodies and for the detection of rubella RNA by in situ hybridization and PCR.

Cases of suspected postnatal or congenital rubella should be reported to the CDC.

PREVENTION

Live attenuated rubella vaccine was licensed in 1969, 7 years after rubella virus was first isolated in culture. This vaccine was developed as a strategy to prevent congenital rubella by ensuring that very few pregnant women would be susceptible and that there would be little circulating wild-type virus. Rubella vaccine induces seroconversion in >95% of recipients. Since its licensure, there have been no major epidemics in the United States, and the number of cases has declined by 98%. The vaccine currently licensed in the United States, RA 27/3, is propagated in human diploid cells and is more immunogenic (particularly with regard to the stimulation of secretory immunity) than previously licensed vaccines. The present vaccination strategy, developed in part when measles was not being adequately controlled, is to immunize all infants at 12–15 months of age with measles-mumps-rubella (MMR) vaccine and to administer a second dose in early childhood. Rubella vaccine may also be administered to anyone who is thought to be susceptible to the infection and is not pregnant; it is particularly important that hospital workers of either sex be immune to rubella so that nosocomial transmission is avoided. Although there has been little change in the prevalence of immunity to rubella among women of childbearing age (~80%), the incidence of congenital rubella is extremely low, with fewer than 10 cases annually. It is likely that, although antibody may be undetectable years after immunization, protection against infection—possibly due to cell-mediated immunity—is the rule. At present, there is little if any evidence of significant waning of clinically important immunity to rubella with time.

On occasion, rubella vaccine may cause arthralgia or arthritis, especially in young women. Very rarely, rubella vaccination results in chronic arthritis; however, even cases of frank arthritis in vaccinees are generally self-limited, lasting only ~1 week.

After investigation of a series of more than 400 women who were inadvertently immunized during pregnancy and who carried their infants to term, the CDC has concluded that vaccine-type rubella virus either does not cause the congenital rubella syndrome at all or does so at an incidence too low to be detected. Nonetheless, rubella vaccine is contraindicated for use in pregnant women, and it is recommended that pregnancy be avoided for at least 3 months after rubella vaccination. It is acceptable for rubella-susceptible children whose mothers also are susceptible to be immunized, as vaccine recipients do not shed rubella virus or transmit it to susceptible individuals. Although it is recommended that rubella vaccine not be given to immunosuppressed persons, the vaccine is given to children infected with HIV. No adverse effects of rubella vaccine have been reported in immunocompromised patients.

℞ Treatment: RUBELLA

There is no specific therapy for rubella. At one time, immune globulin was used in an effort to prevent congenital rubella when pregnant women became infected. However, because administration of immune globulin did not prevent maternal viremia, this approach was discarded. Symptom-based treatment is given for manifestations such as fever, arthralgia, and arthritis.

FURTHER READINGS

Abernathy E et al: Confirmation of rubella within 4 days of rash onset: Comparison of rubella virus RNA detection in oral fluid with immunoglobulin M detection in serum or oral fluid. J Clin Microbiol 47:182, 2009.

Andrade JQ et al: Rubella in pregnancy: Intrauterine transmission and perinatal outcome during a Brazilian epidemic. J Clin Virol 35:285, 2005

Banatvala JE, Brown DWG: Rubella. Lancet 363:1127, 2004

Centers for Disease Control and Prevention: Measles, mumps, and rubella—vaccine use and strategies for elimination of measles, rubella, and congenital rubella syndrome and control of mumps. MMWR Morb Mortal Wkly Rep 47:1, 1998

———: Control and prevention of rubella: Evaluation and management of suspected outbreaks, rubella in pregnant women, and surveillance for congenital rubella syndrome. MMWR Morb Mortal Wkly Rep 50:1, 2001

———: Elimination of rubella and congenital rubella syndrome—United States, 1969–2004. MMWR Morb Mortal Wkly Rep 54:279, 2005

———: Imported case of congenital rubella syndrome—New Hampshire, 2005. MMWR Morb Mortal Wkly Rep 54:1160, 2005

———: Progress toward elimination of rubella and congenital rubella syndrome—the Americas, 2003–2008. MMWR Morb Mortal Wkly Rep 57:1176, 2008

Danavaro-Holliday MC et al: A large rubella outbreak with spread from the workplace to the community. JAMA 284:2733, 2000

Gerber JS, Offit PA: Vaccines and autism: a tale of shifting hypotheses. Clin Infect Dis 48:456, 2009

Plotkin SA, Reef S: Rubella vaccine, in *Vaccines*, SA Plotkin and WA Orenstein (eds). Philadelphia, Saunders, 2004, pp 389–440

Reef SE et al: The changing epidemiology of rubella in the 1990s: On the verge of elimination and new challenges for control and prevention. JAMA 287:464, 2002

Sheridan E: Congenital rubella syndrome: A risk in immigrant populations. Lancet 359:674, 2002

CHAPTER 97

MUMPS

Anne Gershon

DEFINITION

Mumps is an acute, systemic, communicable viral infection whose most distinctive feature is swelling of one or both parotid glands. Involvement of other salivary glands, the meninges, the pancreas, and the gonads also is common.

ETIOLOGIC AGENT

Mumps virus, a paramyxovirus, is pleomorphic and has a diameter ranging from 100 to 300 nm. The virion is composed of RNA and seven proteins. The RNA is surrounded by an envelope composed of glycoproteins, including a hemagglutinin-neuraminidase (HN), a hemolysis cell fusion antigen (F), and a matrix envelope protein (M). A fourth protein (SH) may also be membrane-associated. There are three internal components: a nucleocapsid protein (NP), a phosphoprotein (P), and a large protein (L). There is only one antigenic type of mumps virus. Polymerase chain reaction (PCR) has detected geographic differences among mumps viruses from different locales.

EPIDEMIOLOGY

After the introduction of mumps vaccine in 1967, the incidence of clinical mumps declined significantly in the United States. In 1968 (before widespread immunization), 185,691 cases of mumps were reported in this country. The 231–277 cases reported annually in 2001–2005 represent a >99% reduction from prevaccine levels. Before widespread vaccination, the incidence of mumps was highest in the winter and spring, with epidemics every 2–5 years. At that time, mumps was principally a disease of childhood, although today >50% of cases occur in young adults. Epidemics tended to occur in confined populations (e.g., in schools and the military services).

The incubation period of mumps generally ranges from 14 to 18 days, with extremes of 7 and 23 days. However, because a contact may be shedding virus before the onset of clinical disease or (like one-third of patients) may have subclinical infection, the incubation period in individual cases is often uncertain. One attack of mumps usually confers lifelong immunity. Long-term immunity is also associated with immunization.

PATHOGENESIS

Mumps virus is transmitted by droplet nuclei, saliva, and fomites. Replication of the virus in the epithelium of the upper respiratory tract leads to viremia, which is followed by infection of glandular tissues and/or the central nervous system (CNS).

Little is known of the pathology of mumps since the disease is rarely fatal. The affected glands contain perivascular and interstitial mononuclear cell infiltrates with prominent edema. Necrosis of acinar and epithelial duct cells is evident in the salivary glands and in the germinal epithelium of the seminiferous tubules.

CLINICAL MANIFESTATIONS

The prodrome of mumps consists of fever, malaise, myalgia, and anorexia. Parotitis, if it develops, usually does so within the next 24 h but may be delayed for as long as a week; it is generally bilateral, although the onset on the two sides may not be synchronous and at times only one side is affected. The submaxillary and sublingual glands are involved less often than the parotid and are almost never involved alone. Swelling of the parotid is accompanied by tenderness and obliteration of the space between the ear lobe and the angle of the mandible (Fig. 97-1). The patient frequently reports an earache and finds it difficult to eat, swallow, or talk. Glandular swelling increases for a few days and then gradually subsides, disappearing within a week. The orifice of Stensen's duct is commonly red and swollen. Presternal pitting edema has been described in ~5% of mumps cases, often in association with submandibular adenitis.

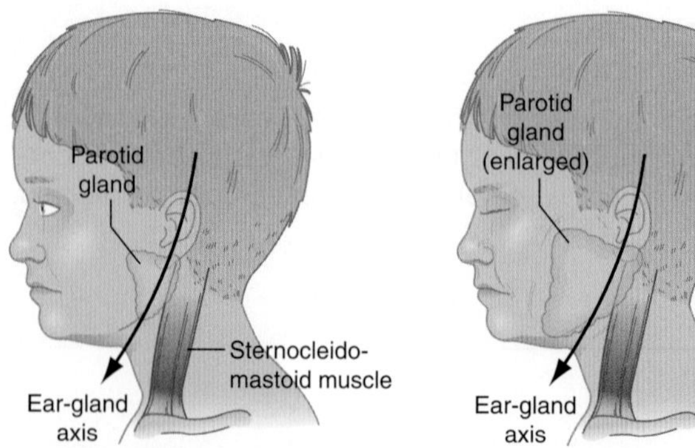

FIGURE 97-1

Schematic drawing of parotid gland infected with mumps virus (*right*) compared with normal gland (*left*). An enlarged cervical lymph node is usually posterior to the imaginary line. *(Reprinted with permission from Gershon A et al: Mumps, in Krugman's Infectious Diseases of Children, 11th ed. Philadelphia, Elsevier, 2004, p 392.)*

Other than parotitis, orchitis is the most common manifestation of mumps among postpubertal males, developing in ~20% of cases. The testis is painful, tender, and enlarged to several times its normal size; accompanying fever is common. Later, testicular atrophy develops in half of the affected men. Since orchitis is bilateral in <15% of cases, sterility after mumps is rare. Oophoritis in women—far less common than orchitis in men—may cause lower abdominal pain but does not lead to sterility.

Aseptic meningitis, which may develop before, during, after, or in the absence of parotitis, is common in both children and adults. Symptoms include stiff neck, headache, and drowsiness. Pleocytosis of the cerebrospinal fluid (CSF), with up to 1000 cells/μL, may develop in up to 50% of cases of clinical mumps, but clinical signs of meningeal irritation are documented in only 5–25% of cases. Within the first 24 h, polymorphonuclear leukocytes may predominate in CSF, but by the second day nearly all the cells are lymphocytes. The glucose level in CSF may be abnormally low, and this finding may arouse suspicion of bacterial meningitis. Aseptic meningitis due to mumps without parotitis is indistinguishable clinically from that caused by other viruses. Mumps meningitis is almost invariably self-limited, although cranial nerve palsies have occasionally led to permanent sequelae, particularly deafness. More rarely, mumps virus may cause encephalitis, which presents as high fever with marked changes in the level of consciousness and frequently results in permanent sequelae in survivors. Other CNS problems occasionally associated with mumps include cerebellar ataxia, facial palsy, transverse myelitis, Guillain-Barré syndrome, and aqueductal stenosis leading to hydrocephalus.

Mumps pancreatitis, which may present as abdominal pain, is difficult to diagnose because an elevated serum amylase level can be associated with either parotitis or pancreatitis. Other unusual complications of mumps include myocarditis, mastitis, thyroiditis, nephritis, arthritis, and thrombocytopenic purpura. An excessive number of spontaneous abortions are associated with gestational mumps when the disease occurs during the first trimester. Mumps in pregnancy does not lead to premature birth or fetal malformations.

TABLE 97-1

DIFFERENTIAL DIAGNOSIS OF PAROTITIS

ETIOLOGY	COMMENTS
Systemic Infections	
Mumps	Rare in countries with vaccination programs
Coxsackievirus infection	Particularly likely in children
HIV infection	In HIV-positive children receiving no antiretroviral therapy; additional disease manifestations likely
Parainfluenza virus type 3 infection	Particularly likely in children; associated with acute respiratory tract symptoms
Influenza A virus infection	Seasonal (winter, spring); associated with acute respiratory tract symptoms
Cat-scratch disease	Unusual but described
Epstein-Barr virus infection	Unusual but described
Systemic Noninfectious Causes	
Sarcoidosis	Additional manifestations of disease likely
Sjögren's syndrome	Additional manifestations of disease likely
Uremia	Additional manifestations of disease likely
Diabetes mellitus	Additional manifestations of disease likely
Drugs	Phenylbutazone, thiouracil
Unilateral Parotitis	
Ductal obstruction due to stones or strictures	Unilateral, gradual onset, suppurative
Parotid cyst	Unilateral, gradual onset
Parotid tumor	Unilateral, gradual onset
Acute Suppurative Parotitis	
Staphylococcus aureus, Streptococcus species, and (rarely) gram-negative bacteria, anaerobes	

Myocarditis as a severe but usually self-limited complication of mumps has been described. Molecular diagnostic assays have implicated mumps virus in some cases of endocardial fibroelastosis following myocarditis.

DIFFERENTIAL DIAGNOSIS

Because of widespread vaccination, mumps is currently a rare disease in the United States. The diagnosis is made easily in patients with acute bilateral parotitis and a history of recent exposure. When parotitis is unilateral or absent or when sites other than the parotid gland are involved, laboratory diagnosis may be required.

The differential diagnosis of parotitis is presented in Table 97-1. Other entities should be considered when manifestations consistent with mumps appear in organs other than the parotid. Testicular torsion may produce a painful scrotal mass resembling that seen in mumps orchitis. Other viruses (e.g., enteroviruses) may cause aseptic meningitis that is clinically indistinguishable from that due to mumps virus.

LABORATORY DIAGNOSIS

Mumps virus is readily isolated after inoculation of appropriate clinical specimens into cell cultures. The virus can be identified rapidly in shell vial cultures by immunofluorescence. Mumps virus may be recovered from saliva, throat, and urine during the first few days of illness and from the CSF of patients with mumps meningitis. Shedding of virus in the urine may persist for as long as 2 weeks. PCR also is used to detect mumps virus in clinical specimens. No particular peripheral blood cell count is characteristic of mumps.

Highly sensitive enzyme-linked immunosorbent assays are useful for serologic diagnosis of mumps and for determination of susceptibility to the disease. Acute mumps can be diagnosed either by the examination of acute- and convalescent-phase sera for a significant increase in IgG antibody levels or by the demonstration of specific IgM in one serum specimen. The mumps skin test is no longer used.

PREVENTION

Live attenuated mumps vaccine (Jeryl Lynn strain) induces antibodies that protect the recipient against infection in >95% of cases. Mumps vaccine is usually administered as part of the measles-mumps-rubella (MMR) vaccine at the age of 12–15 months and again at 4–12 years of age. MMR vaccine will probably be supplanted by MMRV vaccine, which also covers varicella. Licensed by the U.S. Food and Drug Administration in 2005, MMRV is licensed for use only in children 1–13 years of age. Vaccination is also recommended for susceptible older children, adolescents, and adults, particularly male adolescents who have not had mumps. For these patients, either MMR or monovalent mumps vaccine may be given; two doses are preferred. Inadvertent immunization of individuals who are already immune is not associated with significant adverse reactions. Mumps vaccine is not recommended for pregnant women, for patients receiving glucocorticoids, or for other immunocompromised hosts. However, children with HIV infection who are not severely immunocompromised can safely be immunized against mumps; MMR vaccine is usually used for this purpose (Chap. 3). Occasionally, febrile reactions and parotitis have been reported soon after mumps vaccination. Allergic reactions after vaccination, such as rash and pruritus, occur uncommonly and are usually mild and self-limited. In the United States, the incidence of encephalitis during the month after mumps vaccination is no greater than the background incidence rate of encephalitis in the population.

℞ Treatment: MUMPS

Therapy for parotitis and other manifestations of mumps is symptom-based. The administration of analgesics and the application of warm or cold compresses to the parotid area may be helpful. Mumps immune globulin is of no value. Testicular pain may be minimized by the local application of cold compresses and gentle support for the scrotum. Anesthetic blocks also may be used. Neither the administration of glucocorticoids nor incision of the tunica albuginea is of proven value for the treatment of severe orchitis. Anecdotal information on a small number of patients with orchitis suggests that administration of interferon α may be helpful.

FURTHER READINGS

Briss PA et al: Sustained transmission of mumps in a highly vaccinated population: Assessment of primary vaccine failure and waning vaccine-induced immunity. J Infect Dis 169:77, 1994

Centers for Disease Control and Prevention: Measles, mumps, and rubella—vaccine use and strategies for elimination of measles, rubella, and congenital rubella syndrome and control of mumps. MMWR Morb Mortal Wkly Rep 47:1, 1998

———: Mumps epidemic—United Kingdom, 2004–2005. MMWR Morb Mortal Wkly Rep 55:173, 2006

———: Mumps outbreak at a summer camp—New York, 2005. MMWR Morb Mortal Wkly Rep 55:175, 2006

———: Update: Multistate outbreak of mumps—United States, January 1–May 2, 2006. MMWR Morb Mortal Wkly Rep 55:559, 2006

———: Updated recommendations for isolation of persons with mumps. MMWR Morb Mortal Wkly Rep 10;57:1103, 2008

Chaudary S et al: Fulminant mumps myocarditis. Ann Intern Med 110:569, 1989

Cortese MM et al: Mumps vaccine performance among university students during a mumps outbreak. Clin Infect Dis 46:1172, 2008

Davidkin I et al: Etiology of mumps-like illnesses in children and adolescents vaccinated for measles, mumps, and rubella. J Infect Dis 191:719, 2005

Dayan GH, Rubin S: Mumps outbreaks in vaccinated populations: Are available mumps vaccines effective enough to prevent outbreaks? Clin Infect Dis 47:1458, 2008

Gut JP et al: Symptomatic mumps reinfections. J Med Virol 45:17, 1995

McDonald JC et al: Clinical and epidemiologic features of mumps encephalitis and possible causes of vaccine-related disease. Pediatr Infect Dis J 8:751, 1989

Uchida K et al: Rapid and sensitive detection of mumps virus RNA directly from clinical samples by real-time PCR. J Med Virol 75:470, 2005

CHAPTER 98

RABIES AND OTHER RHABDOVIRUS INFECTIONS

Alan C. Jackson ■ Eric C. Johannsen

RABIES

Rabies is an acute viral disease of the central nervous system (CNS) that is transmitted to humans by infected animals. After a prodromal phase, rabies manifests most often as encephalitis—or less frequently as a paralytic form of the disease—and then progresses to coma and death.

ETIOLOGIC AGENT

Rabies virus is a member of the genus *Lyssavirus* in the family Rhabdoviridae, which includes vesicular stomatitis virus (VSV), a bovine pathogen of significant economic importance that can infect humans (see "Other Rhabdoviruses" later in the chapter). *Rhabdos*, meaning "rod-like," refers to the distinctive elongated shape of these viruses. Their enveloped virions contain a single-strand, nonsegmented, negative-sense RNA. The rabies virus genome consists of 11,932 nucleotides and encodes five proteins: nucleocapsid, matrix, phosphoprotein, glycoprotein, and an RNA polymerase. Each animal reservoir harbors one or more distinct rabies virus variants that can be distinguished by the sequence of the nucleocapsid gene.

EPIDEMIOLOGY

Rabies is a zoonosis that is generally transmitted to humans by the bite of a rabid animal. Understanding the epizootiology of rabies is essential in evaluating the need for rabies postexposure prophylaxis (PEP; see "Prevention" later in the chapter). Rabies virus can infect most mammals and is worldwide in distribution.

Historically, dogs were the primary reservoir and vector for rabies, and they remain the major source of transmission to humans in Asia and Africa (see "Global Considerations" later in the chapter). Coordinated vaccination and surveillance programs have essentially eliminated the rabies reservoir in dogs in North America and Europe and have uncovered previously unsuspected reservoirs in wildlife species. Surveillance data from 2006 identified 6940 confirmed animal cases of rabies in the United States. Only 8% of these cases were in domestic animals, including 318 cases in cats, 82 in cattle, and 79 in dogs. Essentially all infections of domestic animals were the result of "spillover" from wildlife reservoirs, not of transmission from one domestic animal to another. In North America, bats, raccoons, skunks, and foxes have endemic rabies virus infection. The importance of each reservoir varies geographically: rabies in raccoons is endemic on the east coast; rabies in skunks occurs predominantly in the Midwest, with another focus in California; and rabies in foxes is found in parts of Texas, Arizona, and Alaska. Rabies in bats is not geographically restricted.

Because each species harbors one or more specific rabies virus variants (or strains), it is possible to trace the source of a human infection even when there is no known exposure. Since 1990, bats have accounted for most cases of human rabies in the United States, with the majority of the remaining cases due to dog exposures occurring in other countries. The majority of human rabies cases acquired from bats have been associated with a single variant (Ln/Ps) harbored by silver-haired and eastern pipistrelle bats. The implication is that the Ln/Ps variant may have particular attributes that render it capable of readily establishing human infections—e.g., an affinity for specific cell receptors or more efficient initial replication in nonneuronal tissues. A contributing factor may be that rabies virus can be transmitted by minor, seemingly unimportant or unrecognized bat bites. In contrast, bites of terrestrial mammals are more likely to receive medical attention. Fatal cases of rabies have resulted when the significance of a known bat exposure was not appreciated. In circumstances where a bat bite or bat salivary contact with broken skin or mucous membranes cannot be excluded (e.g., when a bat is found in a room with an infant or a sleeping adult), the bat should be tested for rabies and expert consultation sought.

Nonbite exposures only rarely transmit rabies virus infection. Exposures to aerosols in the laboratory or in caves containing millions of bats have resulted in human rabies. Transplanted corneal tissue has been the source of eight cases of human rabies, and strict guidelines for donor screening have been adopted in an effort to eliminate this risk. In 2004, three deaths resulted from transplantation of solid organs and another death from transplantation of a vascular conduit from a donor who was initially thought to have died from an intracranial hemorrhage but was retrospectively diagnosed with rabies. Although all organ donors are screened and tested for infectious risks, routine testing of donors for rabies in the absence of epidemiologic risk has not been recommended. There are no known instances in which health care workers have acquired rabies from infected patients. However, standard universal and respiratory precautions should be observed by care givers because contact of the patients' saliva or neuronal tissue with mucous membranes or nonintact skin could result in transmission.

PATHOGENESIS

The incubation period of rabies (defined as the interval between virus exposure and onset of clinical disease) is usually 1–3 months but in rare cases is as short as 2 weeks or >1 year. During most of the incubation period, rabies virus is thought to be present at or close to the site of inoculation (Fig. 98-1), predominantly in muscle cells. Administration of rabies PEP during this incubation period is critical; the benefit of PEP in preventing disease progression once rabies virus has entered peripheral nerves is limited. Several receptors probably account for the ability of rabies virus to infect both sensory and motor neurons. The virus is known to bind to nicotinic acetylcholine receptors, and acetylcholine receptor blockade inhibits rabies virus attachment. Experimental evidence also supports a role for the neural cell adhesion molecule and the $p75^{NTR}$ neurotrophin receptor as receptors for rabies virus. After entering sensory and motor neurons, rabies virus spreads centripetally at a rate of 100–400 mm/d via fast axonal transport to the spinal cord or brainstem. Once the virus enters the CNS, it spreads rapidly throughout the gray matter via established neuroanatomic connections. There are inflammatory changes, but there are few degenerative changes involving neurons and little evidence of neuronal death. These observations have led to the concept that neuronal dysfunction—rather than neuronal death—is responsible for clinical disease in rabies. The basis for the behavioral changes, including aggression, is not well understood. After CNS infection is established, there is centrifugal spread along peripheral nerves to other tissues, including the salivary glands, liver, muscle, skin, adrenal glands, and heart. Rabies virus replication in acinar cells of the salivary glands results in viral excretion in the saliva of rabid animals.

Pathology studies show mild inflammatory changes in the CNS in rabies, with mononuclear inflammatory infiltration in the leptomeninges, perivascular regions, and parenchyma, including microglial nodules called *Babes nodules*. Degenerative neuronal changes are usually not prominent, and neuronophagia is observed occasionally. The most characteristic pathologic finding in rabies is

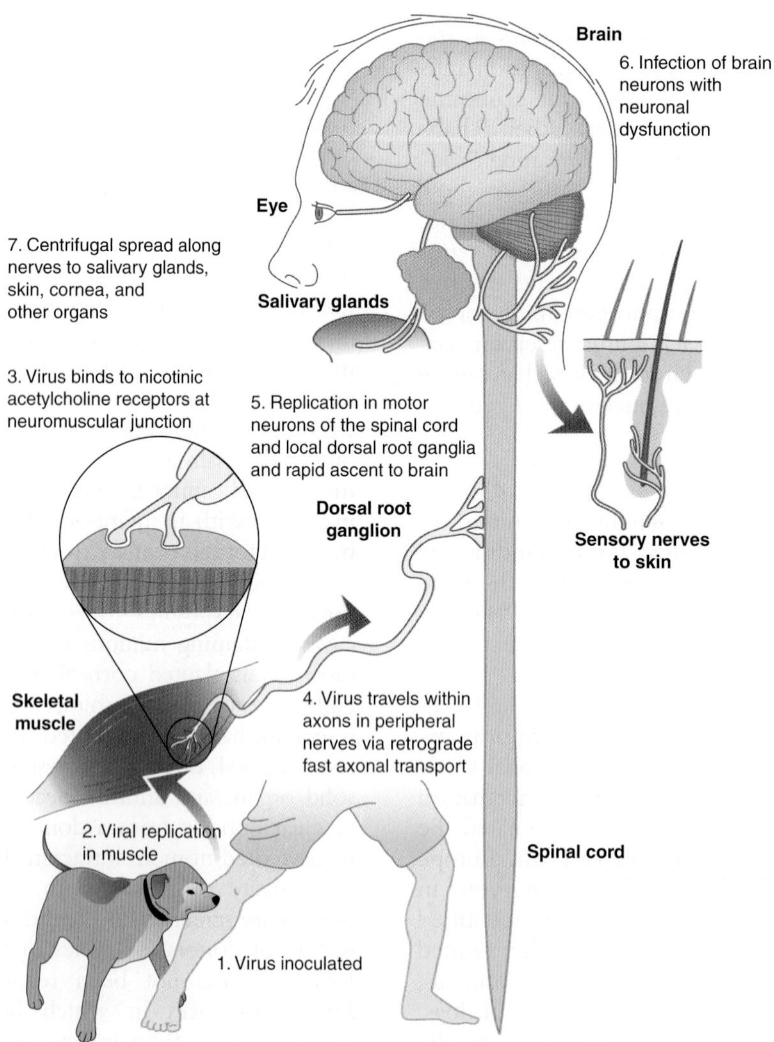

FIGURE 98-1

Schematic representation of the pathogenetic events following peripheral inoculation of rabies virus. *(Adapted from Jackson AC: Human disease, in Rabies, edited by AC Jackson and WH Wunner, 2002, Academic Press, San Diego, pp 219-244; with permission.)*

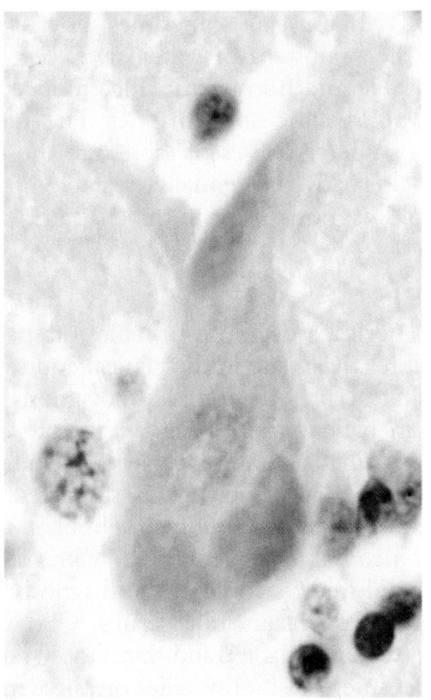

FIGURE 98-2

Three large Negri bodies in the cytoplasm of a cerebellar Purkinje cell from an 8-year-old boy who died of rabies after being bitten by a rabid dog in Mexico. *(From AC Jackson, E Lopez-Corella, N Engl J Med 335:568, 1996. © Massachusetts Medical Society.)*

the *Negri body* (Fig. 98-2). Negri bodies are eosinophilic cytoplasmic inclusions in brain neurons and are composed of randomly oriented rabies virus nucleocapsids embedded in an amorphous substance or matrix. These inclusions occur in a minority of infected cells, are most commonly present in Purkinje cells of the cerebellum and in pyramidal cells in the hippocampus, and are less frequently seen in cortical neurons and in the brainstem. For obscure reasons, Negri bodies are rarely produced in infections caused by laboratory variants of rabies virus, whereas wild, or "street," rabies infection results in Negri bodies in ~80% of cases. Thus, the absence of Negri bodies does not exclude the diagnosis.

CLINICAL MANIFESTATIONS

Rabies has the highest case-fatality rate of any infectious disease. Although the diagnosis of rabies should be considered in any case of unexplained encephalitis or flaccid paralysis accompanied by fever, efforts to prevent the disease are appropriately focused on early identification of rabies exposure and administration of PEP. After an asymptomatic incubation period, clinical rabies progresses through three general phases: a prodrome, an acute neurologic phase, and coma/death (Table 98-1).

Prodromal Features

Clinically apparent rabies infection begins with nonspecific prodromal symptoms, including fever, malaise, headache, nausea, and vomiting. Anxiety or agitation

TABLE 98-1

PROGRESSION OF RABIES VIRUS INFECTION

PHASE	DURATION	SIGNS/SYMPTOMS
Incubation period	1–3 months[a]	None
Prodrome	1–7 days	Fever, malaise, headache, nausea, vomiting, agitation, focal paresthesias, pain
Acute neurologic phase		
Encephalitic (80%)	1–7 days	Fever, confusion, hallucinations, hyperactivity, pharyngeal spasms (hydrophobia/aerophobia), seizures
Paralytic (20%)	2–10 days	Ascending flaccid paralysis
Coma/death	1–14 days	. . .

[a]Typical duration, with a possible range of 2 weeks to >1 year.

may also occur. Paresthesias, pain, or pruritus near the site of the exposure occurs in 50–80% of patients and suggests rabies. The wound has usually healed by this point, and these symptoms may reflect infection of local dorsal root or cranial sensory ganglia.

Encephalitic Rabies

Two acute neurologic forms of rabies are seen in humans: encephalitic (furious) in 80% and paralytic in 20%. Manifestations of encephalitic rabies may be seen in many other viral encephalitides as well. These features include fever, confusion, hallucinations, combativeness, muscle spasms, hyperactivity, and seizures. Autonomic dysfunction is common and may result in hypersalivation, excessive perspiration, gooseflesh, pupillary dilation, and/or priapism. In encephalitic rabies, episodes of hyperexcitability are typically followed by periods of complete lucidity that become shorter as the disease progresses. Rabies encephalitis is most distinguished by early brainstem involvement, which results in the classic symptoms of hydrophobia and aerophobia: involuntary, painful contraction of the diaphragm and accessory respiratory, laryngeal, and pharyngeal muscles in response to swallowing liquids (hydrophobia) or a draft of air (aerophobia). These symptoms are probably due to dysfunction of infected brainstem neurons that normally inhibit inspiratory neurons near the nucleus ambiguus, resulting in exaggerated defense reflexes that protect the respiratory tract. The combination of hypersalivation and pharyngeal dysfunction is also responsible for the classic appearance of "foaming at the mouth" (Fig. 98-3). Brainstem dysfunction progresses rapidly, and coma followed within days by death is the rule unless the course is prolonged by supportive measures. With such measures, late complications can include disturbances of

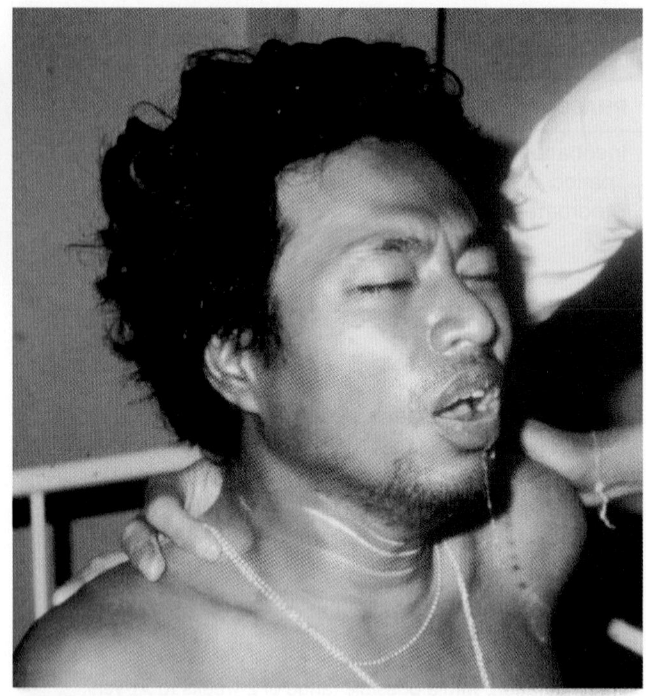

FIGURE 98-3
Hydrophobic spasm of inspiratory muscles associated with terror in a patient with encephalitic (furious) rabies who is attempting to swallow water. *(Copyright DA Warrell, Oxford, UK; with permission.)*

water balance (syndrome of inappropriate antidiuretic hormone secretion or diabetes insipidus), noncardiogenic pulmonary edema, and cardiac arrhythmias due to brainstem dysfunction and/or myocarditis.

Paralytic Rabies
For unknown reasons, muscle weakness predominates and cardinal features of encephalitic rabies (hydrophobia, aerophobia, fluctuating consciousness) are lacking in ~20% of rabies cases. Paralytic rabies is characterized by early and prominent muscle weakness, often beginning in the bitten extremity and spreading to produce quadriparesis and facial weakness. Sphincter involvement is common, but sensory involvement is usually mild. Guillain-Barré syndrome is a common misdiagnosis. Transplantation of corneal tissue from donors in whom paralytic rabies was misdiagnosed as Guillain-Barré syndrome has resulted in clinical rabies and death in recipients. Patients with paralytic rabies generally survive a few days longer than is typical in encephalitic rabies, but multiple-organ failure ensues even with aggressive supportive care.

LABORATORY INVESTIGATIONS
During the early clinical stages of rabies, laboratory findings are nonspecific. Complete blood counts are usually normal. Examination of cerebrospinal fluid (CSF) often reveals mild mononuclear cell pleocytosis with a mildly elevated protein level. Severe pleocytosis (>1000 cells/μL) is unusual and should prompt a search for an alternative diagnosis. CT head scans are usually normal in rabies. MRI brain scans sometimes show signal abnormalities in the brainstem or other areas, but these findings are variable and nonspecific. Electroencephalograms show only nonspecific abnormalities. The most important tests in suspected cases of rabies are those that may identify an alternative, potentially treatable diagnosis (see "Differential Diagnosis" later in the chapter).

DIAGNOSIS
In North America, a diagnosis of rabies often is not considered until relatively late in the clinical course, even with a typical clinical presentation. This diagnosis should be considered in patients presenting with acute encephalitis or with unexplained ascending paralysis, including those in whom Guillain-Barré syndrome is suspected. A lack of animal-bite history or a lack of hydrophobia is not unusual in rabies. Once rabies is suspected, rabies-specific tests should be employed to confirm the diagnosis. Diagnostically useful specimens include serum, CSF, fresh saliva, brain tissue (when available), and skin biopsy samples from the neck. Because skin biopsy relies on the demonstration of rabies virus in cutaneous nerves at the base of hair follicles, samples from the neck should include at least 10 hair follicles. Multiple testing modalities are required to ensure a high negative predictive value. For example, because rabies virus infects immunologically privileged neuronal tissues, serum antibodies often do not develop until very late in the disease.

Rabies Virus–Specific Antibodies
In a previously unimmunized patient, serum neutralizing antibodies to rabies virus are diagnostic. Antibodies may be detected within a few days after the onset of symptoms, but some patients die without detectable antibodies. The presence of rabies virus–specific antibodies in the CSF suggests rabies, regardless of immunization status.

Reverse Transcription Polymerase Chain Reaction (RT-PCR)
Detection of rabies virus RNA by RT-PCR is highly sensitive and specific. This technique can detect virus in fresh saliva samples, CSF, and tissue. In addition, RT-PCR can distinguish between rabies virus variants, permitting the investigator to infer the likely source of an infection.

Direct Fluorescent Antibody (DFA) Testing
DFA testing with rabies antibodies conjugated to fluorescent dyes is highly sensitive and specific and can be applied to brain tissue or skin biopsies from the nape of the neck. In the latter samples, rabies virus can be detected in cutaneous nerves at the base of hair follicles.

DIFFERENTIAL DIAGNOSIS
Early in the course of illness, rabies is frequently indistinguishable from other causes of encephalitis. Herpes simplex virus type 1 and rarely other herpesviruses cause sporadic cases of encephalitis and are important

considerations because they require specific treatment. During summer months, enteroviruses and arthropod-borne viruses are an important diagnostic consideration. PCR testing of CSF for specific viruses should be guided by local epidemiologic patterns. Immune-mediated postviral encephalitis may follow infection with influenza, measles, mumps, varicella-zoster, and other viruses. It is important to recognize that immune-mediated encephalitis may occur as a sequela of immunization with rabies vaccine derived from neural tissues (e.g., Semple vaccine). Drug reactions and vasculitis are other important noninfectious causes of encephalitis that must be considered. A conversion disorder due to an exaggerated fear of rabies ("rabies hysteria") can produce symptoms that closely resemble those of rabies (e.g., aggressive behavior, inability to swallow or communicate); an unusually short "incubation period" can be an important clue to the correct diagnosis.

As previously mentioned, paralytic rabies may mimic Guillain-Barré syndrome. In these cases, the documentation of fever or bladder dysfunction can suggest the diagnosis of rabies. Conversely, Guillain-Barré syndrome may rarely occur as a complication of rabies vaccination and may be mistaken for paralytic rabies (i.e., vaccine failure).

℞ Treatment: RABIES

There is no established treatment for rabies. There have been several recent treatment failures of antiviral therapy, ketamine, and therapeutic coma—measures that were used in a healthy survivor who had rabies virus antibodies present at the time of presentation. Expert opinion should be sought before any course of experimental therapy is embarked upon. A palliative approach may be appropriate for some patients.

PROGNOSIS

Rabies is an almost uniformly fatal disease but is almost always preventable with appropriate postexposure therapy during the incubation period (described in the next section). There are only six well-documented cases of survival after symptomatic rabies infection. All but one of the patients involved had received rabies vaccine before disease onset; these patients represented failures of postexposure rabies prophylaxis. Most patients with rabies die within several days, even with aggressive care in a critical care unit.

PREVENTION

Postexposure Prophylaxis

Since there is no effective therapy for rabies, it is extremely important to prevent the disease after an animal exposure. Figure 98-4 shows the steps involved in making decisions about rabies PEP. On the basis of the history of the exposure and local epidemiologic information, the physician must decide whether initiation of

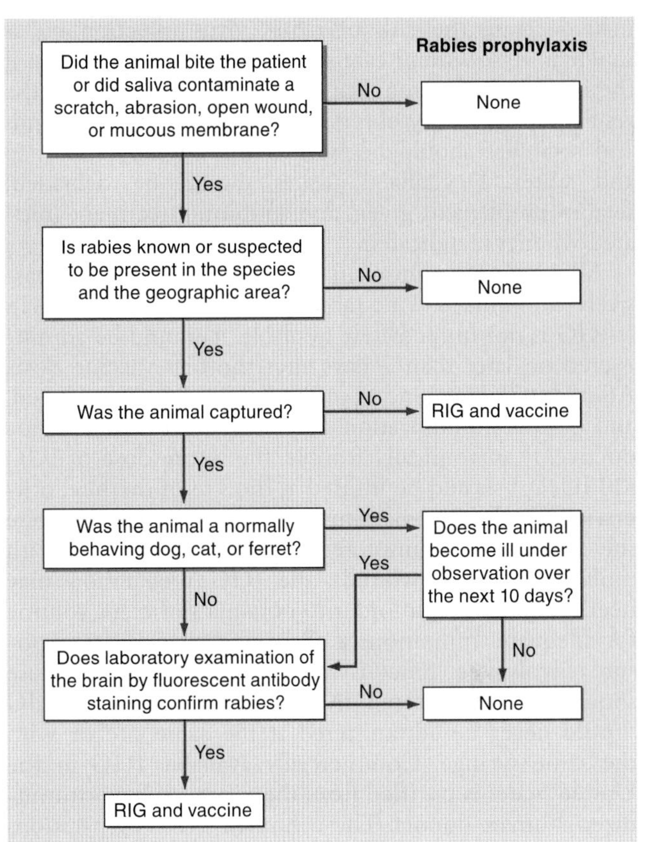

FIGURE 98-4

Algorithm for rabies postexposure prophylaxis. RIG, rabies immune globulin. *[From L Corey, in Harrison's Principles of Internal Medicine, 15th ed. E Braunwald et al (eds): New York, McGraw-Hill, 2001, adapted with permission.]*

PEP is warranted. Healthy dogs, cats, or ferrets may be confined and observed for 10 days. PEP is not necessary if the animal remains healthy. If the animal develops signs of rabies during the observation period, it should be euthanized immediately, and the head should be transported to the laboratory under refrigeration and examined for the presence of rabies virus by DFA testing and viral isolation using cell culture or mouse inoculation. Any animal other than a dog, cat, or ferret should be euthanized immediately and the head submitted for examination. In high-risk exposures and in areas where canine rabies is endemic, rabies prophylaxis should be initiated without waiting for laboratory results. If the laboratory results prove to be negative, it may safely be concluded that the animal's saliva did not contain rabies virus, and immunization should be discontinued. If an animal escapes after an exposure, it must be considered rabid, and PEP must be initiated unless information from public health officials indicates otherwise (i.e., there is no endemic rabies in the area). PEP may be warranted when a person present in the same space as a bat (e.g., a small child or a sleeping adult) cannot reliably rule out contact with an unrecognized bite.

PEP includes local wound care and both active and passive immunization. Local wound care is essential and may decrease the risk of rabies virus infection by as much as 90%. Wound care should not be delayed, even if the initiation of immunization is postponed pending the results of the 10-day observation period. All bite wounds and scratches should be washed thoroughly with soap and water. Devitalized tissues should be debrided, tetanus prophylaxis given, and antibiotic treatment initiated whenever indicated.

All previously unvaccinated persons should be passively immunized with rabies immune globulin (RIG). If RIG is not immediately available, it should be administered no later than 7 days after the first vaccine dose. After day 7, endogenous antibodies are being produced, and passive immunization may actually be counterproductive. If anatomically feasible, the entire dose of RIG (20 IU/kg) should be infused at the site of the bite; otherwise, any RIG remaining after infiltration of the bite site should be administered IM at a distant site. With multiple or large wounds, the RIG preparation may need to be diluted in order to obtain a sufficient volume for adequate infiltration of all wound sites. If the exposure involves a mucous membrane, the entire dose should be administered IM. Rabies vaccine and RIG should never be administered at the same site or with the same syringe. Commercially available RIG in the United States is purified from the serum of hyperimmunized human donors. These human RIG preparations are much better tolerated than are the equine-derived preparations still in use in some countries (see "Global Considerations" later in the chapter). Serious adverse effects of human RIG are uncommon. Local pain and low-grade fever may occur.

Two purified inactivated rabies vaccines are available for rabies PEP in the United States. They are highly immunogenic and remarkably safe compared with earlier vaccines. The traditional recommendation has been to give five 1-mL doses of rabies vaccine IM in the deltoid area on days 3, 7, 14, and 28. (The anterolateral aspect of the thigh is also acceptable in children.) Gluteal injections, which may not always reach muscle, should not be given and have been associated with rare vaccine failures. Ideally, the first dose should be given as soon as possible after exposure; failing that, it should be given without further delay. Pregnancy is not a contraindication for immunization. In June of 2009, the ACIP advised the CDC to change the recommendation to 4 doses of vaccine, administered on days 0, 3, 7, and 14 after exposure. These recommendations will become official once they are accepted by the CDC Director and published in the MMWR. While the new ACIP recommendations are based on evidence that supports a 4-dose regimen, vaccine manufacturers are expected to continue to support the product insert that was developed at the time the product was licensed by the FDA, which instructs providers to administer 5 doses. Glucocorticoids and other immunosuppressive medications may interfere with the development of active immunity and should not be administered during PEP unless they are essential. In several studies, all persons vaccinated with the above schedule developed a serologic response within 2–4 weeks. Routine measurement of serum neutralizing antibody titers is not required, but titers should be measured 2–4 weeks after immunization in immunocompromised persons. Local reactions (pain, erythema, edema, and pruritus) and mild systemic reactions (fever, myalgias, headache, and nausea) are common; anti-inflammatory and antipyretic medications may be used, but immunization should not be discontinued. Systemic allergic reactions are uncommon, but anaphylaxis does occur rarely and can be treated with epinephrine and antihistamines. The risk of rabies development should be carefully considered before the decision is made to discontinue vaccination because of an adverse reaction. Advice and assistance from state health officials or the Centers for Disease Control and Prevention may be helpful in managing adverse reactions to vaccine.

Preexposure Rabies Vaccination

Preexposure rabies prophylaxis should be considered for people with an occupational or recreational risk of rabies exposures, including certain travelers to rabies-endemic areas. This primary schedule consists of three doses of rabies vaccine given on days 0, 7, and 21 or 28. Serum neutralizing antibody tests help determine the need for subsequent booster doses. When a previously immunized individual is exposed to rabies, two booster doses of vaccine should be administered on days 0 and 3. Wound care remains critical. RIG should not be administered to previously vaccinated persons.

GLOBAL CONSIDERATIONS

Worldwide, endemic canine rabies is estimated to cause 55,000 human deaths annually. Most of these deaths occur in Asia and Africa, with rural populations and children most frequently affected. Because of this distribution, most of the burden of rabies PEP is borne by those least able to pay. In Latin America, rabies control efforts in dogs have been quite successful in recent years. In Europe and Canada, an epizootic of rabies in red foxes has been partly controlled by widespread use of baits containing rabies vaccine.

In addition to the rabies vaccines discussed above, vaccines grown in either primary cell lines (hamster or dog kidney) or continuous cell lines (Vero cells) are satisfactory and are available in many countries outside the United States. Less expensive vaccines derived from neural tissues have been used in developing countries; however, these vaccines are associated with serious neuroparalytic complications, and their use should be discontinued as soon as possible. Worldwide, >10 million individuals receive postexposure vaccination against rabies each year.

If human RIG is unavailable, purified equine RIG can be used in the same manner at a dose of 40 IU/kg. Before the administration of equine RIG, hypersensitivity should be assessed by intradermal testing with a 1:10 dilution. The incidence of anaphylactic reactions and serum sickness has been low with recent equine RIG products.

OTHER RHABDOVIRUSES

OTHER LYSSAVIRUSES

A growing number of lyssaviruses other than rabies virus have been discovered to infect bat populations throughout the world. Four of these viruses have produced at least one case of human illness indistinguishable from rabies: European bat lyssaviruses 1 and 2, Australian bat lyssavirus, and the Duvenhage virus (in Africa). Mokola virus, a lyssavirus that has been isolated from shrews with an unknown reservoir species, has also produced human illness in Africa.

VESICULAR STOMATITIS VIRUS

Vesicular stomatitis is a viral disease of cattle, horses, pigs, and some wild mammals. VSV is a member of the genus *Vesiculovirus* in the family Rhabdoviridae. Outbreaks of vesicular stomatitis in animals occur sporadically in the southwestern United States. The infection is associated with severe vesiculation and ulceration of oral tissues, teats, and feet and may be clinically indistinguishable from the more dangerous foot-and-mouth disease. Epidemics are usually seasonal and are probably due to arthropod vectors. Direct animal-to-animal spread can also occur, although the virus cannot penetrate intact skin. Transmission to humans usually results from direct contact with infected animals (particularly cattle) and occasionally follows laboratory exposure. In human disease, early conjunctivitis is followed by an acute influenza-like illness with fever, chills, nausea, vomiting, headache, retrobulbar pain, myalgias, substernal pain, malaise, pharyngitis, and lymphadenitis. Small vesicular lesions may be present on the buccal mucosa or on the fingers. The illness usually lasts 3–6 days, with a subsequent full recovery. Subclinical infections are common. A serologic diagnosis can be made on the basis of a rise in titer of complement-fixing or neutralizing antibodies. Therapy is symptom-based.

FURTHER READINGS

Baer GM (ed): *The Natural History of Rabies*, 2d ed. Boca Raton, CRC Press, 1991

Centers for Disease Control and Prevention: Human rabies prevention—United States, 1999: Recommendations of the Advisory Committee on Immunization Practices (ACIP). MMWR 48(RR-1):1, 1999

———: New [June 24, 2009] ACIP recommendations for human rabies postexposure prophylaxis (*http://www.cdc.gov/rabies/qanda/ACIP4dose.html*).

Hu WT et al: Long-term follow-up after treatment of rabies by induction of coma. N Engl J Med 357:945, 2007

Jackson AC: Rabies: New insights into pathogenesis and treatment. Curr Opin Neurol 19:267, 2006

———, Wunner WH (eds): *Rabies*, 2d ed. London, Elsevier, 2007

Letchworth GJ et al: Vesicular stomatitis. Vet J 157:239, 1999

Warrell MJ, Warrell DA: Rabies and other lyssavirus diseases. Lancet 363:959, 2004

Willoughby RE JR et al: Survival after treatment of rabies with induction of coma. N Engl J Med 352:2508, 2005

World Health Organization: *WHO Expert Consultation on Rabies: First Report*. First Report ed. Geneva, WHO, 2005

CHAPTER 99

INFECTIONS CAUSED BY ARTHROPOD- AND RODENT-BORNE VIRUSES

Clarence J. Peters

Some zoonotic viruses are transmitted in nature without regard to humans and only incidentally infect and produce disease in humans; in addition, a few agents are regularly spread among humans by arthropods. Most of these viruses either are maintained by arthropods or chronically infect rodents. Obviously, the mode of transmission is not a rational basis for taxonomic classification. Indeed, zoonotic viruses from at least seven families act as significant human pathogens (Table 99-1). The virus families differ fundamentally from one another in terms of morphology, replication mechanisms, and genetics. Information on a virus's membership in a family or genus is enlightening with regard to maintenance strategies, sensitivity to antiviral agents, and some aspects of pathogenesis but does not necessarily predict which clinical syndromes (if any) the virus will cause in humans.

FAMILIES OF ARTHROPOD- AND RODENT-BORNE VIRUSES

(Table 99-1)

The Arenaviridae

The Arenaviridae are spherical, 110- to 130-nm particles that bud from the cell's plasma membrane and utilize ambisense RNA genomes with two segments for

TABLE 99-1

MAJOR ZOONOTIC VIRUS FAMILIES AND SOME CHARACTERISTICS OF TYPICAL MEMBERS

FAMILY	GENUS OR GROUP	SYNDROME(S): TYPICAL VIRUSES	MAINTENANCE STRATEGY
Arenaviridae	Old World complex	FM, E: Lymphocytic choriomeningitis virus HF: Lassa fever virus	Chronic infection of rodents, often with persistent viremia; vertical transmission common
	New World or Tacaribe complex	HF: South American HF viruses (Machupo, Junin, Guanarito, Sabia)	Chronic infection of rodents, sometimes with persistent viremia; vertical infection may occur
Bunyaviridae	*Bunyavirus*	E: California serogroup viruses (La Crosse, Jamestown Canyon, California encephalitis) FM: Bunyamwera, group C, Tahyna viruses	Mosquito-vertebrate cycle; transovarial transmission in mosquito common
		FM: Oropouche virus	Transmitted by *Culicoides*
	Phlebovirus	FM: Sandfly fever, Toscana viruses FM: Punta Toro virus	Sandfly transmission between vertebrates, with prominent transovarial component in sandfly
		HF, FM, E: Rift Valley fever virus	Mosquito-vertebrate transmission, with transovarial component in mosquito
	Nairovirus	HF: Crimean-Congo HF virus	Tick-vertebrate, with transovarial transmission in tick
	Hantavirus	HF: Hantaan, Dobrava, Puumala viruses	Rodent reservoir; chronic virus shedding, but chronic viremia unknown
		HF: Sin Nombre and related hantaviruses	Sigmodontine rodent reservoir
Filoviridae[a]	*Ebolavirus, Marburgvirus*	HF: Marburg viruses, Ebola viruses (4 species)	Unknown
Flaviviridae	*Flavivirus* (mosquito-borne)	HF: Yellow fever virus FM, HF: Dengue viruses (4 serotypes) E: St. Louis, Japanese, West Nile, and Murray Valley encephalitis viruses; Rocio viruses	Mosquito-vertebrate; transovarial rare
	Flavivirus (tick-borne)	E: Central European tick-borne encephalitis, Russian spring-summer encephalitis, Powassan viruses HF: Omsk HF, Kyasanur Forest disease viruses	Tick-vertebrate
Reoviridae	*Coltivirus*	FM, E: Colorado tick fever virus	Tick-vertebrate
	Orbivirus	FM, E: Orungo, Kemerovo viruses	Arthropod-vertebrate
Rhabdoviridae[b]	*Vesiculovirus*	FM: Vesicular stomatitis virus (Indiana, New Jersey); Chandipura, Piry viruses	Sandfly-vertebrate, with prominent transovarial component in sandfly
Togaviridae	*Alphavirus*	AR: Sindbis, chikungunya, Mayaro, Ross River, Barmah Forest viruses E: Eastern, western, and Venezuelan equine encephalitis viruses	Mosquito-vertebrate

[a] The Filoviridae are discussed in Chap. 100.
[b] The Rhabdoviridae are discussed in Chap. 98.
Note: Abbreviations refer to the disease syndrome most commonly associated with the virus: FM, fever, myalgia; AR, arthritis, rash; E, encephalitis; HF, hemorrhagic fever.

replication. There are two main phylogenetic branches of Arenaviridae: the Old World viruses, such as Lassa fever and lymphocytic choriomeningitis (LCM) viruses, and the New World viruses, including those causing the South American hemorrhagic fevers (HFs). Arenaviruses persist in nature by chronically infecting rodents with a striking one-virus–one-rodent species relationship. These rodent infections result in long-term virus excretion and perhaps in lifelong viremia; vertical infection is common with some arenaviruses. Humans become infected through the inhalation of aerosols containing arenaviruses, which are then deposited in the terminal air passages, and probably also through close contact with rodents and their excreta, which results in the contamination of mucous membranes or breaks in the skin.

The Bunyaviridae

The family Bunyaviridae includes four medically significant genera. All of these spherical viruses have three negative-sense RNA segments maturing into 90- to 120-nm particles in the Golgi complex and exiting the cell by exocytosis. Viruses of the genus *Bunyavirus* are largely mosquito-borne and have a viremic vertebrate intermediate host; many are also transovarially transmitted in their specific mosquito host. One serologic group also uses biting midges as vectors. Sandflies or mosquitoes are the vectors for the genus *Phlebovirus* (named after phlebotomus fever or sandfly fever, the best-known disease associated with the genus), while ticks serve as vectors for the genus *Nairovirus*. Viruses of both of these genera are also associated with vertical transmission in the arthropod host and with horizontal spread through viremic vertebrate hosts. The genus *Hantavirus* is unique among the Bunyaviridae in that it is not transmitted by arthropods but is maintained in nature by rodent hosts that chronically shed virus. Like the arenaviruses, the hantaviruses usually display striking virus–rodent species specificity. Hantaviruses do not cause chronic viremia in their rodent hosts and are transmitted only horizontally from rodent to rodent.

Other Families

The Flaviviridae are positive-sense, single-strand RNA viruses that form particles of 40–50 nm in the endoplasmic reticulum. The flaviviruses discussed here are from the genus *Flavivirus* and make up two phylogenetically and antigenically distinct divisions transmitted among vertebrates by mosquitoes and ticks, respectively. The mosquito-borne viruses fall into phylogenetic groups that include yellow fever virus, the four dengue viruses, and encephalitis viruses, while the tick-borne group encompasses a geographically varied spectrum of species, some of which are responsible for encephalitis or for hemorrhagic disease with encephalitis. The Reoviridae are double-strand RNA viruses with multisegmented genomes. These 80-nm particles are the only viruses discussed in this chapter that do not have a lipid envelope and thus are insensitive to detergents. The Togaviridae have a single positive-strand RNA genome and bud particles of ~60–70 nm from the plasma membrane. The togaviruses discussed here are all members of the genus *Alphavirus* and are transmitted among vertebrates by mosquitoes in their natural cycle. The Filoviridae and the Rhabdoviridae are discussed in Chaps. 100 and 98, respectively.

PROMINENT FEATURES OF ARTHROPOD- AND RODENT-BORNE VIRUSES

Although this chapter discusses the major features of selected arthropod- and rodent-borne viruses, it does not deal with >500 other distinct recognized zoonotic viruses, about one-fourth of which infect humans. Zoonotic viruses are undergoing genetic evolution, "new" zoonotic viruses are being discovered, and the epidemiology of zoonotic viruses is continuing to evolve through environmental changes affecting vectors, reservoirs, and humans. These zoonotic viruses are most numerous in the tropics but are also found in temperate and frigid climates. Their distribution and seasonal activity may be variable and often depend largely on ecologic conditions such as rainfall and temperature, which in turn affect the density of vectors and reservoirs and the development of infection therein.

Maintenance and Transmission

Arthropod-borne viruses infect their vectors after the ingestion of a blood meal from a viremic vertebrate. The vectors then develop chronic, systemic infection as the viruses penetrate the gut and spread throughout the body. The viruses eventually reach the salivary glands during a period that is referred to as *extrinsic incubation* and that typically lasts 1–3 weeks in mosquitoes. At this point, an arthropod is competent to continue the chain of transmission by infecting another vertebrate when a subsequent blood meal is taken. The arthropod generally is unharmed by the infection, and the natural vertebrate partner usually has only transient viremia with no overt disease. An alternative mechanism for virus maintenance in its arthropod host is transovarial transmission, which is common among members of the family Bunyaviridae.

Rodent-borne viruses such as the hantaviruses and arenaviruses are maintained in nature by chronic infection transmitted between rodents. As in arthropod-borne virus cycles, there is usually a high degree of rodent-virus specificity, and there is no overt disease in the reservoir/vector.

Epidemiology

The distribution of arthropod- and rodent-borne viruses is restricted by the areas inhabited by their reservoir/vectors and provides an important clue in the differential diagnosis. Table 99-2 shows the approximate geographic distribution of the most important of these viruses. Members of each family, each genus, and even each serologically related group usually occur in each area but may not be pathogenic in all areas or may not be a commonly recognized cause of disease in all areas and so may not be included in the table.

Most of these diseases are acquired in a rural setting; a few have urban vectors. Seoul, sandfly fever, and Oropouche viruses are examples of urban viruses, but the most notable are yellow fever, dengue, and chikungunya viruses. A history of mosquito bite has little diagnostic significance in the individual; a history of tick bite is more diagnostically specific. Rodent exposure is often reported by persons infected with an arenavirus or a hantavirus but again has little specificity. Indeed, aerosols may infect persons who have no recollection of having even seen rodents.

Syndromes

Human disease caused by arthropod- and rodent-borne viruses is often subclinical. The spectrum of possible responses to infection is wide, and our knowledge of the outcome of most of these infections is limited. The usual disease syndromes associated with these viruses have been grouped into four categories: fever and myalgia, arthritis and rash, encephalitis, and hemorrhagic fever. Although for the purposes of this discussion most viruses have been placed in a single group, the categories often overlap. For example, West Nile and Venezuelan equine encephalitis viruses are discussed as encephalitis viruses, but during epidemics they may cause many cases

TABLE 99-2

GEOGRAPHIC DISTRIBUTION OF SOME IMPORTANT AND COMMONLY ENCOUNTERED HUMAN ZOONOTIC VIRAL DISEASES

AREA	ARENAVIRIDAE	BUNYAVIRIDAE	FLAVIVIRIDAE	RHABDOVIRIDAE	TOGAVIRIDAE
North America	Lymphocytic choriomeningitis	La Crosse, Jamestown Canyon, California encephalitis; hantavirus pulmonary syndrome	St. Louis, Powassan, West Nile encephalitis; dengue	Vesicular stomatitis	Eastern, western equine encephalitis
South America	Bolivian, Argentine, Venezuelan, and Brazilian HF; lymphocytic choriomeningitis	Oropouche, group C, Punta Toro infection; hantavirus pulmonary syndrome	Yellow fever, dengue, Rocio virus infection	Vesicular stomatitis, Piry virus infection	Mayaro virus infection, Venezuelan equine encephalitis
Europe	Lymphocytic choriomeningitis	Tahyna, Toscana, sandfly fever; HF with renal syndrome	West Nile, Central European tick-borne, Russian spring-summer encephalitis	—	Sindbis virus infection
Middle East	—	Sandfly fever, Crimean-Congo HF	West Nile encephalitis, dengue	—	—
Eastern Asia	—	Sandfly fever; Hantaan, Seoul virus infection	Dengue; Japanese, Russian spring-summer encephalitis; Omsk HF	Chandipura virus infection	—
Southwestern Asia	—	Sandfly fever, Crimean-Congo HF	West Nile, Japanese encephalitis; dengue; Kyasanur Forest disease	—	Chikungunya virus infection
Southeast Asia	—	Seoul virus infection	Japanese encephalitis, dengue	—	Chikungunya virus infection
Africa	Lassa fever	Bunyamwera virus infection, Rift Valley fever	Yellow fever, dengue	—	Sindbis, chikungunya virus infection
Australia	—	—	Murray Valley encephalitis, dengue	—	Ross River, Barmah Forest virus infection

Note: HF, hemorrhagic fever.

of milder febrile syndromes and relatively uncommon cases of encephalitis. Similarly, Rift Valley fever virus is best known as a cause of HF, but the attack rates for febrile disease are far higher, and encephalitis is occasionally seen as well. LCM virus is classified as a cause of fever and myalgia because this syndrome is its most common disease manifestation and because, even when central nervous system (CNS) disease occurs, it is usually mild and is preceded by fever and myalgia. Dengue virus infection is considered as a cause of fever and myalgia (dengue fever) because this is by far the most common manifestation worldwide and is the syndrome most likely to be seen in the United States; however, dengue HF is also discussed in the HF section because of its complicated pathogenesis and importance in pediatric practice in certain areas of the world.

Diagnosis

Laboratory diagnosis is required in any given case, although epidemics occasionally provide clinical and epidemiologic clues on which an educated guess as to etiology can be based. For most arthropod- and rodent-borne viruses, acute-phase serum samples (collected within 3 or 4 days of onset) have yielded isolates, and paired sera have been used to demonstrate rising antibody titers by a variety of tests. Intensive efforts to develop rapid tests for HF have resulted in an antigen-detection enzyme-linked immunosorbent assay (ELISA) and an IgM-capture ELISA that can provide a diagnosis based on a single serum sample within a few hours and are particularly useful in severe cases. More sensitive reverse-transcription polymerase chain reaction (RT-PCR) tests may yield diagnoses based on samples without detectable antigen and may also provide useful genetic information about the virus. Hantavirus infections differ from others discussed here in that severe acute disease is immunopathologic; patients present with serum IgM that serves as the basis for a sensitive and specific test.

At diagnosis, patients with encephalitis are generally no longer viremic or antigenemic and usually do not have virus in cerebrospinal fluid (CSF). In this situation, the value of serologic methods and RT-PCR is being validated. IgM capture is increasingly being used for the simultaneous testing of serum and CSF. IgG ELISA or classic serology is useful in the evaluation of past exposure to the viruses, many of which circulate in areas with a minimal medical infrastructure and sometimes cause mild or subclinical infection.

The remainder of this chapter offers general descriptions of the broad syndromes caused by arthropod- and rodent-borne viruses. Most of the diseases under consideration have not been studied in detail with modern medical approaches; thus available data may be incomplete or biased.

FEVER AND MYALGIA

Fever and myalgia constitute the syndrome most commonly associated with zoonotic virus infection. Many of the numerous viruses belonging to the families listed in Table 99-1 probably cause this syndrome, but several viruses have been selected for inclusion in the table because of their prominent associations with the syndrome and their biomedical importance.

The syndrome typically begins with the abrupt onset of fever, chills, intense myalgia, and malaise. Patients may also report joint pains, but no true arthritis is detectable. Anorexia is characteristic and may be accompanied by nausea or even vomiting. Headache is common and may be severe, with photophobia and retroorbital pain. Physical findings are minimal and are usually confined to conjunctival injection with pain on palpation of muscles or the epigastrium. The duration of symptoms is quite variable but generally is 2–5 days, with a biphasic course in some instances. The spectrum of disease varies from subclinical to temporarily incapacitating.

Less constant findings include a maculopapular rash. Epistaxis may occur but does not necessarily indicate a bleeding diathesis. A minority of the cases caused by some viruses are known or suspected to include aseptic meningitis, but this diagnosis is difficult to make in remote areas, given the patients' photophobia and myalgia as well as the lack of opportunity to examine the CSF. Although pharyngitis may be noted or radiographic evidence of pulmonary infiltrates found in some cases, these viruses are not primary respiratory pathogens. The differential diagnosis includes anicteric leptospirosis, rickettsial diseases, and the early stages of other syndromes discussed in this chapter. These diseases are often described as "flulike," but the usual absence of cough and coryza makes influenza an unlikely confounder except at the earliest stages.

Complete recovery is generally the outcome in this syndrome, although prolonged asthenia and nonspecific symptoms have been described in some cases, particularly after infection with LCM or dengue virus. Treatment is supportive, with aspirin avoided because of the potential for exacerbated bleeding and Reye's syndrome. Efforts at prevention are best based on vector control, which, however, may be expensive or impossible. For mosquito control, destruction of breeding sites is generally the most economically and environmentally sound approach. Measures taken by the individual to avoid the vector can be valuable. Avoiding the vector's habitat and times of peak activity, using screens or other barriers (e.g., permethrin-impregnated bed nets) to prevent the vector from entering dwellings, judiciously applying arthropod repellents such as diethyltoluamide (DEET) to the skin, and wearing permethrin-impregnated clothing are all possible approaches, depending on the vector and its habits.

LYMPHOCYTIC CHORIOMENINGITIS

LCM is transmitted from the common house mouse (*Mus musculus*) to humans by aerosols of excreta and secreta. LCM virus, an arenavirus, is maintained in the mouse mainly by vertical transmission from infected dams. The vertically infected mouse remains viremic for life, with high concentrations of virus in all tissues. Infected colonies of pet hamsters have also served as a link to humans. LCM virus is widely used in immunology laboratories as a model of T-cell function and can silently infect cell cultures and passaged tumor lines, resulting in infections among scientists and animal caretakers. Patients with LCM may have a history of residence in rodent-infested housing or other exposure to rodents. An antibody prevalence of ~5–10% has been reported among adults from the United States, Argentina, and endemic areas of Germany.

LCM differs from the general syndrome of fever and myalgia in that its onset is gradual. Among the conditions occasionally associated with LCM are orchitis, transient alopecia, arthritis, pharyngitis, cough, and maculopapular rash. An estimated one-fourth of patients or fewer experience a febrile phase of 3–6 days and then, after a brief remission, develop renewed fever accompanied by severe headache, nausea and vomiting, and meningeal signs lasting for ~1 week. These patients virtually always recover fully, as do the uncommon patients with clear-cut signs of encephalitis. Recovery may be delayed by transient hydrocephalus.

During the initial febrile phase, leukopenia and thrombocytopenia are common and virus can usually be isolated from blood. During the CNS phase, virus may be found in the CSF, but antibodies are present in blood. The pathogenesis of LCM is thought to resemble that following direct intracranial inoculation of the virus into adult mice; the onset of the immune response leads to T-cell–mediated immunopathologic meningitis. During the meningeal phase, CSF mononuclear-cell counts range from the hundreds to the low thousands per microliter, and hypoglycorrhachia is found in one-third of cases. The IgM-capture ELISA of serum and CSF is usually positive; RT-PCR assays have been developed for application to CSF. Recent infections transmitted by organ transplantation did not include evidence of an immune response, followed a fulminant course (not unlike that of Lassa fever), and required immunohistochemistry or RT-PCR for diagnosis.

Infection with LCM virus should be suspected in acutely ill febrile patients with marked leukopenia and thrombocytopenia. In cases of aseptic meningitis, any of the following should suggest LCM: well-marked febrile prodrome, adult age, autumn seasonality, low CSF glucose levels, or CSF mononuclear cell counts of >1000/μL.

In pregnant women, LCM virus infection may lead to fetal invasion with consequent congenital hydrocephalus and chorioretinitis. Since the maternal infection may be mild, consisting of only a short febrile illness, antibodies to the virus should be sought in both the mother and the fetus in suspicious circumstances, particularly TORCH-negative neonatal hydrocephalus. [TORCH is a battery of tests encompassing *t*oxoplasmosis, *o*ther conditions (congenital syphilis and viral infection), *r*ubella, *c*ytomegalovirus infection, and *h*erpes simplex virus infection.]

BUNYAMWERA VIRUS INFECTION

The mosquito-transmitted Bunyamwera serogroup viruses are found on every continent except Australia and Antarctica. Bunyamwera virus and its close relative Ilesha virus commonly cause febrile disease in Africa. Nigari virus, a reassortant of Bunyamwera virus, has recently been identified as an important human pathogen in Africa. Other related viruses are implicated in such disease in Southeast Asia (Batai virus), Europe (Calovo virus), and South America (Wyeomyia virus). In North America, Cache Valley virus has been implicated in febrile human disease and in rare instances of more serious systemic illness; the presence of serum antibodies to this virus may be associated with congenital malformations. In Central America, the closely related Fort Sherman virus causes the fever-myalgia syndrome.

GROUP C VIRUS INFECTION

The group C viruses include at least 11 agents transmitted by mosquitoes in neotropical forests. These agents are among the most common causes of arboviral infection in humans entering American jungles and cause acute febrile disease.

TAHYNA VIRUS INFECTION

This California serogroup virus (see discussion of California encephalitis later in the chapter) occurs in central and western Europe, and related viruses are emerging in Russia. The significance of Tahyna virus in human health has been well studied only in the Czech and Slovak Republics; there, the virus was found to be a prominent cause of febrile disease, in some cases causing pharyngitis, pulmonary syndromes, and aseptic meningitis. The potential for arboviruses to be unexpectedly involved in such cases in areas of high mosquito prevalence needs to be kept in mind.

OROPOUCHE FEVER

Oropouche virus is transmitted in Central and South America by a biting midge, *Culicoides paraensis*, which often breeds to high density in cacao husks and other vegetable detritus found in towns and cities. Explosive epidemics involving thousands of cases have been reported from several towns in Brazil and Peru. Rash and aseptic meningitis have been detected in a number of cases.

SANDFLY FEVER

The sandfly *Phlebotomus papatasi* transmits sandfly fever. Female sandflies may be infected by the oral route as they take a blood meal and may transmit the virus to offspring when they lay their eggs after a second blood meal. This prominent transovarial pattern was the first to be recognized among dipterans and complicates virus control. A previous designation for sandfly fever, "3-day fever," instructively describes the brief, debilitating course associated with this essentially benign infection. There is neither a rash nor CNS involvement, and complete recovery is the rule.

Sandfly fever is found in the circum-Mediterranean area, extending to the east through the Balkans into China as well as into the Middle East and southwestern Asia. The vector is found in both rural and urban settings and is known for its small size, which enables it to penetrate standard mosquito screens and netting, and for its short flight range. Epidemics have been described in the wake of natural disasters and wars. In parts of Europe, sandfly populations and virus transmission were greatly reduced by the extensive residual spraying conducted after World War II to control malaria, and the incidence continues to be low. A common pattern of disease in endemic areas consists of high attack rates among travelers and military personnel with little or no disease in the local population, who are protected after childhood infection. More than 30 related phleboviruses are transmitted by sandflies and mosquitoes, but most are of unknown significance in terms of human health.

TOSCANA VIRUS DISEASE

Toscana virus is a *Phlebovirus* (family Bunyaviridae) transmitted primarily by the circum-Mediterranean sandfly *P. perniciosus*. The vertebrate amplifying host, if one exists, is unknown. Toscana virus infection is common during the summer among rural residents and vacationers, particularly in Italy, Spain, and Portugal; a number of cases have been identified in travelers returning to Germany and Scandinavia. The disease may manifest as an uncomplicated febrile illness but is often associated with aseptic meningitis, with virus isolated from the CSF.

PUNTA TORO VIRUS DISEASE

Of the several phleboviruses that are associated with New World sandflies and infect humans, Punta Toro virus is the best known. The disease caused by this virus is clinically similar to but epidemiologically different from that caused by the Naples or Sicilian sandfly fever viruses. Punta Toro virus infections are sporadic and are acquired in the tropical forest, where the vectors rest on tree buttresses. Epidemics have not been reported, but antibody prevalences among inhabitants of villages in the endemic areas indicate a cumulative lifetime exposure rate of >50%.

DENGUE FEVER

All four distinct dengue viruses (dengue 1–4) have *Aedes aegypti* as their principal vector, and all cause a similar clinical syndrome. In rare cases, second infection with a serotype of dengue virus different from that involved in the primary infection leads to dengue HF with severe shock (see below). Sporadic cases are seen in the settings of endemic transmission and epidemic disease. Year-round transmission between latitudes 25°N and 25°S has been established, and seasonal forays of the viruses to points as far north as Philadelphia are thought to have taken place in the United States. Dengue fever is seen in the Caribbean region, including Puerto Rico. With increasing spread of the vector mosquito throughout the tropics and subtropics, large areas of the world have become vulnerable to the introduction of dengue viruses, particularly through air travel by infected humans, and both dengue fever and the related dengue HF are becoming increasingly common. Conditions favorable to dengue transmission exist in the southern United States, and bursts of dengue fever activity are to be expected in this region, particularly along the Mexican border, where water may be stored in containers and *A. aegypti* numbers may therefore be greatest. This mosquito, which is also an efficient vector of the yellow fever and chikungunya viruses, typically breeds near human habitation, using relatively fresh water from sources such as water jars, vases, discarded containers, coconut husks, and old tires. *A. aegypti* usually inhabits dwellings and bites during the day.

After an incubation period of 2–7 days, the typical patient experiences the sudden onset of fever, headache, retroorbital pain, and back pain along with the severe myalgia that gave rise to the colloquial designation "break-bone fever." There is often a macular rash on the first day as well as adenopathy, palatal vesicles, and scleral injection. The illness may last a week, with additional symptoms usually including anorexia, nausea or vomiting, marked cutaneous hypersensitivity, and—near the time of defervescence—a maculopapular rash beginning on the trunk and spreading to the extremities and the face. Epistaxis and scattered petechiae are often noted in uncomplicated dengue, and preexisting gastrointestinal lesions may bleed during the acute illness.

Laboratory findings include leukopenia, thrombocytopenia, and, in many cases, serum aminotransferase elevations. The diagnosis is made by IgM ELISA or paired serology during recovery or by antigen-detection ELISA or RT-PCR during the acute phase. Virus is readily isolated from blood in the acute phase if mosquito inoculation or mosquito cell culture is used.

COLORADO TICK FEVER

Several hundred cases of Colorado tick fever are reported annually in the United States. The infection is acquired between March and November through the bite of an infected *Dermacentor andersoni* tick in mountainous western regions at altitudes of 1200–3000 m (4000–10,000 ft). Small mammals serve as the amplifying host. The most common presentation consists of fever and myalgia; meningoencephalitis is not uncommon, and hemorrhagic disease, pericarditis, myocarditis, orchitis, and pulmonary presentations are also reported. Rash develops in a substantial minority of cases. The disease usually lasts 7–10 days and is often biphasic. The most important differential diagnostic considerations since the beginning of the twentieth century have been Rocky Mountain spotted fever and tularemia. In Colorado, Colorado tick fever is much more common than Rocky Mountain spotted fever.

Infection of erythroblasts and other marrow cells by Colorado tick fever virus results in the appearance and persistence (for several weeks) of erythrocytes containing the virus. This feature, detected in smears stained by immunofluorescence, can be diagnostically helpful. The clinical laboratory detects leukopenia and thrombocytopenia.

ORBIVIRUS INFECTION

The orbiviruses encompass many human and veterinary pathogens. For example, Orungo virus is widely transmitted by mosquitoes in tropical Africa and causes febrile disease in humans. The Kemerovo complex includes the Kemerovo, Lipovnik, and Tribec viruses of Russia and central Europe; these viruses are transmitted by ticks and are associated with febrile and neurologic disease.

ENCEPHALITIS

Arboviral encephalitis is a seasonal disease, commonly occurring in the warmer months. Its incidence varies markedly with time and place, depending on ecologic factors. The causative viruses differ substantially in terms of case-infection ratio (i.e., the ratio of clinical to subclinical infections), mortality rate, and residua (Table 99-3). Humans are not an important amplifier of these viruses.

All the viral encephalitides discussed in this section have a similar pathogenesis as far as is known. An infected arthropod ingests a blood meal from a human and infects the host. The initial period of viremia is thought to originate most commonly from the lymphoid system. Viremia leads to CNS invasion, presumably through infection of olfactory neuroepithelium with passage through the cribriform plate or through infection of brain capillaries and multifocal entry into the CNS. During the viremic phase, there may be little or no recognized disease except in the case of tick-borne flaviviral encephalitis, in which there may be a clearly delineated phase of fever and systemic illness. The disease process in the CNS arises partly from direct neuronal infection and subsequent damage and partly from

TABLE 99-3

PROMINENT FEATURES OF ARBOVIRAL ENCEPHALITIS

VIRUS	NATURAL CYCLE	INCUBATION PERIOD, DAYS	ANNUAL NO. OF CASES	CASE-TO-INFECTION RATIO	AGE OF CASES	CASE-FATALITY RATE, %	RESIDUA
La Crosse	*Aedes triseriatus*–chipmunk (transovarial component in mosquito also important)	~3–7	70 (U.S.)	<1:1000	<15 years	<0.5	Recurrent seizures in ~10%; severe deficits in rare cases; decreased school performance and behavioral change suspected in small proportion
St. Louis	*Culex tarsalis*, *C. pipiens*, *C. quinquefasciatus*–birds	4–21	85, with hundreds to thousands in epidemic years (U.S.)	<1:200	Milder cases in the young; more severe cases in adults >40 years old, particularly the elderly	7	Common in the elderly
Japanese	*Culex tritaeniorhynchus*–birds	5–15	>25,000	1:200–300	All ages; children in highly endemic areas	20–50	Common (approximately half of cases); may be severe
West Nile	*Culex* mosquitoes–birds	3–6	?	Very low	Mainly the elderly	5–10	Uncommon
Central European	*Ixodes ricinus*–rodents, insectivores	7–14	Thousands	1:12	All ages; milder in children	1–5	20%
Russian spring-summer	*I. persulcatus*–rodents, insectivores	7–14	Hundreds	—	All ages; milder in children	20	Approximately half of cases; often severe; limb-girdle paralysis
Powassan	*I. cookei*–wild mammals	~10	~1 (U.S.)	—	All ages; some predilection for children	~10	Common (approximately half of cases)
Eastern equine	*Culiseta melanura*–birds	~5–10	5 (U.S.)	1:40 adult 1:17 child	All ages; predilection for children	50–75	Common
Western equine	*Culex tarsalis*–birds	~5–10	~20 (U.S.)	1:1000 adult 1:50 child 1:1 infant	All ages; predilection for children <2 years old (increased mortality in elderly)	3–7	Common only among infants <1 year old
Venezuelan equine (epidemic)	Unknown (multiple mosquito species and horses in epidemics)	1–5	?	1:250 adult 1:25 child (approximate)	All ages; predilection for children	~10	—

edema, inflammation, and other indirect effects. The usual pathologic picture is one of focal necrosis of neurons, inflammatory glial nodules, and perivascular lymphoid cuffing; the severity and distribution of these abnormalities vary with the infecting virus. Involved areas display the "luxury perfusion" phenomenon, with normal or increased total blood flow and low oxygen extraction.

The typical patient presents with a prodrome of nonspecific constitutional symptoms, including fever, abdominal pain, vertigo, sore throat, and respiratory symptoms. Headache, meningeal signs, photophobia, and vomiting follow quickly. Involvement of deeper structures may be signaled by lethargy, somnolence, and intellectual deficit (as disclosed by the mental status examination or failure at serial 7 subtraction); more severely affected patients are obviously disoriented and may be comatose. Tremors, loss of abdominal reflexes, cranial nerve palsies, hemiparesis, monoparesis, difficulty in swallowing, and frontal lobe signs are all common. Spinal and motor neuron diseases are documented with West Nile and Japanese encephalitis viruses. Convulsions and focal signs may be evident early or may appear during the course of the disease. Some patients present with an abrupt onset of fever, convulsions, and other signs of CNS involvement. The results of human infection range from no significant symptoms through febrile headache to aseptic meningitis and finally to full-blown encephalitis; the proportions and severity of these manifestations vary with the infecting virus.

The acute encephalitis usually lasts from a few days to as long as 2–3 weeks, but recovery may be slow, with weeks or months required for the return of maximal recoupable function. Difficulty concentrating, fatigability, tremors, and personality changes are common during recovery. The acute illness requires management of a comatose patient who may have intracranial pressure elevations, inappropriate secretion of antidiuretic hormone, respiratory failure, and convulsions. There is no specific therapy for these viral encephalitides. The only practical preventive measures are vector management and personal protection against the arthropod transmitting the virus; for Japanese encephalitis or tick-borne encephalitis, vaccination should be considered in certain circumstances (see relevant sections below).

The diagnosis of arboviral encephalitis depends on the careful evaluation of a febrile patient with CNS disease, with rapid identification of treatable herpes simplex encephalitis, ruling out of brain abscess, exclusion of bacterial meningitis by serial CSF examination, and performance of laboratory studies to define the viral etiology. Leptospirosis, neurosyphilis, Lyme disease, cat-scratch fever, and newer viral encephalitides such as Nipah virus infection from Malaysia should be considered. The CSF examination usually shows a modest cell count—in the tens or hundreds or perhaps a few thousand. Early in the process, a significant proportion of these cells may be polymorphonuclear leukocytes, but usually there is a mononuclear cell predominance. CSF glucose levels are usually normal. There are exceptions to this pattern of findings. In eastern equine encephalitis, for example, polymorphonuclear leukocytes may predominate during the first 72 h of disease and hypoglycorrhachia may be detected. In LCM, lymphocyte counts may be in the thousands, and the glucose concentration may be diminished. Experience with imaging studies is still evolving; clearly, however, both CT and MRI may be normal, except for evidence of preexisting conditions, or sometimes may suggest diffuse edema. Several patients with eastern equine encephalitis have had focal abnormalities, and individuals with severe Japanese encephalitis have presented with bilateral thalamic lesions that have often been hemorrhagic. Electroencephalography usually shows diffuse abnormalities and is not directly helpful.

A humoral immune response is usually detectable at or near the onset of disease. Both serum and CSF should be examined for IgM antibodies. Virus generally cannot be isolated from blood or CSF, although Japanese encephalitis virus has been recovered from CSF in severe cases. RT-PCR analysis of CSF may yield positive results. Virus can be obtained from and viral antigen is present in brain tissue, although its distribution may be focal.

CALIFORNIA, LA CROSSE, AND JAMESTOWN CANYON VIRUS ENCEPHALITIS

The isolation of California encephalitis virus established the California serogroup of viruses as a cause of encephalitis, and its use as a diagnostic antigen led to the description of many cases of "California encephalitis." In fact, however, this virus has been implicated in only a few cases of encephalitis, and the serologically related La Crosse virus is the major cause of encephalitis among viruses in the California serogroup. "California encephalitis" due to La Crosse virus infection is most commonly reported from the upper Midwest but is also found in other areas of the central and eastern United States, most often in West Virginia, Tennessee, North Carolina, and Georgia. The serogroup includes 13 other viruses, some of which may also be involved in human disease that is misattributed because of the complexity of the group's serology; these viruses include the Jamestown Canyon, snowshoe hare, Inkoo, and Trivittatus viruses, all of which have *Aedes* mosquitoes as their vector and all of which have a strong element of transovarial transmission in their natural cycles.

The mosquito vector of La Crosse virus is *A. triseriatus*. In addition to a prominent transovarial component of transmission, a mosquito can become infected through feeding on viremic chipmunks and other mammals as well as through venereal transmission from another mosquito. The mosquito breeds in sites such as tree holes and abandoned tires and bites during daylight hours. These habits correlate with the risk factors for human cases: recreation in forested areas, residence at the forest's edge, and the presence of abandoned tires around the home. Intensive environmental modification based on these findings has reduced the incidence of disease in a highly endemic area in the Midwest. Most cases occur from July through September. The Asian tiger mosquito, *A. albopictus*, efficiently transmits the virus to mice and also transmits the agent transovarially in the laboratory; this aggressive anthropophilic mosquito has the capacity to urbanize, and its possible impact on transmission to humans is of concern.

An antibody prevalence of ≥20% in endemic areas indicates that infection is common, but CNS disease has been recognized primarily in children <15 years of age. The illness varies from a picture of aseptic meningitis accompanied by confusion to severe and occasionally fatal encephalitis. Although there may be prodromal symptoms, the onset of CNS disease is sudden, with fever, headache, and lethargy often joined by nausea and vomiting, convulsions (in one-half of patients), and coma (in one-third of patients). Focal seizures, hemiparesis, tremor, aphasia, chorea, Babinski signs, and other evidence of significant neurologic dysfunction are common, but residua are not. Perhaps 10% of patients have recurrent seizures in the succeeding months. Other serious sequelae are rare, although a decrease in scholastic standing has been reported and mild personality change has occasionally been suggested. Treatment is supportive over a 1- to 2-week acute phase during which status epilepticus, cerebral edema, and inappropriate secretion of antidiuretic hormone are important concerns. Ribavirin has been used in severe cases, and a clinical trial of this drug is under way.

The blood leukocyte count is commonly elevated, sometimes reaching levels of 20,000/μL, and there is usually a left shift. CSF cell counts are typically 30–500/μL with a mononuclear cell predominance (although 25–90% of cells are polymorphonuclear in some cases). The protein level is normal or slightly increased, and the glucose level is normal. Specific virologic diagnosis based on IgM-capture assays of serum and CSF is efficient. The only human anatomic site from which virus has been isolated is the brain.

Jamestown Canyon virus has been implicated in several cases of encephalitis in adults; in these cases, the disease was usually associated with a significant respiratory illness at onset. Human infection with this virus has been documented in New York, Wisconsin, Ohio, Michigan, Ontario, and other areas of North America where the vector mosquito, *A. stimulans*, feeds on its main host, the white-tailed deer.

ST. LOUIS ENCEPHALITIS

St. Louis encephalitis virus is transmitted between *Culex* mosquitoes and birds. This virus causes low-level endemic infection among rural residents of the western and central United States, where *C. tarsalis* is the vector (see "Western Equine Encephalitis" later in the chapter), but the more urbanized mosquito species *C. pipiens* and *C. quinquefasciatus* have been responsible for epidemics resulting in hundreds or even thousands of cases in cities of the central and eastern United States. Most cases occur in June through October. The urban mosquitoes breed in accumulations of stagnant water and sewage with high organic content and readily bite humans in and around houses at dusk. The elimination of open sewers and trash-filled drainage systems is expensive and may not be possible, but screening of houses and implementation of personal protective measures may be an effective approach for individuals. The rural vector is most active at dusk and outdoors; its bites can be avoided by modification of activities and use of repellents.

Disease severity increases with age: infections that result in aseptic meningitis or mild encephalitis are concentrated in children and young adults, while severe and fatal cases primarily affect the elderly. Infection rates are similar in all age groups; thus the greater susceptibility of older persons to disease is a biologic consequence of aging. The disease has an abrupt onset, sometimes following a prodrome, and begins with fever, lethargy, confusion, and headache. In addition, nuchal rigidity, hypotonia, hyperreflexia, myoclonus, and tremor are common. Severe cases can include cranial nerve palsies, hemiparesis, and convulsions. Patients often report dysuria and may have viral antigen in urine as well as pyuria. The overall mortality rate is generally ~7% but may reach 20% among patients over the age of 60. Recovery is slow. Emotional lability, difficulties in concentration and memory, asthenia, and tremor are commonly prolonged in older patients.

The CSF of patients with St. Louis encephalitis usually contains tens to hundreds of cells, with a lymphocytic predominance and a normal glucose level. Leukocytosis with a left shift is often documented.

JAPANESE ENCEPHALITIS

Japanese encephalitis virus is found throughout Asia, including far eastern Russia, Japan, China, India, Pakistan, and Southeast Asia, and causes occasional epidemics on western Pacific islands. The virus has been detected in the Torres Strait islands, and a human encephalitis case has been identified on the nearby Australian mainland. This flavivirus is particularly common in areas where irrigated rice fields attract the natural avian vertebrate hosts and provide abundant breeding sites for mosquitoes such as *C. tritaeniorhynchus*, which transmit the virus to humans. Additional amplification by pigs, which suffer abortion, and horses, which develop encephalitis, may be significant as well. Vaccination of these additional amplifying hosts may reduce the transmission of the virus. An effective, formalin-inactivated vaccine purified from mouse brain is produced in Japan and licensed for human use in the United States. It is given on days 0, 7, and 30 or—with some sacrifice in serum neutralizing titer—on days 0, 7, and 14. Vaccination is indicated for summer travelers to rural Asia, where the risk of clinical disease may be 0.05–2.1/10,000 per week (Table 3-2). The severe and often fatal disease reported in expatriates must be balanced against the 0.1–1% chance of a late systemic or cutaneous allergic reaction. These reactions are rarely fatal but may be severe and have been known to begin 1–9 days after vaccination, with associated pruritus, urticaria, and angioedema. Live attenuated vaccines are being used in China but are not recommended in the United States at this time.

WEST NILE VIRUS INFECTION

West Nile virus is transmitted among wild birds by *Culex* mosquitoes in Africa, the Middle East, southern Europe, and Asia. It is a common cause of febrile disease without CNS involvement, but it occasionally causes aseptic meningitis and severe encephalitis; these serious infections are particularly common among the elderly. The febrile-myalgic syndrome caused by West Nile virus differs from many others by the frequent appearance of a maculopapular rash concentrated on the trunk and lymphadenopathy. Headache, ocular pain, sore throat, nausea and vomiting, and arthralgia (but not arthritis) are common accompaniments. In addition, the virus has been implicated in severe and fatal hepatic necrosis in Africa.

West Nile virus was introduced into New York City in 1999 and subsequently spread to other areas of the northeastern United States, causing >60 cases of aseptic meningitis or encephalitis among humans as well as die-offs among crows, exotic zoo birds, and other birds. The virus has continued to spread and is now found in almost all states, Canada, and Mexico. *C. pipiens* remains the major vector in the northeastern United States, but several other *Culex* species are also involved, and blue jays compete with crows as amplifiers and lethal targets in other areas of the country. Annually, ~1000–3000 cases of encephalitis with ~100–300 deaths are reported in the United States. The ratio of CNS involvement to infection is thought to be ~1:100; the remainder of patients have subclinical infection or West Nile fever. Encephalitis, sequelae, and death are all more common among the elderly, diabetics, and patients with previous CNS insults. In addition to the more severe motor and cognitive sequelae, milder findings may include tremor, slight abnormalities in motor skills, and loss of executive functions. Intense clinical interest and the availability of laboratory diagnostic methods have made it possible to define a number of unusual clinical features, including chorioretinitis, flaccid paralysis with histologic lesions resembling poliomyelitis, and initial presentation with fever and focal neurologic deficits in the absence of diffuse encephalitis. Immunosuppressed patients may have fulminant courses or develop persistent CNS infection. Virus transmission through both transplantation and blood transfusion has necessitated screening of blood and organ donors by nucleic acid–based tests.

West Nile virus falls into the same phylogenetic group of flaviviruses as St. Louis and Japanese encephalitis viruses, as do Murray Valley and Rocio viruses. The latter two viruses are both maintained in mosquitoes and birds and produce a clinical picture resembling that of Japanese encephalitis. Murray Valley virus has caused occasional epidemics and sporadic cases in Australia. Rocio virus caused recurrent epidemics in a focal area of Brazil in 1975–1977 and then virtually disappeared.

CENTRAL EUROPEAN TICK-BORNE ENCEPHALITIS AND RUSSIAN SPRING-SUMMER ENCEPHALITIS

A spectrum of tick-borne flaviviruses has been identified across the Eurasian land mass. Many are known mainly as agricultural pathogens (e.g., louping ill virus in the United Kingdom). From Scandinavia to the Urals, central European tick-borne encephalitis is transmitted by *Ixodes ricinus*. Human cases occur between April and October, with a peak in June and July. A related and more virulent virus is that of Russian spring-summer encephalitis, which is associated with *I. persulcatus* and is distributed from Europe across the Urals to the Pacific Ocean. The ticks transmit the disease primarily in the spring and early summer, with a lower rate of transmission later in summer. Small mammals are the vertebrate amplifiers for both viruses. The risk varies by geographic area and can be highly localized within a given area; human cases usually follow outdoor activities or consumption of raw milk from infected goats or other infected animals.

After an incubation period of 7–14 days or perhaps longer, the central European viruses classically result in a febrile-myalgic phase that lasts for 2–4 days and is thought to correlate with viremia. A subsequent remission for several days is followed by the recurrence of fever and the onset of meningeal signs. The CNS phase varies from mild aseptic meningitis, which is more common among younger patients, to severe encephalitis with coma, convulsions, tremors, and motor signs lasting for 7–10 days before improvement begins. Spinal and medullary involvement can lead to typical limb-girdle paralysis and to respiratory paralysis. Most patients recover, only a minority with significant deficits. Infections with the Far Eastern viruses generally run a more abrupt course. The encephalitic syndrome caused by these viruses sometimes begins without a remission and has more severe manifestations than the European syndrome. Mortality is high, and major sequelae—most notably, lower motor neuron paralyses of the proximal muscles of the extremities, trunk, and neck—are common.

In the early stage of the illness, virus may be isolated from the blood. In the CNS phase, IgM antibodies are detectable in serum and/or CSF. Thrombocytopenia sometimes develops during the initial febrile illness, which resembles the early hemorrhagic phase of some other tick-borne flaviviral infections, such as Kyasanur Forest disease. Other tick-borne flaviviruses are less common causes of encephalitis, including louping ill virus in the United Kingdom and Powassan virus.

There is no specific therapy for infection with these viruses. However, effective alum-adjuvanted, formalin-inactivated vaccines are produced in Austria, Germany, and Russia. Two doses of the Austrian vaccine separated by an interval of 1–3 months appear to be effective in the field, and antibody responses are similar when vaccine is given on days 0 and 14. Other vaccines have elicited similar neutralizing antibody titers. Since rare cases of postvaccination Guillain-Barré syndrome have been reported, vaccination should be reserved for persons likely to experience rural exposure in an endemic area during the season of transmission. Cross-neutralization for the central European and Far Eastern strains has been established, but there are no published field studies on cross-protection of formalin-inactivated vaccines. Because 0.2–4% of ticks in endemic areas may be infected, tick bites raise the issue of immunoglobulin prophylaxis. Prompt administration of high-titered specific preparations should probably be undertaken, although no controlled data are available to prove the efficacy of this measure. Immunoglobulin should not be administered late because of the risk of antibody-mediated enhancement.

POWASSAN ENCEPHALITIS

Powassan virus is a member of the tick-borne encephalitis virus complex and is transmitted by *I. cookei* among small mammals in eastern Canada and the United States, where it has been responsible for 20 recognized cases of human disease. Other ticks may transmit the virus in a wider geographic area, and there is some concern that *I. scapularis* (also called *I. dammini*), a competent vector in the laboratory, may become involved as it becomes more prominent in the United States. Patients with Powassan encephalitis (many of whom are children) present in May through December after outdoor exposure and an incubation period thought to be ~1 week. Powassan encephalitis is severe, and sequelae are common.

EASTERN EQUINE ENCEPHALITIS

Eastern equine encephalitis is found primarily within endemic swampy foci along the eastern coast of the United States, with a few inland foci as far removed as Michigan. Human cases present from June through October, when the bird–*Culiseta* mosquito cycle spills over into other mosquito species such as *A. sollicitans* or *A. vexans*, which are more likely to bite mammals. There is concern over the potential role of the introduced anthropophilic mosquito species *A. albopictus*, which has been found to be naturally infected and is an effective vector in the laboratory. Horses are a common target for the virus; contact with unvaccinated horses may be associated with human disease, but horses probably do not play a significant role in amplification of the virus.

Eastern equine encephalitis is one of the most destructive of the arboviral conditions, with a brusque onset, rapid progression, high mortality, and frequent residua. This severity is reflected in the extensive necrotic lesions and polymorphonuclear infiltrates found at postmortem examination of the brain and the acute polymorphonuclear CSF pleocytosis often occurring during the first 1–3 days of disease. In addition, leukocytosis with a left shift is a common feature. A formalin-inactivated vaccine has been used to protect laboratory workers but is not generally available or applicable.

WESTERN EQUINE ENCEPHALITIS

The primary maintenance cycle for western equine encephalitis virus in the United States is between *C. tarsalis* and birds, principally sparrows and finches. Equines and humans become infected, and both species suffer encephalitis without amplifying the virus in nature. St. Louis encephalitis is transmitted in a similar cycle in the same region but causes human disease about a month earlier than the period (July through October) in which western equine encephalitis virus is active. Large epidemics of western equine encephalitis took place in the western and central United States and Canada during the 1930s to 1950s, but in recent years the disease has been uncommon. There were 41 reported cases in the United States in 1987 but only 5 reported cases from 1988 to 2001. This decline in incidence may reflect in part the integrated approach to mosquito management that has been employed in irrigation projects and the increasing use of agricultural pesticides; it almost certainly reflects the increased tendency for humans to be indoors behind closed windows at dusk—the peak period of biting by the major vector.

Western equine encephalitis virus causes a typical diffuse viral encephalitis with an increased attack rate and increased morbidity among the young, particularly children <2 years old. In addition, mortality rates are high among the young and the very elderly. One-third of individuals who have convulsions during the acute illness have subsequent seizure activity. Infants <1 year old—particularly those in the first months of life—are at serious risk of motor and intellectual damage. Twice as many males as females develop clinical encephalitis after 5–9 years of age; this difference may be related to greater outdoor exposure of boys to the vector but is also likely to be due in part to biologic differences. A formalin-inactivated vaccine has been used to protect laboratory workers but is not generally available or applicable.

VENEZUELAN EQUINE ENCEPHALITIS

There are six known types of virus in the Venezuelan equine encephalitis complex. An important distinction is between the *epizootic* viruses (subtypes IAB and IC) and the *enzootic* viruses (subtypes ID to IF and types II to VI). The epizootic viruses have an unknown natural cycle but periodically cause extensive epidemics in equines and humans in the Americas. These epidemics rely on the high-level viremia in horses and mules that results in the infection of several species of mosquitoes, which in turn infect humans and perpetuate virus transmission. Humans also have high-level viremia but probably are not important in virus transmission. Enzootic viruses are found primarily in humid tropical forest habitats and are maintained between *Culex* mosquitoes and rodents; these viruses cause human disease but are not pathogenic for horses and do not cause epizootics.

Epizootics of Venezuelan equine encephalitis occurred repeatedly in Venezuela, Colombia, Ecuador, Peru, and other South American countries at intervals of ≤10 years from the 1930s until 1969, when a massive epizootic spread throughout Central America and Mexico, reaching southern Texas in 1972. Genetic sequencing of the virus from the 1969–1972 outbreak suggested that it originated from residual "un-inactivated" virus in veterinary vaccines. The outbreak was terminated in Texas with the use of a live attenuated vaccine (TC-83) originally developed for human use by the U.S. Army; the epizootic virus was then used for further production of inactivated veterinary vaccines. No further epizootic disease was identified until 1995 and subsequently, when additional epizootics took place in Colombia, Venezuela, and Mexico. The viruses involved in these epizootics as well as previously epizootic subtype IC viruses have been shown to be close phylogenetic relatives of known enzootic subtype ID viruses. This finding suggests that active evolution and selection of epizootic viruses are under way in northern South America.

During epizootics, extensive human infection is the rule, with clinical disease in 10–60% of infected individuals. Most infections result in notable acute febrile disease, while relatively few result in encephalitis. A low rate of CNS invasion is supported by the absence of encephalitis among the many infections resulting from exposure to aerosols in the laboratory or from vaccine accidents. The most recent large epizootic of Venezuelan equine encephalitis occurred in Colombia and Venezuela in 1995; of the >85,000 clinical cases, 4% (with a higher proportion among children than adults) included neurologic symptoms and 300 ended in death.

Enzootic strains of Venezuelan equine encephalitis virus are common causes of acute febrile disease, particularly in areas such as the Florida Everglades and the humid Atlantic coast of Central America. Encephalitis has been documented only in the Florida infections; the three cases were caused by type II enzootic virus, also called *Everglades virus*. All three patients had preexisting cerebral disease. Extrapolation from the rate of genetic change suggests that Everglades virus may have been introduced into Florida <200 years ago and that it is most closely related to the ID subtypes that appear to have given evolutionary rise to the epizootic strains active in South America.

The prevention of epizootic Venezuelan equine encephalitis depends on vaccination of horses with the attenuated TC-83 vaccine or with an inactivated vaccine prepared from that strain. Humans can be protected with similar vaccines, but the use of such products is restricted to laboratory personnel because of reactogenicity and limited availability. In addition, wild-type virus and perhaps TC-83 vaccine may have some degree of fetal pathogenicity. Enzootic viruses are genetically and antigenically different from epizootic viruses, and protection against the former with vaccines prepared from the latter is relatively ineffective.

ARTHRITIS AND RASH

True arthritis is a common accompaniment of several viral diseases, such as rubella (caused by a non-alphavirus togavirus), parvovirus B19 infection, and hepatitis B; it is an occasional accompaniment of infection due to mumps virus, enteroviruses, herpesviruses, and adenoviruses. It is not generally appreciated that the alphaviruses are also common causes of arthritis. In fact, the alphaviruses discussed below all cause acute febrile diseases accompanied by the development of true arthritis and a maculopapular rash. Rheumatic involvement includes arthralgia alone, periarticular swelling, and (less commonly) joint effusions. Most of these diseases are less severe and have fewer articular manifestations in children than in adults. In temperate climates, these are summer diseases. No specific therapy or licensed vaccines exist.

SINDBIS VIRUS INFECTION

Sindbis virus is transmitted among birds by mosquitoes. Infections with the northern European strains of this virus (which cause, for example, Pogosta disease in Finland, Karelian fever in the independent states of the former Soviet Union, and Ockelbo disease in Sweden) and with the genetically related southern African strains are particularly likely to result in the arthritis-rash syndrome. Exposure to a rural environment is commonly associated with this infection, which has an incubation period of <1 week.

The disease begins with rash and arthralgia. Constitutional symptoms are not marked, and fever is modest or lacking altogether. The rash, which lasts ~1 week, begins on the trunk, spreads to the extremities, and evolves from macules to papules that often vesiculate. The arthritis of this condition is multiarticular, migratory, and incapacitating, with resolution of the acute phase in a few days. Wrists, ankles, phalangeal joints, knees, elbows, and—to a much lesser extent—proximal and axial joints are involved. Persistence of joint pains and occasionally of arthritis is a major problem and may go on for months or even years despite a lack of deformity.

CHIKUNGUNYA VIRUS INFECTION

It is likely that chikungunya virus ("that which bends up") is of African origin and is maintained among nonhuman primates on that continent by *Aedes* mosquitoes of the subgenus *Stegomyia* in a fashion similar to yellow fever virus. Like yellow fever virus, chikungunya virus is readily transmitted among humans in urban areas by *A. aegypti*. The *A. aegypti*–chikungunya virus transmission cycle has also been introduced into Asia, where it poses a prominent health problem. The disease is endemic in rural areas of Africa, and intermittent epidemics take place in towns and cities of Africa and Asia. In 2004, a massive epidemic in the Indian Ocean region began; it now appears to have been spread totally by travelers. *A. albopictus* was identified as the major vector, and there were multiple exportations to temperate zones and to areas where *A. aegypti* is present. Chikungunya is one more reason (in addition to dengue and yellow fever) that *A. aegypti* must be controlled.

Full-blown disease is most common among adults, in whom the clinical picture may be dramatic. The abrupt onset follows an incubation period of 2–3 days. Fever and severe arthralgia are accompanied by chills and constitutional symptoms such as headache, photophobia, conjunctival injection, anorexia, nausea, and abdominal pain. Migratory polyarthritis mainly affects the small joints of the hands, wrists, ankles, and feet, with lesser involvement of the larger joints. Rash may appear at the outset or several days into the illness; its development often coincides with defervescence, which takes place around day 2 or 3 of disease. The rash is most intense on the trunk and limbs and may desquamate. Petechiae are occasionally seen, and epistaxis is not uncommon, but this virus is not a regular cause of the HF syndrome, even in children. A few patients develop leukopenia. Elevated levels of aspartate aminotransferase (AST) and C-reactive protein have been described, as have mildly decreased platelet counts. Recovery may require weeks. Some older patients continue to experience stiffness, joint pain, and recurrent effusions for several years; this persistence may be especially common in HLA-B27 patients. An investigational live attenuated vaccine has been developed but requires additional testing. It appears to be headed for further development and commercial manufacture stimulated by the Indian Ocean outbreak.

A related virus, O'nyong-nyong, caused a major epidemic of arthritis and rash involving at least 2 million people as it moved across eastern and central Africa in the 1960s. After its mysterious emergence, the virus virtually disappeared, leaving only occasional evidence of its persistence in Kenya until a transient resurgence of epidemic activity in 1997.

MAYARO FEVER

Mayaro virus is maintained in the forests of the Americas by *Haemagogus* mosquitoes and nonhuman primates. It causes a frequently endemic and sometimes epidemic infection of humans and appears to produce a syndrome resembling chikungunya virus infection.

EPIDEMIC POLYARTHRITIS (ROSS RIVER VIRUS INFECTION)

Ross River virus has caused epidemics of distinctive clinical disease in Australia since the beginning of the twentieth century and continues to be responsible for thousands of cases in rural and suburban areas annually. The virus is transmitted by *A. vigilax* and other mosquitoes, and its persistence is thought to involve transovarial transmission. No definitive vertebrate host has been identified, but several mammalian species, including wallabies, have been suggested. Endemic transmission has also been documented in New Guinea, and in 1979 the virus swept through the eastern Pacific Islands, causing hundreds of thousands of illnesses. The virus was carried from island to island by infected humans and was believed to have been transmitted among humans by *A. polynesiensis* and *A. aegypti*.

The incubation period is 7–11 days long, and the onset of illness is sudden, with joint pain usually ushering in the disease. The rash generally develops coincidentally or follows shortly but in some cases precedes joint pains by several days. Constitutional symptoms such as low-grade fever, asthenia, myalgia, headache, and nausea are not prominent and indeed are absent in many cases. Most patients are incapacitated for considerable periods by joint involvement, which interferes with sleeping, walking, and grasping. Wrist, ankle, metacarpophalangeal, interphalangeal, and knee joints are the most commonly involved, although toes, shoulders, and elbows may be affected with some frequency. Periarticular swelling and tenosynovitis are common, and one-third of patients have true arthritis. Only half of all arthritis patients can resume normal activities within 4 weeks, and 10% still must limit their activity at 3 months. Occasional patients are symptomatic for 1–3 years but without progressive arthropathy. Aspirin and nonsteroidal anti-inflammatory drugs are effective for the treatment of symptoms.

Clinical laboratory values are normal or variable in Ross River virus infection. Tests for rheumatoid factor and antinuclear antibodies are negative, and the erythrocyte sedimentation rate is acutely elevated. Joint fluid contains 1000–60,000 mononuclear cells/μL, and Ross River virus antigen is demonstrable in macrophages. IgM antibodies are valuable in the diagnosis of this infection, although they occasionally persist for years. The isolation of the virus from blood by mosquito inoculation or mosquito cell culture is possible early in the illness. Because of the great economic impact of annual epidemics in Australia, an inactivated vaccine is being developed and has been found to be protective in mice.

Perhaps because of the local interest in arboviruses in general and in Ross River virus in particular, other arthritogenic arboviruses have been identified in Australia, including Gan Gan virus, a member of the family Bunyaviridae; Kokobera virus, a flavivirus; and Barmah Forest virus, an alphavirus. The last virus is a common cause of infection and must be differentiated from Ross River virus by specific testing.

HEMORRHAGIC FEVERS

The viral HF syndrome is a constellation of findings based on vascular instability and decreased vascular integrity. An assault, direct or indirect, on the microvasculature leads to increased permeability and (particularly when platelet function is decreased) to actual disruption and local hemorrhage. Blood pressure is decreased, and in severe cases shock supervenes. Cutaneous flushing and conjunctival suffusion are examples of common, observable abnormalities in the control of local circulation. The hemorrhage is inconstant and is in most cases an indication of widespread vascular damage rather than a life-threatening loss of blood volume. Disseminated intravascular coagulation (DIC) is occasionally found in any severely ill patient with HF but is thought to occur regularly only in the early phases of HF with renal syndrome, Crimean-Congo HF, and perhaps some cases of filovirus HF. In some viral HF syndromes, specific organs may be particularly impaired, such as the kidney in HF with renal syndrome, the lung in hantavirus pulmonary syndrome, or the liver in yellow fever, but in all these diseases the generalized circulatory disturbance is critically important.

The pathogenesis of HF is poorly understood and varies among the viruses regularly implicated in the syndrome, which number more than a dozen. In some cases direct damage to the vascular system or even to parenchymal cells of target organs is important, whereas in others soluble mediators are thought to play the major role. The acute phase in most cases of HF is associated with ongoing virus replication and viremia. Exceptions are the hantavirus diseases and dengue HF/dengue shock syndrome (DHF/DSS), in which the immune response plays a major pathogenic role.

The HF syndromes all begin with fever and myalgia, usually of abrupt onset. Within a few days the patient presents for medical attention because of increasing prostration that is often accompanied by severe headache, dizziness, photophobia, hyperesthesia, abdominal or chest pain, anorexia, nausea or vomiting, and other gastrointestinal disturbances. Initial examination often reveals only an acutely ill patient with conjunctival suffusion, tenderness to palpation of muscles or abdomen, and borderline hypotension or postural hypotension, perhaps with tachycardia. Petechiae (often best visualized in the axillae), flushing of the head and thorax, periorbital edema, and proteinuria are common. Levels of AST are usually elevated at presentation or within a day or two thereafter. Hemoconcentration from vascular leakage, which is usually evident, is most marked in hantavirus diseases and in DHF/DSS. The seriously ill patient progresses to more severe symptoms and develops shock and other findings typical of the causative virus. Shock, multifocal bleeding, and CNS involvement (encephalopathy, coma, convulsions) are all poor prognostic signs.

One of the major diagnostic clues is travel to an endemic area within the incubation period for a given syndrome (Table 99-4). Except for Seoul, dengue, and yellow fever virus infections, which have urban vectors, travel to a rural setting is especially suggestive of a diagnosis of HF.

Early recognition is important because of the need for virus-specific therapy and supportive measures, including prompt, atraumatic hospitalization; judicious fluid therapy that takes into account the patient's increased capillary permeability; administration of cardiotonic drugs; use of pressors to maintain blood pressure at levels that will support renal perfusion; treatment of

TABLE 99-4

VIRAL HEMORRHAGIC FEVER (HF) SYNDROMES AND THEIR DISTRIBUTION

DISEASE	INCUBATION PERIOD, DAYS	CASE-INFECTION RATIO	CASE-FATALITY RATE, %	GEOGRAPHIC RANGE	TARGET POPULATION
Lassa fever	5–16	Mild infections probably common	15	West Africa	All ages, both sexes
South American HF	7–14	Most infections (more than half) result in disease	15–30	Selected rural areas of Bolivia, Argentina, Venezuela, and Brazil	Bolivia: Men in countryside; all ages, both sexes in villages Argentina: All ages, both sexes; excess exposure and disease in men Venezuela: All ages, both sexes
Rift Valley fever	2–5	~1:100[a]	~50	Sub-Saharan Africa, Madagascar, Egypt	All ages, both sexes; more often diagnosed in men; preexisting liver disease may predispose
Crimean-Congo HF	3–12	≥1:5	15–30	Africa, Middle East, Turkey, Balkans, southern region of former Soviet Union, western China	All ages, both sexes; men more exposed in some settings
HF with renal syndrome	9–35	Hantaan, >1:1.25; Puumala, 1:20	Hantaan, 5–15; Puumala, <1	Worldwide, depending on rodent reservoir	Excess of male patients (partly due to greater exposure); mainly adults
Hantavirus pulmonary syndrome	~7–28	Very high	40–50	Americas	Excess of male patients due to some occupational exposure; mainly adults
Marburg or Ebola HF	3–16	High	25–90	Sub-Saharan Africa	All ages, both sexes; children less exposed
Yellow fever	3–6	1:2–1:20	20	Africa, South America	All ages, both sexes; adults more exposed in jungle setting; preexisting flavivirus immunity may cross-protect
Dengue HF/ dengue shock syndrome	2–7	Nonimmune, 1:10,000; heterologous immune, 1:100	<1 with supportive treatment	Tropics and subtropics worldwide	Predominantly children; previous heterologous dengue infection predisposes to HF
Kyasanur Forest/ Omsk HF	3–8	Variable	0.5–10	Mysore State, India/ western Siberia	Variable

[a]Figure is for HF cases only. Most infections with Rift Valley fever virus result in fever and myalgia rather than HF.

the relatively common secondary bacterial infections; replacement of clotting factors and platelets as indicated; and the usual precautionary measures used in the treatment of patients with hemorrhagic diatheses. DIC should be treated only if clear laboratory evidence of its existence is found and if laboratory monitoring of therapy is feasible; there is no proven benefit of such therapy. The available evidence suggests that HF patients have a decreased cardiac output and will respond poorly to fluid loading as it is often practiced in the treatment of shock associated with bacterial sepsis. Specific therapy is available for several of the HF syndromes. In addition, several diseases considered in the differential diagnosis—malaria, shigellosis, typhoid, leptospirosis, relapsing fever, and rickettsial disease—are treatable and potentially lethal. Strict barrier nursing and other precautions against infection of medical staff and visitors are indicated in HF except that due to hantaviruses, yellow fever, Rift Valley fever, and dengue.

LASSA FEVER

Lassa virus is known to cause endemic and epidemic disease in Nigeria, Sierra Leone, Guinea, and Liberia, although it is probably more widely distributed in West Africa. This virus and its relatives exist elsewhere in Africa, but their health significance is unknown. Like other arenaviruses, Lassa virus is spread to humans by small-particle aerosols from chronically infected rodents and may also be acquired during the capture or eating of these animals. It can be transmitted by close person-to-person contact. The virus is often present in urine during convalescence and is suspected to be present in seminal fluid early in recovery. Nosocomial spread has occurred but is uncommon if proper sterile parenteral techniques are used. Individuals of all ages and both sexes are affected; the incidence of disease is highest in the dry season, but transmission takes place year-round. In countries where Lassa virus is endemic, Lassa fever can be a prominent cause of febrile disease. For example, in one hospital in Sierra Leone, laboratory-confirmed Lassa fever is consistently responsible for one-fifth of admissions to the medical wards. There are probably tens of thousands of Lassa fever cases annually in West Africa alone.

Among the HF agents, only the arenaviruses are typically associated with a gradual onset of illness. The average case of Lassa fever has a gradual onset that gives way to more severe constitutional symptoms and prostration. Bleeding is seen in only ~15–30% of cases. A maculopapular rash is often noted in light-skinned Lassa patients. Effusions are common, and male-dominant pericarditis may develop late. The fetal death rate is 92% in the last trimester, when the maternal mortality rate is also increased from the usual 15–30%; these figures suggest that interruption of the pregnancy of infected women should be considered. White blood cell counts are normal or slightly elevated, and platelet counts are normal or somewhat low. Deafness coincides with clinical improvement in ~20% of cases and is permanent and bilateral in some. Reinfection may occur but has not been associated with severe disease.

High-level viremia or a high serum concentration of AST statistically predicts a fatal outcome. Thus patients with an AST level of >150 IU/mL should be treated with IV ribavirin. This antiviral nucleoside analogue appears to be effective in reducing mortality rates from the levels documented among retrospective controls, and its only major side effect is reversible anemia that usually does not require transfusion. The drug should be given by slow IV infusion in a dose of 32 mg/kg; this dose should be followed by 16 mg/kg every 6 h for 4 days and then by 8 mg/kg every 8 h for 6 days.

SOUTH AMERICAN HF SYNDROMES (ARGENTINE, BOLIVIAN, VENEZUELAN, AND BRAZILIAN)

These diseases are similar to one another clinically, but their epidemiology differs with the habits of their rodent reservoirs and the interactions of these animals with humans. Person-to-person or nosocomial transmission is rare but has occurred.

The basic disease resembles Lassa fever, with two marked differences. First, thrombocytopenia—often marked—is the rule, and bleeding is quite common. Second, CNS dysfunction is much more common than in Lassa fever and is often manifested by marked confusion, tremors of the upper extremities and tongue, and cerebellar signs. Some cases follow a predominantly neurologic course, with a poor prognosis. The clinical laboratory is helpful in diagnosis since thrombocytopenia, leukopenia, and proteinuria are typical findings.

Argentine HF is readily treated with convalescent-phase plasma given within the first 8 days of illness. In the absence of passive antibody therapy, IV ribavirin in the dose recommended for Lassa fever is likely to be effective in all the South American HF syndromes. The transmission of the disease from men convalescing from Argentine HF to their wives suggests the need for counseling of arenavirus HF patients concerning the avoidance of intimate contacts for several weeks after recovery. A safe, effective, live attenuated vaccine exists for Argentine HF. In experimental animals, this vaccine is cross-protective against the Bolivian HF virus.

RIFT VALLEY FEVER

The mosquito-borne Rift Valley fever virus is also a pathogen of domestic animals such as sheep, cattle, and goats. It is maintained in nature by transovarial transmission in floodwater *Aedes* mosquitoes and presumably also has a vertebrate amplifier. Epizootics and epidemics occur when sheep or cattle become infected during particularly heavy rains; developing high-level viremia, these animals infect many species of mosquitoes. Remote sensing via satellite can detect the ecologic changes associated with high rainfall that predict the likelihood of Rift Valley fever transmission; it can also detect the special depressions from which the floodwater *Aedes* mosquito vectors emerge. In addition, the virus is infectious when transmitted by contact with blood or aerosols from domestic animals or their abortuses. The slaughtered meat is not infectious; anaerobic glycolysis in postmortem tissues results in an acidic environment that rapidly inactivates Bunyaviridae such as Rift Valley fever virus and Crimean-Congo HF virus. The natural range of Rift Valley fever virus is confined to sub-Saharan Africa, where its circulation is markedly enhanced by substantial rainfall such as that which occurred during the El Niño phenomenon of 1997; subsequent spread to the Arabian Peninsula caused epidemic disease in 2000. The virus has also been found in Madagascar and has been introduced into Egypt, where it caused major epidemics in 1977–1979, 1993, and subsequently. Neither person-to-person nor nosocomial transmission has been documented.

Rift Valley fever virus is unusual in that it causes several clinical syndromes. Most infections are manifested as the febrile-myalgic syndrome. A small proportion of infections result in HF with especially prominent liver involvement. Renal failure and DIC are also common features. Perhaps 10% of otherwise mild infections lead to retinal vasculitis; funduscopic examination reveals edema, hemorrhages, and infarction, and some patients have permanently impaired vision. A small proportion of cases (<1 in 200) are followed by typical viral encephalitis. One of the complicated syndromes does not appear to predispose to another.

There is no proven therapy for any of the syndromes described above. Both retinal disease and encephalitis occur after the acute febrile syndrome has ended and serum neutralizing antibody has developed—events suggesting that only supportive care need be given. Epidemic disease is best prevented by vaccination of livestock. The established ability of this virus to propagate after an introduction into Egypt suggests that other potentially receptive areas, including the United States, should have a response ready for such an eventuality. It seems likely that this disease, like Venezuelan equine encephalitis, can be controlled only with adequate stocks of an effective live attenuated vaccine, and there are no such global stocks. A formalin-inactivated vaccine confers immunity to humans, but quantities are limited and three injections are required; this vaccine is recommended for exposed laboratory workers and for veterinarians working in sub-Saharan Africa.

CRIMEAN-CONGO HF

This severe HF syndrome has a wide geographic distribution, potentially being found wherever ticks of the genus *Hyalomma* occur. The propensity of these ticks to feed on domestic livestock and certain wild mammals means that veterinary serosurveys are the most effective mechanism for the surveillance of virus circulation in a region. Human infection is acquired via a tick bite or during the crushing of infected ticks. Domestic animals do not become ill but do develop viremia; thus there is danger of infection at the time of slaughter and for a brief interval thereafter (through contact with hides or carcasses). Cases have followed sheep shearing. An epidemic in South Africa was associated with slaughter of tick-infested ostriches. Nosocomial epidemics are common and are usually related to extensive blood exposure or needle sticks.

Although generally similar to other HF syndromes, Crimean-Congo HF causes extensive liver damage, resulting in jaundice in some cases. Clinical laboratory values indicate DIC and show elevations in AST, creatine phosphokinase, and bilirubin. Patients with fatal cases generally have more marked changes, even in the early days of illness, and also develop leukocytosis rather than leukopenia. In addition, thrombocytopenia is more marked and develops earlier in cases with a fatal outcome.

No controlled trials have been performed with IV ribavirin, but clinical experience and retrospective comparison of patients with ominous clinical laboratory values suggest that ribavirin is efficacious and should be given. No human or veterinary vaccines are recommended.

HF WITH RENAL SYNDROME

This disease, the first to be identified as an HF, is widely distributed over Europe and Asia; the major causative viruses and their rodent reservoirs on these two continents are Puumala virus (bank vole, *Clethrionomys glareolus*) and Hantaan virus (striped field mouse, *Apodemus agrarius*), respectively. Other potential causative viruses exist, including Dobrava virus (yellow-necked field mouse, *A. flavicollis*), which causes severe HF with renal syndrome in the Balkans. Seoul virus is associated with the Norway or sewer rat, *Rattus norvegicus*, and has a worldwide distribution through the migration of the rodent; it is associated with mild or moderate HF with renal syndrome in Asia, but in many areas of the world the human disease has been difficult to identify. Most cases occur in rural residents or vacationers; the exception is Seoul virus disease, which may be acquired in an urban or rural setting or from contaminated laboratory rat colonies. Classic Hantaan disease in Korea (Korean HF) and in rural China (epidemic HF) is most common in spring and fall and is related to rodent density and agricultural practices. Human infection is acquired primarily through aerosols of rodent urine, although virus is also present in saliva and feces. Patients with hantavirus diseases are not infectious. HF with renal syndrome is the most important form of HF today, with >100,000 cases of severe disease in Asia annually and milder Puumala infections numbering in the thousands as well.

Severe cases of HF with renal syndrome caused by Hantaan virus evolve in identifiable stages: the febrile stage with myalgia, lasting 3 or 4 days; the hypotensive stage, often associated with shock and lasting from a few hours to 48 h; the oliguric stage with renal failure, lasting 3–10 days; and the polyuric stage with diuresis and hyposthenuria.

The *febrile stage* is initiated by the abrupt onset of fever, headache, severe myalgia, thirst, anorexia, and often nausea and vomiting. Photophobia, retroorbital pain, and pain on ocular movement are common, and the vision may become blurred with ciliary body inflammation. Flushing over the face, the V area of the neck, and the back is characteristic, as are pharyngeal injection, periorbital edema, and conjunctival suffusion. Petechiae often develop in areas of pressure, the conjunctivae, and the axillae. Back pain and tenderness to percussion at the costovertebral angle reflect massive retroperitoneal edema. Laboratory evidence of mild to moderate DIC is present. Other laboratory findings include proteinuria and an active urinary sediment.

The *hypotensive stage* is ushered in by falling blood pressure and sometimes by shock. The relative bradycardia typical of the febrile phase is replaced by tachycardia. Kinin activation is marked. The rising hematocrit reflects increasing vascular leakage. Leukocytosis with a left shift develops, and thrombocytopenia continues. Atypical lymphocytes—which in fact are activated CD8+ (and, to a lesser extent, CD4+) T cells—circulate. Proteinuria is marked, and the urine's specific gravity falls to 1.010. The renal circulation is congested and compromised from local and systemic circulatory changes resulting in necrosis of tubules, particularly at the corticomedullary junction, and oliguria.

During the *oliguric stage*, hemorrhagic tendencies continue, probably in large part because of uremic bleeding defects. The oliguria persists for 3–10 days before the return of renal function marks the onset of the *polyuric stage*, which carries the danger of dehydration and electrolyte abnormalities.

Mild cases of HF with renal syndrome may be much less stereotypical. The presentation may include only fever, gastrointestinal abnormalities, and transient oliguria followed by hyposthenuria.

HF with renal syndrome should be suspected in patients with rural exposure in an endemic area. Prompt recognition of the disease permits rapid hospitalization and expectant management of shock and renal failure. Useful clinical laboratory parameters include leukocytosis, which may be leukemoid and is associated with a left shift; thrombocytopenia; and proteinuria. Mainstays of therapy are the management of shock, reliance on pressors, modest crystalloid infusion, IV use of human serum albumin, and treatment of renal failure with prompt dialysis for the usual indications. Hydration may result in pulmonary edema, and hypertension should be avoided because of the possibility of intracranial hemorrhage. Use of IV ribavirin has reduced mortality and morbidity in severe cases provided treatment is begun within the first 4 days of illness. The case-fatality ratio may be as high as 15% but with proper therapy should be <5%. Sequelae have not been definitively established, but there is a correlation in the United States between chronic hypertensive renal failure and the presence of antibodies to Seoul virus.

Infections with Puumala virus, the most common cause of HF with renal syndrome in Europe, result in a much attenuated picture but the same general presentation. The syndrome may be referred to by its former name, *nephropathia epidemica*. Bleeding manifestations are found in only 10% of cases, hypotension rather than shock is usually seen, and oliguria is present in only about half of patients. The dominant features may be fever, abdominal pain, proteinuria, mild oliguria, and sometimes blurred vision or glaucoma followed by polyuria and hyposthenuria in recovery. The mortality rate is <1%.

The diagnosis is readily made by IgM-capture ELISA, which should be positive at admission or within 24–48 h thereafter. The isolation of virus is difficult, but RT-PCR of a blood clot collected early in the clinical course or of tissues obtained postmortem will give positive results. Such testing is usually undertaken only if definitive identification of the infecting viral species is required or if molecular epidemiologic questions exist.

HANTAVIRUS PULMONARY SYNDROME

Hantavirus pulmonary syndrome was discovered in 1993, but retrospective identification of cases by immunohistochemistry (1978) and serology (1959) support the idea that it is a newly discovered disease rather than a truly new disease. The causative agents are hantaviruses of a distinct phylogenetic lineage that is associated with the rodent subfamily Sigmodontinae. Sin Nombre virus, which chronically infects the deer mouse (*Peromyscus maniculatus*), is the most important agent of hantavirus pulmonary syndrome in the United States. The disease is also caused by a Sin Nombre virus variant from the white-footed mouse (*P. leucopus*), by Black Creek Canal virus (*Sigmodon hispidus*, the cotton rat), and by Bayou virus (*Oryzomys palustris*, the rice rat). Several other related viruses cause the disease in South America, but Andes virus is unusual in that it, alone among hantaviruses, has been implicated in human-to-human transmission. The disease is linked to rodent exposure and particularly affects rural residents living in dwellings permeable to rodent entry or working at occupations that pose a risk of rodent exposure. Each rodent species has its own particular habits; in the case of the deer mouse, these behaviors include living in and around human habitation.

The disease begins with a prodrome of ~3–4 days (range, 1–11 days) comprising fever, myalgia, malaise, and often gastrointestinal disturbances such as nausea, vomiting, and abdominal pain. Dizziness is common and vertigo occasional. Severe prodromal symptoms bring some individuals to medical attention, but patients are usually recognized as the cardiopulmonary phase begins. Typically, there is slightly lowered blood pressure, tachycardia, tachypnea, mild hypoxemia, and early radiographic signs of pulmonary edema. Physical findings in the chest are often surprisingly scant. The conjunctival and cutaneous signs of vascular involvement seen in other types of HF are absent. During the next few hours, decompensation may progress rapidly to severe hypoxemia and respiratory failure. Most patients surviving the first 48 h of hospitalization are extubated and discharged within a few days, with no apparent residua.

Management during the first few hours after presentation is critical. The goal is to prevent severe hypoxemia by oxygen therapy, with intubation and intensive respiratory management if needed. During this period, hypotension and shock with increasing hematocrit invite aggressive fluid administration, but this intervention should be undertaken with great caution. Because of low cardiac output with myocardial depression and increased pulmonary vascular permeability, shock should be managed expectantly with pressors and modest infusion of fluid guided by the pulmonary capillary wedge pressure. Mild cases can be managed by frequent monitoring and oxygen administration without intubation. Many patients require intubation to manage hypoxemia and also develop shock. Mortality rates remain at ~30–40% even with good management. The antiviral drug ribavirin inhibits the virus in vitro but did not have a marked effect on patients treated in an open-label study.

During the prodrome, the differential diagnosis of hantavirus pulmonary syndrome is difficult, but by the time of presentation or within 24 h thereafter, a number of diagnostically helpful clinical features become apparent. Cough is not usually present at the outset but may develop later. Interstitial edema is evident on the chest x-ray. Later, bilateral alveolar edema with a central distribution develops in the setting of a normal-sized heart; occasionally, the edema is initially unilateral. Pleural effusions are often seen. Thrombocytopenia, circulating atypical lymphocytes, and a left shift (often with leukocytosis) are almost always evident; thrombocytopenia is a particularly important early clue. Hemoconcentration, proteinuria, and hypoalbuminemia should also be sought. Although thrombocytopenia virtually always develops and prolongation of the partial thromboplastin time is the rule, clinical evidence for coagulopathy or laboratory indications of DIC are found in only a minority of cases, usually in severely ill patients. Patients with severe illness also have acidosis and elevated serum levels of lactate. Mildly increased values in renal function tests are common, but patients with severe cases often have markedly elevated concentrations of serum creatinine; some of the viruses other than Sin Nombre virus have been associated with more kidney involvement, but few such cases have been studied. The differential diagnosis includes abdominal surgical conditions and pyelonephritis as well as rickettsial disease, sepsis, meningococcemia, plague, tularemia, influenza, and relapsing fever.

A specific diagnosis is best made by IgM testing of acute-phase serum, which has yielded positive results even in the prodrome. Tests using a Sin Nombre virus antigen detect the related hantaviruses causing the pulmonary syndrome in the Americas. Occasionally, heterologous viruses will react only in the IgG ELISA, but this finding is highly suspicious given the very low seroprevalence of these viruses in normal populations. RT-PCR is usually positive when used to test blood clots obtained in the first 7–9 days of illness as well as tissues; this test is useful in identifying the infecting virus in areas outside the home range of the deer mouse and in atypical cases.

YELLOW FEVER

Yellow fever virus caused major epidemics in the Americas, Africa, and Europe before the discovery of mosquito transmission in 1900 led to its control through attacks on its urban vector, *A. aegypti*. Only then was it found that a jungle cycle also existed in Africa, involving other *Aedes* mosquitoes and monkeys, and that colonization of the New World with *A. aegypti*, originally an African species, had established urban yellow fever as well as an independent sylvatic yellow fever cycle involving *Haemagogus* mosquitoes and New World monkeys in American jungles. Today, urban yellow fever transmission occurs only in some African cities, but the threat exists in the great cities of South America, where reinfestation by *A. aegypti* has taken place and dengue transmission by the same mosquito is common. As late as 1905, New Orleans suffered >3000 cases with 452 deaths from "yellow jack." Despite the existence of a highly effective and safe vaccine, several hundred jungle yellow fever cases occur annually in South America, and thousands of jungle and urban cases occur each year in Africa.

Yellow fever is a typical HF accompanied by prominent hepatic necrosis. A period of viremia, typically lasting 3 or 4 days, is followed by a period of "intoxication." During the latter phase in severe cases, the characteristic jaundice, hemorrhages, black vomit, anuria, and terminal delirium occur, perhaps related in part to extensive hepatic involvement. Blood leukocyte counts may be normal or reduced and are often high in terminal stages. Albuminuria is usually noted and may be marked; as renal function fails in terminal or severe cases, the level of blood urea nitrogen rises proportionately. Abnormalities detected in liver function tests range from modest elevations of AST levels in mild cases to severe derangement.

Urban yellow fever can be prevented by the control of *A. aegypti*. The continuing sylvatic cycle requires vaccination of all visitors to areas of potential transmission. With few exceptions, reactions to vaccine are minimal; immunity is provided within 10 days and lasts for at least 10 years. An egg allergy dictates caution in vaccine administration. Although there are no documented harmful effects of the vaccine on the fetus, pregnant women should be immunized only if they are definitely at risk of yellow fever exposure. Since vaccination has been associated with several cases of encephalitis in children <6 months of age, it should be delayed until after 12 months of age unless the risk of exposure is very high. Rare, serious, multisystemic adverse reactions (occasionally fatal) have been reported, particularly affecting the elderly; nevertheless, the number of deaths of unvaccinated travelers with yellow fever exceeds the number of deaths from vaccination, and a liberal vaccination policy for travelers to involved areas should be pursued. Timely information on changes in yellow fever distribution and yellow fever vaccine requirements can be obtained from Health Information for Travelers, Centers for Disease Control and Prevention, Atlanta, GA 30333; by fax request (404-332-4565; document number 220022); by phone (404-332-4559); or via the Internet (*www.cdc.gov*).

DENGUE HEMORRHAGIC FEVER/DENGUE SHOCK SYNDROME

A syndrome of HF noted in the 1950s among children in the Philippines and Southeast Asia was soon associated with dengue virus infections, particularly those occurring against a background of previous exposure to another dengue-virus serotype. The transient heterotypic protection after dengue virus infection is replaced within several weeks by the potential for heterotypic infection resulting in typical dengue fever (see above) or—uncommonly—in enhanced disease (secondary DHF/DSS). In rare instances, primary dengue infections lead to an HF syndrome, but much less is known about pathogenesis in this situation. In the past 20 years, *A. aegypti* has progressively reinvaded Latin America and other areas, and frequent travel by infected individuals has introduced multiple strains of dengue virus from many geographic areas. Thus the pattern of hyperendemic transmission of multiple dengue serotypes has now been established in the Americas and the Caribbean and has led to the emergence of DHF/DSS as a major problem there as well. Millions of dengue infections, including many thousands of cases of DHF/DSS, occur annually. The severe syndrome is unlikely to be seen in U.S. citizens since few children have the dengue antibodies that can trigger the pathogenetic cascade when a second infection is acquired.

Macrophage/monocyte infection is central to the pathogenesis of dengue fever and to the origin of DHF/DSS. Previous infection with a heterologous dengue-virus serotype may result in the production of nonprotective antiviral antibodies that nevertheless bind to the virion's surface and through interaction with the Fc receptor focus secondary dengue viruses on the target cell, the result being enhanced infection. The host is also primed for a secondary antibody response when viral antigens are released and immune complexes lead to activation of the classic complement pathway, with consequent phlogistic effects. Cross-reactivity at the T-cell level results in the release of physiologically active cytokines, including interferon γ and tumor necrosis factor α. The induction of vascular permeability and shock depends on multiple factors, including the following:

1. *Presence of enhancing and nonneutralizing antibodies*—Transplacental maternal antibody may be present in infants <9 months old, or antibody elicited by previous heterologous dengue infection may be present in older individuals. T-cell reactivity is also intimately involved.
2. *Age*—Susceptibility to DHF/DSS drops considerably after 12 years of age.
3. *Sex*—Females are more often affected than males.
4. *Race*—Caucasians are more often affected than blacks.
5. *Nutritional status*—Malnutrition is protective.
6. *Sequence of infection*—For example, serotype 1 followed by serotype 2 seems to be more dangerous than serotype 4 followed by serotype 2.
7. *Infecting serotype*—Type 2 is apparently more dangerous than other serotypes.

In addition, there is considerable variation among strains of a given serotype, with Southeast Asian serotype 2 strains having more potential to cause DHF/DSS than others.

Dengue HF is identified by the detection of bleeding tendencies (tourniquet test, petechiae) or overt bleeding in the absence of underlying causes such as preexisting gastrointestinal lesions. Dengue shock syndrome, usually accompanied by hemorrhagic signs, is much more serious and results from increased vascular permeability leading to shock. In mild DHF/DSS, restlessness, lethargy, thrombocytopenia (<100,000/μL), and hemoconcentration are detected 2–5 days after the onset of typical dengue fever, usually at the time of defervescence. The maculopapular rash that often develops in dengue fever may also appear in DHF/DSS. In more severe cases, frank shock is apparent, with low pulse pressure, cyanosis, hepatomegaly, pleural effusions, ascites, and in some cases severe ecchymoses and gastrointestinal bleeding. The period of shock lasts only 1 or 2 days, and most patients respond promptly to close monitoring, oxygen administration, and infusion of crystalloid or—in severe cases—colloid. The case-fatality rates reported vary greatly with case ascertainment and the quality of treatment; however, most DHF/DSS patients respond well to supportive therapy, and the overall mortality rate at an experienced center in the tropics is probably as low as 1%.

A virologic diagnosis can be made by the usual means, although multiple flavivirus infections lead to a broad immune response to several members of the group, and this situation may result in a lack of virus specificity of the IgM and IgG immune responses. A secondary antibody response can be sought with tests against several flavivirus antigens to demonstrate the characteristic wide spectrum of reactivity.

The key to control of both dengue fever and DHF/DSS is the control of *A. aegypti*, which also reduces the risk of urban yellow fever and chikungunya virus circulation. Control efforts have been handicapped by the presence of nondegradable tires and long-lived plastic containers in trash repositories, insecticide resistance, urban poverty, and an inability of the public health community to mobilize the populace to respond to the need to eliminate mosquito breeding sites. Live attenuated dengue vaccines are in the late stages of development and have produced promising results in early tests. Whether vaccines can provide safe, durable immunity to an immunopathologic disease such as DHF/DSS in endemic areas is an issue that will have to be tested, but it is hoped that vaccination will reduce transmission to negligible levels.

KYASANUR FOREST DISEASE AND OMSK HEMORRHAGIC FEVER

Kyasanur Forest virus and Omsk HF virus are geographically restricted, tick-borne flaviviruses that cause a syndrome of viral HF during a wave of viremia and that may also enter the CNS to cause subsequent viral encephalitis (see discussion of tick-borne encephalitis earlier in the chapter). There is no therapy for these infections, but an inactivated vaccine has been used in India against Kyasanur Forest disease. A new and related virus isolate has been obtained from butchers with HF in the Middle East; the implication is that there are more agents in this group.

FILOVIRUS HEMORRHAGIC FEVER

See Chap. 100.

FURTHER READINGS

Bruno P et al: The protean manifestations of hemorrhagic fever with renal syndrome. A retrospective review of 26 cases from Korea. Ann Intern Med 113:385, 1990

Calisher CH: Medically important arboviruses of the United States and Canada. Clin Microbiol Rev 7:89, 1994

Centers for Disease Control and Prevention: Update: Management of patients with suspected viral hemorrhagic fever—United States. MMWR 44:475, 1995 (*http://www.cdc.gov/mmwr/preview/mmwrhtml/00038033.htm*)

———: Chikungunya fever diagnosed among international travelers—United States, 2005-2006. MMWR Morb Mortal Wkly Rep 55:1040, 2006

Deresiewicz RL et al: Clinical and neuroradiographic manifestations of eastern equine encephalitis. N Engl J Med 336:1867, 1997

Enria D et al: Arenaviruses, in *Tropical Infectious Diseases: Principles, Pathogens, & Practice*, RL Guerrant et al (eds). New York, Saunders, 1999, pp 1189–1212

Mourya DT, Mishra AC: Chikungunya fever. Lancet 368:186, 2006

Peters CJ, Khan AS: Hantavirus pulmonary syndrome: The new American hemorrhagic fever. Clin Infect Dis 34:1224, 2002

Rivas F et al: Epidemic Venezuelan equine encephalitis in La Guajira, Colombia, 1995. J Infect Dis 175:828, 1997

Solomon SR, Vaughn DW: Pathogenesis and clinical features of Japanese encephalitis and West Nile virus infections. Curr Top Microbiol Immunol 267:171, 2002

Solomon T et al: West Nile encephalitis. BMJ 326:865, 2003

Wurtz R, Paleologos N: La Crosse encephalitis presenting like herpes simplex encephalitis in an immunocompromised adult. Clin Infect Dis 31:1113, 2000

CHAPTER 100

EBOLA AND MARBURG VIRUSES

Clarence J. Peters

DEFINITION

Both Marburg virus and Ebola virus cause an acute febrile illness associated with high mortality. This illness is characterized by multisystem involvement that begins with the abrupt onset of headache, myalgias, and fever and proceeds to prostration, rash, and shock and often to bleeding manifestations. Epidemics usually begin with a single case acquired from an unknown reservoir in nature and spread mainly through close contact with sick persons or their body fluids, either at home or in the hospital.

ETIOLOGY

The family Filoviridae (Fig. 100-1) comprises two antigenically and genetically distinct genera: *Marburgvirus* and *Ebolavirus*. *Ebolavirus* has four readily distinguishable species named for their original sites of recognition: Zaire, Sudan, Côte d'Ivoire, and Reston. Except for the Reston virus, all the Filoviridae are African viruses that cause severe and often fatal disease in humans. The Reston virus, which has been exported from the Philippines on several occasions, has caused fatal infections in monkeys but only subclinical infections in humans. Different strains of the four Ebola species, isolated over time and space, exhibit remarkable sequence conservation, indicating marked genetic stability in their selective niche.

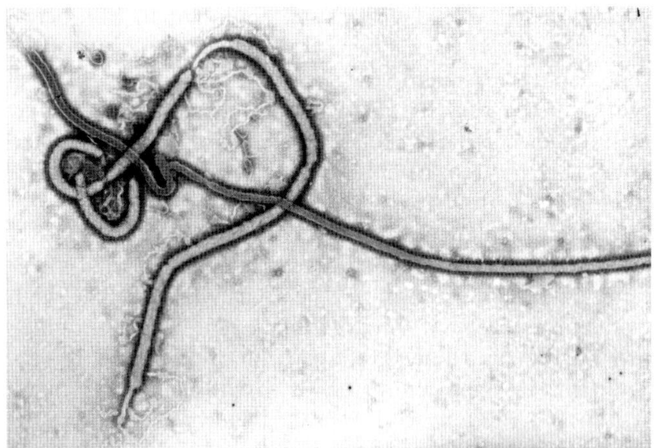

FIGURE 100-1

Ebola virions: diagnostic specimen from the first passage in Vero cells of a blood sample from a patient. Some of the filamentous (negatively stained) virions were fused together, end-to-end, giving the appearance of a "bowl of spaghetti." This image was from the first isolation and visualization of Ebola virus in 1970. *(Courtesy of Fredrick A. Murphy, MD, University of Texas Medical Branch, Galveston, Texas; with permission.)*

Typical filovirus particles contain a single linear, negative-sense, single-stranded RNA arranged in a helical nucleocapsid. The virions are 790–970 nm in length; they may also appear in elongated, contorted forms. The lipid envelope confers sensitivity to lipid solvents and common detergents. The viruses are largely destroyed by heat (60°C, 30 min) and by acidity but may persist for weeks in blood at room temperature. The surface glycoprotein self-associates to form the virion surface spikes, which presumably mediate attachment to cells and fusion. The glycoprotein's high sugar content may contribute to its low capacity to elicit neutralizing antibodies. A smaller form of the glycoprotein, bearing many of its antigenic determinants, is produced by in vitro–infected cells and is found in the circulation in human disease; it has been speculated that this circulating soluble protein may suppress the immune response to the virion surface protein or block antiviral effector mechanisms. Both Marburg virus and Ebola virus are biosafety level 4 pathogens because of their high associated mortality rate and aerosol infectivity.

EPIDEMIOLOGY

Marburg virus was first identified in Germany in 1967, when infected African green monkeys (*Cercopithecus aethiops*) imported from Uganda transmitted the agent to workers in a vaccine laboratory. Of the 25 human cases acquired from monkeys, seven ended in death. The six secondary cases were associated with close contact or parenteral exposure. Secondary spread to the wife of one patient was documented, and virus was isolated from the husband's semen despite the presence of circulating antibodies. Subsequently, isolated cases of Marburg virus infection have been reported from eastern and southern Africa, with limited spread.

In 1999, repeated transmission of Marburg virus to workers in a gold mine in eastern Democratic Republic of the Congo was documented. The secondary spread of the virus among patients' families was more extensive than previously noted, resembling that of Ebola virus and emphasizing the importance of hygiene and proper barrier nursing in the epidemiology of these viruses in Africa.

In 2004–2005, an alarming, massive Marburg virus epidemic, with >250 cases, occurred in Angola. The epidemiologic features resembled those of the Ebola virus epidemics described below, and the case-fatality rate was 90%. This high figure may have been due in part to poor conditions in African hospitals; however, the virus isolated in this epidemic was slightly different phylogenetically from other known strains and exhibited increased virulence in nonhuman primates.

In 1976, epidemics of severe hemorrhagic fever (550 human cases) occurred simultaneously in Zaire and Sudan, and Ebola virus was found to be the etiologic agent. Later, it was shown that different species of virus (with associated mortality rates of 90% and 50%, respectively) had caused the two epidemics. Both epidemics were associated with interhuman spread (particularly in the hospital setting) and the use of unsterilized needles and syringes—a common practice in developing-country hospitals. The epidemics dwindled as the clinics were closed and as people in the endemic area increasingly shunned affected persons and avoided traditional burial practices.

The Zaire Ebola virus recurred in a major epidemic (317 cases, 88% mortality rate) in the Democratic Republic of the Congo in 1995 and in smaller epidemics in Gabon in 1994–1996. Mortality rates were high, transmission to caregivers and others who had direct contact with body fluids was common, and poor hygiene in hospitals exacerbated spread. In the Congo epidemic, an index case was infected in Kikwit in January 1995. The epidemic smoldered until April, when intense nosocomial transmission forced closure of the hospitals; samples were finally sent to the laboratory for Ebola testing, which yielded positive results within a few hours. International assistance, with barrier nursing instruction and materials, was provided; nosocomial transmission ceased, hospitals reopened, and patients were segregated to prevent intrafamilial spread. The last case was reported in June 1995.

Separate emergences of Ebola virus (Zaire) were detected in Gabon in 1994–2003, usually in association with deep-forest exposure and subsequent familial and nosocomial transmission. Die-offs of nonhuman primates were sometimes documented, and Ebola infection was confirmed in at least some animals. In a 1996 episode, a physician exposed to Ebola-infected patients traveled to South Africa with a fever; a nurse who assisted in a cutdown on the physician developed Ebola hemorrhagic fever and died despite intensive care. The index patient was identified retrospectively on the basis of serum antibodies and virus isolation from semen. No additional cases were detected from care of the primary or secondary case, nor were there any secondary cases following care of an unsuspected Côte d'Ivoire Ebola case in Switzerland. Thus, distant transport of Ebola virus is an established risk, but limited nosocomial spread occurs under proper hygienic conditions.

In 2000–2001, an indolent outbreak of Sudan Ebola virus claimed the lives of 224 (53%) of 425 patients with presumptive cases in Uganda.

Reston Ebola virus was first seen in the United States in 1989, when it caused a fatal, highly transmissible disease among cynomolgus macaques imported from the Philippines and quarantined in Reston, Virginia, pending distribution to biomedical researchers. This and other appearances of the Reston virus have been traced to a single export facility in the Philippines, but no source in nature has been established.

Epidemiologic studies (including a specific search in the Kikwit epidemic) have failed to yield evidence for an important role of airborne particles in human disease. This lack of epidemiologic evidence is surprising and seems to conflict with the viruses' classification as biosafety level 4 pathogens (which is based in part on their aerosol infectivity) and with formal laboratory assessments showing a high degree of aerosol infectivity for monkeys. Sick humans apparently do not usually generate sufficient amounts of infectious aerosols to pose a significant hazard to those around them.

Although numerous die-offs have recently been reported among chimpanzees and gorillas (some even threatening the viability of these endangered species), these animals (like humans) appear to be sentinels for virus activity. Speculation about the true reservoirs has centered on bats, and preliminary evidence indicates that bats may indeed be the reservoirs of filoviruses. This evidence includes the detection of antibodies and reverse-transcriptase polymerase chain reaction (RT-PCR) products in bats, the epidemiologic findings in subterranean gold mines in Durba (Democratic Republic of the Congo) where Marburg transmission has occurred, and reported associations of human antibody production with the handling of bats.

PATHOLOGY AND PATHOGENESIS

In humans and in animal models, Ebola and Marburg viruses replicate well in virtually all cell types, including endothelial cells, macrophages, and parenchymal cells of multiple organs. The earliest involvement—that of the mononuclear phagocyte system—is responsible for initiation of the disease process. Viral replication is associated with cellular necrosis both in vivo and in vitro. Significant findings at the light-microscopic level include liver necrosis with Councilman bodies, intracellular inclusions that correlate with extensive collections of viral nucleocapsids, interstitial pneumonitis, cerebral glial nodules, and small infarcts. Antigen and virions are abundant in fibroblasts, interstitium, and (to a lesser extent) the appendages of the subcutaneous tissues in fatal cases; escape through small breaks in the skin or possibly through sweat glands may occur and, if so, may be correlated with the established epidemiologic risk of close contact with patients and the touching of the deceased. Inflammatory cells are not prominent, even in necrotic areas.

In addition to sustaining direct damage from viral infection, patients infected with Ebola virus (Zaire) have high circulating levels of proinflammatory cytokines, which presumably contribute to the severity of the illness. In fact, the virus interacts intimately with the cellular cytokine system. It is resistant to the antiviral effects of interferon α, although this mediator is amply induced. Viral infection of endothelial cells selectively inhibits the expression of major histocompatibility complex class I molecules and blocks the induction of several genes by the interferons. In addition, glycoprotein expression inhibits αV integrin expression, an effect that has been shown to lead to detachment and subsequent death of endothelial cells in vitro.

Acute infection is associated with high levels of circulating virus and viral antigen. Clinical improvement takes place when viral titers decrease concomitantly with the onset of a virus-specific immune response, as detected by enzyme-linked immunosorbent assay (ELISA) or fluorescent antibody testing. In fatal cases, there is usually little evidence of an antibody response, and there is extensive depletion of spleen and lymph nodes. Recovery is apparently mediated by the cellular immune response: convalescent-phase plasma has little in vitro virus-neutralizing capacity and is not protective in passive transfer experiments in monkey and guinea pig models.

CLINICAL MANIFESTATIONS

After an incubation period of ~7–10 days (range, 3–16 days), the patient abruptly develops fever, severe headache, malaise, myalgia, nausea, and vomiting. Continued fever is joined by diarrhea (often severe), chest pain (accompanied by cough), prostration, and depressed mentation. In light-skinned patients (and less often in dark-skinned individuals), a maculopapular rash appears around day 5–7 and is followed by desquamation. Bleeding may begin about this time and is apparent from any mucosal site and into the skin. In some epidemics, fewer than half of patients have had overt bleeding, and this manifestation has been absent even in some fatal cases. Additional findings include edema of the face, neck, and/or scrotum; hepatomegaly; flushing; conjunctival injection; and pharyngitis. Around 10–12 days after the onset of disease, the sustained fever may break, with improvement and eventual recovery of the patient. Recrudescence of fever may be associated with secondary bacterial infections or possibly with localized virus persistence. Late hepatitis, uveitis, and orchitis have been reported, with isolation of virus from semen or detection of PCR products in vaginal secretions for several weeks.

LABORATORY FINDINGS

Leukopenia is common early on; neutrophilia has its onset later. Platelet counts fall below (sometimes much below) 50,000/μL. Laboratory evidence of disseminated intravascular coagulation is found, but its clinical significance and the need for therapy are controversial. Serum levels of alanine and aspartate aminotransferases (particularly the latter) rise progressively, and jaundice develops in some cases. The serum amylase level may be elevated, and this elevation may be associated with abdominal pain, suggesting pancreatitis. Proteinuria is usual; decreased kidney function is proportional to shock.

DIAGNOSIS

Most patients acutely ill as a result of infection with Ebola or Marburg virus have high concentrations of virus in blood. Antigen-detection ELISA is a sensitive, robust diagnostic modality. Virus isolation and RT-PCR are also effective and provide additional sensitivity in some cases. Patients who are recovering develop IgM and IgG antibodies that are best detected by ELISA but are also reactive in the less specific fluorescent antibody test. Skin biopsies are an extremely useful adjunct in postmortem diagnosis of infection with Ebola virus (and, to a lesser extent, Marburg virus) because of the presence of large amounts of viral antigen, the relatively low risk posed by sample collection, and the lack of cold-chain requirements for formalin-fixed tissues.

℞ Treatment: EBOLA AND MARBURG VIRUS INFECTIONS

No virus-specific therapy is available, and—given the extensive viral involvement in fatal cases—supportive treatment may not be as useful as was once hoped. However, recent studies in rhesus monkeys have shown improved survival among animals treated with an inhibitor of factor VIIa/tissue factor or with activated protein C. Vigorous treatment of shock should take into account the likelihood of vascular leak in the pulmonary and systemic circulation and of myocardial functional compromise. The membrane fusion mechanism of Ebola virus resembles that of retroviruses, and the identification of "fusogenic" sequences suggests that inhibitors of cell entry may be developed. Despite the poor neutralizing capacity of polyclonal convalescent-phase sera, phage display of immunoglobulin mRNA from convalescent-phase bone marrow has yielded monoclonal antibodies that have in vitro neutralizing capacity and mediate protection in guinea pig models (but, unfortunately, not in monkey models).

PREVENTION

No vaccine or antiviral drug is currently available, but barrier nursing precautions in African hospitals can greatly decrease the spread of the virus beyond the index case and thus prevent epidemics of infection with filoviruses and with other agents as well. An adenovirus-vectored Ebola glycoprotein gene has proved protective in nonhuman primates and is undergoing phase 1 trials in humans.

FURTHER READINGS

Bray M, Murphy FA: Filovirus research: knowledge expands to meet a growing threat. J Infect Dis 196(Suppl 2):S438, 2007

Feldmann H et al: Proceedings of an international symposium on filoviruses. J Infect Dis Suppl, 2007

Geisbert TW et al: Treatment of Ebola virus infection with a recombinant inhibitor of factor VIIa/tissue factor: A study in rhesus monkeys. Lancet 362:1953, 2003

Peters CJ, LeDuc JW: An introduction to Ebola: The virus and the disease. J Infect Dis 179(Suppl 1):ix, 1999 (Also available at *www.journals.uchicago.edu/JID/*)

Sanchez A et al: Analysis of human peripheral blood samples from fatal and nonfatal cases of Ebola (Sudan) hemorrhagic fever: Cellular responses, virus load, and nitric oxide levels. J Virol 78:10370, 2004

Sullivan NT: Accelerated vaccination for Ebola virus haemorrhagic fever in non-human primates. Nature 424:681, 2003

Towner JS et al: *Marburgvirus* genomics and association with a large hemorrhagic fever outbreak in Angola. J Virol 80:6497, 2006

Tuffs A: Experimental vaccine may have saved Hamburg scientist from Ebola fever. BMJ 338:b1223, 2009

SECTION VI

PRION DISEASES

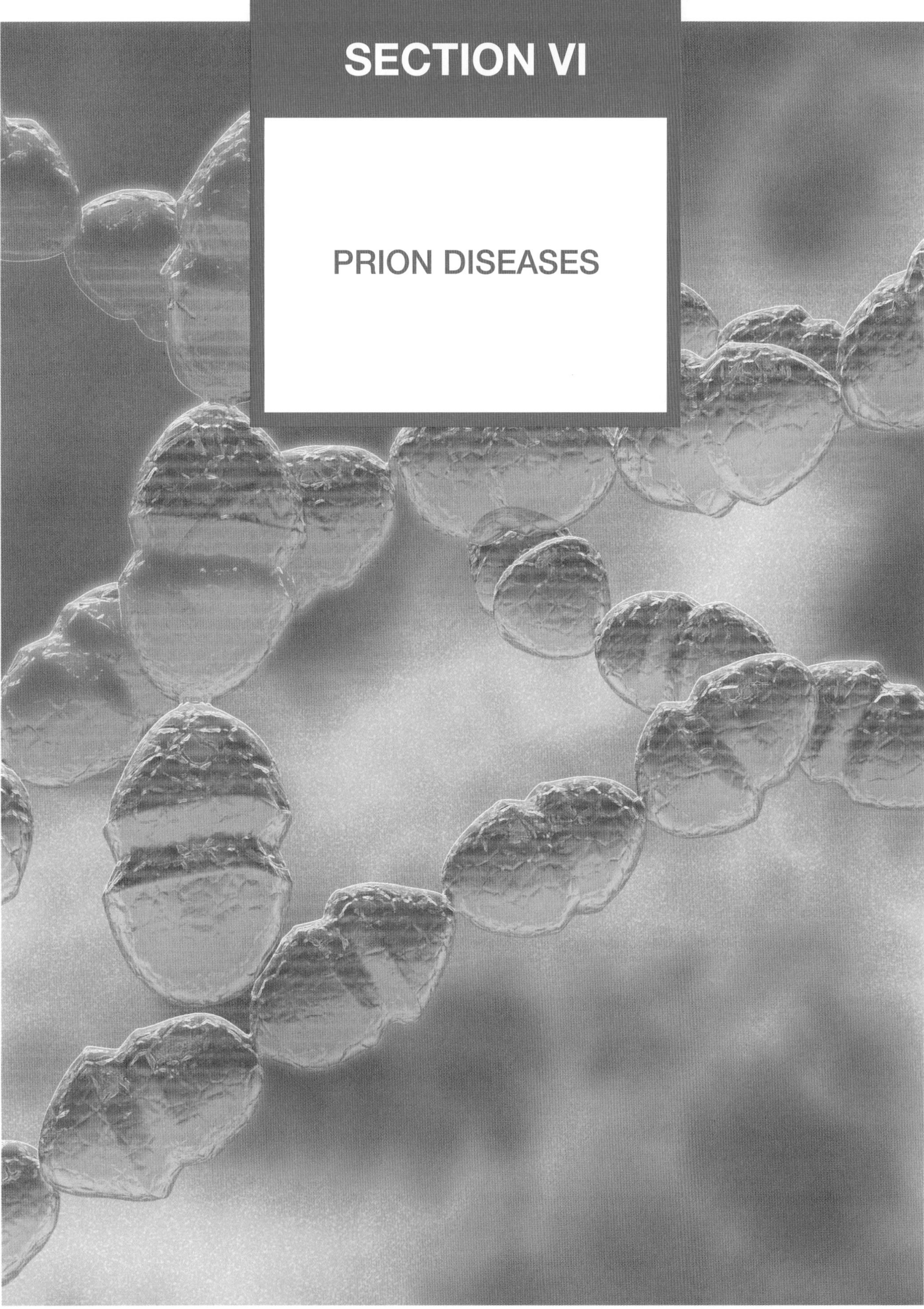

CHAPTER 101

PRION DISEASES

Stanley B. Prusiner ■ Bruce L. Miller

Prions are infectious proteins that cause degeneration of the central nervous system (CNS). Prion diseases are disorders of protein conformation, the most common of which in humans is called Creutzfeldt-Jakob disease (CJD). CJD typically presents with dementia and myoclonus, is relentlessly progressive, and generally causes death within a year of onset. Most CJD patients are between 50 and 75 years of age; however, patients as young as 17 and as old as 83 have been recorded.

In mammals, prions reproduce by binding to the normal, *c*ellular isoform of the *p*rion *p*rotein (PrP^C) and stimulating conversion of PrP^C into the di*s*ease-*c*ausing isoform (PrP^{Sc}). PrP^C is rich in α-helix and has little β-structure, while PrP^{Sc} has less α-helix and a high amount of β-structure (Fig. 101-1). This α-to-β structural transition in the prion protein (PrP) is the fundamental event underlying prion diseases (Table 101-1).

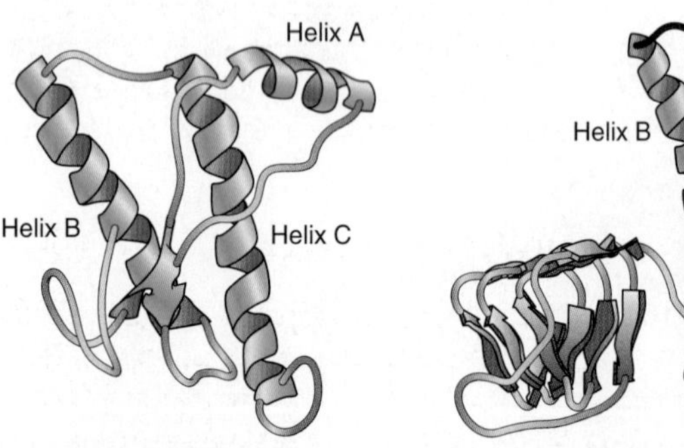

FIGURE 101-1

Structures of prion proteins. *A.* NMR structure of Syrian hamster recombinant (rec) PrP(90–231). Presumably, the structure of the α-helical form of recPrP(90–231) resembles that of PrP^C. recPrP(90–231) is viewed from the interface where PrP^{Sc} is thought to bind to PrP^C. Shown are: α-helices A (residues 144–157), B (172–193), and C (200–227). Flat ribbons depict β-strands S1 (129–131) and S2 (161–163). *(**A,** from SB Prusiner: N Engl J Med 344:1516, 2006; with permission.)* ***B.*** Structural model of PrP^{Sc}. The 90–160 region has been modeled onto a β-helical architecture while the COOH terminal helices B and C are preserved as in PrP^C. *(Image prepared by C. Govaerts.)*

Four new concepts have emerged from studies of prions: (1) Prions are the only known infectious pathogens that are devoid of nucleic acid; all other infectious agents possess genomes composed of either RNA or DNA that direct the synthesis of their progeny. (2) Prion diseases may be manifest as infectious, genetic, and sporadic disorders; no other group of illnesses with a single etiology presents with such a wide spectrum of clinical manifestations. (3) Prion diseases result from the accumulation of PrP^{Sc}, the conformation of which differs substantially from that of its precursor, PrP^C. (4) PrP^{Sc} can exist in a variety of different conformations, each of which seems to specify a particular disease phenotype. How a specific conformation of a PrP^{Sc} molecule is imparted to PrP^C during prion replication to produce nascent PrP^{Sc} with

TABLE 101-1

GLOSSARY OF PRION TERMINOLOGY	
Prion	*Pro*teinaceous *in*fectious particle that lacks nucleic acid. Prions are composed largely, if not entirely, of PrP^{Sc} molecules. They can cause scrapie in sheep and goats, and related neurodegenerative diseases of humans such as Creutzfeldt-Jakob disease (CJD).
PrP^{Sc}	Disease-causing isoform of the prion protein. This protein is the only identifiable macromolecule in purified preparations of scrapie prions.
PrP^C	Cellular isoform of the prion protein. PrP^C is the precursor of PrP^{Sc}.
PrP 27-30	A fragment of PrP^{Sc}, generated by truncation of the NH_2-terminus by limited digestion with proteinase K. PrP 27-30 retains prion infectivity and polymerizes into amyloid.
PRNP	PrP gene located on human chromosome 20.
Prion rod	An aggregate of prions composed largely of PrP 27-30 molecules. Created by detergent extraction and limited proteolysis of PrP^{Sc}. Morphologically and histochemically indistinguishable from many amyloids.
PrP amyloid	Amyloid containing PrP in the brains of animals or humans with prion disease; often accumulates as plaques.

TABLE 101-2

THE PRION DISEASES

DISEASE	HOST	MECHANISM OF PATHOGENESIS
Human		
Kuru	Fore people	Infection through ritualistic cannibalism
iCJD	Humans	Infection from prion-contaminated hGH, dura mater grafts, etc.
vCJD	Humans	Infection from bovine prions
fCJD	Humans	Germ-line mutations in *PRNP*
GSS	Humans	Germ-line mutations in *PRNP*
FFI	Humans	Germ-line mutation in *PRNP* (D178N, M129)
sCJD	Humans	Somatic mutation or spontaneous conversion of PrP^C into PrP^{Sc}?
sFI	Humans	Somatic mutation or spontaneous conversion of PrP^C into PrP^{Sc}?
Animal		
Scrapie	Sheep, goats	Infection in genetically susceptible sheep
BSE	Cattle	Infection with prion-contaminated MBM
TME	Mink	Infection with prions from sheep or cattle
CWD	Mule deer, elk	Unknown
FSE	Cats	Infection with prion-contaminated beef
Exotic ungulate encephalopathy	Greater kudu, nyala, or oryx	Infection with prion-contaminated MBM

Note: BSE, bovine spongiform encephalopathy; CJD, Creutzfeldt-Jakob disease; fCJD, familial Creutzfeldt-Jakob disease; iCJD, iatrogenic Creutzfeldt-Jakob disease; sCJD, sporadic Creutzfeldt-Jakob disease; vCJD, variant Creutzfeldt-Jakob disease; CWD, chronic wasting disease; FFI, fatal familial insomnia; sFI, sporadic fatal insomnia; FSE, feline spongiform encephalopathy; GSS, Gerstmann-Sträussler-Scheinker disease; hGH, human growth hormone; MBM, meat and bone meal; TME, transmissible mink encephalopathy.

the same conformation is unknown. Additionally, it is unclear what factors determine where in the CNS a particular PrP^{Sc} molecule will be deposited.

SPECTRUM OF PRION DISEASES

The sporadic form of CJD is the most common prion disorder in humans. Sporadic CJD (sCJD) accounts for ~85% of all cases of human prion disease, while inherited prion diseases account for 10–15% of all cases (Table 101-2). Familial CJD (fCJD), Gerstmann-Sträussler-Scheinker (GSS) disease, and fatal familial insomnia (FFI) are all dominantly inherited prion diseases that are caused by mutations in the PrP gene.

Although infectious prion diseases account for <1% of all cases and infection does not seem to play an important role in the natural history of these illnesses, the transmissibility of prions is an important biologic feature. *Kuru* of the Fore people of New Guinea is thought to have resulted from the consumption of brains from dead relatives during ritualistic cannibalism. With the cessation of ritualistic cannibalism in the late 1950s, kuru has nearly disappeared, with the exception of a few recent patients exhibiting incubation periods of >40 years. Iatrogenic CJD (iCJD) seems to be the result of the accidental inoculation of patients with prions. Variant CJD (vCJD) in teenagers and young adults in Europe is the result of exposure to tainted beef from cattle with bovine spongiform encephalopathy (BSE).

Six diseases of animals are caused by prions (Table 101-2). Scrapie of sheep and goats is the prototypic prion disease. Mink encephalopathy, BSE, feline spongiform encephalopathy, and exotic ungulate encephalopathy are all thought to occur after the consumption of prion-infected foodstuffs. The BSE epidemic emerged in Britain in the late 1980s and was shown to be due to industrial cannibalism. Whether BSE began as a sporadic case of BSE in a cow or started with scrapie in sheep is unknown. The origin of chronic wasting disease (CWD), a prion disease endemic in deer and elk in regions of North America, is uncertain.

EPIDEMIOLOGY

CJD is found throughout the world. The incidence of sCJD is approximately one case per million population, and thus it accounts for about one in every 10,000 deaths. Because sCJD is an age-dependent neurodegenerative disease, its incidence is expected to increase steadily as older segments of populations in developed and developing countries continue to expand. Although many geographic clusters of CJD have been reported, each has been shown to segregate with a PrP gene mutation. Attempts to identify common exposure to some etiologic agent have been unsuccessful for both the sporadic and familial cases. Ingestion of scrapie-infected sheep or goat meat as a cause of CJD in humans has not been demonstrated by epidemiologic studies, although speculation about this potential route of inoculation continues. Of particular interest are deer hunters who develop CJD, because up to 90% of culled deer in some game herds have been shown to harbor CWD prions. Whether prion disease in deer or elk can be passed to cows, sheep, or directly to humans remains unknown. Studies with Syrian hamsters demonstrate that oral infection with prions can occur, but the process is inefficient compared to intracerebral inoculation.

PATHOGENESIS

The human prion diseases were initially classified as neurodegenerative disorders of unknown etiology on the basis of pathologic changes being confined to the CNS. With the transmission of kuru and CJD to apes, investigators began to view these diseases as infectious CNS illnesses caused by slow viruses. Even though the familial nature of a subset of CJD cases was well described, the significance of this observation became more obscure with the transmission of CJD to animals. Eventually the meaning of heritable CJD became clear with the discovery of mutations in the PRNP gene of these patients. The prion concept explains how a disease can manifest as a heritable as well as an infectious illness. Moreover, the hallmark of all prion diseases, whether sporadic, dominantly inherited, or acquired by infection, is that they involve the aberrant metabolism of PrP.

A major feature that distinguishes prions from viruses is the finding that both PrP isoforms are encoded by a chromosomal gene. In humans, the PrP gene is designated *PRNP* and is located on the short arm of chromosome 20. Limited proteolysis of PrP^{Sc} produces a smaller, protease-resistant molecule of ~142 amino acids designated PrP 27-30; PrP^{C} is completely hydrolyzed under the same conditions (Fig. 101-2). In the presence of detergent, PrP 27-30 polymerizes into amyloid. Prion rods formed by limited proteolysis and detergent extraction are indistinguishable from the filaments that aggregate to form PrP amyloid plaques in the CNS. Both the rods and the PrP amyloid filaments found in brain tissue exhibit similar ultrastructural morphology and green-gold birefringence after staining with Congo red dye.

Prion Strains

The existence of prion strains raised the question of how heritable biologic information can be enciphered in a molecule other than nucleic acid. Various strains of prions have been defined by incubation times and the distribution of neuronal vacuolation. Subsequently, the

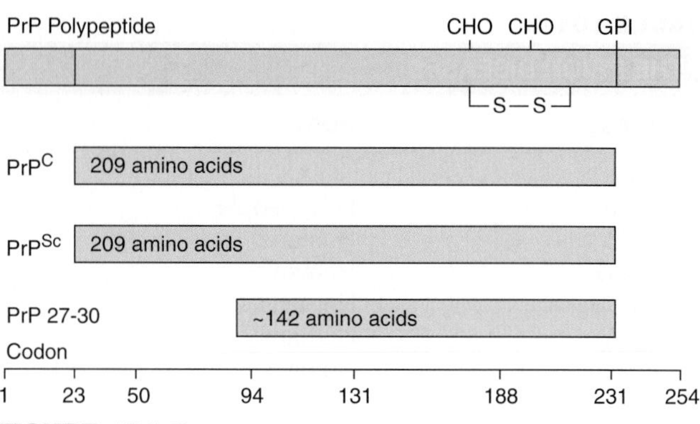

FIGURE 101-2

Prion protein isoforms. Bar diagram of Syrian hamster PrP, which consists of 254 amino acids. After processing of the NH_2 and COOH termini, both PrP^{C} and PrP^{Sc} consist of 209 residues. After limited proteolysis, the NH_2 terminus of PrP^{Sc} is truncated to form PrP 27–30 composed of ~142 amino acids.

patterns of PrP^{Sc} deposition were found to correlate with vacuolation profiles, and these patterns were also used to characterize prion strains.

Persuasive evidence that strain-specific information is enciphered in the tertiary structure of PrP^{Sc} comes from transmission of two different inherited human prion diseases to mice expressing a chimeric human-mouse PrP transgene. In FFI, the protease-resistant fragment of PrP^{Sc} after deglycosylation has a molecular mass of 19 kDa, whereas in fCJD and most sporadic prion diseases, it is 21 kDa (Table 101-3). This difference in molecular mass was shown to be due to different sites of proteolytic cleavage at the NH_2 termini of the two human PrP^{Sc} molecules, reflecting different tertiary structures. These distinct conformations were not unexpected because the amino acid sequences of the PrPs differ.

Extracts from the brains of patients with FFI transmitted disease into mice expressing a chimeric human-mouse PrP transgene and induced formation of the 19-kDa PrP^{Sc}, whereas brain extracts from fCJD and sCJD patients produced the 21-kDa PrP^{Sc} in mice expressing the same transgene. On second passage, these differences were maintained, demonstrating that chimeric PrP^{Sc} can

TABLE 101-3

DISTINCT PRION STRAINS GENERATED IN HUMANS WITH INHERITED PRION DISEASES AND TRANSMITTED TO TRANSGENIC MICE[a]

INOCULUM	HOST SPECIES	HOST PrP GENOTYPE	INCUBATION TIME [DAYS ± SEM] (n/n_0)	PrP^{Sc} (kDa)
None	Human	FFI(D178N, M129)		19
FFI	Mouse	Tg(MHu2M)	206 ± 7 (7/7)	19
FFI → Tg(MHu2M)	Mouse	Tg(MHu2M)	136 ± 1 (6/6)	19
None	Human	fCJD(E200K)		21
fCJD	Mouse	Tg(MHu2M)	170 ± 2 (10/10)	21
fCJD → Tg(MHu2M)	Mouse	Tg(MHu2M)	167 ± 3 (15/15)	21

[a]Tg(MHu2M) mice express a chimeric mouse-human PrP gene.

Note: Clinicopathologic phenotype is determined by the conformation of PrP^{Sc} in accord with the results of the transmission of human prions from patients with FFI to transgenic mice. FFI, fatal familial insomnia; fCJD, familial Creutzfeldt-Jakob disease.

exist in two different conformations based on the sizes of the protease-resistant fragments, even though the amino acid sequence of PrP^{Sc} is invariant.

This analysis was extended when patients with sporadic fatal insomnia (sFI) were identified. Although they did not carry a *PRNP* gene mutation, the patients demonstrated a clinical and pathologic phenotype that was indistinguishable from that of patients with FFI. Furthermore, 19-kDa PrP^{Sc} was found in their brains, and on passage of prion disease to mice expressing a chimeric human-mouse PrP transgene, 19-kDa PrP^{Sc} was also found. These findings indicate that the disease phenotype is dictated by the conformation of PrP^{Sc} and not the amino acid sequence. PrP^{Sc} acts as a template for the conversion of PrP^{C} into nascent PrP^{Sc}. On the passage of prions into mice expressing a chimeric hamster-mouse PrP transgene, a change in the conformation of PrP^{Sc} was accompanied by the emergence of a new strain of prions.

New strains of prions were also generated from recombinant (rec) PrP produced in bacteria. In these studies, recPrP was polymerized into amyloid fibrils and inoculated into transgenic mice expressing very high levels of truncated mouse PrP^{C}; about 500 days later, the mice died of prion disease. These "synthetic prions" were found to be much more stable than any prions previously isolated from animals or humans with naturally occurring prion diseases. Surprisingly, studies of synthetic and naturally occurring prions indicate that the incubation time is directly proportional to the stability of the prion. As the stability increases, the incubation time lengthens; thus, less-stable prions replicate more rapidly. These studies also showed that PrP^{Sc} can adopt a continuum of conformational states, each of which enciphers a distinct incubation-time phenotype.

Species Barrier

Studies on the role of the primary and tertiary structures of PrP in the transmission of prion disease have given new insights into the pathogenesis of these maladies. The amino acid sequence of PrP encodes the species of the prion, and the prion derives its PrP^{Sc} sequence from the last mammal in which it was passaged. While the primary structure of PrP is likely to be the most important or even sole determinant of the tertiary structure of PrP^{C}, PrP^{Sc} seems to function as a template in determining the tertiary structure of nascent PrP^{Sc} molecules as they are formed from PrP^{C}. In turn, prion diversity appears to be enciphered in the conformation of PrP^{Sc}, and thus prion strains seem to represent different conformers of PrP^{Sc}.

In general, transmission of prion disease from one species to another is inefficient, in that not all intracerebrally inoculated animals develop disease, and those that fall ill do so only after long incubation times that can approach the natural life span of the animal. This "species barrier" to transmission is correlated with the degree of similarity between the amino acid sequences of PrP^{C} in the inoculated host and of PrP^{Sc} in the prion inoculum. The importance of sequence similarity between the host and donor PrP argues that PrP^{C} directly interacts with PrP^{Sc} in the prion conversion process.

SPORADIC AND INHERITED PRION DISEASES

Several different scenarios might explain the initiation of sporadic prion disease: (1) A somatic mutation may be the cause and thus follow a path similar to that for germline mutations in inherited disease. In this situation, the mutant PrP^{Sc} must be capable of targeting wild-type PrP^{C}, a process known to be possible for some mutations but less likely for others. (2) The activation barrier separating wild-type PrP^{C} from PrP^{Sc} could be crossed on rare occasions when viewed in the context of a population. Most individuals would be spared while presentations in the elderly with an incidence of ~1 per million would be seen. (3) PrP^{Sc} may be present at very low levels in some normal cells, where it performs some important, as yet unknown, function. The level of PrP^{Sc} in such cells is hypothesized to be sufficiently low as to be not detected by bioassay. In some altered metabolic states, the cellular mechanisms for clearing PrP^{Sc} might become compromised and the rate of PrP^{Sc} formation would then begin to exceed the capacity of the cell to clear it. The third possible mechanism is attractive since it suggests PrP^{Sc} is not simply a misfolded protein, as proposed for the first and second mechanisms, but that it is an alternatively folded molecule with a function. Moreover, the multitude of conformational states that PrP^{Sc} can adopt, as described above, raises the possibility that PrP^{Sc} or another prion-like protein might function in a process like short-term memory where information storage occurs in the absence of new protein synthesis.

More than 30 different mutations resulting in nonconservative substitutions in the human *PRNP* gene have been found to segregate with inherited human prion diseases. Missense mutations and expansions in the octapeptide repeat region of the gene are responsible for familial forms of prion disease. Five different mutations of the *PRNP* gene have been linked genetically to heritable prion disease.

Although phenotypes may vary dramatically within families, specific phenotypes tend to be observed with certain mutations. A clinical phenotype indistinguishable from typical sCJD is usually seen with substitutions at codons 180, 183, 200, 208, 210, and 232. Substitutions at codons 102, 105, 117, 198, and 217 are associated with the GSS variant of prion disease. The normal human PrP sequence contains five repeats of an eight-amino-acid sequence. Insertions from two to nine extra octarepeats frequently cause variable phenotypes ranging from a condition indistinguishable from sCJD to a slowly progressive dementing illness of many years' duration to an early-age-of-onset disorder that is similar to Alzheimer's disease. A mutation at codon 178 resulting in substitution of asparagine for aspartic acid produces FFI if a methionine is encoded at the polymorphic 129 residue on the same allele. Typical CJD is seen if a valine is encoded at position 129 of the same allele.

HUMAN PRNP GENE POLYMORPHISMS

Polymorphisms influence the susceptibility to sporadic, inherited, and infectious forms of prion disease. The methionine/valine polymorphism at position 129 not only modulates the age of onset of some inherited prion diseases but can also determine the clinical phenotype. The finding that homozygosity at codon 129 predisposes to sCJD supports a model of prion production that favors PrP interactions between homologous proteins.

Substitution of the basic residue lysine at position 218 in mouse PrP produced dominant-negative inhibition of prion replication in transgenic mice. This same lysine at position 219 in human PrP has been found in 12% of the Japanese population, and this group appears to be resistant to prion disease. Dominant-negative inhibition of prion replication was also found with substitution of the basic residue arginine at position 171; sheep with arginine are resistant to scrapie prions but are susceptible to BSE prions that were inoculated intracerebrally.

INFECTIOUS PRION DISEASES

IATROGENIC CJD

Accidental transmission of CJD to humans appears to have occurred with corneal transplantation, contaminated electroencephalogram (EEG) electrode implantation, and surgical procedures. Corneas from donors with inapparent CJD have been transplanted to apparently healthy recipients who developed CJD after prolonged incubation periods. The same improperly decontaminated EEG electrodes that caused CJD in two young patients with intractable epilepsy caused CJD in a chimpanzee 18 months after their experimental implantation.

Surgical procedures may have resulted in accidental inoculation of patients with prions, presumably because some instrument or apparatus in the operating theater became contaminated when a CJD patient underwent surgery. Although the epidemiology of these studies is highly suggestive, no proof for such episodes exists.

Dura Mater Grafts

More than 160 cases of CJD after implantation of dura mater grafts have been recorded. All of the grafts were thought to have been acquired from a single manufacturer whose preparative procedures were inadequate to inactivate human prions. One case of CJD occurred after repair of an eardrum perforation with a pericardium graft.

Human Growth Hormone and Pituitary Gonadotropin Therapy

The possibility of transmission of CJD from contaminated human growth hormone (hGH) preparations derived from human pituitaries has been raised by the occurrence of fatal cerebellar disorders with dementia in >180 patients ranging in age from 10 to 41 years. These patients received injections of hGH every 2–4 days for 4–12 years. If it is assumed that these patients developed CJD from injections of prion-contaminated hGH preparations, the possible incubation periods range from 4 to 30 years. Even though several investigations argue for the efficacy of inactivating prions in hGH fractions prepared from human pituitaries with 6 *M* urea, it seems doubtful that such protocols will be used for purifying hGH because recombinant hGH is available. Four cases of CJD have occurred in women receiving human pituitary gonadotropin.

VARIANT CJD

The restricted geographic occurrence and chronology of vCJD raised the possibility that BSE prions have been transmitted to humans through the consumption of tainted beef. More than 190 cases of vCJD have occurred, with >90% of these in Britain. vCJD has also been reported in people either living in or originating from France, Ireland, Italy, the Netherlands, Portugal, Spain, Saudi Arabia, United States, Canada, and Japan.

Because the number of vCJD cases is still small, it not possible to decide if we are at the beginning of a prion disease epidemic in Europe, similar to those seen for BSE and kuru, or if the number of vCJD cases will remain small. What is certain is that prion-tainted meat should be prevented from entering the human food supply.

The most compelling evidence that vCJD is caused by BSE prions was obtained from experiments in mice expressing the bovine PrP transgene. Both BSE and vCJD prions were efficiently transmitted to these transgenic mice and with similar incubation periods. In contrast to sCJD prions, vCJD prions did not transmit disease efficiently to mice expressing a chimeric human-mouse PrP transgene. Earlier studies with nontransgenic mice suggested that vCJD and BSE might be derived from the same source because both inocula transmitted disease with similar but very long incubation periods.

Attempts to determine the origin of BSE and vCJD prions have relied on passaging studies in mice, some of which are described above, as well as studies of the conformation and glycosylation of PrP^{Sc}. One scenario suggests that a particular conformation of bovine PrP^{Sc} was selected for heat resistance during the rendering process and was then reselected multiple times as cattle infected by ingesting prion-contaminated meat and bone meal (MBM) were slaughtered and their offal rendered into more MBM.

NEUROPATHOLOGY

Frequently the brains of patients with CJD have no recognizable abnormalities on gross examination. Patients who survive for several years have variable degrees of cerebral atrophy.

On light microscopy, the pathologic hallmarks of CJD are spongiform degeneration and astrocytic gliosis. The lack of an inflammatory response in CJD and other prion diseases is an important pathologic feature of these degenerative disorders. Spongiform degeneration is characterized by many 1- to 5-μm vacuoles in the neuropil between nerve cell bodies. Generally the spongiform changes occur in the cerebral cortex, putamen, caudate nucleus, thalamus, and molecular layer of the cerebellum. Astrocytic gliosis is a constant but nonspecific feature of prion diseases. Widespread proliferation of fibrous astrocytes is found throughout the gray matter of brains infected with CJD prions. Astrocytic processes filled with glial filaments form extensive networks.

Amyloid plaques have been found in ~10% of CJD cases. Purified CJD prions from humans and animals exhibit the ultrastructural and histochemical characteristics of amyloid when treated with detergents during limited proteolysis. In first passage from some human Japanese CJD cases, amyloid plaques have been found in mouse brains. These plaques stain with antibodies raised against PrP.

The amyloid plaques of GSS disease are morphologically distinct from those seen in kuru or scrapie. GSS plaques consist of a central dense core of amyloid surrounded by smaller globules of amyloid. Ultrastructurally, they consist of a radiating fibrillar network of amyloid fibrils, with scant or no neuritic degeneration. The plaques can be distributed throughout the brain but are most frequently found in the cerebellum. They are often located adjacent to blood vessels. Congophilic angiopathy has been noted in some cases of GSS disease.

In vCJD, a characteristic feature is the presence of "florid plaques." These are composed of a central core of PrP amyloid, surrounded by vacuoles in a pattern suggesting petals on a flower.

CLINICAL FEATURES

Nonspecific prodromal symptoms occur in about a third of patients with CJD and may include fatigue, sleep disturbance, weight loss, headache, malaise, and ill-defined pain. Most patients with CJD present with deficits in higher cortical function. These deficits almost always progress over weeks or months to a state of profound dementia characterized by memory loss, impaired judgment, and a decline in virtually all aspects of intellectual function. A few patients present with either visual impairment or cerebellar gait and coordination deficits. Frequently the cerebellar deficits are rapidly followed by progressive dementia. Visual problems often begin with blurred vision and diminished acuity, rapidly followed by dementia.

Other symptoms and signs include extrapyramidal dysfunction manifested as rigidity, masklike facies, or choreoathetoid movements; pyramidal signs (usually mild); seizures (usually major motor) and, less commonly, hypoesthesia; supranuclear gaze palsy; optic atrophy; and vegetative signs such as changes in weight, temperature, sweating, or menstruation.

Myoclonus

Most patients (~90%) with CJD exhibit myoclonus that appears at various times throughout the illness. Unlike other involuntary movements, myoclonus persists during sleep. Startle myoclonus elicited by loud sounds or bright lights is frequent. It is important to stress that myoclonus is neither specific nor confined to CJD. Dementia with myoclonus can also be due to Alzheimer's disease (AD), dementia with Lewy bodies, cryptococcal encephalitis (Chap. 106), or the myoclonic epilepsy disorder Unverricht-Lundborg disease.

Clinical Course

In documented cases of accidental transmission of CJD to humans, an incubation period of 1.5–2.0 years preceded the development of clinical disease. In other cases, incubation periods of up to 30 years have been suggested. Most patients with CJD live 6–12 months after the onset of clinical signs and symptoms, whereas some live for up to 5 years.

DIAGNOSIS

The constellation of dementia, myoclonus, and periodic electrical bursts in an afebrile 60-year-old patient generally indicates CJD. Clinical abnormalities in CJD are confined to the CNS. Fever, elevated sedimentation rate, leukocytosis in blood, or a pleocytosis in cerebrospinal fluid (CSF) should alert the physician to another etiology to explain the patient's CNS dysfunction.

Variations in the typical course appear in inherited and transmitted forms of the disease. fCJD has an earlier mean age of onset than sCJD. In GSS disease, ataxia is usually a prominent and presenting feature, with dementia occurring late in the disease course. GSS disease typically presents earlier than CJD (mean age 43 years) and is typically more slowly progressive than CJD; death usually occurs within 5 years of onset. FFI is characterized by insomnia and dysautonomia; dementia occurs only in the terminal phase of the illness. Rare sporadic cases have been identified. vCJD has an unusual clinical course, with a prominent psychiatric prodrome that may include visual hallucinations and early ataxia, while frank dementia is usually a late sign of vCJD.

DIFFERENTIAL DIAGNOSIS

Many conditions may mimic CJD superficially. Dementia with Lewy bodies is the most common disorder to be mistaken for CJD. It can present in a subacute fashion with delirium, myoclonus, and extrapyramidal features. Other neurodegenerative disorders to consider include AD, frontotemporal dementia, progressive supranuclear palsy, ceroid lipofuscinosis, and myoclonic epilepsy with Lafora bodies. The absence of abnormalities on diffusion-weighted and FLAIR MRI will usually distinguish these dementing conditions from CJD.

Hashimoto's encephalopathy, which presents as a subacute progressive encephalopathy with myoclonus and periodic triphasic complexes on the EEG, should be excluded in every case of suspected CJD. It is diagnosed by the finding of high titers of antithyroglobulin or antithyroid peroxidase (antimicrosomal) antibodies in the blood and improves with glucocorticoid therapy. Unlike CJD, fluctuations in severity typically occur in Hashimoto's encephalopathy.

Intracranial vasculitides may produce nearly all of the symptoms and signs associated with CJD, sometimes without systemic abnormalities. Myoclonus is exceptional with cerebral vasculitis, but focal seizures may confuse the picture. Prominent headache, absence of myoclonus, stepwise change in deficits, abnormal CSF, and focal white matter changes on MRI or angiographic abnormalities all favor vasculitis.

Paraneoplastic conditions, particularly limbic encephalitis and cortical encephalitis, can also mimic CJD. In many of these patients, dementia appears prior to the diagnosis of a tumor, and in some, no tumor is ever found. Detection of the paraneoplastic antibodies is often the only way to distinguish these cases from CJD.

Other diseases that can simulate CJD include neurosyphilis (Chap. 70), AIDS dementia complex (Chap. 90), progressive multifocal leukoencephalopathy (Chap. 29), subacute sclerosing panencephalitis, progressive rubella panencephalitis, herpes simplex encephalitis, diffuse intracranial tumor (gliomatosis cerebri), anoxic encephalopathy, dialysis dementia, uremia, hepatic encephalopathy, and lithium or bismuth intoxication.

LABORATORY TESTS

The only specific diagnostic tests for CJD and other human prion diseases measure PrP^{Sc}. The most widely used method involves limited proteolysis that generates PrP 27-30, which is detected by immunoassay after denaturation. The conformation-dependent immunoassay (CDI) is based on immunoreactive epitopes that are exposed in PrP^{C} but buried in PrP^{Sc}. The CDI is extremely sensitive and quantitative and is likely to find wide application in both the post- and antemortem detection of prions. In humans, the diagnosis of CJD can be established by brain biopsy if PrP^{Sc} is detected. If no attempt is made to measure PrP^{Sc}, but the constellation of pathologic changes frequently found in CJD is seen in a brain biopsy, then the diagnosis is reasonably secure (see "Neuropathology" earlier in the chapter). Because PrP^{Sc} is not uniformly distributed throughout the CNS, the apparent absence of PrP^{Sc} in a limited sample such as a biopsy does not rule out prion disease. At autopsy, sufficient brain samples should be taken for both PrP^{Sc} immunoassay, preferably by CDI, and immunohistochemistry of tissue sections.

To establish the diagnosis of either sCJD or familial prion disease, sequencing the *PRNP* gene must be performed. Finding the wild-type *PRNP* gene sequence permits the diagnosis of sCJD if there is no history to suggest infection from an exogenous source of prions. The identification of a mutation in the *PRNP* gene sequence that encodes a nonconservative amino acid substitution argues for familial prion disease.

CT may be normal or show cortical atrophy. MRI is valuable for distinguishing sCJD from most other conditions. On FLAIR sequences and diffusion-weighted imaging, ~90% of patients show increased intensity in the basal ganglia and cortical ribboning (Fig. 101-3). This pattern is not seen with other neurodegenerative disorders but has been seen infrequently with viral encephalitis, paraneoplastic syndromes, or seizures. When the typical MRI pattern is present, in the proper clinical setting, diagnosis is facilitated. However, some cases of sCJD do not show this typical pattern, and other early diagnostic approaches are still needed.

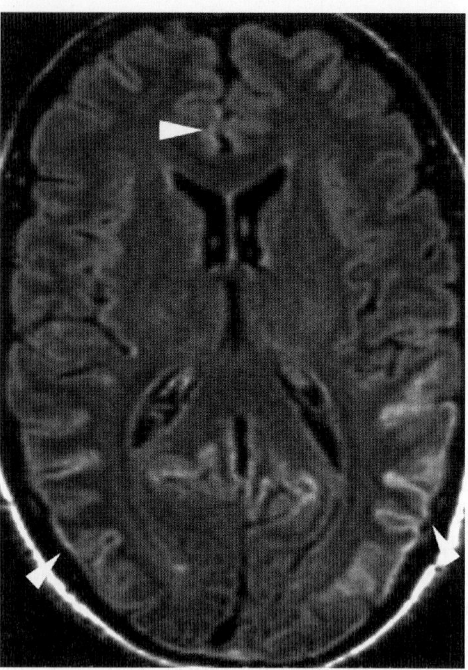

FIGURE 101-3
T2-weighted (FLAIR) MRI showing hyperintensity in the cortex in a patient with sporadic CJD. This so-called "cortical ribboning" along with increased intensity in the basal ganglia on T2 or diffusion-weighted imaging can aid in the diagnosis of CJD.

CSF is nearly always normal but may show protein elevation and, rarely, mild pleocytosis. Although the stress protein 14-3-3 is elevated in the CSF of some patients with CJD, similar elevations of 14-3-3 are found in patients with other disorders; thus this elevation is not specific.

The EEG is often useful in the diagnosis of CJD, although only about 60% of individuals show the typical pattern. During the early phase of CJD, the EEG is usually normal or shows only scattered theta activity. In most advanced cases, repetitive, high-voltage, triphasic, and polyphasic sharp discharges are seen, but in many cases their presence is transient. The presence of these stereotyped periodic bursts of <200 ms duration, occurring every 1–2 s, makes the diagnosis of CJD very likely. These discharges are frequently but not always symmetric; there may be a one-sided predominance in amplitude. As CJD progresses, normal background rhythms become fragmentary and slower.

CARE OF CJD PATIENTS

Although CJD should not be considered either contagious or communicable, it is transmissible. The risk of accidental inoculation by aerosols is very small; nonetheless, procedures producing aerosols should be performed in certified biosafety cabinets. Biosafety level 2 practices, containment equipment, and facilities are recommended by the Centers for Disease Control and Prevention and the National Institutes of Health. The primary problem in caring for patients with CJD is the inadvertent infection of health care workers by needle and stab wounds. The transmission of prions through the air has never been documented. Electroencephalographic and electromyographic needles should not be reused after studies on patients with CJD have been performed.

There is no reason for pathologists or other morgue employees to resist performing autopsies on patients whose clinical diagnosis was CJD. Standard microbiologic practices outlined here, along with specific recommendations for decontamination, seem to be adequate precautions for the care of patients with CJD and the handling of infected specimens.

DECONTAMINATION OF CJD PRIONS

Prions are extremely resistant to common inactivation procedures, and there is some disagreement about the optimal conditions for sterilization. Some investigators recommend treating CJD-contaminated materials once with 1 *N* NaOH at room temperature, but we believe this procedure may be inadequate for sterilization. Autoclaving at 134°C for 5 h or treatment with 2 *N* NaOH for several hours is recommended for sterilization of prions. The term *sterilization* implies complete destruction of prions; any residual infectivity can be hazardous. Recent studies show that sCJD prions bound to stainless steel surfaces are resistant to inactivation by autoclaving at 134°C for 2 h; exposure of bound prions to an acidic detergent solution prior to autoclaving rendered prions susceptible to inactivation.

PREVENTION AND THERAPEUTICS

There is no known effective therapy for preventing or treating CJD. The finding that phenothiazines and acridines inhibit PrP^{Sc} formation in cultured cells led to clinical studies of quinacrine in CJD patients. Although quinacrine seems to slow the rate of decline in some CJD patients, no cure of the disease has been observed. In wild-type mice, quinacrine treatment has been ineffective. Recent studies indicate that inhibition of the P-glycoprotein (Pgp) transport system results in substantially increased quinacrine levels in the brains of mice. Whether such an approach can be used to treat CJD remains to be established.

Like the acridines, anti-PrP antibodies have been shown to eliminate PrP^{Sc} from cultured cells. Additionally, such antibodies in mice, either administered by injection or produced from a transgene, have been shown to prevent prion disease when prions are introduced by a peripheral route, such as intraperitoneal inoculation. Unfortunately, the antibodies were ineffective in mice inoculated intracerebrally with prions. Several drugs, including pentosan polysulfate and porphyrin derivatives, delay the onset of disease in animals inoculated intracerebrally with prions if the drugs are given intracerebrally beginning soon after inoculation.

Structure-based drug design predicated on dominant-negative inhibition of prion formation has produced several promising compounds. Modified quinacrine compounds that are more potent than the parent drug have been found. Whether improving the efficacy of such small molecules will provide general methods for developing novel therapeutics for other neurodegenerative disorders, including AD and Parkinson's disease as well as amyotrophic lateral sclerosis (ALS), remains to be established.

Disclosure: SBP has a financial interest in InPro Biotechnology, Inc.

FURTHER READINGS

Kovacs GG, Budka H: Prion diseases: From protein to cell pathology. Am J Pathol 172:555, 2008

Prusiner SB: Prions, in *Fields Virology*, 5th ed, DM Knipe, PM Howley (eds). Philadelphia, Lippincott Williams & Wilkins, 2007, pp 3059–3092

Safar JG et al: Diagnosis of human prion disease. Proc Natl Acad Sci USA 102:3501, 2005

Stewart LA et al: Systematic review of therapeutic interventions in human prion disease. Neurology 70:1272, 2008

Will RG et al: Diagnosis of new variant Creutzfeldt-Jakob disease. Ann Neurol 47:575, 2000

SECTION VII

FUNGAL AND ALGAL INFECTIONS

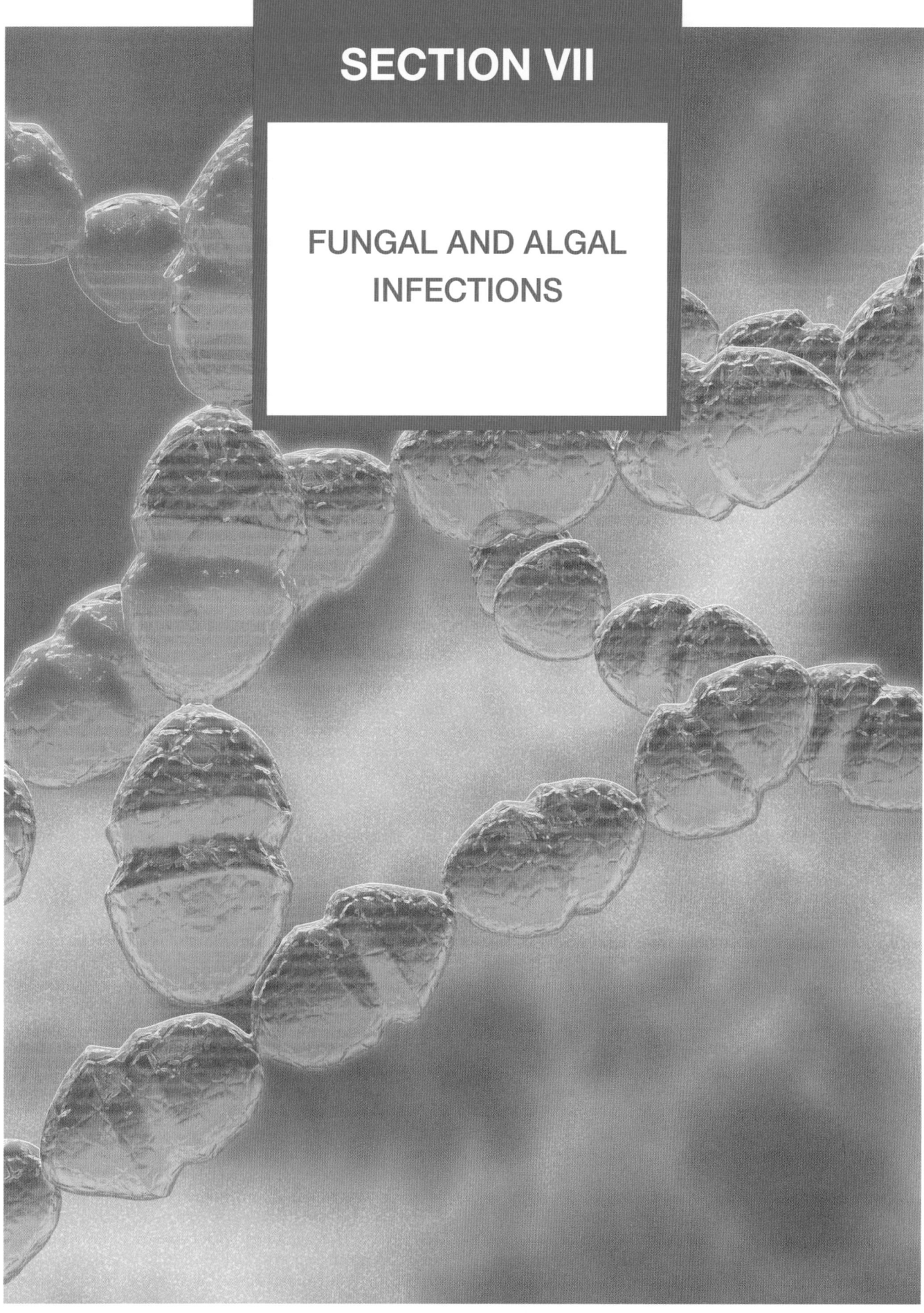

CHAPTER 102

DIAGNOSIS AND TREATMENT OF FUNGAL INFECTIONS

John E. Edwards, Jr.

TERMINOLOGY AND MICROBIOLOGY

Traditionally, fungal infections have been classified into specific categories based on both anatomic location and epidemiology. The most common general anatomic categories are mucocutaneous and deep organ infection; the most common general epidemiologic categories are endemic and opportunistic. Although *mucocutaneous infections* can cause serious morbidity, they are rarely fatal. *Deep organ infections* also cause severe illness in many cases but, in contrast to mucocutaneous infections, are often fatal. The *endemic mycoses* (e.g., coccidioidomycosis) are infections caused by fungal organisms that are not part of the normal human microbial flora and are acquired from environmental sources. In contrast, *opportunistic mycoses* are caused by organisms (e.g., *Candida* and *Aspergillus*) that frequently are components of the normal human flora and whose ubiquity in nature renders them easily acquired by the immunocompromised host. Opportunistic fungi cause serious infections when the immunologic response of the host becomes ineffective, allowing the organisms to transition from harmless commensals to invasive pathogens. Frequently, the diminished effectiveness of the immune system is a result of advanced modern therapies that coincidentally either unbalance the host's microflora or directly interfere with immunologic responses. Endemic mycoses cause more severe illness in immunocompromised patients than in immunocompetent individuals.

Patients acquire infection with endemic fungi almost exclusively by inhalation. The soil is the natural reservoir for the vast majority of endemic mycoses. The dermatophytic fungi may be acquired by human-to-human transmission, but the majority of infections result from environmental contact. In contrast, the opportunistic fungus *Candida* invades the host from normal sites of colonization, usually the mucous membranes of the gastrointestinal tract. In general, innate immunity is the primary defense mechanism against fungi. Although antibodies are formed during many fungal infections (and even during commensalism), they generally do not constitute the primary mode of defense. Nevertheless, in selected infections, as discussed below, measurement of antibody titers may be a useful diagnostic test.

Three other terms frequently used in clinical discussions of fungal infections are *yeast*, *mold*, and *dimorphic fungus*. *Yeasts* are seen as rounded single cells or as budding organisms. *Candida* and *Cryptococcus* are traditionally classified as yeasts. Molds grow as filamentous forms called *hyphae* both at room temperature and when they invade tissue. *Aspergillus*, *Rhizopus* [the species that causes mucormycosis (zygomycosis)], and fungi commonly infecting the skin to cause ringworm and related cutaneous conditions are classified as molds. Variations occur within this classification of yeasts and molds. For instance, when *Candida* infects tissue, both yeasts and filamentous forms may occur (except with *C. glabrata*, which forms only yeasts in tissue); in contrast, *Cryptococcus* exists only in yeast form. *Dimorphic* is the term used to describe fungi that grow as yeasts or large spherical structures in tissue but as filamentous forms at room temperature in the environment. Classified in this group are the organisms causing blastomycosis, paracoccidioidomycosis, coccidioidomycosis, histoplasmosis, blastomycosis, and sporotrichosis.

The incidence of fungal infections has risen substantially over the past several decades. Opportunistic infections have increased in frequency as a consequence of intentional immunosuppression in organ and stem cell transplantation and many other diseases, the administration of cytotoxic chemotherapy for cancers, and the liberal use of antibacterial agents. The incidence of endemic mycoses has increased in geographic locations where there has been substantial population growth.

DIAGNOSIS

The definitive diagnosis of any fungal infection requires histopathologic identification of the fungus invading tissue, accompanied by evidence of an inflammatory response. The identification of an inflammatory response has been especially important with regard to *Aspergillus* infection. *Aspergillus* is ubiquitous and can float from the air onto biopsy material. Therefore, in rare but important instances, this fungus is an ex vivo contaminant during processing of a specimen for microscopy, with a consequent incorrect diagnosis. The stains most commonly used to identify fungi are periodic acid–Schiff and Gomori methenamine silver. *Candida*, unlike other fungi, is visible on gram-stained tissue smears. Hematoxylin and eosin stain is not sufficient to identify *Candida* in tissue specimens. When positive, an India ink preparation of cerebrospinal fluid (CSF) is diagnostic for cryptococcosis. Most laboratories now use calcofluor white staining coupled with fluorescent microscopy to identify fungi in fluid specimens.

Extensive investigations of the diagnosis of deep organ fungal infections have yielded a variety of tests with different degrees of specificity and sensitivity. The most reliable tests are the detection of antibody to *Coccidioides immitis* and *Histoplasma capsulatum* in serum and CSF, the detection of cryptococcal polysaccharide antigen in serum and CSF, and the detection of *Histoplasma* antigen in urine or serum. The test for galactomannan has been used extensively in Europe and is now approved in the United States for diagnosis of aspergillosis. This test requires additional validation before its true usefulness can be determined. Sources of concern are the incidence of false-negative results and the need for multiple serial tests to reduce this incidence. The β-glucan test for *Candida* is also under evaluation but, like the galactomannan test, requires additional validation. Numerous polymerase chain reaction assays to detect antigens are in the developmental stages, as are nucleic acid hybridization techniques; however, these methods are not currently used on a widespread basis in major medical centers.

Of the fungal organisms, *Candida* is by far most frequently recovered from blood. Although *Candida* species can be detected with any of the automated blood culture systems widely used at present, the lysis-centrifugation technique increases the sensitivity of blood cultures for less common organisms (e.g., *H. capsulatum*) and should be used when disseminated fungal infection is suspected.

Except in the cases of coccidioidomycosis, cryptococcosis, and histoplasmosis, there are no fully validated and widely used tests for serodiagnosis of disseminated fungal infection. Skin tests for the endemic mycoses are no longer available.

℞ Treatment: FUNGAL INFECTIONS

This discussion is intended as a brief overview of general strategies for the use of antifungal agents in the treatment of fungal infections. Details on regimens, schedules, and strategies are discussed in the chapters on specific mycoses that follow in this section.

Since fungal organisms are eukaryotic cells that contain most of the same organelles (with many of the same physiologic functions) as human cells, the identification of drugs that selectively kill or inhibit fungi but are not toxic to human cells has been highly problematic. Far fewer antifungal than antibacterial agents have been introduced into clinical medicine.

AMPHOTERICIN B (AmB) The introduction of AmB in the late 1950s revolutionized the treatment of fungal infections in deep organs. Before AmB became available, cryptococcal meningitis and other disseminated fungal infections were nearly always fatal. For nearly a decade after AmB was introduced, it was the only effective agent for the treatment of life-threatening fungal infections. AmB remains the broadest-spectrum antifungal agent but carries several disadvantages, including significant nephrotoxicity, lack of an oral preparation, and unpleasant side effects (fever, chills, and nausea) during treatment. To circumvent nephrotoxicity and infusion side effects, lipid formulations of AmB were developed and have virtually replaced the original colloidal deoxycholate formulation in clinical use (although the older formulation is still available). The lipid formulations include liposomal AmB (L-AB; 435 mg/kg per day) and AmB lipid complex (ABLC; 5 mg/kg per day). A third preparation, AmB colloidal dispersion (ABCD; 3–4 mg/kg per day), is rarely used because of the high incidence of side effects associated with infusion. (The doses listed are standard doses for adults with invasive infection.)

The lipid formulations of AmB have the disadvantage of being considerably more expensive than the deoxycholate formulation. Experience is still accumulating on the comparative efficacy, toxicity, and advantages of the different formulations for specific clinical fungal infections [e.g., central nervous system (CNS) infection]. Whether there is a clinically significant difference in these drugs with respect to CNS penetration or nephrotoxicity remains controversial. Despite these issues and despite the expense, the lipid formulations are now much more commonly used than AmB deoxycholate in the United States.

AZOLES This class of antifungal drugs offers important advantages over AmB: the azoles cause little or no nephrotoxicity and are available in oral preparations. Early azoles included ketoconazole and miconazole, which have been replaced by newer agents for the treatment of deep organ fungal infections. The azoles' mechanism of action is inhibition of ergosterol synthesis in the fungal cell wall. Unlike AmB, these drugs are considered fungistatic, not cidal.

Fluconazole Since its introduction, fluconazole has played an extremely important role in the treatment of a wide variety of serious fungal infections. Its major advantages are the availability of both oral and IV formulations, a long half-life, satisfactory penetration of most body fluids (including ocular fluid and CSF), and minimal toxicity (especially relative to AmB). Its disadvantages include (usually reversible) hepatotoxicity and—at high doses—alopecia, muscle weakness, and dry mouth with a metallic taste. Fluconazole is not effective for the treatment of aspergillosis, mucormycosis, or *Scedosporium apiospermum* infections. It is less effective than the newer azoles against *C. glabrata* and *C. krusei.*

Fluconazole has become the agent of choice for the treatment of coccidioidal meningitis, although relapses have followed therapy with this drug. In addition, fluconazole is useful for both consolidation and maintenance therapy for cryptococcal meningitis. This agent has been shown to be as efficacious as AmB in the treatment of candidemia. The effectiveness of fluconazole in candidemia and the drug's relatively minimal toxicity, in conjunction with the inadequacy of diagnostic tests for widespread hematogenously disseminated candidiasis, have led to a change in the paradigm for candidemia management. The standard of care is now to treat all candidemic patients with an antifungal agent and to change all their intravascular lines, if feasible, rather than merely to remove a singular suspect intravascular line and then observe the patient. The usual fluconazole regimen for treatment of candidemia is 400 mg/d given until 2 weeks after the last positive blood culture.

Fluconazole is considered effective as fungal prophylaxis in bone marrow transplant recipients and high-risk liver transplant patients. Its use for prophylaxis in patients with leukemia, in AIDS patients with low CD4+ T-cell counts, and in patients on surgical intensive care units remains controversial.

Voriconazole Like fluconazole, voriconazole is available in both oral and IV formulations. Voriconazole has a broader spectrum than fluconazole against *Candida* species (including *C. glabrata* and *C. krusei*) and is active against *Aspergillus*, *Scedosporium*, and *Fusarium*. It is generally considered the first-line drug of choice for treatment of aspergillosis. A few case reports have shown voriconazole to be effective in individual patients with coccidioidomycosis, blastomycosis, and histoplasmosis, but (because of limited data) this agent is not recommended for treatment of the endemic mycoses. Among the disadvantages of voriconazole (compared with fluconazole) are its more numerous interactions with many of the drugs used in patients predisposed to fungal infections. Hepatotoxicity, skin rashes (including photosensitivity), and visual disturbances are relatively common. Voriconazole is also considerably more expensive than fluconazole. Moreover, it is advisable to monitor voriconazole levels in certain patients since (1) this drug is completely metabolized in the liver by CYP2C9, CYP3A4, and CYP2C19; and (2) human genetic variability in CYP2C19 activity exists. Dosages should be reduced accordingly in those patients with liver failure. Dose adjustments for renal insufficiency are not necessary; however, because the IV formulation is prepared in cyclodextrin, it should not be given to patients with severe renal insufficiency.

Itraconazole Itraconazole is available in IV and oral (capsule and suspension) formulations. Varying blood levels among patients taking oral itraconazole reflect a disadvantage compared with the other azoles. Itraconazole is the drug of choice for mild to moderate histoplasmosis and blastomycosis and has often been used for chronic mucocutaneous candidiasis. It has been approved by the U.S. Food and Drug Administration (FDA) for use in febrile neutropenic patients. Itraconazole has also proven useful for the treatment of chronic coccidioidomycosis, sporotrichosis, and *S. apiospermum* infection. The mucocutaneous and cutaneous fungal infections that have been treated successfully with itraconazole include oropharyngeal candidiasis (especially in AIDS patients), tinea versicolor, tinea capitis, and onychomycosis. Disadvantages of itraconazole include its poor penetration into the CSF, the use of cyclodextrin in both the oral suspension and the IV preparation, the variable absorption of the capsules, and the need for monitoring of blood levels in patients taking capsules for disseminated mycoses. In recent years, reported cases of severe congestive heart failure in patients taking itraconazole have been a source of concern. Like the other azoles, itraconazole can cause hepatic toxicity.

Posaconazole Posaconazole is approved by the FDA for prophylaxis of aspergillosis and candidiasis in patients at high risk for developing these infections because of severe immunocompromise. This drug has also been evaluated for the treatment of zygomycosis, fusariosis, aspergillosis, and oropharyngeal candidiasis. The relevant studies of posaconazole in zygomycosis, fusariosis, and aspergillosis have examined salvage therapy. A study of >90 patients whose zygomycosis was refractory to other therapy yielded encouraging results. No trials of posaconazole for the treatment of candidemia have yet been reported. Case reports have described the drug's efficacy in coccidioidomycosis and histoplasmosis. Controlled trials have shown its effectiveness as a prophylactic agent in patients with acute leukemia and in bone marrow transplant recipients. In addition, posaconazole has been found to be effective against fluconazole-resistant *Candida* species. The results of a large-scale study of the use of posaconazole as salvage therapy for aspergillosis have been promising but, as of this writing, have not been published in a peer-reviewed format.

ECHINOCANDINS The echinocandins, including the approved drugs caspofungin, anidulafungin, and micafungin, have added considerably to the antifungal armamentarium. All three of these agents inhibit β-1,3-glucan synthase, which is necessary for cell wall synthesis in fungi and is not a component of human cells. None of these agents is available in an oral formulation. The echinocandins are considered fungicidal for *Candida* and fungistatic for *Aspergillus*. Their greatest use to date is against candidal infections. They offer two advantages: broad-spectrum activity against all *Candida* species and relatively low toxicity. The minimum inhibitory concentrations (MICs) of all the echinocandins are highest against *C. parapsilosis*; it is not clear whether these higher MIC values represent less clinical effectiveness against this species. The echinocandins are among the safest antifungal agents.

In controlled trials, *caspofungin* has been at least as efficacious as AmB for the treatment of candidemia and invasive candidiasis and as efficacious as fluconazole for the treatment of candidal esophagitis. In addition, caspofungin has been efficacious as salvage therapy for aspergillosis. At present, it is used most extensively for the treatment of candidemic patients, especially before the infecting species is precisely identified.

Anidulafungin has been approved by the FDA as therapy for candidemia in nonneutropenic patients and for *Candida* esophagitis, intraabdominal infection, and peritonitis. In controlled trials, anidulafungin has been more efficacious than fluconazole against candidemia and invasive candidiasis and as efficacious as fluconazole against candidal esophagitis. When anidulafungin is used with cyclosporine, tacrolimus, or voriconazole, no dosage adjustment is required for either drug in the combination.

Micafungin has been approved for the treatment of esophageal candidiasis and for prophylaxis in patients receiving stem cell transplants. Studies thus far have shown that coadministration of micafungin and cyclosporine does not require dose adjustments for either drug. When micafungin is given with sirolimus, the AUC rises for sirolimus, usually necessitating a reduction in its dose. In open-label trials, favorable results have been obtained with micafungin for the treatment of deep-seated *Aspergillus* and *Candida* infections.

FLUCYTOSINE (5-FLUOROCYTOSINE) The use of flucytosine has diminished in recent years as newer antifungal drugs have been developed. Flucytosine has a unique mechanism of action based on intrafungal conversion to 5-fluorouracil, which is toxic to the cell. Development of resistance to the compound has limited its use as a single agent. Flucytosine is nearly always used in combination with AmB. Its good penetration into the CSF makes it attractive for use with AmB for treatment of cryptococcal meningitis. Flucytosine has also been recommended for the treatment of candidal meningitis in combination with AmB; comparative trials with AmB alone have not been done. Significant and frequent bone marrow depression is seen with flucytosine when this drug is used with AmB.

GRISEOFULVIN AND TERBINAFINE Historically, griseofulvin has been useful primarily for ringworm infection. This agent is usually given for relatively long periods. Terbinafine has been used primarily for onychomycosis but also for ringworm. In comparative studies, terbinafine has been as effective as itraconazole and more effective than griseofulvin for both conditions.

TOPICAL ANTIFUNGAL AGENTS A detailed discussion of the agents used for the treatment of cutaneous fungal infections and onychomycosis is beyond the scope of this chapter; the reader is referred to the dermatology literature. Many classes of compounds have been used to treat the common fungal infections of the skin. Among the azoles used are clotrimazole, econazole, miconazole, oxiconazole, sulconazole, ketoconazole, tioconazole, butoconazole, and terconazole. In general, topical treatment of vaginal candidiasis has been successful. Since there is considered to be little difference in the efficacy of the various vaginal preparations, the choice of agent is made by the physician and/or the patient on the basis of preference and availability. Fluconazole given orally at 150 mg has the advantage of not requiring repeated intravaginal application. Nystatin is a polyene that has been used for both oropharyngeal thrush and vaginal candidiasis. Useful agents in other classes include ciclopirox olamine, haloprogin, terbinafine, naftifine, tolnaftate, and undecylenic acid.

FURTHER READINGS

BATTI Z et al: Review of epidemiology, diagnosis, and treatment of invasive mould infections in allogeneic hematopoietic stem cell transplant recipients. Mycopathologia 162:1, 2006

CHU JH et al: Hospitalizations for endemic mycoses: A population-based national study. Clin Infect Dis 42:822, 2006

DEPAUW BE: Increasing fungal infections in the intensive care unit. Surg Infect (Larchmt) 7(Suppl 2):S93, 2006

DISMUKES WE: Antifungal therapy: Lessons learned over the past 27 years. Clin Infect Dis 42:1289, 2006

ENOCH DA et al: Invasive fungal infections: A review of epidemiology and management options. J Med Microbiol 55:809, 2006

KAUFFMAN CA: Clinical efficacy of new antifungal agents. Curr Opin Microbiol 9:1, 2006

LIPSETT PA: Surgical critical care: Fungal infections in surgical patients. Crit Care Med 34(Suppl):S215, 2006

MANDELL GL et al (eds): Mycoses, in *Principles and Practice of Infectious Diseases*, 6th ed. Elsevier Churchill Livingstone, Philadelphia, 2005, pp 2935–3094

WHEAT LJ: Antigen detection, serology, and molecular diagnosis of invasive mycoses in the immunocompromised host. Transpl Infect Dis 8:128, 2006

CHAPTER 103

HISTOPLASMOSIS

Chadi A. Hage ■ L. Joseph Wheat

ETIOLOGY

Histoplasma capsulatum, a thermal dimorphic fungus, is the etiologic agent of histoplasmosis. In most endemic areas, *H. capsulatum* var. *capsulatum* is the causative agent; in Africa, *H. capsulatum* var. *duboisii* is also found. Mycelia—the naturally infectious form of *Histoplasma*—have a characteristic appearance, with microconidial and macroconidial forms. Microconidia are oval and are small enough (2–5 μm) to reach the terminal bronchioles and alveoli. Shortly after infecting the host, mycelia transform into the yeasts that are found inside macrophages and other phagocytes. The yeast forms are characteristically small (2–5 μm), with occasional narrow budding. In the laboratory, mycelia are best grown at room temperature, whereas yeasts are grown at 37°C on enriched media.

EPIDEMIOLOGY

Histoplasmosis is the most prevalent endemic mycosis in North America. Although this fungal disease has been reported throughout the world, its endemicity is particularly notable in certain parts of North, Central, and South America; Africa; and Asia. In the United States, the endemic areas spread over the Ohio and Mississippi river valleys. This pattern is related to the humid and acidic nature of the soil in these areas. Soil enriched with bird or bat droppings promotes the growth and sporulation of *Histoplasma*. Disruption of soil containing the organism leads to aerosolization of the microconidia and exposure of humans nearby. Activities associated with high-level exposure include spelunking, excavation, cleaning of chicken coops, demolition and remodeling of old buildings, and cutting of dead trees. Most cases seen outside of highly endemic areas represent imported disease—e.g., cases reported in Europe after travel to the Americas, Africa, or Asia.

PATHOGENESIS AND PATHOLOGY

Infection follows inhalation of microconidia (Fig. 103-1). Once they reach the alveolar spaces, microconidia are rapidly recognized and engulfed by alveolar macrophages. At this point, the microconidia transform into budding yeasts (Fig. 103-2), a process that is integral to the pathogenesis of histoplasmosis and is dependent on the availability of calcium and iron inside the phagocytes. The yeasts are capable of growing and multiplying inside resting macrophages. Neutrophils and then lymphocytes are attracted to the site of infection. Before the development of cellular immunity, yeasts use the phagosomes as a vehicle for translocation to local draining lymph nodes, whence they spread hematogenously throughout the reticuloendothelial system. Adequate cellular immunity develops ~2 weeks after infection. T cells produce interferon γ to assist the macrophages in killing the organism and controlling the progression of disease. Interleukin 12 and tumor necrosis factor α (TNF-α) play an essential role in cellular immunity to *H. capsulatum*. In the immunocompetent host, macrophages, lymphocytes, and epithelial cells eventually organize and form granulomas that contain the organisms. These granulomas typically fibrose and calcify; calcified mediastinal lymph nodes and hepatosplenic calcifications are frequently found in healthy individuals from endemic areas. In immunocompetent hosts, infection with *H. capsulatum* confers some immunity to reinfection. In patients with impaired cellular immunity, the infection is not contained and can disseminate. Progressive disseminated histoplasmosis (PDH) can involve multiple organs, most commonly the bone marrow, spleen, liver (Fig. 103-3), adrenal glands, and mucocutaneous membranes. Unlike latent tuberculosis, latent histoplasmosis is rarely reactivated.

Structural lung disease (e.g., emphysema) impairs the clearance of pulmonary histoplasmosis, and chronic pulmonary disease can result. This chronic process is characterized by progressive inflammation, tissue necrosis, and fibrosis mimicking cavitary tuberculosis.

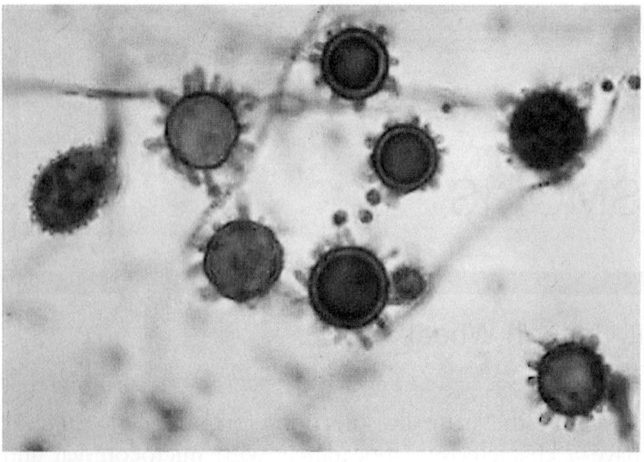

FIGURE 103-1
Spiked spherical conidia of *H. capsulatum* (lactol-phenol cotton blue stain).

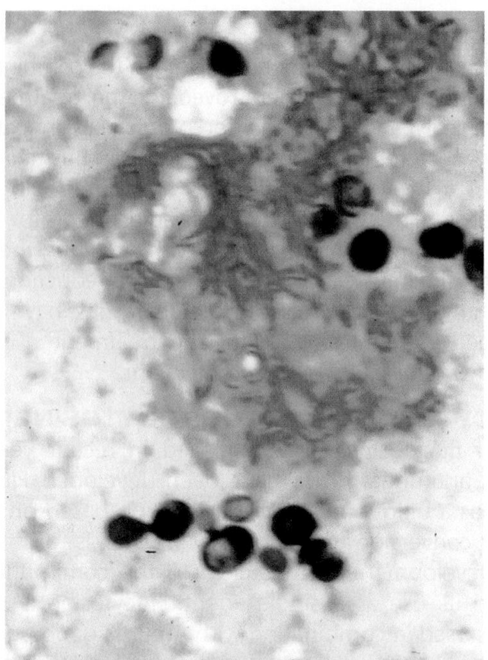

FIGURE 103-2
Small (2–5 μm) narrow budding yeasts of *H. capsulatum* from bronchoalveolar lavage fluid (Grocott's methenamine silver stain).

CLINICAL MANIFESTATIONS

The clinical spectrum of histoplasmosis ranges from asymptomatic infection to life-threatening illness. The attack rate and the extent and severity of the disease depend on the intensity of exposure, the immune status

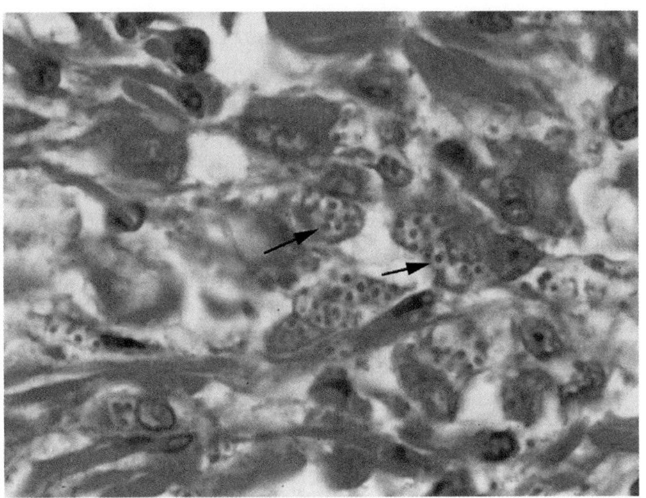

FIGURE 103-3
Intracellular yeasts (*arrows*) of *H. capsulatum* in a liver biopsy specimen (hematoxylin and eosin stain).

of the exposed individual, and the underlying lung architecture of the host.

In immunocompetent individuals with low-level exposure, most *Histoplasma* infections are either asymptomatic or mild and self-limited. Of adults residing in endemic areas, 50–80% have skin-test and/or radiographic evidence of previous infection without clinical manifestations. When symptoms do develop, they usually appear 2–4 weeks after exposure. Heavy exposure leads to a flulike illness with fever, chills, sweats, headache, myalgia, anorexia, cough, dyspnea, and chest pain. Chest radiographs usually show signs of pneumonitis with hilar or mediastinal adenopathy. Pulmonary infiltrates may be focal with light exposure or diffuse with heavy exposure. Rheumatologic symptoms of arthralgia or arthritis, often associated with erythema nodosum, occur in 5–10% of patients with acute histoplasmosis. Pericarditis may also develop. These manifestations represent inflammatory responses to the acute infection rather than its direct effects. Hilar or mediastinal lymph nodes may undergo necrosis and coalesce to form large mediastinal masses that can cause compression of great vessels, proximal airways, and the esophagus. These necrotic lymph nodes also may rupture and create fistulas between mediastinal structures (e.g., bronchoesophageal fistulas).

PDH is typically seen in immunocompromised individuals, who account for ~70% of cases. Common risk factors include AIDS (CD4+ T-cell count, <200/μL), extremes of age, and the use of immunosuppressive medications such as prednisone, methotrexate, and anti-TNF-α agents. The spectrum of PDH ranges from an acute, rapidly fatal course—with diffuse interstitial or reticulonodular lung infiltrates causing respiratory failure, shock, coagulopathy, and multiorgan failure—to a more subacute course with a focal organ distribution. Common manifestations include fever and weight loss. Hepatosplenomegaly is also common. Other findings may include meningitis or focal brain lesions, ulcerations of the oral mucosa, gastrointestinal ulcerations, and adrenal insufficiency. Prompt recognition of this devastating illness is of paramount importance in patients with more severe manifestations or with underlying immunosuppression, especially AIDS (Chap. 90).

Chronic cavitary histoplasmosis is seen in smokers who have structural lung disease (e.g., bullous emphysema). This chronic illness is characterized by productive cough, dyspnea, low-grade fever, night sweats, and weight loss. Chest radiographs usually show upper-lobe infiltrates, cavitation, and pleural thickening—findings resembling those of tuberculosis. Without treatment, the course is slowly progressive.

Fibrosing mediastinitis is an uncommon and serious complication of histoplasmosis. In certain patients, acute infection is followed for unknown reasons by progressive fibrosis around the hilar and mediastinal lymph nodes. Involvement may be unilateral or bilateral; bilateral involvement carries a worse prognosis. Major manifestations include superior vena cava syndrome, obstruction of pulmonary vessels, and recurrent airway obstruction. Patients may experience recurrent pneumonia, hemoptysis, or respiratory failure. Fibrosing mediastinitis is fatal in up to one-third of cases.

In healed histoplasmosis, calcified mediastinal nodes or lung parenchyma may erode through the walls of the airways and cause hemoptysis. This condition is called *broncholithiasis*.

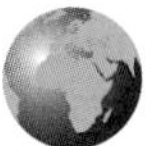
African histoplasmosis caused by *H. capsulatum* var. *duboisii* is clinically distinct and is characterized by frequent skin and bone involvement.

DIAGNOSIS

Fungal culture remains the gold standard diagnostic test for histoplasmosis. However, culture results may not be known for up to 1 month, and cultures are often negative in less severe cases. Cultures are positive in ~75% of cases of PDH and chronic pulmonary histoplasmosis. Cultures of bronchoalveolar lavage (BAL) fluid are positive in about half of patients with acute pulmonary histoplasmosis causing diffuse infiltrates with hypoxemia. In PDH, the culture yield is highest for BAL fluid, bone marrow aspirate, and blood. Cultures of sputum or bronchial washings are usually positive in chronic pulmonary histoplasmosis. Cultures are typically negative, however, in other forms of histoplasmosis.

Fungal stains of cytopathology or biopsy materials showing structures resembling *Histoplasma* yeasts are helpful in the diagnosis of PDH, yielding positive results in about half of cases. Yeasts can be seen in BAL fluid (Fig. 103-2) from patients with diffuse pulmonary infiltrates, in bone marrow biopsy samples, and in biopsy specimens of other involved organs (e.g., the adrenal glands). Occasionally, yeasts are seen in blood smears from patients with severe PDH. However, staining artifacts and other fungal elements may be misidentified as *Histoplasma* yeasts.

The detection of *Histoplasma* antigen in body fluids is extremely useful in the diagnosis of PDH and acute diffuse pulmonary histoplasmosis. The sensitivity of this technique is >90% for urine and 80% for serum from patients with PDH and ~75% for urine from patients with acute pulmonary histoplasmosis. Antigen can be detected in cerebrospinal fluid from patients with meningitis and in BAL fluid from those with pneumonia. Cross-reactivity occurs with African histoplasmosis, blastomycosis, coccidioidomycosis, paracoccidioidomycosis, and *Penicillium marneffei* infection.

Serologic tests, including immunodiffusion and complement fixation, are especially useful for the diagnosis of self-limited acute pulmonary histoplasmosis; however, at least 1 month is required for the production of antibodies after acute infection. A fourfold rise in antibody titer may be seen in patients with acute pulmonary histoplasmosis. Serologic tests are also useful for the diagnosis of chronic pulmonary histoplasmosis. Limitations of serology, however, include insensitivity early in the course of infection in immunosuppressed patients and the persistence of detectable antibody for several years after infection. Positive results from past infection may lead to a misdiagnosis of active histoplasmosis in a patient with another disease process.

℞ Treatment: HISTOPLASMOSIS

Treatment recommendations for histoplasmosis are summarized in Table 103-1.

Treatment is indicated for all patients with PDH or chronic pulmonary histoplasmosis as well as for symptomatic patients with acute pulmonary histoplasmosis causing diffuse infiltrates, especially with hypoxemia. In the vast majority of cases, however, acute pulmonary histoplasmosis resolves without therapy, and treatment is not recommended.

The preferred treatments for histoplasmosis include the lipid formulations of amphotericin B in more severe cases and itraconazole in others. Liposomal amphotericin B has been more effective than the deoxycholate formulation for treatment of PDH in patients with AIDS. The deoxycholate formulation of amphotericin B is an alternative to a lipid formulation in patients who are at a low risk for nephrotoxicity. Posaconazole, voriconazole, and fluconazole are alternatives for patients who cannot take itraconazole.

In severe cases requiring hospitalization, a lipid formulation of amphotericin B is followed by itraconazole. In patients with meningitis, a lipid formulation of amphotericin B should be given for 4–6 weeks before the switch to itraconazole. In immunosuppressed patients, the degree of immunosuppression should be reduced if possible. Antiretroviral treatment improves the outcome of PDH in patients with AIDS and is recommended.

Blood levels of itraconazole should be monitored to ensure adequate drug exposure, and drug interactions should be carefully assessed: itraconazole not only is cleared by cytochrome P450 metabolism but also inhibits cytochrome P450. This profile causes interactions with many other medications.

The duration of treatment for acute pulmonary histoplasmosis is 6–12 weeks, while that for PDH and chronic pulmonary histoplasmosis is ≥1 year. Antigen levels in urine and serum should be monitored during and for at least 1 year after therapy for PDH. Stable or rising antigen levels suggest treatment failure or relapse.

Previously, lifelong itraconazole maintenance therapy was recommended for patients with AIDS once histoplasmosis was diagnosed. Today, however, maintenance therapy is not required for patients who respond well to antiretroviral therapy, with CD4+ T-cell counts of at least 150/μL (preferably >250/μL); who complete at least 1 year of itraconazole therapy; and who exhibit

TABLE 103-1

RECOMMENDATIONS FOR THE TREATMENT OF HISTOPLASMOSIS

TYPE OF HISTOPLASMOSIS	TREATMENT RECOMMENDATIONS	COMMENTS
Acute pulmonary, moderate to severe illness with diffuse infiltrates and/or hypoxemia	Lipid amphotericin B (3–5 mg/kg per day) ± glucocorticoids for 1–2 weeks; then itraconazole (200 mg twice daily) for 12 weeks. Monitor renal and hepatic function.	Patients with mild cases usually recover without therapy, but itraconazole should be considered if the patient's condition has not improved after 1 month.
Chronic/cavitary pulmonary	Itraconazole (200 mg once or twice daily) for at least 12 months. Monitor hepatic function.	Continue treatment until radiographic findings show no further improvement. Monitor for relapse after treatment is stopped.
Progressive disseminated	Lipid amphotericin B (3–5 mg/kg per day) for 1–2 weeks; then itraconazole (200 mg twice daily) for at least 12 months. Monitor renal and hepatic function.	Liposomal amphotericin B is preferred, but the amphotericin B lipid complex may be used because of cost. Chronic maintenance therapy may be necessary if the degree of immunosuppression cannot be reduced.
Central nervous system	Liposomal amphotericin B (5 mg/kg per day) for 4–6 weeks; then itraconazole (200 mg 2 or 3 times daily) for at least 12 months. Monitor renal and hepatic function.	A longer course of lipid amphotericin B is recommended because of the high risk of relapse. Itraconazole should be continued until cerebrospinal fluid or CT abnormalities clear.

neither clinical evidence of active histoplasmosis nor an antigenuria level of >4 ng/mL.

Fibrosing mediastinitis, which represents a chronic fibrotic reaction to past mediastinal histoplasmosis rather than an active infection, does not respond to antifungal therapy. While treatment is often prescribed for patients with acute pulmonary histoplasmosis who have not recovered within 1 month and for those with persistent mediastinal lymphadenopathy, the effectiveness of antifungal therapy in these situations is unknown.

FURTHER READINGS

GOLDMAN M et al: Safety of discontinuation of maintenance therapy for disseminated histoplasmosis after immunologic response to antiretroviral therapy. Clin Infect Dis 38:1485, 2004

GOODWIN R et al: Histoplasmosis in normal hosts. Medicine (Baltimore) 60:231, 1981

JOHNSON PC et al: Safety and efficacy of liposomal amphotericin B compared with conventional amphotericin B for induction therapy of histoplasmosis in patients with AIDS. Ann Intern Med 137:105, 2002

KAUFFMAN CA: Histoplasmosis: A clinical and laboratory update. Clin Microb Rev 20:115, 2007

KENNEDY CC, LIMPER AH: Redefining the clinical spectrum of chronic pulmonary histoplasmosis: a retrospective case series of 46 patients. Medicine (Baltimore) 86:252, 2007

NEWMAN SL: Cell-mediated immunity to *Histoplasma capsulatum*. Semin Respir Infect 16:102, 2001

VAIL GM et al: Incidence of histoplasmosis following allogeneic bone marrow transplant or solid organ transplant in a hyperendemic area. Transpl Infect Dis 4:148, 2002

WHEAT LJ: Histoplasmosis. Experience during outbreaks in Indianapolis and review of the literature. Medicine (Baltimore) 76:339, 1997

———: Current diagnosis of histoplasmosis. Trends Microbiol 11:488, 2003

———: Improvements in diagnosis of histoplasmosis. Expert Opin Biol Ther 6:1207, 2006

——— et al: Pulmonary histoplasmosis syndromes: Recognition, diagnosis, and management. Semin Respir Crit Care Med 25:129, 2004

——— et al: Clinical practice guidelines for the management of patients with histoplasmosis: 2007 update by the Infectious Diseases Society of America. Clin Infect Dis 45:807, 2007

CHAPTER 104

COCCIDIOIDOMYCOSIS

Neil M. Ampel

DEFINITION AND ETIOLOGY

Coccidioidomycosis, commonly known as valley fever, is caused by the dimorphic soil-dwelling fungus *Coccidioides*. Genetic analysis has demonstrated the existence of two species, *C. immitis* and *C. posadasii*. These species are indistinguishable with regard to the clinical disease they cause as well as in routine laboratory tests. Thus, the organism will be referred to simply as *Coccidioides* for the remainder of this chapter.

EPIDEMIOLOGY

Coccidioidomycosis is confined to the Western Hemisphere between the latitudes of 40°N and 40°S. In the United States, areas of high endemicity include the southern portion of the San Joaquin Valley of California, the south-central region of Arizona, and the southwestern Rio Grande Valley. However, infection may be acquired in other areas of the southwestern United States, including the southern coastal counties in California, southern Nevada, and southwestern Utah. Outside the United States, coccidioidomycosis is endemic to northern Mexico as well as to localized regions of Central America. In South America, there are endemic foci in Colombia, Venezuela, northeastern Brazil, Paraguay, Bolivia, and north-central Argentina.

The risk of infection is increased by direct exposure to soil harboring *Coccidioides*. Because of difficulty in isolating *Coccidioides* from the soil, the precise characteristics of potentially infectious soil are not known. In general, *Coccidioides* appears to be supported in previously uncultivated desert soil, such as that found in the Lower Sonoran Life Zone. However, several outbreaks have been associated with soil from archaeologic excavations of Amerindian sites both within and outside of the recognized endemic region.

In endemic areas, many cases of *Coccidioides* infection occur without obvious soil or dust exposure. Climatic factors appear to increase the infection rate in these regions. In particular, periods of dryness after rainy seasons have been associated with marked increases in the number of cases.

Recently, the number of cases of symptomatic coccidioidomycosis has increased dramatically in south-central

Arizona, where most of the state's population resides. The factors causing this increase have not been fully elucidated; however, an influx of older, susceptible individuals into the region as well as increased construction in previously undeveloped desert appear to be involved.

PATHOGENESIS, PATHOLOGY, AND IMMUNE RESPONSE

On agar media and in the soil, *Coccidioides* exists as a filamentous mold. Within this mycelial structure, individual filaments (*hyphae*) elongate and branch, some growing upward. Cells within the hyphae degenerate, leaving alternating barrel-shaped viable cells called *arthroconidia*. Measuring only ~2 × 5 μm, arthroconidia may become airborne for extended periods. The small size of the arthroconidia also allows them to evade initial mechanical mucosal defenses and reach the alveolus, where infection is initiated in the nonimmune host.

Once in a susceptible host, the arthroconidia enlarge, become rounded, and develop internal septations. The resulting structures, called *spherules* (Fig. 104-1), may attain sizes of 80 μm and are unique to *Coccidioides*. The septations encompass uninuclear elements called *endospores*. Spherules may rupture and release packets of endospores that can themselves develop into spherules, thus propagating infection locally. If returned to artificial media or the soil, the fungus reverts to its mycelial stage.

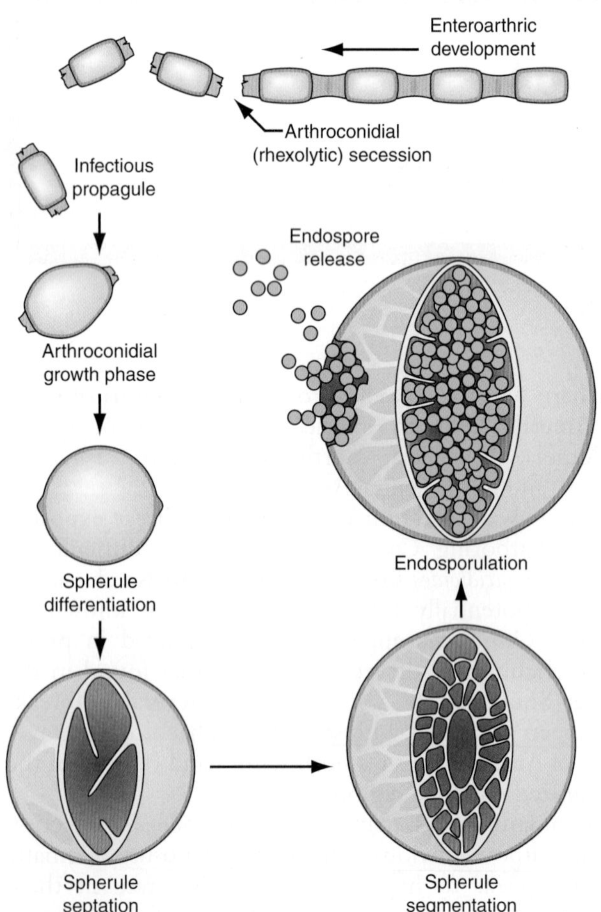

FIGURE 104-1
Life cycle of *Coccidioides*. *(From Kirkland TN, Fierer J: Coccidioidomycosis: A reemerging infectious disease. Emerg Infect Dis 2:192, 1996.)*

Clinical observations and data from studies of animals strongly support the critical role of a robust cellular immune response in the host's control of coccidioidomycosis. Necrotizing granulomas containing spherules are typically identified in patients with resolved pulmonary infection. In disseminated disease, granulomas are generally poorly formed or do not develop at all, and a polymorphonuclear leukocyte response occurs frequently. In patients who are asymptomatic or in whom the initial pulmonary infection resolves, delayed-type hypersensitivity to coccidioidal antigens is routinely documented.

CLINICAL AND LABORATORY MANIFESTATIONS

Coccidioidomycosis is protean in its manifestations. Of infected individuals, 60% are completely asymptomatic, and the remaining 40% have symptoms that are related principally to pulmonary infection, including fever, cough, and pleuritic chest pain. The risk of symptomatic illness increases with age. Coccidioidomycosis is commonly misdiagnosed as community-acquired bacterial pneumonia.

There are several cutaneous manifestations of primary pulmonary coccidioidomycosis. Toxic erythema consisting of a maculopapular rash has been noted in some cases. Erythema nodosum (typically over the lower extremities) or erythema multiforme (usually in a necklace distribution) may occur; these manifestations are seen particularly often in women. Arthralgias and arthritis may develop. The diagnosis of primary pulmonary coccidioidomycosis is suggested by a history of night sweats or profound fatigue as well as by peripheral-blood eosinophilia or hilar or mediastinal lymphadenopathy on chest radiography. While pleuritic chest pain is common, pleural effusion is less so, occurring in fewer than 10% of cases. Such effusions are invariably associated with a pulmonary infiltrate on the same side. The cellular content of these effusions is mononuclear in nature; *Coccidioides* is rarely grown from effusions.

Although primary pulmonary coccidioidomycosis usually resolves without sequelae, several complications may ensue. Pulmonary nodules are residua of primary pneumonia. Generally single, located in the upper lobes, and ≤4 cm in diameter, nodules are often discovered on a routine chest radiograph in an asymptomatic patient. Calcification is uncommon.

Pulmonary cavities occur when a nodule extrudes its contents into the bronchus, resulting in a thin-walled shell. These cavities can be associated with persistent cough, hemoptysis, and pleuritic chest pain. Rarely, a cavity may rupture into the pleural space, causing pyopneumothorax. In such cases, patients present with acute dyspnea, and the chest radiograph reveals a collapsed lung with a pleural air-fluid level. Chronic or persistent pulmonary coccidioidomycosis manifests with prolonged symptoms of fever, cough, and weight loss and is radiographically associated with pulmonary scarring, fibrosis, and cavities. It occurs in fewer than 1% of patients, many of whom already have chronic lung disease of other etiologies.

In some cases, primary pneumonia presents as a diffuse reticulonodular pulmonary process (detected by plain chest radiography) in association with dyspnea and fever. Primary diffuse coccidioidal pneumonia may occur in settings of intense environmental exposure or profoundly suppressed cellular immunity, with unrestrained fungal growth that is frequently associated with fungemia.

Dissemination outside the thoracic cavity occurs in fewer than 1% of infected individuals. Dissemination is more likely to occur in males, particularly those of African-American or Filipino ancestry, and in persons with depressed cellular immunity, including patients with HIV infection and peripheral-blood CD4+ T-cell counts of <250/μL; those receiving chronic glucocorticoid therapy; those with allogeneic solid-organ transplants; and those being treated with tumor necrosis factor α antagonists. Women who acquire infection during the second or third trimester of pregnancy are also at risk for disseminated disease. Common sites for dissemination include the skin, bone, joints, soft tissues, and meninges. Dissemination may follow symptomatic or asymptomatic pulmonary infection and may involve only one site or multiple anatomic foci. When it occurs, clinical dissemination is usually evident within the first few months after primary pulmonary infection.

Meningitis, if untreated, is uniformly fatal. Patients usually present with a persistent headache, which is occasionally accompanied by lethargy and confusion. Nuchal rigidity, if present, is not severe. Examination of cerebrospinal fluid (CSF) demonstrates lymphocytic pleocytosis with profound hypoglycorrhachia and elevated protein levels. CSF eosinophilia is occasionally documented. With or without appropriate therapy, patients may develop hydrocephalus, which presents clinically as a marked decline in mental status, often with gait disturbances.

DIAGNOSIS

As mentioned above, coccidioidomycosis is often misdiagnosed as community-acquired bacterial pneumonia. Serology plays an important role in establishing the diagnosis of coccidioidomycosis. Several techniques are available, including the traditional tube-precipitin (TP) and complement-fixation (CF) assays, immunodiffusion (IDTP and IDCF), and enzyme immunoassay (EIA) to detect IgM and IgG antibodies. TP antibody is found in serum soon after infection and persists for weeks. TP titers are not useful for gauging disease progression, and this antibody is not found in the CSF. Titers of CF antibody generally rise later than do those of TP antibody, and CF antibody usually persists longer. Rising CF titers are associated with clinical progression, and the presence of CF antibody in CSF is an indicator for coccidioidal meningitis.

Because of its commercial availability, the coccidioidal EIA is frequently used as a screening tool for coccidioidal serology. However, the frequent false-positive results obtained with the IgM EIA make this test unreliable. Instead, the traditional TP or IDTP should be used. In addition, while the sensitivity and specificity of the IgG EIA appear to be high when compared with those of the CF and IDCF assays, the optical density obtained in the EIA does not correlate with the serologic titer of either of the latter tests.

Coccidioides grows within 3–7 days at 37°C on a variety of artificial media, including blood agar. Therefore, it is always useful to obtain samples of sputum or other respiratory fluids and tissues for culture in suspected cases of coccidioidomycosis. The clinical laboratory should be alerted to the possibility of this diagnosis, since *Coccidioides* can pose a significant hazard to laboratory workers if it is inadvertently inhaled. *Coccidioides* can also be identified directly. While treatment of samples with potassium hydroxide is rarely fruitful in establishing the diagnosis, examination of sputum or other respiratory fluids after Papanicolaou or Gomori methenamine silver staining reveals spherules in a significant proportion of patients with pulmonary coccidioidomycosis. For fixed tissues (e.g., those obtained from biopsy specimens), spherules with surrounding inflammation can be demonstrated with hematoxylin-eosin or Gomori methenamine silver staining.

℞ Treatment: COCCIDIOIDOMYCOSIS

(Table 104-1) Currently, there are two main classes of antifungals useful for the treatment of coccidioidomycosis. While once routinely prescribed, amphotericin B in all its formulations is now reserved for only the most severe cases of dissemination and for intrathecal or intraventricular administration to patients with coccidioidal meningitis in whom triazole therapy has failed. The original formulation of amphotericin B, which is dispersed with deoxycholate, is usually administered intravenously in doses of 0.7–1.0 mg/kg either daily or three times per week. The newer lipid-based formulations—amphotericin B lipid complex (ABLC), amphotericin B colloidal dispersion (ABCD), and amphotericin B liposomal complex—appear to offer no therapeutic advantage over the deoxycholate formulation but are associated with less renal toxicity. The lipid dispersions are administered intravenously at doses of 5 mg/kg daily or three times per week.

Triazole antifungals are the principal drugs now used to treat most cases of coccidioidomycosis. Clinical trials have demonstrated the usefulness of both fluconazole and itraconazole, and evidence indicates that itraconazole may be more efficacious against bone and joint disease. Because of its demonstrated penetration into CSF, fluconazole is the azole of choice for the treatment of coccidioidal meningitis. For both drugs, a minimal oral adult dosage of 400 mg/d should be used. The maximal dose of itraconazole is 200 mg three times daily, but higher doses of fluconazole may be given. Two newer triazole antifungals, posaconazole and voriconazole, are now available. However, given the paucity of clinical data, the high cost, and (particularly for voriconazole) the potential toxicity, these agents should be reserved for

TABLE 104-1

CLINICAL PRESENTATIONS OF COCCIDIOIDOMYCOSIS, THEIR FREQUENCY, AND RECOMMENDED INITIAL THERAPY FOR THE IMMUNOCOMPETENT HOST

CLINICAL PRESENTATION	FREQUENCY, %	RECOMMENDED THERAPY
Asymptomatic	60	None
Primary pneumonia (focal)	40	In most cases, none[a]
Diffuse pneumonia	<1	Amphotericin B followed by prolonged oral triazole therapy
Pulmonary sequelae	5	
Nodule	—	None
Cavity	—	In most cases, none[b]
Chronic pneumonia	—	Prolonged triazole therapy
Disseminated disease	≤1	
Skin, bone, joint, soft tissue	—	Prolonged triazole therapy[c]
Meningitis	—	Life-long triazole therapy[d]

[a]Treatment is indicated for hosts with depressed cellular immunity as well as for those with prolonged symptoms and signs of increased severity, including night sweats for >3 weeks, weight loss of >10%, a complement-fixation titer of >16, and extensive pulmonary involvement on chest radiography.

[b]Treatment (usually the oral triazoles fluconazole and itraconazole) is recommended for persistent symptoms.

[c]In severe cases, some clinicians would use amphotericin B as initial therapy.

[d]Intraventricular or intrathecal amphotericin B is recommended in cases of triazole failure. Hydrocephalus may occur, requiring a CSF shunt.

cases that remain recalcitrant when treated with fluconazole or itraconazole. High-dose triazole therapy may be teratogenic; thus, amphotericin B should be considered as therapy for coccidioidomycosis in pregnant women.

Most patients with focal primary pulmonary coccidioidomycosis require no therapy. Patients for whom antifungal therapy should be considered include those with underlying cellular immunodeficiencies and those with prolonged symptoms and signs of extensive disease. Specific criteria include symptoms persisting for ≥2 months, night sweats occurring for >3 weeks, weight loss of >10%, a serum CF antibody titer of >1:16, and extensive pulmonary involvement apparent on chest radiograph.

Diffuse pulmonary coccidioidomycosis represents a special situation. Because most patients with this form of disease are profoundly hypoxemic and critically ill, many clinicians favor beginning therapy with amphotericin B and switching to an oral triazole once clinical improvement occurs.

The nodules that may follow primary pulmonary coccidioidomycosis do not require treatment. However, nodules are not easily distinguished from pulmonary malignancies by means of radiographic imaging (including positron emission tomography scans). Close clinical follow-up and biopsy may be required to distinguish these two entities. Most pulmonary cavities do not require therapy. Antifungal treatment should be considered in patients with persistent cough, pleuritic chest pain, and hemoptysis. Occasionally, pulmonary coccidioidal cavities become secondarily infected. This development is usually manifested by an air-fluid level within the cavity. Bacterial flora or *Aspergillus* species are commonly involved, and therapy directed at these organisms should be considered. Surgery is rarely required except in cases of persistent hemoptysis or pyopneumothorax. For chronic pulmonary coccidioidomycosis, prolonged antifungal therapy—lasting for at least 1 year—is usually required, with monitoring of symptoms, radiographic changes, sputum cultures, and serologic titers.

Most cases of disseminated coccidioidomycosis require prolonged antifungal therapy. Duration of treatment is based on resolution of the signs and symptoms of the lesion in conjunction with a significant decline in serum CF antibody titer. Such therapy routinely is continued for at least several years. Relapse occurs in 15–30% of individuals once therapy is discontinued.

Coccidioidal meningitis poses a special challenge. While most patients with this form of disease respond to treatment with oral triazoles, 80% experience relapse when therapy is stopped. Thus, life-long therapy is recommended. In cases of triazole failure, intrathecal or intraventricular amphotericin B may be used. Installation requires considerable expertise and should be performed only by an experienced health care provider. Shunting of CSF in addition to appropriate antifungal therapy is required in cases of meningitis complicated by hydrocephalus. It is prudent to obtain expert consultation in all cases of coccidioidal meningitis.

PREVENTION

There are no proven methods to reduce the risk of acquiring coccidioidomycosis among residents of an endemic region. Avoidance of direct contact with uncultivated soil or with visible dust containing soil presumably reduces the risk. Prophylactic antifungal therapy may be useful in patients who have evidence of active or recent coccidioidomycosis and are about to undergo allogeneic solid-organ transplantation. Data on the use of antifungal agents for prophylaxis in other situations are scanty and do not suggest efficacy.

FURTHER READINGS

BERGSTROM L et al: Increased risk of coccidioidomycosis in patients treated with tumor necrosis factor alpha antagonists. Arthritis Rheum 50:1959, 2004

BLAIR JE et al: The prevention of recrudescent coccidioidomycosis after solid organ transplantation. Transplantation 83:1182, 2007

DiCaudo DJ et al: The exanthem of acute pulmonary coccidioidomycosis: Clinical and histopathologic features of 3 cases and review of the literature. Arch Dermatol 142:744, 2006

Drutz DJ, Catanzaro A: Coccidioidomycosis (parts I and II). Am Rev Respir Dis 117:559 and 727, 1978

Fisher MC et al: Molecular and phenotypic description of *Coccidioides posadasii* sp. nov., previously recognized as the non-California population of *Coccidioides immitis*. Mycologia 94:73, 2002

Galgiani JN et al: Coccidioidomycosis. Clin Infect Dis 41:1217, 2005

——— et al: Comparison of oral fluconazole and itraconazole for progressive, nonmeningeal coccidioidomycosis. A randomized, double-blind trial. Mycoses Study Group. Ann Intern Med 133:676, 2000

Park BJ et al: An epidemic of coccidioidomycosis in Arizona associated with climatic changes, 1998–2001. J Infect Dis 191:1981, 2005

Stevens DA et al: Posaconazole therapy for chronic refractory coccidioidomycosis. Chest 132:952, 2007

Valdivia L et al: Coccidioidomycosis as a common cause of community-acquired pneumonia. Emerg Infect Dis 12:958, 2006

CHAPTER 105

BLASTOMYCOSIS

Stanley W. Chapman ■ Donna C. Sullivan

Blastomycosis is a systemic pyogranulomatous infection, primarily involving the lungs, which arises after inhalation of the conidia of *Blastomyces dermatitidis*. Pulmonary blastomycosis varies from an asymptomatic infection to acute or chronic pneumonia. Hematogenous dissemination occurs frequently. Extrapulmonary disease of the skin, bones, and genitourinary system is common, but almost any organ can be infected.

ETIOLOGIC AGENT

B. dermatitidis is the asexual state of *Ajellomyces dermatitidis*. Two serotypes have been identified on the basis of the presence or absence of the A antigen. *B. dermatitidis* exhibits thermal dimorphism, growing as the mycelial phase at room temperature and as the yeast phase at 37°C. Primary isolation is most dependable for the mycelial phase incubated at 30°C. Definitive identification usually requires conversion to the yeast phase at 37°C or, more commonly, the use of nucleic acid amplification techniques (e.g., AccuProbe, Gen-Probe, San Diego, CA) that detect mycelial-phase growth. Yeast cells are usually 8–15 μm in diameter, have thick refractile cell walls, are multinucleate, and reproduce by a single, large, broad-based bud.

EPIDEMIOLOGY

Most cases of blastomycosis have been reported in North America. Endemic areas include the southeastern and south-central states bordering the Mississippi and Ohio river basins, the midwestern states and Canadian provinces bordering the Great Lakes, and a small area in New York and Canada along the St. Lawrence River. Outside North America, blastomycosis has been reported most frequently in Africa.

Early studies of endemic cases indicated that middle-aged men with outdoor occupations were at greatest risk. Reported outbreaks, however, do not suggest a predilection according to sex, age, race, occupation, or season. *B. dermatitidis* probably grows as microfoci in the warm, moist soil of wooded areas rich in organic debris. Exposure to soil, whether related to work or recreation, appears to be the common factor associated with infection.

PATHOGENESIS

After inhalation, the conidia of *B. dermatitidis* are susceptible to phagocytosis and killing in the lungs by polymorphonuclear leukocytes, monocytes, and alveolar macrophages. This phagocytic response represents innate immunity and probably explains the high frequency of asymptomatic infections in outbreaks. Conidia that escape phagocytosis rapidly convert to the yeast phase in tissue. The greater resistance of the thick-walled yeast form to phagocytosis and killing probably contributes to infection. This yeast-phase conversion also induces the expression of the 120-kDa glycoprotein BAD-1, which is an adhesin, an essential virulence factor, and the major epitope for humoral and cellular immunity. The primary acquired host defense against *B. dermatitidis* is cellular immunity mediated by antigen-specific T cells and lymphokine-activated macrophages.

Approach to the Patient: BLASTOMYCOSIS

Whether acute or chronic, blastomycosis mimics many other disease processes. For example, acute pulmonary blastomycosis may present with signs and symptoms indistinguishable from those of bacterial pneumonia or influenza. Chronic pulmonary blastomycosis most commonly mimics malignancy or tuberculosis. Skin lesions are often misdiagnosed as basal cell or squamous cell carcinoma, pyoderma gangrenosum, or keratoacanthoma. Laryngeal lesions are frequently mistaken for squamous cell carcinoma. Thus, the clinician must maintain a high index of suspicion and perform a careful histologic evaluation of secretions or biopsy material from patients who live in or have visited regions endemic for blastomycosis.

CLINICAL MANIFESTATIONS

Acute pulmonary infection is usually diagnosed in association with point-source outbreaks and is accompanied by the abrupt onset of fever, chills, pleuritic chest pain, arthralgias, and myalgias. Cough is initially nonproductive but frequently becomes purulent as disease progresses. Chest radiographs usually reveal alveolar infiltrates with consolidation. Pleural effusions and hilar adenopathy are uncommon. Most patients diagnosed with pulmonary blastomycosis have chronic indolent pneumonia with signs and symptoms of fever, weight loss, productive cough, and hemoptysis. The most common radiologic findings are alveolar infiltrates with or without cavitation, mass lesions that mimic bronchogenic carcinoma, and fibronodular infiltrates. Respiratory failure (adult respiratory distress syndrome) associated with miliary disease or diffuse pulmonary infiltrates is more common among immunocompromised patients, especially those in the late stages of AIDS (Chap. 90). Mortality rates are ≥50% among these patients, and most deaths occur within the first few days of therapy.

Skin disease is the most common extrapulmonary manifestation of blastomycosis. Two types of skin lesions occur: verrucous (more common) and ulcerative. Osteomyelitis is associated with as many as one-fourth of *B. dermatitidis* infections. The vertebrae, pelvis, sacrum, skull, ribs, or long bones are most frequently involved. Patients with *B. dermatitidis* osteomyelitis often present with contiguous soft-tissue abscesses or chronic draining sinuses. In men, blastomycosis may involve the prostate and epididymis. Central nervous system (CNS) disease occurs in <5% of immunocompetent patients with blastomycosis. In AIDS patients, however, CNS disease has been reported in ~40% of cases, usually presenting as a brain abscess. Less common forms of CNS disease are cranial or spinal epidural abscess and meningitis.

DIAGNOSIS

Definitive diagnosis of blastomycosis requires growth of the organism from sputum, pus, or biopsy material. A presumptive diagnosis is made by visualization of the characteristic broad-based budding yeast in clinical specimens. Serologic diagnosis of blastomycosis is of limited usefulness because of cross-reactivity with other fungal antigens.

A *Blastomyces* antigen assay that detects antigen in urine and serum is commercially available (Mira Vista Diagnostics, Indianapolis, IN). Antigen detection in urine appears to be more sensitive than serum antigen detection. This antigen test may be useful for monitoring of patients during therapy or for early detection of relapse.

℞ Treatment: BLASTOMYCOSIS

The Infectious Diseases Society of America has published guidelines for the treatment of blastomycosis. Selection of an appropriate therapeutic regimen must be based on the clinical form and severity of the disease, the immune status of the patient, and the toxicity of the antifungal agent (Table 105-1). Although spontaneous cures of acute pulmonary infection have been well documented, there are no criteria by which to distinguish patients whose disease will progress or disseminate. Thus, almost all patients with blastomycosis should be treated.

Itraconazole is the agent of choice for immunocompetent patients with mild to moderate pulmonary or non-CNS extrapulmonary disease. Therapy is continued for 6–12 months. Amphotericin B is the preferred initial treatment for patients who are severely immunocompromised, who have life-threatening disease or CNS disease, or whose disease progresses during treatment with itraconazole. Although not rigorously studied, lipid formulations of amphotericin B can provide an alternative for patients who cannot tolerate amphotericin B deoxycholate. Most patients with non-CNS disease whose clinical condition improves after an initial course of amphotericin B (usually 2 weeks in duration) can be switched to itraconazole to complete 6–12 months of therapy. Fluconazole, because of its excellent penetration of the CNS, may have a role in the treatment of patients with brain abscess or meningitis after an initial course of amphotericin B.

The newer triazoles voriconazole and posaconazole have not been studied extensively in human cases of blastomycosis. The echinocandins have variable activity against *B. dermatitidis* and have no place in the treatment of blastomycosis.

PROGNOSIS

Clinical and mycologic response rates are 90–95% among compliant immunocompetent patients given itraconazole for mild to moderate pulmonary and extrapulmonary disease without CNS involvement. Bone and joint disease usually requires 12 months of therapy. The <5% of infections that relapse after an initial course of itraconazole usually respond well to a second treatment course.

TABLE 105-1

TREATMENT OF BLASTOMYCOSIS

DISEASE	PRIMARY THERAPY	ALTERNATIVE THERAPY
Immunocompetent Patient/Life-Threatening Disease		
Pulmonary	AmB,[a] 0.7–1.0 mg/kg qd (total dose: 1.5–2.5 g)	Itraconazole, 200–400 mg/d (once patient's condition has stabilized)
Disseminated		
CNS	AmB, 0.7–1.0 mg/kg qd (total dose: at least 2 g)	Fluconazole, 800 mg/d (if patient is intolerant to full course of AmB)
Non-CNS	AmB, 0.7–1.0 mg/kg qd (total dose: 1.5–2.5 g)	Itraconazole, 200–400 mg/d (once patient's condition has stabilized)
Immunocompetent Patient/Non-Life-Threatening Disease		
Pulmonary or disseminated (non-CNS)	Itraconazole, 200–400 mg/d *or* AmB, 0.5–0.7 mg/kg qd (in patients intolerant to itraconazole or whose disease progresses despite therapy)	Fluconazole, 400–800 mg/d *or* Ketoconazole, 400–800 mg/d
Immunocompromised Patient[b]		
All infections	AmB, 0.7–1.0 mg/kg qd (total dose: 1.5–2.5 g)	Itraconazole, 200–400 mg/d (non-CNS disease, once clinically improved)

[a]In all regimens listed, an AmB lipid formulation (3.0–5.0 mg/kg qd) can be substituted for AmB deoxycholate.

[b]Suppressive therapy with itraconazole may be considered for patients whose immunocompromised state continues. Fluconazole (800 mg/d) may be useful for patients who have CNS disease or are intolerant to itraconazole.

Note: AmB, amphotericin B; CNS, central nervous system.

FURTHER READINGS

Bradsher RW: Blastomycosis, in *Clinical Mycology*, WE Dismukes et al (eds). New York, Oxford University Press, 2003, pp 299–310

——— et al: Blastomycosis. Infect Dis Clin North Am 17:21, 2003

Chapman SW: *Blastomyces dermatitidis*, in *Principles and Practice of Infectious Diseases*, 6th ed, GL Mandell et al (eds). New York, Churchill Livingstone, 2005, pp 3026–3040

———, Sullivan DC: Diagnosis and treatment of blastomycosis, in *Diagnosis and Treatment of Human Mycoses*, D Hospental, M Rinaldi (eds). Totowa, NJ, Humana Press, 2007

——— et al: Practice guidelines for the management of patients with blastomycosis. Clin Infect Dis 30:679, 2000 (updates: *www.idsociety.org*)

Deepe GS et al: Progress in vaccination for histoplasmosis and blastomycosis: Coping with cellular immunity. Med Mycol 43:381, 2005

Hussein R et al: Blastomycosis in the mountainous region of northeast Tennessee. Chest 135:1019, 2009

Lahm T et al: Corticosteroids for blastomycosis-induced ARDS: a report of two patients and review of the literature. Chest 133:1478, 2008

CHAPTER 106

CRYPTOCOCCOSIS

Arturo Casadevall

DEFINITION AND ETIOLOGY

Cryptococcus neoformans, a yeast-like fungus, is the etiologic agent of cryptococcosis. Cryptococcal strains are antigenically and genetically diverse. Both *C. neoformans* and *C. gattii* are pathogenic for humans and can cause cryptococcosis. *C. neoformans* consists of serotypes A and D, and *C. gattii* consists of serotypes B and C. Currently, most authorities further subdivide *C. neoformans* into two varieties: *grubii* (serotype A) and *neoformans* (serotype D). Most clinical microbiology laboratories do not routinely distinguish among cryptococcal species and varieties but rather identify all isolates simply as *C. neoformans.*

EPIDEMIOLOGY

Cryptococcosis was first described in the 1890s but remained relatively rare until the mid-twentieth century, when advances in diagnosis and increases in the number of immunosuppressed individuals markedly raised its reported prevalence. The spectrum of disease caused by *C. neoformans* consists predominantly of meningoencephalitis and pneumonia, but skin and soft tissue infections also occur. Serologic studies have shown that, although cryptococcal *infection* is common among immunocompetent individuals, cryptococcal *disease* (cryptococcosis) is relatively rare in the absence of impaired immunity. Individuals at high risk for cryptococcosis include patients with hematologic malignancies, recipients of solid organ transplants who require ongoing immunosuppressive therapy, persons whose medical conditions necessitate glucocorticoid therapy, and patients with advanced HIV infection and CD4+ T-lymphocyte counts of <200/μL. Since the onset of the HIV pandemic in the early 1980s, the overwhelming majority of cryptococcosis cases have occurred in patients with AIDS (Chap. 90). To understand the impact of HIV infection on the epidemiology of cryptococcosis, it is instructive to note that in the early 1990s there were >1000 cases of cryptococcal meningitis each year in New York City—a figure far exceeding that for all cases of bacterial meningitis. With the advent of effective antiretroviral therapy, the incidence of AIDS-related cryptococcosis has been sharply reduced among treated individuals; however, the disease remains distressingly common in regions where antiretroviral therapy is not readily available, such as Africa and Asia, where up to one-third of patients with AIDS have cryptococcosis.

Cryptococcal infection is acquired from the environment. *C. neoformans* and *C. gattii* inhabit different ecologic niches. *C. neoformans* is frequently found in soils contaminated with avian excreta and can easily be recovered from shaded and humid soils contaminated with pigeon droppings. In contrast, *C. gattii* is not found in bird feces. Instead, it inhabits a variety of arboreal species, including several types of eucalyptus tree. *C. neoformans* strains are found throughout the world; however, var. *grubii* (serotype A) strains are far more common than var. *neoformans* (serotype D) strains among both clinical and environmental isolates. The geographic distribution of *C. gattii* was thought to be largely limited to tropical regions until an outbreak of cryptococcosis caused by a new serotype B strain began in Vancouver in 1999. In addition to the different geographic distributions of the two cryptococcal species, individual susceptibility to these species affects epidemiology. Cryptococcosis caused by the *C. neoformans* varieties occurs mostly in individuals with AIDS (Chap. 90) and other forms of impaired immunity. In contrast, *C. gattii*–related disease is not associated with specific immune deficits and often occurs in immunocompetent individuals.

PATHOGENESIS

Cryptococcal infection is acquired by inhalation of aerosolized infectious particles. The exact nature of these particles is not known; the two leading candidate forms are small desiccated yeast cells and basidiospores. Little is known about the pathogenesis of initial infection. Serologic studies have shown that cryptococcal infection is acquired in childhood, but it is not known whether the initial infection is symptomatic. Given serologic documentation that cryptococcal infection is common yet cryptococcal disease is rare, the consensus is that pulmonary defense mechanisms in immunologically intact individuals are highly effective at containing *C. neoformans*. It is not clear whether initial infection leads to a state of immunity or whether most individuals are subject throughout life to frequent and recurrent infections that resolve without clinical disease. However, evidence indicates that some human cryptococcal infections lead to a state of latency in which viable organisms are harbored for prolonged periods, possibly in granulomas. Thus the inhalation of *C. neoformans* can be followed by clearance of the organism or establishment of the latent state. The consequences of prolonged harboring of *C. neoformans* in the lung are not known, but evidence from animal studies indicates that the organism's prolonged presence could alter the immunologic milieu in the lung and predispose to allergic airway disease.

Cryptococcosis usually presents clinically as chronic meningoencephalitis. The mechanisms by which *C. neoformans* undergoes extrapulmonary dissemination and enters the central nervous system (CNS) remain poorly understood. There is evidence that yeast cells can migrate directly across the endothelium by a mechanism that may be associated with changes in polysaccharide structure. *C. neoformans* has well-defined virulence factors that include the polysaccharide capsule, the ability to make melanin, and the elaboration of enzymes (e.g., phospholipase and urease) that enhance the survival of fungal cells in tissue. Among these virulence factors, the capsule and melanin production have been most extensively studied. The *C. neoformans* capsule is antiphagocytic, and the capsular polysaccharide has been associated with numerous deleterious effects on host immune function. Cryptococcal infections elicit little or no tissue inflammatory response. The immune dysfunction seen in cryptococcosis has been attributed to the release of copious amounts of capsular polysaccharide into tissues, where it probably interferes with local immune responses (Fig. 106-1). In clinical practice, the cryptococcal polysaccharide is the antigen that is measured as a diagnostic marker of *C. neoformans* infection.

Approach to the Patient: CRYPTOCOCCOSIS

Cryptococcosis should be included in the differential diagnosis when any patient presents with findings suggestive of chronic meningitis. Concern about cryptococcosis is heightened by a history of headache and neurologic symptoms in a patient with an underlying immunosuppressive disorder or state that is associated with an increased incidence of cryptococcosis, such as advanced HIV infection or solid organ transplantation.

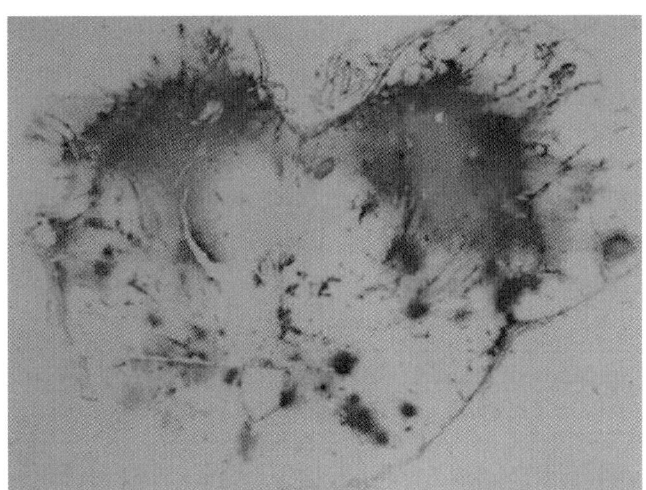

FIGURE 106-1

Cryptococcal antigen in human brain tissue, as revealed by immunohistochemical staining. Brown areas show polysaccharide deposits in the midbrain of a patient who died of cryptococcal meningitis. *(Reprinted with permission from SC Lee et al: Hum Pathol 27:839, 1996.)*

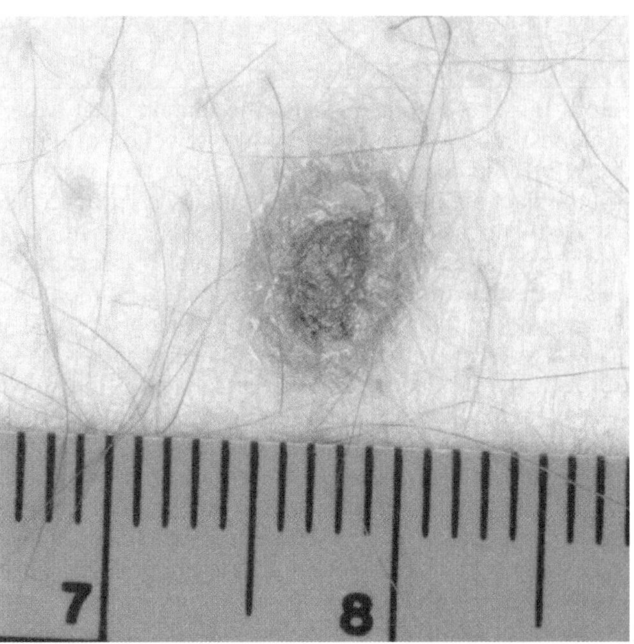

FIGURE 106-2

Disseminated fungal infection. A liver transplant recipient developed six cutaneous lesions similar to the one shown. Biopsy and serum antigen testing demonstrated *Cryptococcus*. Important features of the lesion include a benign-appearing fleshy papule with central umbilication resembling molluscum contagiosum. *(Photo courtesy of Dr. Lindsey Baden; with permission.)*

CLINICAL MANIFESTATIONS

The clinical manifestations of cryptococcosis reflect the site of fungal infection. *C. neoformans* infection can affect any tissue or organ, but the majority of cases that come to clinical attention involve the CNS and/or the lungs. CNS involvement usually presents as signs and symptoms of chronic meningitis, such as headache, fever, lethargy, sensorium deficits, memory deficits, cranial nerve paresis, vision deficits, and meningismus. Cryptococcal meningitis differs from bacterial meningitis in that many *Cryptococcus*-infected patients present with symptoms of several weeks' duration. In addition, classic characteristics of meningeal irritation, such as meningismus, may be absent in cryptococcal meningitis. Indolent cases can present as subacute dementia. Meningeal cryptococcosis can lead to sudden catastrophic vision loss.

Pulmonary cryptococcosis usually presents as cough, increased sputum production, and chest pain. Patients infected with *C. gattii* can present with granulomatous pulmonary masses known as *cryptococcomas*. Fever develops in a minority of cases. Like CNS disease, pulmonary cryptococcosis can follow an indolent course, and the majority of cases probably do not come to clinical attention. In fact, many cases are discovered incidentally during the workup of an abnormal chest radiograph obtained for other diagnostic purposes. Pulmonary cryptococcosis is often associated with antecedent diseases such as malignancy, diabetes, and tuberculosis.

Skin lesions are common in patients with disseminated cryptococcosis and can be highly variable, including papules, plaques, purpura, vesicles, tumor-like lesions, and rashes. The spectrum of cryptococcosis in HIV-infected patients is so varied and has changed so much since the advent of antiretroviral therapy that a distinction between HIV-related and HIV-unrelated cryptococcosis is no longer pertinent. In patients with AIDS and solid organ transplant recipients, the lesions of cutaneous cryptococcosis often resemble those of molluscum contagiosum (Fig. 106-2; Chaps. 84 and 90).

DIAGNOSIS

A diagnosis of cryptococcosis requires the demonstration of *C. neoformans* in normally sterile tissues. Visualization of the capsule of fungal cells in cerebrospinal fluid (CSF) mixed with India ink is a useful rapid diagnostic technique. *C. neoformans* cells in India ink have a distinctive appearance because their capsules exclude ink particles. However, the CSF India ink examination may yield negative results in patients with a low fungal burden. This examination should be performed by a trained individual, since leukocytes and fat globules can sometimes be mistaken for fungal cells. Cultures of CSF and blood that are positive for *C. neoformans* are diagnostic for cryptococcosis. In cryptococcal meningitis, CSF examination usually reveals evidence of chronic meningitis with mononuclear cell pleocytosis and increased protein levels. A particularly useful test is cryptococcal antigen (CRAg) detection in CSF and blood. The assay is based on serologic detection of cryptococcal polysaccharide and is both sensitive and specific. A positive cryptococcal antigen test provides strong presumptive evidence for cryptococcosis; however, because the result is often negative in pulmonary cryptococcosis, the test is less useful in the diagnosis of pulmonary disease.

℞ Treatment: CRYPTOCOCCOSIS

Both the site of infection and the immune status of the host must be considered in the selection of therapy for cryptococcosis. The disease has two general patterns of manifestation: (1) pulmonary cryptococcosis, with no evidence of extrapulmonary dissemination; and (2) extrapulmonary (systemic) cryptococcosis, with or without meningoencephalitis. Pulmonary cryptococcosis in an immunocompetent host sometimes resolves without therapy. However, given the propensity of *C. neoformans* to disseminate from the lung, the inability to gauge the host's immune status precisely, and the availability of low-toxicity therapy in the form of fluconazole, the current recommendation is for pulmonary cryptococcosis in an immunocompetent individual to be treated with fluconazole (200–400 mg/d for 3–6 months). Extrapulmonary cryptococcosis without CNS involvement in an immunocompetent host can be treated with the same regimen, although amphotericin B (AmB; 0.5–1.0 mg/kg daily for 4–6 weeks) may be required for more severe cases. In general, extrapulmonary cryptococcosis without CNS involvement requires less intensive therapy—with the caveat that morbidity and death in cryptococcosis are associated with meningeal involvement. Thus the decision to categorize cryptococcosis as "extrapulmonary without CNS involvement" should be made only after careful evaluation of the CSF reveals no evidence of *C. neoformans* infection. For CNS involvement in a host without AIDS or obvious immune impairment, most authorities recommend initial therapy with AmB (0.5–1.0 mg/kg daily) during an induction phase, which is followed by prolonged therapy with fluconazole (400 mg/d) during a consolidation phase. For cryptococcal meningoencephalitis without a concomitant immunosuppressive condition, the recommended regimen is AmB (0.5–1.0 mg/kg) plus flucytosine (100 mg/kg) daily for 6–10 weeks. Alternatively, patients can be treated with AmB (0.5–1.0 mg/kg) plus flucytosine (100 mg/kg) daily for 2 weeks and then with fluconazole (400 mg/d) for at least 10 weeks. Patients with immunosuppression are treated with the same initial regimens except that consolidation therapy with fluconazole is given for a prolonged period to prevent relapse.

Cryptococcosis in patients with HIV infection always requires aggressive therapy and is considered incurable unless immune function improves. Consequently, therapy for cryptococcosis in the setting of AIDS has two phases: induction therapy (intended to reduce the fungal burden and alleviate symptoms) and lifelong maintenance therapy (to prevent a symptomatic clinical relapse). Pulmonary and extrapulmonary cryptococcosis without evidence of CNS involvement can be treated with fluconazole (200–400 mg/d). In patients who have more extensive disease, flucytosine (100 mg/d) may be added to the fluconazole regimen for 10 weeks, with lifelong fluconazole maintenance therapy thereafter. For HIV-infected patients with evidence of CNS involvement, most authorities recommend induction therapy with AmB. An acceptable regimen is AmB (0.7–1.0 mg/kg) plus flucytosine (100 mg) daily for 2 weeks followed by fluconazole (400 mg/d) for at least 10 weeks and then by lifelong maintenance therapy with fluconazole (200 mg/d). Fluconazole (400–800 mg/d) plus flucytosine (150–100 mg/d) for 6–10 weeks followed by fluconazole (200 mg/d) as maintenance therapy can be used as an alternative. Lipid formulations of AmB can be substituted for AmB deoxycholate in patients with renal impairment. Neither caspofungin nor mycofungin is effective against *C. neoformans*, and neither drug has a role in the treatment of cryptococcosis. Cryptococcal meningoencephalitis is often associated with increased intracranial pressure, which is believed to be responsible for damage to the brain and cranial nerves. Appropriate management of CNS cryptococcosis requires careful attention to the management of intracranial pressure, including the reduction of pressure by repeated therapeutic lumbar puncture and the placement of shunts.

In HIV-infected patients with previously treated cryptococcosis who are receiving fluconazole maintenance therapy, it may be possible to discontinue antifungal drug treatment if antiretroviral therapy results in immunologic improvement. However, certain recipients of maintenance therapy who have a history of successfully treated cryptococcosis can develop a troublesome immune reconstitution syndrome when antiretroviral therapy produces a rebound in immunologic function.

PROGNOSIS AND COMPLICATIONS

Even with antifungal therapy, cryptococcosis is associated with high rates of morbidity and death. For the majority of patients with cryptococcosis, the most important prognostic factor is the extent and the duration of the underlying immunologic deficits that predisposed them to develop the disease. Therefore, cryptococcosis is often curable with antifungal therapy in individuals with no apparent immunologic dysfunction, but, in patients with severe immunosuppression (e.g., those with AIDS), the best that can be hoped for is that antifungal therapy will induce remission, which can then be maintained with lifelong suppressive therapy. Before the advent of antiretroviral therapy, the median overall survival period for AIDS patients with cryptococcosis was <1 year. Cryptococcosis in patients with underlying neoplastic disease has a particularly poor prognosis. For CNS cryptococcosis, poor prognostic markers are a positive CSF assay for yeast cells by initial India ink examination (evidence of a heavy fungal burden), high CSF pressure, low CSF glucose levels, low CSF pleocytosis (<2/μL), recovery of yeast cells from extraneural sites, the absence of antibody to *C. neoformans*, a CSF or serum cryptococcal antigen level of ≥1:32, and concomitant glucocorticoid therapy or hematologic malignancy. A response to treatment does not guarantee cure since relapse of cryptococcosis is common even among patients with relatively intact immune systems. Complications of CNS cryptococcosis include cranial nerve deficits, vision loss, and cognitive impairment.

PREVENTION

No vaccine is available for cryptococcosis. In patients at high risk (e.g., those with advanced HIV infection and CD4+ T lymphocyte counts of <200/μL), primary prophylaxis with fluconazole (200 mg/d) is effective in reducing the prevalence of disease. Since antiretroviral therapy raises the CD4+ T lymphocyte count, it constitutes an immunologic form of prophylaxis. However, cryptococcosis in the setting of immune reconstitution has been reported in patients with HIV infection and recipients of solid organ transplants.

FURTHER READINGS

Abert J et al: A pilot study of the discontinuation of antifungal therapy for disseminated cryptococcal disease in patients with acquired immunodeficiency syndrome, following immunologic response to antiretroviral therapy. J Infect Dis 185:1179, 2002

Chayakulkeeree M, Perfect JP: Cryptococcosis. Infect Dis Clin North Am 20:507, 2006

Liliang P et al: Use of ventriculoperitoneal shunts to treat uncontrollable intracranial hypertension in patients who have cryptococcal meningitis without hydrocephalus. Clin Infect Dis 34:E64, 2002

Lortholary O et al: Incidence and risk factors of immune reconstitution inflammatory syndrome complicating HIV-associated cryptococcosis in France. AIDS 19:1043, 2005

Masur H et al: Guidelines for preventing opportunistic infections among HIV-infected persons—2002. Ann Intern Med 137:435, 2002

Saag MS et al: Practice guidelines for the management of cryptococcal disease. Clin Infect Dis 30:710, 2000

Safdar N et al: Clinical problem-solving. Keeping an open mind. N Engl J Med 360:72, 2009

Singh N et al; Cryptococcal Collaborative Transplant Study Group: *Cryptococcus neoformans* in organ transplant recipients: Impact of calcineurin-inhibitor agents on mortality. J Infect Dis 195:756, 2007

Zonios DI et al: Cryptococcosis and idiopathic CD4 lymphocytopenia. Medicine (Baltimore) 86:78, 2007

CHAPTER 107

CANDIDIASIS

John E. Edwards, Jr.

The genus *Candida* encompasses more than 150 species, only a few of which cause disease in humans. With rare exceptions, the human pathogens are *C. albicans, C. guilliermondii, C. krusei, C. parapsilosis, C. tropicalis, C. kefyr, C. lusitaniae, C. dubliniensis,* and *C. glabrata.* Ubiquitous in nature, these organisms are found on inanimate objects, in foods, and on animals and are normal commensals of humans. They inhabit the gastrointestinal tract (including the mouth and oropharynx), the female genital tract, and the skin. Although cases of candidiasis have been described since antiquity in debilitated patients, the advent of *Candida* species as common human pathogens dates to the introduction of modern therapeutic approaches that suppress normal host defense mechanisms. Of these relatively recent advances, the most important is the use of antibacterial agents that alter the normal human microbial flora and allow nonbacterial species to become more prevalent in the commensal flora. With the introduction of antifungal agents, the causes of *Candida* infections shifted from an almost complete dominance of *C. albicans* to the common involvement of *C. glabrata* and the other species listed above. The non-*albicans* species now account for approximately half of all cases of candidemia and hematogenously disseminated candidiasis. Recognition of this change is clinically important, since the various species differ in susceptibility to the newer antifungal agents. In developed countries, where medical therapeutics are commonly used, *Candida* species are now among the most common nosocomial pathogens. In the United States, these species are the fourth most common isolates from the blood of hospitalized patients.

Candida is a small, thin-walled, ovoid yeast that measures 4–6 μm in diameter and reproduces by budding. Organisms of this genus occur in three forms in tissue: blastospores, pseudohyphae, and hyphae. *Candida* grows readily on simple medium; lysis centrifugation enhances its recovery from blood. Species are identified by biochemical testing (currently with automated devices) or on special agar.

PATHOGENESIS

In the most serious form of *Candida* infection, the organisms disseminate hematogenously and form microabscesses and small macroabscesses in major organs. Although the exact mechanism is not known, *Candida* probably enters the bloodstream from mucosal surfaces after growing to large numbers as a consequence of bacterial suppression by antibacterial drugs; alternatively, in some instances, the organism may enter from the skin. A change from the blastospore stage to the pseudohyphal and hyphal stages is generally considered integral to the organism's penetration into tissue. However, *C. glabrata* can cause extensive infection even though it does not transform into pseudohyphae or hyphae. Numerous reviews of cases of hematogenously disseminated candidiasis have identified the following predisposing factors or conditions: antibacterial agents, indwelling intravascular catheters, hyperalimentation fluids, indwelling urinary catheters, parenteral glucocorticoids, respirators, neutropenia, abdominal and thoracic surgery, cytotoxic chemotherapy, and immunosuppressive agents for organ transplantation. Patients with severe burns, low-birth-weight neonates, and persons using illicit IV drugs are also susceptible. HIV-infected patients with low CD4+ T cell counts and patients with diabetes are susceptible to mucocutaneous infection, which may eventually develop into the disseminated form when other predisposing factors are encountered. Women who receive antibacterial agents may develop vaginal candidiasis.

Innate immunity is the most important defense mechanism against hematogenously disseminated candidiasis, and the neutrophil is the most important component of this defense. Although many immunocompetent individuals have antibodies to *Candida*, the role of these antibodies in defense against the organism is not clear.

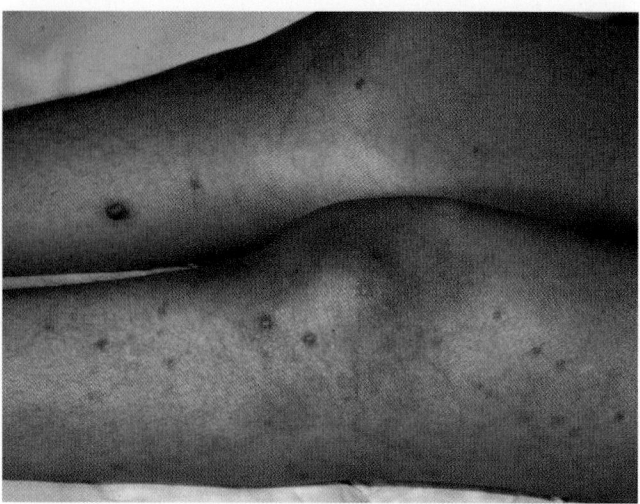

FIGURE 107-1

Macronodular skin lesions associated with hematogenously disseminated candidiasis. *Candida* organisms are usually but not always visible on histopathologic examination. The fungi grow when a portion of the biopsied specimen is cultured. Therefore, for optimal identification, both histopathology and culture should be performed. *(Image courtesy of Dr. Noah Craft and the Victor Newcomer collection at UCLA, archived by Logical Images, Inc.; with permission.)*

CLINICAL MANIFESTATIONS

Mucocutaneous Candidiasis

Thrush is characterized by white, adherent, painless, discrete or confluent patches in the mouth, tongue, or esophagus, occasionally with fissuring at the corners of the mouth. This form of *Candida* disease may also occur at points of contact with dentures. Organisms are identifiable in gram-stained scrapings from lesions. The occurrence of thrush in a young, otherwise healthy-appearing person should prompt an investigation for underlying HIV infection. More commonly, thrush is seen as a nonspecific manifestation of severe debilitating illness. Vulvovaginal candidiasis is accompanied by pruritus, pain, and vaginal discharge that is usually thin but may contain whitish "curds" in severe cases.

Other Candida *skin infections* include paronychia, a painful swelling at the nail-skin interface; onychomycosis, a fungal nail infection rarely caused by this genus; intertrigo, an erythematous irritation with redness and pustules in the skin folds; balanitis, an erythematous-pustular infection of the glans penis; erosio interdigitalis blastomycetica, an infection between the digits of the hands or toes; folliculitis, with pustules developing most frequently in the area of the beard; perianal candidiasis, a pruritic, erythematous, pustular infection surrounding the anus; and diaper rash, a common erythematous-pustular perineal infection in infants. Generalized disseminated cutaneous candidiasis, another form of infection that occurs primarily in infants, is characterized by widespread eruptions over the trunk, thorax, and extremities. The diagnostic macronodular lesions of hematogenously disseminated candidiasis (Fig. 107-1) indicate a high probability for dissemination to multiple organs as well as the skin. While the lesions are seen predominantly in immunocompromised patients treated with cytotoxic drugs, they may also develop in patients without neutropenia.

Chronic mucocutaneous candidiasis is a heterogeneous infection of the hair, nails, skin, and mucous membranes that persists despite intermittent therapy. The onset of disease usually comes in infancy or within the first two decades of life but in rare cases can come in later life. The condition may be mild and limited to a specific area of the skin or nails, or it may take a severely disfiguring form (*Candida* granuloma) characterized by exophytic outgrowths on the skin. The condition is usually associated with specific immunologic dysfunction; most frequently reported is a failure of T lymphocytes to proliferate or to stimulate cytokines in response to stimulation by *Candida* antigens in vitro. Approximately half of patients have associated endocrine abnormalities that together are designated the *a*utoimmune *p*oly*e*ndocrinopathy–*c*andidiasis–*e*ctodermal *d*ystrophy (APECED) syndrome. This syndrome is due to mutations in the autoimmune regulator (*AIRE*) gene and is most prevalent among Finns, Iranian Jews, Sardinians, northern Italians, and Swedes. Conditions that usually follow the onset of the disease include hypoparathyroidism, adrenal insufficiency, autoimmune thyroiditis, Graves' disease, chronic active hepatitis, alopecia, juvenile-onset pernicious anemia, malabsorption, and primary hypogonadism. In addition, dental enamel dysplasia, vitiligo, pitted nail dystrophy, and calcification of the tympanic membranes may occur. Patients with chronic mucocutaneous candidiasis rarely develop hematogenously disseminated candidiasis, probably because their neutrophil function remains intact.

Deeply Invasive Candidiasis

Deeply invasive *Candida* infections may or may not be due to hematogenous seeding. Deep esophageal infection may result from penetration by organisms from superficial esophageal erosions; joint or deep wound infection from contiguous spread of organisms from the skin; kidney infection from catheter-initiated spread of organisms through the urinary tract; infection of intraabdominal organs and the peritoneum from perforation of the gastrointestinal tract; and gallbladder infection from retrograde migration of organisms from the gastrointestinal tract into the biliary drainage system.

However, far more commonly, deeply invasive candidiasis is a result of hematogenous seeding of various organs as a complication of candidemia. Once the organism gains access to the intravascular compartment (either from the gastrointestinal tract or, less often, from the skin through the site of an indwelling intravascular catheter), it may spread hematogenously to a variety of deep organs. The brain, chorioretina (Fig. 107-2), heart, and kidneys are most commonly infected and the liver and spleen less commonly so (most often in neutropenic patients). In fact, nearly any organ can become involved, including the endocrine glands, pancreas, heart valves (native or prosthetic), skeletal muscle, joints (native or prosthetic), bone, and meninges. *Candida* organisms may also spread hematogenously to the skin and cause classic macronodular lesions (Fig. 107-1). Frequently, painful muscular involvement is also evident beneath the area of affected skin. Chorioretinal involvement and skin involvement are highly significant, since both findings are associated with a very high probability of abscess formation in multiple deep organs as a result of generalized hematogenous seeding. Ocular involvement (Fig. 107-2) may require specific treatment, such as partial vitrectomy to prevent permanent blindness. An ocular examination is indicated for all patients with candidemia, whether or not they have ocular manifestations.

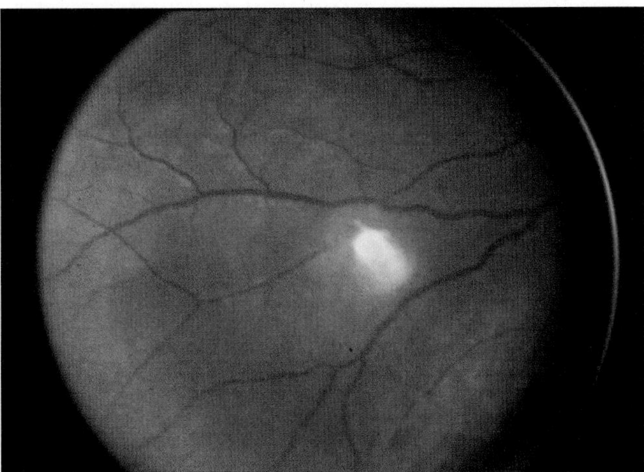

FIGURE 107-2
Hematogenous *Candida* endophthalmitis. A classic off-white lesion projecting from the chorioretina into the vitreous causes the surrounding haze. The lesion is composed primarily of inflammatory cells rather than organisms. Lesions of this type may progress to cause extensive vitreal inflammation and eventual loss of the eye. Partial vitrectomy, combined with IV and possibly intravitreal antifungal therapy, may be helpful in controlling the lesions. *(Image courtesy of Dr. Gary Holland; with permission.)*

DIAGNOSIS

The diagnosis of *Candida* infection is established by visualization of pseudohyphae or hyphae on wet mount (saline and 10% KOH), tissue Gram's stain, periodic acid–Schiff stain, or methenamine silver stain in the presence of inflammation. Absence of organisms on hematoxylin-eosin staining does not reliably exclude *Candida* infection. The most challenging aspect of diagnosis is determining which patients with *Candida* isolates have hematogenously disseminated candidiasis. For instance, recovery of *Candida* from sputum, urine, or peritoneal catheters may indicate mere colonization rather than deep-seated infection, and *Candida* isolation from the blood of patients with indwelling intravascular catheters may reflect inconsequential seeding of the blood from or growth of the organisms on the catheter. Despite extensive research into both antigen and antibody detection systems, there is currently no widely available and validated diagnostic test to distinguish patients with inconsequential seeding of the blood from those whose positive blood cultures represent hematogenous dissemination to multiple organs. Many studies are under way to establish the utility of the β-glucan test. Meanwhile, the presence of ocular or macronodular skin lesions is highly suggestive of widespread infection of multiple deep organs.

℞ Treatment: *CANDIDA* INFECTIONS

MUCOCUTANEOUS *CANDIDA* INFECTION The treatment of mucocutaneous candidiasis is summarized in Table 107-1.

CANDIDEMIA AND SUSPECTED HEMATOGENOUSLY DISSEMINATED CANDIDIASIS All patients with candidemia are now treated with a systemic antifungal agent. A certain percentage of patients, including many of those who have candidemia associated with an indwelling intravascular catheter, probably have "benign" candidemia rather than deep-organ seeding. However, because there is no reliable way to distinguish benign candidemia from deep-organ infection, and because antifungal drugs less toxic than amphotericin B are available, it has become the standard of practice to treat all patients with candidemia, whether or not there is clinical evidence of deep-organ involvement. In addition, if an indwelling intravascular catheter may be involved, it is best to remove or replace the device whenever possible.

TABLE 107-1

TREATMENT OF MUCOCUTANEOUS CANDIDAL INFECTIONS

DISEASE	PREFERRED TREATMENT	ALTERNATIVES
Cutaneous	Topical azole	Topical nystatin
Vulvovaginal	Oral fluconazole (150 mg) or azole cream or suppository	Nystatin suppository
Thrush	Clotrimazole troches	Nystatin
Esophageal	Fluconazole tablets (100–200 mg/d) or itraconazole solution (200 mg/d)	Caspofungin, micafungin, or amphotericin B

The drugs used for the treatment of candidemia and suspected disseminated candidiasis are listed in Table 107-2. Various lipid formulations of amphotericin B, three echinocandins, and the azoles fluconazole and voriconazole are used; no agent within a given class has been clearly identified as superior to the others. Most institutions choose an agent from each class on the basis of their own specific microbial epidemiology, strategies to minimize toxicities, and cost considerations. Unless azole resistance is considered likely, fluconazole is the agent of choice for the treatment of candidemia and suspected disseminated candidiasis in nonneutropenic, hemodynamically stable patients. Initial treatment in the context of likely azole resistance depends, as mentioned above, on the epidemiology of the individual hospital. For example, certain hospitals have a high rate of recovery of *C. glabrata*, while others do not. For hemodynamically unstable or neutropenic patients, initial treatment with broader-spectrum agents is desirable; these drugs include polyenes, echinocandins, or later-generation azoles such as voriconazole. Once the clinical response has been assessed and the pathogen specifically identified, the regimen can be altered accordingly. At present, the vast majority of *C. albicans* isolates are sensitive to fluconazole. Isolates of *C. glabrata* and *C. krusei* are less sensitive to fluconazole and more sensitive to polyenes and echinocandins. *C. parapsilosis* is less sensitive to echinocandins in vitro, although the clinical significance of this finding is not known.

Some generalizations about the management of specific *Candida* infections are possible. Recovery of *Candida* from sputum is almost never indicative of underlying pulmonary candidiasis and does not by itself warrant antifungal treatment. Similarly, *Candida* in the urine of a patient with an indwelling bladder catheter may represent colonization only rather than bladder or kidney infection; however, the threshold for systemic treatment is lower in severely ill patients in this category since it is not possible to distinguish colonization from lower or upper urinary tract infection. If the isolate is *C. albicans*, most clinicians use oral fluconazole rather than a bladder washout with amphotericin, which was more commonly used in the past. The significance of the recovery of *Candida* from abdominal drains in postoperative patients is also unclear, but again, the threshold for treatment is generally low because most of the affected patients have been subjected to factors predisposing to disseminated candidiasis.

Removal of the infected valve and long-term antifungal therapy constitute appropriate treatment for *Candida* endocarditis. Although definitive studies are not available, patients usually are treated for weeks with a systemic antifungal agent and then given chronic suppressive therapy for months or years (and sometimes indefinitely) with an oral azole.

Hematogenous *Candida* endophthalmitis is a special problem requiring ophthalmologic consultation. In lesions that are expanding or that threaten the macula, an IV polyene combined with flucytosine has been the regimen of choice. However, as more data on the azoles

TABLE 107-2

AVAILABLE AGENTS FOR THE TREATMENT OF DISSEMINATED CANDIDIASIS

AGENT	ROUTE OF ADMINISTRATION	COMMENT
Amphotericin B deoxycholate	IV only	Being replaced by lipid formulations
Amphotericin B lipid formulations		Not FDA approved as primary therapy, but used commonly because less toxic than amphotericin B deoxycholate; ABCD associated with frequent infusion reactions
Liposomal (AmBisome, Abelcet)	IV only	
Lipid complex (ABLC)	IV only	
Colloidal dispersion (ABCD)	IV only	
Azoles		
Fluconazole	IV and oral	Most commonly used
Voriconazole	IV and oral	Multiple drug interactions
Echinocandins		Broad spectrum against *Candida* species
Caspofungin	IV only	Approved for disseminated candidiasis
Anidulafungin	IV only	Approved for disseminated candidiasis
Micafungin	IV only	Under evaluation for disseminated candidiasis

Note: Although ketoconazole is approved for the treatment of disseminated candidiasis, it has been replaced by the newer agents listed in this table.

FDA, U.S. Food and Drug Administration.

and echinocandins become available, new strategies may evolve. Of paramount importance is the decision to perform a partial vitrectomy. This procedure debulks the infection and can preserve sight, which may otherwise be lost as a result of vitreal scarring. All patients with candidemia should undergo ophthalmologic examination because of the relatively high frequency of this ocular complication. Not only can this examination detect a developing eye lesion early in its course; in addition, identification of a lesion signifies a probability of ~90% of deep-organ abscesses and may prompt prolongation of therapy for candidemia beyond the recommended 2 weeks after the last positive blood culture.

Although the basis for the consensus is a very small data set, the recommended treatment for *Candida* meningitis is a polyene plus flucytosine. Successful treatment of *Candida*-infected prosthetic material (e.g., an artificial joint) nearly always requires removal of the infected material followed by long-term administration of an antifungal agent selected on the basis of the isolate's sensitivity and the logistics of administration.

PROPHYLAXIS

The use of antifungal agents to prevent *Candida* infections has been controversial, but some general principles have emerged. Most centers administer prophylactic fluconazole (400 mg/d) to recipients of allogeneic stem cell transplants. High-risk liver transplant recipients are also given fluconazole prophylaxis in most centers. The use of prophylaxis for neutropenic patients has varied considerably from center to center; most centers that elect to give prophylaxis to this population use either fluconazole or a comparatively low dose of an IV polyene—either amphotericin B deoxycholate or a lipid formulation of this agent. Some centers have used itraconazole suspension.

Prophylaxis is sometimes given to surgical patients at very high risk. The widespread use of prophylaxis in general surgical or medical intensive care units is not—and should not be—a common practice for three reasons: (1) the incidence of disseminated candidiasis is relatively low, (2) the cost-benefit ratio is suboptimal, and (3) increased resistance with widespread prophylaxis is a valid concern.

Prophylaxis for oropharyngeal or esophageal candidiasis in HIV-infected patients is not recommended unless there are frequent recurrences.

FURTHER READINGS

Edwards JE Jr: Candidiasis, in *Principles and Practice of Infectious Diseases*, 6th ed, GL Mandell et al (eds). Philadelphia, Elsevier Churchill Livingstone, 2005, pp 2938–2973

Falcone M et al: *Candida* infective endocarditis: Report of 15 cases from a prospective multicenter study. Medicine (Baltimore) 88:160, 2009

Gafter-Gvili A et al: Treatment of invasive candidal infections: systematic review and meta-analysis. Mayo Clin Proc 83:1011, 2008

Healy CM et al: Fluconazole prophylaxis in extremely low birth weight neonates reduces invasive candidiasis mortality rates without emergence of fluconazole-resistant *Candida* species. Pediatrics 121:703, 2008

Kauffman CA: Clinical efficacy of new antifungal agents. Curr Opin Microbiol 9:1, 2006

Maschmeyer G: The changing epidemiology of invasive fungal infections: New threats. Int J Antimicrob Agents 27(Suppl 1):3, 2006

Ostrosky-Zeichner L et al: Multicenter clinical evaluation of the (1→3) beta-D-glucan assay as an aid to diagnosis of fungal infections in humans. Clin Infect Dis 41:654, 2005

Pappas PG et al: Guidelines for treatment of candidiasis. Clin Infect Dis 38:161, 2004

Reboli AC et al: Anidulafungin versus fluconazole for invasive candidiasis. N Engl J Med 356:2472, 2007

Ruhnke M: Epidemiology of *Candida albicans* infections and role of non-*Candida-albicans* yeasts. Curr Drug Targets 7:495, 2006

Sobel JD: Current trends and challenges in candidiasis. Oncology (Williston Park) 18(Suppl 13):7, 2004

Spellberg BJ et al: Current treatment strategies for disseminated candidiasis. Clin Infect Dis 42:244, 2006

Tortorano AM et al: Candidaemia in Europe: Epidemiology and resistance. Int J Antimicrob Agents 27:359, 2006

CHAPTER 108

ASPERGILLOSIS

David W. Denning

Aspergillosis is the collective term used to describe all disease entities caused by any one of ~35 pathogenic and allergenic species of *Aspergillus*. Only those species that grow at 37°C can cause invasive infection, although some species without this capability can cause allergic syndromes. *A. fumigatus* is responsible for most cases of invasive aspergillosis, almost all cases of chronic aspergillosis, and most allergic syndromes. *A. flavus* is more prevalent in some hospitals and causes a higher proportion of cases of sinus and cutaneous infection and keratitis than *A. fumigatus*. *A. niger* can cause invasive infection but more commonly colonizes the respiratory tract and causes external otitis. *A. terreus* causes only invasive disease, usually with a poor prognosis. *A. nidulans* occasionally causes invasive infection, primarily in patients with chronic granulomatous disease.

EPIDEMIOLOGY AND ECOLOGY

Aspergillus has a worldwide distribution, most commonly growing in decomposing plant materials (i.e., compost) and in bedding. This hyaline (nonpigmented), septate, branching mold produces vast numbers of conidia (spores) on stalks above the surface of mycelial growth. Aspergilli are found in indoor and outdoor air, on surfaces, and in water from surface reservoirs. Daily exposures vary from a few to many millions of conidia; the latter high numbers of conidia are encountered in hay barns and other very dusty environments. The required size of the infecting inoculum is uncertain; however, only intense exposures (e.g., during construction work, handling of moldy bark or hay, or composting) are sufficient to cause disease in healthy immunocompetent individuals. Allergic syndromes may be exacerbated by continuous antigenic exposure arising from sinus or airway colonization or from nail infection. High-efficiency particulate air (HEPA) filtration is often protective against infection; thus HEPA filters should be installed and monitored for efficiency in operating rooms and in hospital environments that house very–high-risk patients.

The incubation period of invasive aspergillosis after exposure is highly variable, extending in documented cases from 2 to 90 days. Thus community-acquired acquisition of an infecting strain frequently manifests as invasive infection during hospitalization, although nosocomial acquisition is also common. Outbreaks usually are directly related to a contaminated air source in the hospital.

RISK FACTORS AND PATHOGENESIS

The primary risk factors for invasive aspergillosis are profound neutropenia and glucocorticoid use; risk increases with longer duration of these conditions. Higher doses of glucocorticoids increase the risk of both acquisition of invasive aspergillosis and death from the infection. Neutrophil and/or phagocyte dysfunction is also an important risk factor, as evidenced by aspergillosis in chronic granulomatous disease, advanced HIV infection, and relapsed leukemia. An increasing incidence of invasive aspergillosis in medical intensive care units suggests that, in patients who are not immunocompromised, temporary abrogation of protective responses as a result of glucocorticoid use or a general anti-inflammatory state is a significant risk factor. Many patients have some evidence of prior pulmonary disease—typically, a history of pneumonia or chronic obstructive pulmonary disease. Glucocorticoid use does not appear to predispose to invasive *Aspergillus* sinusitis but probably increases the risk of dissemination after pulmonary infection.

Patients with chronic pulmonary aspergillosis have a wide spectrum of underlying pulmonary disease, often tuberculosis or sarcoidosis. Patients are immunocompetent except that a genetic defect in mannose-binding protein is common, as are some cytokine regulation defects, most of which are consistent with an inability to mount an inflammatory immune (T_H1-like) response. Glucocorticoids accelerate disease progression.

Allergic bronchopulmonary aspergillosis (ABPA) is associated with certain HLA class II types; polymorphisms of interleukin (IL) 4Rα, IL-10, and SPA2 genes; and heterozygosity of the cystic fibrosis transmembrane conductance regulator (*CFTR*) gene. These associations suggest a strong genetic basis for the development of a T_H2-like and "allergic" response to *A. fumigatus*; this response probably is also protective against invasive disease, since high-dose glucocorticoid treatment for exacerbations of ABPA almost never leads to invasive aspergillosis.

CLINICAL FEATURES AND APPROACH TO THE PATIENT

(Table 108-1)

Invasive Pulmonary Aspergillosis

Both the frequency of invasive disease and the pace of its progression increase with greater degrees of immunocompromise (Fig. 108-1). Invasive aspergillosis is arbitrarily divided into acute and subacute forms that have courses of ≤1 month and 1–3 months, respectively. More than 80% of cases of invasive aspergillosis involve the lungs. The most common clinical features are no symptoms at all, fever, cough (sometimes productive), nondescript chest discomfort, trivial hemoptysis, and shortness of breath. Although the fever often responds to glucocorticoids, the disease progresses. The keys to early diagnosis in at-risk patients are a high index of suspicion, screening for circulating antigen, and urgent CT of the thorax.

Invasive Sinusitis

The sinuses are involved in 5–10% of cases of invasive aspergillosis, especially in patients with leukemia and recipients of hematopoietic stem cell transplants. In addition to fever, the most common features are nasal or facial discomfort, blocked nose, and nasal discharge (sometimes bloody). Direct examination of the interior of the nose reveals dusky or necrotic-looking tissue in any location. CT or MRI of the sinuses is essential but does not distinguish invasive *Aspergillus* sinusitis from pre-existing allergic sinusitis, bacterial sinusitis, or other fungal sinusitis early in the disease process.

Disseminated Aspergillosis

In the most severely immunocompromised patients, *Aspergillus* disseminates from the lungs to multiple organs—most often to the brain but also to the skin, thyroid, bone, kidney, liver, gastrointestinal tract, eye, and heart valve. Aside from cutaneous lesions, the most common features are gradual clinical deterioration over 1–3 days, with

TABLE 108-1

MAJOR MANIFESTATIONS OF ASPERGILLOSIS

	MAJOR MANIFESTATIONS IN INDICATED TYPE OF DISEASE			
ORGAN	INVASIVE (ACUTE AND SUBACUTE)	CHRONIC	SAPROPHYTIC	ALLERGIC
Lung	Angioinvasive in neutropenia, non-angioinvasive, granulomatous	Chronic cavitary, chronic fibrosing	Aspergilloma (single), airway colonization	Allergic bronchopulmonary, severe asthma with fungal sensitization, extrinsic allergic alveolitis
Sinus	Acute invasive	Chronic invasive, chronic granulomatous	Maxillary fungal ball	Allergic fungal sinusitis, eosinophilic fungal rhinosinusitis
Brain	Abscess, hemorrhagic infarction, meningitis, mycotic cerebral aneurysm	Granulomatous, meningitis	None	None
Skin	Acute disseminated, locally invasive (trauma, burns, IV access)	External otitis, onychomycosis	None	None
Heart	Endocarditis (native or prosthetic), pericarditis	None	None	None
Eye	Keratitis, endophthalmitis (postoperative and disseminated)	None	None	None described

low-grade fever and features of mild sepsis, and multiple nonspecific abnormalities in laboratory tests. In most cases, at least one localization becomes apparent. Blood cultures are not helpful since they are almost always negative.

Cerebral Aspergillosis

Hematogenous dissemination to the brain is a devastating complication of invasive aspergillosis. Single or multiple lesions may develop. In acute disease, hemorrhagic infarction is most typical, and cerebral abscess is common. Rarer manifestations include meningitis, mycotic aneurysm, and cerebral granuloma. Local spread also occurs, resulting in a single abscess. Postoperative infection from cranial sinuses is occasionally recorded and is exacerbated by glucocorticoid use after neurosurgery. The presentation can be either acute or subacute, with mood changes, focal signs, seizures, and decline in mental status. Cerebral granuloma can mimic a primary or secondary tumor. MRI is the most useful immediate

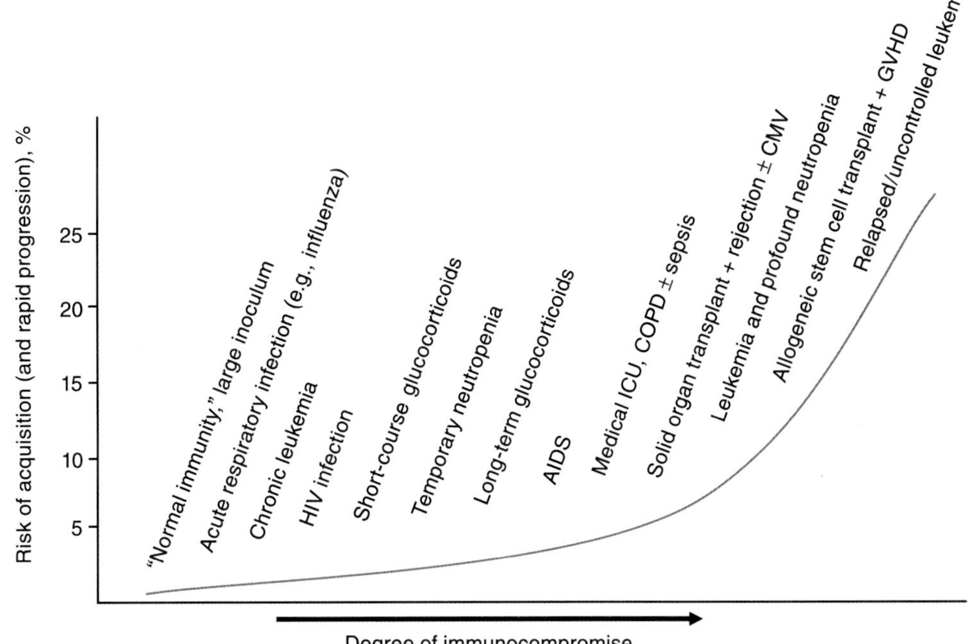

FIGURE 108-1

Invasive aspergillosis: conditions placing patients at elevated risk of acquisition and relatively rapid progression. ICU, intensive care unit; COPD, chronic obstructive pulmonary disease; CMV, cytomegalovirus; GVHD, graft-versus-host disease.

investigation; unenhanced CT of the brain is usually nonspecific, and contrast is often contraindicated in the affected patients because of poor renal function.

Endocarditis

Most cases of *Aspergillus* endocarditis are prosthetic valve infections resulting from contamination during surgery. Native valve disease is reported, especially as a feature of disseminated infection and in persons using illicit IV drugs. Culture-negative endocarditis with large vegetations is the most common presentation, but embolectomy reveals the diagnosis in a few cases.

Cutaneous Aspergillosis

Dissemination of *Aspergillus* occasionally results in cutaneous features, usually an erythematous or purplish nontender area that progresses to a necrotic eschar. Direct invasion of the skin occurs in neutropenic patients at the site of IV catheter insertion and in burn patients. Rapidly progressive local aspergillosis of the skin and underlying tissue may follow trauma, and wounds may become infected with *Aspergillus* after surgery.

Chronic Pulmonary Aspergillosis

The hallmark of chronic cavitary pulmonary aspergillosis (also called semi-invasive aspergillosis, chronic necrotizing aspergillosis, or complex aspergilloma) (Fig. 108-2) is one or more pulmonary cavities expanding over a period of months or years in association with pulmonary symptoms and systemic manifestations such as fatigue and weight loss. (Pulmonary aspergillosis developing over <3 months is better classified as subacute invasive aspergillosis.) Often mistaken initially for tuberculosis, almost all cases occur in patients with prior pulmonary disease (e.g., tuberculosis, atypical mycobacterial infection, sarcoidosis, ankylosing spondylitis, rheumatoid lung disease, pneumothorax, bullae) or prior lung surgery. The onset is insidious, and systemic features are sometimes more prominent than pulmonary symptoms. Cavities may have a fluid level or a well-formed fungal ball, but pericavitary infiltrates and multiple cavities—with or without pleural thickening—are typical. Antibodies to *Aspergillus* are almost always detectable in blood, usually as precipitating antibody and sometimes at high titers. Some patients have concurrent infections—even without a fungal ball—with atypical mycobacteria and/or other bacterial pathogens, such as *Staphylococcus aureus* or *Pseudomonas aeruginosa*. If untreated, chronic pulmonary aspergillosis typically progresses (sometimes relatively rapidly) to unilateral or upper-lobe fibrosis. This end-stage entity is termed *chronic fibrosing pulmonary aspergillosis*.

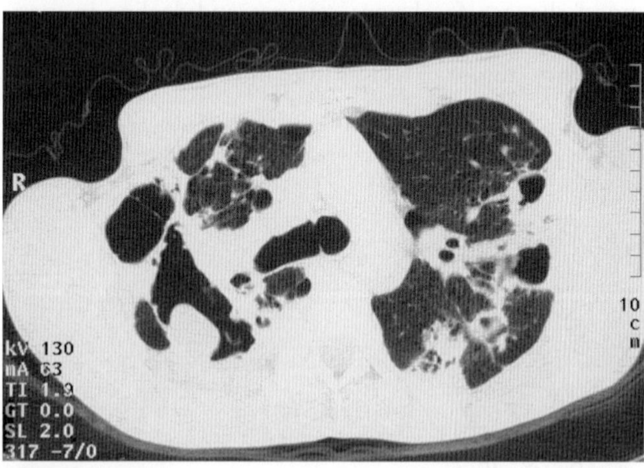

FIGURE 108-2

CT scan image of the chest in a patient with longstanding bilateral chronic cavitary pulmonary aspergillosis. He had a prior history of several bilateral pneumothoraces and required bilateral pleurodesis (1990). CT scan then demonstrated multiple bullae, and sputum cultures grew *A. fumigatus*. The patient had initially weakly and later strongly positive serum *Aspergillus* antibody tests (precipitins). This scan (2003) shows a mixture of thick- and thin-walled cavities in both lungs, with a large cavity containing a probable fungal ball protruding into the large cavity on the right. There is also considerable pleural thickening bilaterally.

Aspergilloma

Aspergilloma (fungal ball) occurs in up to 20% of residual chest cavities ≥2 cm in diameter. Some fungal balls remain stable in a single cavity for many years, and 10% resolve spontaneously. However, aspergillomas are often a feature of chronic pulmonary aspergillosis with its associated features. Signs and symptoms associated with single (simple) aspergillomas are minor, including a cough (sometimes productive), hemoptysis, wheezing, and mild fatigue. More significant signs and symptoms are associated with chronic cavitary pulmonary aspergillosis. The vast majority of fungal balls are caused by *A. fumigatus*, but *A. niger* has been implicated, particularly in diabetic patients; aspergillomas due to *A. niger* can lead to oxalosis with renal dysfunction. The most significant complication of aspergilloma is life-threatening hemoptysis, which may be the presenting manifestation.

Chronic Sinusitis

Three entities are subsumed under this broad label: sinus aspergilloma, chronic invasive sinusitis, and chronic granulomatous sinusitis. *Sinus aspergilloma* is limited to the maxillary sinus and consists of a chronic saprophytic entity in which the sinus cavity is filled with a fungal ball. This form of disease is associated with prior upper-jaw root canal work and chronic (bacterial) sinusitis. About 90% of CT scans show focal hyperattenuation related to concretions; on MRI scans, the T2-weighted signal is decreased, whereas that of bacterial sinusitis is increased. Removal of the fungal ball is curative. No tissue invasion is demonstrable histologically or radiologically.

In contrast, *chronic invasive sinusitis* is a slowly destructive process that most commonly affects the ethmoid and sphenoid sinuses but can involve any sinus. Patients are usually but not always immunocompromised to some degree (e.g., as a result of diabetes or HIV infection). Imaging of the cranial sinuses shows opacification of one or more sinuses, local bone destruction, and invasion of local structures. The differential diagnosis is wide, as numerous other fungi may cause a similar disease and sphenoid sinusitis is often caused by bacteria. Apart from a history of chronic nasal discharge and blockage, loss of the sense of smell, and persistent headache, the usual presenting features are related to local involvement of critical structures. The orbital apex syndrome (blindness and proptosis) is characteristic. Facial swelling, cavernous sinus thrombosis, carotid artery occlusion, pituitary fossa, and brain and skull base invasion have been described.

Chronic granulomatous sinusitis due to *Aspergillus* is most commonly seen in the Middle East and India and is often caused by *A. flavus*. It typically presents late, with facial swelling and unilateral proptosis. The prominent granulomatous reaction histologically distinguishes this disease from chronic invasive sinusitis, in which tissue necrosis with a low-grade mixed-cell infiltrate is typical.

Allergic Bronchopulmonary Aspergillosis

In almost all cases, ABPA represents a hypersensitivity reaction to *A. fumigatus*; rare cases are due to other aspergilli and other fungi. ABPA occurs in ~1% of patients with asthma and in up to 15% of adults with cystic fibrosis, and occasional cases are reported in patients without either of these diseases. Episodes of bronchial obstruction with mucous plugs leading to coughing fits, "pneumonia," consolidation, and breathlessness are typical. Many patients report coughing up thick sputum casts, usually brown or clear. Eosinophilia commonly develops before systemic glucocorticoids are given. The cardinal diagnostic tests include an elevated serum level of total IgE (usually >1000 IU/mL), a positive skin-prick test to *A. fumigatus* extract, or detection of *Aspergillus*-specific IgE and IgG (precipitating) antibodies. Central bronchiectasis is characteristic, but patients may present before it becomes apparent.

Severe Asthma with Fungal Sensitization (SAFS)

Many adults with severe asthma do not fulfill the criteria for ABPA and yet are allergic to fungi. Although *A. fumigatus* is a common allergen, numerous other fungi (e.g., *Cladosporium* and *Alternaria* spp.) are implicated by skin-prick testing and/or specific IgE radioallergosorbent (RAST) testing.

Allergic Sinusitis

Like the lungs, the sinuses manifest allergic responses to *Aspergillus* and other fungi. The affected patients present with chronic (i.e., perennial) sinusitis typically requiring multiple course of antibiotics that are of only limited benefit. Many of these patients have nasal polyps, and all have congested nasal mucosa and sinuses full of mucoid material. The histologic hallmark of allergic fungal sinusitis is local eosinophilia and the breakdown products of eosinophils, Charcot-Leyden crystals. Removal of abnormal mucus and polyps, with local and occasionally systemic administration of glucocorticoids, usually leads to resolution. Persistent or recurrent signs and symptoms may require more extensive surgery (ethmoidectomy) and possibly local antifungal therapy.

Superficial Aspergillosis

Aspergillus can cause keratitis and otitis externa. The former may be difficult to diagnose early enough to save the patient's sight. Treatment requires local surgical debridement as well as both systemic and topical antifungal therapy. Otitis externa is a common problem for which local debridement and local application of antifungal agents constitute the most common approach to treatment.

DIAGNOSIS

Several techniques are required to establish the diagnosis of any form of aspergillosis with confidence. Patients with acute invasive aspergillosis have a relatively heavy load of fungus in the affected organ; thus culture, molecular diagnosis, antigen detection, and histopathology usually confirm the diagnosis. However, the pace of progression leaves only a narrow window for making the diagnosis without losing the patient, and some invasive procedures are not possible because of coagulopathy, respiratory compromise, and other factors. Currently, ~40% of cases of invasive aspergillosis are missed clinically and are diagnosed only at autopsy. Histologic examination of affected tissue reveals either infarction, with invasion of blood vessels by many fungal hyphae, or acute necrosis, with limited inflammation and hyphae. *Aspergillus* hyphae are hyaline, narrow, and septate, with branching at 45°; no yeast forms are present in infected tissue. Hyphae can be seen in cytology or microscopy preparations, which therefore provide a rapid means of presumptive diagnosis.

Culture is important in confirming the diagnosis, given that multiple other (rarer) fungi can mimic *Aspergillus* spp. histologically. Bacterial agar is less sensitive than fungal media for culture. Thus, if physicians do not request fungal culture, the diagnosis may be missed. Culture may be falsely positive (e.g., in patients whose airways are colonized by *Aspergillus*) or falsely negative. Only 10–30% of patients with invasive aspergillosis have a positive culture at any time. Molecular diagnostic techniques promise to be both faster and more sensitive than culture.

The *Aspergillus* antigen test relies on detection of galactomannan release from *Aspergillus* spp. during growth. Antigen testing in high-risk patients is best done prospectively, as positive results usually precede clinical or radiologic features by several days. Antigen testing may be falsely positive in patients receiving certain β-lactam/β-lactamase inhibitor antibiotic combinations, such as tazocillin/sulbactam and amoxicillin/ clavulanic acid; in these cases, a second test is required for confirmation. Antigen testing and molecular testing on bronchoalveolar lavage fluid and cerebrospinal fluid are useful if performed before antifungal therapy has been given for more than a few days. The sensitivity of antigen detection is reduced by antifungal prophylaxis.

Definitive confirmation of the diagnosis requires (1) a positive culture of a sample taken directly from an ordinarily sterile site (e.g., a brain abscess) or (2) positive results of both histologic testing and culture of a sample taken from an affected organ (e.g., sinuses or skin). Most diagnoses of invasive aspergillosis are inferred from fewer data, including the presence of the *halo sign* on a high-resolution thoracic CT scan, in which a localized ground-glass appearance representing hemorrhagic infarction surrounds a nodule. While a halo sign may be produced by other fungi, *Aspergillus* spp. are by far the most common cause. Halo signs are present for ~7 days early in the course of infection in neutropenic patients and are a good prognostic feature. Thick CT sections can give the false appearance of a halo sign, as can other technical factors. Other common radiologic features of invasive pulmonary aspergillosis include pleural-based infarction or cavitation.

For chronic invasive aspergillosis, *Aspergillus* antibody testing is invaluable although relatively imprecise. Titers fall with successful therapy. Cultures are infrequently positive. Some patients with chronic pulmonary aspergillosis also have elevated titers of total serum IgE and *Aspergillus*-specific IgE.

ABPA and SAFS are diagnosed serologically or with skin-prick tests. Allergic *Aspergillus* sinusitis is usually diagnosed histologically, although precipitating antibodies in blood may also be useful.

℞ Treatment: ASPERGILLOSIS

Antifungal drugs active against *Aspergillus* include voriconazole, itraconazole, posaconazole, caspofungin, micafungin, and amphotericin B. Initial IV administration is preferred for acute invasive aspergillosis and oral administration for all other disease that requires antifungal therapy. Current recommendations are shown in Table 108-2. Voriconazole is the preferred agent for invasive aspergillosis; caspofungin, posaconazole, and lipid-associated amphotericin B are second-line agents. Amphotericin B is not active against *A. terreus* or *A. nidulans*. An infectious disease consultation is advised for patients with invasive disease, given the complexity of management. It is not clear whether combination therapy for acute invasive aspergillosis is beneficial, but it is widely used for very ill patients and for those with a poor prognosis. Commonly used combinations include an azole with either caspofungin or micafungin. The interactions of voriconazole and itraconazole with many drugs must be considered before these agents are prescribed. In addition, the effects of both drugs vary substantially from one patient to another, and many authorities recommend monitoring to ensure that drug concentrations are adequate but not excessive. The duration of therapy for invasive aspergillosis varies from ~3 months to several years, depending on the patient's immune status and response to therapy. Relapse occurs if the response is suboptimal and immune reconstitution is not complete.

Itraconazole is the preferred oral agent for chronic and allergic forms of aspergillosis. Voriconazole and posaconazole can be substituted when failure, emergence of resistance, or adverse events occur. An itraconazole dose of 200 mg twice daily is recommended, with monitoring of drug concentrations in the blood. Chronic cavitary pulmonary aspergillosis probably requires lifelong therapy, whereas the duration of treatment for other forms of chronic and allergic aspergillosis requires case-by-case evaluation.

Resistance to one or more azoles, although uncommon, may develop during long-term treatment, and a positive culture during antifungal therapy is an indication for susceptibility testing. Glucocorticoids should be used with caution in chronic cavitary pulmonary aspergillosis.

Surgical treatment is important in several forms of aspergillosis, including maxillary fungal ball and single aspergillomas, in which surgery is curative; invasive aspergillosis involving bone, heart valve, sinuses, proximal areas of the lung, and areas impinging on the great vessels; brain abscess; keratitis; and endophthalmitis. In allergic fungal sinusitis, removal of abnormal mucus and polyps, with local and occasionally systemic glucocorticoid treatment, usually leads to resolution. Persistent or recurrent signs and symptoms may require more extensive surgery (ethmoidectomy) and possibly local antifungal therapy. Surgery is problematic in chronic pulmonary aspergillosis, usually resulting in serious complications. Bronchial artery embolization is preferred for problematic hemoptysis.

PROPHYLAXIS

In situations in which moderate or high risk is predicted (e.g., after induction therapy for acute myeloid leukemia), the need for antifungal prophylaxis for superficial and systemic candidiasis and for invasive aspergillosis is generally accepted. Fluconazole is commonly used in these situations but has no activity against *Aspergillus* spp. Itraconazole capsules are ineffective, and itraconazole solution offers only modest efficacy. Posaconazole solution is probably more effective. Some data support the use of IV low-dose micafungin. No prophylactic regimen is completely successful.

OUTCOME

Invasive aspergillosis is curable if immune reconstitution occurs, whereas allergic and chronic forms are not. The mortality rate for invasive aspergillosis is ~50% if the infection is diagnosed and treated but is 100% if the diagnosis is missed. Cerebral aspergillosis, *Aspergillus* endocarditis, and bilateral extensive invasive pulmonary aspergillosis have very poor outcomes, as does invasive infection in patients with late-stage AIDS, patients with relapsed uncontrolled leukemia, and recipients of allogeneic hematopoietic stem cell transplants.

TABLE 108-2

TREATMENT OF ASPERGILLOSIS

INDICATION	PRIMARY TREATMENT	EVIDENCE LEVEL[a]	PRECAUTIONS	SECONDARY TREATMENT	COMMENTS
Invasive[a]	Voriconazole	AI	Drug interactions (especially with rifampin), renal failure (IV only)	Amphotericin B, caspofungin, posaconazole, micafungin	As primary therapy, voriconazole carries 20% more responses than amphotericin B. If azole prophylaxis fails, it is unclear whether a class change is required for therapy.
Prophylaxis	Itraconazole solution, posaconazole	AI	Diarrhea and vomiting with itraconazole, vincristine interaction	Micafungin, aerosolized amphotericin B	Some centers monitor plasma levels of itraconazole.
ABPA	Itraconazole	AI	Some glucocorticoid interactions, including with inhaled formulations	Voriconazole	Long-term therapy is helpful in most patients. Others can discontinue treatment. No evidence indicates whether or not therapy modifies progression to bronchiectasis/fibrosis.
Single aspergilloma	Surgery	BII	Multicavity disease: poor outcome of surgery; medical therapy preferable	Itraconazole, voriconazole, intracavity amphotericin B	Single large cavities with an aspergilloma are best resected.
Chronic pulmonary[b]	Itraconazole	BII	Poor absorption of capsules with proton pump inhibitors or H_2 blockers	Voriconazole, IV amphotericin B	Resistance may emerge during treatment, especially if plasma drug levels are subtherapeutic.

Note: The oral dose is usually 200 mg bid for voriconazole and itraconazole and 400 mg bid for posaconazole. The IV dose of voriconazole is 6 mg/kg twice at 12-h intervals (loading doses) followed by 4 mg/kg q12h. Plasma monitoring is helpful in optimizing the dosage. Caspofungin is given as a single loading dose of 70 mg, followed by 50 mg/d; some authorities use 70 mg/d for patients weighing >80 kg, and lower doses are required with hepatic dysfunction. Micafungin is given as 50 mg/d for prophylaxis and as at least 150 mg/d for treatment; this drug is not yet approved by the U.S. Food and Drug Administration (FDA) for this indication. Amphotericin B deoxycholate is given at a daily dose of 1 mg/kg if tolerated. Several strategies are available for minimizing renal dysfunction. Lipid-associated amphotericin B is given at 3 mg/kg (AmBisome) or 5 mg/kg (Abelcet). Different regimens are available for aerosolized amphotericin B, but none is FDA approved. Other considerations that may alter dose selection or route include age; concomitant medications; renal, hepatic, or intestinal dysfunction; and drug tolerability.

[a]Evidence levels are those used in treatment guidelines (Stevens DA et al: Practice guidelines for diseases caused by *Aspergillus*. Clin Infect Dis 30:696, 2000).

[b]An infectious disease consultation is appropriate for these patients.

FURTHER READINGS

Agarwal R: Allergic bronchopulmonary aspergillosis. Chest 135:805, 2009

Bochud PY et al: Toll-like receptor 4 polymorphisms and aspergillosis in stem-cell transplantation. N Engl J Med 359:1766, 2008

Camuset J et al: Treatment of chronic pulmonary aspergillosis by voriconazole in nonimmunocompromised patients. Chest 131:1435, 2007

Clancy CJ et al: Bronchoalveolar lavage galactomannan in diagnosis of invasive aspergillosis among solid-organ transplant recipients. J Clin Microbiol 45:1759, 2007

Denning DW et al: The link between fungi and asthma—a summary of the evidence. Eur Respir J 27:615, 2006

Herbrecht R et al: Voriconazole versus amphotericin B for primary therapy of invasive aspergillosis. N Engl J Med 347:408, 2002

Hope WW et al: Laboratory diagnosis of invasive aspergillosis. Lancet Infect Dis 9:609, 2005

——— et al: The invasive and saprophytic syndromes due to *Aspergillus* spp. Med Mycol 43(Suppl 1):S207, 2005

Meersseman W et al: Invasive aspergillosis in the intensive care unit. Clin Infect Dis 45:205, 2007

Moss RB: Pathophysiology and immunology of allergic bronchopulmonary aspergillosis. Med Mycol 43(Suppl 1):S203, 2005

Pasqualotto AC, Denning DW: Post-operative aspergillosis. Clin Microbiol Rev 12:1060, 2006

Tekaia F, Latge JP: *Aspergillus fumigatus*: Saprophyte or pathogen? Curr Opin Microbiol 8:385, 2005

CHAPTER 109

MUCORMYCOSIS

Alan M. Sugar

Mucormycosis (also called *zygomycosis*) is a serious, relatively uncommon invasive fungal infection and one of the most aggressive and lethal invasive mycoses. Physicians caring for patients with diabetes mellitus, immunocompromise (including that following organ transplantation), or iron overload syndromes (particularly those associated with hemodialysis) should be acutely aware of the enhanced susceptibility of these individuals to infection with the Mucorales. Timely diagnosis is critical to survival and minimization of morbidity. Institution of aggressive surgical and medical therapy is critical in maximizing the likelihood of a good outcome. Delay in considering the diagnosis and instituting appropriate therapeutic measures results in increasingly severe disfigurement at best and in death at worst.

ETIOLOGY

Fungi from the order Mucorales are the etiologic agents of mucormycosis. Despite the name of this infection, *Mucor* is not the most common genus recovered from patients. Rather, *Rhizopus* and *Rhizomucor* are the genera usually cultured from tissue samples. Other, less common fungi, including *Absidia*, *Cunninghamella*, *Apophysomyces*, and *Saksenaea*, are increasingly being isolated and, for the most part, cause similar clinical syndromes. Thus, there is no specific clinical feature that permits identification of the precise fungus involved. Submission of appropriate biopsy material to the microbiology laboratory is mandatory to ensure a pathogen's identification.

PATHOGENESIS

Mucorales are found commonly in the environment, and spores of these usually nonpathogenic fungi are likely to be inhaled daily. In the normal human lung, spores are inhibited from germinating into hyphae by alveolar macrophages. However, in diabetic patients, especially those with elevated blood sugar levels and acidemia, the spores germinate, hyphae develop (Fig. 109-1), and the fungi begin an inexorable march throughout the lung tissue, invading blood vessels and surrounding tissues. As blood vessels become involved, thrombosis occurs, tissue necrosis results, and the fungi continue to grow in this devitalized tissue. The use of deferoxamine to treat iron overload is a risk factor for mucormycosis; the siderophore supplies the fungi with iron that enhances their growth.

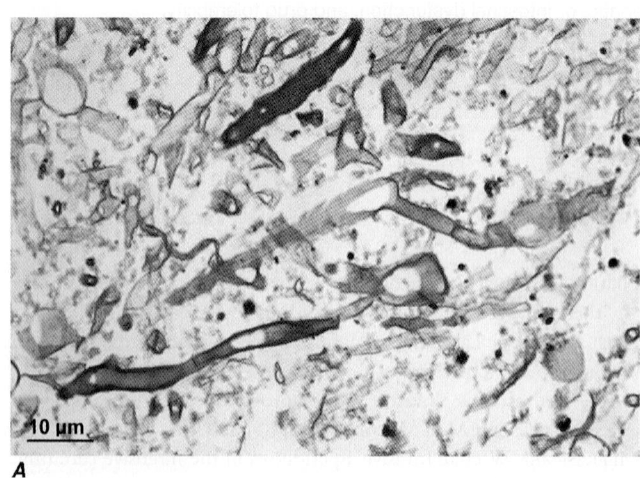

A

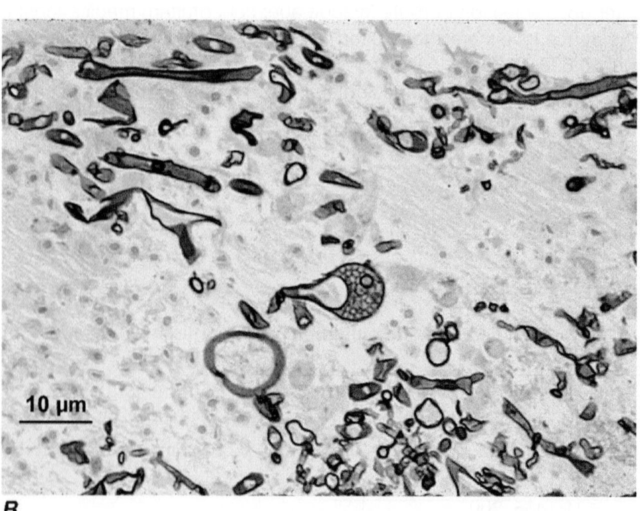

B

FIGURE 109-1

A. Hematoxylin and eosin–stained section of lung tissue showing the broad, infrequently septate, thin-walled hyphae of *Absidia corymbifera*. ***B.*** Grocott's methenamine silver–stained section of lung tissue showing typical zygomycete hyphae of *A. corymbifera. (Courtesy of David Ellis, PhD, Mycology Unit, Women's and Children's Hospital, Adelaide, Australia; with permission.)*

Spores settle in the upper airways, lower airways, or gastrointestinal tract and can spread beyond the initial site of infection, causing disseminated mucormycosis. Increasingly, patients are presenting with extensive cutaneous involvement after direct implantation of spores into the skin as a result of trauma (e.g., that sustained in a motor vehicle accident). The pathology in all these sites is the same, with blood vessel invasion and tissue necrosis as hallmarks and specific organ dysfunction depending on the location of the infection.

CLINICAL MANIFESTATIONS

The manifestations of mucormycosis depend on the site of infection. Patients with *rhinocerebral mucormycosis* may present with symptoms typical of sinusitis. However, progression of symptoms over several days indicates a more serious process than the more common bacterial or viral sinusitis. As the infection spreads, hypesthesia or numbness of the face overlying the infection may develop. Concomitant symptoms include headache, bloody nasal discharge, and changes in mental status. The black eschar of the palate is widely described as a hallmark of rhinocerebral mucormycosis, but the astute clinician will recognize earlier manifestations of this end-stage lesion reflecting invasion of the palate. These subtler lesions, which may consist of discolored, often hyperemic areas on the palate, will, if untreated, progress rapidly to the commonly recognized black eschar, which indicates angioinvasion and tissue necrosis. Involvement of the orbit (Fig. 109-2) compromises proper ocular-muscle function and normal movement of the eye within the skull, resulting in double vision. If the blood supply to the eye is affected by invasion of the retinal artery, blindness develops, often quite rapidly. Proptosis and ptosis are late findings reflecting a mass lesion within the orbit and cranial nerve involvement, respectively. Progression of the infection into the brain results in the formation of brain abscesses and phlegmon; symptoms and signs depend on the location of these lesions. Cavernous sinus thrombosis is an ominous sign. CT and MRI reveal sinus opacification and destruction of contiguous bone, and brain involvement can be readily appreciated.

Pulmonary mucormycosis presents as severe, progressive, tissue-destructive pneumonia. Neutropenia is a common predisposing factor. A high fever and a critical clinical condition are typical. Cavitation of involved lung develops rapidly, and hematogenous spread beyond the lungs to the brain and other organs may occur.

Gastrointestinal mucormycosis occurs primarily in those patients with protein-calorie malnutrition and usually presents as a perforated viscus. Premortem diagnosis is rare, and most patients with this form of mucormycosis do not survive.

Cutaneous mucormycosis is more common than disease at other sites and develops after traumatic injuries in which wounds are contaminated with dirt. Areas of tissue necrosis enlarge rapidly, involving all layers of the skin and underlying structures.

DIAGNOSIS

Laboratory Features

There are no pathognomonic hematologic changes. The abnormalities that are found reflect underlying predisposing conditions (e.g., diabetic ketoacidosis) and general indications of infection, such as elevated white blood cell counts and acute-phase reactant levels. Blood cultures are virtually always negative.

Microscopic examination and culture of biopsy samples from the involved area are critical in making an accurate diagnosis. As much tissue as possible should be submitted to the microbiology and histopathology laboratories.

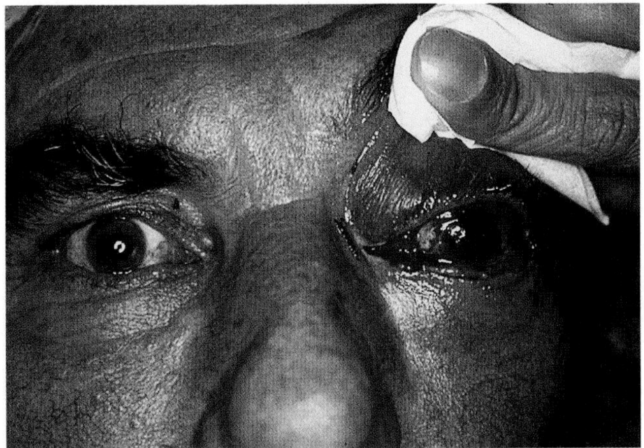

A

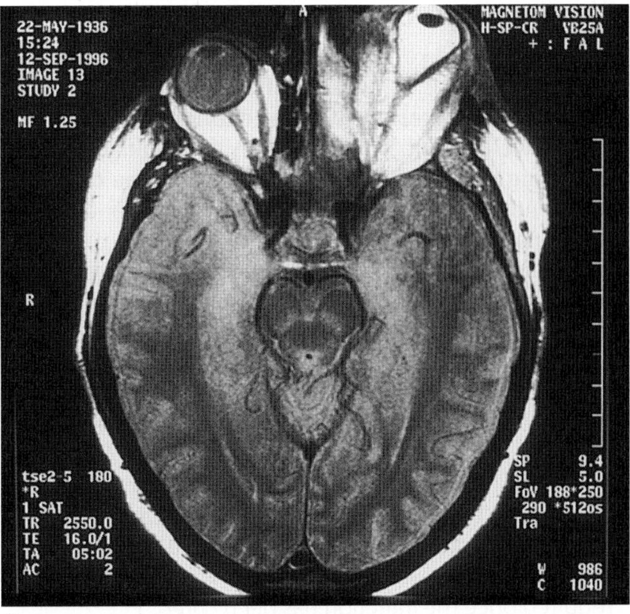

B

FIGURE 109-2

A. Rhinocerebral zygomycosis caused by *Rhizopus oryzae*, with extensive involvement of the orbit. ***B.*** Associated MRI scan. *(Courtesy of David Ellis, PhD, Mycology Unit, Women's and Children's Hospital, Adelaide, Australia; with permission.)*

Swabs are insufficient. These fungi grow rapidly and are usually visible on culture plates within a day or two. Their identification is based on traditional morphologic features. Fixed tissue samples are treated with special stains for fungi; for example, Gomori methenamine silver stains the fungi black against a green background, and periodic acid–Schiff stains the hyphae red. Mucorales appear as broad (diameter, 6–50 μm), usually nonseptate hyphae with branches at right angles; the organisms are often described as ribbon-like. Hyphae cut and viewed on end can deceptively appear yeast-like. The microscopic appearance of the Mucorales is sufficiently different from that of *Aspergillus*, *Fusarium*, and other pathogenic molds (which characteristically appear as narrow, septate hyphae with narrow-angle branching) that a pathologist can readily make a preliminary diagnosis of mucormycosis. Identification of the specific organism requires culture. In the laboratory, each species of Mucorales exhibits characteristic morphologic features that permit specific identification. Molecular methods of speciation are still used only as research tools.

Differential Diagnosis

Other fungal infections, including aspergillosis, fusariosis, and scedosporiosis, must be ruled out by culture and histopathologic analysis. Microscopic examination easily distinguishes the etiologic agents of these infections from the Mucorales. Aggressive pyogenic bacterial infections—e.g., those caused by *Pseudomonas*, *Aeromonas*, or *Vibrio* species; *Staphylococcus aureus*; and a variety of anaerobes—occasionally produce similar clinical presentations but can be ruled out by Gram's staining, culture, and microscopic analysis of tissue samples.

℞ Treatment: MUCORMYCOSIS

Three factors are key to a successful outcome of therapy for mucormycosis: (1) reversal of the underlying predisposition; (2) aggressive surgical debridement; and (3) aggressive antifungal therapy, with early initiation and high drug doses. Failure to undertake all three of these interventions simultaneously has a significant and negative impact on outcome.

Reversal of underlying disease is relatively easy in patients with diabetic ketoacidosis but is more difficult in patients who require continued immunosuppression for control of an underlying disease or after organ transplantation. In all cases, minimization of immunosuppressive medications enhances overall control of the fungal infection.

Aggressive surgical debridement requires the removal of all dead tissue and of tissue that appears to be so severely compromised that its continued viability is in question. Extensive reconstructive surgery may be required once the infection has been cured.

Traditionally, high-dose conventional amphotericin B has been used for the treatment of mucormycosis, but doses have been limited to <1.5 mg/kg per day because of the nearly universal development of nephrotoxicity. Use of lipid formulations at doses of 15–20 mg/kg per day (AmBisome) or 15 mg/kg per day (Abelcet) maximizes the amount of amphotericin B delivered to the tissues as well as the speed of its delivery. At these doses, nephrotoxicity occurs in <50% of patients.

Posaconazole, an experimental triazole antifungal agent, has been shown to be active against mucormycosis in mouse models of infection and in patients who cannot tolerate or do not respond to other antifungal drugs. The precise clinical role for posaconazole in the treatment of mucormycosis is not clear, but this drug may prove to be a valuable alternative to amphotericin B in selected cases. Given the relative rarity of mucormycosis, it is not likely that a randomized study will rigorously compare the roles of the various antifungal agents.

The optimal duration of therapy for mucormycosis is not known precisely. If possible, antifungal administration should be continued for at least 3 months after (1) all clinical abnormalities resolve or stabilize, leaving no clinical evidence of infection at the involved site(s); and (2) scans, x-rays, and laboratory studies yield normal or stable results. Careful follow-up should continue for at least 1 year to confirm that there is no evidence of recurrent infection. With this approach, recurrences should be rare.

FURTHER READINGS

Chayakulkeeree M et al: Zygomycosis: The re-emerging fungal infection. Eur J Clin Microbiol Infect Dis 25:215, 2006

Davari HR et al: Outcome of mucormycosis in liver transplantation: Four cases and a review of literature. Exp Clin Transplant 1:147, 2003

Gonzalez CE et al: Zygomycosis. Infect Dis Clin North Am 16:895, 2002

Greenberg RN et al: Zygomycosis (mucormycosis): Emerging clinical importance and new treatments. Curr Opin Infect Dis 17:517, 2004

——— et al: Posaconazole as salvage therapy for zygomycosis. Antimicrob Agents Chemother 50:126, 2006

Liang KP et al: Rhino-orbitocerebral mucormycosis caused by *Apophysomyces elegans*. J Clin Microbiol 44:892, 2006

O'Neill BM et al: Disseminated rhinocerebral mucormycosis: A case report and review of the literature. J Oral Maxillofac Surg 64:326, 2006

Prabhu RM et al: Mucormycosis and entomophthoramycosis: A review of the clinical manifestations, diagnosis and treatment. Clin Microbiol Infect 10(Suppl 1):31, 2004

Roden MM et al: Epidemiology and outcome of zygomycosis: A review of 929 reported cases. Clin Infect Dis 41:634, 2005

Spellberg B et al: Novel perspectives on mucormycosis: Pathophysiology, presentation, and management. Clin Microbiol Rev 18:556, 2005

CHAPTER 110

MISCELLANEOUS MYCOSES AND ALGAL INFECTIONS

Stanley W. Chapman ■ Donna C. Sullivan

MYCOSES

The clinical spectrum of fungal disease varies from superficial infections of the skin, hair, and nails to life-threatening systemic infections. Superficial infections involve the outermost layers of skin and hair and are associated with little or no inflammation. Cutaneous infections involve deeper layers of the skin, hair follicles, and nails and are accompanied by inflammation. Subcutaneous infections involve the dermis and subcutaneous tissues. Systemic disease involves deep tissue invasion of one or more internal organs and usually follows inhalation of the fungus. In immunocompromised patients, disseminated disease may result from superficial, cutaneous, or subcutaneous fungal infections.

SUPERFICIAL INFECTIONS

Malasseziasis

Tinea (pityriasis) versicolor, caused by lipophilic yeasts of the genus *Malassezia*, is the most common superficial skin infection. The clinical presentation usually consists of scaly hypo- or hyperpigmented macular lesions on the chest, back, neck, and arms.

Etiologic Agents

Malassezia species are components of the human cutaneous flora that are dimorphic, existing in both yeast and mycelial phases. Each phase was originally classified as a separate genus: *Pityrosporum* for the yeast form and *Malassezia* for the mycelial form. The two genera were reclassified in 1986 as a single genus, *Malassezia*. Initially, only one species, *M. furfur*, was recognized, but seven distinct species have since been identified: *M. furfur, M. sympodialis, M. obtusa, M. globosa, M. restricta, M. slooffiae*, and *M. pachydermatis*.

Epidemiology

Malassezia species can be isolated from sebaceous-rich areas of the skin, most frequently from the chest and the midline of the back. The prevalence of tinea versicolor in susceptible age groups (primarily adolescents and young adults) is low in temperate climates but may reach 40–60% in tropical climates.

Pathogenesis

The pathogenesis of tinea versicolor is unclear but may involve the conversion of colonizing yeasts into the mycelial form, which then invades the stratum corneum.

Clinical Manifestations

The lesions of tinea versicolor are usually asymptomatic. Most patients seek medical advice for cosmetic reasons. Lesions typically appear as patches of pink or coppery-brown skin but may appear paler than the surrounding skin, especially in dark-skinned individuals. Although some patients report mild pruritus, the lesions do not usually elicit an immune response. Other cutaneous manifestations associated with *Malassezia* species include seborrheic dermatitis, folliculitis, atopic dermatitis, and dandruff.

Diagnosis

Tinea versicolor is diagnosed on clinical grounds by the characteristic distribution and appearance of skin lesions. Lesions may fluoresce yellow-green under long-wave UVA (Wood's light). Treatment of skin scrapings with potassium hydroxide (KOH) reveals yeasts and hyphal elements with a "spaghetti and meatballs" appearance.

℞ Treatment: MALASSEZIASIS

Malassezia species are susceptible to a variety of topical antifungal agents, including 2.5% selenium sulfide shampoo (a 10- to 15-min application followed by rinsing); topical azoles such as clotrimazole, miconazole, econazole, and ketoconazole; terbinafine gel; and ciclopirox cream/solution. The typical treatment duration is 2 weeks. In patients with extensive or persistent lesions, short-course or pulse therapy with oral ketoconazole (a single 400-mg dose), fluconazole (a single 400-mg dose or 150 mg every week for 4 weeks), or itraconazole (200 mg every other day for 7 days) has proved effective.

Complications

M. furfur is lipophilic and causes catheter-related fungemia in premature neonates and immunocompromised adults receiving IV lipids by central venous catheter. Infection of the lungs is pronounced and frequently results in respiratory failure. *M. pachydermatis*, although not lipophilic, is an increasingly important pathogen in neonatal intensive care units. When its presence is suspected, the microbiology laboratory should be notified because its isolation requires special culture conditions. Catheter-related *Malassezia* infections should be managed with prompt catheter removal and systemic antifungal therapy with amphotericin B or an azole (Table 110-1). Because transmission of both *M. furfur* and *M. pachydermatis* on the hands of health care workers has been documented, a strict hand-washing protocol should be enforced when outbreaks are identified.

Prognosis

In general, the prognosis in tinea versicolor is excellent, but the disease recurs in up to 80% of patients within 2 years after cessation of treatment. Early diagnosis and treatment in patients with disseminated infection improve outcome.

Other Superficial Mycoses

Tinea nigra is a rare infection of the palms caused by the dematiaceous fungus *Hortaea* (formerly *Exophiala*) *werneckii*. Two types of piedra characterized by nodules of fungal elements on the hair shaft have been reported: black piedra caused by *Piedraia hortae* and white piedra caused by *Trichosporon* species (which may also be associated with other superficial infections as well as with invasive trichosporonosis). *T. beigelii* has historically been the most significant pathogen in the genus *Trichosporon*. Recently proposed revisions in classification and nomenclature are based on analysis of 26S rRNA sequences and use of nonmolecular techniques to differentiate 17 species—only 6 of which cause human disease—and 5 varieties of *Trichosporon*. Under this system, *T. beigelii* will be designated *T. cutaneum*. The other five human pathogens included in this revised classification are *T. asteroides, T. ovoides, T. inkin, T. asahii*, and *T. mucoides*. In addition, four serotypes of *Trichosporon* (serotypes I, II, III, and I-III) have been recognized, of which only serotypes I (*T. cutaneum* and *T. mucoides*) and II (*T. asahii, T. asteroides, T. inkin*, and *T. ovoides*) are pathogenic. Given that this revised nomenclature has not been universally adopted, the previous classification system may remain in use for some time and may be a source of confusion.

T. ovoides is usually associated with white piedra of the scalp, whereas *T. inkin* is primarily associated with white piedra of the groin. *T. ovoides* has also been implicated in summer-type hypersensitivity pneumonitis. The treatment of white piedra requires shaving off all the hair in the affected areas and applying a topical azole for 1–4 months.

CUTANEOUS INFECTIONS

The cutaneous mycoses are caused by *dermatophytes*, which infect keratinized tissues, including skin, hair follicles, and nails. These dermatophytic fungi invade the epidermis and elicit an inflammatory reaction, including redness and pruritus. Dermatophytic infections are designated according to the anatomic location of the lesions—e.g., *tinea corporis* (the trunk, shoulders, or limbs), *tinea cruris* (the warm moist areas of the groin, perianal, and perineal areas), *tinea faciei* (the nonhairy areas of the face), *tinea pedis* (the feet), *tinea unguium* (the nails), and *tinea capitis* (the scalp).

Etiologic Agents

Three genera of dermatophytes—*Microsporum, Trichophyton*, and *Epidermophyton*—are associated with human infections. Members of these genera can be divided into three groups according to their natural reservoir and potential for infection: anthropophilic, zoophilic, and geophilic organisms.

Epidemiology

Tinea is common worldwide. It is estimated that more than 8 million office visits to primary care physicians are made annually for tinea-related symptoms.

Pathogenesis

Dermatophytic fungi release proteolytic enzymes and keratinases into the skin. These exocellular enzymes release nutrients and facilitate dissemination through the stratum corneum. A specific host immune response is directed against the organisms.

Clinical Manifestations

Any dermatophyte can cause tinea corporis, which is commonly called "ringworm" because of the typical appearance of lesions: annular scaly patches with raised, erythematous vesicular borders and central clearing. Tinea faciei, like tinea corporis, can be caused by any dermatophyte. *T. rubrum* and *E. floccosum* are common causes of tinea cruris; similar lesions can be caused by *Candida* infection.

Tinea pedis, the most common clinical dermatophytic infection, usually presents with interdigital cracking, scaling, and maceration. Hyperkeratosis and peeling of the soles of the feet are common, with a scaly red "moccasin-like" appearance in chronic cases. The most common cause of tinea pedis is *T. rubrum*. Clinical lesions similar to those of tinea pedis can be caused by nondermatophytic fungi, yeasts, and bacteria.

Tinea unguium is caused by *T. rubrum, T. mentagrophytes*, and *E. floccosum*. The term *onychomycosis* encompasses nail infections due to either dermatophytes or nondermatophytic fungi. Dermatophytes cause 80–90% of cases of onychomycosis. The prevalence of these infections is ~2% among young adults and increases to 20% among individuals 40–60 years of age. Onychomycosis occurs in diabetic patients at the same rate as in the general population but poses a greater risk of bacterial superinfection in diabetes.

Tinea capitis is a common dermatophytic disease of children but is relatively rare among adults. The clinical presentation may vary from a diffuse scaly scalp to scattered areas of scale with or without alopecia. Hair may break off at the scalp ("black-dot ringworm"). Pruritus is not a constant symptom. Inflammatory responses may be minimal or severe, with the formation of a kerion

TABLE 110-1

SYSTEMIC THERAPY FOR MISCELLANEOUS INVASIVE MYCOSES AND THE ALGAL INFECTION PROTOTHECOSIS

TYPE OF INFECTION	FIRST-LINE THERAPY	ALTERNATIVE THERAPY
Malasseziasis		
Central venous catheter–related infections	Removal of central venous catheter AmB[a]	In vitro susceptibility studies indicate that azoles may offer a therapeutic alternative.
Trichosporonosis	AmB in combination with voriconazole[b] (300 mg bid)	GM-CSF or IFN-γ may be a useful therapeutic adjunct.
Sporotrichosis		
Cutaneous/ lymphocutaneous	Itraconazole[c] (100–200 mg/d for 3–6 months)	Terbinafine, 500–1000 mg/d
Non-life-threatening pulmonary, osteoarticular, or disseminated disease	Itraconazole (200 mg bid for 12 months)	AmB (lipid formulation) *or* fluconazole (800 mg/d for 12 months) in patients who cannot tolerate AmB or itraconazole
Life-threatening pulmonary or disseminated disease	AmB	Selected patients may be switched to oral itraconazole (200 mg bid for 12 months)
Eumycetoma	Surgery in combination with: Ketoconazole (200–400 mg/d) *or* Voriconazole (600 mg/d) *or* Terbinafine (500 mg/d)	Posaconazole is currently being evaluated.
Dematiaceous fungal infections	Surgical excision or cryosurgery combined with:	. . .
Chromoblastomycosis	Itraconazole (200–600 mg/d), alone or with 5-fluorocytosine (50–100 mg/kg qd in 3 or 4 divided doses)	
Phaeohyphomycosis		
Cutaneous or subcutaneous disease	Itraconazole (200 mg once or twice daily before surgery and to prevent relapse)	
Systemic/CNS	AmB in combination with itraconazole (200 mg bid) or voriconazole (200 mg bid)	
Paracoccidioidomycosis		
Mild to moderate disease	Itraconazole (200–400 mg/d)	. . .
Severe disease	AmB	Selected patients may be switched to itraconazole after an initial course of AmB.
Penicilliosis		
Mild to moderate disease	Itraconazole (200 mg bid for 2 months)	. . .
Severe disease	AmB	Selected patients may be switched to itraconazole (200 mg bid) after an initial course of AmB. The duration of primary treatment is 2 months.
Suppressive therapy for patients with HIV infection or AIDS	Itraconazole (200 mg/d)	
Fusariosis and pseudallescheriasis/ scedosporiosis	IV voriconazole (6 mg/kg q12h for first 24 h, then 4 mg/kg q12h until neutropenia resolves and clinical response is documented)	Selected patients may be switched to oral voriconazole (200 mg bid) after a clinical response and reversal of neutropenia.
Protothecosis	Itraconazole (200 mg/d for 2 months or until lesions resolve)	Disseminated infections should be treated with IV AmB.

[a]Unless otherwise noted, AmB dosages are 0.6–1.0 mg/kg per day of the deoxycholate formulation or 3–5 mg/kg per day of a lipid formulation.
[b]An initial loading dose of voriconazole is recommended on day 1 for both IV therapy (6 mg/kg q12h) and oral therapy (400 mg q12h).
[c]An initial loading dose of itraconazole is recommended for both IV therapy (200 mg bid for 2 days) and oral therapy (200 mg bid for 2 days).
Note: AmB, amphotericin B; CNS, central nervous system; GM-CSF, granulocyte-macrophage colony-stimulating factor; IFN-γ, interferon γ.

characterized by alopecia, a tender or painful boggy scalp, purulent drainage, and localized lymphadenopathy. *T. tonsurans* is the most common dermatophyte associated with tinea capitis.

Diagnosis

Some skin lesions have distinctive characteristics that allow a presumptive diagnosis, and topical therapy is often initiated solely on the basis of the lesions' appearance. However, the ease of obtaining specimens for microscopic examination and culture should encourage definitive diagnosis. Scrapings of skin lesions can be examined as a wet preparation, with a drop of 10% KOH used to dissolve cells and debris. Samples for fungal cultures should be obtained from patients whose history, physical examination, and KOH-treated specimens are inconclusive with regard to the diagnosis of dermatophytic infection. It is recommended that a definitive diagnosis be established in patients before systemic antifungal agents are administered.

Rx Treatment: CUTANEOUS INFECTIONS

Most tinea infections can be treated with topical agents alone. Many such antifungal agents are widely available as both prescription and over-the-counter products. Topical imidazoles (e.g., clotrimazole, miconazole, econazole, and ketoconazole) are generally well tolerated and efficacious when used twice daily for at least 2 weeks. The allylamines, including terbinafine and naftifine (available in 1% creams or 1% solutions), provide cure rates of ≥75% and require only once-daily application for shorter periods. Tolnaftate powder is best suited for prevention of tinea pedis.

Systemic therapy is indicated for patients who are unresponsive to topical therapy; for those who have infections involving the scalp or bearded areas, who have hyperkeratotic areas on the palms or soles, or who have widespread disease; and for immunocompromised individuals. Once-daily itraconazole (200 mg), terbinafine (250 mg), and griseofulvin (500 mg of the microcrystalline formulation or 375 mg of the ultramicrocrystalline formulation) has proved effective. Treatment should be administered until lesions resolve. For patients with nail disease, itraconazole (200 mg/d) or terbinafine (250 mg/d) is preferred. The duration of therapy is 2–3 months for fingernails and 4–6 months for toenails. Pulse therapy with itraconazole and terbinafine is an option. Relapse of nail disease is common.

Complications

Sites of tinea pedis frequently become superinfected with bacteria. Sometimes these infections are serious, especially in diabetic patients, patients who have undergone saphenous-vein harvest for coronary artery bypass grafts, and patients with any significant venous incompetence.

SUBCUTANEOUS INFECTIONS

Fungal infections that primarily involve the dermis and subcutaneous tissue result from implantation of the organism in the skin through trauma. The major subcutaneous mycoses are sporotrichosis, mycetoma, chromoblastomycosis, and phaeohyphomycosis.

Sporotrichosis

Sporotrichosis most commonly presents as chronic cutaneous, lymphocutaneous, and/or subcutaneous disease. This infection may also be extracutaneous, occurring at pulmonary, osteoarticular, or disseminated sites.

Etiologic Agent

Sporotrichosis is caused by the thermally dimorphic fungus *Sporothrix schenckii*, which is found in soil, plants, and moss and on animals. *S. schenckii* exists worldwide but is most common in tropical and warmer temperate regions, such as Mexico and Central and South America.

Epidemiology

Sporotrichosis is usually an occupational disease of gardeners, farmers, forestry workers, florists, and horticulturists. There have been well-documented epidemics (e.g., among South African gold miners) as well as scattered outbreaks (e.g., among workers handling sphagnum, hay, and wood). Recent reports indicate that infection can be related to zoonotic spread from cats and armadillos.

Pathogenesis

Sporotrichosis most often follows inoculation of the organism into the skin.

Clinical Manifestations

The majority of infections with *S. schenckii* present either as fixed cutaneous sporotrichosis or as lymphangitic or lymphocutaneous disease. Fixed cutaneous disease (plaque sporotrichosis) is limited to the site of inoculation. The primary lesion enlarges and may ulcerate and become verrucous. In lymphocutaneous disease, which accounts for ~80% of cases, secondary lesions ascend along the lymphatics that drain the area, producing small painless nodules that erupt, drain, and ulcerate. Other organisms (e.g., nontuberculous mycobacteria, *Nocardia*, *Leishmania*, and chromoblastomycotic agents) may cause similar lesions. Osteoarticular sporotrichosis is an uncommon complication but may cause granulomatous tenosynovitis and bursitis, particularly in alcoholic patients. Pulmonary sporotrichosis following inhalation of *S. schenckii* conidia has been reported in alcoholic patients with chronic obstructive pulmonary disease. Disseminated disease, including that involving the central nervous system, is most likely to occur in patients who have AIDS or are otherwise immunocompromised.

Diagnosis

A definitive diagnosis is made by culture of *S. schenckii* on any of a variety of media. Histopathologic examination of biopsy material may also contribute to the diagnosis, with detection of the characteristic ovoid or cigar-shaped yeast forms.

℞ Treatment: SPOROTRICHOSIS

Sporotrichosis requires systemic therapy (Table 110-1). Historically, oral therapy with a saturated solution of potassium iodide (SSKI; 5 drops 3 times daily, increasing to 40–50 drops 3 times daily as tolerated) has been successful, but the use of this intervention is often limited by its toxicity. Because it has fewer side effects and is better tolerated, oral itraconazole has replaced SSKI as the treatment of choice for cutaneous and lymphocutaneous sporotrichosis. Terbinafine has also been effective against lymphocutaneous disease, although it has not been approved for this indication by the U.S. Food and Drug Administration. Patients with non-life-threatening pulmonary disease and those with osteoarticular disease should be treated with itraconazole for at least 12 months. Amphotericin B is the preferred agent for patients with life-threatening pulmonary disease or disseminated infection, for patients who cannot tolerate itraconazole, and for patients in whom itraconazole treatment has failed.

Complications

Hematogenous dissemination of *S. schenckii* is most common among immunocompromised patients, including those with HIV infection or AIDS. These patients may develop widespread cutaneous ulcers, granulomas, and systemic disease with pulmonary, meningeal, articular, or generalized infection.

Prognosis

Success rates of 90–100% have been reported for itraconazole treatment of lymphocutaneous sporotrichosis. A clinical response usually occurs within 4–6 weeks of the start of therapy. Patients who relapse usually respond to a second course of itraconazole.

Mycetoma

Mycetoma is a chronic suppurative infection that begins in the subcutaneous tissue and spreads to fascia and bone. Mycetoma due to fungi is called *eumycetoma*, while that caused by actinomycetes is referred to as *actinomycetoma*. Both diseases are characterized by abscesses containing grains composed of large aggregates of filaments (fungal or actinomycete). Traumatic inoculation is responsible for initial infection.

Etiology and Epidemiology

Mycetomas are common in Mexico, Central America, Venezuela, Brazil, Africa, the Middle East, India, Pakistan, and Bangladesh. The most common cause of eumycetoma worldwide is *Madurella mycetomatis*, while the rare cases that occur in the United States are associated with *Pseudallescheria boydii*. Actinomycetoma, the usual form of mycetoma in Mexico and Central America, is associated with *Nocardia brasiliensis, Streptomyces somaliensis, Actinomadura madurae*, and *Actinomadura pelletieri*.

Clinical Manifestations

Clinically, eumycetoma and actinomycetoma are similar, beginning as small, firm, painless subcutaneous plaques or nodules on the foot or leg and, less frequently, on the arms, torso, and scalp. Patients usually present with draining sinus tracts, subcutaneous abscesses, fibrosis with woody induration, and extension to fascia and bone.

Diagnosis

Diagnosis is based on visualization of grains in pus, sinus exudate, or tissue biopsy. Fungal hyphae must be distinguished from the filamentous forms seen in actinomycetoma. Organisms associated with mycetoma, whether fungi or actinomycetes, can be grown on a variety of culture media.

℞ Treatment: MYCETOMA

The treatment of mycetoma is problematic. A combined medical/surgical approach is the option of choice (Table 110-1). Because actinomycetoma does not respond to antifungal agents, the differentiation between eumycetoma and actinomycetoma is crucial. (For the treatment of actinomycetoma, see Chaps. 63 and 64.) Amphotericin B has not generally been effective for the treatment of eumycetoma. A limited number of patients have responded to long-term azole therapy. Posaconazole, an investigational agent, may have a role in the treatment of eumycetoma in the future.

Dematiaceous Fungal Infections

Of the many names applied to infections caused by brown- or black-pigmented soil fungi, *phaeohyphomycosis* and *chromoblastomycosis* are the most widely accepted. Phaeohyphomycosis refers to infections in which the organisms in tissue occur as pigmented yeast-like forms and/or hyphae. Chromoblastomycosis is distinguished by the presence of pigmented sclerotic bodies in tissue.

Chromoblastomycosis is characterized by slow-growing verrucous plaques or nodules, usually on the lower extremities. The most common etiologic agents are *Fonsecaea pedrosoi, F. compacta, Phialophora verrucosa, Rhinocladiella aquaspersa*, and *Cladosporium (Cladophialophora) carrionii*. Most cases affect rural workers living in tropical and subtropical regions, and infection is acquired by traumatic inoculation. Small verrucous papules enlarge slowly but remain painless. Lesions seen in late stages may be superficial or raised purplish irregular plaques; less commonly, they may be nodular, tumorous, verrucous, or cicatricial. In advanced cases, secondary lymphedema, bacterial infections, and keratin necrosis can develop. Although histologic examination of scrapings or biopsy material for characteristic sclerotic bodies can lead to the diagnosis of chromoblastomycosis, culture is required for identification of the causative agent. Treatment is difficult, although many therapeutic interventions have been described (Table 110-1). Results are best when early surgical excision or cryosurgery is used in combination with antifungal therapy. Treatment with itraconazole—either alone or with 5-fluorocytosine—has had some success.

Phaeohyphomycosis presents in four clinical forms: superficial, cutaneous-corneal, subcutaneous, and systemic. *Exophiala jeanselmei, Wangiella dermatitidis*, and *Bipolaris* species are the most common etiologic agents. The route of infection is most likely implantation, with the subsequent formation of an inflammatory cyst. A single inflammatory nondraining cyst located on a proximal limb is the most typical presentation. The diagnosis is usually made by histopathologic detection (in biopsy material) of a fibrous capsule with a granulomatous reaction and a necrotic center. Culture is required to identify specific organisms. Surgical excision of the lesion is essential. Itraconazole treatment reduces the size of large lesions before excision and prevents relapse afterward (Table 110-1). Cerebral phaeohyphomycosis is thought to be due to direct extension from adjacent paranasal sinuses or from a penetrating trauma to the head. Most cases present as a brain abscess with focal neurologic deficits and/or generalized seizures. A review of 101 cases revealed that one-half of patients had no apparent immunocompromising condition. Infections in immunocompromised patients are more likely to disseminate; disseminated infections have been reported in patients with HIV infection, solid-organ transplant recipients, patients with malignancies, and one pregnant woman. Rhinocerebral disease requires surgical drainage along with antifungal therapy. A combination of amphotericin B and itraconazole or voriconazole is recommended.

SYSTEMIC MYCOSES

Paracoccidioidomycosis

Often referred to as South American blastomycosis, paracoccidioidomycosis is a systemic disease caused by the dimorphic fungus *Paracoccidioides brasiliensis*. Pulmonary infection follows inhalation of conidia and may disseminate to other organs, producing secondary lesions in the skin, lymph nodes, and adrenal glands. Subclinical infections have been documented in healthy residents of endemic regions. Paracoccidioidomycosis is most common in Venezuela, Colombia, Ecuador, Argentina, and Brazil. Histopathologic examination of clinical specimens may reveal globose yeast cells with multiple buds. Definitive diagnosis relies on culture of the organism. Itraconazole treatment has been effective (Table 110-1). An initial course of amphotericin B may be required in seriously ill patients.

Penicilliosis

Caused by the thermally dimorphic fungus *Penicillium marneffei*, penicilliosis is a disease of immunocompromised individuals living in or traveling to Southeast Asia. The primary portal of entry is the lungs, and hematologic dissemination follows. Clinical manifestations are similar to those of disseminated histoplasmosis and include fever, chills, weight loss, anemia, generalized lymphadenopathy, and hepatomegaly. Diffuse papular lesions similar to those of molluscum contagiosum are common in patients with HIV infection or AIDS. Small yeast cells may be seen on histopathologic examination of tissue, but definitive diagnosis depends on culture. Amphotericin B is the treatment of choice for severely ill patients (Table 110-1). Patients who have less severe disease or who have responded to an initial course of amphotericin B may be treated with itraconazole. Primary therapy is usually given for 2 months; in patients with HIV infection or AIDS, suppressive therapy with itraconazole may be useful in preventing relapse.

Fusariosis

Fusariosis is an invasive mold infection associated with *Fusarium* species, most commonly *F. solani*. The skin and respiratory tract are the primary portals of entry. Localized skin infections may occur at sites of trauma in immunocompetent hosts. Disease may disseminate from the skin or respiratory tract in immunocompromised patients; 90% of such cases are reported in neutropenic patients with leukemia or recipients of allogeneic bone marrow transplants. The clinical presentation is generally nonspecific, with fever and skin lesions that eventually become necrotic and resemble ecthyma gangrenosum. Clinical, radiographic, and pathologic findings are similar to those in invasive aspergillosis or zygomycosis. Blood cultures are positive in up to 50% of cases, and the presence of a mold in cultured blood from neutropenic patients suggests fusariosis. *Fusarium* species are often resistant to antifungal therapy. High-dose amphotericin B has met with limited success. Therapy with voriconazole (Table 110-1) has been successful in a few patients. Therapy is continued until neutropenia resolves and a clinical response is documented. The prognosis of disseminated infection is related to the reversal of neutropenia and other immunodeficiencies.

Pseudallescheriasis and Scedosporiosis

The emerging pathogens *P. boydii, Scedosporium apiospermum* (the asexual form of *P. boydii*), and *S. prolificans* are molds that cause rare sinopulmonary infections in immunocompetent hosts and that may present as fungus balls in the lungs or paranasal sinuses. Severe pneumonia, invasive sinusitis, and hematogenous dissemination (including brain abscess) occur in immunosuppressed hosts, especially bone marrow transplant recipients. The hyphal elements seen in the tissues of patients with *Pseudallescheria* and *Scedosporium* infections resemble those seen in intravascular invasion by *Aspergillus*. The outcome of treatment is poor, and most patients with disseminated disease die. Amphotericin B is not effective in the treatment of pseudallescheriasis or scedosporiosis. A small number of patients have been cured with voriconazole in the same doses listed for fusariosis (Table 110-1). Surgical debridement and drainage of abscesses may also be necessary.

Trichosporonosis

Trichosporon species, predominantly *T. asahii* and to a lesser extent *T. mucoides*, can cause disseminated trichosporonosis in immunocompromised patients, especially those with profound neutropenia. Unpublished studies describe isolation of *Trichosporon* from pubic sites of white piedra, sputum, skin lesions, and blood. *T. pullulans* (formerly *Monilia pullulans*) is a rare cause of systemic infection. Portals of entry include the skin, gastrointestinal tract, and lungs. The clinical presentation mimics candidiasis. Cultures of blood, skin lesions, or biopsy specimens confirm the diagnosis. *Trichosporon* shares antigens with *Cryptococcus neoformans* and produces positive results in the latex agglutination test. Treatment of *Trichosporon* infections is complicated by resistance to amphotericin B. Mortality rates of >80% have been reported. The azoles, especially voriconazole, have been effective alone or in combination with amphotericin B (Table 110-1). Adjunctive therapy with granulocyte-macrophage colony-stimulating factor or interferon γ may be beneficial. The prognosis, however, is related to the resolution of neutropenia.

ALGAL INFECTIONS

Prototheca, an achlorophyllic alga common in nature, has been associated with rare human infections in Europe, Asia, Oceania, and the United States (particularly the southeastern states). This organism has been isolated from slime flux of trees, industrial ponds, tap water, sewage systems, swimming pools, and soil. Infections with *P. wickerhamii* and *P. zopfii* occur primarily in immunocompromised patients. Protothecosis may present as a cutaneous disease with erythematous nodules, plaques, or superficial ulcers on exposed skin; as olecranon bursitis; or as a systemic infection. Histologic examination of biopsy material may reveal multinucleated giant cells and extra- and intracellular, basophilic to amphiphilic organisms containing endospores. *Prototheca* can be cultured on Sabouraud's agar. The most frequently used therapeutic agent is amphotericin B, which has proved effective even in patients with disseminated protothecosis. Azole antifungal agents such as itraconazole, ketoconazole, and fluconazole have also been used successfully. Surgical excision may play a role in the treatment of localized cutaneous lesions.

FURTHER READINGS

ALY R: Skin, hair, and nail fungal infections. Infect Dis Clin Pract 10:117, 1998

CHAPMAN SW, DANIEL CR III: Cutaneous manifestations of fungal infection. Infect Dis Clin North Am 4:879, 1994

DIGNANI MC et al: Immunomodulation with interferon-gamma and colony-stimulating factors for refractory fungal infections in patients with leukemia. Cancer 104:199, 2005

FLEMING RV, ANAISSIE EJ: Emerging fungal infections, in *Fungal Infections in the Immunocompromised Patient*, JR Wingard, EJ Anaissie (eds). Boca Raton, Taylor & Francis Group, 2005, pp 311–340

——— et al: Emerging and less common fungal pathogens. Infect Dis Clin North Am 16:915, 2002

QUEIROZ-TELLES F et al: Subcutaneous mycoses. Infect Dis Clin North Am 17:59, 2003

SEGAL BH et al: Fungal infections in nontransplant patients with hematologic malignancies. Infect Dis Clin North Am 16:935, 2002

SILVEIRA F, NUCCI M: Emergence of black moulds in fungal disease: Epidemiology and therapy. Curr Opin Infect Dis 14:679, 2001

www.doctorfungus.org

CHAPTER 111

PNEUMOCYSTIS INFECTION

A. George Smulian ■ Peter D. Walzer

DEFINITION AND DESCRIPTION

Pneumocystis is an opportunistic fungal pulmonary pathogen that is an important cause of pneumonia in the immunocompromised host. Although organisms within the *Pneumocystis* genus are morphologically very similar, they are genetically diverse and host-specific. *P. jirovecii* infects humans, whereas *P. carinii*—the original species described in 1909—infects rats. For clarity, only the genus designation *Pneumocystis* will be used in this chapter.

Developmental stages of the organism include the trophic form, the cyst, and the precyst (an intermediate stage). The life cycle of *Pneumocystis* probably involves sexual and asexual reproduction, although definitive proof awaits the development of a reliable culture system.

Pneumocystis contains several different antigen groups, the most prominent of which is the 95- to 140-kDa major surface glycoprotein (MSG). MSG plays a central role in the interaction of *Pneumocystis* with its host.

EPIDEMIOLOGY

Serologic surveys have demonstrated that *Pneumocystis* has a worldwide distribution and that most healthy children have been exposed to the organism by 3–4 years of age. Airborne transmission of *Pneumocystis* has been documented in animal studies; person-to-person transmission has been suggested by hospital outbreaks of *Pneumocystis* pneumonia (PcP) and by molecular epidemiologic analysis of isolates. *Pneumocystis* colonization of immunocompetent individuals has been detected by polymerase chain reaction (PCR) techniques.

PATHOGENESIS AND PATHOLOGY

The host factors that predispose to the development of PcP include defects in cellular and humoral immunity. The risk of PcP among HIV-infected patients rises markedly when circulating CD4+ T-cell counts fall below 200/μL. Other persons at risk for PcP are patients receiving immunosuppressive agents (particularly glucocorticoids) for cancer and organ transplantation; those receiving biologic agents such as infliximab and etanercept for rheumatoid arthritis and inflammatory bowel disease; children with primary immunodeficiency diseases; and premature malnourished infants.

The principal host effector cells against *Pneumocystis* are alveolar macrophages, which ingest and kill the organism, releasing a variety of inflammatory mediators. Proliferating organisms remain extracellular within the alveolus, attaching tightly to type I cells. Alveolar damage results in increased alveolar-capillary permeability and surfactant abnormalities, including a fall in phospholipids and an increase in surfactant proteins A and D. The host inflammatory response to lung injury leads to increases in levels of interleukin 8 and in neutrophil counts in bronchoalveolar lavage (BAL) fluid. These changes correlate with disease severity.

On lung sections stained with hematoxylin and eosin, the alveoli are filled with a typical foamy, vacuolated exudate. Severe disease may include interstitial edema, fibrosis, and hyaline membrane formation. The host inflammatory changes usually consist of hypertrophy of alveolar type II cells, a typical reparative response, and a mild mononuclear cell interstitial infiltrate. Malnourished infants display an intense plasma cell infiltrate that gave the disease its early name: interstitial plasma cell pneumonia.

CLINICAL FEATURES

Patients with PcP develop dyspnea, fever, and nonproductive cough. HIV-infected patients are usually ill for several weeks and may have relatively subtle manifestations. Symptoms in non-HIV-infected patients are of shorter duration and often begin after the glucocorticoid dose has been tapered. A high index of suspicion and a thorough history are key factors in early detection.

Physical findings include tachypnea, tachycardia, and cyanosis, but lung auscultation reveals few abnormalities. Reduced arterial oxygen pressure (Pa_{O_2}), increased alveolar-arterial oxygen gradient ($PA_{O_2} - Pa_{O_2}$), and respiratory alkalosis are evident. Diffusion capacity is reduced, and heightened uptake with nonspecific nuclear imaging techniques (gallium scan) may be noted. Elevated serum concentrations of lactate dehydrogenase, reflecting lung parenchymal damage, have been reported; however, the increase is not specific for PcP.

The classic findings on chest radiography consist of bilateral diffuse infiltrates beginning in the perihilar regions (Fig. 111-1*A*), but various atypical manifestations (nodular densities, cavitary lesions) have also been reported. Pneumothorax occurs, and its management is often difficult. Early in the course of PcP, the chest radiograph may be normal, although high-resolution CT of the lung may reveal ground-glass opacities at this stage (Fig. 111-1*B*).

While *Pneumocystis* usually remains confined to the lungs, cases of disseminated infection have occurred in both HIV-infected and non-HIV-infected patients. Common sites of involvement include the lymph nodes, spleen, liver, and bone marrow.

DIAGNOSIS

Because of the nonspecific nature of the clinical picture, the diagnosis must be based on specific identification of the organism. A definitive diagnosis is made by histopathologic staining. Traditional cell wall stains such as methenamine silver selectively stain the wall of

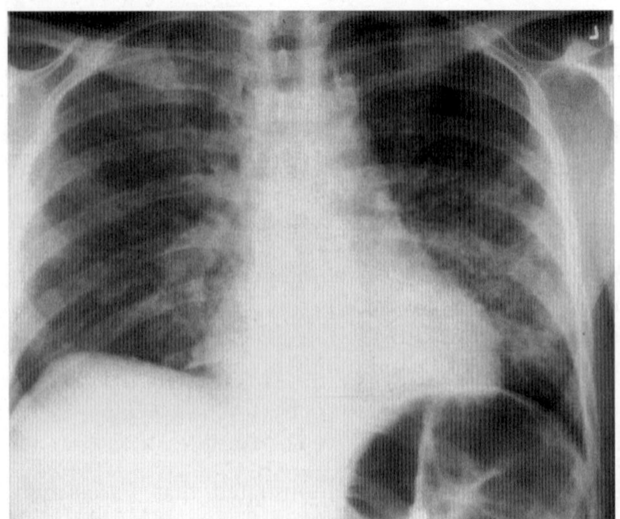

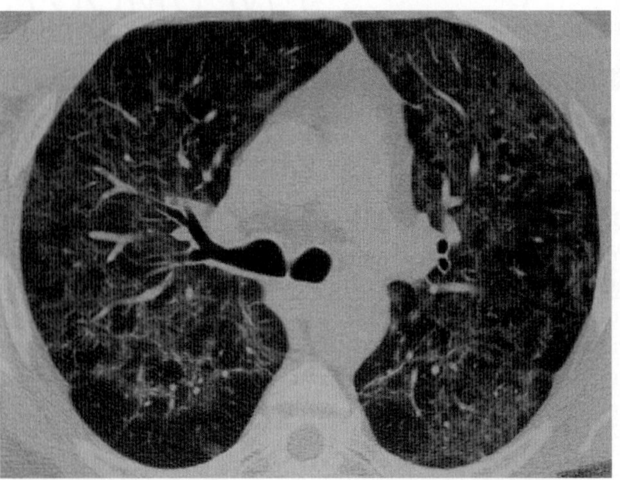

FIGURE 111-1

A. Chest radiograph depicting diffuse infiltrates in an HIV-infected patient with PcP. ***B.*** High-resolution CT of the lung showing ground-glass opacification in an HIV-infected patient with PcP. *(Courtesy of Dr. Cristopher Meyer, with permission.)*

Pneumocystis cysts, while reagents such as Wright-Giemsa stain the nuclei of all developmental stages. Immunofluorescence with monoclonal antibodies is more sensitive and specific than histologic staining. DNA amplification by PCR may become part of routine diagnostics but may not distinguish colonization from infection.

The successful diagnosis of PcP depends on the collection of proper specimens. In general, the yield from different diagnostic procedures is higher in HIV-infected patients than in non-HIV-infected patients because of the higher organism burden in the former group. Sputum induction and oral washes have gained popularity as simple, noninvasive techniques; however, these procedures require trained and dedicated personnel. Fiberoptic bronchoscopy with BAL, which provides information about the organism burden, the host inflammatory response, and the presence of other opportunistic infections, continues to be the mainstay of *Pneumocystis* diagnosis. Transbronchial biopsy and open lung biopsy, the most invasive procedures, are used only when a diagnosis cannot be made by BAL.

COURSE AND PROGNOSIS

In the typical case of untreated PcP, progressive respiratory embarrassment leads to death. Therapy is most effective when instituted early, before there is extensive alveolar damage. If examination of induced sputum is nondiagnostic and BAL cannot be performed in a timely manner, empirical therapy for PcP is reasonable. However, this practice does not eliminate the need for a specific etiologic diagnosis. With improved management of HIV and its complications, mortality from PcP is 15–20% at 1 month and 50–55% at 1 year. Rates of early death remain high among patients who require mechanical ventilation (60%) and among non-HIV-infected patients (40%).

TABLE 111-1

TREATMENT OF PNEUMOCYSTOSIS

DRUG(S), DOSE, ROUTE	ADVERSE EFFECTS
First Choice[a]	
TMP-SMX (5 mg/kg TMP, 25 mg/kg SMX[b]) q6–8h PO or IV	Fever, rash, cytopenias, hepatitis, hyperkalemia, GI disturbances
Other Agents[a]	
TMP, 5 mg/kg q6–8h, plus dapsone, 100 mg qd PO	Hemolysis (G6PD deficiency), methemoglobinemia, fever, rash, GI disturbances
Atovaquone, 750 mg bid PO	Rash, fever, GI and hepatic disturbances
Clindamycin, 300–450 mg q6h PO or 600 mg q6–8h IV, plus primaquine, 15–30 mg qd PO	Hemolysis (G6PD deficiency), methemoglobinemia, rash, colitis, neutropenia
Pentamidine, 3–4 mg/kg qd IV	Hypotension, azotemia, cardiac arrhythmias, pancreatitis, dysglycemias, hypocalcemia, neutropenia, hepatitis
Trimetrexate, 45 mg/m^2 qd IV, plus leucovorin,[c] 20 mg/kg q6h PO or IV	Cytopenias, peripheral neuropathy, hepatic disturbances
Adjunctive Agent	
Prednisone, 40 mg bid × 5 d, 40 mg qd × 5 d, 20 mg qd × 11 d; PO or IV	Immunosuppression, peptic ulcer, hyperglycemia, mood changes, hypertension

[a]Therapy is administered for 14 days to non-HIV-infected patients and for 21 days to HIV-infected patients.

[b]Equivalent of 2 double-strength (DS) tablets. (One DS tablet contains 160 mg of TMP and 800 mg of SMX.)

[c]Leucovorin prevents bone marrow toxicity from trimetrexate.

Note: GI, gastrointestinal; G6PD, glucose-6-phosphate dehydrogenase; TMP-SMX, trimethoprim-sulfamethoxazole.

℞ Treatment: *PNEUMOCYSTIS* INFECTION

Trimethoprim-sulfamethoxazole (TMP-SMX), which acts by inhibiting folic acid synthesis, is considered the drug of choice for all forms of PcP (Table 111-1). Therapy is continued for 14 days in non-HIV-infected patients and for 21 days in persons infected with HIV. Since HIV-infected patients respond more slowly than non-HIV-infected patients, it is prudent to wait at least 7 days after the initiation of treatment before concluding that therapy has failed. TMP-SMX is well tolerated by non-HIV-infected patients, whereas more than half of HIV-infected patients experience serious adverse reactions.

Several alternative regimens are available for the treatment of mild to moderate cases of PcP (a Pa_{O_2} of >70 mmHg or a $PA_{O_2} - Pa_{O_2}$ of <35 mmHg on breathing room air). TMP plus dapsone and clindamycin plus primaquine are about as effective as TMP-SMX. Dapsone and primaquine should not be administered to patients with glucose-6-phosphate dehydrogenase (G6PD) deficiency. Atovaquone is less effective than TMP-SMX but is better tolerated. Since *Pneumocystis* lacks ergosterol, it is not susceptible to antifungal agents that inhibit ergosterol synthesis.

Alternative regimens that are recommended for the treatment of moderate to severe PcP (a Pa_{O_2} of ≤70 mmHg or a $PA_{O_2} - Pa_{O_2}$ of ≥35 mmHg) are parenteral pentamidine, parenteral clindamycin plus primaquine, or trimetrexate plus leucovorin. Parenteral clindamycin plus primaquine may be more efficacious than pentamidine.

Molecular evidence of resistance to sulfonamides and to atovaquone has emerged among human *Pneumocystis* isolates. Although prior sulfonamide exposure is a risk factor, this resistance has also occurred in HIV-infected patients who have never received sulfonamides. The outcome of therapy appears to be linked more strongly to traditional measures—e.g., high Acute Physiology, Age, and Chronic Health Evaluation III (APACHE III) scores, need for positive-pressure ventilation, delayed intubation, and development of pneumothorax—than to the presence of molecular markers of sulfonamide resistance. HIV-infected patients frequently experience deterioration of respiratory function shortly after receiving anti-*Pneumocystis* drugs. The adjunctive administration of tapering doses of glucocorticoids to HIV-infected patients with moderate to severe PcP can prevent this problem and improve the rate of survival (Table 111-1). For maximal benefit, this adjunctive therapy should be started early in the course of the illness. The use of steroids as adjunctive therapy in HIV-infected patients with mild PcP or in non-HIV-infected patients remains to be evaluated.

PREVENTION

Prophylaxis is indicated for HIV-infected patients with CD4+ T-cell counts of <200/μL or a history of oropharyngeal candidiasis and for both HIV-infected and non-HIV-infected patients who have recovered from PcP. Prophylaxis may be discontinued in HIV-infected patients once CD4+ T-cell counts have risen to >200/μL and remained at that level for ≥3 months. Primary prophylaxis guidelines for immunocompromised hosts not infected with HIV are less clear.

TMP-SMX is the drug of choice for primary and secondary prophylaxis (Table 111-2).

This agent also provides protection against toxoplasmosis and some bacterial infections. Alternative regimens are available for individuals intolerant of TMP-SMX (Table 111-2). Although there are no specific recommendations for preventing the spread of *Pneumocystis* in health care facilities, it seems prudent to prevent direct contact between patients with PcP and other susceptible hosts.

TABLE 111-2

PROPHYLAXIS OF PNEUMOCYSTOSIS[a]

DRUG(S), DOSE, ROUTE	COMMENTS
First Choice	
TMP-SMX, 1 DS tablet or 1 SS tablet qd PO[b]	TMP-SMX can be safely reintroduced in some patients who have experienced mild to moderate side effects.
Other Agents	
Dapsone, 50 mg bid or 100 mg qd PO	—
Dapsone, 50 mg qd PO, plus pyrimethamine, 50 mg weekly PO, plus leucovorin, 25 mg weekly PO	Leucovorin prevents bone marrow toxicity from pyrimethamine.
Dapsone, 200 mg weekly PO, plus pyrimethamine, 75 mg weekly PO, plus leucovorin, 25 mg weekly PO	Leucovorin prevents bone marrow toxicity from pyrimethamine.
Pentamidine, 300 mg monthly via Respirgard II nebulizer	Adverse reactions include cough and bronchospasm.
Atovaquone, 1500 mg qd PO	—
TMP-SMX, 1 DS tablet three times weekly PO	TMP-SMX can be safely reintroduced in some patients who have experienced mild to moderate side effects.

[a]For list of adverse effects, see Table 111-1.
[b]One DS tablet contains 160 mg of TMP and 800 mg of SMX.
Note: DS, double-strength; SS, single-strength; TMP-SMX, trimethoprim-sulfamethoxazole.

FURTHER READINGS

Centers for Disease Control and Prevention: Treating opportunistic infections among HIV-infected adults and adolescents: Recommendations from the CDC, the National Institutes of Health and the HIV Medicine Association/Infectious Diseases Society of America. MMWR 53(RR-15):1, 2004

Daly KR et al: Antibody responses to the *Pneumocystis jirovecii* major surface glycoprotein. Emerg Infect Dis 12:1231, 2006

D'Avignon LC et al: *Pneumocystis* pneumonia. Semin Respir Crit Care Med 29:132, 2008

Festic E et al: Acute respiratory failure due to *Pneumocystis* pneumonia in patients without human immunodeficiency virus infection: Outcome and associated features. Chest 128:573, 2005

Green H et al: Prophylaxis of *Pneumocystis* pneumonia in immunocompromised non-HIV-infected patients: Systematic review and meta-analysis of randomized controlled trials. Mayo Clin Proc 82:1052, 2007

Medrano FJ et al: *Pneumocystis jirovecii* in general population. Emerg Infect Dis 11:245, 2005

Miller RF et al: Improved survival for HIV infected patients with severe *Pneumocystis jirovecii* pneumonia is independent of highly active antiretroviral therapy. Thorax 61:716, 2006

Morris A: Is there anything new in *Pneumocystis jirovecii* pneumonia? Changes in *P. jirovecii* pneumonia over the course of the AIDS epidemic. Clin Infect Dis 46:634, 2008

Pisculli ML, Sax PE: Use of a serum beta-glucan assay for diagnosis of HIV-related *Pneumocystis jiroveci* pneumonia in patients with negative microscopic examination results. Clin Infect Dis 46:1928, 2008

Redhead SA et al: *Pneumocystis* and *Trypanosoma cruzi*: Nomenclature and typifications. J Eukaryot Microbiol 53:1, 2006

Tasaka S et al: Serum indicators for the diagnosis of *Pneumocystis* pneumonia. Chest 131:1173, 2007

Thomas CF Jr, Limper AH: *Pneumocystis* pneumonia. N Engl J Med 350:2487, 2004

Zar HJ: Pneumonia in HIV-infected and HIV-uninfected children in developing countries: Epidemiology, clinical features, and management. Curr Opin Pulm Med 10:176, 2004

SECTION VIII

PROTOZOAL AND HELMINTHIC INFECTIONS

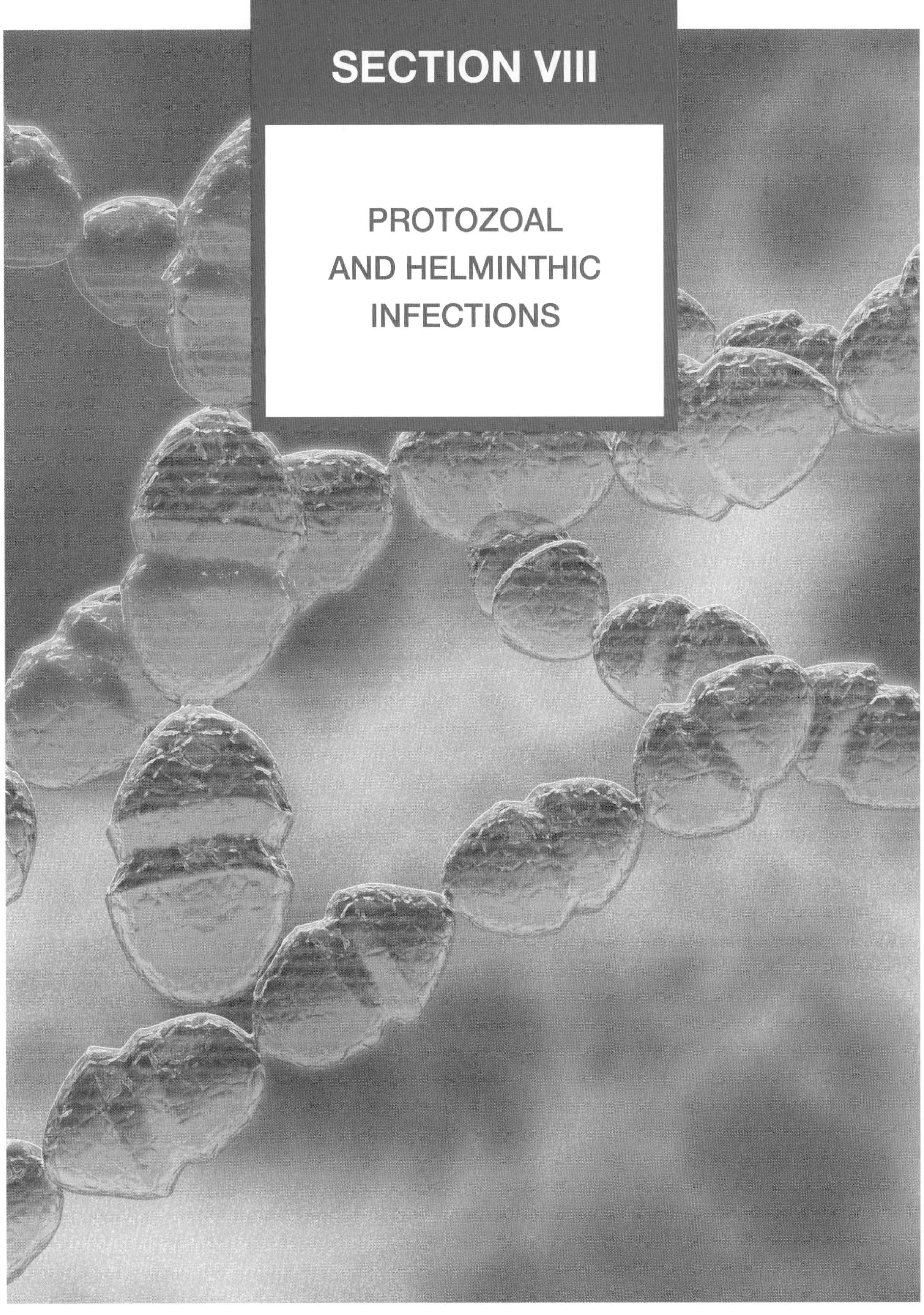

CHAPTER 112

LABORATORY DIAGNOSIS OF PARASITIC INFECTIONS

Sharon L. Reed ■ Charles E. Davis

The cornerstone for the diagnosis of parasitic infections is a thorough history of the patient's illness. Epidemiologic aspects of the illness are especially important because the risks of acquiring many parasites are closely related to occupation, recreation, or travel to areas of high endemicity. Without a basic knowledge of the epidemiology and life cycles of the major parasites, it is difficult to approach the diagnosis of parasitic infections systematically. Accordingly, the medical classification of important human parasites in this chapter emphasizes their geographic distribution, their transmission, and the anatomic location and stages of their life cycle in humans. The text and tables are intended to serve as a guide to the correct diagnostic procedures for the major parasitic infections and to direct the reader to other chapters that contain more comprehensive information about each infection. Tables 112-1 to 112-3 summarize the geographic distributions, anatomic locations, and methods employed for the diagnosis of flatworm, roundworm, and protozoal infections, respectively.

In addition to selecting the correct diagnostic procedures, physicians must counsel their patients to ensure that specimens are collected properly and arrive at the laboratory promptly. For example, the diagnosis of bancroftian filariasis is unlikely to be confirmed by the laboratory unless blood is drawn near midnight, when the nocturnal microfilariae are active. Laboratory personnel and surgical pathologists should be notified in advance when a parasitic infection is suspected. Continuing interaction with the laboratory staff and the surgical pathologists increases the likelihood that parasites in body fluids or biopsy specimens will be examined carefully by the most capable individuals.

INTESTINAL PARASITES

Most helminths and protozoa exit the body in the fecal stream. The patient should be instructed to collect feces in a clean waxed or cardboard container and to record the time of collection on the container. Contamination with water (which could contain free-living protozoa) or with urine (which can damage trophozoites) should be avoided. Fecal samples should be collected before ingestion of barium or other contrast agents for radiologic procedures and before treatment with antidiarrheal agents and antacids, because these substances change the consistency of the feces and interfere with microscopic detection of parasites. Because of the cyclic shedding of most parasites in the feces, a minimum of three samples collected on alternate days should be examined. Examination of a single sample can be up to 50% less sensitive. When delays in transport to the laboratory are unavoidable, fecal samples should be kept in polyvinyl alcohol or another fixative to preserve protozoal trophozoites. New collection kits with instructions for the patient to transfer portions of the sample directly into fixative and bacterial carrier medium may enhance the recovery of trophozoites. Refrigeration will also preserve trophozoites for a few hours and protozoal cysts and helminthic ova for several days.

Analysis of fecal samples entails both macroscopic and microscopic examination. Watery or loose stools are more likely to contain protozoal trophozoites, but protozoal cysts and all stages of helminths may be found in formed feces. If adult worms or tapeworm segments are observed, they should be transported promptly to the laboratory or washed and preserved in fixative for later examination. The only tapeworm with motile segments is *Taenia saginata*, the beef tapeworm, which patients sometimes bring to the physician. Motility is an important distinguishing characteristic, because the ova of *T. saginata* are morphologically indistinguishable from those of *Taenia solium*, the cause of cysticercosis.

Microscopic examination of feces is not complete until direct wet mounts have been evaluated and concentration techniques as well as permanent stains have been applied. Before accepting a report of negativity for ova and parasites as final, the physician should insist that the laboratory undertake each of these procedures. Some intestinal parasites are more readily detected in material other than feces. For example, examination of duodenal

TABLE 112-1

FLATWORM INFECTIONS

PARASITE	GEOGRAPHIC DISTRIBUTION	LIFE-CYCLE HOSTS: INTERMEDIATE (TRANSMISSION)	LIFE-CYCLE HOSTS: DEFINITIVE	DIAGNOSIS: PARASITE STAGE	DIAGNOSIS: BODY FLUID OR TISSUE	DIAGNOSIS: SEROLOGIC TESTS	DIAGNOSIS: OTHER
Tapeworms (Cestodes)							
Intestinal tapeworms							
Taenia saginata (beef tapeworm)	Worldwide	Beef	Humans	Ova, segments	Feces	—	Motile segments
Hymenolepis nana (dwarf tapeworm)	Worldwide	Grain beetles	Humans, mice[a]	Ova	Feces	—	—
Diphyllobothrium latum (fish tapeworm)	Worldwide	Copepods–fish[c]	Humans, other mammals	Ova, segments	Feces	—	Megaloblastic anemia in 1%
T. solium[b] (pork tapeworm)	Worldwide	Swine	Humans	Ova, segments	Feces	WB	Especially Mexico, Central and South America, Africa
Somatic tapeworms							
Echinococcus granulosus (hydatid disease)	Sheep-raising and hunting areas	Sheep, camels, humans, others	Dogs	Hydatid	Lung, liver	WB, EIA	Chest radiography, CT, MRI
E. multilocularis (hydatid disease)	Subarctic areas	Rodents, humans	Foxes, dogs, cats	Hydatid	Liver	—	May resemble cholangiocellular carcinoma
T. solium[b] (pork tapeworm)	Worldwide	Swine, humans	Humans	Cysticercus	Muscles, CNS	WB	CT, MRI, radiography
Flukes (Trematodes)							
Intestinal flukes							
Fasciolopsis buski	China, India	Snails–water chestnuts	Humans	Ova	Feces	—	—
Heterophyes heterophyes	Far East, India	Snails–fish	Humans	Ova	Feces	—	—
Metagonimus yokogawai	Far East, Balkans, North Africa	Snails–fish	Humans	Ova	Feces	—	—
Liver flukes							
Clonorchis sinensis	China, Southeast Asia	Snails–fish	Humans	Ova	Feces, bile	—	Recurrent bacterial cholangitis
Fasciola hepatica	Sheep-raising areas	Snails–watercress	Humans, sheep	Ova	Feces,[d] bile	EIA	Cirrhosis, portal hypertension
Lung flukes							
Paragonimus spp.	Orient, Africa, South America	Snails–crabs/crayfish	Humans, other mammals	Adults, ova	Lung, sputum, feces	WB, EIA	Chest radiography, CT, MRI
Blood flukes							
Schistosoma mansoni	Africa, Central and South America, West Indies	Snails	Humans	Ova, adults	Feces	EIA, WB	Rectal snips, liver biopsy
S. haematobium	Africa	Snails	Humans	Ova, adults	Urine	WB	Liver, urine, or bladder biopsy
S. japonicum	Far East	Snails	Humans	Ova, adults	Feces	WB	Liver biopsy

[a] Larvae also can mature in intestinal villi of humans and mice.

[b] *T. solium* can cause either intestinal infections or cysticercosis. Its ova are identical to those of *T. saginata*; scolices and segments of the two species differ.

[c] When there are two intermediate hosts, the first is separated from the second by a dash. Definitive hosts are infected by the second intermediate host.

[d] Ova seldom reach the fecal stream during acute disease.

Note: WB, western blot; CNS, central nervous system; EIA, enzyme immunoassay. Serologic tests listed in Tables 112-1, 112-2, and 112-3 are available commercially or from the Centers for Disease Control and Prevention, Atlanta, GA.

TABLE 112-2

ROUNDWORM INFECTIONS

PARASITE	GEOGRAPHIC DISTRIBUTION	LIFE-CYCLE HOSTS: INTERMEDIATE (TRANSMISSION)	LIFE-CYCLE HOSTS: DEFINITIVE	DIAGNOSIS: PARASITE STAGE	DIAGNOSIS: BODY FLUID OR TISSUE	DIAGNOSIS: SEROLOGIC TESTS	DIAGNOSIS: OTHER
Intestinal Roundworms							
Enterobius vermicularis (pinworm)	Temperate and tropical zones	Fecal-oral	Humans	Ova	Perianal skin	—	"Cellophane tape" test
Trichuris trichiura (whipworm)	Temperate and tropical zones	Soil, fecal-oral	Humans	Ova	Feces	—	Rectal prolapse
Ascaris lumbricoides (roundworm of humans)	Temperate and tropical zones	Soil, fecal-oral	Humans	Ova	Feces	—	Sx of pulmonary migration
Ancylostoma duodenale (Old World hookworm)	Eurasia, Africa, Pacific	Soil→skin	Humans	Ova/larvae	Feces	—	Sx of pulmonary migration, anemia
Necator americanus (New World hookworm)	U.S., Africa, worldwide	Soil→skin	Humans	Ova/larvae	Feces	—	Sx of pulmonary migration, anemia
Strongyloides stercoralis (strongyloidiasis)	Moist tropics and subtropics	Soil→skin	Humans	Larvae	Feces, sputum, duodenal fluid	EIA	Dissemination in immunodeficiency
Capillaria philippinensis	Southeast Asia, Taiwan, Egypt	Raw fish	Birds	Ova, larvae, adults	Feces	—	Malabsorption/ autoinfection, biopsy
Tissue Roundworms							
Trichinella spiralis (trichinellosis)	Worldwide	Swine/humans	Swine/humans	Larvae	Muscle	EIA	Muscle biopsy
Wuchereria bancrofti (filariasis)	Coastal areas in tropics and subtropics	Mosquitoes	Humans	Microfilariae	Blood, lymph nodes	EIA, RAPID	Nocturnal periodicity[a]
Brugia malayi (filariasis)	Asia, Indian subcontinent	Mosquitoes	Humans	Microfilariae	Blood	EIA, RAPID	Nocturnal
Loa loa (African eye worm)	West and Central Africa	Mango flies (*Chrysops*)	Humans	Microfilariae	Blood	—	May be visible in eye, diurnal
Onchocerca volvulus (river blindness)	Africa, Mexico, Central and South America	Blackflies	Humans	Adults/larvae	Skin/eye	—	Examine nodules or skin snips
Dracunculus medinensis (guinea worm)	Africa	*Cyclops*	Humans	Adults/larvae	Skin	—	May be visible in lesion
Angiostrongylus cantonensis	Southeast Asia, Pacific, Caribbean	Snails/slugs, shrimp/fish	Rats	Larvae	CSF (rarely found)	—	Eosinophilic meningitis
Larva Migrans Syndromes							
Ancylostoma braziliense (creeping eruption)	Tropical and temperate zones	Soil→skin	Dogs/cats, humans	Larvae	Skin	—	Dog and cat hookworm
Toxocara canis and *cati* (visceral larva migrans)	Tropical and temperate zones	Soil, fecal-oral	Dogs/cats, humans	Larvae	Viscera, CNS, eye	EIA[b]	Also caused by roundworms of other species

[a] Blood should be drawn at midnight, except for infection acquired in the South Pacific.

[b] The presence of hemagglutinins is a useful clue.

Note: Sx, signs/symptoms; EIA, enzyme immunoassay; CNS, central nervous system; RAPID, rapid immunographic assay [available at the National Institutes of Health (301-496-5398)].

TABLE 112-3

PROTOZOAL INFECTIONS

PARASITE	GEOGRAPHIC DISTRIBUTION	LIFE-CYCLE HOSTS: INTERMEDIATE (TRANSMISSION)	LIFE-CYCLE HOSTS: DEFINITIVE	DIAGNOSIS: PARASITE STAGE	DIAGNOSIS: BODY FLUID OR TISSUE	DIAGNOSIS: SEROLOGIC TESTS	DIAGNOSIS: OTHER
Intestinal Protozoans							
Entamoeba histolytica (amebiasis)	Worldwide, especially tropics	Fecal-oral	Humans	Troph, cyst	Feces, liver	EIA, antigen detection	Ultrasound, liver CT, PCR
Giardia lamblia (giardiasis)	Worldwide	Fecal-oral	Humans	Troph, cyst	Feces	Antigen detection	String test, DFA, PCR
Isospora belli	Worldwide	Fecal-oral	Humans	Oocyst	Feces	—	Acid-fast[a]
Cryptosporidium	Worldwide	Fecal-oral	Humans, other animals	Oocyst	Feces	Antigen detection	Acid-fast,[a] DFA, biopsy, PCR
Cyclospora cayetanensis	Worldwide?	Fecal-oral	Humans, other animals?	Oocyst	Feces	—	Acid-fast,[a] modified safranin, autofluorescence, biopsy, PCR
Microsporidium (*Enterocytozoon bieneusi*, *Encephalitozoon* spp.) (microsporidiosis)	Worldwide?	?	Animals, humans	Spore	Feces	—	Modified trichrome, acid-fast,[a] biopsy, PCR
Free-Living Amebas							
Naegleria	Worldwide	Warm water	Humans	Troph, cyst	CNS, nares	DFA	Biopsy, nasal swab, culture
Acanthamoeba	Worldwide	Soil, water	Humans	Troph, cyst	CNS, skin, cornea	DFA	Biopsy, scrapings, culture
Blood and Tissue Protozoans							
Plasmodium spp. (malaria)	Subtropics and tropics	Mosquitoes	Humans	Asexual	Blood	Limited use	PCR
Babesia microti (babesiosis)	U.S., especially New England	Ticks	Rodents, humans	Asexual	Blood	IIF	Animal spp. in asplenia, PCR
Trypanosoma rhodesiense (African sleeping sickness)	Sub-Saharan East Africa	Tsetse flies	Humans, herbivores	Tryp	Blood, CSF	IIF[b]	Also chancre, lymph nodes
T. gambiense (African sleeping sickness)	Sub-Saharan West Africa	Tsetse flies	Humans, swine	Tryp	Blood, CSF	Card agglutination, IIF[b,c]	Also chancre, lymph nodes
T. cruzi (Chagas' disease)	Mexico→ South America	Reduviid bugs (triatomes)	Humans, dogs, wild animals	Amastigote, tryp	Multiple organs/ blood	IIF, EIA	Reactivation in immunosuppression
Leishmania tropica, etc.	Widespread in tropics and subtropics	Sandflies (*Phlebotomus*)	Humans, dogs, rodents	Amastigote	Skin	IFA, EIA[d]	Biopsy, scrapings, culture
L. braziliensis (mucocutaneous)	Mexico→ South America	Sandflies (*Lutzomyia*)	Humans, dogs, rodents	Amastigote	Skin, mucous membranes	IFA,[b] EIA	Biopsy, scrapings, culture
L. donovani (kala-azar)	Widespread in tropics and subtropics	Sandflies (*Phlebotomus*)	Humans, dogs, wild animals	Amastigote	RE system	IFA,[b] EIA	Biopsy, culture, PCR
Toxoplasma gondii (toxoplasmosis)	Worldwide	Humans, other mammals	Cats	Cyst, troph	CNS, eye, muscles, other	EIA, IIF	PCR

[a] Acid-fastness is best demonstrated by auramine fluorescence or modified acid-fast stain.
[b] Contact the CDC.
[c] Card agglutination is provided to endemic countries by the World Health Organization.
[d] Limited specificity; most sensitive for *L. donovani*.
Note: troph, trophozoite; tryp, trypomastigote form; IIF, indirect immunofluorescence; RE, reticuloendothelial; PCR, polymerase chain reaction; EIA, enzyme immunoassay; CNS, central nervous system; IFA, indirect fluorescent antibody; CSF, cerebrospinal fluid; DFA, direct fluorescent antibody.

TABLE 112-4

ALTERNATIVE PROCEDURES FOR LABORATORY DIAGNOSIS OF PARASITES FOUND IN FECES[a]

PARASITES AND FECAL STAGES	ALTERNATIVE DIAGNOSTIC PROCEDURES
Tapeworms (Cestodes)	
Taenia saginata ova and segments	Perianal "cellophane tape" test for ova
T. solium ova and segments	Serology; brain biopsy for neurocysticercosis
Flukes (Trematodes)	
Clonorchis (Opisthorchis) sinensis ova	Examination of bile for ova and adults in cholangitis
Fasciola hepatica ova	Examination of bile for ova and adults in cholangitis
Paragonimus spp. ova	Serology; sputum; biopsy of lung or brain for larvae
Schistosoma ova	Serology for all; rectal snips (especially for *S. mansoni*), urine (*S. haematobium*), liver biopsy and liver ultrasound
Roundworms	
Enterobius vermicularis ova and adults	Perianal "cellophane tape" test for ova and adults
Trichuris trichiura ova	None
Ascaris lumbricoides ova and adults	Examination of sputum for larvae in lung disease
Hookworm ova and occasional larvae	Examination of sputum for larvae in lung disease
Strongyloides larvae	Duodenal aspirate or jejunal biopsy; serology; sputum or lung biopsy for filariform larvae in disseminated disease
Protozoans	
Entamoeba histolytica trophozoites and cysts	Serology; liver biopsy for trophozoites
Giardia lamblia trophozoites and cysts	Duodenal aspirate or jejunal biopsy[b]
Isospora belli oocysts	Duodenal aspirate or jejunal biopsy[b]
Cryptosporidium oocysts	Duodenal aspirate or jejunal biopsy[b]
Microsporidium spores	Duodenal aspirate or jejunal biopsy[b]

[a] Stains and concentration techniques are discussed in the text.
[b] Commercial string test is satisfactory; *Isospora* and *Cryptosporidium* are acid-fast.

contents is sometimes necessary to detect *Giardia lamblia*, *Cryptosporidium*, and *Strongyloides* larvae. Use of the "cellophane-tape" technique to detect pinworm ova on the perianal skin sometimes also reveals ova of *T. saginata* deposited perianally when the motile segments disintegrate (Table 112-4).

Two routine solutions are used to make wet mounts for the identification of the various life stages of helminths and protozoa: (1) physiologic saline for trophozoites, cysts, ova, and larvae; and (2) dilute iodine solution for protozoal cysts and ova. Iodine solution must never be used to examine specimens for trophozoites because it kills the parasites and thus eliminates their characteristic motility.

The two most common concentration procedures for detecting small numbers of cysts and ova are formalin-ether sedimentation and zinc sulfate flotation. The formalin-ether technique is preferable, because all parasites sediment but not all float. Slides permanently stained for trophozoites should be prepared before concentration. Additional slides stained for cysts and ova may be made from the concentrate.

In many instances, especially in the differentiation of *Entamoeba histolytica* from other amebas, identification of parasites from wet mounts or concentrates must be considered tentative. Permanently stained smears allow study of the cellular detail necessary for definitive identification. The iron-hematoxylin stain is excellent for critical work, but trichrome staining, which can be completed in 1 h, is a satisfactory alternative that also reveals parasites in specimens preserved in polyvinyl alcohol fixative. Modified acid-fast staining and fluorescent auramine microscopy are useful adjuncts for detection and identification of several intestinal protozoa, including *Cryptosporidium* and *Cyclospora* (Table 112-3).

BLOOD AND TISSUE PARASITES

Invasion of tissue by protozoa and helminths renders the choice of diagnostic techniques more difficult. For example, physicians must understand that aspiration of an amebic liver abscess rarely reveals *E. histolytica* because the trophozoites are located primarily in the abscess wall. They must remember that the urine sediment offers the best opportunity to detect *Schistosoma haematobium* in the young Ethiopian immigrant or the American traveler who returns from Africa with hematuria. Tables 112-1 to 112-3, which offer a quick guide to the geographic distribution and anatomic locations of the major tissue parasites, should help the physician to select the appropriate body fluid or biopsy site for microscopic examination. Tables 112-5 and 112-6 provide additional information about the identification of parasites in samples from specific anatomic locations. The laboratory procedures for

TABLE 112-5

IDENTIFICATION OF PARASITES IN BLOOD AND OTHER BODY FLUIDS

BODY FLUID, PARASITE	ENRICHMENT/STAIN	CULTURE TECHNIQUE
Blood		
Plasmodium spp.	Thick and thin smears/Giemsa or Wright's	Not useful for diagnosis
Leishmania spp.	Buffy coat/Giemsa	Media available from CDC
African trypanosomes[a]	Buffy coat, anion column/wet mount and Giemsa	Mouse or rat inoculation[b]
Trypanosoma cruzi[c]	As for African species	As above and xenodiagnosis
Toxoplasma gondii	Buffy coat/Giemsa	Fibroblast cell lines
Microfilariae[d]	Nuclepore filtration/wet mount and Giemsa	None
Urine		
Schistosoma haematobium	Centrifugation/wet mount	None
Microfilariae (in chyluria)	As for blood	None
Spinal Fluid		
African trypanosomes	Centrifugation, anion column/wet mount and Giemsa	As for blood
Naegleria fowleri	Centrifugation/wet mount and Giemsa or trichrome	Nonnutrient agar overlaid with *Escherichia coli*

[a] *Trypanosoma rhodesiense* and *T. gambiense.*

[b] Inject mice intraperitoneally with 0.2 mL of whole heparinized blood (0.5 mL for rats). After 5 days, tail blood should be checked daily for trypanosomes as described above. Call the CDC (770-488-7775) for information on diagnosis and treatment.

[c] Detectable in blood by conventional techniques only during acute disease. Xenodiagnosis is successful in ~50% of patients with chronic Chagas' disease.

[d] Day (1000–1400 h) and night (2200–0200 h) blood should be drawn to maximize the chance of detecting *Wuchereria* (nocturnal except for Pacific strains), *Brugia* (nocturnal), and *Loa loa* (diurnal).

detection of parasites in other body fluids are similar to those used in the examination of feces. The physician should insist on wet mounts, concentration techniques, and permanent stains for all body fluids. The trichrome or iron-hematoxylin stain is satisfactory for all tissue helminths in body fluids other than blood, but microfilarial worms and blood protozoa are more easily visualized when stained with Giemsa or Wright's stain.

The most common parasites detected in Giemsa-stained blood smears are the plasmodia, microfilariae,

TABLE 112-6

MINOR PROCEDURES FOR DIAGNOSIS OF PARASITIC INFECTIONS

PARASITE(S) AND STAGE	PROCEDURE
Onchocerca volvulus and *Mansonella streptocerca* microfilariae	*Skin snips:* Lift skin with a needle and excise ~1 mg to a depth of 0.5 mm from several sites. Weigh each sample, place it in 0.5 mL of saline for 4 h, and examine wet mounts and Giemsa stains of the saline either directly or after filtration. Count microfilariae.[a]
Loa loa adults and *O. volvulus* adults and microfilariae	*Biopsies of subcutaneous nodules:* Stain routine histopathologic sections and impression smears with Giemsa.
Trichinella spiralis larvae (and perhaps *Taenia solium* cysticerci)	*Muscle biopsies:* Excise ~1.0 g of deltoid or gastrocnemius muscle and squash between two glass slides for direct microscopic examination.
Schistosoma ova of all species, but especially *S. mansoni*	*Rectal snips:* From four areas of mucosa, take 2-mg snips, tease onto a glass slide, and flatten with a second slide before examining directly at 10×. Preparations may be fixed in alcohol or stained.
Trypanosoma gambiense and *T. rhodesiense* trypomastigotes	*Aspirate of chancre or lymph node:*[b] Aspirate center with 18-gauge needle, place a drop on a slide, and examine for motile forms. An otherwise insufficient volume of material may be stained with Giemsa.
Acanthamoeba spp. trophozoites or cysts	*Corneal scrapings:* Obtain sample from ophthalmologist for immediate Giemsa staining and culture on nutrient agar overlaid with *Escherichia coli.*
Cutaneous and mucocutaneous *Leishmania* spp.	*Swabs, aspirates, or punch biopsies of skin lesions:* Obtain specimen from margin of lesion for Giemsa staining of impression smears, and section and culture on special media from CDC.

[a] Counts of >100/mg are associated with significant risk of complications.

[b] Lymph node aspiration is contraindicated in some infections and should be used judiciously.

and African trypanosomes (Table 112-5). Most patients with Chagas' disease present in the chronic phase, when *Trypanosoma cruzi* is no longer microscopically detectable in blood smears. Wet mounts are sometimes more sensitive than stained smears for the detection of microfilariae and African trypanosomes because these active parasites cause noticeable movement of the erythrocytes in the microscopic field. Nuclepore filtration of blood facilitates the detection of microfilariae. The intracellular amastigote forms of *Leishmania* spp. and *T. cruzi* can sometimes be visualized in stained smears of peripheral blood, but aspirates of the bone marrow, liver, and spleen are the best sources for microscopic detection and culture of *Leishmania* in kala-azar and of *T. cruzi* in chronic Chagas' disease. The diagnosis of malaria and the critical distinction among the various *Plasmodium* species are made by microscopic examination of stained thick and thin blood films (Chap. 116).

Although most tissue parasites stain with the traditional hematoxylin and eosin, surgical biopsy specimens should also be stained with appropriate special stains. The surgical pathologist who is accustomed to applying silver stains for *Pneumocystis* to induced sputum and transbronchial biopsies may need to be reminded to examine wet mounts and iron-hematoxylin–stained preparations of pulmonary specimens for helminthic ova and *E. histolytica*. The clinician should also be able to advise the surgeon and pathologist about optimal techniques for the identification of parasites in specimens obtained by certain specialized minor procedures (Table 112-6). For example, the excision of skin snips for the diagnosis of onchocerciasis, the collection of rectal snips for the diagnosis of schistosomiasis, and punch biopsy of skin lesions for the identification and culture of cutaneous and mucocutaneous species of *Leishmania* are simple procedures, but the diagnosis can be missed if the specimens are improperly obtained or processed.

NONSPECIFIC TESTS

Eosinophilia (>500/μL) is a common accompaniment of infections with most of the tissue helminths; absolute numbers of eosinophils may be high in trichinellosis and the migratory phases of filariasis (Table 112-7). Intestinal helminths provoke eosinophilia only during pulmonary migration of the larval stages. Eosinophilia is not a manifestation of protozoal infections, with the possible exceptions of those due to *Isospora* and *Dientamoeba fragilis*.

Like the hypochromic, microcytic anemia of heavy hookworm infections, other nonspecific laboratory abnormalities may suggest parasitic infection in patients with appropriate geographic and/or environmental exposures. Biochemical evidence of cirrhosis or an abnormal urine sediment in an African immigrant certainly raises the possibility of schistosomiasis, and anemia and thrombocytopenia in a febrile traveler or immigrant are among the hallmarks of malaria. CT and MRI also contribute to the diagnosis of infections with many tissue parasites and have become invaluable adjuncts in the diagnosis of neurocysticercosis and cerebral toxoplasmosis.

TABLE 112-7

PARASITES FREQUENTLY ASSOCIATED WITH EOSINOPHILIA[a]

PARASITE	COMMENT
Tapeworms (Cestodes)	
Echinococcus granulosus	When hydatid cyst leaks
Taenia solium	During muscle encystation and in CSF with neurocysticercosis
Flukes (Trematodes)	
Paragonimus spp.	Uniformly high in acute stage
Fasciola hepatica	May be high in acute stage
Clonorchis (Opisthorchis) sinensis	Variable
Schistosoma mansoni	50% of infected travelers
S. haematobium	25% of infected travelers
S. japonicum	Up to 6000/μL in acute infection
Roundworms	
Ascaris lumbricoides	During larval migration
Hookworm species	During larval migration
Strongyloides stercoralis	Profound during migration and early years of infection
Trichinella spiralis	Up to 7000/μL
Filarial species[b]	Varies but can reach 5000–8000/μL
Toxocara spp.	>3000/μL
Ancylostoma braziliense	With extensive cutaneous eruption
Gnathostoma spinigerum	In visceral larva migrans and eosinophilic meningitis
Angiostrongylus cantonensis	In eosinophilic meningitis
A. costaricensis	During larval migration in mesenteric vessels

[a] Virtually every helminth has been associated with eosinophilia. This table includes both common and uncommon parasites that frequently elicit eosinophilia during infection.
[b] *Wuchereria bancrofti*, *Brugia* spp., *Loa loa*, and *Onchocerca volvulus*.

ANTIBODY AND ANTIGEN DETECTION

Useful antibody assays for many of the important tissue parasites are available; most of those listed in Table 112-8 can be obtained from the Centers for Disease Control and Prevention (CDC) in Atlanta. The results of serologic tests not listed in the tables should be interpreted with caution.

The value of antibody assays is limited by several factors. For example, the preparation of thick and thin blood smears remains the procedure of choice for the diagnosis of malaria in individual patients because diagnostic titers to plasmodia develop slowly and do not differentiate

TABLE 112-8

SEROLOGIC AND MOLECULAR TESTS FOR PARASITIC INFECTIONS[a]

PARASITE, INFECTION	ANTIBODY	ANTIGEN OR DNA/RNA
Tapeworms		
Echinococcosis	WB, EIA	
Cysticercosis	WB	
Flukes		
Paragonimiasis	WB, EIA[b]	
Schistosomiasis	EIA, WB	
Fascioliasis	EIA[b]	
Roundworms		
Strongyloidiasis	EIA	
Trichinellosis	EIA	
Toxocariasis	EIA	
Filariasis	EIA[c]	RAPID[c]
Protozoans		
Amebiasis	EIA	EIA,[b] RAPID,[b] PCR
Giardiasis		EIA,[b] RAPID,[b] DFA, PCR
Cryptosporidiosis		EIA,[b] DFA, RAPID,[b] PCR
Malaria (all species)	IIF[d]	PCR
Babesiosis	IIF	PCR
Chagas' disease	IIF, EIA	PCR
Leishmaniasis	IIF, EIA	PCR[b]
Toxoplasmosis	IIF, EIA (IgM)[e]	PCR[b]
Microsporidiosis		PCR
Cyclosporiasis		PCR
Acanthamoebiasis		DFA, PCR
Naegleriasis		DFA, PCR
Balmuthiasis		DFA

[a] Unless otherwise noted, all tests are available at the CDC.
[b] Research or commercial laboratories only.
[c] Available at the NIH (301-496-5398) and commercially.
[d] Of limited use for management of acute disease.
[e] Determination of infection within the last 3 months may require additional tests by a research laboratory.
Note: EIA, enzyme immunoassay; WB, western blot; IIF, indirect immunofluorescence; DFA, direct fluorescent antibody; PCR, polymerase chain reaction; RAPID, rapid immunographic assay. Most antigen and antibody parasite detection kits are available commercially. Most PCRs listed are now available at the CDC and in commercial or research laboratories. Contact the CDC.

species—a critical step in patient management. Filarial antigens cross-react with those from other nematodes; as in assays for antibody to most parasites, the presence of antibody in the filarial assay fails to distinguish between past and current infection. Despite these specific limitations, the restricted geographic distribution of many tropical parasites increases the diagnostic usefulness of both the presence and the absence of antibody in travelers from industrialized countries. In contrast, a large proportion of the world's population has been exposed to *Toxoplasma gondii*, and the presence of IgG antibody to *T. gondii* does not constitute proof of active disease.

Fewer antibody assays are available for the diagnosis of infection with intestinal parasites. *E. histolytica* is the major exception. Sensitive, specific serologic tests are invaluable in the diagnosis of amebiasis. Commercial kits for the detection of antigen by enzyme-linked immunosorbent assay or of whole organisms by fluorescent antibody assay are now available for several protozoan parasites (Table 112-8).

MOLECULAR TECHNIQUES

DNA hybridization with probes that are repeated many times in the genome of a specific parasite and amplification of a specific DNA fragment by the polymerase chain reaction (PCR) have now been established as useful techniques for the diagnosis of several protozoan infections (Table 112-8). Although PCR is very sensitive, it is an adjunct to conventional techniques for parasite detection and should be requested only when microscopic and immunodiagnostic procedures fail to establish the probable diagnosis. For example, only multiple negative blood smears or the failure to identify the infecting species justifies PCR for the diagnosis or proper management of malaria. In addition to PCR of anticoagulated blood, the CDC and several commercial laboratories now perform PCRs for detection of certain specific parasites in stool samples, biopsy specimens, and bronchoalveolar lavage fluid (Table 112-8). Although PCRs are now used primarily for the detection of protozoans, active research efforts are likely to establish their feasibility for the detection of several helminths.

FURTHER READINGS

FLECK SL, MOODY AH: *Diagnostic Techniques in Medical Parasitology*. London, Wright, 1988

FREEDMAN DO et al: Spectrum of disease and relation to place of exposure among ill returned travelers. N Engl J Med 354:119, 2006

GARCIA LS: Laboratory identification of the microsporidia. J Clin Microbiol 40:1892, 2002

——— et al: Algorithms for detection and identification of parasites, in *Manual of Clinical Microbiology*, 9th ed, vol 2, PR Murray et al (eds). Washington, DC, ASM Press, 2007, pp 2020–2039

HERWALDT BL: *Cyclospora cayetanensis*: A review, focusing on the outbreaks of cyclosporiasis in the 1990s. Clin Infect Dis 31:1040, 2000

SEYBOLT LM et al: Diagnostic evaluation of newly arrived asymptomatic refugees with eosinophilia. Clin Infect Dis 42:363, 2006

TANYUKSEL M et al: Laboratory diagnosis of amebiasis. Clin Microbiol Rev 16:713, 2003

WALKER M et al: Parasitic central nervous system infections in immunocompromised hosts: Malaria, microsporidiosis, leishmaniasis, and African trypanosomiasis. Clin Infect Dis 42:115, 2006

WILSON M et al: Molecular immunological approaches to the diagnosis of parasitic infection, in *Manual of Molecular and Clinical Laboratory Immunology,* 7th ed, B Detrick et al (eds). Washington, DC, ASM Press, 2006, pp 557–568

——— et al: *Toxoplasma*, in *Manual of Clinical Microbiology*, 9th ed, vol 2, PR Murray et al (eds). Washington, DC, ASM Press, 2007, pp 2070–2081

CHAPTER 113

AGENTS USED TO TREAT PARASITIC INFECTIONS

Thomas A. Moore

Parasitic infections afflict more than half of the world's population and impose a substantial health burden, particularly in underdeveloped nations, where they are most prevalent. The remarkable success of global campaigns aimed at controlling or eliminating ancient scourges such as dracunculiasis and onchocerciasis has been offset by the spread of other diseases such as trypanosomiasis due to crumbling infrastructures in settings of HIV infection, civil war, and unstable government. The reach of some parasitic diseases, including malaria, has expanded over the past few decades as a result of factors such as deforestation, population shifts, global warming, and other climatic events. Despite major efforts at vaccine development and vector control, chemotherapy remains the single most effective means of controlling parasitic infections. However, efforts to combat the spread of some diseases are hindered by the development and spread of drug resistance, the limited introduction of new antiparasitic agents, and the proliferation of counterfeit medications. Significant advances toward the reduction of the burden of parasitic disease have nevertheless been made, and the significant increase in funding of global health initiatives offers promise for the future.

This chapter deals exclusively with the agents used to treat infections due to parasites. Specific treatment recommendations for the parasitic diseases of humans are listed in subsequent chapters. The pharmacology of the antiparasitic agents is discussed in great detail in Chap. 114.

Table 113-1 presents a brief overview of each agent (including some drugs that are covered in other chapters), along with its major toxicities, spectrum of activity, and safety for use during pregnancy and lactation. Many of the agents are approved by the U.S. Food and Drug Administration but are considered investigational for the treatment of certain infections; these drugs are marked accordingly in the table. In addition, drugs available only through the Centers for Disease Control and Prevention (CDC) Drug Service (telephone: 404-639-3670 or 404-639-2888; *www.cdc.gov/ncidod/dpd/professional/drug_service.htm*) or only through their manufacturers (whose contact information may be available from the CDC) are specified by footnotes in the table.

TABLE 113-1

OVERVIEW OF AGENTS USED FOR THE TREATMENT OF PARASITIC INFECTIONS

DRUGS BY CLASS	PARASITIC INFECTION(S)	ADVERSE EFFECTS	MAJOR DRUG-DRUG INTERACTIONS	PREGNANCY CLASS[a]	BREAST MILK
4-Aminoquinolines					
Amodiaquine	Malaria[b]	Agranulocytosis, hepatotoxicity	No information	Not assigned	No information
Chloroquine	Malaria[b]	*Occasional:* pruritus, nausea, vomiting, headache, hair depigmentation, exfoliative dermatitis, reversible corneal opacity. *Rare:* irreversible retinal injury, nail discoloration, blood dyscrasias	Antacids and kaolin: reduced absorption of chloroquine Ampicillin: bioavailability reduced by chloroquine Cimetidine: increased serum levels of chloroquine Cyclosporine: serum levels increased by chloroquine	Not assigned[c]	Yes
8-Aminoquinolines					
Primaquine	Malaria[b]	*Frequent:* hemolysis in patients with G6PD deficiency. *Occasional:* methemoglobinemia, GI disturbances. *Rare:* CNS symptoms	Quinacrine: potentiated toxicity of primaquine	Contraindicated	No information

(*Continued*)

TABLE 113-1 (*CONTINUED*)

OVERVIEW OF AGENTS USED FOR THE TREATMENT OF PARASITIC INFECTIONS

DRUGS BY CLASS	PARASITIC INFECTION(S)	ADVERSE EFFECTS	MAJOR DRUG-DRUG INTERACTIONS	PREGNANCY CLASS[a]	BREAST MILK
Tafenoquine	Malaria[b]	*Frequent:* hemolysis in patients with G6PD deficiency, mild GI upset. *Occasional:* methemoglobinemia, headaches	No information	Not assigned	No information
Aminoalcohols					
Halofantrine	Malaria[b]	*Frequent:* abdominal pain, diarrhea. *Occasional:* ECG disturbances (dose-related prolongation of QTc and PR interval), nausea, pruritus. Contraindicated in persons who have cardiac disease or who have taken mefloquine in the preceding 3 weeks	Concomitant use of agents that prolong QTc interval contraindicated	C	No information
Lumefantrine	Malaria	*Occasional:* nausea, vomiting, diarrhea, abdominal pain, anorexia, headache, dizziness	No major interactions	Not assigned	No information
Aminoglycosides					
Paromomycin	Amebiasis,[b] infection with *Dientamoeba fragilis,* giardiasis, cryptosporidiosis, leishmaniasis	*Frequent:* GI disturbances (oral dosing only). *Occasional:* nephrotoxicity, ototoxicity, vestibular toxicity (parenteral dosing only)	No major interactions	Not assigned[c]	No information
Amphotericin B Amphotericin B deoxycholate Amphotec (InterMune) Amphotericin B lipid complex, ABLC (Abelcet) Amphotericin B, liposomal (AmBisome)	Leishmaniasis,[d] amebic meningoencephalitis	*Frequent:* fever, chills, hypokalemia, hypomagnesemia, nephrotoxicity. *Occasional:* vomiting, dyspnea, hypotension	Antineoplastic agents: renal toxicity, bronchospasm, hypotension Glucocorticoids, ACTH, digitalis: hypokalemia Zidovudine: increased myelo- and nephrotoxicity	B	No information
Antimonials	Leishmaniasis				
Pentavalent antimony[e]		*Frequent:* arthralgias/myalgias, pancreatitis, ECG changes (QT prolongation, T wave flattening or inversion)	No major interactions	Not assigned	Yes
Meglumine antimonate		*Frequent:* arthralgias/myalgias, pancreatitis, ECG changes (QT prolongation, T wave flattening or inversion)	Antiarrhythmics and tricyclic antidepressants: increased risk of cardiotoxicity	Not assigned	No information
Artemisinin and derivatives	Malaria	*Occasional:* neurotoxicity (ataxia, convulsions), nausea, vomiting, anorexia, contact dermatitis		Not assigned	No information

(*Continued*)

TABLE 113-1 (*CONTINUED*)

OVERVIEW OF AGENTS USED FOR THE TREATMENT OF PARASITIC INFECTIONS

DRUGS BY CLASS	PARASITIC INFECTION(S)	ADVERSE EFFECTS	MAJOR DRUG-DRUG INTERACTIONS	PREGNANCY CLASS[a]	BREAST MILK
Arteether			No information		
Artemether			No clinically significant interactions		
Artesunate			Mefloquine: levels decreased and clearance accelerated by artesunate		
Dihydroartemisinin			Mefloquine: increased absorption		
Atovaquone	Malaria,[a] babesiosis	*Frequent:* nausea, vomiting. *Occasional:* abdominal pain, headache	Plasma levels decreased by rifampin, tetracycline; bioavailability decreased by metoclopramide	C	No information
Azoles Fluconazole Itraconazole Ketoconazole	Leishmaniasis	*Serious:* hepatotoxicity. *Rare:* exfoliative skin disorders, anaphylaxis	Warfarin, oral hypoglycemics, phenytoin, cyclosporine, theophylline, digoxin, dofetilide, quinidine, carbamazepine, rifabutin, busulfan, docetaxel, vinca alkaloids, pimozide, alprazolam, diazepam, midazolam, triazolam, verapamil, atorvastatin, cerivastatin, lovastatin, simvastatin, tacrolimus, sirolimus, indinavir, ritonavir, saquinavir, alfentanil, buspirone, methylprednisolone, trimetrexate: plasma levels increased by azoles Carbamazepine, phenobarbital, phenytoin, isoniazid, rifabutin, rifampin, antacids, H2-receptor antagonists, proton pump inhibitors, nevirapine: decreased plasma levels of azoles Clarithromycin, erythromycin, indinavir, ritonavir: increased plasma levels of azoles	C	Yes
Benzimidazoles					
Albendazole	Ascariasis, capillariasis, clonorchiasis, cutaneous larva migrans, cysticercosis,[b] echinococcosis,[b] enterobiasis, eosinophilic enterocolitis, gnathostomiasis, hookworm, lymphatic filariasis, microsporidiosis, strongyloidiasis, trichinellosis, trichostrongyliasis, trichuriasis, visceral larva migrans	*Occasional:* nausea, vomiting, abdominal pain, headache, reversible alopecia, elevated aminotransferases. *Rare:* leukopenia, rash	Dexamethasone, praziquantel: plasma level of albendazole sulfoxide increased by ~50%	C	Yes[f]

(*Continued*)

TABLE 113-1 (*CONTINUED*)

OVERVIEW OF AGENTS USED FOR THE TREATMENT OF PARASITIC INFECTIONS

DRUGS BY CLASS	PARASITIC INFECTION(S)	ADVERSE EFFECTS	MAJOR DRUG-DRUG INTERACTIONS	PREGNANCY CLASS[a]	BREAST MILK
Mebendazole	Ascariasis,[b] capillariasis, eosinophilic enterocolitis, enterobiasis,[b] hookworm,[b] trichinellosis, trichostrongyliasis, trichuriasis,[b] visceral larva migrans	*Occasional:* diarrhea, abdominal pain, elevated aminotransferases. *Rare:* agranulocytosis, thrombocytopenia, alopecia	Cimetidine: inhibited mebendazole metabolism	C	No information
Thiabendazole	Strongyloidiasis,[b] cutaneous larva migrans,[b] visceral larva migrans[b]	*Frequent:* anorexia, nausea, vomiting, diarrhea, headache, dizziness, asparagus-like urine odor. *Occasional:* drowsiness, giddiness, crystalluria, elevated aminotransferases, psychosis. *Rare:* hepatitis, seizures, angioneurotic edema, Stevens-Johnson syndrome, tinnitus	Theophylline: serum levels increased by thiabendazole	C	No information
Triclabendazole	Fascioliasis, paragonimiasis	*Occasional:* abdominal cramps, diarrhea, biliary colic, transient headache	No information	Not assigned	Yes
Benznidazole	Chagas' disease	*Frequent:* rash, pruritus, nausea, leukopenia, paresthesias	No major interactions	Not assigned	No information
Bithionol[e]	Fascioliasis, paragonimiasis	Diarrhea, abdominal cramps (usually mild and transient)			
Clindamycin	Babesiosis, malaria, toxoplasmosis	*Occasional:* pseudomembranous colitis, abdominal pain, diarrhea, nausea/vomiting. *Rare:* pruritus, skin rashes	No major interactions	B	Yes[f]
Diloxanide furoate	Amebiasis	*Frequent:* flatulence. *Occasional:* nausea, vomiting, diarrhea. *Rare:* pruritus	None reported	Contraindicated	No information
Eflornithine[g] (difluoromethylornithine, DFMO)	Trypanosomiasis	*Frequent:* pancytopenia. *Occasional:* diarrhea, seizures. *Rare:* transient hearing loss	No major interactions	Contraindicated	No information
Emetine and dehydroemetine[e]	Amebiasis, fascioliasis	*Severe:* cardiotoxicity. *Frequent:* pain at injection site. *Occasional:* dizziness, headache, GI symptoms	None reported	X	No information

(Continued)

TABLE 113-1 (*CONTINUED*)

OVERVIEW OF AGENTS USED FOR THE TREATMENT OF PARASITIC INFECTIONS

DRUGS BY CLASS	PARASITIC INFECTION(S)	ADVERSE EFFECTS	MAJOR DRUG-DRUG INTERACTIONS	PREGNANCY CLASS[a]	BREAST MILK
Folate antagonists					
Dihydrofolate reductase inhibitors					
Pyrimethamine	Malaria,[b] isosporiasis, toxoplasmosis[b]	*Occasional:* folate deficiency. *Rare:* rash, seizures, severe skin reactions (toxic epidermal necrolysis, erythema multiforme, Stevens-Johnson syndrome)	Sulfonamides, proguanil, zidovudine: increased risk of bone marrow suppression when used concomitantly	C	Yes
Proguanil and chlorproguanil	Malaria	*Occasional:* urticaria. *Rare:* hematuria, GI disturbances	No major interactions	C	Yes
Trimethoprim	Cyclosporiasis, isosporiasis	Hyperkalemia, GI upset, mild stomatitis	Methotrexate: reduced clearance Warfarin: effect prolonged Phenytoin: hepatic metabolism increased	C	Yes
Dihydropteroate synthetase inhibitors: sulfonamides Sulfadiazine Sulfamethoxazole Sulfadoxine	Malaria,[b] toxoplasmosis[b]	*Frequent:* GI disturbances, allergic skin reactions, crystalluria. *Rare:* severe skin reactions (toxic epidermal necrolysis, erythema multiforme, Stevens-Johnson syndrome), agranulocytosis, aplastic anemia, hypersensitivity of the respiratory tract, hepatitis, interstitial nephritis, hypoglycemia, aseptic meningitis	Thiazide diuretics: increased risk of thrombocytopenia in elderly patients Warfarin: effect prolonged by sulfonamides Methotrexate: levels increased by sulfonamides Phenytoin: metabolism impaired by sulfonamides Sulfonylureas: effect prolonged by sulfonamides	B	Yes
Dihydropteroate synthetase inhibitors: sulfones					
Dapsone	Leishmaniasis, malaria, toxoplasmosis	*Frequent:* rash, anorexia. *Occasional:* hemolysis, methemoglobinemia, neuropathy, allergic dermatitis, anorexia, nausea, vomiting, tachycardia, headache, insomnia, psychosis, hepatitis. *Rare:* agranulocytosis	Rifampin: lowered plasma levels of dapsone	C	Yes
Fumagillin	Microsporidiosis	*Rare:* neutropenia, thrombocytopenia	None reported	No information	No information
Furazolidone	Giardiasis	*Frequent:* nausea/vomiting, brown urine. *Occasional:* rectal itching, headache. *Rare:* hemolytic anemia, disulfiram-like reactions, MAO-inhibitor interactions	Risk of hypertensive crisis when administered for >5 days with MAO inhibitors	C	No information

(*Continued*)

TABLE 113-1 (*CONTINUED*)

OVERVIEW OF AGENTS USED FOR THE TREATMENT OF PARASITIC INFECTIONS

DRUGS BY CLASS	PARASITIC INFECTION(S)	ADVERSE EFFECTS	MAJOR DRUG-DRUG INTERACTIONS	PREGNANCY CLASS[a]	BREAST MILK
Iodoquinol	Amebiasis,[b] balantidiasis, *D. fragilis* infection	*Occasional:* headache, rash, pruritus, thyrotoxicosis, nausea, vomiting, abdominal pain, diarrhea. *Rare:* optic neuritis, peripheral neuropathy, seizures, encephalopathy	No major interactions	C	No information
Ivermectin	Ascariasis, cutaneous larva migrans, gnathostomiasis, loiasis, lymphatic filariases, onchocerciasis,[b] scabies, strongyloidiasis,[b] trichuriasis	*Occasional:* fever, pruritus, headache, myalgias. *Rare:* hypotension	No major interactions	C	Yes[f]
Levamisole	Ascariasis, hookworm	*Frequent:* GI disturbances, dizziness, headache. *Rare:* agranulocytosis, peripheral neuropathy	Alcohol: disulfiram-like effect Warfarin: prolonged prothrombin time	C	No information
Macrolides Azithromycin	Babesiosis	*Occasional:* nausea, vomiting, diarrhea, abdominal pain. *Rare:* angioedema, cholestatic jaundice	Cyclosporine and digoxin: levels increased by azithromycin Nelfinavir: increased levels of azithromycin	B	Yes
Spiramycin[g]	Toxoplasmosis	*Occasional:* GI disturbances, transient skin eruptions. *Rare:* thrombocytopenia, QT prolongation in an infant, cholestatic hepatitis	No major interactions	Not assigned[c]	Yes[f]
Mefloquine	Malaria[b]	*Frequent:* lightheadedness, nausea, headache. *Occasional:* confusion; nightmares; insomnia; visual disturbance; transient and clinically silent ECG abnormalities, including sinus bradycardia, sinus arrhythmia, first-degree AV block, prolongation of QTc interval, and abnormal T waves. *Rare:* psychosis, convulsions, hypotension	Administration of halofantrine <3 weeks after mefloquine use may produce fatal QTc prolongation. Mefloquine may lower plasma levels of anticonvulsants. Levels decreased and clearance accelerated by artesunate	C	Yes
Melarsoprol[e]	Trypanosomiasis	*Frequent:* myocardial injury, encephalopathy, peripheral neuropathy, hypertension. *Occasional:* G6PD-induced hemolysis, erythema nodosum leprosum. *Rare:* hypotension	No major interactions	Not assigned	No information
Metrifonate	Schistosomiasis	*Frequent:* abdominal pain, nausea, vomiting, diarrhea, headache, vertigo, bronchospasm. *Rare:* cholinergic symptoms	No major interactions	B	No

(*Continued*)

TABLE 113-1 (*CONTINUED*)

OVERVIEW OF AGENTS USED FOR THE TREATMENT OF PARASITIC INFECTIONS

DRUGS BY CLASS	PARASITIC INFECTION(S)	ADVERSE EFFECTS	MAJOR DRUG-DRUG INTERACTIONS	PREGNANCY CLASS[a]	BREAST MILK
Miltefosine	Leishmaniasis	*Frequent:* mild and transient (1–2 days) GI disturbances within first 2 weeks of therapy (resolve after treatment completion); motion sickness. *Occasional:* reversible elevations of creatinine and aminotransferases	No major interactions	Not assigned	No information
Niclosamide	Intestinal cestodes[b]	*Occasional:* nausea, vomiting, dizziness, pruritus	No major interactions	B	No information
Nifurtimox[e]	Chagas' disease	*Frequent:* nausea, vomiting, abdominal pain, insomnia, paresthesias, weakness, tremors. *Rare:* seizures (all are reversible and dose-related)	No major interactions	Not assigned	No information
Nitazoxanide	Cryptosporidiosis,[b] giardiasis[b]	*Occasional:* abdominal pain, diarrhea. *Rare:* vomiting, headache	No major interactions	B	No information
Nitroimidazoles					
Metronidazole	Amebiasis,[b] balantidiasis, dracunculiasis, giardiasis, trichomoniasis,[b] *D. fragilis* infection	*Frequent:* nausea, headache, anorexia, metallic aftertaste. *Occasional:* vomiting, insomnia, vertigo, paresthesias, disulfiram-like effects. *Rare:* seizures, peripheral neuropathy	Warfarin: effect enhanced by metronidazole Disulfiram: psychotic reaction Phenobarbital, phenytoin: accelerate elimination of metronidazole Lithium: serum levels elevated by metronidazole Cimetidine: prolonged half-life of metronidazole	B	Yes
Tinidazole	Amebiasis,[b] giardiasis, trichomoniasis	*Occasional:* nausea, vomiting, metallic taste	See metronidazole	C	Yes
Oxamniquine	Schistosomiasis	*Occasional:* dizziness, drowsiness, headache, orange urine, elevated aminotransferases. *Rare:* seizures	No major interactions	C	No information
Paromomycin	Amebiasis,[b] *D. fragilis* infection, giardiasis, cryptosporidiosis, leishmaniasis	*Frequent:* GI disturbances (oral dosing only). *Occasional:* nephrotoxicity, ototoxicity, vestibular toxicity (parenteral dosing only)	No major interactions	Oral: B Parenteral: not assigned[c]	No information
Pentamidine isethionate	Leishmaniasis, trypanosomiasis	*Frequent:* hypotension, hypoglycemia, pancreatitis, sterile abscesses at IM injection sites, GI disturbances, reversible renal failure. *Occasional:* hepatotoxicity, cardiotoxicity, delirium. *Rare:* anaphylaxis	No major interactions	C	No information

(Continued)

TABLE 113-1 (*CONTINUED*)

OVERVIEW OF AGENTS USED FOR THE TREATMENT OF PARASITIC INFECTIONS

DRUGS BY CLASS	PARASITIC INFECTION(S)	ADVERSE EFFECTS	MAJOR DRUG-DRUG INTERACTIONS	PREGNANCY CLASS[a]	BREAST MILK
Piperazine and derivatives					
Piperazine	Ascariasis, enterobiasis	*Occasional:* nausea, vomiting, diarrhea, abdominal pain, headache. *Rare:* neurotoxicity, seizures	None reported	C	No information
Diethylcarbamazine[e]	Lymphatic filariasis, loiasis, tropical pulmonary eosinophilia	*Frequent:* dose-related nausea, vomiting. *Rare:* fever, chills, arthralgias, headaches	None reported	Not assigned[c]	No information
Praziquantel	Clonorchiasis,[b] cysticercosis, diphyllobothriasis, hymenolepiasis, taeniasis, opisthorchiasis, intestinal trematodes, paragonimiasis, schistosomiasis[b]	*Frequent:* abdominal pain, diarrhea, dizziness, headache, malaise. *Occasional:* fever, nausea. *Rare:* pruritus, singultus	No major interactions	B	Yes
Pyrantel pamoate	Ascariasis, eosinophilic enterocolitis, enterobiasis,[b] hookworm, trichostrongyliasis	*Occasional:* GI disturbances, headache, dizziness, elevated aminotransferases	No major interactions	C	No information
Quinacrine[g]	Giardiasis[b]	*Frequent:* headache, nausea, vomiting, bitter taste. *Occasional:* yellow-orange discoloration of skin, sclerae, urine; begins after 1 week of treatment and lasts up to 4 months after drug discontinuation. *Rare:* psychosis, exfoliative dermatitis, retinopathy, G6PD-induced hemolysis, exacerbation of psoriasis, disulfiram-like effects	Primaquine: toxicity potentiated by quinacrine	C	No information
Quinine and quinidine	Malaria, babesiosis	*Frequent:* cinchonism (tinnitus, high-tone deafness, headache, dysphoria, nausea, vomiting, abdominal pain, visual disturbances, postural hypotension), hyperinsulinemia resulting in life-threatening hypoglycemia. *Occasional:* deafness, hemolytic anemia, arrhythmias, hypotension due to rapid IV infusion	Carbonic-anhydrase inhibitors, thiazide diuretics: reduced renal elimination of quinidine Amiodarone, cimetidine: increased quinidine levels Nifedipine: decreased quinidine levels; quinidine slows metabolism of nifedipine Phenobarbital, phenytoin, rifampin: accelerated hepatic elimination of quinidine Verapamil: reduced hepatic clearance of quinidine Diltiazem: decreased clearance of quinidine	X	Yes[f]

(*Continued*)

TABLE 113-1 (*CONTINUED*)

OVERVIEW OF AGENTS USED FOR THE TREATMENT OF PARASITIC INFECTIONS

DRUGS BY CLASS	PARASITIC INFECTION(S)	ADVERSE EFFECTS	MAJOR DRUG-DRUG INTERACTIONS	PREGNANCY CLASS[a]	BREAST MILK
Quinolones					
Ciprofloxacin	Cyclosporiasis, isosporiasis	*Occasional:* nausea, diarrhea, vomiting, abdominal pain/discomfort, headache, restlessness, rash. *Rare:* myalgias/arthralgias, tendon rupture, CNS symptoms (nervousness, agitation, insomnia, anxiety, nightmares or paranoia); convulsions	Probenecid: increased serum levels of ciprofloxacin Theophylline, warfarin: serum levels increased by ciprofloxacin	C	Yes
Suramin[e]	Trypanosomiasis	*Frequent:* immediate: fever, urticaria, nausea, vomiting, hypotension; delayed (up to 24 h): exfoliative dermatitis, stomatitis, paresthesias, photophobia, renal dysfunction. *Occasional:* nephrotoxicity, adrenal toxicity, optic atrophy, anaphylaxis	No major interactions	Not assigned	No information
Tetracyclines	Balantidiasis, *D. fragilis* infection, malaria; lymphatic filariasis (doxycycline)	*Frequent:* GI disturbances. *Occasional:* photosensitivity dermatitis. *Rare:* exfoliative dermatitis, esophagitis, hepatotoxicity	Warfarin: effect prolonged by tetracyclines	D	Yes

[a] Based on U.S. Food and Drug Administration (FDA) pregnancy categories of A–D, X.
[b] Approved by the FDA for this indication.
[c] Use in pregnancy is recommended by international organizations outside the United States.
[d] Only AmBisome has been approved for this indication.
[e] Available through the Centers for Disease Control and Prevention (CDC).
[f] Not believed to be harmful.
[g] Available through the manufacturer.
Note: ACTH, adrenocorticotropic hormone; AV, atrioventricular; CNS, central nervous system; ECG, electrocardiogram; G6PD, glucose 6-phosphate dehydrogenase; MAO, monoamine oxidase.

FURTHER READINGS

Abramowicz M (ed): Drugs for parasitic infections. Med Lett Drugs Ther 46:1, 2004

Moore TA, McCarthy JS: Benzimidazoles (albendazole, mebendazole, thiabendazole, triclabendazole), in *Antimicrobial Therapy and Vaccines*, 2d ed, VL Yu et al (eds). Pittsburgh, ESun Technologies, 2005, pp 1021–1036

Reddy M et al: Oral drug therapy for multiple neglected tropical diseases: A systematic review. JAMA 298:1911, 2007

Shapiro TA, Goldberg DE: Drugs used in the chemotherapy of protozoal infections: Malaria, in *Goodman and Gilman's The Pharmacological Basis of Therapeutics*, 11th ed, L Brunton et al (eds). New York, McGraw-Hill, 2005, pp 1021–1048

Winstanley P, Ward S: Malaria chemotherapy. Adv Parasitol 61:47, 2006

World Health Organization: *Model Prescribing Information: Drugs Used in Parasitic Diseases*, 2d ed. Geneva, WHO, 1995

CHAPTER 114

PHARMACOLOGY OF AGENTS USED TO TREAT PARASITIC INFECTIONS

Thomas A. Moore

This chapter deals exclusively with the pharmacologic properties of the agents used to treat infections due to parasites. Specific treatment recommendations for the parasitic diseases of humans are listed in the chapters on those diseases. Information on these agents' major toxicities, spectrum of activity, and safety for use during pregnancy and lactation is presented in Chap. 113. Many of the agents discussed herein are approved by the U.S. Food and Drug Administration (FDA) but are considered investigational for the treatment of certain infections (see Table 113-1). Drugs marked in the text with an asterisk (*) are available only through the Centers for Disease Control and Prevention (CDC) Drug Service (telephone: 404-639-3670 or 404-639-2888; *www.cdc.gov/ncidod/dpd/professional/drug_service.htm*). Drugs marked with a dagger (†) are available only through their manufacturers; contact information for these manufacturers may be available from the CDC.

ALBENDAZOLE

Like all benzimidazoles, albendazole acts by selectively binding to free β-tubulin in nematodes, inhibiting the polymerization of tubulin and the microtubule-dependent uptake of glucose. Irreversible damage occurs in gastrointestinal (GI) cells of the nematodes, resulting in starvation, death, and expulsion by the host. While highly injurious to nematodes, this fundamental disruption of cellular metabolism also offers treatment for a wide range of parasitic diseases.

Albendazole is poorly absorbed from the GI tract. Administration with a fatty meal increases its absorption by two- to sixfold. Poor absorption may be advantageous for the treatment of intestinal helminths, but successful treatment of tissue helminth infections (e.g., hydatid disease and neurocysticercosis) requires that a sufficient amount of active drug reach the site of infection. The metabolite albendazole sulfoxide is responsible for the drug's therapeutic effect outside the gut lumen. Albendazole sulfoxide crosses the blood-brain barrier, reaching a level significantly higher than that achieved in plasma. The high concentrations of albendazole sulfoxide attained in cerebrospinal fluid (CSF) probably explain the efficacy of albendazole in the treatment of neurocysticercosis.

Albendazole is extensively metabolized in the liver, but there are few data regarding the drug's use in patients with hepatic disease. Single-dose albendazole therapy in humans is largely without side effects (overall frequency, ≤1%). More prolonged courses (e.g., as administered for cystic and alveolar echinococcal disease) have been associated with liver function abnormalities and bone marrow toxicity. Thus, when prolonged use is anticipated, the drug should be administered in treatment cycles of 28 days interrupted by 14 days off therapy. Prolonged therapy with full-dose albendazole (800 mg/d) should be approached cautiously in patients also receiving drugs with known effects on the cytochrome P450 system.

AMODIAQUINE

Amodiaquine has been widely used in the treatment of malaria for >40 years. Like chloroquine (the other major 4-aminoquinoline), amodiaquine is now of limited use because of the spread of resistance. Amodiaquine interferes with hemozoin formation through complexation with heme. Although rapidly absorbed, amodiaquine behaves as a prodrug after oral administration, with the principal plasma metabolite monodesethylamodiaquine as the predominant antimalarial agent. Amodiaquine and its metabolites are all excreted in urine, but there are no recommendations concerning dosage adjustment in patients with impaired renal function. Severe adverse events can occur, albeit rarely (1 case in 2000 treatment courses), with amodiaquine administration. Agranulocytosis and hepatotoxicity can develop with repeated use; therefore, this drug should not be used for prophylaxis.

AMPHOTERICIN B

See Table 113-1 and Chap. 102.

ANTIMONIALS*

Despite associated adverse reactions and the need for prolonged parenteral treatment, the pentavalent antimonial compounds (designated Sb^{V}) have remained the first-line therapy for all forms of leishmaniasis throughout the world, primarily because they are affordable, are effective, and have survived the test of time. Although they have been used for almost 100 years, their mechanism of action against *Leishmania* spp. has only recently come to light. Pentavalent antimonials are active only after bioreduction to the trivalent Sb(III) form. This form inhibits trypanothione reductase, a critical enzyme involved in the oxidative stress management of *Leishmania* spp. The fact that *Leishmania* spp. use trypanothione rather than glutathione (which is used by mammalian cells) may explain the parasite-specific activity of antimonials. The drugs are taken up by the reticuloendothelial system, and their activity against *Leishmania* spp. may be enhanced by this localization. Sodium stibogluconate is the only pentavalent antimonial available in the United States; meglumine antimonate is principally used in francophone countries.

Resistance is a major problem in some areas. Although low-level unresponsiveness to Sb^{v} was identified in India in the 1970s, incremental increases in both the recommended daily dosage (to 20 mg/kg) and the duration of treatment (to 28 days) satisfactorily compensated for the growing resistance until around 1990. There has since been a steady erosion in the capacity of Sb^{v} to induce long-term cure in patients with kala-azar who live in eastern India. Foremost among the many factors that have probably contributed to this failure is the provision of suboptimal treatment for years, which led to the development of drug resistance among parasites. Co-infection with HIV impairs the treatment response.

Sodium stibogluconate is available in aqueous solution and is administered parenterally. Antimony appears to have two elimination phases. When administered IV, the mean half-life of the first phase is <2 h; the mean half-life of the terminal elimination phase is nearly 36 h. This slower phase may be due to conversion of pentavalent antimony to a trivalent form that is the likely cause of the side effects often seen with prolonged therapy.

ARTEMISININ DERIVATIVES

Artesunate, artemether, arteether, and the parent compound artemisinin are sesquiterpene lactones derived from the wormwood plant *Artemisia annua*. These agents are at least 10-fold more potent in vivo than other antimalarial drugs and presently show no cross-resistance with known antimalarial drugs; thus, they have become first-line agents for the treatment of severe falciparum malaria in some areas where multidrug resistance is a major problem. However, to limit the development of resistance, the World Health Organization (WHO) has recommended that artemisinin and its derivatives be used only in areas where there is proven multidrug resistance. Artemether appears to be effective for the treatment of schistosomiasis and is being evaluated for community-based treatment programs.

The artemisinin compounds are rapidly effective against the asexual blood forms of *Plasmodium* spp. but are not active against intrahepatic forms. Artemisinin and its derivatives are highly lipid soluble and readily cross both host and parasite cell membranes. One factor that explains the drugs' highly selective toxicity against malaria is that parasitized erythrocytes concentrate artemisinin and its derivatives to concentrations 100-fold higher than those in uninfected erythrocytes. The antimalarial effect of these agents results primarily from dihydroartemisinin, a compound to which artemether and artesunate are both converted. In the presence of heme or molecular iron, the endoperoxide moiety of dihydroartemisinin decomposes, generating free radicals and other metabolites that damage parasite proteins. Long treatment courses are required. When these agents are used alone, recrudescence may occur. The compounds are available for oral, rectal, IV, or IM administration, depending on the derivative. Artemisinin and its derivatives are cleared rapidly from the circulation. Their short half-lives limit their value for prophylaxis and monotherapy. A combined formulation of artemether and lumefantrine has been developed for the treatment of acute uncomplicated falciparum malaria in areas where *Plasmodium falciparum* is resistant to chloroquine and antifolates.

ATOVAQUONE

Atovaquone is a hydroxynaphthoquinone that exerts broad-spectrum antiprotozoal activity via selective inhibition of parasite mitochondrial electron transport. This agent exhibits potent activity against toxoplasmosis and babesiosis when used with pyrimethamine and azithromycin, respectively. Atovaquone possesses a novel mode of action against *Plasmodium* spp., inhibiting the electron transport system at the level of the cytochrome bc1 complex. The drug is active against both the erythrocytic and the exoerythrocytic stages of *Plasmodium* spp.; however, because it does not eradicate hypnozoites from the liver, patients with *Plasmodium vivax* or *Plasmodium ovale* infections must be given radical prophylaxis.

Malarone is a fixed-dose combination of atovaquone and proguanil used for malaria prophylaxis as well as for the treatment of acute, uncomplicated *P. falciparum* malaria. Malarone has been shown to be effective in regions with multidrug-resistant *P. falciparum*. Resistance to atovaquone has yet to be reported.

The bioavailability of atovaquone varies considerably. Absorption after a single oral dose is slow, increases two- to threefold with a fatty meal, and is dose-limited above 750 mg. The elimination half-life is increased in patients with moderate hepatic impairment. Because of the potential for drug accumulation, the use of atovaquone is contraindicated in persons with severe renal impairment (creatinine clearance rate <30 mL/min). No dosage adjustments are needed in patients with mild to moderate renal impairment. It is unknown if atovaquone is dialyzable.

AZITHROMYCIN

See Table 113-1 and Chap. 33.

AZOLES

See Table 113-1 and Chap. 102.

BENZNIDAZOLE

This oral nitroimidazole derivative is used to treat Chagas' disease, with cure rates of 80–90% recorded in acute infections. Benznidazole is believed to exert its trypanocidal effects by generating oxygen radicals to which the parasites are more sensitive than mammalian cells because of a relative deficiency in antioxidant enzymes. Benznidazole also appears to alter the balance between pro- and anti-inflammatory mediators by downregulating the synthesis of nitrite, interleukin (IL) 6, and IL-10 in macrophages. Benznidazole is highly lipophilic and readily absorbed. The drug is extensively metabolized; only 5% of the dose is excreted unchanged in the urine.

BITHIONOL

Bithionol is a chlorinated bisphenol with activity against trematodes. *Fasciola hepatica* uses fumarate reduction coupled to rhodoquinone for anaerobic energy metabolism. Bithionol competitively inhibits electron transfer to fumarate by rhodoquinone; the result is impaired anaerobic energy metabolism and trematode death. Bithionol is parasite specific for two reasons: (1) Fumarate reductase catalyzes the reverse of the reaction of mammalian succinic dehydrogenase in the Krebs cycle. (2) The rhodoquinone respiratory chain link is unique to the parasite. In the mammalian respiratory chain, the quinone electron carrier is ubiquinone. Bithionol is readily absorbed from the GI tract. It is no longer produced, but limited supplies are available from the CDC.

CHLOROQUINE

This 4-aminoquinoline has marked, rapid schizontocidal and gametocidal activity against blood forms of *P. ovale* and *Plasmodium malariae* and against susceptible strains of *P. vivax* and *P. falciparum*. It is not active against intrahepatic forms (*P. vivax* and *P. ovale*). Parasitized erythrocytes accumulate chloroquine in significantly greater concentrations than do normal erythrocytes. Chloroquine, a weak base, concentrates in the food vacuoles of intraerythrocytic parasites because of a relative pH gradient between the extracellular space and the acidic food vacuole. Once it enters the acidic food vacuole, chloroquine is rapidly converted to a membrane-impermeable protonated form and is trapped. Continued accumulation of chloroquine in the parasite's acidic food vacuoles results in drug levels that are 600-fold higher at this site than in plasma. The high accumulation of chloroquine results in an increase in pH within the food vacuole to a level above that required for the acid proteases' optimal activity, inhibiting parasite heme polymerase; as a result, the parasite is effectively killed with its own metabolic waste. Compared with susceptible strains, chloroquine-resistant plasmodia transport chloroquine out of intraparasitic compartments more rapidly and maintain lower chloroquine concentrations in their acid vesicles. Hydroxychloroquine, a congener of chloroquine, is equivalent to chloroquine in its antimalarial efficacy but is preferred to chloroquine for the treatment of autoimmune disorders because it produces less ocular toxicity when used in high doses.

Chloroquine is well absorbed. However, because it exhibits extensive tissue binding, a loading dose is required to yield effective plasma concentrations. A therapeutic drug level in plasma is reached 2–3 h after oral administration (the preferred route). Chloroquine can be administered IV, but excessively rapid parenteral administration can result in seizures and death from cardiovascular collapse. The mean half-life of chloroquine is 4 days, but the rate of excretion decreases as plasma levels decline, making once-weekly administration possible for prophylaxis in areas with sensitive strains. About half of the parent drug is excreted in urine, but the dose should not be reduced for persons with acute malaria and renal insufficiency.

CIPROFLOXACIN

See Table 113-1 and Chap. 33.

CLINDAMYCIN

See Table 113-1 and Chap. 33.

DAPSONE

See Table 113-1 and Chap. 69.

DEHYDROEMETINE

Emetine is an alkaloid derived from ipecac; dehydroemetine is synthetically derived from emetine and is considered less toxic. Both agents are active against *Entamoeba histolytica* and appear to work by blocking peptide elongation and thus inhibiting protein synthesis. Emetine is rapidly absorbed after parenteral administration, rapidly distributed throughout the body, and slowly excreted in the urine in unchanged form. Both agents are contraindicated in patients with renal disease.

DIETHYLCARBAMAZINE*

A derivative of the antihelmintic agent piperazine with a long history of successful use, diethylcarbamazine (DEC) remains the treatment of choice for lymphatic filariasis and loiasis and has also been used for visceral larva migrans. While piperazine itself has no antifilarial activity, the piperazine ring of DEC is essential for the drug's activity. Although DEC was shown to be an effective agent for treatment of lymphatic filariasis in 1947, its mechanism of action remains to be fully defined. Proposed mechanisms include immobilization due to inhibition of parasite cholinergic muscle receptors, disruption of microtubule formation, and alteration of helminthic surface membranes resulting in enhanced killing by the host's immune system. In addition, DEC enhances adherence properties of eosinophils. The development of resistance under drug pressure (i.e., a progressive decrease in efficacy when the drug is used widely in human populations) has not been observed, although DEC's effect is variable when administered to persons with filariasis. Monthly administration provides effective prophylaxis against both bancroftian filariasis and loiasis.

DEC is well absorbed after oral administration, with peak plasma concentrations reached within 1–2 h. No parenteral form is available. The drug is eliminated largely by renal excretion, with <5% found in feces. If more than one dose is to be administered to an individual with renal dysfunction, the dose should be reduced commensurate with the reduction in creatinine clearance rate. Alkalinization of the urine prevents renal excretion and increases the half-life of DEC. Use in patients with onchocerciasis can precipitate a Mazzotti reaction, with pruritus, fever, and arthralgias. Like other piperazines, DEC is active against *Ascaris* spp. Patients co-infected with this nematode may expel live but paralyzed worms after treatment.

DILOXANIDE FUROATE

Diloxanide furoate, a substituted acetanilide, is a luminally active agent used to eradicate the cysts of *E. histolytica*. After ingestion, diloxanide furoate is hydrolyzed by enzymes in the lumen or mucosa of the intestine, releasing furoic acid and the ester diloxanide; the latter acts directly as an amebicide.

Diloxanide furoate is given alone to asymptomatic cyst passers. For patients with active amebic infections, diloxanide is generally administered in combination with a 5-nitroimidazole such as metronidazole or tinidazole. Diloxanide furoate is rapidly absorbed after oral administration. When coadministered with a 5-nitroimidazole, only diloxanide appears in the systemic circulation; levels peak within 1 h and disappear within 6 h. About 90% of an oral dose is excreted in the urine within 48 h, chiefly as the glucuronide metabolite. Diloxanide furoate is contraindicated in pregnant and breast-feeding women and in children <2 years of age.

EFLORNITHINE†

Eflornithine (difluoromethylornithine, or DFMO) is a fluorinated analogue of the amino acid ornithine. Although originally designed as an antineoplastic agent, eflornithine has proven effective against some trypanosomatids. At one point, the production of this effective agent ceased despite the increasing incidence of human African trypanosomiasis; however, production resumed after eflornithine was discovered to be an effective cosmetic depilatory agent.

Eflornithine has specific activity against all stages of infection with *Trypanosoma brucei gambiense*; however, it is inactive against *T. b. rhodesiense*. The drug acts as an irreversible suicide inhibitor of ornithine decarboxylase, the first enzyme in the biosynthesis of the polyamines putrescine and spermidine. Polyamines are essential for the synthesis of trypanothione, an enzyme required for the maintenance of intracellular thiols in the correct redox state and in the removal of reactive oxygen metabolites. However, polyamines are also essential for cell division in eukaryotes, and ornithine decarboxylase is similar in trypanosomes and mammals. The selective antiparasitic activity of eflornithine is partly explained by the structure of the trypanosomal enzyme, which lacks a 36-amino-acid C-terminal sequence found on mammalian ornithine decarboxylase. This difference results in a lower turnover of ornithine decarboxylase and a more rapid decrease of polyamines in trypanosomes than in the mammalian host. The diminished effectiveness of eflornithine against *T. b. rhodesiense* appears to be due to the parasite's ability to replace the inhibited enzyme more rapidly than *T. b. gambiense*.

Eflornithine is less toxic but more costly than conventional therapy. Eflornithine HCl can be administered IV or PO; however, its bioavailability after oral administration is only 54%. Eflornithine readily crosses the blood-brain barrier; CSF levels are highest in persons with the most severe central nervous system (CNS) involvement. The kidney excretes >80% of the drug dose; therefore, the dosage should be reduced in patients with renal failure.

FUMAGILLIN

Fumagillin is a water-insoluble antibiotic that is derived from the fungus *Aspergillus fumigatus* and is active against microsporidia. This drug is effective when used topically to treat ocular infections due to *Encephalitozoon* spp. When given systemically, fumagillin was effective but caused thrombocytopenia in all recipients in the second week of treatment; this side effect was readily reversed when administration of the drug was stopped. The mechanisms by which fumagillin inhibits microsporidial replication are poorly understood, although the drug may inhibit methionine aminopeptidase 2 by irreversibly blocking the active site.

FURAZOLIDONE

This nitrofuran derivative is an effective alternative agent for the treatment of giardiasis and also exhibits activity against *Isospora belli*. Since it is the only agent active against *Giardia* that is available in liquid form, it is often used to treat young children. Furazolidone undergoes reductive activation in *Giardia lamblia* trophozoites—an event that, unlike the reductive activation of metronidazole, involves an NADH oxidase. The killing effect correlates with the toxicity of reduced products, which damage important cellular components, including DNA. Although furazolidone had been thought to be largely unabsorbed when administered orally, the occurrence of systemic adverse reactions indicates that this is not the case. More than 65% of the drug dose can be recovered from the urine as colored metabolites. Omeprazole reduces the oral bioavailability of furazolidone.

Furazolidone is a monoamine oxidase (MAO) inhibitor; thus caution should be used in its concomitant administration with other drugs (especially indirectly acting sympathomimetic amines) and in the consumption of food and drink containing tyramine during treatment. However, hypertensive crises have not been reported in patients receiving furazolidone, and it has been suggested that—since furazolidone inhibits MAO gradually over several days—the risks are small if treatment is limited to a 5-day course. Because hemolytic anemia can occur in patients with glucose-6-phosphate dehydrogenase (G6PD) deficiency and glutathione instability, furazolidone treatment is contraindicated in mothers who are breast-feeding and in neonates.

HALOFANTRINE

This 9-phenanthrenemethanol is one of three classes of arylaminoalcohols first identified as potential antimalarial agents by the World War II Malaria Chemotherapy Program. Its activity is believed to be similar to that of chloroquine, although it is an oral alternative for the treatment of malaria due to chloroquine-resistant *P. falciparum*. Although the mechanism of action is poorly understood, halofantrine is thought to share mechanism(s) with the 4-aminoquinolines, forming a complex with ferriprotoporphyrin IX and interfering with the degradation of hemoglobin.

Halofantrine exhibits erratic bioavailability, but its absorption is significantly enhanced when it is taken with a fatty meal. The elimination half-life of halofantrine is 1–2 days; it is excreted mainly in feces. Halofantrine is metabolized into *N*-debutyl-halofantrine by the cytochrome P450 enzyme CYP3A4. Grapefruit juice should be avoided during treatment because it increases both halofantrine's bioavailability and halofantrine-induced QT interval prolongation by inhibiting CYP3A4 at the enterocyte level.

IODOQUINOL

Iodoquinol (diiodohydroxyquin), a hydroxyquinoline, is an effective luminal agent for the treatment of amebiasis, balantidiasis, and infection with *Dientamoeba fragilis*. Its mechanism of action is unknown. It is poorly absorbed. Because the drug contains 64% organically bound iodine, it should be used with caution in patients with thyroid disease. Iodine dermatitis occurs occasionally during iodoquinol treatment. Protein-bound serum iodine levels may be increased during treatment and can interfere with certain tests of thyroid function. These effects may persist for as long as 6 months after discontinuation of therapy. Iodoquinol is contraindicated in patients with liver disease. Most serious are the reactions related to prolonged high-dose therapy (optic neuritis, peripheral neuropathy), which should not occur if the recommended dosage regimens are followed.

IVERMECTIN

Ivermectin (22,23-dihydroavermectin) is a derivative of the macrocyclic lactone avermectin produced by the soil-dwelling actinomycete *Streptomyces avermitilis*. Ivermectin is active at low doses against a wide range of helminths and ectoparasites. It is the drug of choice for the treatment of onchocerciasis, strongyloidiasis, cutaneous larva migrans, and scabies. Ivermectin is highly active against microfilariae of the lymphatic filariases but has no macrofilaricidal activity. When ivermectin is used in combination with other agents such as DEC or albendazole for treatment of lymphatic filariasis, synergistic activity is seen. While active against the intestinal helminths *Ascaris lumbricoides* and *Enterobius vermicularis*, ivermectin is only variably effective in trichuriasis and is ineffective against hookworms. Widespread use of ivermectin for treatment of intestinal nematode infections in sheep and goats has led to the emergence of drug resistance in veterinary practice; this development may portend problems in human medical use.

Recent data suggest that ivermectin acts by opening the neuromuscular membrane-associated, glutamate-dependent chloride channels. The influx of chloride ions results in hyperpolarization and muscle paralysis—particularly of the nematode pharynx, with consequent blockage of the oral ingestion of nutrients. Because these chloride channels are present only in invertebrates, the paralysis is seen only in the parasite.

Ivermectin is available only as an oral formulation. The drug is highly protein bound; it is almost completely excreted in feces. The effect of food on bioavailability is unknown. Ivermectin is distributed widely throughout the body; animal studies indicate that it accumulates at the highest concentration in adipose tissue and liver, with little accumulation in the brain. Few data exist to guide therapy in hosts with conditions that may influence drug pharmacokinetics.

Ivermectin is generally administered as a single dose of 150–200 μg/kg. In the absence of parasitic infection, the adverse effects of ivermectin in therapeutic doses are minimal. Adverse effects in patients with filarial infections include fever, myalgia, malaise, lightheadedness, and (occasionally) postural hypotension. The severity of such side effects is related to the intensity of parasite infection, with more symptoms in individuals with a heavy parasite burden. In onchocerciasis, skin edema, pruritus, and mild eye irritation may also occur. The adverse effects are generally self-limiting and only occasionally require symptom-based treatment with antipyretics or antihistamines. More severe complications of ivermectin therapy for onchocerciasis include encephalopathy in patients heavily infected with *Loa loa*. This reaction has led to the suspension of ivermectin distribution for this indication in regions where the two filarial infections are coendemic.

LEVAMISOLE

Levamisole is the levo-isomer of tetramisole and is used to treat ascariasis and hookworm infection. Levamisole appears to act by binding to a distinctive ion channel that forms a nicotinic acetylcholine receptor on nematode muscle. This event causes sustained depolarization of the muscle membrane and results in paralysis of the worm. Levamisole is rapidly absorbed from the GI tract and is extensively metabolized in the liver; the metabolites are excreted in the urine. The use of this drug is contraindicated in patients with preexisting blood disorders (e.g., agranulocytosis) or Sjögren's syndrome. When used for the treatment of helminthic infections, levamisole is well tolerated, with side effects usually limited to GI disturbances.

LUMEFANTRINE

Lumefantrine (benflumetol), a fluorene (benzindene) derivative synthesized in the 1970s by the Chinese Academy of Military Medical Sciences (Beijing), has marked blood schizontocidal activity against a wide range of plasmodia. This agent conforms structurally and in mode of action to the arylaminoalcohol group of antimalarial drugs, including quinine, mefloquine, and halofantrine. Lumefantrine exerts its antimalarial effect as a consequence of its interaction with heme, a degradation product of hemoglobin metabolism. Although its antimalarial activity is slower than that of the artemisinin-based drugs, the recrudescence rate with the recommended lumefantrine regimen is lower. The pharmacokinetic properties of lumefantrine are reminiscent of those of halofantrine, with variable oral bioavailability, considerable augmentation of oral bioavailability by concomitant fat intake, and a terminal elimination half-life of ~4–5 days in patients with malaria.

Artemether and lumefantrine have synergistic activity, and clinical studies in China on several hundred patients show the combination to be safe and well tolerated. The combined formulation of artemether and lumefantrine has been developed for the treatment of falciparum malaria in areas where *P. falciparum* is resistant to chloroquine and antifolates.

MEBENDAZOLE

This benzimidazole is a broad-spectrum antiparasitic agent widely used to treat intestinal helminthiases. Its mechanism of action is similar to that of albendazole; however, it is a more potent inhibitor of parasite malic dehydrogenase and exhibits a more specific and selective effect against intestinal nematodes than the other benzimidazoles.

Mebendazole is available only in oral form but is poorly absorbed from the GI tract; only 5–10% of a standard dose is measurable in plasma. The proportion absorbed from the GI tract is extensively metabolized in the liver. Metabolites appear in the urine and bile; impaired liver or biliary function results in higher plasma mebendazole levels in treated patients. No dose reduction is warranted in patients with renal function impairment. Because mebendazole is poorly absorbed, its incidence of side effects is low. Transient abdominal pain and diarrhea sometimes occur, usually in persons with massive parasite burdens.

MEFLOQUINE

Mefloquine is the preferred drug for prophylaxis of chloroquine-resistant malaria; high doses can be used for treatment. Despite the development of drug-resistant strains of *P. falciparum* in parts of Africa and Southeast Asia, mefloquine is an effective drug throughout most of the world. Cross-resistance of mefloquine with halofantrine and with quinine has been documented in limited areas. Like quinine and chloroquine, this quinoline is active only against the asexual erythrocytic stages of malarial parasites. Unlike quinine, however, mefloquine has a relatively poor affinity for DNA and, as a result, does not inhibit the synthesis of parasitic nucleic acids and proteins. Although both mefloquine and chloroquine inhibit hemozoin formation and heme degradation, mefloquine differs in that it forms a complex with heme that may be toxic to the parasite.

Mefloquine HCl is poorly water soluble and intensely irritating when given parenterally; thus it is available only in tablet form. Its absorption is adversely affected by vomiting and diarrhea but is significantly enhanced when the drug is administered with or after food. About 98% of the drug binds to protein. Mefloquine is excreted mainly in the bile and feces; therefore, no dose adjustment is needed in persons with renal insufficiency. The drug and its main metabolite are not appreciably removed by hemodialysis. No special chemoprophylactic dosage adjustments are indicated for the achievement of plasma concentrations in dialysis patients that are similar to those in healthy persons. Pharmacokinetic differences have been detected among various ethnic populations. In practice, however, these distinctions are of minor importance compared with host immune status and parasite sensitivity. In patients with impaired liver function, the elimination of mefloquine may be prolonged, leading to higher plasma levels.

Mefloquine should be used with caution by individuals participating in activities requiring alertness and fine-motor coordination. If the drug is to be administered for a prolonged period, periodic evaluations are recommended, including liver function tests and ophthalmic examinations. Sleep abnormalities (insomnia, abnormal dreams) have occasionally been reported. Psychosis and seizures occur rarely; mefloquine should not be prescribed to patients with neuropsychiatric conditions, including depression, generalized anxiety disorder, psychosis, schizophrenia, and seizure disorder. If acute anxiety, depression, restlessness, or confusion develops during prophylaxis, these psychiatric symptoms may be considered prodromal to a more serious event, and the drug should be discontinued.

Concomitant use of quinine, quinidine, or drugs producing β-adrenergic blockade may cause significant electrocardiographic abnormalities or cardiac arrest. Halofantrine must not be given simultaneously with or <3 weeks after mefloquine because a potentially fatal prolongation of the QTc interval on electrocardiography may occur. No data exist on mefloquine use after halofantrine use. Administration of mefloquine with quinine or chloroquine may increase the risk of convulsions. Mefloquine may lower plasma levels of anticonvulsants. Caution should be exercised with regard to concomitant antiretroviral therapy, since mefloquine has been shown to exert variable effects on ritonavir pharmacokinetics that are not explained by hepatic CYP3A4 activity or ritonavir protein binding. Vaccinations with attenuated live bacteria should be completed at least 3 days before the first dose of mefloquine.

Women of childbearing age who are traveling to areas where malaria is endemic should be warned against becoming pregnant and encouraged to practice contraception during malaria prophylaxis with mefloquine and for up to 3 months thereafter. However, in the case of unplanned pregnancy, use of mefloquine is not considered an indication for pregnancy termination.

MELARSOPROL*

Melarsoprol has been used since 1949 for the treatment of human African trypanosomiasis (HAT). This trivalent arsenical compound is indicated for the treatment of HAT with neurologic involvement and for the treatment of early HAT that is resistant to suramin or pentamidine. The changing view on the mode of action of arsenicals is well documented. Melarsoprol, like other drugs containing heavy metals, interacts with thiol groups of several different proteins; however, its antiparasitic effects appear to be more specific. Trypanothione reductase is a key enzyme involved in the oxidative stress management of both *Trypanosoma* and *Leishmania* spp., helping to maintain an intracellular reducing environment by reduction of disulfide trypanothione to its dithiol derivative dihydrotrypanothione. Melarsoprol sequesters dihydrotrypanothione, depriving the parasite of its main sulfhydryl antioxidant, and inhibits trypanothione reductase, depriving the parasite of the essential enzyme system that is responsible for keeping trypanothione reduced. These effects are synergistic. The selectivity of arsenical action against trypanosomes is due at least in part to the greater melarsoprol affinity of reduced trypanothione than of other monothiols (e.g., cysteine) on which the mammalian host depends for maintenance of high thiol levels. Melarsoprol enters the parasite via an adenosine transporter; drug-resistant strains lack this transport system.

Melarsoprol is always administered IV. A small but therapeutically significant amount of the drug enters the CSF. The compound is excreted rapidly, with ~80% of the arsenic found in feces.

Melarsoprol is highly toxic. The most serious adverse reaction is reactive encephalopathy, which affects 6% of treated individuals and usually develops within 4 days of the start of therapy, with an average case-fatality rate of 50%. Glucocorticoids are administered with melarsoprol to prevent this development. Because melarsoprol is intensely irritating, care must be taken to avoid infiltration of the drug.

METRIFONATE

Metrifonate has selective activity against *Schistosoma haematobium*. This organophosphorus compound is a prodrug that is converted nonenzymatically to dichlorvos (2,2-dichlorovinyl dimethylphosphate, DDVP), a highly active chemical that irreversibly inhibits the acetylcholinesterase enzyme. Schistosomal cholinesterase is more susceptible to dichlorvos than is the corresponding human enzyme. The exact mechanism of action of metrifonate is uncertain, but the drug is believed to inhibit tegumental acetylcholine receptors that mediate glucose transport.

Metrifonate is administered in a series of three doses at 2-week intervals. After a single oral dose, metrifonate produces a 95% decrease in plasma cholinesterase activity within 6 h, with a fairly rapid return to normal. However, 2.5 months are required for erythrocyte cholinesterase levels to return to normal. Treated persons should not be exposed to neuromuscular blocking agents or organophosphate insecticides for at least 48 h after treatment.

METRONIDAZOLE AND OTHER NITROIMIDAZOLES

See Table 113-1 and Chap. 33.

MILTEFOSINE

In the early 1990s, miltefosine (hexadecylphosphocholine), originally developed as an antineoplastic agent, was discovered to have significant antiproliferative activity against *Leishmania* spp., *Trypanosoma cruzi*, and *T. brucei* parasites in vitro and in experimental animal models. In 1995, Tropical Disease Research, a program sponsored by the WHO and other international groups, entered into an agreement with the company now known as ASTA Medica/Zentaris to develop miltefosine for the treatment of visceral leishmaniasis in India. Miltefosine is the first oral drug that has proved to be highly effective and comparable to amphotericin B against visceral leishmaniasis in India, where antimonial-resistant cases are prevalent. Miltefosine is also effective in previously untreated visceral infections. Cure rates in cutaneous leishmaniasis are comparable to those obtained with antimony.

The activity of miltefosine is attributed to interaction with cell signal transduction pathways and inhibition of phospholipid and sterol biosynthesis. Resistance to miltefosine has not been observed clinically. The drug is readily absorbed from the GI tract, is widely distributed, and accumulates in several tissues. The efficacy of a 28-day treatment course in Indian visceral leishmaniasis is equivalent to that of amphotericin B therapy; however, it appears that a shortened course of 21 days may be equally efficacious.

General recommendations for the use of miltefosine are limited by the exclusion of specific groups from the published clinical trials: persons <12 or >65 years of age, persons with the most advanced disease, breast-feeding women, HIV-infected patients, and individuals with significant renal or hepatic insufficiency.

NICLOSAMIDE

Niclosamide is active against a wide variety of adult tapeworms but not against tissue cestodes. It is also a molluscacide and is used in snail-control programs.

The drug uncouples oxidative phosphorylation in parasite mitochondria, thereby blocking the uptake of glucose by the intestinal tapeworm and resulting in the parasite's death. Niclosamide rapidly causes spastic paralysis of intestinal cestodes in vitro. Its use is limited by its side effects, the necessarily long duration of therapy, the recommended use of purgatives, and—most important—limited availability (i.e., on a named-patient basis from the manufacturer).

Niclosamide is poorly absorbed. Tablets are given on an empty stomach in the morning after a liquid meal the night before, and this dose is followed by another 1 h later. For treatment of hymenolepiasis, the drug is administered for 7 days. A second course is often prescribed. The scolex and proximal segments of the tapeworms are killed on contact with niclosamide and may be digested in the gut. However, disintegration of the adult tapeworm results in the release of viable ova, which theoretically can result in autoinfection. Although fears of the development of cysticercosis in patients with *Taenia solium* infections have proved unfounded, it is still recommended that a brisk purgative be given 2 h after the first dose.

NIFURTIMOX*

This nitrofuran compound is a cheap and effective oral agent for the treatment of acute Chagas' disease. Trypanosomes lack catalase and have very low levels of peroxidase; as a result, they are very vulnerable to by-products of oxygen reduction. When nifurtimox is reduced in the trypanosome, a nitro anion radical is formed and undergoes autooxidation, resulting in the generation of the superoxide anion O_2^-, hydrogen peroxide (H_2O_2), hydroperoxyl radical (HO_2), and other highly reactive and cytotoxic molecules. Despite the abundance of catalases, peroxidases, and superoxide dismutases that neutralize these destructive radicals in mammalian cells, nifurtimox has a poor therapeutic index. Prolonged use is required, but the course may have to be interrupted because of drug toxicity, which develops in 40–70% of recipients. Nifurtimox is well absorbed and undergoes rapid and extensive biotransformation; <0.5% of the original drug is excreted in urine.

NITAZOXANIDE

Nitazoxanide is a 5-nitrothiazole compound used for the treatment of cryptosporidiosis and giardiasis; it is active against other intestinal protozoa as well. The drug is approved for use in children 1–11 years of age.

The antiprotozoal activity of nitazoxanide is believed to be due to interference with the pyruvate-ferredoxin oxidoreductase (PFOR) enzyme–dependent electron transfer reaction that is essential to anaerobic energy metabolism. Studies have shown that the PFOR enzyme from *G. lamblia* directly reduces nitazoxanide by transfer of electrons in the absence of ferredoxin. The DNA-derived PFOR protein sequence of *Cryptosporidium parvum* appears to be similar to that of *G. lamblia*. Interference with the PFOR enzyme–dependent electron transfer reaction may not be the only pathway by which nitazoxanide exerts antiprotozoal activity.

After oral administration, nitazoxanide is rapidly hydrolyzed to an active metabolite, tizoxanide (desacetyl-nitazoxanide). Tizoxanide then undergoes conjugation, primarily by glucuronidation. It is recommended that nitazoxanide be taken with food; however, no studies have been conducted to determine whether the pharmacokinetics of tizoxanide and tizoxanide glucuronide differ in fasted versus fed subjects. Tizoxanide is excreted in urine, bile, and feces, and tizoxanide glucuronide is excreted in urine and bile. The pharmacokinetics of nitazoxanide in patients with impaired hepatic and/or renal function have not been studied. Tizoxanide is highly bound to plasma protein (>99.9%). Therefore, caution should be used when administering this agent concurrently with other highly plasma protein–bound drugs with narrow therapeutic indices, as competition for binding sites may occur.

OXAMNIQUINE

This tetrahydroquinoline derivative is an effective alternative agent for the treatment of *Schistosoma mansoni*, although susceptibility to this drug exhibits regional variation. Oxamniquine exhibits anticholinergic properties, but its primary mode of action seems to rely on ATP-dependent enzymatic drug activation generating an intermediate that alkylates essential macromolecules, including DNA. In treated adult schistosomes, oxamniquine produces marked tegumental alterations that are similar to those seen with praziquantel but that develop less rapidly, becoming evident 4–8 days after treatment.

Oxamniquine is administered orally as a single dose and is well absorbed. Food retards absorption and reduces bioavailability. About 70% of an administered dose is excreted in urine as a mixture of pharmacologically inactive metabolites. Patients should be warned that their urine might have an intense orange-red color. Side effects are uncommon and usually mild, although hallucinations and seizures have been reported.

PAROMOMYCIN (AMINOSIDINE)

First isolated in 1956, this aminoglycoside is an effective oral agent for the treatment of infections due to intestinal protozoa. Parenteral paromomycin appears to be effective against visceral leishmaniasis in India.

Paromomycin inhibits protozoan protein synthesis by binding to the 30S ribosomal RNA in the aminoacyl-tRNA site, causing misreading of mRNA codons. Paromomycin is less active against *G. lamblia* than standard agents; however, like other aminoglycosides, paromomycin is poorly absorbed from the intestinal lumen, and the high levels of drug in the gut compensate for this relatively weak activity. If absorbed or administered systemically, paromomycin can cause ototoxicity and nephrotoxicity. However, systemic absorption is very limited, and toxicity should not be a concern in persons with normal kidneys. Topical formulations are not generally available.

PENTAMIDINE ISETHIONATE

This diamidine is an effective alternative agent for some forms of leishmaniasis and trypanosomiasis. It is available for parenteral and aerosolized administration. While its mechanism of action remains undefined, it is known to exert a wide range of effects, including interaction with trypanosomal kinetoplast DNA; interference with polyamine synthesis by a decrease in the activity of ornithine decarboxylase; and inhibition of RNA polymerase, ribosomal function, and the synthesis of nucleic acids and proteins.

Pentamidine isethionate is well absorbed, is highly tissue bound, and is excreted slowly over several weeks, with an elimination half-life of 12 days. No steady-state plasma concentration is attained in persons given daily injections; the result is extensive accumulation of pentamidine in tissues, primarily the liver, kidney, adrenal, and spleen. Pentamidine does not penetrate well into the CNS. Pulmonary concentrations of pentamidine are increased when the drug is delivered in aerosolized form.

PIPERAZINE

The antihelmintic activity of piperazine is confined to ascariasis and enterobiasis. Piperazine acts as an agonist at extrasynaptic γ-aminobutyric acid (GABA) receptors, causing an influx of chloride ions in the nematode somatic musculature. The ultimate effect is flaccid paralysis of the muscle fibers, leading to the expulsion of live but mostly paralyzed worms. Patients should be warned, as this occurrence can be unsettling.

PRAZIQUANTEL

This heterocyclic pyrazinoisoquinoline derivative is highly active against a broad spectrum of trematodes and cestodes. It is the mainstay of treatment for schistosomiasis and is a critical part of community-based control programs.

All of the effects of praziquantel can be attributed either directly or indirectly to an alteration of intracellular calcium concentrations. Although the exact mechanism of action remains unclear, the major mechanism is disruption of the parasite tegument, causing tetanic contractures with loss of adherence to host tissues and, ultimately, disintegration or expulsion. Praziquantel induces changes in the antigenicity of the parasite by causing the exposure of concealed antigens. Praziquantel also produces alterations in schistosomal glucose metabolism, including decreases in glucose uptake, lactate release, glycogen content, and ATP levels.

Praziquantel exerts its parasitic effects directly and does not need to be metabolized to be effective. It is well absorbed but undergoes extensive first-pass hepatic clearance. Levels of the drug are increased when it is taken with food, particularly carbohydrates, or with cimetidine. Serum levels are reduced by glucocorticoids, chloroquine, carbamazepine, and phenytoin. Praziquantel is completely metabolized in humans, with 80% of the dose recovered as metabolites in urine within 4 days. It is not known to what extent praziquantel crosses the placenta.

Patients with schistosomiasis who have heavy parasite burdens may develop abdominal discomfort, nausea, headache, dizziness, and drowsiness. Symptoms begin 30 min after ingestion, may require spasmolytics for relief, and usually disappear spontaneously after a few hours.

PRIMAQUINE PHOSPHATE

Primaquine, an 8-aminoquinoline, has a broad spectrum of activity against all stages of plasmodial development in humans but has been used most effectively for eradication of the hepatic stage of these parasites. Despite its toxicity, it remains the drug of choice for radical cure of *P. vivax* infections. Primaquine must be metabolized by the host to be effective. It is, in fact, rapidly metabolized; only a small fraction of the dose of the parent drug is excreted unchanged. Although the parasiticidal activity of the three oxidative metabolites remains unclear, they are believed to affect both pyrimidine synthesis and the mitochondrial electron transport chain. The metabolites appear to have significantly less antimalarial activity than primaquine; however, their hemolytic activity is greater than that of the parent drug.

Primaquine causes marked hypotension after parenteral administration and therefore is given only by the oral route. It is rapidly and almost completely absorbed from the GI tract.

Patients should be tested for G6PD deficiency before they receive primaquine. The drug may induce the oxidation of hemoglobin into methemoglobin, irrespective of the G6PD status of the patient. Primaquine is otherwise well tolerated.

PROGUANIL (CHLOROGUANIDE)

Proguanil inhibits plasmodial dihydrofolate reductase and is used with atovaquone for oral treatment of uncomplicated malaria or with chloroquine for malaria prophylaxis in parts of Africa without widespread chloroquine-resistant *P. falciparum*.

Proguanil exerts its effect primarily by means of the metabolite cycloguanil, whose inhibition of dihydrofolate reductase in the parasite disrupts deoxythymidylate synthesis, thus interfering with a key pathway involved in the biosynthesis of pyrimidines required for nucleic acid replication. There are no clinical data indicating that folate supplementation diminishes drug efficacy; women of childbearing age for whom atovaquone/proguanil is prescribed should continue taking folate supplements to prevent neural-tube birth defects.

Proguanil is extensively absorbed regardless of food intake. The drug is 75% protein-bound. The main routes of elimination are hepatic biotransformation and renal excretion; 40–60% of the proguanil dose is excreted by the kidneys. Drug levels are increased and elimination is impaired in patients with hepatic insufficiency.

PYRANTEL PAMOATE

Pyrantel is a tetrahydropyrimidine formulated as pamoate. This safe, well-tolerated, inexpensive drug is used to treat a variety of intestinal nematode infections but is ineffective in trichuriasis. Pyrantel pamoate is usually effective in a single dose. Like levamisole, the drug has as its target the nicotinic acetylcholine receptor on the surface of nematode somatic muscle. Pyrantel depolarizes the neuromuscular junction of the nematode, resulting in its irreversible paralysis and allowing the natural expulsion of the worm.

Pyrantel pamoate is poorly absorbed from the intestine; >85% of the dose is passed unaltered in feces. The absorbed portion is metabolized and excreted in urine. Piperazine, which produces hyperpolarization of muscle cells in intestinal helminths, is antagonistic to pyrantel pamoate and should not be used concomitantly.

Pyrantel pamoate has minimal toxicity at the oral doses used to treat intestinal helminthic infection. It is not recommended for pregnant women or for children <12 months old.

PYRIMETHAMINE

When combined with short-acting sulfonamides, this diaminopyrimidine is effective in malaria, toxoplasmosis, and isosporiasis. Unlike mammalian cells, the parasites that cause these infections cannot utilize preformed pyrimidines obtained through salvage pathways but rather rely completely on de novo pyrimidine synthesis, for which folate derivatives are essential cofactors. The efficacy of pyrimethamine is increasingly limited by the development of resistant strains of *P. falciparum* and *P. vivax*. Single amino acid substitutions to parasite dihydrofolate reductase confer resistance to pyrimethamine by decreasing the enzyme's binding affinity for the drug.

Pyrimethamine is well absorbed; the drug is 87% bound to human plasma proteins. In healthy volunteers, drug concentrations remain at therapeutic levels for up to 2 weeks; drug levels are lower in patients with malaria.

At the usual dosage, pyrimethamine alone causes little toxicity except for occasional skin rashes and, more rarely, blood dyscrasias. Bone marrow suppression sometimes occurs at the higher doses used for toxoplasmosis; at these doses, the drug should be administered with folinic acid.

QUINACRINE*

First introduced as an antimalarial agent in 1930, quinacrine is the only drug approved by the FDA for the treatment of giardiasis. Its production was discontinued in 1992. Although not commercially available, quinacrine can be obtained from alternative sources through the CDC Drug Service. The antiprotozoal mechanism of quinacrine has not been fully elucidated. The drug inhibits NADH oxidase—the same enzyme that activates furazolidone. The differing relative quinacrine uptake rate between human cells and *G. lamblia* may explain the selective toxicity of the drug. Resistance correlates with decreased drug uptake.

Quinacrine is rapidly absorbed from the intestinal tract and is widely distributed in body tissues. Alcohol is best avoided due to a disulfiram-like effect.

QUININE AND QUINIDINE

When combined with another agent, the cinchona alkaloid quinine is effective for the oral treatment of both uncomplicated, chloroquine-resistant malaria and babesiosis. Quinine acts rapidly against the asexual blood stages of all forms of human malaria. For severe malaria, only quinidine (the dextroisomer of quinine) is available in the United States. Quinine concentrates in the acidic food vacuoles of *Plasmodium* spp. The drug inhibits the nonenzymatic polymerization of the highly reactive, toxic heme molecule into the nontoxic polymer pigment hemozoin.

Quinine is readily absorbed when given orally. In patients with malaria, the elimination half-life of quinine increases according to the severity of the infection. However, toxicity is avoided by an increase in the concentration of plasma glycoproteins. The cinchona alkaloids are extensively metabolized, particularly by CYP3A4; only 20% of the dose is excreted unchanged in urine. The drug's metabolites are also excreted in urine and may be responsible for toxicity in patients with renal failure. Renal excretion of quinine is decreased when cimetidine is taken and increased when the urine is acidic. The drug readily crosses the placenta.

Quinidine is both more potent as an antimalarial and more toxic than quinine. Its use requires cardiac monitoring. Dose reduction is necessary in persons with severe renal impairment.

SPIRAMYCIN†

This macrolide is used to treat acute toxoplasmosis in pregnancy and congenital toxoplasmosis. While the mechanism of action is similar to that of other macrolides, the efficacy of spiramycin in toxoplasmosis appears to stem from its rapid and extensive intracellular penetration, which results in macrophage drug concentrations 10–20 times greater than serum concentrations.

Spiramycin is rapidly and widely distributed throughout the body and reaches concentrations in the placenta up to five times those in serum. This agent is excreted mainly in bile. Indeed, in humans, the urinary excretion of active compounds represents only 20% of the administered dose.

Serious reactions to spiramycin are rare. Of the available macrolides, spiramycin appears to have the lowest risk of drug interactions. Complications of treatment are rare but, in neonates, can include life-threatening ventricular arrhythmias that disappear with drug discontinuation.

SULFONAMIDES

See Table 113-1 and Chap. 33.

SURAMIN*

This derivative of urea is the drug of choice for the early stage of African trypanosomiasis. The drug is polyanionic and acts by forming stable complexes with proteins, thus inhibiting multiple enzymes essential to parasite energy metabolism. Suramin appears to inhibit all trypanosome glycolytic enzymes more effectively than it inhibits the corresponding host enzymes.

Suramin is parenterally administered. It binds to plasma proteins and persists at low levels for several weeks after infusion. Its metabolism is negligible. This drug does not penetrate the CNS.

TAFENOQUINE

Tafenoquine is an 8-aminoquinoline with causal prophylactic activity. Its prolonged half-life (2–3 weeks) allows longer dosing intervals when the drug is used for prophylaxis. Tafenoquine has been well tolerated in clinical trials. When tafenoquine is taken with food, its absorption is increased by 50% and the most commonly reported adverse event—mild GI upset—is diminished. Like primaquine, tafenoquine is a potent oxidizing agent, causing hemolysis in patients with G6PD deficiency as well as methemoglobinemia.

TETRACYCLINES

See Table 113-1 and Chap. 33.

THIABENDAZOLE

Discovered in 1961, thiabendazole remains one of the most potent of the numerous benzimidazole derivatives. However, its use has declined significantly because of a higher frequency of adverse effects than is seen with other, equally effective agents.

Thiabendazole is active against most intestinal nematodes that infect humans. Although the exact mechanism of its antihelmintic activity has not been fully elucidated, it is likely to be similar to that of other benzimidazole drugs: namely, inhibition of polymerization of parasite β-tubulin. The drug also inhibits the helminth-specific enzyme fumarate reductase. In animals, thiabendazole has anti-inflammatory, antipyretic, and analgesic effects, which may explain its usefulness in dracunculiasis and trichinosis. Thiabendazole also suppresses egg and/or larval production by some nematodes and may inhibit the subsequent development of eggs or larvae passed in feces. Despite the emergence and global spread of thiabendazole-resistant trichostrongyliasis among sheep, there have been no reports of drug resistance in humans.

Thiabendazole is available in tablet form and as an oral suspension. The drug is rapidly absorbed from the GI tract but can also be absorbed through the skin. Thiabendazole should be taken after meals. This agent is extensively metabolized in the liver before ultimately being excreted; most of the dose is excreted within the first 24 h. The usual dose of thiabendazole is determined by the patient's weight, but some treatment regimens are parasite specific. No particular adjustments are recommended in patients with renal or hepatic failure; only cautious use is advised.

Coadministration of thiabendazole in patients taking theophylline can result in an increase in theophylline levels by >50%. Therefore, serum levels of theophylline should be monitored closely in this situation.

TINIDAZOLE

This nitroimidazole is effective for the treatment of amebiasis, giardiasis, and trichomoniasis. Like metronidazole, tinidazole must undergo reductive activation by the parasite's metabolic system before it can act on protozoal targets. Tinidazole inhibits the synthesis of new DNA in the parasite and causes degradation of existing DNA. The reduced free-radical derivatives alkylate DNA, with consequent cytotoxic damage to the parasite. This damage appears to be produced by short-lived reduction intermediates, resulting in helix destabilization and strain breakage of DNA. The mechanism of action and side effects of tinidazole are similar to those of metronidazole, but adverse events appear to be less frequent and severe with tinidazole. In addition, the significantly longer half-life of tinidazole (>12h) offers potential cure with a single dose.

TRICLABENDAZOLE

While most benzimidazoles have broad-spectrum antihelmintic activity, they exhibit minimal or no activity against *F. hepatica*. In contrast, the antihelmintic activity of triclabendazole is highly specific for *Fasciola* spp. and *Paragonimus* spp., with little activity against nematodes, cestodes, and other trematodes. Triclabendazole is effective against all stages of *Fasciola* spp. The active sulfoxide metabolite of triclabendazole binds to fluke tubulin by assuming a unique nonplanar configuration and disrupts microtubule-based processes. Resistance to triclabendazole in veterinary use has been reported in Australia and Europe; however, no resistance has been documented in humans.

Triclabendazole is rapidly absorbed after oral ingestion; administration with food enhances its absorption and shortens the elimination half-life of the active metabolite. Both the sulfoxide and the sulfone metabolites are highly protein bound (>99%). Treatment with triclabendazole is typically given in one or two doses. No clinical data are available regarding dose adjustment in renal or hepatic insufficiency; however, given the short course of therapy and extensive hepatic metabolism of triclabendazole, dose adjustment is unlikely to be necessary. No information exists on drug interactions.

TRIMETHOPRIM-SULFAMETHOXAZOLE

See Table 113-1 and Chap. 33.

FURTHER READINGS

ABRAMOWICZ M (ed): Drugs for parasitic infections. Med Lett Drugs Ther 46:1, 2004

MOORE TA, MCCARTHY JS: Benzimidazoles (albendazole, mebendazole, thiabendazole, triclabendazole), in *Antimicrobial Therapy and Vaccines*, 2d ed, VL Yu et al (eds). Pittsburgh, ESun Technologies, 2005, pp 1021–1036

SHAPIRO TA, GOLDBERG DE: Drugs used in the chemotherapy of protozoal infections: Malaria, in *Goodman and Gilman's The Pharmacological Basis of Therapeutics*, 11th ed, L Brunton et al (eds). New York, McGraw-Hill, 2005, pp 1021–1048

WARD SA et al: Antimalarial drugs and pregnancy: Safety, pharmacokinetics, and pharmacovigilance. Lancet Infect Dis 7:136, 2007

WINSTANLEY P, WARD S: Malaria chemotherapy. Adv Parasitol 61:47, 2006

WORLD HEALTH ORGANIZATION: *Model Prescribing Information: Drugs Used in Parasitic Diseases*, 2d ed. Geneva, WHO, 1995

PART 2 PROTOZOAL INFECTIONS

CHAPTER 115

AMEBIASIS AND INFECTION WITH FREE-LIVING AMEBAS

Sharon L. Reed

AMEBIASIS

DEFINITION

Amebiasis is an infection with the intestinal protozoan *Entamoeba histolytica*. About 90% of infections are asymptomatic, and the remaining 10% produce a spectrum of clinical syndromes ranging from dysentery to abscesses of the liver or other organs.

LIFE CYCLE AND TRANSMISSION

E. histolytica is acquired by ingestion of viable cysts from fecally contaminated water, food, or hands. Food-borne exposure is most prevalent and is particularly likely when food handlers are shedding cysts or food is being grown with feces-contaminated soil, fertilizer, or water. Besides the drinking of contaminated water, less common means of transmission include oral and anal sexual practices and—in rare instances—direct rectal inoculation through colonic irrigation devices. Motile trophozoites are released from cysts in the small intestine and, in most patients, remain as harmless commensals in the large bowel. After encystation, infectious cysts are shed in the stool and can survive for several weeks in a moist environment. In some patients, the trophozoites invade either the bowel mucosa, causing symptomatic colitis, or the bloodstream, causing distant abscesses of the liver, lungs, or brain. The trophozoites may not encyst in patients with active dysentery, and motile hematophagous trophozoites are frequently present in fresh stools. Trophozoites are rapidly killed by exposure to air or stomach acid, however, and therefore cannot transmit infection.

EPIDEMIOLOGY

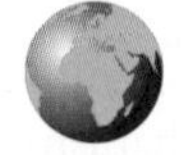

About 10% of the world's population is infected with *Entamoeba*, the majority with noninvasive *Entamoeba dispar*. Amebiasis results from infection with *E. histolytica* and is the third most common cause of death from parasitic disease (after schistosomiasis and malaria). The wide spectrum of clinical disease caused by *Entamoeba* is due in part to the differences between these two infecting species. Cysts of *E. histolytica* and *E. dispar* are morphologically identical, but *E. histolytica* has unique isoenzymes, surface antigens, DNA markers, and virulence properties (Table 115-1). Most asymptomatic carriers, including homosexual men and patients with AIDS, harbor *E. dispar* and have self-limited infections. These observations indicate that *E. dispar* is incapable of causing invasive disease, since *Cryptosporidium* and *Isospora belli*, which also cause only self-limited illnesses in immunocompetent people, cause devastating diarrhea in patients with AIDS. However, host factors play a role as well. In one study, 10% of asymptomatic patients who were colonized with *E. histolytica* went on to develop amebic colitis, while the rest remained asymptomatic and cleared the infection within 1 year.

TABLE 115-1

E. HISTOLYTICA AND E. DISPAR, COMPARED AND CONTRASTED

Similarities
1. Both species are spread through ingestion of infectious cysts.
2. Cysts of the two species are morphologically identical.
3. Both species colonize the large intestine.
Differences
1. Only *E. histolytica* causes invasive disease.
2. Only *E. histolytica* infections elicit a positive amebic serology.
3. The two species have distinct rRNA sequences.
4. The two species have distinct surface antigens and isoenzyme markers.
5. Gal/GalNAc lectin can be used to differentiate the two species in stool ELISA.

Note: ELISA, enzyme-linked immunosorbent assay; Gal/GalNAc, galactose *N*-acetylgalactosamine. See text.

Areas of highest incidence (due to inadequate sanitation and crowding) include most developing countries in the tropics, particularly Mexico, India, and nations of Central and South America, tropical Asia, and Africa. In a 4-year follow-up study of preschool children in a highly endemic area of Bangladesh, 80% of children had at least one episode of infection with *E. histolytica* and 53% had more than one episode. Naturally acquired immunity did develop but was usually short-lived and correlated with the presence in the stool of secretory IgA antibody to the major adherence lectin galactose *N*-acetylgalactosamine (Gal/GalNAc). The main groups at risk for amebiasis in developed countries are returned travelers, recent immigrants, homosexual men, and inmates of institutions.

PATHOGENESIS AND PATHOLOGY

Both trophozoites (Fig. 115-1) and cysts (Fig. 115-2) are found in the intestinal lumen, but only trophozoites of *E. histolytica* invade tissue. The trophozoite is 20–60 μm in diameter and contains vacuoles and a nucleus with a characteristic central nucleolus. In animals, depletion of intestinal mucus, diffuse inflammation, and disruption of the epithelial barrier occur before trophozoites actually come into contact with the colonic mucosa. Trophozoites attach to colonic mucus and epithelial cells by Gal/GalNAc. The earliest intestinal lesions are microulcerations of the mucosa of the cecum, sigmoid colon, or rectum that release erythrocytes, inflammatory cells, and epithelial cells. Proctoscopy reveals small ulcers with heaped-up margins and normal intervening mucosa. Submucosal extension of ulcerations under viable-appearing surface mucosa causes the classic "flask-shaped" ulcer containing trophozoites at the margins of dead and viable tissues. Although neutrophilic infiltrates may accompany the early lesions in animals, human intestinal infection is marked by a paucity of inflammatory cells, probably in part because of the killing of neutrophils by trophozoites (Fig. 115-3).

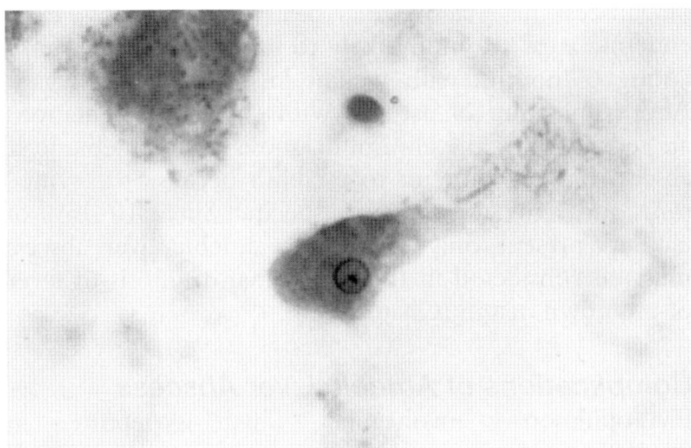

FIGURE 115-1
Trophozoite of *E. histolytica* demonstrating a single nucleus with a central, dot-like nucleolus (trichrome stain).

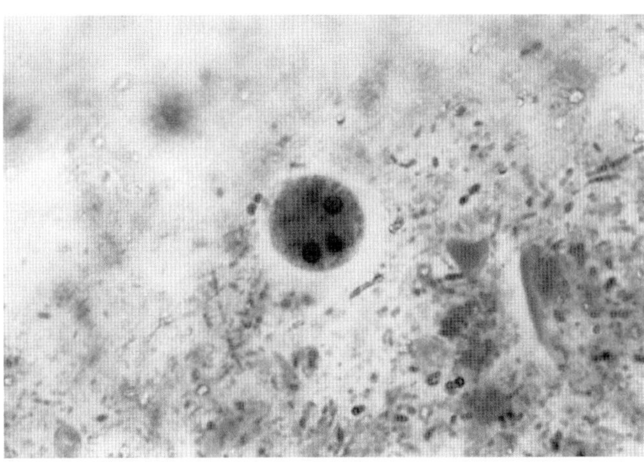

FIGURE 115-2
Cyst of *E. histolytica* showing three of the four nuclei (trichrome stain).

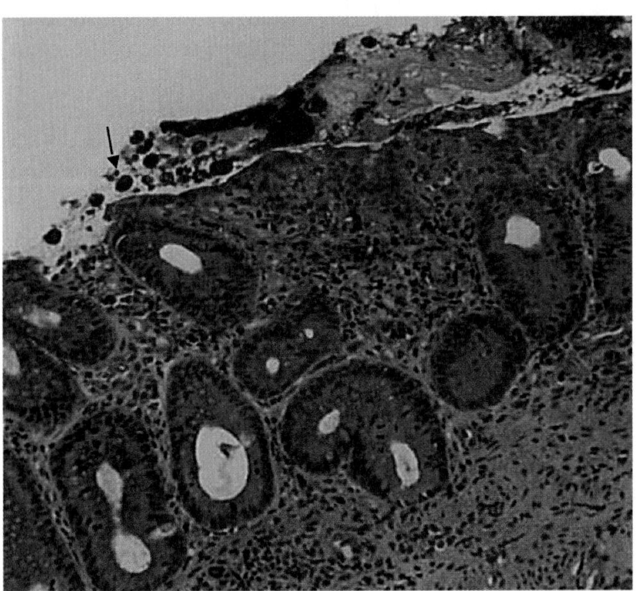

FIGURE 115-3
Pathology of amebic ulcer with colonic invasion. Arrow points to trophozoites (hematoxylin and eosin, 400×).

Treated ulcers characteristically heal with little or no scarring. Occasionally, however, full-thickness necrosis and perforation occur.

Rarely, intestinal infection results in the formation of a mass lesion, or *ameboma*, in the bowel lumen. The overlying mucosa is usually thin and ulcerated, while other layers of the wall are thickened, edematous, and hemorrhagic; this condition results in exuberant formation of granulation tissue with little fibrous-tissue response.

A number of virulence factors have been linked to the ability of *E. histolytica* to invade through the interglandular epithelium. One consists of the extracellular cysteine proteinases that degrade collagen, elastin, IgA, IgG, and the anaphylatoxins C3a and C5a. Other enzymes may disrupt glycoprotein bonds between mucosal epithelial cells in the gut. Amebas can lyse neutrophils, monocytes, lymphocytes, and cells of colonic and hepatic lines. The cytolytic effect of amebas appears to require direct contact with target cells and may be linked to the release of phospholipase A and pore-forming peptides. *E. histolytica* trophozoites also cause apoptosis of human cells.

Liver abscesses are always preceded by intestinal colonization, which may be asymptomatic. Blood vessels may be compromised early by wall lysis and thrombus formation. Trophozoites invade veins to reach the liver through the portal venous system. *E. histolytica* is resistant to complement-mediated lysis—a property critical to survival in the bloodstream. In contrast, *E. dispar* is rapidly lysed by complement and is thus restricted to the bowel lumen. Inoculation of amebas into the portal system of hamsters results in an acute cellular infiltrate consisting predominantly of neutrophils. Later, the neutrophils are lysed by contact with amebas, and the release of neutrophil toxins may contribute to necrosis of hepatocytes. The liver parenchyma is replaced by necrotic material that is surrounded by a thin rim of congested liver tissue. The necrotic contents of a liver abscess are classically described as "anchovy paste," although the fluid is variable in color and is composed of bacteriologically sterile granular debris with few or no cells. Amebas, if seen, tend to be found near the capsule of the abscess.

A study in Bangladeshi schoolchildren revealed that an intestinal IgA response to Gal/GalNAc reduced the risk of new *E. histolytica* infection by 64%. Serum IgG antibody is not protective; titers correlate with the duration of illness rather than with the severity of disease. Indeed, Bangladeshi children with a serum IgG response were more likely than those without such a response to develop new *E. histolytica* infection. Studies of animals suggest that cell-mediated immunity may be important for protection, although patients with AIDS appear not to be predisposed to more severe disease.

CLINICAL SYNDROMES

Intestinal Amebiasis

The most common type of amebic infection is asymptomatic cyst passage. Even in highly endemic areas, most patients harbor *E. dispar*.

Symptomatic amebic colitis develops 2–6 weeks after the ingestion of infectious cysts. A gradual onset of lower abdominal pain and mild diarrhea is followed by malaise, weight loss, and diffuse lower abdominal or back pain. Cecal involvement may mimic acute appendicitis. Patients with full-blown dysentery may pass 10–12 stools per day. The stools contain little fecal material and consist mainly of blood and mucus. In contrast to those with bacterial diarrhea, fewer than 40% of patients with amebic dysentery are febrile. Virtually all patients have heme-positive stools.

More fulminant intestinal infection, with severe abdominal pain, high fever, and profuse diarrhea, is rare and occurs predominantly in children. Patients may develop toxic megacolon, in which there is severe bowel dilation with intramural air. Patients receiving glucocorticoids are at risk for severe amebiasis. Uncommonly, patients develop a chronic form of amebic colitis, which can be confused with inflammatory bowel disease. The association between severe amebiasis complications and glucocorticoid therapy emphasizes the importance of excluding amebiasis when inflammatory bowel disease is suspected. An occasional patient presents with only an asymptomatic or tender abdominal mass caused by an ameboma, which is easily confused with cancer on barium studies. A positive serologic test or biopsy can prevent unnecessary surgery in this setting. The syndrome of postamebic colitis—persistent diarrhea following documented cure of amebic colitis—is controversial; no evidence of recurrent amebic infection can be found, and re-treatment usually has no effect.

Amebic Liver Abscess

Extraintestinal infection by *E. histolytica* most often involves the liver. Of travelers who develop an amebic liver abscess after leaving an endemic area, 95% do so within 5 months. Young patients with an amebic liver abscess are more likely than older patients to present in the acute phase with prominent symptoms of <10 days' duration. Most patients are febrile and have right-upper-quadrant pain, which may be dull or pleuritic in nature and may radiate to the shoulder. Point tenderness over the liver and right-sided pleural effusion is common. Jaundice is rare. Although the initial site of infection is the colon, fewer than one-third of patients with an amebic abscess have active diarrhea. Older patients from endemic areas are more likely to have a subacute course lasting 6 months, with weight loss and hepatomegaly. About one-third of patients with chronic presentations are febrile. Thus, the clinical diagnosis of an amebic liver abscess may be difficult to establish because the symptoms and signs are often nonspecific. Since 10–15% of patients present only with fever, amebic liver abscess must be considered in the differential diagnosis of fever of unknown origin (Chap. 9).

Complications of Amebic Liver Abscess

Pleuropulmonary involvement, which is reported in 20–30% of patients, is the most frequent complication of amebic liver abscess. Manifestations include sterile effusions, contiguous spread from the liver, and rupture into the pleural space. Sterile effusions and contiguous spread usually resolve with medical therapy, but frank rupture into the pleural space requires drainage. A hepatobronchial fistula may cause cough productive of large amounts of necrotic material that may contain amebas. This dramatic complication carries a good prognosis. Abscesses that rupture into the peritoneum may present as an indolent leak or an acute abdomen and require both percutaneous catheter drainage and medical therapy. Rupture into the pericardium, usually from abscesses of the left lobe of the liver, carries the gravest prognosis; it can occur during medical therapy and requires surgical drainage.

Other Extraintestinal Sites

The genitourinary tract may become involved by direct extension of amebiasis from the colon or by hematogenous spread of the infection. Painful genital ulcers, characterized by a punched-out appearance and profuse discharge, may develop secondary to extension from either the intestine or the liver. Both these conditions respond well to medical therapy. Cerebral involvement has been reported in fewer than 0.1% of patients in large clinical series. Symptoms and prognosis depend on the size and location of the lesion.

DIAGNOSTIC TESTS

Laboratory Diagnosis

Stool examinations, serologic tests, and noninvasive imaging of the liver are the most important procedures in the diagnosis of amebiasis. Fecal findings suggestive of amebic colitis include a positive test for heme, a paucity of neutrophils, and amebic cysts or trophozoites. The definitive diagnosis of amebic colitis is made by the demonstration of hematophagous trophozoites of *E. histolytica* (Fig. 115-1). Because trophozoites are killed rapidly by water, drying, or barium, it is important to examine at least three fresh stool specimens. Examination of a combination of wet mounts, iodine-stained concentrates, and trichrome-stained preparations of fresh stool and concentrates for cysts (Fig. 115-2) or trophozoites (Fig. 115-1) confirms the diagnosis in 75–95% of cases. Cultures of amebas are more sensitive but are not routinely available. If stool examinations are negative, sigmoidoscopy with biopsy of the edge of ulcers may increase the yield, but this procedure is dangerous during fulminant colitis because of the risk of perforation. Trophozoites in a biopsy specimen from a colonic mass confirm the diagnosis of ameboma, but trophozoites are rare in liver aspirates because they are found in the abscess capsule and not in the readily aspirated necrotic center. Accurate diagnosis requires experience, since the trophozoites may be confused with neutrophils and the cysts must be differentiated morphologically from *Entamoeba hartmanni*, *Entamoeba coli*, and *Endolimax nana*, which do not cause clinical disease and do not warrant therapy. Unfortunately, the cysts of *E. histolytica* cannot be distinguished microscopically from those of *E. dispar*. Therefore, the microscopic diagnosis of *E. histolytica* can be made only by the detection of *Entamoeba* trophozoites that have ingested erythrocytes.

In terms of sensitivity, stool diagnostic tests based on the detection of the Gal/GalNAc lectin of *E. histolytica* compare favorably with the polymerase chain reaction and with isolation in culture followed by isoenzyme analysis.

Serology is an important addition to the methods used for parasitologic diagnosis of invasive amebiasis. Enzyme-linked immunosorbent assays (ELISAs) and agar gel diffusion assays are positive in more than 90% of patients with colitis, amebomas, or liver abscess. Positive results in conjunction with the appropriate clinical syndrome suggest active disease because serologic findings usually revert to negative within 6–12 months. Even in highly endemic areas such as South Africa, fewer than 10% of asymptomatic individuals have a positive amebic serology. The interpretation of the indirect hemagglutination test is more difficult because titers may remain positive for as long as 10 years.

Up to 10% of patients with acute amebic liver abscess may have negative serologic findings; in suspected cases with an initially negative result, testing should be repeated in a week. In contrast to carriers of *E. dispar*, most asymptomatic carriers of *E. histolytica* develop antibodies. Thus, serologic tests are helpful in assessing the risk of invasive amebiasis in asymptomatic, cyst-passing individuals in nonendemic areas. Serologic tests also should be performed in patients with ulcerative colitis before the institution of glucocorticoid therapy to prevent the development of severe colitis or toxic megacolon owing to unsuspected amebiasis.

Routine hematology and chemistry tests usually are not very helpful in the diagnosis of invasive amebiasis. About three-fourths of patients with an amebic liver abscess have leukocytosis (>10,000 cells/μL); this condition is particularly likely if symptoms are acute or complications have developed. Invasive amebiasis does not elicit eosinophilia. Anemia, if present, is usually multifactorial. Even with large liver abscesses, liver enzyme levels are normal or minimally elevated. The alkaline phosphatase level is most often elevated and may remain so for months. Aminotransferase elevations suggest acute disease or a complication.

Radiographic Studies

Radiographic barium studies are potentially dangerous in acute amebic colitis. Amebomas are usually identified first by a barium enema, but biopsy is necessary for differentiation from carcinoma.

Radiographic techniques such as ultrasonography, CT, and MRI are all useful for detection of the round or oval hypoechoic cyst. More than 80% of patients who have had symptoms for >10 days have a single abscess of the right lobe of the liver (Fig. 115-4). Approximately 50% of patients who have had symptoms for <10 days have multiple abscesses. Findings associated with complications include large abscesses (>10 cm) in the superior part of the right lobe, which may rupture into the pleural space; multiple lesions, which must be differentiated from pyogenic abscesses; and lesions of the left lobe, which may rupture into the

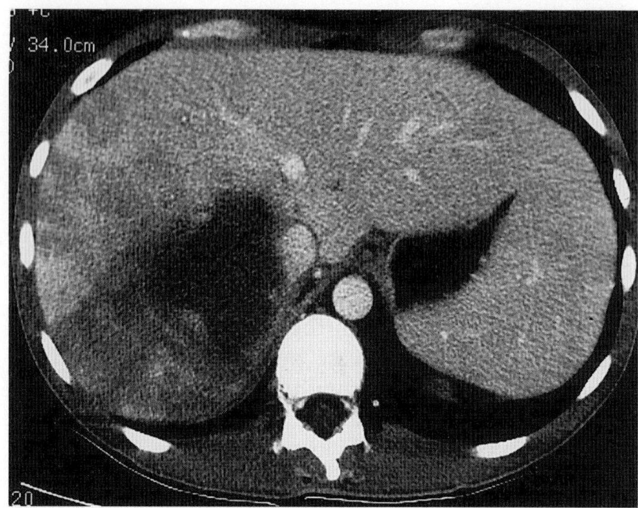

FIGURE 115-4

Abdominal CT scan of a large amebic abscess of the right lobe of the liver. *(Courtesy of the Department of Radiology, UCSD Medical Center, San Diego; with permission.)*

pericardium. Because abscesses resolve slowly and may increase in size in patients who are responding clinically to therapy, frequent follow-up ultrasonography may prove confusing. Complete resolution of a liver abscess within 6 months can be anticipated in two-thirds of patients, but 10% may have persistent abnormalities for a year.

DIFFERENTIAL DIAGNOSIS

The differential diagnosis of intestinal amebiasis includes bacterial diarrheas (Chap. 25) caused by *Campylobacter* (Chap. 56); enteroinvasive *Escherichia coli* (Chap. 51); and species of *Shigella* (Chap. 55), *Salmonella* (Chap. 54), and *Vibrio* (Chap. 57). Although the typical patient with amebic colitis has less prominent fever than in these other conditions as well as heme-positive stools with few neutrophils, correct diagnosis requires bacterial cultures, microscopic examination of stools, and amebic serologic testing. As has already been mentioned, amebiasis must be ruled out in any patient thought to have inflammatory bowel disease.

Because of the variety of presenting signs and symptoms, amebic liver abscess can easily be confused with pulmonary or gallbladder disease or with any febrile illness with few localizing signs, such as malaria (Chap. 116) or typhoid fever (Chap. 54). The diagnosis should be considered in members of high-risk groups who have recently traveled outside the United States (Chap. 4) and in inmates of institutions. Once radiographic studies have identified an abscess in the liver, the most important differential diagnosis is between amebic and pyogenic abscess. Patients with pyogenic abscess typically are older and have a history of underlying bowel disease or recent surgery. Amebic serology is helpful, but aspiration of the abscess, with Gram's staining and culture of the material, may be required for differentiation of the two diseases.

℞ Treatment: AMEBIASIS

INTESTINAL DISEASE (Table 115-2) The drugs used to treat amebiasis can be classified according to their primary site of action. Luminal amebicides are poorly absorbed and reach high concentrations in the bowel, but their activity is limited to cysts and trophozoites close to the mucosa. Only two luminal drugs are available in the United States: iodoquinol and paromomycin. Indications for the use of luminal agents include eradication of cysts in patients with colitis or a liver abscess and treatment of asymptomatic carriers. The majority of asymptomatic individuals who pass cysts are colonized with *E. dispar*, which does not warrant specific therapy. However, it is prudent to treat asymptomatic individuals who pass cysts unless *E. dispar* colonization can be definitively demonstrated by specific antigen-detection tests.

Tissue amebicides reach high concentrations in the blood and tissue after oral or parenteral administration. The development of nitroimidazole compounds, especially metronidazole, was a major advance in the treatment of invasive amebiasis. Patients with amebic colitis should be treated with intravenous or oral metronidazole. Side effects include nausea, vomiting, abdominal discomfort, and a disulfiram-like reaction. Another longer-acting imidazole compound, tinidazole, is also effective and was recently approved in the United States. All patients should also receive a full course of therapy with a luminal agent, since metronidazole does not eradicate cysts. Resistance to metronidazole has been selected in the laboratory but has not been found in clinical isolates. Relapses are not uncommon and probably represent reinfection or failure to eradicate amebas from the bowel because of an inadequate dosage or duration of therapy.

TABLE 115-2

DRUG THERAPY FOR AMEBIASIS

INDICATION	THERAPY
Asymptomatic carriage	Luminal agent: iodoquinol (650-mg tablets), 650 mg tid for 20 days; *or* paromomycin (250-mg tablets), 500 mg tid for 10 days
Acute colitis	Metronidazole (250- or 500-mg tablets), 750 mg PO or IV tid for 5–10 days, *plus* Luminal agent as above
Amebic liver abscess	Metronidazole, 750 mg PO or IV for 5–10 days, *or* Tinidazole, 2 g PO once, *or* Ornidazole,[a] 2 g PO once, *plus* Luminal agent as above

[a]Not available in the United States.

Protozoal and Helminthic Infections SECTION VIII

AMEBIC LIVER ABSCESS Metronidazole is the drug of choice for amebic liver abscess. Longer-acting nitroimidazoles (tinidazole and ornidazole) have been effective as single-dose therapy in developing countries. With early diagnosis and therapy, mortality rates from uncomplicated amebic liver abscess are <1%. The second-line therapeutic agents emetine and chloroquine should be avoided if possible because of the potential cardiovascular and gastrointestinal side effects of the former and the higher relapse rates with the latter. There is no evidence that combined therapy with two drugs is more effective than the single-drug regimen. Studies of South Africans with liver abscesses demonstrated that 72% of patients without intestinal symptoms had bowel infection with *E. histolytica*; thus, all treatment regimens should include a luminal agent to eradicate cysts and prevent further transmission. Amebic liver abscess recurs rarely.

ASPIRATION OF LIVER ABSCESSES More than 90% of patients respond dramatically to metronidazole therapy with decreases in both pain and fever within 72 h. Indications for aspiration of liver abscesses are (1) the need to rule out a pyogenic abscess, particularly in patients with multiple lesions; (2) the lack of a clinical response in 3–5 days; (3) the threat of imminent rupture; and (4) the need to prevent rupture of left-lobe abscesses into the pericardium. There is no evidence that aspiration, even of large abscesses (up to 10 cm), accelerates healing. Percutaneous drainage may be successful even if the liver abscess has already ruptured. Surgery should be reserved for instances of bowel perforation and rupture into the pericardium.

PREVENTION

Amebic infection is spread by ingestion of food or water contaminated with cysts. Since an asymptomatic carrier may excrete up to 15 million cysts per day, prevention of infection requires adequate sanitation and eradication of cyst carriage. In high-risk areas, infection can be minimized by the avoidance of unpeeled fruits and vegetables and the use of bottled water. Because cysts are resistant to readily attainable levels of chlorine, disinfection by iodination (tetraglycine hydroperiodide) is recommended. There is no effective prophylaxis.

INFECTION WITH FREE-LIVING AMEBAS

EPIDEMIOLOGY

Free-living amebas of the genera *Acanthamoeba* and *Naegleria* are distributed throughout the world and have been isolated from a wide variety of fresh and brackish water, including that from lakes, taps, hot springs, swimming pools, and heating and air-conditioning units, and even from the nasal passages of healthy children. Encystation may protect the protozoa from desiccation and food deprivation. The persistence of *Legionella pneumophila* in water supplies may be attributable in part to chronic infection of free-living amebas, particularly *Naegleria*. Free-living amebas of the genus *Balamuthia* have only recently been isolated from soil samples, including a sample from a flowerpot linked to a fatal infection in a child.

NAEGLERIA INFECTIONS

Primary amebic meningoencephalitis caused by *Naegleria fowleri* follows the aspiration of water contaminated with trophozoites or cysts or the inhalation of contaminated dust, leading to invasion of the olfactory neuroepithelium. After an incubation period of 2–15 days, severe headache, high fever, nausea, vomiting, and meningismus develop. Photophobia and palsies of the third, fourth, and sixth cranial nerves are common. Rapid progression to seizures and coma may follow. The prognosis is uniformly poor: most patients die within a week. Only a few survivors, treated with high-dose amphotericin B and rifampin, have been reported. Infection is most common in otherwise-healthy children or young adults, who often report recent swimming in lakes or heated swimming pools.

The diagnosis of *Naegleria* infection should be considered in any patient who has purulent meningitis without evidence of bacteria on Gram's staining, antigen detection assay, and culture. Other laboratory findings resemble those for fulminant bacterial meningitis, with elevated intracranial pressure, high white blood cell counts (up to 20,000/μL), and elevated protein concentrations and low glucose levels in cerebrospinal fluid (CSF). Diagnosis depends on the detection of motile trophozoites in wet mounts of fresh spinal fluid. Antibodies to *Naegleria* spp. have been detected in normal adults; serologic testing is not useful in the diagnosis of acute infection.

ACANTHAMOEBA INFECTIONS

Granulomatous Amebic Encephalitis

Infection with *Acanthamoeba* species follows a more indolent course and typically occurs in chronically ill or debilitated patients. Risk factors include lymphoproliferative disorders, chemotherapy, glucocorticoid therapy, lupus erythematosus, and AIDS. Infection usually reaches the central nervous system (CNS) hematogenously from a primary focus in the sinuses, skin, or lungs. In the CNS, the onset is insidious, and the syndrome often mimics a space-occupying lesion. Altered mental status, headache, and stiff neck may be accompanied by focal findings such as cranial nerve palsies, ataxia, and hemiparesis. Cutaneous ulcers or hard nodules containing amebas are frequently detected in AIDS patients with disseminated *Acanthamoeba* infection.

Examination of the CSF for trophozoites may be diagnostically helpful, but lumbar puncture may be contraindicated because of increased intracerebral pressure. CT frequently reveals cortical and subcortical lesions of decreased density consistent with embolic infarcts. In other patients, multiple enhancing lesions with edema may mimic the computed tomographic appearance of toxoplasmosis (Chap. 121). Demonstration of the trophozoites and cysts of *Acanthamoeba* on wet mounts or in biopsy specimens establishes the diagnosis. Culture on nonnutrient agar plates seeded with *E. coli* may also be helpful.

Fluorescein-labeled antiserum is available from the Centers for Disease Control and Prevention (CDC) for the detection of protozoa in biopsy specimens. Granulomatous amebic encephalitis in patients with AIDS may have an accelerated course (with survival for only 3–40 days) because of the difficulty these individuals have in forming granulomas. Various antimicrobial agents have been used to treat *Acanthamoeba* infection, including pentamidine, trimethoprim-sulfamethoxazole, and fluconazole, but the infection is almost uniformly fatal.

Keratitis

The incidence of keratitis caused by *Acanthamoeba* has increased in the past 20 years, in part as a result of improved diagnosis. Earlier infections were associated with trauma to the eye and exposure to contaminated water. At present, most infections are linked to extended-wear contact lenses, and rare cases are associated with laser-assisted in situ keratomileusis (LASIK). Risk factors include the use of homemade saline, the wearing of lenses while swimming, and inadequate disinfection. Since contact lenses presumably cause microscopic trauma, the early corneal findings may be nonspecific. The first symptoms usually include tearing and the painful sensation of a foreign body. Once infection is established, progression is rapid; the characteristic clinical sign is an annular, paracentral corneal ring representing a corneal abscess. Deeper corneal invasion and loss of vision may follow.

The differential diagnosis includes bacterial, mycobacterial, and herpetic infection. The irregular polygonal cysts of *Acanthamoeba* (Fig. 115-5) may be identified in corneal scrapings or biopsy material, and trophozoites can be grown on special media. Cysts are resistant to available drugs, and the results of medical therapy have been disappointing. Some reports have suggested partial responses to propamidine isethionate eyedrops. Severe infections usually require keratoplasty.

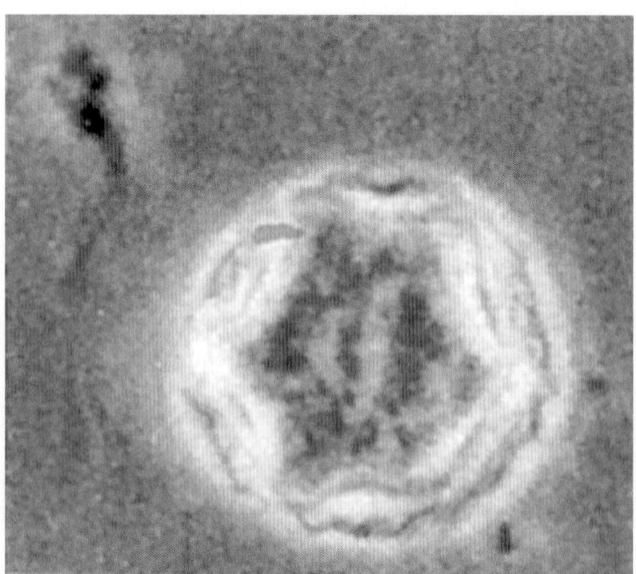

FIGURE 115-5
Double-walled cyst of *Acanthamoeba castellani*, as seen by phase-contrast microscopy. *[From DJ Krogstad et al, in A Balows et al (eds): Manual of Clinical Microbiology, 5th ed. Washington, DC, American Society for Microbiology, 1991.]*

BALAMUTHIA INFECTIONS

Balamuthia mandrillaris, a free-living ameba previously referred to as a leptomyxid ameba, is an important etiologic agent of amebic meningoencephalitis in immunocompetent hosts. The course is typically subacute, with focal neurologic signs, fever, seizures, and headaches leading to death within 1 week to several months after onset. Examination of CSF reveals mononuclear or neutrophilic pleocytosis, elevated protein levels, and normal to low glucose concentrations. Multiple hypodense lesions are usually detected with imaging studies. This mixed picture of space-occupying lesions with CSF pleocytosis is suggestive of *Balamuthia.* Detection of an indirect fluorescent antibody response may be helpful in noninvasive diagnosis, but usually a definitive diagnosis is made post-mortem. Fluorescent antibody is available from the CDC. The variety of drugs used to treat the few surviving patients (numbering fewer than five in the United States) include pentamidine, flucytosine, sulfadiazine, and macrolides. The differential diagnosis includes tuberculomas (Chap. 66) and neurocysticercosis (Chap. 127).

FURTHER READINGS

DEETZ TR et al: Successful treatment of *Balamuthia* amoebic encephalitis: Presentation of two cases. Clin Infect Dis 37:1304, 2003

HAQUE R et al: *Entamoeba histolytica* infection in children and protection from subsequent amebiasis. Infect Immun 37:1304, 2003

HUSTON CD et al: Caspase-3-dependent killing of host cells by the parasite *Entamoeba histolytica*. Cell Microbiol 2:617, 2000

KUMAR R, LLOYD D: Recent advances in the treatment of *Acanthamoeba* keratitis. Clin Infect Dis 35:434, 2002

MARCIANO-CABRAL F: Free-living amoebae as agents of human infection. J Infect Dis 199:1104, 2009

PETRI WA et al: The bittersweet interface of parasite and host lectin-carbohydrate interactions during human invasion by the parasite *Entamoeba histolytica*. Annu Rev Microbiol 56:39, 2002

QUE X, REED SL: Cysteine proteinases and the pathogenesis of amebiasis. Clin Microbiol Rev 13:196, 2002

SANTI-ROCCA J et al: Host-microbe interactions and defense mechanisms in the development of amoebic liver abscesses. Clin Microbiol Rev 22:65, 2009

SCHUSTER FL, VISVESVARA GS: Free-living amoebae as opportunistic and non-opportunistic pathogens of humans and animals. Int J Parasitol 345:1001, 2004

——— et al: Under the radar: *Balamuthia* amebic encephalitis. Clin Infect Dis 48:879, 2009

SOLAYMANI-MOHAMMADI S et al: Comparison of a stool antigen detection kit and PCR for diagnosis of *Entamoeba histolytica* and *Entamoeba dispar* infections in asymptomatic cyst passers in Iran. J Clin Microbiol 44:2258, 2006

STANLEY SL: Amoebiasis. Lancet 361:1025, 2006

———, REED SL: Microbes and microbial toxins: Paradigms for microbial-mucosal interactions. VI. *Entamoeba histolytica*: Parasite-host interactions. Am J Physiol Gastrointest Liver Physiol 280:G1049, 2001

CHAPTER 116

MALARIA

Nicholas J. White ■ Joel G. Breman

Humanity has but three great enemies: Fever, famine and war; of these by far the greatest, by far the most terrible, is fever.

William Osler

Malaria is a protozoan disease transmitted by the bite of infected *Anopheles* mosquitoes. It is the most important of the parasitic diseases of humans, with transmission in 107 countries containing 3 billion people and causing 1–3 million deaths each year. Malaria has now been eliminated from the United States, Canada, Europe, and Russia but, despite enormous control efforts, has resurged in many parts of the tropics. Added to this resurgence are the increasing problems of drug resistance of the parasite and insecticide resistance of the vectors. Occasional local transmission after importation of malaria has occurred recently in several southern and eastern areas of the United States and in Europe, indicating the continual danger to nonmalarious countries. Although there are promising new control and research initiatives, malaria remains today, as it has been for centuries, a heavy burden on tropical communities, a threat to nonendemic countries, and a danger to travelers.

ETIOLOGY AND PATHOGENESIS

Four species of the genus *Plasmodium* cause nearly all malarial infections in humans (although rare infections involve species normally affecting other primates). These are *P. falciparum*, *P. vivax*, *P. ovale*, and *P. malariae* (Table 116-1). Almost all deaths are caused by falciparum malaria. Human infection begins when a female anopheline mosquito inoculates plasmodial *sporozoites* from its salivary gland during a blood meal (Fig. 116-1). These microscopic motile forms of the malarial parasite are carried rapidly via the bloodstream to the liver, where they invade hepatic parenchymal cells and begin a period of asexual reproduction. By this amplification process (known as *intrahepatic* or *preerythrocytic schizogony* or *merogony*), a single sporozoite eventually may produce from 10,000 to >30,000 daughter merozoites. The swollen infected liver cell eventually bursts, discharging motile *merozoites* into the bloodstream. These then invade the red blood cells (RBCs) and multiply six- to twentyfold every 48–72 h. When the parasites reach densities of ~50/μL of blood, the symptomatic stage of the infection

TABLE 116-1

CHARACTERISTICS OF *PLASMODIUM* SPECIES INFECTING HUMANS

	FINDING FOR INDICATED SPECIES			
CHARACTERISTIC	*P. FALCIPARUM*	*P. VIVAX*	*P. OVALE*	*P. MALARIAE*
Duration of intrahepatic phase (days)	5.5	8	9	15
Number of merozoites released per infected hepatocyte	30,000	10,000	15,000	15,000
Duration of erythrocytic cycle (hours)	48	48	50	72
Red cell preference	Younger cells (but can invade cells of all ages)	Reticulocytes and cells up to 2 weeks old	Reticulocytes	Older cells
Morphology	Usually only ring forms[a]; banana-shaped gametocytes	Irregularly shaped large rings and trophozoites; enlarged erythrocytes; Schüffner's dots	Infected erythrocytes, enlarged and oval with tufted ends; Schüffner's dots	Band or rectangular forms of trophozoites common
Pigment color	Black	Yellow-brown	Dark brown	Brown-black
Ability to cause relapses	No	Yes	Yes	No

[a]Parasitemias of >2% are suggestive of *P. falciparum* infection.

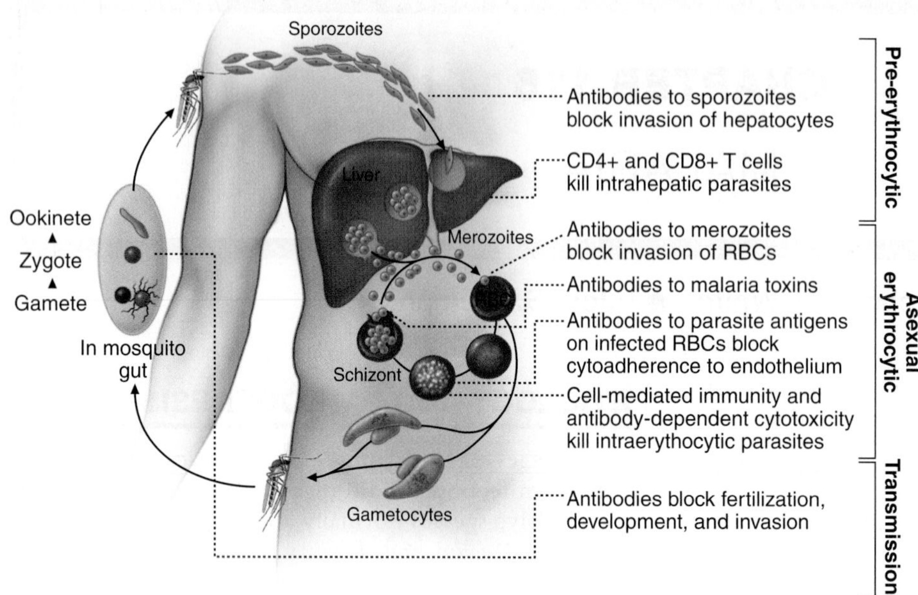
Sporozoites
Antibodies to sporozoites block invasion of hepatocytes
CD4+ and CD8+ T cells kill intrahepatic parasites
Pre-erythrocytic
Liver
Ookinete
Zygote
Gamete
In mosquito gut
Merozoites
Antibodies to merozoites block invasion of RBCs
Antibodies to malaria toxins
Antibodies to parasite antigens on infected RBCs block cytoadherence to endothelium
Asexual erythrocytic
Schizont
Cell-mediated immunity and antibody-dependent cytotoxicity kill intraerythocytic parasites
Gametocytes
Antibodies block fertilization, development, and invasion
Transmission

FIGURE 116-1

The malaria transmission cycle from mosquito to human. RBC, red blood cell.

begins. In *P. vivax* and *P. ovale* infections, a proportion of the intrahepatic forms do not divide immediately but remain dormant for a period ranging from 3 weeks to a year or longer before reproduction begins. These dormant forms, or *hypnozoites*, are the cause of the relapses that characterize infection with these two species.

After entry into the bloodstream, merozoites rapidly invade erythrocytes and become *trophozoites*. Attachment is mediated via a specific erythrocyte surface receptor. In the case of *P. vivax*, this receptor is related to the Duffy blood-group antigen Fy^a or Fy^b. Most West Africans and people with origins in that region carry the Duffy-negative FyFy phenotype and are therefore resistant to *P. vivax* malaria. During the early stage of intraerythrocytic development, the small "ring forms" of the four parasitic species appear similar under light microscopy. As the trophozoites enlarge, species-specific characteristics become evident, pigment becomes visible, and the parasite assumes an irregular or ameboid shape. By the end of the 48-h intraerythrocytic life cycle (72 h for *P. malariae*), the parasite has consumed nearly all the hemoglobin and grown to occupy most of the RBC. It is now called a *schizont*. Multiple nuclear divisions have taken place (*schizogony* or *merogony*), and the RBC then ruptures to release 6–30 daughter merozoites, each potentially capable of invading a new RBC and repeating the cycle. The disease in human beings is caused by the direct effects of RBC invasion and destruction by the asexual parasite and the host's reaction. After a series of asexual cycles (*P. falciparum*) or immediately after release from the liver (*P. vivax, P. ovale, P. malariae*), some of the parasites develop into morphologically distinct, longer-lived sexual forms (*gametocytes*) that can transmit malaria.

After being ingested in the blood meal of a biting female anopheline mosquito, the male and female gametocytes form a zygote in the insect's midgut. This zygote matures into an ookinete, which penetrates and encysts in the mosquito's gut wall. The resulting oocyst expands by asexual division until it bursts to liberate myriad motile sporozoites, which then migrate in the hemolymph to the salivary gland of the mosquito to await inoculation into another human at the next feeding.

EPIDEMIOLOGY

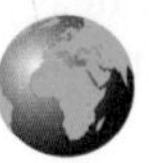

Malaria occurs throughout most of the tropical regions of the world (Fig. 116-2). *P. falciparum* predominates in Africa, New Guinea, and Haiti; *P. vivax* is more common in Central America. The prevalence of these two species is approximately equal in South America, the Indian subcontinent, eastern Asia, and Oceania. *P. malariae* is found in most endemic areas, especially throughout sub-Saharan Africa, but is much less common. *P. ovale* is relatively unusual outside of Africa and, where it is found, comprises <1% of isolates.

The epidemiology of malaria is complex and may vary considerably even within relatively small geographic areas. Endemicity traditionally has been defined in terms of parasitemia rates or palpable-spleen rates in children 2–9 years of age as hypoendemic (<10%), mesoendemic (11–50%), hyperendemic (51–75%), and holoendemic (>75%); however, it is uncommon to use these indices for planning control programs. In holo- and hyperendemic areas (e.g., certain regions of tropical Africa or coastal New Guinea) where there is intense *P. falciparum* transmission, people may sustain more than one infectious mosquito bite per day and are infected repeatedly throughout their lives. In such settings, rates of morbidity and mortality due to malaria are considerable during childhood. Immunity against disease is hard won in these areas, and the burden of disease in young children is high; by adulthood, however, most malarial infections are asymptomatic. Constant, frequent, year-round infection is termed *stable transmission*.

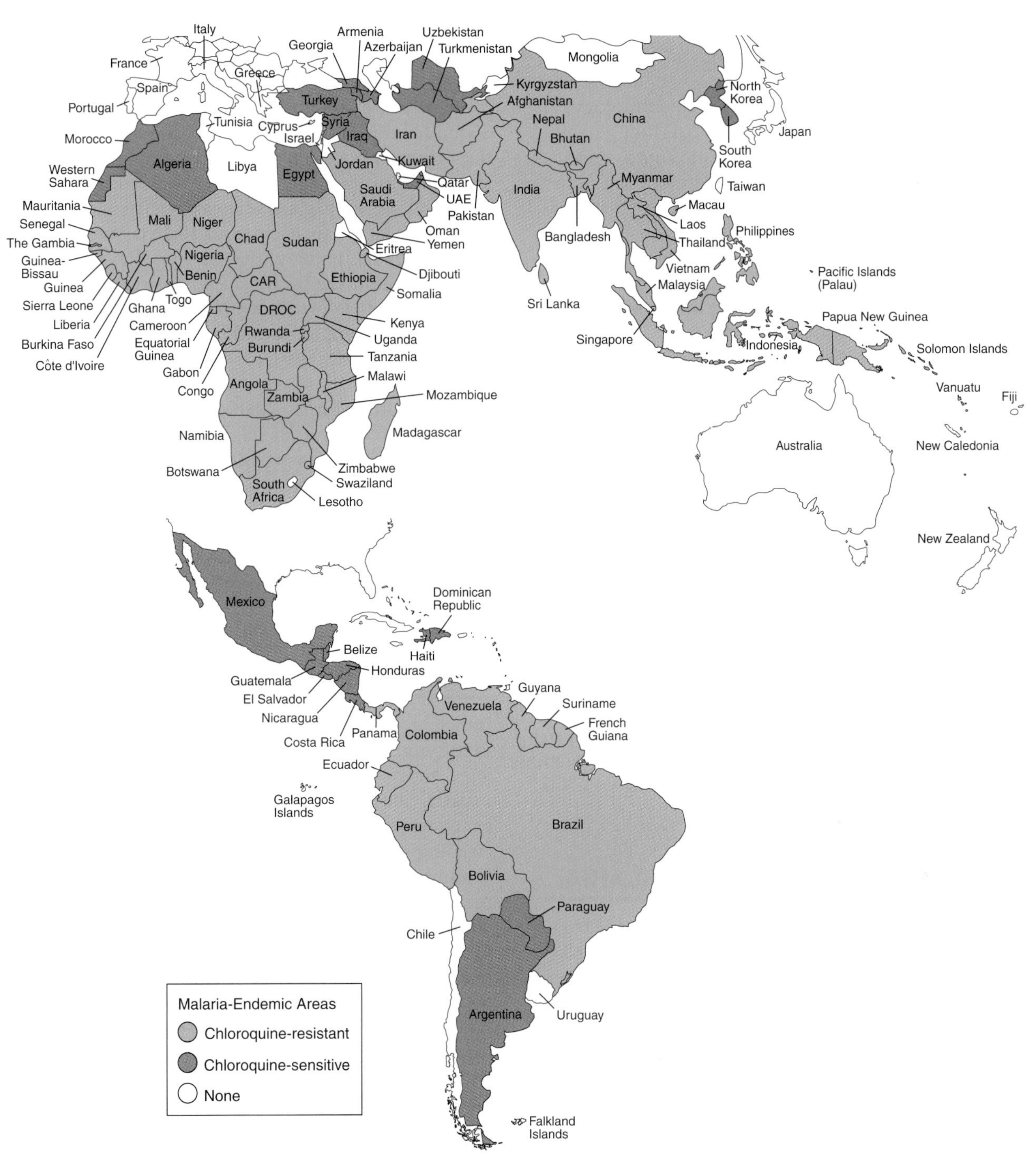

FIGURE 116-2

Malaria-endemic countries in the Americas (***bottom***) and in Africa, the Middle East, Asia, and the South Pacific (***top***), 2007. CAR, Central African Republic; DROC, Democratic Republic of the Congo; UAE, United Arab Emirates.

In areas where transmission is low, erratic, or focal, full protective immunity is not acquired, and symptomatic disease may occur at all ages. This situation usually exists in hypoendemic areas and is termed *unstable transmission*. Even in stable transmission areas, there is often an increased incidence of symptomatic malaria coinciding with increased mosquito breeding and transmission during the rainy season. Malaria behaves like an epidemic disease in some areas, particularly those with unstable malaria, such as northern India, Sri Lanka, Southeast Asia, Ethiopia, Eritrea, Rwanda, Burundi, Southern Africa, and Madagascar. An epidemic can develop when there are changes in environmental, economic, or social conditions, such as heavy rains following drought or migrations (usually of refugees or workers) from a nonmalarious region to an area of high transmission; a breakdown in malaria control and prevention services can intensify epidemic conditions. This situation usually results in considerable mortality among all age groups.

The principal determinants of the epidemiology of malaria are the number (density), the human-biting habits, and the longevity of the anopheline mosquito vectors. Not all of the >400 anophelines can transmit malaria, and those that do vary considerably in their efficiency as malaria vectors. More specifically, the transmission of malaria is directly proportional to the density of the vector, the square of the number of human bites per day per mosquito, and the tenth power of the probability of the mosquito's surviving for 1 day. Mosquito longevity is particularly important, because the portion of the parasite's life cycle that takes place within the mosquito—from gametocyte ingestion to subsequent inoculation (*sporogony*)—lasts 8–30 days, depending on ambient temperature; thus, to transmit malaria, the mosquito must survive for >7 days. In general, at temperatures below 16°–18°C, sporogony is not completed and transmission does not occur, although malaria outbreaks and transmission have recently occurred in the highlands of east Africa—areas (>1500 m) previously free of vectors. The most effective mosquito vectors of malaria are those, such as *Anopheles gambiae* in Africa, which are long-lived, occur in high densities in tropical climates, breed readily, and bite humans in preference to other animals. The entomologic inoculation rate (the number of sporozoite-positive mosquito bites per person per year) is the most common measure of malaria transmission and varies from <1 in some parts of Latin America and Southeast Asia to >300 in parts of tropical Africa.

ERYTHROCYTE CHANGES IN MALARIA

After invading an erythrocyte, the growing malarial parasite progressively consumes and degrades intracellular proteins, principally hemoglobin. The potentially toxic heme is detoxified by polymerization to biologically inert hemozoin (malaria pigment). The parasite also alters the RBC membrane by changing its transport properties, exposing cryptic surface antigens, and inserting new parasite-derived proteins. The RBC becomes more irregular in shape, more antigenic, and less deformable.

In *P. falciparum* infections, membrane protuberances appear on the erythrocyte's surface 12–15 h after the cell's invasion. These "knobs" extrude a high-molecular-weight, antigenically variant, strain-specific erythrocyte membrane adhesive protein (PfEMP1) that mediates attachment to receptors on venular and capillary endothelium—an event termed *cytoadherence*. Several vascular receptors have been identified, of which intercellular adhesion molecule 1 (ICAM-1) is probably the most important in the brain, chondroitin sulfate B in the placenta, and CD36 in most other organs. Thus, the infected erythrocytes stick inside and eventually block capillaries and venules. At the same stage, these *P. falciparum*–infected RBCs may also adhere to uninfected RBCs (to form rosettes) and to other parasitized erythrocytes (agglutination). The processes of cytoadherence, rosetting, and agglutination are central to the pathogenesis of falciparum malaria. They result in the sequestration of RBCs containing mature forms of the parasite in vital organs (particularly the brain), where they interfere with microcirculatory flow and metabolism. Sequestered parasites continue to develop out of reach of the principal host defense mechanism: splenic processing and filtration. As a consequence, only the younger ring forms of the asexual parasites are seen circulating in the peripheral blood in falciparum malaria, and the level of peripheral parasitemia underestimates the true number of parasites within the body. Severe malaria is also associated with reduced deformability of the uninfected erythrocytes, which compromises their passage through the partially obstructed capillaries and venules and shortens RBC survival.

In the other three ("benign") malarias, sequestration does not occur, and all stages of the parasite's development are evident on peripheral blood smears. Whereas *P. vivax*, *P. ovale*, and *P. malariae* show a marked predilection for either young RBCs (*P. vivax*, *P. ovale*) or old cells (*P. malariae*) and produce a level of parasitemia that is seldom >2%, *P. falciparum* can invade erythrocytes of all ages and may be associated with very high levels of parasitemia.

HOST RESPONSE

Initially, the host responds to plasmodial infection by activating nonspecific defense mechanisms. Splenic immunologic and filtrative clearance functions are augmented in malaria, and the removal of both parasitized and uninfected erythrocytes is accelerated. The parasitized cells escaping splenic removal are destroyed when the schizont ruptures. The material released induces the activation of macrophages and the release of proinflammatory mononuclear cell–derived cytokines, which cause fever and exert other pathologic effects. Temperatures of ≥40°C damage mature parasites; in untreated infections, the effect of such temperatures is to further synchronize the parasitic cycle, with eventual production of the regular fever spikes and rigors that originally served to characterize the different malarias. These regular fever patterns (tertian, every 2 days; quartan, every 3 days) are seldom seen today in patients who receive prompt and effective antimalarial treatment.

The geographic distributions of sickle cell disease, ovalocytosis, thalassemia, and glucose-6-phosphate dehydrogenase (G6PD) deficiency closely resemble that of malaria before the introduction of control measures. This similarity suggests that these genetic disorders confer protection against death from falciparum malaria. For example, HbA/S heterozygotes (sickle cell trait) have a sixfold reduction in the risk of dying from severe falciparum malaria. This decrease in risk appears to be related to impaired parasite growth at low oxygen tensions. Parasite multiplication in HbA/E heterozygotes is reduced at high parasite densities. In Melanesia, children with α-thalassemia appear to have more frequent malaria (both vivax and falciparum) in the early years of life, and this pattern of infection appears to protect against severe disease. In Melanesian ovalocytosis, rigid erythrocytes resist merozoite invasion, and the intraerythrocytic milieu is hostile.

Nonspecific host defense mechanisms stop the infection's expansion, and the subsequent specific immune response controls the infection. Eventually, exposure to sufficient strains confers protection from high-level parasitemia and disease but not from infection. As a result of this state of infection without illness (*premunition*), asymptomatic parasitemia is common among adults and older children living in regions with stable and intense transmission (i.e., holo- or hyperendemic areas). Immunity is mainly specific for both the species and the strain of infecting malarial parasite. Both humoral immunity and cellular immunity are necessary for protection, but the mechanisms of each are incompletely understood (Fig. 116-1). Immune individuals have a polyclonal increase in serum levels of IgM, IgG, and IgA, although much of this antibody is unrelated to protection. Antibodies to a variety of parasitic antigens presumably act in concert to limit in vivo replication of the parasite. In the case of falciparum malaria, the most important of these antigens is the surface adhesin—the variant protein PfEMP1 mentioned above. Passively transferred IgG from immune adults has been shown to reduce levels of parasitemia in children; although parasitemia in very young infants can occur, passive transfer of maternal antibody contributes to the relative (but not complete) protection of infants from severe malaria in the first months of life. This complex immunity to disease declines when a person lives outside an endemic area for several months or longer.

Several factors retard the development of cellular immunity to malaria. These factors include the absence of major histocompatibility antigens on the surface of infected RBCs, which precludes direct T cell recognition; malaria antigen–specific immune unresponsiveness; and the enormous strain diversity of malarial parasites, along with the ability of the parasites to express variant immunodominant antigens on the erythrocyte surface that change during the period of infection. Parasites may persist in the blood for months (or, in the case of *P. malariae*, for many years) if treatment is not given. The complexity of the immune response in malaria, the sophistication of the parasites' evasion mechanisms, and the lack of a good in vitro correlate with clinical immunity have all slowed progress toward an effective vaccine.

CLINICAL FEATURES

Malaria is a very common cause of fever in tropical countries. The first symptoms of malaria are nonspecific; the lack of a sense of well-being, headache, fatigue, abdominal discomfort, and muscle aches followed by fever are all similar to the symptoms of a minor viral illness. In some instances, a prominence of headache, chest pain, abdominal pain, arthralgia, myalgia, or diarrhea may suggest another diagnosis. Although headache may be severe in malaria, there is no neck stiffness or photophobia resembling that in meningitis. While myalgia may be prominent, it is not usually as severe as in dengue fever, and the muscles are not tender as in leptospirosis or typhus. Nausea, vomiting, and orthostatic hypotension are common. The classic malarial paroxysms, in which fever spikes, chills, and rigors occur at regular intervals, are relatively unusual and suggest infection with *P. vivax* or *P. ovale*. The fever is irregular at first (that of falciparum malaria may never become regular); the temperature of nonimmune individuals and children often rises above 40°C in conjunction with tachycardia and sometimes delirium. Although childhood febrile convulsions may occur with any of the malarias, generalized seizures are specifically associated with falciparum malaria and may herald the development of cerebral disease. Many clinical abnormalities have been described in acute malaria, but most patients with uncomplicated infections have few abnormal physical findings other than fever, malaise, mild anemia, and (in some cases) a palpable spleen. Anemia is common among young children living in areas with stable transmission, particularly where resistance has compromised the efficacy of antimalarial drugs. In nonimmune individuals with acute malaria, the spleen takes several days to become palpable, but splenic enlargement is found in a high proportion of otherwise healthy individuals in malaria-endemic areas and reflects repeated infections. Slight enlargement of the liver is also common, particularly among young children. Mild jaundice is common among adults; it may develop in patients with otherwise uncomplicated falciparum malaria and usually resolves over 1–3 weeks. Malaria is not associated with a rash like those seen in meningococcal septicemia, typhus, enteric fever, viral exanthems, and drug reactions. Petechial hemorrhages in the skin or mucous membranes—features of viral hemorrhagic fevers and leptospirosis—develop only rarely in severe falciparum malaria.

SEVERE FALCIPARUM MALARIA

Appropriately and promptly treated, uncomplicated falciparum malaria (i.e., the patient can swallow medicines and food) carries a mortality rate of ~0.1%. However, once vital-organ dysfunction occurs or the total proportion of erythrocytes infected increases to >2% (a level corresponding to $>10^{12}$ parasites in an adult), mortality risk rises steeply. The major manifestations of severe falciparum malaria are shown in Table 116-2, and features indicating a poor prognosis are listed in Table 116-3.

Cerebral Malaria

Coma is a characteristic and ominous feature of falciparum malaria and, despite treatment, is associated with death rates of ~20% among adults and 15% among children. Any obtundation, delirium, or abnormal behavior should be taken very seriously. The onset may be gradual or sudden following a convulsion.

Cerebral malaria manifests as diffuse symmetric encephalopathy; focal neurologic signs are unusual. Although some passive resistance to head flexion may be detected, signs of meningeal irritation are lacking. The eyes may be divergent and a pout reflex is common, but

TABLE 116-2

MANIFESTATIONS OF SEVERE FALCIPARUM MALARIA

SIGNS	MANIFESTATIONS
Major	
Unarousable coma/cerebral malaria	Failure to localize or respond appropriately to noxious stimuli; coma persisting for >30 min after generalized convulsion
Acidemia/acidosis	Arterial pH <7.25 or plasma bicarbonate level of <15 mmol/L; venous lactate level of >5 mmol/L; manifests as labored deep breathing, often termed "respiratory distress"
Severe normochromic, normocytic anemia	Hematocrit of <15% or hemoglobin level of <50 g/L (<5 g/dL) with parasitemia level of >100,000/μL
Renal failure	Urine output (24 h) of <400 mL in adults or <12 mL/kg in children; no improvement with rehydration; serum creatinine level of >265 μmol/L (>3.0 mg/dL)
Pulmonary edema/adult respiratory distress syndrome	Noncardiogenic pulmonary edema, often aggravated by overhydration
Hypoglycemia	Plasma glucose level of <2.2 mmol/L (<40 mg/dL)
Hypotension/shock	Systolic blood pressure of <50 mmHg in children 1–5 years or <80 mmHg in adults; core/skin temperature difference of >10°C; capillary refill >2 s
Bleeding/disseminated intravascular coagulation	Significant bleeding and hemorrhage from the gums, nose, and gastrointestinal tract and/or evidence of disseminated intravascular coagulation
Convulsions	More than two generalized seizures in 24 h; signs of continued seizure activity sometimes subtle (e.g., tonic-clonic eye movements without limb or face movement)
Hemoglobinuria[a]	Macroscopic black, brown, or red urine; not associated with effects of oxidant drugs and red blood cell enzyme defects (such as G6PD deficiency)
Other	
Impaired consciousness/ arousable	Unable to sit or stand without support
Extreme weakness	Prostration; inability to sit unaided[b]
Hyperparasitemia	Parasitemia level of >5% in nonimmune patients (>20% in any patient)
Jaundice	Serum bilirubin level of >50 mmol/L (>3.0 mg/dL) if combined with other evidence of vital-organ dysfunction

[a]Hemoglobinuria may occur in uncomplicated malaria.
[b]In a child who is normally able to sit.
Note: G6PD, glucose-6-phosphate dehydrogenase.

other primitive reflexes are usually absent. The corneal reflexes are preserved, except in deep coma. Muscle tone may be either increased or decreased. The tendon reflexes are variable, and the plantar reflexes may be flexor or extensor; the abdominal and cremasteric reflexes are absent. Flexor or extensor posturing may be seen. Approximately 15% of patients have retinal hemorrhages; with pupillary dilatation and indirect ophthalmoscopy, this figure increases to 30–40%. Other funduscopic abnormalities (Fig. 116-3) include discrete spots of retinal opacification (30–60%), papilledema (8% among children, rare among adults), cotton wool spots (<5%), and decolorization of a retinal vessel or segment of vessel (occasional cases). Convulsions, usually generalized and often repeated, occur in up to 50% of children with cerebral malaria. More covert seizure activity is also common, particularly among children, and may manifest as repetitive tonic-clonic eye movements or even hypersalivation. Whereas adults rarely (i.e., in <3% of cases) suffer neurologic sequelae, ~15% of children surviving cerebral malaria—especially those with hypoglycemia, severe anemia, repeated seizures, and deep coma—have some residual neurologic deficit when they regain consciousness; hemiplegia, cerebral palsy, cortical blindness, deafness, and impaired cognition and learning (all of varying duration) have been reported. Approximately 10% of children surviving cerebral malaria have a persistent language deficit. The incidence of epilepsy is increased and the life expectancy decreased among these children.

Hypoglycemia

Hypoglycemia, an important and common complication of severe malaria, is associated with a poor prognosis and is particularly problematic in children and pregnant women. Hypoglycemia in malaria results from a failure of hepatic gluconeogenesis and an increase in the consumption of glucose by both host and, to a much lesser extent, the malaria parasites. To compound the situation, quinine and quinidine—drugs used for the treatment of severe chloroquine-resistant malaria—are powerful stimulants of pancreatic insulin secretion. Hyperinsulinemic hypoglycemia is especially troublesome in pregnant women receiving quinine treatment. In severe disease, the clinical

TABLE 116-3

FEATURES INDICATING A POOR PROGNOSIS IN SEVERE FALCIPARUM MALARIA

Feature
Clinical
Marked agitation
Hyperventilation (respiratory distress)
Hypothermia (<36.5°C)
Bleeding
Deep coma
Repeated convulsions
Anuria
Shock
Laboratory
Biochemistry
Hypoglycemia (<2.2 mmol/L)
Hyperlactatemia (>5 mmol/L)
Acidosis (arterial pH <7.3, serum HCO_3 <15 mmol/L)
Elevated serum creatinine (>265 μmol/L)
Elevated total bilirubin (>50 μmol/L)
Elevated liver enzymes (AST/ALT 3 times upper limit of normal, 5-nucleotidase ↑)
Elevated muscle enzymes (CPK ↑, myoglobin ↑)
Elevated urate (>600 μmol/L)
Hematology
Leukocytosis (>12,000/μL)
Severe anemia (PCV <15%)
Coagulopathy
Decreased platelet count (<50,000/μL)
Prolonged prothrombin time (>3 s)
Prolonged partial thromboplastin time
Decreased fibrinogen (<200 mg/dL)
Parasitology
Hyperparasitemia
Increased mortality at >100,000/μL
High mortality at >500,000/μL
>20% of parasites identified as pigment-containing trophozoites and schizonts
>5% of neutrophils with visible pigment

Note: ALT, alanine aminotransferase; AST, aspartate aminotransferase; CPK, creatine phosphokinase; PCV, packed cell volume.

diagnosis of hypoglycemia is difficult: the usual physical signs (sweating, gooseflesh, tachycardia) are absent, and the neurologic impairment caused by hypoglycemia cannot be distinguished from that caused by malaria.

Acidosis

Acidosis, an important cause of death from severe malaria, results from accumulation of organic acids. Hyperlactatemia commonly coexists with hypoglycemia. In adults, coexisting renal impairment often compounds the acidosis; in children, ketoacidosis may also contribute. Other still-unidentified organic acids are major contributors to acidosis. Acidotic breathing, sometimes called respiratory distress, is a sign of poor prognosis. It is often followed by circulatory failure refractory to volume expansion or inotropic drugs and ultimately by respiratory arrest. The plasma concentrations of bicarbonate or lactate are the best biochemical prognosticators in severe malaria. Lactic acidosis is caused by the combination of anaerobic glycolysis in tissues where sequestered parasites interfere with microcirculatory flow, hypovolemia, lactate production by the parasites, and a failure of hepatic and renal lactate clearance. The prognosis of severe acidosis is poor.

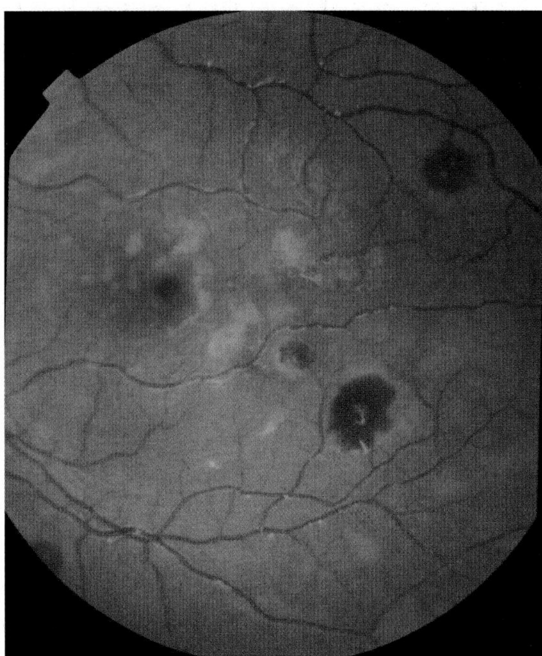

FIGURE 116-3
The eye in cerebral malaria: perimacular whitening and pale-centered retinal hemorrhages. *(Courtesy of N. Beare, T. Taylor, S. Harding, S. Lewallen, and M. Molyneux; with permission.)*

Noncardiogenic Pulmonary Edema

Adults with severe falciparum malaria may develop noncardiogenic pulmonary edema even after several days of antimalarial therapy. The pathogenesis of this variant of the adult respiratory distress syndrome is unclear. The mortality rate is >80%. This condition can be aggravated by overly vigorous administration of IV fluid. Noncardiogenic pulmonary edema can also develop in otherwise uncomplicated vivax malaria, where recovery is usual.

Renal Impairment

Renal impairment is common among adults with severe falciparum malaria but rare among children. The pathogenesis of renal failure is unclear but may be related to erythrocyte sequestration interfering with renal microcirculatory flow and metabolism. Clinically and pathologically, this syndrome manifests as acute tubular necrosis, although renal cortical necrosis never develops. Acute renal failure may occur simultaneously with other vital-organ dysfunction (in which case the mortality risk is high) or may progress as other disease manifestations resolve. In survivors, urine flow resumes in a median of 4 days, and serum creatinine levels return to normal in a mean of 17 days. Early dialysis or hemofiltration considerably enhances the likelihood of a patient's survival, particularly in acute hypercatabolic renal failure.

Hematologic Abnormalities

Anemia results from accelerated RBC removal by the spleen, obligatory RBC destruction at parasite schizogony, and ineffective erythropoiesis. In severe malaria, both infected and uninfected RBCs show reduced deformability, which correlates with prognosis and development of anemia. Splenic clearance of all RBCs is increased. In nonimmune individuals and in areas with unstable transmission, anemia can develop rapidly and transfusion is often required. As a consequence of repeated malarial infections, children in many areas of Africa may develop severe anemia resulting from both shortened RBC survival and marked dyserythropoiesis. Anemia is a common consequence of antimalarial drug resistance, which results in repeated or continued infection.

Slight coagulation abnormalities are common in falciparum malaria, and mild thrombocytopenia is usual. Of patients with severe malaria, <5% have significant bleeding with evidence of disseminated intravascular coagulation. Hematemesis from stress ulceration or acute gastric erosions may also occur.

Liver Dysfunction

Mild hemolytic jaundice is common in malaria. Severe jaundice is associated with *P. falciparum* infections; is more common among adults than among children; and results from hemolysis, hepatocyte injury, and cholestasis. When accompanied by other vital-organ dysfunction (often renal impairment), liver dysfunction carries a poor prognosis. Hepatic dysfunction contributes to hypoglycemia, lactic acidosis, and impaired drug metabolism. Occasional patients with falciparum malaria may develop deep jaundice (with hemolytic, hepatitic, and cholestatic components) without evidence of other vital-organ dysfunction.

Other Complications

Septicemia may complicate severe malaria, particularly in children. In endemic areas, *Salmonella* bacteremia has been associated specifically with *P. falciparum* infections. Chest infections and catheter-induced urinary tract infections are common among patients who are unconscious for >3 days. Aspiration pneumonia may follow generalized convulsions. The frequency of complications of severe falciparum malaria is summarized in Table 116-4.

MALARIA IN PREGNANCY

In heavily endemic (hyper- and holoendemic) areas, falciparum malaria in primi- and secundigravid women is associated with low birth weight (average reduction, ~170 g) and consequently increased infant and childhood mortality. In general, infected mothers in areas of stable transmission remain asymptomatic despite intense accumulation of parasitized erythrocytes in the placental microcirculation. Maternal HIV infection predisposes pregnant women to malaria, predisposes their newborns to congenital malarial infection, and exacerbates the reduction in birth weight associated with malaria.

In areas with unstable transmission of malaria, pregnant women are prone to severe infections and are particularly vulnerable to high-level parasitemia with anemia, hypoglycemia, and acute pulmonary edema. Fetal distress, premature labor, and stillbirth or low birth weight are common results. Fetal death is usual in severe malaria. Congenital malaria occurs in <5% of newborns whose mothers are infected; its frequency and the level of parasitemia are related directly to the parasite density in maternal blood and in the placenta. *P. vivax* malaria in pregnancy is also associated with a reduction in birth weight (average, 110 g), but, in contrast to the situation in falciparum malaria, this effect is more pronounced in multigravid than in primigravid women.

TABLE 116-4

RELATIVE INCIDENCE OF SEVERE COMPLICATIONS OF FALCIPARUM MALARIA

COMPLICATION	NONPREGNANT ADULTS	PREGNANT WOMEN	CHILDREN
Anemia	+	++	+++
Convulsions	+	+	+++
Hypoglycemia	+	+++	+++
Jaundice	+++	+++	+
Renal failure	+++	+++	–
Pulmonary edema	++	+++	+

Key: –, rare; +, infrequent; ++, frequent; +++, very frequent.

MALARIA IN CHILDREN

Most of the estimated 1–3 million persons who die of falciparum malaria each year are young African children. Convulsions, coma, hypoglycemia, metabolic acidosis, and severe anemia are relatively common among children with severe malaria, whereas deep jaundice, acute renal failure, and acute pulmonary edema are unusual. Severely anemic children may present with labored deep breathing, which in the past has been attributed incorrectly to "anemic congestive cardiac failure" but in fact is usually caused by metabolic acidosis, often compounded by hypovolemia. Evidence is accruing that severe malaria can result in long-term neurocognitive and developmental deficits. In general, children tolerate antimalarial drugs well and respond rapidly to treatment.

TRANSFUSION MALARIA

Malaria can be transmitted by blood transfusion, needle-stick injury, sharing of needles by infected injection drug users, or organ transplantation. The incubation period in these settings is often short because there is no preerythrocytic stage of development. The clinical features and management of these cases are the same as for naturally acquired infections. Radical chemotherapy with primaquine is unnecessary for transfusion-transmitted *P. vivax* and *P. ovale* infections.

CHRONIC COMPLICATIONS OF MALARIA

TROPICAL SPLENOMEGALY (HYPERREACTIVE MALARIAL SPLENOMEGALY)

Chronic or repeated malarial infections produce hypergammaglobulinemia; normochromic, normocytic anemia; and, in certain situations, splenomegaly. Some residents of malaria-endemic areas in tropical Africa and Asia exhibit an abnormal immunologic response to repeated infections that is characterized by massive splenomegaly, hepatomegaly, marked elevations in serum titers of IgM and malarial antibody, hepatic sinusoidal lymphocytosis, and (in Africa) peripheral B cell lymphocytosis. This syndrome has been associated with the production of cytotoxic IgM antibodies to CD8+ T lymphocytes, antibodies to CD5+ T lymphocytes, and an increase in the ratio of CD4+ T cells to CD8+ T cells. These events may lead to uninhibited B cell production of IgM and the formation of cryoglobulins (IgM aggregates and immune complexes). This immunologic process stimulates reticuloendothelial hyperplasia and clearance activity and eventually produces splenomegaly. Patients with hyperreactive malarial splenomegaly (HMS) present with an abdominal mass or a dragging sensation in the abdomen and occasional sharp abdominal pains suggesting perisplenitis. Anemia and some degree of pancytopenia are usually evident, and in some cases malarial parasites cannot be found in peripheral-blood smears. Vulnerability to respiratory and skin infections is increased; many patients die of overwhelming sepsis. Persons with HMS who are living in endemic areas should receive antimalarial chemoprophylaxis; the results are usually good. In nonendemic areas, antimalarial treatment is advised. In some cases refractory to therapy, clonal lymphoproliferation may develop and then evolve into a malignant lymphoproliferative disorder.

QUARTAN MALARIAL NEPHROPATHY

Chronic or repeated infections with *P. malariae* (and possibly with other malarial species) may cause soluble immune-complex injury to the renal glomeruli, resulting in the nephrotic syndrome. Other unidentified factors must contribute to this process since only a very small proportion of infected patients develop renal disease. The histologic appearance is that of focal or segmental glomerulonephritis with splitting of the capillary basement membrane. Subendothelial dense deposits are seen on electron microscopy, and immunofluorescence reveals deposits of complement and immunoglobulins; in samples of renal tissue from children, *P. malariae* antigens are often visible. A coarse-granular pattern of basement membrane immunofluorescent deposits (predominantly IgG3) with selective proteinuria carries a better prognosis than a fine-granular, predominantly IgG2 pattern with nonselective proteinuria. Quartan nephropathy usually responds poorly to treatment with either antimalarial agents or glucocorticoids and cytotoxic drugs.

BURKITT'S LYMPHOMA AND EPSTEIN-BARR VIRUS INFECTION

It is possible that malaria-related immunosuppression provokes infection with lymphoma viruses. Burkitt's lymphoma is strongly associated with Epstein-Barr virus. The prevalence of this childhood tumor is high in malarious areas of Africa.

DIAGNOSIS

DEMONSTRATION OF THE PARASITE

The diagnosis of malaria rests on the demonstration of asexual forms of the parasite in stained peripheral-blood smears. After a negative blood smear, repeat smears should be made if there is a high degree of suspicion. Of the Romanowsky stains, Giemsa at pH 7.2 is preferred; Wright's, Field's, or Leishman's stain can also be used. Both thin (Figs. 116-4 and 116-5; see also Figs. 118-1 and 118-2) and thick (Figs. 116-6 to 116-9) blood smears should be examined. The thin blood smear should be rapidly air-dried, fixed in anhydrous methanol, and stained; the RBCs in the tail of the film should then be examined under oil immersion (×1000 magnification). The level of parasitemia is expressed as the number of parasitized erythrocytes per 1000 RBCs. The thick blood film should be of uneven thickness. The smear should be dried thoroughly and stained without fixing. As many layers of erythrocytes overlie one another and are lysed during the staining procedure, the thick film has the advantage of concentrating the parasites (by 40- to 100-fold compared with a thin blood film) and thus increasing diagnostic sensitivity. Both parasites and white blood cells (WBCs) are counted, and the number of parasites per unit volume is calculated from the total leukocyte count. Alternatively, a WBC count of 8000/μL is assumed. This figure is converted to the number of parasitized erythrocytes per microliter. A minimum of 200 WBCs should be counted under oil immersion. Interpretation of blood smear films requires some experience because artifacts are common. Before a thick smear is judged to be negative, 100–200 fields should be examined under oil immersion. In high-transmission areas, the presence of up to 10,000 parasites/μL of blood may be tolerated without symptoms or signs in partially immune individuals. Thus the detection of malaria parasites is sensitive but only poorly specific in identifying malaria as the cause of illness.

Rapid, simple, sensitive, and specific antibody-based diagnostic stick or card tests that detect *P. falciparum*–specific, histidine-rich protein 2 (PfHRP2) or lactate dehydrogenase antigens in finger-prick blood samples have been introduced (Table 116-5). Some of these tests carry a second antibody, which allows falciparum malaria to be distinguished from the less dangerous malarias. Pf HRP2-based tests may remain positive for several

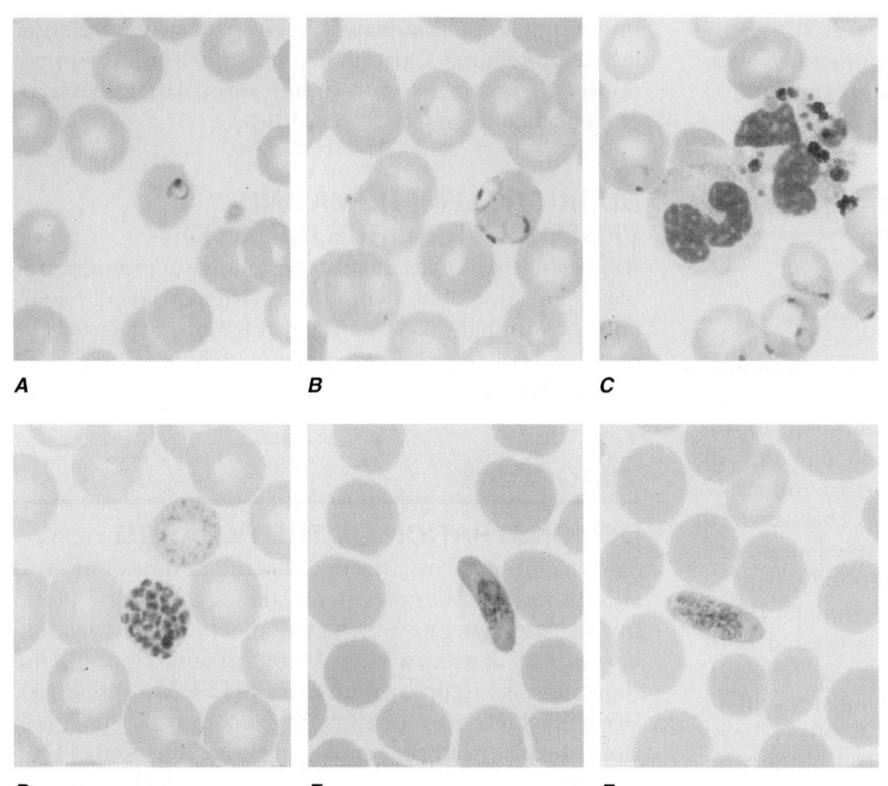

FIGURE 116-4

Thin blood films of *Plasmodium falciparum*. *A.* Young trophozoites. ***B.*** Old trophozoites. ***C.*** Pigment in polymorphonuclear cells and trophozoites. ***D.*** Mature schizonts. ***E.*** Female gametocytes. ***F.*** Male gametocytes. *(Reproduced from Bench Aids for the Diagnosis of Malaria Infections, 2d ed, with the permission of the World Health Organization.)*

weeks after acute infection. This feature is a disadvantage in high-transmission areas where infections are frequent but is of value in the diagnosis of severe malaria in patients who have taken antimalarial drugs and cleared peripheral parasitemia (but in whom the PfHRP2 test remains strongly positive).

The relationship between parasitemia and prognosis is complex; in general, patients with $>10^5$ parasites/μL are at increased risk of dying, but nonimmune patients may die with much lower counts, and partially immune persons may tolerate parasitemia levels many times higher with only minor symptoms. In severe malaria, a poor prognosis

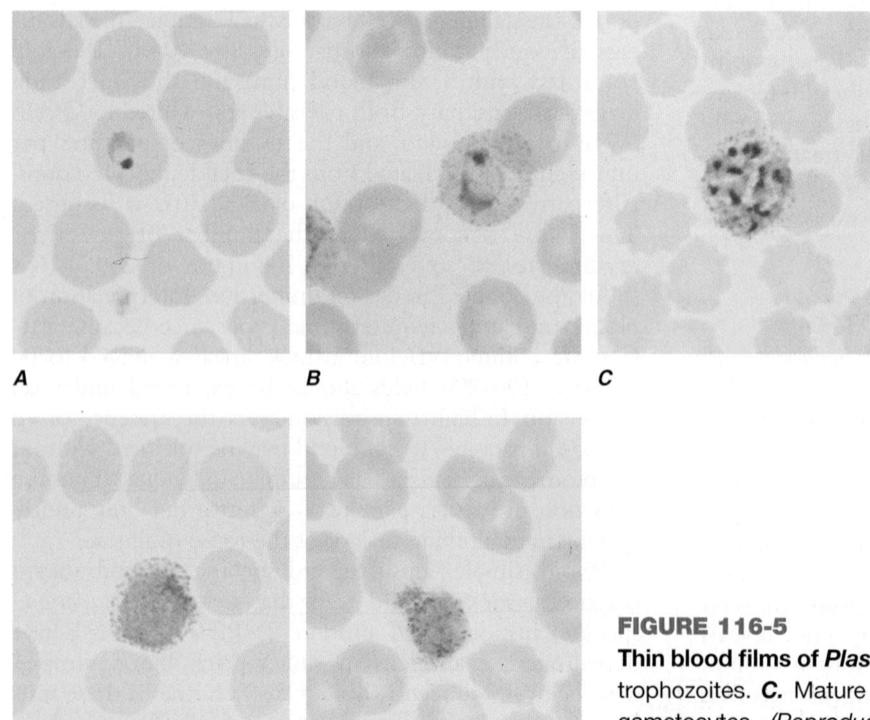

FIGURE 116-5

Thin blood films of *Plasmodium vivax*. *A.* Young trophozoites. ***B.*** Old trophozoites. ***C.*** Mature schizonts. ***D.*** Female gametocytes. ***E.*** Male gametocytes. *(Reproduced from Bench Aids for the Diagnosis of Malaria Infections, 2d ed, with the permission of the World Health Organization.)*

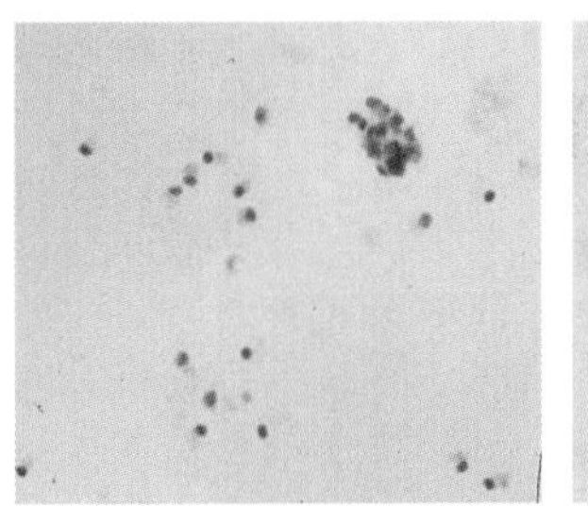

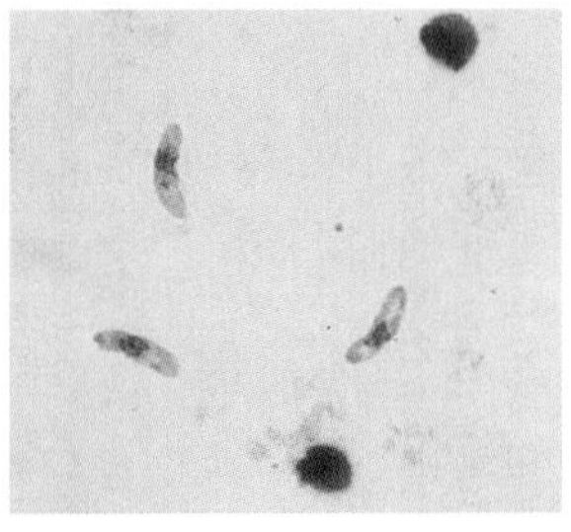

A B

FIGURE 116-6

Thick blood films of *Plasmodium falciparum.* *A.* Trophozoites. ***B.*** Gametocytes. *(Reproduced from Bench Aids for the Diagnosis of Malaria Infections, 2d ed, with the permission of the World Health Organization.)*

is indicated by a predominance of more mature *P. falciparum* parasites (i.e., >20% of parasites with visible pigment) in the peripheral blood film or by the presence of phagocytosed malarial pigment in >5% of neutrophils. In *P. falciparum* infections, gametocytemia peaks 1 week after the peak of asexual parasites. Because the mature gametocytes of *P. falciparum* are not affected by most antimalarial drugs, their persistence does not constitute evidence of drug resistance. Phagocytosed malarial pigment is sometimes seen inside peripheral-blood monocytes or polymorphonuclear leukocytes and may provide a clue to recent infection if malaria parasites are not detectable. After the clearance of the parasites, this intraphagocytic malarial pigment is often evident for several days in the peripheral blood or for longer in bone marrow aspirates or smears of fluid expressed after intradermal puncture. Staining of parasites with the fluorescent dye acridine orange allows more rapid diagnosis of malaria (but not speciation of the infection) in patients with low-level parasitemia.

LABORATORY FINDINGS

Normochromic, normocytic anemia is usual. The leukocyte count is generally normal, although it may be raised in very severe infections. There is slight monocytosis, lymphopenia, and eosinopenia, with reactive lymphocytosis and eosinophilia in the weeks after the acute infection. The erythrocyte sedimentation rate, plasma viscosity, and levels of C-reactive protein and other acute-phase proteins are high. The platelet count is usually reduced to $\sim 10^5/\mu L$.

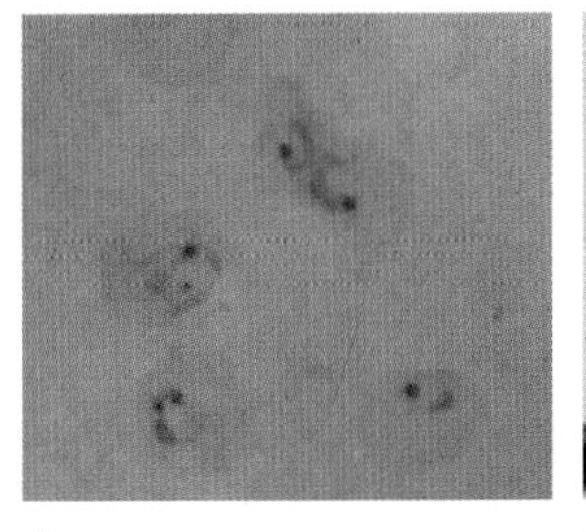

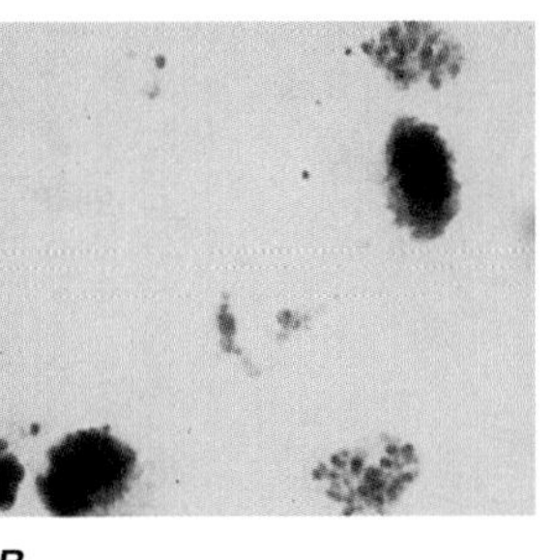

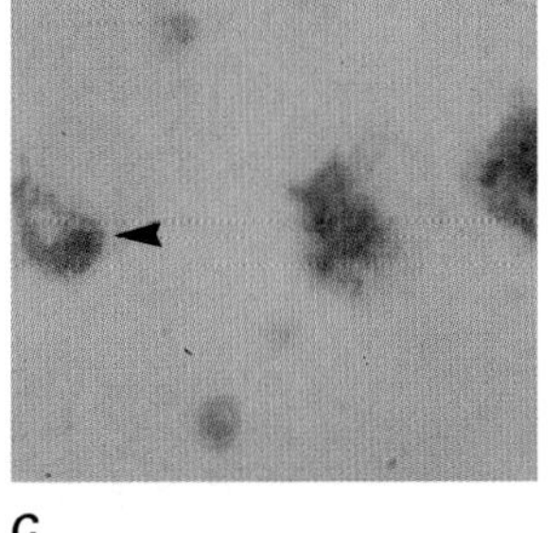

A B C

FIGURE 116-7

Thick blood films of *Plasmodium vivax.* *A.* Trophozoites. ***B.*** Schizonts. ***C.*** Gametocytes. *(Reproduced from Bench Aids for the Diagnosis of Malaria Infections, 2d ed, with the permission of the World Health Organization.)*

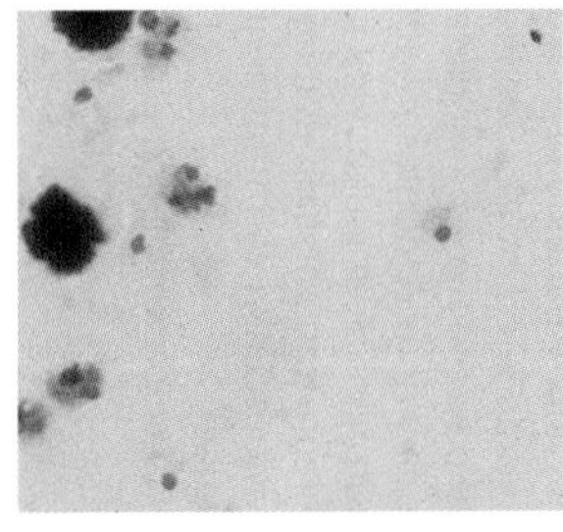

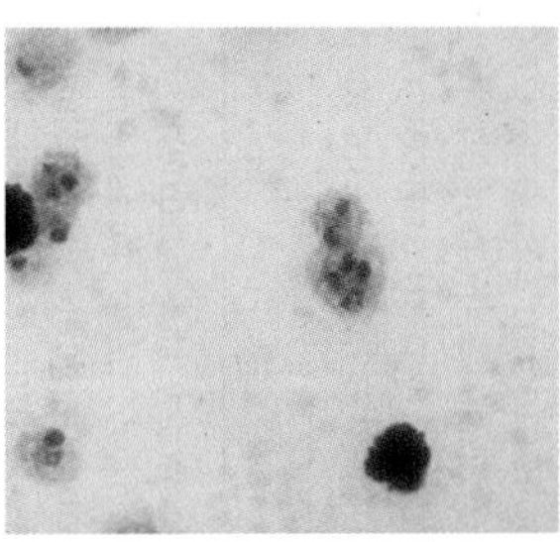

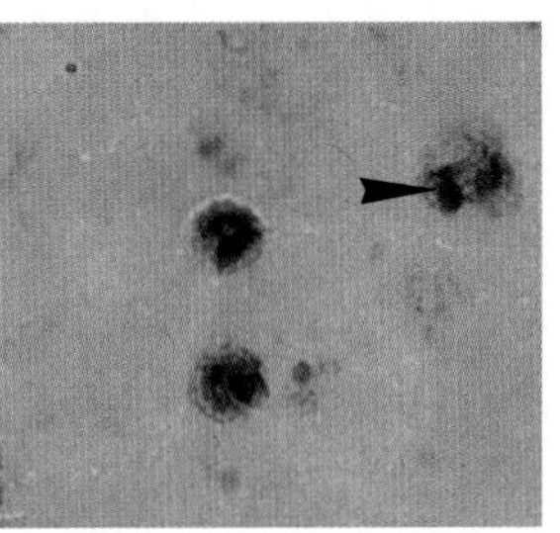

A B C

FIGURE 116-8

Thick blood films of *Plasmodium ovale.* *A.* Trophozoites. ***B.*** Schizonts. ***C.*** Gametocytes. *(Reproduced from Bench Aids for the Diagnosis of Malaria Infections, 2d ed, with the permission of the World Health Organization.)*

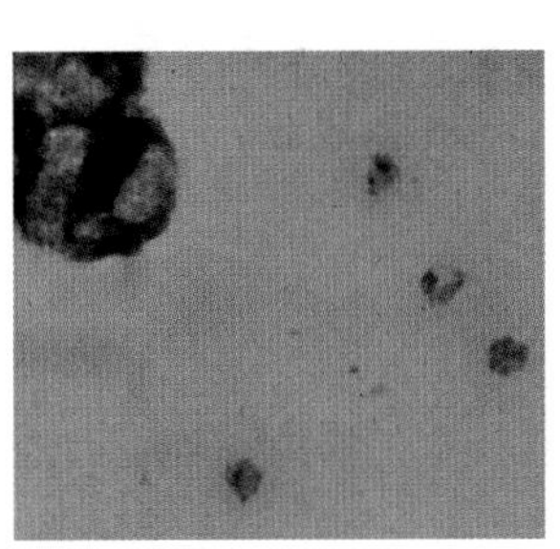

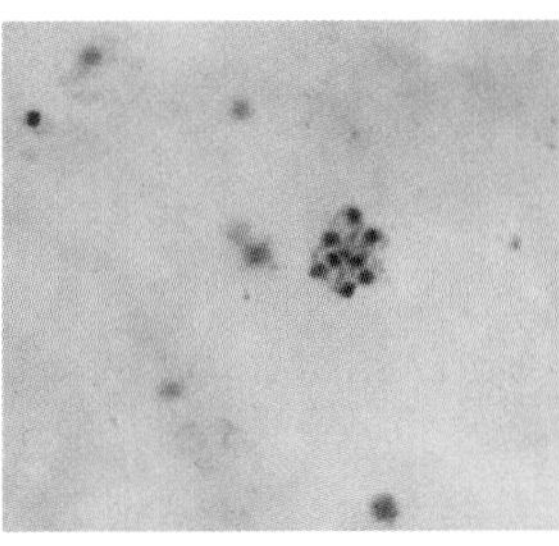

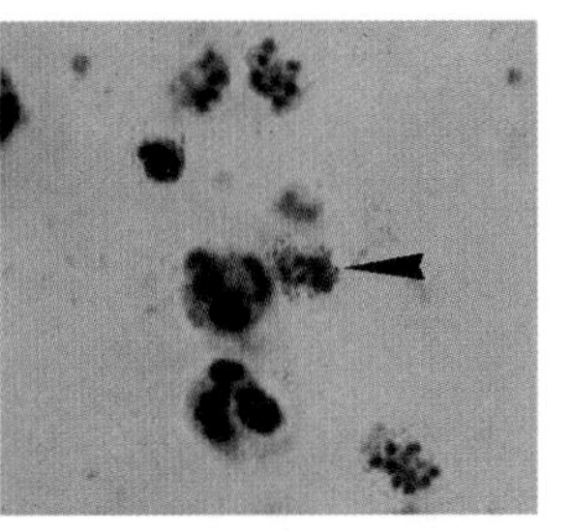

A B C

FIGURE 116-9

Thick blood films of *Plasmodium malariae.* *A.* Trophozoites. ***B.*** Schizonts. ***C.*** Gametocytes. *(Reproduced from Bench Aids for the Diagnosis of Malaria Infections, 2d ed, with the permission of the World Health Organization.)*

TABLE 116-5

METHODS FOR THE DIAGNOSIS OF MALARIA[a]

METHOD	PROCEDURE	ADVANTAGES	DISADVANTAGES
Thick blood film[b]	Blood should be uneven in thickness but sufficiently thin to read watch hands through part of the spot. Stain dried, unfixed blood spot with Giemsa, Field's, or other Romanowsky stain. Count number of asexual parasites per 200 WBCs (or per 500 at low densities). Count gametocytes separately.[c]	Sensitive (0.001% parasitemia); species specific; inexpensive	Requires experience (artifacts may be misinterpreted as low-level parasitemia); underestimates true count
Thin blood film[d]	Stain fixed smear with Giemsa, Field's, or other Romanowsky stain. Count number of RBCs containing asexual parasites per 1000 RBCs. In severe malaria, assess stage of parasite development and count neutrophils containing malaria pigment.[e] Count gametocytes separately.[c]	Rapid; species specific; inexpensive; in severe malaria, provides prognostic information[e]	Insensitive (<0.05% parasitemia); uneven distribution of *P. vivax*, as enlarged infected red cells concentrate at leading edge
PfHRP2 dipstick or card test	A drop of blood is placed on the stick or card, which is then immersed in washing solutions. Monoclonal antibody captures the parasite antigen and reads out as a colored band.	Robust and relatively inexpensive; rapid; sensitivity similar to or slightly lower than that of thick films (~0.001% parasitemia)	Detects only *Plasmodium falciparum*; remains positive for weeks after infection[f]; does not quantitate *P. falciparum* parasitemia
Plasmodium LDH dipstick or card test	A drop of blood is placed on the stick or card, which is then immersed in washing solutions. Monoclonal antibodies capture the parasite antigens and read out as colored bands. One band is genus specific (all malarias), and the other is specific for *P. falciparum.*	Rapid; sensitivity similar to or slightly lower than that of thick films for *P. falciparum* (~0.001% parasitemia)	Slightly more difficult preparation than PfHRP2 tests; may miss low-level parasitemia with *P. vivax*, *P. ovale*, and *P. malariae* and does not speciate these organisms; does not quantitate *P. falciparum* parasitemia
Microtube concentration methods with acridine orange staining	Blood is collected in a specialized tube containing acridine orange, anticoagulant, and a float. After centrifugation, which concentrates the parasitized cells around the float, fluorescence microscopy is performed.	Sensitivity similar or superior to that of thick films (~0.001% parasitemia); ideal for processing large numbers of samples rapidly	Does not speciate or quantitate; requires fluorescence microscopy

[a]Malaria cannot be diagnosed clinically with accuracy, but treatment should be started on clinical grounds if the laboratory confirmation is likely to be delayed. In areas of the world where malaria is endemic and transmission is high, low-level asymptomatic parasitemia is common in otherwise-healthy people. Thus malaria may not be the cause of a fever, although in this context the presence of >10,000 parasites/μL (~0.2% parasitemia) does indicate that malaria is the cause. Antibody and polymerase chain reaction tests have no role in the diagnosis of malaria.

[b]Asexual parasites/200 WBCs × 40 = parasite count/μL (assumes a WBC count of 8000/μL). See Figs. 116-6 to 116-9.

[c]Gametocytemia may persist for days or weeks after clearance of asexual parasites. Gametocytemia without asexual parasitemia does not indicate active infection.

[d]Parasitized RBCs (%) × hematocrit × 1256 = parasite count/μL. See Figs. 116-3 and 116-4.

[e]The presence of >100,000 parasites/μL (~2% parasitemia) is associated with an increased risk of severe malaria, but some patients have severe malaria with lower counts. At any level of parasitemia, the finding that >50% of parasites are tiny rings (cytoplasm width less than half of nucleus width) carries a relatively good prognosis. The presence of visible pigment in >20% of parasites or of phagocytosed pigment in >5% of polymorphonuclear leukocytes (indicating massive recent schizogony) carries a worse prognosis.

[f]Persistence of PfHRP2 is a disadvantage in high-transmission settings, where many asymptomatic people have positive tests, but can be used to diagnostic advantage in low-transmission settings when a sick patient has received previous unknown treatment (which, in endemic areas, often consists of antimalarial drugs). A positive PfHRP2 test indicates that the illness is falciparum malaria, even if the blood smear is negative.

Note: LDH, lactate dehydrogenase; PfHRP2, *P. falciparum* histidine-rich protein 2; RBCs, red blood cells; WBCs, white blood cells.

Severe infections may be accompanied by prolonged prothrombin and partial thromboplastin times and by more severe thrombocytopenia. Levels of antithrombin III are reduced even in mild infection. In uncomplicated malaria, plasma concentrations of electrolytes, blood urea nitrogen (BUN), and creatinine are usually normal. Findings in severe malaria may include metabolic acidosis, with low plasma concentrations of glucose, sodium, bicarbonate, calcium, phosphate, and albumin together with elevations in lactate, BUN, creatinine, urate, muscle and liver enzymes, and conjugated and unconjugated bilirubin. Hypergammaglobulinemia is usual in immune and semi-immune subjects. Urinalysis generally gives normal results. In adults and children with cerebral malaria, the mean opening pressure at lumbar puncture is ~160 mm of cerebrospinal fluid (CSF); usually the CSF is normal or has a slightly elevated total protein level [<1.0 g/L (<100 mg/dL)] and cell count (<20/μL).

℞ Treatment: MALARIA

(Table 116-6) When a patient in or from a malarious area presents with fever, thick and thin blood smears should be prepared and examined immediately to confirm the diagnosis and identify the species of infecting parasite (Figs. 116-4 to 116-9). Repeat blood smears should be performed at least every 12–24 h for 2 days if the first smears are negative and malaria is strongly suspected. Alternatively, a rapid antigen detection card or stick test should be performed. Patients with severe malaria or those unable to take oral drugs should receive parenteral antimalarial therapy. If there is any doubt about the resistance status of the infecting organism, it should be considered resistant. Antimalarial susceptibility testing can be performed but is not generally available and yields results too slowly to influence the choice of treatment. Several drugs are available for oral treatment, and the choice of drug depends on the likely sensitivity of the infecting parasites. Despite recent evidence of chloroquine resistance in *P. vivax* (from parts of Indonesia, Oceania, eastern and southern Asia, and Central and South America), chloroquine remains the treatment of choice for the "benign" human malarias (*P. vivax, P. ovale, P. malariae*) except in Indonesia and Papua New Guinea, where high levels of resistance are prevalent.

The treatment of falciparum malaria has changed radically in recent years. In endemic areas, the World Health Organization now recommends artemisinin-based combinations as first-line treatment for uncomplicated falciparum malaria everywhere. These rapidly and reliably effective drugs are often unavailable in temperate countries (including the United States), where treatment recommendations are limited by the registered available drugs. Fake or substandard drugs, including antimalarial agents, are being sold in many low-income countries; thus, careful attention is required at purchase, especially when the patient fails to respond as expected. Characteristics of antimalarial drugs are shown in Table 116-7.

SEVERE MALARIA In large studies conducted in Asia, parenteral artesunate, a water-soluble artemisinin derivative, has been shown to reduce mortality rates in severe falciparum malaria by 35% from rates obtained with quinine. Artesunate has therefore become the drug of choice. Artesunate is given by the IV route but can also be given by IM injection. Artemether and the closely related drug artemotil (arteether) are oil-based formulations given by IM injection; they are erratically absorbed and do not confer the same survival benefit as artesunate. A rectal formulation of artesunate has been developed as a community-based prereferral treatment for patients in the rural tropics who cannot take oral medications. Although the artemisinin compounds are safer than quinine and considerably safer than quinidine, only one formulation is available in the United States. IV artesunate has recently been approved by the FDA for emergency use for severe malaria through the Centers for Disease Control and Prevention (CDC) Drug Service (see end of chapter for contact information). The antiarrhythmic quinidine gluconate is as effective as quinine and, as it is more readily available, has replaced quinine for the treatment of malaria in the United States. The administration of quinidine must be closely monitored if dysrhythmias and hypotension are to be avoided. Total plasma levels >8 μg/mL, a QT_c interval >0.6 s, or QRS widening beyond 25% of baseline are indications for slowing infusion rates. If arrhythmia or saline-unresponsive hypotension develops, treatment with this drug should be discontinued. Quinine is safer than quinidine; cardiovascular monitoring is not required except when the recipient has cardiac disease.

Severe falciparum malaria constitutes a medical emergency requiring intensive nursing care and careful management. The patient should be weighed and, if comatose, placed on his or her side or prone. Frequent evaluation of the patient's condition is essential. Ancillary drugs such as high-dose glucocorticoids, urea, heparin, dextran, desferrioxamine, antibody to tumor necrosis factor α, and high-dose phenobarbital (20 mg/kg) have proved either ineffective or harmful in clinical trials and should not be used. In acute renal failure or severe metabolic acidosis, hemofiltration or hemodialysis should be started as early as possible.

Parenteral antimalarial treatment should be started as soon as possible. If artemether, quinine, or quinidine is used, an initial loading dose must be given so that therapeutic concentrations are reached as soon as possible. Both quinine and quinidine will cause dangerous hypotension if injected rapidly; when given IV, they must be administered carefully by rate-controlled infusion only. If this approach is not possible, quinine may be given by deep IM injections into the anterior thigh. The optimal therapeutic range for quinine and quinidine in severe malaria is not known with certainty, but

TABLE 116-6

REGIMENS FOR THE TREATMENT OF MALARIA

TYPE OF DISEASE OR TREATMENT	REGIMEN(S)
Uncomplicated Malaria	
Known chloroquine-sensitive strains of *Plasmodium vivax*, *P. malariae*, *P. ovale*, *P. falciparum*[a]	Chloroquine (10 mg of base/kg stat followed by 5 mg/kg at 12, 24, and 36 h or by 10 mg/kg at 24 h and 5 mg/kg at 48 h) *or* Amodiaquine (10–12 mg of base/kg qd for 3 days)
Radical treatment for *P. vivax* or *P. ovale* infection	In addition to chloroquine or amodiaquine as detailed above, primaquine (0.25 mg of base/kg qd; 0.375–0.5 mg of base/kg qd in Southeast Asia and Oceania) should be given for 14 days to prevent relapse. In mild G6PD deficiency, 0.75 mg of base/kg should be given once weekly for 6 weeks. Primaquine should not be given in severe G6PD deficiency.
Sensitive *P. falciparum* malaria[b]	Artesunate (4 mg/kg qd for 3 days) plus sulfadoxine (25 mg/kg)/pyrimethamine (1.25 mg/kg) as a single dose *or* Artesunate (4 mg/kg qd for 3 days) plus amodiaquine (10 mg of base/kg qd for 3 days)[c]
Multidrug-resistant *P. falciparum* malaria	Either artemether-lumefantrine (1.5/9 mg/kg bid for 3 days with food) or artesunate (4 mg/kg qd for 3 days) *plus* Mefloquine (25 mg of base/kg—either 8 mg/kg qd for 3 days or 15 mg/kg on day 2 and then 10 mg/kg on day 3)[c]
Second-line treatment/treatment of imported malaria	Either artesunate (2 mg/kg qd for 7 days) or quinine (10 mg of salt/kg tid for 7 days) *plus 1 of the following 3:* 1. Tetracycline[d] (4 mg/kg qid for 7 days) 2. Doxycycline[d] (3 mg/kg qd for 7 days) 3. Clindamycin (10 mg/kg bid for 7 days) *or* Atovaquone-proguanil (20/8 mg/kg qd for 3 days with food)
Severe Falciparum Malaria[e]	
	Artesunate (2.4 mg/kg stat IV followed by 2.4 mg/kg at 12 and 24 h and then daily if necessary)[f] *or* Artemether (3.2 mg/kg stat IM followed by 1.6 mg/kg qd) *or* Quinine dihydrochloride (20 mg of salt/kg[g] infused over 4 h, followed by 10 mg of salt/kg infused over 2–8 h q8h[h]) *or* Quinidine (10 mg of base/kg[g] infused over 1–2 h, followed by 1.2 mg of base/kg per hour[h] with electrocardiographic monitoring)

[a]Very few areas now have chloroquine-sensitive malaria (Fig. 116-2).
[b]In areas where the partner drug to artesunate is known to be effective.
[c]Fixed-dose coformulated combinations are available.
[d]Tetracycline and doxycycline should not be given to pregnant women or to children <8 years of age.
[e]Oral treatment should be substituted as soon as the patient recovers sufficiently to take fluids by mouth.
[f]Artesunate is the drug of choice when available. The data from large studies in Southeast Asia showed a 35% reduction in mortality rate from that with quinine. Severe malaria in children in high-transmission settings has different characteristics; thus trials are ongoing in Africa comparing artesunate with quinine to determine whether there is a survival benefit in African children.
[g]A loading dose should not be given if therapeutic doses of quinine or quinidine have definitely been administered in the previous 24 h. Some authorities recommend a lower dose of quinidine.
[h]Infusions can be given in 0.9% saline and 5% or 10% dextrose in water. Infusion rates for quinine and quinidine should be carefully controlled.
Note: G6PD, glucose-6-phosphate dehydrogenase.

total plasma concentrations of 8–15 mg/L for quinine and 3.5–8.0 mg/L for quinidine are effective and do not cause serious toxicity. The systemic clearance and apparent volume of distribution of these alkaloids are markedly reduced and plasma protein binding is increased in severe malaria, so that the blood concentrations attained with a given dose are higher. If the patient remains seriously ill or in acute renal failure for >2 days,

TABLE 116-7

PROPERTIES OF ANTIMALARIAL DRUGS

DRUG(S)	PHARMACOKINETIC PROPERTIES	ANTIMALARIAL ACTIVITY	MINOR TOXICITY	MAJOR TOXICITY
Quinine, quinidine	Good oral and IM absorption (quinine); *Cl* and V_d reduced, but plasma protein binding (principally to α-1 acid glycoprotein) increased (90%) in malaria; quinine $t_{1/2}$: 16 h in malaria, 11 h in healthy persons; quinidine $t_{1/2}$: 13 h in malaria, 8 h in healthy persons	Acts mainly on trophozoite blood stage; kills gametocytes of *P. vivax*, *P. ovale*, and *P. malariae* (but not *P. falciparum*); no action on liver stages	*Common:* "Cinchonism": tinnitus, high-tone hearing loss, nausea, vomiting, dysphoria, postural hypotension; ECG QT_c interval prolongation (quinine usually by <10% but quinidine by up to 25%) *Rare:* Diarrhea, visual disturbance, rashes *Note:* Very bitter taste	*Common:* Hypoglycemia *Rare:* Hypotension, blindness, deafness, cardiac arrhythmias, thrombocytopenia, hemolysis, hemolytic-uremic syndrome, vasculitis, cholestatic hepatitis, neuromuscular paralysis *Note:* Quinidine more cardiotoxic
Chloroquine	Good oral absorption, very rapid IM and SC absorption; complex pharmacokinetics; enormous *Cl* and V_d (unaffected by malaria); blood concentration profile determined by distribution processes in malaria; $t_{1/2}$: 1–2 months	As for quinine but acts slightly earlier in asexual cycle	*Common:* Nausea, dysphoria, pruritus in dark-skinned patients, postural hypotension *Rare:* Accommodation difficulties, keratopathy, rash *Note:* Bitter taste, well tolerated	*Acute:* Hypotensive shock (parenteral), cardiac arrhythmias, neuropsychiatric reactions *Chronic:* Retinopathy (cumulative dose, >100 g), skeletal and cardiac myopathy
Amodiaquine	Good oral absorption; largely converted to active metabolite desethylamodiaquine	As for chloroquine	Nausea (tastes better than chloroquine)	Agranulocytosis; hepatitis, mainly with prophylactic use
Mefloquine	Adequate oral absorption; no parenteral preparation; $t_{1/2}$: 14–20 days (shorter in malaria)	As for quinine	Nausea, giddiness, dysphoria, fuzzy thinking, sleeplessness, nightmares, sense of dissociation	Neuropsychiatric reactions, convulsions, encephalopathy
Tetracycline, doxycycline[a]	Excellent absorption; $t_{1/2}$: 8 h for tetracycline, 18 h for doxycycline	Weak antimalarial activity; should not be used alone for treatment	Gastrointestinal intolerance, deposition in growing bones and teeth, photosensitivity, moniliasis, benign intracranial hypertension	Renal failure in patients with impaired renal function (tetracycline)
Halofantrine[b]	Highly variable absorption related to fat intake; $t_{1/2}$: 1–3 days (active desbutyl metabolite $t_{1/2}$: 3–7 days)	As for quinine	Diarrhea	Cardiac conduction disturbances; atrioventricular block; ECG QT_c interval prolongation; potentially lethal ventricular tachyarrhythmias

(*Continued*)

TABLE 116-7 (*CONTINUED*)

PROPERTIES OF ANTIMALARIAL DRUGS

DRUG(S)	PHARMACOKINETIC PROPERTIES	ANTIMALARIAL ACTIVITY	MINOR TOXICITY	MAJOR TOXICITY
Artemisinin and derivatives (artemether, artesunate)	Good oral absorption, slow and variable absorption of IM artemether; artesunate and artemether biotransformed to active metabolite dihydroartemisinin; all drugs eliminated very rapidly; $t_{1/2}$: <1 h	Broader stage specificity and more rapid than other drugs; no action on liver stages; kills all but fully mature gametocytes of *P. falciparum*	Reduction in reticulocyte count (but not anemia)	Anaphylaxis, urticaria, fever
Pyrimethamine	Good oral absorption, variable IM absorption; $t_{1/2}$: 4 days	For blood stages, acts mainly on mature forms; causal prophylactic	Well tolerated	Megaloblastic anemia, pancytopenia, pulmonary infiltration
Proguanil (chloroguanide)	Good oral absorption; biotransformed to active metabolite cycloguanil; $t_{1/2}$: 16 h; biotransformation reduced by oral contraceptive use and in pregnancy	Causal prophylactic; not used alone for treatment	Well tolerated; mouth ulcers and rare alopecia	Megaloblastic anemia in renal failure
Primaquine	Complete oral absorption; active compound not known; $t_{1/2}$: 7 h	Radical cure; eradicates hepatic forms of *P. vivax* and *P. ovale*; kills all stages of gametocyte development of *P. falciparum*	Nausea, vomiting, diarrhea, abdominal pain, hemolysis, methemoglobinemia	Massive hemolysis in subjects with severe G6PD deficiency
Atovaquone	Highly variable absorption related to fat intake; $t_{1/2}$: 30–70 h	Acts mainly on trophozoite blood stage	None identified	None identified
Lumefantrine	Highly variable absorption related to fat intake; $t_{1/2}$: 3–4 days	As for quinine	None identified	None identified

[a] Tetracycline and doxycycline should not be given to pregnant women or to children <8 years of age.

[b] Halofantrine should not be used by patients with long ECG QT_c intervals or known conduction disturbances or by those taking drugs that may affect ventricular repolarization, e.g., quinidine, quinine, mefloquine, chloroquine, neuroleptics, antiarrhythmics, tricyclic antidepressants, terfenadine, or astemizole.

Note: *Cl*, systemic clearance; V_d, total apparent volume of distribution; IM, intramuscular; SC, subcutaneous; ECG, electrocardiogram; G6PD, glucose-6-phosphate dehydrogenase.

maintenance doses of quinine or quinidine should be reduced by 30–50% to prevent toxic accumulation of the drug. The initial doses should never be reduced. If one of the artemisinin derivatives is given, dose reductions are unnecessary, even in renal failure. Exchange transfusion should be considered for severely ill patients, although the precise indications for this procedure have not been agreed upon. It has been recommended that—if safe and feasible—exchange should be considered for patients with severe malaria, but there is no clear evidence that this measure is beneficial. The role of prophylactic anticonvulsants is uncertain. If respiratory support is not available, then a full loading dose of phenobarbital (20 mg/kg) to prevent convulsions should not be given as it may cause respiratory arrest.

When the patient is unconscious, the blood glucose level should be measured every 4–6 h, and values <2.2 mmol/L (40 mg/dL) should mandate treatment with IV dextrose. All patients treated with IV quinine or quinidine should receive a continuous infusion of 5–10% dextrose. The parasite count and hematocrit level should be measured every 6–12 h. Anemia develops rapidly; if the hematocrit falls to <20%, then whole blood (preferably fresh) or packed cells should be transfused slowly, with careful attention to circulatory status. Renal function should be checked daily. Children presenting with severe anemia and acidotic breathing are often hypovolemic; in this situation, resuscitation with crystalloids or blood is indicated. Accurate assessment is vital. Management of fluid balance is difficult in severe malaria, particularly in adults, because of the thin dividing line between overhydration (leading to pulmonary edema) and underhydration (contributing to renal impairment). If necessary, central venous pressures should be measured and maintained in the low-normal range. As soon as the patient can take fluids, oral therapy should be substituted for parenteral treatment.

UNCOMPLICATED MALARIA Infections due to *P. vivax*, *P. malariae*, and *P. ovale* should be treated with oral chloroquine (total dose, 25 mg of base/kg). In much of the tropics, drug-resistant *P. falciparum* has been increasing in distribution, frequency, and intensity. Chloroquine-resistant *P. falciparum* is now present throughout most of the tropical world, and resistance to sulfadoxine/pyrimethamine is widespread and increasing. It is now accepted that, to prevent resistance, falciparum malaria should be treated with drug combinations and not with single drugs in endemic areas; the same rationale has been applied successfully to the treatment of tuberculosis and HIV/AIDS. This combination strategy is based on simultaneous use of two or more drugs with different modes of action: one is usually an artemisinin derivative (artesunate, artemether, or dihydroartemisinin) given for 3 days, and the other is usually a slower-acting antimalarial to which *P. falciparum* is sensitive. Artemisinin combination regimens now constitute first-line recommended treatment for falciparum malaria. In areas with multidrug-resistant falciparum malaria (parts of Asia and South America), either artemether- lumefantrine or artesunate-mefloquine should be used. Although significant resistance to mefloquine has been documented in Thailand, Myanmar, Vietnam, Laos, and Cambodia (Fig. 116-10), mefloquine is usually effective against multidrug-resistant strains of *P. falciparum* outside these areas and, in combination with artesunate, achieves cure rates exceeding 90% nearly everywhere. Atovaquone-proguanil is also highly effective. In areas with more drug-sensitive isolates, atovaquone- proguanil, mefloquine, artesunate-amodiaquine, or artesunate sulfadoxine/pyrimethamine can be used, depending on the prevailing drug susceptibility pattern. These 3-day regimens are all well tolerated, although mefloquine is associated with increased rates of vomiting and dizziness. As second-line treatment for recrudescence following first-line therapy, a 7-day course of either artesunate or quinine plus tetracycline, doxycycline, or clindamycin is effective. Tetracycline and doxycycline cannot be given to pregnant women or to children <8 years of age. Oral quinine is extremely bitter and regularly produces cinchonism comprising tinnitus, high-tone deafness, nausea, vomiting, and dysphoria. Adherence is poor with the required 7-day regimens of quinine.

Patients should be monitored for vomiting for 1 h after the administration of any oral antimalarial drug. If there is vomiting, the dose should be repeated. Symptom-based treatment, with tepid sponging and acetaminophen administration, lowers fever and thereby reduces the

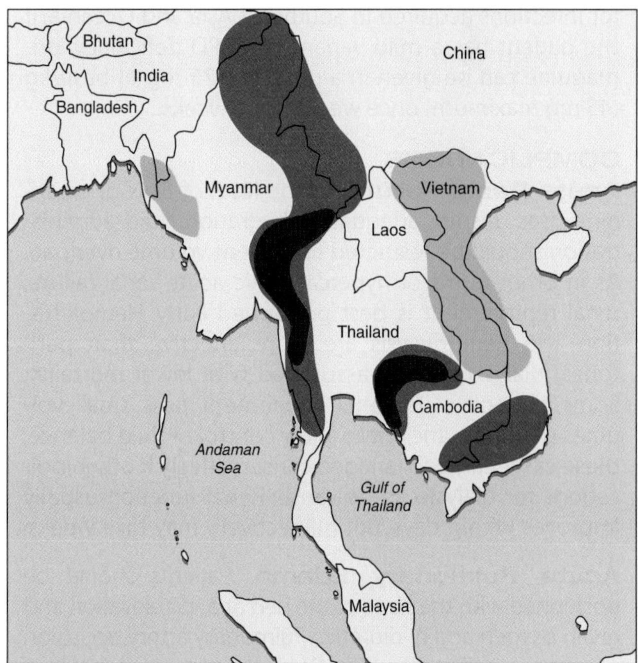

FIGURE 116-10

Mefloquine resistance in *Plasmodium falciparum* in Southeast Asia: high-level mefloquine resistance (*brown*), low-level mefloquine resistance (*red*), and mefloquine sensitivity (failure rate, <20%; *green*). There is insufficient information for the other areas.

patient's propensity to vomit these drugs. Minor central nervous system reactions (nausea, dizziness, sleep disturbances) are common. The incidence of serious adverse neuropsychiatric reactions to mefloquine treatment is ~1 in 1000 in Asia but may be as high as 1 in 200 among Africans and Caucasians. All the antimalarial quinolines (chloroquine, mefloquine, and quinine) exacerbate the orthostatic hypotension associated with malaria, and all are tolerated better by children than by adults. Pregnant women, young children, patients unable to tolerate oral therapy, and nonimmune subjects (e.g., travelers) with suspected malaria should be evaluated carefully and hospitalization considered. If there is any doubt as to the identity of the infecting malarial species, treatment for falciparum malaria should be given. A negative blood smear does not rule out malaria; thick blood films should be checked 1 and 2 days later to exclude the diagnosis. Nonimmune patients receiving treatment for malaria should have daily parasite counts performed until negative thick films indicate clearance of the parasite. If the level of parasitemia does not fall below 25% of the admission value in 48 h or if parasitemia has not cleared by 7 days (and adherence is assured), drug resistance is likely and the regimen should be changed. If treatment failures occur with commonly used antimalarial agents, alternative drugs should be used.

To eradicate persistent liver stages and prevent relapse (radical treatment), primaquine (0.25–0.5 mg of base/kg, adult dose) should be given daily for 14 days to patients with *P. vivax* or *P. ovale* infections after laboratory tests for G6PD deficiency have proved negative. A total dose of 22.5–30 mg for an adult is recommended for infections acquired in Southeast Asia and Oceania. If the patient has a mild variant of G6PD deficiency, primaquine can be given in a dose of 0.75 mg of base/kg (45 mg maximum) once weekly for 6 weeks.

COMPLICATIONS

Acute Renal Failure If the level of BUN or creatinine rises despite adequate rehydration, fluid administration should be restricted to prevent volume overload. As in other forms of hypercatabolic acute renal failure, renal replacement is best performed early. Hemofiltration and hemodialysis are more effective than peritoneal dialysis and are associated with lower mortality. Some patients with renal impairment pass small volumes of urine sufficient to allow control of fluid balance; these cases can be managed conservatively if other indications for dialysis do not arise. Renal function usually improves within days, but full recovery may take weeks.

Acute Pulmonary Edema Patients should be positioned with the head of the bed at a 45° elevation and given oxygen and IV diuretics. Pulmonary artery occlusion pressures may be normal, indicating increased pulmonary capillary permeability. Positive-pressure ventilation should be started early if the immediate measures fail.

Hypoglycemia An initial slow injection of 50% dextrose (0.5 g/kg) should be followed by an infusion of 10% dextrose (0.10 g/kg per hour). The blood glucose level should be checked regularly thereafter as recurrent hypoglycemia is common, particularly among patients receiving quinine or quinidine. In severely ill patients, hypoglycemia commonly occurs together with metabolic (lactic) acidosis and carries a poor prognosis.

Other Complications Patients who develop spontaneous bleeding should be given fresh blood and IV vitamin K. Convulsions should be treated with IV or rectal benzodiazepines and, if necessary, respiratory support. Aspiration pneumonia should be suspected in any unconscious patient with convulsions, particularly with persistent hyperventilation; IV antimicrobial agents and oxygen should be administered, and pulmonary toilet should be undertaken. Hypoglycemia or gram-negative septicemia should be suspected when the condition of any patient suddenly deteriorates for no obvious reason during antimalarial treatment. Systemic *Salmonella* infections are common complications among African children with falciparum malaria.

Antibiotics should be considered for severely ill patients not responding to antimalarial treatment.

PREVENTION

These are halcyon days for malaria prevention and control. New drugs have been discovered and developed; highly effective drugs, insecticide-treated nets, and insecticides for spraying dwellings are being purchased for endemic countries by the Global Fund to Fight HIV/AIDS, Tuberculosis, and Malaria and the President's Malaria Initiative; and even stronger support is being advocated by the Roll Back Malaria Partnership, the Global Health Council, and other supporters of malaria control and research. Still, the eradication of malaria is not yet feasible because of the widespread distribution of *Anopheles* breeding sites; the great number of infected persons; the continued use of ineffective antimalarial drugs; and inadequacies in human and material resources, infrastructure, and control programs. Malaria may be contained by judicious use of insecticides to kill the mosquito vector, rapid diagnosis, appropriate patient management, and—where effective and feasible—administration of intermittent presumptive treatment or chemoprophylaxis to high-risk groups. Malaria researchers are intensifying their efforts to gain a better understanding of parasite-human-mosquito interactions and to develop more effective control and prevention interventions. Despite the enormous investment in efforts to develop a malaria vaccine, no safe, effective, long-lasting vaccine is likely to be available for general use in the near future (Chap. 3). While there is promise for one or more malaria vaccines on the more distant horizon, prevention and control measures continue to rely on antivector and drug-use strategies.

PERSONAL PROTECTION AGAINST MALARIA

Simple measures to reduce the frequency of mosquito bites in malarious areas are very important. These measures include the avoidance of exposure to mosquitoes at their peak feeding times (usually dusk and dawn) and throughout the night as well as the use of insect repellents containing DEET (10–35%) or picaridin (7%; if DEET is unacceptable), suitable clothing, and insecticide-impregnated bed nets or other materials. Widespread use of bed nets treated with residual pyrethroids reduces the incidence of malaria in areas where vectors bite indoors at night and has been shown to reduce mortality rates in western and eastern Africa.

CHEMOPROPHYLAXIS

(Table 116-8; *http://wwwn.cdc.gov/travel/contentMalariaDrugsHC. aspx*; accessed September 13, 2007) Recommendations for prophylaxis depend on knowledge of local patterns of plasmodial drug sensitivity and the likelihood of acquiring malarial infection. When there is uncertainty, drugs effective against resistant *P. falciparum* should be used [atovaquone-proguanil (Malarone), doxycycline, mefloquine, or primaquine]. Chemoprophylaxis is never entirely reliable, and malaria should always be considered in the differential diagnosis of fever in patients who have traveled to endemic areas, even if they are taking prophylactic antimalarial drugs.

Pregnant women traveling to malarious areas should be warned about the potential risks. All pregnant women at risk in endemic areas should be encouraged to attend regular antenatal clinics. Mefloquine is the only drug advised for pregnant women traveling to areas with drug-resistant malaria; this drug is generally considered safe in the second and third trimesters of pregnancy, and the limited data on first-trimester exposure are reassuring. The safety of other prophylactic antimalarial agents in pregnancy has not been established. Antimalarial prophylaxis has been shown to reduce mortality rates among children between the ages of 3 months and 4 years in malaria-endemic areas; however, it is not a logistically or economically feasible option in many countries. The alternative—to give intermittent treatment doses [intermittent preventive treatment (IPT)]—shows promise for more widespread use in infants, young children, and pregnant women. Children born to nonimmune mothers in endemic areas (usually expatriates moving to malaria-endemic areas) should receive prophylaxis from birth.

Travelers should start taking antimalarial drugs 2 days to 1–2 weeks before departure so that any untoward reactions can be detected and so that therapeutic antimalarial blood concentrations will be present when needed (Table 116-8). Antimalarial prophylaxis should continue for 4 weeks after the traveler has left the endemic area, except if atovaquone-proguanil or primaquine has been taken; these drugs have significant activities against the liver stage of the infection (causal prophylaxis) and can be discontinued 1 week after departure from the endemic area. Presumptive self-treatment for malaria with atovaquone-proguanil (for 3 consecutive days) or another drug can be considered under special circumstances; medical advice on self-treatment should be sought before departure for malarious areas and as soon as possible after illness begins.

Atovaquone-proguanil (Malarone; 3.75/1.5 mg/kg or 250/100 mg, daily adult dose) is a fixed-combination, once-daily prophylactic agent that is very well tolerated by adults and children, with fewer adverse gastrointestinal effects than chloroquine-proguanil and fewer adverse central nervous system effects than mefloquine. It is proguanil itself, rather than the antifolate metabolite cycloguanil, that acts synergistically with atovaquone. This combination is effective against all types of malaria, including multidrug-resistant falciparum malaria. Atovaquone-proguanil is best taken with food or a milky drink to optimize absorption. There are insufficient data on the safety of this regimen in pregnancy.

Mefloquine (250 mg of salt weekly, adult dose) has been widely used for malarial prophylaxis because it is usually effective against multidrug-resistant falciparum malaria and is reasonably well tolerated. Mild nausea, dizziness, fuzzy thinking, disturbed sleep patterns, vivid dreams, and malaise are relatively common. Approximately 1 in every 10,000 recipients develops an acute reversible neuropsychiatric reaction manifested by confusion, psychosis, convulsions, or encephalopathy. The role of mefloquine prophylaxis during pregnancy remains uncertain; in studies in Africa, mefloquine prophylaxis was found to be effective and safe during pregnancy. However, in one study from Thailand, treatment of malaria with mefloquine was associated with an increased risk of stillbirth.

Daily administration of doxycycline (100 mg daily, adult dose) is an effective alternative to atovaquone-proguanil or mefloquine. Doxycycline is generally well tolerated but may cause vulvovaginal thrush, diarrhea, and photosensitivity and cannot be used by children <8 years old or by pregnant women.

Chloroquine remains the drug of choice for the prevention of infection with drug-sensitive *P. falciparum* (now found in very few areas of the world) and with the other human malarial species (although chloroquine-resistant *P. vivax* has been reported from parts of eastern Asia, Oceania, and Central and South America). Chloroquine is generally well tolerated, although some patients cannot take the drug because of malaise, headache, visual symptoms (from reversible keratopathy), gastrointestinal intolerance, or (in dark-skinned patients) pruritus. A concomitant filarial infection may provoke or aggravate chloroquine-induced pruritus. Chloroquine is considered safe in pregnancy. With chronic administration for >5 years, a characteristic dose-related retinopathy may develop, but this condition is rare at the doses used for antimalarial prophylaxis. Idiosyncratic or allergic reactions are also rare. Skeletal and cardiac myopathy are potential problems with protracted prophylactic use; they are more likely to occur with the high doses used in the treatment of rheumatoid arthritis. Neuropsychiatric reactions and skin rashes are unusual. When used continuously, amodiaquine, a related aminoquinoline, is associated with a high risk of agranulocytosis (~1 person in 2000) and hepatotoxicity (~1 person in 16,000) and should not be used for prophylaxis.

Primaquine (0.5 mg of base/kg or 30 mg, daily adult dose taken with food) has proved safe and effective in the prevention of drug-resistant falciparum and vivax malaria in adults. This drug can be considered for persons who are traveling to areas with or without drug-resistant *P. falciparum* and who are intolerant to other recommended

TABLE 116-8

DRUGS USED IN THE PROPHYLAXIS OF MALARIA

DRUG	USAGE	ADULT DOSE	PEDIATRIC DOSE	COMMENTS
Atovaquone/proguanil (Malarone)	Prophylaxis in areas with chloroquine- or mefloquine-resistant *Plasmodium falciparum*	1 adult tablet PO[a]	5–8 kg: 1/2 pediatric tablet[b] daily ≥8–10 kg: 3/4 pediatric tablet daily ≥10–20 kg: 1 pediatric tablet daily ≥20–30 kg: 2 pediatric tablets daily ≥30–40 kg: 3 pediatric tablets daily ≥40 kg: 1 adult tablet daily	Begin 1–2 days before travel to malarious areas. Take daily at the same time each day while in the malarious area and for 7 days after leaving such areas. Atovaquone-proguanil is contraindicated in persons with severe renal impairment (creatinine clearance rate <30 mL/min). It is not recommended for children weighing <5 kg, pregnant women, or women breast-feeding infants weighing <5 kg. Atovaquone/proguanil should be taken with food or a milky drink.
Chloroquine phosphate (Aralen and generic)	Prophylaxis only in areas with chloroquine-sensitive *P. falciparum*[c]	300 mg of base (500 mg of salt) PO once weekly	5 mg/kg of base (8.3 mg of salt/kg) PO once weekly, up to a maximum adult dose of 300 mg of base	Begin 1–2 weeks before travel to malarious areas. Take weekly on the same day of the week while in the malarious areas and for 4 weeks after leaving such areas. Chloroquine phosphate may exacerbate psoriasis.
Doxycycline (many brand names and generic)	Prophylaxis in areas with chloroquine- or mefloquine-resistant *P. falciparum*[c]	100 mg PO qd	≥8 years of age: 2 mg/kg, up to adult dose	Begin 1–2 days before travel to malarious areas. Take daily at the same time each day while in the malarious areas and for 4 weeks after leaving such areas. Doxycycline is contraindicated in children <8 years of age and in pregnant women.
Hydroxychloroquine sulfate (Plaquenil)	An alternative to chloroquine for primary prophylaxis only in areas with chloroquine-sensitive *P. falciparum*[c]	310 mg of base (400 mg of salt) PO once weekly	5 mg of base/kg (6.5 mg of salt/kg) PO once weekly, up to maximum adult dose of 310 mg of base	Begin 1–2 weeks before travel to malarious areas. Take weekly on the same day of the week while in the malarious areas and for 4 weeks after leaving such areas. Hydroxychloroquine may exacerbate psoriasis.
Mefloquine (Lariam and generic)	Prophylaxis in areas with chloroquine-resistant *P. falciparum*	228 mg of base (250 mg of salt) PO once weekly	≤9 kg: 4.6 mg of base/kg (5 mg of salt/kg) PO once weekly 10–19 kg: 1/4 tablet once weekly 20–30 kg: 1/2 tablet once weekly 31–45 kg: 3/4 tablet once weekly ≥46 kg: 1 tablet once weekly	Begin 1–2 weeks before travel to malarious areas. Take weekly on the same day of the week while in the malarious areas and for 4 weeks after leaving such areas.Mefloquine is contraindicated in persons allergic to this drug or related compounds (e.g., quinine and quinidine) and in persons with active or recent depression, generalized anxiety disorder, psychosis, schizophrenia, other major psychiatric disorders, or seizures. Use with caution in persons with psychiatric disturbances or a history of depression. Mefloquine is not recommended for persons with cardiac conduction abnormalities.
Primaquine	An option for prophylaxis in special circumstances	30 mg of base (52.6 mg of salt) PO qd	0.5 mg of base/kg (0.8 mg of salt/kg) PO qd, up to adult dose; should be taken with food	Begin 1–2 days before travel to malarious areas. Take daily at the same time each day while in the malarious areas and for 7 days after leaving such areas. Primaquine is contraindicated in persons with G6PD1 deficiency. It is also contraindicated during pregnancy and in lactation unless the infant being breast-fed has a documented normal G6PD level. Use in consultation with malaria experts.
Primaquine	Used for presumptive anti-relapse therapy (terminal prophylaxis) to decrease risk of relapses of *P. vivax* and *P. ovale*.	30 mg of base (52.6 mg of salt) PO qd for 14 days after departure from the malarious area	0.5 mg of base/kg (0.8 mg of salt/kg), up to adult dose, PO qd for 14 days after departure from the malarious area	This therapy is indicated for persons who have had prolonged exposure to *P. vivax* and/or *P. ovale*. It is contraindicated in persons with G6PD1 deficiency as well as during pregnancy and in lactation unless the infant being breast-fed has a documented normal G6PD level.

[a] An adult tablet contains 250 mg of atovaquone and 100 mg of proguanil hydrochloride.
[b] A pediatric tablet contains 62.5 mg of atovaquone and 25 mg of proguanil hydrochloride.
[c] Very few areas now have chloroquine-sensitive malaria (Fig. 116-2).
Source: CDC: *http://wwwn.cdc.gov/travel/contentMalariaDrugsHC.aspx*, accessed September 13, 2007.

drugs. Abdominal pain and oxidant hemolysis—the principal adverse effects—are not common as long as the drug is taken with food and is not given to G6PD-deficient persons. Primaquine should not be given to pregnant women or neonates. Travelers must be tested for G6PD deficiency and be shown to have a level in the normal range before receiving primaquine. In G6PD deficiency, primaquine can cause hemolysis that is sometimes fatal.

In the past, the dihydrofolate reductase inhibitors pyrimethamine and proguanil (chloroguanide) have been administered widely, but the rapid selection of resistance in both *P. falciparum* and *P. vivax* has limited their use. Whereas antimalarial quinolines such as chloroquine act on the erythrocyte stage of parasitic development, the dihydrofolate reductase inhibitors also inhibit preerythrocytic growth in the liver (causal prophylaxis) and development in the mosquito (sporontocidal activity). Proguanil is safe and well tolerated, although mouth ulceration occurs in ~8% of persons using this drug; it is considered safe for antimalarial prophylaxis in pregnancy. The prophylactic use of the combination of pyrimethamine and sulfadoxine is not recommended because of an unacceptable incidence of severe toxicity, principally exfoliative dermatitis and other skin rashes, agranulocytosis, hepatitis, and pulmonary eosinophilia (incidence, 1:7000; fatal reactions, 1:18,000). The combination of pyrimethamine with dapsone (0.2/1.5 mg/kg weekly, 12.5/100 mg, adult dose) is a third-line alternative available in some countries. Dapsone may cause methemoglobinemia and allergic reactions and (at higher doses) may pose a significant risk of agranulocytosis. Proguanil and the pyrimethamine-dapsone combination are not available in the United States.

Because of the increasing spread and intensity of antimalarial drug resistance (Figs. 116-2 and 116-10), the Centers for Disease Control and Prevention (CDC; *http://www.cdc.gov/malaria/index.htm*), which recommends a daily dose of atovaquone-proguanil for all travelers, maintains an updated 24-h travel and malaria information audiotape that can be accessed by touch-tone telephone (877-FYI-TRIP). Regional and disease-specific documents may be requested from the CDC Fax Information Service (888-232-3299). Consultation for the evaluation of prophylaxis failures or treatment of malaria can be obtained from state and local health departments and the CDC Malaria Hotline (770-488-7788) or the CDC Emergency Operations Center (770-488-7100).

FURTHER READINGS

ABDULLA S et al: Safety and immunogenicity of RTS,S/AS02D malaria vaccine in infants. N Engl J Med 359:2533, 2008

BAIRD JK et al: Prevention and treatment of vivax malaria. Curr Infect Dis Rep 9:39, 2007

BEJON P et al: Efficacy of RTS,S/AS01E vaccine against malaria in children 5 to 17 months of age. N Engl J Med 359:2521, 2008

CENTERS FOR DISEASE CONTROL AND PREVENTION: Treatment of malaria (guidelines for clinicians). Atlanta, Department of Health and Human Services, 2000; available online at *http://www.cdc.gov/malaria/diagnosis_treatment/tx_clinicians.htm*

DONDORP A et al: Artesunate versus quinine for treatment of severe falciparum malaria: A randomised trial. Lancet 366:717, 2005

FREEDMAN DO: Clinical practice. Malaria prevention in short-term travelers. N Engl J Med 359:603, 2008

GOMES MF et al: Pre-referral rectal artesunate to prevent death and disability in severe malaria: A placebo-controlled trial. Lancet 373:557, 2009

PHU NH et al: Hemofiltration and peritoneal dialysis in infection-associated acute renal failure in Vietnam. N Engl J Med 347:895, 2002

ROSENTHAL PJ: Artesunate for the treatment of severe falciparum malaria. N Engl J Med 358:1829, 2008

WHITE NJ: The assessment of antimalarial drug efficacy. Trends Parasitol 18:865, 2002

WORLD HEALTH ORGANIZATION: Severe falciparum malaria. Trans R Soc Trop Med Hyg 94(Suppl 1):51, 2000

———: Assessment and monitoring of antimalarial drug efficacy for the treatment of uncomplicated falciparum malaria. WHO/HTM/RBM/2003.50; available online at http://www.who.int/malaria/docs/ProtocolWHO.pdf

———: Guidelines for the treatment of malaria. Geneva, World Health Organization, 2006

CHAPTER 117

BABESIOSIS

Jeffrey A. Gelfand ■ Edouard Vannier

Babesiosis is an emerging infection transmitted by ticks and caused by intraerythrocytic protozoa of the genus *Babesia*. Wild and domestic animals are natural reservoirs of *Babesia* species. Only in the past 50 years has *Babesia* been appreciated to be a pathogen in humans. Usually a mild flulike illness in young and healthy people, babesiosis may develop into a life-threatening malaria-like syndrome in asplenic, immunocompromised, or elderly patients.

ETIOLOGY AND NATURAL CYCLE

In the northeastern United States, *Babesia microti* is transmitted to humans by the hard-bodied tick *Ixodes scapularis* (*I. dammini*). In the fall, adult ticks feed primarily on white-tailed deer. Deer are incompetent reservoirs for *B. microti* but are essential for the maintenance of *I. scapularis*. Adult ticks overwinter and lay eggs in the spring. The eggs hatch into larvae in late July. In August and September, larvae become infected as they feed on *B. microti*–infected white-footed mice. In the spring of the following year, larvae molt into nymphs that remain infected with *B. microti* (transstadial transmission). Early in the summer, these nymphs feed on white-footed mice that become reservoirs of *B. microti*. Transmission of *B. microti* to humans is incidental and occurs primarily at the nymphal stage.

In Europe, *I. ricinus* is regarded as the main vector for infection of humans with *B. divergens*, a pathogen of cattle. *B. divergens* is maintained in the life cycle of the tick by transstadial and transovarial transmission. Nymphs and adults are considered the primary vectors in bovine and human babesiosis.

As ticks feed, *Babesia*-infected red blood cells (RBCs) accumulate in their gut. Gametes fuse into zygotes that translocate across the epithelium, enter the hemolymph, and become kinetes. Some kinetes reach salivary acini and undergo hypertrophy to become dormant sporoblasts. Upon attachment of the tick to the host, sporogony is initiated. In the last hours of feeding, sporozoites are deposited in the host dermis. Once in the blood, sporozoites invade erythrocytes to become trophozoites (see Fig. 118-9). Trophozoites undergo asynchronous schizogony, resulting in the budding of two or four merozoites. Tetrads ("Maltese crosses") are pathognomonic of *B. microti* and other small *Babesia* species (e.g., *B. duncani*) but are seen only rarely in blood smears during infection.

EPIDEMIOLOGY

United States

Babesiosis due to *B. microti* is an emerging infection in the United States. Most of the documented cases have occurred in coastal southern New England (from eastern Connecticut to Cape Cod, MA) and the chain of islands off the coast, particularly Nantucket Island and Martha's Vineyard (MA); Block Island (RI); and eastern Long Island, Shelter Island, and Fire Island (NY). Several cases have been reported from upstate New York, New Jersey, and Pennsylvania and from the upper Midwest (Wisconsin, Minnesota). Because babesiosis is not a notifiable disease in every state and asymptomatic infection is common, the incidence of *B. microti* infection is greatly underestimated. In New York state alone, >800 cases have been reported in the past decade. In Washington state and northern California, nine cases have been attributed to *B. duncani* (isolates WA1 and CA5), *B. duncani*–type parasites (WA2 and CA6), and other closely related babesial parasites (CA1–4). These organisms are antigenically distinct from *B. microti* and belong to the clade of piroplasms found in dogs (*B. conradae*) and wild animals in the western United States. As asymptomatic infection may persist for months without detectable parasitemia, babesiosis may be transmitted by blood transfusion, especially in endemic areas. More than 50 transfusion-transmitted cases have been attributed to *B. microti* and two to *B. duncani* (WA1 and WA2). Neonatal babesiosis is rare and has been acquired by vertical transmission, blood transfusion, or tick bite. Lastly, *B. divergens*–like parasites have been implicated in three cases of acute babesiosis (one each in Missouri, Kentucky, and Washington state).

Other Countries

Babesiosis is rare in Europe, with half of >35 cases documented in France and the British Isles. In addition to the original case from Croatia, cases have been reported from the central Alpine region (Austria, Italy, Switzerland) and from southern Europe (Spain, Portugal). Most cases have involved asplenic patients and have been attributed to *B. divergens*. *B. microti* has been implicated in only a handful of cases, although serologic evidence of *B. microti* infection has emerged from Switzerland and midwestern Germany. A study of two patients from Austria and Italy has identified *Babesia* EU1 as a novel pathogen that belongs to the *B. divergens* clade and is closely related to *B. odocoilei*, a parasite of white-tailed deer.

Sporadic cases of human babesiosis have been described in Mexico, Colombia, the Canary Islands, Ivory Coast, Egypt, Mozambique, South Africa, and India. Cases due to *B. microti*–like piroplasms have been reported from Taiwan and Japan.

CLINICAL PRESENTATION

Infections with *B. microti* vary in severity. Asymptomatic infection or self-limiting flulike illness occurs in ~25% of adults and ~50% of children. The incubation period lasts 1–6 weeks. Onset is gradual. The most common manifestations are fever (intermittent or sustained, with temperatures sometimes reaching 40°C), fatigue, malaise, shaking chills, sweats, myalgias, and arthralgias. Less frequent symptoms include shortness of breath, headache, anorexia, and nausea. Malaise, myalgias, arthralgias, and shortness of breath may help differentiate babesiosis from other febrile illnesses. Fever is the salient feature on physical examination. Mild splenomegaly and hepatomegaly may be noted. Jaundice is rare.

Low hematocrit, low hemoglobin, and hemoglobinuria are consistent with hemolytic anemia. The parasitemia level is usually 1–10% in immunocompetent hosts but can reach 85% in asplenic patients. Reticulocyte counts are elevated, white blood cell (WBC) counts are normal or slightly low, and thrombocytopenia is common. Levels of liver enzymes (including alkaline phosphatase, lactate dehydrogenase, aspartate and alanine aminotransferases, and bilirubin) are elevated. With hemolysis, the serum haptoglobin concentration is low, and urinalysis may show hemoglobinuria and proteinuria.

Complications of babesiosis include acute respiratory failure, disseminated intravascular coagulation, congestive heart failure, and renal failure. *B. microti* infection may be fatal in 5–10% of cases in hospitalized patients. Severe anemia (hemoglobin concentration, <10 g/dL) and high-level parasitemia (>10%) are risk factors for complications. Alkaline phosphatase levels of >125 U/L, WBC counts of $>5 \times 10^9$/L, and male gender are strong predictors of severe disease, as defined by death, hospitalization for >2 weeks, or admission to an intensive care unit for >2 days. Severe babesiosis is common among asplenic patients, patients co-infected with *Borrelia burgdorferi* (i.e., those with Lyme disease), persons >50 years of age, and individuals with comorbidities, including HIV infection, cancer, and other diseases associated with immunosuppression. Infection may recrudesce after splenectomy or immunosuppressive therapy.

Babesiosis due to *B. divergens* occurs most often in asplenic patients. After an incubation period of 1–3 weeks, disease suddenly appears. Hemoglobinuria—the presenting symptom—is followed by jaundice, persistent high fever (40°–41°C), myalgias, shaking chills, and drenching sweats. Babesiosis may evolve into a shocklike syndrome, with renal failure and pulmonary edema. The parasitemia level can reach 80%. Hemoglobin levels may plunge to 4–8 g/dL. The mortality rate remains high (42%).

Infections with *B. duncani* and related parasites range from asymptomatic to severe and are sometimes fatal.

DIAGNOSIS

A diagnosis of babesiosis should be considered for any symptomatic patient who resides or travels in endemic areas. The tick bite often goes unnoticed. Because symptoms are nonspecific, the diagnosis requires laboratory testing. Babesiosis is diagnosed by microscopic examination of Giemsa-stained thin blood smears (see Fig. 118-9). *Babesia* spp. appear annular, oval, or piriform. Ring forms are most common and do not contain the central brownish deposits (hemozoin) typical of *Plasmodium falciparum*. Tetrads are indicative of small babesial parasites, such as *B. microti* and *B. duncani*. An indirect immunofluorescent antibody test (IFAT) for *B. microti* is available from the Centers for Disease Control and Prevention. A serum IgG titer of ≥1:64 is diagnostic. The latter test has good predictive value for infection but must be interpreted in the clinical context; antibodies do not develop until at least 1 week into the illness, and serologic testing does not distinguish prior infection from active infection. Thus, IFAT is ideal for detection of past or persistent infection but not of fulminant acute infection. Antibodies to *B. microti* do not react with *B. divergens* or *B. duncani*. The persistence of low-grade infection is best diagnosed by polymerase chain reaction (PCR)–based amplification of the babesial 18S rRNA gene in blood samples. As primers are species-specific, this assay is a valuable adjunct in the diagnosis of babesiosis.

℞ Treatment: BABESIOSIS

(See Table 117-1) Whether *B. microti* infection should be treated depends on the clinical context. Asymptomatic infections need not be treated, but if *Babesia* organisms continue to be seen on blood smear or by PCR for >3 months, treatment should be considered. Symptomatic infections should not be treated if blood smear and PCR are both negative for *Babesia*. If *Babesia* is detected in blood samples from symptomatic patients, treatment should be initiated.

A combination of atovaquone and azithromycin, given for 7–10 days, constitutes initial therapy for non-life-threatening (mild) babesiosis due to *B. microti*. For immunocompromised patients, higher doses of azithromycin (600–1000 mg/d) than those listed in the table are used. A combination of clindamycin and quinine is given for 7–10 days to patients with severe *B. microti* babesiosis; whenever possible, clindamycin should be given IV rather than PO. Partial or complete RBC exchange

TABLE 117-1

ANTIBIOTIC REGIMENS FOR THE TREATMENT OF BABESIOSIS

ORGANISM	SEVERITY	ADULTS	CHILDREN
B. microti	Mild[a]	Atovaquone (750 mg q12h PO) *plus* Azithromycin (500–1000 mg/d PO on day 1, 250 mg/d PO thereafter)	Atovaquone (20 mg/kg q12h PO; maximum, 750 mg/dose) *plus* Azithromycin [10 mg/kg qd PO on day 1 (maximum, 500 mg/dose), 5 mg/kg qd PO thereafter (maximum, 250 mg/dose)]
	Severe[a]	Clindamycin (300–600 mg q6h IV or 600 mg q8h PO) *plus* Quinine (650 mg q6–8h PO) *plus* Consider RBC exchange transfusion	Clindamycin (7–10 mg/kg q6–8h IV or 7–10 mg/kg q6–8h PO; maximum, 600 mg/dose) *plus* Quinine (8 mg/kg q8h PO; maximum, 650 mg/dose) *plus* Consider RBC exchange transfusion
B. divergens	Mild or severe[b]	Immediate complete RBC exchange transfusion *plus* Clindamycin (600 mg q6–8h IV) *plus* Quinine (650 mg q8h PO)	Immediate complete RBC exchange transfusion *plus* Clindamycin (7–10 mg/kg q6–8h IV; maximum, 600 mg/dose) *plus* Quinine (8 mg/kg q8h PO; maximum, 650 mg/dose)

[a] Treatment duration: 7–10 days.
[b] Treatment duration: generally 7–10 days, but may vary.
Note: RBC, red blood cell.

transfusion is advised in severe babesiosis, which is defined as a parasitemia level of >10%; significant hemolysis; or renal, hepatic, or pulmonary compromise. Treatment failures have been described with the recommended medical regimens. Other combination therapies may be used. A combination of azithromycin and quinine was effective in two patients with infection refractory to clindamycin plus quinine. One patient with AIDS and chronic babesiosis was treated successfully with a combination of clindamycin, doxycycline, and azithromycin after becoming allergic to quinine.

In patients with mild *B. microti* babesiosis, symptoms should improve within the first 48 h of therapy and should resolve within 3 months. In patients with severe babesiosis, hematocrit and parasitemia should be monitored each day or every other day until symptoms recede and the parasitemia level is <5%. Re-treatment may be required if the babesial parasite or amplifiable babesial DNA is detected for >3 months after initial therapy, but routine testing is not needed for immunocompetent patients who are asymptomatic. Underlying immunodeficiency (such as malignancy or HIV infection) should be considered in patients with severe or prolonged episodes of babesiosis.

There is increasing evidence that immunosuppressed patients may need treatment for considerably longer periods.

Patients with babesiosis should be evaluated for Lyme disease (Chap. 166) and human granulocytotropic anaplasmosis (Chap. 167), as all three infections may be acquired from the same tick vector. In endemic areas for these infections, relevant antimicrobial therapy should be considered when an intercurrent infection is strongly suspected.

B. divergens infection is often severe and progresses rapidly. The recommended treatment is immediate complete blood exchange transfusion and medical therapy with IV clindamycin plus oral quinine. Exchange transfusion ensures a complete and rapid removal of parasitized RBCs, RBC debris, and inflammatory mediators. Although uninfected RBCs are introduced by exchange transfusion, anemia may persist for >1 month. If so, additional transfusion is needed.

PREVENTION

Individuals who live or travel in endemic areas, especially those at increased risk for severe babesiosis, should be advised to avoid tick exposure by wearing protective clothing (long sleeves/long pants, with pants tucked into socks); applying tick repellents (such as DEET) to clothing; and limiting outdoor activities, especially between May and September, when infection risk is highest. Thorough skin examination after outdoor exposure allows removal of ticks within 24 h of attachment—i.e., before transmission can occur.

FURTHER READINGS

Aguilar-Delfin I et al: Resistance to acute babesiosis is associated with interleukin-12 and gamma interferon–mediated responses and requires macrophages and natural killer cells. Infect Immun 71:2002, 2003

Gubernot DM et al: *Babesia* infection through blood transfusions: reports received by the US Food and Drug Administration, 1997–2007. Clin Infect Dis 48:25, 2009

Holman PJ: Phylogenetic and biologic evidence that *Babesia divergens* is not endemic in the United States. Ann NY Acad Sci 1081:518, 2006

Krause PJ et al: Persistent and relapsing babesiosis in immunocompromised patients. Clin Infect Dis 46:370, 2008

Kuwayama DP, Briones RJ: Spontaneous splenic rupture caused by *Babesia microti* infection. Clin Infect Dis 46:e92, 2008

Thompson C et al: Coinfecting deer-associated zoonoses: Lyme disease, babesiosis, and ehrlichiosis. Clin Infect Dis 33:676, 2001

Vannier E et al: Human babesiosis. Infect Dis Clin North Am 22:469, viii-ix, 2008

Yokoyama N et al: Erythrocyte invasion by *Babesia* parasites: Current advances in the elucidation of the molecular interactions between the protozoan ligands and host receptors in the invasion stage. Vet Parasitol 138:22, 2006

CHAPTER 118

ATLAS OF BLOOD SMEARS OF MALARIA AND BABESIOSIS

Nicholas J. White ■ Joel G. Breman

Four species of blood protozoan parasites cause human malaria: the potentially lethal and often drug-resistant *Plasmodium falciparum*; the relapsing parasites *P. vivax* and *P. ovale*; and *P. malariae*, which can persist at low densities for years. Occasional infections in individuals who have been in tropical forests may be caused by monkey parasites—notably, *P. knowlesi*.

The malaria parasites are readily seen under the microscope (×1000 magnification) in thick and thin blood smears stained with supravital dyes (e.g., Giemsa's, Field's,

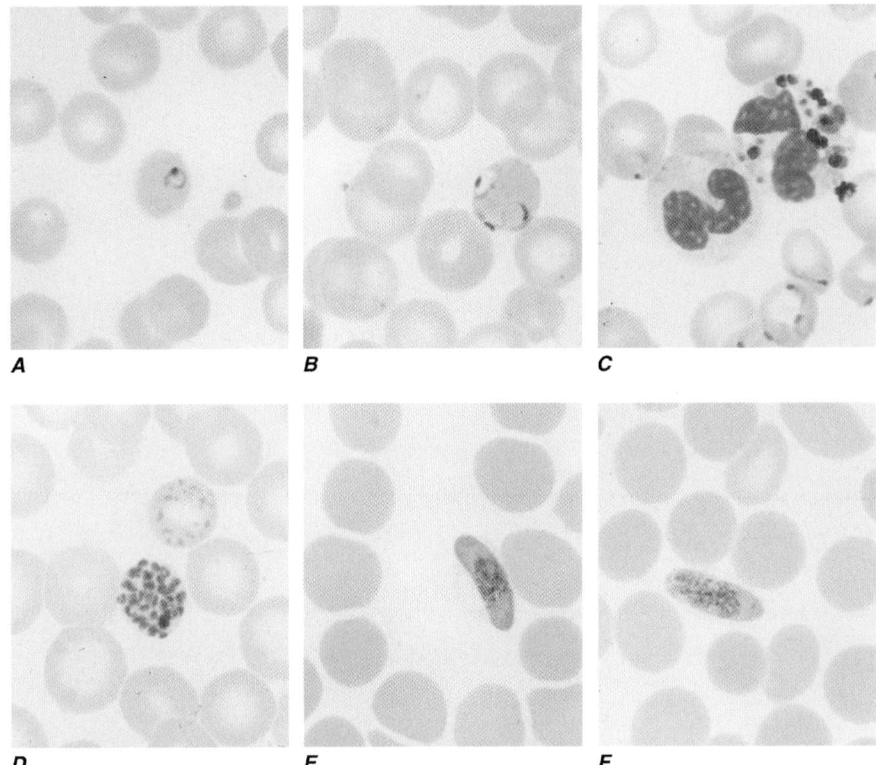

FIGURE 118-1
Thin blood films of *Plasmodium falciparum*. *A.* Young trophozoites. ***B.*** Old trophozoites. ***C.*** Pigment in polymorphonuclear cells and trophozoites. ***D.*** Mature schizonts. ***E.*** Female gametocytes. ***F.*** Male gametocytes. *(Reproduced from Bench Aids for the Diagnosis of Malaria Infections, 2d ed, with the permission of the World Health Organization.)*

Wright's, Leishman's). Thin film smears are shown in Figs. 118-1 to 118-4; thick film smears are shown in Figs. 118-5 to 118-8. The morphologic characteristics of the parasites are summarized in Table 118-1. In the thick film, lysis of red blood cells by water leaves the stained white cells and parasites, allowing detection of densities as low as 50 parasites/μL. This degree of sensitivity is up to 100 times greater than that of the thin film, in which the red cells are fixed and the malaria parasites are seen inside the cells. The thin film is better for speciation and provides useful prognostic information in severe falciparum malaria. Several findings are associated with increased mortality risk: high parasite counts, more mature parasites (>20% containing visible malaria pigment), and phagocytosed malaria pigment in >5% of neutrophils.

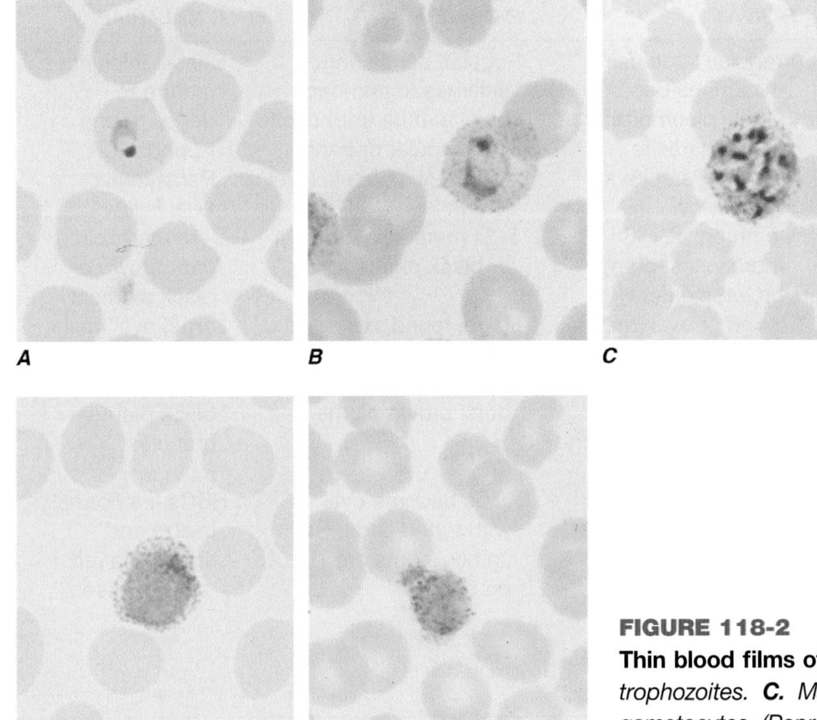

FIGURE 118-2
Thin blood films of *Plasmodium vivax*. *A.* *Young trophozoites.* **B.** *Old trophozoites.* ***C.*** *Mature schizonts.* ***D.*** *Female gametocytes.* ***E.*** *Male gametocytes. (Reproduced from Bench Aids for the Diagnosis of Malaria Infections, 2d ed, with the permission of the World Health Organization.)*

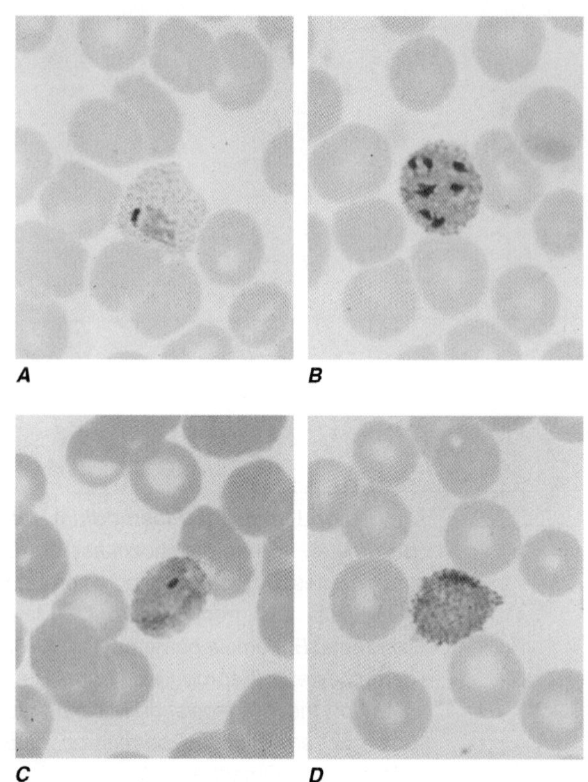

FIGURE 118-3

Thin blood films of *Plasmodium ovale*. *A.* Old trophozoites. ***B.*** Mature schizonts. ***C.*** Male gametocytes. ***D.*** Female gametocytes. *(Reproduced from Bench Aids for the Diagnosis of Malaria Infections, 2d ed, with the permission of the World Health Organization.)*

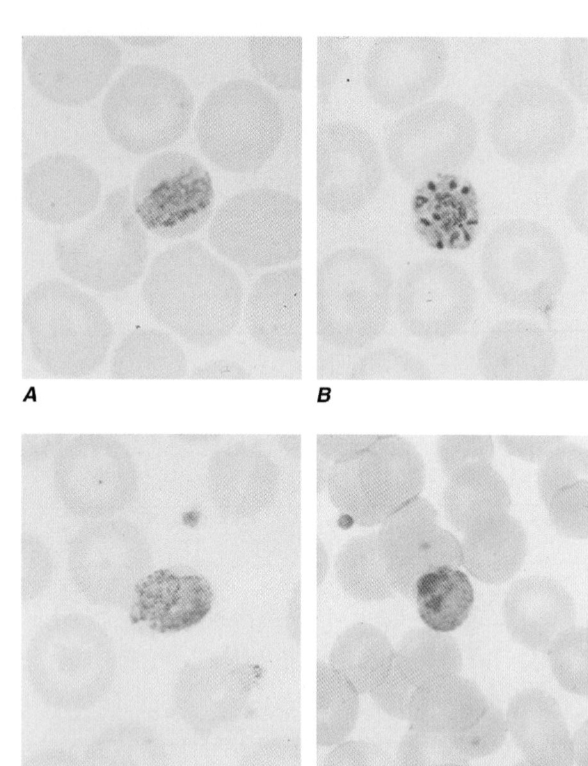

FIGURE 118-4

Thin blood films of Plasmodium malariae. *A.* Old trophozoites. ***B.*** Mature schizonts. ***C.*** Male gametocytes. ***D.*** Female gametocytes. *(Reproduced from Bench Aids for the Diagnosis of Malaria Infections, 2d ed, with the permission of the World Health Organization.)*

TABLE 118-1

MORPHOLOGIC CHARACTERISTICS OF HUMAN MALARIA PARASITES

	P. FALCIPARUM	*P. VIVAX*	*P. OVALE*	*P. MALARIAE*
Asexual parasites	Usually only fine blue ring forms (some resembling stereo headsets) are seen. Parasitemia level may exceed 2%.	Irregular, large, fairly thick rings become highly pleomorphic as the parasite grows. Parasitemia level is low.	Regular, dense ring enlarges to compact, blue, mature trophozoite (rectangular or band-form). Parasitemia level is low.	Dense, thick rings mature to dense, round trophozoites. Parasitemia level is low.
Schizonts	Rare in peripheral blood; 8–32 merozoites, dark brown-black pigment	Common; 12–18 merozoites, orange-brown pigment	8–14 merozoites, brown or black pigment	8–10 merozoites, dark brown or black pigment
Gametocytes	Banana-shaped; male: light blue; female: darker blue; a few scattered blue-black pigment granules in cytoplasm	Round or oval; male: round, pale blue; female: oval, dark blue; triangular nucleus, a few orange pigment granules	Large, round, dense, and blue (like *P. malariae*), but prominent James's dots; brown pigment	Large, oval; male: pale blue; female: dense blue; large black pigment granules
RBC changes	RBCs are normal in size. As the parasite matures, the RBC cytoplasm becomes pale, the cells become crenated, and a few small red dots may appear over the cytoplasm (Maurer's clefts).	RBCs are enlarged. Pale red Schüffner's dots increase in number as the parasite matures.	RBCs become oval with tufted ends. Red James's dots are prominent.	RBCs are normal in size and shape. No red dots are seen.

Note: RBC, red blood cell.

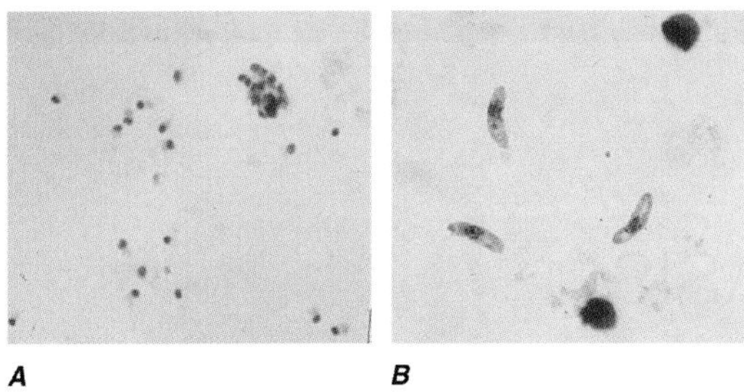

FIGURE 118-5

Thick blood films of *Plasmodium falciparum*. *A.* Trophozoites. ***B.*** Gametocytes. *(Reproduced from Bench Aids for the Diagnosis of Malaria Infections, 2d ed, with the permission of the World Health Organization.)*

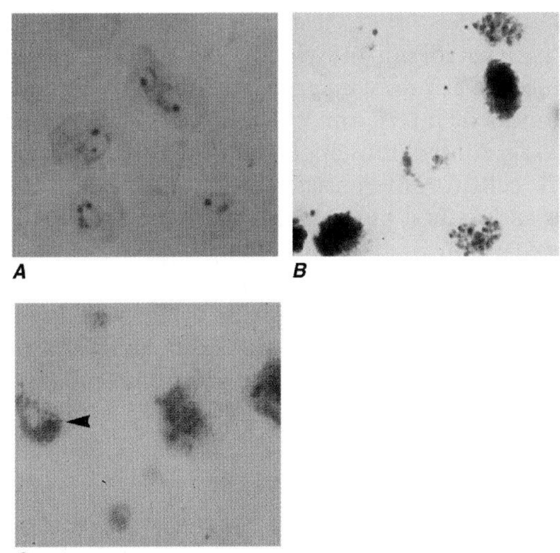

FIGURE 118-6

Thick blood films of *Plasmodium vivax*. *A.* Trophozoites. ***B.*** Schizonts. ***C.*** Gametocytes. *(Reproduced from Bench Aids for the Diagnosis of Malaria Infections, 2d ed, with the permission of the World Health Organization.)*

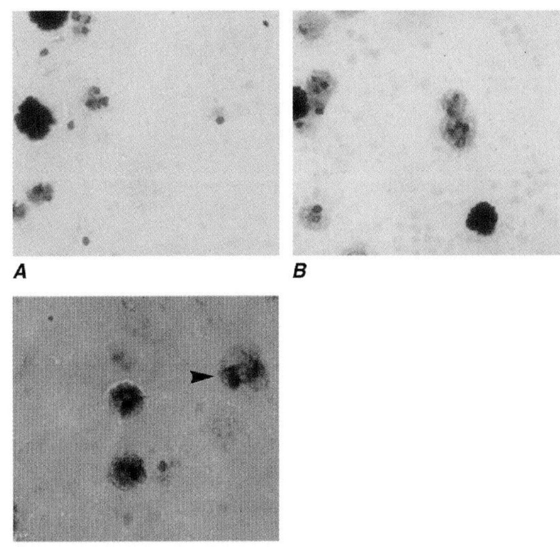

FIGURE 118-7

Thick blood films of *Plasmodium ovale*. *A.* Trophozoites. ***B.*** Schizonts. ***C.*** Gametocytes. *(Reproduced from Bench Aids for the Diagnosis of Malaria Infections, 2d ed, with the permission of the World Health Organization.)*

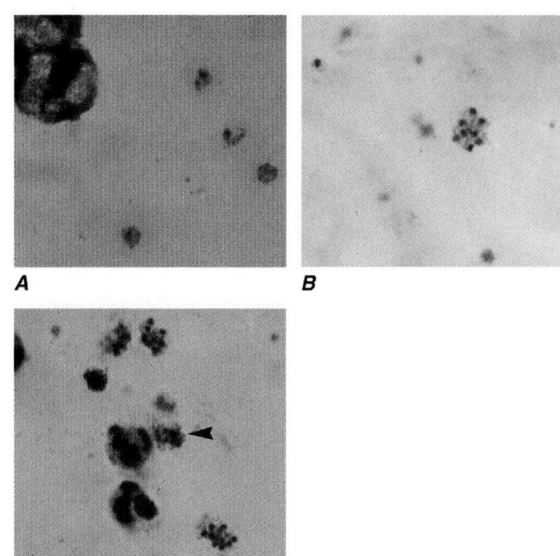

FIGURE 118-8

Thick blood films of *Plasmodium malariae*. *A.* Trophozoites. ***B.*** Schizonts. ***C.*** Gametocytes. *(Reproduced from Bench Aids for the Diagnosis of Malaria Infections, 2d ed, with the permission of the World Health Organization.)*

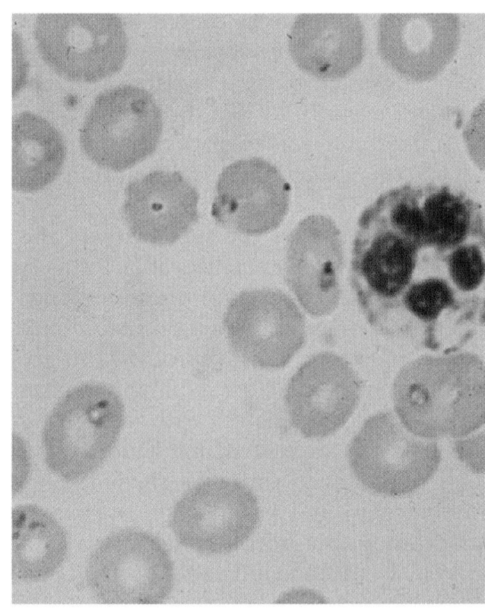

FIGURE 118-9

Thin blood film showing trophozoites of *Babesia*. *(Reproduced from Bench Aids for the Diagnosis of Malaria Infections, 2d ed, with the permission of the World Health Organization.)*

Babesia microti appears as a small ring form resembling *P. falciparum*. Unlike *Plasmodium*, *Babesia* does not cause the production of pigment in parasites, nor are schizonts or gametocytes formed. Figure 118-9 shows a thin blood film of trophozoites of *Babesia*.

FURTHER READINGS

Warhurst C, Williams JE: Laboratory procedures for diagnosis of malaria, in Abdalla SH, Pasvol G (series eds): *Malaria: A Hematological Perspective*. G Pasvol, SL Hoffman (eds): *Tropical Medicine: Science and Practice*, vol 4. London, Imperial College Press, 2004

CHAPTER 119

LEISHMANIASIS

Barbara L. Herwaldt

The term *leishmaniasis* encompasses multiple clinical syndromes. Most notable are visceral, cutaneous, and mucosal leishmaniasis, which result from infection of macrophages throughout the reticuloendothelial system, in the dermis, and in the naso-oropharyngeal mucosa, respectively.

Leishmaniasis, a vector-borne disease caused by obligate intracellular protozoa, is characterized by vast diversity and by specificity within that diversity. The disease is endemic in focal areas of ~90 countries in the tropics, subtropics, and southern Europe, in settings that range from deserts to rain forests and from rural to urban areas. Infection in humans is caused by ~20 *Leishmania* species (*Leishmania* and *Viannia* subgenera) (Table 119-1), which are transmitted by ~30 species of phlebotomine sandflies (*Phlebotomus* [Old World] and *Lutzomyia* [New World]). Amid this diversity, particular parasite, vector, and host species maintain the transmission cycle in a given setting.

Both the diversity and the specificity of the disease confound attempts to generalize about any aspect of leishmaniasis, including control measures and clinical management. The multitudinous possible combinations of *Leishmania* species/strains, syndromes, and geographic areas—modified by host factors and immunoinflammatory responses—may be associated with clinically relevant differences, such as diverse manifestations of infection and diverse responses to particular therapies. It is essential that clinicians understand the dangers associated with extrapolating data from one setting to another and the importance of individualizing patient care, with expert consultation.

LIFE CYCLE AND IMMUNOREGULATION

Leishmania parasites, which target and persist in tissue macrophages, are transmitted by the bite of female phlebotomine sandflies. While probing for a blood meal, sandflies regurgitate the parasite's flagellated promastigote stage into the host's skin; sandfly salivary components with immunomodulating effects have been shown to promote experimental infection. Promastigotes bind to receptors on macrophages, are phagocytized, and transform within phagolysosomes into nonflagellated amastigotes (Fig. 119-1), which replicate and infect additional macrophages. Amastigotes ingested by sandflies transform back into infective promastigotes. Other modes of transmission include congenital and parenteral (e.g., by blood transfusion or needle sharing).

Leishmaniasis is viewed as a model system for exploring immunoregulatory responses to intracellular pathogens. Murine models of *L. major* infection exemplify the T_H1/T_H2 paradigm, in which polarized T_H1 and T_H2 responses govern resistance and susceptibility, respectively. Production of interferon γ (IFN-γ) by T_H1 and natural killer cells confers resistance; interleukin (IL) 12 induces naïve T cells to differentiate into T_H1 cells and induces T cells and natural killer cells to produce IFN-γ. In contrast, expansion of IL-4-producing T_H2 cells and IL-10 mediate susceptibility.

Although the immunoregulatory responses are more complex and less polarized in humans than in inbred mice, key principles are evident. The immunoinflammatory response is central to pathogenesis, healing is associated

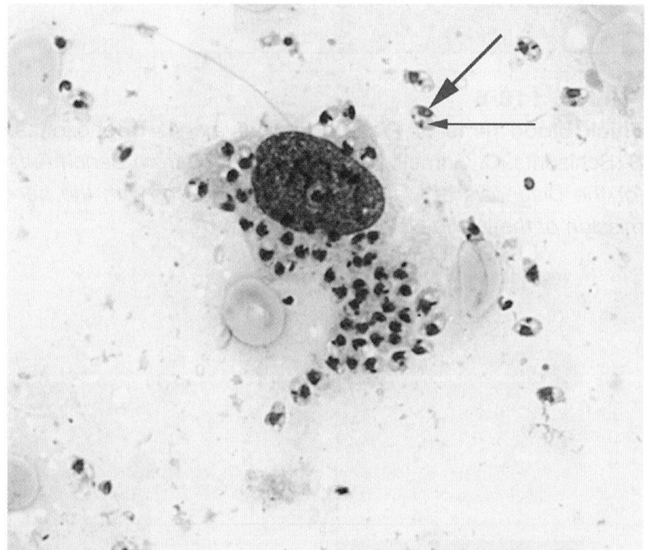

FIGURE 119-1

Amastigotes (the tissue stage of *Leishmania* parasites) in a Giemsa-stained impression smear of tissue from a patient with cutaneous leishmaniasis. Amastigotes are oval or egg shaped and ~2–4 μm in length. Their internal organelles include a nucleus (*larger arrow*) and rod-shaped kinetoplast (*smaller arrow*). In particular, the kinetoplast, a specialized mitochondrial structure that contains extranuclear DNA, should be visualized. The extracellular amastigotes probably were released from macrophages during manipulation of the specimen. Magnification: ×1000, obtained using a ×100 oil-immersion objective. *(Photograph courtesy of H. Bishop; with permission.)*

TABLE 119-1

LEISHMANIA SPECIES THAT CAUSE DISEASE IN HUMANS

SPECIES[a]	CLINICAL SYNDROME[b]	GEOGRAPHIC DISTRIBUTION[c]
Subgenus *Leishmania*		
L. donovani complex		
L. donovani sensu stricto	VL (PKDL, OWCL)	China, Indian subcontinent (southern Asia), southwestern Asia, Ethiopia,[d] Kenya, Somalia, Sudan, Uganda; possibly sporadic elsewhere in sub-Saharan Africa
L. infantum sensu stricto[e]	VL (OWCL)	China, central and southwestern Asia, Middle East, southern Europe, northern Africa, Ethiopia,[d] Sudan; sporadic elsewhere in sub-Saharan Africa
L. chagasi[e]	VL (NWCL)	Central and South America
L. mexicana complex		
L. mexicana	NWCL (DCL)	Mexico, Central and South America; sporadic in Texas and Oklahoma
L. amazonensis	NWCL (ML, DCL, VL)	Panama and South America
L. tropica	OWCL (VL)[f]	Central Asia, India, Pakistan, southwestern Asia, Middle East, Turkey, Greece, northern Africa, Ethiopia,[d] Kenya, Namibia
L. major	OWCL	Central Asia, India, Pakistan, southwestern Asia, Middle East, Turkey, northern Africa, Sahel region of north-central Africa, Ethiopia,[d] Sudan, Kenya
L. aethiopica	OWCL (DCL)	Ethiopia,[d] Kenya, Uganda
Subgenus *Viannia*		
L. (V.) braziliensis	NWCL (ML)	Central and South America
L. (V.) guyanensis	NWCL (ML)	South America
L. (V.) panamensis	NWCL (ML)	Central America, Venezuela, Colombia, Ecuador, Peru
L. (V.) peruviana	NWCL[g]	Peru (western slopes of Andes)

[a]Species other than those listed here have been reported to infect humans.
[b]DCL, diffuse cutaneous leishmaniasis; ML, mucosal leishmaniasis; NWCL, New World (American) cutaneous leishmaniasis; OWCL, Old World cutaneous leishmaniasis; PKDL, post–kala-azar dermal leishmaniasis; VL, visceral leishmaniasis. Clinical syndromes less frequently associated with the various species are shown in parentheses.
[c]The geographic distribution is highly focal within countries/regions, and the order in which areas are listed does not reflect the level of endemicity. (See text for further information.) The geographic distribution of cases evaluated in countries such as the United States reflects travel and immigration patterns.
[d]Cutaneous and visceral leishmaniasis also are endemic in parts of Eritrea, but the causative species have not been well established.
[e]"*L. infantum*" and "*L. chagasi*" are considered synonymous.
[f]*L. tropica* also causes leishmaniasis recidivans and viscerotropic leishmaniasis.
[g]The cutaneous leishmaniasis syndrome caused by this species is called *uta*.

with activation of macrophages to kill intracellular amastigotes, and persistent infection is characteristic. Although the correlates of immunity are not fully defined and may differ between treated and untreated persons, nonsterile cure is a mixed blessing: quiescent parasites may help the host maintain a protective T cell–mediated immune response but may also serve as a source for activation of latent or clinically cured infection if the protective mechanisms fail.

EPIDEMIOLOGY, PREVENTION, AND CONTROL

Leishmaniasis is endemic or emerging in focal areas of ~90 countries in Asia, the Middle East, southern Europe, and Africa (Old World disease) and the Americas (New World disease) (Table 119-1). Upwards of several hundred thousand cases of visceral leishmaniasis and 1–1.5 million cases of cutaneous leishmaniasis occur annually. Leishmaniasis is associated with the loss of ~2.4 million disability-adjusted life-years.

More than 90% of the world's cases of visceral leishmaniasis occur in three regions: (1) southern Asia or the Indian subcontinent, particularly in Bihar State in northeastern India and in foci in Bangladesh and Nepal; (2) eastern Africa (Sudan and neighboring countries); and (3) the Americas, particularly in periurban areas of northeastern Brazil. The predominant etiologic agents are *L. donovani* in southern Asia and eastern Africa and *L. infantum/L. chagasi* elsewhere in the Old and New Worlds. These organisms can also cause cutaneous leishmaniasis.

More than 90% of the world's cases of cutaneous leishmaniasis occur in Afghanistan (Fig. 119-2), Algeria, Iran, Iraq, Pakistan, Saudi Arabia, and Syria (Old World)

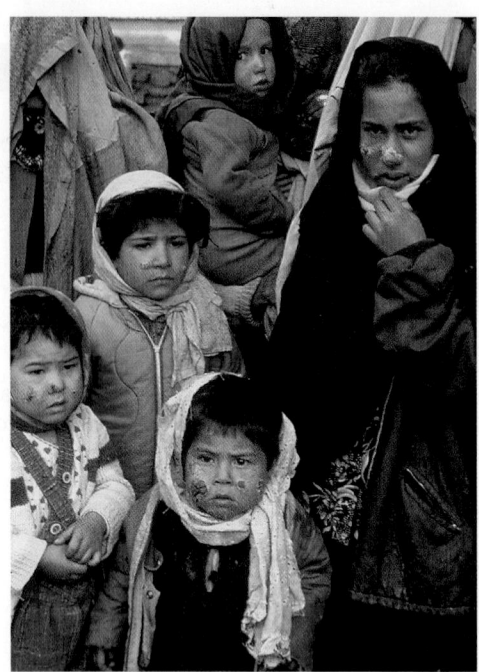

FIGURE 119-2

People in Kabul, Afghanistan, standing in line for hours on a bitterly cold day in February 1997 at a treatment center for cutaneous leishmaniasis. Kabul is experiencing a prolonged epidemic of anthroponotic cutaneous leishmaniasis caused by *Leishmania tropica. [Photograph courtesy of Dr. R. Ashford and reprinted with permission from Elsevier Science (Lancet 354:1193, 1999).]*

and in Brazil and Peru (New World). The predominant etiologic agents are *L. tropica*, *L. major*, and *L. aethiopica* (Old World) and species of the *L. mexicana* complex and the *Viannia* subgenus (New World).

In general, prevention and control measures are difficult to sustain and must be tailored to the setting. Vaccine strategies are being explored. Vector characteristics contribute to the focality of transmission in time and place and have implications for preventive measures. Sandflies are nocturnal (i.e., most active from dusk to dawn), have a limited flight range (usually remaining within a few hundred meters of their breeding site), and are small (about one-third the size of mosquitoes). Personal protective measures include minimizing nocturnal outdoor activities, wearing protective clothing, and applying insect repellent to exposed skin. In settings with domiciliary transmission, spraying dwellings with residual-action insecticides and using bed nets treated with long-lasting insecticides may be protective.

Most transmission cycles traditionally have been classified as zoonotic, except for the anthroponotic cycles of *L. donovani* (in southern Asia and potentially in eastern Africa) and *L. tropica*. However, some zoonotic cycles may be partially anthroponotic (and vice versa), and transmission patterns can evolve (e.g., from predominantly sylvatic to include domiciliary transmission) in the context of environmental and epidemiologic changes.

If transmission is exclusively or partially anthroponotic, treatment of infected persons can serve as a control measure, and suboptimal treatment can lead to dissemination of drug resistance. In southern Asia, which arguably carries ~70% of the global burden of visceral leishmaniasis, transmission of *L. donovani* is anthroponotic and largely intra- or peridomiciliary. In 2005, India, Nepal, and Bangladesh resolved to collaborate to reduce the annual incidence of visceral leishmaniasis to <1 case per 10,000 persons by the year 2015. For areas where canids are reservoir hosts (*L. infantum*/*L. chagasi*–endemic regions), various control strategies are being explored (e.g., insecticide- impregnated dog collars and vaccine candidates).

CLINICAL MANIFESTATIONS AND DIFFERENTIAL DIAGNOSIS

VISCERAL LEISHMANIASIS

The general term *visceral leishmaniasis* encompasses a broad spectrum of severity and manifestations, with a chronic, subacute, or acute onset and an incubation period of weeks, months, or sometimes years. In contrast, the term *kala-azar* typically is reserved for advanced, life-threatening disease. Although *kala-azar* means black [*kala*] fever [*azar*] in Hindi, darkening of the skin is uncommon. The classic manifestations of advanced disease include prolonged fever; cachexia (malnutrition being both a risk factor for and a sequela of visceral leishmaniasis); hepatosplenomegaly (with splenomegaly usually predominant and the spleen sometimes massive); anemia; leukopenia (neutropenia, marked eosinopenia, and relative lymphocytosis and monocytosis); thrombocytopenia, sometimes associated with bleeding; hypergammaglobulinemia (chiefly IgG, from polyclonal B cell activation); and hypoalbuminemia. The differential diagnosis includes tropical and infectious diseases that cause fever or organomegaly (e.g., typhoid fever, subacute bacterial endocarditis, miliary tuberculosis, brucellosis, histoplasmosis, tropical splenomegaly syndrome, and schistosomiasis) and myeloproliferative diseases (e.g., leukemia and lymphoma).

Post–kala-azar dermal leishmaniasis (PKDL) is a syndrome characterized by skin lesions (including macules, papules, nodules, and patches) that are typically most prominent on the face and that develop during or after therapy for visceral leishmaniasis. In Sudan, PKDL is noted in ~50% of patients from 0 to 6 months after therapy and usually heals spontaneously. In contrast, in India, PKDL is noted in ~5–10% of patients, occurring several years after treatment and usually requiring further therapy. PKDL can be confused with miliaria rubra, syphilis, yaws, and leprosy.

The diagnosis of visceral leishmaniasis should be considered for HIV-infected patients who have ever been in leishmaniasis-endemic areas and have manifestations consistent with visceral infection. The leishmanial infection may have been acquired recently (e.g., from a contaminated syringe) or may represent activation of latent infection acquired in the distant past; most co-infected patients with clinically evident visceral infection have CD4+ T lymphocyte counts of <200/μL.

Most cases of *Leishmania*-HIV co-infection have been reported from southern Europe (particularly Spain, France,

Italy, and Portugal). Whereas antiretroviral therapy has decreased the incidence of clinically manifest leishmanial infection in Europe, increasing numbers of co-infected cases are being reported in resource-poor countries.

CUTANEOUS LEISHMANIASIS

Typically, the incubation period of cutaneous leishmaniasis ranges from weeks to months. Lesions progress from papules to plaques (which can be smooth or scaly and develop central ulceration; Fig. 119-3) to atrophic scars. The spectrum includes papulonodular, nodular, and noduloulcerative lesions. Multiple primary lesions, satellite lesions, regional adenopathy, nodular lymphangitis, secondary bacterial infection, and thick hemorrhagic crusts or verrucous (wart-like) scale are variably present. Both active and healed lesions can cause considerable morbidity. Spontaneous resolution does not preclude reactivation of infection, dissemination to mucous membranes (see below), or reinfection.

Cutaneous leishmaniasis can be confused with tropical, traumatic, and venous-stasis ulcers; foreign-body reactions; myiasis; infected insect bites; impetigo, ecthyma, and pyoderma gangrenosum; superficial and deep fungal, mycobacterial, and spirochetal infections; and cutaneous sarcoidosis and neoplasms.

The polyparasitic and oligoparasitic ends of the disease spectrum are represented by diffuse cutaneous leishmaniasis (DCL) and leishmaniasis recidivans, respectively. DCL, which typically is caused by *L. aethiopica* (Old World) and *L. mexicana* species (New World), develops in the context of *Leishmania*-specific anergy and is manifested by chronic, disseminated, nonulcerative lesions, with abundant parasites but few lymphocytes. DCL should be differentiated from benign disseminated cutaneous leishmaniasis, lepromatous leprosy, and PKDL. Leishmaniasis recidivans, which most characteristically is caused by *L. tropica*, is a hyperergic variant with scarce parasites. It resembles lupus vulgaris and is characterized by a chronic, solitary plaque (typically on the cheek) that heals centrally but slowly expands at the periphery.

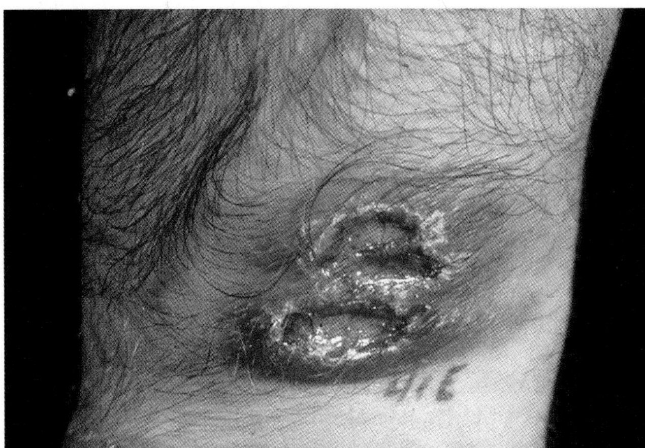

FIGURE 119-3
Ulcerative skin lesions with raised outer borders on the arm of a patient with New World (American) cutaneous leishmaniasis acquired in Costa Rica. *(Photograph courtesy of Dr. A. Wright; with permission.)*

MUCOSAL LEISHMANIASIS

Traditionally, the term *mucosal leishmaniasis* (or *espundia*) refers to a potentially disfiguring sequela of New World cutaneous leishmaniasis that results from dissemination of parasites from the skin to the naso-oropharyngeal mucosa. Mucosal leishmaniasis is caused by species in the *Viannia* subgenus [especially *L. (V.) braziliensis* and *L. (V.) panamensis* but also *L. (V.) guyanensis*] and by *L. amazonensis* (Table 119-1).

The magnitudes and the determinants (both parasite- and host-related) of the risks for mucosal dissemination and mucosal disease are poorly defined. Overall risk estimates for mucosal disease typically are ≤5% (~1–10%). The risk appears to be higher in South America and southern Central America than in *L. Viannia*–endemic regions further north (e.g., in Guatemala and Mexico). Mucosal and cutaneous lesions can be noted concomitantly or appear decades apart. Mucosal disease typically is noted within several years after the resolution of the original cutaneous lesions, which usually were not treated or were treated suboptimally.

The initial manifestations of mucosal disease typically are persistent, unusual nasal symptoms (e.g., epistaxis and stuffiness), with erythema and edema of the nasal mucosa, which can be followed by progressive, ulcerative destruction of the naso-oropharyngeal mucosa and surrounding tissues in the context of a hyperactive immune response. The differential diagnosis includes other infectious diseases (e.g., rhinoscleroma, paracoccidioidomycosis, histoplasmosis, leprosy, syphilis, and tertiary yaws), sarcoidosis, neoplasms, and mucosal ulceration from cocaine use.

DIAGNOSIS

PRINCIPLES AND PERSPECTIVE

Leishmaniasis often is diagnosed presumptively by clinical and epidemiologic criteria. Definitive diagnosis requires demonstration of the parasite in specimens from infected sites, which typically relies on classic microbiologic methods—i.e., detection of amastigotes by light microscopic examination of stained slides or detection of promastigotes by in vitro culture. In general, amastigotes, including their characteristic internal organelles (Fig. 119-1), are more easily recognizable on Giemsa-stained smears (e.g., thin smears of dermal scrapings or bone marrow aspirates and impression smears of biopsy specimens) than in tissue sections, particularly if organisms are rare.

Leishmania species can be distinguished by isoenzyme analysis of cultured promastigotes or determination of monoclonal antibody specificity. Molecular techniques of assorted types, with diverse genetic markers, are at various stages of development and validation for diagnosis of leishmaniasis and identification of species. Analyses of the genomes and the proteome profiles of *Leishmania* species may lead to novel diagnostic approaches.

Immunologic diagnostic methods include serologic assays and tests for *Leishmania*-specific cell-mediated immunity (e.g., skin testing for delayed-type hypersensitivity reactions). The utility of such methods depends in part on the syndrome. Most serologic assays do not reliably distinguish active from quiescent infection. No leishmanin skin-test preparation has been approved for use in the United States.

VISCERAL LEISHMANIASIS

Patients with advanced visceral leishmaniasis commonly have relatively heavy parasite burdens and high-level antibody responses that are not protective but are useful diagnostically; skin-test reactivity develops after recovery. Aspirates and biopsy specimens (e.g., of spleen, bone marrow, liver, or lymph node) are useful for parasitologic confirmation by traditional and molecular methods. Although the diagnostic yield is highest for splenic aspirates (>95%), bone marrow aspiration is safer.

In the appropriate setting, seropositivity is often the diagnostic standard. Although test performance can vary by region, approaches that offer the potential for improved field applicability include direct agglutination testing with freeze-dried antigen and immunochromatographic dipstick testing of fingerstick blood for antibody to recombinant antigens or synthetic peptides (e.g., rK39). In addition, assays for detection of leishmanial antigen in urine are being evaluated.

The sensitivity of serologic methods is lower in HIV-infected patients than in persons not infected with HIV (~50% vs. >90%). In contrast, the parasites may be abundant in typical sites (e.g., bone marrow), in atypical sites (e.g., gastrointestinal tissue), and in circulating monocytes—a circumstance that facilitates parasitologic diagnosis. The sensitivities of peripheral-blood smear and buffy-coat culture are ~50% and ~70%, respectively. PCR may be even more sensitive.

CUTANEOUS AND MUCOSAL LEISHMANIASIS

Aspirates and biopsy specimens of skin lesions and lymph nodes are useful for parasitologic confirmation of cutaneous and mucosal leishmaniasis by traditional and molecular methods. Parasitologic confirmation of mucosal leishmaniasis—a pauciparasitic syndrome—by traditional methods can be difficult. Serologic testing usually is not helpful for patients with cutaneous leishmaniasis; except in patients with DCL and some patients with mucosal leishmaniasis, antibody is either undetectable or present at low levels. In contrast, skin-test reactivity usually develops during active infection except in patients with DCL.

℞ Treatment: LEISHMANIASIS

PRINCIPLES AND PERSPECTIVE (Table 119-2)

Decisions about whether and how to treat leishmaniasis should be individualized. For cases in which systemic treatment is indicated, the parenterally administered pentavalent antimonial (Sb^V) compounds sodium stibogluconate and meglumine antimonate have been the mainstays of therapy for more than half a century. Manifestations of toxicity (e.g., body aches, malaise, elevated aminotransferase levels, chemical pancreatitis, and electrocardiographic abnormalities) are commonly noted but usually do not limit therapy and are reversible.

Conventional amphotericin B deoxycholate and pentamidine isethionate, the traditional parenteral alternatives to Sb^V, were previously relegated to second-line status, largely because of less experience with their use for the treatment of leishmaniasis and greater concern about their induction of potentially serious or irreversible toxicities (e.g., renal impairment). Amphotericin B, which has high-level, broad-spectrum antileishmanial activity, has been upgraded to first-line status in settings in which its benefits outweigh its risks (e.g., for Sb^V-resistant visceral leishmaniasis).

Lipid formulations of amphotericin B passively target the agent to macrophage-rich organs, resulting in less renal and other toxicity and permitting the use of higher daily doses and shorter courses of therapy. Targeting of drug to the reticuloendothelial system is ideal for visceral leishmaniasis but may not be advantageous for other syndromes. For amphotericin B and other antileishmanial agents, various delivery/targeting mechanisms and formulations are being explored.

Although some alternative therapies may have utility in particular settings, even data from well-conducted clinical trials cannot necessarily be generalized to other contexts. Of particular note, data from the many clinical trials of therapy for visceral leishmaniasis in foci in northeastern India are not necessarily directly applicable to visceral leishmaniasis caused by *L. donovani* in other foci in southern Asia or elsewhere (e.g., eastern Africa) or to visceral infection caused by *L. infantum/chagasi*—let alone to other leishmanial syndromes.

Except for the development of resistance to Sb^V and pentamidine, Indian kala-azar typically is easier to treat than visceral leishmaniasis elsewhere: i.e., it is more responsive to therapy, even with lower total doses. Counterintuitively, visceral leishmaniasis often is easier to treat than cutaneous or mucosal leishmaniasis. Achieving adequate drug levels in the phagolysosomes of dermal and mucosal macrophages can be challenging, and the difficulty can be compounded by the fact that some dermotropic species are intrinsically less sensitive than *L. donovani* to particular drugs.

Some of these issues are exemplified by miltefosine, the first highly active oral agent for visceral leishmaniasis. Both experimental (in vitro) and clinical data indicate that *L. donovani* (the agent of Indian visceral leishmaniasis) is highly sensitive to miltefosine, whereas other species are variably responsive. In addition, the long half-life of the drug and suboptimal treatment predispose to the development of resistance. The most common side effects of therapy include gastrointestinal symptoms and reversible elevations in creatinine and aminotransferase levels. Miltefosine's teratogenicity in animals has

TABLE 119-2

PARENTERAL AND ORAL DRUG REGIMENS FOR TREATMENT OF LEISHMANIASIS[a]

CLINICAL SYNDROME, DRUG	ROUTE OF ADMINISTRATION	REGIMEN
Visceral Leishmaniasis		
Parenteral therapy		
Pentavalent antimony[b]	IV, IM	20 mg Sb^V/kg qd for 28 days
Amphotericin B, lipid formulation[c]	IV	2–5 mg/kg qd (total: usually ~15–21 mg/kg)
Amphotericin B (deoxycholate)	IV	0.5–1 mg/kg qod or qd (total: usually ~15–20 mg/kg)
Paromomycin sulfate[d]	IV, IM	15–20 mg/kg qd for ~21 days
Pentamidine isethionate	IV, IM	4 mg/kg qod or thrice weekly for ~15–30 doses
Oral therapy		
Miltefosine[d,e]	PO	2.5 mg/kg qd for 28 days
Cutaneous Leishmaniasis		
Parenteral therapy		
Pentavalent antimony[b]	IV, IM	20 mg Sb^V/kg qd for 10–20 days (standard recommendation: 20 days)
Pentamidine isethionate	IV, IM	2 mg/kg qod for 7 doses
Amphotericin B (deoxycholate)	IV	0.5–1 mg/kg qod or qd (total: up to ~20 mg/kg)
Oral therapy		
Fluconazole	PO	200 mg qd for 6 weeks[f]
Ketoconazole	PO	600 mg qd for 28 days[f]
Itraconazole	PO	200 mg bid for 28 days[f]
Miltefosine[d,e]	PO	2.5 mg/kg qd for 28 days
Mucosal Leishmaniasis		
Pentavalent antimony[b]	IV, IM	20 mg Sb^V/kg qd for 28 days
Amphotericin B (deoxycholate)	IV	1 mg/kg qod or qd (total: usually ~20–40 mg/kg)
Pentamidine isethionate	IV, IM	2–4 mg/kg qod or thrice weekly for ≥15 doses

[a]See text for additional details and perspective about the drugs and regimens in this table and about treatment of leishmaniasis in general. Some of the listed drugs are effective only against certain *Leishmania* species/strains and only in certain areas of the world. Classification of drugs/regimens in such categories as first-line, alternative, (in)effective, investigational, (un)available, and cost-prohibitive is highly dependent on the setting. Ranges shown for doses and durations of therapy reflect variability both in dosage regimens among clinical trials and in responsiveness in different settings. To maximize effectiveness and minimize toxicity, the listed regimens should be individualized according to the particularities of the case and in consultation with an expert. Children may need different dosage regimens. Except for liposomal amphotericin B (see footnote *c*), as of this writing, none of the drugs listed is licensed by the U.S. Food and Drug Administration (FDA) for the treatment of leishmaniasis per se.

[b]The Centers for Disease Control and Prevention (CDC) provides the pentavalent antimonial (Sb^V) compound sodium stibogluconate (Pentostam; Glaxo Operations UK Limited, Barnard Castle, United Kingdom; 100 mg Sb^V/mL) to U.S.-licensed physicians through the CDC Drug Service (404-639-3670) under an IND mechanism with the FDA. The other widely used Sb^V compound, meglumine antimonate (Glucantime; typically, ~85 mg Sb^V/mL), is available primarily in Spanish- and French-speaking areas of the world. Locally made (generic) Sb^V preparations may have different Sb^V concentrations and may vary in quality and safety.

[c]The lipid formulations of amphotericin B include liposomal amphotericin B and amphotericin B lipid complex. In 1997, the FDA approved the following regimen of liposomal amphotericin B for immunocompetent patients with visceral leishmaniasis: 3 mg/kg qd on days 1–5, 14, and 21, for a total of 21 mg/kg. For immunosuppressed patients, the approved regimen is 4 mg/kg qd on days 1–5, 10, 17, 24, 31, and 38, for a total of 40 mg/kg. Many alternative regimens have been proposed for immunocompetent patients in various regions of the world; the regimens vary with respect to total and daily doses, number of doses, and intervals between doses. See text for perspective on the use of lipid formulations of amphotericin B for treatment of cutaneous and mucosal leishmaniasis.

[d]Not commercially available in the United States as of this writing.

[e]Miltefosine, which is teratogenic in animals, should not be used to treat pregnant women. Women of child-bearing age should use effective birth control during treatment and for 2 months thereafter. See text regarding the treatment of mucosal leishmaniasis.

[f]Adult dosage.

implications for its use in women of child-bearing age (Table 119-2).

VISCERAL LEISHMANIASIS The primary goal of treatment for visceral leishmaniasis is to prevent death. Highly effective antileishmanial therapy is essential, as is supportive care (e.g., therapy for malnutrition, anemia, bleeding, and intercurrent infections). In most regions, Sb^V therapy remains highly effective. However, use of an alternative agent should be considered if high-level Sb^V resistance is prevalent or if non-Sb^V therapy is advantageous for other reasons (e.g., duration, cost, or tolerability). In general, most patients feel better and become afebrile during the first week of therapy;

resolution of splenomegaly and hematologic abnormalities may require weeks or months.

In northeastern India, districts of Bihar State north of the Ganges River constitute the epicenter of the epidemic of Sb^V resistance, which is spreading—to varying degrees—to contiguous areas of India and southern Nepal. Conventional amphotericin B has become first-line therapy where Sb^V and pentamidine are no longer effective. Lipid formulations of amphotericin B, which are cost-prohibitive where they are most needed, are increasingly being used in southern Europe.

The anthroponotic transmission of *L. donovani* in southern Asia is both a blessing and a curse: a blessing because treatment can serve as a control measure, and a curse because suboptimal treatment can and does lead to the development and dissemination of drug resistance and thereby to the elimination of drugs from the limited armamentarium and to the demise of patients who cannot afford or access the few alternatives. In this context, the oral agent miltefosine, which is registered for commercial use in India and some other countries, has great potential but also is highly vulnerable. The advent of oral therapy translates into unsupervised outpatient treatment, in which patients buy the quantity of drug they can afford and prematurely stop therapy when their supply is depleted or their symptoms are alleviated. Unless protective measures are implemented (e.g., with directly observed or multidrug therapy), drug resistance almost assuredly will develop and spread. The oral agent sitamaquine, an 8-amino-quinoline, is being field-tested in various regions but appears to have a narrow therapeutic window and can cause nephrotoxicity.

The aminoglycoside paromomycin (the chemical equivalent of aminosidine) is a candidate parenteral agent for use alone or in drug combinations. To date, the rates of response in field tests have been variable; response rates may be higher in India than in eastern Africa.

Patients who are co-infected with HIV may initially respond well to standard therapy but typically experience more toxicity. Antiretroviral therapy delays but does not prevent relapses. Consensus approaches to treatment and secondary prophylaxis have not been established.

CUTANEOUS LEISHMANIASIS Decisions about clinical management of cutaneous leishmaniasis should be based on consideration of goals (e.g., accelerating the healing of skin lesions, decreasing morbidity, decreasing risks for local and mucosal dissemination and relapse), parasite factors (e.g., tissue tropisms and drug sensitivities), and the extent to which the lesions are of concern or are bothersome because of their location (e.g., on the face or near joints), number, size, persistence, or other features (e.g., nodular lymphangitis). When optimal effectiveness is important, parenteral Sb^V therapy is generally recommended. The first sign of a clinical response typically is decreasing induration, and relapses usually are noted first at the margins of healed lesions.

Although clinical trials of conventional amphotericin B for cutaneous leishmaniasis have not been conducted and standard dosage regimens have not been established, this agent almost assuredly is highly and broadly effective, albeit potentially toxic. Conflicting, limited data are available for lipid formulations. Pentamidine was effective in Colombia [predominantly against *L. (V.) panamensis*] but not in Peru [against *L. (V.) braziliensis*].

The effectiveness of the oral agent miltefosine is species and strain dependent. For example, this drug has been effective against *L. (V.) panamensis* in Colombia but ineffective against *L. (V.) braziliensis* in Guatemala. At best, azoles have shown modest activity against particular species in isolated studies—e.g., ketoconazole and itraconazole against *L. mexicana* in Guatemala, ketoconazole against *L. (V.) panamensis* in Panama, and fluconazole against *L. major* in Saudi Arabia. Itraconazole has been ineffective against *L. (V.) panamensis* in Colombia.

Local therapy can be considered for some cases without demonstrable local dissemination or risk of mucosal dissemination (e.g., for relatively benign lesions caused by *L. mexicana* or *L. major*). Examples of approaches being used or evaluated in some settings include intralesional Sb^V, various formulations of paromomycin ointments, topical immunomodulators, thermotherapy, and cryotherapy.

MUCOSAL LEISHMANIASIS The traditional treatment options for mucosal leishmaniasis include Sb^V and conventional amphotericin B; conflicting, limited data are available for lipid formulations of the latter drug. The response rates approach those for cutaneous leishmaniasis if mucosal disease is detected and treated at early stages, whereas advanced disease may be unresponsive or relapse repeatedly. Oral miltefosine therapy shows promise, on the basis of a clinical trial in Bolivia. Adjunctive immunotherapy is being evaluated. Concomitant glucocorticoid therapy is indicated if respiratory compromise develops after initiation of therapy.

FURTHER READINGS

ALVAR J et al: Chemotherapy in the treatment and control of leishmaniasis. Adv Parasitol 61:223, 2006

AMATO VS et al: Treatment of mucosal leishmaniasis in Latin America: Systematic review. Am J Trop Med Hyg 77:266, 2007

COLER RN, REED SG: Second-generation vaccines against leishmaniasis. Trends Parasitol 21:244, 2005

CROFT SL et al: Drug resistance in leishmaniasis. Clin Microbiol Rev 19:111, 2006

CRUZ I et al: *Leishmania*/HIV co-infections in the second decade. Indian J Med Res 123:357, 2006

HERWALDT BL: Leishmaniasis. Lancet 354:1191, 1999

MURRAY HW et al: Advances in leishmaniasis. Lancet 366:1561, 2005

SMITH DF et al: Comparative genomics: From genotype to disease phenotype in the leishmaniases. Int J Parasitol 37:1173, 2007

SUNDAR S et al: Injectable paromomycin for visceral leishmaniasis in India. N Engl J Med 356:2571, 2007

CHAPTER 120

TRYPANOSOMIASIS

Louis V. Kirchhoff

The genus *Trypanosoma* contains many species of protozoans. *Trypanosoma cruzi*, the cause of Chagas' disease in the Americas, and the two trypanosome subspecies that cause human African trypanosomiasis, *Trypanosoma brucei gambiense* and *T. brucei rhodesiense*, are the only members of the genus that cause disease in humans.

CHAGAS' DISEASE

DEFINITION

Chagas' disease, or American trypanosomiasis, is a zoonosis caused by the protozoan parasite *T. cruzi*. Acute Chagas' disease is usually a mild febrile illness that results from initial infection with the organism. After spontaneous resolution of the acute illness, most infected persons remain for life in the indeterminate phase of chronic Chagas' disease, which is characterized by subpatent parasitemia, easily detectable antibodies to *T. cruzi*, and an absence of symptoms. In a minority of chronically infected patients, cardiac and gastrointestinal lesions develop that can result in serious morbidity and even death.

LIFE CYCLE AND TRANSMISSION

T. cruzi is transmitted among its mammalian hosts by hematophagous triatomine insects, often called *reduviid bugs*. The insects become infected by sucking blood from animals or humans who have circulating parasites. Ingested organisms multiply in the gut of the triatomines, and infective forms are discharged with the feces at the time of subsequent blood meals. Transmission to a second vertebrate host occurs when breaks in the skin, mucous membranes, or conjunctivae become contaminated with bug feces that contain infective parasites. *T. cruzi* can also be transmitted by the transfusion of blood donated by infected persons, by organ transplantation, from mother to fetus, and in laboratory accidents.

PATHOLOGY

An indurated inflammatory lesion called a *chagoma* often appears at the parasites' portal of entry. Local histologic changes include the presence of parasites within leukocytes and cells of subcutaneous tissues and the development of interstitial edema, lymphocytic infiltration, and reactive hyperplasia of adjacent lymph nodes. After dissemination of the organisms through the lymphatics and the bloodstream, muscles (including the myocardium) may become heavily parasitized (Fig. 120-1). The characteristic pseudocysts present in sections of infected tissues are intracellular aggregates of multiplying parasites.

In the minority of persons with chronic *T. cruzi* infections who develop related clinical manifestations, the heart is the organ most commonly affected. Changes include thinning of the ventricular walls, biventricular enlargement, apical aneurysms, and mural thrombi. Widespread lymphocytic infiltration, diffuse interstitial fibrosis, and atrophy of myocardial cells are often apparent, but parasites are difficult to find in myocardial tissue. Conduction-system involvement often affects the right branch and the left anterior branch of the bundle of His. In chronic Chagas' disease of the gastrointestinal tract (megadisease), the esophagus and colon may exhibit varying degrees of dilatation. On microscopic examination, focal inflammatory lesions with lymphocytic infiltration are seen, and the number of neurons in the myenteric plexus may be markedly reduced. Accumulating experimental evidence implicates the persistence of parasites and the accompanying chronic inflammation—rather than autoimmune mechanisms—as the basis for the pathology in patients with chronic *T. cruzi* infection.

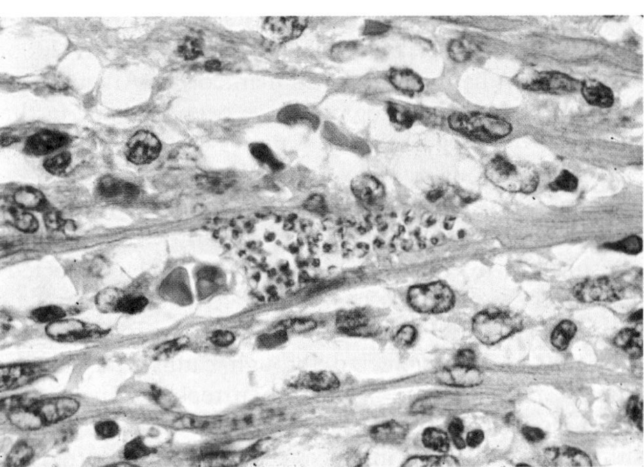

FIGURE 120-1
Trypanosoma cruzi in the heart muscle of a child who died of acute Chagas' myocarditis. An infected myocyte containing several dozen *T. cruzi* amastigotes is in the center of the field (hematoxylin and eosin, ×900).

EPIDEMIOLOGY

T. cruzi is found only in the Americas. Wild and domestic mammals harboring *T. cruzi* and infected triatomines are found in spotty distributions from the southern United States to southern Argentina. Humans become involved in the cycle of transmission when infected vectors take up residence in the primitive wood, adobe, and stone houses common in much of Latin America. Thus human *T. cruzi* infection is a health problem primarily among the poor in rural areas of Mexico and Central and South America. Most new *T. cruzi* infections in rural settings occur in children, but the incidence is unknown because most cases go undiagnosed. Historically, transfusion-associated transmission of *T. cruzi* has been a serious public health problem in many endemic countries. However, with some notable exceptions, transmission by this route has been markedly reduced as effective programs for the screening of donated blood have been implemented. Several dozen patients with HIV and chronic *T. cruzi* infections who underwent acute recrudescence of the latter have been described. These patients generally presented with *T. cruzi* brain abscesses, a manifestation of the illness that does not occur in immunocompetent persons. Currently, it is estimated that 12 million people are chronically infected with *T. cruzi* and that 25,000 deaths due to the illness occur each year. Of chronically infected persons, 10–30% eventually develop symptomatic cardiac lesions or gastrointestinal disease. The resulting morbidity and mortality make Chagas' disease the most important parasitic disease burden in Latin America.

In recent years, the rate of *T. cruzi* transmission has decreased markedly in several endemic countries as a result of successful programs involving vector control, blood-bank screening, and education of at-risk populations. A major program begun in 1991 in the "southern cone" nations of South America (Uruguay, Paraguay, Bolivia, Brazil, Chile, and Argentina) has provided the framework for much of this progress. Uruguay and Chile were certified transmission-free in the late 1990s, and Brazil was declared free of transmission in 2006. Transmission has been reduced markedly in Argentina as well. Similar control programs have been initiated in the countries of northern South America and in the Central American nations.

Acute Chagas' disease is rare in the United States. Five cases of autochthonous transmission and five instances of transmission by blood transfusion have been reported. Moreover, *T. cruzi* was transmitted to five recipients of organs from three *T. cruzi*–infected donors. Two of these recipients became infected through cardiac transplants. Acute Chagas' disease has not been reported in tourists returning to the United States from Latin America, although two such instances have been reported in Europe. In contrast, the prevalence of chronic *T. cruzi* infections in the United States has increased considerably in recent years. Data from the 2000 census indicate that >12 million immigrants from Chagas'-endemic countries currently live in the United States, ~8 million of whom are Mexicans. The prevalence of *T. cruzi* infection in Mexico is 0.5–1.0%, and most of the 4 million immigrants from Chagas'-endemic nations who are not Mexicans come from countries in which the prevalence of *T. cruzi* infection is greater than it is in Mexico. The total number of *T. cruzi*–infected persons living in the United States can be estimated reasonably to be 80,000–120,000. The number of instances of transfusion-associated transmission in this country is likely to be considerably greater than the number reported. Screening of the U.S. blood supply for evidence of *T. cruzi* infection has recently begun (see "Diagnosis" later in the chapter).

CLINICAL COURSE

The first signs of acute Chagas' disease develop at least 1 week after invasion by the parasites. When the organisms enter through a break in the skin, an indurated area of erythema and swelling (the chagoma), accompanied by local lymphadenopathy, may appear. *Romaña's sign*—the classic finding in acute Chagas' disease, which consists of unilateral painless edema of the palpebrae and periocular tissues—can result when the conjunctiva is the portal of entry (Fig. 120-2). These initial local signs may be followed by malaise, fever, anorexia, and edema of the face and lower extremities. A morbilliform rash may also appear. Generalized lymphadenopathy and hepatosplenomegaly may develop. Severe myocarditis develops rarely; most deaths in acute Chagas' disease are due to heart failure. Neurologic signs are not common, but meningoencephalitis occurs occasionally. The acute symptoms resolve spontaneously in virtually all patients, who then enter the asymptomatic or indeterminate phase of chronic *T. cruzi* infection.

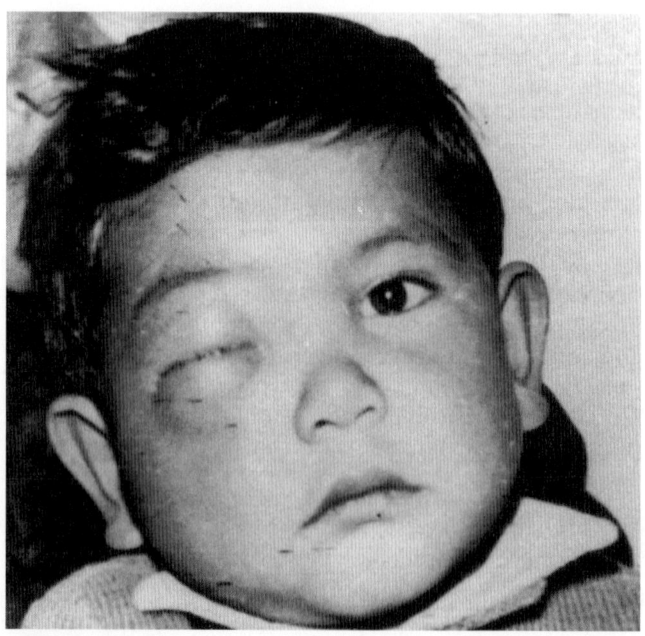

FIGURE 120-2
Romaña's sign in an Argentinean patient with acute *T. cruzi* infection. *(Courtesy of Dr. Humberto Lugones, Centro de Chagas, Santiago del Estero, Argentina; with permission.)*

Symptomatic chronic Chagas' disease becomes apparent years or even decades after the initial infection. The heart is commonly involved, and symptoms are caused by rhythm disturbances, dilated cardiomyopathy, and thromboembolism. Right bundle-branch block is a common electrocardiographic abnormality, but other types of atrioventricular block, premature ventricular contractions, and tachy- and bradyarrhythmias occur frequently. Cardiomyopathy often results in right-sided or biventricular heart failure. Embolization of mural thrombi to the brain or other areas may take place. Patients with megaesophagus suffer from dysphagia, odynophagia, chest pain, and regurgitation. Aspiration can occur (especially during sleep) in patients with severe esophageal dysfunction, and repeated episodes of aspiration pneumonitis are common. Weight loss, cachexia, and pulmonary infection can result in death. Patients with megacolon are plagued by abdominal pain and chronic constipation, and advanced megacolon can cause obstruction, volvulus, septicemia, and death.

DIAGNOSIS

The diagnosis of acute Chagas' disease requires the detection of parasites. Microscopic examination of fresh anticoagulated blood or of the buffy coat is the simplest way to see the motile organisms. Parasites also can be seen in Giemsa-stained thin and thick blood smears. Microhematocrit tubes containing acridine orange as a stain can be used for the same purpose. When repeated attempts to visualize the organisms are unsuccessful, polymerase chain reaction (PCR) or hemoculture in special media can be performed. When used by experienced personnel, all of these methods yield positive results in a high proportion of cases of acute Chagas' disease. Hemoculture has the disadvantage of taking several weeks to give positive results. Serologic testing plays no role in diagnosing acute Chagas' disease.

Chronic Chagas' disease is diagnosed by the detection of specific antibodies that bind to *T. cruzi* antigens. Demonstration of the parasite is not of primary importance. In Latin America, ~20 assays are commercially available, including several based on recombinant antigens. Unfortunately, these tests have varying levels of sensitivity and specificity, and false-positive reactions are a particular problem—typically with samples from patients who have other infectious and parasitic diseases or autoimmune disorders. In addition, confirmatory testing has presented a persistent challenge. For these reasons, it is generally recommended that specimens be tested in at least two assays and that well-characterized positive and negative comparison samples be included in each run. The radioimmune precipitation assay (Chagas' RIPA) is a highly sensitive and specific confirmatory method for detecting antibodies to *T. cruzi* [approved under the Clinical Laboratory Improvement Amendment (CLIA) and available in the author's laboratory]. In December 2006, the U.S. Food and Drug Administration (FDA) approved a test to screen blood and organ donors for *T. cruzi* infection (Ortho *T. cruzi* ELISA Test System, Ortho-Clinical Diagnostics, Raritan, NJ). In late January 2007, the American Red Cross and Blood Systems, Inc.—blood-collection agencies that together account for ~65% of the U.S. blood supply—initiated screening of all the donations they process for *T. cruzi*. The Chagas' RIPA is being used as the confirmatory assay. Data generated during the first 2 months of screening suggest that if 65% of the blood supply continues to be tested, ~1500 Ortho-reactive donors will be identified annually, ~350 of whom will be RIPA-positive; these figures reflect an overall prevalence of ~1 in 30,000 donors. The use of PCR assays to detect *T. cruzi* DNA in chronically infected persons has been studied extensively. The sensitivity of this approach has not been shown to be reliably greater than that of serology, and no PCR assays are commercially available.

Rx Treatment: CHAGAS' DISEASE

Therapy for Chagas' disease is unsatisfactory. For many years, only two drugs—nifurtimox and benznidazole—have been available for this purpose. Unfortunately, both drugs lack efficacy and often cause severe side effects.

In acute Chagas' disease, nifurtimox markedly reduces the duration of symptoms and parasitemia and decreases the mortality rate. Nevertheless, limited studies have shown that only ~70% of acute infections are cured parasitologically by a full course of treatment. Despite its limitations, treatment with nifurtimox should be initiated as early as possible in acute Chagas' disease. Common adverse effects of nifurtimox include abdominal pain, anorexia, nausea, vomiting, and weight loss. Neurologic reactions to the drug may include restlessness, disorientation, insomnia, twitching, paresthesia, polyneuritis, and seizures. These symptoms usually disappear when the dosage is reduced or treatment is discontinued. The recommended daily dosage is 8–10 mg/kg for adults, 12.5–15 mg/kg for adolescents, and 15–20 mg/kg for children 1–10 years of age. The drug should be given orally in four divided doses each day, and therapy should be continued for 90–120 days. Nifurtimox is available from the Drug Service of the Centers for Disease Control and Prevention (CDC) in Atlanta (telephone number, 770-639-3670).

The efficacy of benznidazole is similar to that of nifurtimox; a cure rate of 90% among congenitally infected infants treated before their first birthday has been reported. Adverse effects include peripheral neuropathy, rash, and granulocytopenia. The recommended oral dosage is 5 mg/kg per day for 60 days. Benznidazole is generally considered the drug of choice in Latin America.

The question of whether patients in the indeterminate or chronic symptomatic phase of Chagas' disease should be treated with nifurtimox or benznidazole has been debated for years. The fact that parasitologic cure rates in chronically infected persons may be <10% is central to this controversy. There is no convincing evidence from properly controlled trials that treatment of adults with long-standing *T. cruzi* infections with either of the drugs is beneficial. The current consensus of Latin American authorities is that all *T. cruzi*–infected persons up to 18 years old should be given benznidazole or nifurtimox.

The usefulness of allopurinol, fluconazole, and itraconazole for the treatment of acute Chagas' disease has been studied in laboratory animals and to a lesser extent in humans. None of these drugs has exhibited a level of anti–*T. cruzi* activity that warrants its use in patients. Several newer antifungal azoles have shown promise in animal studies but have not yet been tested in humans.

Patients who develop cardiac and/or gastrointestinal disease in association with *T. cruzi* infection should be referred to appropriate subspecialists for further evaluation and treatment. Cardiac transplantation is an option for patients with end-stage chagasic cardiopathies, and >100 such transplantations have been done in Brazil and the United States. The survival rate among Chagas' disease cardiac transplant recipients is higher than that among persons receiving cardiac transplants for other reasons. This better outcome may be due to the fact that lesions are limited to the heart in most patients with symptomatic chronic Chagas' disease.

PREVENTION

Since drug therapy is unsatisfactory and vaccines are not available, the control of *T. cruzi* transmission in endemic countries must depend on reduction of domiciliary vector populations by spraying of insecticides, improvements in housing, and education of at-risk persons. As noted above, these measures, coupled with serologic screening of blood donors, have markedly reduced transmission of the parasite in many endemic countries. Tourists would be wise to avoid sleeping in dilapidated houses in rural areas of endemic countries. Mosquito nets and insect repellent provide additional protection.

In view of the possibly serious consequences of chronic *T. cruzi* infection, it would be prudent for all immigrants from endemic regions living in the United States to be tested for evidence of infection. Identification of persons harboring the parasite would permit periodic electrocardiographic monitoring, which can be important because pacemakers benefit some patients who develop ominous rhythm disturbances. The possibility of congenital transmission is yet another justification for screening. Guidance for the evaluation and long-term monitoring of *T. cruzi*–infected persons is being developed by staff at the CDC.

Laboratory personnel should wear gloves and eye protection when working with *T. cruzi* and infected vectors.

SLEEPING SICKNESS

DEFINITION

Sleeping sickness, or human African trypanosomiasis (HAT), is caused by flagellated protozoan parasites that belong to the *T. brucei* complex and are transmitted to humans by tsetse flies. In untreated patients, the trypanosomes first cause a febrile illness that is followed months or years later by progressive neurologic impairment and death.

THE PARASITES AND THEIR TRANSMISSION

The East African (*rhodesiense*) and the West African (*gambiense*) forms of sleeping sickness are caused, respectively, by two trypanosome subspecies: *T. brucei rhodesiense* and *T. brucei gambiense*. These subspecies are morphologically indistinguishable but cause illnesses that are epidemiologically and clinically distinct (Table 120-1). The parasites are transmitted by blood-sucking tsetse flies of the genus *Glossina*. The insects acquire the infection when they ingest blood from infected mammalian hosts. After many cycles of multiplication in the midgut of the vector, the parasites migrate to the salivary glands. Their transmission takes place when they are inoculated into a mammalian host during a subsequent blood meal. The injected trypanosomes multiply in the blood (Fig. 120-3) and other extracellular spaces and evade immune destruction for long periods by undergoing antigenic variation, a process driven by gene switching in which the antigenic structure of the organisms' surface coat of glycoproteins changes periodically.

PATHOGENESIS AND PATHOLOGY

A self-limited inflammatory lesion (trypanosomal chancre) may appear a week or so after the bite of an infected

TABLE 120-1

COMPARISON OF WEST AFRICAN AND EAST AFRICAN TRYPANOSOMIASES

POINT OF COMPARISON	WEST AFRICAN (*GAMBIENSE*)	EAST AFRICAN (*RHODESIENSE*)
Organism	*T. b. gambiense*	*T. b. rhodesiense*
Vectors	Tsetse flies (palpalis group)	Tsetse flies (morsitans group)
Primary reservoir	Humans	Antelope and cattle
Human illness	Chronic (late CNS disease)	Acute (early CNS disease)
Duration of illness	Months to years	<9 months
Lymphadenopathy	Prominent	Minimal
Parasitemia	Low	High
Diagnosis by rodent inoculation	No	Yes
Epidemiology	Rural populations	Workers in wild areas, rural populations, tourists in game parks

Note: CNS, central nervous system.
Source: Reprinted with permission from LV Kirchhoff in GL Mandell et al (eds): *Principles and Practice of Infectious Diseases*, 6th ed. Philadelphia, Elsevier Churchill Livingstone, 2005.

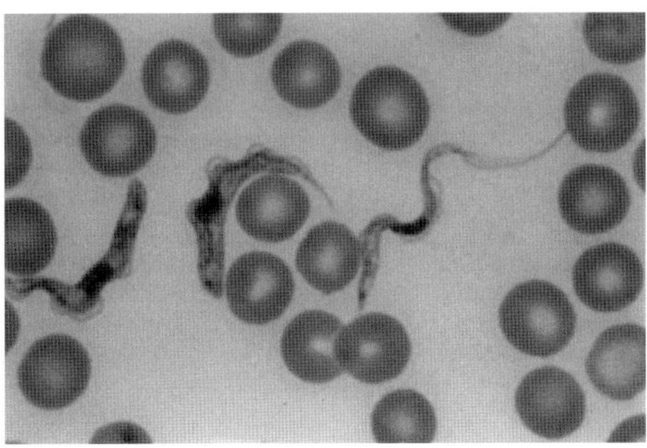

FIGURE 120-3
Trypanosoma brucei rhodesiense forms in rat blood. The slender parasite is thought to be the form that multiplies in mammalian hosts, while the stumpy forms are nondividing and are capable of infecting insect vectors (Giemsa, ×1200). *(Courtesy of Dr. G. A. Cook, Madison, WI; with permission.)*

tsetse fly. A systemic febrile illness then evolves as the parasites are disseminated through the lymphatics and bloodstream. Systemic HAT without central nervous system (CNS) involvement is generally referred to as *stage I disease*. In this stage, widespread lymphadenopathy and splenomegaly reflect marked lymphocytic and histiocytic proliferation and invasion of morular cells, which are plasmacytes that may be involved in the production of IgM. Endarteritis, with perivascular infiltration of both parasites and lymphocytes, may develop in lymph nodes and the spleen. Myocarditis develops frequently in patients with stage I disease and is especially common in *T. b. rhodesiense* infections.

Hematologic manifestations that accompany stage I HAT include moderate leukocytosis, thrombocytopenia, and anemia. High levels of immunoglobulins, consisting primarily of polyclonal IgM, are a constant feature, and heterophile antibodies, antibodies to DNA, and rheumatoid factor are often detected. High levels of antigen-antibody complexes may play a role in the tissue damage and increased vascular permeability that facilitate dissemination of the parasites.

Stage II disease involves invasion of the CNS. The presence of trypanosomes in perivascular areas is accompanied by intense infiltration of mononuclear cells. Abnormalities in cerebrospinal fluid (CSF) include increased pressure, elevated total protein concentration, and pleocytosis. In addition, trypanosomes are frequently found in CSF.

EPIDEMIOLOGY

The trypanosomes that cause sleeping sickness are found only in Africa. Approximately 50 million persons are at risk of acquiring HAT, and tens of thousands of new cases occur every year. Precise data are not available because health statistics are often incomplete in the developing countries where HAT is endemic. Sleeping sickness has undergone a resurgence in recent years, with major epidemics in the Sudan, Ivory Coast, Chad, the Central African Republic, and several other endemic countries.

Humans are the only reservoir of *T. b. gambiense*, which occurs in widely distributed foci in tropical rain forests of Central and West Africa. *Gambiense* trypanosomiasis is primarily a problem in rural populations; tourists rarely become infected. Trypanotolerant antelope species in savanna and woodland areas of Central and East Africa are the principal reservoir of *T. b. rhodesiense*. Cattle can also be infected with this and other trypanosome species but generally succumb to the infection. Since risk results for the most part from contact with tsetse flies that feed on wild animals, humans acquire *T. b. rhodesiense* infection only incidentally, usually while visiting or working in areas where infected game and vectors are present. Roughly one or two patients with HAT acquired in East African game parks (and typically caused by *T. b. rhodesiense*) are reported to the CDC each year.

CLINICAL COURSE

A painful trypanosomal chancre appears in some patients at the site of inoculation of the parasite. Hematogenous and lymphatic dissemination (stage I disease) is marked by the onset of fever. Typically, bouts of high temperatures lasting several days are separated by afebrile periods. Lymphadenopathy is prominent in *T. b. gambiense* trypanosomiasis. The nodes are discrete, movable, rubbery, and nontender. Cervical nodes are often visible, and enlargement of the nodes of the posterior cervical triangle, or *Winterbottom's sign*, is a classic finding. Pruritus and maculopapular rashes are common. Inconstant findings include malaise, headache, arthralgias, weight loss, edema, hepatosplenomegaly, and tachycardia. The differential diagnosis of stage I HAT includes many diseases that are common in the tropics and are associated with fevers. HIV infection, malaria, and typhoid fever are common in populations at risk for HAT and need to be considered.

CNS invasion (stage II disease) is characterized by the insidious development of protean neurologic manifestations that are accompanied by progressive abnormalities in the CSF. A picture of progressive indifference and daytime somnolence develops (hence the designation "sleeping sickness"), sometimes alternating with restlessness and insomnia at night. A listless gaze accompanies a loss of spontaneity, and speech may become halting and indistinct. Extrapyramidal signs may include choreiform movements, tremors, and fasciculations. Ataxia is frequent, and the patient may appear to have Parkinson's disease, with a shuffling gait, hypertonia, and tremors. In the final phase, progressive neurologic impairment ends in coma and death.

The most striking difference between the West African and East African trypanosomiases is that the latter illness tends to follow a more acute course. Typically, in tourists with *T. b. rhodesiense* disease, systemic signs of infection, such as fever, malaise, and headache, appear before the end of the trip or shortly after the return home. Persistent tachycardia unrelated to fever is common early in the course of *T. b. rhodesiense* trypanosomiasis, and death may result from arrhythmias and congestive heart failure before CNS disease develops. In general, untreated *T. b. rhodesiense* trypanosomiasis leads to death in a matter of weeks to months, often without a clear distinction between the hemolymphatic and CNS stages. In contrast, *T. b. gambiense* disease can smolder for many months or even for years.

DIAGNOSIS

A definitive diagnosis of HAT requires detection of the parasite. If a chancre is present, fluid should be expressed and examined directly by light microscopy for the highly motile trypanosomes. The fluid also should be fixed and stained with Giemsa. Material obtained by needle aspiration of lymph nodes early in the illness should be examined similarly. Examination of wet preparations and Giemsa-stained thin and thick films of serial blood samples is also useful. If parasites are not seen initially in blood, efforts should be made to concentrate the organisms; the simplest method involves the use of microhematocrit tubes containing acridine orange. In these tubes the parasites are separated from blood cells by centrifugation and are easily seen under light microscopy because of the stain. Alternatively, the buffy coat from 10–15 mL of anticoagulated blood can be examined directly under a microscope. The likelihood of finding parasites in blood is higher in stage I than in stage II disease and in patients infected with *T. b. rhodesiense* rather than *T. b. gambiense*. Trypanosomes may also be seen in material aspirated from the bone marrow; the aspirate can be inoculated into liquid culture medium, as can blood, buffy coat, lymph node aspirates, and CSF. Finally, *T. b. rhodesiense* infection can be detected by inoculation of these specimens into mice or rats, which—when positive—results in patent parasitemias in a week or two. Although this method is highly sensitive for the detection of *T. b. rhodesiense*, it does not detect *T. b. gambiense* because of host specificity.

It is essential to examine CSF from all patients in whom HAT is suspected. Abnormalities in the CSF that may be associated with stage II disease include an increase in the CSF mononuclear cell count as well as increases in opening pressure and in levels of total protein and IgM. Trypanosomes may be seen in the sediment of centrifuged CSF. Any CSF abnormality in a patient in whom trypanosomes have been found at other sites must be viewed as pathognomonic for CNS involvement and thus must prompt specific treatment for CNS disease. In patients with CSF pleocytosis in whom parasites are not found, tuberculous meningitis and HIV-associated CNS infections such as cryptococcosis should be considered in the differential diagnosis.

A number of serologic assays are available to aid in the diagnosis of HAT, but their variable sensitivity and specificity mandate that decisions about treatment be based on demonstration of the parasite. These tests are of value for epidemiologic surveys. PCR assays for detecting African trypanosomes in humans have been developed, but none is commercially available.

TABLE 120-2

TREATMENT OF HUMAN AFRICAN TRYPANOSOMIASES[a]

CAUSATIVE ORGANISM	CLINICAL STAGE: I (NORMAL CSF)	CLINICAL STAGE: II (ABNORMAL CSF)
T. brucei gambiense (West African)	Pentamidine Alternative: Suramin	Eflornithine Alternative: Melarsoprol
T. brucei rhodesiense (East African)	Suramin	Melarsoprol

[a]For doses and duration, see text.

Note: CSF, cerebrospinal fluid.

℞ Treatment: SLEEPING SICKNESS

The drugs used for treatment of HAT are suramin, pentamidine, eflornithine, and the organic arsenical melarsoprol. In the United States these drugs can be obtained from the CDC. Therapy for HAT must be individualized on the basis of the infecting subspecies, the presence or absence of CNS disease, adverse reactions, and occasionally drug resistance. The choices of drugs for the treatment of HAT are summarized in Table 120-2.

Suramin is highly effective against stage I East African disease. However, it can cause serious adverse effects and must be administered under the close supervision of a physician. A 100- to 200-mg IV test dose should be given to detect hypersensitivity. The dosage for adults is 20 mg/kg on days 1, 5, 12, 18, and 26. The drug is given by slow IV infusion of a freshly prepared 10% aqueous solution. Approximately 1 patient in 20,000 has an immediate, severe, and potentially fatal reaction to the drug, developing nausea, vomiting, shock, and seizures. Less severe reactions include fever, photophobia, pruritus, arthralgias, and skin eruptions. Renal damage is the most common important adverse effect of suramin. Transient proteinuria often appears during treatment. A urinalysis should be done before each dose, and treatment should be discontinued if proteinuria increases or if casts and red cells appear in the sediment. Suramin should not be given to patients with renal insufficiency.

Eflornithine is highly effective for treatment of both stages of West African trypanosomiasis. In the trials on which the FDA based its approval, this agent cured >90% of 600 patients with stage II disease. The recommended treatment schedule is 400 mg/kg per day, given intravenously in four divided doses, for 2 weeks. Adverse reactions include diarrhea, anemia, thrombocytopenia, seizures, and hearing loss. The high dosage and duration of therapy required are disadvantages that make widespread use of eflornithine difficult.

Pentamidine is the first-line drug for patients with stage I West African HAT. The dose for both adults and children is 4 mg/kg per day, given intramuscularly or intravenously, for 10 days. Frequent, immediate adverse reactions include nausea, vomiting, tachycardia, and hypotension. These reactions are usually transient and do not warrant cessation of therapy. Other adverse reactions include nephrotoxicity, abnormal liver function tests, neutropenia, rashes, hypoglycemia, and sterile abscesses.

The arsenical melarsoprol is the drug of choice for the treatment of East African trypanosomiasis with CNS involvement and is an alternative agent for stage II West African disease. Melarsoprol cures both stages of the disease and therefore is also indicated for the treatment of stage I disease in patients who fail to respond to or cannot tolerate suramin or pentamidine. However, because of its relatively high toxicity, melarsoprol is never the first choice for the treatment of stage I disease. For East African disease, the drug should be given to adults in three courses of 3 days each. The dosage is 2–3.6 mg/kg per day, given intravenously in three divided doses for 3 days, followed 1 week later by 3.6 mg/kg per day, also in three divided doses and for 3 days. The latter course is repeated 7 days later. In debilitated patients, suramin is administered for 2–4 days before therapy with melarsoprol is initiated; an 18-mg initial dose of the latter drug, followed by progressive increases to the standard dose, has been recommended. For children, a total of 18–25 mg/kg should be given over 1 month. An IV starting dose of 0.36 mg/kg should be increased gradually to a maximum of 3.6 mg/kg at 1- to 5-day intervals, for a total of 9 or 10 doses. The regimen for West African disease is 2.2 mg/kg per day, given intravenously for 10 days.

Melarsoprol is highly toxic and should be administered with great care. To reduce the likelihood of drug-induced encephalopathy, all patients receiving melarsoprol should be given prednisolone at a dose of 1 mg/kg (up to 40 mg) per day, beginning 1–2 days before the first dose of melarsoprol and continuing through the last dose. Without prednisolone prophylaxis, the incidence of reactive encephalopathy has been reported to be as high as 18% in some series. Clinical manifestations of reactive encephalopathy include high fever, headache, tremor, impaired speech, seizures, and even coma and death. Treatment with melarsoprol should be discontinued at the first sign of encephalopathy but may be restarted cautiously at lower doses a few days after signs have resolved. Extravasation of the drug results in intense local reactions. Vomiting, abdominal pain, nephrotoxicity, and myocardial damage can occur.

PREVENTION

HAT poses complex public-health and epizootic problems in Africa. Considerable progress has been made in some areas through control programs that focus on eradication of vectors and drug treatment of infected humans; however, there is no consensus on the best approach to solving the overall problem, and major epidemics continue to occur. Individuals can reduce their risk of acquiring trypanosomiasis by avoiding areas known to harbor infected insects, by wearing protective clothing, and by using insect repellent. Chemoprophylaxis is not recommended, and no vaccine is available to prevent transmission of the parasites.

FURTHER READINGS

Bisser S et al: Equivalence trial of melarsoprol and nifurtimox monotherapy and combination therapy for the treatment of second-stage *Trypanosoma brucei gambiense* sleeping sickness. J Infect Dis 195:322, 2007

Chang CD et al: Evaluation of a prototype *Trypanosoma cruzi* antibody assay with recombinant antigens on a fully automated chemiluminescence analyzer for blood donor screening. Transfusion 46:1737, 2006

Fiorelli AI et al: Later evolution after cardiac transplantation in Chagas' disease. Transplant Proc 37:2793, 2005

Kirchhoff LV et al: Transfusion-associated Chagas' disease (American trypanosomiasis) in Mexico: Implications for transfusion medicine in the United States. Transfusion 46:298, 2006

Lambert N et al: Chagasic encephalitis as the initial manifestation of AIDS. Ann Intern Med 144:941, 2006

Mascola L et al: Chagas disease after organ transplantation—Los Angeles, California, 2006. MMWR 55:798, 2006

Rassi A Jr et al: Development and validation of a risk score for predicting death in Chagas' heart disease. N Engl J Med 355:799, 2006

Sartori AM et al: Exacerbation of HIV viral load simultaneous with asymptomatic reactivation of chronic Chagas' disease. Am J Trop Med Hyg 67:521, 2002

Schmunis GA, Cruz JR: Safety of the blood supply in Latin America. Clin Microbiol Rev 18:12, 2005

Welburn SC et al: Crisis, what crisis? Control of Rhodesian sleeping sickness. Trends Parasitol 22:123, 2006

CHAPTER 121

TOXOPLASMA INFECTIONS

Lloyd H. Kasper

DEFINITION

Toxoplasmosis is caused by infection with the obligate intracellular parasite *Toxoplasma gondii*. Acute infection acquired after birth may be asymptomatic but frequently results in the chronic persistence of cysts in the host's tissues. In both acute and chronic toxoplasmosis, the parasite is responsible for clinically evident disease, including lymphadenopathy, encephalitis, myocarditis, and pneumonitis. Congenital toxoplasmosis is an infection of newborns that results from the transplacental passage of parasites from an infected mother to the fetus. These infants usually are asymptomatic at birth but later manifest a wide range of signs and symptoms, including chorioretinitis, strabismus, epilepsy, and psychomotor retardation.

ETIOLOGY

T. gondii is an intracellular coccidian that infects both birds and mammals. There are two distinct stages in the life cycle of *T. gondii* (Fig. 121-1). In the *nonfeline* stage, tissue cysts that contain bradyzoites or sporulated oocysts are ingested by an intermediate host (e.g., a human, mouse, sheep, pig, or bird). The cyst is rapidly digested by the acidic-pH gastric secretions. Bradyzoites or sporozoites are released, enter the small-intestinal epithelium, and transform into rapidly dividing tachyzoites. The tachyzoites can infect and replicate in all mammalian cells except red blood cells. Once attached to the host cell, the parasite penetrates the cell and forms a parasitophorous vacuole within which it divides. Parasite replication continues until the number of parasites

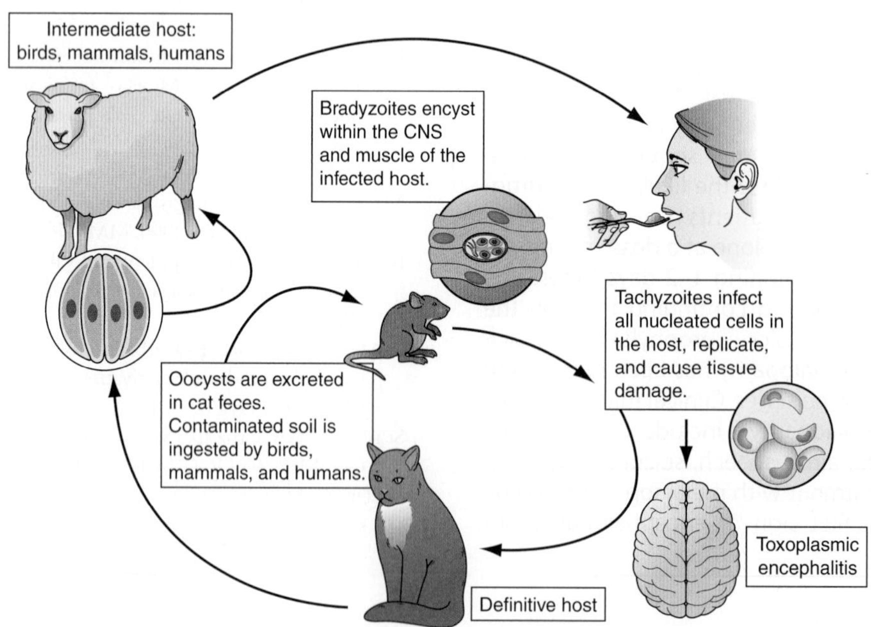

FIGURE 121-1

Life cycle of *Toxoplasma gondii*. The cat is the definitive host in which the sexual phase of the cycle is completed. Oocysts shed in cat feces can infect a wide range of animals, including birds, rodents, grazing domestic animals, and humans. The bradyzoites found in the muscle of food animals may infect humans who eat insufficiently cooked meat products, particularly lamb and pork. Although human disease can take many forms, congenital infection and encephalitis from reactivation of latent infection in the brains of immunosuppressed persons are the most important manifestations. CNS, central nervous system. *(Courtesy of Dominique Buzoni-Gatel, Institut Pasteur, Paris; with permission.)*

within the cell approaches a critical mass and the cell ruptures, releasing parasites that infect adjoining cells.

As a result of this process, an infected organ soon shows evidence of cytopathology. Most tachyzoites are eliminated by the host's humoral and cell-mediated immune responses. Tissue cysts containing many bradyzoites develop 7–10 days after systemic tachyzoite infection. These tissue cysts occur in various host organs but persist principally within the central nervous system (CNS) and muscle. The development of this chronic stage completes the nonfeline portion of the life cycle. Active infection in the immunocompromised host is most likely to be due to the spontaneous release of encysted parasites that undergo rapid transformation into tachyzoites within the CNS.

The principal (*feline*) stage in the life cycle takes place in the cat (the definitive host) and its prey. The parasite's sexual phase is defined by the formation of oocysts within the feline host. This enteroepithelial cycle begins with the ingestion of the bradyzoite tissue cysts and culminates (after several intermediate stages) in the production of gametes. Gamete fusion produces a zygote, which envelops itself in a rigid wall and is secreted in the feces as an unsporulated oocyst. After 2–3 days of exposure to air at ambient temperature, the noninfectious oocyst sporulates to produce eight sporozoite progeny. The sporulated oocyst can be ingested by an intermediate host, such as a person emptying a cat's litter box or a pig rummaging in a barnyard. It is in the intermediate host that *T. gondii* completes its life cycle.

EPIDEMIOLOGY

T. gondii infects a wide range of mammals and birds. Its seroprevalence depends on the locale and the age of the population. Generally, hot arid climatic conditions are associated with a low prevalence of infection. In the United States and most European countries, the seroprevalence increases with age and exposure. For example, in the United States, 5–30% of individuals 10–19 years old and 10–67% of those >50 years old have serologic evidence of exposure; seroprevalence increases by ~1% per year. In Central America, France, Turkey, and Brazil, the seroprevalence is higher. There may be as many as 2100 cases of toxoplasmic encephalitis (TE) each year in the United States.

TRANSMISSION

Oral Transmission

The principal source of human *Toxoplasma* infection remains uncertain. Transmission usually takes place by the oral route and can be attributable to ingestion of either sporulated oocysts from contaminated soil or bradyzoites from undercooked meat. During acute feline infection, a cat may excrete as many as 100 million parasites per day. These very stable sporozoite-containing oocysts are highly infectious and may remain viable for many years in the soil. Humans infected during a well-documented outbreak of oocyst-transmitted infection develop stage-specific antibodies to the oocyst/sporozoite.

Children and adults also can acquire infection from tissue cysts containing bradyzoites. The ingestion of a single cyst is all that is required for human infection. Undercooking or insufficient freezing of meat is an important source of infection in the developed world. In the United States, 10–20% of lamb products and 25–35% of pork products show evidence of cysts that contain bradyzoites. The incidence in beef is much lower—perhaps as low as 1%. Direct ingestion of bradyzoite cysts in these various meat products leads to acute infection.

Transmission via Blood or Organs

In addition to oral transmission, direct transmission of the parasite by blood or organ products during transplantation takes place at a low rate. Viable parasites can be cultured from refrigerated anticoagulated blood, which may be a source of infection in individuals receiving blood transfusions. *T. gondii* infection also has been reported in kidney and heart transplant recipients who were uninfected before transplantation.

Transplacental Transmission

About one-third of all women who acquire infection with *T. gondii* during pregnancy transmit the parasite to the fetus; the remainder give birth to normal, uninfected babies. Of the various factors that influence fetal outcome, gestational age at the time of infection is the most critical (see below). Few data support a role for recrudescent maternal infection as the source of congenital disease. Thus, women who are seropositive before pregnancy usually are protected against acute infection and do not give birth to congenitally infected neonates.

The following general guidelines can be used to evaluate congenital infection. There is essentially no risk if the mother becomes infected ≥6 months before conception. If infection is acquired <6 months before conception, the likelihood of transplacental infection increases as the interval between infection and conception decreases. In pregnancy, if the mother becomes infected during the first trimester, the incidence of transplacental infection is lowest (~15%), but the disease in the neonate is most severe. If maternal infection occurs during the third trimester, the incidence of transplacental infection is greatest (65%), but the infant is usually asymptomatic at birth. Infected infants who are normal at birth may have a higher incidence of learning disabilities and chronic neurologic sequelae than uninfected children. Only a small proportion (20%) of women infected with *T. gondii* develop clinical signs of infection. Often the diagnosis is first appreciated when routine postconception serologic tests show evidence of specific antibody.

PATHOGENESIS

Upon the host's ingestion of either tissue cysts containing bradyzoites or oocysts containing sporozoites, the parasites are released from the cysts by a digestive process. Bradyzoites are resistant to the effect of pepsin and invade the host's gastrointestinal tract. Within enterocytes (or other gut-associated cells), the parasites undergo morphologic transformation, giving rise to invasive tachyzoites. These tachyzoites induce a parasite-specific secretory IgA response. From the gastrointestinal tract, parasites are disseminated to a variety of organs, particularly lymphatic tissue, skeletal muscle, myocardium, retina, placenta, and the CNS. At these sites, the parasite infects host cells, replicates, and invades the adjoining cells. In this fashion, the hallmarks of the infection develop: cell death and focal necrosis surrounded by an acute inflammatory response.

In the immunocompetent host, both the humoral and the cellular immune responses control infection; parasite virulence and tissue tropism may be strain specific. Tachyzoites are sequestered by a variety of immune mechanisms, including induction of parasiticidal antibody, activation of macrophages with radical intermediates, production of interferon γ (IFN-γ), and stimulation of cytotoxic T lymphocytes of the CD8+ phenotype. These antigen-specific lymphocytes are capable of killing both extracellular parasites and target cells infected with parasites. As tachyzoites are cleared from the acutely infected host, tissue cysts containing bradyzoites begin to appear, usually within the CNS and the retina. In the immunocompromised or fetal host, the immune factors necessary to control the spread of tachyzoite infection are lacking. This altered immune state allows the persistence of tachyzoites and gives rise to progressive focal destruction that results in organ failure (i.e., necrotizing encephalitis, pneumonia, and myocarditis).

Persistence of infection with cysts containing bradyzoites is common in the immunocompetent host. This lifelong infection usually remains subclinical. Although bradyzoites are in a slow metabolic phase, cysts do degenerate and rupture within the CNS. This degenerative process, with the development of new bradyzoite-containing cysts, is the most probable source of recrudescent infection in immunocompromised individuals and the most likely stimulus for the persistence of antibody titers in the immunocompetent host.

PATHOLOGY

Cell death and focal necrosis due to replicating tachyzoites induce an intense mononuclear inflammatory response in any tissue or cell type infected. Tachyzoites rarely can be visualized by routine histopathologic staining of these inflammatory lesions. However, immunofluorescent staining with parasitic antigen–specific antibodies can reveal either the organism itself or evidence of antigen. In contrast to this inflammatory process caused by tachyzoites, bradyzoite-containing cysts cause inflammation only at the early stages of development, and even this inflammation may be a response to the presence of tachyzoite antigens. Once the cysts reach maturity, the inflammatory process can no longer be detected, and the cysts remain immunologically quiescent within the brain matrix until they rupture.

Lymph Nodes

During acute infection, lymph node biopsy demonstrates characteristic findings, including follicular hyperplasia and irregular clusters of tissue macrophages with eosinophilic cytoplasm. Granulomas rarely are evident in these specimens. Although tachyzoites are not usually visible, they can be sought either by subinoculation of infected tissue into mice, with resultant disease, or by polymerase chain reaction (PCR). PCR amplification of DNA fragments representing either p30 (SAG-1) or p22 (SAG-2) surface antigen or B1 antigen is an effective and sensitive assay for establishing lymph node infection by tachyzoites.

Eyes

In the eye, infiltrates of monocytes, lymphocytes, and plasma cells may produce uni- or multifocal lesions. Granulomatous lesions and chorioretinitis can be observed in the posterior chamber after acute necrotizing retinitis. Other ocular complications include iridocyclitis, cataracts, and glaucoma.

Central Nervous System

During CNS involvement, both focal and diffuse meningoencephalitis can be documented, with evidence of necrosis and microglial nodules. Necrotizing encephalitis in patients without AIDS is characterized by small diffuse lesions with perivascular cuffing in contiguous areas. In the AIDS population, polymorphonuclear leukocytes may be present in addition to monocytes, lymphocytes, and plasma cells. Cysts containing bradyzoites frequently are found contiguous with the necrotic tissue border. As stated previously, it is estimated that there are as many as 2100 cases of TE in the United States each year.

Lungs and Heart

Among patients with AIDS who die of toxoplasmosis, 40–70% have involvement of the lungs and heart. Interstitial pneumonitis can develop in neonates and immunocompromised patients. Thickened and edematous alveolar septa infiltrated with mononuclear and plasma cells are apparent. This inflammation may extend to the endothelial walls. Tachyzoites and bradyzoite-containing cysts have been observed within the alveolar membrane. Superimposed bronchopneumonia can be caused by other microbial agents. Cysts and aggregates of parasites in cardiac muscle tissue are evident in patients with AIDS who die of toxoplasmosis. Focal necrosis surrounded by inflammatory cells is associated with hyaline necrosis and disrupted myocardial cells. Pericarditis is associated with toxoplasmosis in some patients.

Gastrointestinal Tract

Acute infection in certain strains of inbred mice (B6) results in lethal ileitis within 7–9 days. This inflammatory bowel disease has been recognized in several mammalian species, including pigs and nonhuman primates. The association between human inflammatory bowel disease and either acute or recurrent *Toxoplasma* infection has not been established.

Other Sites

Pathologic changes during disseminated infection are similar to those described for the lymph nodes, eyes, and CNS. In patients with AIDS, the skeletal muscle, pancreas, stomach, and kidneys can be involved, with necrosis, invasion by inflammatory cells, and (rarely) tachyzoites detectable by routine staining. Large necrotic lesions may cause direct tissue destruction. In addition, secondary effects from acute infection of these various organs, including pancreatitis, myositis, and glomerulonephritis, have been reported.

HOST IMMUNE RESPONSE

Acute *Toxoplasma* infection evokes a cascade of protective immune responses in the immunocompetent host. *Toxoplasma* enters the host at the gut mucosal level and evokes a mucosal immune response that includes the production of antigen-specific secretory IgA. Titers of serum IgA antibody directed at p30 (SAG-1) are a useful marker for congenital and acute toxoplasmosis. Milk-whey IgA from acutely infected mothers contains a high titer of antibody to *T. gondii* and can block infection of enterocytes in vitro. In mice, IgA intestinal secretions directed at the parasite are abundant and are associated with the induction of mucosal T cells.

Within the host, *T. gondii* rapidly induces detectable levels of both IgM and IgG serum antibodies. Monoclonal gammopathy of the IgG class can occur in congenitally infected infants. IgM levels may be increased in newborns with congenital infection. The polyclonal IgG antibodies evoked by infection are parasiticidal in vitro in the presence of serum complement and are the basis for the Sabin-Feldman dye test. However, cell-mediated immunity is the major protective response evoked by the parasite during host infection. Macrophages are activated after phagocytosis of antibody-opsonized parasites. This activation can lead to death of the parasite by either an oxygen-dependent or an oxygen-independent process. If the parasite is not phagocytosed and enters the macrophage by active penetration, it continues to replicate, and this replication may represent the mechanism for transport and dissemination to distant organs. *Toxoplasma* stimulates a robust interleukin (IL) 12 response by human dendritic cells. The requirement for costimulation via CD40/154 has been established. The CD4+ and CD8+ T-cell responses are antigen-specific and further stimulate the production of a variety of important lymphokines that expand the T-cell and natural killer cell repertoire. *T. gondii* is a potent inducer of a T_H1 phenotype, with IL-12 and IFN-γ playing an essential role in the control of the parasites' growth in the host. Regulation of the inflammatory response is at least partially under the control of a T_H2 response that includes the production of IL-4 and IL-10 in seropositive individuals. Both asymptomatic patients and those with active infection may have a depressed CD4+ to CD8+ ratio. This shift may be correlated with a disease syndrome but is not necessarily correlated with disease outcome. Human T-cell clones of both the CD4+ and the CD8+ phenotypes are cytolytic against parasite-infected macrophages. These T-cell clones produce cytokines that are "microbistatic." IL-18, IL-7, and IL-15 upregulate the production of IFN-γ and may be important during acute and chronic infection. The effect of IFN-γ may be paradoxical, with stimulation of a host downregulatory response as well.

Although in patients with AIDS *T. gondii* infection is believed to be recrudescent, determination of antibody titers is not helpful in establishing reactivation. Because of the severe depletion in CD4+ T cells, quite frequently there is no observed increase in antibody titer during exacerbation of infection. T cells from AIDS patients with reactivation of toxoplasmosis fail to secrete both IFN-γ and IL-2. This alteration in the production of these critical immune cytokines contributes to the persistence of infection. *Toxoplasma* infection frequently develops late in the course of AIDS, when the loss of T-cell–dependent protective mechanisms, particularly CD8+ T cells, becomes most pronounced.

CLINICAL MANIFESTATIONS

In persons whose immune systems are intact, acute toxoplasmosis is usually asymptomatic and self-limited. This condition can go unrecognized in 80–90% of adults and children with acquired infection. The asymptomatic nature of this infection makes diagnosis difficult in mothers infected during pregnancy. In contrast, the wide range of clinical manifestations in congenitally infected children includes severe neurologic complications such as hydrocephalus, microcephaly, mental retardation, and chorioretinitis. If prenatal infection is severe, multiorgan failure and subsequent intrauterine fetal death can occur. In children and adults, chronic infection can persist throughout life, with little consequence to the immunocompetent host.

Toxoplasmosis in Immunocompetent Patients

The most common manifestation of acute toxoplasmosis is cervical lymphadenopathy. The nodes may be single or multiple, are usually nontender, are discrete, and vary in firmness. Lymphadenopathy also may be found in suboccipital, supraclavicular, inguinal, and mediastinal areas. Generalized lymphadenopathy occurs in 20–30% of symptomatic patients. Between 20 and 40% of patients with lymphadenopathy also have headache, malaise, fatigue, and fever [usually with a temperature of <40°C (<104°F)]. A smaller proportion of symptomatic individuals have myalgia, sore throat, abdominal pain, maculopapular rash, meningoencephalitis, and confusion. Rare complications associated with infection in the normal immune host include pneumonia, myocarditis, encephalopathy, pericarditis, and polymyositis. Symptoms associated with acute infection usually resolve within several weeks, although the lymphadenopathy may persist for some months. In one epidemic, toxoplasmosis was diagnosed correctly in only 3 of the 25 patients who consulted physicians. If toxoplasmosis is considered in the differential diagnosis, routine laboratory and serologic screening should precede node biopsy.

The results of routine laboratory studies are usually unremarkable except for minimal lymphocytosis, an elevated erythrocyte sedimentation rate, and a nominal increase in liver aminotransferases. Evaluation of cerebrospinal fluid (CSF) in cases with evidence of encephalopathy or meningoencephalitis shows an elevation of intracranial pressure, mononuclear pleocytosis (10–50 cells/mL), a slight increase in protein concentration, and (occasionally) an increase in the gamma globulin level. PCR amplification of the *Toxoplasma* DNA target sequence in CSF may be beneficial. The CSF of chronically infected individuals is normal.

Infection of Immunocompromised Patients

Patients with AIDS and those receiving immunosuppressive therapy for lymphoproliferative disorders are at greatest risk for developing acute toxoplasmosis. This predilection may be due either to reactivation of latent infection or to acquisition of parasites from exogenous sources such as blood or transplanted organs. In individuals with AIDS, >95% of cases of TE are believed to be due to recrudescent infection. In most of these cases, encephalitis develops when the CD4+ T-cell count falls below 100/μL. In immunocompromised hosts, the disease may be rapidly fatal if untreated. Thus accurate diagnosis and initiation of appropriate therapy are necessary to prevent fulminant infection.

Toxoplasmosis is a principal opportunistic infection of the CNS in persons with AIDS. Although geographic origin may be related to frequency of infection, it has no correlation with the severity of disease in immunocompromised hosts. Individuals with AIDS who are seropositive for *T. gondii* are at very high risk for encephalitis. In the United States, about one-third of the 15–40% of adult AIDS patients who are latently infected with *T. gondii* develop TE.

The signs and symptoms of acute toxoplasmosis in immunocompromised patients principally involve the CNS (Fig. 121-2). More than 50% of patients with clinical manifestations have intracerebral involvement. Clinical findings at presentation range from nonfocal to focal dysfunction. CNS findings include encephalopathy, meningoencephalitis, and mass lesions. Patients may present with altered mental status (75%), fever (10–72%), seizures (33%), headaches (56%), and focal neurologic findings (60%), including motor deficits, cranial nerve palsies, movement disorders, dysmetria, visual-field loss, and aphasia. Patients who present with evidence of diffuse cortical dysfunction develop evidence of focal neurologic disease as infection progresses. This altered condition is due not only to the necrotizing encephalitis caused by direct invasion by the parasite but also to secondary effects, including vasculitis, edema, and hemorrhage. The onset of infection can range from an insidious process over several weeks to an acute confusional state with fulminant focal deficits, including hemiparesis, hemiplegia, visual-field defects, localized headache, and focal seizures.

Although lesions can occur anywhere in the CNS, the areas most often involved appear to be the brainstem, basal ganglia, pituitary gland, and corticomedullary junction. Brainstem involvement gives rise to a variety of neurologic dysfunctions, including cranial nerve palsy, dysmetria, and ataxia. With basal ganglionic infection, patients may develop hydrocephalus, choreiform movements, and choreoathetosis. Because *Toxoplasma* usually causes encephalitis, meningeal involvement is uncommon, and thus CSF findings may be unremarkable or may include a modest increase in cell count and in protein—but not glucose—concentration.

Cerebral toxoplasmosis must be differentiated from other opportunistic infections or tumors in the CNS of AIDS patients. The differential diagnosis includes herpes simplex encephalitis, cryptococcal meningitis, progressive multifocal leukoencephalopathy, and primary CNS lymphoma. Involvement of the pituitary gland can give rise to panhypopituitarism and hyponatremia from inappropriate secretion of vasopressin (antidiuretic hormone). AIDS-dementia complex may present as cognitive impairment, attention loss, and altered memory. Brain biopsy in patients who have been treated for TE but who continue to exhibit neurologic dysfunction often fails to identify organisms.

Autopsies of *Toxoplasma*-infected patients have demonstrated the involvement of multiple organs, including the lungs, gastrointestinal tract, pancreas, skin, eyes, heart, and liver. *Toxoplasma* pneumonia can be confused with *Pneumocystis* pneumonia (PcP). Respiratory involvement usually presents as dyspnea, fever, and a nonproductive cough and may rapidly progress to acute respiratory failure with hemoptysis, metabolic acidosis, hypotension, and (occasionally) disseminated intravascular coagulation. Histopathologic studies demonstrate necrosis and a mixed

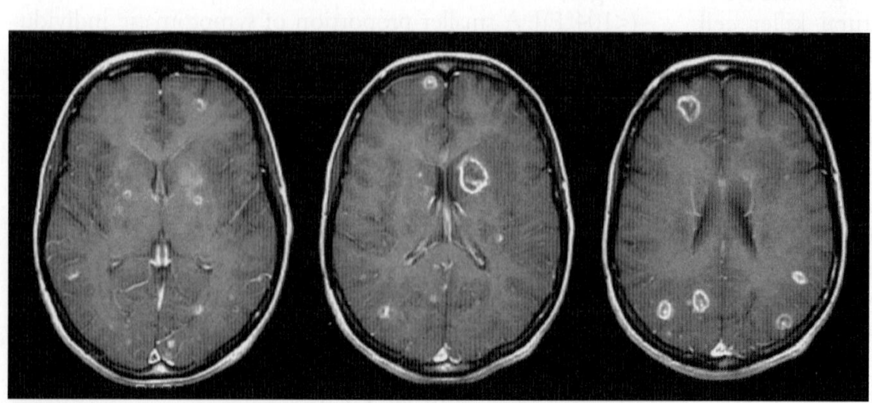

FIGURE 121-2
Toxoplasmic encephalitis in a 36-year-old patient with AIDS. The multiple lesions are demonstrated by magnetic resonance scanning (T1 weighted with gadolinium enhancement). *(Courtesy of Clifford Eskey, Dartmouth Hitchcock Medical Center, Hanover, NH; with permission.)*

cellular infiltrate. The presence of organisms is a helpful diagnostic indicator, but organisms can also be found in healthy tissue. Infection of the heart is usually asymptomatic but can be associated with cardiac tamponade or biventricular failure. Infections of the gastrointestinal tract and the liver have been documented.

Congenital Toxoplasmosis

Between 400 and 4000 infants born each year in the United States are affected by congenital toxoplasmosis. Infection of the placenta leads to hematogenous infection of the fetus. As stated earlier, the proportion of fetuses that become infected increases but the clinical severity of the infection declines as gestation proceeds. Persistence of *T. gondii* can ultimately result in reactivation and further damage decades later. Factors associated with relatively severe disabilities include delays in diagnosis and in initiation of therapy, neonatal hypoxia and hypoglycemia, profound visual impairment (see "Ocular Infection," below), uncorrected hydrocephalus, and increased intracranial pressure. If treated appropriately, upwards of 70% of children have normal developmental, neurologic, and ophthalmologic findings at follow-up evaluations. Treatment for 1 year with pyrimethamine and a sulfonamide is tolerated with minimal toxicity (see "Treatment" later in the chapter).

Ocular Infection

Infection with *T. gondii* is estimated to cause 35% of all cases of chorioretinitis in the United States and Europe. Most ocular involvement is believed to be due to congenital infection, with a very low incidence following acquired infection. Between 1 and 3% of all patients with AIDS develop debilitating chorioretinitis due to *T. gondii*. A variety of ocular manifestations are documented, including blurred vision, scotoma, photophobia, and eye pain. Macular involvement occurs with loss of central vision, and nystagmus is secondary to poor fixation. Involvement of the extraocular muscles may lead to disorders of convergence and to strabismus. Ophthalmologic examination should be undertaken in newborns with suspected congenital infection. As the inflammation resolves, vision improves, but episodic flare-ups of chorioretinitis, which progressively destroy retinal tissue and lead to glaucoma, are common.

The ophthalmologic examination reveals yellow-white, cotton-like patches with indistinct margins of hyperemia. As the lesions age, white plaques with distinct borders and black spots within the retinal pigment become more apparent. Lesions usually are located near the posterior pole of the retina; they may be single but are more commonly multiple. Congenital lesions may be unilateral or bilateral and show evidence of massive chorioretinal degeneration with extensive fibrosis. Surrounding these areas of involvement are a normal retina and vasculature. In patients with AIDS, retinal lesions are often large, with diffuse retinal necrosis, and include both free tachyzoites and cysts containing bradyzoites. Toxoplasmic chorioretinitis may be a prodrome to the development of encephalitis.

DIAGNOSIS

Tissue and Body Fluids

The differential diagnosis of acute toxoplasmosis can be made by appropriate culture, serologic testing, and PCR (Table 121-1). Although difficult, the isolation of *T. gondii* from blood or other body fluids can be accomplished after subinoculation of the sample into the peritoneal cavity of mice. Mice should be tested for organisms in the peritoneal fluid 6–10 days after inoculation. If no parasites are found in the mouse's peritoneal fluid, its anti-*Toxoplasma* serum titer can be evaluated 4–6 weeks after inoculation. Isolation of *T. gondii* from the patient's body fluids reflects acute infection, whereas isolation from biopsied tissue is an indication only of the presence of tissue cysts and should not be misinterpreted as evidence of acute toxoplasmosis. Persistent parasitemia in patients with latent, asymptomatic infection is rare. Histologic examination of lymph nodes may suggest the characteristic changes described above. Demonstration of tachyzoites in lymph nodes establishes the diagnosis

TABLE 121-1

DIFFERENTIAL LABORATORY DIAGNOSIS OF TOXOPLASMOSIS

CLINICAL SETTING	ALTERNATIVE DIAGNOSIS	DISTINGUISHING CHARACTERISTICS
Mononucleosis syndrome	Epstein-Barr virus	Serologic test
	Cytomegalovirus	Serologic test
	HIV	Serologic test
Congenital infection	Cytomegalovirus	Viral culture
	Herpes simplex virus	Viral culture
	Rubella virus	Viral culture/serologic test
	Syphilis	Serologic test
	Listeriosis	Bacterial culture
Retinochoroiditis in immuno-competent individual	Tuberculosis	Bacterial culture
	Syphilis	Serologic test
	Histoplasmosis	Serologic test/culture
Retinochoroiditis in AIDS	Cytomegalovirus	Viral culture/PCR
	Syphilis	Serologic test
	Herpes simplex virus	Viral culture/PCR
	Varicella-zoster virus	Viral culture/PCR
	Fungal infection	Culture
CNS lesions in AIDS	Lymphoma or metastatic tumor	Tissue biopsy
	Brain abscess	Bacterial culture
	Progressive multifocal leukoen-cephalopathy	PCR
	Fungal/mycobacterial infection	Biopsy and culture

Source: Adapted from Schwartzman JD: Toxoplasmosis, in *Principles and Practice of Clinical Parasitology.* Hoboken, Wiley, 2001.

of acute toxoplasmosis. Like subinoculation into mice, histologic demonstration of cysts containing bradyzoites confirms prior infection with *T. gondii* but is nondiagnostic for acute infection.

Serology

The procedures just described have great diagnostic value but are limited by difficulties encountered either in the growth of parasites in vivo or in the identification of tachyzoites by histochemical methods. Serologic testing has become the routine method of diagnosis. A wide range of serologic tests that can be used to measure antibody to *T. gondii* are available commercially.

Diagnosis of acute infection with *T. gondii* can be established by detection of the simultaneous presence of IgG and IgM antibodies to *Toxoplasma* in serum. The presence of circulating IgA favors the diagnosis of an acute infection. The Sabin-Feldman dye test, the indirect fluorescent antibody test, and the enzyme-linked immunosorbent assay (ELISA) all satisfactorily measure circulating IgG antibody to *Toxoplasma*. Positive IgG titers (>1:10) can be detected as early as 2–3 weeks after infection. These titers usually peak at 6–8 weeks and decline slowly to a new baseline level that persists for life. It is necessary to measure the serum IgM titer in concert with the IgG titer to better establish the time of infection. The methods currently available for this determination are the double-sandwich IgM-ELISA and the IgM-immunosorbent assay (IgM-ISAGA). Both of these assays are specific and sensitive, and their use precludes the false-positive results associated with tests for rheumatoid factor and antinuclear antibody. The double-sandwich IgA-ELISA is more sensitive than the IgM-ELISA for detecting congenital infection in the fetus and newborn.

Recently, the results obtained with PCR have suggested high sensitivity, specificity, and clinical utility in the diagnosis of TE in resource-poor settings.

Molecular Diagnostics

Molecular approaches can directly detect *T. gondii* in biologic samples independent of the serologic response. Specific molecular analysis for either the B1 gene or the 529-bp sequence is useful. Real-time PCR is a promising technique that can provide quantitative results. Isolates can be genotyped and polymorphic sequences can be obtained, with the consequent identification of the precise strain. Knowledge of the correct sequence is important in studies on the correlation of clinical signs and symptoms of disease with the *T. gondii* genotype.

The Immunocompetent Adult or Child

For the patient who presents with lymphadenopathy only, a positive IgM titer is an indication of acute infection—and an indication for therapy, if that is clinically warranted (see "Treatment" later in the chapter). The serum IgM titer should be determined again in 3 weeks. An elevation in the IgG titer without an increase in the IgM titer suggests that infection is present but is not acute. If there is a borderline increase in either IgG or IgM, the titers should be reassessed in 3–4 weeks.

The Immunocompromised Host

A presumptive clinical diagnosis of TE in patients with AIDS is based on clinical presentation, history of exposure (as evidenced by positive serology), and radiologic evaluation. To detect latent infection with *T. gondii*, HIV-infected persons should be tested for IgG antibody to *Toxoplasma* soon after HIV infection is diagnosed. When these criteria are used, the predictive value is as high as 80%. More than 97% of patients with AIDS and toxoplasmosis have IgG antibody to *T. gondii* in serum. IgM serum antibody usually is not detectable. Attempts to evaluate rising IgG titers or to determine whether IgM is present are not productive. Serologic evidence of infection virtually always precedes the development of TE. It is therefore important to determine the *Toxoplasma* antibody status of all patients infected with HIV. Antibody titers may range from negative to 1:1024 in patients with AIDS and TE. Fewer than 3% of patients have no demonstrable antibody to *Toxoplasma* at diagnosis. Intrathecal antibody to *T. gondii* may be present; determination of the titer may help identify prior infection.

Patients with TE have focal or multifocal abnormalities demonstrable by CT or MRI. Neuroradiologic evaluation should include double-dose contrast CT of the head. By this test, single and frequently multiple contrast-enhancing lesions (<2 cm) may be identified. MRI usually demonstrates multiple lesions located in both hemispheres, with the basal ganglia and corticomedullary junction most commonly involved; MRI provides a more sensitive evaluation of the efficacy of therapy than does CT (Fig. 121-2). These findings are not pathognomonic of *Toxoplasma* infection, since 40% of CNS lymphomas are multifocal and 50% are ring-enhancing. For both MRI and CT scans, the rate of false-negative results is ~10%. The finding of a single lesion on an MRI scan increases the likelihood of primary CNS lymphoma (in which solitary lesions are four times more likely than in TE) and strengthens the argument for the performance of a brain biopsy. A therapeutic trial of anti-*Toxoplasma* medications is frequently used to assess the diagnosis. Treatment of presumptive TE with pyrimethamine plus clindamycin results in quantifiable clinical improvement in >50% of patients by day 3. By day 7, >90% of treated patients show evidence of improvement. In contrast, if patients fail to respond or have lymphoma, clinical signs and symptoms worsen by day 7. Patients in this category require brain biopsy with or without a change in therapy. This procedure can now be performed by a stereotactic CT-guided method that reduces the potential for complications. Brain biopsy for *T. gondii* identifies organisms in 50–75% of cases. PCR amplification of genetic material of the parasite found in the CSF may prove diagnostically beneficial in the future.

Now used in some centers, single-photon emission CT (SPECT) has been touted as a definitive means of detecting or ruling out *Toxoplasma* infection when a

CNS lesion is suspected. In the future, SPECT may well be widely used for this purpose.

As in other conditions, the radiologic response may lag behind the clinical response. Resolution of lesions may take from 3 weeks to 6 months. Some patients show clinical improvement despite worsening radiographic findings.

Congenital Infection

The issue of concern when a pregnant woman has evidence of recent *T. gondii* infection is obviously whether the fetus is infected. PCR analysis of the amniotic fluid for the B1 gene of *T. gondii* has replaced fetal blood sampling. Serologic diagnosis is based on the persistence of IgG antibody or a positive IgM titer after the first week of life (a time frame that excludes placental leak). The IgG determination should be repeated every 2 months. An increase in IgM beyond the first week of life is indicative of acute infection. However, up to 25% of infected newborns may be seronegative and have normal routine physical examinations. Thus assessment of the eye and the brain, with ophthalmologic testing, CSF evaluation, and radiologic studies, is important in establishing the diagnosis.

Ocular Toxoplasmosis

Because of the congenital nature of ocular toxoplasmosis, the serum antibody titer may not correlate with the presence of active lesions in the fundus. In general, a positive IgG titer (measured in undiluted serum if necessary) in conjunction with typical lesions establishes the diagnosis. Antibody production is expressed in terms of the Goldmann-Witmer coefficient (C), in which C = [anti-*Toxoplasma* IgG (aqueous humor/serum)]/[total IgG (serum/aqueous humor)]. The positive cutoff of 3 is the generally accepted discrimination level. The sensitivity of this index as a diagnostic tool lies between 60 and 85%, with a specificity close to 90% in persons of European or North American origin. Confirmation of local specific antibody production in the eye indicates that the site of inflammatory activity is localized to this organ. However, two-thirds of patients without evidence of specific antibody production at initial clinical presentation later develop a detectable titer. If lesions are atypical and the titer is in the low-positive range, the diagnosis is presumptive. The parasitic antigen–specific polyclonal IgG assay as well as parasitic antigen–specific PCR may facilitate the diagnosis. Accordingly, the clinical diagnosis of ocular toxoplasmosis can be supported in 60–90% of cases by laboratory tests, depending on the time of anterior chamber puncture and the panel of antibody analyses used. In the remaining cases, the possibility of a falsely negative laboratory diagnosis or of an incorrect clinical diagnosis cannot be clarified further.

℞ Treatment: TOXOPLASMOSIS

CONGENITAL INFECTION Congenitally infected neonates are treated with daily oral pyrimethamine (0.5–1 mg/kg) and sulfadiazine (100 mg/kg) for 1 year. In addition, therapy with spiramycin (100 mg/kg per day) plus prednisone (1 mg/kg per day) is efficacious for congenital infection.

INFECTION IN IMMUNOCOMPETENT PATIENTS Immunologically competent adults and older children who have only lymphadenopathy do not require specific therapy unless they have persistent, severe symptoms. Patients with ocular toxoplasmosis should be treated for 1 month with pyrimethamine plus either sulfadiazine or clindamycin. Prenatal antibiotic therapy can reduce the number of infants severely affected by *Toxoplasma* infection.

INFECTION IN IMMUNOCOMPROMISED PATIENTS

Primary Prophylaxis Patients with AIDS should be treated for acute toxoplasmosis; in immunocompromised patients, toxoplasmosis is rapidly fatal if untreated. Before the introduction of antiretroviral therapy (ART), the median survival time was >1 year for patients who could tolerate treatment for TE. Despite their toxicity, the drugs used to treat TE were required for survival prior to ART. The incidence of TE has declined as survival of patients with HIV infection has increased as a result of ART.

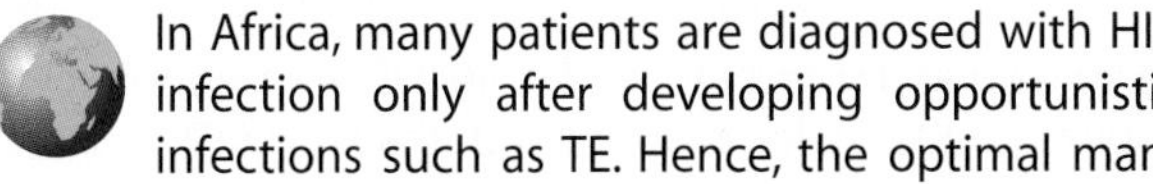

In Africa, many patients are diagnosed with HIV infection only after developing opportunistic infections such as TE. Hence, the optimal management of these opportunistic infections is important if the benefits of subsequent ART are to be realized. AIDS patients who are seropositive for *T. gondii* and who have a CD4+ T-lymphocyte count of <100/μL should receive prophylaxis against TE. A recent Cochrane analysis of clinical trials of TE treatment failed to document the superiority of any one regimen. Of the currently available agents, trimethoprim-sulfamethoxazole (TMP-SMX) appears to be an effective alternative for TE in resource-poor settings where the preferred combination of pyrimethamine plus sulfadiazine is not available. The daily dose of TMP-SMX recommended as the preferred regimen for PcP prophylaxis (one double-strength tablet) is effective against TE. If patients cannot tolerate TMP-SMX, the recommended alternative is dapsone-pyrimethamine, which is also effective against PcP. Atovaquone with or without pyrimethamine also can be considered. Prophylactic monotherapy with dapsone, pyrimethamine, azithromycin, clarithromycin, or aerosolized pentamidine is probably insufficient. AIDS patients who are seronegative for *Toxoplasma* and are not receiving prophylaxis for PcP should be retested for IgG antibody to *Toxoplasma* if their CD4+ T-cell count drops to <100/μL. If seroconversion has taken place, then the patient should be given prophylaxis as described above.

Discontinuing Primary Prophylaxis Some current studies indicate that prophylaxis against TE can be discontinued in patients who have responded to ART and whose CD4+ T-lymphocyte count has been >200/μL for 3 months. Although patients with CD4+ T-lymphocyte counts of <100/μL are at greatest risk for developing TE, the risk that this condition will develop when the count has increased to 100–200/μL has not been established. Thus, prophylaxis should indeed be discontinued only when the count has increased to >200/μL. Continued prophylaxis at a CD4+ count of >200/μL has only a limited preventive effect against TE. Discontinuation of therapy reduces the pill burden; the potential for drug toxicity, drug interaction, or selection of drug-resistant pathogens; and cost. Prophylaxis should be recommenced if the CD4+ T-lymphocyte count again decreases to <100–200/μL.

Individuals who have completed initial therapy for TE should receive treatment indefinitely unless immune reconstitution, with a CD4+ T-cell count of >200/μL, occurs as a consequence of ART. Combination therapy with pyrimethamine plus sulfadiazine plus leucovorin is effective for this purpose. An alternative to sulfadiazine in this regimen is clindamycin. Unfortunately, only the combination of pyrimethamine plus sulfadiazine provides protection against PcP as well.

Discontinuing Secondary Prophylaxis (Chronic Maintenance Therapy) Patients receiving secondary prophylaxis for TE are at low risk for recurrence when they have completed initial therapy for TE, remain asymptomatic, and have a CD4+ T-lymphocyte count of >200/μL for at least 6 months after ART. This recommendation is based on recent observations in a large cohort (381 patients) and is consistent with more extensive data indicating the safety of discontinuing secondary prophylaxis for other opportunistic infections during advanced HIV disease. Discontinuation of chronic maintenance therapy among these patients appears reasonable. A repeat MRI brain scan is recommended. Secondary prophylaxis should be reintroduced if the CD4+ T-lymphocyte count decreases to <200/μL.

PREVENTION

All HIV-infected persons, including those who lack IgG antibody to *Toxoplasma*, should be counseled regarding sources of *Toxoplasma* infection. The chances of primary infection with *Toxoplasma* can be reduced by not eating undercooked meat and by avoiding oocyst-contaminated material (i.e., a cat's litter box). Specifically, lamb, beef, and pork should be cooked to an internal temperature of 165°–170°F; from a more practical perspective, meat cooked until it is no longer pink inside usually satisfies this requirement. Hands should be washed thoroughly after work in the garden, and all fruits and vegetables should be washed. If the patient owns a cat, the litter box should be cleaned or changed daily, preferably by an HIV-negative, nonpregnant person; alternatively, patients should wash their hands thoroughly after changing the litter box. Patients should be encouraged to keep their cats inside and not to adopt or handle stray cats. Cats should be fed only canned or dried commercial food or well-cooked table food, not raw or undercooked meats. Patients need not be advised to part with their cats or to have their cats tested for toxoplasmosis. Blood intended for transfusion into *Toxoplasma*-seronegative immunocompromised individuals should be screened for antibody to *T. gondii*. Although such serologic screening is not routinely performed, seronegative women should be screened for evidence of infection several times during pregnancy if they are exposed to environmental conditions that put them at risk for infection with *T. gondii*. HIV-positive individuals should adhere closely to these preventive measures.

FURTHER READINGS

Dedicoat M: Management of toxoplasmic encephalitis in HIV-infected adults (with an emphasis on resource-poor settings). Cochrane Database Syst Rev 3:CD005420, 2006

Garweg JG: Determinants of immunodiagnostic success in human ocular toxoplasmosis. Parasite Immunol 27:61, 2005

Jones JL et al: *Toxoplasma gondii* infection in the United States, 1999–2004, decline from the prior decade. Am J Trop Med Hyg 77:405, 2007

Lehmann T et al: Globalization and the population structure of *Toxoplasma gondii*. Proc Natl Acad Sci USA 103:11423, 2006

Masur H et al: Guidelines for preventing opportunistic infections among HIV-infected persons—2002. Ann Intern Med 137:435, 2002

McLeod R et al: Outcome of treatment for congenital toxoplasmosis, 1981–2004: The National Collaborative Chicago-Based, Congenital Toxoplasmosis Study. Clin Infect Dis 42:1383, 2006

Miro JM et al: Discontinuation of primary and secondary *Toxoplasma gondii* prophylaxis is safe in HIV-infected patients after immunological restoration with highly active antiretroviral therapy: Results of an open, randomized, multicenter clinical trial. Clin Infect Dis 43:79, 2006

Mocroft A et al: Decline in the AIDS and death rates in the EuroSIDA study: An observational study. Lancet 362:22, 2003

Schmidt DR et al: The national neonatal screening programme for congenital toxoplasmosis in Denmark: Results from the initial four years, 1999–2002. Arch Dis Child 91:661, 2006

Switaj K et al: Recent trends in molecular diagnostics for *Toxoplasma gondii* infections. Clin Microbiol Infect 11:170, 2005

SYROCOT (Systematic Review on Congenital Toxoplasmosis) Study Group et al: Effectiveness of prenatal treatment for congenital toxoplasmosis: a meta-analysis of individual patients' data. Lancet 369:115, 2007

Tan HK et al: Risk of visual impairment in children with congenital toxoplasmic retinochoroiditis. Am J Ophthalmol 144:648, 2007

CHAPTER 122

PROTOZOAL INTESTINAL INFECTIONS AND TRICHOMONIASIS

Peter F. Weller

PROTOZOAL INFECTIONS

GIARDIASIS

Giardia lamblia (also known as *G. intestinalis*) is a cosmopolitan protozoal parasite that inhabits the small intestines of humans and other mammals.

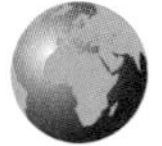

Giardiasis is one of the most common parasitic diseases in both developed and developing countries worldwide, causing both endemic and epidemic intestinal disease and diarrhea.

Life Cycle and Epidemiology

(Fig. 122-1) Infection follows the ingestion of environmentally hardy cysts, which excyst in the small intestine, releasing flagellated trophozoites (Fig. 122-2) that multiply by binary fission. *Giardia* remains a pathogen of the proximal small bowel and does not disseminate hematogenously. Trophozoites remain free in the lumen or attach to the mucosal epithelium by means of a ventral sucking disk. As a trophozoite encounters altered conditions, it forms a morphologically distinct cyst, which is the stage of the parasite usually found in the feces. Trophozoites may be present and even predominate in loose or watery stools, but it is the resistant cyst that survives outside the body and is responsible for transmission. Cysts do not tolerate heating, desiccation, or continued exposure to feces but do remain viable for months in cold fresh water. The number of cysts excreted varies widely but can approach 10^7 per gram of stool.

Ingestion of as few as 10 cysts is sufficient to cause infection in humans. Because cysts are infectious when excreted, person-to-person transmission occurs where fecal hygiene is poor. Giardiasis, as symptomatic or asymptomatic infections, is especially prevalent in day-care centers; person-to-person spread also takes place in other institutional settings with poor fecal hygiene and during anal-oral contact. If food is contaminated with *Giardia* cysts after cooking or preparation, food-borne transmission can occur. Waterborne transmission accounts for episodic infections (e.g., in campers and travelers) and for major epidemics in metropolitan areas. Surface water, ranging from mountain streams to large municipal reservoirs, can become contaminated with fecally derived *Giardia* cysts; outmoded water systems are subject to cross-contamination from leaking sewer lines. The efficacy of water as a means of transmission is enhanced by the small infectious inoculum of *Giardia*, the prolonged survival of cysts in cold water, and the resistance of cysts to killing by routine chlorination methods that are adequate

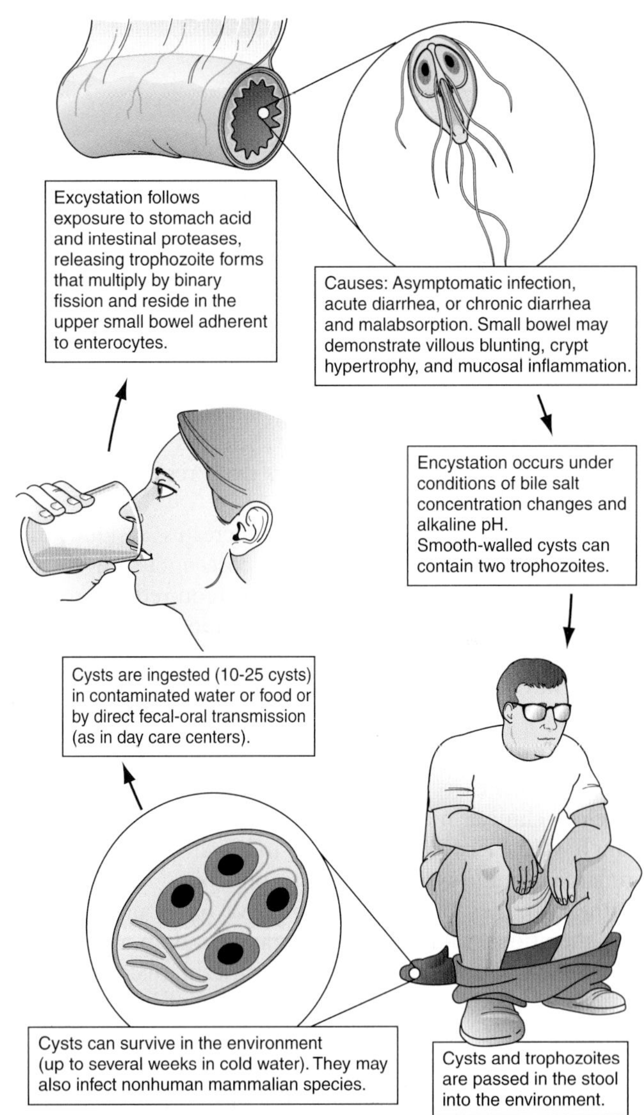

Excystation follows exposure to stomach acid and intestinal proteases, releasing trophozoite forms that multiply by binary fission and reside in the upper small bowel adherent to enterocytes.
Causes: Asymptomatic infection, acute diarrhea, or chronic diarrhea and malabsorption. Small bowel may demonstrate villous blunting, crypt hypertrophy, and mucosal inflammation.
Encystation occurs under conditions of bile salt concentration changes and alkaline pH. Smooth-walled cysts can contain two trophozoites.
Cysts are ingested (10-25 cysts) in contaminated water or food or by direct fecal-oral transmission (as in day care centers).
Cysts can survive in the environment (up to several weeks in cold water). They may also infect nonhuman mammalian species.
Cysts and trophozoites are passed in the stool into the environment.

FIGURE 122-1

Life cycle of *Giardia*. *(Reprinted from RL Guerrant et al: Tropical Infectious Disease: Principles, Pathogens and Practice, 2d ed, 2006, p 987, with permission from Elsevier Science.)*

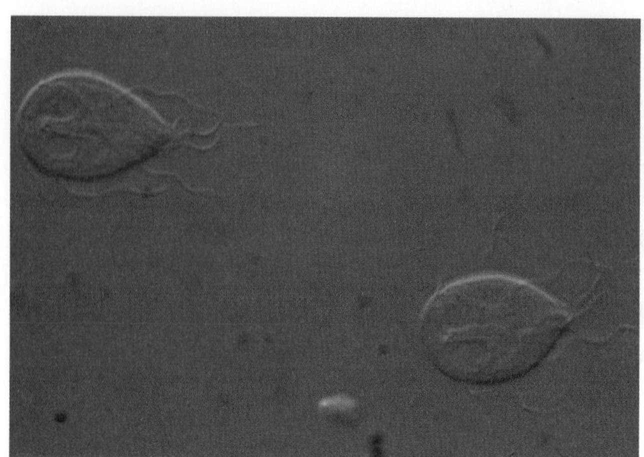

FIGURE 122-2
Flagellated, binucleate ***Giardia*** **trophozoite.**

for controlling bacteria. Viable cysts can be eradicated from water by either boiling or filtration. In the United States, *Giardia* (like *Cryptosporidium*; see below) is a common cause of waterborne epidemics of gastroenteritis. *Giardia* is common in developing countries, and infections may be acquired by travelers.

The importance of animal reservoirs as sources of infection for humans is unclear. *Giardia* parasites morphologically similar to those in humans are found in many mammals, including beavers from reservoirs implicated in epidemics, dogs, and cats.

Giardiasis, like cryptosporidiosis, creates a significant economic burden because of the costs incurred in the installation of water filtration systems required to prevent waterborne epidemics, in the management of epidemics that involve large communities, and in the evaluation and treatment of endemic infections.

Pathophysiology

The reasons that some, but not all, infected patients develop clinical manifestations and the mechanisms by which *Giardia* causes alterations in small-bowel function are largely unknown. Although trophozoites adhere to the epithelium, they do not cause invasive or locally destructive alterations. The lactose intolerance and, in a minority of infected adults and children, significant malabsorption that develop are clinical signs of the loss of brush-border enzyme activities. In most infections, the morphology of the bowel is unaltered; however, in a few cases (usually in chronically infected, symptomatic patients), the histopathologic findings (including flattened villi) and the clinical manifestations resemble those of tropical sprue and gluten-sensitive enteropathy. The pathogenesis of diarrhea in giardiasis is not known.

The natural history of *Giardia* infection varies markedly. Infections may be aborted, transient, recurrent, or chronic. Parasite as well as host factors may be important in determining the course of infection and disease. Both cellular and humoral responses develop in human infections, but their precise roles in the control of infection and/or disease are unknown. Because patients with hypogammaglobulinemia suffer from prolonged, severe infections that are poorly responsive to treatment, humoral immune responses appear to be important. The greater susceptibility of the young than of the old and of newly exposed persons than of chronically exposed populations suggests that at least partial protective immunity may develop. *Giardia* isolates vary genotypically, biochemically, and biologically, and variations among isolates may contribute to different courses of infection.

Clinical Manifestations

Disease manifestations of giardiasis range from asymptomatic carriage to fulminant diarrhea and malabsorption. Most infected persons are asymptomatic, but in epidemics the proportion of symptomatic cases may be higher. Symptoms may develop suddenly or gradually. In persons with acute giardiasis, symptoms develop after an incubation period that lasts at least 5–6 days and usually 1–3 weeks. Prominent early symptoms include diarrhea, abdominal pain, bloating, belching, flatus, nausea, and vomiting. Although diarrhea is common, upper intestinal manifestations such as nausea, vomiting, bloating, and abdominal pain may predominate. The duration of acute giardiasis is usually >1 week, although diarrhea often subsides. Individuals with chronic giardiasis may present with or without having experienced an antecedent acute symptomatic episode. Diarrhea is not necessarily prominent, but increased flatus, loose stools, sulfurous belching, and (in some instances) weight loss occur. Symptoms may be continual or episodic and can persist for years. Some persons who have relatively mild symptoms for long periods recognize the extent of their discomfort only in retrospect. Fever, the presence of blood and/or mucus in the stools, and other signs and symptoms of colitis are uncommon and suggest a different diagnosis or a concomitant illness. Symptoms tend to be intermittent yet recurring and gradually debilitating, in contrast with the acute disabling symptoms associated with many enteric bacterial infections. Because of the less severe illness and the propensity for chronic infections, patients may seek medical advice late in the course of the illness; however, disease can be severe, resulting in malabsorption, weight loss, growth retardation, and dehydration. A number of extraintestinal manifestations have been described, such as urticaria, anterior uveitis, and arthritis; whether these are caused by giardiasis or concomitant processes is unclear.

Giardiasis can be severe in patients with hypogammaglobulinemia and can complicate other preexisting intestinal diseases, such as that occurring in cystic fibrosis. In patients with AIDS, *Giardia* can cause enteric illness that is refractory to treatment.

Diagnosis

(Table 122-1) Giardiasis is diagnosed by detection of parasite antigens in the feces or by identification of cysts in the feces or of trophozoites in the feces or small intestines. Cysts are oval, measure 8–12 μm × 7–10 μm, and characteristically contain four nuclei. Trophozoites are pear-shaped, dorsally convex, flattened parasites with

TABLE 122-1

DIAGNOSIS OF INTESTINAL PROTOZOAL INFECTIONS

PARASITE	STOOL O+P[a]	FECAL ACID-FAST STAIN	STOOL ANTIGEN IMMUNO-ASSAYS	OTHER
Giardia	+		+	
Cryptosporidium	–	+	+	
Isospora	–	+		
Cyclospora	–	+		
Microsporidia	–			Special fecal stains, tissue biopsies

[a]O+P, ova and parasites.

two nuclei and four pairs of flagella (Fig. 122-2). The diagnosis is sometimes difficult to establish. Direct examination of fresh or properly preserved stools as well as concentration methods should be used. Because cyst excretion is variable and may be undetectable at times, repeated examination of stool, sampling of duodenal fluid, and biopsy of the small intestine may be required to detect the parasite. Tests for parasitic antigens in stool are at least as sensitive and specific as good microscopic examinations and are easier to perform. All of these methods occasionally yield false-negative results.

℞ Treatment: GIARDIASIS

Cure rates with metronidazole (250 mg thrice daily for 5 days) are usually >90%. Tinidazole (2 g once by mouth) is reportedly more effective than metronidazole. Nitazoxanide (500 mg twice daily for 3 days) is an alternative agent for treatment of giardiasis. Paromomycin, an oral aminoglycoside that is not well absorbed, can be given to symptomatic pregnant patients, although information is limited on how effectively this agent eradicates infection.

Almost all patients respond to therapy and are cured, although some with chronic giardiasis experience delayed resolution of symptoms after eradication of *Giardia*. For many of the latter patients, residual symptoms probably reflect delayed regeneration of intestinal brush-border enzymes. Continued infection should be documented by stool examinations before treatment is repeated. Patients who remain infected after repeated treatments should be evaluated for reinfection through family members, close personal contacts, and environmental sources as well as for hypogammaglobulinemia. In cases refractory to multiple treatment courses, prolonged therapy with metronidazole (750 mg thrice daily for 21 days) has been successful.

Prevention

Although *Giardia* is extremely infectious, disease can be prevented by consumption of noncontaminated food and water and by personal hygiene when caring for infected children. Boiling or filtering potentially contaminated water prevents infection.

CRYPTOSPORIDIOSIS

The coccidian parasite *Cryptosporidium* causes diarrheal disease that is self-limited in immunocompetent human hosts but can be severe in persons with AIDS or other forms of immunodeficiency. Two species of *Cryptosporidium, C. hominis* and *C. parvum,* cause most human infections.

Life Cycle and Epidemiology

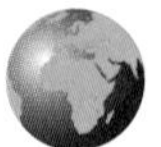

Cryptosporidium species are widely distributed in the world. Cryptosporidiosis is acquired by the consumption of oocysts (50% infectious dose: ~132 oocysts in nonimmune individuals), which excyst to liberate sporozoites that in turn enter and infect intestinal epithelial cells. The parasite's further development involves both asexual and sexual cycles, which produce forms capable of infecting other epithelial cells and of generating oocysts that are passed in the feces. *Cryptosporidium* species infect a number of animals, and *C. parvum* can spread from infected animals to humans. Since oocysts are immediately infectious when passed in feces, person-to-person transmission takes place in day-care centers and among household contacts and medical providers. Waterborne transmission (especially that of *C. hominis*) accounts for infections in travelers and for common-source epidemics. Oocysts are quite hardy and resist killing by routine chlorination. Both drinking water and recreational water (e.g., pools, waterslides) have been increasingly recognized as sources of infection.

Pathophysiology

Although intestinal epithelial cells harbor cryptosporidia in an intracellular vacuole, the means by which secretory diarrhea is elicited remain uncertain. No characteristic pathologic changes are found by biopsy. The distribution of infection can be spotty within the principal site of infection, the small bowel. Cryptosporidia are found in the pharynx, stomach, and large bowel of some patients and at times in the respiratory tract. Especially in patients with AIDS, involvement of the biliary tract can cause papillary stenosis, sclerosing cholangitis, or cholecystitis.

Clinical Manifestations

Asymptomatic infections can occur in both immunocompetent and immunocompromised hosts. In immunocompetent persons, symptoms develop after an incubation period of ~1 week and consist principally of watery nonbloody diarrhea, sometimes in conjunction with abdominal pain, nausea, anorexia, fever, and/or weight loss. In these hosts, the illness usually subsides after 1–2 weeks. In contrast, in immunocompromised hosts (especially those with AIDS and CD4+ T cell counts <100/μL), diarrhea can be chronic, persistent, and remarkably profuse, causing clinically significant fluid and electrolyte depletion. Stool volumes may range from 1 to 25 L/d. Weight loss, wasting, and abdominal pain may be severe. Biliary tract involvement can manifest as midepigastric or right upper quadrant pain.

Diagnosis

(Table 122-1) Evaluation starts with fecal examination for small oocysts, which are smaller (4–5 μm in diameter) than the fecal stages of most other parasites. Because conventional stool examination for ova and parasites does not detect *Cryptosporidium*, specific testing must be requested. Detection is enhanced by evaluation of stools (obtained on multiple days) by several techniques, including modified acid-fast and direct immunofluorescent stains and enzyme immunoassays. Cryptosporidia can also be identified by light and electron microscopy at the apical surfaces of intestinal epithelium from biopsy specimens of the small bowel and, less frequently, the large bowel.

℞ Treatment: CRYPTOSPORIDIOSIS

Nitazoxanide is approved by the U.S. Food and Drug Administration for the treatment of cryptosporidiosis and is available in tablet form for adults (500 mg twice daily for 3 days) and as an elixir for children. To date, however, this agent has not been effective for the treatment of HIV-infected patients, in whom improved immune status due to antiretroviral therapy can lead to amelioration of cryptosporidiosis. Otherwise, treatment includes supportive care with replacement of fluids and electrolytes and administration of antidiarrheal agents. Biliary tract obstruction may require papillotomy or T-tube placement. Prevention requires minimizing exposure to infectious oocysts in human or animal feces. Use of submicron water filters may minimize acquisition of infection from drinking water.

ISOSPORIASIS

The coccidian parasite *Isospora belli* causes human intestinal disease. Infection is acquired by the consumption of oocysts, after which the parasite invades intestinal epithelial cells and undergoes both sexual and asexual cycles of development. Oocysts excreted in stool are not immediately infectious but must undergo further maturation.

Although *I. belli* infects many animals, little is known about the epidemiology or prevalence of this parasite in humans. It appears to be most common in tropical and subtropical countries. Acute infections can begin abruptly with fever, abdominal pain, and watery nonbloody diarrhea and can last for weeks or months. In patients who have AIDS or are immunocompromised for other reasons, infections often are not self-limited but rather resemble cryptosporidiosis, with chronic, profuse watery diarrhea. Eosinophilia, which is not found in other enteric protozoan infections, may be detectable. The diagnosis (Table 122-1) is usually made by detection of the large (~25-μm) oocysts in stool by modified acid-fast staining. Oocyst excretion may be low-level and intermittent; if repeated stool examinations are unrevealing, sampling of duodenal contents by aspiration or small-bowel biopsy (often with electron-microscopic examination) may be necessary.

℞ Treatment: ISOSPORIASIS

Trimethoprim-sulfamethoxazole (TMP-SMX; 160/800 mg four times daily for 10 days, and for HIV-infected patients, then three times daily for 3 weeks) is effective. For patients intolerant of sulfonamides, pyrimethamine (50–75 mg/d) can be used. Relapses can occur in persons with AIDS and necessitate maintenance therapy with TMP-SMX (160/800 mg three times per week).

CYCLOSPORIASIS

Cyclospora cayetanensis, a cause of diarrheal illness, is globally distributed: illness due to *C. cayetanensis* has been reported in the United States, Asia, Africa, Latin America, and Europe. The epidemiology of this parasite has not yet been fully defined, but waterborne transmission and food-borne transmission by basil and imported raspberries have been recognized. The full spectrum of illness attributable to *Cyclospora* has not been delineated. Some patients may harbor the infection without symptoms, but many have diarrhea, flulike symptoms, and flatulence and belching. The illness can be self-limited, can wax and wane, or in many cases can involve prolonged diarrhea, anorexia, and upper gastrointestinal symptoms, with sustained fatigue and weight loss in some instances. Diarrheal illness may persist for >1 month. *Cyclospora* can cause enteric illness in patients infected with HIV.

The parasite is detectable in epithelial cells of small-bowel biopsy samples and elicits secretory diarrhea by unknown means. The absence of fecal blood and leukocytes indicates that disease due to *Cyclospora* is not caused by destruction of the small-bowel mucosa. The diagnosis (Table 122-1) can be made by detection of spherical 8- to 10-μm oocysts in the stool, although routine stool O and P examinations are not sufficient. Specific fecal examinations must be requested to detect the oocysts, which are variably acid-fast and are fluorescent when viewed with ultraviolet light microscopy. Cyclosporiasis should be considered in the differential diagnosis of prolonged diarrhea, with or without a history of travel by the patient to other countries.

℞ Treatment: CYCLOSPORIASIS

Cyclosporiasis is treated with TMP-SMX (160/800 mg twice daily for 7 days). HIV-infected patients may experience relapses after such treatment and thus may require longer-term suppressive maintenance therapy.

MICROSPORIDIOSIS

Microsporidia are obligate intracellular spore-forming protozoa that infect many animals and cause disease in humans, especially as opportunistic pathogens in AIDS. Microsporidia are members of a distinct phylum, Microspora, which contains dozens of genera and hundreds of species. The various microsporidia are differentiated by their developmental life cycles, ultrastructural features, and molecular taxonomy based on ribosomal RNA. The complex life cycles of the organisms result in the production of infectious spores (Fig. 122-3). Currently, eight genera of microsporidia—*Encephalitozoon, Pleistophora, Nosema, Vittaforma, Trachipleistophora, Brachiola, Microsporidium,* and *Enterocytozoon*—are recognized as causes of human disease. Although some microsporidia are probably prevalent causes of self-limited or asymptomatic infections in immunocompetent patients, little is known about how microsporidiosis is acquired.

Microsporidiosis is most common among patients with AIDS, less common among patients with other types of immunocompromise, and rare among immunocompetent hosts. In patients with AIDS, intestinal infections with *Enterocytozoon bieneusi* and *Encephalitozoon* (formerly *Septata*) *intestinalis* are recognized to contribute to chronic diarrhea and wasting; these infections are found in 10–40% of patients with chronic diarrhea. Both organisms have been found in the biliary tracts of patients with cholecystitis. *E. intestinalis* may also disseminate to cause fever, diarrhea, sinusitis, cholangitis, and bronchiolitis. In patients with AIDS, *Encephalitozoon hellem* has caused superficial keratoconjunctivitis as well as sinusitis, respiratory tract disease, and disseminated infection. Myositis due to *Pleistophora* has been documented. *Nosema, Vittaforma,* and *Microsporidium* have caused stromal keratitis associated with trauma in immunocompetent patients.

Microsporidia are small gram-positive organisms with mature spores measuring 0.5–2 μm × 1–4 μm. Diagnosis of microsporidial infections in tissue often requires electron microscopy, although intracellular spores can be visualized by light microscopy with hematoxylin and eosin, Giemsa, or tissue Gram's stain. For the diagnosis of intestinal microsporidiosis, modified trichrome or chromotrope

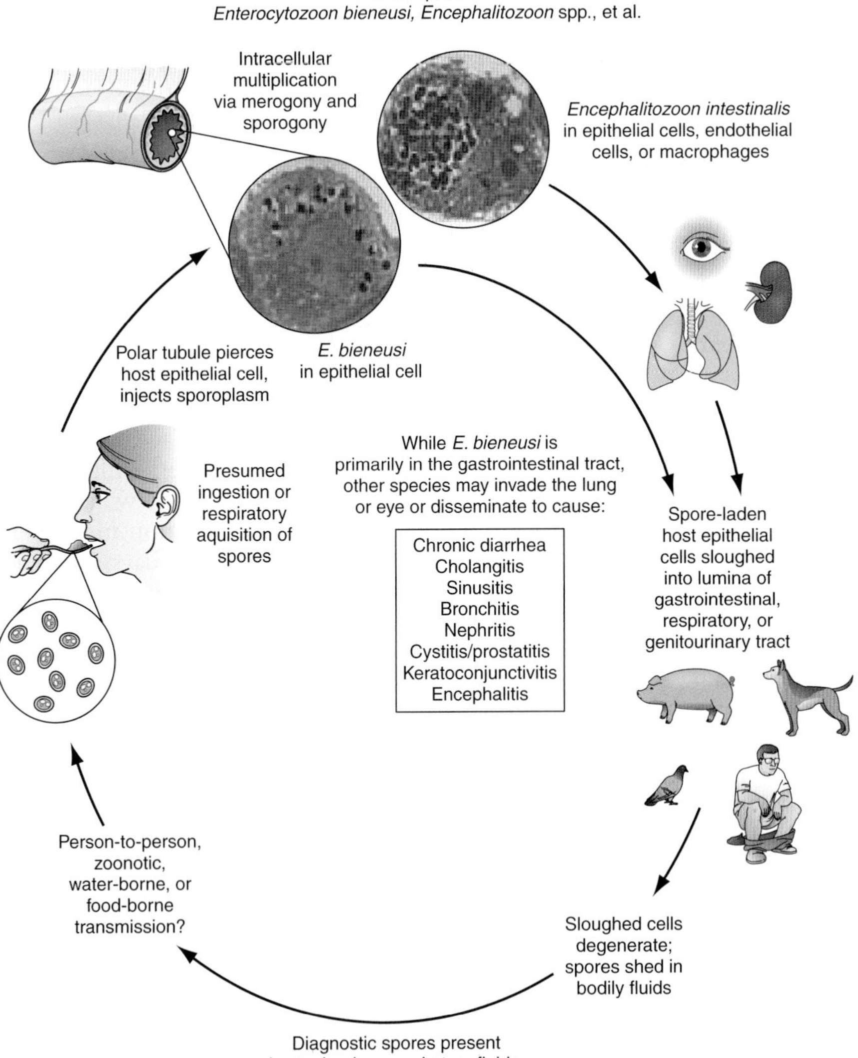

FIGURE 122-3

Life cycle of microsporidia. *(Reprinted from RL Guerrant et al: Tropical Infectious Disease: Principles, Pathogens and Practice, 2d ed, 2006, p 1128, with permission from Elsevier Science.)*

2R-based staining and Uvitex 2B or calcofluor fluorescent staining reveal spores in smears of feces or duodenal aspirates. Definitive therapies for microsporidial infections remain to be established. For superficial keratoconjunctivitis due to *E. hellem*, topical therapy with fumagillin suspension has shown promise (Chap. 113). For enteric infections with *E. bieneusi* and *E. intestinalis* in HIV-infected patients, therapy with albendazole may be efficacious (Chap. 113).

OTHER INTESTINAL PROTOZOA

Balantidiasis

Balantidium coli is a large ciliated protozoal parasite that can produce a spectrum of large-intestinal disease analogous to amebiasis.

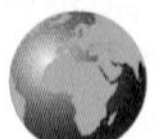

The parasite is widely distributed in the world. Since it infects pigs, cases in humans are more common where pigs are raised. Infective cysts can be transmitted from person to person and through water, but many cases are due to the ingestion of cysts derived from porcine feces in association with slaughtering, with use of pig feces for fertilizer, or with contamination of water supplies by pig feces.

Ingested cysts liberate trophozoites, which reside and replicate in the large bowel. Many patients remain asymptomatic, but some have persisting intermittent diarrhea, and a few develop more fulminant dysentery. In symptomatic individuals, the pathology in the bowel—both gross and microscopic—is similar to that seen in amebiasis, with varying degrees of mucosal invasion, focal necrosis, and ulceration. Balantidiasis, unlike amebiasis, does not spread hematogenously to other organs. The diagnosis is made by detection of the trophozoite stage in stool or sampled colonic tissue. Tetracycline (500 mg four times daily for 10 days) is an effective therapeutic agent.

Blastocystis Hominis *Infection*

B. hominis, while believed by some to be a protozoan capable of causing intestinal disease, remains an organism of uncertain pathogenicity. Some patients who pass *B. hominis* in their stools are asymptomatic, whereas others have diarrhea and associated intestinal symptoms. Diligent evaluation reveals other potential bacterial, viral, or protozoal causes of diarrhea in some but not all patients with symptoms. Because the pathogenicity of *B. hominis* is uncertain and because therapy for *Blastocystis* infection is neither specific nor uniformly effective, patients with prominent intestinal symptoms should be fully evaluated for other infectious causes of diarrhea. If diarrheal symptoms associated with *Blastocystis* are prominent, either metronidazole (750 mg thrice daily for 10 days) or TMP-SMX (160 mg/800 mg twice daily for 7 days) can be used.

Dientamoeba Fragilis *Infection*

D. fragilis is unique among intestinal protozoa in that it has a trophozoite stage but not a cyst stage. How trophozoites survive to transmit infection is not known. When symptoms develop in patients with *D. fragilis* infection, they are generally mild and include intermittent diarrhea, abdominal pain, and anorexia. The diagnosis is made by the detection of trophozoites in stool; the lability of these forms accounts for the greater yield when fecal samples are preserved immediately after collection. Since fecal excretion rates vary, examination of several samples obtained on alternate days increases the rate of detection. Iodoquinol (650 mg three times daily for 20 days), paromomycin (25–35 mg/kg per day in three doses for 7 days), metronidazole (500–750 mg three times daily for 10 days), or tetracycline (500 mg four times daily for 10 days) is appropriate for treatment.

TRICHOMONIASIS

Various species of trichomonads can be found in the mouth (in association with periodontitis) and occasionally in the gastrointestinal tract. *Trichomonas vaginalis*—one of the most prevalent protozoal parasites in the United States—is a pathogen of the genitourinary tract and a major cause of symptomatic vaginitis.

LIFE CYCLE AND EPIDEMIOLOGY

T. vaginalis is a pear-shaped, actively motile organism that measures about 10 × 7 μm, replicates by binary fission, and inhabits the lower genital tract of females and the urethra and prostate of males. In the United States, it accounts for ~3 million infections per year in women. While the organism can survive for a few hours in moist environments and could be acquired by direct contact, person-to-person venereal transmission accounts for virtually all cases of trichomoniasis. Its prevalence is greatest among persons with multiple sexual partners and among those with other sexually transmitted diseases (Chap. 28).

CLINICAL MANIFESTATIONS

Many men infected with *T. vaginalis* are asymptomatic, although some develop urethritis and a few have epididymitis or prostatitis. In contrast, infection in women, which has an incubation period of 5–28 days, is usually symptomatic and manifests with malodorous vaginal discharge (often yellow), vulvar erythema and itching, dysuria or urinary frequency (in 30–50% of patients), and dyspareunia. These manifestations, however, do not clearly distinguish trichomoniasis from other types of infectious vaginitis.

DIAGNOSIS

Detection of motile trichomonads by microscopic examination of wet mounts of vaginal or prostatic secretions has been the conventional means of diagnosis. Although this approach provides an immediate diagnosis, its sensitivity for the detection of *T. vaginalis* is only ~50–60% in routine evaluations of vaginal secretions. Direct immunofluorescent antibody staining is more sensitive (70–90%) than wet-mount examinations. *T. vaginalis* can be recovered from the urethra of both males and females and is detectable in males after prostatic massage. Culture of the parasite is the most sensitive means of detection; however, the facilities for culture are not generally available, and detection of the organism takes 3–7 days.

℞ Treatment: TRICHOMONIASIS

Metronidazole, given either as a single 2-g dose or in 500-mg doses twice daily for 7 days, is usually effective. Tinidazole (a single 2-g dose) is also effective. All sexual partners must be treated concurrently to prevent reinfection, especially from asymptomatic males. In males with persistent symptomatic urethritis after therapy for nongonococcal urethritis, metronidazole therapy should be considered for possible trichomoniasis. Alternatives to metronidazole for treatment during pregnancy are not readily available, although use of 100-mg clotrimazole vaginal suppositories nightly for 2 weeks may cure some infections in pregnant women. Reinfection often accounts for apparent treatment failures, but strains of *T. vaginalis* exhibiting high-level resistance to metronidazole have been encountered. Treatment of these resistant infections with higher oral doses, parenteral doses, or concurrent oral and vaginal doses of metronidazole or with tinidazole has been successful.

FURTHER READINGS

Centers for Disease Control and Prevention, Division of Parasitic Diseases: *http://www.cdc.gov/ncidod/dpd/default.htm*

Chex XM et al: Cryptosporidiosis. N Engl J Med 346:1723, 2002

Didier ES: Microsporidiosis: An emerging and opportunistic infection in humans and animals. Acta Trop 94:61, 2005

Hlavsa MC et al: Giardiasis surveillance—United States, 1998–2002. MMWR Surveill Summ 54:9, 2005

——— et al: Cryptosporidiosis surveillance—United States, 1999–2002. MMWR Surveill Summ 54:1, 2005

Leder K et al: No correlation between clinical symptoms and *Blastocystis hominis* in immunocompetent individuals. J Gastroenterol Hepatol 20:1390, 2005

Pattullo L et al: Stepwise diagnosis of *Trichomonas vaginalis* infection in adolescent women. J Clin Microbiol 47:59, 2009

Pierce KK, Kirkpatrick BD: Update on human infections caused by intestinal protozoa. Curr Opin Gastroenterol 25:12, 2009

Roxstrom-Lindquist K et al: Giardia immunity—an update. Trends Parasitol 22:26, 2006

Shafir SC et al: Current issues and considerations regarding trichomoniasis and human immunodeficiency virus in African-Americans. Clin Microbiol Rev 22:37, 2009

Sutton M et al: The prevalence of *Trichomonas vaginalis* infection among reproductive-age women in the United States, 2001–2004. Clin Infect Dis 45:1319, 2007

Vandenberg O et al: Clinical and microbiological features of dientamoebiasis in patients suspected of suffering from a parasitic gastrointestinal illness: A comparison of *Dientamoeba fragilis* and *Giardia lamblia* infections. Int J Infect Dis 10:255, 2006

Van Der Pol B et al: Prevalence, incidence, natural history, and response to treatment of *Trichomonas vaginalis* infection among adolescent women. J Infect Dis 192:2039, 2005

Weiss LM, Schwartz DA: Microsporidiosis, in *Tropical Infectious Diseases: Principles, Pathogens and Practice*, 2d ed, RL Guerrant et al (eds). Elsevier, Philadelphia, 2006, pp 1126–1140

Weitzel T et al: Epidemiological and clinical features of travel-associated cryptosporidiosis. Clin Microbiol Infect 12:921, 2006

Yoder JS, Beach MJ: Cryptosporidiosis surveillance—United States, 2003–2005. MMWR Surveill Summ 56:1, 2007

——— et al: Giardiasis surveillance—United States, 2003–2005. MMWR Surveill Summ 56:11, 2007

PART 3 HELMINTHIC INFECTIONS

CHAPTER 123

TRICHINELLA AND OTHER TISSUE NEMATODES

Peter F. Weller

Nematodes are elongated, symmetric roundworms. Parasitic nematodes of medical significance may be broadly classified as either predominantly intestinal or tissue nematodes. This chapter covers trichinellosis, visceral and ocular larva migrans, cutaneous larva migrans, cerebral angiostrongyliasis, and gnathostomiasis. All are zoonotic infections caused by incidental exposure to infectious nematodes. The clinical symptoms of these infections are due largely to invasive larval stages that (except in the case of *Trichinella*) do not reach maturity in humans.

TRICHINELLOSIS

Trichinellosis develops after the ingestion of meat containing cysts of *Trichinella*—for example, pork or other meat from a carnivore. Although most infections are mild and asymptomatic, heavy infections can cause severe enteritis, periorbital edema, myositis, and (infrequently) death.

Life Cycle and Epidemiology

Eight species of *Trichinella* are recognized as causes of infection in humans. Two species are distributed worldwide: *T. spiralis*, which is found in a great variety of carnivorous and omnivorous animals, and *T. pseudospiralis*, which is found in mammals and birds.

T. nativa is present in Arctic regions and infects bears; *T. nelsoni* is found in equatorial eastern Africa, where it is common among felid predators and scavengers such as hyenas and bush pigs; and *T. britovi* is found in Europe, western Africa, and western Asia among carnivores but not among domestic swine. *T. murrelli* is present in North American game animals.

After human consumption of trichinous meat, encysted larvae are liberated by digestive acid and pepsin (Fig. 123-1). The larvae invade the small-bowel mucosa and mature into adult worms. After ~1 week, female worms release newborn larvae that migrate via the circulation to striated muscle. The larvae of all species except *T. pseudospiralis*, *T. papuae*, and *T. zimbabwensis* then encyst by inducing a radical transformation in the muscle cell architecture. Although host immune responses may help to expel intestinal adult worms, they have little effect on muscle-dwelling larvae.

Human trichinellosis is often caused by the ingestion of infected pork products and thus can occur in almost any location where the meat of domestic or wild swine is eaten. Human trichinellosis also may be acquired from the meat of other animals, including dogs (in parts of Asia and Africa), horses (in Italy and France), and bears and walruses (in northern regions). Although cattle (being herbivores) are not natural hosts of *Trichinella*, beef has been implicated in outbreaks when contaminated or adulterated with trichinous pork. Laws that prohibit the feeding of uncooked garbage to pigs have greatly reduced the transmission of trichinellosis in the United States. About 12 cases of trichinellosis are reported annually in this country, but most mild cases probably remain undiagnosed. Recent U.S. and Canadian outbreaks have been attributable to consumption of wild game (especially bear meat) and, less frequently, of pork.

Pathogenesis and Clinical Features

Clinical symptoms of trichinellosis arise from the successive phases of parasite enteric invasion, larval migration, and muscle encystment (Fig. 123-1). Most light infections (those with <10 larvae per gram of muscle) are asymptomatic, whereas heavy infections (which can involve >50 larvae per gram of muscle) can be life-threatening. Invasion of the gut by large numbers of parasites occasionally provokes diarrhea during the first week after infection. Abdominal pain, constipation, nausea, or vomiting also may be prominent.

Symptoms due to larval migration and muscle invasion begin to appear in the second week after infection. The

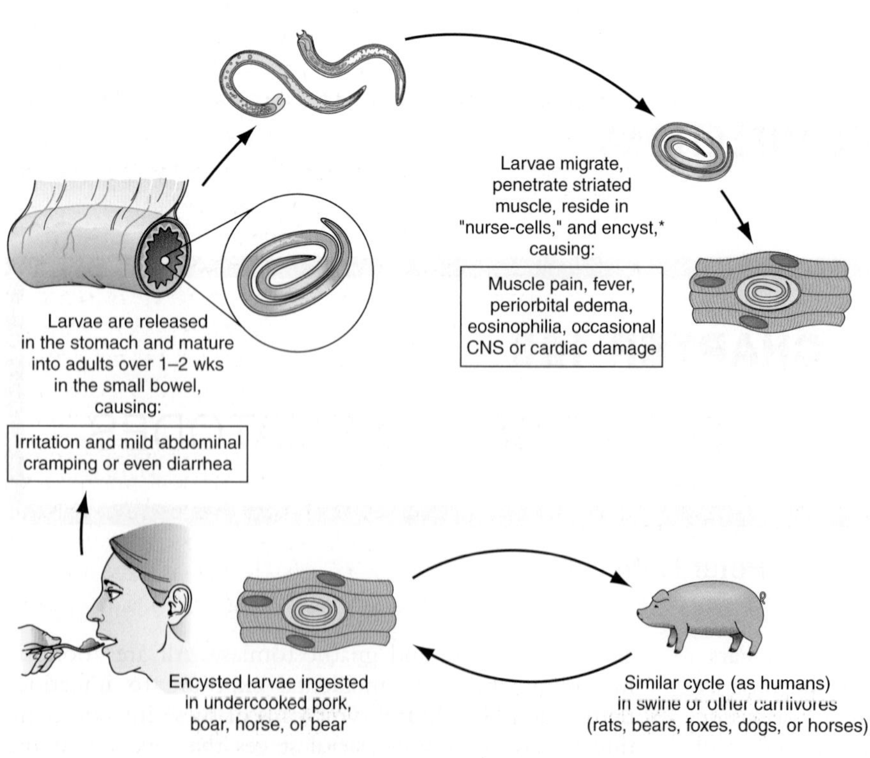
Larvae migrate, penetrate striated muscle, reside in "nurse-cells," and encyst,* causing:
Muscle pain, fever, periorbital edema, eosinophilia, occasional CNS or cardiac damage
Larvae are released in the stomach and mature into adults over 1–2 wks in the small bowel, causing:
Irritation and mild abdominal cramping or even diarrhea
Encysted larvae ingested in undercooked pork, boar, horse, or bear
Similar cycle (as humans) in swine or other carnivores (rats, bears, foxes, dogs, or horses)
*T. papuae, T. zimbabwensis, and T. pseudospiralis do not encyst.

FIGURE 123-1

Life cycle of *Trichinella spiralis* (cosmopolitan); *nelsoni* (equatorial Africa); *britovi* (Europe, western Africa, western Asia); *nativa* (Arctic); *murrelli* (North America); *papuae* (Papua New Guinea); *zimbabwensis* (Tanzania); and *pseudospiralis* (cosmopolitan). *[Reprinted from Guerrant RL et al (eds): Tropical Infectious Diseases: Principles, Pathogens and Practice, 2d ed, p 1218. © 2006, with permission from Elsevier Science.]*

migrating *Trichinella* larvae provoke a marked local and systemic hypersensitivity reaction, with fever and hypereosinophilia. Periorbital and facial edema is common, as are hemorrhages in the subconjunctivae, retina, and nail beds ("splinter" hemorrhages). A maculopapular rash, headache, cough, dyspnea, or dysphagia sometimes develops. Myocarditis with tachyarrhythmias or heart failure—and, less commonly, encephalitis or pneumonitis—may develop and accounts for most deaths of patients with trichinellosis.

Upon onset of larval encystment in muscle 2–3 weeks after infection, symptoms of myositis with myalgias, muscle edema, and weakness develop, usually overlapping with the inflammatory reactions to migrating larvae. The most commonly involved muscle groups include the extraocular muscles; the biceps; and the muscles of the jaw, neck, lower back, and diaphragm. Peaking ~3 weeks after infection, symptoms subside only gradually during a prolonged convalescence. Uncommon infections with *T. pseudospiralis*, whose larvae do not encapsulate in muscles, elicit prolonged polymyositis-like illness.

Laboratory Findings and Diagnosis

Blood eosinophilia develops in >90% of patients with symptomatic trichinellosis and may peak at a level of >50% between 2 and 4 weeks after infection. Serum levels of muscle enzymes, including creatine phosphokinase, are elevated in most symptomatic patients. Patients should be questioned thoroughly about their consumption of pork or wild-animal meat and about illness in other individuals who ate the same meat. A presumptive clinical diagnosis can be based on fevers, eosinophilia, periorbital edema, and myalgias after a suspect meal. A rise in the titer of parasite-specific antibody, which usually does not occur until after the third week of infection, confirms the diagnosis. Alternatively, a definitive diagnosis requires surgical biopsy of at least 1 g of involved muscle; the yields are highest near tendon insertions. The fresh muscle tissue should be compressed between glass slides and examined microscopically (Fig. 123-2), because larvae may be overlooked by examination of routine histopathologic sections alone.

℞ Treatment: TRICHINELLOSIS

Most lightly infected patients recover uneventfully with bed rest, antipyretics, and analgesics. Glucocorticoids like prednisone (Table 123-1) are beneficial for severe myositis and myocarditis. Mebendazole and albendazole are active against enteric stages of the parasite, but their efficacy against encysted larvae has not been conclusively demonstrated.

Prevention

Larvae may be killed by cooking pork until it is no longer pink or by freezing it at –15°C for 3 weeks. However, Arctic *T. nativa* larvae in walrus or bear meat are relatively resistant and may remain viable despite freezing.

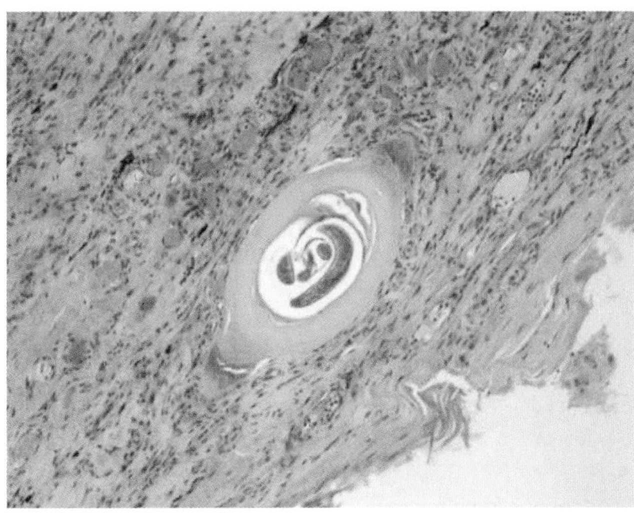

FIGURE 123-2
***Trichinella* larva** encysted in a characteristic hyalinized capsule in striated muscle tissue. *(Photo/Wadsworth Center, New York State Department of Health. Reprinted from CDC MMWR 53:606, 2004; public domain.)*

VISCERAL AND OCULAR LARVA MIGRANS

Visceral larva migrans is a syndrome caused by nematodes that are normally parasitic for nonhuman host species. In humans, the nematode larvae do not develop into adult worms but instead migrate through host tissues and elicit eosinophilic inflammation. The more common form of visceral larva migrans is toxocariasis due to larvae of the canine ascarid *Toxocara canis*, less commonly to the feline ascarid *T. cati*, and even less commonly to the pig ascarid *Ascaris suum*. Rare cases with eosinophilic meningoencephalitis have been caused by the raccoon ascarid *Baylisascaris procyonis*.

Life Cycle and Epidemiology

The canine roundworm *T. canis* is distributed among dogs worldwide. Ingestion of infective eggs by dogs is followed by liberation of *Toxocara* larvae, which penetrate the gut wall and migrate intravascularly into canine tissues, where most remain in a developmentally arrested state. During pregnancy, some larvae resume migration in bitches and infect puppies prenatally (through transplacental transmission) or after birth (through suckling). Thus, in lactating bitches and puppies, larvae return to the intestinal tract and develop into adult worms, which produce eggs that are released in the feces. Humans acquire toxocariasis mainly by eating soil contaminated by puppy feces that contains infective *T. canis* eggs. Visceral larva migrans is most common among children who habitually eat dirt.

Pathogenesis and Clinical Features

Clinical disease most commonly afflicts preschool children. After humans ingest *Toxocara* eggs, the larvae hatch

TABLE 123-1

THERAPY FOR TISSUE NEMATODE INFECTIONS

INFECTION	SEVERITY	TREATMENT
Trichinellosis	Mild	Supportive
	Moderate	Albendazole (400 mg bid × 8–14 days) *or* Mebendazole (200–400 mg tid × 3 days, then 400 mg tid × 8–14 days)
	Severe	Add glucocorticoids (e.g., prednisone, 1 mg/kg qd × 5 days)
Visceral larva migrans	Mild to moderate	Supportive
	Severe	Glucocorticoids (as above)
	Ocular	Not fully defined; albendazole (800 mg bid for adults, 400 mg bid for children) with glucocorticoids × 5–20 days has been effective
Cutaneous larva migrans		Ivermectin (single dose, 200 μg/kg) *or* Albendazole (200 mg bid × 3 days)
Angiostrongyliasis	Mild to moderate	Supportive
	Severe	Glucocorticoids (as above)
Gnathostomiasis		Ivermectin (200 μg/kg per day × 2 days) *or* Albendazole (400 mg bid × 21 days)

and penetrate the intestinal mucosa, from which they are carried by the circulation to a wide variety of organs and tissues. The larvae invade the liver, lungs, central nervous system (CNS), and other sites, provoking intense local eosinophilic granulomatous responses. The degree of clinical illness depends on larval number and tissue distribution, reinfection, and host immune responses. Most light infections are asymptomatic and may be manifest only by blood eosinophilia. Characteristic symptoms of visceral larva migrans include fever, malaise, anorexia and weight loss, cough, wheezing, and rashes. Hepatosplenomegaly is common. These features are often accompanied by extraordinary peripheral eosinophilia, which may approach 90%. Uncommonly, seizures or behavioral disorders develop. Rare deaths are due to severe neurologic, pneumonic, or myocardial involvement.

The ocular form of the larva migrans syndrome occurs when *Toxocara* larvae invade the eye. An eosinophilic granulomatous mass, most commonly in the posterior pole of the retina, develops around the entrapped larva. The retinal lesion can mimic retinoblastoma in appearance, and mistaken diagnosis of the latter condition can lead to unnecessary enucleation. The spectrum of eye involvement also includes endophthalmitis, uveitis, and chorioretinitis. Unilateral visual disturbances, strabismus, and eye pain are the most common presenting symptoms. In contrast to visceral larva migrans, ocular toxocariasis usually develops in older children or young adults with no history of pica; these patients seldom have eosinophilia or visceral manifestations.

Diagnosis

In addition to eosinophilia, leukocytosis and hypergammaglobulinemia may be evident. Transient pulmonary infiltrates are apparent on chest x-rays of about half of patients with symptoms of pneumonitis. The clinical diagnosis can be confirmed by an enzyme-linked immunosorbent assay for toxocaral antibodies. Stool examination for parasite eggs, while important in the evaluation of unexplained eosinophilia, is worthless for toxocariasis, since the larvae do not develop into egg-producing adults in humans.

℞ Treatment: VISCERAL AND OCULAR LARVA MIGRANS

The vast majority of *Toxocara* infections are self-limited and resolve without specific therapy. In patients with severe myocardial, CNS, or pulmonary involvement, glucocorticoids may be employed to reduce inflammatory complications. Available anthelmintic drugs, including mebendazole and albendazole, have not been shown conclusively to alter the course of larva migrans. Control measures include prohibiting dog excreta in public parks and playgrounds, deworming dogs, and preventing pica in children. Treatment of ocular disease is not fully defined, but the administration of albendazole in conjunction with glucocorticoids has been effective (Table 123-1).

CUTANEOUS LARVA MIGRANS

Cutaneous larva migrans ("creeping eruption") is a serpiginous skin eruption caused by burrowing larvae of animal hookworms, usually the dog and cat hookworm *Ancylostoma braziliense*. The larvae hatch from eggs passed in dog and cat feces and mature in the soil. Humans become infected after skin contact with soil in areas frequented by dogs and cats, such as areas underneath house porches. Cutaneous larva migrans is prevalent among children and travelers in regions with warm humid climates, including the southeastern United States.

After larvae penetrate the skin, erythematous lesions form along the tortuous tracks of their migration through the dermal-epidermal junction; the larvae advance several centimeters in a day. The intensely pruritic lesions may occur anywhere on the body and can be numerous if the patient has lain on the ground. Vesicles and bullae may form later. The animal hookworm larvae do not mature in humans and, without treatment, will die after an interval ranging from weeks to a couple of months, with resolution of skin lesions. The diagnosis is made on clinical grounds. Skin biopsies only rarely detect diagnostic larvae. Symptoms can be alleviated by ivermectin or albendazole (Table 123-1).

ANGIOSTRONGYLIASIS

Angiostrongylus cantonensis, the rat lungworm, is the most common cause of human eosinophilic meningitis (Fig. 123-3).

Life Cycle and Epidemiology

This infection occurs principally in Southeast Asia and the Pacific Basin but has spread to other areas of the world. *A. cantonensis* larvae produced by adult worms in the rat lung migrate to the gastrointestinal tract and are expelled with the feces. They develop into infective larvae in land snails and slugs. Humans acquire the infection by ingesting raw infected mollusks; vegetables contaminated by mollusk slime; or crabs, freshwater shrimp, and certain marine fish that have themselves eaten infected mollusks. The larvae then migrate to the brain.

Pathogenesis and Clinical Features

The parasites eventually die in the CNS, but not before initiating pathologic consequences that, in heavy infections, can result in permanent neurologic sequelae or death. Migrating larvae cause marked local eosinophilic inflammation and hemorrhage, with subsequent necrosis and granuloma formation around dying worms. Clinical symptoms develop 2–35 days after the ingestion of larvae. Patients usually present with an insidious or abrupt excruciating frontal, occipital, or bitemporal headache. Neck stiffness, nausea and vomiting, and paresthesias are also common. Fever, cranial and extraocular nerve palsies, seizures, paralysis, and lethargy are uncommon.

Laboratory Findings

Examination of cerebrospinal fluid (CSF) is mandatory in suspected cases and usually reveals an elevated opening pressure, a white blood cell count of 150–2000/μL, and an eosinophilic pleocytosis of >20%. The protein concentration is usually elevated and the glucose level normal. The larvae of *A. cantonensis* are only rarely seen in CSF. Peripheral-blood eosinophilia may be mild. The diagnosis is generally based on the clinical presentation of eosinophilic meningitis together with a compatible epidemiologic history.

℞ Treatment: ANGIOSTRONGYLIASIS

Specific chemotherapy is not of benefit in angiostrongyliasis; larvicidal agents may exacerbate inflammatory brain lesions. Management consists of supportive measures, including the administration of analgesics, sedatives, and—in severe cases—glucocorticoids (Table 123-1). Repeated lumbar punctures with removal of CSF can relieve symptoms. In most patients,

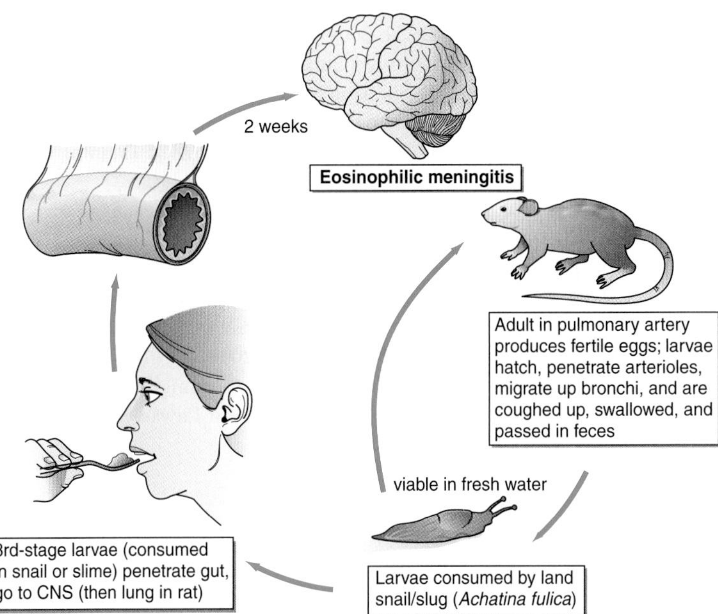
2 weeks
Eosinophilic meningitis
Adult in pulmonary artery produces fertile eggs; larvae hatch, penetrate arterioles, migrate up bronchi, and are coughed up, swallowed, and passed in feces
viable in fresh water
3rd-stage larvae (consumed in snail or slime) penetrate gut, go to CNS (then lung in rat)
Larvae consumed by land snail/slug (*Achatina fulica*)

FIGURE 123-3

Life cycle of *Angiostrongylus cantonensis* (rat lung worm). Also found in Southeast Asia, Pacific Islands, Cuba, Australia, Japan, China, Mauritius, and U.S. ports. *[Reprinted from Guerrant RL et al (eds): Tropical Infectious Diseases: Principles, Pathogens and Practice, 2d ed, p 1225. (c) 2006, with permission from Elsevier Science.]*

cerebral angiostrongyliasis has a self-limited course, and recovery is complete. The infection may be prevented by adequately cooking snails, crabs, and prawns and inspecting vegetables for mollusk infestation. Other parasitic or fungal causes of eosinophilic meningitis in endemic areas may include gnathostomiasis (see below), paragonimiasis (Chap. 126), schistosomiasis (Chap. 126), neurocysticercosis (Chap. 127), and coccidioidomycosis (Chap. 104).

GNATHOSTOMIASIS

Infection of human tissues with larvae of *Gnathostoma spinigerum* can cause eosinophilic meningoencephalitis, migratory cutaneous swellings, or invasive masses of the eye and visceral organs.

Life Cycle and Epidemiology

Human gnathostomiasis occurs in many countries and is notably endemic in Southeast Asia and parts of China and Japan. In nature, the mature adult worms parasitize the gastrointestinal tract of dogs and cats. First-stage larvae hatch from eggs passed into water and are ingested by *Cyclops* species (water fleas). Infective third-stage larvae develop in the flesh of many animal species (including fish, frogs, eels, snakes, chickens, and ducks) that have eaten either infected *Cyclops* or another infected second intermediate host. Humans typically acquire the infection by eating raw or undercooked fish or poultry. Raw fish dishes, such as *som fak* in Thailand and *sashimi* in Japan, account for many cases of human gnathostomiasis. Some cases in Thailand result from the local practice of applying frog or snake flesh as a poultice.

Pathogenesis and Clinical Features

Clinical symptoms are due to the aberrant migration of a single larva into cutaneous, visceral, neural, or ocular tissues. After invasion, larval migration may cause local inflammation, with pain, cough, or hematuria accompanied by fever and eosinophilia. Painful, itchy, migratory swellings may develop in the skin, particularly in the distal extremities or periorbital area. Cutaneous swellings usually last ~1 week but often recur intermittently over many years. Larval invasion of the eye can provoke a sight-threatening inflammatory response. Invasion of the CNS results in eosinophilic meningitis with myeloencephalitis, a serious complication due to ascending larval migration along a large nerve track. Patients characteristically present with agonizing radicular pain and paresthesias in the trunk or a limb, which are followed shortly by paraplegia. Cerebral involvement, with focal hemorrhages and tissue destruction, is often fatal.

Diagnosis and Treatment

Cutaneous migratory swellings with marked peripheral eosinophilia, supported by an appropriate geographic and dietary history, generally constitute an adequate basis for a clinical diagnosis of gnathostomiasis. However, patients may present with ocular or cerebrospinal involvement without antecedent cutaneous swellings. In the latter case, eosinophilic pleocytosis is demonstrable (usually along with hemorrhagic or xanthochromic CSF), but worms are almost never recovered from CSF. Surgical removal of the parasite from subcutaneous or ocular tissue, though rarely feasible, is both diagnostic and therapeutic. Albendazole or ivermectin may be helpful (Table 123-1). At present, cerebrospinal involvement is managed with supportive measures and generally with a course of glucocorticoids. Gnathostomiasis can be prevented by adequate cooking of fish and poultry in endemic areas.

FURTHER READINGS

Barisani-Asenbauer T et al: Treatment of ocular toxocariasis with albendazole. J Ocul Pharmacol Ther 17:287, 2001

Bouchard O et al: Cutaneous larva migrans in travelers: A prospective study, with assessment of therapy with ivermectin. Clin Infect Dis 31:493, 2000

CDC Division of Parasitic Diseases. *www.cdc.gov/ncidod/dpd/default.htm*

Cianferoni A et al: Visceral larva migrans associated with earthworm ingestion: Clinical evolution in an adolescent patient. Pediatrics 117:e336, 2006

Gottstein B et al: Epidemiology, diagnosis, treatment, and control of trichinellosis. Clin Microbiol Rev 22:127, 2009

Ligon BL: Gnathostomiasis: A review of a previously localized zoonosis now crossing numerous geographical boundaries. Semin Pediatr Infect Dis 16:137, 2005

Madariaga MG et al: A probable case of human neurotrichinellosis in the United States. Am J Trop Med Hyg 77:347, 2007

Magana M et al: Gnathostomiasis: Clinicopathologic study. Am J Dermatopathol 26:91, 2004

Menard A et al: Imported cutaneous gnathostomiasis: Report of five cases. Trans R Soc Trop Med Hyg 97:200, 2003

Puljiz I et al: Electrocardiographic changes in trichinellosis: A retrospective study of 154 patients. Ann Trop Med Parasitol 99:403, 2005

Sakai S et al: Pulmonary lesions associated with visceral larva migrans due to *Ascaris suum* or *Toxocara canis*: Imaging of six cases. AJR Am J Roentgenol 186:1697, 2006

Slom TJ et al: An outbreak of eosinophilic meningitis caused by *Angiostrongylus cantonensis* in travelers returning from the Caribbean. N Engl J Med 346:668, 2002

Tsai HC et al: Outbreak of eosinophilic meningitis associated with drinking raw vegetable juice in southern Taiwan. Am J Trop Med Hyg 71:222, 2004

CHAPTER 124
INTESTINAL NEMATODES

Peter F. Weller ■ Thomas B. Nutman

More than a billion persons worldwide are infected with one or more species of intestinal nematodes. Table 124-1 summarizes biologic and clinical features of infections due to the major intestinal parasitic nematodes. These parasites are most common in regions with poor fecal sanitation, particularly in resource-poor countries in the tropics and subtropics, but they have also been seen with increasing frequency among immigrants and refugees to resource-rich countries. Although nematode infections are not usually fatal, they contribute to malnutrition and diminished work capacity. It is interesting that these helminth infections may protect some individuals from allergic disease. Humans may on occasion be infected with nematode parasites that ordinarily infect animals; these zoonotic infections produce diseases such as trichostrongyliasis, anisakiasis, capillariasis, and abdominal angiostrongyliasis.

Intestinal nematodes are roundworms; they range in length from 1 mm to many centimeters when mature (Table 124-1). Their life cycles are complex and highly varied; some species, including *Strongyloides stercoralis* and *Enterobius vermicularis*, can be transmitted directly from person to person, while others, such as *Ascaris lumbricoides, Necator americanus*, and *Ancylostoma duodenale*, require a soil phase for development. Because most helminth parasites do not self-replicate, the acquisition of a heavy burden of adult worms requires repeated exposure to the parasite in its infectious stage, whether larva or egg. Hence, clinical disease, as opposed to asymptomatic infection, generally develops only with prolonged residence in an endemic area. In persons with marginal nutrition, intestinal helminth infections may impair growth and development. Eosinophilia and elevated serum IgE levels are features of many helminthic infections and, when unexplained, should always prompt a search for occult helminthiasis. Significant protective immunity to intestinal nematodes appears not to develop in humans, although mechanisms of parasite immune evasion and host immune responses to these infections have not been elucidated in detail.

ASCARIASIS

A. lumbricoides is the largest intestinal nematode parasite of humans, reaching up to 40 cm in length. Most infected individuals have low worm burdens and are asymptomatic. Clinical disease arises from larval migration in the lungs or effects of the adult worms in the intestines.

Life Cycle

Adult worms live in the lumen of the small intestine. Mature female *Ascaris* worms are extraordinarily fecund, each producing up to 240,000 eggs a day, which pass with the feces. Ascarid eggs, which are remarkably resistant to environmental stresses, become infective after several weeks of maturation in the soil and can remain infective for years. After infective eggs are swallowed, larvae hatched in the intestine invade the mucosa, migrate through the circulation to the lungs, break into the alveoli, ascend the bronchial tree, and return via swallowing to the small intestine, where they develop into adult worms. Between 2 and 3 months elapse between initial infection and egg production. Adult worms live for 1–2 years.

Epidemiology

Ascaris is widely distributed in tropical and subtropical regions as well as in other humid areas, including the rural southeastern United States. Transmission typically occurs through fecally contaminated soil and is due either to a lack of sanitary facilities or to the use of human feces as fertilizer. With their propensity for hand-to-mouth fecal carriage, younger children are most affected. Infection outside endemic areas, though uncommon, can occur when eggs on transported vegetables are ingested.

Clinical Features

During the lung phase of larval migration, ~9–12 days after egg ingestion, patients may develop an irritating nonproductive cough and burning substernal discomfort that is aggravated by coughing or deep inspiration. Dyspnea and blood-tinged sputum are less common. Fever is usually reported. Eosinophilia develops during this symptomatic phase and subsides slowly over weeks. Chest x-rays may reveal evidence of eosinophilic pneumonitis (Löffler's syndrome), with rounded infiltrates a few millimeters to several centimeters in size. These infiltrates may be transient and intermittent, clearing after several weeks. Where there is seasonal transmission of the parasite, seasonal pneumonitis with eosinophilia may develop in previously infected and sensitized hosts.

TABLE 124-1

MAJOR HUMAN INTESTINAL PARASITIC NEMATODES

	PARASITIC NEMATODE				
FEATURE	***ASCARIS LUMBRICOIDES*** **(ROUNDWORM)**	***NECATOR AMERICANUS, ANCYLOSTOMA DUODENALE*** **(HOOKWORM)**	***STRONGYLOIDES STERCORALIS***	***TRICHURIS TRICHIURA*** **(WHIPWORM)**	***ENTEROBIUS VERMICULARIS*** **(PINWORM)**
Global prevalence in humans (millions)	1221	740	50	795	300
Endemic areas	Worldwide	Hot, humid regions	Hot, humid regions	Worldwide	Worldwide
Infective stage	Egg	Filariform larva	Filariform larva	Egg	Egg
Route of infection	Oral	Percutaneous	Percutaneous or autoinfection	Oral	Oral
Gastrointestinal location of worms	Jejunal lumen	Jejunal mucosa	Small-bowel mucosa	Cecum, colonic mucosa	Cecum, appendix
Adult worm size	15–40 cm	7–12 mm	2 mm	30–50 mm	8–13 mm (female)
Pulmonary passage of larvae	Yes	Yes	Yes	No	No
Incubation period[a] (days)	60–75	40–100	17–28	70–90	35–45
Longevity	1 y	*N. americanus*: 2–5 y *A. duodenale*: 6–8 y	Decades (owing to autoinfection)	5 y	2 months
Fecundity (eggs/day/worm)	240,000	*N. americanus*: 4000–10,000 *A. duodenale*: 10,000–25,000	5000–10,000	3000–7000	2000
Principal symptoms	Rarely gastrointestinal or biliary obstruction	Iron-deficiency anemia in heavy infection	Gastrointestinal symptoms; malabsorption or sepsis in hyperinfection	Gastrointestinal symptoms, anemia	Perianal pruritus
Diagnostic stage	Eggs in stool	Eggs in fresh stool, larvae in old stool	Larvae in stool or duodenal aspirate; sputum in hyperinfection	Eggs in stool	Eggs from perianal skin on cellulose acetate tape
Treatment	Mebendazole Albendazole Pyrantel pamoate Ivermectin	Mebendazole Pyrantel pamoate Albendazole	1. Ivermectin 2. Albendazole	Mebendazole Albendazole Ivermectin	Mebendazole Pyrantel pamoate Albendazole

[a]Time from infection to egg production by mature female worm.

In established infections, adult worms in the small intestine usually cause no symptoms. In heavy infections, particularly in children, a large bolus of entangled worms can cause pain and small-bowel obstruction, sometimes complicated by perforation, intussusception, or volvulus. Single worms may cause disease when they migrate into aberrant sites. A large worm can enter and occlude the biliary tree, causing biliary colic, cholecystitis, cholangitis, pancreatitis, or (rarely) intrahepatic abscesses. Migration of an adult worm up the esophagus can provoke coughing and oral expulsion of the worm. In highly endemic areas, intestinal and biliary ascariasis can rival acute appendicitis and gallstones as causes of surgical acute abdomen.

Laboratory Findings

Most cases of ascariasis can be diagnosed by microscopic detection of characteristic *Ascaris* eggs (65 by 45 μm) in fecal samples. Occasionally, patients present after passing an adult worm—identifiable by its large size and smooth cream-colored surface—in the stool or through the mouth or nose. During the early transpulmonary migratory phase, when eosinophilic pneumonitis occurs, larvae can be found in sputum or gastric aspirates before diagnostic eggs appear in the stool. The eosinophilia that is prominent during this early stage usually decreases to minimal levels in established infection. Adult worms may be visualized, occasionally serendipitously, on contrast studies of the gastrointestinal tract. A plain abdominal film may reveal masses of worms in gas-filled loops of bowel in patients with intestinal obstruction. Pancreaticobiliary worms can be detected by ultrasound and endoscopic retrograde cholangiopancreatography; the latter method also has been used to extract biliary *Ascaris* worms.

℞ Treatment: ASCARIASIS

Ascariasis should always be treated to prevent potentially serious complications. Albendazole (400 mg once), mebendazole (500 mg once), or ivermectin (150–200 μg/kg once) is effective. These medications are contraindicated in pregnancy, however. Pyrantel pamoate (11 mg/kg once; maximum, 1 g) is safe in pregnancy. Mild diarrhea and abdominal pain are uncommon side effects of these agents. Partial intestinal obstruction should be managed with nasogastric suction, IV fluid administration, and instillation of piperazine through the nasogastric tube, but complete obstruction and its severe complications require immediate surgical intervention.

HOOKWORM

Two hookworm species (*A. duodenale* and *N. americanus*) are responsible for human infections. Most infected individuals are asymptomatic. Hookworm disease develops from a combination of factors—a heavy worm burden, a prolonged duration of infection, and an inadequate iron intake—and results in iron-deficiency anemia and, on occasion, hypoproteinemia.

Life Cycle

Adult hookworms, which are ~1 cm long, use buccal teeth (*Ancylostoma*) or cutting plates (*Necator*) to attach to the small-bowel mucosa and suck blood (0.2 mL/d per *Ancylostoma* adult) and interstitial fluid. The adult hookworms produce thousands of eggs daily. The eggs are deposited with feces in soil, where rhabditiform larvae hatch and develop over a 1-week period into infectious filariform larvae. Infective larvae penetrate the skin and reach the lungs by way of the bloodstream. There they invade alveoli and ascend the airways before being swallowed and reaching the small intestine. The prepatent period from skin invasion to appearance of eggs in the feces is ~6–8 weeks, but it may be longer with *A. duodenale*. Larvae of *A. duodenale*, if swallowed, can survive and develop directly in the intestinal mucosa. Adult hookworms may survive over a decade but usually live ~6–8 years for *A. duodenale* and 2–5 years for *N. americanus*.

Epidemiology

A. duodenale is prevalent in southern Europe, North Africa, and northern Asia, and *N. americanus* is the predominant species in the western hemisphere and equatorial Africa. The two species overlap in many tropical regions, particularly Southeast Asia. In most areas, older children have the highest incidence and greatest intensity of hookworm infection. In rural areas where fields are fertilized with human feces, older working adults also may be heavily affected.

Clinical Features

Most hookworm infections are asymptomatic. Infective larvae may provoke pruritic maculopapular dermatitis ("ground itch") at the site of skin penetration as well as serpiginous tracks of subcutaneous migration (similar to those of cutaneous larva migrans; Chap. 123) in previously sensitized hosts. Larvae migrating through the lungs occasionally cause mild transient pneumonitis, but this condition develops less frequently in hookworm infection than in ascariasis. In the early intestinal phase, infected persons may develop epigastric pain (often with postprandial accentuation), inflammatory diarrhea, or other abdominal symptoms accompanied by eosinophilia. The major consequence of chronic hookworm infection is iron deficiency. Symptoms are minimal if iron intake is adequate, but marginally nourished individuals develop symptoms of progressive iron-deficiency anemia and hypoproteinemia, including weakness and shortness of breath.

Laboratory Findings

The diagnosis is established by the finding of characteristic 40- by 60-μm oval hookworm eggs in the feces. Stool-concentration procedures may be required to detect light infections. Eggs of the two species are indistinguishable by light microscopy. In a stool sample that is not fresh, the eggs may have hatched to release rhabditiform larvae, which need to be differentiated from those of *S. stercoralis*. Hypochromic microcytic anemia, occasionally with eosinophilia or hypoalbuminemia, is characteristic of hookworm disease.

℞ Treatment: HOOKWORM INFECTION

Hookworm infection can be eradicated with several safe and highly effective anthelmintic drugs, including albendazole (400 mg once), mebendazole (500 mg once), and pyrantel pamoate (11 mg/kg for 3 days). Mild iron-deficiency anemia can often be treated with oral iron alone. Severe hookworm disease with protein loss and malabsorption necessitates nutritional support and oral iron replacement along with deworming.

Ancylostoma Caninum *and* Ancylostoma Braziliense

A. caninum, the canine hookworm, has been identified as a cause of human eosinophilic enteritis, especially in northeastern Australia. In this zoonotic infection, adult hookworms attach to the small intestine (where they may be visualized by endoscopy) and elicit abdominal pain and intense local eosinophilia. Treatment with mebendazole (100 mg twice daily for 3 days) or albendazole (400 mg once) or endoscopic removal is effective. Both of these animal hookworm species can cause cutaneous larva migrans ("creeping eruption"; Chap. 123).

STRONGYLOIDIASIS

S. stercoralis is distinguished by its ability—unusual among helminths—to replicate in the human host. This capacity permits ongoing cycles of autoinfection as infective larvae are internally produced. Strongyloidiasis can thus persist for decades without further exposure of the host to exogenous infective larvae. In immunocompromised hosts, large numbers of invasive *Strongyloides* larvae can disseminate widely and can be fatal.

Life Cycle

In addition to a parasitic cycle of development, *Strongyloides* can undergo a free-living cycle of development in the soil (Fig. 124-1). This adaptability facilitates the parasite's survival in the absence of mammalian hosts. Rhabditiform larvae passed in feces can transform into infectious filariform larvae either directly or after a free-living phase of development. Humans acquire strongyloidiasis when filariform larvae in fecally contaminated soil penetrate the skin or mucous membranes. The larvae then travel through the bloodstream to the lungs, where they break into the alveolar spaces, ascend the bronchial tree, are swallowed, and thereby reach the small intestine. There the larvae mature into adult worms that penetrate the mucosa of the proximal small bowel. The minute (2-mm-long) parasitic adult female worms reproduce by parthenogenesis; adult males do not exist. Eggs hatch in the intestinal mucosa, releasing rhabditiform larvae that migrate to the lumen and pass with the feces into soil. Alternatively, rhabditiform larvae in the bowel can develop directly into filariform larvae that penetrate the colonic wall or perianal skin and enter the circulation to repeat the migration that establishes ongoing internal reinfection. This autoinfection cycle allows strongyloidiasis to persist for decades.

Epidemiology

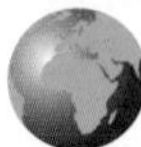

S. stercoralis is spottily distributed in tropical areas and other hot, humid regions and is particularly common in Southeast Asia, sub-Saharan Africa,

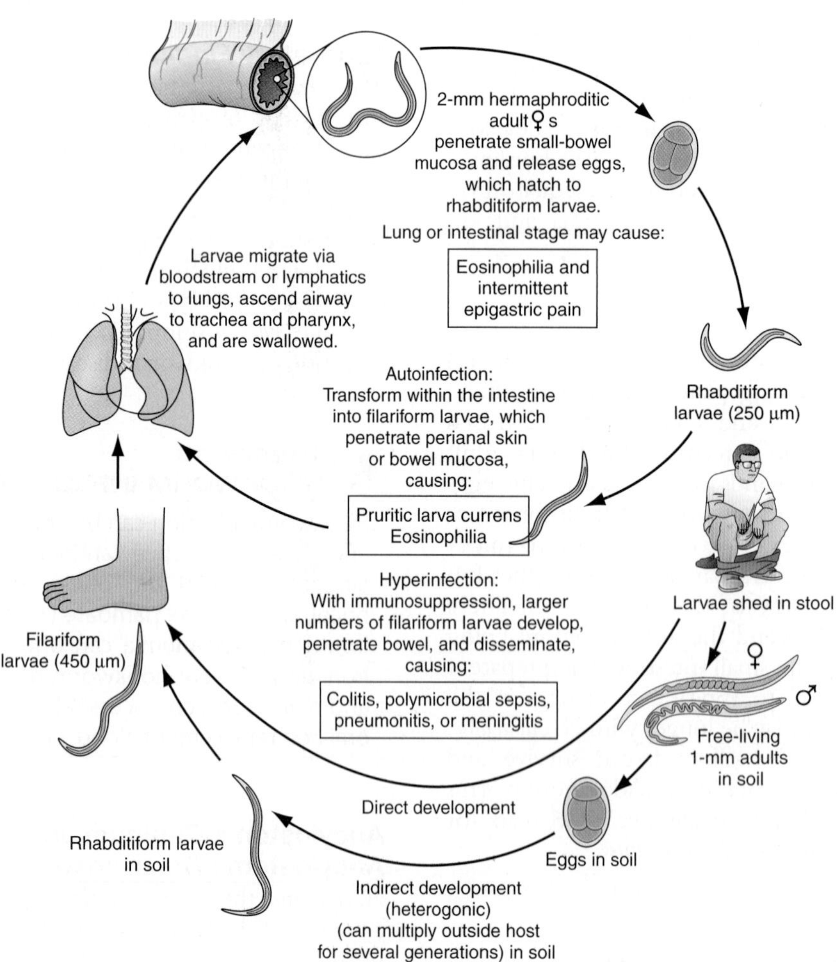

FIGURE 124-1
Life cycle of *Strongyloides stercoralis*. *[Adapted from Guerrant RL et al (eds): Tropical Infectious Diseases: Principles, Pathogens and Practice, 2d ed, p 1276. © 2006, with permission from Elsevier Science.]*

and Brazil. In the United States, the parasite is endemic in parts of the South and is found in immigrants and military veterans who have lived in endemic areas abroad.

Clinical Features

In uncomplicated strongyloidiasis, many patients are asymptomatic or have mild cutaneous and/or abdominal symptoms. Recurrent urticaria, often involving the buttocks and wrists, is the most common cutaneous manifestation. Migrating larvae can elicit a pathognomonic serpiginous eruption, *larva currens* ("running larva"). This pruritic, raised, erythematous lesion advances as rapidly as 10 cm/h along the course of larval migration. Adult parasites burrow into the duodenojejunal mucosa and can cause abdominal (usually midepigastric) pain, which resembles peptic ulcer pain except that it is aggravated by food ingestion. Nausea, diarrhea, gastrointestinal bleeding, mild chronic colitis, and weight loss can occur. Small-bowel obstruction may develop with early, heavy infection. Pulmonary symptoms are rare in uncomplicated strongyloidiasis. Eosinophilia is common, with levels fluctuating over time.

The ongoing autoinfection cycle of strongyloidiasis is normally contained by unknown factors of the host's immune system. Abrogation of host immunity, especially with glucocorticoid therapy and much less commonly with other immunosuppressive medications, leads to hyperinfection, with the generation of large numbers of filariform larvae. Colitis, enteritis, or malabsorption may develop. In disseminated strongyloidiasis, larvae may invade not only gastrointestinal tissues and the lungs but also the central nervous system, peritoneum, liver, and kidneys. Moreover, bacteremia may develop because of the passage of enteric flora through disrupted mucosal barriers. Gram-negative sepsis, pneumonia, or meningitis may complicate or dominate the clinical course. Eosinophilia is often absent in severely infected patients. Disseminated strongyloidiasis, particularly in patients with unsuspected infection who are given glucocorticoids, can be fatal. Strongyloidiasis is a frequent complication of infection with human T-cell lymphotropic virus type I, but disseminated strongyloidiasis is not common among patients infected with HIV.

Diagnosis

In uncomplicated strongyloidiasis, the finding of rhabditiform larvae in feces is diagnostic. Rhabditiform larvae are ~250 μm long, with a short buccal cavity that distinguishes them from hookworm larvae. In uncomplicated infections, few larvae are passed and single stool examinations detect only about one-third of cases. Serial examinations and the use of the agar plate detection method improve the sensitivity of stool diagnosis. In uncomplicated strongyloidiasis (but not in hyperinfection), stool examinations may be repeatedly negative. *Strongyloides* larvae may also be found by sampling of the duodenojejunal contents by aspiration or biopsy. An enzyme-linked immunosorbent assay for serum antibodies to antigens of *Strongyloides* is a sensitive method of diagnosing uncomplicated infections. Such serologic testing should be performed for patients whose geographic histories indicate potential exposure, especially those who exhibit eosinophilia and/or are candidates for glucocorticoid treatment of other conditions. In disseminated strongyloidiasis, filariform larvae should be sought in stool as well as in samples obtained from sites of potential larval migration, including sputum, bronchoalveolar lavage fluid, or surgical drainage fluid.

℞ Treatment: STRONGYLOIDIASIS

Even in the asymptomatic state, strongyloidiasis must be treated because of the potential for subsequent fatal hyperinfection. Ivermectin (200 μg/kg daily for 2 days) is more effective than albendazole (400 mg daily for 3 days). For disseminated strongyloidiasis, treatment with ivermectin should be extended for at least 5–7 days or until the parasites are eradicated.

TRICHURIASIS

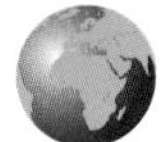

Most infections with the *Trichuris trichiura* are asymptomatic, but heavy infections may cause gastrointestinal symptoms. Like the other soil-transmitted helminths, whipworm is distributed globally in the tropics and subtropics and is most common among poor children from resource-poor regions of the world.

Life Cycle

Adult *Trichuris* worms reside in the colon and cecum, the anterior portions threaded into the superficial mucosa. Thousands of eggs laid daily by adult female worms pass with the feces and mature in the soil. After ingestion, infective eggs hatch in the duodenum, releasing larvae that mature before migrating to the large bowel. The entire cycle takes ~3 months, and adult worms may live for several years.

Clinical Features

Tissue reactions to *Trichuris* are mild. Most infected individuals have no symptoms or eosinophilia. Heavy infections may result in abdominal pain, anorexia, and bloody or mucoid diarrhea resembling inflammatory bowel disease. Rectal prolapse can result from massive infections in children, who often suffer from malnourishment and other diarrheal illnesses. Moderately heavy *Trichuris* burdens also contribute to growth retardation.

Diagnosis and Treatment

The characteristic 50- by 20-μm lemon-shaped *Trichuris* eggs are readily detected on stool examination. Adult worms, which are 3–5 cm long, are occasionally seen on proctoscopy. Mebendazole (500 mg once) or albendazole (400 mg daily for 3 doses) is safe and effective for treatment. Ivermectin (200 μg/kg daily for 3 doses) is also safe but is not quite as efficacious as the benzimidazoles.

ENTEROBIASIS (PINWORM)

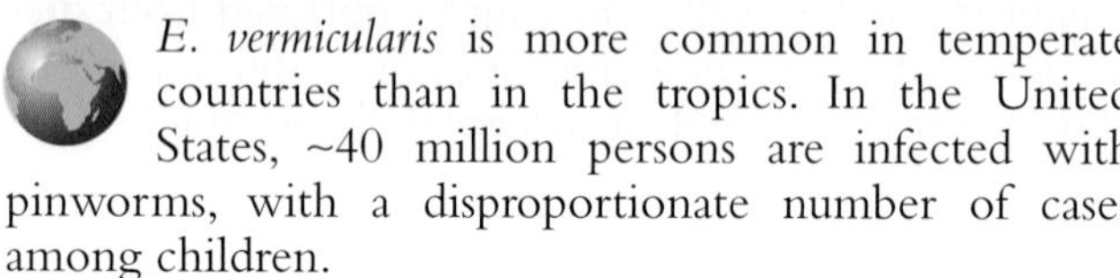

E. vermicularis is more common in temperate countries than in the tropics. In the United States, ~40 million persons are infected with pinworms, with a disproportionate number of cases among children.

Life Cycle and Epidemiology

Enterobius adult worms are ~1 cm long and dwell in the cecum. Gravid female worms migrate nocturnally into the perianal region and release up to 10,000 immature eggs each. The eggs become infective within hours and are transmitted by hand-to-mouth passage. From ingested eggs, larvae hatch and mature into adults. This life cycle takes ~1 month, and adult worms survive for ~2 months. Self-infection results from perianal scratching and transport of infective eggs on the hands or under the nails to the mouth. Because of the ease of person-to-person spread, pinworm infections are common among family members.

Clinical Features

Most pinworm infections are asymptomatic. Perianal pruritus is the cardinal symptom. The itching, which is often worse at night as a result of the nocturnal migration of the female worms, may lead to excoriation and bacterial superinfection. Heavy infections have been claimed to cause abdominal pain and weight loss. On rare occasions, pinworms invade the female genital tract, causing vulvovaginitis and pelvic or peritoneal granulomas. Eosinophilia is uncommon.

Diagnosis

Since pinworm eggs are not released in feces, the diagnosis cannot be made by conventional fecal ova and parasites tests. Instead, eggs are detected by the application of clear cellulose acetate tape to the perianal region in the morning. After the tape is transferred to a slide, microscopic examination will detect pinworm eggs, which are oval, measure 55 by 25 μm, and are flattened along one side.

℞ Treatment: ENTEROBIASIS

Infected children and adults should be treated with mebendazole (100 mg once), albendazole (400 mg once), or pyrantel pamoate (11 mg/kg once; maximum, 1 g), with the same treatment repeated after 2 weeks. Treatment of household members is advocated to eliminate asymptomatic reservoirs of potential reinfection.

TRICHOSTRONGYLIASIS

Trichostrongylus species, which are normally parasites of herbivorous animals, occasionally infect humans, particularly in Asia and Africa. Humans acquire the infection by accidentally ingesting *Trichostrongylus* larvae on contaminated leafy vegetables. The larvae do not migrate in humans but mature directly into adult worms in the small bowel. These worms ingest far less blood than hookworms; most infected persons are asymptomatic, but heavy infections may give rise to mild anemia and eosinophilia. *Trichostrongylus* eggs in stool examinations resemble those of hookworms but are larger (85 by 115 μm). Treatment consists of mebendazole or albendazole (Chap. 113).

ANISAKIASIS

Anisakiasis is a gastrointestinal infection caused by the accidental ingestion in uncooked saltwater fish of nematode larvae belonging to the family Anisakidae. The incidence of anisakiasis in the United States has increased as a result of the growing popularity of raw fish dishes. Most cases occur in Japan, the Netherlands, and Chile, where raw fish—sashimi, pickled green herring, and ceviche, respectively—are national culinary staples. Anisakid nematodes parasitize large sea mammals such as whales, dolphins, and seals. As part of a complex parasitic life cycle involving marine food chains, infectious larvae migrate to the musculature of a variety of fish. Both *Anisakis simplex* and *Pseudoterranova decipiens* have been implicated in human anisakiasis, but an identical gastric syndrome may be caused by the red larvae of eustrongylid parasites of fish-eating birds.

When humans consume infected raw fish, live larvae may be coughed up within 48 h. Alternatively, larvae may immediately penetrate the mucosa of the stomach. Within hours, violent upper abdominal pain accompanied by nausea and occasionally vomiting ensues, mimicking an acute abdomen. The diagnosis can be established by direct visualization on upper endoscopy, outlining of the worm by contrast radiographic studies, or histopathologic examination of extracted tissue. Extraction of the burrowing larvae during endoscopy is curative. In addition, larvae may pass to the small bowel, where they penetrate the mucosa and provoke a vigorous eosinophilic granulomatous response. Symptoms may appear 1–2 weeks after the infective meal, with intermittent abdominal pain, diarrhea, nausea, and fever resembling the manifestations of Crohn's disease. The diagnosis may be suggested by barium studies and confirmed by curative surgical resection of a granuloma in which the worm is embedded. Anisakid eggs are not found in the stool, since the larvae do not mature in humans. Anisakid larvae in saltwater fish are killed by cooking to 60°C, freezing at –20°C for 3 days, or commercial blast freezing, but not usually by salting, marinating, or cold smoking. No medical treatment is available; surgical or endoscopic removal should be undertaken.

CAPILLARIASIS

Intestinal capillariasis is caused by ingestion of raw fish infected with *Capillaria philippinensis*. Subsequent autoinfection can lead to a severe wasting syndrome. The disease occurs in the Philippines and Thailand and, on occasion, elsewhere in Asia. The natural cycle of *C. philippinensis* involves fish from fresh and brackish water. When humans eat infected raw fish, the larvae mature in the intestine into adult worms, which produce invasive larvae that cause intestinal inflammation and villus loss. Capillariasis has an insidious onset with nonspecific abdominal pain and watery diarrhea. If untreated, progressive autoinfection can lead to protein-losing enteropathy and severe malabsorption and ultimately to death from cachexia, cardiac failure, or superinfection. The diagnosis is established by identification of the characteristic peanut-shaped (20- by 40-μm) eggs on stool examination. Severely ill patients require hospitalization and supportive therapy in addition to prolonged anthelmintic treatment with mebendazole or albendazole (Chap. 113).

ABDOMINAL ANGIOSTRONGYLIASIS

Abdominal angiostrongyliasis is found in Latin America and Africa. The zoonotic parasite *Angiostrongylus costaricensis* causes eosinophilic ileocolitis after the ingestion of contaminated vegetation. *A. costaricensis* normally parasitizes the cotton rat and other rodents, with slugs and snails serving as intermediate hosts. Humans become infected by accidentally ingesting infective larvae in mollusk slime deposited on fruits and vegetables; children are at highest risk. The larvae penetrate the gut wall and migrate to the mesenteric artery, where they develop into adult worms. Eggs deposited in the gut wall provoke an intense eosinophilic granulomatous reaction, and adult worms may cause mesenteric arteritis, thrombosis, or frank bowel infarction. Symptoms may mimic those of appendicitis, including abdominal pain and tenderness, fever, vomiting, and a palpable mass in the right iliac fossa. Leukocytosis and eosinophilia are prominent. A barium enema may reveal ileocecal-filling defects, but a definitive diagnosis is usually made surgically with partial bowel resection. Pathologic study reveals a thickened bowel wall with eosinophilic granulomas surrounding the *Angiostrongylus* eggs. In nonsurgical cases, the diagnosis rests solely on clinical grounds because larvae and eggs cannot be detected in the stool. Medical therapy for abdominal angiostrongyliasis (mebendazole, thiabendazole; Chap. 113) is of uncertain efficacy. Careful observation and surgical resection for severe symptoms are the mainstays of treatment.

FURTHER READINGS

Bethony J et al: Soil-transmitted helminth infections: Ascariasis, trichuriasis, and hookworm. Lancet 367:1521, 2006

Biggs BA et al: Management of chronic strongyloidiasis in immigrants and refugees: Is serologic testing useful? Am J Trop Med Hyg 80:788, 2009

Hotez PJ et al: Hookworm infection. N Engl J Med 351:799, 2004

Keiser PB et al: *Strongyloides stercoralis* in the immunocompromised population. Clin Microbiol Rev 17:208, 2004

Lam CS et al: Disseminated strongyloidiasis: A retrospective study of clinical course and outcome. Eur J Clin Microbiol Infect Dis 25:14, 2006

Lim S et al: Complicated and fatal *Strongyloides* infection in Canadians: Risk factors, diagnosis and management. CMAJ 171:479, 2004

Lu LH et al: Human intestinal capillariasis (*Capillaria philippinensis*) in Taiwan. Am J Trop Med Hyg 74:810, 2006

Marcos LA et al: *Strongyloides* hyperinfection syndrome: an emerging global infectious disease. Trans R Soc Trop Med Hyg 102:314, 2008

Shah OJ et al: Biliary ascariasis: A review. World J Surg 30:1500, 2006

CHAPTER 125

FILARIAL AND RELATED INFECTIONS

Thomas B. Nutman ■ Peter F. Weller

Filarial worms are nematodes that dwell in the subcutaneous tissues and the lymphatics. Eight filarial species infect humans (Table 125-1); of these, four—*Wuchereria bancrofti*, *Brugia malayi*, *Onchocerca volvulus*, and *Loa loa*—are responsible for most serious filarial infections. Filarial parasites, which infect an estimated 170 million persons worldwide, are transmitted by specific species of mosquitoes or other arthropods and have a complex life cycle including infective larval stages carried by insects and adult worms that reside in either lymphatic or subcutaneous tissues of humans. The offspring of adults are microfilariae, which, depending on their species, are 200–250 μm long and 5–7 μm wide, may or may not be enveloped in a loose sheath, and either circulate in the

TABLE 125-1

CHARACTERISTICS OF THE FILARIAE

ORGANISM	PERIODICITY	DISTRIBUTION	VECTOR	LOCATION OF ADULT	MICROFILARIAL LOCATION	SHEATH
Wuchereria bancrofti	Nocturnal	Cosmopolitan areas worldwide, including South America and Africa	*Culex* (mosquitoes)	Lymphatic tissue	Blood	+
		Mainly India	*Anopheles* (mosquitoes)			
		China, Indonesia	*Aedes* (mosquitoes)			
	Subperiodic	Eastern Pacific	*Aedes* (mosquitoes)	Lymphatic tissue	Blood	+
Brugia malayi	Nocturnal	Southeast Asia, Indonesia, India	*Mansonia, Anopheles* (mosquitoes)	Lymphatic tissue	Blood	+
	Subperiodic	Indonesia, Southeast Asia	*Coquillettidia, Mansonia* (mosquitoes)	Lymphatic tissue	Blood	+
B. timori	Nocturnal	Indonesia	*Anopheles* (mosquitoes)	Lymphatic tissue	Blood	+
Loa loa	Diurnal	West and Central Africa	*Chrysops* (deerflies)	Subcutaneous tissue	Blood	+
Onchocerca volvulus	None	South and Central America, Africa	*Simulium* (blackflies)	Subcutaneous tissue	Skin, eye	–
Mansonella ozzardi	None	South and Central America	*Culicoides* (midges)	Undetermined site	Blood	–
		Caribbean	*Simulium* (blackflies)			
M. perstans	None	South and Central America, Africa	*Culicoides* (midges)	Body cavities, mesentery, perirenal tissue	Blood	–
M. streptocerca	None	West and Central Africa	*Culicoides* (midges)	Subcutaneous tissue	Skin	–

blood or migrate through the skin (Table 125-1). To complete the life cycle, microfilariae are ingested by the arthropod vector and develop over 1–2 weeks into new infective larvae. Adult worms live for many years, whereas microfilariae survive for 3–36 months. The *Rickettsia*-like endosymbiont *Wolbachia* has been found intracellularly in all stages of *Brugia, Wuchereria, Mansonella,* and *Onchocerca* and is viewed as a possible target for antifilarial chemotherapy.

Usually, infection is established only with repeated, prolonged exposures to infective larvae. Since the clinical manifestations of filarial diseases develop relatively slowly, these infections should be considered to induce chronic diseases with possible long-term debilitating effects. In terms of the nature, severity, and timing of clinical manifestations, patients with filarial infections who are native to endemic areas and undergo lifelong exposure may differ significantly from those who are travelers or who have recently moved to these areas. Characteristically, filarial disease is more acute and intense in newly exposed individuals than in natives of endemic areas.

LYMPHATIC FILARIASIS

Lymphatic filariasis is caused by *W. bancrofti, B. malayi,* or *B. timori*. The threadlike adult parasites reside in lymphatic channels or lymph nodes, where they may remain viable for more than two decades.

EPIDEMIOLOGY

W. bancrofti, the most widely distributed human filarial parasite, affects an estimated 115 million people and is found throughout the tropics and subtropics, including Asia and the Pacific Islands, Africa, areas of South America, and the Caribbean basin. Humans are the only definitive host for the parasite. Generally, the subperiodic form is found only in the Pacific Islands; elsewhere, *W. bancrofti* is nocturnally periodic. (Nocturnally periodic forms of microfilariae are scarce in peripheral blood by day and increase at night, whereas subperiodic forms are present in peripheral blood at all times and reach maximal levels in the afternoon.) Natural vectors for *W. bancrofti* are *Culex fatigans* mosquitoes in urban settings and anopheline or aedean mosquitoes in rural areas.

Brugian filariasis due to *B. malayi* occurs primarily in China, India, Indonesia, Korea, Japan, Malaysia, and the Philippines. *B. malayi* also has two forms distinguished by the periodicity of microfilaremia. The more common nocturnal form is transmitted in areas of coastal rice fields, while the subperiodic form is found in forests. *B. malayi* naturally infects cats as well as humans. *B. timori* exists only on islands of the Indonesian archipelago.

PATHOLOGY

The principal pathologic changes result from inflammatory damage to the lymphatics, which is typically caused by adult worms and not by microfilariae. Adult worms live in afferent lymphatics or sinuses of lymph nodes and cause lymphatic dilatation and thickening of the vessel walls. The infiltration of plasma cells, eosinophils, and macrophages in and around the infected vessels, along with endothelial and connective tissue proliferation, leads to tortuosity of the lymphatics and damaged or incompetent lymph valves. Lymphedema and chronic-stasis changes with hard or brawny edema develop in the overlying skin. These consequences of filariasis are due both to direct effects of the worms and to the inflammatory response of the host to the parasite. Inflammatory responses are believed to cause the granulomatous and proliferative processes that precede total lymphatic obstruction. It is thought that the lymphatic vessel remains patent as long as the worm remains viable and that the death of the worm leads to enhanced granulomatous reaction and fibrosis. Lymphatic obstruction results, and, despite collateralization of the lymphatics, lymphatic function is compromised.

CLINICAL FEATURES

The most common presentations of the lymphatic filariases are asymptomatic (or subclinical) microfilaremia, hydrocele (Fig. 125-1), acute adenolymphangitis (ADL), and chronic lymphatic disease. In areas where *W. bancrofti* or *B. malayi* is endemic, the overwhelming majority of infected individuals have few overt clinical manifestations of filarial infection despite large numbers of circulating microfilariae in the peripheral blood. Although they may be clinically asymptomatic, virtually all persons with *W. bancrofti* or *B. malayi* microfilaremia have some degree of subclinical disease that includes microscopic hematuria and/or proteinuria, dilated (and tortuous) lymphatics (visualized by imaging), and—in men—scrotal lymphangiectasia (detectable by ultrasound). In spite of these findings, the majority of individuals appear to remain clinically asymptomatic for years; relatively few progress to either acute or chronic disease.

ADL is characterized by high fever, lymphatic inflammation (lymphangitis and lymphadenitis), and transient local edema. The lymphangitis is retrograde, extending peripherally from the lymph node draining the area where the adult parasites reside. Regional lymph nodes are often enlarged, and the entire lymphatic channel can

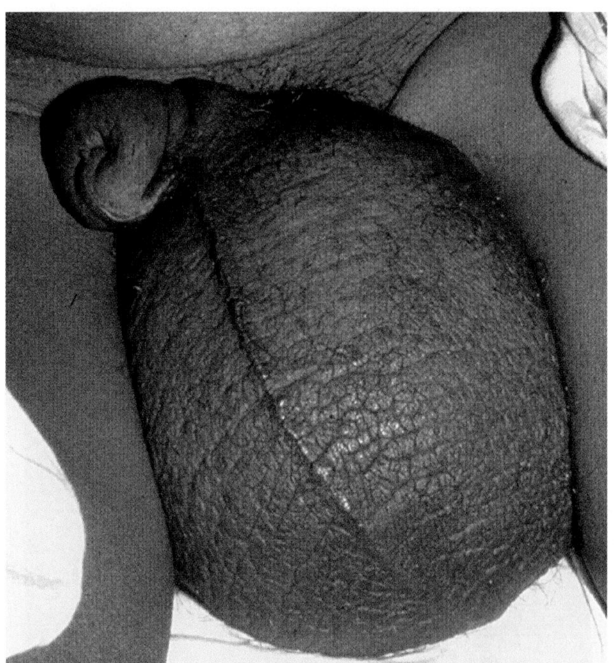

FIGURE 125-1
Hydrocele associated with *Wuchereria bancrofti* infection.

become indurated and inflamed. Concomitant local thrombophlebitis can occur as well. In brugian filariasis, a single local abscess may form along the involved lymphatic tract and subsequently rupture to the surface. The lymphadenitis and lymphangitis can involve both the upper and lower extremities in both bancroftian and brugian filariasis, but involvement of the genital lymphatics occurs almost exclusively with *W. bancrofti* infection. This genital involvement can be manifested by funiculitis, epididymitis, and scrotal pain and tenderness. In endemic areas, another type of acute disease—dermatolymphangioadenitis (DLA)—is recognized as a syndrome that includes high fever, chills, myalgias, and headache. Edematous inflammatory plaques clearly demarcated from normal skin are seen. Vesicles, ulcers, and hyperpigmentation may also be noted. There is often a history of trauma, burns, radiation, insect bites, punctiform lesions, or chemical injury. Entry lesions, especially in the interdigital area, are common. DLA is often diagnosed as cellulitis.

If lymphatic damage progresses, transient lymphedema can develop into lymphatic obstruction and the permanent changes associated with elephantiasis (Fig. 125-2). Brawny edema follows early pitting edema, and thickening of the subcutaneous tissues and hyperkeratosis occur. Fissuring of the skin develops, as do hyperplastic changes. Superinfection of these poorly vascularized tissues becomes a problem. In bancroftian filariasis, in which genital involvement is common, hydroceles may develop (Fig. 125-1); in advanced stages, this condition may evolve into scrotal lymphedema and scrotal elephantiasis. Furthermore, if there is obstruction of the retroperitoneal lymphatics, the increased renal lymphatic pressure leads to rupture of the renal lymphatics and the development of

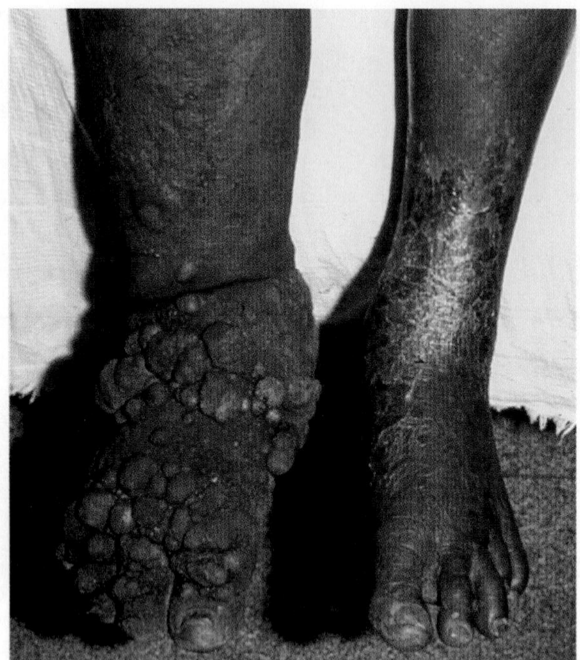

FIGURE 125-2
Elephantiasis of the lower extremity associated with *Wuchereria bancrofti* infection.

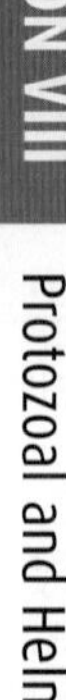

chyluria, which is usually intermittent and most prominent in the morning.

The clinical manifestations of filarial infections in travelers or transmigrants who have recently entered an endemic region are distinctive. Given a sufficient number of bites by infected vectors, usually over a 3- to 6-month period, recently exposed patients can develop acute lymphatic or scrotal inflammation with or without urticaria and localized angioedema. Lymphadenitis of epitrochlear, axillary, femoral, or inguinal lymph nodes is often followed by retrogradely evolving lymphangitis. Acute attacks are short-lived and are not usually accompanied by fever. With prolonged exposure to infected mosquitoes, these attacks, if untreated, become more severe and lead to permanent lymphatic inflammation and obstruction.

DIAGNOSIS

A definitive diagnosis can be made only by detection of the parasites and hence can be difficult. Adult worms localized in lymphatic vessels or nodes are largely inaccessible. Microfilariae can be found in blood, in hydrocele fluid, or (occasionally) in other body fluids. Such fluids can be examined microscopically, either directly or—for greater sensitivity—after concentration of the parasites by the passage of fluid through a polycarbonate cylindrical pore filter (pore size, 3 μm) or by the centrifugation of fluid fixed in 2% formalin (Knott's concentration technique). The timing of blood collection is critical and should be based on the periodicity of the microfilariae in the endemic region involved. Many infected individuals do not have microfilaremia, and definitive diagnosis in such cases can be difficult. Assays for circulating antigens of *W. bancrofti* permit the diagnosis of microfilaremic and cryptic (amicrofilaremic) infection. Two tests are commercially available: an enzyme-linked immunosorbent assay (ELISA) and a rapid-format immunochromatographic card test. Both assays have sensitivities of 96–100% and specificities approaching 100%. There are currently no tests for circulating antigens in brugian filariasis.

Polymerase chain reaction (PCR)–based assays for DNA of *W. bancrofti* and *B. malayi* in blood have been developed. A number of studies indicate that this diagnostic method is of equivalent or greater sensitivity compared with parasitologic methods, detecting patent infection in almost all infected individuals.

In cases of suspected lymphatic filariasis, examination of the scrotum or the female breast by means of high-frequency ultrasound in conjunction with Doppler techniques may result in the identification of motile adult worms within dilated lymphatics. Worms may be visualized in the lymphatics of the spermatic cord in up to 80% of infected men. Live adult worms have a distinctive pattern of movement within the lymphatic vessels (termed the *filaria dance sign*). Radionuclide lymphoscintigraphic imaging of the limbs reliably demonstrates widespread lymphatic abnormalities in both asymptomatic microfilaremic persons and those with clinical manifestations of lymphatic pathology. While of potential utility in the delineation of anatomic changes associated with infection, lymphoscintigraphy is unlikely to assume primacy in the diagnostic evaluation of individuals with suspected infection; it is principally a research tool, although it has been used more widely for assessment of lymphedema of any cause. Eosinophilia and elevated serum concentrations of IgE and antifilarial antibody support the diagnosis of lymphatic filariasis. There is, however, extensive cross-reactivity between filarial antigens and antigens of other helminths, including the common intestinal roundworms; thus, interpretations of serologic findings can be difficult. In addition, residents of endemic areas can become sensitized to filarial antigens (and thus be serologically positive) through exposure to infected mosquitoes without having patent filarial infections.

The ADL associated with lymphatic filariasis must be distinguished from thrombophlebitis, infection, and trauma. Retrogradely evolving lymphangitis is a characteristic feature that helps distinguish filarial lymphangitis from ascending bacterial lymphangitis. Chronic filarial lymphedema must also be distinguished from the lymphedema of malignancy, postoperative scarring, trauma, chronic edematous states, and congenital lymphatic system abnormalities.

℞ Treatment: LYMPHATIC FILARIASIS

With newer definitions of clinical syndromes in lymphatic filariasis and new tools to assess clinical status (e.g., ultrasound, lymphoscintigraphy, circulating filarial antigen assays, PCR), approaches to treatment based on infection status can be considered. Diethylcarbamazine (DEC, 6 mg/kg daily for 12 days), which has both macro- and microfilaricidal properties, remains the treatment of choice for the individual with active lymphatic filariasis (microfilaremia, antigen positivity, or adult worms on ultrasound). An alternative treatment is albendazole (400 mg bid for 21 days), although this drug's macrofilaricidal efficacy may be less than that of DEC. An 8-week course of daily doxycycline (targeting the intracellular *Wolbachia* endosymbiont) has significant macrofilaricidal activity, as does a 7-day course of daily DEC/albendazole.

As has already been mentioned, a growing body of evidence indicates that, although they may be asymptomatic, virtually all persons with *W. bancrofti* or *B. malayi* microfilaremia have some degree of subclinical disease (hematuria, proteinuria, abnormalities on lymphoscintigraphy). Thus, early treatment of asymptomatic persons is recommended to prevent further lymphatic damage. For ADL, supportive treatment (including the administration of antipyretics and analgesics) is recommended, as is antibiotic therapy if secondary bacterial infection is likely. Similarly, because lymphatic disease is associated with the presence of adult worms, treatment with DEC is recommended for microfilaria-negative adult-worm carriers.

In persons with chronic manifestations of lymphatic filariasis, treatment regimens that emphasize hygiene, prevention of secondary bacterial infections, and physiotherapy have gained wide acceptance for morbidity control. These regimens are similar to those recommended for lymphedema of most nonfilarial causes and known by a variety of names, including *complex decongestive physiotherapy* and *complex lymphedema therapy*. Hydroceles (Fig. 125-1) can be drained repeatedly or managed surgically. With chronic manifestations of lymphatic filariasis, drug treatment should be reserved for individuals with evidence of active infection; therapy has been associated with clinical improvement and, in some cases, reversal of lymphedema.

The recommended course of DEC treatment (12 days; total dose, 72 mg/kg) has remained standard for many years. However, data indicate that single-dose DEC treatment with 6 mg/kg may be equally efficacious. The 12-day course provides more rapid short-term microfilarial suppression. Regimens that use combinations of single doses of albendazole and either DEC or ivermectin all have a sustained microfilaricidal effect. As mentioned above, an 8-week course of daily doxycycline (200 mg/d) or a 7-day course of daily DEC/albendazole has both significant macrofilaricidal activity and sustained microfilaricidal activity.

Side effects of DEC treatment include fever, chills, arthralgias, headaches, nausea, and vomiting. Both the development and the severity of these reactions are directly related to the number of microfilariae circulating in the bloodstream. The adverse reactions may represent either an acute hypersensitivity reaction to the antigens being released by dead and dying parasites or an inflammatory reaction induced by lipopolysaccharides from the intracellular *Wolbachia* endosymbionts freed from their intracellular niche. Ivermectin has a side effect profile similar to that of DEC when used in lymphatic filariasis. In patients infected with *L. loa*, who have high levels of *Loa* microfilaremia, DEC—like ivermectin (see "Loiasis" later in the chapter)—can elicit severe encephalopathic complications. When used in single-dose regimens for the treatment of lymphatic filariasis, albendazole is associated with relatively few side effects.

PREVENTION AND CONTROL

Avoidance of mosquito bites usually is not feasible for residents of endemic areas, but visitors should make use of insect repellent and mosquito nets. Impregnated bednets have a salutary effect. DEC can kill developing forms of filarial parasites and is useful as a prophylactic agent in humans.

Community-based intervention is the current approach to elimination of lymphatic filariasis as a public health problem. The underlying tenet of this approach is that mass annual distribution of antimicrofilarial chemotherapy—albendazole with either DEC (for all areas except those where onchocerciasis is coendemic) or ivermectin—will profoundly suppress microfilaremia. If the suppression is sustained, then transmission can be interrupted. As an added benefit, these combinations have secondary effects on gastrointestinal helminths. An alternative approach to the control of lymphatic filariasis is the use of salt fortified with DEC. Community use of DEC-fortified salt dramatically reduces microfilarial density with no apparent adverse reactions. Community education and clinical care for persons already suffering from the chronic sequelae of lymphatic filariasis are important components of filariasis control and elimination programs.

TROPICAL PULMONARY EOSINOPHILIA

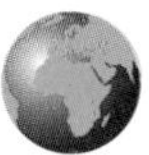

Tropical pulmonary eosinophilia (TPE) is a distinct syndrome that develops in some individuals infected with lymphatic filarial species. This syndrome affects males and females in a ratio of 4:1, often during the third decade of life. The majority of cases have been reported from India, Pakistan, Sri Lanka, Brazil, Guyana, and Southeast Asia.

CLINICAL FEATURES

The main features include a history of residence in filarial-endemic regions, paroxysmal cough and wheezing (usually nocturnal and probably related to the nocturnal periodicity of microfilariae), weight loss, low-grade fever, adenopathy, and pronounced blood eosinophilia (>3000 eosinophils/μL). Chest x-rays or CT scans may be normal but generally show increased bronchovascular markings. Diffuse miliary lesions or mottled opacities may be present in the middle and lower lung fields. Tests of pulmonary function show restrictive abnormalities in most cases and obstructive defects in half. Characteristically, total serum IgE levels (10,000–100,000 ng/mL) and antifilarial antibody titers are markedly elevated.

PATHOLOGY

In TPE, microfilariae and parasite antigens are rapidly cleared from the bloodstream by the lungs. The clinical symptoms result from allergic and inflammatory reactions elicited by the cleared parasites. In some patients, trapping of microfilariae in other reticuloendothelial organs can cause hepatomegaly, splenomegaly, or lymphadenopathy. A prominent, eosinophil-enriched, intraalveolar infiltrate is often reported, and with it comes the release of cytotoxic proinflammatory granular proteins that may mediate some of the pathology seen in TPE. In the absence of successful treatment, interstitial fibrosis can lead to progressive pulmonary damage.

DIFFERENTIAL DIAGNOSIS

TPE must be distinguished from asthma, Löffler's syndrome, allergic bronchopulmonary aspergillosis, allergic granulomatosis with angiitis (Churg-Strauss syndrome), the systemic vasculitides (most notably periarteritis nodosa and Wegener's granulomatosis), chronic eosinophilic pneumonia, and the idiopathic hypereosinophilic syndrome. In addition to a geographic history of filarial exposure, useful features for distinguishing TPE include wheezing that is solely nocturnal, very high levels of antifilarial antibodies, and a rapid initial response to treatment with DEC.

℞ Treatment: TROPICAL PULMONARY EOSINOPHILIA

DEC is used at a daily dosage of 4–6 mg/kg for 14 days. Symptoms usually resolve within 3–7 days after the initiation of therapy. Relapse, which occurs in ~12–25% of cases (sometimes after an interval of years), requires retreatment.

ONCHOCERCIASIS

Onchocerciasis ("river blindness") is caused by the filarial nematode *O. volvulus*, which infects an estimated 13 million individuals. The majority of individuals infected with *O. volvulus* live in the equatorial region of Africa extending from the Atlantic coast to the Red Sea. About 70,000 persons are infected in Guatemala and Mexico, with smaller foci in Venezuela, Colombia, Brazil, Ecuador, Yemen, and Saudi Arabia. Onchocerciasis is the second leading cause of infectious blindness worldwide.

ETIOLOGY AND EPIDEMIOLOGY

Infection in humans begins with the deposition of infective larvae on the skin by the bite of an infected blackfly. The larvae develop into adults, which are typically found in subcutaneous nodules. About 7 months to 3 years after infection, the gravid female releases microfilariae that migrate out of the nodule and throughout the tissues, concentrating in the dermis. Infection is transmitted to other persons when a female fly ingests microfilariae from the host's skin and these microfilariae then develop into infective larvae. Adult *O. volvulus* females and males are ~40–60 cm and ~3–6 cm in length, respectively. The life span of adults can be as long as 18 years, with an average of ~9 years. Because the blackfly vector breeds along free-flowing rivers and streams (particularly in rapids) and generally restricts its flight to an area within several kilometers of these breeding sites, both biting and disease transmission are most intense in these locations.

PATHOLOGY

Onchocerciasis primarily affects the skin, eyes, and lymph nodes. In contrast to the pathology in lymphatic filariasis, the damage in onchocerciasis is elicited by microfilariae and not by adult parasites. In the skin, there are mild but chronic inflammatory changes that can result in loss of elastic fibers, atrophy, and fibrosis. The subcutaneous nodules, or onchocercomata, consist primarily of fibrous tissues surrounding the adult worm, often with a peripheral ring of inflammatory cells. In the eye, neovascularization and corneal scarring lead to corneal opacities and blindness. Inflammation in the anterior and posterior chambers frequently results in anterior uveitis, chorioretinitis, and optic atrophy. Although punctate opacities are due to an inflammatory reaction surrounding dead or dying microfilariae, the pathogenesis of most manifestations of onchocerciasis is still unclear.

CLINICAL FEATURES

Skin

Pruritus and rash are the most frequent manifestations of onchocerciasis. The pruritus can be incapacitating; the rash is typically a papular eruption (Fig. 125-3) that is generalized rather than localized to a particular region of the body. Long-term infection results in exaggerated and premature wrinkling of the skin, loss of elastic fibers, and epidermal atrophy that can lead to loose, redundant skin and hypo- or hyperpigmentation. Localized eczematoid dermatitis can cause hyperkeratosis, scaling, and pigmentary changes. In an immunologically hyperreactive form of onchodermatitis (commonly termed *sowdah*, from the Yemeni word meaning "black"), the affected skin darkens as a consequence of the profound inflammation that occurs as microfilariae in the skin are cleared.

Onchocercomata

These subcutaneous nodules, which can be palpable and/or visible, contain the adult worm. In African patients, they are common over the coccyx and sacrum, the trochanter of the femur, the lateral anterior crest, and other bony prominences; in patients from South and Central America, nodules tend to

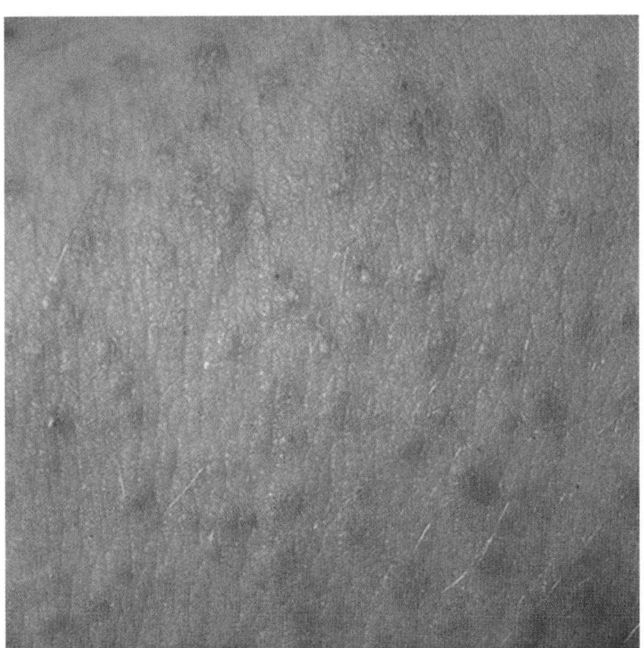

FIGURE 125-3
Papular eruption as a consequence of onchocerciasis.

develop preferentially in the upper part of the body, particularly on the head, neck, and shoulders.

Nodules vary in size and characteristically are firm and not tender. It has been estimated that, for every palpable nodule, there are four deeper nonpalpable ones.

Ocular Tissue

Visual impairment is the most serious complication of onchocerciasis and usually affects only those persons with moderate or heavy infections. Lesions may develop in all parts of the eye. The most common early finding is conjunctivitis with photophobia. Punctate keratitis—acute inflammatory reactions surrounding dying microfilariae and manifested as "snowflake" opacities—is common among younger patients and resolves without apparent complications.

Sclerosing keratitis occurs in 1–5% of infected persons and is the leading cause of onchocercal blindness in Africa. Anterior uveitis and iridocyclitis develop in ~5% of infected persons in Africa. In Latin America, complications of the anterior uveal tract (pupillary deformity) may cause secondary glaucoma. Characteristic chorioretinal lesions develop as a result of atrophy and hyperpigmentation of the retinal pigment epithelium. Constriction of the visual fields and frank optic atrophy may occur.

Lymph Nodes

Mild to moderate lymphadenopathy is common, particularly in the inguinal and femoral areas, where the enlarged nodes may hang down in response to gravity ("hanging groin"), sometimes predisposing to inguinal and femoral hernias.

Systemic Manifestations

Some heavily infected individuals develop cachexia with loss of adipose tissue and muscle mass. Among adults who become blind, there is a three- to fourfold increase in the mortality rate.

DIAGNOSIS

Definitive diagnosis depends on the detection of an adult worm in an excised nodule or, more commonly, of microfilariae in a skin snip. Skin snips are obtained with a corneal-scleral punch, which collects a blood-free skin biopsy sample extending to just below the epidermis, or by lifting of the skin with the tip of a needle and excision of a small (1- to 3-mm) piece with a sterile scalpel blade. The biopsy tissue is incubated in tissue culture medium or in saline on a glass slide or flat-bottomed microtiter plate. After incubation for 2–4 h (or occasionally overnight in light infections), microfilariae emergent from the skin can be seen by low-power microscopy.

Eosinophilia and elevated serum IgE levels are common but, because they occur in many parasitic infections, are not diagnostic in themselves. Assays to detect specific antibodies to *Onchocerca* and PCR to detect onchocercal DNA in skin snips are used in specialized laboratories and are highly sensitive and specific.

The *Mazzotti test* is a provocative technique that can be used in cases where the diagnosis of onchocerciasis is still in doubt (i.e., when skin snips and ocular examination reveal no microfilariae). A small dose of DEC (0.5–1.0 mg/kg) is given orally; the ensuing death of any dermal microfilariae elicits the development or exacerbation of pruritus or dermatitis within hours—an event that strongly suggests onchocerciasis.

℞ Treatment: ONCHOCERCIASIS

The main goals of therapy are to prevent the development of irreversible lesions and to alleviate symptoms. Surgical excision is recommended when nodules are located on the head (because of the proximity of microfilaria-producing adult worms to the eye), but chemotherapy is the mainstay of management. Ivermectin, a semisynthetic macrocyclic lactone active against microfilariae, is the first-line agent for the treatment of onchocerciasis. It is given orally in a single dose of 150 μg/kg, either yearly or semiannually. Recently, more frequent ivermectin administration (every 3 months) has been suggested to ameliorate pruritus and skin disease. Moreover, quadrennial administration of ivermectin has some macrofilaricidal activity.

After treatment, most individuals have few or no reactions. Pruritus, cutaneous edema, and/or maculopapular rash occurs in ~1–10% of treated individuals. In areas of Africa co-endemic for *O. volvulus* and *L. loa*, however, ivermectin is contraindicated (as it is for pregnant or breast-feeding women) because of severe posttreatment encephalopathy seen in patients, especially children, who are heavily microfilaremic for *L. loa* (2000–5000 microfilariae/mL). Although ivermectin treatment results in a marked drop in microfilarial density, its effect can be short-lived (<3 months in some cases). Thus, it is occasionally necessary to give ivermectin more frequently for persistent symptoms. A 6-week course of doxycycline is macrofilaristatic, rendering female adult worms sterile for long periods. Because this agent targets the *Wolbachia* endosymbiont of the filarial parasite, new approaches for definitive treatment (i.e., cure) may become available.

PREVENTION

Vector control has been beneficial in highly endemic areas in which breeding sites are vulnerable to insecticide spraying, but most areas endemic for onchocerciasis are not suited to this type of control. Community-based administration of ivermectin every 6–12 months is being used to interrupt transmission in endemic areas. This measure, in conjunction with vector control, has already helped reduce the prevalence of disease in endemic foci in Africa and Latin America. No drug has proved useful for prophylaxis of *O. volvulus* infection.

LOIASIS

ETIOLOGY AND EPIDEMIOLOGY

Loiasis is caused by *L. loa* (the African eye worm), which is present in the rain forests of West and Central Africa. Adult parasites (females, 50–70 mm long and 0.5 mm wide; males, 25–35 mm long and 0.25 mm wide) live in subcutaneous tissues. Microfilariae circulate in the blood with a diurnal periodicity that peaks between 12:00 noon and 2:00 P.M.

CLINICAL FEATURES

Manifestations of loiasis in natives of endemic areas may differ from those in temporary residents or visitors. Among the indigenous population, loiasis is often an asymptomatic infection with microfilaremia. Infection may be recognized only after subconjunctival migration of an adult worm (Fig. 125-4) or may be manifested by episodic Calabar swellings—evanescent localized areas of angioedema and erythema developing on the extremities and less frequently at other sites. Nephropathy, encephalopathy, and cardiomyopathy are rare. In patients who are not residents of endemic areas, allergic symptoms predominate, episodes of Calabar swelling tend to be more frequent and debilitating, microfilaremia is rare, and eosinophilia and increased levels of antifilarial antibodies are characteristic.

PATHOLOGY

The pathogenesis of the manifestations of loiasis is poorly understood. Calabar swellings are thought to result from a hypersensitivity reaction to adult worm antigens.

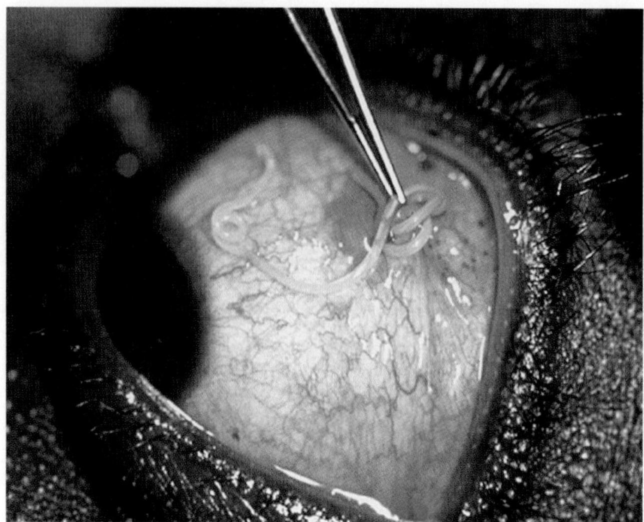

FIGURE 125-4
Adult *Loa loa* being surgically removed after its subconjunctival migration.

DIAGNOSIS

Definitive diagnosis of loiasis requires the detection of microfilariae in the peripheral blood or the isolation of the adult worm from the eye (Fig. 125-4) or from a subcutaneous biopsy specimen from a site of swelling developing after treatment. PCR-based assays for the detection of *L. loa* DNA in blood are available in specialized laboratories and are highly sensitive and specific. In practice, the diagnosis must often be based on a characteristic history and clinical presentation, blood eosinophilia, and elevated levels of antifilarial antibodies, particularly in travelers to an endemic region, who are usually amicrofilaremic. Other clinical findings in the latter individuals include hypergammaglobulinemia, elevated levels of serum IgE, and elevated leukocyte and eosinophil counts.

℞ Treatment: LOIASIS

DEC (8–10 mg/kg per day for 21 days) is effective against both the adult and the microfilarial forms of *L. loa*, but multiple courses are frequently necessary before loiasis resolves completely. In cases of heavy microfilaremia, allergic or other inflammatory reactions can take place during treatment, including central nervous system involvement with coma and encephalitis. Heavy infections can be treated initially with apheresis to remove the microfilariae and with glucocorticoids (40–60 mg of prednisone per day) followed by doses of DEC (0.5 mg/kg per day). If antifilarial treatment has no adverse effects, the prednisone dose can be rapidly tapered and the dose of DEC gradually increased to 8–10 mg/kg per day.

Albendazole or ivermectin is effective in reducing microfilarial loads, although neither is approved for this purpose by the U.S. Food and Drug Administration. DEC (300 mg weekly) is an effective prophylactic regimen for loiasis.

STREPTOCERCIASIS

Mansonella streptocerca, found mainly in the tropical forest belt of Africa from Ghana to the Democratic Republic of the Congo, is transmitted by biting midges. The major clinical manifestations involve the skin and include pruritus, papular rashes, and pigmentation changes. Many infected individuals have inguinal adenopathy, although most are asymptomatic. The diagnosis is made by detection of the characteristic microfilariae in skin snips. DEC (6 mg/kg per day in divided doses for 14–21 days) effectively kills both microfilariae and adult worms. As in onchocerciasis, treatment is sometimes accompanied by urticaria, arthralgias, myalgias, headaches, and abdominal discomfort. Ivermectin at a single dose of 150 μg/kg leads to sustained suppression of microfilariae in the skin and is likely to assume primacy in the treatment of streptocerciasis.

MANSONELLA PERSTANS INFECTION

Mansonella perstans, distributed across the center of Africa and in northeastern South America, is transmitted by midges. Adult worms reside in serous cavities—pericardial, pleural, and peritoneal—as well as in the mesentery and the perirenal and retroperitoneal tissues. Microfilariae circulate in the blood without periodicity. The clinical and pathologic features of the infection are poorly defined. Most patients appear to be asymptomatic, but manifestations may include transient angioedema and pruritus of the arms, face, or other parts of the body (analogous to the Calabar swellings of loiasis); fever; headache; arthralgias; and right-upper-quadrant pain. Occasionally, pericarditis and hepatitis occur. The diagnosis is based on the demonstration of microfilariae in blood or serosal effusions. Perstans filariasis is often associated with peripheral-blood eosinophilia and antifilarial antibody elevations. Although DEC (8–10 mg/kg per day for 21 days) is the standard therapeutic agent, there is little evidence that it is effective. Cure is indicated by the disappearance of symptoms and eosinophilia; multiple courses of therapy are usually required. Ivermectin, used in frequent repeated doses, can reduce blood microfilarial levels. Both mebendazole (100 mg bid for 30 days) and albendazole (400 mg bid for 10 days) have occasionally been reported to be effective.

MANSONELLA OZZARDI INFECTION

The distribution of *Mansonella ozzardi* is restricted to Central and South America and certain Caribbean islands. Adult worms are rarely recovered from humans. Microfilariae circulate in the blood without periodicity. Although this organism has often been considered nonpathogenic, headache, articular pain, fever, pulmonary symptoms, adenopathy, hepatomegaly, pruritus, and eosinophilia have been ascribed to *M. ozzardi* infection. The diagnosis is made by detection of microfilariae in peripheral blood. Ivermectin (a single dose of 6 mg) is effective in treating this infection.

DRACUNCULIASIS (GUINEA WORM INFECTION)

ETIOLOGY AND EPIDEMIOLOGY

The incidence of dracunculiasis, caused by *Dracunculus medinensis*, has declined dramatically because of global eradication efforts. Current estimates suggest that there are slightly more than 10,000 cases worldwide, the majority in Sudan, Ghana, and Mali. Asia has now been deemed dracunculiasis-free.

Humans acquire *D. medinensis* when they ingest water containing infective larvae derived from *Cyclops*, a crustacean that is the intermediate host. Larvae penetrate the stomach or intestinal wall, mate, and mature. The adult male probably dies; the female worm develops over a year and migrates to subcutaneous tissues, usually in the lower extremity. As the thin female worm, ranging in length from 30 cm to 1 m, approaches the skin, a blister forms that, over days, breaks down and forms an ulcer. When the blister opens, large numbers of motile, rhabditiform larvae can be released into stagnant water; ingestion by *Cyclops* completes the life cycle.

CLINICAL FEATURES

Few or no clinical manifestations of dracunculiasis are evident until just before the blister forms, when there is an onset of fever and generalized allergic symptoms, including periorbital edema, wheezing, and urticaria. The emergence of the worm is associated with local pain and swelling. When the blister ruptures (usually as a result of immersion in water) and the adult worm releases larva-rich fluid, symptoms are relieved. The shallow ulcer surrounding the emerging adult worm heals over weeks to months. Such ulcers, however, can become secondarily infected, the result being cellulitis, local inflammation, abscess formation, or (uncommonly) tetanus. Occasionally, the adult worm does not emerge but becomes encapsulated and calcified.

DIAGNOSIS

The diagnosis is based on the findings developing with the emergence of the adult worm, as described above.

Rx Treatment: DRACUNCULIASIS

Gradual extraction of the worm by winding of a few centimeters on a stick each day remains the common and effective practice. Worms may be excised surgically. The administration of metronidazole (250 mg tid for 10 days) may relieve symptoms but has no proven activity against the worm.

PREVENTION

Prevention, which remains the only real control measure, depends on the provision of safe drinking water.

ZOONOTIC FILARIAL INFECTIONS

Dirofilariae that affect primarily dogs, cats, and raccoons occasionally infect humans incidentally, as do *Brugia* and *Onchocerca* parasites that affect small mammals. Because humans are an abnormal host, the parasites never develop fully. Pulmonary dirofilarial infection caused by the canine heartworm *Dirofilaria immitis* generally presents in humans as a solitary pulmonary nodule. Chest pain, hemoptysis, and cough are uncommon. Infections with *D. repens* (from dogs) or *D. tenuis* (from raccoons) can cause local subcutaneous nodules in humans. Zoonotic *Brugia* infection can produce isolated lymph node enlargement, whereas zoonotic *Onchocerca* can cause subconjunctival masses. Eosinophilia levels and antifilarial antibody titers are not commonly elevated. Excisional biopsy is both diagnostic and curative. These infections usually do not respond to chemotherapy.

FURTHER READINGS

Bockarie MJ et al: Mass treatment to eliminate filariasis in Papua New Guinea. N Engl J Med 347:1841, 2002

Boussinesq M et al: Clinical picture, epidemiology and outcome of *Loa*-associated serious adverse events related to mass ivermectin treatment of onchocerciasis in Cameroon. Filaria J 2(Suppl 1):S4, 2003

Dreyer G et al: Acute attacks in the extremities of persons living in an area endemic for bancroftian filariasis: Differentiation of two syndromes. Trans R Soc Trop Med Hyg 93:413, 1999

Gardon J et al: Serious reactions after mass treatment of onchocerciasis with ivermectin in an area endemic for *Loa loa* infection. Lancet 350:18, 1997

Hoerauf A et al: Depletion of *Wolbachia* endobacteria in *Onchocerca* volvulus by doxycycline and microfilaridermia after ivermectin treatment. Lancet 357:1415, 2001

——— et al: Onchocerciasis. BMJ 326:207, 2003

Kyelem D et al: Determinants of success in national programs to eliminate lymphatic filariasis: A perspective identifying essential elements and research needs. Am J Trop Med Hyg 79:480, 2008

McPherson T et al: Interdigital lesions and frequency of acute dermatolymphangioadenitis in lymphoedema in a filariasis-endemic area. Br J Dermatol 154:933, 2006

Ottesen EA: Lymphatic filariasis: Treatment, control and elimination. Adv Parasitol 61:395, 2006

Walther M, Muller R: Diagnosis of human filariases (except onchocerciasis). Adv Parasitol 53:149, 2003

WHO Expert Committee on Onchocerciasis: Onchocerciasis and its control: Fourth report. Tech Rep Ser No 852. Geneva, World Health Organization, 1995

CHAPTER 126

SCHISTOSOMIASIS AND OTHER TREMATODE INFECTIONS

Adel A.F. Mahmoud

Trematodes, or flatworms, are a group of morphologically and biologically heterogeneous organisms that belong to the phylum Platyhelminthes. Human infection with trematodes occurs in many geographic areas and can cause considerable morbidity and mortality. For clinical purposes, significant trematode infections of humans may be divided according to tissues invaded by adult flukes: blood, biliary tree, intestines, and lungs (Table 126-1).

Trematodes share some common morphologic features, including macroscopic size (from 1 cm to several cm); dorsoventral, flattened, bilaterally symmetric bodies (adult worms); and the prominence of two suckers. Except for schistosomes, all human parasitic trematodes are hermaphroditic. Their life cycle involves a definitive host (mammalian/human), in which adult worms initiate sexual reproduction, and an intermediate host (snails), in which asexual multiplication of larvae occurs. More than one intermediate host may be necessary for some species of trematodes. Human infection is initiated either by direct penetration of intact skin or by ingestion. Upon maturation within humans, adult flukes initiate sexual reproduction and egg production. Helminth ova leave the definitive host in excreta or sputum and, upon reaching suitable environmental conditions, they hatch, releasing free-living miracidia that seek specific snail intermediate hosts. After asexual reproduction, cercariae are released from infected snails. In certain species, these organisms infect humans; in others, they find a second intermediate host to allow encystment into metacercariae—the infective stage.

TABLE 126-1

MAJOR HUMAN TREMATODE INFECTIONS

TREMATODE	TRANSMISSION	ENDEMIC AREA(S)
Blood Flukes		
Schistosoma mansoni	Skin penetration by cercariae released from snails	Africa, South America, Middle East
S. japonicum	Skin penetration by cercariae released from snails	China, Philippines, Indonesia
S. intercalatum	Skin penetration by cercariae released from snails	West Africa
S. mekongi	Skin penetration by cercariae released from snails	Southeast Asia
S. haematobium	Skin penetration by cercariae released from snails	Africa, Middle East
Biliary (Hepatic) Flukes		
Clonorchis sinensis	Ingestion of metacercariae in freshwater fish	Far East
Opisthorchis viverrini	Ingestion of metacercariae in freshwater fish	Far East, Thailand
O. felineus	Ingestion of metacercariae in freshwater fish	Far East, Europe
Fasciola hepatica	Ingestion of metacercariae on aquatic plants or in water	Worldwide
F. gigantica	Ingestion of metacercariae on aquatic plants or in water	Sporadic, Africa
Intestinal Flukes		
Fasciolopsis buski	Ingestion of metacercariae on aquatic plants	Southeast Asia
Heterophyes heterophyes	Ingestion of metacercariae in freshwater or brackish-water fish	Far East, North Africa
Lung Flukes		
Paragonimus westermani	Ingestion of metacercariae in crayfish or crabs	Global except North America and Europe

The host-parasite relationship in trematode infections is a product of certain biologic features of these organisms: they are multicellular, undergo several developmental changes within the host, and usually result in chronic infections. In general, the distribution of worm infections in human populations is *overdispersed*; i.e., it follows a negative binomial mathematical relationship in which most infected individuals harbor low worm burdens while a small percentage are heavily infected. It is the heavily infected minority who are particularly prone to disease sequelae and who constitute an epidemiologically significant reservoir of infection in endemic areas. Equally important is an appreciation that worms do not multiply within the definitive host and that they have a relatively long life span, ranging from a few months to a few years. Morbidity and death due to trematode infections reflect a multifactorial process that results from the tipping of a delicate balance between intensity of infection and host reactions, which initiate and modulate immunologic and pathologic outcome. Furthermore, the genetics of the parasite and of the human host contribute to the outcome of infection and disease. Infections with trematodes that migrate through or reside in host tissues are associated with a moderate to high degree of peripheral blood eosinophilia; this association is of significance in protective and immunopathologic sequelae and is a useful clinical indicator of infection.

Approach to the Patient: TREMATODE INFECTION

The approach to individuals with suspected trematode infection begins with a question: Where have you been? Details of geographic history, exposure to freshwater bodies, and indulgence in local eating habits without ensuring safety of food and drink are all essential elements in the history. The workup plan must include a detailed physical examination and tests appropriate for the suspected infection. Diagnosis is based either on detection of the relevant stage of the parasite in excreta, sputum, or (rarely) tissue samples or on sensitive and specific serologic tests. Consultation with physicians familiar with these infections or with the U.S. Centers for Disease Control and Prevention (CDC) is helpful in guiding diagnosis and selecting therapy.

BLOOD FLUKES: SCHISTOSOMIASIS

Human schistosomiasis is caused by five species of the parasitic trematode genus *Schistosoma*: the intestinal species *S. mansoni*, *S. japonicum*, *S. mekongi*, and *S. intercalatum* and the urinary species *S. haematobium*. Infection may cause considerable morbidity in the intestines, liver, and urinary tract, and a proportion of affected individuals die. Other schistosomes (e.g., avian species) may invade human skin but then die in subcutaneous tissue, producing only self-limiting cutaneous manifestations.

ETIOLOGY

Human infection is initiated by penetration of intact skin with infective cercariae. These organisms, which are released from infected snails in freshwater bodies, measure ~2 mm in length and possess an anterior and a ventral sucker that attach to the skin and facilitate penetration. Once in subcutaneous tissue, cercariae transform into schistosomula, with morphologic, membrane, and immunologic changes. The cercarial outer membrane changes from a trilaminar to a heptalaminar structure that is then maintained throughout the organism's life span in humans. This transformation is thought to be the schistosome's main adaptive mechanism for survival in humans. Schistosomula begin their migration within 2–4 days via venous or lymphatic vessels, reaching the lungs and finally the liver parenchyma. Sexually mature worms descend into the venous system at specific anatomic locations: intestinal veins (*S. mansoni, S. japonicum, S. mekongi,* and *S. intercalatum*) and vesical veins (*S. haematobium*). After mating, adult gravid females travel against venous blood flow to small tributaries, where they deposit their ova intravascularly. Schistosome ova (Fig. 126-1) have specific morphologic features that vary with the species. Aided by enzymatic secretions through minipores in eggshells, ova move through the venous wall, traversing host tissues to reach the lumen of the intestinal or urinary tract, and are voided with stools or urine. Approximately 50% of ova are retained in host tissues locally (intestines or urinary tract) or are carried by venous blood flow to the liver and other organs. Schistosome ova that reach freshwater

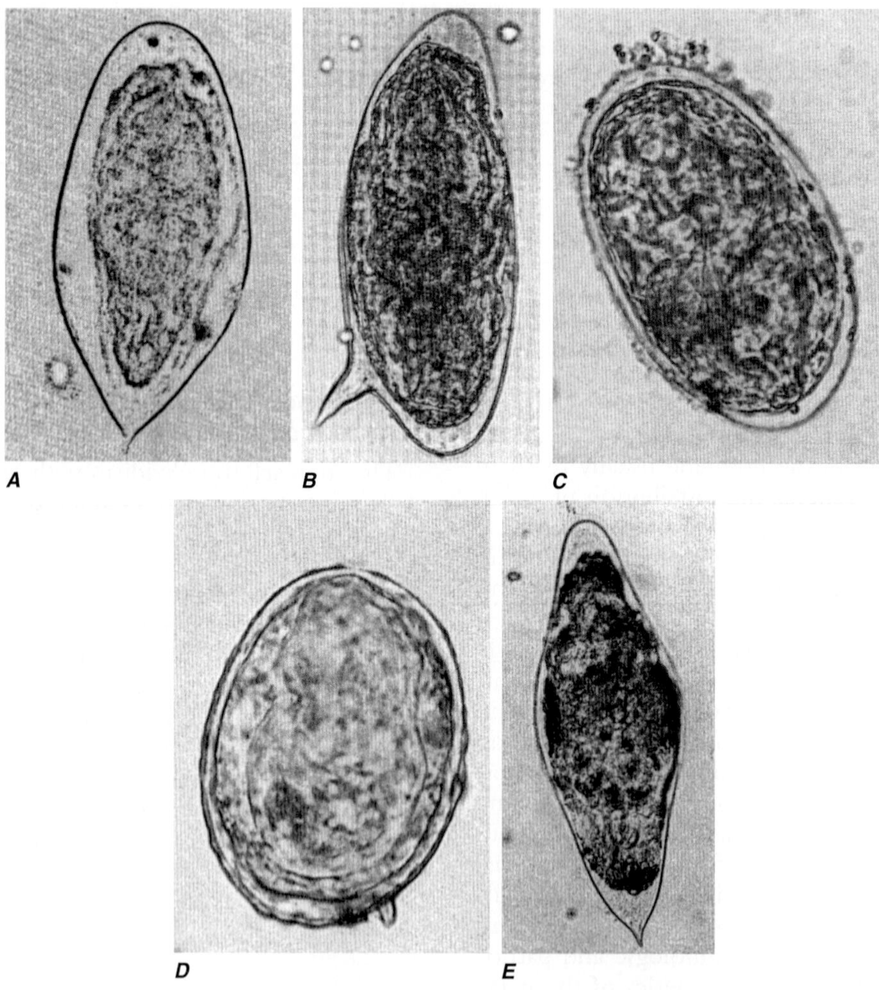

FIGURE 126-1

Morphology of schistosome eggs, the diagnostic stage of the parasite's life cycle. ***A.*** *S. haematobium* egg found in urine sample. Egg is large (~140 μm long), with a terminal spine. ***B.*** *S. mansoni* egg found in feces. Egg is large (~150 μm long), with a thin shell and lateral spine. ***C.*** *S. japonicum* egg found in feces. Egg is smaller than that of *S. mansoni* (~90 μm long), with a small spine or hooklike structure. ***D.*** *S. mekongi* egg found in feces. Egg is similar to that of *S. japonicum* but smaller (~65 μm long). ***E.*** *S. intercalatum* egg found in feces. Egg is larger than that of *S. haematobium* (~190 μm long), with a longer, sharply pointed spine. *(From LR Ash, TC Orihel: Atlas of Human Parasitology, 3d ed. Chicago, ASCP Press, 1990; with permission.)*

bodies hatch, releasing free-living miracidia that seek the snail intermediate host and undergo several asexual multiplication cycles. Finally, infective cercariae are shed from snails.

Adult schistosomes are ~1–2 cm long. Males are slightly shorter than females, with flattened bodies and anteriorly curved edges forming the gynecophoral canal, in which mature adult females are usually held. Females are longer, slender, and rounded in cross-section. The precise nature of biochemical and reproductive exchanges between the two sexes is unknown, as are the regulatory mechanisms for pairing. Adult schistosomes parasitize specific sites in the host venous system. What guides adult intestinal schistosomes to branches of the superior or inferior mesenteric veins or adult *S. haematobium* worms to the vesical plexus is unknown. In addition, adult worms inhibit the coagulation cascade and evade the effector arms of the host immune responses by still-undetermined mechanisms. The genome of schistosomes is relatively large (~270 Mb) and is arrayed on seven pairs of autosomes and one pair of sex chromosomes. For *S. mansoni*, a total of ~14,000 genes have been estimated; some are species-conserved. The complete sequence of the schistosome genome should be available soon.

EPIDEMIOLOGY

The global distribution of schistosome infection in human populations (Fig. 126-2) is dependent on both parasite and host factors. Information on prevalence and global distribution is inexact. The five *Schistosoma* species are estimated to infect 200–300 million individuals in South America, the Caribbean, Africa, the Middle East, and Southeast Asia. The total population living under conditions favoring transmission approximates double or triple that number—a fact reflecting the public health significance of schistosomiasis.

In endemic areas, the rate of yearly onset of new infection, or incidence, is generally low. Prevalence, on the other hand, starts to be appreciable by the age of 3–4 years and builds to a maximum that varies by endemic region (up to 100%) in the 15- to 20-year age group. Prevalence then stabilizes or decreases slightly in older age groups (>40 years). Intensity of infection (as measured by fecal or urinary egg counts, which correlate with adult worm burdens in most circumstances) follows the increase in prevalence up to the age of 15–20 years and then declines markedly in older age groups. This decline may reflect acquisition of resistance or may be due to changes in water contact patterns, since older people have less exposure. Furthermore, the overdispersed distribution of schistosomes in human populations may be due to the heterogeneity of worm populations, with some more invasive than others; alternatively, it may be due to the demonstrated differences in genetic susceptibility of host populations.

Disease due to schistosome infection is the outcome of parasitologic, host, and additional infectious, nutritional, and environmental factors. Most disease syndromes relate to the presence of one or more of the parasite stages in humans. Disease manifestations in the populations of endemic areas correlate, in general, with the intensity and

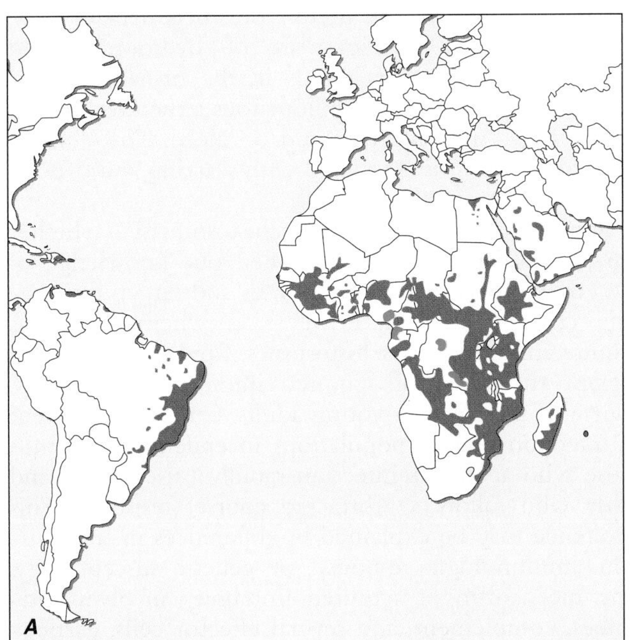

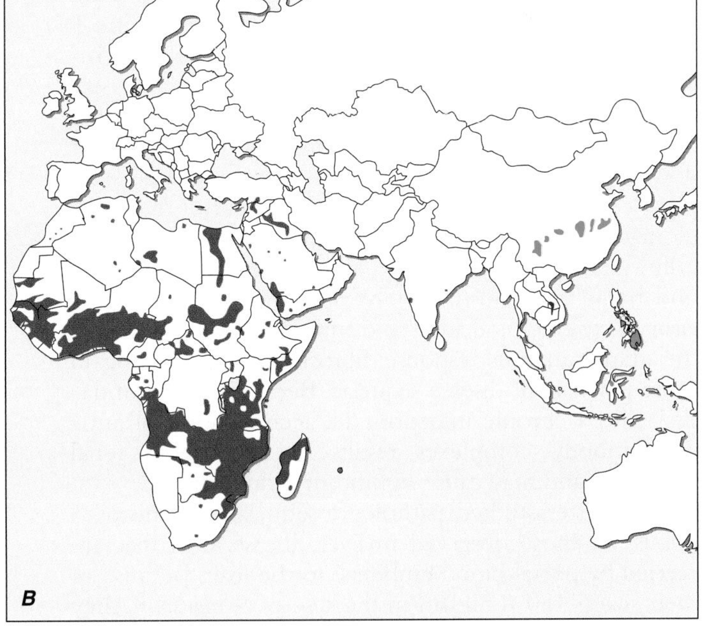

FIGURE 126-2

Global distribution of schistosomiasis. ***A.*** *S. mansoni* infection (*dark blue*) is endemic in Africa, the Middle East, South America, and a few Caribbean countries. *S. intercalatum* infection (*green*) is endemic in sporadic foci in West and Central Africa. ***B.*** *S. haematobium* infection (*purple*) is endemic in Africa and the Middle East. The major endemic countries for *S. japonicum* infection (*green*) are China, the Philippines, and Indonesia. *S. mekongi* infection (*red*) is endemic in sporadic foci in Southeast Asia.

duration of infection as well as with the age and genetic susceptibility of the host. Overall, disease manifestations are clinically relevant in only a small proportion of persons infected with any of the intestinal schistosomes. In contrast, urinary schistosomiasis manifests clinically in most infected individuals. Recent estimates of total morbidity due to chronic schistosomiasis indicate a significantly greater burden than was previously appreciated.

Patients with both HIV infection and schistosomiasis excrete far fewer eggs in their stools than those infected with *S. mansoni* alone; the mechanism underlying this difference is unknown. Treatment with praziquantel may result in reduced HIV replication and increased CD4+ T lymphocyte counts.

PATHOGENESIS AND IMMUNITY

Cercarial invasion is associated with dermatitis arising from dermal and subdermal inflammatory responses, both humoral and cell-mediated. As the parasites approach sexual maturity and with the commencement of oviposition, acute schistosomiasis or Katayama fever (a serum sickness–like illness; see "Clinical Features" next in the chapter) may occur. The associated antigen excess results in formation of soluble immune complexes, which may be deposited in several tissues, initiating multiple pathologic events. In chronic schistosomiasis, most disease manifestations are due to eggs retained in host tissues. The granulomatous response around these ova is cell-mediated and is regulated both positively and negatively by a cascade of cytokine, cellular, and humoral responses. Granuloma formation begins with recruitment of a host of inflammatory cells in response to antigens secreted by the living organism within the ova. Cells recruited initially include phagocytes, antigen-specific T cells, and eosinophils. Fibroblasts, giant cells, and B lymphocytes predominate later. These lesions reach a size many times that of parasite eggs, thus inducing organomegaly and obstruction. Immunomodulation or downregulation of host responses to schistosome eggs plays a significant role in limiting the extent of the granulomatous lesions—and consequently disease—in chronically infected experimental animals or humans. The underlying mechanisms involve another cascade of regulatory cytokines and idiotypic antibodies. Subsequent to the granulomatous response, fibrosis sets in, resulting in more permanent disease sequelae. Because schistosomiasis is also a chronic infection, the accumulation of antigen-antibody complexes results in deposits in renal glomeruli and may cause significant kidney disease.

The better-studied pathologic sequelae in schistosomiasis are those observed in liver disease. Ova that are carried by portal blood embolize to the liver. Because of their size (~150 × 60 μm in the case of *S. mansoni*), they lodge at presinusoidal sites, where granulomas are formed. These granulomas contribute to the hepatomegaly observed in infected individuals. Schistosomal liver enlargement is also associated with certain class I and class II human leukocyte antigen (HLA) haplotypes and markers; its genetic basis appears to be multigenic. Presinusoidal portal blockage causes several hemodynamic changes, including portal hypertension and associated development of portosystemic collaterals at the esophagogastric junction and other sites. Esophageal varices are most likely to break and cause repeated episodes of hematemesis. Because changes in hepatic portal blood flow occur slowly, compensatory arterialization of the blood flow through the liver is established. While this compensatory mechanism may be associated with certain metabolic side effects, retention of hepatocyte perfusion permits maintenance of normal liver function for several years.

The second most significant pathologic change in the liver relates to fibrosis. It is characteristically periportal (Symmers' clay pipe–stem fibrosis) but may be diffuse. Fibrosis, when diffuse, may be seen in areas of egg deposition and granuloma formation but is also seen in distant locations such as portal tracts. Schistosomiasis results in pure fibrotic lesions in the liver; cirrhosis occurs when other nutritional factors or infectious agents (e.g., hepatitis B or C virus) are involved. In recent years, it has been recognized that deposition of fibrotic tissue in the extracellular matrix results from the interaction of T lymphocytes with cells of the fibroblast series; several cytokines, such as interleukin (IL) 2, IL-4, IL-1, and transforming growth factor β (TGF-β), are known to stimulate fibrogenesis. The process may be dependent on the genetic constitution of the host. Furthermore, regulatory cytokines that can suppress fibrogenesis, such as interferon γ (IFN-γ) or IL-12, may play a role in modulating the response.

While the above description focuses on granuloma formation and fibrosis of the liver, similar processes occur in urinary schistosomiasis. Granuloma formation at the lower end of the ureters obstructs urinary flow, with subsequent development of hydroureter and hydronephrosis. Similar lesions in the urinary bladder cause the protrusion of papillomatous structures into its cavity; these may ulcerate and/or bleed. The chronic stage of infection is associated with scarring and deposition of calcium in bladder wall.

Studies on immunity to schistosomiasis, whether innate or adaptive, have expanded our knowledge of the components of these responses and target antigens. The critical question, however, is whether humans acquire immunity to schistosomes. Epidemiologic data suggest the onset of acquired immunity during the course of infection in young adults. Curative treatment of infection divides populations in endemic areas into those who acquire reinfection rapidly (susceptible) and those who follow a protracted course (resistant). This difference may be explained by differences in transmission, immunologic response, or genetic susceptibility. The mechanism of acquired immunity involves antibodies, complement, and several effector cells, particularly eosinophils. Furthermore, the intensity of schistosome infection has been correlated with a region in chromosome 5. In several studies, a few protective schistosome antigens have been identified as vaccine candidates, but none has been evaluated in human populations to date.

CLINICAL FEATURES

In general, disease manifestations of schistosomiasis occur in three stages, which vary not only by species but also by intensity of infection and other host factors, such as age and genetics. During the phase of cercarial invasion, a form of dermatitis may be observed. This so-called swimmers' itch occurs most often with *S. mansoni* and *S. japonicum* infections, manifesting 2 or 3 days after invasion as an itchy maculopapular rash on the affected areas of the skin. The condition is particularly severe when humans are exposed to avian schistosomes. This form of cercarial dermatitis is also seen around freshwater lakes in the northern United States, particularly in the spring. Cercarial dermatitis is a self-limiting clinical entity. During worm maturation and at the beginning of oviposition (i.e., 4–8 weeks after skin invasion), acute schistosomiasis or Katayama fever—a serum sickness–like syndrome with fever, generalized lymphadenopathy, and hepatosplenomegaly—may develop. Individuals with acute schistosomiasis show a high degree of peripheral blood eosinophilia. Parasite-specific antibodies may be detected before schistosome eggs are identified in excreta. Acute schistosomiasis has become an important clinical entity worldwide because of increased travel to endemic areas. Travelers are exposed to parasites while swimming or wading in freshwater bodies and upon their return present with the acute manifestations. The course of acute schistosomiasis is generally benign, but deaths are occasionally reported in association with heavy exposure to schistosomes.

The main clinical manifestations of chronic schistosomiasis are species-dependent. Intestinal species (*S. mansoni, S. japonicum, S. mekongi*, and *S. intercalatum*) cause intestinal and hepatosplenic disease as well as several manifestations associated with portal hypertension. During the intestinal phase, which may begin a few months after infection and may last for years, symptomatic patients characteristically have colicky abdominal pain, bloody diarrhea, and anemia. Patients may also report fatigue and an inability to perform daily routine functions and may show evidence of growth retardation. It has been demonstrated that schistosomiasis morbidity is generally underappreciated. The severity of intestinal schistosomiasis is often related to the intensity of the worm burden. The disease runs a chronic course and may result in colonic polyposis, which has been reported from some endemic areas, such as Egypt.

The hepatosplenic phase of disease manifests early (during the first year of infection, particularly in children) with liver enlargement due to parasite-induced granulomatous lesions. Hepatomegaly is seen in ~15–20% of infected individuals; it correlates roughly with intensity of infection, occurs more often in children, and may be related to specific HLA haplotypes. In subsequent phases of infection, presinusoidal blockage of blood flow leads to portal hypertension and splenomegaly. Moreover, portal hypertension may lead to varices at the lower end of the esophagus and at other sites. Patients with schistosomal liver disease may have right-upper-quadrant "dragging" pain during the hepatomegaly phase, and this pain may move to the left upper quadrant as splenomegaly progresses. Bleeding from esophageal varices may, however, be the first clinical manifestation of this phase. Patients may experience repeated bleeding but seem to tolerate its impact, since an adequate total hepatic blood flow permits normal liver function for a considerable duration. In late-stage disease, typical fibrotic changes occur along with liver function deterioration and the onset of ascites, hypoalbuminemia, and defects in coagulation. Intercurrent viral infections of the liver (especially hepatitis B and C) or nutritional deficiencies may well accelerate or exacerbate the deterioration of hepatic function.

The extent and severity of intestinal and hepatic disease in schistosomiasis mansoni and japonica have been well described. While it was originally thought that *S. japonicum* might induce more severe disease manifestations because the adult worms can produce 10 times more eggs than *S. mansoni*, subsequent field studies have not supported this claim. Clinical observations of individuals infected with *S. mekongi* or *S. intercalatum* have been less detailed, partly because of the limited geographic distribution of these organisms.

The clinical manifestations of *S. haematobium* infection occur relatively early and involve a high percentage of infected individuals. Up to 80% of children infected with *S. haematobium* have dysuria, frequency, and hematuria, which may be terminal. Urine examination reveals blood and albumin as well as an unusually high frequency of bacterial urinary tract infection and urinary sediment cellular metaplasia. These manifestations correlate with intensity of infection, the presence of urinary bladder granulomas, and subsequent ulceration. Along with local effects of granuloma formation in the urinary bladder, obstruction of the lower end of the ureters results in hydroureter and hydronephrosis, which may be seen in 25–50% of infected children. As infection progresses, bladder granulomas undergo fibrosis, which results in typical sandy patches visible on cystoscopy. In many endemic areas, an association between squamous cell carcinoma of the bladder and *S. haematobium* infection has been observed. Such malignancy is detected in a younger age group than is transitional cell carcinoma. In fact, *S. haematobium* has now been classified as a human carcinogen.

Significant disease may occur in other organs during chronic schistosomiasis. Most important are the lungs and central nervous system (CNS); other locations, such as the skin and the genital organs, are far less frequently affected. In pulmonary schistosomiasis, embolized eggs lodge in small arterioles, producing acute necrotizing arteriolitis and granuloma formation. During *S. mansoni* and *S. japonicum* infection, schistosome eggs reach the lungs after the development of portosystemic collateral circulation; in *S. haematobium* infection, ova may reach the lungs directly via connections between the vesical and systemic circulation. Subsequent fibrous tissue deposition leads to endarteritis obliterans, pulmonary hypertension, and cor pulmonale. The most common symptoms are cough, fever, and dyspnea. Cor pulmonale may be diagnosed radiologically on the basis of prominent right side of the heart and dilation of the pulmonary artery. Frank evidence of right-sided heart failure may be seen in late cases.

CNS schistosomiasis is important but less common than pulmonary schistosomiasis. It characteristically occurs as cerebral disease due to *S. japonicum* infection. Migratory worms deposit eggs in the brain and induce a granulomatous response. The frequency of this manifestation among infected individuals in some endemic areas (e.g., the Philippines) is calculated at 2–4%. Jacksonian epilepsy due to *S. japonicum* infection is the second most common cause of epilepsy in these areas. *S. mansoni* and *S. haematobium* infections have been associated with transverse myelitis. This syndrome is thought to be due to eggs traveling to the venous plexus around the spinal cord. In schistosomiasis mansoni, transverse myelitis is usually seen in the chronic stage after the development of portal hypertension and portosystemic shunts, which allow ova to travel to the spinal cord veins. This proposed sequence of events has been challenged because of a few reports of transverse myelitis occurring early in the course of *S. mansoni* infection. More information is needed to confirm these observations. During schistosomiasis haematobia, ova may travel through communication between vesical and systemic veins, resulting in spinal cord disease that may be detected at any stage of infection. Pathologic study of lesions in schistosomal transverse myelitis may reveal eggs along with necrotic or granulomatous lesions. Patients usually present with acute or rapidly progressing lower-leg weakness accompanied by sphincter dysfunction.

DIAGNOSIS

Physicians in areas not endemic for schistosomiasis face considerable diagnostic challenges. In the most common clinical presentation, a traveler returns with symptoms and signs of acute syndromes of schistosomiasis—namely, cercarial dermatitis or Katayama fever. Central to correct diagnosis is a thorough inquiry into travel history and exposure to freshwater bodies, whether slow or fast running. Differential diagnosis of fever in returned travelers includes a spectrum of infections whose etiologies are viral (e.g., Dengue fever), bacterial (e.g., enteric fever, leptospirosis), rickettsial, or protozoal (e.g., malaria). In cases of Katayama fever, prompt diagnosis is essential and is based on clinical presentation, high-level peripheral blood eosinophilia, and a positive serologic assay for schistosomal antibodies. Two tests are available at the CDC: the Falcon assay screening test/enzyme-linked immunosorbent assay (FAST-ELISA) and the confirmatory enzyme-linked immunoelectrotransfer blot (EITB). Both tests are highly sensitive and ~96% specific. In some instances, examination of stool or urine for ova may yield positive results.

Individuals with established infection are diagnosed by a combination of geographic history, characteristic clinical presentation, and presence of schistosome ova in excreta. The diagnosis may also be established with the serologic assays mentioned above or with those that detect circulating schistosome antigens. These assays can be applied either to blood or to other body fluids (e.g., cerebrospinal fluid). For suspected schistosome infection, stool examination by the Kato thick smear or any other concentration method generally identifies all but the most lightly infected individuals. For *S. haematobium*, urine may be examined by microscopy of sediment or by filtration of a known volume through Nuclepore filters. Kato thick smear and Nuclepore filtration provide quantitative data on the intensity of infection, which is of value in assessing the degree of tissue damage and in monitoring the effect of chemotherapy. Schistosome infection may also be diagnosed by examination of tissue samples, typically rectal biopsies; other biopsy procedures (e.g., liver biopsy) are not needed, except in rare circumstances.

Differential diagnosis of schistosomal hepatomegaly must include viral hepatitis of all etiologies, miliary tuberculosis, malaria, visceral leishmaniasis, ethanol abuse, and causes of hepatic and portal vein obstruction. Differential diagnosis of hematuria in *S. haematobium* infection includes bacterial cystitis, tuberculosis, urinary stones, and malignancy.

Rx Treatment: SCHISTOSOMIASIS

Treatment of schistosomiasis depends on stage of infection and clinical presentation. Other than topical dermatologic applications for relief of itching, no specific treatment is indicated for cercarial dermatitis caused by avian schistosomes. Therapy for acute schistosomiasis or Katayama fever needs to be adjusted appropriately for each case. While antischistosomal chemotherapy may be used, it does not have a significant impact on maturing worms. In severe acute schistosomiasis, management in an acute-care setting is necessary, with supportive measures and consideration of glucocorticoid treatment. Once the acute critical phase is over, specific chemotherapy is indicated for parasite elimination. For all individuals with established infection, treatment to eradicate the parasite should be administered. The drug of choice is praziquantel, which—depending on the infecting species (Table 126-2)—is administered PO as a total of 40 or 60 mg/kg in two or three doses over a single day. Praziquantel treatment results in parasitologic cure in ~85% of cases and reduces egg counts by >90%. Few side effects have been encountered, and those that do develop usually do not interfere with completion of treatment. Dependence on a single chemotherapeutic agent has raised the possibility of development of resistance in schistosomes; to date, such resistance does not seem to be clinically significant. The effect of antischistosomal treatment on disease manifestations varies by stage. Early hepatomegaly and bladder lesions are known to resolve after chemotherapy, but the late established manifestations, such as fibrosis, do not recede. Additional management modalities are needed for individuals with other manifestations, such as hepatocellular failure or recurrent hematemesis. The use of these interventions is guided by general medical and surgical principles.

PREVENTION AND CONTROL

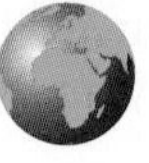

Transmission of schistosomiasis is dependent on human behavior. Since the geographic distribution of infections in endemic regions of the world

TABLE 126-2

DRUG THERAPY FOR HUMAN TREMATODE INFECTIONS

INFECTION	DRUG OF CHOICE	ADULT DOSE AND DURATION
Blood Flukes		
S. mansoni, S. intercalatum, S. haematobium	Praziquantel	20 mg/kg, 2 doses in 1 day
S. japonicum, S. mekongi	Praziquantel	20 mg/kg, 3 doses in 1 day
Biliary (Hepatic) Flukes		
C. sinensis, O. viverrini, O. felineus	Praziquantel	25 mg/kg, 3 doses in 1 day
F. hepatica, F. gigantica	Triclabendazole	10 mg/kg once
Intestinal Flukes		
F. buski, H. heterophyes	Praziquantel	25 mg/kg, 3 doses in 1 day
Lung Flukes		
P. westermani	Praziquantel	25 mg/kg, 3 doses per day for 2 days

is not clearly demarcated, it is prudent for travelers to avoid contact with all freshwater bodies, irrespective of the speed of water flow or unsubstantiated claims of safety. Some topical agents, when applied to skin, may inhibit cercarial penetration, but none is currently available. If exposure occurs, a follow-up visit with a health care provider is strongly recommended. Prevention of infection in inhabitants of endemic areas is a significant challenge. Residents of these regions use freshwater bodies for sanitary, domestic, recreational, and agricultural purposes. Several control measures have been used, including application of molluscicides, provision of sanitary water and sewage disposal, chemotherapy, and health education. Current recommendations to countries endemic for schistosomiasis emphasize the use of multiple approaches. With the advent of an oral, safe, and effective antischistosomal agent, chemotherapy has been most successful in reducing intensity of infection and reversing disease. The duration of this positive impact depends on transmission dynamics of the parasite in any specific endemic region. The ultimate goal of research on prevention and control is development of a vaccine. Although there are a few promising leads, this goal is probably not within reach during the next decade or so.

LIVER (BILIARY) FLUKES

Several species of biliary fluke infecting humans are particularly common in Southeast Asia and Russia. Other species are transmitted in Europe, Africa, and the Americas. On the basis of their migratory pathway in humans, these infections may be divided into the *Clonorchis* and *Fasciola* groups (Table 126-1).

CLONORCHIASIS AND OPISTHORCHIASIS

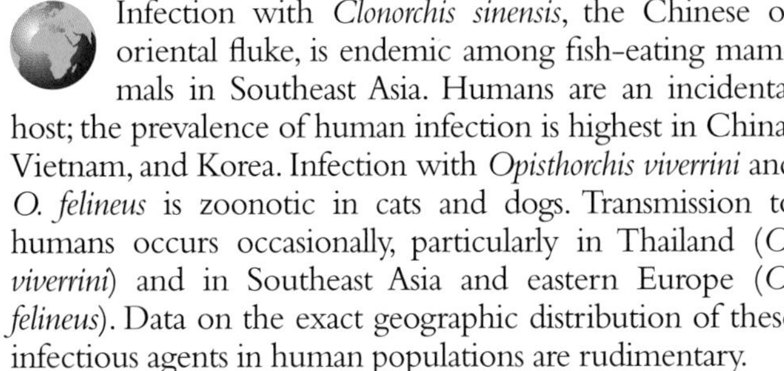

Infection with *Clonorchis sinensis*, the Chinese or oriental fluke, is endemic among fish-eating mammals in Southeast Asia. Humans are an incidental host; the prevalence of human infection is highest in China, Vietnam, and Korea. Infection with *Opisthorchis viverrini* and *O. felineus* is zoonotic in cats and dogs. Transmission to humans occurs occasionally, particularly in Thailand (*O. viverrini*) and in Southeast Asia and eastern Europe (*O. felineus*). Data on the exact geographic distribution of these infectious agents in human populations are rudimentary.

Infection with any of these three species is established by ingestion of raw or inadequately cooked freshwater fish harboring metacercariae. These organisms excyst in the duodenum, releasing larvae that travel through the ampulla of Vater and mature into adult worms in bile canaliculi. Mature flukes are flat and elongated, measuring 1–2 cm in length. The hermaphroditic worms reproduce by releasing small operculated eggs, which pass with bile into the intestines and are voided with stools. The life cycle is completed in the environment in specific freshwater snails (the first intermediate host) and encystment of metacercariae in freshwater fish.

Except for late sequelae, the exact clinical syndromes caused by clonorchiasis and opisthorchiasis are not well defined. Since most infected individuals harbor a low worm burden, many are asymptomatic. Moderate to heavy infection may be associated with vague right-upper-quadrant pain. In contrast, chronic or repeated infection is associated with manifestations such as cholangitis, cholangiohepatitis, and biliary obstruction. Cholangiocarcinoma is epidemiologically related to *C. sinensis* infection in China and to *O. viverrini* infection in northeastern Thailand. This association has resulted in classification of these infectious agents as human carcinogens.

FASCIOLIASIS

Infections with *Fasciola hepatica* and *F. gigantica* are worldwide zoonoses that are particularly endemic in sheep-raising countries. Human cases have been reported in South America, Europe, Africa, Australia, and the Far East. Recent estimates indicate a worldwide prevalence of 17 million cases. High endemicity has been reported in certain areas of Peru and Bolivia. In most endemic areas the predominant species is *F. hepatica*, but in Asia and Africa a varying degree of overlap with *F. gigantica* has been observed.

Humans acquire fascioliasis by ingestion of metacercariae attached to certain aquatic plants, such as watercress. Infection may also be acquired by consumption of contaminated water or ingestion of food items washed with such water. Acquisition of human infection through consumption of freshly prepared raw liver containing immature flukes has been reported. Infection is initiated when metacercariae excyst, penetrate the gut wall, and travel through the peritoneal cavity to invade the liver capsule. Adult worms finally reach bile ducts, where they produce large operculated eggs, which are voided in bile through the gastrointestinal tract to the outside environment. The flukes' life cycle is completed in specific snails (the first intermediate host) and encystment on aquatic plants.

Clinical features of fascioliasis relate to the stage and intensity of infection. Acute disease develops during parasite migration (1–2 weeks after infection) and includes fever, right-upper-quadrant pain, hepatomegaly, and eosinophilia. CT of the liver may show migratory tracks. Symptoms and signs usually subside as the parasites reach their final habitat. In individuals with chronic infection, bile duct obstruction and biliary cirrhosis are infrequently demonstrated. No relation to hepatic malignancy has been ascribed to fascioliasis.

DIAGNOSIS

Diagnosis of infection with any of the biliary flukes depends on a high degree of suspicion, elicitation of an appropriate geographic history, and stool examination for characteristically shaped parasite ova. Additional evidence may be obtained by documenting peripheral blood eosinophilia or imaging the liver. Serologic testing is helpful, particularly in lightly infected individuals.

℞ Treatment: BILIARY FLUKES

Drug therapy (praziquantel or triclabendazole) is summarized in Table 126-2. Patients with anatomic lesions in the biliary tract or malignancy are managed according to general medical guidelines.

INTESTINAL FLUKES

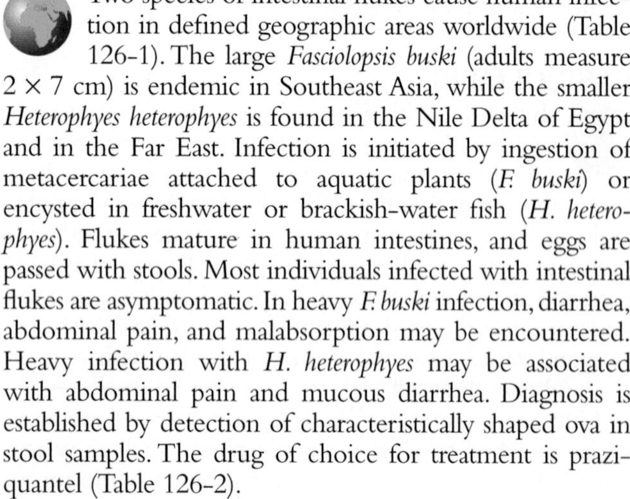

Two species of intestinal flukes cause human infection in defined geographic areas worldwide (Table 126-1). The large *Fasciolopsis buski* (adults measure 2 × 7 cm) is endemic in Southeast Asia, while the smaller *Heterophyes heterophyes* is found in the Nile Delta of Egypt and in the Far East. Infection is initiated by ingestion of metacercariae attached to aquatic plants (*F. buski*) or encysted in freshwater or brackish-water fish (*H. heterophyes*). Flukes mature in human intestines, and eggs are passed with stools. Most individuals infected with intestinal flukes are asymptomatic. In heavy *F. buski* infection, diarrhea, abdominal pain, and malabsorption may be encountered. Heavy infection with *H. heterophyes* may be associated with abdominal pain and mucous diarrhea. Diagnosis is established by detection of characteristically shaped ova in stool samples. The drug of choice for treatment is praziquantel (Table 126-2).

LUNG FLUKES

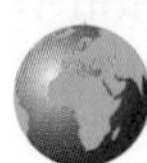

Infection with the lung fluke *Paragonimus westermani* (Table 126-1) and related species (e.g., *P. africanus*) is endemic in many parts of the world, excluding North America and Europe. Endemicity is particularly noticeable in West Africa, Central and South America, and Asia. In nature, the reservoir hosts of *P. westermani* are wild and domestic felines. In Africa, *P. africanus* has been found in other species, such as dogs. Adult lung flukes, which are 7–12 mm in length, are found encapsulated in the lungs of infected persons. In rare circumstances, flukes are found encysted in the CNS (cerebral paragonimiasis) or abdominal cavity. Humans acquire lung fluke infection by ingesting infective metacercariae encysted in the muscles and viscera of crayfish and freshwater crabs. In endemic areas, these crustaceans are consumed either raw or pickled. Once the organisms reach the duodenum, they excyst, penetrate the gut wall, and travel through the peritoneal cavity, diaphragm, and pleural space to reach the lungs. Mature flukes are found in the bronchioles surrounded by cystic lesions. Parasite eggs are either expectorated with sputum or swallowed and passed to the outside environment with feces. The life cycle is completed in snails and freshwater crustacea.

When maturing flukes lodge in lung tissues, they cause hemorrhage and necrosis, resulting in cyst formation. The adjacent lung parenchyma shows evidence of inflammatory infiltration, predominantly by eosinophils. Cysts usually measure 1–2 cm in diameter and may contain one or two worms each. With the onset of oviposition, cysts usually rupture in adjacent bronchioles—an event allowing ova to exit the human host. Older cysts develop thickened walls, which may undergo calcification. During the active phase of paragonimiasis, lung tissues surrounding parasite cysts may contain evidence of pneumonia, bronchitis, bronchiectasis, and fibrosis.

Pulmonary paragonimiasis is particularly symptomatic in persons with moderate to heavy infection. Productive cough with brownish sputum or frank hemoptysis associated with peripheral blood eosinophilia is usually the presenting feature. Chest examination may reveal signs of pleurisy. In chronic cases, bronchitis or bronchiectasis may predominate, but these conditions rarely proceed to lung abscess. Imaging of the lungs demonstrates characteristic features, including patchy densities, cavities, pleural effusion, and ring shadows. Cerebral paragonimiasis presents as either space-occupying lesions or epilepsy.

DIAGNOSIS

Pulmonary paragonimiasis is diagnosed by detection of parasite ova in sputum and/or stools. Serology is of considerable help in egg-negative cases and in cerebral paragonimiasis.

℞ Treatment: LUNG FLUKES

The drug of choice for treatment is praziquantel (Table 126-2). Other medical or surgical management may be needed for pulmonary or cerebral lesions.

CONTROL AND PREVENTION OF TISSUE FLUKES

For residents of nonendemic areas who are visiting an endemic region, the only effective preventive measure is to avoid ingestion of local plants, fish, or crustaceans; if their ingestion is necessary, these items should be washed or cooked thoroughly. Instruction on water and food preparation and consumption should be included in physicians' advice to travelers (Chap. 4). Interruption of transmission among residents of endemic areas depends on avoiding ingestion of infective stages and disposing of feces and sputum appropriately to prevent hatching of eggs in the environment. These two approaches rely greatly on socioeconomic development and health education. In countries where economic progress has resulted in financial and social improvements, transmission has decreased. The third approach to control in endemic communities entails selective use of chemotherapy for individuals posing the highest risk of transmission—i.e., those with heavy infections. The availability of praziquantel—a broad-spectrum, safe, and effective anthelmintic agent—provides a means for reducing the reservoirs of infection in human populations. However, the existence of most of these helminths as zoonoses in several animal species complicates control efforts.

FURTHER READINGS

Alves Oliveira LF et al: Cytokine production associated with peripheral fibrosis during chronic schistosomiasis mansoni in humans. Infect Immun 74:1215, 2006

Caffrey CR: Chemotherapy of schistosomiasis: Present and future. Curr Opin Chem Biol 11:433, 2007

Centers for Disease Control and Prevention: *http://www.cdc.gov/ncidod/dpd*

Doenhoff MJ et al: Praziquantel: Mechanisms of action, resistance and new derivatives for schistosomiasis. Curr Opin Infect Dis 21:659, 2008

Drugs for Parasitic Infections. Med Lett Drugs Ther, August 1, 2004

Jia TW et al: Assessment of the age-specific disability weight of chronic schistosomiasis japonica. Bull World Health Organ 85:458, 2007

Kallestrup P et al: Schistosomiasis and HIV-1 infection in rural Zimbabwe: Effect of treatment of schistosomiasis on CD4 cell count and plasma HIV-1 RNA load. J Infect Dis 192:1956, 2005

King CH: Lifting the burden of schistosomiasis—defining elements of infection-associated disease and the benefits of antiparasite treatment. J Infect Dis 196:653, 2007

Lapa M et al: Cardiopulmonary manifestations of hepatosplenic schistosomiasis. Circulation 119:1518, 2009

Leshem E et al: Acute schistosomiasis outbreak: Clinical features and economic impact. Clin Infect Dis 47:1499, 2008

Lim JH et al: Parasitic diseases of the biliary tract. AJR Am J Roentgenol 188:1596, 2007

Lun ZR et al: Clonorchiasis: A key foodborne zoonosis in China. Lancet Infect Dis 5:31, 2005

Mahmoud AAFM (ed): Schistosomiasis, in *Tropical Medicine: Science and Practice*, G Pasvol, S Hoffman (eds). London, Imperial College Press, 2001, pp 1–510

Nicolls DJ et al: Characteristics of schistosomiasis in travelers reported to the GeoSentinel Surveillance Network 1997–2008. Am J Trop Med Hyg 79:729, 2008

Stauffer WM et al: Biliary liver flukes (opisthorchiasis and clonorchiasis) in immigrants in the United States: Often subtle and diagnosed years after arrival. J Travel Med 11:157, 2004

Toward the elimination of schistosomiasis. N Engl J Med 360:106, 2009

Wang LD et al: A strategy to control transmission of *Schistosoma japonicum* in China. N Engl J Med 360:121, 2009

CHAPTER 127
CESTODES

A. Clinton White, Jr. ■ Peter F. Weller

Cestodes, or tapeworms, are segmented worms. The adults reside in the gastrointestinal tract, but the larvae can be found in almost any organ. Human tapeworm infections can be divided into two major clinical groups. In one group, humans are the definitive hosts, with the adult tapeworms living in the gastrointestinal tract (*Taenia saginata*, *Diphyllobothrium*, *Hymenolepis*, and *Dipylidium caninum*). In the other, humans are intermediate hosts, with larval-stage parasites present in the tissues; diseases in this category include echinococcosis, sparganosis, and coenurosis. For *Taenia solium*, the human may be either the definitive or the intermediate host.

The ribbon-shaped tapeworm attaches to the intestinal mucosa by means of sucking cups or hooks located on the scolex. Behind the scolex is a short, narrow neck from which proglottids (segments) form. As each proglottid matures, it is displaced further back from the neck by the formation of new, less mature segments. The progressively elongating chain of attached proglottids, called the *strobila*, constitutes the bulk of the tapeworm.

The length varies among species. In some, the tapeworm may consist of more than 1000 proglottids and may be several meters long. The mature proglottids are hermaphroditic and produce eggs, which are subsequently released. Since eggs of the different *Taenia* species are morphologically identical, differences in the morphology of the scolex or proglottids provide the basis for diagnostic identification to the species level.

Most human tapeworms require at least one intermediate host for complete larval development. After ingestion of the eggs or proglottids by an intermediate host, the larval oncospheres are activated, escape the egg, and penetrate the intestinal mucosa. The oncosphere migrates to tissues and develops into an encysted form known as a *cysticercus* (single scolex), a *coenurus* (multiple scolices), or a *hydatid* (cyst with daughter cysts, each containing several protoscolices). Ingestion by the definitive host of tissues containing a cyst enables a scolex to develop into a tapeworm.

TAENIASIS SAGINATA

The beef tapeworm *T. saginata* occurs in all countries where raw or undercooked beef is eaten. It is most prevalent in sub-Saharan African and Middle Eastern countries. *T. saginata asiatica* is a variant of *T. saginata* that is found in Asia and for which pigs are the intermediate host.

Etiology and Pathogenesis

Humans are the only definitive host for the adult stage of *T. saginata*. This tapeworm, which can reach 8 m in length, inhabits the upper jejunum and has a scolex with four prominent suckers and 1000–2000 proglottids. Each gravid segment has 15–30 uterine branches (in contrast to 8–12 for *T. solium*). The eggs are indistinguishable from those of *T. solium*; they measure 30–40 μm, contain the oncosphere, and have a thick brown striated shell. Eggs deposited on vegetation can live for months or years until they are ingested by cattle or other herbivores. The embryo released after ingestion invades the intestinal wall and is carried to striated muscle, where it transforms into a cysticercus. When ingested in raw or undercooked beef, this form can infect humans. After the cysticercus is ingested, it takes ~2 months for the mature adult worm to develop.

Clinical Manifestations

Patients become aware of the infection most commonly by noting passage of proglottids in their feces. The proglottids are often motile, and patients may experience perianal discomfort when proglottids are discharged. Mild abdominal pain or discomfort, nausea, change in appetite, weakness, and weight loss can occur with *T. saginata* infection.

Diagnosis

The diagnosis is made by the detection of eggs or proglottids in the stool. Eggs may also be present in the perianal area; thus, if proglottids or eggs are not found in the stool, the perianal region should be examined with use of a cellophane-tape swab (as in pinworm infection; Chap. 124). Distinguishing *T. saginata* from *T. solium* requires examination of mature proglottids or the scolex. Serologic tests are not helpful diagnostically. Eosinophilia and elevated levels of serum IgE may be detected.

℞ Treatment: TAENIASIS SAGINATA

A single dose of praziquantel (10 mg/kg) is highly effective.

Prevention

The major method of preventing infection is the adequate cooking of beef; exposure to temperatures as low as 56°C for 5 min will destroy cysticerci. Refrigeration or salting for long periods or freezing at −10°C for 9 days also kills cysticerci in beef. General preventive measures include inspection of beef and proper disposal of human feces.

TAENIASIS SOLIUM AND CYSTICERCOSIS

The pork tapeworm *T. solium* can cause two distinct forms of infection in humans: adult tapeworms in the intestine or larval forms in the tissues (cysticercosis). Humans are the only definitive hosts for *T. solium*; pigs are the usual intermediate hosts, although other animals may harbor the larval forms.

T. solium exists worldwide but is most prevalent in Latin America, sub-Saharan Africa, China, southern and Southeast Asia, and eastern Europe. Cysticercosis occurs in industrialized nations largely as a result of the immigration of infected persons from endemic areas.

Etiology and Pathogenesis

The adult tapeworm generally resides in the upper jejunum. The scolex attaches by both sucking disks and two rows of hooklets. Often only one adult worm is present, but that worm may live for years. The tapeworm, usually ~3 m in length, may have as many as 1000 proglottids, each of which produces up to 50,000 eggs. Groups of 3–5 proglottids are generally released and excreted into the feces, and the eggs in these proglottids are infective for both humans and animals. The eggs may survive in the environment for several months. After ingestion of eggs by the pig intermediate host, the larvae are activated, escape the egg, penetrate the intestinal wall, and are carried to many tissues, with a predilection for striated muscle of the neck, tongue, and trunk. Within 60–90 days, the encysted larval stage develops. These cysticerci can survive for months to years. By ingesting undercooked pork containing cysticerci, humans acquire infections that lead to intestinal tapeworms. Infections that cause human cysticercosis follow the ingestion of *T. solium* eggs, usually from close contact with a tapeworm carrier. Autoinfection may

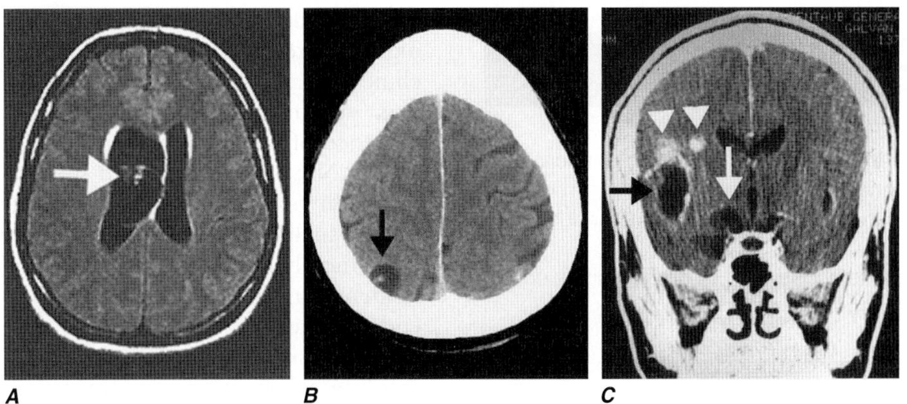

FIGURE 127-1

Neurocysticercosis is caused by *Taenia solium*. Neurologic infection can be classified on the basis of the location and viability of the parasites. When the parasites are in the ventricles, they often cause obstructive hydrocephalus. ***A.*** MRI showing a cysticercus in the lateral ventricle, with resultant hydrocephalus. The arrow points to the scolex within the cystic parasite. ***B.*** CT showing a parenchymal cysticercus, with enhancement of the cyst wall and an internal scolex (*arrow*). ***C.*** Multiple cysticerci, including calcified lesions from prior infection (*arrowheads*), viable cysticerci in the basilar cisterns (*white arrow*), and a large degenerating cysticercus in the Sylvian fissure (*black arrow*). *(Modified with permission from JC Bandres et al: Clin Infect Dis 15:799, 1992. © The University of Chicago Press.)*

occur if an individual with an egg-producing tapeworm ingests eggs derived from his or her own feces.

Clinical Manifestations

Intestinal infections with *T. solium* may be asymptomatic. Fecal passage of proglottids may be noted by patients. Other symptoms are infrequent.

In cysticercosis, the clinical manifestations are variable. Cysticerci can be found anywhere in the body but are most commonly detected in the brain, cerebrospinal fluid (CSF), skeletal muscle, subcutaneous tissue, or eye. The clinical presentation of cysticercosis depends on the number and location of cysticerci as well as the extent of associated inflammatory responses or scarring. Neurologic manifestations are the most common (Fig. 127-1). Seizures are associated with inflammation surrounding cysticerci in the brain parenchyma. These seizures may be generalized, focal, or Jacksonian. Hydrocephalus results from obstruction of CSF flow by cysticerci and accompanying inflammation or by CSF outflow obstruction from arachnoiditis. Signs of increased intracranial pressure, including headache, nausea, vomiting, changes in vision, dizziness, ataxia, or confusion, are often evident. Patients with hydrocephalus may develop papilledema or display altered mental status. When cysticerci develop at the base of the brain or in the subarachnoid space, they may cause chronic meningitis or arachnoiditis, communicating hydrocephalus, or strokes.

Diagnosis

The diagnosis of intestinal *T. solium* infection is made by the detection of eggs or proglottids, as described for *T. saginata*. In cysticercosis, diagnosis can be difficult. A consensus conference has delineated absolute, major, minor, and epidemiologic criteria for diagnosis (Table 127-1). Diagnostic certainty is possible only with definite demonstration of the parasite (absolute criteria). This task can be accomplished by histologic observation of the parasite in excised tissue, by funduscopic visualization of the parasite in the eye (in the anterior chamber, vitreous, or subretinal spaces), or by neuroimaging studies demonstrating cystic lesions containing a characteristic scolex. In most cases, diagnostic certainty is not possible. Instead, a clinical diagnosis is made on the basis of a combination of clinical presentation, radiographic studies, serologic tests, and exposure history.

Neuroimaging findings suggestive of neurocysticercosis constitute the primary major diagnostic criterion. These findings include cystic lesions with or without enhancement (e.g., ring enhancement), one or more nodular calcifications (which may also have associated enhancement), or focal enhancing lesions. Cysticerci in the brain parenchyma are usually 5–20 mm in diameter and rounded. Cystic lesions in the subarachnoid space or fissures may enlarge up to 6 cm in diameter and may be lobulated. For cysticerci within the subarachnoid space or ventricles, the walls may be very thin and the cyst fluid is often isodense with CSF. Thus, obstructive hydrocephalus or enhancement of the basilar meninges may be the only finding on CT in extraparenchymal neurocysticercosis. Cysticerci in the ventricles or subarachnoid space are usually visible to an experienced neuroradiologist on MRI or on CT with intraventricular contrast injection. CT is more sensitive than MRI in identifying calcified lesions, whereas MRI is better for identifying cystic lesions and enhancement.

The second major diagnostic criterion is detection of specific antibodies to cysticerci. While most tests employing unfractionated antigen have high rates of false-positive and false-negative results, this problem can be overcome by using the more specific immunoblot assay. An immunoblot assay using lentil-lectin purified glycoproteins has >99% specificity and is highly sensitive. However,

TABLE 127-1

DIAGNOSTIC CRITERIA FOR HUMAN CYSTICERCOSIS[a]

1. Absolute criteria
   a. Demonstration of cysticerci by histologic or microscopic examination of biopsy material
   b. Visualization of the parasite in the eye by funduscopy
   c. Neuroradiologic demonstration of cystic lesions containing a characteristic scolex
2. Major criteria
   a. Neuroradiologic lesions suggestive of neurocysticercosis
   b. Demonstration of antibodies to cysticerci in serum by enzyme-linked immunoelectrotransfer blot
   c. Resolution of intracranial cystic lesions spontaneously or after therapy with albendazole or praziquantel alone
3. Minor criteria
   a. Lesions compatible with neurocysticercosis detected by neuroimaging studies
   b. Clinical manifestations suggestive of neurocysticercosis
   c. Demonstration of antibodies to cysticerci or cysticercal antigen in cerebrospinal fluid by ELISA
   d. Evidence of cysticercosis outside the central nervous system (e.g., cigar-shaped soft tissue calcifications)
4. Epidemiologic criteria
   a. Residence in a cysticercosis-endemic area
   b. Frequent travel to a cysticercosis-endemic area
   c. Household contact with an individual infected with *Taenia solium*

[a]Diagnosis is confirmed by either one absolute criterion or a combination of two major criteria, one minor criterion, and one epidemiologic criterion. A probable diagnosis is supported by the fulfillment of (1) one major criterion plus two minor criteria; (2) one major criterion plus one minor criterion and one epidemiologic criterion; or (3) three minor criteria plus one epidemiologic criterion.
Note: ELISA, enzyme-linked immunosorbent assay.
Source: Modified from Del Brutto et al.

patients with single intracranial lesions or with calcifications may be seronegative. With this assay, serum samples provide greater diagnostic sensitivity than CSF. All of the diagnostic antigens have been cloned, and enzyme-linked immunosorbent assays (ELISAs) using recombinant antigens are being developed. Antigen detection assays employing monoclonal antibodies to detect parasite antigen in the blood or spinal fluid may also facilitate diagnosis. However, these assays are not widely available.

Studies have demonstrated that clinical criteria can aid in the diagnosis in selected cases. In patients from endemic areas who had single enhancing lesions presenting with seizures, a normal physical examination, and no evidence of systemic disease (e.g., no fever, adenopathy, or abnormal chest radiograph), the constellation of rounded CT lesions 5–20 mm in diameter with no midline shift was almost always caused by neurocysticercosis. Finally, spontaneous resolution or resolution after therapy with albendazole alone is consistent with neurocysticercosis.

Minor diagnostic criteria include neuroimaging findings consistent with but less characteristic of cysticercosis, clinical manifestations suggestive of neurocysticercosis (e.g., seizures, hydrocephalus, or altered mental status), evidence of cysticercosis outside the central nervous system (CNS; e.g., cigar-shaped soft tissue calcifications), or detection of antibody in CSF by ELISA. Epidemiologic criteria include exposure to a tapeworm carrier or household member infected with *T. solium*, current or prior residence in an endemic area, and frequent travel to an endemic area.

Diagnosis is confirmed in patients with either one absolute criterion or a combination of two major criteria, one minor criterion, and one epidemiologic criterion (Table 127-1). A probable diagnosis is supported by the fulfillment of (1) one major criterion plus two minor criteria; (2) one major criterion plus one minor criterion and one epidemiologic criterion; or (3) three minor criteria plus one epidemiologic criterion. While the CSF is usually abnormal in neurocysticercosis, CSF abnormalities are not pathognomonic. Patients may have CSF pleocytosis with a predominance of lymphocytes, neutrophils, or eosinophils. The protein level in CSF may be elevated; the glucose concentration is usually normal but may be depressed.

℞ Treatment: TAENIASIS SOLIUM AND CYSTICERCOSIS

Intestinal *T. solium* infection is treated with a single dose of praziquantel (10 mg/kg). However, praziquantel occasionally evokes an inflammatory response in the CNS if concomitant cryptic cysticercosis is present. Niclosamide (2 g) is also effective but is not widely available.

The initial management of neurocysticercosis should focus on symptom-based treatment of seizures or hydrocephalus. Seizures can usually be controlled with antiepileptic treatment. If parenchymal lesions resolve without development of calcifications and patients remain free of seizures, antiepileptic therapy can usually be discontinued after 1–2 years. Placebo-controlled trials are beginning to clarify the clinical advantage of antiparasitic drugs for parenchymal neurocysticercosis. Trends toward faster resolution of neuroradiologic abnormalities have been observed in most studies. The clinical benefits are less dramatic and consist mainly of shortening the period during which recurrent seizures occur and decreasing the number of patients who have many recurrent seizures. For the treatment of patients with brain parenchymal cysticerci, most authorities favor antiparasitic drugs, including praziquantel (50–60 mg/kg daily in three divided doses for 15–30 days) or albendazole (15 mg/kg per day for 8–28 days). Both agents may exacerbate the inflammatory response around the dying parasite, thereby exacerbating seizures or hydrocephalus as well. Thus, patients receiving these drugs should be carefully monitored, and high-dose glucocorticoids should be used during treatment. Since glucocorticoids induce first-pass metabolism of praziquantel and may decrease its antiparasitic effect, cimetidine should be coadministered to inhibit praziquantel metabolism.

For patients with hydrocephalus, the emergent reduction of intracranial pressure is the mainstay of therapy. In the case of obstructive hydrocephalus, the preferred approach is removal of the cysticercus via endoscopic surgery. However, this intervention is not always possible. An alternative approach is initially to perform a diverting procedure, such as ventriculoperitoneal shunting. Historically, shunts have usually failed, but low failure rates have been attained with administration of antiparasitic drugs and glucocorticoids. Open craniotomy to remove cysticerci is now required only infrequently. For patients with subarachnoid cysts or giant cysticerci, glucocorticoids are needed to reduce arachnoiditis and accompanying vasculitis. Most authorities recommend prolonged courses of antiparasitic drugs and shunting when hydrocephalus is present. In patients with diffuse cerebral edema and elevated intracranial pressure due to multiple inflamed lesions, glucocorticoids are the mainstay of therapy, and antiparasitic drugs should be avoided. For ocular and spinal medullary lesions, drug-induced inflammation may cause irreversible damage. Most patients should be managed surgically, although case reports have described cures with medical therapy.

Prevention

Measures for the prevention of intestinal *T. solium* infection consist of the application to pork of precautions similar to those described above for beef with regard to *T. saginata* infection. The prevention of cysticercosis involves minimizing the opportunities for ingestion of fecally derived eggs by means of good personal hygiene, effective fecal disposal, and treatment and prevention of human intestinal infections. Mass chemotherapy has been administered to human and porcine populations in efforts at disease eradication.

ECHINOCOCCOSIS

Echinococcosis is an infection caused in humans by the larval stage of the *Echinococcus granulosus* complex, *E. multilocularis*, or *E. vogeli*. *E. granulosus* complex parasites, which produce unilocular cystic lesions, are prevalent in areas where livestock is raised in association with dogs.

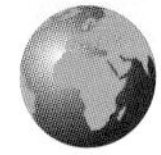

These parasites are found on all continents, with areas of high prevalence in China, central Asia, the Middle East, the Mediterranean region, eastern Africa, and parts of South America. Molecular evidence suggests that *E. granulosus* strains may actually belong to more than one species; specifically, strains from sheep, cattle, pigs, horses, and camels probably represent separate species. *E. multilocularis*, which causes multilocular alveolar lesions that are locally invasive, is found in Alpine, sub-Arctic, or Arctic regions, including Canada, the United States, and central and northern Europe; China; and central Asia. *E. vogeli* causes polycystic hydatid disease and is found only in Central and South America.

Like other cestodes, echinococcal species have both intermediate and definitive hosts. The definitive hosts are canines that pass eggs in their feces. After the ingestion of eggs, cysts develop in the intermediate hosts—sheep, cattle, humans, goats, camels, and horses for the *E. granulosus* complex and mice and other rodents for *E. multilocularis*. When a dog (*E. granulosus*) or fox (*E. multilocularis*) ingests infected meat containing cysts, the life cycle is completed.

Etiology

The small (5-mm-long) adult *E. granulosus* worm, which lives for 5–20 months in the jejunum of dogs, has only three proglottids: one immature, one mature, and one gravid. The gravid segment splits to release eggs that are morphologically similar to *Taenia* eggs and are extremely hardy. After humans ingest the eggs, embryos escape from the eggs, penetrate the intestinal mucosa, enter the portal circulation, and are carried to various organs, most commonly the liver and lungs. Larvae develop into fluid-filled unilocular hydatid cysts that consist of an external membrane and an inner germinal layer. Daughter cysts develop from the inner aspect of the germinal layer, as do germinating cystic structures called *brood capsules*. New larvae, called *protoscolices*, develop in large numbers within the brood capsule. The cysts expand slowly over a period of years.

The life cycle of *E. multilocularis* is similar except that wild canines, such as foxes, serve as the definitive hosts and small rodents serve as the intermediate hosts. The larval form of *E. multilocularis*, however, is quite different in that it remains in the proliferative phase, the parasite is always multilocular, and vesicles without brood capsule or protoscolices progressively invade the host tissue by peripheral extension of processes from the germinal layer.

Clinical Manifestations

Slowly enlarging echinococcal cysts generally remain asymptomatic until their expanding size or their space-occupying effect in an involved organ elicits symptoms. The liver and the lungs are the most common sites of these cysts. The liver is involved in about two-thirds of *E. granulosus* infections and in nearly all *E. multilocularis* infections. Since a period of years elapses before cysts enlarge sufficiently to cause symptoms, they may be discovered incidentally on a routine x-ray or ultrasound study.

Patients with hepatic echinococcosis who are symptomatic most often present with abdominal pain or a palpable mass in the right upper quadrant. Compression of a bile duct or leakage of cyst fluid into the biliary tree may mimic recurrent cholelithiasis, and biliary obstruction can result in jaundice. Rupture of or episodic leakage from a hydatid cyst may produce fever, pruritus, urticaria, eosinophilia, or anaphylaxis. Pulmonary hydatid cysts may rupture into the bronchial tree or peritoneal cavity and produce cough, dyspnea, chest pain, or hemoptysis. Rupture of hydatid cysts, which can occur spontaneously or at surgery, may lead to multifocal dissemination of protoscolices, which can form additional cysts. Other presentations are due to the involvement of bone (invasion of the medullary cavity with slow bone erosion producing pathologic fractures), the CNS (space-occupying lesions), the heart (conduction defects, pericarditis), and the pelvis (pelvic mass).

The larval forms of *E. multilocularis* characteristically present as a slowly growing hepatic tumor, with progressive destruction of the liver and extension into vital structures. Patients commonly report upper quadrant and epigastric pain. Liver enlargement and obstructive jaundice may be apparent. The lesions may infiltrate adjoining organs (e.g., diaphragm, kidneys, or lungs) or may metastasize to the spleen, lungs, or brain.

Diagnosis

Radiographic and related imaging studies are important in detecting and evaluating echinococcal cysts. Plain films will define pulmonary cysts of *E. granulosus*—usually as rounded masses of uniform density—but may miss cysts in other organs unless there is cyst wall calcification (as occurs in the liver). MRI, CT, and ultrasound reveal well-defined cysts with thick or thin walls. When older cysts contain a layer of hydatid sand that is rich in accumulated protoscolices, these imaging methods may detect this fluid layer of different density. However, the most pathognomonic finding, if demonstrable, is that of daughter cysts within the larger cyst. This finding, like eggshell or mural calcification on CT, is indicative of *E. granulosus* infection and helps to distinguish the cyst from carcinomas, bacterial or amebic liver abscesses, or hemangiomas. In contrast, ultrasound or CT of alveolar hydatid cysts reveals indistinct solid masses with central necrosis and plaquelike calcifications.

A specific diagnosis of *E. granulosus* infection can be made by the examination of aspirated fluids for protoscolices or hooklets, but diagnostic aspiration is not usually recommended because of the risk of fluid leakage resulting in either dissemination of infection or anaphylactic reactions. Serodiagnostic assays can be useful, although a negative test does not exclude the diagnosis of echinococcosis. Cysts in the liver elicit positive antibody responses in ~90% of cases, whereas up to 50% of individuals with cysts in the lungs are seronegative. Detection of antibody to specific echinococcal antigens by immunoblotting has the highest degree of specificity.

℞ Treatment: ECHINOCOCCOSIS

Therapy for cystic echinococcosis is based on considerations of the size, location, and manifestations of cysts and the overall health of the patient. Surgery has traditionally been the principal definitive method of treatment. Currently, ultrasound staging is recommended for *E. granulosus* infections (Fig. 127-2). For CE1 lesions, uncomplicated CE3 lesions, and some CE2 lesions, PAIR (*p*ercutaneous *a*spiration, *i*nfusion of scolicidal agents,

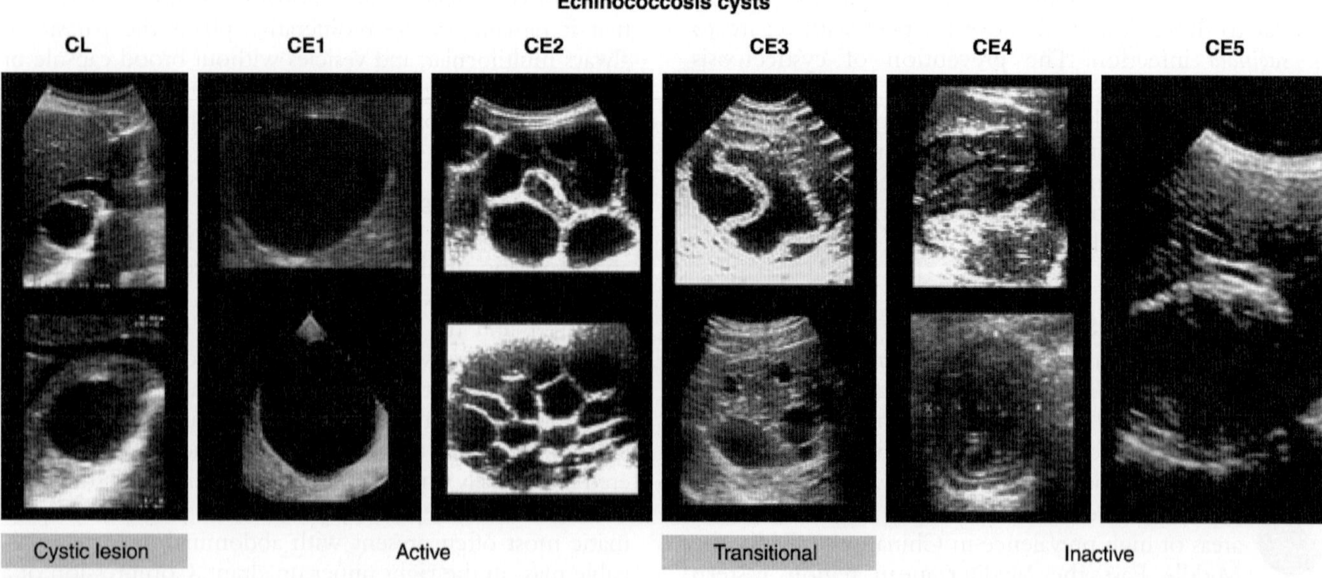

FIGURE 127-2

Management of cystic hydatid disease caused by *Echinococcus granulosus* should be based on viability of the parasite, which can be estimated from radiographic appearance. The ultrasound appearance includes lesions classified as active, transitional, and inactive. *Active* cysts include types CL (with a cystic lesion and no visible cyst wall), CE1 [with a visible cyst wall and internal echoes (snowflake sign)], and CE2 (with a visible cyst wall and internal septation). *Transitional cysts* (CE3) may have detached laminar membranes or may be partially collapsed. *Inactive cysts* include types CE4 (a nonhomogeneous mass) and CE5 (a cyst with a thick calcified wall). *[Adapted from RL Guerrant et al (eds): Tropical Infectious Diseases: Principles, Pathogens and Practice, 2d ed, p 1312. © 2005, with permission from Elsevier Science.]*

and reaspiration) is now recommended instead of surgery. PAIR is contraindicated for superficially located cysts (because of the risk of rupture), for cysts with multiple thick internal septal divisions (honeycombing pattern), and for cysts communicating with the biliary tree. For prophylaxis of secondary peritoneal echinococcosis due to inadvertent spillage of fluid during PAIR, the administration of albendazole (15 mg/kg daily in two divided doses) should be initiated at least 4 days before the procedure and continued for at least 4 weeks afterward. Ultrasound- or CT-guided aspiration allows confirmation of the diagnosis by demonstration of protoscolices in the aspirate. After aspiration, contrast material should be injected to detect occult communications with the biliary tract. Alternatively, the fluid should be checked for bile staining by dipstick. If no bile is found and no communication visualized, the contrast material is reaspirated, with subsequent infusion of scolicidal agents (usually 95% ethanol; alternatively, hypertonic saline). Daughter cysts within the primary cyst may need to be punctured separately. In experienced hands, this approach yields rates of cure and relapse equivalent to those following surgery, with less perioperative morbidity and shorter hospitalization.

Surgery remains the treatment of choice for complicated *E. granulosus* cysts (e.g., those communicating with the biliary tract) or for areas where PAIR is not possible. For *E. granulosus*, the preferred surgical approach is pericystectomy, in which the entire cyst and the surrounding fibrous tissue are removed. The risks posed by leakage of fluid during surgery or PAIR include anaphylaxis and dissemination of infectious protoscolices. The latter complication has been minimized by careful attention to the prevention of spillage of the cyst and by soaking of the drapes with hypertonic saline. Infusion of scolicidal agents is no longer recommended because of problems with hypernatremia, intoxication, or sclerosing cholangitis. Albendazole, which is active against *Echinococcus*, should be administered adjunctively, beginning several days before resection and continuing for several weeks for *E. granulosus*. Praziquantel (50 mg/kg daily for 2 weeks) may hasten the death of the protoscolices. Medical therapy with albendazole alone for 12 weeks to 6 months results in cure in ~30% of cases and in improvement in another 50%. In many instances of treatment failure, *E. granulosus* infections are subsequently treated successfully with PAIR or additional courses of medical therapy. Response to treatment is best assessed by serial imaging studies, with attention to cyst size and consistency. Some cysts may not demonstrate complete radiologic resolution even though no viable protoscolices are present. Some of these cysts with partial radiologic resolution (e.g., CE4) can be managed with observation only.

Surgical resection remains the treatment of choice for *E. multilocularis* infection. Complete removal of the parasite continues to offer the best chance for cure. Ongoing therapy with albendazole for at least 2 years after presumptively curative surgery is recommended. Most cases are diagnosed at a stage at which complete resection is not possible; in these cases, albendazole treatment should be continued indefinitely, with careful monitoring. In some cases, liver transplantation has been used because of the size of the necessary liver resection. However, continuous immunosuppression favors the proliferation of *E. multilocularis* larvae and reinfection of the transplant. Thus, indefinite treatment with albendazole is required.

Prevention

In endemic areas, echinococcosis can be prevented by administering praziquantel to infected dogs, by denying dogs access to infected animals, or by vaccinating sheep. Limitation of the number of stray dogs is helpful in reducing the prevalence of infection among humans.

HYMENOLEPIASIS NANA

Infection with *Hymenolepis nana*, the dwarf tapeworm, is the most common of all the cestode infections. *H. nana* is endemic in both temperate and tropical regions of the world. Infection is spread by fecal/oral contamination and is common among institutionalized children.

Etiology and Pathogenesis

H. nana is the only cestode of humans that does not require an intermediate host. Both the larval and adult phases of the life cycle take place in the human. The adult—the smallest tapeworm parasitizing humans—is ~2 cm long and dwells in the proximal ileum. Proglottids, which are quite small and are rarely seen in the stool, release spherical eggs 30–44 μm in diameter, each of which contains an oncosphere with six hooklets. The eggs are immediately infective and are unable to survive for >10 days in the external environment. H. nana can also be acquired by the ingestion of infected insects (especially larval meal-worms and larval fleas). When the egg is ingested by a new host, the oncosphere is freed and penetrates the intestinal villi, becoming a cysticercoid larva. Larvae migrate back into the intestinal lumen, attach to the mucosa, and mature into adult worms over 10–12 days. Eggs may also hatch before passing into the stool, causing internal autoinfection with increasing numbers of intestinal worms. Although the life span of adult H. nana worms is only ~4–10 weeks, the autoinfection cycle perpetuates the infection.

Clinical Manifestations

H. nana infection, even with many intestinal worms, is usually asymptomatic. When infection is intense, anorexia, abdominal pain, and diarrhea develop.

Diagnosis

Infection is diagnosed by the finding of eggs in the stool.

Treatment: HYMENOLEPIASIS NANA

Praziquantel (25 mg/kg once) is the treatment of choice, since it acts against both the adult worms and the cysticercoids in the intestinal villi. Nitazoxanide (500 mg bid for 3 days) may be used as an alternative.

Prevention

Good personal hygiene and improved sanitation can eradicate the disease. Epidemics have been controlled by mass chemotherapy coupled with improved hygiene.

HYMENOLEPIASIS DIMINUTA

Hymenolepis diminuta, a cestode of rodents, occasionally infects small children, who ingest the larvae in uncooked cereal foods contaminated by fleas and other insects in which larvae develop. Infection is usually asymptomatic and is diagnosed by the detection of eggs in the stool. Treatment with praziquantel results in cure in most cases.

DIPHYLLOBOTHRIASIS

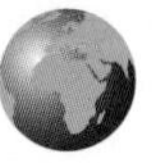

Diphyllobothrium latum and other *Diphyllobothrium* species are found in the lakes, rivers, and deltas of the northern hemisphere, Central Africa, and Chile.

Etiology and Pathogenesis

The adult worm—the longest tapeworm (up to 25 m)—attaches to the ileal and occasionally to the jejunal mucosa by its suckers, which are located on its elongated scolex. The adult worm has 3000–4000 proglottids, which release ~1 million eggs daily into the feces. If an egg reaches water, it hatches and releases a free-swimming embryo that can be eaten by small freshwater crustaceans (*Cyclops* or *Diaptomus* species). After an infected crustacean containing a developed procercoid is swallowed by a fish, the larva migrates into the fish's flesh and grows into a plerocercoid, or sparganum larva. Humans acquire the infection by ingesting infected raw or smoked fish. Within 3–5 weeks, the tapeworm matures into an adult in the human intestine.

Clinical Manifestations

Most *D. latum* infections are asymptomatic, although manifestations may include transient abdominal discomfort, diarrhea, vomiting, weakness, and weight loss. Occasionally, infection can cause acute abdominal pain and intestinal obstruction; in rare cases, cholangitis or cholecystitis may be produced by migrating proglottids. Because the tapeworm absorbs large quantities of vitamin B_{12} and interferes with ileal B_{12} absorption, vitamin B_{12} deficiency can develop. Up to 2% of infected patients, especially the elderly, have megaloblastic anemia resembling pernicious anemia and may exhibit neurologic sequelae of B_{12} deficiency.

Diagnosis

The diagnosis is made readily by the detection of the characteristic eggs in the stool. The eggs possess a single shell with an operculum at one end and a knob at the other. Mild to moderate eosinophilia may be detected.

Treatment: DIPHYLLOBOTHRIASIS

Praziquantel (5–10 mg/kg once) is highly effective. Parenteral vitamin B_{12} should be given if B_{12} deficiency is manifest.

Prevention

Infection can be prevented by heating fish to 54°C for 5 min or by freezing it at −18°C for 24 h. Placing fish in brine with a high salt concentration for long periods kills the eggs.

DIPYLIDIASIS

Dipylidium caninum, a common tapeworm of dogs and cats, may accidentally infect humans. Dogs, cats, and occasionally humans become infected by ingesting fleas harboring cysticercoids. Children are more likely to become infected than adults. Most infections are asymptomatic, but abdominal pain, diarrhea, anal pruritus, urticaria, eosinophilia, or passage of segments in the stool may occur. The diagnosis is made by the detection of proglottids or ova in the stool. As in D. latum infection, therapy consists of praziquantel. Prevention requires anthelmintic treatment and flea control for pet dogs or cats.

SPARGANOSIS

Humans can be infected by the sparganum, or plerocercoid larva, of a diphyllobothrid tapeworm of the genus *Spirometra.* Infection can be acquired by the consumption of water containing infected *Cyclops*; by the ingestion of infected snakes, birds, or mammals; or by the application of infected flesh as poultices. The worm migrates slowly in tissues, and infection commonly presents as a subcutaneous swelling. Periorbital tissues can be involved, and ocular sparganosis may destroy the eye. Surgical excision is used to treat localized sparganosis.

COENUROSIS

This rare infection of humans by the larval stage (coenurus) of the dog tapeworm *Taenia multiceps* or *T. serialis* results in a space-occupying cystic lesion. As in cysticercosis, involvement of the CNS and subcutaneous tissue is most common. Both definitive diagnosis and treatment require surgical excision of the lesion. Chemotherapeutic agents generally are not effective.

FURTHER READINGS

Centers for Disease Control and Prevention, Division of Parasitic Diseases: *www.cdc.gov/ncidod/dpd/default.htm*

Del Brutto OH et al: Proposed diagnostic criteria for neurocysticercosis. Neurology 57:177, 2001

Eckert J, Deplazes P: Biological, epidemiological, and clinical aspects of echinococcosis, a zoonosis of increasing concern. Clin Microbiol Rev 17:107, 2004

Garcia HH et al: Current consensus guidelines for treatment of neurocysticercosis. Clin Microbiol Rev 15:747, 2002

——— et al: A trial of antiparasitic treatment to reduce the rate of seizures due to cerebral cysticercosis. N Engl J Med 350:249, 2004

Nash TE et al: Treatment of neurocysticercosis: Current status and future research needs. Neurology 67:1120, 2006

Pawlowski ZS et al: Echinococcosis in humans: Clinical aspects, diagnosis, and treatment, in *WHO/OIE Manual on Echinococcosis in Humans and Animals: A Public Health Problem of Global Concern*, J Eckert et al (eds). Paris, World Organization for Animal Health, 2001

Schantz PM et al: Echinococcosis, in *Tropical Infectious Diseases: Principles, Pathogens and Practice*, 2d ed, RL Guerrant et al (eds). Philadelphia, Churchill Livingstone, 2005, p 1304

Scholz T et al: Update on the human broad tapeworm (genus diphyllobothrium), including clinical relevance. Clin Microbiol Rev 22:146, 2009

Singh G, Prabhakar S: *Taenia solium Cysticercosis: From Basic Science to Clinical Science.* Wallingford, UK, CABI Publishing, 2002

World Health Organization Informal Working Group on Echinococcosis: Pair: puncture, aspiration, injection, re-aspiration: An option for the treatment of cystic echinococcosis. WHO/CDS/CSR/APH/2001.6. Geneva, WHO, 2001

———: International classification of ultrasound images in cystic echinococcosis for application in clinical and field epidemiological settings. Acta Tropica 85:253, 2003

APPENDIX

LABORATORY VALUES OF CLINICAL IMPORTANCE

Alexander Kratz ■ Michael A. Pesce ■ Daniel J. Fink†

INTRODUCTORY COMMENTS

The following are tables of reference values for laboratory tests, special analytes, and special function tests. A variety of factors can influence reference values. Such variables include the population studied, the duration and means of specimen transport, laboratory methods and instrumentation, and even the type of container used for the collection of the specimen. The reference or "normal" ranges given in this Appendix may therefore not be appropriate for all laboratories, and these values should only be used as general guidelines. Whenever possible, reference values provided by the laboratory performing the testing should be utilized in the interpretation of laboratory data. Values supplied in this Appendix reflect typical reference ranges in adults. Pediatric reference ranges may vary significantly from adult values.

In preparing the Appendix, the authors have taken into account the fact that the system of international units (SI, système international d'unités) is used in most countries and in some medical journals. However, clinical laboratories may continue to report values in "conventional" units. Therefore, both systems are provided in the Appendix. The dual system is also used in the text except for (1) those instances in which the numbers remain the same but only the terminology is changed (mmol/L for meq/L or IU/L for mIU/mL), when only the SI units are given; and (2) most pressure measurements (e.g., blood and cerebrospinal fluid pressures), when the conventional units (mmHg, mmH_2O) are used. In all other instances in the text the SI unit is followed by the traditional unit in parentheses.

†Deceased.

TABLE A-1

HEMATOLOGY AND COAGULATION

ANALYTE	SPECIMEN[a]	SI UNITS	CONVENTIONAL UNITS
Activated clotting time	WB	70–180 s	70–180 s
Activated protein C resistance (Factor V Leiden)	P	Not applicable	Ratio > 2.1
Alpha$_2$ antiplasmin	P	0.87–1.55	87–155%
Antiphospholipid antibody panel			
PTT-LA (Lupus anticoagulant screen)	P	Negative	Negative
Platelet neutralization procedure	P	Negative	Negative
Dilute viper venom screen	P	Negative	Negative
Anticardiolipin antibody	S		
IgG		0–15 arbitrary units	0–15 GPL
IgM		0–15 arbitrary units	0–15 MPL
Antithrombin III	P		
Antigenic		220–390 mg/L	22–39 mg/dL
Functional		0.7–1.30 U/L	70–130%
Anti-Xa assay (heparin assay)	P		
Unfractionated heparin		0.3–0.7 kIU/L	0.3–0.7 IU/mL
Low-molecular-weight heparin		0.5–1.0 kIU/L	0.5–1.0 IU/mL
Danaparoid (Orgaran)		0.5–0.8 kIU/L	0.5–0.8 IU/mL
Autohemolysis test	WB	0.004–0.045	0.4–4.50%
Autohemolysis test with glucose	WB	0.003–0.007	0.3–0.7%
Bleeding time (adult)		<7.1 min	<7.1 min
Bone marrow: see **Table A-8**			
Clot retraction	WB	0.50–1.00/2 h	50–100%/2 h
Cryofibrinogen	P	Negative	Negative
D-Dimer	P	0.22–0.74 μg/mL	0.22–0.74 μg/mL
Differential blood count	WB		
Neutrophils		0.40–0.70	40–70%
Bands		0.0–0.05	0–5%
Lymphocytes		0.20–0.50	20–50%
Monocytes		0.04–0.08	4–8%
Eosinophils		0.0–0.6	0–6%
Basophils		0.0–0.02	0–2%
Eosinophil count	WB	150–300/μL	150–300/mm^3
Erythrocyte count	WB		
Adult males		4.30–5.60 × 10^{12}/L	4.30–5.60 × 10^6/mm^3
Adult females		4.00–5.20 × 10^{12}/L	4.00–5.20 × 10^6/mm^3
Erythrocyte life span	WB		
Normal survival		120 days	120 days
Chromium labeled, half life ($t_{1/2}$)		25–35 days	25–35 days
Erythrocyte sedimentation rate	WB		
Females		0–20 mm/h	0–20 mm/h
Males		0–15 mm/h	0–15 mm/h
Euglobulin lysis time	P	7200–14,400 s	120–240 min
Factor II, prothrombin	P	0.50–1.50	50–150%
Factor V	P	0.50–1.50	50–150%
Factor VII	P	0.50–1.50	50–150%
Factor VIII	P	0.50–1.50	50–150%
Factor IX	P	0.50–1.50	50–150%
Factor X	P	0.50–1.50	50–150%
Factor XI	P	0.50–1.50	50–150%
Factor XII	P	0.50–1.50	50–150%
Factor XIII screen	P	Not applicable	Present
Factor inhibitor assay	P	<0.5 Bethesda Units	<0.5 Bethesda Units

(Continued)

TABLE A-1 (*CONTINUED*)

HEMATOLOGY AND COAGULATION

ANALYTE	SPECIMEN[a]	SI UNITS	CONVENTIONAL UNITS
Fibrin(ogen) degradation products	P	0–1 mg/L	0–1 μg/mL
Fibrinogen	P	2.33–4.96 g/L	233–496 mg/dL
Glucose-6-phosphate dehydrogenase (erythrocyte)	WB	<2400 s	<40 min
Ham's test (acid serum)	WB	Negative	Negative
Hematocrit	WB		
Adult males		0.388–0.464	38.8–46.4
Adult females		0.354–0.444	35.4–44.4
Hemoglobin			
Plasma	P	6–50 mg/L	0.6–5.0 mg/dL
Whole blood	WB		
Adult males		133–162 g/L	13.3–16.2 g/dL
Adult females		120–158 g/L	12.0–15.8 g/dL
Hemoglobin electrophoresis	WB		
Hemoglobin A		0.95–0.98	95–98%
Hemoglobin A_2		0.015–0.031	1.5–3.1%
Hemoglobin F		0–0.02	0–2.0%
Hemoglobins other than A, A_2, or F		Absent	Absent
Heparin-induced thrombocytopenia antibody	P	Negative	Negative
Joint fluid crystal	JF	Not applicable	No crystals seen
Joint fluid mucin	JF	Not applicable	Only type I mucin present
Leukocytes			
Alkaline phosphatase (LAP)	WB	0.2–1.6 μkat/L	13–100 μ/L
Count (WBC)	WB	3.54–9.06 × 10^9/L	3.54–9.06 × 10^3/mm^3
Mean corpuscular hemoglobin (MCH)	WB	26.7–31.9 pg/cell	26.7–31.9 pg/cell
Mean corpuscular hemoglobin concentration (MCHC)	WB	323–359 g/L	32.3–35.9 g/dL
Mean corpuscular hemoglobin of reticulocytes (CH)	WB	24–36 pg	24–36 pg
Mean corpuscular volume (MCV)	WB	79–93.3 fL	79–93.3 μm^3
Mean platelet volume (MPV)	WB	9.00–12.95 fL	9.00–12.95 μm^3
Osmotic fragility of erythrocytes	WB		
Direct		0.0035–0.0045	0.35–0.45%
Index		0.0030–0.0065	0.30–0.65%
Partial thromboplastin time, activated	P	26.3–39.4 s	26.3–39.4 s
Plasminogen	P		
Antigen		84–140 mg/L	8.4–14.0 mg/dL
Functional		0.70–1.30	70–130%
Plasminogen activator inhibitor 1	P	4–43 μg/L	4–43 ng/mL
Platelet aggregation	PRP	Not applicable	>65% aggregation in response to adenosine diphosphate, epinephrine, collagen, ristocetin, and arachidonic acid
Platelet count	WB	165–415 × 10^9/L	165–415 × 10^3/mm^3
Platelet, mean volume	WB	6.4–11 fL	6.4–11.0 μm^3
Prekallikrein assay	P	0.50–1.5	50–150%
Prekallikrein screen	P		No deficiency detected
Protein C	P		
Total antigen		0.70–1.40	70–140%
Functional		0.70–1.30	70–130%
Protein S	P		
Total antigen		0.70–1.40	70–140%
Functional		0.65–1.40	65–140%
Free antigen		0.70–1.40	70–140%
Prothrombin gene mutation G20210A	WB	Not applicable	Not present
Prothrombin time	P	12.7–15.4 s	12.7–15.4 s

(*Continued*)

TABLE A-1 (CONTINUED)

HEMATOLOGY AND COAGULATION			
ANALYTE	SPECIMEN[a]	SI UNITS	CONVENTIONAL UNITS
Protoporphyrin, free erythrocyte	WB	0.28–0.64 μmol/L of red blood cells	16–36 μg/dL of red blood cells
Red cell distribution width	WB	<0.145	<14.5%
Reptilase time	P	16–23.6 s	16–23.6 s
Reticulocyte count	WB		
Adult males		0.008–0.023 red cells	0.8–2.3% red cells
Adult females		0.008–0.020 red cells	0.8–2.0% red cells
Reticulocyte hemoglobin content	WB	>26 pg/cell	>26 pg/cell
Ristocetin cofactor (functional von Willebrand factor)	P		
Blood group O		0.75 mean of normal	75% mean of normal
Blood group A		1.05 mean of normal	105% mean of normal
Blood group B		1.15 mean of normal	115% mean of normal
Blood group AB		1.25 mean of normal	125% mean of normal
Sickle cell test	WB	Negative	Negative
Sucrose hemolysis	WB	<0.1	<10% hemolysis
Thrombin time	P	15.3–18.5 s	15.3–18.5 s
Total eosinophils	WB	150–300 × 10^6/L	150–300/mm^3
Transferrin receptor	S, P	9.6–29.6 nmol/L	9.6–29.6 nmol/L
Viscosity			
Plasma	P	1.7–2.1	1.7–2.1
Serum	S	1.4–1.8	1.4–1.8
Von Willebrand factor (vWF) antigen (factor VIII:R antigen)	P		
Blood group O		0.75 mean of normal	75% mean of normal
Blood group A		1.05 mean of normal	105% mean of normal
Blood group B		1.15 mean of normal	115% mean of normal
Blood group AB		1.25 mean of normal	125% mean of normal
Von Willebrand factor multimers	P	Normal distribution	Normal distribution
White blood cells: see "leukocytes"			

[a]P, plasma; JF, joint fluid; PRP, platelet-rich plasma; S, serum; WB, whole blood.

TABLE A-2

CLINICAL CHEMISTRY AND IMMUNOLOGY			
ANALYTE	SPECIMEN[a]	SI UNITS	CONVENTIONAL UNITS
Acetoacetate	P	20–99 μmol/L	0.2–1.0 mg/dL
Adrenocorticotropin (ACTH)	P	1.3–16.7 pmol/L	6.0–76.0 pg/mL
Alanine aminotransferase (AST, SGPT)	S	0.12–0.70 μkat/L	7–41 U/L
Albumin	S		
Female		41–53 g/L	4.1–5.3 g/dL
Male		40–50 g/L	4.0–5.0 g/L
Aldolase	S	26–138 nkat/L	1.5–8.1 U/L
Aldosterone (adult)	S, P		
Supine, normal sodium diet		55–250 pmol/L	2–9 ng/dL
Upright, normal sodium diet			2–5-fold increase over supine value
Supine, low-sodium diet			2–5-fold increase over normal sodium diet level
	U	6.38–58.25 nmol/d	2.3–21.0 μg/24 h
Alpha fetoprotein (adult)	S	0–8.5 μg/L	0–8.5 ng/mL
$Alpha_1$ antitrypsin	S	1.0–2.0 g/L	100–200 mg/dL
Ammonia, as NH_3	P	11–35 μmol/L	19–60 μg/dL
Amylase (method dependent)	S	0.34–1.6 μkat/L	20–96 U/L
Androstenedione (adult)	S	1.75–8.73 nmol/L	50–250 ng/dL

(Continued)

CLINICAL CHEMISTRY AND IMMUNOLOGY

ANALYTE	SPECIMEN[a]	SI UNITS	CONVENTIONAL UNITS
Angiotensin-converting enzyme (ACE)	S	0.15–1.1 μkat/L	9–67 U/L
Anion gap	S	7–16 mmol/L	7–16 mmol/L
Apo B/Apo A-1 ratio		0.35–0.98	0.35–0.98
Apolipoprotein A-1	S	1.19–2.40 g/L	119–240 mg/dL
Apolipoprotein B	S	0.52–1.63 g/L	52–163 mg/dL
Arterial blood gases			
$[HCO_3^-]$		22–30 mmol/L	22–30 meq/L
P_{CO_2}		4.3–6.0 kPa	32–45 mmHg
pH		7.35–7.45	7.35–7.45
P_{O_2}		9.6–13.8 kPa	72–104 mmHg
Aspartate aminotransferase (AST, SGOT)	S	0.20–0.65 μkat/L	12–38 U/L
Autoantibodies			
Anti-adrenal antibody	S	Not applicable	Negative at 1:10 dilution
Anti-double-strand (native) DNA	S	Not applicable	Negative at 1:10 dilution
Anti–glomerular basement membrane antibodies	S		
Qualitative		Negative	Negative
Quantitative		<5 kU/L	<5 U/mL
Anti-granulocyte antibody	S	Not applicable	Negative
Anti-Jo-1 antibody	S	Not applicable	Negative
Anti-La antibody	S	Not applicable	Negative
Anti-mitochondrial antibody	S	Not applicable	Negative
Antineutrophil cytoplasmic autoantibodies, cytoplasmic (C-ANCA)	S		
Qualitative		Negative	Negative
Quantitative (antibodies to proteinase 3)		<2.8 kU/L	<2.8 U/mL
Antineutrophil cytoplasmic autoantibodies, perinuclear (P-ANCA)	S		
Qualitative		Negative	Negative
Quantitative (antibodies to myeloperoxidase)		<1.4 kU/L	<1.4 U/mL
Antinuclear antibody	S	Not applicable	Negative at 1:40
Anti–parietal cell antibody	S	Not applicable	Negative at 1:20
Anti-Ro antibody	S	Not applicable	Negative
Anti-platelet antibody	S	Not applicable	Negative
Anti-RNP antibody	S	Not applicable	Negative
Anti-Scl 70 antibody	S	Not applicable	Negative
Anti-Smith antibody	S	Not applicable	Negative
Anti-smooth-muscle antibody	S	Not applicable	Negative at 1:20
Anti-thyroglobulin	S	Not applicable	Negative
Anti-thyroid antibody	S	<0.3 kIU/L	<0.3 IU/mL
B type natriuretic peptide (BNP)	P	Age and gender specific: <167 ng/L	Age and gender specific: <167 pg/mL
Bence Jones protein, serum	S	Not applicable	None detected
Bence Jones protein, urine, qualitative	U	Not applicable	None detected in 50 × concentrated urine
Bence Jones Protein, urine, quantitative	U		
Kappa		<25 mg/L	<2.5 mg/dL
Lambda		<50 mg/L	<5.0 mg/dL
β_2-Microglobulin			
	S	<2.7 mg/L	<0.27 mg/dL
	U	<120 μg/d	<120 μg/day
Bilirubin	S		
Total		5.1–22 μmol/L	0.3–1.3 mg/dL
Direct		1.7–6.8 μmol/L	0.1–0.4 mg/dL
Indirect		3.4–15.2 μmol/L	0.2–0.9 mg/dL
C peptide (adult)	S, P	0.17–0.66 nmol/L	0.5–2.0 ng/mL
C1-esterase-inhibitor protein	S		
Antigenic		124–250 mg/L	12.4–24.5 mg/dL
Functional		Present	Present

(Continued)

TABLE A-2 (CONTINUED)

CLINICAL CHEMISTRY AND IMMUNOLOGY

ANALYTE	SPECIMEN[a]	SI UNITS	CONVENTIONAL UNITS
CA 125	S	0–35 kU/L	0–35 U/mL
CA 19-9	S	0–37 kU/L	0–37 U/mL
CA 15-3	S	0–34 kU/L	0–34 U/mL
CA 27-29	S	0–40 kU/L	0–40 U/mL
Calcitonin	S		
Male		3–26 ng/L	3–26 pg/mL
Female		2–17 ng/L	2–17 pg/mL
Calcium	S	2.2–2.6 mmol/L	8.7–10.2 mg/dL
Calcium, ionized	WB	1.12–1.32 mmol/L	4.5–5.3 mg/dL
Carbon dioxide content (TCO_2)	P (sea level)	22–30 mmol/L	22–30 meq/L
Carboxyhemoglobin (carbon monoxide content)	WB		
Nonsmokers		0–0.04	0–4%
Smokers		0.04–0.09	4–9%
Onset of symptoms		0.15–0.20	15–20%
Loss of consciousness and death		>0.50	>50%
Carcinoembryonic antigen (CEA)	S		
Nonsmokers		0.0–3.0 μg/L	0.0–3.0 ng/mL
Smokers		0.0–5.0 μg/L	0.0–5.0 ng/mL
Ceruloplasmin	S	250–630 mg/L	25–63 mg/dL
Chloride	S	102–109 mmol/L	102–109 meq/L
Cholesterol: see **Table A-5**			
Cholinesterase	S	5–12 kU/L	5–12 U/mL
Complement			
C3	S	0.83–1.77 g/L	83–177 mg/dL
C4	S	0.16–0.47 g/L	16–47 mg/dL
Total hemolytic complement (CH50)	S	50–150%	50–150%
Factor B	S	0.17–0.42 g/L	17–42 mg/dL
Coproporphyrins (types I and III)	U	150–470 μmol/d	100–300 μg/d
Cortisol			
Fasting, 8 A.M.–12 noon	S	138–690 nmol/L	5–25 μg/dL
12 noon–8 P.M.		138–414 nmol/L	5–15 μg/dL
8 P.M.–8 A.M.		0–276 nmol/L	0–10 μg/dL
Cortisol, free	U	55–193 nmol/24 h	20–70 μg/24 h
C-reactive protein	S	0.2–3.0 mg/L	0.2–3.0 mg/L
Creatine kinase (total)	S		
Females		0.66–4.0 μkat/L	39–238 U/L
Males		0.87–5.0 μkat/L	51–294 U/L
Creatine kinase-MB	S		
Mass		0.0–5.5 μg/L	0.0–5.5 ng/mL
Fraction of total activity (by electrophoresis)		0–0.04	0–4.0%
Creatinine	S		
Female		44–80 μmol/L	0.5–0.9 ng/mL
Male		53–106 μmol/L	0.6–1.2 ng/mL
Cryoproteins	S	Not applicable	None detected
Dehydroepiandrosterone (DHEA) (adult)	S		
Male		6.2–43.4 nmol/L	180–1250 ng/dL
Female		4.5–34.0 nmol/L	130–980 ng/dL
Dehydroepiandrosterone (DHEA) sulfate	S		
Male (adult)		100–6190 μg/L	10–619 μg/dL
Female (adult, premenopausal)		120–5350 μg/L	12–535 μg/dL
Female (adult, postmenopausal)		300–2600 μg/L	30–260 μg/dL
Deoxycorticosterone (DOC) (adult)	S	61–576 nmol/L	2–19 ng/dL
11-Deoxycortisol (adult) (compound S) (8:00 A.M.)	S	0.34–4.56 nmol/L	12–158 ng/dL
Dihydrotestosterone			
Male	S, P	1.03–2.92 nmol/L	30–85 ng/dL
Female		0.14–0.76 nmol/L	4–22 ng/dL
Dopamine	P	<475 pmol/L	<87 pg/mL

(*Continued*)

TABLE A-2 (*CONTINUED*)

CLINICAL CHEMISTRY AND IMMUNOLOGY

ANALYTE	SPECIMEN[a]	SI UNITS	CONVENTIONAL UNITS
Dopamine	U	425–2610 nmol/d	65–400 μg/d
Epinephrine	P		
Supine (30 min)		<273 pmol/L	<50 pg/mL
Sitting		<328 pmol/L	<60 pg/mL
Standing (30 min)		<491 pmol/L	<90 pg/mL
Epinephrine	U	0–109 nmol/d	0–20 μg/d
Erythropoietin	S	4–27 U/L	4–27 U/L
Estradiol	S, P		
Female			
Menstruating:			
Follicular phase		74–532 pmol/L	<20–145 pg/mL
Mid-cycle peak		411–1626 pmol/L	112–443 pg/mL
Luteal phase		74–885 pmol/L	<20–241 pg/mL
Postmenopausal		217 pmol/L	<59 pg/mL
Male		74 pmol/L	<20 pg/mL
Estrone	S, P		
Female			
Menstruating:			
Follicular phase		55–555 pmol/L	15–150 pg/mL
Luteal phase		55–740 pmol/L	15–200 pg/mL
Postmenopausal		55–204 pmol/L	15–55 pg/mL
Male		55–240 pmol/L	15–65 pg/mL
Fatty acids, free (nonesterified)	P	<0.28–0.89 mmol/L	<8–25 mg/dL
Ferritin	S		
Female		10–150 μg/L	10–150 ng/mL
Male		29–248 μg/L	29–248 ng/mL
Follicle stimulating hormone (FSH)	S, P		
Female			
Menstruating:			
Follicular phase		3.0–20.0 IU/L	3.0–20.0 mIU/mL
Ovulatory phase		9.0–26.0 IU/L	9.0–26.0 mIU/mL
Luteal phase		1.0–12.0 IU/L	1.0–12.0 mIU/mL
Postmenopausal		18.0–153.0 IU/L	18.0–153.0 mIU/mL
Male		1.0–12.0 IU/L	1.0–12.0 mIU/mL
Free testosterone, adult	S		
Female		2.1–23.6 pmol/L	0.6–6.8 pg/mL
Male		163–847 pmol/L	47–244 pg/mL
Fructosamine	S	<285 μmol/L	<285 μmol/L
Gamma glutamyltransferase	S	0.15–0.99 μkat/L	9–58 U/L
Gastrin	S	<100 ng/L	<100 pg/mL
Glucagon	P	20–100 ng/L	20–100 pg/mL
Glucose (fasting)	P		
Normal		4.2–6.1 mmol/L	75–110 mg/dL
Impaired glucose tolerance		6.2–6.9 mmol/L	111–125 mg/dL
Diabetes mellitus		>7.0 mmol/L	>125 mg/dL
Glucose, 2 h postprandial	P	3.9–6.7 mmol/L	70–120 mg/dL
Growth hormone (resting)	S	0.5–17.0 μg/L	0.5–17.0 ng/mL
Hemoglobin A_{lc}	WB	0.04–0.06 Hb fraction	4.0–6.0%
High-density lipoprotein (HDL) (see **Table A-5**)			
Homocysteine	P	4.4–10.8 μmol/L	4.4–10.8 μmol/L
Human chorionic gonadotropin (hCG)	S		
Non-pregnant female		<5 IU/L	<5 mIU/mL
1–2 weeks postconception		9–130 IU/L	9–130 mIU/mL
2–3 weeks postconception		75–2600 IU/L	75–2600 mIU/mL
3–4 weeks postconception		850–20,800 IU/L	850–20,800 mIU/mL
4–5 weeks postconception		4000–100,200 IU/L	4000–100,200 mIU/mL

(*Continued*)

CLINICAL CHEMISTRY AND IMMUNOLOGY

ANALYTE	SPECIMEN[a]	SI UNITS	CONVENTIONAL UNITS
5–10 weeks postconception		11,500–289,000 IU/L	11,500–289,000 mIU/mL
10–14 weeks postconception		18,300–137,000 IU/L	18,300–137,000 mIU/mL
Second trimester		1400–53,000 IU/L	1400–53,000 mIU/mL
Third trimester		940–60,000 IU/L	940–60,000 mIU/mL
β-Hydroxybutyrate	P	0–290 μmol/L	0–3 mg/dL
5-Hydroindoleacetic acid [5-HIAA]	U	10.5–36.6 μmol/d	2–7 mg/d
17-Hydroxyprogesterone (adult)	S		
Male		0.15–7.5 nmol/L	5–250 ng/dL
Female			
Follicular phase		0.6–3.0 nmol/L	20–100 ng/dL
Midcycle peak		3–7.5 nmol/L	100–250 ng/dL
Luteal phase		3–15 nmol/L	100–500 ng/dL
Postmenopausal		≤2.1 nmol/L	≤70 ng/dL
Hydroxyproline	U, 24 h	38–500 μmol/d	38–500 μmol/d
Immunofixation	S	Not applicable	No bands detected
Immunoglobulin, quantitation (adult)	S		
IgA		0.70–3.50 g/L	70–350 mg/dL
IgD		0–140 mg/L	0–14 mg/dL
IgE		24–430 μg/L	10–179 IU/mL
IgG		7.0–17.0 g/L	700–1700 mg/dL
IgG_1		2.7–17.4 g/L	270–1740 mg/dL
IgG_2		0.3–6.3 g/L	30–630 mg/dL
IgG_3		0.13–3.2 g/L	13–320 mg/dL
IgG_4		0.11–6.2 g/L	11–620 mg/dL
IgM		0.50–3.0 g/L	50–300 mg/dL
Insulin	S, P	14.35–143.5 pmol/L	2–20 μU/mL
Iron	S	7–25 μmol/L	41–141 μg/dL
Iron-binding capacity	S	45–73 μmol/L	251–406 μg/dL
Iron-binding capacity saturation	S	0.16–0.35	16–35%
Joint fluid crystal	JF	Not applicable	No crystals seen
Joint fluid mucin	JF	Not applicable	Only type I mucin present
Ketone (acetone)	S, U	Negative	Negative
17 Ketosteroids	U	0.003–0.012 g/d	3–12 mg/d
Lactate	P, arterial	0.5–1.6 mmol/L	4.5–14.4 mg/dL
	P, venous	0.5–2.2 mmol/L	4.5–19.8 mg/dL
Lactate dehydrogenase	S	2.0–3.8 μkat/L	115–221 U/L
Lactate dehydrogenase isoenzymes	S		
Fraction 1 (of total)		0.14–0.26	14–26%
Fraction 2		0.29–0.39	29–39%
Fraction 3		0.20–0.25	20–26%
Fraction 4		0.08–0.16	8–16%
Fraction 5		0.06–0.16	6–16%
Lipase (method dependent)	S	0.51–0.73 μkat/L	3–43 U/L
Lipids: see **Table A-5**			
Lipoprotein (a)	S	0–300 mg/L	0–30 mg/dL
Low-density lipoprotein (LDL) (see **Table A-5**)			
Luteinizing hormone (LH)	S, P		
Female			
Menstruating			
Follicular phase		2.0–15.0 U/L	2.0–15.0 U/L
Ovulatory phase		22.0–105.0 U/L	22.0–105.0 U/L
Luteal phase		0.6–19.0 U/L	0.6–19.0 U/L
Postmenopausal		16.0–64.0 U/L	16.0–64.0 U/L
Male		2.0–12.0 U/L	2.0–12.0 U/L
Magnesium	S	0.62–0.95 mmol/L	1.5–2.3 mg/dL
Metanephrine	P	<0.5 nmol/L	<100 pg/mL

(Continued)

TABLE A-2 (*CONTINUED*)

CLINICAL CHEMISTRY AND IMMUNOLOGY

ANALYTE	SPECIMEN[a]	SI UNITS	CONVENTIONAL UNITS
Metanephrine	U	30–211 mmol/mol creatinine	53–367 µg/g creatinine
Methemoglobin	WB	0.0–0.01	0–1%
Microalbumin urine	U		
24-h urine		0.0–0.03 g/d	0–30 mg/24 h
Spot urine		0.0–0.03 g/g creatinine	0–30 µg/mg creatinine
Myoglobin	S		
Male		19–92 µg/L	19–92 µg/L
Female		12–76 µg/L	12–76 µg/L
Norepinephrine	U	89–473 nmol/d	15–80 µg/d
Norepinephrine	P		
Supine (30 min)		650–2423 pmol/L	110–410 pg/mL
Sitting		709–4019 pmol/L	120–680 pg/mL
Standing (30 min)		739–4137 pmol/L	125–700 pg/mL
N-telopeptide (cross linked), NTx	S		
Female, premenopausal		6.2–19.0 nmol BCE	6.2–19.0 nmol BCE
Male		5.4–24.2 nmol BCE	5.4–24.2 nmol BCE
Bone collagen equivalent (BCE)			
N-telopeptide (cross linked), NTx	U		
Female, premenopausal		17–94 nmol BCE/mmol creatinine	17–94 nmol BCE/mmol creatinine
Female, postmenopausal		26–124 nmol BCE/mmol creatinine	26–124 nmol BCE/mmol creatinine
Male		21–83 nmol BCE/mmol creatinine	21–83 nmol BCE/mmol creatinine
Bone collagen equivalent (BCE)			
5′ Nucleotidase	S	0.02–0.19 µkat/L	0–11 U/L
Osmolality	P	275–295 mOsmol/kg serum water	275–295 mOsmol/kg serum water
	U	500–800 mOsmol/kg water	500–800 mOsmol/kg water
Osteocalcin	S	11–50 µg/L	11–50 ng/mL
Oxygen content	WB		
Arterial (sea level)		17–21	17–21 vol%
Venous (sea level)		10–16	10–16 vol%
Oxygen percent saturation (sea level)	WB		
Arterial		0.97	94–100%
Venous, arm		0.60–0.85	60–85%
Parathyroid hormone (intact)	S	8–51 ng/L	8–51 pg/mL
Phosphatase, alkaline	S	0.56–1.63 µkat/L	33–96 U/L
Phosphorus, inorganic	S	0.81–1.4 mmol/L	2.5–4.3 mg/dL
Porphobilinogen	U	None	None
Potassium	S	3.5–5.0 mmol/L	3.5–5.0 meq/L
Prealbumin	S	170–340 mg/L	17–34 mg/dL
Progesterone	S, P		
Female			
Follicular		<3.18 nmol/L	<1.0 ng/mL
Midluteal		9.54–63.6 nmol/L	3–20 ng/mL
Male		<3.18 nmol/L	<1.0 ng/mL
Prolactin	S	0–20 µg/L	0–20 ng/mL
Prostate-specific antigen (PSA)	S		
Male			
<40 years		0.0–2.0 µg/L	0.0–2.0 ng/mL
>40 years		0.0–4.0 µg/L	0.0–4.0 ng/mL
PSA, free; in males 45–75 years, with PSA values between 4 and 20 µg/mL	S	>0.25 associated with benign prostatic hyperplasia	>25% associated with benign prostatic hyperplasia

(*Continued*)

TABLE A-2 (CONTINUED)

CLINICAL CHEMISTRY AND IMMUNOLOGY

ANALYTE	SPECIMEN[a]	SI UNITS	CONVENTIONAL UNITS
Protein fractions	S		
Albumin		35–55 g/L	3.5–5.5 g/dL (50–60%)
Globulin		20–35 g/L	2.0–3.5 g/dL (40–50%)
$Alpha_1$		2–4 g/L	0.2–0.4 g/dL (4.2–7.2%)
$Alpha_2$		5–9 g/L	0.5–0.9 g/dL (6.8–12%)
Beta		6–11 g/L	0.6–1.1 g/dL (9.3–15%)
Gamma		7–17 g/L	0.7–1.7 g/dL (13–23%)
Protein, total	S	67–86 g/L	6.7–8.6 g/dL
Pyruvate	P, arterial	40–130 μmol/L	0.35–1.14 mg/dL
	P, venous	40–130 μmol/L	0.35–1.14 mg/dL
Rheumatoid factor	S, JF	<30 kIU/L	<30 IU/mL
Serotonin	WB	0.28–1.14 μmol/L	50–200 ng/mL
Serum protein electrophoresis	S	Not applicable	Normal pattern
Sex hormone binding globulin (adult)	S		
Male		13–71 nmol/L	13–71 nmol/L
Female		18–114 nmol/L	18–114 nmol/L
Sodium	S	136–146 mmol/L	136–146 meq/L
Somatomedin-C (IGF-1) (adult)	S		
16–24 years		182–780 μg/L	182–780 ng/mL
25–39 years		114–492 μg/L	114–492 ng/mL
40–54 years		90–360 μg/L	90–360 ng/mL
>54 years		71–290 μg/L	71–290 ng/mL
Somatostatin	P	<25 ng/L	<25 pg/mL
Testosterone, total, morning sample	S		
Female		0.21–2.98 nmol/L	6–86 ng/dL
Male		9.36–37.10 nmol/L	270–1070 ng/dL
Thyroglobulin	S	0.5–53 μg/L	0.5–53 ng/mL
Thyroid-binding globulin	S	13–30 mg/L	1.3–3.0 mg/dL
Thyroid-stimulating hormone	S	0.34–4.25 mIU/L	0.34–4.25 μIU/mL
Thyroxine, free (fT_4)	S	10.3–21.9 pmol/L	0.8–1.7 ng/dL
Thyroxine, total (T_4)	S	70–151 nmol/L	5.4–11.7 μg/dL
(Free) thyroxine index	S	6.7–10.9	6.7–10.9
Transferrin	S	2.0–4.0 g/L	200–400 mg/dL
Triglycerides	S	0.34–2.26 mmol/L	30–200 mg/dL
Triiodothyronine, free (fT_3)	S	3.7–6.5 pmol/L	2.4–4.2 pg/mL
Triiodothyronine, total (T_3)	S	1.2–2.1 nmol/L	77–135 ng/dL
Troponin I	S		
Normal population, 99 %tile		0–0.08 μg/L	0–0.08 ng/mL
Cut-off for MI		>0.4 μg/L	>0.4 ng/mL
Troponin T	S		
Normal population, 99 %tile		0–0.1 μg/L	0–0.01 ng/mL
Cut-off for MI		0–0.1 μg/L	0–0.1 ng/mL
Urea nitrogen	S	2.5–7.1 mmol/L	7–20 mg/dL
Uric acid	S		
Females		0.15–0.33 μmol/L	2.5–5.6 mg/dL
Males		0.18–0.41 μmol/L	3.1–7.0 mg/dL
Urobilinogen	U	0.09–4.2 μmol/d	0.05–25 mg/24 h
Vanillylmandelic acid (VMA)	U, 24h	<30 μmol/d	<6 mg/d
Vasoactive intestinal polypeptide	P	0–60 ng/L	0–60 pg/mL

[a]P, plasma; S, serum; U, urine; WB, whole blood; JF, joint fluid.

TABLE A-3

TOXICOLOGY AND THERAPEUTIC DRUG MONITORING

	THERAPEUTIC RANGE		TOXIC LEVEL	
DRUG	**SI UNITS**	**CONVENTIONAL UNITS**	**SI UNITS**	**CONVENTIONAL UNITS**
Acetaminophen	66–199 μmol/L	10–30 μg/mL	>1320 μmol/L	>200 μg/mL
Amikacin				
Peak	34–51 μmol/L	20–30 μg/mL	>60 μmol/L	>35 μg/mL
Trough	0–17 μmol/L	0–10 μg/mL	>17 μmol/L	>10 μg/mL
Amitriptyline/nortriptyline (total drug)	430–900 nmol/L	120–250 ng/mL	>1800 nmol/L	>500 ng/mL
Amphetamine	150–220 nmol/L	20–30 ng/mL	>1500 nmol/L	>200 ng/mL
Bromide	1.3–6.3 mmol/L 9.4–18.8 mmol/L	Sedation: 10–50 mg/dL Epilepsy: 75–150 mg/dL	6.4–18.8 mmol/L >18.8 mmol/L >37.5 mmol/L	51–150 mg/dL: mild toxicity >150 mg/dL: severe toxicity >300 mg/dL: lethal
Carbamazepine	17–42 μmol/L	4–10 μg/mL	85 μmol/L	>20 μg/mL
Chloramphenicol				
Peak	31–62 μmol/L	10–20 μg/mL	>77 μmol/L	>25 μg/mL
Trough	15–31 μmol/L	5–10 μg/mL	>46 μmol/L	>15 μg/mL
Chlordiazepoxide	1.7–10 μmol/L	0.5–3.0 μg/mL	17 μmol/L	>5.0 μg/mL
Clonazepam	32–240 nmol/L	10–75 ng/mL	>320 nmol/L	>100 ng/mL
Clozapine	0.6–2.1 μmol/L	200–700 ng/mL	>3.7 μmol/L	>1200 ng/mL
Cocaine			>3.3 μmol/L	>1.0 μg/mL
Codeine	43–110 nmol/mL	13–33 ng/mL	>3700 nmol/mL	>1100 ng/mL (lethal)
Cyclosporine				
Renal transplant				
0–6 months	208–312 nmol/L	250–375 ng/mL	>312 nmol/L	>375 ng/mL
6–12 months after transplant	166–250 nmol/L	200–300 ng/mL	>250 nmol/L	>300 ng/mL
>12 months	83–125 nmol/L	100–150 ng/mL	>125 nmol/L	>150 ng/mL
Cardiac transplant				
0–6 months	208–291 nmol/L	250–350 ng/mL	>291 nmol/L	>350 ng/mL
6–12 months after transplant	125–208 nmol/L	150–250 ng/mL	>208 nmol/L	>250 ng/mL
>12 months	83–125 nmol/L	100–150 ng/mL	>125 nmol/L	150 ng/mL
Lung transplant				
0–6 months	250–374 nmol/L	300–450 ng/mL	>374 nmol/L	>450 ng/mL
Liver transplant				
0–7 days	249–333 nmol/L	300–400 ng/mL	>333 nmol/L	>400 ng/mL
2–4 weeks	208–291 nmol/L	250–350 ng/mL	>291 nmol/L	>350 ng/mL
5–8 weeks	166–249 nmol/L	200–300 ng/mL	>249 nmol/L	>300 ng/mL
9–52 weeks	125–208 nmol/L	150–250 ng/mL	>208 nmol/L	>250 ng/mL
>1 year	83–166 nmol/L	100–200 ng/mL	>166 nmol/L	>200 ng/mL
Desipramine	375–1130 nmol/L	100–300 ng/mL	>1880 nmol/L	>500 ng/mL
Diazepam (and metabolite)				
Diazepam	0.7–3.5 μmol/L	0.2–1.0 μg/mL	>7.0 μmol/L	>2.0 μg/mL
Nordiazepam	0.4–6.6 μmol/L	0.1–1.8 μg/mL	>9.2 μmol/L	>2.5 μg/mL
Digoxin	0.64–2.6 nmol/L	0.5–2.0 ng/mL	>3.1 nmol/L	>2.4 ng/mL
Disopyramide	>7.4 μmol/L	2.5 μg/mL	20.6 μmol/L	>7 μg/mL
Doxepin and nordoxepin				
Doxepin	0.36–0.98 μmol/L	101–274 ng/mL	>1.8 μmol/L	>503 ng/mL
Nordoxepin	0.38–1.04 μmol/L	106–291 ng/mL	>1.9 μmol/L	>531 ng/mL
Ethanol				
Behavioral changes			>4.3 mmol/L	>20 mg/dL
Legal limit			≥17 mmol/L	≥80 mg/dL
Critical with acute exposure			>54 mmol/L	>250 mg/dL

(Continued)

TABLE A-3 (*CONTINUED*)

TOXICOLOGY AND THERAPEUTIC DRUG MONITORING

	THERAPEUTIC RANGE		TOXIC LEVEL	
DRUG	SI UNITS	CONVENTIONAL UNITS	SI UNITS	CONVENTIONAL UNITS
Ethylene glycol				
Toxic			>2 mmol/L	>12 mg/dL
Lethal			>20 mmol/L	>120 mg/dL
Ethosuximide	280–700 μmol/L	40–100 μg/mL	>700 μmol/L	>100 μg/mL
Flecainide	0.5–2.4 μmol/L	0.2–1.0 μg/mL	>3.6 μmol/L	>1.5 μg/mL
Gentamicin				
Peak	10–21 μmol/mL	5–10 μg/mL	>25 μmol/mL	>12 μg/mL
Trough	0–4.2 μmol/mL	0–2 μg/mL	>4.2 μmol/mL	>2 μg/mL
Heroin (diacetyl morphine)			>700 μmol/L	>200 ng/mL (as morphine)
Ibuprofen	49–243 μmol/L	10–50 μg/mL	>97 μmol/L	>200 μg/mL
Imipramine (and metabolite)				
Desimipramine	375–1130 nmol/L	100–300 ng/mL	>1880 nmol/L	>500 ng/mL
Total imipramine + desimipramine	563–1130 nmol/L	150–300 ng/mL	>1880 nmol/L	>500 ng/mL
Lidocaine	5.1–21.3 μmol/L	1.2–5.0 μg/mL	>38.4 μmol/L	>9.0 μg/mL
Lithium	0.5–1.3 meq/L	0.5–1.3 meq/L	>2 mmol/L	>2 meq/L
Methadone	1.3–3.2 μmol/L	0.4–1.0 μg/mL	>6.5 μmol/L	>2 μg/mL
Methamphetamine		20–30 ng/mL		0.1–1.0 μg/mL
Methanol			>6 mmol/L	>20 mg/dL
			>16 mmol/L	>50 mg/dL, severe toxicity
			>28 mmol/L	>89 mg/dL, lethal
Methotrexate				
Low-dose	0.01–0.1 μmol/L	0.01–0.1 μmol/L	>0.1 mmol/L	>0.1 mmol/L
High-dose (24 h)	<5.0 μmol/L	<5.0 μmol/L	>5.0 μmol/L	>5.0 μmol/L
High-dose (48 h)	<0.50 μmol/L	<0.50 μmol/L	>0.5 μmol/L	>0.5 μmol/L
High-dose (72 h)	<0.10 μmol/L	<0.10 μmol/L	>0.1 μmol/L	>0.1 μmol/L
Morphine	35–250 μmol/L	10–70 ng/mL	180–14000 μmol/L	50–4000 ng/mL
Nitroprusside (as thiocyanate)	103–499 μmol/L	6–29 μg/mL	860 μmol/L	>50 μg/mL
Nortriptyline	190–569 nmol/L	50–150 ng/mL	>1900 nmol/L	>500 ng/mL
Phenobarbital	65–172 μmol/L	15–40 μg/mL	>215 μmol/L	>50 μg/mL
Phenytoin	40–79 μmol/L	10–20 μg/mL	>118 μmol/L	>30 μg/mL
Phenytoin, free	4.0–7.9 μg/mL	1–2 μg/mL	>13.9 μg/mL	>3.5 μg/mL
% Free	0.08–0.14	8–14		
Primidone and metabolite				
Primidone	23–55 μmol/L	5–12 μg/mL	>69 μmol/L	>15 μg/mL
Phenobarbital	65–172 μmol/L	15–40 μg/mL	>215 μmol/L	>50 μg/mL
Procainamide				
Procainamide	17–42 μmol/L	4–10 μg/mL	>51 μmol/L	>12 μg/mL
NAPA (*N*-acetylprocainamide)	22–72 μmol/L	6-20 μg/mL	>126 μmol/L	>35 μg/mL
Quinidine	>6.2–15.4 μmol/L	2.0 -5.0 μg/mL	>31 μmol/L	>10 μg/mL
Salicylates	145–2100 μmol/L	2–29 mg/dL	>2172 μmol/L	>30 mg/dL
Sirolimus (trough level)				
Kidney transplant	4.4–13.1 nmol/L	4–12 ng/mL	>16 nmol/L	>15 ng/mL
Tacrolimus (FK506) (trough)				
Kidney and liver				
0–2 months posttransplant	12–19 nmol/L	10–15 ng/mL	>25 nmol/L	>20 ng/mL
>2 months posttransplant	6–12 nmol/L	5–10 ng/mL		
Heart				
0–2 months posttransplant	19–25 nmol/L	15–20 ng/mL	>25 nmol/L	>20 ng/mL
3–6 months posttransplant	12–19 nmol/L	10–15 ng/mL		
>6 months posttransplant	10–12 nmol/L	8–10 ng/mL		
Theophylline	56–111 μg/mL	10–20 μg/mL	>140 μg/mL	>25 μg/mL

(*Continued*)

TABLE A-3 (CONTINUED)

TOXICOLOGY AND THERAPEUTIC DRUG MONITORING

	THERAPEUTIC RANGE		TOXIC LEVEL	
DRUG	SI UNITS	CONVENTIONAL UNITS	SI UNITS	CONVENTIONAL UNITS
Thiocyanate				
After nitroprusside infusion	103–499 μmol/L	6–29 μg/mL	860 μmol/L	>50 μg/mL
Nonsmoker	17–69 μmol/L	1–4 μg/mL		
Smoker	52–206 μmol/L	3–12 μg/mL		
Tobramycin				
Peak	11–22 μg/L	5–10 μg/mL	>26 μg/L	>12 μg/mL
Trough	0–4.3 μg/L	0–2 μg/mL	>4.3 μg/L	>2 μg/mL
Valproic acid	350–700 μmol/L	50–100 μg/mL	>1000 μmol/L	>150 μg/mL
Vancomycin				
Peak	14–28 μmol/L	20–40 μg/mL	>55 μmol/L	>80 μg/mL
Trough	3.5–10.4 μmol/L	5–15 μg/mL	>14 μmol/L	>20 μg/mL

TABLE A-4

VITAMINS AND SELECTED TRACE MINERALS

		REFERENCE RANGE	
SPECIMEN	ANALYTE[a]	SI UNITS	CONVENTIONAL UNITS
Aluminum	S	<0.2 μmol/L	<5.41μg/L
	U, random	0.19–1.11 μmol/L	5–30 μg/L
Arsenic	WB	0.03–0.31 μmol/L	2–23 μg/L
	U, 24 h	0.07–0.67 μmol/d	5–50 μg/d
Cadmium	WB	<44.5 nmol/L	<5.0 μg/L
Coenzyme Q10 (ubiquinone)	P	433–1532 μg/L	433–1532 μg/L
B carotene	S	0.07–1.43 μmol/L	4–77 μg/dL
Copper			
	S	11–22 μmol/L	70–140 μg/dL
	U, 24 h	<0.95 μmol/d	<60 μg/d
Folic acid	RC	340–1020 nmol/L cells	150–450 ng/mL cells
Folic acid	S	12.2–40.8 nmol/L	5.4–18.0 ng/mL
Lead (adult)	S	<0.5 μmol/L	<10 μg/dL
Mercury			
	WB	3.0–294 nmol/L	0.6–59 μg/L
	U, 24 h	<99.8 nmol/L	<20 μg/L
Selenium	S	0.8–2.0 μmol/L	63–160 μg/L
Vitamin A	S	0.7–3.5 μmol/L	20–100 μg/dL
Vitamin B_1 (thiamine)	S	0–75 nmol/L	0–2 μg/dL
Vitamin B_2 (riboflavin)	S	106–638 nmol/L	4–24 μg/dL
Vitamin B_6	P	20–121 nmol/L	5–30 ng/mL
Vitamin B_{12}	S	206–735 pmol/L	279–996 pg/mL
Vitamin C (ascorbic acid)	S	23–57 μmol/L	0.4–1.0 mg/dL
Vitamin D_3, 1,25-dihydroxy	S	60–108 pmol/L	25–45 pg/mL
Vitamin D_3, 25-hydroxy	P		
Summer		37.4–200 nmol/L	15–80 ng/mL
Winter		34.9–105 nmol/L	14–42 ng/mL
Vitamin E	S	12–42 μmol/L	5–18 μg/mL
Vitamin K	S	0.29–2.64 nmol/L	0.13–1.19 ng/mL
Zinc	S	11.5–18.4 μmol/L	75–120 μg/dL

[a]P, plasma; RC, red cells; S, serum; WB, whole blood; U, urine.

TABLE A-5

CLASSIFICATION OF LDL, TOTAL, AND HDL CHOLESTEROL

LDL Cholesterol, mg/dL (mmol/L)	
<70 (<1.81)	Therapeutic option for very high risk patients
<100 (<2.59)	Optimal
100–129 (2.59–3.34)	Near optimal/above optimal
130–159 (3.36–4.11)	Borderline high
160–189 (4.14–4.89)	High
≥190 (≥4.91)	Very high
Total Cholesterol, mg/dL (mmol/L)	
<200 (<5.17)	Desirable
200–239 (5.17–6.18)	Borderline high
≥240 (≥6.21)	High
HDL Cholesterol, mg/dL (mmol/L)	
<40 (<1.03)	Low
≥60 (≥1.55)	High

Note: LDL, low-density lipoprotein; HDL, high-density lipoprotein
Source: Executive summary of the third report of the National Cholesterol Education Program (NCEP) expert panel on detection, evaluation, and treatment of high blood cholesterol in adults (adult treatment panel III). JAMA 285:2486, 2001; and implications of recent clinical trials for the National Cholesterol Education Program Adult Treatment Panel III Guidelines: SM Grundy et al for the Coordinating Committee of the National Cholesterol Education Program. Circulation 110:227, 2004.

REFERENCE VALUES FOR SPECIFIC ANALYTES

TABLE A-6

CEREBROSPINAL FLUID (CSF)[a]

	REFERENCE RANGE	
CONSTITUENT	**SI UNITS**	**CONVENTIONAL UNITS**
Osmolarity	292–297 mmol/kg water	292–297 mOsmol/L
Electrolytes		
Sodium	137–145 mmol/L	137–145 meq/L
Potassium	2.7–3.9 mmol/L	2.7–3.9 meq/L
Calcium	1.0–1.5 mmol/L	2.1–3.0 meq/L
Magnesium	1.0–1.2 mmol/L	2.0–2.5 meq/L
Chloride	116–122 mmol/L	116–122 meq/L
CO_2 content	20–24 mmol/L	20–24 meq/L
P_{CO_2}	6–7 kPa	45–49 mmHg
pH	7.31–7.34	
Glucose	2.22–3.89 mmol/L	40–70 mg/dL
Lactate	1–2 mmol/L	10–20 mg/dL
Total protein		
Lumbar	0.15–0.5 g/L	15–50 mg/dL
Cisternal	0.15–0.25 g/L	15–25 mg/dL
Ventricular	0.06–0.15 g/L	6–15 mg/dL
Albumin	0.066–0.442 g/L	6.6–44.2 mg/dL
IgG	0.009–0.057 g/L	0.9–5.7 mg/dL
IgG index[b]	0.29–0.59	

(*Continued*)

TABLE A-6 (*CONTINUED*)

CEREBROSPINAL FLUID (CSF)[a]

CONSTITUENT	REFERENCE RANGE	
	SI UNITS	CONVENTIONAL UNITS
Total protein (*Continued*)		
Oligoclonal bands	<2 bands not present in matched serum sample	
Ammonia	15–47 μmol/L	25–80 μg/dL
Creatinine	44–168 μmol/L	0.5–1.9 mg/dL
Myelin basic protein	<4 μg/L	
CSF pressure		50–180 mmH_2O
CSF volume (adult)	~150 mL	
Red blood cells	0	0
Leukocytes		
Total	0–5 mononuclear cells per μL	0–5 mononuclear cells per mm^3
Differential		
Lymphocytes	60–70%	
Monocytes	30–50%	
Neutrophils	None	

[a]Since cerebrospinal fluid concentrations are equilibrium values, measurements of the same parameters in blood plasma obtained at the same time are recommended. However, there is a time lag in attainment of equilibrium, and cerebrospinal levels of plasma constituents that can fluctuate rapidly (such as plasma glucose) may not achieve stable values until after a significant lag phase.
[b]IgG index = CSF IgG(mg/dL) × serum albumin(g/dL)/Serum IgG(g/dL) × CSF albumin(mg/dL).

TABLE A-7

URINE ANALYSIS

	REFERENCE RANGE	
	SI UNITS	CONVENTIONAL UNITS
Acidity, titratable	20–40 mmol/d	20–40 meq/d
Ammonia	30–50 mmol/d	30–50 meq/d
Amylase		4–400 U/L
Amylase/creatinine clearance ratio $[(Cl_{am}/Cl_{cr}) \times 100]$	1–5	1–5
Calcium (10 meq/d or 200 mg/d dietary calcium)	<7.5 mmol/d	<300 mg/d
Creatine, as creatinine		
Female	<760 μmol/d	<100 mg/d
Male	<380 μmol/d	<50 mg/d
Creatinine	8.8–14 mmol/d	1.0–1.6 g/d
Eosinophils	<100,000 eosinophils/L	<100 eosinophils/mL
Glucose (glucose oxidase method)	0.3–1.7 mmol/d	50–300 mg/d
5-Hydroxyindoleacetic acid (5-HIAA)	10–47 μmol/d	2–9 mg/d
Iodine, spot urine		
WHO classification of iodine deficiency		
Not iodine deficient	>100 μg/L	>100 μg/L
Mild iodine deficiency	50–100 μg/L	50–100 μg/L
Moderate iodine deficiency	20–49 μg/L	20–49 μg/L
Severe iodine deficiency	<20 μg/L	<20 μg/L

(*Continued*)

TABLE A-7(*CONTINUED*)

URINE ANALYSIS

	REFERENCE RANGE	
	SI UNITS	CONVENTIONAL UNITS
Microalbumin		
Normal	0.0–0.03 g/d	0–30 mg/d
Microalbuminuria	0.03–0.30 g/d	30–300 mg/d
Clinical albuminuria	>0.3 g/d	>300 mg/d
Microalbumin/creatinine ratio		
Normal	0–3.4 g/mol creatinine	0–30 μg/mg creatinine
Microalbuminuria	3.4–34 g/mol creatinine	30–300 μg/mg creatinine
Clinical albuminuria	>34 g/mol creatinine	>300 μg/mg creatinine
Oxalate		
Male	80–500 μmol/d	7–44 mg/d
Female	45–350 μmol/d	4–31 mg/d
pH	5.0–9.0	5.0–9.0
Phosphate (phosphorus) (varies with intake)	12.9–42.0 mmol/d	400–1300 mg/d
Potassium (varies with intake)	25–100 mmol/d	25–100 meq/d
Protein	<0.15 g/d	<150 mg/d
Sediment		
Red blood cells	0–2/high power field	
White blood cells	0–2/high power field	
Bacteria	None	
Crystals	None	
Bladder cells	None	
Squamous cells	None	
Tubular cells	None	
Broad casts	None	
Epithelial cell casts	None	
Granular casts	None	
Hyaline casts	0–5/low power field	
Red blood cell casts	None	
Waxy casts	None	
White cell casts	None	
Sodium (varies with intake)	100–260 mmol/d	100–260 meq/d
Specific gravity	1.001–1.035	1.001–1.035
Urea nitrogen	214–607 mmol/d	6–17 g/d
Uric acid (normal diet)	1.49–4.76 mmol/d	250–800 mg/d

Note: WHO, World Health Organization.

TABLE A-8

DIFFERENTIAL NUCLEATED CELL COUNTS OF BONE MARROW ASPIRATES[a]

	OBSERVED RANGE, %	95% CONFIDENCE INTERVALS, %	MEAN, %
Blast cells	0–3.2	0–3.0	1.4
Promyelocytes	3.6–13.2	3.2–12.4	7.8
Neutrophil myelocytes	4–21.4	3.7–10.0	7.6
Eosinophil myelocytes	0–5.0	0–2.8	1.3
Metamyelocytes	1–7.0	2.3–5.9	4.1
Neutrophils			
Males	21.0–45.6	21.9–42.3	32.1
Females	29.6–46.6	28.8–45.9	37.4
Eosinophils	0.4–4.2	0.3–4.2	2.2
Eosinophils plus eosinophil myelocytes	0.9–7.4	0.7–6.3	3.5
Basophils	0–0.8	0–0.4	0.1
Erythroblasts			
Males	18.0–39.4	16.2–40.1	28.1
Females	14.0–31.8	13.0–32.0	22.5
Lymphocytes	4.6–22.6	6.0–20.0	13.1
Plasma cells	0–1.4	0–1.2	0.6
Monocytes	0–3.2	0–2.6	1.3
Macrophages	0–1.8	0–1.3	0.4
M:E ratio			
Males	1.1–4.0	1.1–4.1	2.1
Females	1.6–5.4	1.6–5.2	2.8

[a]Based on bone marrow aspirate from 50 healthy volunteers (30 men, 20 women).
Source: From BJ Bain: The bone marrow aspirate of healthy subjects. Br J Haematol 94:206, 1996.

TABLE A-9

STOOL ANALYSIS

	REFERENCE RANGE	
	SI UNITS	CONVENTIONAL UNITS
Amount	0.1–0.2 kg/d	100–200 g/24 h
Coproporphyrin	611–1832 nmol/d	400–1200 μg/24 h
Fat		
Adult		<7 g/d
Adult on fat-free diet		<4 g/d
Fatty acids	0–21 mmol/d	0–6 g/24 h
Leukocytes	None	None
Nitrogen	<178 mmol/d	<2.5 g/24 h
pH	7.0–7.5	
Occult blood	Negative	Negative
Trypsin		20–95 U/g
Urobilinogen	85–510 μmol/d	50–300 mg/24 h
Uroporphyrins	12–48 nmol/d	10–40 μg/24 h
Water	<0.75	<75%

Source: Modified from FT Fishbach, MB Dunning III: *A Manual of Laboratory and Diagnostic Tests*, 7th ed., Lippincott Williams & Wilkins, Philadelphia, 2004.

TABLE A-10

RENAL FUNCTION TESTS

	REFERENCE RANGE	
	SI UNITS	**CONVENTIONAL UNITS**
Clearances (corrected to 1.72 m^2 body surface area)		
Measures of glomerular filtration rate		
Inulin clearance (Cl)		
Males (mean ± 1 SD)	2.1 ± 0.4 mL/s	124 ± 25.8 mL/min
Females (mean ± 1 SD)	2.0 ± 0.2 mL/s	119 ± 12.8 mL/min
Endogenous creatinine clearance	1.5–2.2 mL/s	91–130 mL/min
Measures of effective renal plasma flow and tubular function		
p-Aminohippuric acid clearance (Cl_{PAH})		
Males (mean ± 1 SD)	10.9 ± 2.7 mL/s	654 ± 163 mL/min
Females (mean ± 1 SD)	9.9 ± 1.7 mL/s	594 ± 102 mL/min
Concentration and dilution test		
Specific gravity of urine		
After 12-h fluid restriction	>1.025	>1.025
After 12-h deliberate water intake	≤1.003	≤1.003
Protein excretion, urine	<0.15 g/d	<150 mg/d
Specific gravity, maximal range	1.002–1.028	1.002–1.028
Tubular reabsorption, phosphorus	0.79–0.94 of filtered load	79–94% of filtered load

TABLE A-11

CIRCULATORY FUNCTION TESTS

	RESULTS: REFERENCE RANGE	
TEST	**SI UNITS (RANGE)**	**CONVENTIONAL UNITS (RANGE)**
Arteriovenous oxygen difference	30–50 mL/L	30–50 mL/L
Cardiac output (Fick)	2.5–3.6 L/m^2 of body surface area per min	2.5–3.6 L/m^2 of body surface area per min
Contractility indexes		
Max. left ventricular *dp/dt*(*dp/dt*)/DP when DP = 5.3 kPa (40 mmHg) (DP, diastolic pressure)	220 kPa/s (176–250 kPa/s) (37.6 ± 12.2)/s	1650 mmHg/s (1320–1880 mmHg/s) (37.6 ± 12.2)/s
Mean normalized systolic ejection rate (angiography)	3.32 ± 0.84 end-diastolic volumes per second	3.32 ± 0.84 end-diastolic volumes per second
Mean velocity of circumferential fiber shortening (angiography)	1.83 ± 0.56 circumferences per second	1.83 ± 0.56 circumferences per second
Ejection fraction: stroke volume/end-diastolic volume (SV/EDV)	0.67 ± 0.08 (0.55–0.78)	0.67 ± 0.08 (0.55–0.78)
End-diastolic volume	70 ± 20.0 mL/m^2 (60–88 mL/m^2)	70 ± 20.0 mL/m^2 (60–88 mL/m^2)
End-systolic volume	25 ± 5.0 mL/m^2 (20–33 mL/m^2)	25 ± 5.0 mL/m^2 (20–33 mL/m^2)
Left ventricular work		
Stroke work index	50 ± 20.0 (g·m)/m^2 (30–110)	50 ± 20.0 (g·m)/m^2 (30–110)
Left ventricular minute work index	1.8–6.6 [(kg·m)/m^2]/min	1.8–6.6 [(kg·m)/m^2]/min
Oxygen consumption index	110–150 mL	110–150 mL
Maximum oxygen uptake	35 mL/min (20–60 mL/min)	35 mL/min (20–60 mL/min)
Pulmonary vascular resistance	2–12 (kPa·s)/L	20–130 (dyn·s)/cm^5
Systemic vascular resistance	77–150 (kPa·s)/L	770–1600 (dyn·s)/cm^5

Source: E Braunwald et al: *Heart Disease*, 6th ed, Philadelphia, Saunders, 2001.

TABLE A-12

GASTROINTESTINAL TESTS

TEST	RESULTS	
	SI UNITS	CONVENTIONAL UNITS
Absorption tests		
D-Xylose: after overnight fast, 25 g xylose given in oral aqueous solution		
Urine, collected for following 5 h	25% of ingested dose	25% of ingested dose
Serum, 2 h after dose	2.0–3.5 mmol/L	30–52 mg/dL
Vitamin A: a fasting blood specimen is obtained and 200,000 units of vitamin A in oil is given orally	Serum level should rise to twice fasting level in 3–5 h	Serum level should rise to twice fasting level in 3–5 h
Bentiromide test (pancreatic function): 500 mg bentiromide (chymex) orally; *p*-aminobenzoic acid (PABA) measured		
Plasma		>3.6 (±1.1) μg/mL at 90 min
Urine	>50% recovered in 6 h	>50% recovered in 6 h
Gastric juice		
Volume		
24 h	2–3 L	2–3 L
Nocturnal	600–700 mL	600–700 mL
Basal, fasting	30–70 mL/h	30–70 mL/h
Reaction		
pH	1.6–1.8	1.6–1.8
Titratable acidity of fasting juice	4–9 μmol/s	15–35 meq/h
Acid output		
Basal		
Females (mean ± 1 SD)	0.6 ± 0.5 μmol/s	2.0 ± 1.8 meq/h
Males (mean ± 1 SD)	0.8 ± 0.6 μmol/s	3.0 ± 2.0 meq/h
Maximal (after SC histamine acid phosphate, 0.004 mg/kg body weight, and preceded by 50 mg promethazine, or after betazole, 1.7 mg/kg body weight, or pentagastrin, 6 μg/kg body weight)		
Females (mean ± 1 SD)	4.4 ± 1.4 μmol/s	16 ± 5 meq/h
Males (mean ± 1 SD)	6.4 ± 1.4 μmol/s	23 ± 5 meq/h
Basal acid output/maximal acid output ratio	≤0.6	≤0.6
Gastrin, serum	0–200 μg/L	0–200 pg/mL
Secretin test (pancreatic exocrine function): 1 unit/kg body weight, IV		
Volume (pancreatic juice) in 80 min	>2.0 mL/kg	>2.0 mL/kg
Bicarbonate concentration	>80 mmol/L	>80 meq/L
Bicarbonate output in 30 min	>10 mmol	>10 meq

TABLE A-13

NORMAL VALUES OF DOPPLER ECHOCARDIOGRAPHIC MEASUREMENTS IN ADULTS

	RANGE	MEAN
RVD (cm), measured at the base in apical 4-chamber view	2.6–4.3	3.5 ± 0.4
LVID (cm), measured in the parasternal long axis view	3.6–5.4	4.7 ± 0.4
Posterior LV wall thickness (cm)	0.6–1.1	0.9 ± 0.4
IVS wall thickness (cm)	0.6–1.1	0.9 ± 0.4
Left atrial dimension (cm), antero-posterior dimension	2.3–3.8	3.0 ± 0.3
Aortic root dimension (cm)	2.0–3.5	2.4 ± 0.4
Aortic cusps separation (cm)	1.5–2.6	1.9 ± 0.4
Percentage of fractional shortening	34–44%	36%
Mitral flow (m/s)	0.6–1.3	0.9
Tricuspid flow (m/s)	0.3–0.7	0.5
Pulmonary artery (m/s)	0.6–0.9	0.75
Aorta (m/s)	1.0–1.7	1.35

Note: RVD, right ventricular dimension; LVID, left ventricular internal dimension; LV, left ventricle; IVS, interventricular septum.
Source: From A Weyman: *Principles and Practice of Echocardiography*, 2d ed., Philadelphia, Lea & Febiger, 1994.

TABLE A-14

SUMMARY OF VALUES USEFUL IN PULMONARY PHYSIOLOGY

SPECIMEN	SYMBOL	TYPICAL VALUES: MAN, AGE 40, 75 kg, 175 cm TALL	TYPICAL VALUES: WOMAN, AGE 40, 60 kg, 160 cm TALL
Pulmonary Mechanics			
Spirometry—volume-time curves			
Forced vital capacity	FVC	5.1 L	3.6 L
Forced expiratory volume in 1 s	FEV_1	4.1 L	2.9 L
FEV_1/FVC	FEV_1%	80%	82%
Maximal midexpiratory flow	MMF (FEF 25–27)	4.8 L/s	3.6 L/s
Maximal expiratory flow rate	MEFR (FEF 200–1200)	9.4 L/s	6.1 L/s
Spirometry—flow-volume curves			
Maximal expiratory flow at 50% of expired vital capacity	V_{max} 50 (FEF 50%)	6.1 L/s	4.6 L/s
Maximal expiratory flow at 75% of expired vital capacity	V_{max} 75 (FEF 75%)	3.1 L/s	2.5 L/s
Resistance to airflow			
Pulmonary resistance	RL (R_L)	<3.0 (cmH_2O/s)/L	
Airway resistance	Raw	<2.5 (cmH_2O/s)/L	
Specific conductance	SGaw	>0.13 cmH_2O/s	
Pulmonary compliance			
Static recoil pressure at total lung capacity	Pst TLC	25 ± 5 cmH_2O	
Compliance of lungs (static)	CL	0.2 L cmH_2O	
Compliance of lungs and thorax	C(L + T)	0.1 L cmH_2O	
Dynamic compliance of 20 breaths per minute	C dyn 20	0.25 ± 0.05 L/cmH_2O	
Maximal static respiratory pressures			
Maximal inspiratory pressure	MIP	>90 cmH_2O	>50 cmH_2O
Maximal expiratory pressure	MEP	>150 cmH_2O	>120 cmH_2O
Lung Volumes			
Total lung capacity	TLC	6.7 L	4.9 L
Functional residual capacity	FRC	3.7 L	2.8 L
Residual volume	RV	2.0 L	1.6 L
Inspiratory capacity	IC	3.3 L	2.3 L
Expiratory reserve volume	ERV	1.7 L	1.1 L
Vital capacity	VC	5.0 L	3.4 L
Gas Exchange (Sea Level)			
Arterial O_2 tension	Pa_{O_2}	12.7 ± 0.7 kPa (95 ± 5 mmHg)	
Arterial CO_2 tension	Pa_{CO_2}	5.3 ± 0.3 kPa (40 ± 2 mmHg)	
Arterial O_2 saturation	Sa_{O_2}	0.97 ± 0.02 (97 ± 2%)	
Arterial blood pH	pH	7.40 ± 0.02	
Arterial bicarbonate	HCO_3^-	24 + 2 meq/L	
Base excess	BE	0 ± 2 meq/L	
Diffusing capacity for carbon monoxide (single breath)	DL_{CO}	0.42 mL CO/s per mmHg (25 mL CO/min per mmHg)	
Dead space volume	V_D	2 mL/kg body wt	
Physiologic dead space; dead space-tidal volume ratio	V_D/V_T		
Rest		≤35% V_T	
Exercise		≤20% V_T	
Alveolar-arterial difference for O_2	$P(A - a)_{O_2}$	≤2.7 kPa ≤20 kPa (≤20 mmHg)	

TABLE A-15

BODY FLUIDS AND OTHER MASS DATA

	REFERENCE RANGE	
	SI UNITS	CONVENTIONAL UNITS
Body fluid		
Total volume (lean) of body weight	50% (in obese) to 70%	
Intracellular	0.3–0.4 of body weight	
Extracellular	0.2–0.3 of body weight	
Blood		
Total volume		
Males	69 mL per kg body weight	
Females	65 mL per kg body weight	
Plasma volume		
Males	39 mL per kg body weight	
Females	40 mL per kg body weight	
Red blood cell volume		
Males	30 mL per kg body weight	1.15–1.21 L/m^2 of body surface area
Females	25 mL per kg body weight	0.95–1.00 L/m^2 of body surface area
Body mass index	18.5–24.9 kg/m^2	18.5–24.9 kg/m^2

TABLE A-16

RADIATION-DERIVED UNITS

QUANTITY	OLD UNIT	SI UNITS	NAME FOR SI UNIT (and Abbreviation)	CONVERSION
Activity	Curie (Ci)	Disintegrations per second (dps)	Becquerel (Bq)	1 Ci = 3.7×10^{10} Bq 1 mCi = 37 mBq 1 μCi = 0.037 MBq or 37 GBq 1 Bq = 2.703×10^{-11} Ci
Absorbed dose	Rad	Joule per kilogram (J/kg)	Gray (Gy)	1 Gy = 100 rad 1 rad = 0.01 Gy 1 mrad = 10^{-3} cGy
Exposure	Roentgen (R)	Coulomb per kilogram (C/kg)	—	1 C/kg = 3876 R 1 R = 2.58×10^{-4} C/kg 1 mR = 258 pC/kg
Dose equivalent	Rem	Joule per kilogram (J/kg)	Sievert (Sv)	1 Sv = 100 rem 1 rem = 0.01 Sv 1 mrem = 10 μSv

ACKNOWLEDGMENT

The authors acknowledge the contributions of Dr. Patrick M. Sluss, Dr. James L. Januzzi, and Dr. Kent B. Lewandrowski to this chapter in previous editions of Harrison's Principles of Internal Medicine.

FURTHER READINGS

KRATZ A et al: Case records of the Massachusetts General Hospital. Weekly clinicopathological exercises. Laboratory reference values. N Engl J Med 351:1548, 2004

LEHMAN HP, HENRY JB: SI units, in *Henry's Clinical Diagnosis and Management by Laboratory Methods*, 21st ed, RC McPherson, MR Pincus (eds). Philadelphia, Elsevier Saunders, 2007, pp 1404–1418

PESCE MA: Reference ranges for laboratory tests and procedures, in *Nelson's Textbook of Pediatrics*, 18th ed, RM Klegman et al (eds). Philadelphia, Elsevier Saunders, 2007, pp 2943–2949

SOLBERG HE: Establishment and use of reference values, in *Tietz Textbook of Clinical Chemistry and Molecular Diagnostics*, 4th ed, CA Burtis et al (eds). Philadelphia, Elsevier Saunders, 2006, pp 425–448

REVIEW AND SELF-ASSESSMENT*

Charles Wiener ■ Gerald Bloomfield ■ Cynthia D. Brown ■ Joshua Schiffer ■ Adam Spivak

QUESTIONS

DIRECTIONS: Choose the **one best** response to each question.

1. Which type of bite represents a potential medical emergency in an asplenic patient?

   A. Cat bite
   B. Dog bite
   C. Fish bite
   D. Human bite

2. A 24-year-old man with advanced HIV infection presents to the emergency department with a tan painless nodule on the lower extremity (Fig. 2). He is afebrile and has no other lesions. He does not take antiretroviral therapy, and his last CD4+ T-cell count was 20/μL. He lives with a friend who has cats and kittens. A biopsy shows lobular proliferation of blood vessels lined by enlarged endothelial cells and a mixed acute and chronic inflammatory infiltrate. Tissue stains show gram-negative bacilli. Which of the following is most likely to be effective therapy for the lesion?

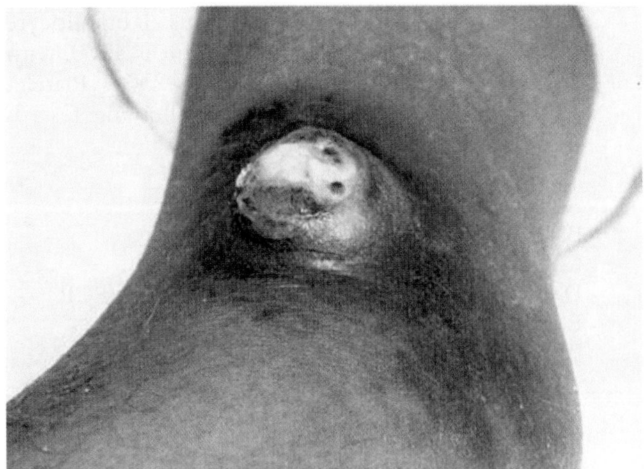

FIGURE 2

2. (*Continued*)

   A. Azithromycin
   B. Cephazolin
   C. Interferon α
   D. Penicillin
   E. Vancomycin

3. A 26-year-old woman comes to your clinic complaining of 3–4 weeks of a malodorous white vaginal discharge. She recently began having unprotected sexual intercourse with a new male partner. He is asymptomatic. Her only medication is oral contraceptives. Examination reveals a thin white discharge that evenly coats the vagina. Further examination of the discharge reveals that it has a pH of 5.0 and has a "fishy" odor when 10% KOH is added to the discharge. Microscopic examination reveals vaginal cells coated with coccobacillary organisms. Which of the following therapies is indicated?

   A. Acyclovir, 400 mg PO tid × 7 days
   B. Metronidazole, 2 g PO × 1
   C. Metronidazole, 500 mg PO bid × 7 days
   D. Fluconazole, 100 mg PO × 1
   E. Vaginal douching

4. All of the following infections associated with sexual activity correlate with increased acquisition of HIV infection in women *except*

   A. bacterial vaginosis
   B. *Chlamydia*
   C. gonorrhea
   D. herpes simplex virus-2
   E. *Trichomonas vaginalis*
   F. all of the above are associated with increased acquisition

5. A 9-year-old boy is brought to a pediatric emergency room by his father. He has had 2 days of headache, neck stiffness, and photophobia and this morning had a temperature of 38.9°C (102°F). He has also had several episodes of vomiting and diarrhea

*Questions and answers were selected by Miriam J. Baron, MD, from Wiener C, et al (eds). *Harrison's Principles of Internal Medicine Self-Assessment and Board Review*, 17th ed. New York: McGraw-Hill, 2008.

5. (*Continued*)
overnight. A lumbar puncture is performed, which reveals pleocytosis in the cerebrospinal fluid (CSF). Which of the following is true regarding enteroviruses as a cause of aseptic meningitis?

A. An elevated CSF protein rules out enteroviruses as a cause of meningitis.
B. Enteroviruses are responsible for up to 90% of aseptic meningitis in children.
C. Lymphocytes will predominate in the CSF early on, with a shift to neutrophils at 24 h.
D. Symptoms are more severe in children than in adults.
E. They occur more commonly in the winter and spring.

6. A 48-year-old female presents to her physician with a 2-day history of fever, arthralgias, diarrhea, and headache. She recently returned from an eco-tour in tropical sub-Saharan Africa, where she went swimming in inland rivers. Notable findings on physical examination include a temperature of 38.7°C (101.7°F); 2-cm tender mobile lymph nodes in the axilla, cervical, and femoral regions; and a palpable spleen. Her white blood cell count is 15,000/μL with 50% eosinophils. She should receive treatments with which of the following medications?

A. Chloroquine
B. Mebendazole
C. Metronidazole
D. Praziquantel
E. Thiabendazole

7. A 39-year-old woman received a liver transplant 2 years ago and is maintained on prednisone, 5 mg, and cyclosporine A, 8 mg/kg per day. She has had two episodes of rejection since transplant, as well an episode of cytomegalovirus syndrome and *Nocardia* pneumonia. She intends to take a 2-week gorilla-watching trip to Rwanda and seeks your advice regarding her health while abroad. Which of the following potential interventions is strictly contraindicated?

A. Malaria prophylaxis
B. Meningococcal vaccine
C. Rabies vaccine
D. Typhoid purified polysaccharide vaccine
E. Yellow fever vaccine

8. A 17-year-old woman presents to the clinic complaining of vaginal itchiness and malodorous discharge. She is sexually active with multiple partners, and she is interested in getting tested for sexually transmitted diseases. A wet-mount microscopic examination is performed, and trichomonal parasites are identified. Which of the following statements regarding trichomoniasis is true?

8. (*Continued*)
A. A majority of women are asymptomatic.
B. No treatment is necessary as disease is self-limited.
C. The patient's sexual partner need not be treated.
D. Trichomoniasis can only be spread sexually.
E. Trichomoniasis is 100% sensitive to metronidazole.

9. The most common clinical presentation of infection with *Babesia microti* is

A. acute hepatitis
B. chronic meningitis
C. generalized lymphadenopathy
D. overwhelming hemolysis, high-output congestive heart failure, respiratory failure, and disseminated intravascular coagulation
E. self-limited flulike illness

10. When given as a first-line agent for invasive *Aspergillus* infection, voriconazole commonly causes all of the following side effects *except*

A. drug-drug interactions
B. hepatotoxicity
C. photosensitivity skin rashes
D. renal toxicity
E. visual disturbances

11. A 42-year-old man with AIDS and a CD4+ lymphocyte count of 23 presents with shortness of breath and fatigue in the absence of fevers. On examination, he appears chronically ill with pale conjunctiva. Hematocrit is 16%. Mean corpuscular volume is 84. Red cell distribution width is normal. Bilirubin, lactose dehydrogenase, and haptoglobin are all within normal limits. Reticulocyte count is zero. White blood cell count is 4300, with an absolute neutrophil count of 2500. Platelet count is 105,000. Which of the following tests is most likely to produce a diagnosis?

A. Bone marrow aspirate and biopsy
B. Iron studies
C. Parvovirus B19 IgG
D. Parvovirus B19 polymerase chain reaction (PCR)
E. Parvovirus B19 IgM
F. Peripheral blood smear

12. While attending the University of Georgia, a group of friends go on a 5-day canoeing and camping trip in rural southern Georgia. A few weeks later, one of the campers develops a serpiginous, raised, pruritic, erythematous eruption on the buttocks. *Strongyloides* larvae are found in his stool. Three of his companions, who are asymptomatic, are also found to have strongyloides larvae in their stool. Which of the following is indicated in the asymptomatic carriers?

12. (*Continued*)
    A. Fluconazole
    B. Ivermectin
    C. Mebendazole
    D. Mefloquine
    E. Treatment only for symptomatic illness

13. A 79-year-old man has had a diabetic foot ulcer overlying his third metatarsal head for 3 months but has not been compliant with his physician's request to offload the affected foot. He presents with dull, throbbing foot pain and subjective fevers. Examination reveals a putrid-smelling wound notable also for a pus-filled 2.5-cm wide ulcer. A metal probe is used to probe the wound and it detects bone as well as a 3-cm deep cavity. Gram stain of the pus shows gram-positive cocci in chains, gram-positive rods, gram-negative diplococci, enteric-appearing gram-negative rods, tiny pleomorphic gram-negative rods, and a predominance of neutrophils. Which of the following empirical antibiotic regimens is recommended while blood and drainage cultures are processed?

    A. Ampicillin/sulbactam, 1.5 g IV q6h
    B. Clindamycin, 600 mg PO tid
    C. Linezolid, 600 mg IV bid
    D. Metronidazole, 500 mg PO qid
    E. Vancomycin, 1g IV bid

14. You are a physician working on a cruise ship traveling from Miami to the Yucatán Peninsula. In the course of 24 h, 32 people are seen with acute gastrointestinal illness that is marked by vomiting and watery diarrhea. The most likely causative agent of the illness is

    A. enterohemorrhagic *Escherichia coli*
    B. norovirus
    C. rotavirus
    D. *Shigella*
    E. *Salmonella*

15. The standard starting regimen for acid-fast bacilli smear–positive active pulmonary tuberculosis is

    A. isoniazid
    B. isoniazid, rifampin
    C. isoniazid, moxifloxacin, pyrazinamide, ethambutol
    D. isoniazid, rifampin, pyrazinamide, ethambutol
    E. rifampin, moxifloxacin, pyrazinamide, ethambutol

16. All of the following are common manifestations of cytomegalovirus (CMV) infection following lung transplantation *except*

    A. bronchiolitis obliterans
    B. CMV esophagitis
    C. CMV pneumonia
    D. CMV retinitis
    E. CMV syndrome (fever, malaise, cytopenias, transaminitis, and CMV viremia)

17. Which of the following statements regarding severe acute respiratory syndrome (SARS) is true?

    A. SARS displays poor human-to-human transmission.
    B. SARS is more severe among children than adults.
    C. The etiologic agent of SARS is in the Adenovirus family.
    D. There have been no reported cases of SARS since 2004.
    E. There is no known environmental reservoir for the virus causing SARS.

18. A 72-year-old woman is admitted to the intensive care unit with respiratory failure. She has fever, obtundation, and bilateral parenchymal consolidation on chest imaging. Which of the following is true regarding the diagnosis of *Legionella* pneumonia?

    A. Acute and convalescent antibodies are not helpful due to the presence of multiple serotypes.
    B. *Legionella* can never be seen on a Gram stain.
    C. *Legionella* cultures grow rapidly on the proper media.
    D. *Legionella* urinary antigen maintains utility after antibiotic use.
    E. Polymerase chain reaction (PCR) for *Legionella* DNA is the "gold standard" diagnostic test.

19. A 23-year-old woman is newly diagnosed with genital herpes simplex virus (HSV)-2 infection. What can you tell her that the chance of reactivation disease will be during the first year after infection?

    A. 5%
    B. 25%
    C. 50%
    D. 75%
    E. 90%

20. The most common cause of traveler's diarrhea in Mexico is

    A. *Campylobacter jejuni*
    B. *Entamoeba histolytica*
    C. enterotoxigenic *Escherichia coli*
    D. *Giardia lamblia*
    E. *Vibrio cholerae*

21. A patient comes to clinic and describes progressive muscle weakness over several weeks. He has also experienced nausea, vomiting, and diarrhea. One month ago he had been completely healthy and describes a bear hunting trip in Alaska, where they ate some of the game they killed. Soon after he returned, his gastrointestinal (GI) symptoms began, followed by muscle weakness in his jaw and neck that has now spread to his arms and lower back. Examination confirms decreased muscle strength in the upper extremities and neck. He also has slowed extraocular movements. Laboratory examination

21. (*Continued*)
shows panic values for elevated eosinophils and serum creatine phosphokinase. Which of the following organisms is most likely the cause of his symptoms?

A. *Campylobacter*
B. Cytomegalovirus
C. *Giardia*
D. *Taenia solium*
E. *Trichinella*

22. Abacavir is a nucleoside transcription inhibitor that carries which side effect unique for HIV antiretroviral agents?

A. Fanconi's anemia
B. Granulocytopenia
C. Lactic acidosis
D. Lipoatrophy
E. Severe hypersensitivity reaction

23. A 30-year-old healthy woman presents to the hospital with severe dyspnea, confusion, productive cough, and fevers. She had been ill 1 week prior with a flu-like illness characterized by fever, myalgias, headache, and malaise. Her illness almost entirely improved without medical intervention until 36 h ago, when she developed new rigors followed by progression of the respiratory symptoms. On initial examination, her temperature is 39.6°C, pulse is 130 beats per minute, blood pressure is 95/60 mmHg, respiratory rate is 40, and oxygen saturation is 88% on 100% face mask. On examination she is clammy, confused, and very dyspneic. Lung examination reveals amphoric breath sounds over her left lower lung fields. She is intubated and resuscitated with fluid and antibiotics. Chest CT scan reveals necrosis of her left lower lobe. Blood and sputum cultures grow *Staphylococcus aureus*. This isolate is likely to be resistant to which of the following antibiotics?

A. Doxycycline
B. Linezolid
C. Methicillin
D. Trimethoprim/sulfamethoxazole (TMP/SMX)
E. Vancomycin

24. A 24-year-old woman presents with diffuse arthralgias and morning stiffness in her hands, knees, and wrists. Two weeks earlier she had a self-limited febrile illness notable for a red facial rash and lacy reticular rash on her extremities. On examination, her bilateral wrists, metacarpophalangeal joints, and proximal interphalangeal joints are warm and slightly boggy. What test is most likely to reveal her diagnosis?

A. Antinuclear antibody
B. *Chlamydia trachomatis* ligase chain reaction of the urine
C. Joint aspiration for crystals and culture

24. (*Continued*)
D. Parvovirus B19 IgM
E. Rheumatoid factor

25. *Candida albicans* is isolated from the following patients. Rate the likelihood in order from *greatest to least* that the positive culture represents true infection rather than contaminant or noninfectious colonization?

Patient X: A 63-year-old man admitted to the intensive care unit (ICU) with pneumonia who has recurrent fevers after receiving 5 days of levofloxacin for pneumonia. A urinalysis drawn from a Foley catheter shows positive leukocyte esterase, negative nitrite, 15 white blood cells/hpf, 10 red blood cells/hpf, and 10 epithelial cells/hpf. Urine culture grows *Candida albicans*.

Patient Y: A 38-year-old female on hemodialysis presents with low-grade fevers and malaise. Peripheral blood cultures grow *Candida albicans* in one out of a total of three sets of blood cultures in the aerobic bottle only.

Patient Z: A 68-year-old man presents with a 2-day history of fever, productive cough, and malaise. Chest roentgenogram reveals a left lower lobe infiltrate. A sputum Gram stain shows many PMNs, few epithelial cells, moderate gram-positive cocci in chains, and yeast consistent with *Candida*.

A. Patient X > patient Z > patient Y
B. Patient Y > patient Z > patient X
C. Patient Y > patient X > patient Z
D. Patient X > patient Y > patient Z
E. Patient Z > patient X > patient Y

26. A 38-year-old man with HIV/AIDS presents with 4 weeks of diarrhea, fever, and weight loss. Which of the following tests makes the diagnosis of cytomegalovirus (CMV) colitis?

A. CMV IgG
B. Colonoscopy with biopsy
C. Serum CMV polymerase chain reaction (PCR)
D. Stool CMV antigen
E. Stool CMV culture

27. A 46-year-old veterinary researcher who frequently operates on rats presents to the emergency room with jaundice and scant hemoptysis. She recalls having a fairly deep cut on her hand during an operation about 14 days prior. She has had no recent travel or other animal exposures. Her illness started ~9 days prior with fever, chills, severe headache, intense myalgias, and nausea. She also noted bilateral conjunctival injection. Thinking that she had influenza infection, she stayed home from work and started to feel better 5 days into the illness. However, within a day her symptoms had returned with worsening headache, and

27. (*Continued*)
soon thereafter she developed jaundice. On initial evaluation, her temperature is 38.6°C, pulse is 105 beats per minute, and blood pressure is 156/89 mmHg with O_2 saturations of 92% on room air. She appears acutely ill and is both icteric and profoundly jaundiced. Her liver is enlarged and tender, but there are no palpable masses and she has no splenomegaly. Laboratory results are notable for a BUN of 64, creatinine of 3.6, total bilirubin of 64.8 (direct 59.2), AST = 84, ALT = 103, alkaline phosphatase = 384, white blood cell (WBC) count is 11,000 with 13% bands and 80% polymorphonuclear forms, hematocrit of 33%, and platelets = 142. Urinalysis reveals 20 WBCs/hpf, 3+ protein, and granular casts. Coagulation studies are within normal limits. Lumbar puncture reveals a sterile pleocytosis. CT scan of the chest shows diffuse flame-like infiltrates consistent with pulmonary hemorrhage. What is the likely diagnosis?

A. Acute interstitial pneumonitis
B. Acute myeloid leukemia
C. Polyarteritis nodosum
D. Rat bite fever (*Streptobacillus moniliformis* infection)
E. Weil's syndrome (*Leptospira interrogans* infection)

28. A 17-year-old boy in Arkansas presents to a clinic in August with fever, headache, myalgias, nausea, and anorexia 8 days after returning from a 1-week camping trip. Physical examination is remarkable for a temperature of 38.6°C and a generally fatigued but nontoxic appearing, well-developed young man. He does not have a rash, and orthostatic vital sign measurements are negative. What would be a reasonable course of action?

A. Initiate ceftriaxone, 1g IM × 1
B. Initiate doxycycline, 100 mg PO bid
C. Initiate oseltamivir, 75 mg PO qd
D. Reassure the patient and order a heterophile antibody titer (Monospot)
E. Reassure the patient and order rickettsial serologies

29. A patient presents to the clinic complaining of nausea, vomiting, crampy abdominal pain, and markedly increased flatus. The patient has not experienced any diarrhea or vomiting but notes that he has been belching more than usual and he describes a "sulfur-like" odor when he does so. He returned from a 3-week trip to Peru and Ecuador several days ago and notes that his symptoms began about a week ago. Giardiasis is considered in the differential. Which of the following is true regarding *Giardia*?

A. Boiling water prior to ingestion will not kill *Giardia* cysts.
B. *Giardia* is a disease of developing nations; if this patient had not travelled, there would be no likelihood of giardiasis.

29. (*Continued*)
C. Hematogenous dissemination and eosinophilia are common.
D. Ingestion of as few as 10 cysts can cause human disease.
E. Lack of diarrhea makes the diagnosis of *Giardia* very unlikely.

30. An 18-year-old man presents with a firm, nontender lesion around his anal orifice. The lesion is about 1.5 cm in diameter and has a cartilaginous feel on clinical examination. The patient reports that it has progressed to this stage from a small papule. It is not tender. He reports recent unprotected anal intercourse. Bacterial culture of the lesion is negative. A rapid plasmin reagin (RPR) test is also negative. Therapeutic interventions should include

A. IM ceftriaxone, 1g
B. IM penicillin G benzathine, 2.4 million U
C. oral acyclovir, 200 mg 5 times per day
D. observation
E. surgical resection with biopsy

31. One month after receiving a 14-day course of omeprazole, clarithromycin, and amoxicillin for *Helicobacter pylori*–associated gastric ulcer disease, a 44-year-old woman still has mild dyspepsia and pain after meals. What is the appropriate next step in management?

A. Empirical long-term proton pump inhibitor therapy
B. Endoscopy with biopsy to rule out gastric adenocarcinoma
C. *H. pylori* serology testing
D. Reassurance
E. Second-line therapy for *H. pylori* with omeprazole, bismuth subsalicylate, tetracycline, and metronidazole
F. Urea breath test

32. Which of the following statements regarding the currently licensed human papillomavirus (HPV) vaccine (Gardasil) is true?

A. It does not protect against genital warts.
B. It is an inactivated live virus vaccine.
C. It is targeted toward all oncogenic strains of HPV but is only 70% effective at decreasing infection in an individual.
D. Once sexually active, women will derive little protective benefit from the vaccine.
E. Vaccinees should continue to receive standard Pap smear testing.

33. A 25-year-old woman presents with 1 day of fever to 38.3°C (101°F), sore throat, dysphagia, and a number of grayish-white papulovesicular lesions on the soft palate, uvula, and anterior pillars of the tonsils (Fig. 33). The patient is most likely infected with which of the following?

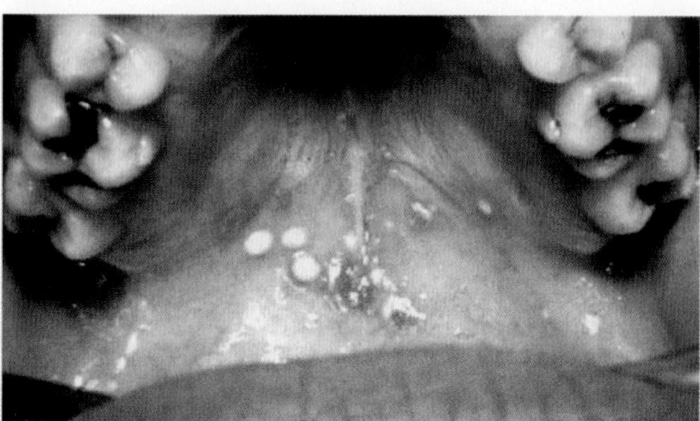

FIGURE 33

33. (*Continued*)
    A. *Candida albicans*
    B. Coxsackievirus
    C. Herpesvirus
    D. HIV
    E. *Staphylococcus lugdunensis*

34. A 19-year-old female from Guatemala presents to your office for a routine screening physical examination. At age 4 she was diagnosed with acute rheumatic fever. She does not recall the specifics of her illness and remembers only that she was required to be on bed rest for 6 months. She has remained on penicillin V orally at a dose of 250 mg bid since that time. She asks if she can safely discontinue this medication. She has had only one other flare of her disease, at age 8, when she stopped taking penicillin at the time of her emigration to the United States. She is currently working as a day care provider. Her physical examination is notable for normal point of maximal impulse (PMI) with a grade III/VI holosystolic murmur that is heard best at the apex of the heart and radiates to the axilla. What do you advise the patient to do?

    A. An echocardiogram should be performed to determine the extent of valvular damage before deciding if penicillin can be discontinued.
    B. Penicillin prophylaxis can be discontinued because she has had no flares in 5 years.
    C. She should change her dosing regimen to IM benzathine penicillin every 8 weeks.
    D. She should continue on penicillin indefinitely as she had a previous recurrence, has presumed rheumatic heart disease, and is working in a field with high occupational exposure to group A streptococcus.
    E. She should replace penicillin prophylaxis with polyvalent pneumococcal vaccine every 5 years.

35. In a patient with bacterial endocarditis, which of the following echocardiographic lesions is most likely to lead to embolization?

35. (*Continued*)
    A. 5-mm mitral valve vegetation
    B. 5-mm tricuspid valve vegetation
    C. 11-mm aortic valve vegetation
    D. 11-mm mitral valve vegetation
    E. 11-mm tricuspid valve vegetation

36. A 19-year-old man presents to the emergency department with 4 days of watery diarrhea, nausea, vomiting, and low-grade fever. He recalls no unusual meals, sick contacts, or travel. He is hydrated with IV fluid, given antiemetics, and discharged home after feeling much better. Three days later two out of three blood cultures are positive for *Clostridium perfringens*. He is called at home and says that he feels fine and is back to work. What should your next instruction to the patient be?

    A. Return for IV penicillin therapy
    B. Return for IV penicillin therapy plus echocardiogram
    C. Return for IV penicillin therapy plus colonoscopy
    D. Return for surveillance blood culture
    E. Reassurance

37. All of the following are clinical manifestations of *Ascaris lumbricoides* infection *except*

    A. asymptomatic carriage
    B. fever, headache, photophobia, nuchal rigidity, and eosinophilia
    C. nonproductive cough and pleurisy with eosinophilia
    D. right upper quadrant pain and fever
    E. small-bowel obstruction

38. An 87-year-old nursing home resident is brought by ambulance to a local emergency room. He is obtunded and ill-appearing. Per nursing home staff, the patient has experienced low-grade temperatures, poor appetite, and lethargy over several days. A lumbar puncture is performed, and the Gram stain returns gram-positive rods and many white blood cells. *Listeria* meningitis is diagnosed and appropriate antibiotics are begun. Which of the following best describes a clinical difference between *Listeria* and other causes of bacterial meningitis?

    A. More frequent nuchal rigidity.
    B. More neutrophils are present on the cerebrospinal fluid (CSF) differential.
    C. Photophobia is more common.
    D. Presentation is often more subacute.
    E. White blood cell (WBC) count is often more elevated in the CSF.

39. All of the following statements regarding human T cell lymphotropic virus-I (HTLV-I) infection are true *except*

39. (*Continued*)
   A. Acute T cell leukemia is associated with HTLV-I infection.
   B. HTLV-I endemic regions include southern Japan, the Caribbean, and South America.
   C. HTLV-I infection is associated with a gradual decline in T cell function and immunosuppression.
   D. HTLV-I is transmitted parenterally, sexually, and from mother to child.
   E. Tropical spastic paraparesis is associated with HTLV-I infection.

40. A 3-year-old boy is brought by his parents to clinic. They state that he has experienced fevers, anorexia, weight loss, and, most recently, has started wheezing at night. He had been completely healthy until these symptoms started 2 months ago. The family had travelled through Europe several months prior and reported no unusual exposures or exotic foods. They have a puppy at home. On examination, the child is ill-appearing and is noted to have hepatosplenomegaly. Laboratory results show a panic value of 82% eosinophils. Total white blood cells are elevated. A complete blood count is repeated to rule out a laboratory error and eosinophils are 78%. Which of the following is the most likely organism or process?

   A. *Cysticercus*
   B. Giardiasis
   C. *Staphylococcus lugdunensis*
   D. Toxocariasis
   E. Trichinellosis

41. An otherwise healthy 5-year-old child presents with low-grade fevers, sore throat, and red, itchy eyes. He attends summer camp, where several other campers were ill. On examination, the patient is noted to have pharyngitis and bilateral conjunctivitis. Which of the following is the most likely etiologic agent?

   A. Adenovirus
   B. Enterovirus
   C. Influenza virus
   D. Metapneumovirus
   E. Rhinovirus

42. A 35-year-old male is seen 6 months after a cadaveric renal allograft. The patient has been on azathioprine and prednisone since that procedure. He has felt poorly for the past week with fever to 38.6°C (101.5°F), anorexia, and a cough productive of thick sputum. Chest x-ray reveals a left lower lobe (5 cm) nodule with central cavitation. Examination of the sputum reveals long, crooked, branching, beaded gram-positive filaments. The most appropriate initial therapy would include the administration of which of the following antibiotics?

42. (*Continued*)
   A. Ceftazidime
   B. Erythromycin
   C. Penicillin
   D. Sulfisoxazole
   E. Tobramycin

43. A 53-year-old male with a history of alcoholism presents with an enlarging mass at the angle of the jaw. The patient describes the mass slowly enlarging over a period of 6 weeks with occasional associated pain. He has also noted intermittent fevers throughout this period. Recently, he has developed yellowish drainage from the inferior portion of the mass. He takes no medications and has no other past history. He drinks six beers daily. On physical examination, the patient has a temperature of 37.9°C (100.2°F). His dentition is poor. There is diffuse soft tissue swelling and induration at the angle of the mandible on the left. It is mildly tender, and no discrete mass is palpable. The area of swelling is ~8 × 8 cm. An aspirate is sent for Gram stain and culture. The culture initially grows *Eikenella corrodens*. After 7 days you receive a call reporting growth of a gram-positive bacillus branching at acute angles on anaerobic media. What organism is causing this man's clinical presentation?

   A. *Actinomyces*
   B. *Eikenella corrodens*
   C. *Mucormycosis*
   D. *Nocardia*
   E. *Peptostreptococcus*

44. A 19-year-old man presents to an urgent care clinic with urethral discharge. He reports three new female sexual partners over the past 2 months. What should his management be?

   A. Nucleic acid amplification test for *Neisseria gonorrhoeae* and *Chlamydia trachomatis* and return to clinic in 2 days
   B. Cefpodoxime, 400 mg PO × 1, and azithromycin, 1g PO × 1 for the patient and his partners
   C. Nucleic acid amplification test for *N. gonorrhoeae* and *C. trachomatis plus* cefpodoxime, 400 mg PO × 1, and azithromycin, 1 g PO × 1, for the patient
   D. Nucleic acid amplification test for *N. gonorrhoeae* and *C. trachomatis plus* cefpodoxime, 400 mg PO × 1, and azithromycin, 1g PO × 1, for the patient and his recent partners
   E. Nucleic acid amplification test for *N. gonorrhoeae* and *C. trachomatis plus* cefpodoxime, 400 mg PO × 1, azithromycin, 1g PO × 1, and flagyl, 2 g PO × 1, for the patient and his partners

45. A 19-year-old college student is brought to the emergency department by friends from his dormitory for confusion and altered mental status. They state that many colleagues have upper respiratory

45. (*Continued*)
tract infections. He does not use alcohol or illicit drugs. His physical examination is notable for confusion, fever, and a rigid neck. Cerebrospinal fluid (CSF) examination reveals a white blood cell count of 1800 cells/μL with 98% neutrophils, glucose of 1.9 mmol/L (35 mg/dL), and protein of 1.0 g/L (100 mg/dL). Which of the following antibiotic regimens is most appropriate as initial therapy?

A. Ampicillin plus vancomycin
B. Ampicillin plus gentamicin
C. Cefazolin plus doxycycline
D. Cefotaxime plus doxycycline
E. Cefotaxime plus vancomycin

46. A 38-year-old woman presents to the emergency department with severe abdominal pain. She has no past medical or surgical history. She recalls no recent history of abdominal discomfort, diarrhea, melena, bright red blood per rectum, nausea, or vomiting prior to this acute episode. She ate ceviche (lime-marinated raw fish) at a Peruvian restaurant 3 h prior to presentation. On examination, she is in terrible distress and has dry heaves. Temperature is 37.6°C; heart rate is 128 beats per minute; blood pressure is 174/92 mmHg. Examination is notable for an extremely tender abdomen with guarding and rebound tenderness. Bowel sounds are present and hyperactive. Rectal examination is normal and guaiac test is negative. Pelvic examination is unremarkable. White blood cell count is 6738/μL; hematocrit is 42%. A complete metabolic panel and lipase and amylase levels are all within normal limits. CT of the abdomen shows no abnormality. What is the next step in her management?

A. CT angiogram of the abdomen
B. Pelvic ultrasonography
C. Proton pump inhibitor therapy and observation
D. Right upper quadrant ultrasonography
E. Upper endoscopy

47. Which of the following clinical features can be used to rule out malaria in favor of another tropical febrile illness in a returning traveler?

A. Diarrhea
B. Lack of paroxysmal nature of the fevers
C. Lack of splenomegaly
D. Severe myalgias and retroorbital headache
E. None of the above

48. Which of the following statements regarding liver abscesses is true?

A. Amebic liver abscess should be ruled out only by direct sampling and culture of pus.
B. Alkaline phosphatase is the most likely liver function test to be abnormal in the presence of a liver abscess.
C. *Candida* species are most commonly isolated from patients with abscesses that develop as a result of peritoneal or pelvic pathology.
D. Patients with liver abscesses nearly always have right upper quadrant pain.
E. All of the above are true.

49. A 40-year-old male is admitted to the hospital with 2–3 weeks of fever, tender lymph nodes, and right upper quadrant abdominal pain. He reports progressive weight loss and malaise over a year. On examination, he is found to be febrile and frail with temporal wasting and oral thrush. Matted, tender anterior cervical lymphadenopathy <1 cm and tender hepatomegaly are noted. He is diagnosed with AIDS (CD4+ lymphocyte count = 12/μL and HIV RNA 650,000 copies/mL). Blood cultures grow *Mycobacterium avium*. He is started on rifabutin and clarithromycin, as well as dapsone for *Pneumocystis* prophylaxis, and discharged home 2 weeks later after his fevers subside. He follows up with an HIV provider 4 weeks later and is started on tenofovir, emtricitabine, and efavirenz. Two weeks later he returns to clinic with fevers, neck pain, and abdominal pain. His temperature is 39.2°C, heart rate is 110 beats per minute, blood pressure is 110/64 mmHg, and oxygen saturations are normal. His cervical nodes are now 2 cm in size and extremely tender, and one has fistulized to his skin and is draining yellow pus that is acid-fast bacillus stain–positive. His hepatomegaly is pronounced and tender. What is the *most likely* explanation for his presentation?

A. Cryptococcal meningitis
B. HIV treatment failure
C. Immune reconstitution syndrome to *Mycobacterium avium*
D. Kaposi's sarcoma
E. *Mycobacterium avium* treatment failure due to drug resistance

50. Which of the following statements regarding prevention of human respiratory syncytial virus (HRSV) infection in children is true?

A. All children who are admitted to the hospital more than twice a year should be vaccinated against HRSV.
B. Barrier precautions remain the only effective means of prevention.
C. Children should be vaccinated at birth.
D. Inactivated, whole-virus vaccine should be considered in children <2 years old.
E. RSV immune globulin should be given monthly to children <2 years old who were born prematurely.

51. A 52-year-old woman with alcoholic cirrhosis, portal hypertension, esophageal varices, and history of hepatic encephalopathy presents to the hospital with confusion over several days. Her husband remarks that

51. (*Continued*)
the patient has been adherent to her medicines. These medicines include labetalol, furosemide, aldactone, and lactulose. Physical examination is notable for temperature of 38.3°C, heart rate of 115 beats per minute, blood pressure of 105/62 mmHg, respiratory rate of 12 breaths per minute, and oxygen saturation of 96% on room air. The patient is extremely drowsy, only intermittently able to answer questions, and disoriented. She has slight asterixis. Lungs are clear. Cardiac examination is unremarkable. Her abdomen is distended and tense but non-tender. She has 3+ lower extremity edema extending to her thighs. She is guaiac negative. Her cranial nerves and extremity strength are symmetric and normal. Laboratory studies reveal a leukocyte count of 4830/μL, hematocrit = 33% (baseline = 30%), and platelet count of 94,000/μL. Basic metabolic panel is unremarkable. What is an essential component of the diagnostic workup?

A. CT scan of the head
B. Esophagogastroduodenoscopy
C. Paracentesis
D. Therapeutic trial of lactulose
E. Serum ammonia level

52. A 34-year-old immigrant from Burundi presents with fever, headache, severe myalgias, photophobia, conjunctival injection, and prostration. He lived in a refugee camp for the previous 10 years. In the camp, he was treated for several unknown febrile illnesses. Since arriving in the United States 7 years ago, he has worked as a computer analyst and lived only in a metropolitan Northwest city with no significant travel. Initial blood cultures are negative. Five days into the illness he develops hypotension, pneumonitis, encephalopathy, and gangrene of his distal digits as well as a petechial, hemorrhagic rash over his entire body except for his face. A biopsy of his rash reveals immunohistochemical changes consistent with a rickettsial infection. Which of the following rickettsial pathogens is most likely in this patient?

A. *Coxiella burnetii* (Q fever)
B. *Rickettsia africae* (African tick-borne fever)
C. *Rickettsia prowazekii* (Louse-borne typhus)
D. *Rickettsia rickettsii* (Rocky Mountain spotted fever)
E. *Rickettsia typhi* (Murine typhus)

53. *Borrelia burgdorferi* serology testing is indicated for which of the following patients, all of whom reside in Lyme-endemic regions?

A. A 19-year-old female camp counselor who presents with her second episode of an inflamed, red and tender left knee and right ankle
B. A 23-year-old male house painter who presents with a primary erythema migrans lesion at the site of a witnessed tick bite
C. A 36-year-old female state park ranger who presents with a malar rash, diffuse arthralgias/arthritis of her shoulders, knees, metacarpophalangeal and proximal interphalangeal joints; pericarditis; and acute glomerulonephritis
D. A 42-year-old woman with chronic fatigue, myalgias, and arthralgias
E. A 46-year-old male gardener who presents with fevers, malaise, migratory arthralgias/myalgias, and three erythema migrans lesions

54. A 39-year-old injection drug user with a history of right-sided endocarditis and HIV infection notes back pain and fevers over the past week. He had an abscess recently on his right arm that he drained on his own. He is part of a needle-exchange program and always cleans his arm before shooting heroin into the vein in his antecubital fossa. On physical examination, he has a temperature of 38.1°C, heart rate of 124 beats per minute, and blood pressure of 75/30 mmHg. He is in a great deal of distress and is slightly confused. He has a 4/6 left lower sternal border murmur that varies with the respiratory cycle. His jugular venous pressure is monophasic and to the jaw when seated at 90°. Lung examination is clear. Abdomen is benign. He is very tender over his lower spine. His extremities are warm. Leg strength is 5/5 on the right, with 4/5 left hip flexion and extension, 3/5 left knee flexion and extension, and 3/5 left foot extension. His Babinski reflex is upgoing on the left and downgoing on the right. What is the next step in management?

A. Avoidance of antibiotics until more definitive culture data is obtained; serial neurologic examinations
B. Urgent MRI and neurosurgical consultation; vancomycin after blood cultures are drawn
C. Urgent MRI and neurosurgical consultation; vancomycin plus cefepime after blood cultures are drawn
D. Urgent MRI and neurosurgical consultation; avoidance of antibiotics until more definitive culture data are obtained
E. Vancomycin plus cefepime after blood cultures are drawn; serial neurologic examinations

55. An HIV-positive patient with a CD4 count of 110/μL who is not taking any medications presents to an urgent care center with complaints of a headache for the past week. He also notes nausea and intermittently blurred vision. Examination is notable for normal vital signs without fever but mild papilledema. Head CT does not show dilated ventricles. The definitive diagnostic test for this patient is

A. cerebrospinal fluid (CSF) culture
B. MRI with gadolinium imaging

55. (*Continued*)
   C. ophthalmologic examination including visual field testing
   D. serum cryptococcal antigen testing
   E. urine culture

56. Current Centers for Disease Control and Prevention (CDC) recommendations are that screening for HIV be performed in which of the following?

   A. All high-risk groups (injection drug users, men who have sex with men, and high-risk heterosexual women)
   B. All U.S. adults
   C. Injection drug users
   D. Men who have sex with men
   E. Women who have sex with more than two men per year

57. A 26-year-old woman presents late in the third trimester of her pregnancy with high fevers, myalgias, backache, and malaise. She is admitted and started on empirical broad-spectrum antibiotics. Blood cultures return positive for *Listeria monocytogenes*. She delivers a 5-lb infant 24 h after admission. Which of the following statements regarding antibiotic treatment for this infection is true?

   A. Clindamycin should be used in patients with penicillin allergy.
   B. Neonates should receive weight-based ampicillin and gentamicin.
   C. Penicillin plus gentamicin is first-line therapy for the mother.
   D. Quinolones should be used for *Listeria* bacteremia in late-stage pregnancy.
   E. Trimethoprim-sulfamethoxazole has no efficacy against *Listeria*.

58. A 23-year-old previously healthy female letter carrier works in a suburb in which the presence of rabid foxes and skunks has been documented. She is bitten by a bat, which then flies away. Initial examination reveals a clean break in the skin in the right upper forearm. She has no history of receiving treatment for rabies and is unsure about vaccination against tetanus. The physician should

   A. clean the wound with a 20% soap solution
   B. clean the wound with a 20% soap solution and administer tetanus toxoid
   C. clean the wound with a 20% soap solution, administer tetanus toxoid, and administer human rabies immune globulin intramuscularly
   D. clean the wound with a 20% soap solution, administer tetanus toxoid, administer human rabies immune globulin IM, and administer human diploid cell vaccine
   E. clean the wound with a 20% soap solution and administer human diploid cell vaccine

59. A 23-year-old woman develops cytomegalovirus (CMV) pneumonitis 5 months after a lung transplant. She developed severe side effects from ganciclovir while receiving prophylaxis. Foscarnet is prescribed for this episode. Which of the following side effects is most likely?

   A. Bone marrow suppression
   B. Electrolyte wasting
   C. Embryotoxic
   D. Lethargy and tremors
   E. Hyperkalemia

60. A 38-year-old woman is seen in clinic for a decrease in cognitive and executive function. Her husband is concerned because she is no longer able to pay bills, keep appointments, or remember important dates. She also seems to derive considerably less pleasure from caring for her children and her hobbies. She is unable to concentrate for long enough to enjoy movies. This is a clear change from her functional status 6 months prior. A workup reveals a positive HIV antibody by enzyme immunoassay and Western blot. Her CD4+ lymphocyte count is 378/μL with a viral load of 78,000/mL. She is afebrile with normal vital signs. Her affect is blunted, and she seems disinterested in the medical interview. Neurologic examination for strength, sensation, cerebellar function, and cranial nerve function is nonfocal. Fundoscopic examination is normal. Mini-Mental Status Examination score is 22/30. A serum rapid plasmin reagin (RPR) test is negative. MRI of the brain shows only cerebral atrophy disproportionate to her age but no focal lesions. What is the next step in her management?

   A. Antiretroviral therapy
   B. Cerebrospinal fluid (CSF) JV virus polymerase chain reaction (PCR)
   C. CSF mycobacterial PCR
   D. CSF VDRL test
   E. Serum cryptococcal antigen
   F. *Toxoplasma* IgG

61. A 72-year-old male is admitted to the hospital with bacteremia and pyelonephritis. He is HIV-negative and has no other significant past medical history. Two weeks into his treatment with antibiotics a fever evaluation reveals a blood culture positive for *Candida albicans*. Examination is unremarkable. White blood cell count is normal. The central venous catheter is removed, and systemic antifungal agents are initiated. What further evaluation is recommended?

   A. Abdominal CT scan to evaluate for abscess
   B. Chest x-ray
   C. Funduscopic examination
   D. Repeat blood cultures
   E. Transthoracic echocardiogram

62. A 40-year-old man with HIV (CD4+ lymphocyte count = 180, viral load = 1000 copies/mL) was treated for secondary syphilis based on generalized painless lymphadenopathy, a diffuse maculopapular rash that included his palms and soles, and a preceding primary genital chancre. He reported no neurologic or ophthalmic symptoms at the time and received one dose of IM penicillin G benzathine. At the time of diagnosis, his rapid plasmin reagin (RPR) titer was 1:64 and fluorescent treponemal antibody-absorption (FTA-ABS) test was positive. He follows up a year later and is found to have an RPR titer of 1:64 and his FTA-ABS remains positive. What is the appropriate intervention at this time?

A. Aqueous penicillin G 24 mU/d IV given as 4 mU q4h × 10 days
B. Doxycycline, 100 mg PO bid
C. Lumbar puncture
D. Penicillin desensitization
E. Penicillin G benzathine 2.4 mU IM weekly × 3 doses

63. A person with liver disease caused by *Schistosoma mansoni* would be most likely to have

A. ascites
B. esophageal varices
C. gynecomastia
D. jaundice
E. spider nevi

64. A previously healthy 28-year-old male describes several episodes of fever, myalgia, and headache that have been followed by abdominal pain and diarrhea. He has experienced up to 10 bowel movements per day. Physical examination is unremarkable. Laboratory findings are notable only for a slightly elevated leukocyte count and an elevated erythrocyte sedimentation rate. Wright's stain of a fecal sample reveals the presence of neutrophils. Colonoscopy reveals inflamed mucosa. Biopsy of an affected area discloses mucosal infiltration with neutrophils, monocytes, and eosinophils; epithelial damage, including loss of mucus; glandular degeneration; and crypt abscesses. The patient notes that several months ago he was at a church barbecue where several people contracted a diarrheal illness. Although this patient could have inflammatory bowel disease, which of the following pathogens is most likely to be responsible for his illness?

A. *Campylobacter*
B. *Escherichia coli*
C. Norwalk agent
D. *Staphylococcus aureus*
E. *Salmonella*

65. Deficits in the complement membrane attack complex (C5-8) are associated with recurrent infections of what variety?

A. *Pseudomonas aeruginosa*
B. Catalase-positive bacteria
C. *Streptococcus pneumoniae*
D. *Salmonella* spp.
E. *Neisseria meningitis*

66. Which of the following pathogens are cardiac transplant patients at unique risk for acquiring from the donor heart early after transplant when compared to other solid organ transplant patients?

A. *Cryptococcus neoformans*
B. Cytomegalovirus
C. *Pneumocystis jiroveci*
D. *Staphylococcus aureus*
E. *Toxoplasma gondii*

67. A 68-year-old woman has been in the medical intensive care unit for 10 days with a chronic obstructive pulmonary disease flare and pneumonia, including the initial 6 days on a mechanical ventilator. She just finished a course of moxifloxacin and glucocorticoid taper when she develops abdominal discomfort over 2 days. Vital signs reveal a temperature of 38.2°C, heart rate of 94 beats per minute, blood pressure of 162/94 mmHg, respiratory rate of 18 per minute, and oxygen saturation of 90%. On examination, she is in moderate distress. She is not using accessory muscles but is tachypneic. She has a slight bilateral wheeze with good air movement. Heart sounds are distant and unchanged. Her abdomen is moderately distended and tense, with scant bowel sounds present. There is no guarding or rebound, but she is tender throughout. Review of her records reveals no bowel movement over the past 72 h and no stool is palpable in the rectal vault. White blood cell count has increased from 7100/μL to 38,000/μL over the past 2 days. Abdominal plain film shows what is read as a probable ileus in the right lower quadrant. Aside from nasogastric (NG) tube placement with suction and NPO status, which of the following should your management also include?

A. Intravenous immunoglobulin (IVIg)
B. Metronidazole, 500 mg IV tid
C. Piperacillin/tazobactam, 3.37 g IV q6h
D. Restart moxifloxacin, 400 PO qd
E. Vancomycin, 500 mg PO qid

68. Regarding the epidemiology of influenza viruses, which of the following is true?

A. Antigenic drift requires a change in both hemagglutinin (H) and neuraminidase (N) antigens.
B. Antigenic shift is defined by an exchange of hemagglutinin (H) and neuraminidase (N) antigens between influenza A and influenza B viruses.

68. (*Continued*)
    C. Avian influenza outbreaks in humans occur when human influenza A viruses undergo antigenic shifts with influenza A from poultry.
    D. Influenza C virus infections, while uncommon, are more virulent on a population basis due to its increased ability to undergo antigenic shift.
    E. The lethality associated with avian influenza is related to its ability to spread via person-to-person contact.

69. A 62-year-old man returns from a vacation to Arizona with fever, pleurisy, and a nonproductive cough. All of the following factors on history and laboratory examination favor a diagnosis of pulmonary coccidioidomycosis rather than community-acquired pneumonia *except*

    A. eosinophilia
    B. erythema nodosum
    C. mediastinal lymphadenopathy on chest roentgenogram
    D. positive *Coccidioides* complement fixation titer
    E. travel limited to Northern Arizona (Grand Canyon area)

70. A sputum culture from a patient with cystic fibrosis showing which of the following organisms has been associated with a rapid decline in pulmonary function and a poor clinical prognosis?

    A. *Burkholderia cepacia*
    B. *Pseudomonas aeruginosa*
    C. *Staphylococcus aureus*
    D. *Staphylococcus epidermidis*
    E. *Stenotrophomonas maltophilia*

71. A 34-year-old injection drug user presents with a 2-day history of slurred speech, blurry vision that is worse with bilateral gaze deviation, dry mouth, and difficulty swallowing both liquids and solids. He states that his arms feel weak as well but denies any sensory deficits. He has had no recent illness but does describe a chronic ulcer on his left lower leg that has felt slightly warm and tender of late. He frequently injects heroin into the edges of the ulcer. On review of systems, he reports mild shortness of breath but denies any gastrointestinal symptoms, urinary retention, or loss of bowel or bladder continence. Physical examination reveals a frustrated, nontoxic appearing man who is alert and oriented but noticeably dysarthric. He is afebrile with stable vital signs. Cranial nerve examination reveals bilateral cranial nerve six deficits and an inability to maintain medial gaze in both eyes. He has mild bilateral ptosis, and both pupils are reactive but sluggish. His strength is 5/5 in all extremities except for his shoulder shrug, which is 4/5. Sensory examination and deep tendon reflexes are within normal limits in all four extremities. His oropharynx is dry. Cardiopulmonary and abdominal examinations are normal. He has a 4 cm × 5 cm well-granulated lower extremity ulcer with redness, warmth, and erythema noted on the upper margin of the ulcer. What is the treatment of choice?

    A. Glucocorticoids
    B. Equine antitoxin to *Clostridium botulinum* neurotoxin
    C. Intravenous heparin
    D. Naltrexone
    E. Plasmapheresis

72. In an HIV-infected patient, *Isospora belli* infection is different from *Cryptosporidium* infection in which of the following ways?

    A. *Isospora* causes a more fulminant diarrheal syndrome leading to rapid dehydration and even death in the absence of rapid rehydration.
    B. *Isospora* infection may cause biliary tract disease, whereas cryptosporidiosis is strictly limited to the lumen of the small and large bowel.
    C. *Isospora* is more likely to infect immunocompetent hosts than *Cryptosporidium*.
    D. *Isospora* is less challenging to treat and generally responds well to trimethoprim/sulfamethoxazole treatment.
    E. *Isospora* occasionally causes large outbreaks among the general population.

73. A 27-year-old man presents to your clinic with 2 weeks of sore throat, malaise, myalgias, night sweats, fevers, and chills. He visited an urgent care center and was told that he likely had the flu. He was told that he had a "negative test for mono." The patient is homosexual, states that he is in a monogamous relationship and has unprotected receptive and insertive anal and oral intercourse with one partner. He had several partners prior to his current partner 4 years ago but none recently. He reports a negative HIV-1 test 2 years ago and recalls being diagnosed with *Chlamydia* infection 4 years ago. He is otherwise healthy with no medical problems. You wish to rule out the diagnosis of acute HIV. Which blood test should you order?

    A. CD4+ lymphocyte count
    B. HIV enzyme immunoassay (EIA)/Western blot combination testing
    C. HIV resistance panel
    D. HIV RNA by polymerase chain reaction (PCR)
    E. HIV RNA by ultrasensitive PCR

74. A 20-year-old female is 36 weeks pregnant and presents for her first evaluation. She is diagnosed with *Chlamydia trachomatis* infection of the cervix. Upon delivery, what complication is her infant most at risk for?

74. (*Continued*)
A. Jaundice
B. Hydrocephalus
C. Hutchinson triad
D. Conjunctivitis
E. Sensorineural deafness

75. A 45-year-old woman with known HIV infection and medical nonadherence to therapy is admitted to the hospital with 2–3 weeks of increasing dyspnea on exertion and malaise. Chest radiograph shows bilateral alveolar infiltrates and induced sputum is positive for *Pneumocystis jiroveci*. Which of the following clinical conditions is an indication for administration of adjunct glucocorticoids?

A. Acute respiratory distress syndrome
B. CD4+ lymphocyte count < 100/μL
C. No clinical improvement 5 days into therapy
D. Pneumothorax
E. Room air Pa_{O_2} <70 mmHg

76. Caspofungin is a first-line agent for which of the following conditions?

A. Candidemia
B. Histoplasmosis
C. Invasive aspergillosis
D. Mucormycosis
E. Paracoccidioidomycosis
F. Tinidazole

77. What is the most common side effect of oral ribavirin when used with pegylated interferon for the treatment of hepatitis C?

A. Drug-associated lupus
B. Hemolytic anemia
C. Hyperthyroidism
D. Leukopenia
E. Rash

78. A previously unvaccinated health care worker incurs a needle stick from a patient with known active hepatitis B infection. What is the appropriate management for the health care worker?

A. Hepatitis B immunoglobulins
B. Hepatitis B vaccine
C. Hepatitis B vaccine plus hepatitis B immunoglobulins
D. Hepatitis B vaccine plus lamivudine
E. Lamivudine plus tenofovir

79. A 55-year-old male is admitted to the hospital with aspiration pneumonia. Over the past 8 months he has had a relentless neurologic decline characterized by dementia with severe memory loss and decline in intellectual function. These symptoms were preceded by 2–3 months of labile mood, weight loss, and headache. Currently he is awake but unable to answer questions. Neurologic examination is notable for normal cranial nerves and sensation. He has marked myoclonus provoked by startle or bright lights, but it also occurs spontaneously during sleep. Prior evaluation revealed normal serum chemistries, negative serologic tests for syphilis, and normal cerebrospinal fluid (CSF) studies. Head CT scan is normal. The infectious agent that caused his neurologic syndrome is most likely a(n)

A. DNA virus
B. fungus
C. protein lacking nucleic acid
D. protozoan
E. RNA virus

80. A previously healthy 19-year-old man presents with several days of headache, cough with scant sputum, and fever of 38.6°C. On examination, pharyngeal erythema is noted and lung fields are clear. Chest radiograph reveals focal bronchopneumonia in the lower lobes. His hematocrit is 24.7%, down from a baseline measure of 46%. The only other laboratory abnormality is an indirect bilirubin of 3.4. A peripheral smear reveals no abnormalities. A cold agglutinin titer is measured at 1:64. What is the most likely infectious agent?

A. *Coxiella burnetii*
B. *Legionella pneumophila*
C. Methicillin-resistant *Staphylococcus aureus*
D. *Mycoplasma pneumoniae*
E. *Streptococcus pneumoniae*

81. A 79-year-old Filipino-American man with diabetes mellitus, coronary artery disease, and emphysema develops the acute onset of low back pain and night sweats. Ten days prior, he underwent a prolonged lithotripsy procedure for septic ureteral stones. He was treated for a positive PPD 23 years ago. He moved to the United States 20 years ago and was a rice farmer in the Philippines prior to moving. Examination reveals tenderness over the lumbar spine. He has 5/5 strength in his lower extremities. MRI shows findings consistent with osteomyelitis of L3 and L4, with narrowing of the disc space and a small contiguous epidural abscess that is not compressing his spinal cord. A needle culture of the epidural abscess drawn prior to administration of antibiotics will most likely reveal which of the following?

A. *Brucella melitensis*
B. *Escherichia coli*
C. *Mycobacterium tuberculosis*
D. *Staphylococcus aureus*
E. Polymicrobial content with gram-positive cocci in chains, enteric gram-negative rods, and anaerobic pleomorphic forms

82. A 64-year-old man in Wisconsin develops a high fever and malaise over 2 days. He has spent his weekends over the past month chopping wood in his backyard. Initial laboratory examination reveals a neutrophil count of 1000/μL, platelet count of 84,000/μL, AST of 140 U/L, and ALT of 183 U/L. A peripheral blood smear reveals prominent morulae in neutrophils. What is the most likely diagnosis?

A. Anaplasmosis
B. Human monocytotropic ehrlichiosis
C. Lyme disease
D. Rocky Mountain spotted fever
E. Systemic lupus erythematosus

83. A 26-year-old asthmatic continues to have coughing fits and dyspnea despite numerous steroid tapers and frequent use of albuterol over the past few months. Persistent infiltrates are seen on chest roentgenogram. A pulmonary consultation suggests an evaluation for allergic bronchopulmonary aspergillosis. What is the diagnostic test of choice?

A. Bronchoalveolar lavage (BAL) with fungal culture
B. Galactomannan enzyme immunoassay (EIA)
C. High-resolution CT
D. Pulmonary function tests
E. Serum IgE level

84. A patient who has undergone prosthetic valve surgery 6 weeks ago is readmitted with signs and symptoms consistent with infective endocarditis. Which of the following is the most likely etiologic organism?

A. *Candida albicans*
B. Coagulase-negative staphylococci
C. *Enterococcus*
D. *Escherichia coli*
E. *Pseudomonas aeruginosa*

85. A 47-year-old woman with known HIV/AIDS (CD4+ lymphocyte = 106/μL and viral load = 35,000/mL) presents with painful growths on the side of her tongue (Fig. 85). What is the most likely diagnosis?

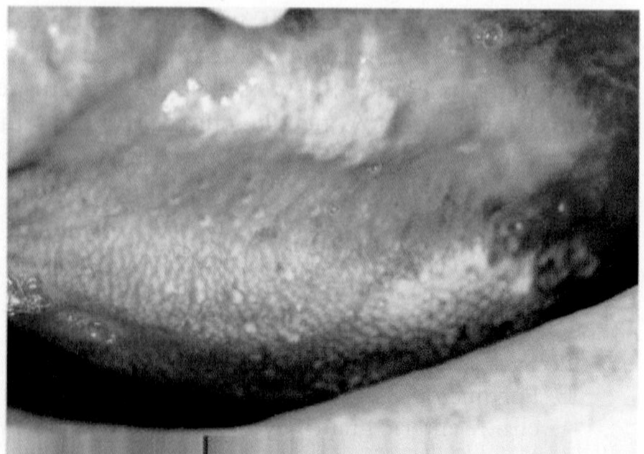

FIGURE 85

85. (*Continued*)
A. Aphthous ulcers
B. Hairy leukoplakia
C. Herpes stomatitis
D. Oral candidiasis
E. Oral Kaposi's sarcoma

86. A 25-year-old male is seen in the emergency department for symptoms of fevers and abdominal swelling, early satiety, and weight loss. His symptoms began abruptly 2 weeks ago. He was previously healthy and is taking no medications. He denies illicit drug use and recently immigrated to the United States from Bangladesh. On physical examination, temperature is 39.0°C (102.2°F) and pulse is 120, with normal blood pressure and respiratory rate. The remainder of the exam is notable for cachexia and a distended abdomen with a massively enlarged spleen. The spleen is tender and soft. The liver is not palpable. Mild peripheral adenopathy is present. Which of the following statements is correct regarding this patient with presumed kala azar leishmaniasis?

A. He probably has normal cell counts on peripheral blood smear.
B. *Leishmania donovani* is not endemic in Bangladesh.
C. *Leishmania*-specific cell-mediated immunity probably is present.
D. Splenic aspiration offers the highest diagnostic yield.
E. Treatment can be delayed until the diagnosis is confirmed.

87. All of the following are examples of an indication for checking an HIV-resistance genotype *except*

A. a 23-year-old man presents to the clinic with a new diagnosis of HIV infection.
B. a 34-year-old man with HIV-1 infection was started on antiretroviral therapy (ART) [tenofovir (TDF), emtricitabine (FTC), efavirenz (EFV)] 1 month ago. At that time his CD4+ lymphocyte count was 213/μL and HIV-1 viral load was 65,000 (4.8 log). On recheck 1 month later, his HIV-1 viral load is 37,000 (4.6 log). He states that he is taking his medicine 100% of the time.
C. a 42-year-old man with HIV/AIDS who was started on ART [TDF, FTC, and ritonavir-boosted atazanavir (ATV/r)] 1 year ago was lost to follow-up. Originally his HIV-1 viral load was 197,000 (5.3 log) and CD4+ lymphocyte count was 11/μL. He was 100% compliant with his pills until he ran out of medicines 2 months ago. Viral load on recheck is 184,000 (log 5.3) with CD4+ lymphocyte count of 138/μL.
D. a 52-year-old woman who has had full viral suppression (HIV-1 viral load <30/mL) and 100% medical compliance on ART [zidovudine (AZT), lamivudine (3TC), EFV] for 2 years has relapsed on IV heroin over the past 3 months. She states that she continued to take her ART with "a few missed doses here and there." Repeat viral load is 3800/mL and CD4+ lymphocyte count is stable at 413/μL.

88. Patients with which of the following have the *lowest* risk of invasive pulmonary *Aspergillus* infection?

A. Allogeneic stem cell transplant with graft-vs-host disease
B. HIV infection
C. Long-standing high-dose glucocorticoids
D. Post-solid organ transplant with multiple episodes of rejection
E. Relapsed/uncontrolled leukemia

89. Rifampin lowers serum levels of all of the following medicines *except*

A. amiodarone
B. anticonvulsants
C. oyclosporine
D. hormonal contraceptives
E. protease inhibitors
F. warfarin

90. Which single clinical feature has the most specificity in differentiating *Pseudomonas aeruginosa* sepsis from other causes of severe sepsis in a hospitalized patient?

A. Ecthyma gangrenosum
B. Hospitalization for severe burn
C. Profound bandemia
D. Recent antibiotic exposure
E. Recent mechanical ventilation for >14 days

91. Which of the following individuals with a known history of prior latent tuberculosis infection (without therapy) has the greatest likelihood of developing reactivation tuberculosis?

A. A 28-year-old woman with anorexia nervosa, a body mass index of 16 kg/m^2, and a serum albumin of 2.3 g/dL
B. A 36-year-old intravenous drug user who does not have HIV but is homeless
C. A 42-year-old man who is HIV-positive with a CD4 count of 350/μL on highly active antiretroviral therapy
D. A 68-year-old man who worked as a stone mason for many years and has silicosis
E. A 73-year-old man who was infected while stationed in Korea in 1958

92. A 42-year-old Nigerian man comes to the emergency room because of fevers, fatigue, weight loss, and cough for 3 weeks. He complains of fevers and a 4.5-kg weight loss. He describes his sputum as yellow in color. It has rarely been blood streaked. He immigrated to the United States 1 year ago and is an undocumented alien. He has never been treated for tuberculosis, has never had a purified protein derivative (PPD) skin test placed, and does not recall receiving BCG vaccination. He denies HIV risk factors. He is married and reports no ill contacts. He smokes a pack of cigarettes daily and

92. (*Continued*)
drinks a pint of vodka on a daily basis. On physical examination, he appears chronically ill with temporal wasting. His body mass index is 21 kg/m^2. Vital signs are: blood pressure 122/68 mmHg, heart rate 89 beats per minute, respiratory rate 22 breaths per minute, Sa_{O_2} 95% on room air, and temperature 37.9°C. There are amphoric breath sounds posteriorly in the right upper lung field with a few scattered crackles in this area. No clubbing is present. The examination is otherwise unremarkable. The portion of the CT scan of his lungs is shown in Fig. 92.

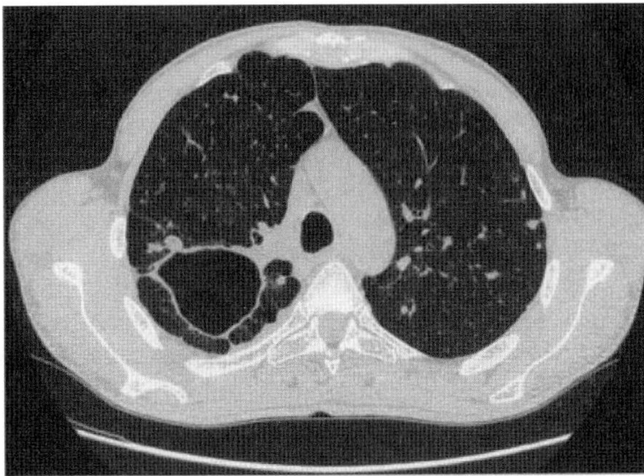

FIGURE 92

A stain for acid-fast bacilli is negative. What is the most appropriate approach to the ongoing care of this patient?

A. Admit the patient on airborne isolation until three expectorated sputums show no evidence of acid-fast bacilli.
B. Admit the patient without isolation as he is unlikely to be infectious with a negative acid-fast smear.
C. Perform a biopsy of the lesion and consult oncology.
D. Place a PPD test on his forearm and have him return for evaluation in 3 days.
E. Start a 6-week course of antibiotic treatment for anaerobic bacterial abscess.

93. A 34-year-old man seeks the advice of his primary care physician because of an asymptomatic rash on his chest. There are coalescing light brown to salmon-colored macules present on the chest. A scraping of the lesions is viewed after a wet preparation with 10% potassium hydroxide solution. There are both hyphal and spore forms present, giving the slide an appearance of "spaghetti and meatballs." In addition, the lesions fluoresce to a yellow-green appearance under a Wood's lamp. Tinea versicolor is diagnosed. Which of the following microorganisms is responsible for this skin infection?

A. *Fusarium solani*
B. *Malassezia furfur*
C. *Sporothrix schenkii*
D. *Trichophyton rubrum*

94. A 68-year-old woman seeks evaluation for an ulcerative lesion on her right hand. She reports the area on the back of her right hand was initially red and not painful. There appeared to be a puncture wound in the center of the area, and she thought she had a simple scratch acquired while gardening. Over the next several days, the lesion became verrucous and ulcerated. Now, the patient has noticed several nodular areas along the arm, one of which ulcerated and began draining a serous fluid today. She is also noted to have an enlarged and tender epitrochlear lymph node on the right arm. A biopsy of the edge of the lesion shows ovoid and cigar-shaped yeasts. Sporotrichosis is diagnosed. What is the most appropriate therapy for this patient?

A. Amphotericin B intravenously
B. Caspofungin intravenously
C. Clotrimazole topically
D. Itraconazole orally
E. Selenium sulfide topically

95. A 44-year-old man presents to the emergency room for evaluation of a severe sore throat. His symptoms began this morning with mild irritation on swallowing and have gotten progressively severe over the course of 12 h. He has been experiencing a fever to as high as 39°C at home and also reports progressive shortness of breath. He denies antecedent rhinorrhea or tooth or jaw pain. He has had no ill contacts. On physical examination, the patient appears flushed and in respiratory distress with use of accessory muscles of respiration. Inspiratory stridor is present. He is sitting leaning forward and is drooling with his neck extended. His vital signs are as follows: temperature 39.5°C, blood pressure 116/60 mmHg, heart rate 118 beats per minute, respiratory rate 24 breaths per minute, Sa_{O_2} 95% on room air. Examination of his oropharynx shows erythema of the posterior oropharynx without exudates or tonsillar enlargement. The uvula is midline. There is no sinus tenderness and no cervical lymphadenopathy. His lung fields are clear to auscultation, and cardiovascular examination reveals a regular tachycardia with a II/VI systolic ejection murmur heard at the upper right sternal border. Abdominal, extremity, and neurologic examinations are normal. Laboratory studies reveal a white blood cell count of 17,000 μL with a differential of 87% neutrophil, 8% band forms, 4% lymphocytes, and 1% monocytes. Hemoglobin is 13.4 g/dL with a hematocrit of 44.2%. An arterial blood gas on room air has a pH of 7.32, a Pa_{CO_2} of 48 mmHg, and Pa_{O_2} of 92 mmHg. A lateral neck film shows an edematous epiglottis. What is the next most appropriate step in evaluation and treatment of this individual?

A. Ampicillin, 500 mg IV q6h
B. Ceftriaxone, 1 g IV q24h

95. (*Continued*)
C. Endotracheal intubation and ampicillin, 500 mg IV q6h
D. Endotracheal intubation, ceftriaxone, 1 g IV q24h, and clindamycin, 600 mg IV q6h
E. Laryngoscopy and close observation

96. A 45-year-old man from western Kentucky presents to the emergency room in September complaining of fevers, headaches, and muscle pains. He recently had been on a camping trip with several friends during which they hunted for their food, including fish, squirrels, and rabbits. He did not recall any tick bites during the trip, but does recall having several mosquito bites. For the past week, he has had an ulceration on his right hand with redness and pain surrounding it. He also has noticed some pain and swelling near his right elbow. None of the friends he camped with have been similarly ill. His vital signs are blood pressure 106/65 mmHg, heart rate 116 beats per minute, respiratory rate 24 breaths per minute, and temperature 38.7°C. His oxygen saturation is 93% on room air. He appears mildly tachypneic and flushed. His conjunctiva are not injected and his mucous membranes are dry. The chest examination reveals crackles in the right mid-lung field and left base. His heart rate is tachycardic but regular. There is a II/VI systolic ejection murmur heard best at the lower left sternal border. His abdominal examination is unremarkable. On the right hand, there is an erythematous ulcer with a punched-out center covered by a black eschar. He has no cervical lymphadenopathy, but there are markedly enlarged and tender lymph nodes in the right axillae and epitrochlear regions. The epitrochlear node has some fluctuance with palpation. A chest x-ray shows fluffy bilateral alveolar infiltrates. Over the first 12 h of his hospitalization, the patient becomes progressively hypotensive and hypoxic, requiring intubation and mechanical ventilation. What is the most appropriate therapy for this patient?

A. Ampicillin, 2 g IV q6h
B. Ceftriaxone, 1 g IV daily
C. Ciprofloxacin, 400 mg IV twice daily
D. Doxycycline, 100 mg IV twice daily
E. Gentamicin, 5 mg/kg twice daily

97. A 24-year-old man seeks evaluation for painless penile ulcerations. He noted the first lesion about 2 weeks ago, and since that time, two adjacent areas have also developed ulceration. He states that there has been blood staining his underwear from slight oozing of the ulcers. He has no past medical history and takes no medication. He returned 5 weeks ago from a vacation in Brazil where he did have unprotected sexual intercourse with a local woman. He denies other high-risk sexual behaviors and has never had sex with prostitutes. He was last tested for

97. (*Continued*)
HIV 2 years ago. He has never had a chlamydial or gonococcal infection. On examination, there are three well-defined red, friable lesions measuring 5 mm or less on the penile shaft. They bleed easily with any manipulation. There is no pain with palpation. There is shotty inguinal lymphadenopathy. On biopsy of one lesion, there is a prominent intracytoplasmic inclusion of bipolar organisms in an enlarged mononuclear cell. Additionally, there is epithelial cell proliferation with an increased number of plasma cells and few neutrophils. A rapid plasma reagin test is negative. Cultures grow no organisms. What is the most likely causative organism?

A. *Calymmatobacterium granulomatis* (donovanosis)
B. *Chlamydia trachomatis* (lymphogranuloma venereum)
C. *Haemophilus ducreyi* (chancroid)
D. *Leishmania amazonensis* (cutaneous leishmaniasis)
E. *Treponema pallidum* (secondary syphilis)

98. A 19-year-old man plans on traveling through Central America by bus. He comes to clinic interested in travel advice and any vaccinations he may need. He has no medical history and takes no medicines. In addition to DEET and mosquito netting, which of the following recommendations would be important for prophylaxis against malaria?

A. Atovaquone
B. Chloroquine
C. Doxycycline
D. Mefloquine
E. Primaquine

99. Which of the following is the most common source of fever in travelers returning from Southeast Asia?

A. Dengue fever
B. Malaria
C. Mononucleosis
D. Salmonella
E. Yellow fever

100. A 54-year-old woman presents to the emergency room complaining of pain and redness of her left face and cheek. The area of redness began abruptly yesterday. At that time, the area was about 5 mm^2 near the nasolabial fold. There was rapid progression of the redness to an area that is now about 5 cm^2. In addition, she is complaining of intense pain in this area. On examination, there is a well-demarcated 5 cm^2 area of erythema along her left nasolabial fold. The borders are raised and indurated. The entire area is very tender to touch. Over the next 24 h, the affected area begins to develop a flaccid bullae. What is the most appropriate treatment for this patient?

100. (*Continued*)
A. Acyclovir
B. Clindamycin
C. Clindamycin and penicillin
D. Penicillin
E. Trimethoprim and sulfamethoxazole

101. In the urgent care clinic, you are evaluating a 47-year-old woman with poorly controlled diabetes who has a chief complaint of "sinusitis." She does not have a history of atopy. She first noticed a headache 2 days ago and now feels very congested in her upper nasal passages. She has hyperesthesia over her nasal bridge as well and is inquiring about antibiotics to treat her infection. She has a bloody nasal discharge with occasional black specks. On examination, the sinuses are full and tender. She has a temperature of 38.3°C. Oral examination shows a black eschar on the roof of her mouth surrounded by discolored hyperemic areas on the palate. What is the most appropriate intervention at this time?

A. Ciprofloxacin and quarantine for possible anthrax
B. ENT consultation if no improvement with oral antibiotics
C. Immediate biopsy of the involved areas and lipid amphotericin
D. Immediate biopsy of the lesion and voriconazole
E. Intranasal decongestants and close follow-up

102. A 63-year-old man from Mississippi comes to your office for evaluation of a chronic sore on his thigh. He has an open sore on his anterior thigh that has been draining purulent material for many months. The thigh is non-tender but is warm to touch. The material is purulent and foul-smelling. He has been given multiple antibiotic courses and recently finished a course of itraconazole without relief of his symptoms. He has an intact neurovascular examination of his lower extremities. His erythrocyte sedimentation rate is 64, white blood cell count is 15,000/μL, and hemoglobin is 8 mg/dL. A plain radiograph of the affected thigh shows a periosteal reaction of the femur with osteopenia. There is suggestion of a sinus tract between the femur and the skin. A Gram stain of the pus shows broad-based budding yeast and you make a presumptive diagnosis of blastomyces osteomyelitis. What is the treatment of choice for this patient?

A. Amphotericin B
B. Caspofungin
C. Itraconazole
D. Moxifloxacin
E. Voriconazole

ANSWERS

1. The answer is B.
(Chap. 14) Cat bites are the most likely animal bites to lead to cellulitis due to deep inoculation and the frequent presence of *Pasteurella multicoda*. In the immunocompetent host, only cat bites warrant empirical antibiotics. Often the first dose is given parenterally. Ampicillin/sulbactam followed by oral amoxicillin/clavulanate is effective empirical therapy for cat bites. However, in the asplenic patient, a dog bite can lead to rapid overwhelming sepsis as a result of *Capnocytophaga canimorsus* bacteremia. These patients should be followed closely and given third-generation cephalosporins early in the course of infection. Empirical therapy should also be considered for dog bites in the elderly, for deep bites, and for bites on the hand.

2. The answer is A.
(Chap. 61) This patient has bacillary angiomatosis due to cutaneous infection with *Bartonella quintana* or *B. henselae*. Kittens are the likely source of the infection in this case. Bacillary angiomatosis occurs in HIV-infected patients with CD4+ T cell counts <100/μL. The cutaneous lesions of bacillary angiomatosis are typically painless cutaneous lesions but may appear as subcutaneous nodules, ulcerated plaques, or verrucous growths. They may be single or multiple. The differential diagnosis includes Kaposi's sarcoma, pyogenic granuloma, and tumors. Biopsy findings are as described in this case, and the diagnosis is best made with histology. Treatment is with azithromycin or doxycycline. Oxacillin or vancomycin is the treatment for staphylococcal or streptococcal skin infections.

3. The answer is C.
(Chap. 28) This patient has a classic presentation and microscopic examination of bacterial vaginosis. Bacterial vaginosis, which is linked with HIV acquisition, herpes simplex virus (HSV) 2 shedding and acquisition, gonorrhea and *Chlamydia* acquisition, increased risk of preterm delivery, and subacute pelvic inflammatory disease, is unfortunately very difficult to treat. With the best available regimens, women recur at a rate of about 25%. Metronidazole, either as an oral formulation or vaginal gel, is recommended for at least 7 days for primary infection and 10–14 days for recurrence. Intravaginal clindamycin for this duration is also an option but has been associated with more anaerobic drug resistance. Treatment of male partners with metronidazole does not prevent recurrence of bacterial vaginosis. Metronidazole, 2 g PO × 1, is standard treatment for *Trichomonas* but is too short a duration for bacterial vaginosis. Fluconazole is used for vaginal candidiasis. Douching has no proven role in bacterial vaginosis infection. Acyclovir is the recommended treatment for HSV-2 genital infection.

4. The answer is F.
(Chap. 28) HIV is the leading cause of death in some developing countries. Efforts to decrease transmission include screening and treatment of sexually associated infections. All of the listed conditions have been linked with higher acquisition of HIV, based on epidemiologic studies and high biologic plausibility. Up to 50% of women of reproductive age in developing countries have bacterial vaginosis. All of the bacterial infections are curable, and treatment can decrease the frequency of genital herpes recurrences. This highlights an additional reason that primary care doctors should screen for each of these infections in female patients with detailed historic questions, genitourinary and rectal examinations, and evidence-based routine screening for these infections based on age and risk category.

5. The answer is B.
(Chap. 94) Enteroviruses are responsible for up to 90% of aseptic meningitis in which an etiologic agent can be identified. Symptoms are typically more severe in adults than children. Illness is more frequent in the summer and fall in temperate climates, whereas other causes of viral meningitis are more common in winter and spring. CSF analysis always shows an elevated (though usually <1000 cells/μL) white blood cell count. Early, there may be a neutrophil predominance; however, this typically shifts toward lymphocyte predominance by 24 h. CSF glucose and protein are usually normal, though the latter can sometimes be elevated. The illness is typically self-limiting and prognosis is excellent.

6. The answer is D.
(Chaps. 113 and 126) This patient has Katayama fever caused by infection with *Schistosoma mansoni*. Approximately 4–8 weeks after exposure the parasite migrates through the portal and pulmonary circulations. This phase of the illness may be asymptomatic but in some cases evokes a hypersensitivity response and a serum sickness–type illness. Eosinophilia is usual. Since there is not a large enteric burden of parasites during this phase of the illness, stool studies may not be positive and serology may be helpful, particularly in patients from nonendemic areas. Praziquantel is the treatment of choice because Katayama fever may progress to include neurologic complications. Chloroquine is used for treatment of malaria; mebendazole for ascariasis, hookworm, trichinosis, and visceral larval migrans; metronidazole for amebiasis, giardiasis, and trichomoniasis; and thiabendazole for strongyloides.

7. The answer is E.
(Chap. 3) Live attenuated viruses are generally contraindicated as vaccines for immunocompromised hosts for fear of vaccine-induced disease. The most cited example of this is smallpox vaccine resulting in disseminated vaccinia infection. However, yellow fever vaccine is another example of a live virus vaccine. The other examples listed in this example are inactivated organisms (rabies, IM typhoid) or polysaccharide (meningococcal) and are therefore noninfectious. Oral typhoid vaccine is a live attenuated strain, so the IM form is likely preferable in this host. Malaria prophylaxis currently involves chemoprophylaxis rather than vaccination. While safe from an infectious standpoint, potential interactions with cyclosporine should be monitored.

8. The answer is D.
(*Chap. 122*) Trichomoniasis is transmitted via sexual contact with an infected partner. Many men are asymptomatic but may have symptoms of urethritis, epididymitis, or prostatitis. Most women will have symptoms of infection that include vaginal itching, dyspareunia, and malodorous discharge. These symptoms do not distinguish *Trichomonas* infection from other forms of vaginitis, such as bacterial vaginosis. Trichomoniasis is not a self-limited infection and should be treated for symptomatic and public health reasons. Wet-mount examination for motile trichomonads has a sensitivity of 50–60% in routine examination. Direct immunofluorescent antibody staining of secretions is more sensitive and can also be performed immediately. Culture is not widely available and takes 3–7 days. Treatment should consist of metronidazole either as a single 2-g dose or 500-mg doses twice daily for 7 days; all sexual partners should be treated. Trichomoniasis resistant to metronidazole has been reported and is managed with increased doses of metronidazole or with tinidazole.

9. The answer is E.
(*Chap. 117*) Babesiosis due to *B. microti* is transmitted to humans by the hard-bodied tick. The infection occurs mostly in coastal southern New England and eastern Long Island; however, cases have been reported in New York, Pennsylvania, Wisconsin, and Minnesota. Most cases of babesiosis are probably never recognized because the most common (25% of adults) presentation is either asymptomatic or indistinguishable from many other self-limited acute febrile illnesses. After an incubation of 1–6 weeks after a tick bite, patients may develop fever (intermittent or sustained as high as 40°C), malaise, shaking chills, myalgias, and arthralgias. Severe infection is most common in asplenic patients and the elderly and in immunosuppressed patients (HIV, malignancy, immunosuppressive medications). Patients co-infected with *Borrelia burgdorferi* (Lyme disease) are also at risk of severe infection. It is notable for an enormous parasitemia that can reach as high as 85% and is associated with hemolysis, high-output congestive heart failure, and renal and respiratory failure.

10. The answer is D.
(*Chap. 102*) Voriconazole is an azole antifungal with a broader spectrum of activity than fluconazole against *Candida* species (including *C. glabrata* and *C. krusei*) and has activity against *Aspergillus* species. It is available in oral and parenteral forms. Voriconazole's visual disturbances are common, transient, and harmless, but patients should be warned to expect them. Voriconazole interacts significantly with many other medications, including immunosuppressive agents, such as tacrolimus, that are often used in patients at risk for systemic fungal infections. Voriconazole may also cause liver toxicity and photosensitivity. Renal toxicity is an issue with amphotericin B products rather than the azoles.

11. The answer is D.
(*Chap. 85*) Immunocompromised patients occasionally cannot clear parvovirus infection due to lack of T-cell function. As parvovirus B19 selectively infects red cell precursors, persistent infection can lead to a prolonged red cell aplasia and persistent drop in hematocrit, with low or absent reticulocytes. Pure red cell aplasia has been reported in HIV infection, lymphoproliferative diseases, and after transplantation. Iron studies will show adequate iron but decreased utilization. The peripheral smear usually shows no abnormalities other than normocytic anemia and the absence of reticulocytes. Antibody tests are not useful in this setting as immunocompromised patients do not produce adequate antibodies against the virus. Therefore, a PCR is the most useful diagnostic test. Bone marrow biopsy may be suggestive as it will show no red cell precursors, but usually a less invasive PCR test is adequate. Immediate therapy is with red cell transfusion, followed by IV immunoglobulins, which contain adequate titers of antibody against parvovirus B19.

12. The answer is B.
(*Chap. 124*) Strongyloides is the only helminth that can replicate in the human host, allowing autoinfection. Humans acquire strongyloides when larvae in fecally contaminated soil penetrate the skin or mucus membranes. The larvae migrate to the lungs via the bloodstream, break through the alveolar spaces, ascend the respiratory airways, and are swallowed to reach the small intestine where they mature into adult worms. Adult worms may penetrate the mucosa of the small intestine. Strongyloides is endemic in Southeast Asia, Sub-Saharan Africa, Brazil, and the Southern United States. Many patients with strongyloides are asymptomatic or have mild gastrointestinal symptoms or the characteristic cutaneous eruption, larval currens, as described in this case. Small-bowel obstruction may occur with early heavy infection. Eosinophilia is common with all clinical manifestations. In patients with impaired immunity, particularly glucocorticoid therapy, hyperinfection or dissemination may occur. This may lead to colitis, enteritis, meningitis, peritonitis, and acute renal failure. Bacteremia or gram-negative sepsis may develop due to bacterial translocation through disrupted enteric mucosa. Because of the risk of hyperinfection, all patients with strongyloides, even asymptomatic carriers, should be treated with ivermectin, which is more effective than albendazole. Fluconazole is used to treat candidal infections. Mebendazole is used to treat trichuriasis, enterobiasis (pinworm), ascariasis, and hookworm. Mefloquine is used for malaria prophylaxis.

13. The answer is A.
(*Chap. 22*) The Gram stain is polymicrobial and the putrid smell is very specific for anaerobic organisms. The diagnosis of acute osteomyelitis is also very likely based on the positive probe to bone test and wide ulcer. Broad-spectrum antibiotics are indicated. Vancomycin and linezolid cover methicillin-resistant *Staphylococcus aureus* (MRSA) and streptococcal isolates but would miss gram-negative rods and anaerobic bacteria. Metronidazole covers only anaerobes, missing gram-positives that are key in the initiation of diabetic foot infections. Clindamycin covers gram-positives and anaerobes but misses gram-negative rods. Ampicillin-sulbactam is broad

spectrum and covers all three classes of organism. If the patient has a history of MRSA or MRSA risk factors, then the addition of vancomycin or linezolid is a strong consideration.

14. The answer is B.
(Chap. 25) Norovirus, or the so-called Norwalk-like agent, was initially described as a cause of food-borne illness in Norwalk, Ohio, in 1968. Since that time the virus responsible has been identified as a small RNA virus of the Caliciviridae family. The initial detection of the Norwalk agent was poor, relying on electron microscopy or immune electron microscopy. Using these techniques, the Norwalk agent was identified as the causative agent in 19–42% of nonbacterial diarrheal outbreaks. With the development of more sensitive molecular assays (reverse transcriptase PCR, enzyme-linked immunosorbent assay), Norwalk-like viruses are being found as increasingly frequent causes of diarrheal outbreaks. Treatment is supportive as symptoms improve within 10–51 h. Rotavirus is the most common cause of viral diarrhea in infants but is uncommon in adults. Salmonella, shigella, and *E. coli* present with more colonic and systemic manifestations.

15. The answer is D.
(Chap. 69) Drugs used to treat *Mycobacterium tuberculosis* are classified as first-line or second-line. First-line agents, which are proven most effective and are necessary for any short-course treatment regimen, include isoniazid, rifampin, ethambutol, and pyrazinamide. First-line supplemental agents, which are highly effective with acceptable toxicity, include rifabutin, rifapentine, and streptomycin. Second-line agents, which are either less clinically active or have greater toxicity, include para-aminosalicylic acid, ethionamide, cycloserine, amikacin, and capreomycin. The fluoroquinolones, levofloxacin and moxifloxacin, are active against *M. tuberculosis* but are not yet considered first-line therapy. While not approved for treatment of *M. tuberculosis* in the United States, promising trials are underway. Some experts consider moxifloxacin a supplemental first-line therapy. It is necessary to have at least three active agents during the 2-month induction phase of active tuberculosis therapy. Ethambutol is initially used as a fourth agent to account for the possibility of drug resistance to one of the other agents. Consolidation phase includes rifampin and isoniazid, and is 4–7 months in length, depending on anatomic location of infection as well as clearance of sputum cultures at 2 months.

16. The answer is D.
(Chaps. 12 and 83) CMV retinitis, a common CMV infection in HIV patients, occurs very rarely in solid organ transplant patients. CMV does affect the lung in a majority of transplant patients if either donor or recipient is CMV-seropositive pretransplant. CMV disease in transplant recipients typically develops 30–90 days post-transplant. It rarely occurs within 2 weeks of transplantation. CMV very commonly causes a pneumonitis that clinically is difficult to distinguish from acute rejection. Prior CMV infection has been associated with bronchiolitis obliterans syndrome (chronic rejection) in lung transplant recipients. As with HIV, the gastrointestinal tract is commonly involved with CMV infection. Endoscopy with biopsy showing characteristic giant cells, not serum polymerase chain reaction (PCR), is necessary to make this diagnosis. The CMV syndrome is also common in lung transplant patients. Serum CMV PCR should be sent as part of the workup for all nonspecific fevers, worsening lung function, liver function abnormalities, or falling leukocyte counts occurring more than a couple of weeks after transplant.

17. The answer is D.
(Chap. 87) In 2002, an outbreak of a severe systemic illness, named *severe acute respiratory syndrome*, or SARS, began in China. Ultimately 8000 cases were recorded in 28 countries. The etiologic agent proved to be a virus associated with the Coronavirus family, now named *SARS-CoV*. The natural reservoir appears to be the horseshoe bat, though human exposure may have come from domesticated animals such as the palm civet. While some patients acquired the virus from animals or the environment, the majority appear to have contracted the illness from other people. Human-to-human transmission, either by aerosol or fecal-oral routes, is efficient. Environmental transmission (water, sewage) may also have played a role, particularly in the outbreak centered in an apartment complex. In the outbreak, children had a much less severe clinical course compared to adults. In 2003 the outbreak ceased, and no new cases have arisen since 2004. Many unanswered questions linger in the wake of this illness.

18. The answer is D.
(Chap. 49) *Legionella* urine antigen is detectable within 3 days of symptoms and will remain positive for 2 months. It is not affected by antibiotic use. The urinary antigen test is formulated to detect only *L. pneumophilia* (which causes 80% of *Legionella* infections) but cross-reactivity with other *Legionella* species has been reported. The urinary test is sensitive and highly specific. Typically, Gram's staining of specimens from sterile sites such as pleural fluid show numerous white blood cells but no organisms. However, *Legionella* may appear as faint, pleomorphic gram-negative bacilli. *Legionella* may be cultured from sputum even when epithelial cells are present. Cultures, grown on selective media, take 3–5 days to show visible growth. Antibody detection using acute and convalescent serum is an accurate means of diagnosis. A fourfold rise is diagnostic, but this takes up to 12 weeks so is most useful for epidemiologic investigation. *Legionella* PCR has not been shown to be adequately sensitive and specific for clinical use. It is used for environmental sampling.

19. The answer is E.
(Chap. 80) Primary genital herpes due to HSV-2 is characterized by fever, headache, malaise, inguinal lymphadenopathy, and diffuse genital lesions of varying stage.

The cervix and urethra are usually involved in women. While both HSV-2 and HSV-1 can involve the genitals, the recurrence rate of HSV-2 is much higher (90% in the first year) than with HSV-1 (55% in the first year). The rate of reactivation for HSV-2 is very high. Acyclovir (or its cogeners valacyclovir and famciclovir) is effective in shortening the duration of symptoms and lesions in genital herpes. Chronic daily therapy can reduce the frequency of recurrences in those with frequent reactivation. Valacyclovir has been shown to reduce transmission of HSV-2 between sexual partners.

20. The answer is C.
(Chap. 25) Enterotoxigenic *E. coli* is responsible for 50% of traveler's diarrhea in Latin America and 15% in Asia. Enterotoxigenic and enteroaggregative *E. coli* are the most common isolates from persons with classic secretory traveler's diarrhea. Treatment of frequent watery stools due to presumed *E. coli* infection may be with ciprofloxacin, or because of concerns regarding increasing ciprofloxacin resistance, azithromycin. *E. histolytica* and *V. cholerae* account for smaller percentages of traveler's diarrhea in Mexico. *Campylobacter* is more common in Asia and during the winter in subtropical areas. *Giardia* is associated with contaminated water supplies and in campers who drink from freshwater streams.

21. The answer is E.
(Chap. 123) Trichinellosis occurs when infected meat products are eaten, most frequently pork. The organism can also be transmitted through the ingestion of meat from dogs, horses, and bears. Recent outbreaks in the United States and Canada have been related to consumption of wild game, particularly bear meat. During the first week of infection, diarrhea, nausea, and vomiting are prominent features. As the parasites migrate from the GI tract, fever and eosinophilia are often present. Larvae encyst after 2–3 weeks in muscle tissue, leading to myositis and weakness. Myocarditis and maculopapular rash are less common features of this illness. *Giardia* and *Campylobacter* are organisms that are frequently acquired by drinking contaminated water; neither will produce this pattern of disease. While both will cause GI symptoms (and *Campylobacter* will cause fever), neither will cause eosinophilia or myositis. *Taenia solium*, or pork tape-worm, shares a similar pathogenesis to *Trichinella* but does not cause myositis. Cytomegalovirus has varied presentations but none that lead to this presentation.

22. The answer is E.
(Chap. 90) Abacavir use is associated with a potentially severe hypersensitivity reaction in about 5% of patients. There is likely a genetic component, with HLAB*5701 being a significant risk factor for hypersensitivity syndrome. Symptoms, which usually occur within 2 weeks of therapy but can take >6 weeks to emerge, include fever, maculopapular rash, fatigue, malaise, gastrointestinal symptoms, and/or dyspnea. Once a diagnosis is suspected, the drug should be stopped and never given again because rechallenge can be fatal. For this reason, both the diagnosis and patient education once the diagnosis is made must be performed thoroughly and carefully. It is important to note that two available combination pills contain abacavir (epzicom, trizivir), so patients must know to avoid these as well. Fanconi's anemia is a rare disorder associated with tenofovir. Zidovudine causes anemia and sometimes granulocytopenia. Stavudine and other nucleoside reverse transcriptase inhibitors are associated with lipoatrophy of the face and legs.

23. The answer is C.
(Chap. 35) In recent years, the emergence of "community acquired" methicillin-resistant *Staphylococcus aureus* (CA-MRSA) in numerous populations has been well documented. This pathogen most commonly leads to pyogenic infections of the skin but has also been associated with necrotizing fasciitis, infectious pyomyositis, endocarditis, and osteomyelitis. The most feared complication is a necrotizing pneumonia that often follows influenza upper respiratory infection and can affect previously healthy people. This pathogen produces the Panton-Valentine leukocidin protein that forms holes in the membranes of neutrophils as they arrive at the site of infection, and serves as marker for this pathogen. An easy way to identify this strain of MRSA is its sensitivity profile. Unlike MRSA isolates of the past, which were sensitive only to vancomycin, daptomycin, quinupristin/dalfopristin, and linezolid, CA-MRSA are almost uniformly susceptible to TMP/SMX and doxycycline as well. The organism is also usually sensitive to clindamycin. The term *community-acquired* has probably outlived its usefulness as this isolate has become the most common *S. aureus* isolate causing infection in many hospitals around the world.

24. The answer is D.
(Chap. 85) The most likely diagnosis based on her antecedent illness with a facial rash is parvovirus infection. Parvovirus commonly leads to a diffuse symmetric arthritis in the immune phase of illness when IgM antibodies are developed. Occasionally the arthritis persists over months and can mimic rheumatoid arthritis. The acute nature of these complaints makes systemic lupus erythematosus and rheumatoid arthritis less likely. Reactive arthritis due to *Chlamydia* or a list of other bacterial pathogens tends to effect large joints such as the sacroiliac joints and spine. It is also sometimes accompanied by uveitis and urethritis. The large number of joints involved with a symmetric distribution argues against crystal or septic arthropathy.

25. The answer is C.
(Chap. 107) Isolation of yeast from the blood stream can virtually never be considered a contaminant. Presentation may be indolent with malaise only, or fulminant with overwhelming sepsis in the neutropenic host. All indwelling catheters need to be removed to ensure clearance of infection, and evaluation for endocarditis and endophthalmitis should be strongly considered, particularly in patients with persistently positive cultures or

fever. Both of these complications of fungemia often entail surgical intervention for cure. A positive yeast culture in the urine is often difficult to interpret, particularly in patients on antibiotics and in the ICU. Most frequently, a positive culture for yeast represents contamination, even if the urinalysis suggests bladder inflammation. An attractive option is to remove the Foley catheter and recheck a culture. Antifungals are indicated if the patient appears ill, in the context of renal transplant where fungal balls can develop in the graft, and often in neutropenic patients. *Candida* pneumonia is uncommon, even in immunocompromised patients. A positive yeast culture of the sputum is usually representative of commensal oral flora and should not be managed as an infection, particularly as in this case where acute bacterial pneumonia is likely.

26. The answer is B.
(Chap. 90) CMV colitis should be considered in AIDS patients with CD4+ lymphocyte count <50/μL, fevers, and diarrhea. Diarrhea is often bloody but can be watery. Initial evaluation often involves stool studies to rule out other parasitic or bacterial causes of diarrhea in AIDS patients. A standard panel will include some or all of the following depending on epidemiologic and historical data: *Clostridium difficile* stool antigen, stool culture, stool *Mycobacterium avium intracellulare* culture, stool ova and parasite examination and special stains for *Cryptosporidium, Isospora, Cyclospora,* and *Microsporidium*. There is no stool or serum test that is useful for the evaluation of CMV colitis in an HIV-infected patient. A positive CMV IgG is merely a marker of past infection. If this test is negative, then the pretest probability of developing active CMV decreases substantially. Serum CMV PCR has gained utility in solid organ and bone marrow transplant patients for following treatment response for invasive CMV infection. However, in HIV-infected patients, CMV viremia correlates imprecisely with colitis. Further, because CMV is a latent-lytic herpesvirus, a positive serum PCR does not imply disease unless drawn in the right clinical context, for which there is none in HIV infection. Colonic histology is sensitive and specific for the diagnosis of CMV colitis, with large-cell inclusion bodies being diagnostic.

27. The answer is E.
(Chap. 72) The patient has Weil's syndrome due to infection with *Leptospira interrogans* as evidenced by her flu-like prodrome followed by profound hyperbilirubinemia with only minor hepatocellular dysfunction as well as renal failure. Rats are the most important reservoir. The organism is excreted in urine and can survive in water for months. Important sources of exposure include occupational, recreation in contaminated waters, and being homeless in contaminated living areas. Weil's represents the immune phase of the disease in its most severe form. A bleeding diathesis is common, as is pulmonary hemorrhage. The conjunctival suffusion during the initial spirochetemic phase of the disease is an important diagnostic clue. Penicillin G is appropriate therapy for severe leptospirosis, but its comparative efficacy is not yet proven in the literature. Acute myelogenous leukemia would likely cause more characteristic abnormalities in blood counts with this degree of illness. Acute interstitial pneumonitis (Haman-Rich syndrome) affects only the lung and would not be associated with the severe increases in bilirubin. Polyarteritis nodosa rarely involved the lung and would not be expected to cause such a high bilirubin, even in the setting of hepatic ischemia. Rat-bite fever causes intermittent fevers, polyarthritis, and a nonspecific rash.

28. The answer is B.
(Chap. 75) Rocky Mountain spotted fever, caused by *Rickettsia rickettsii*, occurs throughout the United States, Canada, Mexico, Central America, and South America. It is transmitted by the dog tick in the eastern two-thirds of the United States and by the wood tick in the western United States. Humans are typically infected during tick season from May through September. In the preantibiotic era, the case fatality rate approached 25%. Currently the mortality remains ~5%, mostly due to delayed recognition and therapy. The incubation period after a tick bite is approximately 1 week. The initial signs and symptoms of Rocky Mountain spotted fever are entirely nonspecific, and the typical rash is often not seen in early disease. It may be difficult to distinguish from many self-limited viral syndromes. Only 60% of patients recall a tick bite, and only 3% of patients have the classic history of tick bite, fever, and rash. Therefore, assessment for this potentially deadly disease should be based on epidemiologic grounds. His recent high-risk travel period for tick bite in a highly endemic region makes this patient a high pretest probability. Empirical treatment is warranted and will not affect the diagnostic workup. A diagnostic indirect immunofluorescent antibody test will not be positive (≥1:64 titer) until 7–10 days after symptoms. The only diagnostic test that is useful during the acute illness is immunohistochemical staining for *R. rickettsii* of a biopsy from a skin rash. Doxycycline is effective therapy and should be continued until the patient is afebrile and improving.

29. The answer is D.
(Chap. 122) Giardia lamblia is one of the most common parasitic diseases, with worldwide distribution. It occurs in developed and developing countries. Infection follows ingestion of environmental cysts, which excyst in the small intestine releasing flagellated trophozoites. *Giardia* does not disseminate hematogenously; it remains in the small intestine. Cysts are excreted in stool, which accounts for person-to-person spread; however, they do not survive for prolonged periods in feces. Ingestion of contaminated water sources is another major form of infection. *Giardia* cysts can thrive in cold water for months. Filtering or boiling water will remove cysts. As few as 10 cysts can cause human disease, which has a broad spectrum of presentations. Most infected patients are asymptomatic. Symptoms in infected patients are due to small-intestinal dysfunction. Typical early symptoms include diarrhea, abdominal pain, bloating, nausea, vomiting, flatus, and belching. Diarrhea is a very common

complaint, particularly early, but in some patients constipation will occur. Later, diarrhea may resolve, with malabsorption symptoms predominating. The presence of fever, eosinophilia, blood or mucus in stools, or colitis symptoms should suggest an alternative diagnosis. Diagnosis is made by demonstrating parasite antigens, cysts, or trophozoites in the stool.

30. The answer is B.
(Chap. 70) The patient's clinical examination is consistent with primary syphilis and he should receive appropriate therapy. In primary syphilis, 25% of patients will have negative nontreponemal tests for syphilis (RPR or VDRL). A single dose of long-acting benzathine penicillin is the recommended treatment for primary, secondary, and early latent syphilis. Ceftriaxone is the treatment of choice for gonorrhea, but this lesion is not consistent with that diagnosis. Ceftriaxone given daily for 7–10 days is an alternative treatment for primary and secondary syphilis. Acyclovir is the drug of choice for genital herpes. Herpetic lesions are classically multiple and painful. Observation is not an option because the chancre will resolve spontaneously without treatment and the patient will remain infected and infectious.

31. The answer is F.
(Chap. 52) It is impossible to know whether the patient's continued dyspepsia is due to persistent *H. pylori* as a result of treatment failure or to some other cause. A quick noninvasive test to look for the presence of *H. pylori* is a urea breath test. This test can be done as an outpatient and gives a rapid, accurate response. Patients should not have received any proton pump inhibitors or antimicrobials in the meantime. Stool antigen test is another good option if urea breath testing is not available. If the urea breath test is positive >1 month after completion of first-line therapy, second-line therapy with a proton pump inhibitor, bismuth subsalicylate, tetracycline, and metronidazole may be indicated. If the urea breath test is negative, the remaining symptoms are unlikely due to persistent *H. pylori* infection. Serology is useful only for diagnosing infection initially, but it can remain positive and therefore misleading in those who have cleared *H. pylori*. Endoscopy is a consideration to rule out ulcer or upper gastrointestinal malignancy but is generally preferred after two failed attempts to eradicate *H. pylori*. (See Fig. 52-1.)

32. The answer is E.
(Chap. 86) Genital human papilloma virus is thought to be the most common sexually transmitted infection in the United States. A recent study of initially seronegative college-aged women found 60% became infected within 5 years. This underscores the importance of the recent development of effective vaccines and continued cervical cancer screening strategies. Approximately 20–25% of the U.S. population past 11–12 years old is seropositive for HSV-2. The high prevalence of this infection in the general population is due to several factors including lifelong infection, ongoing transmission during latent infection due to asymptomatic shedding of HSV-2 in the genital mucosa, and high rates of transmission within monogamous partnerships. These features are markedly different than those associated with bacterial STIs such as gonorrhea and syphilis, which require high rates of partner change to persist in subpopulations. HIV-1 infections are still concentrated within high-risk populations (men who sleep with men, injection drug users, high-risk heterosexuals, and immigrants from high prevalence regions).

There are two available HPV vaccines. Gardasil (Merck) is currently licensed and contains HPV types 6, 11, 16, and 18; Cervarix (Glaxo-SmithKline) is pending final regulatory approval and contains HPV types 16 and 18. HPV types 6 and 11 cause 90% of anogenital warts. HPV 16 and 18 cause 70% of cervical cancers. Both vaccines consist of virus-like particles without any viral nucleic acid, therefore are not active. Both provide nearly 100% protection against two common oncogenic strains of HPV (16 and 18) but neglect to cover the other strains that cause up to 30% of cervical cancer. Because the vaccines do not protect against all oncogenic HPV serotypes, it is recommended that Pap screening of women for cervical cancer continue according to prior schedules. The vaccine should be given to girls and young women between the ages of 9 and 26 provided that they do not have evidence of infection with both HPV 16 and 18 already.

33. The answer is B.
(Chap. 94) These lesions are diagnostic of herpangina, which is caused by coxsackievirus A. They are typically round and discrete, which helps differentiate them from thrush caused by *Candida* species. Unlike HSV stomatitis, herpangina lesions are not associated with gingivitis. Herpangina usually presents with dysphagia, odynophagia, and fever; these lesions can persist for several weeks. The lesions do not ulcerate.

34. The answer is D.
(Chap. 36) Recurrent episodes of rheumatic fever are most common in the first 5 years after the initial diagnosis. Penicillin prophylaxis is recommended for at least this period. After the first 5 years secondary prophylaxis is determined on an individual basis. Ongoing prophylaxis is currently recommended for patients who have had recurrent disease, have rheumatic heart disease, or work in occupations that have a high risk for reexposure to group A streptococcal infection. Prophylactic regimens are penicillin V, PO 250 mg bid, benzathine penicillin, 1.2 million units IM every 4 weeks, and sulfadiazine, 1 g PO daily. Polyvalent pneumococcal vaccine has no cross-reactivity with group A streptococcus.

35. The answer is D.
(Chap. 19) While any valvular vegetation can embolize, vegetations located on the mitral valve and vegetations >10 mm are at the greatest risk of embolizing. Of the choices given, C, D, and E are large enough to increase the

risk of embolization. However, only choice D demonstrates the risks of both size and location. Hematogenously seeded infection from an embolized vegetation may involve any organ, but particularly affects those organs with the highest blood flow. Embolisms are seen in up to 50% of patients with endocarditis. Tricuspid lesions will lead to pulmonary septic emboli, common in injection drug users. Mitral and aortic lesions can lead to embolic infections in the skin, spleen, kidneys, meninges, and skeletal system. A dreaded neurologic complication is mycotic aneurysm, focal dilations of arteries at points in the arterial wall that have been weakened by infection in the vasa vasorum or septic emboli, leading to hemorrhage.

36. The answer is E.
(Chap. 42) Clostridia are gram-positive spore-forming obligate anaerobes that reside normally in the gastrointestinal (GI) tract. Several clostridial species can cause severe disease. *C. perfringens,* which is the second most common clostridial species to normally colonize the GI tract, is associated with food poisoning, gas gangrene, and myonecrosis. *C. septicum* is seen often in conjunction with GI tumors. *C. sordellii* is associated with septic abortions. All can cause a fulminant overwhelming bacteremia, but this condition is rare. The fact that this patient is well several days after his acute complaints rules out this fulminant course. A more common scenario is transient, self-limited bacteremia due to transient gut translocation during an episode of gastroenteritis. There is no need to treat when this occurs, and no further workup is necessary. *Clostridium* spp. sepsis rarely causes endocarditis because overwhelming disseminated intravascular coagulation and death occur so rapidly. Screening for GI tumor is warranted when *C. septicum* is cultured from the blood or a deep wound infection.

37. The answer is B.
(Chap. 124) Ascaris lumbricoides is the longest nematode (15–40 cm) parasite of humans. It resides in tropical and subtropical regions. In the United States, it is found mostly in the rural Southeast. Transmission is through fecally contaminated soil. Most commonly the worm burden is low and it causes no symptoms. Clinical disease is related to larval migration to the lungs or to adult worms in the gastrointestinal tract. The most common complications occur due to a high gastrointestinal adult worm burden leading to small-bowel obstruction (most often in children with a narrow-caliber small-bowel lumen) or migration leading to obstructive complications such as cholangitis, pancreatitis, or appendicitis. Rarely, adult worms can migrate to the esophagus and be orally expelled. During the lung phase of larval migration (9–12 days after egg ingestion) patients may develop a nonproductive cough, fever, eosinophilia, and pleuritic chest pain. Eosinophilic pneumonia syndrome (Löffler's syndrome) is characterized by symptoms and lung infiltrates. Meningitis is not a known complication of ascariasis but can occur with disseminated strongyloidiasis in an immunocompromised host.

38. The answer is D.
(Chap. 39) Listeria meningitis typically affects the elderly and the chronically ill. It is frequently a more subacute (developing over days) illness than other etiologies of bacterial meningitis. It may be mistaken for aseptic meningitis. Meningeal signs, including nuchal rigidity, are less common, as is photophobia, than in other, more acute causes of bacterial meningitis. Typically WBC counts in the CSF range from 100–5000/μL with a less pronounced neutrophilia. 75% of patients will have a WBC count <1000/μL. Gram's stain is only positive in 30–40% of cases. Case fatality rates are ~20%.

39. The answer is C.
(Chap. 89) HTLV-I is a retrovirus that is a chronic infection like HIV, but it does not cause similar sequelae. It was the first identified human retrovirus. Gradual decline of CD4+ lymphocyte number and function is a feature of HIV but not of HTLV-I. While many people in endemic areas have serologic evidence of infection, most do not develop disease. The two major complications of HTLV-I are tropical spastic paraparesis and acute T cell leukemia. Tropical spastic paraparesis is an upper motor neuron disease of insidious onset leading to weakness, lower extremity stiffness, urinary incontinence, and eventually a thoracic myelopathy, leading to a bedridden state in about a third of patients after 10 years. It is more common in women than men. It can easily be confused with multiple sclerosis; this is why it is important to be able to recall the geographic regions where HTLV-I is endemic when evaluating a myelopathy. Acute T cell leukemia is a difficult-to-treat leukemia that is specific to chronic HTLV-I infection. HTLV-I is thought to be transmitted in a similar fashion to HIV.

40. The answer is D.
(Chap. 123) Visceral larva migrans, caused in this case by the canine roundworm *Toxocara canis*, most commonly affects young children who are exposed to canine stool. *Toxocara* eggs are ingested and begin their life cycle in the small intestine. They migrate to many tissues in the body. Particularly characteristic of this illness are hepatosplenomegaly and profound eosinophilia, at times close to 90% of the total white blood cell count. Staphylococci will not typically cause eosinophilia. Trichinellosis, caused by ingesting meat from carnivorous animals that has been infected with *Trichinella* cysts, does not cause hepatosplenomegaly and is uncommon without eating a suspicious meal. Giardiasis is characterized by profuse diarrhea and abdominal pain without systemic features or eosinophilia. Cysticercosis typically causes myalgias and can spread to the brain, where it is often asymptomatic but can lead to seizures.

41. The answer is A.
(Chap. 87) While most of the choices listed above can cause pharyngitis in children, adenovirus classically presents with bilateral granular conjunctivitis as well as pharyngitis, and is frequently the cause of an outbreak among children who are in close contact with one another. Symptom-based and supportive therapies are

indicated for all infections other than disseminated infections in immunocompromised patients. Rhinovirus infections manifest clinically as a common cold with sore throat and rhinorrhea. Human metapneumovirus (HMPV) is a recently described respiratory pathogen. Infections usually occur in winter, and antibodies are present in most children by age 5. Clinically HMPV appears similar to human respiratory syncytial virus, with upper and lower respiratory symptoms. Serious infections may occur in immunocompromised patients. Parainfluenza predominantly is a mild coldlike illness in older children and adults, presenting with hoarseness often without cough. Enteroviruses most frequently cause an acute undifferentiated febrile illness but may cause rhinitis, pharyngitis, and pneumonia.

42. The answer is D.
(Chaps. 12 and 63) This patient is chronically immunosuppressed from his antirejection prophylactic regimen, which includes both glucocorticoids and azathioprine. However, the finding of a cavitary lesion on chest x-ray considerably narrows the possibilities and increases the likelihood of nocardial infection. The other clinical findings, including production of profuse thick sputum, fever, and constitutional symptoms, are also quite common in patients who have pulmonary nocardiosis. The Gram stain, which demonstrates filamentous branching gram-positive organisms, is characteristic. Most species of *Nocardia* are acid-fast if a weak acid is used for decolorization (e.g., modified Kinyoun method). These organisms can also be visualized by silver staining. They grow slowly in culture, and the laboratory must be alerted to the possibility of their presence on submitted specimens. Once the diagnosis, which may require an invasive approach, is made, sulfonamides are the drugs of choice. Sulfadiazine or sulfisoxazole from 6–8 g/d in four divided doses generally is administered, but doses up to 12 g/d have been given. The combination of sulfamethoxazole and trimethoprim has also been used, as have the oral alternatives minocycline and ampicillin and IV amikacin. There is little experience with the newer β-lactam antibiotics, including the third-generation cephalosporins and imipenem. Erythromycin alone is not effective, although it has been given successfully along with ampicillin. In addition to appropriate antibiotic therapy, the possibility of disseminated nocardiosis must be considered; sites include brain, skin, kidneys, bone, and muscle.

43. The answer is A.
(Chap. 64) The most common site of actinomycosis infection is the craniofacial area. Often the infection is associated with poor dentition, facial trauma, or tooth extraction. Clinically this presents as a chronic cellulitis of the face, often with drainage through sinus tracts. The infection may spread without regard for tissue planes, and adjacent bony structures may be involved. Diagnosis requires a high degree of suspicion. The drainage is frequently contaminated with other organisms, especially gram-negative rods. The characteristic sulfur granules may not be seen unless deep tissue is sampled. On Gram's stain, the characteristic appearance shows an intense gram-positive center and branching rods at the periphery. As opposed to the strictly aerobic *Nocardia* species, *Actinomyces* grows slowly in anaerobic and microaerobic conditions. Therapy requires a long course of antibiotics, even though the organism is very sensitive to penicillin therapy. This is presumed to be due to the difficulty of using antibiotics to penetrate the thick-walled masses and sulfur granules. Current recommendations are for penicillin IV for 2–6 weeks followed by oral therapy for a total of 6–12 months. Surgery should be reserved for patients who are not responsive to medical therapy.

44. The answer is D.
(Chap. 28) Urethritis in men causes dysuria with or without discharge, usually without frequency. The most common causes of urethritis in men include *N. gonorrhoeae, C. trachomatis, Mycoplasma genitalium, Ureaplasma urealyticum, Trichomonas vaginalis,* herpes simplex virus, and possibly adenovirus. Until recently, *C. trachomatis* accounted for 30–40% of cases; however, this number may be falling. Recent studies suggest that *M. genitalium* is a common cause of non-chlamydial cases. Currently, the initial diagnosis of urethritis in men includes specific tests only for *N. gonorrhoeae* and *C. trachomatis*. Tenets of urethral discharge treatment include providing treatment for the most common causes of urethritis with the assumption that the patient may be lost to follow up. Therefore, prompt empirical treatment for gonorrhea and *Chlamydia* infections should be given on the day of presentation to the clinic. Azithromycin will also be effective for *M. genitalium*. If pus can be milked from the urethra, cultures should be sent for definitive diagnosis and to allow for contact tracing by the health department, as both of the above are reportable diseases. Urine nucleic acid amplification tests are an acceptable substitute in the absence of pus. It is also critical to provide empirical treatment for at-risk sexual contacts. If symptoms do not respond to the initial empirical therapy, patients should be reevaluated for compliance with therapy, reexposure, and *T. vaginalis* infection.

45. The answer is E.
(Chaps. 36, 44, and 29) In a previously healthy student, particularly one living in a dormitory, *Staphylococcus pneumoniae* and *Neisseria meningitides* are the pathogens most likely to be causing community-acquired bacterial meningitis. As a result of the increasing prevalence of penicillin- and cephalosporin-resistant streptococci, initial empirical therapy should include a third- or fourth-generation cephalosporin plus vancomycin. Dexamethasone has been shown in children and adults to decrease meningeal inflammation and unfavorable outcomes in acute bacterial meningitis. In a recent study of adults the effect on outcome was most notable in patients with *S. pneumoniae* infection. The first dose (10 mg IV) should be administered 15–20 min before or with the first dose of antibiotics and is unlikely to be of benefit unless it is begun 6 h after the initiation of antibiotics. Dexamethasone may decrease the penetration of vancomycin into the CSF.

46. The answer is E.
(Chap. 124) This patient's most likely diagnosis is anisakiasis. This is a nematode infection where humans are an accidental host. It occurs hours to days after ingesting eggs that previously settled into the muscles of fish. The main risk factor for infection is eating raw fish. Presentation mimics an acute abdomen. History is critical as upper endoscopy is both diagnostic and curative. The implicated nematodes burrow into the mucosa of the stomach causing intense pain and must be manually removed by endoscope or, on rare occasion, surgery. There is no medical agent known to cure anisakiasis.

47. The answer is E.
(Chap. 116) All febrile travelers returning from, or immigrants arriving from, *Plasmodium falciparum*– endemic regions should be assumed to have infection with this most severe form of malaria until proven otherwise. *P. falciparum* is the most common infection in returning travelers, may be fatal if not treated, and none of the listed features have sufficient predictive value to rule out malaria. Splenomegaly is a common feature of malaria but is not present in all cases. *P. vivax* and *P. ovale* infections often have paroxysmal fevers but not enough so as to carry significant predictive value; this feature is rarely present in *P. falciparum*–infected persons. Severe myalgias and retroorbital headache often appropriately prompt interest in a diagnosis of dengue fever, but these symptoms are common in malaria as well. Abdominal pain is a very common feature of malaria, and diarrhea can also occur.

48. The answer is B.
(Chap. 24) Microbiologic data are critical in establishing the source of a liver abscess. Polymicrobial samples of pus or blood cultures with gram-negative rods, enterococcus, and anaerobes suggest an abdominal or pelvic source. Hepatosplenic candidiasis once commonly occurred in leukemia or stem cell transplant patients not receiving antifungal prophylaxis. Fungemia was thought to develop in the portal vasculature with poor clearance of yeast during neutropenia. The rejuvenation of neutrophils correlated with symptoms of hepatic abscess. Hepatosplenic candidiases is now quite rare, given the widespread use of fluconazole prophylaxis in patients with prolonged neutropenia. Certain species such as *Streptococcus milleri* or *Staphylococcus aureus* likely indicate a primary bacteremia and warrant a search for the source of this, depending on the typical ecologic niche of the organism isolated. Amebic abscesses should be considered in the context of host epidemiology: those with a low to medium pretest probability based on travel history, who also have a negative amebic serology, are effectively ruled out for disease, without needing to sample the abscess percutaneously. Fever is the most common presenting sign of liver abscess. Only 50% of patients with liver abscess have right upper quadrant pain, hepatomegaly, or jaundice. Therefore, half of patients may have no signs localizing to the liver. An elevated alkaline phosphatase level is the most sensitive laboratory finding in liver abscess, present in ~70% of cases. Other liver function abnormalities are less common.

49. The answer is C.
(Chap. 90) Immune reconstitution syndrome (IRIS) is commonly seen after the initiation of antiretroviral therapy (ART) in patients with AIDS and a concomitant opportunistic infection (OI). It is a syndrome where either a previously recognized OI worsens after ART despite an initial period of improvement after standard therapy for that particular infection, or when an OI that was not previously recognized is unmasked after ART therapy. The latter scenario occurs presumably as immune cells become reactivated and recognize the presence of a pathogen that disseminated in the absence of adequate T cell response with the patient remaining subclinical prior to ART. Many opportunistic pathogens are known to behave this way but *Cryptococcus*, *Mycobacterium tuberculosis*, and *Mycobacterium avium* complex (MAI/MAC) are the most likely to be associated with IRIS. Risk factors for IRIS are low CD4+ lymphocyte count at ART initiation, initiation of ART within 2 months of treatment initiation for the OI, adequate virologic response to ART, and increase in CD4+ lymphocyte count as a result of ART. IRIS can be diagnostically challenging and is very diverse in terms of clinical presentation and severity. Depending on the organ system and pathogen involved, drug-resistant OI and new OI must be considered, sometimes necessitating invasive biopsies and cultures. In this case, the overlap of organ system with the original presentation, low likelihood of MAI drug resistance, and timing of the syndrome favor IRIS. Therapy is with nonsteroidal anti-inflammatory drugs and sometimes glucocorticoids. OI treatment is continued, and all efforts are made to continue ART as well, except under the most dire of clinical circumstances.

50. The answer is E.
(Chap. 87) Human respiratory syncytial virus (HRSV), previously known as RSV, is an RNA paramyxovirus. HRSV is the major respiratory pathogen in children, the foremost cause of lower respiratory illness in infants, and a cause of a common cold–like syndrome. It is a common and important nosocomial pathogen. RSV Ig, also known as *palivizumab*, has been approved as a monthly injection for children <2 years old who have congenital heart or lung disease or who were born prematurely as a means of preventing RSV infection. It has not been shown to be beneficial in HRSV pneumonia. Barrier precautions should be used, especially in locations where there are high transmission rates; however, with the advent of RSV Ig this is not the only means of prevention. An inactivated, whole-virus RSV vaccine trial found that patients receiving the vaccine appeared more likely to acquire RSV infection. An adequate vaccine has not been developed to date.

51. The answer is C.
(Chap. 24) Primary bacterial peritonitis is a complication of ascites associated with cirrhosis. Clinical presentation can be misleading as only 80% of patients have fever, and abdominal symptoms are only variably present. Therefore, when patients with known cirrhosis

develop worsening encephalopathy, fever, and/or malaise, the diagnosis should strongly be considered and ruled out. In this case, a peritoneal polymorphonuclear leukocyte count of >250/μL would be diagnostic of bacterial peritonitis even if Gram's stain were negative. The paracentesis also might provide microbiologic confirmation. CT of the head would be useful for the diagnosis of cerebral edema associated with severe hepatic encephalopathy or in the presence of focal neurologic findings suggesting an epidural bleed. Cirrhotic patients are at great risk of gastrointestinal (GI) bleeding and it may worsen hepatic encephalopathy by increasing the protein load in the colon. Esophagastroduodenoscopy would be a reasonable course of action, particularly if stools were guaiac positive or there was gross evidence of hematemesis or melena. In this case, there is no evidence of GI bleeding and there is mild hemoconcentration, possibly from peritonitis. Lactulose, and possibly neomycin or rifaximin, is a logical therapeutic trial in this patient if peritonitis is not present. Serum ammonia level may suggest hepatic encephalopathy, if elevated, but does not have sufficient predictive value on its own to rule in or rule out this diagnosis.

52. The answer is C.
(Chap. 75) Only two rickettsial infections, *R. prowazekii* and *C. burnetii*, have a recrudescent or chronic stage. This patient has louse-borne (epidemic) typhus caused by *R. prowazekii*. Louse-borne typhus occurs most commonly in outbreaks in overcrowded, poorly hygienic areas such as refugee camps. There was an outbreak of ~100,000 people living in refugee camps in Burundi in 1997. It is the second most severe form of rickettsial disease and can recur years after acute infection, as in this patient. This is thought to occur as a result of waning immunity. Rocky Mountain spotted fever would be consistent with this patient's presentation but he has no epidemiologic risk factors apparent for this disease. African tick-borne fever is considerably less severe and is often associated with a black eschar at the site of a tick bite. Murine typhus is usually less severe and does not exist in a recrudescent form. Q fever can cause chronic disease but this is almost always in the form of endocarditis.

53. The answer is A.
(Chap. 74) Lyme serology tests should be done only in patients with an intermediate pretest probability of having Lyme disease. The presence of erythema migrans in both patient B and patient E is diagnostic of Lyme disease in the correct epidemiologic context. The diagnosis is entirely clinical. Patient C's clinical course sounds more consistent with systemic lupus erythematosus, and initial laboratory evaluation should focus on this diagnosis. Patients with chronic fatigue, myalgias, and cognitive change are occasionally concerned about Lyme disease as a potential etiology for their symptoms. However, the pretest probability of Lyme is low in these patients, assuming the absence of antecedent erythema migrans, and a positive serology is unlikely to be a true positive test. Lyme arthritis typically occurs months after the initial infection and occurs in ~60% of untreated patients. The typical attack is large joint, oligoarticular, and intermittent, lasting weeks at a time. Oligoarticular arthritis carries a broad differential diagnosis including sarcoidosis, spondyloarthropathy, rheumatoid arthritis, psoriatic arthritis, and Lyme disease. Lyme serology is appropriate in this situation. Patients with Lyme arthritis usually have the highest IgG antibody responses seen in the infection.

54. The answer is C.
(Chap. 22) This patient has at minimum severe sepsis and has a very high pretest probability of an epidural abscess compressing his spinal cord, based on the development of weakness and upper motor neuron signs. Both represent true emergencies. From a sepsis standpoint, the most likely organisms are gram-positive skin flora with methicillin-resistant or sensitive *Staphylococcus aureus* representing a distinct possibility. Vancomycin given intravenously is therefore imperative. However, other gram-negative organisms such as *Pseudomonas* and the HACEK organisms are sometimes causes of bacteremia and endocarditis in injection drug users. Given this patient's unstable hemodynamic state, it would be sensible to empirically cover gram-negative rods as well with cefepime. As the infection is life threatening, it would not be prudent to await operative culture data prior to starting broad-spectrum antibiotics. An epidural abscess needs to be diagnosed and surgically decompressed as rapidly as possible to prevent permanent loss of neurologic function.

55. The answer is A.
(Chap. 106) Cryptococcal meningoencephalitis presents with early manifestations of headache, nausea, gait disturbance, confusion, and visual changes. Fever and nuchal rigidity are often mild or absent. Papilledema is present in ~30% of cases. Asymmetric cranial nerve palsies occur in 25% of cases. Neuroimaging is often normal. If there are focal neurologic findings, an MRI may be used to diagnose cryptococcomas in the basal ganglia or caudate nucleus, although they are more common in immunocompetent patients with *C. neoformans* var. *gattii*. Imaging does not make the diagnosis. The definitive diagnosis remains CSF culture. However, capsular antigen testing in both the serum and the CSF is very sensitive and can provide a presumptive diagnosis. Approximately 90% of patients, including all with a positive CSF smear, and the majority of AIDS patients have detectable cryptococcal antigen. The result is often negative in patients with pulmonary disease. However, because of a very small false-positive rate in antigen testing, CSF culture remains the definitive diagnostic test. In this condition *C. neoformans* often can also be cultured from the urine; however, other testing methods are more rapid and useful.

56. The answer is B.
(Chap. 90) CDC guidelines now state that all adults should receive HIV testing, with the availability of a

patient opt-out mechanism rather than informed consent. The basis for this is that ~25% of the 1 million Americans infected with HIV are unaware of their status, there is good available treatment for HIV that serves to extend the lifespan and decrease HIV transmission, and HIV testing is shown to correlate with a decrease in risk-taking behaviors. Cost-benefit analysis has suggested this approach has advantages to current approaches focusing on screening high-risk populations. Pretest counseling is desirable but not always built into the testing process so physicians should provide some degree of preparation for a positive test. If the diagnosis is made, support systems should be activated that may include trained nurses, social workers, or community support centers.

57. The answer is B.
(Chap. 39) *Listeria* bacteremia in pregnancy is a relatively rare but serious infection both for mother and fetus. Vertical transmission may occur, with 70–90% of fetuses developing infection from the mother. Preterm labor is common. Prepartum treatment of the mother increases the chances of a healthy delivery. Mortality among fetuses approaches 50% and is much lower in neonates receiving appropriate antibiotics. First-line therapy is with ampicillin, with gentamicin often added for synergy. This recommendation is the same for mother and child. In patients with true penicillin allergy, the therapy of choice is trimethoprim-sulfamethoxazole. Quinolones have shown animal model and in vitro efficacy against *Listeria*, but there is not enough clinical evidence to recommend these agents as first-line therapy.

58. The answer is D.
(Chap. 98) The patient has been bitten by a member of a species known to carry rabies in an area in which rabies is endemic. Based on the animal vector and the facts that the skin was broken and that saliva possibly containing the rabies virus was present, postexposure rabies prophylaxis should be administered. If an animal involved in an unprovoked bite can be captured, it should be killed humanely and the head should be sent immediately to an appropriate laboratory for rabies examination by the technique of fluorescent antibody staining for viral antigen. If a healthy dog or cat bites a person in an endemic area, the animal should be captured, confined, and observed for 10 days. If the animal remains healthy for this period, the bite is highly unlikely to have transmitted rabies. Postexposure prophylactic therapy includes vigorous cleaning of the wound with a 20% soap solution to remove any virus particles that may be present. Tetanus toxoid and antibiotics should also be administered. Passive immunization with anti-rabies antiserum in the form of human rabies immune globulin (rather than the corresponding equine antiserum because of the risk of serum sickness) is indicated at a dose of 10 units/kg into the wound and 10 units/kg IM into the gluteal region. Second, one should actively immunize with an antirabies vaccine [either human diploid cell vaccine or rabies vaccine absorbed (RVA)] in four 1-mL doses given IM, preferably in the deltoid or anterior lateral thigh area. The four doses are given over a 28-day period. The administration of either passive or active immunization without the other modality results in a higher failure rate than does the combination therapy.

59. The answer is B.
(Chap. 79) Foscarnet is a potent agent used for drug-resistant CMV, herpes simplex virus (HSV) and varicella-zoster virus (VZV), or for patients who are intolerant of first-line agents. It may cause acute renal failure. It also binds divalent metals, commonly causing hypokalemia, hypocalcemia, hypophosphatemia, and hyperphosphatemia. It is often poorly tolerated as a result of nausea and malaise as well. Ganciclovir commonly causes bone marrow suppression and potential significant neutropenia when used for CMV infections, necessitating a switch to foscarnet. Foscarnet commonly causes renal failure. Acyclovir (used for HSV and VZV) is generally very well tolerated but may cause lethargy and tremors. Aerosolized ribavirin is used to treat respiratory syncytial virus infection in infants. It is a mutagen and teratogen and is embryotoxic.

60. The answer is A.
(Chap. 90) This patient most likely has HIV encephalopathy of moderate severity. Other neurologic conditions associated with HIV may be considered with a broad initial workup, but her reasonably high CD4+ count, lack of focal deficits and lack of mass lesions on high-resolution brain imaging makes toxoplasmosis, central nervous system (CNS) tuberculoma, progressive multifocal leukoencephalopathy (PML), or CNS lymphoma all less unlikely. Immediate highly active antiretroviral therapy is the treatment of choice for HIV encephalopathy, and she warrants this despite her CD4+ lymphocyte count placing her in a gray zone according to current guidelines in regard to starting therapy. A lumbar puncture looking for VDRL is unnecessary as a serum RPR test is a very good screening test for any type of syphilis; JC virus detected in the CSF would suggest PML, but her pretest probability for this is low because it usually affects patients with a low CD4+ T-cell count. Serum cryptococcal antigen has excellent performance characteristics, but there is little reason to suspect cryptococcal meningitis in the absence of headache or elevated intracerebral pressure.

61. The answer is C.
(Chap. 107) *Candidemia* may lead to seeding of other organs. Among nonneutropenic patients up to 10% develop retinal lesions; therefore, it is very important to perform thorough funduscopy. Focal seeding can occur within 2 weeks of the onset of candidemia and may occur even if the patient is afebrile or the infection clears. The lesions may be unilateral or bilateral and are typically small white retinal exudates. However, retinal infection may progress to retinal detachment, vitreous abscess, or extension into the anterior chamber of the eye. Patients may be asymptomatic initially but may also report blurring, ocular pain, or scotoma. Abdominal abscess are possible but usually occur in patients

recovering from profound neutropenia. Fungal endocarditis is also possible but is more common in patients who use IV drugs and may have a murmur on cardiac examination. Fungal pneumonia and pulmonary abscesses are very rare and are not likely in this patient.

62. The answer is C.
(Chap. 70) This patient has failed therapy for syphilis as his RPR titer has not decreased fourfold over the course of a year. The FTA-ABS may remain positive even after effective treatment. There is no indication for penicillin desensitization. A lumbar puncture is indicated when there is not a fourfold decrease in RPR titre 6–12 months after appropriate therapy, particularly in patients with HIV. A lumbar puncture showing pleocytosis, elevated protein, and/or a positive VDRL will confirm the diagnosis and the need for 10–14 days of IV penicillin. If the CSF is negative, re-treatment with three doses of IM penicillin for late latent syphilis is adequate. There is no reason to begin treatment for neurosyphilis until the diagnosis is made. Doxycycline, 100 mg PO bid for 30 days, is an alternative treatment for syphilis of unknown duration or >1 year duration, but not for neurosyphilis.

63. The answer is B.
(Chap. 126) Schistosoma mansoni infection of the liver causes cirrhosis from vascular obstruction resulting from periportal fibrosis but relatively little hepatocellular injury. Hepatosplenomegaly, hypersplenism, and esophageal varices develop quite commonly, and schistosomiasis is usually associated with eosinophilia. Spider nevi, gynecomastia, jaundice, and ascites are observed less commonly than they are in alcoholic and postnecrotic fibrosis.

64. The answer is A.
(Chap. 56) Campylobacters are motile, curved gram-negative rods. The principal diarrheal pathogen is *C. jejuni*. This organism is found in the gastrointestinal tract of many animals used for food production and is usually transmitted to humans in raw or undercooked food products or through direct contact with infected animals. Over half the cases are due to insufficiently cooked contaminated poultry. *Campylobacter* is a common cause of diarrheal disease in the United States. The illness usually occurs within 2–4 days after exposure to the organism in food or water. Biopsy of an affected patient's jejunum, ileum, or colon reveals findings indistinguishable from those of Crohn's disease and ulcerative colitis. Although the diarrheal illness is usually self-limited, it may be associated with constitutional symptoms, lasts more than 1 week, and recurs in 5–10% of untreated patients. Complications include pancreatitis, cystitis, arthritis, meningitis, and Guillain-Barré syndrome. The symptoms of *Campylobacter* enteritis are similar to those resulting from infection with *Salmonella, Shigella*, and *Yersinia*; all these agents cause fever and the presence of fecal leukocytes. The diagnosis is made by isolating *Campylobacter* from the stool, which requires selective media. *E. coli* (enterotoxigenic) generally is not associated with the finding of fecal leukocytes; nor is the Norwalk agent. *Campylobacter* is a far more common cause of a recurrent relapsing diarrheal illness that could be pathologically confused with inflammatory bowel disease than are *Yersinia, Salmonella, Shigella*, and enteropathogenic *E. coli*.

65. The answer is E.
(Chap. 1) Deficiencies in the complement system predispose patients to a variety of infections. Most of these deficits are congenital. Patients with sickle cell disease have acquired functional defects in the alternative complement pathway. They are at risk of infection from *S. pneumoniae* and *Salmonella* spp. Patients with liver disease, nephrotic syndrome, and systemic lupus erythematosus may have defects in C3. They are at particular risk for infections with *Staphylococcus aureus, S. pneumoniae, Pseudomonas* spp, and *Proteus* spp. Patients with congenital or acquired (usually systemic lupus erythematosus) deficiencies in the terminal complement cascade (C5-8) are at particular risk of infection from *Neisseria* spp such as *N. meningitis* or *N. gonorrhoeae*.

66. The answer is E.
(Chaps. 12 and 121) T. gondii commonly achieves latency in cysts during acute infection. Reactivation in the central nervous system in AIDS patients is well known. However, *Toxoplasma* cysts also reside in the heart. Thus, transplanting a *Toxoplasma*-positive heart into a negative recipient may cause reactivation in the months after transplant. Serologic screening of cardiac donors and recipients for *T. gondii* is important. To account for this possibility, prophylactic doses of trimethoprim-sulfamethoxazole, which is also effective prophylaxis against *Pneumocystis* and *Nocardia*, is standard after cardiac transplantation. Cardiac transplant recipients, similar to all other solid organ transplant recipients, are at risk of developing infections related to impaired cellular immunity, particularly >1 month to 1 year posttransplant. Wound infections or mediastinitis from skin organisms may complicate the early transplant (<1 month) period.

67. The answer is B.
(Chap. 43) Severe *C. difficile*–associated disease may mimic a surgical abdomen and patients may not have diarrhea. The lack of diarrhea should not overshadow the other signs and risk factors that are suggestive of *C. difficile*–associated disease, including significant leukocytosis, long hospitalization, prior antibiotics, and probable enteral tube feeds while on the ventilator. Adynamic ileus is a serious and well-known complication of *C. difficile*–associated disease. All potentially serious manifestations that could be *C. difficile*–associated disease should be empirically treated as such until stool antigen tests are negative and an alternative clinical explanation is found. Intravenous metronidazole may be less optimal than oral vancomycin for severe cases, and this patient may fail therapy. However, oral medicines are less likely to reach the target organ in the presence of an adynamic ileus, necessitating IV metronidazole. Some advocate combining administration of oral vancomycin by

NG tube with IV metronidazole. All potentially offending antibiotics should be stopped (if possible, as is the case here with the patient having recovered from her pneumonia) rather than continued. Surgical colectomy may be necessary in fulminant cases when there is no response to medical therapy. Intravenous immunoglobulins, which may provide antibodies to *C. difficile* toxin, are reserved for severe or multiple recurrent cases of *C. difficile*–associated disease.

68. The answer is C.
(Chap. 88) Avian influenza epidemics occur when human influenza A undergoes an antigenic exchange with influenza found in poultry. Recent outbreaks have not been associated with effective human-to-human spread; nearly all patients reported exposure to infected poultry. Past influenza pandemics, including the 1918–1919 pandemic, appear to have originated from antigenic exchange between human and avian influenza viruses. Antigenic shifts are defined as major changes in the hemagglutinin (H) and neuraminidase (N) antigens and occur only with influenza A. Minor antigenic changes are known as antigenic drift and can occur with hemagglutinin alone or with both hemagglutinin (H) and neuraminidase (N). While influenza A and B are genetically and morphologically similar, the latter virus' inability to undergo antigenic shifts lessens its virulence and involvement in pandemic flu. Influenza C is a rare cause of disease in humans and is typically a clinically mild, self-limited infection.

69. The answer is E.
(Chap. 104) There is no *Coccidioides* in Northern Arizona (i.e., the Grand Canyon region). The organism can be cultured from dry top soil in the high desert of Southern Arizona surrounding Phoenix and Tucson. Eosinophilia is a common laboratory finding in acute coccidioidomycosis and erythema nodosum is a common cutaneous clinical feature. Mediastinal lymphadenopathy is more commonly seen on radiographs for all acute pneumonias due to endemic mycoses, including *Coccidioides*, rather than due to bacterial pneumonia. A positive complement fixation test is one method to definitively diagnose acute infection.

70. The answer is A.
(Chaps. 53) *B. cepacia* is an opportunistic pathogen that has been responsible for nosocomial outbreaks. It also colonizes and infects the lower respiratory tract of patients with cystic fibrosis, chronic granulomatous disease, and sickle cell disease. In patients with cystic fibrosis it portends a rapid decline in pulmonary function and a poor clinical prognosis. It also may cause a resistant necrotizing pneumonia. *B. cepacia* is often intrinsically resistant to a variety of antimicrobials, including many β-lactams and aminoglycosides. Trimethoprim-sulfamethoxazole (TMP/SMX) is usually the first-line treatment. *P. aeruginosa* and *S. aureus* are common colonizers and pathogens in patients with cystic fibrosis. *Stenotrophomonas maltophilia* is the pathogen, particularly in patients with cancer, transplants, and critical illness. *S. maltophilia* is a cause of pneumonia, urinary tract infection, wound infection, and bacteremia. TMP/SMX is usually the treatment of choice for *Stenotrophomonas.*

71. The answer is B.
(Chap. 41). This patient most likely has wound botulism. The use of "black-tar" heroin has been identified as a risk factor for this form of botulism. Typically the wound appears benign, and unlike in other forms of botulism, gastrointestinal symptoms are absent. Symmetric *descending* paralysis suggests botulism, as does cranial nerve involvement. This patient's ptosis, diplopia, dysarthria, dysphagia, lack of fevers, normal reflexes, and lack of sensory deficits are all suggestive. Botulism can be easily confused with Guillain-Barré syndrome (GBS), which is often characterized by an antecedent infection and rapid, symmetric *ascending* paralysis and treated with plasmapheresis. The Miller Fischer variant of GBS is known for cranial nerve involvement with ophthalmoplegia, ataxia, and areflexia being the most prominent features. Elevated protein in the cerebrospinal fluid also favors GBS over botulism. Both botulism and GBS can progress to respiratory failure, so making a diagnosis by physical examination is critical. Other diagnostic modalities that may be helpful are wound culture, serum assay for toxin, and examination for decreased compound muscle action potentials on routine nerve stimulation studies. Patients with botulism are at risk of respiratory failure due to respiratory muscle weakness or aspiration. They should be followed closely with oxygen saturation monitoring and serial measurement of forced vital capacity.

72. The answer is D.
(Chap. 90) *Isospora* and *Cryptosporidium* cause very similar clinical disease in AIDS patients that ranges from intermittent, self-resolved watery diarrhea with abdominal cramping and sometimes nausea, to a potentially fatal cholera-like presentation in the most immunocompromised hosts. *Cryptosporidium* may cause biliary disease and can lead to cholangitis. *Isospora* is limited to the gut lumen. *Cryptosporidium* is not always an opportunistic infection and has led to widespread community outbreaks. *Isospora* is not seen in immunocompetent hosts. Finally, treatment for *Isospora* is usually successful. In fact, this infection is rarely seen in the developed world because trimethoprim/sulfamethoxazole, which is commonly used for *Pneumocystis* prophylaxis, tends to eradicate *Isospora*. Cryptosporidiosis, on the other hand, is very difficult to cure and interventions are controversial. Some clinicians favor nitazoxanone, but cure rates are mediocre and immune reconstitution with antiretroviral therapy is ultimately critical to cure the gastrointestinal disease.

73. The answer is D.
(Chap. 90) Acute HIV should be suspected in any at-risk person who presents with a mono-like illness; it is diagnosed by positive plasma RNA PCR. Patients typically have not developed sufficient antibodies to the virus yet to develop a positive EIA, and the diagnosis

of HIV is usually missed if this test is sent within the first 2 months of HIV acquisition. It is tempting for clinicians to send an ultrasensitive PCR, but this only decreases specificity (false-positive tests with detection of very low levels of HIV are possible due to cross contamination in the laboratory) with no other benefit. There is typically a massive amount of HIV virus in the plasma during acute infection, and the ultrasensitive assay is never required for detection at this stage of disease. Ultra-sensitive assays are helpful in the context of therapy to ensure that there is not persistence of low-level viremia. CD4+ lymphocyte count decreases during many acute infections, including HIV, and is therefore not diagnostically appropriate. CD4+ lymphocyte counts are useful to risk stratify for opportunistic infection in stable patients with known HIV infection. Resistance tests are sent only when the diagnosis is confirmed.

74. The answer is D.
(Chap. 77) Congenital infection from maternal transmission can lead to severe consequences for the neonate; thus, prenatal care and screening for infection are very important. *C. trachomatis* is associated with up to 25% of exposed neonates who develop inclusion conjunctivitis. It can also be associated with pneumonia and otitis media in the newborn. Pneumonia in the newborn has been associated with later development of bronchitis and asthma. Hydrocephalus can be associated with toxoplasmosis. Hutchinson triad, which is Hutchinson teeth (blunted upper incisors), interstitial keratitis, and eighth nerve deafness, is due to congenital syphilis. Sensorineural deafness can be associated with congenital rubella exposure. Treatment of *C. trachomatis* in the infant consists of oral erythromycin.

75. The answer is E.
(Chap. 90) P. jiroveci lung infection is known to worsen after initiation of treatment, likely due to lysis of organism and immune response to its intracellular contents. It is thought that adjunct administration of glucocorticoids may reduce inflammation and subsequent lung injury in patients with moderate to severe pneumonia due to *P. jiroveci*. Adjunct administration of glucocorticoids in patients with moderate to severe disease as determined by a room air Pa_{O_2} <70 mmHg or an A – a gradient >35 mmHg decrease mortality. Glucocorticoids should be given for a total duration of 3 weeks. Patients often do not improve until many days into therapy and often initially worsen; steroids should be used as soon as hypoxemia develops rather than wait for lack of improvement. Pneumothoraces and adult respiratory distress syndrome (ARDS) are common feared complications of *Pneumocystis* infection. If patients present with ARDS due to *Pneumocystis* pneumonia, they would meet the criterion for adjunct glucocorticoids due to the severe nature of disease.

76. The answer is A.
(Chap. 102) Caspofungin and the other echinocandins (anidulafungin, micafungin) inhibit fungal synthesis of B-1,3-glucan synthase, a necessary enzyme for fungal cell wall synthesis that does not have a human correlate. These agents are available only parentally, not orally. They are fungicidal for *Candida* species and fungistatic against *Aspergillus* species. Caspofungin is as at least equivalently effective as amphotericin B for disseminated candidiasis and is as effective as fluconazole for candidal esophagitis. It is not a first-line therapy for *Aspergillus* infection but may be used as salvage therapy. The echinocandins, including caspofungin, have an extremely high safety profile. They do not have activity against mucormycosis, paracoccidiomycosis, or histoplasmosis.

77. The answer is B.
(Chap. 79) Oral ribavirin combined with pegylated interferon appears to be the most effective regimen for treating hepatitis C. Ribavirin does not exert antiviral effect but may be an immune modulator in combination with the interferon. Hemolytic anemia occurs in nearly 25% of patients receiving this therapy. Common approaches to this problem are dose reduction, cessation of ribavirin therapy, or use of red cell growth factors. Rash can occur but is less common. Interferon has common side effects as well, including flulike symptoms, depression, sleep disturbances, personality change, leukopenia, and thrombocytopenia.

78. The answer is C.
(Chap. 3) Hepatitis B is efficiently spread as a blood-borne pathogen. In approximately one-third of needle stick cases where the victim is not immunized (either by vaccine or prior clearance of infection), hepatitis B transmission will occur. This is in comparison to 3% for hepatitis C and 0.3% for HIV-1 infections. Moreover, hepatitis B, because it is a DNA virus, can survive for prolonged amount of times on unsterilized surfaces. This speaks to the goal of 100% vaccination against hepatitis B for all health care workers. Rapid administration of both hepatitis B vaccine and immunoglobulins are the most effective way to prevent transmission if a high-risk stick occurs to a nonimmune health care worker. No data exist to support the use of antiviral therapy for hepatitis B needle sticks, though this strategy has proven effective for HIV-1 associated needle sticks.

79. The answer is C.
(Chap. 101) Prions are infectious proteins that lack nucleic acids and cause neurodegenerative diseases. The most common prion disease in humans is sporadic Creutzfeldt-Jakob disease (s-CJD). Others include familial CJD, fatal familial insomnia, kuru, and iatrogenic CJD. Prions result when an abnormal prion protein binds to a normal isoform of the prion protein, stimulating its conversion into the abnormal isoform. Abnormal prion isoforms have a greater proportion of β-structure and less a–helix than do normal isoforms. The α-to-β structural transition underlies the etiology of the central nervous system degeneration. The patient described has a typical presentation of s-CJD with sleep disturbance, fatigue, and defects in higher cortical functions. CJD

progresses quickly to dementia. Over 90% of patients with CJD exhibit myoclonus during the illness. Typically the myoclonus is provoked by startle, loud noises, or bright lights and will occur even during sleep. The diagnosis requires an appropriate clinical presentation and no other etiologies on CSF examination. There is no widely available laboratory test for diagnosis. Brain biopsy may demonstrate spongiform degeneration and the presence of prion proteins.

80. The answer is D.
(Chap. 76) Mycoplasma pneumoniae is a common cause of pneumonia that is often underdiagnosed based on difficult and time-consuming culture techniques, it likely causes mild respiratory symptoms, and because it is adequately treated with standard antibiotic regimens for community-acquired pneumonia. It is spread easily person-to-person, and outbreaks in crowded conditions are common. Most patients develop a cough without radiographic abnormalities. Pharyngitis, rhinitis, and ear pain are also common. *M. pneumoniae* commonly induces the production of cold agglutinins, which in turn can cause an IgM- and complement-mediated intravascular hemolytic anemia. The presence of cold agglutinins is specific for *M. pneumoniae* infection only in the context of a consistent clinical picture for infection, as in this patient. Cold agglutinins are more common in children. Blood smear shows no abnormality, which is in contrast to IgG or warm-type hemolytic anemia where spherocytes are seen. Since there is no easy diagnostic test, empirical therapy is often administered.

81. The answer is B.
(Chap. 22) The most common overall cause of acute bacterial osteomyelitis of the spine is *S. aureus*, accounting for ~50% of cases due to a single organism, introduced via the bloodstream in patients at risk for bloodstream infections (injecting drug users, hemodialysis patients, open postoperative wounds). However, in older male patients with lumbar osteomyelitis, genitourinary or enteric pathogens, such as *E. coli*, are common, particularly after recent urinary tract infections and/or urologic surgeries, accounting for up to 25% of cases of vertebral osteomyelitis. Pathogenesis may occur via retrograde introduction of organism into the spine via the spinal venous plexus. Polymicrobial osteomyelitis is most often due to contiguous infection, such as a decubitus ulcer or diabetic foot infection, rather than bloodstream introductions that are more typical in the spine. Tuberculosis (Pott's disease) is always a consideration for osteomyelitis of the spine. However, this patient's presentation is likely too acute for tuberculosis, and the thoracic spine is a slightly more typical location than the lumbar spine. Brucellosis commonly involves the spine, but this patient's potential exposure to *Brucella* spp. is dated and the course of the infection is too acute for brucellosis. Hypothetically each of the listed infections is possible, highlighting the importance of holding antibiotics before culturing the epidural space, provided that the patient does not have sepsis on original presentation.

82. The answer is A.
(Chap. 75) Anaplasmosis (formerly human granulocytic ehrlichiosis) occurs mostly in the northeastern and upper midwestern United States. It shares the *Ixodes* tick vector with Lyme disease. It is typically a disease of older males (median age 51 years). Because seroprevalence rates are high in endemic areas, subclinical infection is likely common. The disease typically presents with fever (>90% of cases), myalgias, headache, and malaise. Thrombocytopenia, leukopenia, and elevated aminotransaminase activity is common. Adult respiratory distress syndrome, toxic shock–like syndrome, and opportunistic infections may occur, particularly in the elderly. Human granulocytotropic anaplasmosis should be considered on the differential of a flulike illness during May through December in endemic regions. Morulae, intracytoplasmic inclusions, are seen in the neutrophils of up to 80% of cases of human granulocytotropic anaplasmosis on peripheral blood smear and are diagnostic in the appropriate clinical context. This patient has high epidemiologic risk based on his long periods of time outside in an endemic region. Human monocytotropic ehrlichiosis, which can be a more severe illness, has morulae in mononuclear cells (not neutrophils) in a minority of cases. Lyme disease, which may be difficult to distinguish from human granulocytotropic anaplasmosis or human monocytotropic ehrlichiosis, will not cause morulae. Treatment of human granulocytotropic anaplasmosis is with doxycycline.

83. The answer is E.
(Chap. 108) Allergic bronchopulmonary aspergillosis (ABPA) is not a true infection but rather a hypersensitivity immune response to colonizing *Aspergillus* species. It occurs in ~1% of patients with asthma and in up to 15% of patients with cystic fibrosis. Patients typically have wheezing that is difficult to control with usual agents, infiltrates on chest radiographs due to mucus plugging of airways, a productive cough often with mucus casts, and bronchiectasis. Eosinophilia is common if glucocorticoids have not been administered. The total IgE is of value if >1000 IU/mL in that it represents a significant allergic response and is very suggestive of ABPA. In the proper clinical context, a positive skin test for *Aspergillus* antigen or detection of serum *Aspergillus*-specific IgG or IgE precipitating antibodies are supportive of the diagnosis. Galactomannan EIA is useful for invasive aspergillosis but has not been validated for ABPA. There is no need to try to culture an organism via BAL to make the diagnosis of ABPA. Chest CT, which may reveal bronchiectasis, or pulmonary function testing, which will reveal an obstructive defect, will not be diagnostic.

84. The answer is B.
(Chap. 19) Prosthetic cardiac valves are at high risk of developing endocarditis after bacteremia. Patients who develop endocarditis within 2 months of valve surgery most likely have acquired their infection nosocomially as a result of intra-operative contamination of the prosthesis or of a bacteremic postoperative event. Coagulase-negative staphylococci are the most common (33%)

nosocomial pathogens during this time frame, followed by *Staphylococcus aureus* (22%), facultative gram-negative bacilli (13%), enterococci (8%), diphtheroids (6%), and fungi (6%) (see Table 19-1). The modes of infection and typical organisms causing prosthetic valve endocarditis >12 months after surgery are similar to those in community-acquired endocarditis. Both sets of pathogens must be considered in the intermediate 2–12 months after surgery.

85. The answer is B.
(Chap. 90) Oral hairy leukoplakia is due to severe overgrowth of Epstein-Barr virus infection in T cell–deficient patients. It is not premalignant, is often unrecognized by the patient, but is sometimes a cosmetic, symptomatic, and therapeutic nuisance. The white thickened folds on the side of the tongue can be pruritic or painful and sometimes resolve with acyclovir derivatives or topical podophyllin resin. Ultimate resolution occurs after immune reconstitution with antiretroviral therapy. Oral candidiasis or thrush is a very common, relatively easy-to-treat condition in HIV patients and takes on an appearance of white plaques on the tongue, palate, and buccal mucosa that bleed with blunt removal. Herpes simplex virus (HSV) recurrences or aphthous ulcers present as painful ulcerating lesions. The latter should be considered when oral ulcers persist, do not respond to acyclovir, and do not culture HSV. Kaposi's sarcoma is uncommon in the oropharynx and takes on a violet hue, suggesting its highly vascularized content.

86. The answer is D.
(Chap. 119) This patient comes from an area endemic for visceral leishmaniasis that includes Bangladesh, India, Nepal, Sudan, and Brazil. Although many species can cause cutaneous or mucosal disease, the *L. donovani* complex generally is associated with visceral leishmaniasis. The organism is transmitted by the bite of the sand-fly in the majority of cases. Although many patients remain asymptomatic, malnourished persons are at particular risk for progression to symptomatic disease or kala azar, the life-threatening form. The presentation of this disease generally includes fever, cachexia, and splenomegaly. Hepatomegaly is rare compared with other tropical diseases associated with organomegaly, such as malaria, miliary tuberculosis, and schistosomiasis. Pancytopenia is associated with severe disease, as are hypergammaglobulinemia and hypoalbuminemia. Although active investigation is under way to determine a means of diagnosing leishmaniasis by molecular techniques, the current standard remains demonstration of the organism on a stained slide or in tissue culture of a biopsy specimen. Splenic aspiration has the highest yield, with reported sensitivity of 98%. In light of the high mortality associated with this disease, treatment should not be delayed. The mainstay of therapy is a pentavalent antimonial, but newer therapies including amphotericin and pentamidine can be indicated in certain situations. In this case it would be prudent to rule out malaria with a thick and a thin smear. Rarely, the intracellular amastigote forms of *Leishmania* spp. can be seen on a peripheral smear.

87. The answer is C.
(Chap. 90) HIV resistance testing is recommended in selecting initial ART where the prevalence of resistance is high (such as in the United States or Europe) and in determining new therapy for patients with virologic failure while on ART. In the United States, the predominant virus in up to 12% of new cases has one major genotypic resistance mutation (patient A). In the patient failing ART, a resistance genotype should be performed while the patient is on therapy. In the absence of ART, the majority of virus reverts to wild type and the genotype appears normal (genotypes only sample the dominant viral form, though many exist); however, archived viruses in latent pools that are not accessible with current commercially available assays may in fact harbor resistance. Therefore a genotype for patient C is likely to be of little value. Following the initiation of therapy the patient should have a 1 log (tenfold) reduction in plasma HIV RNA levels within 1–2 months. Failure to achieve this response (patient B) may warrant a change in therapy. Patient D has breakthrough failure after a period of intermittent compliance. To determine if she has developed a new resistance pattern, she should have a genotype performed while on therapy to allow for adequate selection pressure from the antiviral agents to select the resistant virus leading to failure as the dominant strain.

88. The answer is B.
(Chap. 108) The primary risk factor for developing invasive *Aspergillus* infection is neutropenia and glucocorticoid use. Risk is proportional to the degree and length of neutropenia and the dose of glucocorticoid. HIV patients rarely develop invasive aspergillosis, and if they do, it is in the context of prolonged neutropenia and/or advanced disease. Patients with graft-vs-host disease and uncontrolled leukemia are at particularly elevated risk. The infection is seen in solid organ transplant patients, particularly those requiring high cumulative doses of glucocorticoids for graft rejection. (See Fig. 108-1.)

89. The answer is A.
(Chap. 69) Rifampin is considered the most potent and important antituberculosis drug. It is also active against other organisms, including some gram-positive and gram-negative organisms, as well as against *Legionella* spp, *Mycobacterium marinum*, and *M. kansasii*. It is notable for turning body fluids a red-orange color. Its use should be avoided or carefully monitored in patients with severe hepatic disease, but it does not need to be dose-adjusted in renal failure. Rifampin is a potent P450 CY3PA inducer and may lower the half-life and therefore effective levels of many important drugs, including anticonvulsants, cyclosporine, hormonal contraceptives, protease inhibitors, narcotics, tricyclic antidepressants, azole antifungals, beta blockers, and many antibiotics. Patients need to be monitored for the effects of subtherapeutic levels whether by directly measuring drug levels (anticonvulsants, cyclosporine), direct effects of the drug (warfarin), or with clinical adjustment (contraceptives, protease inhibitors). While not studied extensively, rifabutin has

a similar, although likely lesser, effect on the same medications as rifampin. Amiodarone is not metabolized by CY3PA.

90. The answer is A.
(Chap. 53) Ecthyma gangrenosum is a disseminated collection of geographic, painful, reddish, maculopapular lesions that rapidly progress from pink to purple and finally to a black, dry necrosis. They are teeming with causative bacteria. In reviews on ecthyma, *Pseudomonas aeruginosa* is the most common isolate from blood and skin lesions. However, many organisms can cause this foreboding rash. Neutropenic patients and AIDS patients are at highest risk, but diabetics and intensive care unit (ICU) patients are also affected. Pseudomonal sepsis is severe with a high mortality. Its presentation is otherwise difficult to discern from other severe sepsis syndromes, with hypothermia, fever, hypotension, organ damage, encephalopathy, bandemia, and shock being common findings. Though antibiotic use, severe burns, and long ICU stays increase the risk for *Pseudomonas* infection, these exposures are also risk factors for other bacterial infections, many of which also carry daunting resistant profiles. Because of *P. aeruginosa*'s propensity for multidrug resistance, two agents (usually an antipseudomonal β-lactam plus an aminoglycoside or ciprofloxacin) are warranted until culture data return confirming sensitivity to one or both agents. At this point the choice to narrow to one antibiotic or not is still debated and is largely physician preference.

91. The answer is C.
(Chap. 66) While all the patients listed have an increased risk of developing reactivation tuberculosis, the greatest risk factor for development of active tuberculosis is HIV positivity. The risk of developing active infection is greatest in those with the lowest CD4 counts; however, having a CD4 count above a threshold value does not negate the risk of developing an active infection. The reported incidence of developing active tuberculosis in HIV-positive individuals with a positive PPD is 10% per year, compared to a lifetime risk of 10% in immunocompetent individuals. The relative risk of developing active tuberculosis in an HIV-positive individual is 100 times that of an immunocompetent individual. All of the individuals listed as choices have risk factors for developing active tuberculosis. Malnutrition and severe underweight confers a twofold greater risk of developing active tuberculosis, whereas IV drug use increases the risk 10–30 times. Silicosis also increases the risk of developing active tuberculosis 30 times. While the risk of developing active tuberculosis is greatest in the first year after exposure, the risk also increases in the elderly.

92. The answer is A.
(Chap. 66) The CT scan shows a large cavitary lesion in the right upper lobe of the lung. In this man from an endemic area for tuberculosis, this finding should be treated as active pulmonary tuberculosis until proven otherwise. In addition, this patient's symptoms suggest a chronic illness with low-grade fevers, weight loss, and temporal wasting that would be consistent with active pulmonary tuberculosis. If a patient is suspected of having active pulmonary tuberculosis, the initial management should include documentation of disease while protecting health care workers and the population in general. This patient should be hospitalized in a negative-pressure room on airborne isolation until three expectorated sputum samples have been demonstrated to be negative. The samples should preferably be collected in the early morning as the burden of organisms is expected to be higher on a more concentrated sputum. The sensitivity of a single sputum for the detection of tuberculosis in confirmed cases is only 40–60%. Thus, a single sputum sample is inadequate to determine infectivity and the presence of active pulmonary tuberculosis. Skin testing with a PPD of the tuberculosis mycobacterium is used to detect latent infection with tuberculosis and has no role in determining whether active disease is present.

The cavitary lung lesion shown on the CT imaging of the chest could represent malignancy or a bacterial lung abscess, but given that the patient is from a high-risk area for tuberculosis, tuberculosis would be considered the most likely diagnosis until ruled out by sputum testing.

93. The answer is B.
(Chap. 110) Tinea versicolor is the most common superficial skin infection. It is caused by lipophilic yeasts of the genus *Malassezia*, most commonly *M. furfur*. In tropical areas, the prevalence of tinea versicolor is 40–60%, whereas in temperate areas it is about 1%. In general, most individuals seek evaluation for cosmetic reasons as the lesions in tinea versicolor are asymptomatic or only mildly pruritic. The lesions typically appear as patches of pink or coppery-brown skin, but the areas may be hypopigmented in dark-skinned individuals. Diagnosis can be made by demonstrating the organism on potassium hydroxide preparation where a typical "spaghetti and meatballs" appearance may be seen. This is due to the presence of both spore forms and hyphal forms within the skin. Under long-wave UVA light (Wood's lamp), the affected areas fluoresce to yellow-green. The organism is sensitive to a variety of antifungals. Selenium sulfide shampoo, topical azoles, terbinafine, and ciclopirox have all been used with success. A 2-week treatment regimen typically shows good results, but the infection typically recurs within 2 years of initial treatment.

94. Answer is D.
(Chap. 110) Sporothrix schenkii is a thermally dimorphic fungus found in soil, plants, and moss and occurs most commonly in gardeners, farmers, florists, and forestry workers. Sporotrichosis develops after inoculation of the organism into the skin with a contaminated puncture or scratch. The disease typically presents as a fixed cutaneous lesion or with lymphocutaneous spread. The initial lesion typically ulcerates and become verrucous in appearance. The draining lymphatic channels become

affected in up to 80% of cases. This presents as painless nodules along the lymphatic channel, which ulcerate. A definitive diagnosis is made by culturing the organism. A biopsy of the lesion may show ovoid or cigar-shaped yeast forms. Treatment for sporotrichosis is systemic therapy. Options include oral itraconazole, saturated solution of potassium iodide, and terbinafine. However, terbinafine has not been approved for this indication in the United States. Topical antifungals are not effective. In cases of serious system disease such as pulmonary sporotrichosis, amphotericin B is the treatment of choice. Caspofungin is not effective against *S. schenkii*.

95. The answer is D.

(Chap. 47) Generally thought of as a disease of children, epiglottitis is increasingly becoming a disease of adults since the wide use of *Haemophilus influenzae* type B vaccination. Epiglottitis can cause life-threatening airway obstruction due to cellulitis of the epiglottis and supraglottic tissues, classically due to *H. influenzae* type B infection. However, other organisms are also common causes including nontypeable *H. influenzae, Streptococcus pneumoniae, H. parainfluenzae, Staphylococcus aureus*, and viral infection. The initial evaluation and treatment for epiglottitis in adults includes airway management and intravenous antibiotics. The patient presented here is demonstrating signs of impending airway obstruction with stridor, inability to swallow secretions, and use of accessory muscles of inspiration. A lateral neck x-ray shows the typical thumb sign indicative of a swollen epiglottis. In addition, the patient has evidence of hypoventilation with carbon dioxide retention. Thus, in addition to antibiotics, this patient should also be intubated and mechanically ventilated electively under a controlled setting as he is at high risk for mechanical airway obstruction. Antibiotic therapy should cover the typical organisms outlined above and include coverage for oral anaerobes.

In adults presenting without overt impending airway obstruction, laryngoscopy would be indicated to assess airway patency. Endotracheal intubation would be recommended for those with >50% airway obstruction. In children, endotracheal intubation is often recommended as laryngoscopy in children has provoked airway obstruction to a much greater degree than adults, and increased risk of mortality has been demonstrated in some series in children when the airway is managed expectantly.

96. The answer is E.

(Chap. 59) The most likely infecting organism in this patient is *Francisella tularensis*. Gentamicin is the antibiotic of choice for the treatment of tularemia. Fluoroquinolones have shown in vitro activity against *F. tularensis* and have successfully been used in a few cases of tularemia. Currently, however, it cannot be recommended as first-line therapy as data are limited in regard to its efficacy relative to gentamicin, but can be considered if an individual is unable to tolerate gentamicin. To date, there have been no clinical trials of fluoroquinolones to definitively demonstrate equivalency with gentamicin. Third-generation cephalosporins have in vitro activity against *F. tularensis*. However, use of ceftriaxone in children with tularemia resulted in almost universal failure. Likewise, tetracycline and chloramphenicol also have limited usefulness with a higher relapse rate (up to 20%) when compared to gentamicin. *F. tularensis* is a small gram-negative, pleomorphic bacillus that is found both intra- and extracellularly. It is found in mud, water, and decaying animal carcasses, and ticks and wild rabbits are the source for most human infections in the southeast United States and Rocky Mountains. In western states, tabanid flies are the most common vectors. The organisms usually enter the skin through the bite of a tick or through an abrasion. On further questioning, the patient above reported that during the camping trip he was primarily responsible for skinning the animals and preparing dinner. He did suffer a small cut on his right hand at the site where the ulceration is apparent. The most common clinical manifestations of *F. tularensis* are ulceroglandular and glandular disease, accounting for 75–85% of cases. The ulcer appears at the site of entry of the bacteria and lasts for 1–3 weeks and may develop a black eschar at the base. The draining lymph nodes become enlarged and fluctuant. They may drain spontaneously. In a small percentage of patients, the disease becomes systemically spread, as is apparent in this case, with pneumonia, fevers, and sepsis syndrome. When this occurs, the mortality rate approaches 30% if untreated. However, with appropriate antibiotic therapy the prognosis is very good. Diagnosis requires a high clinical suspicion as demonstration of the organism is difficult. It rarely seen on Gram's stain because the organisms stain weakly and are so small that they are difficult to distinguish from background material. On polychromatically stained tissue, they may be seen both intra- and extracellularly, singly, or in clumps. Moreover, *F. tularensis* is a difficult organism to culture and requires cysteine-glucose–blood agar. However, most labs do not attempt to culture the organism because of the risk of infection in laboratory workers, requiring biosafety level 2 practices. Usually the diagnosis is confirmed by agglutination testing with titers >1:160 confirming diagnosis.

97. The answer is A.

(Chap. 62) Donovanosis is caused by the intracellular organism *Calymmatobacterium granulomatis* and most often presents as a painless erythematous genital ulceration after a 1–4 week incubation period. However, incubation periods can be as long as 1 year. The infection is predominantly sexually transmitted, and autoinoculation can lead to formation of new lesions by contact with adjacent infected skin. Typically the lesion is painless but bleeds easily. Complications include phimosis in men and pseudo-elephantiasis of the labia in women. If the infection is untreated, it can lead to progressive destruction of the penis or other organs. Diagnosis is made by demonstration of *Donovan bodies* within large mononuclear cells on smears from the lesion. Donovan bodies refers to the appearance of multiple intracellular organisms within the cytoplasm of mononuclear cells. These

organisms are bipolar and have an appearance similar to a safety pin. On histologic examination, there is an increase in the number of plasma cells with few neutrophils; additionally, epithelial hyperplasia is present and can resemble neoplasia. A variety of antibiotics can be used to treat donovanosis including macrolides, tetracyclines, trimethoprim-sulfamethoxazole, and chloramphenicol. Treatment should be continued until the lesion has healed, often requiring ≥5 weeks of treatment.

All of the choices listed in the question above are in the differential diagnosis of penile ulcerations. Lymphogranuloma venereum is endemic in the Caribbean. The ulcer of primary infection heals spontaneously, and the second phase of the infection results in markedly enlarged inguinal lymphadenopathy, which may drain spontaneously. *H. ducreyi* results in painful genital ulcerations, and the organism can be cultured from the lesion. The painless ulcerations of cutaneous leishmaniasis can appear similarly to those of donovanosis but usually occur on exposed skin. Histologic determination of intracellular parasites can distinguish leishmaniasis definitively from donovanosis. Finally, it is unlikely that the patient has syphilis in the setting of a negative rapid plasma reagin test, and the histology is inconsistent with this diagnosis.

98. The answer is B.
(Chap. 4) Malaria prophylaxis recommendations vary by region. Currently the recommended malaria prophylaxis for Central America is chloroquine. In contrast, due to chloroquine resistance of falciparum malaria, prophylaxis in India and most areas in Africa is with atovaquone/proguanil, doxycycline, or mefloquine. Table 4-2 represents the chemoprophylaxis regimens for malaria arranged by country as currently recommended by the Centers for Disease Control and Prevention.

99. The answer is A.
(Chap. 4) The causes of fever in travelers vary by geography. In general, all febrile travelers returning from malaria-endemic regions should be assumed to have malaria until ruled out or another diagnosis established, since falciparum malaria may be life-threatening and effective therapy is available. Dengue is particularly common in Southeast Asia. Most cases are self-limited and require supportive therapy. A small proportion, however, can develop hemorrhagic fever or a shock syndrome. Table 4-3 lists the most common causes of febrile illness in returning travelers by country.

100. The answer is D.
(Chap. 21) Erysipelas is a soft tissue infection caused by *Streptococcus pyogenes* that occurs most frequently on the face or extremities. The infection is marked by abrupt onset of fiery-red swelling with intense pain. The infection progresses rapidly and is marked by well-defined and indurated margins. Flaccid bullae may develop on the second or third day. Only rarely does the infection involve the deeper soft tissues. Penicillin is the treatment of choice. However, swelling may progress despite appropriate treatment with desquamation of the affected area.

101. The answer is C.
(Chap. 109) This patient has signs and symptoms of mucormycosis. Although mucormycosis is a relatively uncommon invasive fungal infection, patients with poorly controlled diabetes, patients receiving glucocorticoids, immunocompromised patients, or patients with iron overload syndromes receiving desferrioxamine have an enhanced susceptibility to this devastating infection. The "gold standard" diagnosis is tissue culture, but a common hallmark is the black eschar noted on the palate, which represents invasion of the fungus into tissue, with necrosis. The black eschar in this scenario should prompt the clinician to do more than prescribe treatment for sinusitis. Black eschars on the extremities can be found with anthrax infection or spider bites. Given the mortality associated with this infection and the rapidity with which it progresses, it is not prudent to wait for an ENT consultation after a course of antibiotics. The infection is usually fatal. Successful therapy requires reversal of the underlying predisposition (glucose control in this case), aggressive surgical debridement, and early initiation of antifungal therapy. Voriconazole is not thought to be effective in the treatment of mucormycosis. Posaconazole, an experimental azole antifungal, has been shown to be effective in mouse models of the disease and has been used in patients unable to tolerate amphotericin.

102. The answer is A.
(Chap. 105) Although spontaneous cures of pulmonary infection with *Blastomyces dermatitidis* have been well documented, almost all patients with blastomycosis should be treated since there is no way to distinguish which patients will progress or disseminate. Extrapulmonary disease should always be treated, especially if the patient is immunocompromised. Itraconazole is indicated for non-central nervous system extra-pulmonary disease in mild to moderate cases. Otherwise, amphotericin B is the treatment of choice, especially if there has been treatment failure with itraconazole. The echinocandins have variable activity against *B. dermatitidis* and are not recommended for blastomycosis. The triazole antifungals have not been studied extensively in human cases of blastomycosis. Fluoroquinolones have activity against many mycobacterial species, but do not have activity against fungi, including *B. dermatitidis*.

INDEX

Bold number indicates the start of the main discussion of the topic; numbers with "f " and "t" refer to figure and table pages.